SUBJECT ENTRY SECTION

Sample Entry

GENETIC COUNSELING

Rhodes, Rosamond. Genetic links, family ties, and social bonds: rights and responsibilities in the face of genetic knowledge. *Journal of Medicine and Philosophy.* 1998 Feb; 23(1): 10-30. 42 refs. 19 fn. BE57518.

> *autonomy; beneficence; case studies; confidentiality; decision making; directive counseling; disclosure; *family members; family relationship; friends; *genetic counseling; genetic disorders; *genetic information; genetic research; *genetic screening; Huntington's disease; *moral obligations; *moral policy; *obligations to society; patient participation; *patients; privacy; rights; social interaction; Tay Sachs disease; *truth disclosure; volunteers; pedigree studies; population genetics; *right not to know

Currently, some of the most significant moral issues involving genetic links relate to genetic knowledge. In this paper, instead of looking at the frequently addressed issues of responsibilities professionals or institutions have to individuals, I take up the question of what responsibilities individuals have to one another with respect to genetic knowledge. I address the questions of whether individuals have a moral right to pursue their own goals without contributing to society's knowledge of population genetics, without adding to their family's knowledge of its genetic history, and without discovering genetic information about themselves and their offspring. These questions lead to an examination of the presumed right to genetic ignorance and an exploration of a variety of social bonds. Analyzing cases in light of these considerations leads to a surprising conclusion about a widely accepted precept of genetic counseling, to some ethical insights into typical problems, and to some further unanswered questions about personal responsibility in the face of genetic knowledge.

BIBLIOGRAPHY
OF
BIOETHICS

BIBLIOGRAPHY
OF
BIOETHICS

Volume 25

Editors

LeRoy Walters
Tamar Joy Kahn

Associate Editors
Frances Amitay Abramson
Hannelore S. Ninomiya
Cecily Orr

KENNEDY INSTITUTE OF ETHICS
GEORGETOWN UNIVERSITY
Box 571212
WASHINGTON, DC 20057-1212

This *Bibliography of Bioethics* is an ongoing project
of the Kennedy Institute of Ethics. New volumes
of the *Bibliography* are published annually.

ISSN 0363-0161
ISBN 1-883913-05-5

This publication was supported by funds provided under
Contract N01 LM73514 with the National Library of Medicine,
and under Grant 5 P41 HG01115-05 from the National
Human Genome Research Institute.

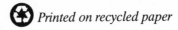 *Printed on recycled paper*

Contents

CONTENTS

CONTENTS

*The subheading *Special Populations* includes such groups as the aged, the mentally disabled, the terminally ill, prisoners, minority groups, and women.

Staff

LeRoy Walters, Ph.D.
Tamar Joy Kahn, M.L.S.
Editors

Doris M. Goldstein, M.A., M.L.S.
Director of Library and Information Services

Frances Amitay Abramson, M.A., M.S.
Hannelore S. Ninomiya, M.A., M.L.S.
Cecily Orr, M.L.S., M.A.
Bibliographers

Patricia C. Martin, M.A.
Data Entry Coordinator

Susan Cartier Poland, J.D.
Legal Research Associate

Laura Jane Bishop, Ph.D.
Research Associate

Jonathan J. Boyles, B.A.
Legal Research Assistant

Kathleen Reynolds, MAT, M.A.
Administrative Officer

Margaret Moral
Student Assistant

Editorial Advisory Board

INTRODUCTION

INTRODUCTION

The Field of Bioethics

Bioethics can be defined as the systematic study of value questions that arise in health care delivery and in biomedicine. Specific bioethical issues that have recently received national and international attention include euthanasia, assisted suicide, new reproductive technologies, cloning, human experimentation, genetic engineering, abortion, informed consent, acquired immunodeficiency syndrome (AIDS), organ donation and transplantation, and managed care and other concerns in the allocation of health care resources.

As this list of topics suggests, the field of bioethics includes several dimensions. The first is the ethics of the professional patient relationship. Traditionally, the accent has been on the duties of health professionals—duties that, since the time of Hippocrates, have frequently been delineated in codes of professional ethics. In more recent times the rights of patients have also received considerable attention. Research ethics, the study of value problems in biomedical and behavioral research, constitutes a second dimension of bioethics. During the 20th century, as both the volume and visible achievements of such research have increased, new questions have arisen concerning the investigator-subject relationship and the potential social impact of biomedical and behavioral research and technology. In recent years a third dimension of bioethics has emerged— the quest to develop reasonable public policy guidelines for both the delivery of health care and the allocation of health care resources, as well as for the conduct of research.

No single academic discipline is adequate to discuss these various dimensions of bioethics. For this reason bioethics has been, since its inception in the late 1960s, a cross-disciplinary field. The primary participants in the interdisciplinary discussion have been physicians and other health professionals, biologists, psychologists, sociologists, lawyers, historians, and philosophical and religious ethicists.

During the past thirty years there has been a rapid growth of academic, professional, and public interest in the field of bioethics. One evidence of this interest is the establishment of numerous research institutes and teaching programs in bioethics, both in the United States and abroad. In recent years, professional societies, federal and state legislatures, and the courts have also turned increasing attention to problems in the field. In addition, during the past several years there has been a veritable explosion of literature on bioethical issues.

The literature of bioethics appears in widely scattered sources and is reported in diverse indexes which employ a bewildering variety of subject headings. This *Bibliography* is the product of a unique information retrieval system designed to identify the central issues of bioethics, to develop an indexing language appropriate to the field, and to provide comprehensive, cross-disciplinary coverage of current English-language materials on bioethical topics.

The Scope of the Bibliography

This twenty-fifth volume of the *Bibliography of Bioethics* includes materials which discuss the ethical aspects of the following major topics and subtopics:[1]

BIOETHICS, IN GENERAL
PROFESSIONAL ETHICS
  Codes of Ethics
  Medical Ethics
  Nursing Ethics
ETHICISTS AND ETHICS COMMITTEES
  Clinical Ethics Committees
  Research Ethics Committees
PROFESSIONAL PATIENT RELATIONSHIP
  Confidentiality
  Informed Consent
  Patients' Rights
  Treatment Refusal
  Truth Disclosure
HEALTH CARE AND PUBLIC HEALTH
  AIDS
  Care of Special Populations
  Managed Care
  Resource Allocation
REPRODUCTION
  Abortion
  Contraception
  Prenatal Diagnosis
  Prenatal Injuries
  Sterilization
REPRODUCTIVE TECHNOLOGIES
  Artificial Insemination
  Cloning
  In Vitro Fertilization
  Surrogate Mothers
GENETIC INTERVENTION AND RESEARCH
  Eugenics
  Gene Therapy
  Genetic Counseling

Genetic Screening
Genome Mapping
Patenting Life Forms
Recombinant DNA Research
ORGAN AND TISSUE DONATION AND TRANSPLANTATION
  Fetal Tissue Donation
DEATH AND DYING
  Active Euthanasia
  Advance Directives
  Allowing to Die
  Assisted Suicide
  Determination of Death
  Resuscitation Orders
  Terminal Care
MENTAL HEALTH THERAPIES
  Behavior Control
  Electroconvulsive Therapy
  Involuntary Commitment
  Psychoactive Drugs
  Psychosurgery
HUMAN EXPERIMENTATION
  Behavioral Research
  Embryo and Fetal Research
  Informed Consent
  Regulation
  Research on Special Populations
ANIMAL EXPERIMENTATION
BIOMEDICAL RESEARCH
  Fraud and Misconduct
BIOMEDICINE AND VIOLENCE
  Biological and Nuclear Warfare
  Torture.

The *Bibliography* seeks to cite all substantive English-language materials that discuss ethical aspects of the topics and subtopics listed above. It therefore incorporates a variety of media and literary forms, including journal and newspaper articles, monographs, essays in books, court decisions, bills, laws, audiovisual materials, and unpublished documents. This twenty-fifth volume of the *Bibliography* indexes documents[2] that were published since 1977, concentrating primarily on documents published in 1997 and 1998.

A cross-disciplinary monitoring system has been devised in an effort to secure documents falling within the subject-matter scope outlined above. Among the reference tools and databases the staff searches for pertinent citations are the following:

Abortion Law Reporter
AGRICOLA
All England Law Reports (subject index)
Australian National Bibliography
BioLaw
Booklist

Books in Print® *PLUS*™
Canadian Books in Print
Catholic Periodical and Literature Index
CATLINE
Choice
Clearinghouse Review

---

[1] Several additional topics are closely related to the field of bioethics but have not been included in the *Bibliography*. Among these are human sexuality, ecology, and world hunger.

[2] In this Introduction the word "document" is used to refer to both print and nonprint materials.

Cumulative Index to Nursing and Allied Health
   Literature
Current Contents: Clinical Medicine
Current Contents: Social and Behavioral Sciences
Current Work in the History of Medicine
DISSERTATION ABSTRACTS ONLINE
Dominion Law Reports (subject index)
GAO Reports, Testimony, Correspondence and
   Other Publications
HSTAR
Humanities Index
Index to Canadian Legal Periodical Literature
Index to Foreign Legal Periodicals
LegalTrac
Library Journal
MEDLINE

Mental and Physical Disability Law Reporter
Monthly Catalog of U.S. Government Publications
New Titles in Bioethics
PAIS INTERNATIONAL
PHILOSOPHER'S INDEX
POPLINE
PsycINFO®
Readers' Guide to Periodical Literature
RELIGION INDEX
Right-to-Die Law Digest
Science Books and Films
Social Sciences Index
SOCIOLOGICAL ABSTRACTS
Specialty Law Digest: Health Care Law
Whitaker's Books in Print
WorldCat.

In addition, the *Bibliography* staff directly monitors over 130 journals and newspapers for articles and citations falling within the scope of bioethics. Please note, however, that the journal articles cited in this volume are actually drawn from 507 journals, not limited to the following directly monitored publications:

Academic Medicine
Accountability in Research
AIDS and Public Policy Journal
AIDS Policy and Law
America
American Journal of Human Genetics
American Journal of Law and Medicine
American Journal of Nursing
American Journal of Psychiatry
American Journal of Public Health
Annals of Health Law
Annals of Internal Medicine
Annals of the Royal College of Physicians and
   Surgeons of Canada
Archives of Family Medicine
Archives of Internal Medicine
Assia—Jewish Medical Ethics
ATLA: Alternatives to Laboratory Animals
Bioethics
BMJ (British Medical Journal)
Brandeis Law Journal
Bulletin of Medical Ethics
California Law Review
Cambridge Quarterly of Healthcare Ethics
Canadian Medical Association Journal
Christian Bioethics
Christian Century
Clinical Ethics Report
Columbia Law Review
Death Studies
Ethics
Ethics and Behavior
Ethics and Medicine: A Christian Perspective
Eubios Journal of Asian and International
   Bioethics
European Journal of Health Law
First Things: A Monthly Journal of Religion and
   Public Life
Gene Therapy

Georgetown Law Journal
Harvard Law Review
Hastings Center Report
Health
Health Affairs
Health and Human Rights
Health Care Analysis: Journal of Health Philosophy
   and Policy
Health Law in Canada
Health Matrix
Health Policy
Health Progress
HEC (HealthCare Ethics Committee) Forum
Human Gene Therapy
Human Life Review
Human Reproduction
Human Reproduction and Genetic Ethics: An
   International Journal
Humane Health Care International
International Digest of Health Legislation
International Journal of Bioethics
International Journal of Health Services
International Journal of Law and Psychiatry
International Journal of Technology Assessment in
   Health Care
IRB: A Review of Human Subjects Research
Issues in Law and Medicine
Issues in Science and Technology
JAMA
Joint Commission Journal on Quality Improvement
Journal of Advanced Nursing
Journal of Clinical Ethics
Journal of Contemporary Health Law and Policy
Journal of Ethics, Law and Aging
Journal of Genetic Counseling
Journal of Halacha and Contemporary Society
Journal of Health Politics, Policy and Law
Journal of Law, Medicine and Ethics
Journal of Legal Medicine

Journal of Medical Ethics
Journal of Medical Genetics
Journal of Medical Humanities
Journal of Medicine and Philosophy
Journal of Palliative Care
Journal of Psychiatry and Law
Journal of Public Health Policy
Journal of Religion and Health
Journal of Religious Ethics
Journal of Social Philosophy
Journal of the American Academy of Psychiatry
    and the Law
Journal of the American Geriatrics Society
Kennedy Institute of Ethics Journal
Lancet
Linacre Quarterly
Literature and Medicine
M&GS (Medicine and Global Survival)
Medical Humanities Review
Medical Law International
Medical Law Review
Medical Trial Technique Quarterly
Medicine and Law
Medicine, Conflict and Survival
Michigan Law Review
Milbank Quarterly
Minnesota Medicine
Nature
Nature Biotechnology
Nature Genetics
Nature Medicine
NCEHR Communiqué (National Council on

Ethics in Human Research)
New England Journal of Medicine
New Scientist
New York Times
New York University Law Review
Newsweek
Notre Dame Journal of Law, Ethics and Public Policy
Nursing Ethics
Omega: Journal of Death and Dying
Perspectives in Biology and Medicine
Pharos
Philosophy and Public Affairs
Philosophy and Public Policy
Politics and the Life Sciences
Psychiatric Services
Public Affairs Quarterly
Science
Science News
Science, Technology, and Human Values
The Sciences
Social Philosophy and Policy
Social Science and Medicine
Stanford Law Review
Theoretical Medicine and Bioethics (formerly
    Theoretical Medicine)
Time
UCLA Law Review
University of Chicago Law Review
Virginia Law Review
Western Journal of Medicine
Women's Health Issues
Yale Law Journal.

This twenty-fifth volume of the *Bibliography* includes bibliographic data for 3,612 documents, published between 1977 and 1998. Most were published in 1997 (1,494) and 1998 (1,025).

All documents cited by the *Bibliography* are in the collection of the National Reference Center for Bioethics Literature (NRCBL). For information on ordering photocopies, contact the NRCBL at the Kennedy Institute of Ethics, Georgetown University, Box 571212, Washington, DC 20057-1212; telephone 202-687-3885 or 800-MED-ETHX; e-mail: medethx@gunet.georgetown.edu.

Arrangement of the Bibliography

This volume of the *Bibliography of Bioethics* is divided into four parts:

1. Introduction
2. List of Journals Cited
3. Subject Entry Section
4. Author Index.

Part 3, the Subject Entry Section, constitutes the core of the *Bibliography*.

List of Journals Cited

The second part of the *Bibliography,* the List of Journals Cited, records the title of each journal cited in the Subject Entry Section. When available, the International Standard Serial Number (ISSN) of the journal is also listed. The dual purpose of this list is to indicate precisely which journal is designated by each journal title and to obviate the need to include an ISSN number with each citation.

Subject Entry Section

The Subject Entry Section, the main part of the *Bibliography,* contains one or more entries for each of the documents processed by the bioethics information retrieval system during the preceding year. In Volume 25 of the *Bibliography,* entries for 3,612 documents have been included in the Subject Entry Section. By form, these 3,612 documents can be categorized as follows:

Journal articles	2,450
Essays in books	724
Monographs	269
Newspaper articles	74
Court decisions	40
Bills or laws	27
Unpublished documents	25
Audiovisual materials	3

The Subject Entry Section is organized under 78 major subject headings, of which 23 are further divided by subheadings. Each subheading is separated from the major subject term by a slash.

Readers of the *Bibliography* should first scan the alphabetic list of subject headings in the Table of Contents to determine where citations of interest to them are likely to be found. Only subject headings actually occurring in Volume 25 are included on this list.

The Subject Entry Section includes cross references of three types. *See* cross references lead the reader from terms that are not used as subject headings to terms that are used. *See under* cross references are generated from subheadings and guide the reader to the applicable major term in the alphabetical sequence of subject headings. *See also* cross references suggest additional subject headings where the reader may find citations of related interest.

Citation formats in the Subject Entry Section are based on the ANSI[3] standard for bibliographic references. As explained below, the citations are accompanied by indexing terms known as Keywords; in addition, 626 of the citations are accompanied by brief abstracts.

A sample subject heading and a sample entry for a journal article follow:

GENETIC COUNSELING

Rhodes, Rosamond. Genetic links, family ties, and social bonds: rights and responsibilities in the face of genetic knowledge. *Journal of Medicine and Philosophy.* 1998 Feb; 23(1): 10-30. 42 refs. 19 fn. BE57518.

*autonomy; beneficence; case studies; confidentiality; decision making; directive counseling; disclosure; *family members; family relationship; friends; *genetic counseling; genetic disorders; *genetic information; genetic research; *genetic screening; Huntington's disease; *moral obligations; *moral policy; *obligations to society; patient participation; *patients; privacy; rights; social interaction; Tay Sachs disease; *truth disclosure; volunteers; pedigree studies; population genetics; *right not to know

Currently, some of the most significant moral issues involving genetic links relate to genetic knowledge. In this paper, instead of looking at the frequently addressed issues of responsibilities professionals or institutions have to individuals, I take up the question of what responsibilities individuals have to one another with respect to genetic knowledge. I address the questions of whether individuals have a moral right to pursue their own goals without contributing to society's knowledge of population genetics, without adding to their family's knowledge of its genetic history, and without discovering genetic information about themselves and their offspring. These questions lead to an examination of the presumed right to genetic ignorance and an exploration of a variety of social bonds. Analyzing cases in light of these considerations leads to a surprising conclusion about a widely accepted precept of genetic counseling, to some ethical insights into typical problems, and to some further unanswered questions about personal responsibility in the face of genetic knowledge.

---

[3] *American National Standard for Bibliographic References,* ANSI Z39.29-1977 (New York: American National Standards Institute; 1977).

BIBLIOGRAPHY OF BIOETHICS

Eleven data elements may appear in an entry for a journal article:

1. Subject heading: **GENETIC COUNSELING**
2. Author(s): **Rhodes, Rosamond**
3. Title of article: Genetic links, family ties, and social bonds. . . .
4. Name of journal[4]: *Journal of Medicine and Philosophy*
5. Date of publication: 1998 Feb
6. Volume and issue number: 23(1)
7. Pagination: 10-30
8. Number of references and/or footnotes: 42 refs. 19 fn.
9. Bioethics Accession Number[5]. BE57518
10. Keywords: *autonomy; beneficence, etc.
11. Abstract: Currently, some. . . .

Keywords (element 10) consist of descriptors, proposed descriptors, and identifiers. Descriptors (*autonomy; etc.) are indexing terms chosen from a controlled vocabulary, the *Bioethics Thesaurus,* to represent the concepts in each document. Proposed descriptors (pedigree studies; etc.) are trial indexing terms that are being considered for possible inclusion in the *Thesaurus.* Identifiers, of which there are none in the sample entry, are proper nouns which are not part of the *Bioethics Thesaurus.* In most cases identifiers refer to a particular person, organization, legal decision, corporate body, geographic location, or time period.

Descriptor Keywords are listed first in alphabetical order in a paragraph that follows the Bioethics Accession Number. Proposed descriptors are listed next, also in alphabetical order. Identifiers are listed in alphabetical sequence following the last descriptor or proposed descriptor. Descriptors appear with every citation in the *Bibliography of Bioethics.* Proposed descriptors and identifiers are added to records as needed.

Approximately 10-20 Keywords are assigned to each document, and the general indexing policy is to employ the most specific term available. The most important concepts are designated by asterisks: *autonomy; etc. Keywords are included with each citation in the *Bibliography* to serve as guides to the subject content of a record.

Abstracts (element 11) appear in citations for some journal articles and all court decisions in the *Bibliography.* The abstracts in journal article citations are reprinted from journals that are major sources of information in the field of bioethics with permission from the source journals[6]. The abstracts in court decision citations were written by *Bibliography* staff, as indicated by the annotation "(KIE abstract)", to provide a brief summary of the decision.

The sample entry presented above displays the format and elements which appear in a journal article entry. Distinctive formats are used for each of the major forms of material encountered, for example, monographs, essays in monographs, and court decisions. Letters to the editor, editorials, news articles, and specific types of audiovisual materials are also identified in the bibliographic data.

Several print and nonprint forms contain data elements which do not appear in journal article entries. Among these additional elements the most important are the following:

1. Monographs
   Author or editor of book
   Title of book
   International Standard Book Number (ISBN)

---

[4] International Standard Serial Numbers (ISSNs) are not included in individual entries. Instead, the ISSNs of all journals cited in the Subject Entry Section are included in the part of the *Bibliography* entitled "List of Journals Cited."

[5] The Bioethics Accession Number may be used when ordering copies of hard-to-locate documents from the National Reference Center for Bioethics Literature.

[6] *American Journal of Law and Medicine; American Journal of Public Health; Annals of Internal Medicine; Archives of Internal Medicine; Bioethics; BMJ (British Medical Journal); Cambridge Quarterly of Healthcare Ethics; Christian Bioethics; Ethics; Ethics and Behavior; Hastings Center Report; Health Care Analysis; HEC (HealthCare Ethics Committee) Forum; Human Gene Therapy; International Journal of Bioethics; JAMA; Journal of Clinical Ethics; Journal of Health Politics, Policy and Law; Journal of Law, Medicine and Ethics; Journal of Medical Ethics; Journal of Medical Humanities; Journal of Medicine and Philosophy; Kennedy Institute of Ethics Journal; Lancet; Milbank Quarterly; Nature; New England Journal of Medicine; Nursing Ethics; Philosophy and Public Affairs; Science; Social Science and Medicine; and Theoretical Medicine and Bioethics.*

    2. Essays in monographs (analytics)
        Author(s) of essay
        Title of essay
        Author(s)/editor(s) of monograph
          in which essay appears
    3. Court decisions
        Date of decision
        Abstract.

Author Index

Citations in the Author Index are followed by one or more subject headings in parentheses. Readers interested in finding related citations, or in seeing the indexing Keywords, and perhaps abstracts for particular citations, can turn to an applicable subject heading in the Subject Entry Section. Citations that have no personal or corporate author are listed at the end of the Author Index under ANONYMOUS.

The *Bibliography of Bioethics* on the World Wide Web via BIOETHICSLINE®

The entries published in all of the annual volumes of the *Bibliography of Bioethics* are available in the database BIOETHICS-LINE, which is updated bimonthly. BIOETHICSLINE is produced for the U.S. National Library of Medicine (NLM), with additional support from the National Human Genome Research Institute, by the Bioethics Information Retrieval Project, part of the National Reference Center for Bioethics Literature at the Kennedy Institute of Ethics, Georgetown University. Free searching of BIOETHICSLINE via Internet Grateful Med (IGM), an NLM World Wide Web application, is available at http://igm.nlm.nih.gov. Access to the database, together with an online *Searcher's Guide* and an annotated list of Keywords (see paragraph below on the *Bioethics Thesarus*), is available also through the Web gateway page of the Kennedy Institute of Ethics at http://bioethics.georgetown.edu.

Bioethics Thesaurus

The *Bioethics Thesaurus* is an indexing language developed by the *Bibliography* staff specifically for the cross-disciplinary field of bioethics. Keywords from the *Thesaurus,* which accompany all citations in the *Bibliography,* are used for searching the BIOETHICSLINE database. The main part of the *Thesaurus,* an annotated alphabetic list of Keywords, is available on the World Wide Web at http://bioethics.georgetown.edu. Copies of the full *Thesaurus,* which includes several appendixes, may be purchased by contacting the Administrative Officer, *Bibliography of Bioethics,* Kennedy Institute of Ethics, Georgetown University, Box 571212, Washington, DC 20057-1212; telephone 202-687-6689 or 800-MED-ETHX; fax 200-687-6770; e-mail: medethx@gunet.georgetown.edu.

Acknowledgments

It is a pleasure to acknowledge the assistance of numerous persons who played a major role in the production of this twenty-fifth volume of the *Bibliography of Bioethics.*

The Bibliographers, Frances Amitay Abramson, Hannelore S. Ninomiya, and Cecily Orr, monitored journals, indexed documents, and continued to develop the language of the Bioethics Thesaurus. Patricia C. Martin, Data Entry Coordinator, organized and supervised data entry. Susan Cartier Poland, Legal Research Associate, acquired legal materials and edited abstracts written for court decisions by Jonathan J. Boyle, Legal Research Assistant. Laura Jane Bishop, Research Associate, monitored the indexes and many of the journals listed in the Introduction. In addition, Ms. Bishop and her student assistants played significant roles in securing documents. Margaret Moral assumed responsibility for the input of data. Kathleen Reynolds, Administrative Officer, provided administrative support for the project. and oversaw sales and distribution of the *Bibliography.*

The Director of Library and Information Services at the Kennedy Institute of Ethics, Doris Goldstein, provided general coordination for the project and, together with her staff, secured many of the documents which are included in the *Bibliography.* We wish to thank Librarians Martina Darragh, Lucinda Fitch Huttlinger, and Pat Milmoe McCarrick, who monitored numerous journals.

This twenty-fifth volume of the *Bibliography* has been produced with the aid of computer programs developed by Natalie A. Arluk and Karen A. Kraly, Office of Computer and Communications Systems, the National Library of Medicine.

The staff wishes to thank Stuart J. Nelson, M.D., Head of the Medical Subject Headings Section at the National Library of Medicine, who generously shared his expertise. The members of our Editorial Advisory Board contributed numerous valuable suggestions that have been incorporated into the *Bibliography.*

Funding for the costs of this twenty-fifth volume was provided through Contract N01 LM73514 with the National Library of Medicine (NLM). We wish to thank NLM for its long-term financial support, and to express our appreciation to our NLM Project Officer, Sheldon Kotzin, and to our Assistant Project Officer, Lou Knecht, for their excellent advice. We also thank Mary Smith, our Contracting Officer, and Liem T. Nguyen, Contract Specialist, for their efficiency and helpfulness. Additional funding for this volume of the *Bibliography* was provided through Grant 5 P41 HG01115-05 from the National Human Genome Research Institute (NHGRI). We thank Elizabeth Thomson, Program Director, ELSI Branch, NHGRI, for her interest and support.

Inquiries about purchasing Volumes 10-25 of the *Bibliography* should be directed to the Administrative Officer, *Bibliography of Bioethics,* Kennedy Institute of Ethics, Georgetown University, Box 571212, Washington, DC 20057-1212, telephone 202-687-6689 or 800-MED-ETHX; fax 202-687-6770, e-mail: medethx@gunet.georgetown.edu. Earlier volumes are out of print.

The bibliographic information published in volumes 1-25 of the *Bibliography of Bioethics* is also available as a National Library of Medicine database, BIOETHICSLINE®. For further information about free World Wide Web access to BIOETHICSLINE via Internet Grateful Med, contact the MEDLARS Management Section, National Library of Medicine, 8600 Rockville Pike, Bethesda, Maryland 20894; telephone 301-496-6193 or 888-FIND-NLM/888-346-3656; e-mail: mms@nlm.nih.gov; Internet: http://igm.nlm.nih.gov. BIOETHICSLINE access and search aids are also available through the Web gateway of the Kennedy Institute of Ethics at http://bioethics.georgetown.edu.

The database has also been issued in CD-ROM format from two sources: BIOETHICSLINE® *Plus* is available from SilverPlatter Information, Inc., 1-800-343-0064 or www.silverplatter.com/usa, and BioethicsLine is available from OVID Technologies, Inc., 1-800-950-2035 Ext. 249 or www.ovid.com.

*   *   *

The staff welcomes suggestions for the improvement of future volumes of the *Bibliography of Bioethics.* Please send all comments to:

Editors, *Bibliography of Bioethics*
Kennedy Institute of Ethics
Box 571212
Georgetown University
Washington, DC 20057-1212.

May 12, 1999

LeRoy Walters
Tamar Joy Kahn

LIST OF JOURNALS CITED

LIST OF JOURNALS CITED

A

AACN Clinical Issues in Critical Care Nursing ISSN 1046–7467

ABA Journal: The Lawyer's Magazine ISSN 0747–0088

Academic Emergency Medicine ISSN 1069–6563

Academic Medicine ISSN 1040–2446

Academic Psychiatry ISSN 1042–9670

ACOG Committee Opinions ISSN 1074–861X

Administration in Mental Health ISSN 0090–1180

Advances in Nursing Science ISSN 0161–9268

Age and Ageing ISSN 0002–0729

AIDS and Public Policy Journal ISSN 0887–3852

AIDS Policy and Law ISSN 0887–1493

Alberta Law Review ISSN 0002–4821

Alcohol and Alcoholism ISSN 0735–0414

All England Law Reports ISSN 0002–5569

Alzheimer Disease and Associated Disorders ISSN 0893–0341

America ISSN 0002–7049

American Biology Teacher ISSN 0002–7685

American Family Physician ISSN 0002–838X

American Journal of Criminal Law ISSN 0537–3549

American Journal of Diseases of Children ISSN 0002–922X

American Journal of Emergency Medicine ISSN 0735–6757

American Journal of Epidemiology ISSN 0002–9262

American Journal of Health–System Pharmacy ISSN 1079–2082

American Journal of Hospice and Palliative Care ISSN 1049–9091

American Journal of Human Genetics ISSN 0002–9297

American Journal of Kidney Diseases ISSN 0272–6386

American Journal of Legal History ISSN 0002–9319

American Journal of Medical Genetics ISSN 0148–7299

American Journal of Medicine ISSN 0002–9343

American Journal of Nursing ISSN 0002–936X

American Journal of Obstetrics and Gynecology ISSN 0002–9378

American Journal of Orthopsychiatry ISSN 0002–9432

American Journal of Otolaryngology ISSN 0196–0709

American Journal of Perinatology ISSN 0735–1631

American Journal of Preventive Medicine ISSN 0749–3797

American Journal of Psychiatry ISSN 0002–953X

American Journal of Public Health ISSN 0090–0036

American Journal of Respiratory and Critical Care Medicine ISSN 1073–449X

American Medical Record Association Journal ISSN 0273–9976

American Philosophical Association Newsletter on Philosophy and Medicine

American Psychologist ISSN 0003–066X

American Surgeon ISSN 0003–1348

Anesthesiology ISSN 0003–3022

Annals of Emergency Medicine ISSN 0196–0644

Annals of Health Law ISSN 1075–2994

Annals of Internal Medicine ISSN 0003–4819

Annals of Oncology ISSN 0923–7534

Annals of Plastic Surgery ISSN 0148–7043

Annals of Science ISSN 0003–3790

Annals of the New York Academy of Sciences ISSN 0077–8923

Annals of the Royal College of Surgeons of England ISSN 0035–8843

Annual Review of Medicine ISSN 0066–4219

AORN Journal (Association of Operating Room Nurses) ISSN 0001–2092

Applied Nursing Research ISSN 0897–1897

Archives of Dermatology ISSN 0003–987X

Archives of Disease in Childhood ISSN 0003–9888

Archives of Family Medicine ISSN 1063–3987

Archives of General Psychiatry ISSN 0003–990X

Archives of Internal Medicine ISSN 0003–9926

Archives of Neurology ISSN 0003–9942

Archives of Ophthalmology ISSN 0003–9950

Archives of Pathology and Laboratory Medicine ISSN 0003–9985

Archives of Psychiatric Nursing ISSN 0883–9417

Archives of Surgery ISSN 0004–0010

Arctic Medical Research ISSN 0782–226X

ATLA: Alternatives to Laboratory Animals ISSN 0261–1929

Atlantic Monthly ISSN 1072–7825

Atlantic Reporter, 2d Series

Australian and New Zealand Journal of Medicine ISSN 0004–8291

Australian and New Zealand Journal of Obstetrics and Gynaecology ISSN 0004–8666

Australian and New Zealand Journal of Psychiatry ISSN 0004–8674

Australian and New Zealand Journal of Public Health ISSN 1326–0200

Australian and New Zealand Journal of Surgery ISSN 0004–8682

Australian Critical Care ISSN 1036–7314

Australian Family Physician ISSN 0300–8495

Australian Journal of Social Issues ISSN 0004–9557

Australian Journal on Ageing ISSN 0726–4240

Aviation, Space, and Environmental Medicine ISSN 0095–6562

B

Behavioral Sciences and the Law ISSN 0735–3936

Berkeley Municipal Code

Between the Species
Bio/Technology   ISSN 0733-222X
Bioethics   ISSN 0269-9702
Bioethics Forum   ISSN 1065-7274
BMJ (British Medical Journal)   ISSN 0959-8138
Boston College Environmental Affairs Law Review
    ISSN 0190-7034
British Heart Journal   ISSN 0007-0769
British Journal of General Practice   ISSN 0960-1643
British Journal of Medical Psychology   ISSN
    0007-1129
British Journal of Nursing   ISSN 0966-0461
British Journal of Obstetrics and Gynaecology   ISSN
    0306-5456
British Journal of Social Psychology   ISSN 0144-6665
British Journal of Social Work   ISSN 0045-3102
British Journal of Theatre Nursing   ISSN 0027-6049
Bulletin of Medical Ethics   ISSN 0269-1485
Bulletin of the American Academy of Psychiatry and
    the Law   ISSN 0091-634X
Bulletin of the Atomic Scientists   ISSN 0096-3402
Bulletin of the New York Academy of Medicine   ISSN
    0028-7091
Burns, Including Thermal Injury   ISSN 0305-4179
Business and Professional Ethics Journal   ISSN
    0277-2027

C

Caduceus   ISSN 0882-6447
California Health and Safety Code (West)
California Reporter, 2d Series   ISSN 8750-2623
Cambridge Law Journal   ISSN 0008-1973
Cambridge Quarterly of Healthcare Ethics   ISSN
    0963-1801
Canadian Bar Review   ISSN 0008-3003
Canadian Journal of Psychiatry   ISSN 0706-7437
Canadian Medical Association Journal   ISSN
    0008-4409
Canadian Psychology   ISSN 0708-5591
Cancer   ISSN 0008-543X
Cancer Epidemiology, Biomarkers and Prevention
    ISSN 1055-9965
Cancer Treatment Reports   ISSN 0361-5960
Chest   ISSN 0012-3692
Child: Care, Health and Development ISSN 0305-1862
Children's Legal Rights Journal   ISSN 0278-7210
Child's Nervous System   ISSN 0256-7040
Christian Bioethics   ISSN 1380-3603
Christian Century   ISSN 0009-5281
Christian Science Monitor   ISSN 0882-245X
Cleveland Clinic Journal of Medicine ISSN 0891-1150
Clinical and Investigative Medicine   ISSN 0147-958X
Clinical Genetics   ISSN 0009-9163
Clinical Obstetrics and Gynecology   ISSN 0009-9201
Clinical Oncology (Royal College of Radiologists)
    ISSN 0936-6555
Clinical Research   ISSN 0009-9279
Clinical Transplantation   ISSN 0902-0063
Clinics in Laboratory Medicine   ISSN 0272-2712
Code of Virginia Annotated
Colorado Journal of International Environmental Law
    and Policy   ISSN 1050-0391

Columbia Journal of Law and Social Problems   ISSN
    0010-1923
Commentary   ISSN 0010-2601
Connecticut Medicine   ISSN 0010-6178
Controlled Clinical Trials   ISSN 0197-2456
Critical Care Clinics   ISSN 0749-0704
Critical Care Medicine   ISSN 0090-3493
Critical Care Nursing Quarterly   ISSN 0887-9303
Cytokines and Molecular Therapy   ISSN 1355-6568

D

Dauphin County Reports
Death Studies   ISSN 0748-1187
Dialog: A Journal of Theology   ISSN 0012-2033
Dialysis and Transplantation   ISSN 0090-2934
Dimensions of Critical Care Nursing ISSN 0730-4625
Discover   ISSN 0274-7529
Dolentium Hominum: Church and Health in the World
Dominion Law Reports, 4th Series   ISSN 0012-5350
Drug and Alcohol Dependence   ISSN 0376-8716

E

East African Medical Journal   ISSN 0012-835X
Educational Gerontology   ISSN 0360-1277
Environmental Values   ISSN 0963-2719
Epidemiology   ISSN 1044-3983
Ethics   ISSN 0014-1704
Ethics and Behavior   ISSN 1050-8422
Ethics and Medicine   ISSN 0266-688X
European Journal of Cancer   ISSN 0959-8049
European Journal of Cancer Care   ISSN 0961-5423
European Psychiatry   ISSN 0924-9338

F

Family Law Reports   ISSN 0261-4375
Family Planning Perspectives   ISSN 0014-7354
Family Practice Research Journal   ISSN 0270-2304
Federal Register   ISSN 0097-6326
Federal Reporter, 2d Series   ISSN 1048-3888
Federal Reporter, 3d Series   ISSN 1048-3888
Federal Supplement   ISSN 1047-7306
Fertility and Sterility   ISSN 0015-0282
Focus on Critical Care   ISSN 0736-3605
Free Inquiry   ISSN 0272-0701

G

Gender and Society   ISSN 0891-2432
Gene Therapy   ISSN 0969-7128
General Hospital Psychiatry   ISSN 0163-8343
GenEthics News   ISSN 1354-1366
Genetic Resource
GeneWATCH   ISSN 0740-9737
Genome Science and Technology   ISSN 1070-2830
Georgetown Law Journal   ISSN 0016-8092

H

Hastings Center Report   ISSN 0093-0334
Health Affairs   ISSN 0278-2715

Health Care Analysis   ISSN 1065-3058
Health Care for Women International   ISSN 0739-9332
Health Communication   ISSN 1041-0236
Health Matrix   ISSN 0748-383X
Health Policy   ISSN 0168-8510
Health Progress   ISSN 0882-1577
Healthcare Forum Journal   ISSN 0899-9287
Heart and Lung   ISSN 0147-9563
HEC (HealthCare Ethics Committee) Forum   ISSN 0956-2737
High Technology Law Journal   ISSN 0885-2715
Home Healthcare Nurse   ISSN 0884-741X
Hospital and Community Psychiatry ISSN 0022-1597
Hospital and Health Services Administration   ISSN 8750-3735
Hospital Practice (Office Edition)   ISSN 8750-2836
Hospital Progress   ISSN 0018-5817
Hospital Topics   ISSN 0018-5868
Hospitals   ISSN 0018-5973
Hospitals and Health Networks   ISSN 1068-8838
Houston Law Review   ISSN 0018-6694
Human Life Review   ISSN 0097-9783
Human Reproduction   ISSN 0268-1161
Human Research Report   ISSN 0885-0615
Human Rights   ISSN 0046-8185

I

IEEE Engineering in Medicine and Biology Magazine   ISSN 0739-5175
Image: The Journal of Nursing Scholarship   ISSN 0743-5150
Indian Heart Journal   ISSN 0019-4832
Indiana Medicine   ISSN 0746-8288
Infection Control and Hospital Epidemiology   ISSN 0899-823X
Intensive Care Medicine   ISSN 0342-4642
International Digest of Health Legislation   ISSN 0020-6563
International Journal of Bioethics   ISSN 1145-0762
International Journal of Epidemiology   ISSN 0300-5771
International Journal of Geriatric Psychiatry   ISSN 0885-6230
International Journal of Gynaecology and Obstetrics   ISSN 0020-7292
International Journal of Health Services   ISSN 0020-7314
International Journal of Law and Psychiatry   ISSN 0160-2527
International Journal of Nursing Studies   ISSN 0020-7489
International Journal of Technology Assessment in Health Care   ISSN 0266-4623
International Philosophical Quarterly   ISSN 0019-0365
International Psychogeriatrics   ISSN 1041-6102
Iowa Medicine   ISSN 0746-8709
IRB: A Review of Human Subjects Research   ISSN 0193-7758
Issues in Law and Medicine   ISSN 8756-8160
Issues in Mental Health Nursing   ISSN 0161-2840

J

JAMA   ISSN 0098-7484
Journal of Acquired Immune Deficiency Syndromes   ISSN 0894-9255
Journal of Addictive Diseases   ISSN 1055-0887
Journal of Adolescent Health   ISSN 1054-139X
Journal of Advanced Nursing   ISSN 0309-2402
Journal of Allied Health   ISSN 0090-7421
Journal of Assisted Reproduction and Genetics   ISSN 1058-0468
Journal of Biosocial Science   ISSN 0021-9320
Journal of Business Ethics   ISSN 0167-4544
Journal of Christian Nursing   ISSN 0743-2550
Journal of Clinical Endocrinology and Metabolism   ISSN 0021-972X
Journal of Clinical Ethics   ISSN 1046-7890
Journal of Clinical Nursing   ISSN 0962-1067
Journal of Clinical Oncology   ISSN 0732-183X
Journal of Community and Applied Social Psychology   ISSN 1052-9284
Journal of Consumer Research   ISSN 0093-5301
Journal of Contemporary Health Law and Policy   ISSN 0882-1046
Journal of Contemporary Law   ISSN 0097-9937
Journal of Craniofacial Genetics and Developmental Biology   ISSN 0270-4145
Journal of Critical Care   ISSN 0883-9441
Journal of Dental Education   ISSN 0022-0337
Journal of Dental Research   ISSN 0022-0345
Journal of Emergency Nursing   ISSN 0099-1767
Journal of Epidemiology and Biostatistics   ISSN 1359-5229
Journal of Ethics, Law, and Aging   ISSN 1076-1616
Journal of Evaluation in Clinical Practice   ISSN 1356-1294
Journal of Family Law   ISSN 0022-1066
Journal of Family Practice   ISSN 0094-3509
Journal of Forensic Sciences   ISSN 0022-1198
Journal of General Internal Medicine ISSN 0884-8734
Journal of Genetic Counseling   ISSN 1059-7700
Journal of Geriatric Psychiatry   ISSN 0022-1414
Journal of Gerontological Nursing   ISSN 0098-9134
Journal of Halacha and Contemporary Society   ISSN 0730-2614
Journal of Health and Social Behavior   ISSN 0022-1465
Journal of Health Care for the Poor and Underserved   ISSN 1049-2089
Journal of Health Politics, Policy and Law   ISSN 0361-6878
Journal of Holistic Nursing   ISSN 0898-0101
Journal of Human Resources   ISSN 0022-166X
Journal of Intensive Care Medicine   ISSN 0885-0666
Journal of Internal Medicine   ISSN 0954-6820
Journal of Investigative Medicine   ISSN 1081-5589
Journal of Laboratory and Clinical Medicine   ISSN 0022-2143
Journal of Law and Health   ISSN 1044-6419
Journal of Legal Medicine   ISSN 0194-7648
Journal of Long-Term Care Administration   ISSN 0093-4445

Journal Of Long Term Home Health Care ISSN 1072–4281

Journal of Marital and Family Therapy ISSN 0194–472X

Journal of Medical Education ISSN 0022–2577

Journal of Medical Ethics ISSN 0306–6800

Journal of Medical Genetics ISSN 0022–2593

Journal of Medical Humanities ISSN 1041–3545

Journal of Medicine and Philosophy ISSN 0360–5310

Journal Of Mental Health Administration ISSN 0092–8623

Journal Of Molecular Medicine ISSN 0946–2716

Journal of NIH Research ISSN 1043–609X

Journal of Nursing Administration ISSN 0002–0443

Journal of Nursing Education ISSN 0148–4834

Journal of Nursing Management ISSN 0966–0429

Journal of Obstetric, Gynecologic and Neonatal Nursing ISSN 0884–2175

Journal of Occupational and Environmental Medicine ISSN 1076–2752

Journal of Occupational Medicine ISSN 0096–1736

Journal of Pain and Symptom Management ISSN 0885–3924

Journal of Palliative Care ISSN 0825–8597

Journal of Pediatric Surgery ISSN 0022–3468

Journal of Pediatrics ISSN 0022–3476

Journal of Perinatal Medicine ISSN 0300–5577

Journal of Perinatology ISSN 0743–8346

Journal of Pharmacy and Law ISSN 1062–4546

Journal of Professional Nursing ISSN 8755–7223

Journal of Psychiatry and Neuroscience ISSN 1180–4882

Journal of Psychosocial Nursing and Mental Health Services ISSN 0279–3695

Journal of the American Academy of Child Psychiatry ISSN 0002–7138

Journal of the American Academy of Psychiatry and the Law ISSN 1093–6793

Journal of the American College of Dentists ISSN 0002–7979

Journal of the American Dental Association ISSN 0002–8177

Journal of the American Dietetic Association ISSN 0002–8223

Journal of the American Geriatrics Society ISSN 0002–8614

Journal of the American Optometric Association ISSN 0003–0244

Journal of the American Veterinary Medical Association ISSN 0003–1488

Journal of the Medical Association of Georgia ISSN 0025–7028

Journal of the National Medical Association ISSN 0027–9684

Journal of the Royal College of Physicians of London ISSN 0035–8819

Journal of the Royal Society of Medicine ISSN 0141–0768

Journal Of The Society For Gynecologic Investigation ISSN 1071–5576

Journal of Women and Aging ISSN 0895–2841

JPMA: Journal of the Pakistan Medical Association ISSN 0030–9982

Jurimetrics Journal ISSN 0022–6793

K

Kennedy Institute of Ethics Journal ISSN 1054–6863

L

Lancet ISSN 0023–7507

Laryngoscope ISSN 0023–852X

Law and Mental Health ISSN 0890–5037

Law and Philosophy ISSN 0167–5249

Law and Policy ISSN 0265–8240

Law and Psychology Review ISSN 0098–5961

Law, Medicine and Health Care ISSN 0277–8459

Legal Medical Quarterly ISSN 0703–1211

Liberty, Life and Family

Linacre Quarterly ISSN 0024–3639

M

Managed Care ISSN 1062–3388

McGill Law Journal ISSN 0024–9041

McKinney's Consolidated Laws of New York Annotated

Medical Anthropology Quarterly ISSN 0745–5194

Medical Care ISSN 0025–7079

Medical Decision Making ISSN 0272–989X

Medical Education ISSN 0308–0110

Medical Ethics Newsletter

Medical Group Management Journal ISSN 0899–8949

Medical Humanities Review ISSN 0892–2772

Medical Journal of Australia ISSN 0025–729X

Medical Law Review ISSN 0967–0742

Medsurg Nursing ISSN 1092–0811

Mental and Physical Disability Law Reporter ISSN 0883–7902

Mental Retardation ISSN 0047–6765

Microbial and Comparative Genomics ISSN 1090–6592

Minerva ISSN 0026–4695

Minnesota Medicine ISSN 0026–556X

Mount Sinai Journal of Medicine ISSN 0027–2507

N

N and HC Perspectives on Community ISSN 1081–8731

National Black Law Journal ISSN 0896–0194

Nature ISSN 0028–0836

Nature Biotechnology ISSN 1087–0156

Nature Medicine ISSN 1078–8956

NCCE News (Veterans Health Administration National Center for Clinical Ethics)

Nephrology, Dialysis, Transplantation ISSN 0931–0509

Neurology ISSN 0028–3878

New England Journal of Medicine ISSN 0028–4793

New England Journal on Criminal and Civil Confinement ISSN 0740–8994

New Hampshire Revised Statutes Annotated

New Jersey Medicine ISSN 0885–842X

New Law Journal ISSN 0306–6479

New Republic   ISSN 0028-6583
New Scientist   ISSN 0262-4079
New York Law School Journal of Human Rights   ISSN 8756-8926
New York Review of Books   ISSN 0028-7504
New York State Journal of Medicine   ISSN 0028-7628
New York Supplement, 2d Series   ISSN 1048-3624
New York Times   ISSN 0362-4331
New York Times Magazine   ISSN 0028-7822
New Zealand Medical Journal   ISSN 0028-8446
Newsweek   ISSN 0028-9604
Nichibunken Newsletter   ISSN 0914-6482
North Carolina Law Review   ISSN 0029-2524
North Eastern Reporter, 2d Series   ISSN 1048-3632
North Western Reporter, 2d Series   ISSN 1048-3640
Notre Dame Law Review   ISSN 0745-3515
Nursing Economics   ISSN 0746-1739
Nursing Ethics   ISSN 0969-7330
Nursing Life   ISSN 0279-3091
Nursing Management   ISSN 0744-6314
Nursing Outlook   ISSN 0029-6554
Nursing Science Quarterly   ISSN 0894-3184
Nursing Standard   ISSN 0029-6570

O

Obstetrics and Gynecology   ISSN 0029-7844
Occupational Medicine   ISSN 0885-114X
Omega: A Journal of Death and Dying   ISSN 0030-2228
Oncology   ISSN 0890-9091
Oncology Nursing Forum   ISSN 0190-535X
Origins   ISSN 0093-609X

P

Pacific Law Journal   ISSN 0030-8757
Pacific Reporter, 2d Series   ISSN 1044-9442
Paediatric and Perinatal Epidemiology   ISSN 0269-5022
Palliative Medicine   ISSN 0269-2163
Patient Education and Counseling   ISSN 0738-3991
Pediatric AIDS and HIV Infection   ISSN 1045-5418
Pediatric Clinics of North America   ISSN 0031-3955
Pediatric Nursing   ISSN 0097-9805
Pediatrics   ISSN 0031-4005
Pepperdine Law Review   ISSN 0092-430X
Perceptual and Motor Skills   ISSN 0031-5125
Personalist   ISSN 0031-5621
Perspectives in Biology and Medicine   ISSN 0031-5982
Pharos   ISSN 0031-7179
Philosophical Quarterly   ISSN 0031-8094
Philosophy   ISSN 0031-8191
Philosophy and Public Affairs   ISSN 0049-3915
Philosophy and Public Policy   ISSN 1067-2478
Plastic and Reconstructive Surgery   ISSN 0032-1052
Plastic Surgical Nursing   ISSN 0741-5206
Politics and the Life Sciences   ISSN 0730-9384
Polity   ISSN 0032-3497
Postgraduate Medical Journal   ISSN 0032-5473
Professional Ethics   ISSN 1063-6579
Professional Nurse (London)   ISSN 0266-8130
Professional Psychology: Research and Practice   ISSN 0735-7028

Psychiatric Annals   ISSN 0048-5713
Psychiatric Clinics of North America   ISSN 0193-953X
Psychiatric Quarterly   ISSN 0033-2720
Psychiatric Services   ISSN 1075-2730
Psychiatry   ISSN 0033-2747
Psycho-Oncology   ISSN 1057-9249
Psychological Reports   ISSN 0033-2941
Psychopharmacology (Berlin)   ISSN 0033-3158
Psychosomatics   ISSN 0033-3182
Psychotherapy   ISSN 0090-144X
Psychotherapy and Psychosomatics   ISSN 0033-3190
Public Health   ISSN 0033-3506
Public Understanding of Science   ISSN 0963-6625

Q

QRB/Quality Review Bulletin   ISSN 0097-5990
Quality in Health Care   ISSN 0963-8172
Quality of Life Research   ISSN 0962-9343

R

Responsive Community   ISSN 1053-0754
Review of Religious Research   ISSN 0034-673X
Rhode Island Medical Journal   ISSN 0363-7913
Risk: Health, Safety and Environment   ISSN 1073-8673
RN   ISSN 0033-7021
Rutgers Law Review   ISSN 0036-0465

S

Sangyo Ika Daigaku Zasshi/Journal of University of Occupational and Environmental Health   ISSN 0387-821X
Scandinavian Journal of Caring Sciences   ISSN 0283-9318
Scandinavian Journal of Gastroenterology   ISSN 0036-5521
Scandinavian Journal of Social Medicine   ISSN 0300-8037
SCI Nursing   ISSN 0888-8299
Science   ISSN 0036-8075
Science and Engineering Ethics   ISSN 1353-3452
Science News   ISSN 0036-8423
Science, Technology, and Human Values   ISSN 0162-2439
Scientific American   ISSN 0036-8733
Seminars in Dialysis   ISSN 0894-0959
Seminars in Oncology   ISSN 0093-7754
Seminars in Oncology Nursing   ISSN 0749-2081
Seminars in Perinatology   ISSN 0146-0005
Seminars in Reproductive Endocrinology   ISSN 0734-8630
Singapore Medical Journal   ISSN 0037-5675
Social History of Medicine   ISSN 0951-631X
Social Philosophy and Policy   ISSN 0265-0525
Social Science and Medicine   ISSN 0277-9536
Social Work   ISSN 0037-8046
Society   ISSN 0147-2011
Sociology of Health and Illness   ISSN 0141-9889
Sociology of Religion   ISSN 1069-4404
South African Medical Journal   ISSN 0038-2469

South Eastern Reporter, 2d Series ISSN 1042–6531
Southern California Law Review ISSN 0038–3910
Southern California Review of Law and Women's Studies
Southern Medical Journal ISSN 0038–4348
Southwestern Law Journal ISSN 0038–4836
Stanford Law and Policy Review ISSN 1044–4386
Studies in Christian Ethics ISSN 0953–9468
Studies in Family Planning ISSN 0039–3665
Supreme Court Reporter

T

Teaching and Learning in Medicine ISSN 1040–1334
Teaching of Psychology ISSN 0098–6283
Technology in Society ISSN 0160–791X
Texas Dental Journal ISSN 0040–4284
Texas Journal of Women and the Law ISSN 1058–5427
Texas Law Review ISSN 0040–4411
Theoretical Medicine ISSN 0167–9902
Theoretical Medicine and Bioethics ISSN 1386–7415
Theoretical Surgery ISSN 0179–8669
Time ISSN 0040–781X
Today's OR Nurse ISSN 0194–5181
Tradition: A Journal of Orthodox Jewish Thought ISSN 0041–0608
Transfusion ISSN 0041–1132
Transfusion Medicine Reviews ISSN 0887–7963
Transfusion Science ISSN 0955–3886
Transplantation ISSN 0041–1337
Transplantation Proceedings ISSN 0041–1345
Transplantation Reviews ISSN 0955–470X
Trial ISSN 0041–2538
Tulane Law Review ISSN 0041–3992

U

UCLA Law Review ISSN 0041–5650
Ultrasound in Obstetrics and Gynecology ISSN 0960–7692
U.S. News and World Report ISSN 0041–5537
University of Kansas Law Review ISSN 0083–4025
University of Michigan Journal of Law Reform ISSN 0033–1546
University of Pittsburgh Law Review ISSN 0041–9915
University of San Francisco Law Review ISSN 0042–0018
UNOS Update ISSN 1077–8268
Update [Loma Linda University Center for Christian Bioethics]
USA Weekend

V

Vanderbilt Law Review ISSN 0042–2533
Vard i Norden ISSN 0107–4083
Veterinary Quarterly ISSN 0165–2176
Veterinary Record ISSN 0042–4900

W

Wall Street Journal ISSN 0099–9660
Washington Post ISSN 0190–8286

Washington University Law Quarterly ISSN 0043–0862
West Indian Medical Journal ISSN 0043–3144
West Virginia Law Review ISSN 0043–3268
Western Journal of Nursing Research ISSN 0193–9459
Women and Health ISSN 0363–0242
Women's Health Issues ISSN 1049–3867
Women's Rights Law Reporter ISSN 0085–8269
Women's Studies International Forum ISSN 0277–5395
World Journal of Surgery ISSN 0364–2313

Y

Yale Law and Policy Review ISSN 0740–8048
Yale Law Journal ISSN 0044–0094

SUBJECT ENTRY SECTION

SUBJECT ENTRY SECTION

ABORTION

See also FETUSES

Alan Guttmacher Institute. Induced Abortion. [Fact sheet]. New York, NY: Alan Guttmacher Institute; 1996. 2 p. BE57382.
*abortion, induced; age factors; childbirth; contraception; government financing; government regulation; health insurance; legal aspects; minors; motivation; risk; socioeconomic factors; *statistics; women's health services; United States

Bausola, Adriano. The cultural anthropology of the right to life. *Dolentium Hominum: Church and Health in the World.* 1996; 31(11th Yr., No. 1): 146–149. BE57367.
*abortion on demand; aged; attitudes; capitalism; Christian ethics; chronically ill; commodification; cultural pluralism; euthanasia; fetuses; historical aspects; humanism; *libertarianism; moral obligations; morality; rights; secularism; sexuality; social worth; socialism; *value of life; *values; women's rights; *Western World

Beckwith, Francis J. Personal bodily rights, abortion, and unplugging the violinist. *International Philosophical Quarterly.* 1992 Mar; 32(1, Issue 125): 105–118. 28 fn. BE57774.
abortion on demand; *abortion, induced; autonomy; childbirth; *fetuses; killing; libertarianism; *moral obligations; *moral policy; mortality; mother fetus relationship; parent child relationship; personhood; *pregnant women; rape; *rights; value of life; women's rights

Boonin–Vail, David. A defense of "A defense of abortion": on the responsibility objection to Thomson's argument. *Ethics.* 1997 Jan; 107(2): 286–313. 42 fn. BE55689.
*abortion, induced; *fetuses; intention; *moral obligations; *moral policy; mother fetus relationship; negligence; philosophy; *pregnant women; presumed consent; rape; rights; value of life; Thomson, Judith

Budziszewski, J. Why we kill the weak. *Human Life Review.* 1997 Fall; 23(4): 67–74. BE57427.
*abortion, induced; *active euthanasia; *allowing to die; compassion; conscience; family relationship; justice; *killing; love; moral development; moral obligations; motivation; *vulnerable populations; withholding treatment; duty to die

Calhoun, Byron C.; Reitman, James S.; Hoeldtke, Nathan J. Perinatal hospice: a response to partial birth abortion for infants with congenital defects. *Issues in Law and Medicine.* 1997 Fall; 13(2): 125–143. 86 fn. BE57805.
allowing to die; *alternatives; autonomy; *childbirth; *chromosome abnormalities; *congenital disorders; conscience; counseling; death; decision making; *fetal development; fetuses; health personnel; hospices; informed consent; methods; *newborns; *palliative care; parents; personhood; pregnant women; privacy; psychological stress; *selective abortion; suffering; theology; value of life; viability; *pregnancy trimesters

Callahan, Joan C. Birth control ethics. *In:* Chadwick, Ruth, ed. Encyclopedia of Applied Ethics, Volume 1. San Diego, CA: Academic Press; 1998: 335–351. 17 refs. ISBN 0–12–227066–5. BE56371.
abortion on demand; *abortion, induced; attitudes; autonomy; beginning of life; coercion; congenital disorders; *contraception; drug abuse; eugenics; family planning; females; fetuses; government regulation; hormones; infanticide; international aspects; involuntary sterilization; males; medical devices; *methods; *moral policy; *morality; multiple pregnancy; personhood; physicians; politics; *population control; pregnant women; prenatal diagnosis; prenatal injuries; *public policy; religion; *reproduction; selective abortion; sex determination; sexuality; *social control; socioeconomic factors; voluntary sterilization; wedge argument; women's rights

Cavanagh, Denis. Legal abortion in America: factors in the dynamics of change. *Liberty, Life and Family.* 1996; 2(2): 309–317. 14 fn. BE56932.
*abortion on demand; *abortion, induced; attitudes; beginning of life; Christian ethics; congenital disorders; decision making; fetuses; financial support; internship and residency; legal aspects; medical education; obstetrics and gynecology; organizational policies; physicians; political activity; pregnant women; professional organizations; public policy; rape; selective abortion; survey; therapeutic abortion; value of life; viability; women's rights; American Association of Pro-Life Obstetricians and Gynecologists; American College of Obstetricians and Gynecologists; American Council for Graduate Medical Education; Right to Life Movement; Roe v. Wade; *United States

Davis, Anne J.; Aroskar, Mila A.; Liaschenko, Joan, et al. Abortion. *In: their* Ethical Dilemmas and Nursing Practice. Fourth Edition. Stamford, CT: Appleton and Lange; 1997: 135–157. 95 fn. ISBN 0–8385–2283–1. BE58596.
*abortion, induced; attitudes; case studies; conscience; fetuses; historical aspects; legal aspects; moral obligations; *nurses; nursing ethics; obligations of society; personhood; physicians; political activity; pregnant women; religion; rights; selective abortion; Supreme Court decisions; United States

Devine, Philip E. 'Conservative' views of abortion. *In:* Edwards, Rem B., ed. Advances in Bioethics. Volume 2: New Essays on Abortion and Bioethics. Greenwich, CT: JAI Press; 1997: 183–202. 58 refs. ISBN 0–7623–0194–5. BE56794.
*abortion, induced; attitudes; contraception; embryos; fetuses; freedom; killing; legal aspects; moral obligations; *moral policy; personhood; political activity; *public policy; rape; religion; selective abortion; therapeutic abortion; violence; women's rights; potentiality; United States

Devine, Philip E. Homicide, criminal versus justifiable. *In:* Chadwick, Ruth, ed. Encyclopedia of Applied Ethics, Volume 2. San Diego, CA: Academic Press; 1998: 587–595. 14 refs. ISBN 0–12–227067–3. BE56396.
*abortion, induced; *active euthanasia; assisted suicide; Christian ethics; criminal law; double effect; intention; involuntary euthanasia; *killing; moral policy; personhood; philosophy; public policy; secularism; speciesism; *suicide;

BE = bioethics accession number   fn. = footnotes   refs. = references

theology; utilitarianism; voluntary euthanasia; wedge argument

Dwyer, Susan; Feinberg, Joel. The Problem of Abortion. Third Edition. Belmont, CA: Wadsworth; 1997. 243 p. Bibliography: p. 236–243. ISBN 0–534–50514–7. BE56241.

*abortion, induced; autonomy; beginning of life; ethical theory; feminist ethics; fetal development; *fetuses; human characteristics; infanticide; killing; legal aspects; *moral obligations; *moral policy; morality; personhood; philosophy; pregnant women; public policy; rights; Roman Catholic ethics; self concept; standards; Supreme Court decisions; value of life; viability; virtues; Canada; United States

Edwards, Rem B., ed. Advances in Bioethics. Volume 2: New Essays on Abortion and Bioethics. Greenwich, CT: JAI Press; 1997. 346 p. (Advances in bioethics; v.2). 670 refs. 24 fn. ISBN 0–7623–0194–5. BE56788.

*abortion, induced; anencephaly; attitudes; brain death; counseling; determination of death; fetal development; *fetuses; government financing; government regulation; indigents; killing; legal aspects; legal rights; methods; moral obligations; moral policy; personhood; political activity; politics; privacy; Protestant ethics; public policy; religious ethics; Roman Catholic ethics; standards; Supreme Court decisions; terminology; women's rights; Right to Life Movement; United States

Ewart, Wendy R.; Winikoff, Beverly. Toward safe and effective medical abortion. *Science.* 1998 Jul 24; 281(5376): 520–521. 7 refs. BE58908.

*abortion, induced; biomedical research; developing countries; drug industry; *drugs; health care delivery; *international aspects; morbidity; mortality; public policy; risks and benefits; surgery; therapeutic research; *women's health; methotrexate; misoprostol; RU–486

Gert, Heather J. Viability. *In:* Dwyer, Susan; Feinberg, Joel, eds. The Problem of Abortion. Third Edition. Belmont, CA: Wadsworth; 1997: 118–126. 16 fn. Reprinted from *International Journal of Philosophical Studies,* 1995; 3: 133–142. ISBN 0–534–50514–7. BE56086.

abortion on demand; *abortion, induced; autonomy; biomedical technologies; childbirth; congenital disorders; *fetal development; *fetuses; government regulation; infanticide; killing; legal obligations; *moral obligations; *moral policy; *pregnant women; public policy; *rights; standards; state interest; Supreme Court decisions; value of life; *viability; dependency; *pregnancy trimesters; Roe v. Wade; United States

Gibson, Susanne. Abortion. *In:* Chadwick, Ruth, ed. Encyclopedia of Applied Ethics, Volume 1. San Diego, CA: Academic Press; 1998: 1–8. 18 refs. ISBN 0–12–227066–5. BE56362.

aborted fetuses; *abortion, induced; biomedical technologies; embryo research; feminist ethics; fetal development; fetal research; fetal tissue donation; fetuses; *moral policy; personhood; pregnant women; review; rights; utilitarianism; value of life; viability

Harris, John. Should we attempt to eradicate disability? *In:* Morscher, Edgar; Neumaier, Otto; Simons, Peter, eds. Applied Ethics in a Troubled World. Boston, MA: Kluwer Academic; 1998: 105–114. 24 fn. ISBN 0–7923–4965–2. BE58585.

active euthanasia; allowing to die; *congenital disorders; *disabled; embryo transfer; embryos; eugenics; fetuses; in vitro fertilization; *infanticide; intention; maternal health; newborns; personhood; political activity; quality of life; reproduction; *selective abortion; *social discrimination; therapeutic abortion; value of life; International Wittgenstein

Symposium

Hemminki, Elina; Santalahti, Päivi; Louhiala, Pekka. Ethical conflicts in regulating the start of life. *Perspectives in Biology and Medicine.* 1997 Summer; 40(4): 586–591. 21 refs. BE56604.

abortion on demand; *abortion, induced; allowing to die; *beginning of life; biomedical technologies; congenital disorders; disabled; embryos; eugenics; fetuses; *intensive care units; multiple pregnancy; *newborns; patient care; personhood; prematurity; *prenatal diagnosis; *reproductive technologies; selective abortion; values

Hodgson, Jane E. Abortion procedures and abortifacients. *In:* Edwards, Rem B., ed. Advances in Bioethics. Volume 2: New Essays on Abortion and Bioethics. Greenwich, CT: JAI Press; 1997: 75–106. 50 refs. ISBN 0–7623–0194–5. BE56790.

*abortion, induced; contraception; counseling; drugs; fetal development; fetuses; government regulation; health care; health care delivery; historical aspects; informed consent; international aspects; legal aspects; medical education; medical fees; *methods; minors; organizational policies; parental consent; parental notification; personhood; physician's role; professional organizations; psychology; risks and benefits; violence; women's rights; postcoital contraceptives; American College of Obstetricians and Gynecologists; Bangladesh; United States

Holt, Janet. Screening and the perfect baby. *In:* Frith, Lucy, ed. Ethics and Midwifery: Issues in Contemporary Practice. Boston, MA: Butterworth–Heinemann; 1996: 140–155. 14 refs. ISBN 0–7506–3056–6. BE58637.

attitudes; *congenital disorders; decision making; disabled; economics; eugenics; fetuses; genetic disorders; genetic predisposition; genetic screening; legal aspects; mass screening; nurse midwives; pregnant women; *prenatal diagnosis; public policy; risk; selection for treatment; *selective abortion; sex determination; social discrimination; social impact; teleological ethics; wedge argument; Great Britain

Hurry, Stephanie. Termination of pregnancy -- a nurse's right to choose. *British Journal of Theatre Nursing.* 1997 Oct; 7(7): 18–22. 15 refs. BE58357.

*abortion, induced; accountability; *conscience; emergency care; historical aspects; legal aspects; nurse patient relationship; *nurses; *nursing ethics; patient care; standards; Great Britain

Johnston, S.R.D.; Broadley, K.; Henson, G., et al. Management of metastatic melanoma during pregnancy. [Case study and commentaries]. *BMJ (British Medical Journal).* 1998 Mar 14; 316(7134): 848–851. 13 refs. BE57757.

altruism; *cancer; case studies; cesarean section; *childbirth; *decision making; drugs; fetal development; *fetuses; maternal health; morbidity; mortality; parents; *patient care; *pregnant women; *prognosis; radiology; *risks and benefits; terminally ill; *therapeutic abortion; viability

Kavanaugh, John F. Partial truths. *America.* 1997 Apr 5; 176(11): 24. BE55786.

*abortion, induced; beginning of life; *fetal development; killing; *methods; personhood; Roman Catholic ethics; *pregnancy trimesters

Lewin, Tamar. A new technique makes abortions possible earlier. [News]. *New York Times.* 1997 Dec 21: 1, 30. BE56777.

*abortion, induced; beginning of life; contraception; drugs; *fetal development; *methods; political activity; Roman Catholic ethics; surgery; *pregnancy trimesters; Planned Parenthood; Right to Life Movement; RU–486; United

---

BE = bioethics accession number   fn. = footnotes   refs. = references

States

Lewin, Tamar. Abortion fell again in 1995, U.S. says, but rose in some areas last year. [News]. *New York Times.* 1997 Dec 5: A14. BE58241.
  *abortion, induced; age factors; contraception; females; fetal development; socioeconomic factors; statistics; trends; geographic factors; *United States

Marquis, Don. Abortion. *In:* Borchert, Donald M., ed. The Encyclopedia of Philosophy. Supplement. New York, NY: Simon and Schuster Macmillan; 1996: 1–3. 19 refs. ISBN 0–02–864629–0. BE57219.
  *abortion, induced; beginning of life; ethical analysis; fetuses; *moral policy; personhood; philosophy; pregnant women; religion; value of life

Matteo, Anthony M. Beyond the impasse: making moral sense of abortion. *In:* Gottfried, Paul, ed. Religion and Public Life. Volume 29: Theologies and Moral Concern. New Brunswick, NJ: Transaction Publishers; 1995: 21–32. 15 fn. ISBN 1–56000–823–7. BE57282.
  *abortion on demand; *abortion, induced; adoption; animal rights; attitudes; autonomy; consensus; cultural pluralism; ethical relativism; fetuses; killing; legal aspects; *moral policy; personhood; political activity; pregnant women; *public policy; rights; selective abortion; social impact; Supreme Court decisions; therapeutic abortion; value of life; values; Right to Life Movement; United States

Nelson, James Lindemann. The meaning of the act: reflections on the expressive force of reproductive decision making and policies. *Kennedy Institute of Ethics Journal.* 1998 June; 8(2): 165–182. 9 refs. 3 fn. BE58375.
  abortion on demand; *congenital disorders; *decision making; *disabled; fetuses; genetic disorders; genetic screening; intention; *motivation; *pregnant women; *prenatal diagnosis; quality of life; reproduction; rights; *selective abortion; social worth; *stigmatization; values; voluntary sterilization; ELSI–funded publication; Buchanan, Allen

Prenatal and preconceptual testing and screening programs provide information on the basis of which people can choose to avoid the birth of children likely to face disabilities. Some disabilities advocates have objected to such programs and to the decisions made within them, on the grounds that measures taken to avoid the birth of children with disabilities have an "expressive force" that conveys messages disrespectful to people with disabilities. Assessing such a claim requires careful attention to general considerations relating meaning, intention, and social practices; it has only begun to receive such attention. Building on work by Allen Buchanan, who has challenged this claim, I further consider the disabilities advocates' objection, ultimately concluding that it is misplaced; neither individual actions nor general practices of this type necessarily express disrespectful messages.

Nisand, I.; Shenfield, F. Multiple pregnancies and embryo reduction: ethical and legal issues. *In:* Shenfield, F.; Sureau, C., eds. Ethical Dilemmas in Assisted Reproduction. New York, NY: Parthenon Pub. Group; 1997: 67–75. 19 refs. ISBN 1–85070–916–5. BE57948.
  legal aspects; *multiple pregnancy; prematurity; reproductive technologies; risk; risks and benefits; *selective abortion; twins; France; Great Britain

Peters, Ted. Designer genes and selective abortion. *In: his* For the Love of Children: Genetic Technology and the Future of the Family. Louisville, KY: Westminster John Knox Press; 1996: 85–118, 193–199. 63 fn. ISBN 0–664–25468–3. BE55697.
  adoption; beginning of life; coercion; confidentiality; decision making; disabled; employment; eugenics; fetal development; *fetuses; genetic counseling; *genetic disorders; genetic information; *genetic predisposition; *genetic screening; government regulation; insurance; killing; legal rights; *personhood; pregnant women; prenatal diagnosis; privacy; Protestant ethics; public policy; risk; *Roman Catholic ethics; *selective abortion; *social discrimination; value of life; viability; dignity; Genetic Privacy Act 1994; United States

Riddle, John M. Eve's Herbs: A History of Contraception and Abortion in the West. Cambridge, MA: Harvard University Press; 1997. 341 p. 1,330 fn. ISBN 0–674–27024–X. BE56628.
  *abortion, induced; *alternative therapies; ancient history; attitudes; *contraception; drugs; *females; fetuses; health personnel; *historical aspects; infanticide; information dissemination; international aspects; legal aspects; literature; nurse midwives; population control; religion; reproduction; technical expertise; *folk medicine; *plants; *Western World; Eighteenth Century; Europe; Middle Ages; Nineteenth Century; Seventeenth Century; Sixteenth Century; Twentieth Century; United States

Rodgers, Bruce D.; Rodgers, Diane E. Abortion: the seduction of medicine. *Liberty, Life and Family.* 1996; 2(2): 285–308. 49 fn. BE56041.
  aborted fetuses; *abortion, induced; compassion; disabled; eugenics; fetal research; fetal therapy; fetuses; health facilities; malpractice; medical education; medical ethics; medicine; morality; organizational policies; physicians; population control; pregnant women; prenatal diagnosis; professional organizations; psychological stress; quality of life; remuneration; reproduction; selective abortion; sexuality; social discrimination; suffering; technical expertise; therapeutic abortion; unwanted children; value of life; violence; women's health services; women's rights; United States

Rorty, Mary V.; Pinkerton, JoAnn V. Elective fetal reduction: the ultimate elective surgery. *Journal of Contemporary Health Law and Policy.* 1996 Fall; 13(1): 53–77. 64 fn. BE55793.
  case studies; congenital disorders; *decision making; disclosure; drugs; embryo transfer; genetic disorders; guidelines; informed consent; institutional policies; international aspects; morality; morbidity; mortality; *multiple pregnancy; newborns; patient participation; physicians; pregnant women; prematurity; prenatal diagnosis; reproductive technologies; *risk; *selective abortion; sex determination; socioeconomic factors; treatment outcome; twins; United States

Russo, Nancy Felipe; Dabul, Amy J. The relationship of abortion to well–being: do race and religion make a difference? *Professional Psychology: Research and Practice.* 1997 Feb; 28(1): 23–31. 48 refs. BE58315.
  *abortion, induced; attitudes; *blacks; comparative studies; *counseling; disclosure; education; evaluation studies; females; government regulation; informed consent; mental health; *psychological stress; psychotherapy; quality of life; *religion; risks and benefits; Roman Catholics; self concept; *socioeconomic factors; state government; *whites; self–help groups; United States

Schwartz, Lewis M. An essay on the moral status question. *In:* Edwards, Rem B., ed. Advances in Bioethics. Volume 2: New Essays on Abortion and Bioethics. Greenwich, CT: JAI Press; 1997: 267–301. 11 refs. ISBN 0–7623–0194–5. BE56797.
  *abortion, induced; adults; *fetal development; *fetuses; *killing; *moral obligations; *moral policy; pain; persistent vegetative state; *personhood; philosophy

---

BE = bioethics accession number   fn. = footnotes   refs. = references

Shanahan, Timothy; Wang, Robin. Abortion. *In: their* Reason and Insight: Western and Eastern Perspectives on the Pursuit of Moral Wisdom. Belmont, CA: Wadsworth; 1996: 359–395. Includes references, readings, and discussion questions. Designed as a textbook for college students. ISBN 0–534–23167–5. BE56141.
> *abortion, induced; attitudes; Buddhist ethics; fetal development; fetuses; international aspects; killing; *moral policy; *morality; personhood; physicians; pregnant women; public policy; rights; value of life; values; non-Western World; pregnancy trimesters; Western World; China; Japan; Thailand

Sherlock, Kevin. The Scarlet Survey: An Accounting from Courthouses, Health Agencies, Police Blotters, and Morgues Across America of Women and Girls Exploited by Abortion on Demand. Akron, OH: Brennyman Books; 1997. 272 p. Bibliography: p. 270. ISBN 0–9654036–1–0. BE57387.
> *abortion on demand; abortion, induced; blacks; breast cancer; coercion; criminal law; federal government; fraud; health facilities; killing; malpractice; misconduct; morbidity; mortality; newborns; physicians; political activity; politics; pregnant women; professional competence; sex offenses; social discrimination; statistics; Planned Parenthood Federation of America; Right to Life Movement; United States

Simms, Madeleine; Chervenak, Frank A.; McCullough, Laurence B., et al. Is third trimester abortion justified? [Letters and responses]. *British Journal of Obstetrics and Gynaecology.* 1996 Feb; 103(2): 187–189. 12 refs. BE56562.
> community services; disabled; *fetal development; fetuses; killing; legal aspects; moral obligations; moral policy; obligations of society; obligations to society; parents; physicians; pregnant women; prenatal diagnosis; prognosis; quality of life; resource allocation; *selective abortion; *pregnancy trimesters; Great Britain

Simpson, Joe Leigh; Carson, Sandra A. Multifetal reduction in high-order gestations: a nonelective procedure? [Editorial]. *Journal Of The Society For Gynecologic Investigation.* 1996 Jan–Feb; 3(1): 1–2. 8 refs. BE57915.
> counseling; directive counseling; embryo transfer; genetic screening; informed consent; *multiple pregnancy; prenatal diagnosis; reproductive technologies; *selective abortion

Stein, Edward. Choosing the sexual orientation of children. *Bioethics.* 1998 Jan; 12(1): 1–24. 57 fn. BE58483.
> females; genetic determinism; genetic intervention; genetic research; *homosexuals; international aspects; justice; legal aspects; males; *moral policy; *parents; preimplantation diagnosis; prenatal diagnosis; *public policy; reproduction; reproductive technologies; rights; *selective abortion; *sex determination; *sex preselection; sexuality; social discrimination; social impact; *stigmatization; suffering; women's rights; India; United States

Strasser, Mark. Dependence, reliance and abortion. *Philosophical Quarterly.* 1985 Jan; 35(138): 73–82. 6 fn. Commentary on M. Davis, "Foetuses, famous violinists, and the right to continued aid," *PQ* 1983 Jul; 33(132): 259–278. BE57840.
> *abortion, induced; altruism; *fetuses; justice; killing; *moral obligations; *moral policy; *mother fetus relationship; personhood; *pregnant women; rights; viability

Struve, James K. The consultation: a patient's request to be referred for an abortion sends this physician into an ethical tailspin. *Minnesota Medicine.* 1996 Aug; 79(8):

12–13. 3 refs. BE55595.
> abortion on demand; *abortion, induced; attitudes; childbirth; community services; counseling; *physicians; pregnant women; public policy; referral and consultation; value of life; United States

Sumner, L.W. A third way. *In:* Dwyer, Susan; Feinberg, Joel, eds. The Problem of Abortion. Third Edition. Belmont, CA: Wadsworth; 1997: 98–117. 18 fn. Revised version of his *Abortion and Moral Theory*, Princeton Press; 1981: 124–160. ISBN 0–534–50514–7. BE56091.
> abortion on demand; *abortion, induced; beginning of life; brain; congenital disorders; conscience; contraception; emotions; *fetal development; *fetuses; human characteristics; infanticide; intelligence; killing; maternal health; *moral obligations; *moral policy; morality; pain; personhood; pregnant women; *public policy; *rights; risks and benefits; selective abortion; self concept; sex offenses; socioeconomic factors; speciesism; *standards; therapeutic abortion; *value of life; viability; *pregnancy trimesters; rationality

Sumner, L.W. Moderate views of abortion. *In:* Edwards, Rem B., ed. Advances in Bioethics. Volume 2: New Essays on Abortion and Bioethics. Greenwich, CT: JAI Press; 1997: 203–226. 26 refs. ISBN 0–7623–0194–5. BE56795.
> *abortion, induced; *fetal development; *fetuses; government regulation; informed consent; killing; legal aspects; *moral obligations; *moral policy; morality; policy analysis; politics; pregnant women; *public policy; time factors; value of life; viability; women's rights; United States

Timpson, Joanne. Abortion: the antithesis of womanhood? *Journal of Advanced Nursing.* 1996 Apr; 23(4): 776–785. 121 refs. BE57511.
> *abortion, induced; autonomy; contraception; *females; *feminist ethics; human body; international aspects; legal aspects; mortality; mothers; parent child relationship; pregnant women; reproduction; social control; social discrimination; value of life; *women's health services; *women's rights; Abortion Act 1967 (Great Britain); Great Britain; National Health Service

Warren, Mary Anne. Abortion and human rights. *In: her*: Moral Status: Obligations to Persons and Other Living Things. New York, NY: Oxford University Press; 1997: 201–223. 36 fn. ISBN 0–19–823668–9. BE56998.
> *abortion, induced; autonomy; beginning of life; coercion; contraception; decision making; embryos; fetal development; fetuses; future generations; *human rights; legal aspects; moral obligations; *moral policy; mother fetus relationship; parent child relationship; personhood; population control; pregnant women; prenatal injuries; privacy; public policy; reproduction; self concept; treatment refusal; value of life; viability; *women's rights; potentiality; United States

Weiss, Gail. Sex-selective abortion: a relational approach. *In:* DiQuinzio, Patrice; Young, Iris Marion, eds. Feminist Ethics and Social Policy. Bloomington, IN: Indiana University Press; 1997: 274–290. 16 refs. 11 fn. ISBN 0–253–21125–5. BE57288.
> abortion, induced; autonomy; coercion; *decision making; family members; family relationship; *females; *feminist ethics; infanticide; international aspects; moral policy; mother fetus relationship; mothers; motivation; pregnant women; prenatal diagnosis; public policy; *selective abortion; *sex determination; social control; social dominance; *socioeconomic factors; values; China; India; Ruddick, Sara; Warren, Mary Anne

White, Robert J. Partial–birth abortion: a neurosurgeon speaks. *America.* 1997 Oct 18; 177(11): 4–5. BE56599.
> *abortion, induced; attitudes; brain; *fetal development; fetuses; *methods; pain; physicians; *neurosurgery;

BE = bioethics accession number   fn. = footnotes   refs. = references

*pregnancy trimesters

ABORTION/ATTITUDES

Beckman, Linda J.; Harvey, S. Marie. Experience and acceptability of medical abortion with mifepristone and misoprostol among U.S. women. *Women's Health Issues.* 1997 Jul–Aug; 7(4): 253–262. 24 refs. BE55705.
*abortion, induced; *attitudes; *drugs; females; fetal development; human experimentation; knowledge, attitudes, practice; *methods; motivation; *pregnant women; risks and benefits; surgery; survey; women's health services; pregnancy trimesters; Oregon; RU–486; *United States; Vermont; Washington

Cook, Elizabeth Adell; Jelen, Ted G.; Wilcox, Clyde. Measuring public attitudes on abortion: methodological and substantive considerations. *Family Planning Perspectives.* 1993 May–Jun; 25(3): 118–121, 145. 9 fn. BE56027.
*abortion, induced; consensus; evaluation; government regulation; mass media; political activity; *public opinion; *public policy; state government; *survey; *questionnaires; *United States

Davis, N. Ann. Not drowning but waving: reflections on swimming through the shark–infested waters of the abortion debate. *In:* Edwards, Rem B., ed. Advances in Bioethics. Volume 2: New Essays on Abortion and Bioethics. Greenwich, CT: JAI Press; 1997: 227–265. 42 refs. 24 fn. ISBN 0–7623–0194–5. BE56796.
abortion on demand; *abortion, induced; *attitudes; autonomy; conscience; decision making; *dissent; females; feminist ethics; fetuses; government regulation; libertarianism; males; moral development; moral policy; *morality; mother fetus relationship; personhood; *political activity; pregnant women; *public policy; quality of life; socioeconomic factors; terminology; utilitarianism; value of life; women's rights; liberalism; Right to Life Movement; United States

Drake, Harriet; Reid, Margaret; Marteau, Theresa. Attitudes towards termination for fetal abnormality: comparisons in three European countries. *Clinical Genetics.* 1996 Mar; 49(3): 134–140. 16 refs. BE57055.
abortion on demand; abortion, induced; anencephaly; *attitudes; chromosome abnormalities; comparative studies; *congenital disorders; cystic fibrosis; dementia; Down syndrome; *genetic disorders; genetic screening; genetics; *health personnel; Huntington's disease; *international aspects; mentally retarded; obstetrics and gynecology; physically disabled; physicians; *pregnant women; prenatal diagnosis; *public opinion; public policy; *selective abortion; sex determination; spina bifida; survey; *Europe; *Germany; *Great Britain; *Portugal

Finlay, Barbara. Gender differences in attitudes toward abortion among Protestant seminarians. *Review of Religious Research.* 1996 Jun; 37(4): 354–360. 14 refs. 1 fn. BE57690.
*abortion, induced; *attitudes; *clergy; comparative studies; *females; *males; *Protestants; selective abortion; students; survey; therapeutic abortion; Presbyterian Church

Furedi, Ann. Many people who disapprove of abortion nevertheless think it should be legal. [Letter]. *BMJ (British Medical Journal).* 1997 Nov 1; 315(7116): 1165. 3 refs. BE58208.
abortion on demand; *abortion, induced; minors; *public opinion; *public policy; selective abortion; survey; *Great Britain

Goldberg, Carey; Elder, Janet. Public still backs

abortion, but wants limits, poll says. [News]. *New York Times.* 1998 Jan 16: A1, A16. BE58040.
abortion on demand; *abortion, induced; drugs; government regulation; legal aspects; motivation; political activity; politics; *public opinion; selective abortion; state government; survey; therapeutic abortion; trends; postcoital contraceptives; RU–486; *United States

Goldfarb, James; Kinzer, Donna J.; Boyle, Marian, et al. Attitudes of in vitro fertilization and intrauterine insemination couples toward multiple gestation pregnancy and multifetal pregnancy reduction. *Fertility and Sterility.* 1996 Apr; 65(4): 815–820. 18 refs. BE56462.
artificial insemination; *attitudes; embryo transfer; females; hormones; in vitro fertilization; males; *married persons; *multiple pregnancy; *patients; *reproductive technologies; *selective abortion; survey; treatment outcome; Ohio; University Hospitals of Cleveland

Hardacre, Helen. Marketing the Menacing Fetus in Japan. Berkeley, CA: University of California Press; 1997. 310 p. (Twentieth–century Japan; 7). Bibliography: p. 265–293. ISBN 0–520–20553–7. BE56521.
*aborted fetuses; *abortion, induced; advertising; *attitudes; Buddhist ethics; childbirth; females; historical aspects; *industry; males; mass media; mother fetus relationship; personhood; political activity; psychological stress; public policy; *religion; reproduction; sexuality; social discrimination; stigmatization; trends; ethnographic studies; guilt; *Japan; Shintoism; Twentieth Century

Lewin, Tamar. Debate distant for many having abortions. [News]. *New York Times.* 1998 Jan 17: A1, A9. BE57598.
abortion on demand; *abortion, induced; *attitudes; contraception; government regulation; legal aspects; political activity; *pregnant women; public opinion; socioeconomic factors; Supreme Court decisions; Roe v. Wade; United States

Norup, Michael. Attitudes towards abortion in the Danish population. *Bioethics.* 1997 Oct; 11(5): 439–449. 14 fn. BE56336.
*abortion on demand; *abortion, induced; age factors; *attitudes; chromosome abnormalities; *congenital disorders; cystic fibrosis; Down syndrome; females; fetal development; fetuses; kidney diseases; males; morality; *public opinion; religion; *selective abortion; socioeconomic factors; survey; value of life; pregnancy trimesters; *Denmark
This article reports the results of a survey, by mailed questionnaire, of the attitudes among a sample of the Danish population towards abortion for social and genetic reasons. Of 1080 questionnaires sent to a random sample of persons between 18 and 45 years, 731 (68%) were completed and returned. A great majority of the respondents were liberal towards early abortion both for social reasons and in case of minor disease. In contrast, there was controversy about late abortions for social reasons and in the case of Down syndrome. Further there was strong reluctance to accept late abortion in case of minor disease. An analysis of the response patterns showed that most of the respondents had gradualist views on abortion, i.e. they would allow all early abortions, but only abortions for some reasons later in pregnancy. It was also found that the number who would find an early abortion acceptable in general was much higher than the number who would accept it in their own case. These findings suggest that a great part of the resistance towards abortion does not rest on a concern for the rights and interests for the fetus. Instead it may be explained on a view according to which fetal life is ascribed intrinsic moral value.

Viljoen, D.; Oosthuizen, C.; van der Westhuizen, S.

BE = bioethics accession number   fn. = footnotes   refs. = references

Patient attitudes to prenatal screening and termination of pregnancy at Groote Schuur Hospital: a two year prospective study. *East African Medical Journal.* 1996 May; 73(5): 327–329. 6 refs. BE55535.
    *attitudes; *congenital disorders; genetic counseling; genetic disorders; *pregnant women; *prenatal diagnosis; religion; *selective abortion; socioeconomic factors; survey; Muslims; prospective studies; Groote Schuur Hospital (Cape Town); *South Africa

ABORTION/FINANCIAL SUPPORT

Edwards, Rem B. Public funding of abortions and abortion counseling for poor women. *In:* Edwards, Rem B., ed. Advances in Bioethics. Volume 2: New Essays on Abortion and Bioethics. Greenwich, CT: JAI Press; 1997: 303–334. 60 refs. ISBN 0–7623–0194–5. BE56798.
    *abortion, induced; attitudes; conscience; *counseling; economics; eugenics; family planning; freedom; *government financing; human rights; *indigents; informed consent; legal aspects; legal rights; minority groups; obligations of society; *public policy; religion; religious ethics; resource allocation; values; United States

Haas–Wilson, Deborah. Women's reproductive choices: the impact of Medicaid funding restrictions. *Family Planning Perspectives.* 1997 Sep–Oct; 29(5): 228–233. 53 fn. BE58461.
    *abortion, induced; childbirth; decision making; evaluation studies; *government financing; *government regulation; indigents; pregnant women; public policy; *social impact; *state government; statistics; *Medicaid; *United States

Sloan, Laura Curry. Constitutional law –– state impediments to abortion funding –– National Education Association of Rhode Island v. Garrahy. [Note]. *University of Kansas Law Review.* 1985 Winter; 34(2): 387–409. 186 fn. BE57049.
    *abortion, induced; constitutional law; equal protection; government financing; *government regulation; *health insurance reimbursement; *legal aspects; *legal rights; privacy; state government; Harris v. McRae; Maher v. Roe; *National Education Association of Rhode Island v. Garrahy; *Rhode Island; Roe v. Wade; United States

U.S. District Court, D. Utah, C.D. Utah Women's Clinic, Inc. v. Graham. *Federal Supplement.* 1995 Jun 20 (date of decision). 892: 1379–1385. BE56138.
    *abortion, induced; *federal government; *government financing; *government regulation; rape; sex offenses; *state government; therapeutic abortion; incest; Hyde Amendment; *Medicaid; *United States; *Utah; *Utah Women's Clinic, Inc. v. Graham
The U.S. District Court, Utah, enjoined state officials from enforcing Utah's abortion funding restriction to the extent that it conflicts with federal Medicaid law. As long as Utah accepts federal Medicaid funds, the state is required to participate in the program on the terms established by Congress. Accordingly, Utah cannot deny Medicaid funding for "medically necessary" abortions to eligible women pregnant through rape or incest, so long as federal matching funds are available for such abortions. (KIE abstract)

An H.M.O., Catholic–run, bars coverage for abortions. [News]. *New York Times.* 1997 Nov 17: B5. BE56181.
    *abortion, induced; contraception; family planning; federal government; females; *government financing; government regulation; *health insurance reimbursement; *health maintenance organizations; indigents; *institutional policies; refusal to treat; *Roman Catholics; state government; women's health services; *religious health facilities; *Fidelis Care (NY); *Medicaid; *New York

ABORTION/FOREIGN COUNTRIES

Birchard, Karen. Rape sparks abortion row in Ireland. [News]. *Lancet.* 1997 Dec 6; 350(9092): 1688. BE56922.
    *abortion, induced; adolescents; *legal aspects; *rape; therapeutic abortion; *Ireland

Church of England. Board for Social Responsibility. Abortion and the Church: What are the Issues? London: Church House Publishing; 1993 Jan. 31 p. Bibliography: p. 22. Pub. No. GS Misc 408. Published for the General Synod of the Church of England. ISBN 0–7151–6578–X. BE57740.
    *abortion, induced; beginning of life; childbirth; *Christian ethics; congenital disorders; conscience; cultural pluralism; drugs; fetal development; fetuses; health personnel; killing; *legal aspects; *morality; personhood; pregnant women; *Protestant ethics; *public policy; secularism; selective abortion; therapeutic abortion; *value of life; viability; Abortion Act 1967 (Great Britain); *Anglican Church; *Great Britain; Human Fertilisation and Embryology Act 1990; National Health Service; RU–486

Clarity, James F. Irish girl, 13, to abort baby in England. [News]. *New York Times.* 1997 Dec 2: A7. BE58235.
    *abortion, induced; adolescents; *government regulation; *international aspects; *legal aspects; parents; rape; Roman Catholics; socioeconomic factors; Supreme Court decisions; Great Britain; *Ireland

Cordner, Stephen; Ettershank, Kathy. Australian doctors charged over abortion. [News]. *Lancet.* 1998 Feb 21; 351(9102): 578. BE58505.
    *abortion, induced; *legal aspects; *legal liability; *physicians; Australia; *Western Australia

Csordas, Thomas J. A handmaid's tale: the rhetoric of personhood in American and Japanese healing of abortions. *In:* Sargent, Carolyn F.; Brettell, Caroline B., eds. Gender and Health: An International Perspective. Upper Saddle River, NJ: Prentice Hall; 1996: 227–241. 23 refs. 5 fn. ISBN 0–13–079427–9. BE58095.
    *aborted fetuses; *abortion, induced; *Buddhist ethics; comparative studies; emotions; *females; international aspects; mother fetus relationship; *personhood; *psychological stress; psychology; *religion; *Roman Catholics; grief; guilt; *Japan; *Pentecostal Christians; *United States

David, Henry P.; Baban, Adriana. Women's health and reproductive rights: Romanian experience. *Patient Education and Counseling.* 1996 Aug; 28(3): 235–245. 25 refs. BE57259.
    *abortion, induced; adults; coercion; contraception; decision making; *family planning; *females; *government regulation; historical aspects; *illegal abortion; *knowledge, attitudes, practice; morbidity; mortality; mothers; motivation; *population control; pregnant women; psychological stress; *public policy; reproduction; sexuality; social control; *social impact; socioeconomic factors; survey; women's health; *women's rights; qualitative research; *Romania; Twentieth Century

Dillon, Michele. Cultural differences in the abortion discourse of the Catholic Church: evidence from four countries. *Sociology of Religion.* 1996 Spring; 57(1): 25–36. 26 refs. BE58118.
    *abortion, induced; communication; comparative studies; cultural pluralism; *international aspects; law; morality; *organizational policies; *political activity; public policy; *Roman Catholic ethics; secularism; socioeconomic factors; value of life; women's rights; *Great Britain; *Ireland; *Poland; *United States

---

BE = bioethics accession number   fn. = footnotes   refs. = references

Drake, Harriet; Reid, Margaret; Marteau, Theresa. Attitudes towards termination for fetal abnormality: comparisons in three European countries. *Clinical Genetics.* 1996 Mar; 49(3): 134–140. 16 refs. BE57055.
> abortion on demand; abortion, induced; anencephaly; *attitudes; chromosome abnormalities; comparative studies; *congenital disorders; cystic fibrosis; dementia; Down syndrome; *genetic disorders; genetic screening; genetics; *health personnel; Huntington's disease; *international aspects; mentally retarded; obstetrics and gynecology; physically disabled; physicians; *pregnant women; prenatal diagnosis; *public opinion; public policy; *selective abortion; sex determination; spina bifida; survey; *Europe; *Germany; *Great Britain; *Portugal

Furedi, Ann. Many people who disapprove of abortion nevertheless think it should be legal. [Letter]. *BMJ (British Medical Journal).* 1997 Nov 1; 315(7116): 1165. 3 refs. BE58208.
> abortion on demand; *abortion, induced; minors; *public opinion; *public policy; selective abortion; survey; *Great Britain

Hardacre, Helen. Marketing the Menacing Fetus in Japan. Berkeley, CA: University of California Press; 1997. 310 p. (Twentieth-century Japan; 7). Bibliography: p. 265–293. ISBN 0-520-20553-7. BE56521.
> *aborted fetuses; *abortion, induced; advertising; *attitudes; Buddhist ethics; childbirth; females; historical aspects; *industry; males; mass media; mother fetus relationship; personhood; political activity; psychological stress; public policy; *religion; *reproduction; sexuality; social discrimination; stigmatization; trends; ethnographic studies; guilt; *Japan; Shintoism; Twentieth Century

Human Rights Watch Women's Rights Project. Abortion policy and restrictions on women's rights in post-communist Poland. *In: its* The Human Rights Watch Global Report on Women's Human Rights. New York, NY: Human Rights Watch; 1995 Aug: 451–456. 14 fn. ISBN 0-300-06546-9. BE56088.
> *abortion, induced; codes of ethics; equal protection; *government regulation; *legal aspects; legislation; medical fees; physicians; political activity; politics; pregnant women; selective abortion; therapeutic abortion; *women's rights; *Poland; Polish Medical College

Human Rights Watch Women's Rights Project. The abortion debate and violations of civil liberties in Ireland. *In: its* The Human Rights Watch Global Report on Women's Human Rights. New York, NY: Human Rights Watch; 1995 Aug: 444–451. 29 fn. ISBN 0-300-06546-9. BE56087.
> *abortion, induced; counseling; government regulation; information dissemination; international aspects; *legal aspects; legal rights; legislation; minors; pregnant women; rape; Abortion Information Bill 1995 (Ireland); Attorney General v. X; European Court of Human Rights; European Court of Justice; International Convention on Civil and Political Rights; *Ireland; Open Door Counselling v. Ireland

Hungary. Law No. 79 of 17 December 1992 on the protection of the life of the fetus. *International Digest of Health Legislation.* 1993; 44(2): 249–253. BE57186.
> abortion on demand; *abortion, induced; conscience; contraception; family planning; fetal development; *fetuses; *legal aspects; maternal health; patient care; pregnant women; standards; therapeutic abortion; value of life; *Hungary

Ibrahim, Youssef M. Algeria to permit abortions for rape victims. [News]. *New York Times.* 1998 Apr 14: A6. BE57920.
> *abortion, induced; *females; Islamic ethics; political activity; *public policy; *rape; *violence; *Algeria

Kovac, Carl. Abortion stirs up controversy in Hungary. [News]. *BMJ (British Medical Journal).* 1998 Apr 4; 316(7137): 1038. BE58121.
> *abortion, induced; autonomy; fetuses; hospitals; *legal aspects; minors; political activity; refusal to treat; *Hungary; Right to Life Movement

Loff, Bebe; Cordner, Stephen. Abortion bills introduced to Western Australian parliament. [News]. *Lancet.* 1998 Mar 21; 351(9106): 892. BE58858.
> *abortion, induced; counseling; informed consent; legal liability; *legislation; physicians; pregnant women; *Western Australia

Mao, Xin; Wertz, Dorothy C. China's genetic services providers' attitudes towards several ethical issues: a cross-cultural survey. *Clinical Genetics.* 1997 Aug; 52(2): 100–109. 38 refs. BE57506.
> *attitudes; common good; confidentiality; congenital disorders; developing countries; *directive counseling; *disclosure; *DNA data banks; DNA fingerprinting; duty to warn; eugenics; *genetic counseling; *genetic disorders; *genetic information; genetic materials; genetic predisposition; genetic services; genome mapping; government regulation; *health personnel; informed consent; law enforcement; minority groups; population control; public policy; reproductive technologies; *selective abortion; *sex determination; socioeconomic factors; survey; *China

Montgomery, Jonathan. Health care law and ethics: abortion; fertility; maternity care; selective treatment of the newborn; transplantation; terminal care and euthanasia. *In: his* Health Care Law. New York, NY: Oxford University Press; 1997: 357–456. 503 fn. ISBN 0-19-876260-7. BE56245.
> *abortion, induced; active euthanasia; *adults; *allowing to die; assisted suicide; body parts and fluids; cadavers; childbirth; congenital disorders; conscience; contraception; family planning; fetuses; health personnel; *legal aspects; legal liability; legislation; living wills; maternal health; minors; *newborns; *organ donation; organ donors; organ transplantation; *patient care; persistent vegetative state; *pregnant women; prenatal injuries; remuneration; *reproductive technologies; selective abortion; spousal consent; sterilization (sexual); surrogate mothers; terminal care; therapeutic abortion; treatment refusal; *Great Britain

Murphy, Denis. Ireland faces a "first". *Human Life Review.* 1997 Spring; 23(2): 45–52. BE57430.
> *abortion, induced; constitutional amendments; double effect; health facilities; legal aspects; mass media; minors; physicians; *political activity; *politics; pregnant women; rape; suicide; Supreme Court decisions; therapeutic abortion; women's health services; women's rights; Attorney General v. X; Dublin; *Ireland; Marie Stopes Reproductive Choices; Right to Life Movement

Norup, Michael. Attitudes towards abortion in the Danish population. *Bioethics.* 1997 Oct; 11(5): 439–449. 14 fn. BE56336.
> *abortion on demand; *abortion, induced; age factors; *attitudes; chromosome abnormalities; *congenital disorders; cystic fibrosis; Down syndrome; females; fetal development; fetuses; kidney diseases; males; morality; *public opinion; religion; *selective abortion; socioeconomic factors; survey; value of life; pregnancy trimesters; *Denmark

This article reports the results of a survey, by mailed questionnaire, of the attitudes among a sample of the Danish population towards abortion for social and genetic reasons. Of 1080 questionnaires sent to a random sample of persons between 18 and 45 years, 731 (68%) were completed and returned. A great majority of the

---

respondents were liberal towards early abortion both for social reasons and in case of minor disease. In contrast, there was controversy about late abortions for social reasons and in the case of Down syndrome. Further there was strong reluctance to accept late abortion in case of minor disease. An analysis of the response patterns showed that most of the respondents had gradualist views on abortion, i.e. they would allow all early abortions, but only abortions for some reasons later in pregnancy. It was also found that the number who would find an early abortion acceptable in general was much higher than the number who would accept it in their own case. These findings suggest that a great part of the resistance towards abortion does not rest on a concern for the rights and interests for the fetus. Instead it may be explained on a view according to which fetal life is ascribed intrinsic moral value.

Petersen, Kerry. Medical negligence and wrongful birth actions: Australian developments. *Journal of Medical Ethics.* 1997 Oct; 23(5): 319–322. 17 fn. BE57108.
   *abortion, induced; childbirth; diagnosis; health facilities; *legal aspects; *legal liability; *negligence; physicians; *pregnant women; quality of health care; social discrimination; state government; time factors; *wrongful life; diagnostic errors; *Australia; *CES v. Superclinics; New South Wales

Wrongful birth actions aim to compensate litigants who are negligently deprived by health professionals of their right to reproductive choice. Access to safe and legal abortion is integral to the action and wrongful birth claims in the United Kingdom have been facilitated by the Abortion Act 1967 (as amended). The recent Australian case CES v Superclinics (1995) 38 NSWLR 47 shows how judicial confusion about the legality of abortion can result in judges condoning medical negligence. The Superclinics case also suggests that doctors are not required to provide pregnant women with the same standard of care as other patients. These developments show that law can become incoherent and health professionals can act negligently with impunity when reproductive choice does not have a secure legal foundation.

Poland. Law of 7 January 1993 on family planning, protection of human fetuses, and the conditions under which pregnancy termination is permissible. *International Digest of Health Legislation.* 1993; 44(2): 253–255. BE57185.
   *abortion, induced; family planning; fetuses; genetic screening; health education; health personnel; *legal aspects; legal liability; patient care; pregnant women; prenatal diagnosis; value of life; *Poland

Shepherd, John Robert. Marriage and Mandatory Abortion among the 17th-Century Siraya. Arlington, VA: American Anthropological Association; 1995. 99 p. (American Ethnological Society monograph series; no. 6) Bibliography: p. 87–99. ISBN 0-913167-71-1. BE58899.
   *abortion, induced; age factors; anthropology; *historical aspects; *mandatory programs; marital relationship; *minority groups; population control; pregnant women; *Seventeenth Century; *Taiwan

Sidley, Pat. South Africa's liberal abortion laws challenged. [News]. *BMJ (British Medical Journal).* 1998 Jun 6; 316(7146): 1696. BE58244.
   *abortion, induced; *legal aspects; political activity; socioeconomic factors; value of life; *South Africa

Spurgeon, David. Canadian doctor calls for more education on abortion. [News]. *BMJ (British Medical Journal).* 1997 Nov 15; 315(7118): 1251. BE56917.
   *abortion, induced; medical education; methods; *physicians; political activity; *violence; *Canada; Romalis, Garson

Tu, Ping; Smith, Herbert L. Determinants of induced abortion and their policy implications in four counties in North China. *Studies in Family Planning.* 1995 Sep–Oct; 26(5): 278–286. 54 refs. 5 fn. BE57424.
   *abortion, induced; family planning; females; males; population control; pregnant women; *public policy; socioeconomic factors; standards; statistics; survey; geographic factors; *China

Viljoen, D.; Oosthuizen, C.; van der Westhuizen, S. Patient attitudes to prenatal screening and termination of pregnancy at Groote Schuur Hospital: a two year prospective study. *East African Medical Journal.* 1996 May; 73(5): 327–329. 6 refs. BE55535.
   *attitudes; *congenital disorders; genetic counseling; genetic disorders; *pregnant women; *prenatal diagnosis; religion; *selective abortion; socioeconomic factors; survey; Muslims; prospective studies; Groote Schuur Hospital (Cape Town); *South Africa

Williams, A. Susan. Investigating abortion. *In: her* Women and Childbirth in the Twentieth Century: A History of the National Birthday Trust Fund 1928–93. Phoenix Mill, Gloucestershire, Eng.: Sutton; 1997: 99–123, 286–289. 134 fn. ISBN 0-7509-1209-X. BE56548.
   *abortion, induced; contraception; females; government regulation; *historical aspects; *illegal abortion; *legal aspects; methods; morbidity; mortality; nurse midwives; physicians; political activity; population control; public policy; socioeconomic factors; survey; questionnaires; *England; Great Britain; Joint Council of Midwifery (Great Britain); Twentieth Century

ABORTION/LEGAL ASPECTS

Annas, George J. Partial-birth abortion, Congress, and the Constitution. *New England Journal of Medicine.* 1998 Jul 23; 339(4): 279–283. 28 refs. BE59073.
   *abortion, induced; *constitutional law; criminal law; *decision making; federal government; *fetal development; fetuses; *government regulation; *legal rights; maternal health; mental health; *methods; *organizational policies; *physicians; *politics; pregnant women; professional organizations; state interest; Supreme Court decisions; viability; *American College of Obstetricians and Gynecologists; *American Medical Association; Doe v. Bolton; *Partial-Birth Abortion Ban Act (1997 bill); Planned Parenthood of Southeastern Pennsylvania v. Casey; Roe v. Wade; *U.S. Congress; *United States

Appleton, Susan Frelich. Doctors, patients and the Constitution: a theoretical analysis of the physician's role in "private" reproductive decisions. *Washington University Law Quarterly.* 1985 Summer; 63(2): 183–236. 387 fn. BE56653.
   *abortion, induced; *constitutional law; contraception; counseling; *decision making; females; fetal development; fetuses; financial support; *government regulation; historical aspects; illegal abortion; informed consent; *legal aspects; *legal rights; physician patient relationship; physician's role; *physicians; *pregnant women; *privacy; professional autonomy; public policy; reproduction; social discrimination; state government; state interest; *Supreme Court decisions; viability; women's health services; women's rights; pregnancy trimesters; City of Akron v. Akron Center for Reproductive Health; Doe v. Bolton; Nineteenth Century; Planned Parenthood of Kansas City v. Ashcroft; Roe v.

BE = bioethics accession number   fn. = footnotes   refs. = references

Wade; Twentieth Century; *United States

Bopp, James; Coleson, Richard E. Roe v. Wade and the euthanasia debate. *Issues in Law and Medicine.* 1997 Spring; 12(4): 343–354. 38 fn. BE57802.
abortion on demand; *abortion, induced; *assisted suicide; constitutional law; *due process; freedom; *government regulation; *legal aspects; legal rights; pregnant women; privacy; *right to die; state government; state interest; Supreme Court decisions; terminally ill; *wedge argument; Fourteenth Amendment; *Planned Parenthood of Southeastern Pennsylvania v. Casey; *Roe v. Wade; *United States

Church of England. Board for Social Responsibility. Abortion and the Church: What are the Issues? London: Church House Publishing; 1993 Jan. 31 p. Bibliography: p. 22. Pub. No. GS Misc 408. Published for the General Synod of the Church of England. ISBN 0-7151-6578-X. BE57740.
*abortion, induced; beginning of life; childbirth; *Christian ethics; congenital disorders; conscience; cultural pluralism; drugs; fetal development; fetuses; health personnel; killing; *legal aspects; *morality; personhood; pregnant women; *Protestant ethics; *public policy; secularism; selective abortion; therapeutic abortion; *value of life; viability; Abortion Act 1967 (Great Britain); *Anglican Church; *Great Britain; Human Fertilisation and Embryology Act 1990; National Health Service; RU-486

Cordner, Stephen; Ettershank, Kathy. Australian doctors charged over abortion. [News]. *Lancet.* 1998 Feb 21; 351(9102): 578. BE58505.
*abortion, induced; *legal aspects; *legal liability; *physicians; Australia; *Western Australia

Devins, Neal. Shaping Constitutional Values: Elected Government, the Supreme Court, and the Abortion Debate. Baltimore, MD: Johns Hopkins University Press; 1996. 193 p. 550 fn. ISBN 0-8018-5285-4. BE56139.
*abortion, induced; *constitutional law; democracy; federal government; government financing; government regulation; judicial action; *legal aspects; legislation; political activity; *politics; public opinion; state government; *Supreme Court decisions; Roe v. Wade; U.S. Congress; *United States

Eller, Thomas R. Informed consent civil actions for post-abortion psychological trauma. *Notre Dame Law Review.* 1996; 71(4): 639–670. 214 fn. BE56659.
*abortion, induced; alternatives; coercion; counseling; *disclosure; fetal development; government regulation; *informed consent; *legal aspects; *legal liability; legal rights; maternal health; mental health; paternalism; *physicians; *pregnant women; *psychological stress; *risk; state government; Supreme Court decisions; *Planned Parenthood of Southeastern Pennsylvania v. Casey; *United States

Ginsburg, Ruth Bader. Some thoughts on autonomy and equality in relation to Roe v. Wade. *North Carolina Law Review.* 1985 Jan; 63(2): 375–386. 83 fn. The William T. Joyner Lecture on Constitutional Law at the University of North Carolina School of Law, 6 Apr 1984. BE56674.
*abortion, induced; *autonomy; *constitutional law; due process; employment; *equal protection; *females; fetal development; fetuses; financial support; *government regulation; indigents; *legal aspects; *legal rights; males; minority groups; *pregnant women; reproduction; social discrimination; state government; state interest; *Supreme Court decisions; viability; women's rights; pregnancy trimesters; *Roe v. Wade; *United States

Greenhouse, Linda. Overturning of late-term abortion ban is let stand. [News]. *New York Times.* 1998 Mar 24: A15. BE57919.
*abortion, induced; *fetal development; *government regulation; *legal aspects; *methods; state government; Supreme Court decisions; *Ohio; *United States; *Voinovich v. Women's Medical Professional Corp.

Greenhouse, Linda. U.S. appellate panel rules Ohio ban on late-term abortion is unconstitutional. [News]. *New York Times.* 1997 Nov 19: A24. BE56183.
*abortion, induced; constitutional law; fetal development; *government regulation; *legal aspects; *methods; pregnant women; state government; viability; women's health; *pregnancy trimesters; *Ohio; *Women's Medical Professional Corp. v. Voinovich

Haas-Wilson, Deborah. The impact of state abortion restrictions on minors' demand for abortions. *Journal of Human Resources.* 1996 Winter; 31(1): 140–158. 33 refs. BE57992.
*abortion, induced; government financing; *government regulation; *legal aspects; *minors; *parental consent; *parental notification; pregnant women; *social impact; state government; statistics; Medicaid; *United States

Haas-Wilson, Deborah. Women's reproductive choices: the impact of Medicaid funding restrictions. *Family Planning Perspectives.* 1997 Sep–Oct; 29(5): 228–233. 53 fn. BE58461.
*abortion, induced; childbirth; decision making; evaluation studies; *government financing; *government regulation; indigents; pregnant women; public policy; *social impact; *state government; statistics; *Medicaid; *United States

Human Rights Watch Women's Rights Project. Abortion policy and restrictions on women's rights in post-communist Poland. *In: its* The Human Rights Watch Global Report on Women's Human Rights. New York, NY: Human Rights Watch; 1995 Aug: 451–456. 14 fn. ISBN 0-300-06546-9. BE56088.
*abortion, induced; codes of ethics; equal protection; *government regulation; *legal aspects; legislation; medical fees; physicians; political activity; politics; pregnant women; selective abortion; therapeutic abortion; *women's rights; *Poland; Polish Medical College

Human Rights Watch Women's Rights Project. The abortion debate and violations of civil liberties in Ireland. *In: its* The Human Rights Watch Global Report on Women's Human Rights. New York, NY: Human Rights Watch; 1995 Aug: 444–451. 29 fn. ISBN 0-300-06546-9. BE56087.
*abortion, induced; counseling; government regulation; information dissemination; international aspects; *legal aspects; legal rights; legislation; minors; pregnant women; rape; Abortion Information Bill 1995 (Ireland); Attorney General v. X; European Court of Human Rights; European Court of Justice; International Convention on Civil and Political Rights; *Ireland; Open Door Counselling v. Ireland

Hungary. Law No. 79 of 17 December 1992 on the protection of the life of the fetus. *International Digest of Health Legislation.* 1993; 44(2): 249–253. BE57186.
abortion on demand; *abortion, induced; conscience; contraception; family planning; fetal development; *fetuses; *legal aspects; maternal health; patient care; pregnant women; standards; therapeutic abortion; value of life; *Hungary

Hyde, Henry J. The acceptable time. *Human Life Review.* 1997 Spring; 23(2): 75–78. Text of a speech in the U.S. House of Representatives on 20 Mar 1997, during the debate on the Partial Birth Abortion Ban Act of 1997. BE57429.

BE = bioethics accession number   fn. = footnotes   refs. = references

*abortion, induced; fetuses; government regulation; *killing; *legislation; *methods; *value of life; viability; U.S. Congress; *United States

Klasing, Murphy S. Death of an unborn child: jurisprudential inconsistencies in wrongful death, criminal homicide, and abortion cases. *Pepperdine Law Review.* 1995; 22(3): 933–979. 385 fn. BE56670.
*abortion, induced; *beginning of life; criminal law; fetal development; *fetuses; judicial action; killing; *legal aspects; *legal liability; negligence; newborns; *personhood; prenatal injuries; *state government; Supreme Court decisions; torts; *viability; *wrongful death; *United States

Lester, David. Abortion laws and infanticide. *Psychological Reports.* 1995 Jun; 76(3, pt. 2): 1370. 3 refs. BE55513.
*abortion, induced; comparative studies; government regulation; *infanticide; infants; *international aspects; killing; *legal aspects; newborns; *social impact; statistics

McDonagh, Eileen L. Breaking the Abortion Deadlock: From Choice to Consent. New York, NY: Oxford University Press; 1996. 280 p. 873 fn. ISBN 0–19–509142–6. BE55804.
abortion on demand; *abortion, induced; altruism; due process; equal protection; females; fetuses; freedom; government financing; government regulation; indigents; informed consent; *legal rights; males; maternal health; moral policy; obligations of society; personhood; policy analysis; political activity; politics; pregnant women; privacy; *public policy; rape; rights; risk; social discrimination; state interest; Supreme Court decisions; therapeutic abortion; value of life; viability; *women's rights; Medicaid; Right to Life Movement; *United States

Marsh, Frank H. Abortion and the law: the Supreme Court, privacy, and abortion. *In:* Edwards, Rem B., ed. Advances in Bioethics. Volume 2: New Essays on Abortion and Bioethics. Greenwich, CT: JAI Press; 1997: 107–123. 33 refs. ISBN 0–7623–0194–5. BE56791.
*abortion, induced; confidentiality; constitutional law; due process; *fetuses; freedom; government financing; *government regulation; indigents; *legal aspects; *legal rights; mandatory reporting; medical records; *politics; pregnant women; privacy; *public policy; review; *standards; state government; state interest; *Supreme Court decisions; *women's rights; Planned Parenthood of Southeastern Pennsylvania v. Casey; Roe v. Wade; *United States; Webster v. Reproductive Health Services

Montgomery, Jonathan. Health care law and ethics: abortion; fertility; maternity care; selective treatment of the newborn; transplantation; terminal care and euthanasia. *In:* his Health Care Law. New York, NY: Oxford University Press; 1997: 357–456. 503 fn. ISBN 0–19–876260–7. BE56245.
*abortion, induced; active euthanasia; *adults; *allowing to die; assisted suicide; body parts and fluids; cadavers; childbirth; congenital disorders; conscience; contraception; family planning; fetuses; health personnel; *legal aspects; legal liability; legislation; living wills; maternal health; minors; *newborns; *organ donation; organ donors; organ transplantation; *patient care; persistent vegetative state; *pregnant women; prenatal injuries; remuneration; *reproductive technologies; selective abortion; spousal consent; sterilization (sexual); surrogate mothers; terminal care; therapeutic abortion; treatment refusal; *Great Britain

Petersen, Kerry. Medical negligence and wrongful birth actions: Australian developments. *Journal of Medical Ethics.* 1997 Oct; 23(5): 319–322. 17 fn. BE57108.
*abortion, induced; childbirth; diagnosis; health facilities; *legal aspects; *legal liability; *negligence; physicians; *pregnant women; quality of health care; social discrimination; state government; time factors; *wrongful

life; diagnostic errors; *Australia; *CES v. Superclinics; New South Wales
Wrongful birth actions aim to compensate litigants who are negligently deprived by health professionals of their right to reproductive choice. Access to safe and legal abortion is integral to the action and wrongful birth claims in the United Kingdom have been facilitated by the Abortion Act 1967 (as amended). The recent Australian case CES v Superclinics (1995) 38 NSWLR 47 shows how judicial confusion about the legality of abortion can result in judges condoning medical negligence. The Superclinics case also suggests that doctors are not required to provide pregnant women with the same standard of care as other patients. These developments show that law can become incoherent and health professionals can act negligently with impunity when reproductive choice does not have a secure legal foundation.

Poland. Law of 7 January 1993 on family planning, protection of human fetuses, and the conditions under which pregnancy termination is permissible. *International Digest of Health Legislation.* 1993; 44(2): 253–255. BE57185.
*abortion, induced; family planning; fetuses; genetic screening; health education; health personnel; *legal aspects; legal liability; patient care; pregnant women; prenatal diagnosis; value of life; *Poland

Scoglio, Stefano. Abortion and the new privacy paradigm. *In:* his Transforming Privacy: A Transpersonal Philosophy of Rights. Westport, CT: Praeger; 1998: 153–185. 73 fn. ISBN 0–275–95607–5. BE57284.
*abortion, induced; allowing to die; autonomy; Christian ethics; constitutional law; counseling; decision making; disclosure; due process; fetal development; fetuses; freedom; government financing; government regulation; *legal aspects; *legal rights; *pregnant women; *privacy; state interest; *Supreme Court decisions; third party consent; value of life; viability; pregnancy trimesters; Harris v. McRae; Italy; Planned Parenthood of Southeastern Pennsylvania v. Casey; Roe v. Wade; *United States; Webster v. Reproductive Health Services

Seelye, Katharine Q. Advocates of abortion rights report a rise in restrictions. [News]. *New York Times.* 1998 Jan 15: A16. BE57599.
*abortion, induced; *government regulation; political activity; state government; statistics; Right to Life Movement; *United States

Segers, Mary C.; Byrnes, Timothy A., eds. Abortion Politics in American States. Armonk, NY: M.E. Sharpe; 1995. 279 p. 880 fn. ISBN 1–56324–449–7. BE57799.
abortion on demand; *abortion, induced; comparative studies; conscience; federal government; females; freedom; government financing; *government regulation; health facilities; historical aspects; legal aspects; legal rights; parental consent; parental notification; political activity; *politics; pregnant women; public opinion; public participation; *public policy; Roman Catholics; sex offenses; *state government; Supreme Court decisions; therapeutic abortion; violence; women's rights; Arizona; California; Louisiana; Maryland; Massachusetts; Minnesota; North Carolina; Ohio; Pennsylvania; Right to Life Movement; *United States; Washington

Sensibaugh, Christine Cregan; Allgeier, Elizabeth Rice. Factors considered by Ohio juvenile court judges in judicial bypass judgments: a policy–capturing approach. *Politics and the Life Sciences.* 1996 Mar; 15(1): 35–47. 37 refs. BE55643.
*abortion, induced; age factors; case studies; coercion; comparative studies; competence; comprehension; *decision

---

BE = bioethics accession number   fn. = footnotes   refs. = references

making; evaluation studies; guidelines; *judicial action; *minors; parental notification; risks and benefits; third party consent; *judges; *Ohio

Sidley, Pat. South Africa's liberal abortion laws challenged. [News]. *BMJ (British Medical Journal).* 1998 Jun 6; 316(7146): 1696. BE58244.
*abortion, induced; *legal aspects; political activity; socioeconomic factors; value of life; *South Africa

Sloan, Laura Curry. Constitutional law -- state impediments to abortion funding -- National Education Association of Rhode Island v. Garrahy. [Note]. *University of Kansas Law Review.* 1985 Winter; 34(2): 387–409. 186 fn. BE57049.
*abortion, induced; constitutional law; equal protection; government financing; *government regulation; *health insurance reimbursement; *legal aspects; *legal rights; privacy; state government; Harris v. McRae; Maher v. Roe; *National Education Association of Rhode Island v. Garrahy; *Rhode Island; Roe v. Wade; United States

Sollom, Terry. State actions on reproductive health issues in 1996. *Family Planning Perspectives.* 1997 Jan–Feb; 29(1): 35–40. 4 fn. BE58462.
*abortion, induced; AIDS serodiagnosis; childbirth; contraception; counseling; *family planning; fetal development; government financing; *government regulation; health facilities; health insurance reimbursement; hospitals; indigents; methods; mothers; newborns; parental consent; parental notification; patient care; political activity; *state government; Medicaid; *United States

U.S. Congress. House. Committee on the Judiciary. Subcommittee on the Constitution. Partial–Birth Abortion. Hearing, 15 Jun 1995. Washington, DC: U.S. Government Printing Office; 1995. 142 p. Serial No. 31. ISBN 0–16–052345–1. BE56099.
*abortion, induced; federal government; *fetal development; fetuses; *government regulation; killing; *legal aspects; legislation; maternal health; *methods; morbidity; pain; physicians; pregnant women; *pregnancy trimesters; *Partial–Birth Abortion Ban Act (1995 bill); *United States

U.S. Congress. Senate. A bill to amend Title 18, United States Code, to ban partial–birth abortions [Partial–Birth Abortion Ban Act of 1995]. S. 939, 104th Cong., 1st Sess. Introduced by Robert C. Smith and Phil Gramm; 1995 Jun 19. 3 p. The Senate version of this bill was not used. The Senate amended the House version of the bill, H.R. 1833, and passed the amended version. This bill was vetoed by President Clinton on 10 Apr 1996. BE55612.
*abortion, induced; fetal development; *legal aspects; legal liability; legislation; *methods; physicians; pregnant women; pregnancy trimesters; *Partial–Birth Abortion Ban Act (1995 bill); *United States

U.S. District Court, D. Montana, Great Falls Division. Armstrong v. Mazurek. *Federal Supplement.* 1995 Sep 29 (date of decision). 906: 561–569. BE58896.
*abortion, induced; equal protection; *government regulation; *legal aspects; legal rights; physicians; pregnant women; standards; state government; state interest; Supreme Court decisions; *Armstrong v. Mazurek; *Montana
The U.S. District Court for the District of Montana enjoined Montana's enforcement of provisions of a state law that required abortions after the first trimester to be performed in a licensed hospital and prohibited the advertisement of services of a physician or facility performing abortion services. The court refused to enjoin provisions of the law that required abortions to be performed by licensed physicians only. The suit was

brought by three Montana physicians who perform abortions, three Montana physicians who routinely refer patients to other abortion providers, and a physician assistant–certified, the only physician assistant–certified in the state who performs abortions. The court found that the hardship of the "physicians only" provision of the law placed on the physician assistant–certified was insufficient for a preliminary injunction. The court also found that the law was not an undue burden on a woman's right to choose to abort or restrict access to abortion, did not violate the Equal Protection Clause, and did not constitute a bill of attainder (a law enacted in the form of retroactive legislation to impose punishment on specific individuals), as the law advanced the state's legitimate interest in protecting the health of its citizens. (KIE abstract)

U.S. District Court, D. South Dakota, W.D. Planned Parenthood, Sioux Falls Clinic v. Miller. *Federal Supplement.* 1994 Aug 22 (date of decision). 860: 1409–1421. BE55972.
*abortion, induced; constitutional law; counseling; criminal law; *government regulation; informed consent; judicial action; *legal aspects; legal liability; legislation; minors; parental notification; pregnant women; state government; *Planned Parenthood, Sioux Falls Clinic v. Miller; *South Dakota
The U.S. District Court for the District of South Dakota ruled constitutionally valid those parts of a South Dakota statute requiring that a minor give one parent 48 hours notice prior to having an abortion and specifying information to be disclosed to a woman seeking an abortion. The court found that information required for informed consent to an abortion amounted to reasonable disclosure. Other state abortion requirements, however, were found to be invalid. These included a provision permitting bypass of parental notification, because the provision applied to only abused or neglected minors and in effect made any pregnant teenager who wished to bypass parental notification an abused or neglected minor. Provisions in the law for financial penalties for persons performing or attempting to perform an abortion without following state law were determined to be an impermissible obstacle to the right to an abortion, particularly in this case where only one physician in the state and within a 235–mile radius performs abortions. (KIE abstract)

U.S. District Court, D. Utah, C.D. Utah Women's Clinic, Inc. v. Graham. *Federal Supplement.* 1995 Jun 20 (date of decision). 892: 1379–1385. BE56138.
*abortion, induced; *federal government; *government financing; *government regulation; rape; sex offenses; *state government; therapeutic abortion; incest; Hyde Amendment; *Medicaid; *United States; *Utah; *Utah Women's Clinic, Inc. v. Graham
The U.S. District Court, Utah, enjoined state officials from enforcing Utah's abortion funding restriction to the extent that it conflicts with federal Medicaid law. As long as Utah accepts federal Medicaid funds, the state is required to participate in the program on the terms established by Congress. Accordingly, Utah cannot deny Medicaid funding for "medically necessary" abortions to eligible women pregnant through rape or incest, so long as federal matching funds are available for such abortions. (KIE abstract)

ABORTION/MINORS

Haas–Wilson, Deborah. The impact of state abortion restrictions on minors' demand for abortions. *Journal of*

Human Resources. 1996 Winter; 31(1): 140–158. 33 refs. BE57992.
  *abortion, induced; government financing; *government regulation; *legal aspects; *minors; *parental consent; *parental notification; pregnant women; *social impact; state government; statistics; Medicaid; *United States

Pierson, Vicky Howell. Missouri's parental consent law and teen pregnancy outcomes. *Women and Health.* 1995; 22(3): 47–58. 14 refs. 3 fn. BE55609.
  *abortion, induced; *adolescents; adoption; age factors; alternatives; blacks; childbirth; *government regulation; *minors; *parental consent; pregnant women; *social impact; state government; *statistics; time factors; whites; geographic factors; *Missouri

Sensibaugh, Christine Cregan; Allgeier, Elizabeth Rice. Factors considered by Ohio juvenile court judges in judicial bypass judgments: a policy–capturing approach. *Politics and the Life Sciences.* 1996 Mar; 15(1): 35–47. 37 refs. BE55643.
  *abortion, induced; age factors; case studies; coercion; comparative studies; competence; comprehension; *decision making; evaluation studies; guidelines; *judicial action; *minors; parental notification; risks and benefits; third party consent; *judges; *Ohio

ABORTION/RELIGIOUS ASPECTS

Alvare, Helen M. A response to Leslie Griffin. *In:* Wildes, Kevin Wm.; Mitchell, Alan C., eds. Choosing Life: A Dialogue on *Evangelium Vitae.* Washington, DC: Georgetown University Press; 1997: 179–185. 8 fn. ISBN 0–87840–646–8. BE56687.
  *abortion, induced; beginning of life; embryos; human rights; killing; legal aspects; mass media; natural law; personhood; politics; public policy; *Roman Catholic ethics; theology; women's rights; Evangelium Vitae; United States

Barry, Robert. The Roman Catholic position on abortion. *In:* Edwards, Rem B., ed. Advances in Bioethics. Volume 2: New Essays on Abortion and Bioethics. Greenwich, CT: JAI Press; 1997: 151–182. 58 refs. ISBN 0–7623–0194–5. BE56793.
  *abortion, induced; aggression; beginning of life; contraception; double effect; fetal development; fetuses; historical aspects; intention; killing; marital relationship; moral obligations; motivation; personhood; pregnant women; *Roman Catholic ethics; sexuality; therapeutic abortion; United States

Bernardin, Joseph. The consistent ethic of life after *Webster.* *In:* Langan, John P., ed. Joseph Cardinal Bernardin: A Moral Vision for America. Washington, DC: Georgetown University Press; 1998: 79–92. Address at the Woodstock Theological Center, Georgetown University, 20 May 1990. ISBN 0–87840–675–1. BE58524.
  abortion on demand; *abortion, induced; government regulation; justice; *moral policy; obligations of society; political activity; politics; public opinion; *public policy; *Roman Catholic ethics; Roman Catholics; social impact; state government; Supreme Court decisions; *value of life; vulnerable populations; Roe v. Wade; *United States; Webster v. Reproductive Health Services

Church of England. Board for Social Responsibility. Abortion and the Church: What are the Issues? London: Church House Publishing; 1993 Jan. 31 p. Bibliography: p. 22. Pub. No. GS Misc 408. Published for the General Synod of the Church of England. ISBN 0–7151–6578–X. BE57740.
  *abortion, induced; beginning of life; childbirth; *Christian

ethics; congenital disorders; conscience; cultural pluralism; drugs; fetal development; fetuses; health personnel; killing; *legal aspects; *morality; personhood; pregnant women; *Protestant ethics; *public policy; secularism; selective abortion; therapeutic abortion; *value of life; viability; Abortion Act 1967 (Great Britain); *Anglican Church; *Great Britain; Human Fertilisation and Embryology Act 1990; National Health Service; RU–486

Csordas, Thomas J. A handmaid's tale: the rhetoric of personhood in American and Japanese healing of abortions. *In:* Sargent, Carolyn F.; Brettell, Caroline B., eds. Gender and Health: An International Perspective. Upper Saddle River, NJ: Prentice Hall; 1996: 227–241. 23 refs. 5 fn. ISBN 0–13–079427–9. BE58095.
  *aborted fetuses; *abortion, induced; *Buddhist ethics; comparative studies; emotions; *females; international aspects; mother fetus relationship; *personhood; *psychological stress; psychology; *religion; *Roman Catholics; grief; guilt; *Japan; *Pentecostal Christians; *United States

Dillon, Michele. Cultural differences in the abortion discourse of the Catholic Church: evidence from four countries. *Sociology of Religion.* 1996 Spring; 57(1): 25–36. 26 refs. BE58118.
  *abortion, induced; communication; comparative studies; cultural pluralism; *international aspects; law; morality; *organizational policies; *political activity; public policy; *Roman Catholic ethics; secularism; socioeconomic factors; value of life; women's rights; *Great Britain; *Ireland; *Poland; *United States

Fein, Esther B. Hospital deals raise concern on abortion. [News]. *New York Times.* 1997 Oct 14: B1, B10. BE57985.
  *abortion, induced; contraception; economics; health care delivery; *health facilities; hospitals; *institutional policies; political activity; public participation; *religious hospitals; reproductive technologies; *Roman Catholic ethics; sterilization (sexual); women's health services; *health facility mergers; Benedictine Hospital (Kingston, NY); Cross River Health Company (Kingston, NY)

Finlay, Barbara. Gender differences in attitudes toward abortion among Protestant seminarians. *Review of Religious Research.* 1996 Jun; 37(4): 354–360. 14 refs. 1 fn. BE57690.
  *abortion, induced; *attitudes; *clergy; comparative studies; *females; *males; *Protestants; selective abortion; students; survey; therapeutic abortion; Presbyterian Church

Fisher, Ian. Casualty of the abortion debate: a doctor, aiming at conciliation, instead loses a post. [News]. *New York Times.* 1998 Mar 24: B1, B7. BE57986.
  *abortion, induced; dissent; *employment; faculty; *hospitals; *medical schools; *physicians; *religious hospitals; *Roman Catholics; women's health services; *health facility mergers; *Mesches, David; *New York Medical College (Valhalla)

Fournier, Keith A.; Watkins, William D. In Defense of Life. Colorado Springs, CO: NavPress; 1996. 159 p. 352 fn. ISBN 08910–98801. BE56728.
  aborted fetuses; *abortion, induced; *active euthanasia; aged; *allowing to die; *assisted suicide; beginning of life; body parts and fluids; brain death; *Christian ethics; commodification; congenital disorders; death; determination of death; disabled; economics; eugenics; fetal tissue donation; fetuses; government regulation; health personnel; historical aspects; human experimentation; infanticide; international aspects; judicial action; *killing; legal aspects; love; *morality; *newborns; organ donation; *political activity; population control; pregnant women; psychological stress; public policy; quality of life; rights; *value of life; *values;

BE = bioethics accession number   fn. = footnotes   refs. = references

violence; hope; Humphry, Derek; Kevorkian, Jack; *Right to Life Movement; Roe v. Wade; Smith, Susan; United States

Griffin, Leslie C. Evangelium Vitae: abortion. *In:* Wildes, Kevin Wm.; Mitchell, Alan C., eds. Choosing Life: A Dialogue on *Evangelium Vitae.* Washington, DC: Georgetown University Press; 1997: 159–173. 18 fn. ISBN 0–87840–646–8. BE56685.
  *abortion, induced; beginning of life; conscience; contraception; democracy; health personnel; killing; law; legal aspects; moral complicity; natural law; personhood; politics; population control; *Roman Catholic ethics; *theology; *value of life; *Evangelium Vitae; United States

Grisez, Germain. Difficult moral questions: may a physician remain in a group that provides immoral services? *Linacre Quarterly.* 1997 May; 64(2): 21–25. BE55616.
  *abortion, induced; *conscience; *contraception; drugs; employment; family planning; family practice; health maintenance organizations; intention; interprofessional relations; *moral complicity; obstetrics and gynecology; *physicians; *referral and consultation; *Roman Catholic ethics; *Roman Catholics; voluntary sterilization; group practice

Hardacre, Helen. Marketing the Menacing Fetus in Japan. Berkeley, CA: University of California Press; 1997. 310 p. (Twentieth–century Japan; 7). Bibliography: p. 265–293. ISBN 0–520–20553–7. BE56521.
  *aborted fetuses; *abortion, induced; advertising; *attitudes; Buddhist ethics; childbirth; females; historical aspects; *industry; males; mass media; mother fetus relationship; personhood; political activity; psychological stress; public policy; *religion; reproduction; sexuality; social discrimination; stigmatization; trends; ethnographic studies; guilt; *Japan; Shintoism; Twentieth Century

Howell, Nancy R. Abortion and religion. *In:* Edwards, Rem B., ed. Advances in Bioethics. Volume 2: New Essays on Abortion and Bioethics. Greenwich, CT: JAI Press; 1997: 125–149. 34 refs. ISBN 0–7623–0194–5. BE56792.
  *abortion, induced; autonomy; Buddhist ethics; Christian ethics; common good; contraception; cultural pluralism; ecology; fetal development; *fetuses; Hindu ethics; indigents; Islamic ethics; Jewish ethics; *moral policy; morality; obligations of society; personhood; population control; pregnant women; *Protestant ethics; *religious ethics; rights; sterilization (sexual); theology; value of life; women's rights; Right to Life Movement; United States

Kopfensteiner, Thomas R. A response to Leslie Griffin's essay. *In:* Wildes, Kevin Wm.; Mitchell, Alan C., eds. Choosing Life: A Dialogue on *Evangelium Vitae.* Washington, DC: Georgetown University Press; 1997: 174–178. ISBN 0–87840–646–8. BE56686.
  *abortion, induced; embryos; killing; moral obligations; personhood; *Roman Catholic ethics; value of life; Declaration on Abortion; Evangelium Vitae

Peters, Ted. Designer genes and selective abortion. *In: his* For the Love of Children: Genetic Technology and the Future of the Family. Louisville, KY: Westminster John Knox Press; 1996: 85–118, 193–199. 63 fn. ISBN 0–664–25468–3. BE55697.
  adoption; beginning of life; coercion; confidentiality; decision making; disabled; employment; eugenics; fetal development; *fetuses; genetic counseling; *genetic disorders; genetic information; *genetic predisposition; *genetic screening; government regulation; insurance; killing; legal rights; *personhood; pregnant women; prenatal diagnosis; privacy; Protestant ethics; public policy; risk; *Roman Catholic ethics; *selective abortion; *social

discrimination; value of life; viability; dignity; Genetic Privacy Act 1994; United States

Rae, Scott B. Prenatal genetic testing, abortion, and beyond. *In:* Kilner, John F.; Pentz, Rebecca D.; Young, Frank E., eds. Genetic Ethics: Do the Ends Justify the Genes? Grand Rapids, MI: W.B. Eerdmans; 1997: 136–145. 12 fn. ISBN 0–8028–4428–6. BE56721.
  *Christian ethics; disabled; embryos; fetal therapy; fetuses; genetic counseling; *genetic disorders; *genetic screening; genome mapping; late–onset disorders; personhood; *preimplantation diagnosis; *prenatal diagnosis; quality of life; *selective abortion; sex determination; uncertainty; value of life; United States

Salihu, Hamisu Mohammed. Genetic counselling among Muslims: questions remain unanswered. [Letter]. *Lancet.* 1997 Oct 4; 350(9083): 1035–1036. 2 refs. BE57359.
  clergy; fetal development; *genetic counseling; genetic disorders; *genetic screening; *Islamic ethics; *preimplantation diagnosis; *prenatal diagnosis; *selective abortion; socioeconomic factors; Cameroon; Great Britain

Stallsworth, Paul T., ed. The Right Choice: Pro–Life Sermons from Elizabeth Achtemeier [and Others]. Nashville, TN: Abingdon Press; 1997. 118 p. 25 fn. ISBN 0–687–05079–0. BE57640.
  *abortion, induced; adoption; autonomy; beginning of life; *Christian ethics; clergy; embryos; family relationship; fathers; fetuses; freedom; killing; love; morality; personhood; political activity; pregnant women; secularism; Supreme Court decisions; *theology; unwanted children; *value of life; women's rights; Planned Parenthood of Southeastern Pennsylvania v. Casey; Right to Life Movement; Roe v. Wade; United States

Weatherford, Roy. Philippa Foot and the doctrine of double effect. *Personalist.* 1979 Jan; 60(1): 105–113. 20 fn. Commentary on P. Foot, "The problem of abortion and the doctrine of the double effect," *Oxford Review* 1967; 5. BE57437.
  *abortion, induced; *double effect; fetuses; intention; *killing; moral obligations; *moral policy; pregnant women; *Roman Catholic ethics; *therapeutic abortion; hysterectomy; *Foot, Philippa

An H.M.O., Catholic–run, bars coverage for abortions. [News]. *New York Times.* 1997 Nov 17: B5. BE56181.
  *abortion, induced; contraception; family planning; federal government; females; *government financing; government regulation; *health insurance reimbursement; *health maintenance organizations; indigents; *institutional policies; refusal to treat; *Roman Catholics; state government; women's health services; *religious health facilities; *Fidelis Care (NY); *Medicaid; *New York

ACCESS TO HEALTH CARE *See* HEALTH CARE, RESOURCE ALLOCATION

ACQUIRED IMMUNODEFICIENCY SYNDROME *See* AIDS

ADVANCE DIRECTIVES

See also TREATMENT REFUSAL

Ackerman, Terrence F. Forsaking the spirit for the letter of the law: advance directives in nursing homes. *Journal of the American Geriatrics Society.* 1997 Jan; 45(1): 114–116. 1 ref. Commentary on M. Mezey et al., "Implementation of the Patient Self–Determination Act

---

BE = bioethics accession number   fn. = footnotes   refs. = references

(PSDA) in nursing homes in New York City," p. 43–49. BE55751.

*advance care planning; *advance directives; allowing to die; dementia; disclosure; *evaluation; family members; goals; *institutional policies; legal aspects; legislation; living wills; medical records; nurse's role; nurses; *nursing homes; patient education; patient transfer; patients; physician's role; proprietary health facilities; resuscitation orders; risks and benefits; *social workers; state government; technical expertise; third party consent; time factors; values; withholding treatment; *New York City; *Patient Self–Determination Act 1990

Alpert, Hillel R.; Hoijtink, Herbert; Fischer, Gary S., et al. Psychometric analysis of an advance directive. *Medical Care.* 1996 Oct; 34(10): 1057–1065. 16 refs. BE59002.

*advance care planning; *advance directives; allowing to die; artificial feeding; *attitudes; biomedical technologies; chronically ill; comparative studies; critically ill; decision making; dementia; diagnosis; drugs; *evaluation; evaluation studies; palliative care; *patients; persistent vegetative state; *physicians; prognosis; prolongation of life; *public opinion; quality of life; renal dialysis; resuscitation; standards; surgery; survey; terminally ill; treatment refusal; ventilators; coma; Massachusetts

Asai, Atsushi; Fukuhara, Shunichi; Inoshita, Osamu, et al. Medical decisions concerning the end of life: a discussion with Japanese physicians. *Journal of Medical Ethics.* 1997 Oct; 23(5): 323–327. 5 refs. BE57101.

*advance directives; *allowing to die; *attitudes; cancer; *decision making; diagnosis; family members; knowledge, attitudes, practice; organizational policies; *physicians; professional organizations; prognosis; *prolongation of life; *resuscitation; resuscitation orders; survey; *terminally ill; *truth disclosure; *withholding treatment; patient abandonment; qualitative research; *Japan; Japan Medical Association

OBJECTIVES: Life–sustaining treatment at the end of life gives rise to many ethical problems in Japan. Recent surveys of Japanese physicians suggested that they tend to treat terminally ill patients aggressively. We studied why Japanese physicians were reluctant to withhold or withdraw life–support from terminally ill patients and what affected their decisions. DESIGN AND PARTICIPANTS: A qualitative study design was employed, using a focus group interview with seven physicians, to gain an in–depth understanding of attitudes and rationales in Japan regarding medical care at the end of life. RESULTS: Analysis revealed that physicians and patients' family members usually make decisions about life–sustaining treatment, while the patients' wishes are unavailable or not taken into account. Both physicians and family members tend to consider withholding or withdrawing life–sustaining treatment as abandonment or even killing. The strongest reason to start cardiopulmonary resuscitation -- and to continue it until patients' family members arrive -- seems to be the family members' desire to be at the bedside at the time of death. All physicians participating in our study regarded advance directives that provide information as to patients' wishes about life–sustaining treatment desirable. All expressed concern, however, that it would be difficult to forego or discontinue life–support based on a patient's advance directive, particularly when the patient's family opposed the directive. CONCLUSION: Our group interview suggested several possible barriers to death with dignity and the appropriate use of advance directives in Japan. Further qualitative and quantitative research in this regard is needed.

Berger, Jeffrey T. Cultural discrimination in mechanisms for health decisions: a view from New York. *Journal of Clinical Ethics.* 1998 Summer; 9(2): 127–131. 31 fn. BE58958.

advance care planning; *advance directives; *allowing to die; artificial feeding; attitudes; autonomy; *cultural pluralism; *decision making; empirical research; family members; family relationship; *legal aspects; *minority groups; *prolongation of life; *public policy; social discrimination; state government; third party consent; trust; values; withholding treatment; *New York

Berghmans, R.L.P. Advance directives for non–therapeutic dementia research: some ethical and policy considerations. *Journal of Medical Ethics.* 1998 Feb; 24(1): 32–37. 25 refs. BE57403.

*advance directives; *competence; decision making; *dementia; *human experimentation; informed consent; moral policy; *nontherapeutic research; personhood; research subjects; selection of subjects; self concept; third party consent

This paper explores the use of advance directives in clinical dementia research. The focus is on advance consent to participation of demented patients in non–therapeutic research involving more than minimal risks and/or burdens. First, morally relevant differences between advance directives for treatment and care, and advance directives for dementia research are discussed. Then attention is paid to the philosophical issue of dementia and personal identity, and the implications for the moral authority of research advance directives. Thirdly, a number of practical shortcomings of advance directives for non–therapeutic dementia research are explored and attention is paid to the role of proxies. It is concluded that upon a closer look the initial attractiveness of advance directives for dementia research is lessened, and that it is doubtful whether these instruments can compensate for the lack of subject consent in case of non–therapeutic dementia research involving more than minimal risks and/or burdens for the incompetent demented subject.

Bradley, Elizabeth; Walker, Leslie; Blechner, Barbara, et al. Assessing capacity to participate in discussions of advance directives in nursing homes: findings from a study of the Patient Self–Determination Act. *Journal of the American Geriatrics Society.* 1997 Jan; 45(1): 79–83. 33 refs. BE55758.

administrators; *advance care planning; *advance directives; *aged; attitudes; autonomy; communication; *competence; *decision making; *family members; health personnel; institutional policies; legislation; living wills; medical records; nurses; *nursing homes; patient admission; *patient education; *patient participation; *patients; psychological stress; social workers; survey; third party consent; time factors; qualitative research; retrospective studies; *Connecticut; *Patient Self–Determination Act 1990

Canada. Alberta. Advance Directives Act. Bill 58, 23rd Legislature, 2d Sess. Introduced by Ms. Haley.; 1994. 16 p. BE57698.

*advance directives; competence; decision making; *legal aspects; legal guardians; patient care; psychosurgery; standards; sterilization (sexual); third party consent; tissue donation; *Advance Directives Act 1994 (AB); *Alberta

Canada. Manitoba. Health Care Directives Act. 1993 Jul 26 (date of proclamation). *International Digest of Health Legislation.* 1995; 46(2): 195–196. BE57180.

*advance directives; *legal aspects; *Health Care Directives Act (MB); *Manitoba

Dexter, Paul R.; Wolinsky, Fredric D.; Gramelspacher, Gregory P., et al. Effectiveness of computer–generated

---

BE = bioethics accession number					fn. = footnotes					refs. = references

reminders for increasing discussions about advance directives and completion of advance directive forms: a randomized, controlled trial. *Annals of Internal Medicine.* 1998 Jan 15; 128(2): 102–110. 55 refs. BE57908.

advance care planning; *advance directives; age factors; *communication; *computers; evaluation studies; patients; *physicians; primary health care; Indiana

BACKGROUND: Physicians can increase the rate of completion of advance directive forms by discussing directives with their patients, but the means by which physicians can be induced to initiate these discussions are unclear. Computer-generated reminders have been shown to increase physician compliance with practice guidelines. OBJECTIVE: To determine the effects of computer-generated reminders to physicians on the frequency of advance directive discussions between patients and their primary caregivers and the frequency of consequent establishment of advance directives. DESIGN: Randomized, controlled trial with a 2 x 2 factorial design. SETTING: An outpatient general medicine practice associated with an urban public hospital. PARTICIPANTS: Participants were 1) 1009 patients who were at least 75 years of age or were at least 50 years of age with serious underlying disease and 2) 147 primary care physicians (108 housestaff and 39 faculty). INTERVENTION: Computer-generated reminders that recommended discussion of one or both of two types of advance directives compared with no reminders. MEASUREMENTS: Discussions about advance directives, determined by patient interviews after all scheduled patient-physician outpatient encounters, and completed advance directive forms. The study period was approximately 1 year. RESULTS: Physicians who did not receive reminders (controls) discussed advance directives with 4% of the study patients compared with 24% for physicians who received both types of reminders (adjusted odds ratio, 7.7 [95% CI, 3.4 to 18]; P less than 0.001). Physicians who did not receive reminders completed advance directive forms with only 4% of their study patients compared with 15% for physicians who received both types of reminders (adjusted odds ratio, 7.0 [CI, 2.9 to 17]; P less than 0.001). Overall, 45% of patients with whom advance directives were discussed completed at least one type of advance directive. CONCLUSIONS: Simple computer-generated reminders aimed at primary caregivers can increase the rates of discussion of advance directives and completion of advance directive forms among elderly outpatients with serious illnesses.

Docker, Chris. Advance directives/living wills. *In:* McLean, Sheila A.M., ed. Contemporary Issues in Law, Medicine and Ethics. Brookfield, VT: Dartmouth; 1996: 179–214. 194 fn. ISBN 1-85521-586-1. BE57796.

*advance directives; advisory committees; allowing to die; *alternatives; assisted suicide; clinical ethics committees; communication; competence; decision making; family members; *international aspects; judicial action; *legal aspects; legislation; *living wills; medical records; patients; physicians; review; *risks and benefits; state government; Supreme Court decisions; third party consent; treatment refusal; voluntary euthanasia; withholding treatment; values histories; Airedale NHS Trust v. Bland; Australia; Canada; Cruzan v. Director, Missouri Department of Health; Finland; *Great Britain; House of Lords Select Committee on Medical Ethics; Law Commission (Great Britain); Netherlands; Patient Self-Determination Act 1990; United States

Docker, Christopher. The way forward? *In:* McLean, Sheila A.M., ed. Death, Dying and the Law. Brookfield, VT: Dartmouth; 1996: 129–160. 99 fn. ISBN

1-85521-657-4. BE57217.

*active euthanasia; *advance directives; aged; *allowing to die; *assisted suicide; decision making; double effect; economics; hospices; legal aspects; living wills; pain; *palliative care; *persistent vegetative state; physicians; public policy; *resource allocation; selection for treatment; terminal care; withholding treatment; *Great Britain; National Health Service; Netherlands; United States

Dresser, Rebecca; Astrow, Alan B. An alert and incompetent self: the irrelevance of advance directives. [Case study and commentaries]. *Hastings Center Report.* 1998 Jan–Feb; 28(1): 28–30. BE57295.

*advance directives; *allowing to die; autonomy; case studies; clinical ethics committees; *competence; *critically ill; *decision making; *dissent; emotions; friends; *living wills; love; *patient care team; patient participation; patient transfer; physicians; professional patient relationship; prognosis; *prolongation of life; *third party consent; time factors; treatment refusal; *uncertainty; *ventilators

Dyer, Clare. Living wills put on statutory footing. [News]. *BMJ (British Medical Journal).* 1998 Jan 3; 316(7124): 9. 1 ref. BE58102.

active euthanasia; *advance directives; competence; *legal aspects; legislation; living wills; patients; third party consent; *Great Britain

Dyer, Clare. UK public calls for legislation over living wills. [News]. *BMJ (British Medical Journal).* 1998 Mar 28; 316(7136): 959. BE58080.

*advance directives; judicial action; legal obligations; *legislation; *living wills; physicians; *public opinion; public policy; treatment refusal; *Great Britain

Emson, Harry E. The right to die: withdrawal of tube feeding in the persistent vegetative state in Canada. *In:* Grubb, Andrew, ed. Decision-Making and Problems of Incompetence. New York, NY: Wiley; 1994: 181–186. 9 fn. ISBN 0-471-94236-7. BE57135.

*advance directives; *allowing to die; *artificial feeding; autonomy; clinical ethics committees; competence; cultural pluralism; *decision making; family members; hospitals; informed consent; *knowledge, attitudes, practice; *legal aspects; patients; *persistent vegetative state; physicians; right to die; third party consent; treatment refusal; *withholding treatment; *Canada

Fins, Joseph J. Advance directives and SUPPORT. [Editorial]. *Journal of the American Geriatrics Society.* 1997 Apr; 45(4): 519–520. 23 refs. BE57114.

*advance care planning; *advance directives; communication; control groups; decision making; economics; *evaluation studies; family members; hospitals; medical records; palliative care; physician patient relationship; physician's role; *research design; resuscitation orders; social impact; *terminal care; treatment refusal; continuity of patient care; *Study to Understand Prognoses and Preferences for Outcomes and Risks of Treatments (SUPPORT)

FitzGerald, John; Wenger, Neil. The invalid advance directive. *Bioethics Forum.* 1997 Summer; 13(2): 32–34. 5 refs. BE58280.

advance care planning; *advance directives; case studies; *communication; competence; *decision making; evaluation; family members; hospitals; *patients; physicians; terminal care; terminally ill; treatment refusal; withholding treatment

Friedland, Steven I. The health care proxy and the narrative of death. *Journal of Law and Health.* 1995–1996; 10(1): 95–151. 277 fn. BE57144.

administrators; *advance directives; *allowing to die; attitudes; *attitudes to death; autonomy; biomedical technologies; communication; *death; determination of

---

BE = bioethics accession number   fn. = footnotes   refs. = references

death; evaluation studies; government regulation; historical aspects; hospitals; knowledge, attitudes, practice; *legal aspects; legal rights; living wills; medicine; physicians; prolongation of life; right to die; state government; survey; treatment refusal; Health Care Proxy Law 1990 (NY); New York; *United States

Gadd, Elaine. Changing the law on decision making for mentally incapacitated adults: should advance directives have a statutory basis? [Editorial]. *BMJ (British Medical Journal).* 1998 Jan 10; 316(7125): 90. 8 refs. BE57306.
    *advance directives; advisory committees; allowing to die; autonomy; *decision making; *informed consent; *legal aspects; *mentally disabled; nontherapeutic research; public policy; risks and benefits; *third party consent; treatment refusal; *Great Britain; Law Commission (Great Britain)

Ghusn, Husam F.; Teasdale, Thomas A.; Jordan, Darlene. Continuity of do–not resuscitate orders between hospital and nursing home settings. *Journal of the American Geriatrics Society.* 1997 Apr; 45(4): 465–469. 9 refs. BE57115.
    *advance directives; aged; *communication; comparative studies; diagnosis; *hospitals; institutional policies; medical records; *nursing homes; *patient discharge; *patient transfer; *resuscitation orders; treatment refusal; continuity of patient care; Houston (TX); Texas

Gross, Mortimer D. What do patients express as their preferences in advance directives? *Archives of Internal Medicine.* 1998 Feb 23; 158(4): 363–365. 16 refs. BE57960.
    *advance directives; *allowing to die; artificial feeding; *attitudes; *decision making; hospitals; institutionalized persons; living wills; *patients; *prolongation of life; resuscitation orders; risks and benefits; survey; treatment refusal; coma; outpatients; Illinois
BACKGROUND: Since the passage of the Patient Self–Determination Act in 1991, there has been interest in urging patients to execute advance directives (ADs) for medical care. There are not much data, however, as to what the ADs that patients execute actually specify. I have investigated the percentage of inpatients and outpatients who are admitted to a community hospital who have executed ADs, and I have tabulated what preferences are actually expressed in the ADs that are in hospital records. METHODS: A questionnaire is filled out by each patient admitted to this hospital, and their response recorded as to whether they have executed an AD. I have tabulated these responses for inpatients and outpatients for the calendar year 1994. I have also examined the ADs in all available hospital records, and tabulated the wishes expressed in these directives. RESULTS: For inpatient admissions during the calendar year 1994, of 8727 questionnaires completed, 11% of patients indicated that they had executed an AD. For outpatients, the corresponding figures are 22,966 and 15%. A total of 343 hospital records containing ADs were examined. Of these, 15 were nonmedical directives and were excluded. Of the 328 medical ADs, 86 (26%) were living wills, expressing the wish that if the individual had an incurable disease or irreversible injury that he or she not be given any treatment that would only delay death. There were 210 power of attorney for health care forms completed; these were 64% of all the medical ADs. Of these, 7 did not specify any preference that patients wanted their proxy to follow. The remaining 203 forms were divided as follows: 189 individuals requested that they did not want life–sustaining treatment if the burdens of treatment outweighed the expected benefits; 12 wanted their lives to be prolonged unless they were in an irreversible coma; and 2 wanted their lives to be prolonged to the greatest

possible extent regardless of the chances for recovery or the cost. There were 32 do not resuscitate forms executed exclusively by residents of nursing homes that specified that they did not want cardiopulmonary resuscitation or artificial feeding. CONCLUSIONS: The overwhelming desire expressed by the patients in the ADs was not to have their lives prolonged if their medical condition were such that treatment would merely delay death. Only a minuscule number of patients, less than 0.7%, wanted everything done to prolong life regardless of the chance for improvement or the cost. Because such a small percentage of patients have ADs, it is recommended that each hospital appoint a committee on ADs to do everything possible to encourage patients to execute an AD. A second mission of this committee would be to do everything possible to encourage physicians to pay close attention to their patients' wishes for medical care at the end of life.

Hammes, Bernard J.; Rooney, Brenda L. Death and end–of–life planning in one midwestern community. *Archives of Internal Medicine.* 1998 Feb 23; 158(4): 383–390. 20 refs. BE57961.
    *advance care planning; *advance directives; aged; allowing to die; artificial feeding; death; *decision making; drugs; education; evaluation studies; family members; health facilities; medical records; palliative care; physicians; quality of life; resuscitation; statistics; survey; *terminal care; treatment refusal; ventilators; withholding treatment; retrospective studies; Wisconsin
BACKGROUND: The major health care organizations in a geographically defined area implemented an extensive, collaborative advance directive education program approximately 2 years prior to this study. OBJECTIVES: To determine for a geographically defined population the prevalence and type of end–of–life planning and the relationship between end–of–life plans and decisions in all local health care organizations, including hospitals, medical clinics, long–term care facilities, home health agencies, hospices, and the county health department. METHODS: For more than 11 months, end–of–life planning and decisions were retrospectively studied for all adult decedents residing in areas within 5 ZIP codes. These decedents were mentally capable in the 10 years prior to death and died while under the care of the participating health care organizations. Data were collected from medical records and death certificates. Treating physicians and decedent proxies were also contacted for interviews. RESULTS: A total of 540 decedents were included in this study. The prevalence of written advance directives was 85%. Almost all these documents (95%) were in the decedent's medical record. The median time between advance directive documentation and death was 1.2 years. Almost all advance directive documents requested that treatment be forgone as death neared. Treatment was forgone in 98% of the deaths. Treatment preferences expressed in advance directives seemed to be consistently followed while making end–of–life decisions. CONCLUSIONS: This study provides a more complete picture of death, end–of–life planning, and decision making in a geographic area where an extensive advance directive education program exists. It indicates that advance planning can be prevalent and can effectively guide end–of–life decisions.

Harrison, Helen. Need exists for advance directives from parents. [Letter; title supplied]. *Journal of Perinatology.* 1995 Nov–Dec; 15(6): 522. 1 ref. BE55936.
    *advance directives; *allowing to die; congenital disorders; *decision making; *newborns; *parents; *physicians;

---

*prolongation of life; psychological stress; resuscitation; withholding treatment

Huber, Ruth; Evans, Virginia Cox. Trust in physicians to honor death related instructions. *Omega: A Journal of Death and Dying.* 1997–1998; 36(1): 9–21. 39 refs. BE57720.
*advance directives; age factors; *aged; *allowing to die; assisted suicide; attitudes to death; comparative studies; *decision making; *institutionalized persons; *knowledge, attitudes, practice; *physician patient relationship; *physicians; *prolongation of life; *public opinion; residential facilities; *right to die; survey; *terminal care; treatment refusal; *trust; voluntary euthanasia; Kentucky

Johns, Jeanine L. Advance directives and opportunities for nurses. *Image: The Journal of Nursing Scholarship.* 1996 Summer; 28(2): 149–153. 52 refs. BE55874.
*advance directives; allowing to die; attitudes; decision making; evaluation; family members; health personnel; legal aspects; living wills; *nurses; nursing research; organizational policies; patient education; patients; professional organizations; risks and benefits; statistics; United States

Kaplan, Richard S.; Tuennerman, Jill A. Advance directives. [Letter]. *Journal of the American Geriatrics Society.* 1997 Sep; 45(9): 1156–1157. BE56310.
*advance directives; *patient education

Kimura, Rihito. Death, dying, and advance directives in Japan: sociocultural and legal points of view. *In:* Sass, Hans–Martin; Veatch, Robert M.; Kimura, Rihito, eds. Advance Directives and Surrogate Decision Making in Health Care: United States, Germany, and Japan. Baltimore, MD: Johns Hopkins University Press; 1998: 187–208. 29 refs. ISBN 0–8018–5831–3. BE59042.
*active euthanasia; *advance directives; *allowing to die; assisted suicide; attitudes; *attitudes to death; cancer; common good; criminal law; decision making; diagnosis; drugs; family members; *family relationship; historical aspects; *legal aspects; living wills; model legislation; national health insurance; organ donation; organizational policies; pain; palliative care; paternalism; patient advocacy; physician patient relationship; physicians; professional organizations; prognosis; prolongation of life; public opinion; *public policy; resuscitation orders; social dominance; *terminal care; terminally ill; third party consent; trends; trust; truth disclosure; *values; voluntary euthanasia; withholding treatment; oral directives; *Japan; Japan Medical Association; Japan Science Council; Japanese Society for Dying with Dignity

Koch, Hans–Georg. The decision to aid dying and related legal issues: advance directives and durable powers of attorney under German law. *In:* Sass, Hans–Martin; Veatch, Robert M.; Kimura, Rihito, eds. Advance Directives and Surrogate Decision Making in Health Care: United States, Germany, and Japan. Baltimore, MD: Johns Hopkins University Press; 1998: 114–135. 46 refs. 1 fn. ISBN 0–8018–5831–3. BE59039.
*advance directives; *allowing to die; artificial feeding; autonomy; case studies; competence; *decision making; family members; guidelines; judicial action; *legal aspects; living wills; model legislation; *physicians; prolongation of life; suffering; suicide; terminal care; *terminally ill; terminology; third party consent; treatment refusal; withholding treatment; oral directives; values histories; *Germany

Kohut, Nitsa; Sam, Mehran; O'Rourke, Keith, et al. Stability of treatment preferences: although most preferences do not change, most people change some of their preferences. *Journal of Clinical Ethics.* 1997

Summer; 8(2): 124–135. 25 fn. BE56356.
*advance directives; allowing to die; artificial feeding; *decision making; drugs; evaluation studies; HIV seropositivity; *patients; prognosis; prolongation of life; resuscitation; third party consent; *time factors; treatment refusal; ventilators; antibiotics; follow-up studies; outpatients; prospective studies; questionnaires; Ontario; *Toronto

Lane, Arline; Dubler, Nancy Neveloff. The health care agent: selected but neglected. *Bioethics Forum.* 1997 Summer; 13(2): 17–21. 3 refs. BE58282.
*advance directives; aged; allowing to die; artificial feeding; case studies; communication; *decision making; dementia; ethicists; *family members; legal aspects; patient care team; physicians; professional family relationship; prolongation of life; quality of life; risks and benefits; *third party consent; uncertainty; New York

Laurence, D.R. Wills, living wills and enduring powers of attorney. *Journal of the Royal College of Physicians of London.* 1995 Nov–Dec; 29(6): 488–489. BE55568.
*advance directives; aged; family members; forms; legal aspects; *living wills; Great Britain

Link, Ronald C. Recent American developments in the right to die: the *Cruzan* case, living wills, durable powers and family consent statutes. *In:* Grubb, Andrew, ed. Decision–Making and Problems of Incompetence. New York, NY: Wiley; 1994: 127–172. 169 fn. ISBN 0–471–94236–7. BE57134.
*advance directives; *allowing to die; artificial feeding; *decision making; *family members; federal government; freedom; *legal aspects; legal rights; legislation; living wills; patient care; patients; persistent vegetative state; physicians; prolongation of life; right to die; state government; state interest; Supreme Court decisions; terminally ill; *third party consent; treatment refusal; value of life; *withholding treatment; Cruzan v. Director, Missouri Department of Health; Patient Self–Determination Act 1990; *United States

Loewy, Erich H. Ethical considerations in executing and implementing advance directives. [Editorial]. *Archives of Internal Medicine.* 1998 Feb 23; 158(4): 321–324. 20 refs. BE57962.
*advance directives; allowing to die; attitudes; competence; *decision making; economics; goals; living wills; patients; physician patient relationship; physicians; prolongation of life; quality of life; ventilators; personal identity

Lynn, Joanne; Teno, Joan. A care provider perspective on advance directives and surrogate decision making for incompetent adults in the United States. *In:* Sass, Hans–Martin; Veatch, Robert M.; Kimura, Rihito, eds. Advance Directives and Surrogate Decision Making in Health Care: United States, Germany, and Japan. Baltimore, MD: Johns Hopkins University Press; 1998: 3–33. 65 refs. ISBN 0–8018–5831–3. BE59035.
advance care planning; *advance directives; aged; allowing to die; artificial feeding; case studies; chronically ill; communication; *competence; cultural pluralism; *decision making; empirical research; evaluation; *family members; legal aspects; *living wills; persistent vegetative state; physicians; prolongation of life; public policy; resuscitation orders; *risks and benefits; terminally ill; *third party consent; uncertainty; values; withholding treatment; cognition disorders; Patient Self–Determination Act 1990; United States

McCanna, Tony. A practical advance directive survey. *Bioethics Forum.* 1997 Summer; 13(2): 44–46. BE58281.
adults; *advance directives; *hospitals; institutional policies; living wills; medical records; patients; social workers; statistics; survey; Kansas; *Kansas City; Missouri

---

McCarrick, Pat Milmoe, comp. Bibliography [advance directives]. *In:* Sass, Hans–Martin; Veatch, Robert M.; Kimura, Rihito, eds. Advance Directives and Surrogate Decision Making in Health Care: United States, Germany, and Japan. Baltimore, MD: Johns Hopkins University Press; 1998: 279–302. ISBN 0-8018-5831-3. BE59045.
 *advance directives; allowing to die; cultural pluralism; decision making; *international aspects; legal aspects; living wills; terminal care; third party consent; treatment refusal; Germany; Japan; United States

McLean, Sheila A.M., ed. Death, Dying and the Law. Brookfield, VT: Dartmouth; 1996. 185 p. (Medico–legal series). 531 fn. ISBN 1-85521-657-4. BE57209.
 *active euthanasia; *advance directives; *allowing to die; *assisted suicide; competence; decision making; disabled; futility; international aspects; legal aspects; palliative care; persistent vegetative state; *physicians; prognosis; public policy; resource allocation; suffering; *terminal care; treatment refusal; *voluntary euthanasia; withholding treatment; Airedale NHS Trust v. Bland; Death with Dignity Act (OR); *Great Britain; Netherlands; United States

McLean, Sheila A.M. Transplantation and the 'nearly dead': the case of elective ventilation. *In:* McLean, Sheila A.M., ed. Contemporary Issues in Law, Medicine and Ethics. Brookfield, VT: Dartmouth; 1996: 143–162. 80 fn. ISBN 1-85521-586-1. BE57794.
 *advance directives; altruism; beneficence; body parts and fluids; decision making; gifts; informed consent; intention; *legal aspects; moral policy; *organ donation; patients; physicians; *prolongation of life; public policy; resuscitation; risks and benefits; scarcity; *ventilators; *Great Britain; House of Lords Select Committee on Medical Ethics; Human Tissue Act 1961 (Great Britain); Law Commission (Great Britain)

Markson, Lawrence; Clark, Jack; Glantz, Leonard, et al. The doctor's role in discussing advance preferences for end–of–life care: perceptions of physicians practicing in the VA. *Journal of the American Geriatrics Society.* 1997 Apr; 45(4): 399–406. 44 refs. BE57118.
 *advance care planning; *advance directives; age factors; communication; *decision making; federal government; incentives; *knowledge, attitudes, practice; moral obligations; *physician's role; physicians; *primary health care; public hospitals; survey; terminal care; *Department of Veterans Affairs; United States

Marshall, Patricia A.; Koenig, Barbara A.; Barnes, Donelle M., et al. Multiculturalism, bioethics, and end–of–life care: case narratives of Latino cancer patients. *In:* Monagle, John F.; Thomasma, David C., eds. Health Care Ethics: Critical Issues for the 21st Century. Gaithersburg, MD: Aspen Publishers; 1998: 421–431. 30 fn. ISBN 0-8342-0911-X. BE56293.
 *advance care planning; *advance directives; Asian Americans; *attitudes; blacks; *cancer; case studies; communication; comprehension; *cultural pluralism; decision making; diagnosis; empirical research; family members; family relationship; females; *Hispanic Americans; males; minority groups; narrative ethics; physicians; prognosis; psychological stress; religion; resuscitation orders; *terminally ill; third party consent; truth disclosure; *values; whites; ethnographic studies; United States

Meisel, Alan. Legal issues in decision making for incompetent patients: advance directives and surrogate decision making. *In:* Sass, Hans–Martin; Veatch, Robert M.; Kimura, Rihito, eds. Advance Directives and Surrogate Decision Making in Health Care: United States, Germany, and Japan. Baltimore, MD: Johns

Hopkins University Press; 1998: 34–65. 62 refs. 11 fn. References include separate lists of court cases and legislation. ISBN 0-8018-5831-3. BE59036.
 *advance directives; *allowing to die; artificial feeding; case studies; *competence; conflict of interest; constitutional law; critically ill; *decision making; dementia; equal protection; *family members; futility; judicial action; *legal aspects; legal rights; legislation; *living wills; patients; persistent vegetative state; physically disabled; physicians; pregnant women; privacy; prolongation of life; right to die; risks and benefits; standards; state government; terminally ill; *third party consent; treatment refusal; uncertainty; values; withholding treatment; Patient Self-Determination Act 1990; *United States

Meran, Johannes Gobertus; Poliwoda, Hubert. Clinical perspectives on advance directives and surrogate decision making. *In:* Sass, Hans–Martin; Veatch, Robert M.; Kimura, Rihito, eds. Advance Directives and Surrogate Decision Making in Health Care: United States, Germany, and Japan. Baltimore, MD: Johns Hopkins University Press; 1998: 95–113. 37 refs. ISBN 0-8018-5831-3. BE59038.
 *advance directives; alternatives; attitudes; autonomy; case studies; chronically ill; communication; competence; comprehension; critically ill; *decision making; disclosure; family members; informed consent; legal aspects; living wills; physician patient relationship; *physicians; prognosis; recall; resuscitation; resuscitation orders; risks and benefits; suicide; terminally ill; third party consent; treatment refusal; uncertainty; withholding treatment; Austria; *Germany; United States

Mezey, Mathy; Mitty, Ethel; Rappaport, Michael, et al. Implementation of the Patient Self–Determination Act (PSDA) in nursing homes in New York City. *Journal of the American Geriatrics Society.* 1997 Jan; 45(1): 43–49. 34 refs. Commented on by T.F. Ackerman, p. 114–116. BE55767.
 *advance directives; aged; allowing to die; attitudes; clinical ethics committees; community services; *competence; continuing education; cultural pluralism; decision making; *evaluation; evaluation studies; family members; health personnel; *institutional policies; *knowledge, attitudes, practice; legislation; living wills; medical records; *nursing homes; *patient education; patient transfer; *patients; proprietary health facilities; resuscitation orders; *social workers; statistics; survey; third party consent; withholding treatment; voluntary health facilities; *New York City; *Patient Self-Determination Act 1990

Michel, Vicki. Reflections on cultural difference and advance directives. *Bioethics Forum.* 1997 Summer; 13(2): 22–26. 11 refs. 1 fn. BE58283.
 *advance care planning; *advance directives; allowing to die; Asian Americans; *attitudes; autonomy; blacks; comparative studies; *cultural pluralism; decision making; family members; family relationship; Hispanic Americans; *minority groups; prolongation of life; trust; whites; United States

Morrison, R. Sean; Zayas, Luis H.; Mulvihill, Michael, et al. Barriers to completion of healthcare proxy forms: a qualitative analysis of ethnic differences. *Journal of Clinical Ethics.* 1998 Summer; 9(2): 118–126. 28 fn. BE58957.
 advance care planning; *advance directives; *aged; *attitudes; attitudes to death; *blacks; communication; comparative studies; comprehension; counseling; *cultural pluralism; decision making; disadvantaged; family members; family relationship; *Hispanic Americans; *knowledge, attitudes, practice; *minority groups; motivation; physicians; survey; terminal care; third party consent; trust; *whites; withholding treatment; absence of proxy; qualitative research; *New York City

---

BE = bioethics accession number   fn. = footnotes   refs. = references

Murphy, G. Don; Schenkenberg, Tom; Hunter, Jeff S., et al. Advance directives: a computer assisted approach to assuring patients' rights and compliance with PSDA (Patient Self-Determination Act) and JCAHO standards. *HEC (HealthCare Ethics Committee) Forum.* 1997 Sep; 9(3): 247–255. 14 refs. BE56175.
    *advance directives; communication; *computers; *hospitals; *institutional policies; medical records; patient admission; patient education; public hospitals; standards; Salt Lake City VA Medical Center

National Kidney Foundation. Implementing Advance Directives: Suggested Guidelines for Dialysis Facilities. [Pamphlet]. New York, NY: National Kidney Foundation; 1993 Dec. 16 p. 10 fn. BE57744.
    *advance directives; communication; conscience; forms; *guidelines; *health facilities; health personnel; information dissemination; *institutional policies; legal aspects; medical records; patient admission; patient care; patient transfer; referral and consultation; religion; *renal dialysis; time factors; Patient Self-Determination Act 1990; United States

New York. Health care agents and proxies. *McKinney's Consolidated Laws of New York Annotated.* 1994 Mar 28 (date effective). Sects. 2980 to 2992. 26 p. BE58575.
    *advance directives; competence; *legal aspects; state government; third party consent; *New York

Ohi, Gen. Advance directives and the Japanese ethos. *In:* Sass, Hans-Martin; Veatch, Robert M.; Kimura, Rihito, eds. Advance Directives and Surrogate Decision Making in Health Care: United States, Germany, and Japan. Baltimore, MD: Johns Hopkins University Press; 1998: 175–186. 7 refs. ISBN 0-8018-5831-3. BE59041.
    *advance directives; *attitudes; autonomy; cancer; case studies; common good; *communication; cultural pluralism; diagnosis; *family relationship; physician patient relationship; physicians; privacy; prognosis; psychological stress; *social interaction; socioeconomic factors; terminally ill; trust; *truth disclosure; *non-Western World; oral directives; Western World; Asia; *Japan

Pearlman, Robert A.; Cole, William G.; Patrick, Donald L., et al. Advance care planning: eliciting patient preferences for life-sustaining treatment. *Patient Education and Counseling.* 1995 Sep; 26(1–3): 353–361. 65 refs. BE55575.
    *advance care planning; *advance directives; allowing to die; autonomy; *communication; counseling; decision making; empirical research; health personnel; living wills; patient care; *patient education; patients; prolongation of life; quality of life; teaching methods; terminal care; values; United States

Phillips, Jennifer M. Reducing postmortem examination refusal by families of research subjects. *IRB: A Review of Human Subjects Research.* 1997 Sep–Oct; 19(5): 10–11. BE57139.
    *advance directives; *autopsies; *consent forms; death; family members; patients; *research subjects; *third party consent

Post, Stephen G. Physician-assisted suicide in Alzheimer's disease. *Journal of the American Geriatrics Society.* 1997 May; 45(5): 647–651. 26 refs. BE55843.
    active euthanasia; *advance directives; aged; *assisted suicide; attitudes; autonomy; beneficence; chronically ill; competence; *dementia; economics; health personnel; *hospices; international aspects; legal aspects; *long-term care; managed care programs; *palliative care; physicians; policy analysis; public opinion; *public policy; quality of life; resource allocation; self concept; social discrimination; social impact; suffering; *terminal care; terminally ill; wedge argument; withholding treatment; *United States

Rabbinical Assembly. Committee on Jewish Law and Standards. Jewish Medical Directives for Health Care. New York, NY: The Assembly; 1994 Jan. 16 p. Edited by Aaron L. Mackler, chairman of the Law Committee's Subcommittee on Biomedical Ethics, based on papers by Avram I. Reisner and Elliot N. Dorff. BE57997.
    active euthanasia; *advance directives; allowing to die; artificial feeding; assisted suicide; autopsies; clergy; communication; competence; decision making; diagnosis; double effect; drugs; family members; forms; home care; hospices; *Jewish ethics; legal aspects; living wills; organ donation; pain; patient care; persistent vegetative state; physicians; prognosis; prolongation of life; resuscitation; state government; surgery; terminal care; terminally ill; third party consent; treatment refusal; truth disclosure; value of life; values; ventilators; withholding treatment; amputation; *Conservative Judaism; United States

Rich, Ben A. Advance directives: the next generation. *Journal of Legal Medicine.* 1998 Mar; 19(1): 63–97. 100 fn. BE58900.
    *advance care planning; *advance directives; allowing to die; artificial feeding; attitudes to death; autonomy; communication; *decision making; evaluation; forms; informed consent; judicial action; *legal aspects; legislation; living wills; palliative care; physician's role; *physicians; review; *terminal care; third party consent; treatment refusal; uncertainty; oral directives; values histories; Patient Self-Determination Act 1990; Study to Understand Prognoses and Preferences for Outcomes and Risks of Treatments (SUPPORT); United States

Rich, Ben A. Prospective autonomy and critical interests: a narrative defense of the moral authority of advance directives. *Cambridge Quarterly of Healthcare Ethics.* 1997 Spring; 6(2): 138–147. 24 fn. BE56435.
    *advance directives; allowing to die; *autonomy; competence; *dementia; *moral policy; *narrative ethics; paternalism; *personhood; prolongation of life; public policy; quality of life; right to die; *self concept; treatment refusal; *personal identity; rationality; Dresser, Rebecca; Dworkin, Ronald; Parfit, Derek

In the mid to late 1980s a debate arose over the moral and legal authority of advance medical directives. At the center of this debate were two point-counterpoint law journal articles by Rebecca Dresser and Nancy Rhoden. What appeared to have the makings of an ongoing critical dialogue ended with the untimely death of Nancy Rhoden. Rebecca Dresser, however, has continued her challenge of advance directives in numerous publications, most recently in a critique of Ronald Dworkin's *Life's Dominion*. Like Rhoden, Dworkin has been a staunch advocate of advance directives as an exercise of what has come to be referred to as prospective or precedent autonomy. In this paper I will consider a number of the issues that Dresser has repeatedly raised about the infirmities of advance directives, and suggest that it is from an understanding of and appreciation for the narrative dimension of the life of a person that advance directives draw one of their most powerful justifications.

Rich, Ben A. The values history: restoring narrative identity to long-term care. *Journal of Ethics, Law, and Aging.* 1996 Fall–Winter; 2(2): 75–84. 29 refs. 7 fn. BE57143.
    *advance directives; *aged; autonomy; *communication; competence; dehumanization; dementia; family members; health personnel; institutionalized persons; *long-term care; narrative ethics; *nursing homes; patient care; personhood; physician patient relationship; privacy; *quality of health care; *quality of life; self concept; time factors; value of life; *values; dignity; *personal identity; *values histories

---

BE = bioethics accession number   fn. = footnotes   refs. = references

Rye, Patricia D.; Wallston, Kenneth A.; Wallston, Barbara Strudler, et al. The desire to control terminal health care and attitudes toward living wills. *American Journal of Preventive Medicine.* 1985 May–Jun; 1(3): 56–60. 14 refs. BE56749.
    *adults; *attitudes; *autonomy; decision making; intention; *living wills; patients; survey; *terminal care; Tennessee

Sansone, Paulette; Phillips, Michael. Advance directives for elderly people: worthwhile cause or wasted effort? *Social Work.* 1995 May; 40(3): 397–401. 16 refs. BE55580.
    *advance directives; *aged; *allowing to die; artificial feeding; *attitudes; cancer; *communication; comparative studies; consensus; dementia; drugs; evaluation studies; *family members; Jews; knowledge, attitudes, practice; living wills; nursing homes; *prolongation of life; renal dialysis; residential facilities; Roman Catholics; social workers; survey; third party consent; withholding treatment; coma; professional role; New York City

Sansone, Paulette; Schmitt, Louise. Assessing values: the neglected dimension in long-term care. *HEC (HealthCare Ethics Committee) Forum.* 1997 Sep; 9(3): 264–275. 34 refs. BE56179.
    advance care planning; *advance directives; *aged; attitudes to death; autonomy; clinical ethics committees; decision making; dementia; institutionalized persons; legislation; long-term care; *nursing homes; patient care; patient discharge; social workers; terminal care; *values; *values histories; Patient Self-Determination Act 1990

Sass, Hans–Martin. Advance directives. *In:* Chadwick, Ruth, ed. Encyclopedia of Applied Ethics, Volume 1. San Diego, CA: Academic Press; 1998: 41–49. 17 refs. ISBN 0-12-227066-5. BE56364.
    *advance directives; allowing to die; attitudes; autonomy; beneficence; competence; forms; legal aspects; living wills; palliative care; paternalism; personhood; physicians; review; risks and benefits; standards; third party consent; time factors; values histories

Sass, Hans–Martin; Veatch, Robert M.; Kimura, Rihito, eds. Advance Directives and Surrogate Decision Making in Health Care: United States, Germany, and Japan. Baltimore, MD: Johns Hopkins University Press; 1998. 311 p. Includes references. ISBN 0-8018-5831-3. BE59034.
    advance care planning; *advance directives; allowing to die; attitudes to death; autonomy; beneficence; brain death; common good; competence; *cultural pluralism; *decision making; family members; family relationship; forms; historical aspects; informed consent; *international aspects; justice; legal aspects; living wills; organ donation; palliative care; paternalism; patient participation; physician patient relationship; physicians; privacy; prolongation of life; *public policy; religion; review; terminal care; third party consent; treatment refusal; trends; truth disclosure; *values; withholding treatment; oral directives; values histories; *Germany; *Japan; *United States

Sass, Hans–Martin. Images of killing and letting-die, of self-determination and beneficence: the ethical debate on advance directives and surrogate decision making in Germany. *In:* Sass, Hans-Martin; Veatch, Robert M.; Kimura, Rihito, eds. Advance Directives and Surrogate Decision Making in Health Care: United States, Germany, and Japan. Baltimore, MD: Johns Hopkins University Press; 1998: 136–172. 129 refs. ISBN 0-8018-5831-3. BE59040.
    active euthanasia; *advance directives; *allowing to die; attitudes; *autonomy; beneficence; case studies; competence; cultural pluralism; *decision making; dissent; family members; guidelines; killing; legal aspects; living wills; National Socialism; palliative care; patient advocacy;

physicians; professional organizations; prolongation of life; quality of life; right to die; risks and benefits; suffering; suicide; terminally ill; terminology; third party consent; truth disclosure; uncertainty; values; withholding treatment; oral directives; values histories; German Society for Humane Dying; *Germany

Sass, Hans–Martin, comp. Model forms of advance directives and advance care documents. *In:* Sass, Hans–Martin; Veatch, Robert M.; Kimura, Rihito, eds. Advance Directives and Surrogate Decision Making in Health Care: United States, Germany, and Japan. Baltimore, MD: Johns Hopkins University Press; 1998: 223–278. This appendix consists of an introduction and the text of seventeen advance directive forms. ISBN 0-8018-5831-3. BE59044.
    *advance directives; allowing to die; biomedical technologies; competence; decision making; *forms; *international aspects; *living wills; mentally disabled; models, theoretical; narrative ethics; organ donation; patient care; persistent vegetative state; physically disabled; pregnant women; prolongation of life; religious ethics; terminal care; terminally ill; third party consent; treatment refusal; values; withholding treatment; values histories; *Germany; *Japan; *United States

Schirm, Victoria; Stachel, Luisa. The values history as a nursing intervention to encourage use of advance directives among older adults. *Applied Nursing Research.* 1996 May; 9(2): 93–96. 17 refs. BE57975.
    *advance care planning; *advance directives; *aged; information dissemination; *knowledge, attitudes, practice; living wills; *nurse's role; *values histories; United States

Sechriest, Kay; Payne, John; Jordan, Lynn, et al. Confronting the right to die: caught between a patient's will and a doctor's order. [Case study and commentaries]. *Journal of Christian Nursing.* 1985 Fall; 2(4): 5–10. BE56974.
    attitudes; case studies; Christian ethics; *decision making; interprofessional relations; legal aspects; *living wills; *nurses; *patient advocacy; *physicians; *prolongation of life; *resuscitation orders; right to die

Singer, Peter A.; Martin, Douglas K.; Lavery, James V., et al. Reconceptualizing advance care planning from the patient's perspective. *Archives of Internal Medicine.* 1998 Apr 27; 158(8): 879–884. 37 refs. BE58308.
    *advance care planning; *advance directives; allowing to die; autonomy; *communication; competence; death; decision making; *family members; family relationship; *goals; *knowledge, attitudes, practice; living wills; *patients; renal dialysis; survey; terminal care; third party consent; treatment refusal; withholding treatment; qualitative research; Toronto
    BACKGROUND: Traditional academic assumptions about advance care planning (ACP) include the following: (1) the purpose of ACP is preparing for incapacity; (2) ACP is based on the ethical principle of autonomy and the exercise of control; (3) the focus of ACP is completing written advance directive forms; and (4) ACP occurs within the context of the physician–patient relationship. These assumptions about ACP have never been empirically validated. OBJECTIVE: To examine the traditional academic assumptions by exploring ACP from the perspective of patients actively participating in the planning process. METHODS: Forty-eight patients (30 men and 18 women with a mean age of 48.3 years) who were undergoing hemodialysis were interviewed 6 months after receiving an advance directive form. Their experience of ACP was noted in interviews that were audiotaped, transcribed, and analyzed. RESULTS: The

---

BE = bioethics accession number   fn. = footnotes   refs. = references

participants said that their purpose in ACP was to prepare for death and dying, and their underlying goals included the exercise of control and an attempt to relieve burdens placed on loved ones. Advance care planning was viewed as a social process, and completing a written advance directive form was often regarded as unnecessary. Participants often involved close loved ones, but physicians infrequently. CONCLUSIONS: The traditional academic assumptions are not fully supported from the perspective of patients involved in ACP. The patients we interviewed stated that (1) the purpose of ACP is not only preparing for incapacity but also preparing for death; (2) ACP is not based solely on autonomy and the exercise of control, but also on personal relationships and relieving burdens placed on others; (3) the focus of ACP is not only on completing written advance directive forms but also on the social process; and (4) ACP does not occur solely within the context of the physician–patient relationship but also within relationships with close loved ones.

Sommerville, Ann; British Medical Association. Advance Statements about Medical Treatment: Code of Practice with Explanatory Notes. London: BMJ Publishing Group; 1995. 39 p. 11 fn. Includes 16 page booklet in back pocket. ISBN 0-7279-0914-2. BE58947.
*advance directives; communication; competence; conscience; decision making; *guidelines; health personnel; informed consent; legal aspects; legal liability; patient care; physicians; *practice guidelines; professional organizations; public policy; records; *standards; treatment refusal; oral directives; *British Medical Association; Great Britain

Sommerville, Ann. Are advance directives really the answer? And what was the question? In: McLean, Sheila A.M., ed. Death, Dying and the Law. Brookfield, VT: Dartmouth; 1996: 29–47. 41 fn. ISBN 1-85521-657-4. BE57212.
*advance directives; allowing to die; autonomy; competence; decision making; dementia; evaluation; international aspects; legal aspects; organizational policies; persistent vegetative state; personhood; physicians; professional organizations; prolongation of life; psychiatric wills; public policy; *risks and benefits; terminally ill; treatment refusal; British Medical Association; *Great Britain; House of Lords; House of Lords Select Committee on Medical Ethics; Law Commission (Great Britain); United States

Spike, Jeffrey. A paradox about capacity, alcoholism, and noncompliance. Journal of Clinical Ethics. 1997 Fall; 8(3): 303–306. 4 fn. BE57567.
*advance directives; *alcohol abuse; *autonomy; *competence; *decision making; family members; *paternalism; *patient care; *patient compliance; *patient participation; physician patient relationship; *physicians; *surgery; third party consent; time factors; *treatment refusal; values; rationality; Ulysses contracts

Steinberg, M.A.; Cartwright, C.M.; Parker, M.H., et al. Patient Self-Determination in Terminal Care: Phase 2. Designing "Useful" Advance Directives and Proxies. Report to the Commonwealth Department of Human Services and Health, Research and Development Grants Program. Brisbane, QLD: University of Queensland Medical School, Department of Social and Preventive Medicine; 1997 May. 130 p. 29 refs. BE58986.
advance care planning; *advance directives; aged; *evaluation; evaluation studies; *forms; health personnel; legal aspects; living wills; nurses; physicians; primary health care; terminal care; third party consent; focus groups; Australia

Steinberg, M.A.; Cartwright, C.M.; MacDonald, S.M.,

et al. Self-determination in terminal care: a comparison of GP and community members' responses. Australian Family Physician. 1997 Jun; 26(6): 703–705, 707. 11 refs. 8 fn. BE57552.
*advance directives; age factors; *attitudes; autonomy; comparative studies; decision making; home care; hospices; hospitals; legal aspects; patient participation; *physicians; *public opinion; survey; *terminal care; Australia; *Queensland

Stryker, Jeff. Ethical issues in treating incompetent patients with HIV disease. In: Cohen, P.T.; Sande, Merle A.; Volberding, Paul A., eds. The AIDS Knowledge Base: A Textbook on HIV Disease from the University of California, San Francisco, and the San Francisco General Hospital. Second Edition. Boston, MA: Little, Brown; 1994: 11.3–1 to 11.3–4. 17 refs. ISBN 0-316-77067-1. BE56642.
*adults; *advance directives; *AIDS; allowing to die; competence; *decision making; dementia; futility; *HIV seropositivity; legal aspects; living wills; mothers; *newborns; patients; physicians; prolongation of life; third party consent; withholding treatment; United States

Tamburini, Joan Killion. Lessons on a minimally acceptable quality of life. Bioethics Forum. 1997 Summer; 13(2): 38–41. Followed by a list of Websites and an "Advance directives timeline" compiled by Don Reynolds. BE58285.
*advance directives; aged; historical aspects; information dissemination; legal aspects; living wills; *quality of life; right to die; terminally ill; Midwest Bioethics Center; Twentieth Century; United States

Teno, Joan; Lynn, Joanne; Wenger, Neil, et al. Advance directives for seriously ill hospitalized patients: effectiveness with the Patient Self-Determination Act and the SUPPORT intervention. [For the SUPPORT Investigators]. Journal of the American Geriatrics Society. 1997 Apr; 45(4): 500–507. 23 refs. BE57122.
advance care planning; *advance directives; *communication; comparative studies; *critically ill; *decision making; *evaluation; evaluation studies; family members; hospitals; living wills; medical records; patient education; patients; physician patient relationship; physician's role; physicians; prognosis; *resuscitation orders; terminal care; third party consent; retrospective studies; seriously ill; *Patient Self-Determination Act 1990; *Study to Understand Prognoses and Preferences for Outcomes and Risks of Treatments (SUPPORT); United States

Teno, Joan; Lynn, Joanne; Connors, Alfred F., et al. The illusion of end-of-life resource savings with advance directives. [For the SUPPORT Investigators]. Journal of the American Geriatrics Society. 1997 Apr; 45(4): 513–518. 15 refs. BE57124.
*advance directives; communication; comparative studies; control groups; *critically ill; *economics; *evaluation; evaluation studies; *hospitals; *medical records; patient admission; patients; research design; resource allocation; resuscitation; resuscitation orders; social impact; socioeconomic factors; *terminal care; treatment refusal; *seriously ill; Patient Self-Determination Act 1990; *Study to Understand Prognoses and Preferences for Outcomes and Risks of Treatments (SUPPORT); United States

Teno, Joan M.; Licks, Sandra; Lynn, Joanne, et al. Do advance directives provide instructions that direct care? [For the SUPPORT Investigators]. Journal of the American Geriatrics Society. 1997 Apr; 45(4): 508–512. 12 refs. BE57123.
*advance directives; *allowing to die; biomedical technologies; *communication; *critically ill; *decision making; *evaluation; evaluation studies; hospitals; living

---

BE = bioethics accession number   fn. = footnotes   refs. = references

wills; medical records; patient care; prognosis; prolongation of life; third party consent; treatment refusal; *seriously ill; *Study to Understand Prognoses and Preferences for Outcomes and Risks of Treatments (SUPPORT); United States

Terrence Higgins Trust (Great Britain). Living Will Project. Advance directives and AIDS. *In:* Grubb, Andrew, ed. Decision–Making and Problems of Incompetence. New York, NY: Wiley; 1994: 187–196. 20 fn. ISBN 0–471–94236–7. BE57136.
*advance directives; *AIDS; *attitudes; competence; *HIV seropositivity; international aspects; *legal aspects; *living wills; organizational policies; patients; physicians; professional organizations; *program descriptions; public opinion; survey; terminal care; third party consent; British Medical Association; *Great Britain; London; Terrence Higgins Trust

Tonelli, Mark. Beyond living wills. *Bioethics Forum.* 1997 Summer; 13(2): 6–12. 13 refs. 4 fn. BE58286.
advance care planning; *advance directives; allowing to die; autonomy; decision making; evaluation; family members; futility; *living wills; physicians; prolongation of life; quality of health care; quality of life; resuscitation orders; standards; *terminal care; treatment refusal; withholding treatment

Tsuchida, Tomoaki. A differing perspective on advance directives. *In:* Sass, Hans-Martin; Veatch, Robert M.; Kimura, Rihito, eds. Advance Directives and Surrogate Decision Making in Health Care: United States, Germany, and Japan. Baltimore, MD: Johns Hopkins University Press; 1998: 209–221. 10 refs. 2 fn. ISBN 0–8018–5831–3. BE59043.
*advance directives; attitudes; *attitudes to death; *brain death; Buddhist ethics; *common good; decision making; determination of death; family members; *family relationship; guidelines; living wills; national health insurance; organ donation; paternalism; physician patient relationship; physicians; public opinion; religion; terminal care; third party consent; truth disclosure; *values; Confucian ethics; dependency; *Japan; Japanese Society for Dying with Dignity

U.S. General Accounting Office. Patient Self-Determination Act: Providers Offer Information on Advance Directives but Effectiveness Uncertain. Report to the Ranking Minority Member, Subcommittee on Health, Committee on Ways and Means, House of Representatives. Washington, DC: U.S. General Accounting Office; 1995 Aug 28. 48 p. 47 fn. GAO/HEHS-95-135. Appendixes include sample advance directive forms, and developments in state law regarding advance directives. BE57389.
*advance directives; allowing to die; attitudes; communication; conscience; decision making; emergency care; *evaluation; federal government; forms; *government regulation; *hospitals; *information dissemination; *institutional policies; legislation; living wills; medical records; patient care; patient transfer; physicians; professional autonomy; state government; terminal care; third party consent; oral directives; values histories; Department of Health and Human Services; *Patient Self-Determination Act 1990; Uniform Health-Care Decisions Act 1993; *United States

Veatch, Robert M. Ethical dimensions of advance directives and surrogate decision making in the United States. *In:* Sass, Hans-Martin; Veatch, Robert M.; Kimura, Rihito, eds. Advance Directives and Surrogate Decision Making in Health Care: United States, Germany, and Japan. Baltimore, MD: Johns Hopkins University Press; 1998: 66–91. 72 refs. 7 fn. ISBN 0–8018–5831–3. BE59037.

adults; *advance directives; aged; *allowing to die; anencephaly; artificial feeding; *autonomy; beneficence; brain pathology; competence; consensus; *decision making; family members; freedom; futility; historical aspects; informed consent; judicial action; justice; *legal rights; living wills; mentally retarded; minors; moral policy; parents; paternalism; patients' rights; persistent vegetative state; physician patient relationship; physicians; professional autonomy; prolongation of life; refusal to treat; religion; *risks and benefits; Roman Catholic ethics; *third party consent; *treatment refusal; trends; ventilators; withholding treatment; liberalism; oral directives; values histories; Hippocratic Oath; In re Baby K; In re Conroy; In re Phillip B.; In re Quinlan; Twentieth Century; *United States

Weir, Robert F.; Peters, Charles. Affirming the decisions adolescents make about life and death. *Hastings Center Report.* 1997 Nov–Dec; 27(6): 29–40. 22 fn. BE57858.
*adolescents; *advance care planning; *advance directives; *age factors; allowing to die; autonomy; chronically ill; *communication; *competence; counseling; critically ill; *decision making; disclosure; dissent; empirical research; guidelines; *informed consent; legal aspects; legislation; organizational policies; parents; *patient advocacy; *patient care; *patient participation; pediatrics; physician patient relationship; physicians; practice guidelines; professional family relationship; professional organizations; prolongation of life; risks and benefits; state government; *terminal care; terminally ill; *treatment refusal; trust; American Academy of Pediatrics; Patient Self-Determination Act 1990; United States
Adolescents who are critically, chronically, and terminally ill traditionally have been given little voice in their health care treatment. But over the last three decades attitudes have begun to shift. The legal and medical professions as well as parents and children's advocates have started to recognize that cognitively normal adolescents have decisionmaking capacity and believe these patients ought to have the opportunity to participate in even the toughest of health treatment decisions. Advances directives, if used with sensitivity and care, could prove a valuable means of giving these older pediatric patients a say in their care.

Wellman, Carl. The inalienable right to life and the durable power of attorney. *Law and Philosophy.* 1995; 14(2): 245–269. BE55598.
*advance directives; *allowing to die; communication; decision making; *freedom; informed consent; killing; legal rights; moral obligations; *moral policy; patient care; physicians; privacy; prolongation of life; right to die; *rights; third party consent; *treatment refusal; *value of life; withholding treatment

Worth–Staten, Patricia A.; Poniatowski, Larry. Advance directives and patient rights: a Joint Commission perspective. *Bioethics Forum.* 1997 Summer; 13(2): 47–50. 2 refs. BE58287.
*advance directives; decision making; family members; *hospitals; informed consent; *institutional policies; patient participation; *patients' rights; *standards; terminal care; withholding treatment; *Joint Commission on Accreditation of Healthcare Organizations; United States

Youngner, Stuart J.; Shuck, Jerry M. Advance directives and the determination of death. *In:* McCullough, Laurence B.; Jones, James W.; Brody, Baruch A., eds. Surgical Ethics. New York, NY: Oxford University Press; 1998: 57–77. 49 refs. ISBN 0–19–510347–5. BE58340.
advance care planning; *advance directives; brain death; cardiac death; *communication; decision making; *determination of death; family members; goals; guidelines; living wills; organ donation; palliative care; *physicians; professional autonomy; prolongation of life; quality of life;

BE = bioethics accession number   fn. = footnotes   refs. = references

*resuscitation orders; *surgery; terminally ill; third party consent; treatment refusal; values; withholding treatment; Patient Self-Determination Act 1990; United States

Zaman, Syed; Battcock, Timothy. Doctors need to know more about advance directives. [Letter]. *BMJ (British Medical Journal).* 1998 Jul 11; 317(7151): 146–147. 5 refs. BE58815.
> *advance directives; *knowledge, attitudes, practice; *physicians; survey; *England

AGED
See under
PATIENT CARE/AGED

AIDS

See also PUBLIC HEALTH

Arno, Peter S.; Bonuck, Karen. The economics and financing of HIV disease. *In:* Cohen, P.T.; Sande, Merle A.; Volberding, Paul A., eds. The AIDS Knowledge Base: A Textbook on HIV Disease from the University of California, San Francisco, and the San Francisco General Hospital. Second Edition. Boston, MA: Little, Brown; 1994: 9.3–1 to 9.3–12. 79 refs. ISBN 0-316-77067-1. BE56645.
> *AIDS; children; chronically ill; community services; critically ill; drugs; *economics; females; government financing; health care; *HIV seropositivity; home care; hospitals; long-term care; males; patient care; social impact; terminally ill; trends; outpatients; undertreatment; Medicaid; Orphan Drug Act 1983; United States

Bayer, Ronald; Stryker, Jeff. Ethical challenges posed by clinical progress in AIDS. *American Journal of Public Health.* 1997 Oct; 87(10): 1599–1602. 28 refs. BE56202.
> *AIDS; autonomy; common good; developing countries; disadvantaged; *drugs; *economics; federal government; government financing; health care delivery; health insurance; *HIV seropositivity; *justice; paternalism; *patient care; *patient compliance; public health; public policy; *refusal to treat; socioeconomic factors; state government; withholding treatment; Medicaid; United States

Casarett, David J.; Lantos, John D. Have we treated AIDS too well? Rationing and the future of AIDS exceptionalism. *Annals of Internal Medicine.* 1998 May 1; 128(9): 756–759. 29 refs. BE57906.
> *AIDS; biomedical research; drugs; *economics; government financing; health care reform; health insurance; justice; patient care; political activity; *public policy; *resource allocation; stigmatization; AZT; Ryan White Comprehensive AIDS Resources Emergency Act 1990; *United States

During the past decade, medical therapy for AIDS has become more effective but also prohibitively expensive. A medical tragedy has been transformed into a financial crisis, and society has responded by establishing special programs and sources of funding for AIDS. These maneuvers parallel earlier approaches to HIV testing and reporting that have collectively come to be known as 'exceptionalism.' This paper suggests that exceptionalism in resource allocation is a fragile, short-term solution. In the long run, AIDS exceptionalism will create growing injustice and should be avoided. However, we should not eliminate the advances that this exceptionalism has already achieved. Instead, we need a working dialogue between these advances and public policy.

Chervenak, Frank A.; McCullough, Laurence B. Common ethical dilemmas encountered in the management of HIV-infected women and newborns. *Clinical Obstetrics and Gynecology.* 1996 Jun; 39(2): 411–419. 16 refs. BE56746.
> adolescents; advance directives; AIDS serodiagnosis; autonomy; *beneficence; children; communicable diseases; competence; confidentiality; contact tracing; contraception; counseling; decision making; disadvantaged; disclosure; drugs; fetuses; health facilities; *HIV seropositivity; informed consent; interprofessional relations; *moral obligations; *newborns; obligations to society; parental notification; patient advocacy; *patient care; patient care team; patient participation; patients; *physicians; *pregnant women; public health; rights; selective abortion; social discrimination; terminal care; AZT; United States

Chochinov, Harvey Max; Wilson, Keith G.; Breitbart, William, et al. Assisted suicide for HIV patients. [Letter and response]. *American Journal of Psychiatry.* 1997 Feb; 154(2): 294–295. 2 refs. BE55813.
> AIDS; *assisted suicide; *attitudes; depressive disorder; *HIV seropositivity; pain; palliative care; *patients; psychological stress; stigmatization; terminally ill; ambulatory care; undertreatment

Coles, Matthew. Discrimination, insurance, health care decisions, and wills. *In:* Cohen, P.T.; Sande, Merle A.; Volberding, Paul A., eds. The AIDS Knowledge Base: A Textbook on HIV Disease from the University of California, San Francisco, and the San Francisco General Hospital. Second Edition. Boston, MA: Little, Brown; 1994: 9.2–1 to 9.2–13. 12 refs. ISBN 0-316-77067-1. BE56637.
> advance directives; *AIDS; AIDS serodiagnosis; allowing to die; competence; confidentiality; decision making; disabled; disclosure; employment; federal government; *government regulation; health facilities; *health insurance; health insurance reimbursement; health personnel; *HIV seropositivity; homosexuals; insurance selection bias; investigational drugs; *legal aspects; mandatory testing; medical records; *social discrimination; state government; third party consent; treatment refusal; *United States

Cooke, Molly; Gourlay, Linda; Collette, Linda, et al. Informal caregivers and the intention to hasten AIDS-related death. *Archives of Internal Medicine.* 1998 Jan 12; 158(1): 69–75. 35 refs. BE56300.
> *active euthanasia; *AIDS; assisted suicide; *drugs; evaluation studies; family members; friends; HIV seropositivity; home care; homosexuals; hospices; hospitals; *intention; males; motivation; *palliative care; physician's role; psychological stress; survey; *terminal care; terminally ill; voluntary euthanasia; *caregivers; narcotics; prospective studies; sedatives; San Francisco

OBJECTIVES: To determine the extent to which homosexual men dying of the acquired immunodeficiency syndrome (AIDS) receive medication intended to hasten death. To assess the impact on caregivers of administering medications intended to hasten death. METHODS: In a prospective study of caregiving partners of men with AIDS (n = 140), characteristics of the ill partner, the caregiver, and the relationship were assessed at baseline and 1 month before the ill partner's death. Three months after the death, caregivers were asked if they had increased their partner's narcotic and/or sedative-hypnotic medication dose and if so, what had been the objective of the increase, and their comfort with their medication decisions. RESULTS: Of 140 ill partners who died of AIDS, 17 (12.1%) received an increase in the use of medications immediately before death intended to hasten death. Diagnoses and care needs of ill partners who

---

received increases in the use of medications to hasten death did not differ from those of ill partners receiving medication for symptoms. Fourteen increases (10%) in use of medications were administered by caregivers. These caregivers did not differ from those administering medication for symptom control in level of distress, caregiving burden, relationship characteristics, or comfort with the medication decision, but they reported more social support and positive meaning in caregiving. CONCLUSION: The decision to hasten death is not a rare event in this group of men. There is no evidence that it is the result of caregiver distress, poor relationship quality, or intolerable caregiving burden; and it does not cause excessive discomfort in the surviving partner. This study, although small, has implications for the policy debate on assisted suicide.

David, Lori A. The legal ramifications in criminal law of knowingly transmitting AIDS. *Law and Psychology Review.* 1995 Spring; 19: 259–271. 96 fn. BE56029.
  *AIDS; *criminal law; *HIV seropositivity; killing; *legal liability; *patients; state government; United States

Dorozynski, Alexander. Scandal unfolds over blood donation in French prisons. [News]. *BMJ (British Medical Journal).* 1998 Jan 17; 316(7126): 171. BE57958.
  *administrators; blood donation; *blood transfusions; disclosure; *HIV seropositivity; legal liability; *misconduct; *physicians; prisoners; risk; *France

Elliott, Richard; Canadian HIV/AIDS Legal Network and Canadian AIDS Society. Joint Project on Legal and Ethical Issues. Criminal Law and HIV/AIDS: Final Report. Montreal, PQ: Canadian HIV/AIDS Legal Network and the Canadian AIDS Society; 1997 Mar. 181 p. Bibliography: p. 111–119. ISBN 1–896735–08–8. BE57887.
  *AIDS; confidentiality; *criminal law; disclosure; drug abuse; *HIV seropositivity; international aspects; killing; *legal aspects; *legal liability; legislation; *patients; pregnant women; prenatal injuries; public health; public policy; sexuality; Australia; *Canada; Criminal Code of Canada; Europe; New Zealand; South Africa; United States

Fishman, Rachelle H.B. Israeli courts intervene in medical issues. [News]. *Lancet.* 1997 Sep 20; 350(9081): 874. BE56489.
  adults; allowing to die; children; compensation; *HIV seropositivity; hospitals; *judicial action; *legal aspects; mentally retarded; negligence; parents; renal dialysis; suffering; *treatment refusal; truth disclosure; *Israel

Fuller, Jon. AIDS prevention: a challenge to the Catholic moral tradition. *America.* 1996 Dec 28; 175(20): 13–20. BE56084.
  adults; *AIDS; children; contraception; developing countries; drug abuse; females; health education; *HIV seropositivity; international aspects; minority groups; moral obligations; *moral policy; morbidity; mortality; *preventive medicine; public health; *public policy; *Roman Catholic ethics; *social impact; *vulnerable populations; war; *condoms; *needle–exchange programs; Africa; Asia; United States

Ginzburg, Harold M. The legal perspective: the duty to notify. *Pediatric AIDS and HIV Infection.* 1996 Aug; 7(4): 269–272. 16 refs. BE57069.
  AIDS serodiagnosis; blood banks; *blood transfusions; contact tracing; *disclosure; *duty to warn; *HIV seropositivity; *hospitals; *legal liability; negligence; *physicians; *California; *Reisner v. Regents of the University of California; United States

Gostin, Lawrence O.; Webber, David W. HIV infection and AIDS in the public health and health care systems: the role of law and litigation. *JAMA.* 1998 Apr 8; 279(14): 1108–1113. 102 refs. BE57333.
  *AIDS; AIDS serodiagnosis; anonymous testing; compensation; confidentiality; counseling; diagnosis; disabled; disclosure; duty to warn; employment; federal government; health care delivery; health insurance; health personnel; *HIV seropositivity; iatrogenic disease; informed consent; judicial action; *legal aspects; legal liability; legal rights; legislation; mandatory reporting; mandatory testing; negligence; occupational exposure; patient care; patients; pregnant women; preventive medicine; prisoners; privacy; psychological stress; public health; *public policy; social discrimination; standards; state government; voluntary programs; needle–exchange programs; AIDS Litigation Project; Americans with Disabilities Act 1990; *United States

The AIDS Litigation Project has reviewed nearly 600 reported cases involving individuals with human immunodeficiency virus (HIV) infection and acquired immunodeficiency syndrome (AIDS) in the federal and state courts in the United States between 1991 and 1997. Cases were identified through a federal and 50–state computer and library search. An important subset of litigation relates to HIV/AIDS in the public health and health care systems, since the law affects health care institutions and professionals, patients, and public health policy in America. This subset of HIV/AIDS litigation includes testing and reporting; privacy, the duty to warn, and the right to know; physician standards of care in prevention and treatment; and discrimination and access to health care. In broad terms, the review demonstrates a reliance on voluntary testing and protection of patient privacy through HIV–specific statutes and the common law. Negligence with potential civil and criminal liability has been alleged in cases of erroneous or missed diagnosis of HIV infection. In the first AIDS case to be considered by the Supreme Court, the Court will decide whether patients with asymptomatic HIV infection are protected under the Americans With Disabilities Act. Considerable progress has been made, both socially and legally, during the first 2 decades of the epidemic, but much still needs to be accomplished to protect privacy, prevent discrimination, and promote tolerance.

Hein, Karen. Aligning science with politics and policy in HIV prevention. *Science.* 1998 Jun 19; 280(5371): 1905–1906. 5 refs. BE58268.
  *AIDS; costs and benefits; empirical research; federal government; government financing; health education; *HIV seropositivity; international aspects; mass media; *politics; prevalence; *preventive medicine; public health; *public policy; resource allocation; condoms; needle–exchange programs; Thailand; *United States

Illingworth, Patricia. Warning: AIDS health promotion programs may be hazardous to your autonomy. *In:* Overall, Christine and Zion, William P., eds. Perspectives on AIDS: Ethical and Social Issues. New York, NY: Oxford University Press; 1991: 138–154. 39 fn. ISBN 0–19–540749–0. BE58292.
  *AIDS; attitudes; *autonomy; *behavior control; *coercion; common good; drug abuse; *health education; *health promotion; HIV seropositivity; *information dissemination; methods; motivation; operant conditioning; preventive medicine; *public health; public policy; self concept; sexuality; social discrimination; social impact; Canada

Kaplan, Edward H. Israel's ban on use of Ethiopians' blood: how many infectious donations were prevented? *Lancet.* 1998 Apr 11; 351(9109): 1127–1128. 15 refs. BE58309.

BE = bioethics accession number   fn. = footnotes   refs. = references

aliens; blood banks; *blood donation; *deception; *HIV seropositivity; prevalence; *preventive medicine; *public policy; risk; statistics; *stigmatization; *emigration and immigration; Ethiopia; *Israel

Lamke, Celia. Distributive justice and HIV disease in intensive care. *Critical Care Nursing Quarterly.* 1996 May; 19(1): 55–64. 23 refs. BE55724.
  *AIDS; *decision making; *HIV seropositivity; *intensive care units; *justice; nurses; patient admission; patient care team; patients; physicians; *resource allocation; *selection for treatment; standards

Magnusson, R.S. Australian HIV/AIDS legislation: a review for doctors. *Australian and New Zealand Journal of Medicine.* 1996 Jun; 26(3): 396–406. 47 refs. BE57503.
  *AIDS; AIDS serodiagnosis; coercion; confidentiality; contact tracing; criminal law; disclosure; duty to warn; government regulation; *HIV seropositivity; informed consent; *legal aspects; mandatory testing; privacy; refusal to treat; social discrimination; voluntary programs; *Australia

Mehuron, Kate. "Undemocratic afflictions": a feminist response to the AIDS epidemic. *In:* DiQuinzio, Patrice; Young, Iris Marion, eds. Feminist Ethics and Social Policy. Bloomington, IN: Indiana University Press; 1997: 208–225. 83 refs. 12 fn. ISBN 0–253–21125–5. BE57286.
  *AIDS; attitudes; biological warfare; *blacks; community services; drug abuse; federal government; *females; *feminist ethics; guidelines; *health care delivery; historical aspects; HIV seropositivity; *homosexuals; human experimentation; *indigents; males; mass media; metaphor; minority groups; morality; *political activity; preventive medicine; *public policy; resource allocation; selection of subjects; sexuality; social control; *social discrimination; *socioeconomic factors; *stigmatization; trust; values; women's health; women's health services; empowerment; *genocide; Centers for Disease Control and Prevention; The Social Impact of AIDS in the United States (National Research Council); *United States

Murphy, Timothy F. AIDS. *In:* Chadwick, Ruth, ed. Encyclopedia of Applied Ethics, Volume 1. San Diego, CA: Academic Press; 1998: 111–122. 10 refs. ISBN 0–12–227066–5. BE56365.
  *AIDS; AIDS serodiagnosis; alternative therapies; confidentiality; drug abuse; duty to warn; employment; epidemiology; females; health care; health insurance; health personnel; *HIV seropositivity; homosexuals; human experimentation; indigents; males; obligations of society; occupational exposure; patient care; privacy; public policy; refusal to treat; reproduction; resource allocation; self induced illness; sexuality; stigmatization; needle–exchange programs; United States

New York. Court of Appeals. North Shore University Hospital v. Rosa. *North Eastern Reporter, 2d Series.* 1995 Oct 24 (date of decision). 657: 483–486. BE58829.
  *dentistry; *HIV seropositivity; homosexuals; *hospitals; human rights; *institutional policies; *legal rights; males; *social discrimination; state government; *infection control; *New York; *North Shore University Hospital v. Rosa
  The New York Court of Appeals upheld the lower appellate court's decision that a dental clinic's "isolation treatment" protocol did not violate the state human rights law. The clinic's protocol applied to any patient either known or perceived to be an intravenous drug abuser, a recipient of multiple blood transfusions, a hemodialysis patient, a male homosexual, a prostitute, or patient infected with HIV, hepatitis B, mononucleosis or tuberculosis. Under the protocol, the patient was placed in an examination room marked with a small "x," the

room contents were draped with plastic, and the physicians and staff wore additional protection. The clinic established the protocol in 1983, three years prior to the CDC's release of its "Recommended Infection Control Practices for Dentistry." The court found that the "isolation treatment" did not block a patient's access to care and was not a pretext for discrimination, because the protocol, based on prevailing medical knowledge in 1985, was a *bona fide* effort to protect both patients and staff. (KIE abstract)

Onwuteaka–Philipsen, B.D.; van der Wal, G. Cases of euthanasia and physician assisted suicide among AIDS patients reported to the Public Prosecutor in North Holland. *Public Health.* 1998 Jan; 112(1): 53–56. 17 refs. BE58216.
  *AIDS; *assisted suicide; evaluation studies; females; males; mandatory reporting; medical specialties; mortality; *patients; physicians; referral and consultation; statistics; trends; *voluntary euthanasia; retrospective studies; *Netherlands

O'Toole, Erin M. HIV–specific crime legislation: targeting an epidemic for criminal prosecution. *Journal of Law and Health.* 1995–1996; 10(1): 183–208. 141 fn. BE57434.
  AIDS serodiagnosis; anonymous testing; confidentiality; *criminal law; disclosure; equal protection; federal government; *government regulation; health personnel; *HIV seropositivity; informed consent; *legal liability; legal rights; *legislation; mandatory testing; military personnel; *patients; privacy; public health; quarantine; social discrimination; state government; state interest; voluntary programs; Fourteenth Amendment; *United States

Overall, Christine; Zion, William P., eds. Perspectives on AIDS: Ethical and Social Issues. New York, NY: Oxford University Press; 1991. 179 p. Bibliography: p. 174–175. ISBN 0–19–540749–0. BE58288.
  *AIDS; AIDS serodiagnosis; attitudes; autonomy; behavior control; Christian ethics; coercion; common good; confidentiality; duty to warn; females; health care; health education; health personnel; health promotion; *HIV seropositivity; homosexuals; human experimentation; informed consent; investigational drugs; Jewish ethics; mandatory testing; metaphor; moral obligations; *moral policy; *obligations of society; occupational exposure; patient care; physically disabled; public health; *public policy; quarantine; refusal to treat; research design; resource allocation; rights; risk; Roman Catholic ethics; sexuality; social discrimination; social problems; stigmatization; terminally ill; values; *Canada; United States

Pan–European Consultation on HIV/AIDS in the Context of Public Health and Human Rights, Prague, 26–27 Nov 1991. HIV/AIDS in the Context of Public Health and Human Rights: Report of a Pan–European Consultation. London: International Association of Rights and Humanity, on behalf of the World Health Organization Regional Office for Europe; 1993[?]. 65 p. Includes references. ISBN 1–874680–00–0. BE55802.
  *AIDS; AIDS serodiagnosis; biomedical research; community services; confidentiality; contact tracing; guidelines; health care; health education; health personnel; *HIV seropositivity; human experimentation; *human rights; *international aspects; mandatory testing; moral obligations; occupational exposure; patient care; prevalence; privacy; professional ethics; public health; public policy; social discrimination; socioeconomic factors; *Europe; World Health Organization

Rubenstein, William B.; Eisenberg, Ruth; Gostin, Lawrence O. The Rights of People Who Are HIV

Positive: The Authoritative ACLU Guide to the Rights of People Living with HIV Disease and AIDS. Carbondale, IL: Southern Illinois University Press; 1996. 384 p. (An American Civil Liberties Union handbook). Includes references. Appendices include a brief bibliography; selected organizations providing legal assistance to people with HIV disease; national, regional, and state offices of the ACLU; and the legal system. ISBN 0–8093–1992–6. BE56515.

advance directives; *AIDS; AIDS serodiagnosis; aliens; alternative therapies; anonymous testing; blood transfusions; competence; confidentiality; contact tracing; disclosure; drug abuse; drugs; duty to warn; employment; federal government; government regulation; health care delivery; health facilities; health insurance; health personnel; *HIV seropositivity; human experimentation; *human rights; iatrogenic disease; informed consent; *legal aspects; legal liability; legal obligations; *legal rights; mandatory reporting; mandatory testing; medical records; military personnel; patient access to records; patient care; prisoners; public health; quarantine; refusal to treat; schools; sex offenses; social discrimination; third party consent; treatment refusal; Americans with Disabilities Act 1990; Medicaid; Medicare; Rehabilitation Act 1973; *United States

Schüklenk, Udo; del Rio, Carlos; Magis, Carlos, et al. AIDS in the developing world. *In:* Chadwick, Ruth, ed. Encyclopedia of Applied Ethics, Volume 1. San Diego, CA: Academic Press; 1998: 123–127. 5 refs. ISBN 0–12–227066–5. BE56366.

*AIDS; comprehension; confidentiality; *developing countries; drug industry; drugs; economics; health care; health education; health promotion; HIV seropositivity; human experimentation; human rights; immunization; informed consent; international aspects; patient care; preventive medicine; public policy; religion; research subjects; resource allocation; sexuality; social discrimination; Africa; Asia; Latin America

Sher, Ruben. AIDS treatment and bioethics in South Africa. *In:* Chadwick, Ruth, ed. Encyclopedia of Applied Ethics, Volume 1. San Diego, CA: Academic Press; 1998: 129–135. ISBN 0–12–227066–5. BE56367.

active euthanasia; *AIDS; AIDS serodiagnosis; allowing to die; *alternative therapies; assisted suicide; blacks; confidentiality; cultural pluralism; developing countries; disclosure; drugs; education; family members; health personnel; *HIV seropositivity; human experimentation; iatrogenic disease; occupational exposure; patient care; physicians; placebos; professional competence; professional ethics; refusal to treat; sociology of medicine; terminally ill; *folk medicine; *South Africa

Smith, Katharine V.; Russell, Jan. Ethical issues experienced by HIV–infected African–American women. *Nursing Ethics.* 1997 Sep; 4(5): 394–402. 35 refs. BE56884.

AIDS serodiagnosis; *attitudes; *blacks; disclosure; family members; *females; *HIV seropositivity; reproduction; social impact; survey; truth disclosure; ethnographic studies; United States

Stein, Michael D.; Freedberg, Kenneth A.; Sullivan, Lisa M., et al. Sexual ethics: disclosure of HIV–positive status to partners. *Archives of Internal Medicine.* 1998 Feb 9; 158(3): 253–257. 21 refs. BE57976.

blacks; *contact tracing; contraception; *disclosure; drug abuse; females; Hispanic Americans; *HIV seropositivity; homosexuals; knowledge, attitudes, practice; males; *patients; preventive medicine; *sexuality; stigmatization; survey; whites; condoms; Boston; Providence (RI); United States

OBJECTIVE: To determine factors associated with disclosure of human immunodeficiency virus (HIV)–positive status to sexual partners. METHODS:

We interviewed 203 consecutive patients presenting for primary care for HIV at 2 urban hospitals. One hundred twenty–nine reported having sexual partners during the previous 6 months. The primary outcome of interest was whether patients had told all the sexual partners they had been with over the past 6 months that they were HIV positive. We analyzed the relationships between sociodemographic, alcohol and drug use, social support, sexual practice, and clinical variables; and whether patients had told their partners that they were HIV positive was analyzed by using multiple logistic regression. RESULTS: Study patients were black (46%), Latino (23%), white (27%), and the majority were men (69%). Regarding risk of transmission, 41% were injection drug users, 20% were homosexual or bisexual men, and 39% were heterosexually infected. Sixty percent had disclosed their HIV status to all sexual partners. Of the 40% who had not disclosed, half had not disclosed to their one and only partner. Among patients who did not disclose, 57% used condoms less than all the time. In multiple logistic regression analysis, the odds that an individual with 1 sexual partner disclosed was 3.2 times the odds that a person with multiple sexual partners disclosed. The odds that an individual with high spousal support disclosed was 2.8 times the odds of individuals without high support, and the odds that whites or Latinos disclosed was 3.1 times the odds that blacks disclosed. CONCLUSIONS: Many HIV–infected individuals do not disclose their status to sexual partners. Nondisclosers are not more likely to regularly use condoms than disclosers. Sexual partners of HIV–infected persons continue to be at risk for HIV transmission.

Stryker, Jeff. Ethical issues in public health policy toward HIV disease. *In:* Cohen, P.T.; Sande, Merle A.; Volberding, Paul A., eds. The AIDS Knowledge Base: A Textbook on HIV Disease from the University of California, San Francisco, and the San Francisco General Hospital. Second Edition. Boston, MA: Little, Brown; 1994: 11.6–1 to 11.6–4. 17 refs. ISBN 0–316–77067–1. BE56644.

*AIDS; AIDS serodiagnosis; confidentiality; contact tracing; duty to warn; employment; *HIV seropositivity; mandatory reporting; moral obligations; physicians; *public health; *public policy; quarantine; risks and benefits; schools; social discrimination; United States

Stryker, Jeff. Ethical issues in treating competent patients with HIV disease. *In:* Cohen, P.T.; Sande, Merle A.; Volberding, Paul A., eds. The AIDS Knowledge Base: A Textbook on HIV Disease from the University of California, San Francisco, and the San Francisco General Hospital. Second Edition. Boston, MA: Little, Brown; 1994: 11.2–1 to 11.2–5. 19 refs. ISBN 0–316–77067–1. BE56641.

advance directives; *AIDS; *allowing to die; *assisted suicide; communication; compassion; competence; *decision making; depressive disorder; drug abuse; futility; HIV seropositivity; homosexuals; intensive care units; *palliative care; *patient participation; patients; physicians; *prolongation of life; resuscitation orders; socioeconomic factors; *suicide; *terminally ill; treatment refusal; ventilators; withholding treatment; United States

Stryker, Jeff. Ethical issues in treating incompetent patients with HIV disease. *In:* Cohen, P.T.; Sande, Merle A.; Volberding, Paul A., eds. The AIDS Knowledge Base: A Textbook on HIV Disease from the University of California, San Francisco, and the San Francisco General Hospital. Second Edition. Boston, MA: Little, Brown; 1994: 11.3–1 to 11.3–4. 17 refs. ISBN

BE = bioethics accession number   fn. = footnotes   refs. = references

0–316–77067–1. BE56642.
*adults; *advance directives; *AIDS; allowing to die; competence; *decision making; dementia; futility; *HIV seropositivity; legal aspects; living wills; mothers; *newborns; patients; physicians; prolongation of life; third party consent; withholding treatment; United States

Terrence Higgins Trust (Great Britain). Living Will Project. Advance directives and AIDS. *In:* Grubb, Andrew, ed. Decision–Making and Problems of Incompetence. New York, NY: Wiley; 1994: 187–196. 20 fn. ISBN 0–471–94236–7. BE57136.
*advance directives; *AIDS; *attitudes; competence; *HIV seropositivity; international aspects; *legal aspects; *living wills; organizational policies; patients; physicians; professional organizations; *program descriptions; public opinion; survey; terminal care; third party consent; British Medical Association; *Great Britain; London; Terrence Higgins Trust

Thompson, Carolyn R. HIV and the blood supply: assessing MANTRA [mandatory notification of transfusion alternatives] legislation. *Politics and the Life Sciences.* 1995 Aug; 14(2): 221–228. 33 refs. 12 fn. Includes list of cited legislation. BE55639.
AIDS; *alternatives; blood donation; *blood transfusions; directed donation; *disclosure; economics; *government regulation; *HIV seropositivity; *informed consent; *legislation; mandatory programs; organizational policies; physicians; psychological stress; risk; *social impact; standards; *state government; voluntary programs; autologous blood transfusion; American Red Cross; United States

Tulsky, James A.; Cassileth, Barrie R.; Bennett, Charles L. The effect of ethnicity on ICU use and DNR orders in hospitalized AIDS patients. *Journal of Clinical Ethics.* 1997 Summer; 8(2): 150–157. 18 fn. BE55777.
advance care planning; *AIDS; allowing to die; attitudes; *blacks; comparative studies; *Hispanic Americans; hospitals; *intensive care units; males; medical records; *minority groups; mortality; *patient admission; *patient care; patients; prolongation of life; *resuscitation orders; statistics; *terminal care; *time factors; treatment outcome; *whites; multicenter studies; retrospective studies; severity of illness index; Chicago; Los Angeles; Miami

U.S. Court of Appeals, Fifth Circuit. Deramus v. Jackson National Life Insurance Company. *Federal Reporter, 3d Series.* 1996 Aug 7 (date of decision). 92: 274–283. BE56197.
AIDS; AIDS serodiagnosis; *diagnosis; *disclosure; *duty to warn; *HIV seropositivity; industry; *legal aspects; *legal liability; *legal obligations; *life insurance; patient access to records; spousal notification; truth disclosure; *Deramus v. Jackson National Life Insurance Co.; *Mississippi
The U.S. Court of Appeals for the Fifth Circuit affirmed the lower court's dismissal of a claim by the widow of a man who died of AIDS that the insurer had owed her husband the duty to inform him of his positive HIV status. In 1988 while undergoing tests for increased insurance coverage, the husband tested positive for HIV. He was told that the insurer refused to increase coverage but was not told the specific medical reason for the denial. The wife, now widow, did not test positive for HIV in 1988 and continues to test negative. The court declined to hold an insurance company to the same burden of care as a physician. (KIE abstract)

Webber, David W., ed. AIDS and the Law. Third Edition. New York, NY: Wiley Law Publications; 1997. 624 p. Includes references. Kept up to date by pocket parts. ISBN 0–471–13542–9. BE56520.
*AIDS; AIDS serodiagnosis; aliens; coercion;

confidentiality; criminal law; disabled; duty to warn; education; employment; *federal government; financial support; government financing; government regulation; health care; *HIV seropositivity; indigents; international aspects; judicial action; *legal aspects; legal liability; legal rights; mandatory testing; military personnel; public health; public policy; quarantine; social discrimination; *state government; torts; voluntary programs; emigration and immigration; Americans with Disabilities Act 1990; Medicaid; Rehabilitation Act 1973; *United States

Hospital must notify third party if it suspects patient has HIV [Garcia v. Santa Rosa Health Care Corp.]. *AIDS Policy and Law.* 1996 Jul 26; 11(13): 13. 1 ref. BE56229.
contact tracing; *disclosure; *duty to warn; hemophilia; *HIV seropositivity; *hospitals; *legal aspects; *legal obligations; married persons; patients; *Garcia v. Santa Rosa Health Care Corp.; *Texas

AIDS/CONFIDENTIALITY

Altman, Lawrence K. Sex, privacy and tracking H.I.V. infections. [News]. *New York Times.* 1997 Nov 4: F1, F2. BE57732.
*AIDS; confidentiality; *contact tracing; disclosure; *HIV seropositivity; mandatory programs; patients; preventive medicine; public health; sexually transmitted diseases; United States

Bassford, H.A. HIV testing and confidentiality. *In:* Overall, Christine and Zion, William P., eds. Perspectives on AIDS: Ethical and Social Issues. New York, NY: Oxford University Press; 1991: 106–121. 17 fn. ISBN 0–19–540749–0. BE58290.
*AIDS serodiagnosis; *confidentiality; contact tracing; duty to warn; health education; *HIV seropositivity; mandatory testing; patient compliance; physician patient relationship; physicians; public health; public policy; quarantine; social discrimination; stigmatization; voluntary programs; Canada; United States

Burr, Chandler. The AIDS exception: privacy vs. public health. *Atlantic Monthly.* 1997 June; 279(6): 57–67. BE57989.
*AIDS; AIDS serodiagnosis; anonymous testing; blood donation; *confidentiality; contact tracing; counseling; drugs; epidemiology; federal government; historical aspects; *HIV seropositivity; homosexuals; informed consent; *legal rights; mandatory reporting; mandatory testing; newborns; patient care; patients; *political activity; pregnant women; *privacy; *public health; *public policy; sexually transmitted diseases; social discrimination; state government; stigmatization; voluntary programs; Americans with Disabilities Act 1990; Centers for Disease Control and Prevention; United States

Coles, Matthew. The law and health care workers: confidentiality, testing, and treatment. *In:* Cohen, P.T.; Sande, Merle A.; Volberding, Paul A., eds. The AIDS Knowledge Base: A Textbook on HIV Disease from the University of California, San Francisco, and the San Francisco General Hospital. Second Edition. Boston, MA: Little, Brown; 1994: 9.1–1 to 9.1–11. 11 refs. ISBN 0–316–77067–1. BE56638.
*AIDS; *AIDS serodiagnosis; *confidentiality; contact tracing; disclosure; duty to warn; federal government; government regulation; *health facilities; health insurance; *health personnel; *HIV seropositivity; informed consent; *legal aspects; mandatory reporting; occupational exposure; *refusal to treat; social discrimination; state government; *United States

Fein, Esther B. Medical professionals with H.I.V. keep silent, fearing reprisals. [News]. *New York Times.* 1997

Dec 21: 41, 45. BE56775.
*confidentiality; *disclosure; employment; health insurance; *HIV seropositivity; iatrogenic disease; occupational exposure; *physicians; social discrimination; United States

Gelo, Florence; O'Connor, Bonnie; Vaught, Wayne. Should we protect families from patients? [Case study and commentaries]. *Hastings Center Report.* 1998 May–Jun; 28(3): 18–21. BE58608.
attitudes to death; cadavers; case studies; *communicable diseases; competence; confidentiality; cultural pluralism; *death; decision making; *duty to warn; *emotions; *family members; health personnel; hepatitis; *HIV seropositivity; minority groups; privacy; risk; grief; *infection control

Jürgens, Ralf; Palles, Michael. HIV Testing and Confidentiality: A Discussion Paper. Montreal: Canadian HIV/AIDS Legal Network; 1997. 317 p. Includes references. Prepared for the Canadian HIV/AIDS Legal Network and the Canadian AIDS Society. ISBN 1-896735-06-1. BE58162.
advisory committees; AIDS; *AIDS serodiagnosis; aliens; anonymous testing; coercion; *confidentiality; contact tracing; counseling; *disclosure; duty to warn; guidelines; health personnel; *HIV seropositivity; informed consent; legal aspects; mandatory reporting; *mandatory testing; newborns; organizational policies; pregnant women; prisoners; privacy; professional organizations; public policy; risks and benefits; sex offenses; *voluntary programs; diagnostic kits; emigration and immigration; partner notification; prostitution; *Canada

Kovac, Carl. Anonymous AIDS testing in Hungary to end. [News]. *BMJ (British Medical Journal).* 1997 Sep 6; 315(7108): 567. BE56873.
*AIDS serodiagnosis; *anonymous testing; *confidentiality; *disclosure; *HIV seropositivity; legislation; *public policy; *Hungary

McGuire, John; Nieri, Deborah; Abbott, David, et al. Do Tarasoff principles apply in AIDS–related psychotherapy? Ethical decision making and the role of therapist homophobia and perceived client dangerousness. *Professional Psychology: Research and Practice.* 1995 Dec; 26(6): 608–611. 34 refs. BE55625.
*attitudes; *confidentiality; dangerousness; *duty to warn; *health personnel; hemophilia; *HIV seropositivity; *homosexuals; *knowledge, attitudes, practice; legal aspects; patient care; professional ethics; professional patient relationship; psychology; *psychotherapy; sexuality; social discrimination; state government; *stigmatization; survey; prostitution; Florida; Tarasoff v. Regents

Pochard, Frédéric; Grassin, Marc; Le Roux, Nadège, et al. Medical secrecy or disclosure in HIV transmission: a physician's ethical conflict. [Letter]. *Archives of Internal Medicine.* 1998 Aug 10–24; 158(14–15): 1716, 1719. 5 refs. BE58950.
beneficence; *confidentiality; *disclosure; double effect; *HIV seropositivity; justice; *patients; physician patient relationship; *physicians; *sexuality; values; *partner notification; *sexual partners

Purtilo, Ruth; Sonnabend, Joseph; Purtilo, David T. Confidentiality, informed consent and untoward social consequences in research on a "new killer disease" (AIDS). *Clinical Research.* 1983 Oct; 31(4): 462–472. 31 refs. BE57233.
*AIDS; communication; *confidentiality; *epidemiology; *homosexuals; *informed consent; investigator subject relationship; investigators; public participation; research design; research subjects; *stigmatization; trust; *life style; United States

Richardson, Lynda. AIDS group opposes use of names in H.I.V. reports. [News]. *New York Times.* 1998 Jan 17: B6. BE57734.
attitudes; *confidentiality; data banks; *HIV seropositivity; *mandatory reporting; organizational policies; physicians; public policy; registries; state government; Gay Men's Health Crisis; *New York

Richardson, Lynda. Albany likely to get names of people with H.I.V. [News]. *New York Times.* 1998 Jan 14: B5. BE57733.
attitudes; *confidentiality; data banks; *HIV seropositivity; *mandatory reporting; patients; physicians; *public policy; registries; state government; *New York

Schlossberger, Eugene; Hecker, Lorna. HIV and family therapists' duty to warn: a legal and ethical analysis. *Journal of Marital and Family Therapy.* 1996 Jan; 22(1): 27–40. 63 refs. BE57065.
autonomy; *confidentiality; disclosure; *duty to warn; government regulation; health personnel; *HIV seropositivity; informed consent; *legal aspects; legal liability; *psychotherapy; sexuality; state government; *family therapy; Tarasoff v. Regents of the University of California; United States

Shaw, M.; Tomlinson, D.; Higginson, I. Survey of HIV patients' views on confidentiality and non-discrimination policies in general practice. *BMJ (British Medical Journal).* 1996 Jun 8; 312(7044): 1463–1464. 5 refs. BE57053.
administrators; *attitudes; blacks; *confidentiality; *diagnosis; *disclosure; drug abuse; *HIV seropositivity; homosexuals; *institutional policies; *patient care team; *patients; physicians; primary health care; *social discrimination; survey; group practice; outpatients; London

Simini, Bruno. Public warned about HIV-1-positive prostitute in Italy. [News]. *Lancet.* 1998 Feb 21; 351(9102): 580. BE58472.
*confidentiality; disclosure; *duty to warn; females; *HIV seropositivity; mass media; public health; sex offenses; *prostitution; *Italy

Sizemore, James Paul. Alabama's confidentiality quagmire: psychotherapists, AIDS, mandatory reporting, and *Tarasoff.* *Law and Psychology Review.* 1995 Spring; 19: 241–257. 85 fn. BE56043.
*AIDS; *confidentiality; *duty to warn; health personnel; *HIV seropositivity; *legal aspects; legislation; *mandatory reporting; *privileged communication; professional patient relationship; *psychotherapy; state government; *Alabama; Tarasoff v. Regents

Tracking H.I.V. infections in New York. [Editorial]. *New York Times.* 1998 Jan 15: A20. BE57735.
*confidentiality; *HIV seropositivity; *mandatory reporting; physicians; *public policy; state government; *New York

AIDS/HEALTH PERSONNEL

Akinsanya, J.A.; Rouse, Paul. Who Will Care? A Survey of the Knowledge and Attitudes of Hospital Nurses to People with HIV/AIDS: Report Submitted to the Department of Health. Chelmsford, Eng.: Anglia Polytechnic University, Faculty of Health and Social Work; 1991. 146 p. 80 refs. BE56146.
*AIDS; AIDS serodiagnosis; confidentiality; disclosure; *HIV seropositivity; hospitals; *knowledge, attitudes, practice; morality; *nurses; occupational exposure; patient care; quarantine; refusal to treat; risk; survey; infection control; questionnaires; *Great Britain

---

BE = bioethics accession number   fn. = footnotes   refs. = references

American Nurses Association. American Nurses Association position statements on bloodborne and airborne diseases. *In: its* Compendium of American Nurses Association Position Statements. Washington, DC: American Nurses Publishing; 1996: 1–65. Includes references. ISBN 1-55810-123-3. BE57451.
    adolescents; *AIDS; AIDS serodiagnosis; communicable diseases; confidentiality; disclosure; drug abuse; duty to warn; employment; females; health care delivery; *HIV seropositivity; iatrogenic disease; *nurses; nursing education; nursing ethics; occupational exposure; *organizational policies; primary health care; prisoners; professional organizations; public health; rape; sexually transmitted diseases; socioeconomic factors; standards; students; infection control; needle–exchange programs; tuberculosis; *American Nurses Association; United States

Bayer, Ronald. Discrimination, informed consent, and the HIV infected clinician. [Editorial]. *BMJ (British Medical Journal).* 1997 Mar 29; 314(7085): 915–916. 5 refs. BE58403.
    AIDS serodiagnosis; disclosure; *HIV seropositivity; iatrogenic disease; informed consent; mandatory testing; patient care; *physicians; risk; social discrimination

Birchard, Karen. Ireland rules out compulsory HIV testing. [News]. *Lancet.* 1997 Oct 25; 350(9086): 1232. BE56921.
    advisory committees; *AIDS serodiagnosis; compensation; employment; *HIV seropositivity; iatrogenic disease; *mandatory testing; *physicians; *public policy; *voluntary programs; Advisory Group on the Transmission of Blood–Borne Diseases (Ireland); *Department of Health (Ireland); *Ireland

Coles, Matthew. The law and health care workers: confidentiality, testing, and treatment. *In:* Cohen, P.T.; Sande, Merle A.; Volberding, Paul A., eds. The AIDS Knowledge Base: A Textbook on HIV Disease from the University of California, San Francisco, and the San Francisco General Hospital. Second Edition. Boston, MA: Little, Brown; 1994: 9.1-1 to 9.1-11. 11 refs. ISBN 0-316-77067-1. BE56638.
    *AIDS; *AIDS serodiagnosis; *confidentiality; contact tracing; disclosure; duty to warn; federal government; government regulation; *health facilities; health insurance; *health personnel; *HIV seropositivity; informed consent; *legal aspects; mandatory reporting; occupational exposure; *refusal to treat; social discrimination; state government; *United States

Combs, Elmer W. Home health, AIDS, and refusal to care. *Home Healthcare Nurse.* 1996 Mar; 14(3): 188–194. 32 refs. BE55846.
    attitudes; beneficence; guidelines; *HIV seropositivity; *home care; justice; *nurses; nursing ethics; occupational exposure; professional autonomy; professional organizations; *refusal to treat; risk; risks and benefits; self induced illness; stigmatization; American Nurses Association

Curran, William J. Legal history of emergency medicine from medieval common law to the AIDS epidemic. *American Journal of Emergency Medicine.* 1997 Nov; 15(7): 658–670. 88 refs. BE58355.
    *AIDS; *emergency care; federal government; government regulation; *historical aspects; *HIV seropositivity; *hospitals; judicial action; *legal aspects; *legal liability; *legal obligations; malpractice; organizational policies; patient admission; patient transfer; *physicians; professional organizations; *refusal to treat; review; social discrimination; standards; state government; torts; traffic accidents; Eighteenth Century; Emergency Medical Treatment and Active Labor Act 1986; England; Good Samaritanism; Nineteenth Century; *Twentieth Century; *United States

Epstein, Ronald M.; Morse, Diane S.; Frankel, Richard M., et al. Awkward moments in patient–physician communication about HIV risk. *Annals of Internal Medicine.* 1998 Mar 15; 128(6): 435–442. 50 refs. BE57305.
    *communication; *counseling; emotions; evaluation studies; family practice; *HIV seropositivity; internal medicine; knowledge, attitudes, practice; patients; *physician patient relationship; *physicians; *professional competence; *risk; New York
    BACKGROUND: Physicians frequently encounter patients who are at risk for HIV infection, but they often evaluate risk behaviors ineffectively. OBJECTIVE: To describe the barriers to and facilitators of comprehensive HIV risk evaluation in primary care office visits. DESIGN: Qualitative thematic and sequential analysis of videotaped patient–physician discussions about HIV risk. Tapes were reviewed independently by physician and patient and were coded by the research team. SETTING: Physicians' offices. PARTICIPANTS: Convenience sample of 17 family physicians and general internists. Twenty–six consenting patients 18 to 45 years of age who indicated concern about or risks for HIV infection on a 10–item questionnaire administered before the physician visit were included. MEASUREMENTS: A thematic coding scheme and a five–level description of the depth of HIV–related discussion. RESULTS: In 73% of the encounters, physicians did not elicit enough information to characterize patients' HIV risk status. The outcome of HIV–related discussions was substantially influenced by the manner in which the physician introduced the topic, handled awkward moments, and dealt with problematic language and the extent to which the physician sought the patient's perspective. Feelings of ineffectiveness and strong emotions interfered with some physicians' ability to assess HIV risk. Physicians easily recognized problematic communication during reviews of their own videotapes. CONCLUSIONS: Comprehensive HIV risk discussions included providing a rationale for discussion, effectively negotiating awkward moments, repairing problematic language, persevering with the topic, eliciting the patient's perspective, responding to fears and expectations, and being empathic. Educational programs should use videotape review and should concentrate on physicians' personal reactions to discussing emotionally charged topics.

Farthing, Charles F. A necessary risk: why we doctors should volunteer to try an AIDS vaccine. *Washington Post.* 1997 Oct 19: C1, C6. BE57845.
    *AIDS; *autoexperimentation; historical aspects; *human experimentation; *immunization; *physicians; professional organizations; risks and benefits; *volunteers; International Association of Physicians in AIDS Care

Fein, Esther B. Medical professionals with H.I.V. keep silent, fearing reprisals. [News]. *New York Times.* 1997 Dec 21: 41, 45. BE56775.
    *confidentiality; *disclosure; employment; health insurance; *HIV seropositivity; iatrogenic disease; occupational exposure; *physicians; social discrimination; United States

Freedman, Benjamin. Health-care workers' occupational exposure to HIV: obligations and entitlements. *In:* Overall, Christine; Zion, William P., eds. Perspectives on AIDS: Ethical and Social Issues. New York, NY: Oxford University Press; 1991: 91–105. 36 fn. ISBN 0-19-540749-0. BE58289.
    employment; *health personnel; *HIV seropositivity; medical ethics; *moral obligations; *occupational exposure; organizational policies; *patient care; *physicians;

BE = bioethics accession number   fn. = footnotes   refs. = references

professional organizations; *refusal to treat; remuneration; *risk; virtues; Canada; United States

General Medical Council (Great Britain). Duties of a Doctor: Guidance from the General Medical Council. [Booklets]. London: The Council; 1995. portfolio of 4 booklets. BE57156.

advertising; AIDS serodiagnosis; biomedical research; *confidentiality; conflict of interest; disclosure; duty to warn; family practice; gifts; *guidelines; *HIV seropositivity; iatrogenic disease; informed consent; *interprofessional relations; *medical ethics; medical fees; medical specialties; occupational exposure; patient care; *physician patient relationship; *physicians; professional competence; referral and consultation; refusal to treat; self regulation; traffic accidents; *General Medical Council (Great Britain); *Great Britain

Illinois. Appellate Court, First District, Sixth Division. Doe v. Noe. *North Eastern Reporter, 2d Series.* 1997 Dec 26 (date of decision). 690: 1012–1023. BE58578.

confidentiality; *disclosure; *HIV seropositivity; iatrogenic disease; informed consent; *legal aspects; *legal liability; legal obligations; obstetrics and gynecology; *physicians; psychological stress; *surgery; *Doe v. Noe; Faya v. Almaraz; *Illinois

The Appellate Court of Illinois, First District, Sixth Division held that a physician has a legal duty to disclose his or her HIV–positive status when seeking a patient's informed consent prior to an invasive medical procedure. The court dismissed the patient's claim of battery, as the patient had consented to the procedure, and the patient's claim of malpractice based on informed consent, as the patient could not prove injury, meaning transmission of the disease during the surgeries. The court also dismissed the patient's claims against the physician's partner, the physician's employer, and the hospital in which the procedure was performed, as they had no duty to know or disclose the physician's HIV status. (KIE abstract)

Irvin, Susan M. The great dilemma [AIDS]. *Nursing Standard.* 1995 Sep 27–Oct 3; 10(1): 50–53. 22 refs. BE55872.

*AIDS serodiagnosis; confidentiality; duty to warn; *health personnel; *HIV seropositivity; *hospitals; informed consent; *institutional policies; *mandatory testing; nurses; occupational exposure; *patients; refusal to treat; risks and benefits; values; *voluntary programs; universal precautions; United States

McCarthy, Michael. AIDS doctors push for live–virus vaccine trials. *Lancet.* 1997 Oct 11; 350(9084): 1082. BE56930.

*AIDS; attitudes; autoexperimentation; dissent; HIV seropositivity; *human experimentation; *immunization; *physicians; preventive medicine; professional organizations; *risks and benefits; *volunteers; *International Association of Physicians in AIDS Care; United States

McGuire, John; Nieri, Deborah; Abbott, David, et al. Do Tarasoff principles apply in AIDS–related psychotherapy? Ethical decision making and the role of therapist homophobia and perceived client dangerousness. *Professional Psychology: Research and Practice.* 1995 Dec; 26(6): 608–611. 34 refs. BE55625.

*attitudes; *confidentiality; dangerousness; *duty to warn; *health personnel; hemophilia; *HIV seropositivity; *homosexuals; *knowledge, attitudes, practice; legal aspects; patient care; professional ethics; professional patient relationship; psychology; *psychotherapy; sexuality; social discrimination; state government; *stigmatization; survey; prostitution; Florida; Tarasoff v. Regents

Rom, Mark Carl. Fatal Extraction: The Story Behind the Florida Dentist Accused of Infecting His Patients with HIV and Poisoning Public Health. San Francisco, CA: Jossey–Bass Publishers; 1997. 226 p. 443 fn. ISBN 0–7879–0991–2. BE57924.

*AIDS; AIDS serodiagnosis; confidentiality; decision making; *dentistry; disclosure; family members; federal government; guidelines; *health personnel; *HIV seropositivity; *iatrogenic disease; *investigators; judicial action; legal aspects; mandatory testing; mass media; patient care; *patients; political activity; politics; professional competence; *public health; public policy; state government; trust; voluntary programs; infection control; retrospective studies; *Acer, David; *Bergalis, Kimberly; *Centers for Disease Control and Prevention; Florida; United States

Sadowsky, Donald; Kunzel, Carol. Measuring dentists' willingness to treat HIV–positive patients. *Journal of the American Dental Association.* 1994 Jun; 125(6): 705–710. 23 refs. BE55593.

*AIDS; *attitudes; *dentistry; *health personnel; *HIV seropositivity; *knowledge, attitudes, practice; occupational exposure; *patient care; *refusal to treat; survey; private practice; New York City

Slome, Lee; Moulton, Jeffrey; Huffine, Carol, et al. Physicians' attitudes toward assisted suicide in AIDS. *Journal of Acquired Immune Deficiency Syndromes.* 1992; 5(7): 712–718. 30 refs. BE56238.

*AIDS; *assisted suicide; comparative studies; drugs; emotions; HIV seropositivity; homosexuals; intention; *knowledge, attitudes, practice; legal aspects; medical specialties; mental health; physician patient relationship; physician's role; *physicians; referral and consultation; suffering; survey; terminally ill; values; Hemlock Society; San Francisco; United States

Steele, A.; Melby, V. Nurses' knowledge and beliefs about AIDS: comparing nurses in hospital, community and hospice settings. *Journal of Advanced Nursing.* 1995 Nov; 22(5): 879–887. 37 refs. BE57510.

*AIDS; *attitudes; *community services; comparative studies; HIV seropositivity; *hospices; *hospitals; *knowledge, attitudes, practice; *nurses; nursing education; *occupational exposure; patient care; professional competence; refusal to treat; stigmatization; *Northern Ireland

Stryker, Jeff. Health care workers and HIV disease: an ethical overview. *In:* Cohen, P.T; Sande, Merle A.; Volberding, Paul A., eds. The AIDS Knowledge Base: A Textbook on HIV Disease from the University of California, San Francisco, and the San Francisco General Hospital. Second Edition. Boston, MA: Little, Brown; 1994: 11.1–1 to 11.1–6. 40 refs. ISBN 0–316–77067–1. BE56639.

*AIDS; attitudes; disclosure; drug abuse; *health facilities; *health personnel; *HIV seropositivity; homosexuals; iatrogenic disease; *institutional ethics; moral obligations; morality; occupational exposure; professional ethics; refusal to treat; risk; social worth; infection control; United States

U.S. District Court, W.D. Michigan, S.D. Mauro v. Borgess Medical Center. *Federal Supplement.* 1995 May 4 (date of decision). 886: 1349–1356. BE56137.

disabled; *employment; federal government; government regulation; *health personnel; *HIV seropositivity; hospitals; *legal rights; *social discrimination; state government; Americans with Disabilities Act 1990; *Mauro v. Borgess Medical Center; Michigan; United States

The U.S. District Court for the Western District of Michigan dismissed an employee's claim of discrimination by his hospital employer based on his positive HIV status. Mauro worked as a surgical

---

technician at Borgess Medical Center. When he refused to submit to HIV testing or to take a position as case cart/instrument coordinator with similar pay and benefits but without the risk of direct exposure of the patient to the infection, he was laid off. The court found that the hospital's offer was a reasonable accommodation. Because the infrequent hands-on assistance of a surgical technician in emergency matters was an essential task, restructuring the position to avoid patient contact meant requiring an additional person in the operating room, which was unreasonable. (KIE abstract)

U.S. Supreme Court. Bragdon v. Abbott. *Supreme Court Reporter.* 1998 Jun 25 (date of decision). 118: 2196–2218. BE56299.
*dentistry; disabled; federal government; females; government regulation; guidelines; *health personnel; *HIV seropositivity; *legal aspects; *legal obligations; legal rights; legislation; occupational exposure; *patient care; patients; professional organizations; *refusal to treat; reproduction; social discrimination; American Dental Association; *Americans with Disabilities Act 1990; *Bragdon v. Abbott; Maine; Rehabilitation Act 1973; *United States
Abbott was an asymptomatic HIV-infected patient whose dentist, Bragdon, refused to fill a cavity for her in his office. The dentist offered to fill the cavity in a hospital, which would have required the patient to pay for incidental hospital charges. Abbott brought charges under the Americans with Disabilities Act of 1990 alleging discrimination on the basis of a disability which substantially limited a major life activity, her ability to reproduce and bear children. The U.S. Supreme Court held that asymptomatic HIV infection, because of its predictable course and the immediacy with which the virus begins to damage the infected person's white blood cells, is a disability that affects the major life activity of reproduction from the moment of infection. The Court rejected the dentist's argument that major life activities must have a public, economic, or daily character. The dissent argued that reproduction is not a major life activity and that the patient did not present evidence that her asymptomatic HIV status substantially limited her ability to reproduce. The case was remanded for a determination whether the dentist had raised a triable issue of fact to warrant a trial on the merits. (KIE abstract)

Yedidia, Michael J.; Berry, Carolyn A.; Barr, Judith K. Changes in physicians' attitudes toward AIDS during residency training: a longitudinal study of medical school graduates. *Journal of Health and Social Behavior.* 1996 Jun; 37(2): 179–191. 32 refs. BE56899.
*AIDS; *attitudes; drug abuse; evaluation studies; faculty; homosexuals; *internship and residency; *medical education; medical specialties; *physicians; *refusal to treat; *students; survey; prospective studies; New York

Suit says patient was denied heart surgery because of HIV. [News]. *AIDS Policy and Law.* 1997 May 16; 12(9): 3. BE58479.
alternatives; heart diseases; *HIV seropositivity; *hospitals; *legal aspects; legal liability; occupational exposure; *physicians; referral and consultation; *refusal to treat; risk; *social discrimination; *surgery; *District of Columbia; *Flowers v. George Washington University Medical Center

AIDS/HUMAN EXPERIMENTATION

Aaby, Peter; Babiker, Abdel; Darbyshire, Janet, et al. Ethics of HIV trials. [Letters]. *Lancet.* 1997 Nov 22; 350(9090): 1546–1547. 5 refs. BE58468.

*control groups; *developing countries; *drugs; economics; *HIV seropositivity; *human experimentation; international aspects; *placebos; *pregnant women; random selection; *research design; Africa; AZT

Altman, Lawrence K. AIDS experts leave journal after studies are criticized. [News]. *New York Times.* 1997 Oct 15: A10. BE57899.
*developing countries; disclosure; *drugs; *editorial policies; federal government; government financing; *HIV seropositivity; *human experimentation; immunization; international aspects; investigators; *placebos; pregnant women; research design; scientific misconduct; AZT; *Ho, David; *New England Journal of Medicine; United States; Wenzel, Richard; *Wilfert, Catherine

Ault, Alicia. USA accused of funding placebo-controlled AIDS trials. [News]. *Lancet.* 1997 May 3; 349(9061): 1305. BE56073.
AIDS; *developing countries; drugs; federal government; government financing; *HIV seropositivity; *human experimentation; *newborns; *placebos; *pregnant women; public policy; withholding treatment; AZT; Centers for Disease Control and Prevention; National Institutes of Health; *United States

Benatar, David; Benatar, Solomon R. Informed consent and research. *BMJ (British Medical Journal).* 1998 Mar 28; 316(7136): 1008. 2 refs. BE57553.
*AIDS serodiagnosis; *anonymous testing; biomedical research; confidentiality; epidemiology; *HIV seropositivity; *human experimentation; *informed consent; medical records; patients; research design; research subjects; South Africa

Bhagwanjee, Satish; Muckart, David J.J.; Jeena, Prakash M., et al. Does HIV status influence the outcome of patients admitted to a surgical intensive care unit? A prospective double blind study. [Article, commentaries, and response]. *BMJ (British Medical Journal).* 1997 Apr 12; 314(7087): 1077–1084. 26 refs. BE55661.
*AIDS serodiagnosis; anonymous testing; blacks; comparative studies; confidentiality; critically ill; developing countries; disadvantaged; disclosure; empirical research; *epidemiology; futility; *HIV seropositivity; hospitals; human experimentation; *informed consent; injuries; *intensive care units; justice; morbidity; mortality; patient admission; patient discharge; patients; research design; research ethics committees; *research subjects; resource allocation; scientific misconduct; *selection for treatment; surgery; *treatment outcome; prospective studies; *South Africa
OBJECTIVES: (a) To assess the impact of HIV status (HIV negative, HIV positive, AIDS) on the outcome of patients admitted to intensive care units for diseases unrelated to HIV; (b) to decide whether a positive test result for HIV should be a criterion for excluding patients from intensive care for diseases unrelated to HIV. DESIGN: A prospective double blind study of all admissions over six months. HIV status was determined in all patients by enzyme linked immunosorbent assay (ELISA), immunofluorescence assay, western blotting, and flow cytometry. The ethics committee considered the clinical implications of the study important enough to waive patients' right to informed consent. Staff and patients were blinded to HIV results. On discharge patients could be advised of their HIV status if they wished. SETTING: A 16 bed surgical intensive care unit. SUBJECTS: All 267 men and 135 women admitted to the unit during the study period. INTERVENTIONS: None. MAIN OUTCOME MEASURES: APACHE II score (acute physiological, age, and chronic health evaluation), organ failure, septic

---

BE = bioethics accession number   fn. = footnotes   refs. = references

shock, durations of intensive care unit and hospital stay, and intensive care unit and hospital mortality. RESULTS: No patient had AIDS. 52 patients were tested positive for HIV and 350 patients were tested negative. The two groups were similar in sex distribution but differed significantly in age, incidence of organ failure (37 (71%) v 171 (49%) patients), and incidence of septic shock (20 (38%) v 54 (15%)). After adjustment for age there were no differences in intensive care unit or hospital mortality or in the durations of stay in the intensive care unit or hospital. CONCLUSIONS: Morbidity was higher in HIV positive patients but there was no difference in mortality. In this patient population a positive HIV test result should not be a criterion for excluding a patient from intensive care.

Bloom, Barry R. The highest attainable standard: ethical issues in AIDS vaccines. *Science.* 1998 Jan 9; 279(5348): 186–188. 15 fn. BE58034.
  *AIDS; codes of ethics; *developing countries; drugs; economics; ethical review; goals; guidelines; *human experimentation; *immunization; informed consent; *international aspects; placebos; preventive medicine; research design; standards; *therapeutic research; Council for International Organizations of Medical Sciences; Declaration of Helsinki; International Ethical Guidelines for Biomedical Research Involving Human Subjects; UNAIDS; United Nations; World Health Organization

Brody, Baruch A. Research on the vulnerable sick. *In:* Kahn, Jeffrey P.; Mastroianni, Anna C.; Sugarman, Jeremy, eds. Beyond Consent: Seeking Justice in Research. New York, NY: Oxford University Press; 1998: 32–46. 24 fn. ISBN 0-19-511353-5. BE58842.
  autonomy; *cancer; *critically ill; disclosure; *emergency care; federal government; government regulation; *HIV seropositivity; *human experimentation; *informed consent; investigational drugs; *justice; *nontherapeutic research; *patients; placebos; research design; research subjects; risks and benefits; terminally ill; *therapeutic research; third party consent; time factors; trends; values; vulnerable populations; deferred consent; Food and Drug Administration; United States

Clark, Peter A. The ethics of placebo-controlled trials for perinatal transmission of HIV in developing countries. *Journal of Clinical Ethics.* 1998 Summer; 9(2): 156–166. 44 fn. BE58961.
  AIDS; alternatives; autonomy; beneficence; common good; comprehension; *control groups; costs and benefits; *developing countries; drugs; ethical analysis; ethical relativism; guidelines; *HIV seropositivity; *human experimentation; human rights; informed consent; international aspects; justice; *moral policy; morbidity; *newborns; patient care; *placebos; *pregnant women; prevalence; public policy; *research design; research subjects; risks and benefits; socioeconomic factors; standards; vulnerable populations; AZT; United States

Cleaton–Jones, Peter E.; Busse, Peter; Emery, Sean, et al. Availability of antiretroviral therapy after clinical trials with HIV infected patients are ended: an ethical dilemma. [Article and commentaries]. *BMJ (British Medical Journal).* 1997 Mar 22; 314(7084): 887–891. 7 refs. BE58772.
  *AIDS; communication; *developing countries; *drug industry; *drugs; economics; *financial support; government financing; guidelines; health care delivery; *HIV seropositivity; *human experimentation; *institutional ethics; investigators; patient advocacy; *patient care; private sector; research ethics committees; *research subjects; resource allocation; *therapeutic research; *continuity of patient care; Declaration of Helsinki; Medical Research Council (South Africa); *South Africa

Dixon, John. Catastrophic rights: vital public interests and civil liberties in conflict. *In:* Overall, Christine and Zion, William P., eds. Perspectives on AIDS: Ethical and Social Issues. New York, NY: Oxford University Press; 1991: 122–137. 9 refs. ISBN 0-19-540749-0. BE58291.
  *AIDS; *autonomy; beneficence; coercion; *common good; control groups; government regulation; *HIV seropositivity; *human experimentation; *investigational drugs; investigators; *paternalism; patients; physicians; political activity; *public policy; random selection; *research design; resource allocation; *rights; *terminally ill; therapeutic research; treatment refusal; investigational therapies; AZT; Canada; United States

Farthing, Charles F. A necessary risk: why we doctors should volunteer to try an AIDS vaccine. *Washington Post.* 1997 Oct 19: C1, C6. BE57845.
  *AIDS; *autoexperimentation; historical aspects; *human experimentation; *immunization; *physicians; professional organizations; risks and benefits; *volunteers; International Association of Physicians in AIDS Care

Halsey, Neal A.; Sommer, Alfred; Henderson, Donald A., et al. Ethics and international research. [Editorial]. *BMJ (British Medical Journal).* 1997 Oct 18; 315(7114): 965–966. 8 refs. BE55908.
  *developing countries; *drugs; economics; *ethical relativism; guidelines; health care delivery; *HIV seropositivity; *human experimentation; *international aspects; *newborns; *placebos; *pregnant women; *research design; standards; *AZT; Centers for Disease Control and Prevention; Council for International Organizations of Medical Sciences; United States; World Health Organization

Josefson, Debbie. US journal attacks unethical HIV trials. [News]. *BMJ (British Medical Journal).* 1997 Sep 27; 315(7111): 765. BE56928.
  *developing countries; *drugs; economics; editorial policies; *HIV seropositivity; *human experimentation; *placebos; pregnant women; public policy; *research design; Africa; Asia; AZT; Latin America; New England Journal of Medicine; United States

Josefson, Deborah. Doctors volunteer to be guinea pigs for AIDS vaccine. [News]. *BMJ (British Medical Journal).* 1997 Oct 4; 315(7112): 833. BE56068.
  AIDS; attitudes; *autoexperimentation; federal government; government regulation; *HIV seropositivity; *human experimentation; *immunization; international aspects; investigators; *physicians; risks and benefits; *volunteers; *International Association of Physicians in AIDS Care; National Institute of Allergy and Infectious Diseases; United Nations; United States

Kaiser, Jocelyn. Bangkok study adds fuel to AIDS ethics debate. [News]. *Science.* 1997 Nov 28; 278(5343): 1553. BE56906.
  AIDS; developing countries; *drugs; *HIV seropositivity; *human experimentation; *placebos; pregnant women; *research design; AZT; *Thailand

Kaiser, Jocelyn. Flap on NEJM board over ethics articles. [News]. *Science.* 1997 Oct 10; 278(5336): 211. BE56066.
  *developing countries; dissent; *editorial policies; *HIV seropositivity; *human experimentation; interprofessional relations; investigators; *newborns; *placebos; *pregnant women; scientific misconduct; withholding treatment; *Ho, David; *New England Journal of Medicine; *Wilfert, Catherine

Kaiser, Jocelyn. UNAIDS to weigh vaccine ethics. [News]. *Science.* 1997 Sep 19; 277(5333): 1751. BE56067.
  *developing countries; drugs; *HIV seropositivity; *human experimentation; *immunization; *international aspects;

BE = bioethics accession number   fn. = footnotes   refs. = references

newborns; patient care; placebos; pregnant women; AZT; *UNAIDS; United Nations

Kerns, Thomas A. Ethical Issues in HIV Vaccine Trials. New York, NY: St. Martin's Press; 1997. 249 p. Bibliography: p. 239–244. Appendices include texts of the Nuremberg Code, the International Ethical Guidelines for Biomedical Research Involving Human Subjects, a proposed Bill of Rights and Responsibilities for Participants in HIV Vaccine Trials, a test of understanding for informed consent, and proposed application forms for ethical review. ISBN 0–312–16397–5. BE57278.

*AIDS; autonomy; beneficence; coercion; common good; compensation; comprehension; confidentiality; control groups; counseling; developing countries; disclosure; economics; ethical review; forms; goals; guidelines; *HIV seropositivity; *human experimentation; *immunization; incentives; informed consent; injuries; investigators; justice; *moral policy; motivation; placebos; preventive medicine; research design; research ethics committees; research subjects; review; *risks and benefits; selection of subjects; social discrimination; third party consent; *volunteers; vulnerable populations; Brazil; Council for International Organizations of Medical Sciences; International Ethical Guidelines for Biomedical Research Involving Human Subjects; Nuremberg Code; Thailand; Uganda; World Health Organization

Kigotho, Anderson Wachira. Another HIV–1 trial loses placebo control. [News]. *Lancet.* 1997 Dec 20–27; 350(9094): 1831. BE57861.

control groups; *developing countries; *drugs; females; *HIV seropositivity; *human experimentation; *international aspects; mothers; newborns; *placebos; *pregnant women; *research design; *therapeutic research; AZT; *Ethiopia; Johns Hopkins University; United States

Levine, Carol. Changing views of justice after Belmont: AIDS and the inclusion of "vulnerable" subjects. *In:* Vanderpool, Harold Y., ed. The Ethics of Research Involving Human Subjects: Facing the 21st Century. Frederick, MD: University Publishing Group; 1996: 105–126. 37 fn. ISBN 1–55572–036–6. BE56984.

advisory committees; *AIDS; autonomy; beneficence; children; federal government; females; fetuses; government financing; government regulation; guidelines; *HIV seropositivity; *human experimentation; informed consent; investigational drugs; *justice; minority groups; patients; pregnant women; *public policy; research ethics committees; research subjects; risks and benefits; scientific misconduct; *selection of subjects; trends; *vulnerable populations; Belmont Report; Food and Drug Administration; National Commission for the Protection of Human Subjects; National Institutes of Health; Tuskegee Syphilis Study; United States

Levine, Robert J. The "best proven therapeutic method" standard in clinical trials in technologically developing countries. [Editorial]. *IRB: A Review of Human Subjects Research.* 1998 Jan–Feb; 20(1): 5–9. 19 fn. BE58519.

*control groups; *developing countries; *drugs; economics; guidelines; *HIV seropositivity; *human experimentation; international aspects; newborns; patient care; *placebos; *pregnant women; *research design; *standards; *AZT; Declaration of Helsinki

McCarthy, Michael. AIDS doctors push for live-virus vaccine trials. *Lancet.* 1997 Oct 11; 350(9084): 1082. BE56930.

*AIDS; attitudes; autoexperimentation; dissent; HIV seropositivity; *human experimentation; *immunization; *physicians; preventive medicine; professional organizations; *risks and benefits; *volunteers; *International Association of Physicians in AIDS Care; United States

Marshall, Eliot. AIDS therapy: controversial trial offers hopeful result. [News]. *Science.* 1998 Feb 27; 279(5355): 1299. BE57260.

costs and benefits; *developing countries; *drugs; *HIV seropositivity; *human experimentation; international aspects; newborns; *placebos; *pregnant women; *research design; therapeutic research; time factors; *Africa; *AZT; *Thailand

Marwick, Charles. Bioethics group considers transnational research. [News]. *JAMA.* 1998 May 13; 279(18): 1425. BE57862.

advisory committees; *developing countries; *drugs; federal government; government financing; guidelines; *HIV seropositivity; *human experimentation; *international aspects; newborns; *placebos; *pregnant women; *public policy; *research design; scientific misconduct; *therapeutic research; *Africa; AZT; Declaration of Helsinki; National Bioethics Advisory Commission; *United States

Mbidde, Edward. Bioethics and local circumstances. [Editorial]. *Science.* 1998 Jan 9; 279(5348): 155. 5 fn. BE58030.

*developing countries; guidelines; health care; *HIV seropositivity; *human experimentation; international aspects; pregnant women; regulation; research design; socioeconomic factors; standards; Africa; Council for International Organizations of Medical Sciences; International Ethical Guidelines for Biomedical Research Involving Human Subjects

Phanuphak, Praphan; Vermund, Sten H. Ethical issues for perinatal HIV trials in developing countries. [Editorial]. *Pediatric AIDS and HIV Infection.* 1996 Aug; 7(4): 236–238. 15 refs. BE57070.

control groups; costs and benefits; *developing countries; drugs; ethical relativism; *HIV seropositivity; *human experimentation; *newborns; placebos; *pregnant women; preventive medicine; research design; therapeutic research; AZT

Phanuphak, Praphan. Ethical issues in studies in Thailand of the vertical transmission of HIV. *New England Journal of Medicine.* 1998 Mar 19; 338(12): 834–835. 5 refs. BE57707.

AIDS; alternatives; control groups; *developing countries; *drugs; government financing; *HIV seropositivity; *human experimentation; international aspects; *newborns; *nontherapeutic research; *placebos; *pregnant women; *preventive medicine; private sector; *public policy; *research design; resource allocation; scientific misconduct; *therapeutic research; time factors; withholding treatment; *AZT; Centers for Disease Control and Prevention; National Institutes of Health; *Thailand; United States; Walter Reed Army Institute of Research

Purtilo, Ruth; Sonnabend, Joseph; Purtilo, David T. Confidentiality, informed consent and untoward social consequences in research on a "new killer disease" (AIDS). *Clinical Research.* 1983 Oct; 31(4): 462–472. 31 refs. BE57233.

*AIDS; communication; *confidentiality; *epidemiology; *homosexuals; *informed consent; investigator subject relationship; investigators; public participation; research design; research subjects; *stigmatization; trust; *life style; United States

Robb, Merlin L.; Khambaroong, Chirasak; Nelson, Kenrad E., et al. Studies in Thailand of the vertical transmission of HIV. [Letters]. *New England Journal of Medicine.* 1998 Mar 19; 338(12): 843–844. 2 refs. BE57708.

AIDS; *drugs; financial support; health care delivery; *HIV seropositivity; *human experimentation; informed consent;

BE = bioethics accession number   fn. = footnotes   refs. = references

newborns; *nontherapeutic research; patient care; *pregnant women; *standards; *therapeutic research; time factors; *AZT; Chiang Mai University; Department of Defense; Johns Hopkins University; Ministry of Health (Thailand); National Institutes of Health; *Thailand; United States; Walter Reed Army Institute of Research

Schüklenk, Udo; Hogan, Carlton. AIDS clinical trials: ethical and design issues. *International Journal of Bioethics.* 1997 Sep; 8(3): 127–132. 29 fn. BE57432.
  *AIDS; autonomy; coercion; *drugs; *human experimentation; patient compliance; patient participation; patients; political activity; random selection; *research design; research subjects; selection of subjects; terminally ill; *therapeutic research; uncertainty; volunteers

Sidley, Pat. AIDS drug scandal in South Africa continues. [News]. *BMJ (British Medical Journal).* 1998 Mar 14; 316(7134): 800. BE57761.
  administrators; *AIDS; conflict of interest; drug industry; *drugs; economics; ethical review; government financing; government regulation; *human experimentation; investigators; legal aspects; *politics; *scientific misconduct; *South Africa; *Virodene; Zuma, Nkosazana

Stryker, Jeff. Ethical issues in HIV disease research. *In:* Cohen, P.T.; Sande, Merle A.; Volberding, Paul A., eds. The AIDS Knowledge Base: A Textbook on HIV Disease from the University of California, San Francisco, and the San Francisco General Hospital. Second Edition. Boston, MA: Little, Brown; 1994: 11.5–1 to 11.5–6. 29 refs. 0-316-77067–1. BE56643.
  *AIDS; children; confidentiality; control groups; drug abuse; females; *HIV seropositivity; *human experimentation; indigents; informed consent; *investigational drugs; minority groups; patient advocacy; patient care; patients; placebos; prisoners; random selection; research design; *research subjects; *selection of subjects; vulnerable populations; expedited review; United States

Tindall, Brett; Forde, Sally; Ross, Michael W., et al. Effects of two formats of informed consent on knowledge amongst persons with advanced HIV disease in a clinical trial of didanosine. *Patient Education and Counseling.* 1994 Dec; 24(3): 261–266. 14 refs. BE55776.
  *AIDS; *communication; comparative studies; *comprehension; *consent forms; decision making; *drugs; evaluation; homosexuals; human experimentation; *informed consent; *knowledge, attitudes, practice; males; *methods; patient care; *patient education; *patients; physicians; recall; *research subjects; survey; *therapeutic research; Australia; DDI

Varmus, Harold; Satcher, David. Ethical complexities of conducting research in developing countries. *New England Journal of Medicine.* 1997 Oct 2; 337(14): 1003–1005. 6 refs. BE55835.
  AIDS; autonomy; beneficence; *control groups; *developing countries; *drugs; economics; ethical review; federal government; *HIV seropositivity; *human experimentation; international aspects; justice; *moral policy; *newborns; *placebos; *pregnant women; *preventive medicine; *public policy; *research design; risks and benefits; *therapeutic research; *AZT; Centers for Disease Control and Prevention; National Institutes of Health; *United States

Wadman, Meredith. Controversy flares over AIDS prevention trials in Third World. [News]. *Nature.* 1997 Oct 30; 389(6654): 894. BE56162.
  *developing countries; *drugs; federal government; government financing; government regulation; *HIV seropositivity; *human experimentation; investigators; newborns; *placebos; *pregnant women; preventive medicine; *research design; therapeutic research; *AZT; Department of Health and Human Services; Johns Hopkins

University; National Institutes of Health; Public Citizen; *United States

Wadman, Meredith. US dispute over live AIDS vaccine trials. [News]. *Nature.* 1997 Oct 2; 389(6650): 426. BE56061.
  *attitudes; *autoexperimentation; federal government; government regulation; *HIV seropositivity; *human experimentation; *immunization; *investigators; physicians; public policy; risks and benefits; *volunteers; *International Association of Physicians in AIDS Care; *National Institute of Allergy and Infectious Diseases; *United States

Wehrwein, Peter; Morris, Kelly. HIV-1-vaccine-trial go-ahead reawakens ethics debate. [News]. *Lancet.* 1998 Jun 13; 351(9118): 1789. BE58863.
  control groups; *developing countries; drug abuse; economics; federal government; government regulation; *HIV seropositivity; *human experimentation; *immunization; industry; *international aspects; placebos; preventive medicine; needle–exchange programs; Food and Drug Administration; Thailand; United States; VaxGen

AIDS/TESTING AND SCREENING

American Academy of Pediatrics; American College of Obstetricians and Gynecologists. Joint Statement on Human Immunodeficiency Virus Screening. Issued by the American Academy of Pediatrics [and] by the American College of Obstetricians and Gynecologists, Washington, DC; 1995 Aug. 1 p. BE57275.
  *AIDS serodiagnosis; counseling; *HIV seropositivity; informed consent; *newborns; obstetrics and gynecology; *organizational policies; parental consent; patient education; pediatrics; physicians; *pregnant women; professional organizations; *American Academy of Pediatrics; *American College of Obstetricians and Gynecologists

American Academy of Pediatrics. Task Force on Pediatric AIDS. Perinatal human immunodeficiency virus (HIV) testing. *Pediatrics.* 1992 Apr; 89(4, Pt.2): 791–794. 34 refs. BE57988.
  *AIDS serodiagnosis; anonymous testing; counseling; economics; females; guidelines; *HIV seropositivity; infants; informed consent; mandatory testing; mothers; *newborns; *organizational policies; parental consent; patient care; pediatrics; pregnant women; preventive medicine; professional organizations; risks and benefits; voluntary programs; *American Academy of Pediatrics; United States

Bassford, H.A. HIV testing and confidentiality. *In:* Overall, Christine and Zion, William P., eds. Perspectives on AIDS: Ethical and Social Issues. New York, NY: Oxford University Press; 1991: 106–121. 17 fn. ISBN 0–19–540749–0. BE58290.
  *AIDS serodiagnosis; *confidentiality; contact tracing; duty to warn; high education; *HIV seropositivity; mandatory testing; patient compliance; physician patient relationship; physicians; public health; public policy; quarantine; social discrimination; stigmatization; voluntary programs; Canada; United States

Benatar, David; Benatar, Solomon R. Informed consent and research. *BMJ (British Medical Journal).* 1998 Mar 28; 316(7136): 1008. 2 refs. BE57553.
  *AIDS serodiagnosis; *anonymous testing; biomedical research; confidentiality; epidemiology; *HIV seropositivity; *human experimentation; *informed consent; medical records; patients; research design; research subjects; South Africa

Bhagwanjee, Satish; Muckart, David J.J.; Jeena, Prakash M., et al. Does HIV status influence the

---

outcome of patients admitted to a surgical intensive care unit? A prospective double blind study. [Article, commentaries, and response]. *BMJ (British Medical Journal)*. 1997 Apr 12; 314(7087): 1077-1084. 26 refs. BE55661.

> *AIDS serodiagnosis; anonymous testing; blacks; comparative studies; confidentiality; critically ill; developing countries; disadvantaged; disclosure; empirical research; *epidemiology; futility; *HIV seropositivity; hospitals; human experimentation; *informed consent; injuries; *intensive care units; justice; morbidity; mortality; patient admission; patient discharge; patients; research design; research ethics committees; *research subjects; resource allocation; scientific misconduct; *selection for treatment; surgery; *treatment outcome; prospective studies; *South Africa

OBJECTIVES: (a) To assess the impact of HIV status (HIV negative, HIV positive, AIDS) on the outcome of patients admitted to intensive care units for diseases unrelated to HIV; (b) to decide whether a positive test result for HIV should be a criterion for excluding patients from intensive care for diseases unrelated to HIV. DESIGN: A prospective double blind study of all admissions over six months. HIV status was determined in all patients by enzyme linked immunosorbent assay (ELISA), immunofluorescence assay, western blotting, and flow cytometry. The ethics committee considered the clinical implications of the study important enough to waive patients' right to informed consent. Staff and patients were blinded to HIV results. On discharge patients could be advised of their HIV status if they wished. SETTING: A 16 bed surgical intensive care unit. SUBJECTS: All 267 men and 135 women admitted to the unit during the study period. INTERVENTIONS: None. MAIN OUTCOME MEASURES: APACHE II score (acute physiological, age, and chronic health evaluation), organ failure, septic shock, durations of intensive care unit and hospital stay, and intensive care unit and hospital mortality. RESULTS: No patient had AIDS. 52 patients were tested positive for HIV and 350 patients were tested negative. The two groups were similar in sex distribution but differed significantly in age, incidence of organ failure (37 (71%) v 171 (49%) patients), and incidence of septic shock (20 (38%) v 54 (15%)). After adjustment for age there were no differences in intensive care unit or hospital mortality or in the durations of stay in the intensive care unit or hospital. CONCLUSIONS: Morbidity was higher in HIV positive patients but there was no difference in mortality. In this patient population a positive HIV test result should not be a criterion for excluding a patient from intensive care.

Birchard, Karen. Ireland rules out compulsory HIV testing. [News]. *Lancet.* 1997 Oct 25; 350(9086): 1232. BE56921.

> advisory committees; *AIDS serodiagnosis; compensation; employment; *HIV seropositivity; iatrogenic disease; *mandatory testing; *physicians; *public policy; *voluntary programs; Advisory Group on the Transmission of Blood-Borne Diseases (Ireland); *Department of Health (Ireland); *Ireland

Burris, Scott. Driving the epidemic underground? A new look at law and the social risk of HIV testing. *AIDS and Public Policy Journal.* 1997 Summer; 12(2): 66-78. 48 fn. BE58478.

> *AIDS serodiagnosis; attitudes; confidentiality; disadvantaged; drug abuse; *HIV seropositivity; homosexuals; *legal aspects; minority groups; physicians; primary health care; privacy; psychology; public policy; *risk; *social discrimination; social impact; *socioeconomic factors; stigmatization; *vulnerable populations; United

States

Coles, Matthew. The law and health care workers: confidentiality, testing, and treatment. *In:* Cohen, P.T.; Sande, Merle A.; Volberding, Paul A., eds. The AIDS Knowledge Base: A Textbook on HIV Disease from the University of California, San Francisco, and the San Francisco General Hospital. Second Edition. Boston, MA: Little, Brown; 1994: 9.1-1 to 9.1-11. 11 refs. ISBN 0-316-77067-1. BE56638.

> *AIDS; *AIDS serodiagnosis; *confidentiality; contact tracing; disclosure; duty to warn; federal government; government regulation; *health facilities; health insurance; *health personnel; *HIV seropositivity; informed consent; *legal aspects; mandatory reporting; occupational exposure; *refusal to treat; social discrimination; state government; *United States

Danziger, Renée; Gill, Nöel. HIV testing and HIV prevention in Sweden. [Article and commentary]. *BMJ (British Medical Journal).* 1998 Jan 24; 316(7127): 293-296. 13 refs. BE57701.

> *AIDS; *AIDS serodiagnosis; common good; contact tracing; disadvantaged; disclosure; females; *HIV seropositivity; *legal aspects; males; *mandatory programs; mandatory reporting; mandatory testing; moral obligations; *patients; pregnant women; *prevalence; *preventive medicine; public health; *public policy; quarantine; risks and benefits; statistics; *Communicable Diseases Act 1988 (Sweden); Great Britain; *Sweden

De Cock, Kevin M.; Johnson, Anne M. From exceptionalism to normalisation: a reappraisal of attitudes and practice around HIV testing. *BMJ (British Medical Journal).* 1998 Jan 24; 316(7127): 290-293. 39 refs. BE57703.

> *AIDS; *AIDS serodiagnosis; anonymous testing; confidentiality; drug abuse; drugs; females; health facilities; *HIV seropositivity; homosexuals; informed consent; knowledge, attitudes, practice; males; mortality; newborns; patient care; patients; patients' rights; *physician's role; political activity; pregnant women; *prevalence; preventive medicine; public health; *risks and benefits; social discrimination; stigmatization; *voluntary programs; *Great Britain; United States

Ingram, Miranda. Russia delays HIV testing for foreigners. [News]. *BMJ (British Medical Journal).* 1995 Aug 12; 311(7002): 407. BE56105.

> *AIDS serodiagnosis; aliens; *HIV seropositivity; international aspects; *legal aspects; legislation; *mandatory testing; physicians; public policy; *Russia

Irvin, Susan M. The great dilemma [AIDS]. *Nursing Standard.* 1995 Sep 27-Oct 3; 10(1): 50-53. 22 refs. BE55872.

> *AIDS serodiagnosis; confidentiality; duty to warn; *health personnel; *HIV seropositivity; *hospitals; informed consent; *institutional policies; *mandatory testing; nurses; occupational exposure; *patients; refusal to treat; risks and benefits; values; *voluntary programs; universal precautions; United States

Jürgens, Ralf; Palles, Michael. HIV Testing and Confidentiality: A Discussion Paper. Montreal: Canadian HIV/AIDS Legal Network; 1997. 317 p. Includes references. Prepared for the Canadian HIV/AIDS Legal Network and the Canadian AIDS Society. ISBN 1-896735-06-1. BE58162.

> advisory committees; AIDS; *AIDS serodiagnosis; aliens; anonymous testing; coercion; *confidentiality; contact tracing; counseling; *disclosure; duty to warn; guidelines; health personnel; *HIV seropositivity; informed consent; legal aspects; mandatory reporting; *mandatory testing;

BE = bioethics accession number   fn. = footnotes   refs. = references

newborns; organizational policies; pregnant women; prisoners; privacy; professional organizations; public policy; risks and benefits; sex offenses; *voluntary programs; diagnostic kits; emigration and immigration; partner notification; prostitution; *Canada

Kovac, Carl. Anonymous AIDS testing in Hungary to end. [News]. *BMJ (British Medical Journal).* 1997 Sep 6; 315(7108): 567. BE56873.
    *AIDS serodiagnosis; *anonymous testing; *confidentiality; *disclosure; *HIV seropositivity; legislation; *public policy; *Hungary

Leary, Warren E. Panel urges H.I.V. tests for all pregnant women. [News]. *New York Times.* 1998 Oct 15: A22. BE58994.
    advisory committees; *AIDS serodiagnosis; costs and benefits; *counseling; drugs; HIV seropositivity; *mandatory testing; newborns; patient care; *pregnant women; preventive medicine; *public policy; AZT; Institute of Medicine; *United States

Magnusson, Roger S. Testing for HIV without specific consent: a short review. *Australian and New Zealand Journal of Public Health.* 1996 Feb; 20(1): 57–60. 33 refs. BE57964.
    *AIDS serodiagnosis; anonymous testing; autonomy; disclosure; epidemiology; *HIV seropositivity; *informed consent; legal aspects; patients; pregnant women; privacy; research subjects; Australia; New Zealand

Mayor, Susan. Pregnant women should routinely be offered HIV tests. [News]. *BMJ (British Medical Journal).* 1998 May 2; 316(7141): 1333. 1 ref. BE58700.
    advisory committees; *AIDS serodiagnosis; cesarean section; drugs; fetuses; HIV seropositivity; information dissemination; patient care; *pregnant women; preventive medicine; public policy; *voluntary programs; *Great Britain

Minkoff, Howard; O'Sullivan, Mary Jo. The case for rapid HIV testing during labor. *JAMA.* 1998 Jun 3; 279(21): 1743–1744. 25 refs. BE58421.
    *AIDS serodiagnosis; *childbirth; counseling; drugs; *HIV seropositivity; informed consent; minority groups; newborns; patient care; *pregnant women; preventive medicine; syphilis; AZT

Nakchbandi, Inaam A.; Longenecker, J. Craig; Ricksecker, M. Ann, et al. A decision analysis of mandatory compared with voluntary HIV testing in pregnant women. *Annals of Internal Medicine.* 1998 May 1; 128(9): 760–767. 21 refs. BE57914.
    *AIDS serodiagnosis; comparative studies; *decision analysis; drugs; *HIV seropositivity; *mandatory testing; mortality; newborns; patient care; *pregnant women; public policy; *risks and benefits; social impact; *voluntary programs; AZT; United States
    BACKGROUND: The benefit of antiretroviral therapy in reducing maternal–fetal transmission of HIV during pregnancy has caused a public policy debate about the relative benefits of mandatory HIV screening and voluntary HIV screening in pregnant women. OBJECTIVE: To evaluate the benefits and risks of mandatory compared with voluntary HIV testing of pregnant women to help guide research and policy. DESIGN: A decision analysis that incorporated the following variables: acceptance and benefit of prenatal care, acceptance and benefit of zidovudine therapy in HIV–infected women, prevalence of HIV infection, and mandatory compared with voluntary HIV testing. MEASUREMENTS: The threshold deterrence rate (defined as the percentage of women who, if deterred

from seeking prenatal care because of a mandatory HIV testing policy, would offset the benefit of zidovudine in reducing vertical HIV transmission) and the difference between a policy of mandatory testing and a policy of voluntary testing in the absolute number of HIV–infected infants or dead infants. RESULTS: Voluntary HIV testing was preferred over a broad range of values in the model. At baseline, the threshold deterrence rate was 0.4%. At a deterrence rate of 0.5%, the number of infants (n = 167) spared HIV infection annually in the United States under a mandatory HIV testing policy would be lower than the number of perinatal deaths (n = 189) caused by lack of prenatal care. CONCLUSIONS: The most important variables in the model were voluntary HIV testing, the deterrence rate associated with mandatory testing compared with voluntary testing, and the prevalence of HIV infection in women of child–bearing age. At high levels of acceptance of voluntary HIV testing, the benefits of a policy of mandatory testing are minimal and may create the potential harms of avoiding prenatal care to avoid mandatory testing.

Segal, Arthur I.; Macer, James A.; Pillsbury, S. Gainer, et al. Physician attitudes toward human immunodeficiency virus testing in pregnancy. [Article and commentaries]. *American Journal of Obstetrics and Gynecology.* 1996 Jun; 174(6): 1750–1756. 11 refs. BE55922.
    *AIDS serodiagnosis; *attitudes; confidentiality; costs and benefits; counseling; drugs; guidelines; *HIV seropositivity; knowledge, attitudes, practice; legal aspects; mandatory reporting; *mandatory testing; newborns; obstetrics and gynecology; organizational policies; patient care; *physicians; *pregnant women; professional organizations; state government; survey; *voluntary programs; American Academy of Pediatrics; American College of Obstetricians and Gynecologists; AZT; *California; Centers for Disease Control and Prevention; United States

Stryker, Jeff. Ethical issues in the use of tests for HIV infection. *In:* Cohen, P.T.; Sande, Merle A.; Volberding, Paul A., eds. The AIDS Knowledge Base: A Textbook on HIV Disease from the University of California, San Francisco, and the San Francisco General Hospital. Second Edition. Boston, MA: Little, Brown; 1994: 11.4–1 to 11.4–5. 11 refs. ISBN 0–316–77067–1. BE56640.
    *AIDS; *AIDS serodiagnosis; autonomy; behavior control; contact tracing; counseling; drugs; employment; health insurance; *HIV seropositivity; informed consent; patient care; psychological stress; public health; risks and benefits; social discrimination; stigmatization

U.S. Court of Appeals, Third Circuit. United States v. Ward. *Federal Reporter, 3d Series.* 1997 Nov 13 (date of decision). 131: 335–343. BE58832.
    *AIDS serodiagnosis; confidentiality; *criminal law; disclosure; HIV seropositivity; *legal aspects; *mandatory testing; prisoners; *rape; United States; *United States v. Ward; Violence Against Women Act
    The U.S. Court of Appeals for the Third Circuit held that a district court order requiring a criminal defendant to provide a blood sample to test for HIV antibodies did not violate his Fourth Amendment rights. Ward, an interstate truck driver, abducted a woman from a New Jersey parking lot and repeatedly raped her in his truck over the next three days until she escaped in Illinois. The court had ordered Ward to provide a blood sample for HIV–AIDS testing under the federal Violence Against Women Act. Under the Act, a blood test is permissible only when the accused is charged with sexual assault that poses a risk of HIV transmission, probable

---

BE = bioethics accession number   fn. = footnotes   refs. = references

cause exists that the accused committed the assault, the victim requests the test, and the test would provide information necessary for the victim's health. Pursuant to the Act, the lower court also directed that the results would remain confidential except for disclosure to the victim and the defendant and their respective doctors. (KIE abstract)

D.C. hospital must pay $400,000 for forced test and denial of care. [News]. *AIDS Policy and Law.* 1997 May 2; 12(8): 1, 8–9. 2 fn. BE56405.
   *AIDS serodiagnosis; coercion; *compensation; disclosure; employment; *HIV seropositivity; *homosexuals; *hospitals; institutional policies; *legal aspects; *legal liability; *mandatory testing; medical records; psychological stress; *refusal to treat; social discrimination; *District of Columbia; *Estate of Doe v. Howard University Hospital

Informed consent needed before HIV testing of pregnant mothers: CMA. [News]. *Canadian Medical Association Journal.* 1997 Apr 15; 156(8): 1108. BE57355.
   *AIDS serodiagnosis; guidelines; informed consent; mass screening; *organizational policies; physicians; *pregnant women; professional organizations; voluntary programs; *Canadian Medical Association

ALLOWING TO DIE

See also EUTHANASIA, RESUSCITATION ORDERS, SELECTION FOR TREATMENT, TERMINAL CARE, TREATMENT REFUSAL

Alderson, Priscilla; Nicholson, Richard. Deciding when to withhold or withdraw life-sustaining treatment for children. *Bulletin of Medical Ethics.* 1997 Apr; No. 127: 13–20. 43 fn. BE57586.
   *allowing to die; autopsies; *children; communication; *decision making; futility; infants; legal aspects; newborns; palliative care; parents; patient care team; patient participation; persistent vegetative state; quality of life; risks and benefits; terminally ill; treatment refusal; uncertainty; *withholding treatment; Great Britain

Angell, Marcia. Helping desperately ill people to die. *In:* Emanuel, Linda L., ed. Regulating How We Die: The Ethical, Medical, and Legal Issues Surrounding Physician–Assisted Suicide. Cambridge, MA: Harvard University Press; 1998: 3–20, 263–264. 19 fn. ISBN 0–674–66654–2. BE58531.
   *active euthanasia; *allowing to die; *assisted suicide; attitudes; autonomy; competence; critically ill; decision making; family members; government regulation; legal aspects; persistent vegetative state; physician's role; *physicians; public opinion; public policy; right to die; standards; state government; suffering; terminally ill; third party consent; treatment refusal; *voluntary euthanasia; wedge argument; withholding treatment; Brophy v. New England Sinai Hospital; In re Quinlan; Lane v. Candura; Netherlands; *United States

Appelbaum, Paul S. Let my wife bleed to death. *Medical Ethics Newsletter.* 1997 Fall; 3(3): 3, 7. 2 refs. BE58114.
   *allowing to die; case studies; competence; *critically ill; *depressive disorder; *emergency care; *family members; legal aspects; *mentally ill; physicians; spousal consent; suicide; *treatment refusal; withholding treatment

Arnold, Denis G.; Menzel, Paul T. When comes "the end of the day?" A comment on the dialogue between Dax Cowart and Robert Burt. *Hastings Center Report.* 1998 Jan–Feb; 28(1): 25–27. 2 fn. Commentary on D. Cowart and R. Burt, p. 14–24. BE57293.
   *allowing to die; *autonomy; burns; *communication;

competence; *decision making; *dissent; *pain; palliative care; paternalism; patient advocacy; physician patient relationship; prognosis; *prolongation of life; *right to die; *time factors; *treatment refusal; Cowart, Dax

Australia. New South Wales. Department of Health. Dying with Dignity: Interim Guidelines on Management. North Sydney, NSW: NSW Health; 1993 Mar 1. 6 p. 2 refs. State Health Publication No. (HPA) 93–33. BE57383.
   advance care planning; advance directives; *allowing to die; autonomy; communication; counseling; double effect; drugs; family members; futility; guidelines; health personnel; legal aspects; medical records; palliative care; *practice guidelines; resuscitation orders; state government; terminally ill; withholding treatment; Australia; *New South Wales

Battin, Margaret P. Euthanasia: the way we do it, the way they do it. [Revised]. *In:* Monagle, John F.; Thomasma, David C., eds. Health Care Ethics: Critical Issues for the 21st Century. Gaithersburg, MD: Aspen Publishers; 1998: 311–322. 15 fn. ISBN 0–8342–0911–X. BE56288.
   active euthanasia; advance directives; *allowing to die; *assisted suicide; autonomy; *international aspects; involuntary euthanasia; legal aspects; national health insurance; physician patient relationship; physicians; policy analysis; *public policy; resource allocation; risks and benefits; *socioeconomic factors; standards; suffering; *terminally ill; third party consent; treatment refusal; *voluntary euthanasia; wedge argument; withholding treatment; German Society for Humane Dying; *Germany; *Netherlands; *United States

Beauchamp, Tom L. Physician–assisted suicide: a response to Edmund Pellegrino. *In:* Wildes, Kevin Wm.; Mitchell, Alan C., eds. Choosing Life: A Dialogue on *Evangelium Vitae.* Washington, DC: Georgetown University Press; 1997: 254–258. 3 fn. ISBN 0–87840–646–8. BE56692.
   *allowing to die; *assisted suicide; autonomy; intention; *killing; moral obligations; *moral policy; physician patient relationship; physicians; Protestant ethics; risks and benefits; Roman Catholic ethics; treatment refusal; *voluntary euthanasia; withholding treatment; Evangelium Vitae

Beecham, Linda. BMA to consult on withdrawing treatment. [News]. *BMJ (British Medical Journal).* 1998 Jul 18; 317(7152): 165. BE58509.
   *allowing to die; decision making; guidelines; mentally disabled; physicians; professional organizations; public participation; withholding treatment; *British Medical Association; *Great Britain

Berger, Jeffrey T.; Rosner, Fred; Potash, Joel, et al. Medical futility: towards consensus on disagreement. *HEC (HealthCare Ethics Committee) Forum.* 1998 Mar; 10(1): 102–118. 51 refs. BE59062.
   aged; *allowing to die; anencephaly; autonomy; case studies; communication; consensus; *decision making; dissent; economics; family members; *futility; *goals; infants; legal aspects; moral obligations; moral policy; patient care; patients; *physicians; prognosis; prolongation of life; refusal to treat; resource allocation; *risks and benefits; standards; terminology; treatment outcome; *values; ventilators; withholding treatment; United States

Berkowitz, Kenneth A. End-of-life decisionmaking in the Veterans Health Administration. *HEC (HealthCare Ethics Committee) Forum.* 1997 Jun; 9(2): 169–181. 19 refs. BE55965.
   *allowing to die; autonomy; case studies; clinical ethics committees; competence; decision making; *ethics consultation; federal government; futility; institutional policies; physicians; prognosis; *public hospitals; *public policy; renal dialysis; resuscitation; terminally ill; third party

---

consent; withholding treatment; *New York Department of Veterans Affairs Medical Center; Veterans Health Administration

Berkowitz, Sheldon T.; Boisaubin, Eugene V.; Perkins, Henry S., et al. Race and the delivery of care. [Letters and response]. *Hastings Center Report.* 1998 Jan–Feb; 28(1): 5–6. BE57289.
    *allowing to die; *blacks; communication; *critically ill; *cultural pluralism; *decision making; *dissent; economics; emergency care; *family members; *futility; minority groups; *physicians; *professional family relationship; *prolongation of life; *social discrimination; *trust; whites; *United States

Borthwick, Christian J. The permanent vegetative state: ethical crux, medical fiction? *Issues in Law and Medicine.* 1996 Fall; 12(2): 167–185. 68 fn. BE58761.
    allowing to die; brain pathology; consensus; *diagnosis; economics; pain; *persistent vegetative state; professional organizations; prognosis; *standards; time factors; *uncertainty; locked-in syndrome; Multi-Society Task Force on PVS

Bradley, Peter; Przygoda, Pablo; Saimovici, Javier, et al. Physician assisted suicide, euthanasia, and withdrawal of treatment. [Letters]. *BMJ (British Medical Journal).* 1998 Jan 3; 316(7124): 71–72. 9 refs. BE57955.
    *active euthanasia; *allowing to die; *assisted suicide; attitudes; double effect; intention; moral policy; *physicians; survey; terminal care; terminology; wedge argument; withholding treatment; Argentina; Great Britain

Brock, Dan W. An ethical framework for surrogate decision-making. *In:* Grubb, Andrew, ed. Decision-Making and Problems of Incompetence. New York, NY: Wiley; 1994: 41–52. 9 fn. ISBN 0-471-94236-7. BE57128.
    adults; advance directives; *allowing to die; autonomy; *competence; *decision making; family members; informed consent; legal aspects; moral policy; patient care; physician's role; prolongation of life; quality of life; risks and benefits; *standards; *third party consent; treatment refusal; value of life; values; withholding treatment; *United States

Brody, Howard. Bringing clarity to the futility debate: don't use the wrong cases. *Cambridge Quarterly of Healthcare Ethics.* 1998 Summer; 7(3): 269–273. 15 fn. Commented on by L.J. Schneiderman, p. 273–278. BE58555.
    *allowing to die; *anencephaly; *decision making; dissent; *family members; *futility; *goals; *persistent vegetative state; personhood; *physicians; *prolongation of life; technical expertise; *values; withholding treatment; In re Baby K; In re Wanglie

Brody, Howard. Medical futility: a useful concept? *In:* Zucker, Marjorie B.; Zucker, Howard D., eds. Medical Futility and the Evaluation of Life-Sustaining Interventions. New York, NY: Cambridge University Press; 1997: 1–14. 14 refs. ISBN 0-521-56877-3. BE55975.
    *allowing to die; autonomy; *communication; *decision making; disclosure; dissent; family members; *futility; goals; hospitals; informed consent; institutional policies; justice; medical ethics; *patient participation; *patients; *physicians; prognosis; quality of life; resource allocation; resuscitation orders; risks and benefits; *technical expertise; terminology; treatment outcome; uncertainty; *values; withholding treatment; *professional integrity; United States

Brophy, Patricia. Death with dignity. [Personal narrative]. *In:* Zucker, Marjorie B.; Zucker, Howard D., eds. Medical Futility and the Evaluation of Life-Sustaining

Interventions. New York, NY: Cambridge University Press; 1997: 15–23. 3 refs. ISBN 0-521-56877-3. BE55974.
    *allowing to die; *artificial feeding; attitudes to death; clergy; *decision making; *dissent; *family members; *futility; *hospitals; institutional policies; judicial action; married persons; patient advocacy; patient transfer; *persistent vegetative state; professional family relationship; prolongation of life; quality of life; third party consent; withholding treatment; Brophy v. New England Sinai Hospital; *Brophy, Patricia; *Brophy, Paul; Massachusetts

Budziszewski, J. Why we kill the weak. *Human Life Review.* 1997 Fall; 23(4): 67–74. BE57427.
    *abortion, induced; *active euthanasia; *allowing to die; compassion; conscience; family relationship; justice; *killing; love; moral development; moral obligations; motivation; *vulnerable populations; withholding treatment; duty to die

Byrne, Paul A.; Kurt, Edward J.; Campbell, Donald D., et al. Quinlan re-examined. *Linacre Quarterly.* 1997 May; 64(2): 58–65. 28 refs. BE55620.
    *allowing to die; autopsies; brain death; brain pathology; *diagnosis; euthanasia; family members; judicial action; *legal aspects; legal rights; *persistent vegetative state; privacy; prognosis; right to die; *social impact; social worth; third party consent; trends; withholding treatment; *In re Quinlan; *Quinlan, Karen; United States

Castellani, Betty C. Medical ethics: prolonging life or protracting death? *Journal of the Medical Association of Georgia.* 1990 Nov; 79(11): 835–837. 4 refs. BE55635.
    *allowing to die; attitudes to death; decision making; legal aspects; legal liability; literature; patients; physician patient relationship; physicians; prolongation of life; quality of life; *right to die; suffering; third party consent; treatment refusal; Georgia; Gulliver's Travels (Swift, J.)

Cohen–Almagor, Raphael. Autonomy, life as an intrinsic value, and the right to die in dignity. *Science and Engineering Ethics.* 1995; 1(3): 261–272. 33 fn. BE56026.
    abortion, induced; aged; *allowing to die; assisted suicide; *autonomy; competence; decision making; family members; futility; legal aspects; moral policy; paternalism; persistent vegetative state; physicians; *prolongation of life; *quality of life; resource allocation; *right to die; suffering; terminology; treatment refusal; *value of life; voluntary euthanasia; withholding treatment; dignity; Great Britain; United States

Cowart, Dax; Burt, Robert. Confronting death: who chooses, who controls? A dialogue between Dax Cowart and Robert Burt. *Hastings Center Report.* 1998 Jan–Feb; 28(1): 14–24. 1 ref. Commented on by D.G. Arnold and P.T. Menzel, p. 25–27. BE57292.
    *allowing to die; attitudes; *autonomy; *beneficence; *burns; *communication; competence; *decision making; *dissent; freedom; human rights; informed consent; nurses; *pain; palliative care; *paternalism; patient advocacy; *physically disabled; *physician patient relationship; physician's role; *prolongation of life; quality of life; *right to die; self concept; suffering; *time factors; *treatment refusal; values; *Cowart, Dax
On 21 November 1996, Dax Cowart and Robert Burt jointly delivered the Heather Koller Memorial Lecture at Pacific Lutheran University. This was the first time that they spoke together in a public forum. Dax Cowart now lives and practices law in Corpus Christi, Texas. In the summer of 1973, he was critically injured in a propane gas explosion that took his father's life and very deeply burned more than two-thirds of his own body. He was left blind and without the use of his hands. For more than a year Dax underwent extraordinarily painful treatments in the acute burn ward of two hospitals.

BE = bioethics accession number   fn. = footnotes   refs. = references

Throughout his ordeal he demanded to die by refusing consent to his disinfectant treatments. Despite repeated declarations of competence by his psychiatrist, all his pleas were rejected. In 1974, while still hospitalized, he helped make the famous "Please Let Me Die" video, and in 1984 a second video, "Dax's Case." In 1986 Dax Cowart received a law degree from Texas Tech University. Burt and Cowart have corresponded over the course of several years on the subject of Dax's case and related issues. They met for the first time during their trip to Tacoma, Washington for the Koller Memorial Lecture. The following is an edited transcript of their public remarks.

Davis, Anne J.; Aroskar, Mila A.; Liaschenko, Joan, et al. Dying and death. *In: their* Ethical Dilemmas and Nursing Practice. Fourth Edition. Stamford, CT: Appleton and Lange; 1997: 159–183. 58 fn. ISBN 0–8385–2283–1. BE58597.
    *active euthanasia; adults; advance directives; *allowing to die; assisted suicide; caring; case studies; decision making; determination of death; hospices; legal aspects; newborns; *nurses; nursing ethics; resuscitation orders; right to die; suffering; suicide; *terminal care; third party consent; treatment refusal; withholding treatment; United States

Docker, Christopher. The way forward? *In:* McLean, Sheila A.M., ed. Death, Dying and the Law. Brookfield, VT: Dartmouth; 1996: 129–160. 99 fn. ISBN 1–85521–657–4. BE57217.
    *active euthanasia; *advance directives; aged; *allowing to die; *assisted suicide; decision making; double effect; economics; hospices; legal aspects; living wills; pain; *palliative care; *persistent vegetative state; physicians; public policy; *resource allocation; selection for treatment; terminal care; withholding treatment; *Great Britain; National Health Service; Netherlands; United States

Dorner, Becky; Gallagher-Allred, Charlette; Deering, Carole P., et al. The "to feed or not to feed" dilemma. *Journal of the American Dietetic Association.* 1997 Oct; 97(10, Suppl. 2): S172–S176. 19 refs. BE58257.
    advance directives; aged; allied health personnel; *allowing to die; *artificial feeding; *guidelines; *institutional policies; legal aspects; *nursing homes; *nutrition; *practice guidelines; risks and benefits; withholding treatment

Dowey, J.A. Child B: A Personal View. *BMJ (British Medical Journal).* 1997 Jan 18; 314(7075): 200. BE58833.
    *allowing to die; children; death; decision making; dissent; futility; government financing; parents; physicians; prognosis; *prolongation of life; refusal to treat; surgery; treatment outcome; withholding treatment; Bowen, Jaymee; Great Britain

Drane, James F. Caring to the End: Policy Suggestions and Ethics Education for Hospice and Home Health-Care Agencies. Erie, PA: Lake Area Health Education Center; 1997. 308 p. Includes references. Appendices include sample advance directives; a model for competency evaluation; what one hospice/home health-care agency did with the policy suggestions; and a glossary of terms. ISBN 0–9658342–0–4. BE58161.
    advance directives; *allowing to die; artificial feeding; assisted suicide; blood transfusions; clinical ethics committees; competence; confidentiality; *decision making; double effect; economics; education; futility; health care delivery; health facilities; health personnel; *home care; *hospices; informed consent; *institutional policies; intention; killing; legal aspects; patient admission; patient transfer; physicians; prolongation of life; quality of life; religious ethics; renal dialysis; resuscitation orders; *terminal care; third party consent; values; ventilators; wedge

argument; withholding treatment; United States

Draper, Heather. Euthanasia. *In:* Chadwick, Ruth, ed. Encyclopedia of Applied Ethics, Volume 2. San Diego, CA: Academic Press; 1998: 175–187. 5 refs. ISBN 0–12–227067–3. BE56382.
    *active euthanasia; *allowing to die; artificial feeding; autonomy; beneficence; competence; deontological ethics; double effect; drugs; *euthanasia; futility; informed consent; intention; involuntary euthanasia; killing; *moral policy; motivation; pain; palliative care; persistent vegetative state; physicians; public policy; quality of life; resource allocation; resuscitation; review; right to die; risks and benefits; suffering; suicide; terminology; third party consent; treatment refusal; utilitarianism; value of life; voluntary euthanasia; wedge argument; withholding treatment; culpability

Dresser, Rebecca; Astrow, Alan B. An alert and incompetent self: the irrelevance of advance directives. [Case study and commentaries]. *Hastings Center Report.* 1998 Jan–Feb; 28(1): 28–30. BE57295.
    *advance directives; *allowing to die; autonomy; case studies; clinical ethics committees; *competence; *critically ill; *decision making; *dissent; emotions; friends; *living wills; love; *patient care team; patient participation; patient transfer; physicians; professional patient relationship; prognosis; *prolongation of life; *third party consent; time factors; treatment refusal; *uncertainty; *ventilators

Dyer, Clare. Hillsborough survivor emerges from permanent vegetative state. [News]. *BMJ (British Medical Journal).* 1997 Apr 5; 314(7086): 996. BE55817.
    allowing to die; artificial feeding; diagnosis; legal aspects; *persistent vegetative state; *prognosis; *prolongation of life; time factors; *treatment outcome; withholding treatment; Bland, Tony; *Devine, Andrew; Great Britain

Eiser, Arnold R. Withdrawal from dialysis: the role of autonomy and community-based values. *American Journal of Kidney Diseases.* 1996 Mar; 27(3): 451–457. 39 refs. BE56568.
    *allowing to die; *autonomy; *beneficence; bioethical issues; *common good; *communitarianism; competence; consensus; *cultural pluralism; *decision making; dissent; ethics consultation; family members; futility; guidelines; international aspects; judicial action; legal aspects; *libertarianism; minority groups; moral policy; paternalism; patients; persistent vegetative state; physician patient relationship; *physician's role; physicians; *prolongation of life; public participation; quality of life; *renal dialysis; *standards; third party consent; *treatment refusal; *values; *withholding treatment; undertreatment; Europe; *United States

Engelhardt, H. Tristram. Medical decisions in a context of conflicts. *Chest.* 1985 Sep; 88(3, Suppl.): 172S–174S. 11 refs. BE56703.
    advance directives; *allowing to die; autonomy; biomedical technologies; extraordinary treatment; palliative care; prolongation of life; resource allocation; right to die; treatment refusal; withholding treatment; United States

Fenigsen, Richard. Physician-assisted death in the Netherlands: impact on long-term care. *Issues in Law and Medicine.* 1995 Winter; 11(3): 283–297. 59 fn. BE58820.
    *active euthanasia; adults; age factors; *aged; *allowing to die; assisted suicide; attitudes; children; congenital disorders; decision making; *disabled; Down syndrome; hospitals; infants; *involuntary euthanasia; *long-term care; mentally retarded; newborns; nurses; nursing homes; physicians; public opinion; *public policy; quality of health care; *social impact; *voluntary euthanasia; *withholding treatment; *Netherlands

---

BE = bioethics accession number   fn. = footnotes   refs. = references

Frader, Joel E.; Watchko, Jon. Futility issues in pediatrics. *In:* Zucker, Marjorie B.; Zucker, Howard D., eds. Medical Futility and the Evaluation of Life-Sustaining Interventions. New York, NY: Cambridge University Press; 1997: 48–57. 19 refs. ISBN 0–521–56877–3. BE55978.

*allowing to die; *children; clinical ethics committees; communication; conflict of interest; *decision making; *dissent; economics; federal government; *futility; government regulation; hospitals; institutional policies; intensive care units; legal aspects; *newborns; *parents; *pediatrics; *physicians; *prematurity; professional family relationship; prognosis; *prolongation of life; resource allocation; socioeconomic factors; treatment outcome; *uncertainty; values; viability; withholding treatment; Child Abuse Prevention and Treatment Act 1984; United States

Gelder, Mark S. Life and death decisions in the intensive care unit. *Cancer.* 1995 Nov 15; 76(10, Suppl.): 2171–2175. 61 refs. BE56865.

age factors; aged; *allowing to die; *cancer; communication; costs and benefits; *decision making; family members; females; *intensive care units; mortality; patient admission; patient care; patient care team; physician patient relationship; prognosis; prolongation of life; resource allocation; resuscitation; *selection for treatment; treatment outcome; withholding treatment; severity of illness index; United States

Gert, Bernard; Culver, Charles M.; Clouser, K. Danner. An alternative to physician–assisted suicide: a conceptual and moral analysis. *In:* Battin, Margaret P.; Rhodes, Rosamond; Silvers, Anita, eds. Physician Assisted Suicide: Expanding the Debate. New York, NY: Routledge; 1998: 182–202. 25 fn. ISBN 0–415–92003–5. BE58789.

*active euthanasia; *allowing to die; alternatives; artificial feeding; *assisted suicide; competence; double effect; drugs; food; freedom; government regulation; informed consent; intention; *killing; legal aspects; model legislation; *moral obligations; *moral policy; pain; *palliative care; *physicians; policy analysis; prolongation of life; public policy; right to die; state government; suffering; suicide; Supreme Court decisions; terminal care; terminally ill; time factors; treatment refusal; *voluntary euthanasia; withholding treatment; analgesia; dehydration; rationality; United States; Vacco v. Quill; Washington v. Glucksberg

Gert, Bernard. Euthanasia. *In:* Borchert, Donald M., ed. The Encyclopedia of Philosophy. Supplement. New York, NY: Simon and Schuster Macmillan; 1996: 155–158. 12 refs. ISBN 0–02–864629–0. BE57221.

*active euthanasia; advance directives; *allowing to die; competence; killing; moral policy; patient participation; physicians; public policy; suffering; treatment refusal; withholding treatment

Gibson, Susanne. Acts and omissions. *In:* Chadwick, Ruth, ed. Encyclopedia of Applied Ethics, Volume 1. San Diego, CA: Academic Press; 1998: 23–28. 8 refs. ISBN 0–12–227066–5. BE56363.

*active euthanasia; *allowing to die; deontological ethics; *ethical analysis; ethical theory; *killing; moral obligations; moral policy; rights; teleological ethics; virtues; culpability

Gillis, Jonathan. When lifesaving treatment in children is not the answer. [Editorial]. *BMJ (British Medical Journal).* 1997 Nov 15; 315(7118): 1246–1247. 5 refs. BE57167.

*allowing to die; *children; decision making; dissent; futility; *guidelines; legal aspects; *organizational policies; palliative care; parents; *pediatrics; physicians; professional organizations; suffering; *withholding treatment; *Great Britain; *Royal College of Paediatrics and Child Health

Godfrey, Nelda S.; Kuehne, Dale S.; Wildes, Kevin Wm. In the care of a nurse. [Case study and commentaries]. *Hastings Center Report.* 1997 Sep-Oct; 27(5): 23–24. BE56125.

active euthanasia; advance directives; *allowing to die; autonomy; case studies; *conscience; *deception; *decision making; *dissent; drugs; family members; hospitals; institutional ethics; institutional policies; intensive care units; *misconduct; moral obligations; *nurses; *nursing ethics; patient advocacy; *patient care team; *prolongation of life; terminally ill; treatment refusal; withholding treatment

Goodhall, Lesley. Tube feeding dilemmas: can artificial nutrition and hydration be legally or ethically withheld or withdrawn? *Journal of Advanced Nursing.* 1997 Feb; 25(2): 217–222. 19 refs. BE57509.

advance directives; aged; *allowing to die; *artificial feeding; autonomy; competence; decision making; deontological ethics; legal aspects; legal liability; nurse's role; persistent vegetative state; physicians; quality of life; teleological ethics; third party consent; utilitarianism; withholding treatment; Airedale NHS Trust v. Bland; Great Britain

Haddad, Amy. Ethics in action: you've recently been assigned to care for a post–trauma patient who has been in a persistent vegetative state for a month -- what would you do? *RN.* 1996 May; 59(5): 21–22, 24. 4 refs. BE56866.

*allowing to die; case studies; decision making; *dissent; *family members; futility; *nurse's role; *persistent vegetative state; professional family relationship; prognosis; *prolongation of life; time factors; withholding treatment

Herb, Alice; Lazar, Eliot J. Ethics committees and end–of–life decision making. *In:* Zucker, Marjorie B.; Zucker, Howard D., eds. Medical Futility and the Evaluation of Life–Sustaining Interventions. New York, NY: Cambridge University Press; 1997: 110–122. 13 refs. ISBN 0–521–56877–3. BE55984.

advance directives; *allowing to die; case studies; *clinical ethics committees; committee membership; *decision making; *dissent; education; ethicist's role; *family members; hospitals; institutional policies; interdisciplinary communication; legal aspects; *mediation; organization and administration; patient care; *physicians; prognosis; prolongation of life; *referral and consultation; resuscitation orders; uncertainty; withholding treatment; Joint Commission on the Accreditation of Healthcare Organizations; United States

Hesse, Katherine A. Ethical issues and terminal management of the old old. *Journal of Geriatric Psychiatry.* 1995; 28(1): 75–95. 64 refs. Paper presented at a meeting of the Boston Society for Gerontologic Psychiatry, Inc., "Older, Old People," 30 Oct 1993. BE55558.

advance directives; *age factors; *aged; *allowing to die; attitudes; autonomy; chronically ill; competence; decision making; dementia; family members; futility; patient participation; physicians; prognosis; prolongation of life; quality of life; refusal to treat; resuscitation; right to die; *terminal care; terminally ill; third party consent; treatment refusal; ventilators; withholding treatment; dignity

Hoefler, James M. Managing Death: The First Guide for Patients, Family Members, and Care Providers on Forgoing Treatment at the End of Life. Boulder, CO: Westview Press; 1997. 206 p. Includes references. ISBN 0–8133–2816–0. BE57922.

advance directives; advisory committees; aged; *allowing to die; artificial feeding; consensus; *decision making; dementia; drugs; economics; extraordinary treatment; family members; futility; guidelines; health personnel; hospices; legal aspects; legal rights; persistent vegetative state;

---

physicians; professional organizations; prolongation of life; Protestant ethics; public opinion; quality of health care; resource allocation; right to die; Roman Catholic ethics; standards; *terminal care; treatment refusal; withholding treatment; antibiotics; dehydration; starvation; In re Fiori; United States

Holm, Søren. The medical hierarchy and perceived influence on technical and ethical decisions. *Journal of Internal Medicine.* 1995 May; 237(5): 487–492. 5 refs. BE56003.
*allowing to die; attitudes; cancer; conscience; *decision making; dissent; evaluation studies; hospitals; institutional policies; *internal medicine; interprofessional relations; knowledge, attitudes, practice; medical ethics; nurse's role; nurses; patient care team; physician nurse relationship; *physicians; prolongation of life; referral and consultation; *social dominance; *sociology of medicine; statistics; survey; technical expertise; *terminally ill; withholding treatment; *Denmark

Jaffe, Allan S.; Landau, William M. Death after death: the presumption of informed consent for cardiopulmonary resuscitation -- ethical paradox and clinical conundrum. *Neurology.* 1993 Nov; 43(11): 2173–2178. 32 refs. BE58497.
*allowing to die; artificial feeding; *decision making; family members; informed consent; persistent vegetative state; physicians; *prognosis; prolongation of life; quality of life; resuscitation; third party consent; treatment outcome; treatment refusal; uncertainty; withholding treatment

Johnson, Linda; Potter, Robert Lyman. Professional and public community projects for developing medical futility guidelines. *In:* Zucker, Marjorie B.; Zucker, Howard D., eds. Medical Futility and the Evaluation of Life–Sustaining Interventions. New York, NY: Cambridge University Press; 1997: 155–167. 5 refs. ISBN 0–521–56877–3. BE55987.
advance directives; *allowing to die; clinical ethics committees; communication; consensus; cultural pluralism; *decision making; democracy; education; family members; *futility; goals; *guidelines; home care; hospices; *hospitals; *institutional policies; intensive care units; nursing homes; *organizational policies; *palliative care; patients; physicians; *program descriptions; *public participation; *public policy; refusal to treat; resource allocation; standards; *terminal care; terminally ill; terminology; withholding treatment; *community policies; Citywide Task Force on Medical Futility (Houston, TX); Collaborative Bioethics Working Group (Akron, OH); Colorado Collective for Medical Decisions; Extreme Care: Humane Options (ECHO) (Sacramento, CA); Guidelines for the Responsible Utilization of Intensive Care (Appleton, WI); Minnesota Center for Health Care Ethics; North Carolina Consortium to Set Limits in Medicine; Santa Monica UCLA Medical Center; Study to Understand Prognoses and Preferences for Outcomes and Risks of Treatments (SUPPORT); United States

Kamm, Frances M. Physician–assisted suicide, euthanasia, and intending death. *In:* Battin, Margaret P.; Rhodes, Rosamond; Silvers, Anita, eds. Physician Assisted Suicide: Expanding the Debate. New York, NY: Routledge; 1998: 28–62. 53 fn. ISBN 0–415–92003–5. BE58779.
accountability; *active euthanasia; *allowing to die; *assisted suicide; beneficence; *death; deontological ethics; *double effect; *drugs; *ethical analysis; *euthanasia; *intention; involuntary euthanasia; *killing; *moral obligations; *moral policy; morality; *pain; *palliative care; paralysis; personhood; *physicians; psychological stress; quality of life; right to die; suffering; suicide; terminal care; terminally ill; terminology; treatment refusal; value of life; *voluntary euthanasia; withholding treatment

Kaplan, Karen Orloff. Not quite the last word: scenarios and solutions. *In:* Zucker, Marjorie B.; Zucker, Howard D., eds. Medical Futility and the Evaluation of Life–Sustaining Interventions. New York, NY: Cambridge University Press; 1997: 179–192. 6 refs. ISBN 0–521–56877–3. BE55989.
advance care planning; *allowing to die; communication; consensus; *decision making; economics; family members; *futility; legal aspects; palliative care; patient advocacy; patients; physicians; professional patient relationship; refusal to treat; resource allocation; selection for treatment; terminal care; time factors; *trends; values; vulnerable populations; withholding treatment; United States

Kelly, David F. Alternatives to physician–assisted suicide. *American Journal of Otolaryngology.* 1995 May–Jun; 16(3): 181–185. BE56211.
active euthanasia; *allowing to die; *assisted suicide; drugs; economics; killing; legal aspects; morality; pain; *palliative care; public policy; Roman Catholic ethics; *terminal care; terminally ill; treatment refusal; voluntary euthanasia; wedge argument; withholding treatment; analgesia; United States

Kemp, Virginia H. The role of critical care nurses in the ethical decision–making process. *Dimensions of Critical Care Nursing.* 1985 Nov–Dec; 4(6): 354–359. 10 refs. BE56493.
*allowing to die; case studies; clinical ethics committees; communication; competence; *critically ill; *decision making; ethical analysis; evaluation; family members; guidelines; health personnel; institutional policies; intensive care units; interprofessional relations; legal aspects; *nurse's role; *nurses; patient care; patients; resuscitation orders; withholding treatment

Keyserlingk, Edward W. Quality of life decisions and the hopelessly ill patient: the physician as moral agent and truth teller. *In:* Hoshino, Kazumasa, ed. Japanese and Western Bioethics: Studies in Moral Diversity. Boston, MA: Kluwer Academic; 1997: 103–116. 20 refs. ISBN 0–7923–4112–0. BE57086.
*allowing to die; *communication; *decision making; disclosure; extraordinary treatment; *family members; *futility; goals; medicine; paternalism; patients; *persistent vegetative state; *physician's role; physicians; professional family relationship; prognosis; prolongation of life; *quality of life; refusal to treat; risks and benefits; suffering; *terminally ill; treatment outcome; treatment refusal; *truth disclosure; *values; withholding treatment; Canada; Japan; United States

Kmietowicz, Zosia. Woman dies two months after food withdrawal. [News]. *BMJ (British Medical Journal).* 1997 May 24; 314(7093): 1503. BE56466.
aged; *allowing to die; brain pathology; decision making; family members; *food; killing; legal aspects; physicians; quality of life; third party consent; voluntary euthanasia; *withholding treatment; cerebrovascular disorders; *Great Britain; *Ormerod, May; Taylor, Ken; Voluntary Euthanasia Society (Great Britain)

Kopelman, Loretta M. Medical futility. *In:* Chadwick, Ruth, ed. Encyclopedia of Applied Ethics, Volume 3. San Diego, CA: Academic Press; 1998: 185–196. 18 refs. ISBN 0–12–227068–1. BE56253.
allowing to die; autonomy; consensus; costs and benefits; *decision making; disabled; dissent; family members; *futility; goals; *models, theoretical; paternalism; patients; physicians; professional autonomy; professional organizations; prolongation of life; public participation; quality of life; resource allocation; social discrimination; *standards; suffering; value of life; values; hope

Kowalski, Susan D. Assisted suicide: is there a future?

Ethical and nursing considerations. *Critical Care Nursing Quarterly.* 1996 May; 19(1): 45–54. 10 refs. BE55723.
*active euthanasia; *allowing to die; artificial feeding; *assisted suicide; autonomy; case studies; chronically ill; common good; competence; double effect; economics; guidelines; *nurses; organizational policies; pain; palliative care; persistent vegetative state; physicians; professional organizations; professional patient relationship; quality of life; *right to die; suffering; terminal care; terminally ill; terminology; third party consent; treatment refusal; ventilators; *voluntary euthanasia; wedge argument; withholding treatment; American Nurses Association; Netherlands; United States

Kuhse, Helga. From intention to consent: learning from experience with euthanasia. *In:* Battin, Margaret P.; Rhodes, Rosamond; Silvers, Anita, eds. Physician Assisted Suicide: Expanding the Debate. New York, NY: Routledge; 1998: 252–266. 38 fn. ISBN 0–415–92003–5. BE58792.
*allowing to die; *assisted suicide; autonomy; comparative studies; *double effect; drugs; empirical research; informed consent; *intention; international aspects; involuntary euthanasia; killing; *knowledge, attitudes, practice; legal aspects; *moral policy; *palliative care; *physicians; policy analysis; *public policy; statistics; terminal care; *terminally ill; treatment refusal; *voluntary euthanasia; wedge argument; *withholding treatment; sedatives; *Australia; *Euthanasia Laws Act 1996 (Australia); *Netherlands; New York State Task Force on Life and the Law; United States

Lafrance, W. André; Singer, Peter A. Is it ethical to forgo treatment? [Letter and response]. *Canadian Medical Association Journal.* 1997 Dec 15; 157(12): 1740–1741. 1 ref. BE59053.
active euthanasia; *allowing to die; artificial feeding; assisted suicide; extraordinary treatment; *palliative care; quality of health care; *terminal care; *withholding treatment; Canada

Lanken, Paul N. Ethical considerations in pulmonary intensive care. *In:* Fishman, Alfred P., ed. Pulmonary Rehabilitation. New York, NY: Marcel Dekker; 1996: 289–308. 19 refs. (Lung biology in health and disease; v. 91). ISBN 082479673X. BE57281.
*allowing to die; autonomy; beneficence; communication; competence; decision making; family members; futility; *intensive care units; justice; legal aspects; paternalism; patient admission; prognosis; prolongation of life; refusal to treat; resource allocation; resuscitation orders; third party consent; treatment refusal; withholding treatment; United States

McLean, Sheila A.M., ed. Death, Dying and the Law. Brookfield, VT: Dartmouth; 1996. 185 p. (Medico–legal series). 531 fn. ISBN 1–85521–657–4. BE57209.
*active euthanasia; *advance directives; *allowing to die; *assisted suicide; competence; decision making; disabled; futility; international aspects; legal aspects; palliative care; persistent vegetative state; *physicians; prognosis; public policy; resource allocation; suffering; *terminal care; treatment refusal; *voluntary euthanasia; withholding treatment; Airedale NHS Trust v. Bland; Death with Dignity Act (OR); *Great Britain; Netherlands; United States

Mazur, Dennis J. How older patient preferences are influenced by consideration of future health outcomes. *Journal of the American Geriatrics Society.* 1997 Jun; 45(6): 725–728. 11 refs. BE55727.
advance care planning; *aged; *allowing to die; *attitudes; brain pathology; decision making; family members; health; *males; married persons; mentally disabled; morbidity; *patient care; *patients; physically disabled; physicians; *prolongation of life; *quality of life; resuscitation; survey; *treatment outcome; *treatment refusal; *ventilators;

withholding treatment; cerebrovascular disorders; *intubation; Oregon

Moretti, Anna. Advocating for the dying: the view of family and friends. *Bioethics Forum.* 1997 Summer; 13(2): 27–31. BE58284.
advance directives; *allowing to die; attitudes; case studies; *decision making; dissent; *family members; futility; hospitals; legal aspects; nurses; *patient advocacy; physicians; prolongation of life; right to die; terminal care; *terminally ill; treatment refusal; withholding treatment

Norris, Patrick F. Palliative care and killing: understanding ethical distinctions. *Bioethics Forum.* 1997 Fall; 13(3): 25–30. 6 refs. 1 fn. BE57529.
*active euthanasia; *allowing to die; *assisted suicide; *double effect; drugs; *intention; *killing; moral policy; pain; *palliative care; suicide; *terminal care; terminally ill; withholding treatment; sedatives

Pace, Nicholas A. Law and ethics at the end of life: the practitioner's view. *In:* McLean, Sheila A.M., ed. Death, Dying and the Law. Brookfield, VT: Dartmouth; 1996: 3–18. 44 fn. ISBN 1–85521–657–4. BE57210.
advance directives; aged; *allowing to die; autonomy; case studies; competence; *decision making; double effect; drugs; emergency care; extraordinary treatment; family members; futility; intensive care units; intention; international aspects; legal aspects; physicians; prognosis; quality of life; resource allocation; risks and benefits; Roman Catholic ethics; *terminal care; terminally ill; third party consent; withholding treatment; *Great Britain; United States

Pondělíček, Ivo; Königova, Radana. The problem of euthanasia and dysthanasia in burns. *Burns, Including Thermal Injury.* 1983 Sep; 10(1): 61–63. 5 refs. BE57496.
active euthanasia; aged; *allowing to die; *burns; *critically ill; prognosis; prolongation of life; quality of life; suffering

Quill, Timothy E.; Kimsma, Gerrit. End–of–life care in the Netherlands and the United States: a comparison of values, justifications, and practices. *Cambridge Quarterly of Healthcare Ethics.* 1997 Spring; 6(2): 189–204. 127 fn. BE56476.
*allowing to die; *assisted suicide; autonomy; case studies; common good; comparative studies; competence; consensus; decision making; dissent; double effect; drugs; freedom; government regulation; guidelines; health care delivery; hospices; intention; *international aspects; *knowledge, attitudes, practice; legal aspects; mass media; obligations of society; *palliative care; physician patient relationship; *physicians; policy analysis; public opinion; *public policy; social control; socioeconomic factors; statistics; *suffering; *terminal care; *values; *voluntary euthanasia; *Netherlands; *United States
Voluntary active euthanasia (VAE) and physician–assisted suicide (PAS) remain technically illegal in the Netherlands, but the practices are openly tolerated provided that physicians adhere to carefully constructed guidelines. Harsh criticism of the Dutch practice by authors in the United States and Great Britain has made achieving a balanced understanding of its clinical, moral, and policy implications very difficult. Similar practice patterns probably exist in the United States, but they are conducted in secret because of a more uncertain legal and ethical climate. In this manuscript, we plan to compare end–of–life care in the United States and the Netherlands with regard to underlying values, justifications, and practices. We will explore the risks and benefits of each system for a real patient who was faced with a common end–of–life clinical dilemma, and close with challenges for public policies in both countries.

BE = bioethics accession number   fn. = footnotes   refs. = references

Quill, Timothy E.; Lo, Bernard; Brock, Dan W. Palliative options of last resort: a comparison of voluntarily stopping eating and drinking, terminal sedation, physician-assisted suicide, and voluntary active euthanasia. *JAMA.* 1997 Dec 17; 278(23): 2099-2104. 70 refs. BE56434.

> *active euthanasia; *allowing to die; artificial feeding; *assisted suicide; autonomy; beneficence; chronically ill; comparative studies; competence; conscience; diagnosis; double effect; *drugs; ethical analysis; family members; food; guidelines; informed consent; intention; legal aspects; *moral policy; pain; *palliative care; physician's role; physicians; prognosis; *public policy; suffering; *terminal care; terminally ill; treatment refusal; *voluntary euthanasia; *sedatives; United States

Palliative care is generally agreed to be the standard of care for the dying, but there remain some patients for whom intolerable suffering persists. In the face of ethical and legal controversy about the acceptability of physician-assisted suicide and voluntary active euthanasia, voluntarily stopping eating and drinking and terminal sedation have been proposed as ethically superior responses of last resort that do not require changes in professional standards or the law. The clinical and ethical differences and similarities between these 4 practices are critically compared in light of the doctrine of double effect, the active/passive distinction, patient voluntariness, proportionality between risks and benefits, and the physician's potential conflict of duties. Terminal sedation and voluntarily stopping eating and drinking would allow clinicians to remain responsive to a wide range of patient suffering, but they are ethically and clinically more complex and closer to physician-assisted suicide and voluntary active euthanasia than is ordinarily acknowledged. Safeguards are presented for any medical action that may hasten death, including determining that palliative care is ineffective, obtaining informed consent, ensuring diagnostic and prognostic clarity, obtaining an independent second opinion, and implementing reporting and monitoring processes. Explicit public policy about which of these practices are permissible would reassure the many patients who fear a bad death in their future and allow for a predictable response for the few whose suffering becomes intolerable in spite of optimal palliative care.

Rafkin, Harry S.; Rainey, Thomas. Physicians and medical futility: experience in the critical care setting. *In:* Zucker, Marjorie B.; Zucker, Howard D., eds. Medical Futility and the Evaluation of Life-Sustaining Interventions. New York, NY: Cambridge University Press; 1997: 24-35. 17 refs. ISBN 0-521-56877-3. BE55976.

> advance directives; age factors; AIDS; *allowing to die; cancer; *communication; *critically ill; *decision making; dissent; *family members; forms; *futility; hospitals; informed consent; institutional policies; *intensive care units; *patients; *physicians; *prognosis; quality of life; resuscitation orders; terminal care; third party consent; *treatment outcome; uncertainty; values; withholding treatment; St. Francis Hospital (Pittsburgh, PA); United States

Rapin, M. The ethics of intensive care. [Editorial]. *Intensive Care Medicine.* 1987; 13(5): 300-303. 7 refs. BE56631.

> *allowing to die; *decision making; diagnosis; economics; family members; futility; *intensive care units; palliative care; *patient admission; patient care; patient care team; physicians; *prognosis; prolongation of life; resource allocation; *selection for treatment; *withholding treatment; *France

Reitman, James S. The dilemma of "medical futility": a "wisdom model" for decisionmaking. *Issues in Law and Medicine.* 1996 Winter; 12(3): 231-264. 144 fn. BE58464.

> advance directives; aged; *allowing to die; anencephaly; attitudes to death; autonomy; biomedical technologies; competence; consensus; *decision making; dissent; family members; *futility; informed consent; legal aspects; models, theoretical; *moral policy; newborns; patients; persistent vegetative state; physicians; *prolongation of life; quality of life; resource allocation; resuscitation; rights; risks and benefits; standards; terminal care; third party consent; treatment outcome; uncertainty; value of life; withholding treatment; hope; In re Baby K; In re Wanglie; United States

Rhodes, Rosamond. Futility and the goals of medicine. *Journal of Clinical Ethics.* 1998 Summer; 9(2): 194-205. 33 fn. BE58966.

> aged; *allowing to die; *autonomy; case studies; conscience; *decision making; dissent; family members; *futility; *goals; intensive care units; legal aspects; *medicine; *moral obligations; palliative care; patient discharge; physician patient relationship; physician's role; *physicians; *professional autonomy; *prolongation of life; quality of life; *refusal to treat; resource allocation; *terminally ill; value of life; values; *withholding treatment; coma; United States

Rubin, Susan B. When Doctors Say No: The Battleground of Medical Futility. Bloomington, IN: Indiana University Press; 1998. 191 p. (Medical ethics series). Bibliography: p. 163-185. ISBN 0-253-33463-2. BE59106.

> *allowing to die; autonomy; case studies; consensus; *decision making; *dissent; ethical analysis; *family members; *futility; goals; guidelines; justice; legal aspects; medicine; models, theoretical; moral obligations; *moral policy; patient participation; *patients; physician patient relationship; *physicians; professional organizations; *prolongation of life; public policy; quality of life; refusal to treat; resource allocation; resuscitation; resuscitation orders; review; standards; technical expertise; terminology; uncertainty; *values; withholding treatment; United States

Sass, Hans-Martin. Images of killing and letting-die, of self-determination and beneficence: the ethical debate on advance directives and surrogate decision making in Germany. *In:* Sass, Hans-Martin; Veatch, Robert M.; Kimura, Rihito, eds. Advance Directives and Surrogate Decision Making in Health Care: United States, Germany, and Japan. Baltimore, MD: Johns Hopkins University Press; 1998: 136-172. 129 refs. ISBN 0-8018-5831-3. BE59040.

> active euthanasia; *advance directives; *allowing to die; attitudes; *autonomy; beneficence; case studies; competence; cultural pluralism; *decision making; dissent; family members; guidelines; killing; legal aspects; living wills; National Socialism; palliative care; patient advocacy; physicians; professional organizations; prolongation of life; quality of life; right to die; risks and benefits; suffering; suicide; terminally ill; terminology; third party consent; truth disclosure; uncertainty; values; withholding treatment; oral directives; values histories; German Society for Humane Dying; *Germany

Schneiderman, Lawrence J. Commentary: bringing clarity to the futility debate: are the cases wrong? *Cambridge Quarterly of Healthcare Ethics.* 1998 Summer; 7(3): 273-278. 14 fn. Commentary on H. Brody, "Bringing clarity to the futility debate: don't use the wrong cases," p. 269-273. BE58571.

> *allowing to die; alternative therapies; *anencephaly; *decision making; dissent; *family members; *futility; *goals; medicine; *persistent vegetative state; personhood; *physicians; *prolongation of life; technical expertise; *values; withholding treatment; evidence-based medicine; In re Baby K; In re Wanglie

---

BE = bioethics accession number   fn. = footnotes   refs. = references

Shanahan, Timothy; Wang, Robin. Suicide and euthanasia. *In: their* Reason and Insight: Western and Eastern Perspectives on the Pursuit of Moral Wisdom. Belmont, CA: Wadsworth; 1996: 396–425. Includes references, readings, and discussion questions. Designed as a textbook for college students. ISBN 0–534–23167–5. BE56142.
> *active euthanasia; *allowing to die; attitudes; attitudes to death; brain death; Buddhist ethics; determination of death; Hindu ethics; international aspects; *moral policy; *morality; physician's role; *suicide; non–Western World; rationality; Western World; India; Japan

Sheldon, Tony. Row over force feeding of patients with Alzheimer's disease. [News]. *BMJ (British Medical Journal).* 1997 Aug 9; 315(7104): 327. BE57353.
> *allowing to die; *artificial feeding; attitudes; decision making; *dementia; euthanasia; family members; food; force feeding; institutional policies; killing; *nursing homes; patient care team; physicians; terminally ill; treatment refusal; *withholding treatment; dehydration; *Netherlands

Smith, George P. Final Exits: Safeguarding Self–Determination and the Right to Be Free from Cruel and Unusual Punishment. Chicago, IL: Northwestern University Medical School; 1997. 15 p. 88 fn. BE57696.
> *allowing to die; autonomy; costs and benefits; *decision making; family members; *futility; guidelines; human characteristics; justice; legal aspects; palliative care; patients; persistent vegetative state; *physicians; practice guidelines; prolongation of life; *quality of life; refusal to treat; resuscitation; rights; risks and benefits; utilitarianism; withholding treatment; Eighth Amendment; United States

Spielman, Bethany. Community futility policies: the illusion of consensus? *In:* Zucker, Marjorie B.; Zucker, Howard D., eds. Medical Futility and the Evaluation of Life–Sustaining Interventions. New York, NY: Cambridge University Press; 1997: 168–178. 44 refs. ISBN 0–521–56877–3. BE55988.
> *allowing to die; autonomy; clinical ethics committees; communitarianism; consensus; cultural pluralism; *decision making; *dissent; economics; family members; *futility; hospitals; *institutional policies; judicial action; legal aspects; legal liability; legislation; patient transfer; patients; physicians; professional autonomy; *prolongation of life; *public participation; refusal to treat; selection for treatment; standards; state government; terminology; values; withholding treatment; *community policies; United States

Spritz, Norton. Physicians and medical futility: experience in the setting of general medical care. *In:* Zucker, Marjorie B.; Zucker, Howard D., eds. Medical Futility and the Evaluation of Life–Sustaining Interventions. New York, NY: Cambridge University Press; 1997: 36–47. 10 refs. ISBN 0–521–56877–3. BE55977.
> *allowing to die; autonomy; chronically ill; communication; consensus; *decision making; dementia; economics; family members; *futility; institutional policies; patients; persistent vegetative state; physicians; prognosis; prolongation of life; quality of life; renal dialysis; resource allocation; risks and benefits; treatment outcome; values; withholding treatment; United States

Sprung, Charles L.; Eidelman, Leonid A.; Steinberg, Avraham. Is the patient's right to die evolving into a duty to die?: Medical decision making and ethical evaluations in health care. *Journal of Evaluation in Clinical Practice.* 1997 Feb; 3(1): 69–75. 49 refs. BE59069.
> *allowing to die; coercion; conflict of interest; *decision making; dissent; economics; family members; *futility; managed care programs; moral obligations; obligations to society; patient advocacy; patients; physician patient relationship; *physicians; *prolongation of life; resource

allocation; right to die; treatment refusal; trends; values; wedge argument; withholding treatment; *duty to die; United States

Stead, Eugene A. Cognitive brain death: the major ethical issue of our time. [Editorial]. *Journal of the Medical Association of Georgia.* 1990 Nov; 79(11): 814–815. BE55641.
> *aged; *allowing to die; brain; brain death; *brain pathology; decision making; *dementia; economics; family members; nursing homes; quality of health care; standards; *withholding treatment; personal financing; United States

Stell, Lance K. Physician–assisted suicide: to decriminalize or legalize, that is the question. *In:* Battin, Margaret P.; Rhodes, Rosamond; Silvers, Anita, eds. Physician Assisted Suicide: Expanding the Debate. New York, NY: Routledge; 1998: 225–251. 49 fn. ISBN 0–415–92003–5. BE58791.
> *allowing to die; *assisted suicide; autonomy; competence; criminal law; ethical analysis; government regulation; *intention; *killing; *legal aspects; *moral policy; physician patient relationship; physician's role; *physicians; policy analysis; *public policy; right to die; state interest; *suicide; Supreme Court decisions; terminally ill; treatment refusal; withholding treatment; Cruzan v. Director, Missouri Department of Health; United States; Vacco v. Quill; Washington v. Glucksberg

Strain, James J.; Snyder, Stephen L.; Drooker, Martin. Conflict resolution: experience of consultation–liaison psychiatrists. *In:* Zucker, Marjorie B.; Zucker, Howard D., eds. Medical Futility and the Evaluation of Life–Sustaining Interventions. New York, NY: Cambridge University Press; 1997: 98–109. 8 refs. ISBN 0–521–56877–3. BE55983.
> *allowing to die; caring; case studies; decision making; *dissent; emotions; *family members; *futility; goals; mediation; motivation; patient care team; patient transfer; *patients; *physician patient relationship; *physicians; professional family relationship; *prolongation of life; psychiatric diagnosis; *psychiatry; psychological stress; *psychology; *referral and consultation; refusal to treat; resource allocation; retreatment; terminal care; *treatment refusal; trust; guilt; health services misuse; patient abandonment; United States

Stryker, Jeff. Ethical issues in treating competent patients with HIV disease. *In:* Cohen, P.T.; Sande, Merle A.; Volberding, Paul A., eds. The AIDS Knowledge Base: A Textbook on HIV Disease from the University of California, San Francisco, and the San Francisco General Hospital. Second Edition. Boston, MA: Little, Brown; 1994: 11.2–1 to 11.2–5. 19 refs. ISBN 0–316–77067–1. BE56641.
> advance directives; *AIDS; *allowing to die; *assisted suicide; communication; compassion; competence; *decision making; depressive disorder; drug abuse; futility; HIV seropositivity; homosexuals; intensive care units; *palliative care; *patient participation; patients; physicians; *prolongation of life; resuscitation orders; socioeconomic factors; *suicide; *terminally ill; treatment refusal; ventilators; withholding treatment; United States

Sullivan, Lucy G. Euthanasia: wrong problem, wrong answer. *Medical Journal of Australia.* 1996 Nov 18; 165(10): 558–560. 21 refs. BE57360.
> active euthanasia; aged; *allowing to die; *decision making; family members; futility; guidelines; legal aspects; *paralysis; *persistent vegetative state; physically disabled; physicians; public participation; quality of life; suicide; terminally ill; treatment refusal; value of life; withholding treatment; *quadriplegia

---

BE = bioethics accession number   fn. = footnotes   refs. = references

Teno, Joan M.; Licks, Sandra; Lynn, Joanne, et al. Do advance directives provide instructions that direct care? [For the SUPPORT Investigators]. *Journal of the American Geriatrics Society.* 1997 Apr; 45(4): 508–512. 12 refs. BE57123.

> *advance directives; *allowing to die; biomedical technologies; *communication; *critically ill; *decision making; *evaluation; evaluation studies; hospitals; living wills; medical records; patient care; prognosis; prolongation of life; third party consent; treatment refusal; *seriously ill; *Study to Understand Prognoses and Preferences for Outcomes and Risks of Treatments (SUPPORT); United States

Thomasma, David C. Ensuring a good death. *Bioethics Forum.* 1997 Winter; 13(4): 7–17. 50 refs. BE58913.

> active euthanasia; advance directives; *allowing to die; assisted suicide; attitudes to death; autonomy; biomedical technologies; double effect; economics; family members; *moral obligations; pain; palliative care; patients' rights; *physicians; *prolongation of life; *suffering; *terminal care; terminally ill; value of life; withholding treatment; United States

Tripp, Glenn; McCotter, Patricia I. Ethics committee consultation: a case. *HEC (HealthCare Ethics Committee) Forum.* 1997 Dec; 9(4): 389–392. BE58090.

> *allowing to die; brain pathology; cancer; case studies; *clinical ethics committees; competence; *critically ill; *decision making; *ethicist's role; hospitals; legal aspects; legal guardians; palliative care; prognosis; resuscitation orders; third party consent; time factors

Our hospital's Medical Ethics Committee (HEC) is routinely asked by attending physicians for advice regarding the ethical approach to difficult treatment decisions in patient care. As a result of several recent cases, the HEC is reevaluating its role during *ad hoc* consultations. At issue is whether the HEC should function in an advisory capacity only, or upon request, as a surrogate decisionmaker when urgent medical treatment decisions are needed.

Trnobranski, Philippa H. The decision to prolong life: ethical perspectives of a clinical dilemma. *Journal of Clinical Nursing.* 1996 Jul; 5(4): 233–240. 28 refs. BE56888.

> active euthanasia; *allowing to die; *decision making; ethical theory; extraordinary treatment; health personnel; legal aspects; moral policy; persistent vegetative state; personhood; professional ethics; *prolongation of life; quality of life; resource allocation; terminally ill; value of life; withholding treatment; Airedale NHS Trust v. Bland; Great Britain

Ubel, Peter A.; Asch, David A. Semantic and moral debates about hastening death: a survey of bioethicists. *Journal of Clinical Ethics.* 1997 Fall; 8(3): 242–249. 24 fn. BE57617.

> *active euthanasia; *allowing to die; artificial feeding; *assisted suicide; *attitudes; case studies; competence; *consensus; *dissent; *double effect; *drugs; *ethicists; family members; intention; involuntary euthanasia; killing; *moral policy; *morality; pain; palliative care; physicians; survey; *terminology; third party consent; treatment refusal; ventilators; *voluntary euthanasia; *withholding treatment; American Association of Bioethics; United States

Uhlmann, Michael M., ed. Last Rights? Assisted Suicide and Euthanasia Debated. Washington, DC: Ethics and Public Policy Center; Grand Rapids, MI: W.B. Eerdmans; 1998. 667 p. 511 fn. ISBN 0-8028-4199-6. BE57202.

> *active euthanasia; *allowing to die; *assisted suicide; attitudes to death; autonomy; Christian ethics; coercion; compassion; competence; double effect; drugs; freedom; government regulation; historical aspects; intention; Jewish ethics; killing; legal aspects; medical ethics; model legislation; *moral policy; morality; natural law; pain; personhood; philosophy; physician's role; physicians; quality of life; review; *right to die; Roman Catholic ethics; state interest; suffering; *suicide; Supreme Court decisions; theology; treatment refusal; utilitarianism; value of life; vulnerable populations; wedge argument; withholding treatment; rationality; Western World; American Medical Association; Netherlands; United States; Vacco v. Quill; Washington v. Glucksberg

van der Maas, Paul J. End of life decisions in mentally disabled people: protecting vulnerable life does not mean prolonging it regardless of suffering. [Editorial]. *BMJ (British Medical Journal).* 1997 Jul 12; 315(7100): 73. 10 refs. BE55597.

> *active euthanasia; *allowing to die; *decision making; drugs; *mentally retarded; patient care team; *physicians; statistics; *terminally ill; withholding treatment; *Netherlands

van Thiel, G.J.M.W.; van Delden, J.J.M.; de Haan, K., et al. Retrospective study of doctors' "end of life decisions" in caring for mentally handicapped people in institutions in the Netherlands. *BMJ (British Medical Journal).* 1997 Jul 12; 315(7100): 88–91. 8 refs. BE55583.

> *active euthanasia; *allowing to die; communication; competence; *decision making; drugs; family members; *institutionalized persons; *mentally retarded; mortality; motivation; nurses; *palliative care; *physicians; referral and consultation; statistics; suffering; survey; *terminal care; *terminally ill; withholding treatment; retrospective studies; *Netherlands

OBJECTIVES: To gain insight into the reasons behind and the prevalence of doctors' decisions at the end of life that might hasten a patient's death ("end of life decisions") in institutions caring for mentally handicapped people in the Netherlands, and to describe important aspects of the decisions making process. DESIGN: Survey of random sample of doctors caring for mentally handicapped people by means of self completed questionnaires and structured interviews. SUBJECTS: 89 of the 101 selected doctors completed the questionnaire. 67 doctors had taken an end of life decision and were interviewed about their most recent case. MAIN OUTCOME MEASURES: Prevalence of end of life decisions; types of decisions; characteristics of patients; reasons why the decision was taken; and the decision making process. RESULTS: The 89 doctors reported 222 deaths for 1995. An end of life decision was taken in 97 cases (44%); in 75 the decision was to withdraw or withhold treatment, and in 22 it was to relieve pain or symptoms with opiates in dosages that may have shortened life. In the 67 most recent cases with an end of life decision the patients were mostly incompetent (63) and under 65 years old (51). Only two patients explicitly asked to die, but in 23 cases there had been some communication with the patient. In 60 cases the doctors discussed the decision with nursing staff and in 46 with a colleague. CONCLUSIONS: End of life decisions are an important aspect of the institutionalised care of mentally handicapped people. The proportion of such decisions in the total number of deaths is similar to that in other specialties. However, the discussion of such decisions is less open in the care of mental handicap than in other specialties. Because of distinctive features of care in this specialty an open debate about end of life decisions should not be postponed.

Veatch, Robert M. Autonomy and communitarianism: the ethics of terminal care in cross-cultural perspective. *In:*

CENTER: BE = bioethics accession number   fn. = footnotes   refs. = references

Hoshino, Kazumasa, ed. Japanese and Western Bioethics: Studies in Moral Diversity. Boston, MA: Kluwer Academic; 1997: 119–129. 36 refs. 2 fn. ISBN 0-7923-4112-0. BE57087.

advance directives; *allowing to die; *autonomy; Christian ethics; common good; *communitarianism; comparative studies; *competence; constitutional law; critically ill; *cultural pluralism; *decision making; family members; freedom; historical aspects; international aspects; medical ethics; moral obligations; paternalism; patients; patients' rights; physicians; privacy; prolongation of life; refusal to treat; secularism; *terminally ill; third party consent; treatment refusal; withholding treatment; liberalism; Western World; Hippocratic Oath; Japan; *United States

Veatch, Robert M., ed. The ethics of death and dying. *In:* Jonsen, Albert R.; Veatch, Robert M.; Walters, LeRoy, eds. Source Book in Bioethics: A Documentary History. Washington, DC: Georgetown University Press; 1998: 111–252. 14 fn. ISBN 0-87840-683-2. BE57891.

adults; advisory committees; age factors; *allowing to die; anencephaly; artificial feeding; attitudes to death; brain death; competence; *determination of death; family members; federal government; futility; government regulation; guidelines; historical aspects; *legal aspects; mentally disabled; model legislation; moral policy; newborns; persistent vegetative state; prolongation of life; public policy; standards; state government; third party consent; ventilators; *Cruzan v. Director, Missouri Department of Health; *In re Baby K; *In re Conroy; *In re Quinlan; Natural Death Act (CA); *President's Commission for the Study of Ethical Problems; *Superintendent v. Saikewicz; *Twentieth Century; *United States

Warren, Mary Anne. Euthanasia and the moral status of human beings. *In: her*: Moral Status: Obligations to Persons and Other Living Things. New York, NY: Oxford University Press; 1997: 185–200. 13 fn. ISBN 0-19-823668-9. BE56997.

*active euthanasia; adults; advance directives; *allowing to die; anencephaly; *assisted suicide; brain death; children; coercion; competence; *euthanasia; *human rights; *involuntary euthanasia; killing; legal aspects; *moral obligations; *moral policy; newborns; persistent vegetative state; prolongation of life; public policy; quality of life; suffering; suicide; terminally ill; terminology; third party consent; treatment refusal; *value of life; *voluntary euthanasia; Netherlands; United States

Wellman, Carl. The inalienable right to life and the durable power of attorney. Law and Philosophy. 1995; 14(2): 245–269. BE55598.

*advance directives; *allowing to die; communication; decision making; *freedom; informed consent; killing; legal rights; moral obligations; *moral policy; patient care; physicians; privacy; prolongation of life; right to die; *rights; third party consent; *treatment refusal; *value of life; withholding treatment

Williams, Christopher J.; Pieri, Lorenzo; Sims, Andrew, et al. Does palliative care have a role in treatment of anorexia nervosa? We should strive to keep patients alive [and] Palliative care does not mean giving up. BMJ (British Medical Journal). 1998 Jul 18; 317(7152): 195–197. 10 refs. BE58817.

*allowing to die; artificial feeding; *behavior disorders; chronically ill; competence; depressive disorder; drugs; force feeding; hospices; hospitals; *palliative care; *patient care; prognosis; *prolongation of life; terminally ill; treatment refusal; *anorexia nervosa; opiates

Wise, Jacqui. When life saving treatment should be withdrawn in children. [News]. BMJ (British Medical

Journal). 1997 Oct 4; 315(7112): 834. BE56060.

*allowing to die; brain death; *children; communication; *decision making; disabled; *organizational policies; palliative care; parental consent; persistent vegetative state; physicians; professional organizations; prognosis; prolongation of life; *standards; suffering; withholding treatment; *Great Britain; *Royal College of Paediatrics and Child Health

Zeman, Adam. Persistent vegetative state. Lancet. 1997 Sep 13; 350(9080): 795–799. 64 refs. BE56321.

allowing to die; brain death; brain pathology; diagnosis; paralysis; patient care; *persistent vegetative state; *prognosis; terminology; time factors; treatment outcome; uncertainty; coma

Zoloth-Dorfman, Laurie; Rubin, Susan B. "Medical futility": managed care and the powerful new vocabulary for clinical and public policy discourse. Healthcare Forum Journal. 1997 Mar–Apr; 40(2): 28, 30–33. BE57057.

AIDS; allowing to die; biomedical technologies; case studies; clinical ethics committees; costs and benefits; cultural pluralism; *decision making; dissent; family members; *futility; *goals; health facilities; institutional policies; justice; *managed care programs; medicine; patient care team; persistent vegetative state; physicians; practice guidelines; *prolongation of life; public policy; *resource allocation; terminally ill; *values; *withholding treatment; evidence-based medicine; United States

Zucker, Marjorie B.; Zucker, Howard D., eds. Medical Futility and the Evaluation of Life-Sustaining Interventions. New York, NY: Cambridge University Press; 1997. 201 p. 332 refs. 14 fn. ISBN 0-521-56877-3. BE55973.

advance directives; aged; *allowing to die; alternative therapies; attitudes to death; autonomy; children; clinical ethics committees; common good; communication; consensus; cultural pluralism; *decision making; *dissent; economics; family members; *futility; guidelines; intensive care units; judicial action; legal aspects; legislation; medicine; newborns; nursing homes; *palliative care; patients; physicians; professional autonomy; *prolongation of life; psychiatry; public participation; referral and consultation; refusal to treat; religion; resource allocation; resuscitation orders; *terminal care; terminology; treatment outcome; values; vulnerable populations; withholding treatment; community policies; United States

Doctors not obliged to accede to patients' requests to die. [BMA Annual Meeting, July 1998]. BMJ (British Medical Journal). 1998 Jul 18; 317(7152): 217–218. BE58512.

*allowing to die; autonomy; moral obligations; organizational policies; palliative care; *physicians; professional organizations; right to die; treatment refusal; British Medical Association; Great Britain

Philosophers reflect on suicide. [Editorial]. America. 1997 Apr 5; 176(11): 3. BE56235.

*allowing to die; *assisted suicide; attitudes; competence; drugs; ethicists; legal aspects; moral policy; *physicians; public policy; terminally ill; withholding treatment; United States

ALLOWING TO DIE/ATTITUDES

Asai, Atsushi; Fukuhara, Shunichi; Inoshita, Osamu, et al. Medical decisions concerning the end of life: a discussion with Japanese physicians. Journal of Medical Ethics. 1997 Oct; 23(5): 323–327. 5 refs. BE57101.

*advance directives; *allowing to die; *attitudes; cancer; *decision making; diagnosis; family members; knowledge, attitudes, practice; organizational policies; *physicians;

BE = bioethics accession number   fn. = footnotes   refs. = references

professional organizations; prognosis; *prolongation of life; *resuscitation; resuscitation orders; survey; *terminally ill; *truth disclosure; *withholding treatment; patient abandonment; qualitative research; *Japan; Japan Medical Association

OBJECTIVES: Life–sustaining treatment at the end of life gives rise to many ethical problems in Japan. Recent surveys of Japanese physicians suggested that they tend to treat terminally ill patients aggressively. We studied why Japanese physicians were reluctant to withhold or withdraw life–support from terminally ill patients and what affected their decisions. DESIGN AND PARTICIPANTS: A qualitative study design was employed, using a focus group interview with seven physicians, to gain an in–depth understanding of attitudes and rationales in Japan regarding medical care at the end of life. RESULTS: Analysis revealed that physicians and patients' family members usually make decisions about life–sustaining treatment, while the patients' wishes are unavailable or not taken into account. Both physicians and family members tend to consider withholding or withdrawing life–sustaining treatment as abandonment or even killing. The strongest reason to start cardiopulmonary resuscitation –– and to continue it until patients' family members arrive –– seems to be the family members' desire to be at the bedside at the time of death. All physicians participating in our study regarded advance directives that provide information as to patients' wishes about life–sustaining treatment desirable. All expressed concern, however, that it would be difficult to forego or discontinue life–support based on a patient's advance directive, particularly when the patient's family opposed the directive. CONCLUSION: Our group interview suggested several possible barriers to death with dignity and the appropriate use of advance directives in Japan. Further qualitative and quantitative research in this regard is needed.

Asch, David A.; Hansen–Flaschen, John; Lanken, Paul N. Decisions to limit or continue life–sustaining treatment by critical care physicians in the United States: conflicts between physicians' practices and patients' wishes. *American Journal of Respiratory and Critical Care Medicine.* 1995 Feb; 151(2, Pt. 1): 288–292. 35 refs. BE56549.
    adults; age factors; *allowing to die; artificial feeding; *attitudes; *decision making; *dissent; evaluation studies; family members; *futility; informed consent; intensive care units; internal medicine; motivation; paternalism; *patients; *physicians; prognosis; *prolongation of life; renal dialysis; statistics; survey; third party consent; treatment refusal; ventilators; *withholding treatment; United States

Berger, Douglas; Fukunishi, Isao; O'Dowd, Mary Alice, et al. A comparison of Japanese and American psychiatrists' attitudes towards patients wishing to die in the general hospital. *Psychotherapy and Psychosomatics.* 1997; 66(6): 319–328. 27 refs. BE59010.
    *active euthanasia; *allowing to die; *assisted suicide; *attitudes; comparative studies; competence; depressive disorder; hospitals; international aspects; mental health; motivation; *physicians; *psychiatry; quality of life; referral and consultation; right to die; suicide; survey; terminally ill; treatment refusal; truth disclosure; values; *voluntary euthanasia; rationality; *Japan; *United States

Berger, Douglas; Takahashi, Yoshitomo; Fukunishi, Isao, et al. Japanese psychiatrists' attitudes toward patients wishing to die in the general hospital: a cultural perspective. *Cambridge Quarterly of Healthcare Ethics.* 1997 Fall; 6(4): 470–479. 44 fn. BE56456.
    active euthanasia; *allowing to die; *assisted suicide;

*attitudes; competence; *depressive disorder; *euthanasia; family members; family relationship; hospitals; patients; persistent vegetative state; *physicians; prolongation of life; *psychiatric diagnosis; *psychiatry; *quality of life; resuscitation orders; *right to die; suffering; *suicide; survey; terminally ill; third party consent; treatment refusal; voluntary euthanasia; withholding treatment; rationality; *Japan

Brody, Baruch. Medical futility: philosophical reflections on death. *In:* Hoshino, Kazumasa, ed. Japanese and Western Bioethics: Studies in Moral Diversity. Boston, MA: Kluwer Academic; 1997: 135–144. 10 refs. ISBN 0–7923–4112–0. BE57089.
    advance directives; *allowing to die; *attitudes; *attitudes to death; biomedical technologies; competence; consensus; *decision making; dissent; family members; *futility; legal rights; patients; physicians; *prolongation of life; refusal to treat; risks and benefits; terminally ill; third party consent; treatment refusal; value of life; values; withholding treatment; United States

Crain, Madeleine. A cross–cultural study of beliefs, attitudes and values in Chinese–born American and non–Chinese frail homebound elderly. *Journal Of Long Term Home Health Care.* 1996 Winter; 15(1): 9–18. 25 refs. BE58902.
    *aged; *allowing to die; *Asian Americans; *attitudes; *attitudes to death; comparative studies; *cultural pluralism; decision making; health; home care; quality of life; survey; *values; *whites; New York City

Gross, Mortimer D. What do patients express as their preferences in advance directives? *Archives of Internal Medicine.* 1998 Feb 23; 158(4): 363–365. 16 refs. BE57960.
    *advance directives; *allowing to die; artificial feeding; *attitudes; *decision making; hospitals; institutionalized persons; living wills; *patients; *prolongation of life; resuscitation orders; risks and benefits; survey; treatment refusal; coma; outpatients; Illinois

BACKGROUND: Since the passage of the Patient Self–Determination Act in 1991, there has been interest in urging patients to execute advance directives (ADs) for medical care. There are not much data, however, as to what the ADs that patients execute actually specify. I have investigated the percentage of inpatients and outpatients who are admitted to a community hospital who have executed ADs, and I have tabulated what preferences are actually expressed in the ADs that are in hospital records. METHODS: A questionnaire is filled out by each patient admitted to this hospital, and their response recorded as to whether they have executed an AD. I have tabulated these responses for inpatients and outpatients for the calendar year 1994. I have also examined the ADs in all available hospital records, and tabulated the wishes expressed in these directives. RESULTS: For inpatient admissions during the calendar year 1994, of 8727 questionnaires completed, 11% of patients indicated that they had executed an AD. For outpatients, the corresponding figures are 22,966 and 15%. A total of 343 hospital records containing ADs were examined. Of these, 15 were nonmedical directives and were excluded. Of the 328 medical ADs, 86 (26%) were living wills, expressing the wish that if the individual had an incurable disease or irreversible injury that he or she not be given any treatment that would only delay death. There were 210 power of attorney for health care forms completed; these were 64% of all the medical ADs. Of these, 7 did not specify any preference that patients wanted their proxy to follow. The remaining 203 forms were divided as follows: 189 individuals requested that they did not want life–sustaining treatment if the burdens of treatment

---

BE = bioethics accession number   fn. = footnotes   refs. = references

outweighed the expected benefits; 12 wanted their lives to be prolonged unless they were in an irreversible coma; and 2 wanted their lives to be prolonged to the greatest possible extent regardless of the chances for recovery or the cost. There were 32 do not resuscitate forms executed exclusively by residents of nursing homes that specified that they did not want cardiopulmonary resuscitation or artificial feeding. CONCLUSIONS: The overwhelming desire expressed by the patients in the ADs was not to have their lives prolonged if their medical condition were such that treatment would merely delay death. Only a minuscule number of patients, less than 0.7%, wanted everything done to prolong life regardless of the chance for improvement or the cost. Because such a small percentage of patients have ADs, it is recommended that each hospital appoint a committee on ADs to do everything possible to encourage patients to execute an AD. A second mission of this committee would be to do everything possible to encourage physicians to pay close attention to their patients' wishes for medical care at the end of life.

Grubb, Andrew; Walsh, Pat; Lambe, Neil, et al. Doctors' Views on the Management of Patients in Persistent Vegetative State (PVS): A UK Study. London: Kings College London, Centre of Medical Law and Ethics; 1997. 68 p. (Occasional papers series; 1). 175 fn. ISBN 1-898484-20-1. BE59108.
advance directives; age factors; *allowing to die; artificial feeding; *attitudes; brain pathology; comparative studies; *decision making; diagnosis; drugs; family members; home care; hospitals; knowledge, attitudes, practice; legal aspects; medical specialties; nursing homes; *patient care; patient care team; *persistent vegetative state; *physicians; prognosis; quality of life; rehabilitation; resource allocation; *selection for treatment; statistics; surgery; survey; terminology; time factors; treatment outcome; *withholding treatment; antibiotics; questionnaires; Airedale NHS Trust v. Bland; *Great Britain

Hassan, Riaz. Euthanasia and the medical profession: an Australian study. *Australian Journal of Social Issues.* 1996 Aug; 31(3): 239-252. 12 refs. BE58274.
*active euthanasia; *allowing to die; *assisted suicide; *attitudes; family members; *knowledge, attitudes, practice; legal aspects; motivation; patients; *physicians; survey; *voluntary euthanasia; *Australia; Netherlands; *South Australia

Huber, Ruth; Evans, Virginia Cox. Trust in physicians to honor death related instructions. *Omega: A Journal of Death and Dying.* 1997-1998; 36(1): 9-21. 39 refs. BE57720.
*advance directives; age factors; *aged; *allowing to die; assisted suicide; attitudes to death; comparative studies; *decision making; *institutionalized persons; *knowledge, attitudes, practice; *physician patient relationship; *physicians; *prolongation of life; *public opinion; residential facilities; *right to die; survey; *terminal care; treatment refusal; *trust; voluntary euthanasia; Kentucky

Hui, Elsie; Ho, Suzanne C.; Tsang, June, et al. Attitudes toward life-sustaining treatment of older persons in Hong Kong. *Journal of the American Geriatrics Society.* 1997 Oct; 45(10): 1232-1236. 27 refs. BE56464.
age factors; *aged; *allowing to die; *attitudes; biomedical technologies; *decision making; disclosure; females; *hospitals; knowledge, attitudes, practice; *patients; *prolongation of life; *residential facilities; *resuscitation; resuscitation orders; single persons; survey; treatment outcome; treatment refusal; *Hong Kong

O'Brien, Linda A.; Siegert, Elisabeth A.; Grisso, Jeane

Ann, et al. Tube feeding preferences among nursing home residents. *Journal of General Internal Medicine.* 1997 Jun; 12(6): 364-371. 38 refs. BE58361.
advance directives; *aged; *allowing to die; *artificial feeding; *attitudes; blacks; brain pathology; communication; decision making; family members; females; health personnel; institutionalized persons; males; *nursing homes; *patient care; *patients; persistent vegetative state; physical restraint; *prolongation of life; survey; treatment refusal; whites; withholding treatment; Delaware; New Jersey; Pennsylvania

Parkash, Ravi; Burge, Frederick. The family's perspective on issues of hydration in terminal care. *Journal of Palliative Care.* 1997 Winter; 13(4): 23-27. 16 refs. BE58823.
*allowing to die; *artificial feeding; *attitudes; cancer; decision making; emotions; *family members; *palliative care; risks and benefits; suffering; survey; *terminal care; terminally ill; values; withholding treatment; *dehydration; qualitative research; Nova Scotia

Sansone, Paulette; Phillips, Michael. Advance directives for elderly people: worthwhile cause or wasted effort? *Social Work.* 1995 May; 40(3): 397-401. 16 refs. BE55580.
*advance directives; *aged; *allowing to die; artificial feeding; *attitudes; cancer; *communication; comparative studies; consensus; dementia; drugs; evaluation studies; *family members; Jews; knowledge, attitudes, practice; living wills; nursing homes; *prolongation of life; renal dialysis; residential facilities; Roman Catholics; social workers; survey; third party consent; withholding treatment; coma; professional role; New York City

Schneiderman, Lawrence J.; Kaplan, Robert M.; Rosenberg, Esther, et al. Do physicians' own preferences for life-sustaining treatment influence their perceptions of patients' preferences? A second look. *Cambridge Quarterly of Healthcare Ethics.* 1997 Spring; 6(2): 131-137. 18 refs. BE56437.
advance directives; AIDS; *allowing to die; *attitudes; biomedical technologies; brain pathology; cancer; comparative studies; *consensus; *decision making; evaluation studies; pain; *patients; physician patient relationship; *physicians; prognosis; *prolongation of life; quality of life; survey; terminally ill; *third party consent; treatment refusal; values; withholding treatment; coma; California; University of California, San Diego Medical Center
Previous studies have documented the fallibility of attempts by surrogates and physicians to act in a substituted judgment capacity and predict end-of-life treatment decisions on behalf of patients. We previously reported that physicians misperceive their patients' preferences and substitute their own preferences for those of their patients with respect to four treatments: cardiopulmonary resuscitation (CPR) in the event of cardiac arrest, ventilator for an indefinite period of time, medical nutrition and hydration for an indefinite period of time, and hospitalization in the event of pneumonia. This paper extends our previous observations and reports on a different and larger population of subjects, employing a more detailed procedure-oriented advance directive instrument as well as a quality-of-life questionnaire. Our hypothesis remains the same, namely, that physicians' predictions of their patients' end-of-life treatment choices are closer to the choices they would make for themselves than to the choices expressed by their patients. Since physicians are the ones who ultimately exercise control over these important decisions, any unrecognized projection of personal preferences onto their patients would raise serious concerns about physicians acting in a substituted judgment capacity. It would also emphasize the

---

BE = bioethics accession number   fn. = footnotes   refs. = references

importance of patients choosing surrogate decisionmakers carefully and, even more important, explicating clearly their directive instructions as part of advance care planning.

Steiber, Steven R. Right to die: public balks at deciding for others. *Hospitals.* 1987 Mar 5; 61(5): 72. BE56669.
   age factors; *allowing to die; family members; females; hospitals; living wills; males; persistent vegetative state; *public opinion; *right to die; third party consent; treatment refusal; withholding treatment; Gallup poll; *United States

Sullivan, Mark; Rapp, Suzanne; Fitzgibbon, Dermot, et al. Pain and the choice to hasten death in patients with painful metastatic cancer. *Journal of Palliative Care.* 1997 Autumn; 13(3): 18–28. 34 refs. BE58070.
   *active euthanasia; *allowing to die; artificial feeding; *assisted suicide; *attitudes; *cancer; depressive disorder; double effect; drugs; hospitals; living wills; *pain; *palliative care; *patients; physicians; *quality of life; resuscitation orders; right to die; suicide; survey; *terminal care; *terminally ill; treatment refusal; values; voluntary euthanasia; withholding treatment; analgesia; outpatients; United States; University of Washington Medical Center

Sulmasy, Daniel P.; Terry, Peter B.; Weisman, Carol S., et al. The accuracy of substituted judgments in patients with terminal diagnoses. *Annals of Internal Medicine.* 1998 Apr 15; 128(8): 621–629. 34 refs. BE57916.
   age factors; allowing to die; *attitudes; comparative studies; *consensus; *decision making; dementia; *evaluation; evaluation studies; *family members; *patients; prognosis; *prolongation of life; resuscitation; socioeconomic factors; *terminal care; *terminally ill; *third party consent; ventilators; coma; Baltimore; District of Columbia
BACKGROUND: Patients' loved ones often make end-of-life treatment decisions, but the accuracy of their substituted judgments and the factors associated with accuracy are poorly understood. OBJECTIVE: To assess the accuracy of judgments made by surrogate decision makers; ascertain the beliefs, practices, and clinical and sociodemographic factors associated with accuracy of surrogates' decisions; assess the preferences of patients for life-sustaining treatments; and compare differences in accuracy across diagnoses. DESIGN: Cross-sectional paired interviews. SETTING: Outpatient practices of three university hospitals. PATIENTS: 250 patients with terminal diagnoses of congestive heart failure, AIDS, amyotrophic lateral sclerosis, lung cancer, and chronic obstructive pulmonary disease (50 patient–surrogate pairs in each group) and 50 general medical patients and their surrogates. MEASUREMENTS: The accuracy of surrogate predictions was measured by using scales based on 10 potential treatments in each of three hypothetical clinical scenarios. RESULTS: Preferences varied according to mode of treatment and scenario. On average, surrogates made correct predictions in 66% of instances. Accuracy was better for the permanent coma scenario than for the scenarios of severe dementia or coma with a small chance of recovery (P less than 0.001). In a binary logit model, the accuracy of substituted judgments was positively associated with the patient having spoken with the surrogate about end-of-life issues (odds ratio [OR], 1.9 [95% CI, 1.6 to 2.3]), the patient having private insurance (OR, 1.4 [CI, 1.1 to 1.7]), the surrogate's level of education (OR, 1.5 [CI, 1.2 to 1.9]), and the patient's level of education (OR, 1.7 [CI, 1.4 to 2.2]). Accuracy was negatively associated with the patient's belief that he or she would live longer than 10 years (OR, 0.6 [CI, 0.5 to 0.7]), surrogate experience

with life-sustaining treatment (OR, 0.4 [CI, 0.3 to 0.5]), surrogate participation in religious services (OR, 0.67 [CI, 0.50 to 0.91]), and a diagnosis of heart failure (OR, 0.6 [CI, 0.5 to 0.8]). Age, ethnicity, marital status, religion, and advance directives were not associated with accuracy. CONCLUSIONS: The accuracy of substituted judgments is associated with multiple clinically apparent patient and surrogate factors. This information can help clinicians identify conditions under which substituted judgments are likely to be accurate or inaccurate and can help target populations for education designed to improve the accuracy of surrogate decision making.

Walker, Gail C. The right to die: healthcare workers' attitudes compared with a national public poll. *Omega: A Journal of Death and Dying.* 1997; 35(4): 339–345. 4 refs. BE57722.
   *active euthanasia; advance directives; *allowing to die; *attitudes; autonomy; clinical ethics committees; comparative studies; competence; congenital disorders; *decision making; drugs; family members; hospitals; newborns; *nurses; pain; palliative care; parents; patients; *public opinion; quality of life; *right to die; suffering; *suicide; survey; terminally ill; third party consent; treatment refusal; withholding treatment; dependency; New York; Times Mirror Center; United States

Weeks, Jane C.; Cook, E. Francis; O'Day, Steven J., et al. Relationship between cancer patients' predictions of prognosis and their treatment preferences. *JAMA.* 1998 Jun 3; 279(21): 1709–1714. 31 refs. BE58433.
   adults; *allowing to die; *attitudes; *cancer; comparative studies; comprehension; *decision making; evaluation studies; hospitals; mortality; *palliative care; patient participation; *patients; physicians; *prognosis; *prolongation of life; risk; survey; *terminal care; *terminally ill; treatment outcome; truth disclosure; teaching hospitals; Study to Understand Prognoses and Preferences for Outcomes and Risks of Treatments (SUPPORT); United States
CONTEXT: Previous studies have documented that cancer patients tend to overestimate the probability of long-term survival. If patient preferences about the trade-offs between the risks and benefits associated with alternative treatment strategies are based on inaccurate perceptions of prognosis, then treatment choices may not reflect each patient's true values. OBJECTIVE: To test the hypothesis that among terminally ill cancer patients an accurate understanding of prognosis is associated with a preference for therapy that focuses on comfort over attempts at life extension. DESIGN: Prospective cohort study. SETTING: Five teaching hospitals in the United States. PATIENTS: A total of 917 adults hospitalized with stage III or IV non–small cell lung cancer or colon cancer metastatic to liver in phases 1 and 2 of the Study to Understand Prognoses and Preferences for Outcomes and Risks of Treatments (SUPPORT). MAIN OUTCOME MEASURES: Proportion of patients favoring life-extending therapy over therapy focusing on relief of pain and discomfort, patient and physician estimates of the probability of 6-month survival, and actual 6-month survival. RESULTS: Patients who thought they were going to live for at least 6 months were more likely (odds ratio [OR], 2.6; 95% confidence interval [CI], 1.8–3.7) to favor life-extending therapy over comfort care compared with patients who thought there was at least a 10% chance that they would not live 6 months. This OR was highest (8.5; 95% CI, 3.0–24.0) among patients who estimated their 6-month survival probability at greater than 90% but whose physicians estimated it at 10% or less. Patients overestimated their chances of surviving 6 months, while

---

BE = bioethics accession number   fn. = footnotes   refs. = references

physicians estimated prognosis quite accurately. Patients who preferred life–extending therapy were more likely to undergo aggressive treatment, but controlling for known prognostic factors, their 6–month survival was no better. CONCLUSIONS: Patients with metastatic colon and lung cancer overestimate their survival probabilities and these estimates may influence their preferences about medical therapies.

Wurzbach, Mary Ellen. Long–term care nurses' ethical convictions about tube feeding. *Western Journal of Nursing Research.* 1996 Feb; 18(1): 63–76. 27 refs. BE56898.
> aged; *allowing to die; *artificial feeding; *attitudes; decision making; education; family members; *knowledge, attitudes, practice; *long–term care; *nurses; nursing homes; physicians; survey; *uncertainty; withholding treatment; qualitative research; Wisconsin

ALLOWING TO DIE/INFANTS

American Academy of Pediatrics. Committee on Bioethics. Ethics and the care of critically ill infants and children. *Pediatrics.* 1996 Jul; 98(1): 149–152. 58 refs. BE55656.
> *allowing to die; children; congenital disorders; *critically ill; *decision making; federal government; futility; government regulation; *infants; *intensive care units; legal aspects; low birth weight; *newborns; *organizational policies; *parents; *patient care; *pediatrics; *physicians; prematurity; professional organizations; prognosis; *prolongation of life; public policy; resource allocation; selection for treatment; terminally ill; treatment outcome; uncertainty; withholding treatment; *American Academy of Pediatrics; United States

American Association on Mental Deficiency; Association for Persons with Severe Handicaps; American Association of University Affiliated Programs for the Developmentally Disabled; et al. Brief of Amici Curiae in Support of Petitioner: Margaret M. Heckler v. American Hospital Association, No. 84–1529, on Writ of Certiorari to the U.S. Court of Appeals for the Second Circuit. Washington, DC: Filed in the Supreme Court of the United States, October term, 1985; 1985. 27 p. 44 fn. BE57849.
> *allowing to die; *congenital disorders; decision making; *disabled; Down syndrome; federal government; *government regulation; *legal aspects; legal rights; mentally retarded; *newborns; professional organizations; *quality of life; selection for treatment; *social discrimination; value of life; withholding treatment; Child Abuse Amendments 1984; *Heckler v. American Hospital Association; Rehabilitation Act 1973; United States

Brawn, W.J.; De Giovanni, J.V.; Hutchinson, S., et al. Hypoplastic left heart syndrome. [Letters]. *BMJ (British Medical Journal).* 1997 May 10; 314(7091): 1414. 4 refs. BE56855.
> *allowing to die; *congenital disorders; *decision making; diagnosis; disabled; *heart diseases; mortality; *newborns; *palliative care; *parents; prenatal diagnosis; prognosis; program descriptions; *quality of life; selective abortion; *surgery; terminal care; *treatment outcome; uncertainty; *Great Britain; New York

Caniano, Donna A.; Hazebroek, Frans W.J.; DenBesten, Karen E., et al. End–of–life decisions for surgical neonates: experience in the Netherlands and United States. *Journal of Pediatric Surgery.* 1995 Oct; 30(10): 1420–1424. 13 refs. BE55659.
> *allowing to die; artificial feeding; chromosome abnormalities; comparative studies; *congenital disorders; *decision making; drugs; evaluation studies; futility; *intensive care units; *international aspects; mortality; *newborns; nurses; parents; physicians; *prognosis; quality of life; *resuscitation orders; *surgery; time factors; treatment outcome; ventilators; *withholding treatment; antibiotics; *Netherlands; *United States

Coon, Stephanie M.; Keyes, Denis W. Attitudes and Opinions of Preservice Professionals: Withholding Life–Sustaining Treatment from Infants with Severe Disabilities. Available from ERIC Document Reproduction Service, DYNCORP I&ET, 7420 Fullerton Rd., Suite 110, Springfield, VA 22153–2852; Document No. ED374635; EC303360; 1994 Jun 2. 55 p. 22 refs. Paper presented at the 118th Annual Meeting of the American Association on Mental Retardation, Boston, MA, 2 Jun 1994. BE57739.
> age factors; *allowing to die; *attitudes; comparative studies; *congenital disorders; decision making; disabled; education; medical education; mentally retarded; *newborns; nursing education; parents; prognosis; *prolongation of life; quality of life; *students; surgery; survey; treatment refusal; universities; *withholding treatment; College of Charleston; Medical University of South Carolina; South Carolina

Dyer, Clare. British court allows terminally ill baby to die. [News]. *BMJ (British Medical Journal).* 1997 Nov 29; 315(7120): 1398. BE57172.
> *allowing to die; decision making; *dissent; *infants; Jewish ethics; Jews; judicial action; *legal aspects; palliative care; *parents; physicians; *religion; resuscitation orders; right to die; *value of life; *ventilators; *withholding treatment; *Great Britain; *Orthodox Judaism

Dyer, Clare. Scottish inquiry vindicates decision not to resuscitate baby. [News]. *BMJ (British Medical Journal).* 1997 Jul 5; 315(7099): 9. BE56079.
> *allowing to die; *decision making; *dissent; futility; *legal aspects; low birth weight; *newborns; *parents; *physicians; *prematurity; *resuscitation; viability; withholding treatment; *al–Zidgali, Faisal; *Cassidy, Rebecca; *Great Britain; *Scotland

Fournier, Keith A.; Watkins, William D. In Defense of Life. Colorado Springs, CO: NavPress; 1996. 159 p. 352 fn. ISBN 08910–99801. BE56728.
> aborted fetuses; *abortion, induced; *active euthanasia; aged; *allowing to die; *assisted suicide; beginning of life; body parts and fluids; brain death; *Christian ethics; commodification; congenital disorders; death; determination of death; disabled; economics; eugenics; fetal tissue donation; fetuses; government regulation; health personnel; historical aspects; human experimentation; infanticide; international aspects; judicial action; *killing; legal aspects; love; *morality; *newborns; organ donation; *political activity; population control; pregnant women; psychological stress; public policy; quality of life; rights; *value of life; *values; violence; hope; Humphry, Derek; Kevorkian, Jack; *Right to Life Movement; Roe v. Wade; Smith, Susan; United States

Frader, Joel E.; Watchko, Jon. Futility issues in pediatrics. *In:* Zucker, Marjorie B.; Zucker, Howard D., eds. Medical Futility and the Evaluation of Life–Sustaining Interventions. New York, NY: Cambridge University Press; 1997: 48–57. 19 refs. ISBN 0–521–56877–3. BE55978.
> *allowing to die; *children; clinical ethics committees; communication; conflict of interest; *decision making; *dissent; economics; federal government; *futility; government regulation; hospitals; institutional policies; intensive care units; legal aspects; *newborns; *parents; *pediatrics; *physicians; *prematurity; professional family relationship; prognosis; *prolongation of life; resource allocation; socioeconomic factors; treatment outcome;

BE = bioethics accession number   fn. = footnotes   refs. = references

*uncertainty; values; viability; withholding treatment; Child Abuse Prevention and Treatment Act 1984; United States

Georgia. Court of Appeals. Velez v. Bethune. *South Eastern Reporter, 2d Series.* 1995 Dec 5 (date of decision). 466: 627–635. BE56739.

*allowing to die; *decision making; *legal aspects; *legal liability; *newborns; parental consent; *physicians; prematurity; terminally ill; ventilators; *withholding treatment; *wrongful death; Georgia; *Velez v. Bethune

The Georgia Court of Appeals overturned the lower court and allowed parents to proceed against the physician and hospital with a claim of wrongful death of their infant, whose life support was unilaterally withdrawn. Nine-day-old Mary Elizabeth Bethune had been born at twenty-four weeks and was dying due to severe prematurity. The court held that the doctor had no right to decide unilaterally to discontinue treatment, even if the infant were dying, without the consent of the parents. In the opinion of the chief judge, wrongful death includes wrongful hastening of death. (KIE abstract)

Great Britain. England. Court of Appeal, Civil Division. Re B (A Minor) (Wardship: Medical Treatment). *All England Law Reports.* 1981 Aug 7 (date of decision). [1990] 3: 927–930. BE57394.

*allowing to die; congenital disorders; *decision making; *Down syndrome; *judicial action; *legal aspects; *newborns; parents; physicians; *quality of life; refusal to treat; *surgery; third party consent; treatment refusal; *withholding treatment; *Great Britain; *Re B (A Minor) (Wardship: Medical Treatment)

The British Court of Appeal, Civil Division, allowed the appeal of the local NHS health authority and authorized life-saving surgery for a mentally retarded infant against her parents' wishes. B was born with Down syndrome and an intestinal blockage. Without an operation, she would die within days; with an operation and without other complications, her life expectancy was between 20 and 30 years. Acting in what they saw as their child's best interests, her parents refused to consent to the operation. The appellate court's decision to authorize surgery was based on the welfare of the child. The judges held that if the operation were successful the girl could live the normal life span of a Down syndrome child with the handicaps of such a child, and "it is not for this court to say that life of that description ought to be extinguished." (KIE abstract)

Great Britain. England. Court of Appeal, Civil Division. Re J (A Minor) (Wardship: Medical Treatment). *All England Law Reports.* 1992 Jun 10 (date of decision). [1992] 4: 614–626. BE58577.

*allowing to die; *brain pathology; critically ill; *decision making; *disabled; dissent; extraordinary treatment; *infants; injuries; intensive care units; *judicial action; *legal aspects; *minors; parents; patient admission; physicians; *prognosis; *prolongation of life; *ventilators; *withholding treatment; *Great Britain; National Health Service; *Re J (A Minor) (Wardship: Medical Treatment)

The Civil Division of England's Court of Appeal overturned the lower court's order of mechanical ventilation for a profoundly handicapped sixteen-month-old child against the clinical judgment of the child's doctors. Since hitting his head in a fall at age four weeks, J had not mentally developed past that time and he was blind and he suffered from severe cerebral palsy and epilepsy. He required nasogastric tubal feeding and, although he occasionally responded to sound, whether or not he recognized his caregivers was uncertain. His divorced mother and the local

authority shared parental authority over J, who resided with foster parents. The consultant pediatrician reported that if J were to suffer a life-threatening event, ordinary resuscitation, antibiotics and physiotherapy would be appropriate, but intervention with intensive measures including mechanical ventilation would be medically inappropriate. Two other specialists agreed with those findings, but another consultant found mechanical ventilation not to be cruel and thought J could be weaned from it if it became so. The mother and local health authority asked the court to require the health authority to continue all treatment, including mechanical ventilation, of J. The Official Solicitor and the health authority opposed such an order. The lower court granted an interim order requiring mechanical ventilation if necessary over the five weeks prior to the main hearing. The appellate court viewed such an order as an abuse of judicial power and held that the physician's duty to the patient is to treat with the necessary consent in accord with the best clinical judgment and that, as long as those with parental authority consent to J's treatment by the health authority, he must be treated in accord with the best clinical judgment of that authority's personnel. (KIE abstract)

Harrison, Helen. Need exists for advance directives from parents. [Letter; title supplied]. *Journal of Perinatology.* 1995 Nov–Dec; 15(6): 522. 1 ref. BE55936.

*advance directives; *allowing to die; congenital disorders; *decision making; *newborns; *parents; *physicians; *prolongation of life; psychological stress; resuscitation; withholding treatment

Howard, Philip J.; Cole, A.P.; Grassin, Marc, et al. End-of-life decisions in Dutch paediatric practice. [Letters]. *Lancet.* 1997 Sep 13; 350(9080): 816–817. 5 refs. BE57165.

*active euthanasia; *allowing to die; artificial feeding; *decision making; drugs; *infants; *intention; killing; *knowledge, attitudes, practice; legal aspects; legal liability; mandatory reporting; *newborns; parental consent; parents; *paternalism; *pediatrics; peer review; *physicians; *professional autonomy; psychological stress; referral and consultation; regulation; wedge argument; *withholding treatment; neonatology; France; Great Britain; *Netherlands; United States

Jain, Renu; Thomasma, David C.; Ragas, Rasa. Response to "Ethics and drug infants," by Michelle Oberman (*CQ* Vol. 6, No. 2): points of variance. *Cambridge Quarterly of Healthcare Ethics.* 1998 Winter; 7(1): 94–96. BE58456.

*allowing to die; child abuse; competence; congenital disorders; *decision making; disadvantaged; *dissent; *drug abuse; emotions; ethics consultation; *mothers; *newborns; parental consent; parents; *paternalism; patient advocacy; *patient compliance; physicians; pregnant women; prenatal injuries; prognosis; *prolongation of life; rehabilitation; stigmatization; treatment refusal; withholding treatment; homeless persons

Kinlaw, Kathy. Is it ethical to provide futile care? *Journal of the Medical Association of Georgia.* 1990 Nov; 79(11): 839–842. 3 refs. BE55630.

*allowing to die; communication; *decision making; dissent; extraordinary treatment; family members; *futility; legal aspects; physicians; prognosis; *prolongation of life; quality of life; suffering; terminology; values; withholding treatment; United States

Koch, Tom; Ridgley, Mark. Distanced perspectives: AIDS, anencephaly, and AHP [Analytic Hierarchy Process]. *Theoretical Medicine and Bioethics.* 1998 Jan;

19(1): 47–58. 26 fn. BE57311.
  AIDS; *allowing to die; *anencephaly; *bioethical issues; brain pathology; *decision analysis; *decision making; equal protection; *futility; infants; *law; legal aspects; medicine; models, theoretical; *newborns; *personhood; prolongation of life; *quality of life; self concept; social interaction; speciesism; *standards; value of life; ventilators; withholding treatment; In re Baby K; In re T.A.C.P.; United States

Lowenthal, Barbara; Getz, Marjorie; Kaye, Celia. The special educator and the hospital ethics committee. Available from the ERIC Document Reproduction Service, DYNCORP I&ET, 7420 Fullerton Rd., Suite 110, Springfield, VA 22153-2852; Document No. ED320338; EC231146; 1990 Feb. 40 p. 34 refs. Paper presented at the Conference of the Learning Disabilities Association, Anaheim, CA, 1990 February 21–24. BE57693.
  *allowing to die; biomedical technologies; brain death; case studies; child abuse; children; *clinical ethics committees; committee membership; *congenital disorders; *decision making; determination of death; disabled; dissent; education; *ethics consultation; federal government; government regulation; hospitals; *infants; *institutional policies; legislation; low birth weight; mentally retarded; *newborns; organ donation; parents; *patient care; persistent vegetative state; *prolongation of life; psychological stress; *quality of life; suffering; surgery; treatment refusal; *value of life; ventilators; *withholding treatment; Department of Health and Human Services; Education of the Handicapped Act Amendments 1986; *Lutheran General Hospital (Park Ridge, IL); United States

Lusthaus, Evelyn W. Involuntary euthanasia and current attempts to define persons with mental retardation as less than human. *Mental Retardation.* 1985 Jun; 23(3): 148–154. 46 refs. BE56962.
  *allowing to die; children; congenital disorders; *dehumanization; human characteristics; *involuntary euthanasia; legal aspects; *mentally retarded; *newborns; parents; *personhood; *quality of life; selection for treatment; treatment refusal; *value of life; withholding treatment; United States

Miller, Pam. Ethical issues in neonatal intensive care. *In:* Frith, Lucy, ed. Ethics and Midwifery: Issues in Contemporary Practice. Boston, MA: Butterworth–Heinemann; 1996: 123–139. 24 refs. ISBN 0-7506-3056-6. BE58636.
  *allowing to die; artificial feeding; biomedical technologies; case studies; communication; *congenital disorders; *decision making; *intensive care units; moral policy; mothers; *newborns; *nurse midwives; *nurse's role; nurses; parents; patient advocacy; patient care; personhood; physicians; *prematurity; professional family relationship; prognosis; quality of life; resource allocation; risks and benefits; *selection for treatment; suffering; terminal care; treatment outcome; value of life; withholding treatment; Great Britain

Minow, Martha. Beyond state intervention in the family: for Baby Jane Doe. *University of Michigan Journal of Law Reform.* 1985 Summer; 18(4): 933–1014. 192 fn. BE56969.
  *allowing to die; *congenital disorders; decision making; federal government; *government regulation; judicial action; *legal aspects; *newborns; parent child relationship; parents; quality of life; state government; trust; value of life; withholding treatment; *Baby Jane Doe; New York; *United States

New York. Supreme Court, Queens County. In re Long Island Jewish Medical Center. *New York Supplement, 2d Series.* 1996 Feb 28 (date of decision). 641: 989–992. BE56740.

*allowing to die; *brain death; *decision making; *determination of death; dissent; *hospitals; *infants; institutional policies; *legal aspects; *parents; physicians; religion; ventilators; withholding treatment; *In re Long Island Jewish Medical Center; New York
The New York Supreme Court for Queens County authorized hospital withdrawal of a respirator from a brain dead infant. Three experts, two board certified pediatric specialists, retained by the hospital and another medical expert retained by the parents, certified the brain death of the five-month-old infant. Although hospital policy did not provide in writing for "reasonable accommodation" of religious or moral objections to determinations of death by the patient or the patient's family, the court found that the hospital did provide reasonable accommodation by keeping the parents informed, having its doctors available for consultation, encouraging a second opinion, and seeking judicial intervention. (KIE abstract)

Norup, Michael. Limits of neonatal treatment: a survey of attitudes in the Danish population. *Journal of Medical Ethics.* 1998 Jun; 24(3): 200–206. 18 refs. BE59117.
  active euthanasia; *allowing to die; *attitudes; congenital disorders; critically ill; decision making; diagnosis; morbidity; mortality; *newborns; parents; prematurity; prognosis; prolongation of life; *public opinion; quality of life; religion; risk; socioeconomic factors; survey; treatment outcome; treatment refusal; *withholding treatment; *Denmark
  OBJECTIVES: To study attitudes in the Danish population towards treatment of severely handicapped and extremely preterm infants and to define areas of consensus and controversy. DESIGN: Mail-delivered questionnaire. SETTING: Denmark. Survey sample––A random sample of 1080 persons aged from 18 to 45 years. RESULTS: The overall response rate was 68%. There was strong consensus (more than 75% agreement) that life–prolonging treatment should be provided for an infant born after 24 weeks' gestation with respiratory distress and, for an infant with myelomeningocele, when the parents were in favour of treatment. Further, there was almost uniform agreement that not all infants should be treated no matter how serious the condition. Major controversies concerned the severity of a condition needed to justify omission of life-prolonging treatment, the role of parental attitude and the options in non-treatment cases. Forty-six per cent thought it ought to be legal to kill the infant in at least some of these cases. CONCLUSION: Although the study revealed wide divergences of opinion with regard to questions about limits of treatment and about end–of–life decisions it also showed that there was general acceptance both that life–prolonging treatment ought to be provided even in relatively severe cases if this was in accordance with parental wishes, and that life should not be saved at all costs.

Oberman, Michelle. Response to "Discontinuing life support in an infant of a drug addicted mother: whose decision is it?" by Renu Jain and David C. Thomasma. *Cambridge Quarterly of Healthcare Ethics.* 1997 Spring; 6(2): 235–239. 5 fn. BE56432.
  *allowing to die; child abuse; competence; *congenital disorders; *decision making; disadvantaged; *dissent; *drug abuse; *emotions; legal guardians; morality; *mothers; *newborns; parents; patient advocacy; *physicians; pregnant women; prematurity; prenatal injuries; prolongation of life; United States

Rhoden, Nancy K. Treatment dilemmas for imperiled newborns: why quality of life counts. *Southern California*

BE = bioethics accession number   fn. = footnotes   refs. = references

Law Review. 1985 Sep; 58(6): 1283–1347. 360 fn. BE56666.

advisory committees; *allowing to die; artificial feeding; *brain pathology; chromosome abnormalities; clinical ethics committees; *congenital disorders; *decision making; disabled; drugs; federal government; futility; genetic disorders; *government regulation; *guidelines; intensive care units; judicial action; *legal aspects; mentally retarded; *newborns; parents; physicians; *prematurity; *prognosis; prolongation of life; *quality of life; risks and benefits; selection for treatment; social discrimination; social interaction; *standards; state government; suffering; surgery; terminally ill; treatment refusal; ventilators; *withholding treatment; antibiotics; coma; American Academy of Pediatrics v. Heckler; *Child Abuse Prevention and Treatment Act 1984; Department of Health and Human Services; President's Commission for the Study of Ethical Problems; Rehabilitation Act 1973; *United States

Schenker, Joseph G.; International Federation of Gynecology and Obstetrics. Committee for the Study of Ethical Aspects of Human Reproduction. Report of the FIGO Committee for the Study of Ethical Aspects of Human Reproduction. *International Journal of Gynaecology and Obstetrics.* 1997 Jun; 57(3): 333–337. 1 fn. BE57508.

*allowing to die; confidentiality; *congenital disorders; contraception; gene therapy; genetic enhancement; *genetic intervention; genetic materials; germ cells; guidelines; HIV seropositivity; informed consent; *newborns; organizational policies; quality of health care; remuneration; *reproduction; sexuality; withholding treatment; women's health services; women's rights; International Federation of Gynecology and Obstetrics

van der Heide, A.; van der Maas, P.J.; Kollée, L.A.A. End-of-life decisions in Dutch paediatric practice. [Letter]. *Lancet.* 1997 Dec 6; 350(9092): 1711. 2 refs. BE58154.

*active euthanasia; *allowing to die; attitudes; *decision making; drugs; *infants; legal aspects; *newborns; parents; *pediatrics; peer review; *physicians; *Netherlands

Watchko, Jon F. Decision making on critically ill infants by parents. *American Journal of Diseases of Children.* 1983 Aug; 137(8): 795–798. 17 refs. BE57228.

*allowing to die; clinical ethics committees; communication; critically ill; *decision making; judicial action; models, theoretical; *newborns; parents; physicians; referral and consultation

Yellin, Paul B.; Fleischman, Alan R. DNR in the DR? *Journal of Perinatology.* 1995 May–Jun; 15(3): 232–236. 16 refs. BE57700.

advance directives; *allowing to die; beneficence; *congenital disorders; *decision making; futility; moral policy; *newborns; parents; pediatrics; physicians; prematurity; prenatal diagnosis; prognosis; prolongation of life; *resuscitation; *resuscitation orders; uncertainty; *withholding treatment; neonatology

ALLOWING TO DIE/LEGAL ASPECTS

American Association on Mental Deficiency; Association for Persons with Severe Handicaps; American Association of University Affiliated Programs for the Developmentally Disabled; et al. Brief of Amici Curiae in Support of Petitioner: Margaret M. Heckler v. American Hospital Association, No. 84–1529, on Writ of Certiorari to the U.S. Court of Appeals for the Second Circuit. Washington, DC: Filed in the Supreme Court of the United States, October term, 1985; 1985. 27 p. 44 fn. BE57849.

*allowing to die; *congenital disorders; decision making; *disabled; Down syndrome; federal government; *government regulation; *legal aspects; legal rights; mentally retarded; *newborns; professional organizations; *quality of life; selection for treatment; *social discrimination; value of life; withholding treatment; Child Abuse Amendments 1984; *Heckler v. American Hospital Association; Rehabilitation Act 1973; United States

Arras, John D. Physician-assisted suicide: a tragic view. *Journal of Contemporary Health Law and Policy.* 1997 Spring; 13(2): 361–389. 94 fn. BE56000.

advance directives; *allowing to die; *assisted suicide; autonomy; *chronically ill; coercion; competence; constitutional law; cultural pluralism; decision making; depressive disorder; due process; economics; equal protection; freedom; government regulation; intention; judicial action; killing; *legal aspects; legal rights; legislation; managed care programs; *moral policy; pain; *palliative care; physically disabled; physician patient relationship; *physicians; *public policy; religion; review; *right to die; secularism; *social impact; state government; suffering; terminally ill; third party consent; *voluntary euthanasia; vulnerable populations; *wedge argument; withholding treatment; Compassion in Dying v. State of Washington; Quill v. Vacco; *United States

Berger, Jeffrey T. Cultural discrimination in mechanisms for health decisions: a view from New York. *Journal of Clinical Ethics.* 1998 Summer; 9(2): 127–131. 31 fn. BE58958.

advance care planning; *advance directives; *allowing to die; artificial feeding; attitudes; autonomy; *cultural pluralism; *decision making; empirical research; family members; family relationship; *legal aspects; *minority groups; *prolongation of life; *public policy; social discrimination; state government; third party consent; trust; values; withholding treatment; *New York

Bopp, James; Coleson, Richard E. A critique of family members as proxy decisionmakers without legal limits. *Issues in Law and Medicine.* 1996 Fall; 12(2): 133–165. 232 fn. BE58760.

adults; *allowing to die; artificial feeding; *autonomy; competence; *conflict of interest; congenital disorders; *decision making; *disabled; economics; emotions; *evaluation; *family members; family relationship; *legal aspects; legal rights; minors; motivation; newborns; parental consent; persistent vegetative state; physicians; prolongation of life; quality of life; *standards; state interest; *third party consent; value of life; withholding treatment; adult offspring; In re Lawrance; United States

Bourke, Leon H. Couture v. Couture. [Note]. *Issues in Law and Medicine.* 1990 Fall; 6(2): 201–204. BE56611.

advance directives; *allowing to die; beneficence; decision making; family members; *food; *government regulation; *legal aspects; legal guardians; prognosis; prolongation of life; *public policy; state government; state interest; *terminally ill; third party consent; *withholding treatment; *coma; *Couture v. Couture; *Ohio

Buchanan, Allen E. The limits of proxy decisionmaking for incompetents. *UCLA Law Review.* 1981; 29(2): 386–408. 58 fn. BE56486.

*allowing to die; *autonomy; brain death; *competence; *decision making; dementia; determination of death; family members; *judicial action; legal aspects; legal rights; *mentally retarded; *persistent vegetative state; personhood; physicians; resuscitation; right to die; *standards; state interest; *terminally ill; third party consent; treatment refusal; withholding treatment; In re Dinnerstein; In re Quinlan; In re Spring; Superintendent v. Saikewicz; *United States

Cantor, Norman L. Can healthcare providers obtain

judicial intervention against surrogates who demand "medically inappropriate" life support for incompetent patients? *Critical Care Medicine.* 1996 May; 24(5): 883–887. 28 fn. BE57957.

> *allowing to die; attitudes; competence; conscience; *decision making; dissent; economics; *family members; futility; hospitals; *judicial action; *legal aspects; persistent vegetative state; physicians; *prolongation of life; quality of life; resource allocation; suffering; value of life; withholding treatment; Hamilton, Teresa; In re Baby K; In re Jane Doe; In re Wanglie; *United States

Delany, Linda. Withholding life–sustaining treatment: the case of Miss D. *Health Care Analysis.* 1997 Sep; 5(3): 237–238, 242. 9 fn. BE55822.

> *allowing to die; artificial feeding; *brain pathology; *decision making; *diagnosis; guidelines; judicial action; *legal aspects; persistent vegetative state; physicians; professional organizations; *uncertainty; withholding treatment; coma; *England; *Great Britain; *In re a Ward of Court; *Ireland; *Re Miss D; Royal College of Physicians

Delaware. Supreme Court. In re Tavel. *Atlantic Reporter, 2d Series.* 1995 Aug 2 (date of decision). 661: 1061–1072. BE56248.

> aged; *allowing to die; *artificial feeding; autonomy; competence; *decision making; family members; *legal aspects; *legal guardians; legislation; living wills; *persistent vegetative state; state government; third party consent; treatment refusal; withholding treatment; Death with Dignity Act (DE); *Delaware; *In re Tavel

The Supreme Court of Delaware upheld the lower court decision to permit removal of a feeding tube from a patient who was in a form of persistent vegetative state and who did not have a written advance directive. At age 88, Rose Tavel suffered a stroke which paralyzed one side of her body and left the other side unresponsive. Over the next three and a half years she deteriorated into a "coma vigil," which is a fixed neurological state where the patient appears to be awake yet is noncommunicative and unable to control bodily functions. Tavel's daughter sought to remove the gastrostomy tube which kept her mother alive. The court granted her the authority to do so after it found that a living will under the state Death with Dignity Act was not required. As guardian the daughter could substitute her judgment in the decision making after she considered the values and statements of her incompetent mother and provided that the evidence was clear and convincing. (KIE abstract)

Devlin, Maureen M. In re Fiori. [Note]. *Issues in Law and Medicine.* 1996 Fall; 12(2): 189–190. BE58762.

> *allowing to die; autonomy; *decision making; *family members; *legal aspects; *persistent vegetative state; state government; state interest; third party consent; treatment refusal; withholding treatment; *In re Fiori; Pennsylvania

Dresser, Rebecca. Missing persons: legal perceptions of incompetent patients. *Rutgers Law Review.* 1994 Winter; 46(2): 609–719. 385 fn. BE56656.

> advance directives; aged; *allowing to die; *autonomy; compassion; *competence; *decision making; *dementia; family members; judicial action; *legal aspects; mentally ill; mentally retarded; models, theoretical; persistent vegetative state; *prolongation of life; *quality of life; right to die; *risks and benefits; self concept; *standards; suffering; third party consent; treatment refusal; withholding treatment; empathy; In re Conroy; In re Quinlan; In re Spring; In re Storar; *United States

Dyer, Clare. PVS criteria put under spotlight. [News]. *BMJ (British Medical Journal).* 1997 Mar 29; 314(7085): 919. BE58513.

> *allowing to die; artificial feeding; *diagnosis; *legal aspects; *persistent vegetative state; physicians; professional organizations; *standards; withholding treatment; *Great Britain; Royal College of Physicians

Emson, Harry E. The right to die: withdrawal of tube feeding in the persistent vegetative state in Canada. *In:* Grubb, Andrew, ed. Decision–Making and Problems of Incompetence. New York, NY: Wiley; 1994: 181–186. 9 fn. ISBN 0–471–94236–7. BE57135.

> *advance directives; *allowing to die; *artificial feeding; autonomy; clinical ethics committees; competence; cultural pluralism; *decision making; family members; hospitals; informed consent; *knowledge, attitudes, practice; *legal aspects; patients; *persistent vegetative state; physicians; right to die; third party consent; treatment refusal; *withholding treatment; *Canada

Evans, Jennifer L. Are children competent to make decisions about their own deaths? *Behavioral Sciences and the Law.* 1995 Winter; 13(1): 27–41. 58 refs. BE55784.

> age factors; *allowing to die; autonomy; case studies; *competence; *decision making; *legal aspects; legislation; *minors; *parents; *patient participation; physicians; psychological stress; standards; state interest; terminally ill; *treatment refusal; truth disclosure; withholding treatment; United States

Fenwick, Andrea J. Applying best interests to persistent vegetative state -- a principled distortion? *Journal of Medical Ethics.* 1998 Apr; 24(2): 86–92. 45 fn. Commented on by R. Gillon, p. 75–76. This paper won the 1997 UK Forum Essay Competition, organized in collaboration with the *JME.* BE58076.

> active euthanasia; *allowing to die; *artificial feeding; chronically ill; death; *decision making; intention; *judicial action; *legal aspects; legal guardians; patients; *persistent vegetative state; physicians; prognosis; *quality of life; resource allocation; risks and benefits; *standards; state interest; terminology; third party consent; *withholding treatment; *England; *Ireland; *Scotland

"Best interests" is widely accepted as the appropriate foundation principle for medico–legal decisions concerning treatment withdrawal from patients in persistent vegetative state (PVS). Its application appears to progress logically from earlier use regarding legally incompetent patients. This author argues, however, that such confidence in the relevance of the principle of best interests to PVS is misplaced, and that current construction in this context is questionable on four specific grounds. Furthermore, it is argued that the resulting legal inconsistency is distorting both the principle itself and, more particularly, individual patient interests.

Ferguson, Pamela R. Causing death or allowing to die? Developments in the law. *Journal of Medical Ethics.* 1997 Dec; 23(6): 368–372. 19 fn. Commented on by F. Randall, p. 373–376. BE57658.

> *active euthanasia; *allowing to die; artificial feeding; *criminal law; decision making; *double effect; drugs; futility; *intention; *killing; law; *legal aspects; *legal liability; moral obligations; moral policy; *morality; motivation; pain; patients; *persistent vegetative state; *physicians; public policy; quality of life; *terminally ill; voluntary euthanasia; *withholding treatment; *Airedale NHS Trust v. Bland; *Great Britain; *Law Hospital NHS Trust v. Lord Advocate; *R v. Cox

Several cases which have been considered by the courts in recent years have highlighted the legal dilemmas facing doctors whose decisions result in the ending of a patient's life. This paper considers the case of Dr Cox, who was convicted of attempting to murder one of his patients, and explores the roles of motive, diminished responsibility and consent in cases of "mercy killing". The Cox decision is compared to that of Tony Bland and Janet Johnstone, in which the patients were in a persistent vegetative state. In all three cases, the doctors believed that their patients' quality of life was so poor that their continued existence was of no benefit to them, and decided that their lives should not be unduly prolonged, yet the doctor who was prosecuted was the one whose dying patient had requested that her death be hastened. The paper examines the law's seemingly contradictory approaches to such cases.

Friedland, Steven I. The health care proxy and the narrative of death. *Journal of Law and Health.* 1995–1996; 10(1): 95–151. 277 fn. BE57144.
administrators; *advance directives; *allowing to die; attitudes; *attitudes to death; autonomy; biomedical technologies; communication; *death; determination of death; evaluation studies; government regulation; historical aspects; hospitals; knowledge, attitudes, practice; *legal aspects; legal rights; living wills; medicine; physicians; prolongation of life; right to die; state government; survey; treatment refusal; Health Care Proxy Law 1990 (NY); New York; *United States

Garwin, Mark. The duty to care -- the right to refuse: changing roles of patients and physicians in end-of-life decision making. *Journal of Legal Medicine.* 1998 Mar; 19(1): 99–125. 95 fn. BE58901.
advance directives; *allowing to die; autonomy; beneficence; coercion; communication; competence; *decision making; disclosure; economics; emergency care; incentives; informed consent; judicial action; *legal aspects; *legal liability; legal rights; models, theoretical; physician patient relationship; *physicians; *prolongation of life; resuscitation orders; standards; state interest; terminal care; third party consent; torts; *treatment refusal; withholding treatment; directive adherence; Anderson v. St. Francis-St. George Hospital; *United States

George, James E.; Quattrone, Madelyn S.; Goldstone, Marc. A pediatric right to die? *Journal of Emergency Nursing.* 1995 Aug; 21(4): 341–342. 1 ref. BE56603.
*allowing to die; children; *legal aspects; parents; persistent vegetative state; *right to die; treatment refusal; ventilators; withholding treatment; Michigan; *Rosebush v. Oakland County Prosecutor

Georgia. Court of Appeals. Velez v. Bethune. *South Eastern Reporter, 2d Series.* 1995 Dec 5 (date of decision). 466: 627–635. BE56739.
*allowing to die; *decision making; *legal aspects; *legal liability; *newborns; parental consent; *physicians; prematurity; terminally ill; ventilators; *withholding treatment; *wrongful death; Georgia; *Velez v. Bethune
The Georgia Court of Appeals overturned the lower court and allowed parents to proceed against the physician and hospital with a claim of wrongful death of their infant, whose life support was unilaterally withdrawn. Nine-day-old Mary Elizabeth Bethune had been born at twenty-four weeks and was dying due to severe prematurity. The court held that the doctor had no right to decide unilaterally to discontinue treatment, even if the infant were dying, without the consent of the parents. In the opinion of the chief judge, wrongful death includes wrongful hastening of death. (KIE abstract)

Gillon, Raanan. Persistent vegetative state, withdrawal of artificial nutrition and hydration, and the patient's "best interests". [Editorial]. *Journal of Medical Ethics.* 1998 Apr; 24(2): 75–76. 2 refs. Commentary on A. Fenwick, p. 86–92. BE58078.
*allowing to die; *artificial feeding; beneficence; death; *decision making; intention; justice; *legal aspects; legal obligations; moral obligations; patients; *persistent vegetative state; physicians; resource allocation; risks and benefits; *standards; *withholding treatment; England

Glantz, Leonard H. Legal issues in withholding or withdrawing medical treatment. [Article and discussion]. *Chest.* 1985 Sep; 88(3, Suppl.): 175S–182S. 18 fn. BE56954.
advance directives; *allowing to die; case studies; competence; *decision making; informed consent; *legal aspects; physicians; quality of life; right to die; third party consent; treatment refusal; ventilators; withholding treatment; *United States

Gostin, Lawrence O. Deciding life and death in the courtroom: from Quinlan to Cruzan, Glucksberg, and Vacco -- a brief history and analysis of constitutional protection of the 'right to die'. *JAMA.* 1997 Nov 12; 278(18): 1523–1528. 60 refs. BE57164.
advance directives; *allowing to die; artificial feeding; *assisted suicide; autonomy; coercion; competence; *constitutional law; criminal law; decision making; double effect; drugs; due process; economics; equal protection; freedom; *historical aspects; intention; judicial action; killing; *legal aspects; legal liability; legal rights; legislation; *palliative care; patients; physician patient relationship; physician's role; *physicians; public opinion; review; *right to die; risks and benefits; social worth; state government; *state interest; *Supreme Court decisions; *terminally ill; third party consent; treatment refusal; value of life; values; vulnerable populations; wedge argument; withholding treatment; *Cruzan v. Director, Missouri Department of Health; Fourteenth Amendment; *In re Quinlan; New Jersey; New York; Patient Self-Determination Act 1990; *Twentieth Century; *United States; *Vacco v. Quill; Washington; *Washington v. Glucksberg
This article analyzes judicial determinations on the "right to die" from Quinlan to Cruzan, Glucksberg, and Vacco. The body of law known as right-to-die cases extends ordinary treatment refusal doctrine to end-of-life decisions. The courts, having affirmed a right to refuse life-sustaining treatment, held that certain categorical distinctions that had been drawn lacked a rational basis. No rational distinction could be made between competent vs incompetent patients, withholding vs withdrawing treatment, and ordinary vs extraordinary treatment. The courts, however, had persistently affirmed one categorical distinction: between withdrawing life-sustaining treatment on the one hand and active euthanasia or physician-assisted dying on the other. In Washington v Glucksberg and Vacco v Quill, the Supreme Court unanimously held that physician-assisted suicide is not a fundamental liberty interest protected by the Constitution. Notably, five members of the Court wrote or joined in concurring opinions that took a more liberal view. The Court powerfully approved aggressive palliation of pain. The Supreme Court, hinting that it would find state legalization of physician-assisted suicide constitutional, invited the nation to pursue an earnest debate on physician assistance in the dying process.

Great Britain. England. Court of Appeal, Civil Division. Re B (A Minor) (Wardship: Medical Treatment). *All England Law Reports.* 1981 Aug 7 (date of decision). [1990] 3: 927–930. BE57394.
*allowing to die; congenital disorders; *decision making; *Down syndrome; *judicial action; *legal aspects; *newborns; parents; physicians; *quality of life; refusal to treat; *surgery; third party consent; treatment refusal; *withholding treatment; *Great Britain; *Re B (A Minor) (Wardship: Medical Treatment)

BE = bioethics accession number   fn. = footnotes   refs. = references

The British Court of Appeal, Civil Division, allowed the appeal of the local NHS health authority and authorized life–saving surgery for a mentally retarded infant against her parents' wishes. B was born with Down syndrome and an intestinal blockage. Without an operation, she would die within days; with an operation and without other complications, her life expectancy was between 20 and 30 years. Acting in what they saw as their child's best interests, her parents refused to consent to the operation. The appellate court's decision to authorize surgery was based on the welfare of the child. The judges held that if the operation were successful the girl could live the normal life span of a Down syndrome child with the handicaps of such a child, and "it is not for this court to say that life of that description ought to be extinguished." (KIE abstract)

Great Britain. England. Court of Appeal, Civil Division. Re J (A Minor) (Wardship: Medical Treatment). *All England Law Reports.* 1992 Jun 10 (date of decision). [1992] 4: 614–626. BE58577.
  *allowing to die; *brain pathology; critically ill; *decision making; *disabled; dissent; extraordinary treatment; *infants; injuries; intensive care units; *judicial action; *legal aspects; *minors; parents; patient admission; physicians; *prognosis; *prolongation of life; *ventilators; *withholding treatment; *Great Britain; National Health Service; *Re J (A Minor) (Wardship: Medical Treatment)

The Civil Division of England's Court of Appeal overturned the lower court's order of mechanical ventilation for a profoundly handicapped sixteen–month–old child against the clinical judgment of the child's doctors. Since hitting his head in a fall at age four weeks, J had not mentally developed past that time and he was blind and he suffered from severe cerebral palsy and epilepsy. He required nasogastric tubal feeding and, although he occasionally responded to sound, whether or not he recognized his caregivers was uncertain. His divorced mother and the local authority shared parental authority over J, who resided with foster parents. The consultant pediatrician reported that if J were to suffer a life–threatening event, ordinary resuscitation, antibiotics and physiotherapy would be appropriate, but intervention with intensive measures including mechanical ventilation would be medically inappropriate. Two other specialists agreed with those findings, but another consultant found mechanical ventilation not to be cruel and thought J could be weaned from it if it became so. The mother and local health authority asked the court to require the health authority to continue all treatment, including mechanical ventilation, of J. The Official Solicitor and the health authority opposed such an order. The lower court granted an interim order requiring mechanical ventilation if necessary over the five weeks prior to the main hearing. The appellate court viewed such an order as an abuse of judicial power and held that the physician's duty to the patient is to treat with the necessary consent in accord with the best clinical judgment and that, as long as those with parental authority consent to J's treatment by the health authority, he must be treated in accord with the best clinical judgment of that authority's personnel. (KIE abstract)

Grubb, Andrew. Incompetent patient (PVS): decision-making, courts and the family -- In re Tavel. [Comment]. *Medical Law Review.* 1997 Summer; 5(2): 245–250. BE57869.
  *allowing to die; artificial feeding; *decision making; family members; *legal aspects; legal guardians; *persistent vegetative state; standards; third party consent; withholding

treatment; *Delaware; Great Britain; *In re Tavel

Grubb, Andrew. Incompetent patient (PVS): withdrawal of feeding and compliance with RCP guidelines -- Re D. [Comment]. *Medical Law Review.* 1997 Summer; 5(2): 225–227. BE57868.
  *allowing to die; artificial feeding; diagnosis; guidelines; *legal aspects; *persistent vegetative state; professional organizations; uncertainty; withholding treatment; *Great Britain; *Re D; Royal College of Physicians

Hanafin, Patrick. Last Rights: Death, Dying and the Law in Ireland. Cork, Ireland: Cork University Press; 1997. 114 p. (Undercurrents; 12). 255 fn. ISBN 1-85918-156-2. BE57047.
  advance directives; *allowing to die; artificial feeding; assisted suicide; attitudes; attitudes to death; *autonomy; beneficence; brain pathology; clergy; constitutional law; criminal law; *decision making; dissent; family members; *international aspects; judicial action; killing; legal rights; legislation; natural law; persistent vegetative state; physicians; privacy; *right to die; Roman Catholic ethics; Supreme Court decisions; terminally ill; third party consent; treatment refusal; trends; *value of life; *voluntary euthanasia; withholding treatment; Australia; Canada; Great Britain; In re a Ward of Court; *Ireland; *Medical Council (Ireland); Netherlands; Northern Territory; Right to Life Movement; United States

Hanley, Ruth Ann. Hoffmeister v. Satz. [Note]. *Issues in Law and Medicine.* 1990 Fall; 6(2): 205–206. BE56615.
  *allowing to die; decision making; dementia; family members; *food; *government regulation; *legal aspects; legal rights; *nursing homes; patient compliance; patient discharge; physicians; prolongation of life; *public policy; state government; terminally ill; third party consent; treatment refusal; *withholding treatment; coma; *Florida; *Hoffmeister v. Satz

Hodgson, John. Rights of the terminally ill patient. *Annals of Health Law.* 1996; 5: 169–191. 93 fn. BE58364.
  *active euthanasia; adults; advance directives; *allowing to die; artificial feeding; assisted suicide; competence; *decision making; family members; informed consent; judicial action; *legal aspects; legal liability; *legal rights; minors; palliative care; *persistent vegetative state; physicians; quality of life; right to die; standards; *terminally ill; *third party consent; *treatment refusal; withholding treatment; Airedale NHS Trust v. Bland; *Great Britain; House of Lords Select Committee on Medical Ethics; Law Commission (Great Britain)

Jennett, Bryan. Managing patients in a persistent vegetative state since *Airedale NHS Trust v. Bland.* In: McLean, Sheila A.M., ed. Death, Dying and the Law. Brookfield, VT: Dartmouth; 1996: 19–28. 32 fn. ISBN 1-85521-657-4. BE57211.
  *allowing to die; artificial feeding; decision making; family members; futility; intention; international aspects; judicial action; *legal aspects; *persistent vegetative state; physicians; prognosis; prolongation of life; religious ethics; resource allocation; time factors; value of life; withholding treatment; Airedale NHS Trust v. Bland; *Great Britain; Netherlands; New Zealand; United States

Keown, John. Life and death in Dublin. *Cambridge Law Journal.* 1996 Mar; 55(1): 6–8. BE55937.
  *allowing to die; *artificial feeding; autonomy; *brain pathology; competence; constitutional law; *decision making; family members; iatrogenic disease; *legal aspects; legal rights; patients' rights; privacy; prolongation of life; quality of life; risks and benefits; state interest; suicide; third party consent; treatment refusal; withholding treatment; *In re a Ward of Court; *Ireland

Kimura, Rihito. Death, dying, and advance directives in Japan: sociocultural and legal points of view. *In:* Sass, Hans-Martin; Veatch, Robert M.; Kimura, Rihito, eds. Advance Directives and Surrogate Decision Making in Health Care: United States, Germany, and Japan. Baltimore, MD: Johns Hopkins University Press; 1998: 187–208. 29 refs. ISBN 0–8018–5831–3. BE59042.
*active euthanasia; *advance directives; *allowing to die; assisted suicide; attitudes; *attitudes to death; cancer; common good; criminal law; decision making; diagnosis; drugs; family members; *family relationship; historical aspects; *legal aspects; living wills; model legislation; national health insurance; organ donation; organizational policies; pain; palliative care; paternalism; patient advocacy; physician patient relationship; physicians; professional organizations; prognosis; prolongation of life; public opinion; *public policy; resuscitation orders; social dominance; *terminal care; terminally ill; third party consent; trends; trust; truth disclosure; *values; voluntary euthanasia; withholding treatment; oral directives; *Japan; Japan Medical Association; Japan Science Council; Japanese Society for Dying with Dignity

Koch, Hans–Georg. The decision to aid dying and related legal issues: advance directives and durable powers of attorney under German law. *In:* Sass, Hans-Martin; Veatch, Robert M.; Kimura, Rihito, eds. Advance Directives and Surrogate Decision Making in Health Care: United States, Germany, and Japan. Baltimore, MD: Johns Hopkins University Press; 1998: 114–135. 46 refs. 1 fn. ISBN 0–8018–5831–3. BE59039.
*advance directives; *allowing to die; artificial feeding; autonomy; case studies; competence; *decision making; family members; guidelines; judicial action; *legal aspects; living wills; model legislation; *physicians; prolongation of life; suffering; suicide; terminal care; *terminally ill; terminology; third party consent; treatment refusal; withholding treatment; oral directives; values histories; *Germany

Kondro, Wayne. Murder–or–mercy case tested in Canada. [News]. *Lancet.* 1997 May 17; 349(9063): 1458. BE55824.
*active euthanasia; cancer; *criminal law; family members; hospitals; intensive care units; *killing; *legal liability; patients; *physicians; right to die; third party consent; *withholding treatment; *Canada; Mills, Paul; *Morrison, Nancy; Nova Scotia; Victoria General Hospital (Halifax, NS)

Link, Ronald C. Recent American developments in the right to die: the *Cruzan* case, living wills, durable powers and family consent statutes. *In:* Grubb, Andrew, ed. Decision–Making and Problems of Incompetence. New York, NY: Wiley; 1994: 127–172. 169 fn. ISBN 0–471–94236–7. BE57134.
*advance directives; *allowing to die; artificial feeding; *decision making; *family members; federal government; freedom; *legal aspects; legal rights; legislation; living wills; patient care; patients; persistent vegetative state; physicians; prolongation of life; right to die; state government; state interest; Supreme Court decisions; terminally ill; *third party consent; treatment refusal; value of life; *withholding treatment; Cruzan v. Director, Missouri Department of Health; Patient Self–Determination Act 1990; *United States

McLean, Sheila A.M. Law at the end of life: what next? *In:* McLean, Sheila A.M., ed. Death, Dying and the Law. Brookfield, VT: Dartmouth; 1996: 49–66. 56 fn. ISBN 1–85521–657–4. BE57213.
*active euthanasia; advance directives; advisory committees; *allowing to die; assisted suicide; autonomy; congenital disorders; decision making; double effect; *legal aspects; newborns; palliative care; persistent vegetative state; *public policy; quality of life; state interest; terminal care; treatment refusal; value of life; withholding treatment; Airedale NHS Trust v. Bland; *Great Britain; *House of Lords Select Committee on Medical Ethics

McLean, Sheila A.M. Letting die or assisting death: how should the law respond to the patient in a persistent vegetative state? *In:* Petersen, Kerry, ed. Intersections: Women on Law, Medicine and Technology. Brookfield, VT: Ashgate; 1997: 167–184. 26 refs. 5 fn. ISBN 1–85521–882–8. BE57491.
*allowing to die; artificial feeding; clinical ethics committees; *decision making; judicial action; killing; *legal aspects; legislation; *persistent vegetative state; quality of life; *standards; third party consent; *withholding treatment; *Airedale NHS Trust v. Bland; *Great Britain; Law Hospital NHS Trust v. The Lord Advocate; Scotland

Meisel, Alan. Legal issues in decision making for incompetent patients: advance directives and surrogate decision making. *In:* Sass, Hans–Martin; Veatch, Robert M.; Kimura, Rihito, eds. Advance Directives and Surrogate Decision Making in Health Care: United States, Germany, and Japan. Baltimore, MD: Johns Hopkins University Press; 1998: 34–65. 62 refs. 11 fn. References include separate lists of court cases and legislation. ISBN 0–8018–5831–3. BE59036.
*advance directives; *allowing to die; artificial feeding; case studies; *competence; conflict of interest; constitutional law; critically ill; *decision making; dementia; equal protection; *family members; futility; judicial action; *legal aspects; legal rights; legislation; *living wills; patients; persistent vegetative state; physically disabled; physicians; pregnant women; privacy; prolongation of life; right to die; risks and benefits; standards; state government; terminally ill; *third party consent; treatment refusal; uncertainty; values; withholding treatment; Patient Self–Determination Act 1990; *United States

Minow, Martha. Beyond state intervention in the family: for Baby Jane Doe. *University of Michigan Journal of Law Reform.* 1985 Summer; 18(4): 933–1014. 192 fn. BE56969.
*allowing to die; *congenital disorders; decision making; federal government; *government regulation; judicial action; *legal aspects; *newborns; parent child relationship; parents; quality of life; state government; trust; value of life; withholding treatment; *Baby Jane Doe; New York; *United States

Montgomery, Jonathan. Health care law and ethics: abortion; fertility; maternity care; selective treatment of the newborn; transplantation; terminal care and euthanasia. *In: his* Health Care Law. New York, NY: Oxford University Press; 1997: 357–456. 503 fn. ISBN 0–19–876260–7. BE56245.
*abortion, induced; active euthanasia; *adults; *allowing to die; assisted suicide; body parts and fluids; cadavers; childbirth; congenital disorders; conscience; contraception; family planning; fetuses; health personnel; *legal aspects; legal liability; legislation; living wills; maternal health; minors; *newborns; *organ donation; organ donors; organ transplantation; *patient care; persistent vegetative state; *pregnant women; prenatal injuries; remuneration; *reproductive technologies; selective abortion; spousal consent; sterilization (sexual); surrogate mothers; terminal care; therapeutic abortion; treatment refusal; *Great Britain

National Legal Center for the Medically Dependent and Disabled, Inc. Amicus Curiae Brief of the Ethics and Advocacy Task Force of the Nursing Home Action Group in Support of the Commonwealth of Pennsylvania, Attorney General, in re: Daniel Joseph Fiori, an Adjudged Incompetent, No. 0006 E.D. Appeal Docket 1995. Filed in the Supreme Court of Pennsylvania; 1995 Mar 16. 42 p. 17 fn. Appeal from judgment of Superior Court in No. 00737 Philadelphia 1993, entered 17 Jan 1995, affirming the judgment of the Court of Common Pleas of Bucks County, Orphans' Court Division, at No. 49355, entered 3 Feb 1993. BE56342.

> *allowing to die; artificial feeding; *decision making; disabled; due process; equal protection; *family members; *judicial action; *legal aspects; *legal guardians; *legal rights; nursing homes; *patient advocacy; *persistent vegetative state; *prolongation of life; quality of life; social discrimination; standards; state government; state interest; third party consent; treatment refusal; withholding treatment; *In re Fiori; *Pennsylvania

Oddi, Samuel. The tort of interference with the right to die: the wrongful living cause of action. *Georgetown Law Journal.* 1986 Dec; 75(2): 625–665. 180 fn. BE56700.

> allowing to die; compensation; hospitals; *legal aspects; *legal liability; negligence; physicians; *prolongation of life; *right to die; state interest; *torts; treatment refusal; *wrongful life; *United States

Orentlicher, David. The Supreme Court and terminal sedation: an ethically inferior alternative to physician–assisted suicide. *In:* Battin, Margaret P.; Rhodes, Rosamond; Silvers, Anita, eds. Physician Assisted Suicide: Expanding the Debate. New York, NY: Routledge; 1998: 301–311. 29 fn. ISBN 0–415–92003–5. BE58795.

> active euthanasia; *allowing to die; *artificial feeding; *assisted suicide; competence; double effect; drugs; food; *intention; involuntary euthanasia; *legal aspects; moral policy; *palliative care; *physicians; right to die; suffering; *Supreme Court decisions; terminally ill; vulnerable populations; wedge argument; *withholding treatment; *sedatives; United States; *Vacco v. Quill; *Washington v. Glucksberg

Pennsylvania. Court of Common Pleas, Dauphin County. Rideout v. Hershey Medical Center. *Dauphin County Reports.* 1995 Dec 29 (date of decision). 115: 472–498. BE57098.

> *allowing to die; *children; *decision making; *dissent; futility; *hospitals; *legal aspects; *legal liability; *legal rights; parental consent; *parents; physicians; *prolongation of life; psychological stress; *refusal to treat; terminally ill; *ventilators; *withholding treatment; Pennsylvania; *Rideout v. Hershey Medical Center

The Pennsylvania Court of Common Pleas for Dauphin County allowed the parents of Brianne Rideout to sue the Hershey Medical Center under the common law for taking their daughter off assisted breathing without their consent. In this case the parents were acting as if they were the state in an attempt to preserve life while the hospital acted as if it were the patient by unilaterally usurping Brianne's right to refuse treatment. Brianne, age 2, suffered from a malignant brain tumor and her condition was terminal. Three days before she was taken off life support, her pupils had become fixed and dilated. Upon removal of the ventilator, she breathed on her own for the next two days prior to her death from lack of oxygen and subsequent cardiopulmonary failure. Under common law the hospital had committed battery, defined as unauthorized touching, when its doctors disconnected Brianne's ventilator because Brianne's surrogate decision makers, her parents, did not consent. The parents were also deprived of the parental right to make medical decisions for their child. They did not have a right to insist on medical treatment nor did the hospital need to require parental approval for all medical treatment. But where the treatment was life–sustaining and thus involved the child's own right to life, their parental right to make those medical decisions for

Brianne was violated. However, neither the state privacy interest nor the federal liberty interest had been violated, because, as the court reasoned, the decision to withdraw treatment has always been defined as a right to refuse treatment, not as a right to demand or to continue treatment. (KIE abstract)

Pennsylvania. Supreme Court, E.D. In re Fiori. *Atlantic Reporter, 2d Series.* 1996 Apr 2 (date of decision). 673: 905–914. BE55971.

> *allowing to die; artificial feeding; autonomy; *decision making; *family members; *legal aspects; nursing homes; *persistent vegetative state; state government; third party consent; treatment refusal; withholding treatment; *In re Fiori; *Pennsylvania

The Supreme Court of Pennsylvania, Eastern District, upheld a Superior Court ruling that consent of a close family member, with approval of two qualified physicians, is sufficient to terminate life–sustaining treatment of an incompetent adult in a long–term persistent vegetative state who has not previously expressed a view regarding life–sustaining treatment. The Superior Court rejected the Attorney General's argument that a guardian ad litem must be appointed and clear and convincing evidence must be shown that the patient would have withdrawn treatment under the circumstances presented, requiring a court proceeding in every case. (KIE abstract)

Prip, William; Moretti, Anna. Medical futility: a legal perspective. *In:* Zucker, Marjorie B.; Zucker, Howard D., eds. Medical Futility and the Evaluation of Life–Sustaining Interventions. New York, NY: Cambridge University Press; 1997: 136–154. 51 refs. 14 fn. ISBN 0–521–56877–3. BE55986.

> advance directives; *allowing to die; anencephaly; autonomy; *decision making; *dissent; emergency care; *family members; federal government; *futility; infants; judicial action; *legal aspects; legal liability; legal rights; legislation; newborns; *patients; *physicians; *prolongation of life; *refusal to treat; resuscitation orders; *right to treatment; state government; ventilators; withholding treatment; Child Abuse Amendments 1984; Gilgunn v. Massachusetts General Hospital; In re Baby K; In re Wanglie; Uniform Health–Care Decisions Act 1993; *United States

Quinn, Kevin P. Assisted suicide and equal protection: in defense of the distinction between killing and letting die. *Issues in Law and Medicine.* 1997 Fall; 13(2): 145–171. 129 fn. BE57806.

> *allowing to die; *assisted suicide; constitutional law; double effect; due process; *equal protection; government regulation; *intention; *killing; *legal aspects; legal rights; *moral policy; physicians; public policy; *right to die; state government; Supreme Court decisions; terminally ill; treatment refusal; withholding treatment; Compassion in Dying v. State of Washington; Cruzan v. Director, Missouri Department of Health; Fourteenth Amendment; *New York; *Quill v. Vacco; *United States; *Vacco v. Quill; *Washington; Washington v. Glucksberg

Randall, Fiona. Why causing death is not necessarily morally equivalent to allowing to die — a response to Ferguson. *Journal of Medical Ethics.* 1997 Dec; 23(6): 373–376. 1 ref. Commentary on P.R. Ferguson, "Causing death or allowing to die? Developments in the law," p. 368–372. BE57665.

> *active euthanasia; *allowing to die; artificial feeding; *criminal law; futility; *intention; involuntary euthanasia; *killing; law; *legal aspects; legal liability; moral obligations; *moral policy; *morality; pain; patients; *persistent vegetative state; *physicians; public policy; quality of life; terminally ill; *withholding treatment; Airedale NHS Trust

---

BE = bioethics accession number   fn. = footnotes   refs. = references

v. Bland; *Great Britain; Law Hospital NHS Trust v. Lord Advocate; R v. Cox

Rhoden, Nancy K. Treatment dilemmas for imperiled newborns: why quality of life counts. *Southern California Law Review.* 1985 Sep; 58(6): 1283–1347. 360 fn. BE56666.
advisory committees; *allowing to die; artificial feeding; *brain pathology; chromosome abnormalities; clinical ethics committees; *congenital disorders; *decision making; disabled; drugs; federal government; futility; genetic disorders; *government regulation; *guidelines; intensive care units; judicial action; *legal aspects; mentally retarded; *newborns; parents; physicians; *prematurity; *prognosis; prolongation of life; *quality of life; risks and benefits; selection for treatment; social discrimination; social interaction; *standards; state government; suffering; surgery; terminally ill; treatment refusal; ventilators; *withholding treatment; antibiotics; coma; American Academy of Pediatrics v. Heckler; *Child Abuse Prevention and Treatment Act 1984; Department of Health and Human Services; President's Commission for the Study of Ethical Problems; Rehabilitation Act 1973; *United States

Stell, Lance K. Physician–assisted suicide: to decriminalize or legalize, that is the question. *In:* Battin, Margaret P.; Rhodes, Rosamond; Silvers, Anita, eds. Physician Assisted Suicide: Expanding the Debate. New York, NY: Routledge; 1998: 225–251. 49 fn. ISBN 0-415-92003-5. BE58791.
*allowing to die; *assisted suicide; autonomy; competence; criminal law; ethical analysis; government regulation; *intention; *killing; *legal aspects; *moral policy; physician patient relationship; physician's role; *physicians; policy analysis; *public policy; right to die; state interest; *suicide; Supreme Court decisions; terminally ill; treatment refusal; withholding treatment; Cruzan v. Director, Missouri Department of Health; United States; Vacco v. Quill; Washington v. Glucksberg

Towner, Henry. In re Martin. [Note]. *Issues in Law and Medicine.* 1996 Winter; 12(3): 267–271. BE58465.
advance directives; *allowing to die; artificial feeding; *competence; *decision making; *disabled; dissent; family members; *legal aspects; *standards; third party consent; treatment refusal; withholding treatment; oral directives; *In re Martin; Michigan

Veatch, Robert M. Ethical dimensions of advance directives and surrogate decision making in the United States. *In:* Sass, Hans–Martin; Veatch, Robert M.; Kimura, Rihito, eds. Advance Directives and Surrogate Decision Making in Health Care: United States, Germany, and Japan. Baltimore, MD: Johns Hopkins University Press; 1998: 66–91. 72 refs. 7 fn. ISBN 0-8018-5831-3. BE59037.
adults; *advance directives; aged; *allowing to die; anencephaly; artificial feeding; *autonomy; beneficence; brain pathology; competence; consensus; *decision making; family members; freedom; futility; historical aspects; informed consent; judicial action; justice; *legal rights; living wills; mentally retarded; minors; moral policy; parents; paternalism; patients' rights; persistent vegetative state; physician patient relationship; physicians; professional autonomy; prolongation of life; refusal to treat; religion; *risks and benefits; Roman Catholic ethics; *third party consent; *treatment refusal; trends; ventilators; withholding treatment; liberalism; oral directives; values histories; Hippocratic Oath; In re Baby K; In re Conroy; In re Phillip B.; In re Quinlan; Twentieth Century; *United States

Veatch, Robert M., ed. The ethics of death and dying. *In:* Jonsen, Albert R.; Veatch, Robert M.; Walters, LeRoy, eds. Source Book in Bioethics: A Documentary History. Washington, DC: Georgetown University

Press; 1998: 111–252. 14 fn. ISBN 0-87840-683-2. BE57891.
adults; advisory committees; age factors; *allowing to die; anencephaly; artificial feeding; attitudes to death; brain death; competence; *determination of death; family members; federal government; futility; government regulation; guidelines; historical aspects; *legal aspects; mentally disabled; model legislation; moral policy; newborns; persistent vegetative state; prolongation of life; public policy; standards; state government; third party consent; ventilators; withholding treatment; *Cruzan v. Director, Missouri Department of Health; *In re Baby K; *In re Conroy; *In re Quinlan; Natural Death Act (CA); *President's Commission for the Study of Ethical Problems; *Superintendent v. Saikewicz; *Twentieth Century; *United States

Yount, Lisa. Should doctors ever hasten patients' deaths? [Juvenile literature]. *In: her* Issues in Biomedical Ethics. San Diego, CA: Lucent Books; 1998: 36–55, 101–102. 29 fn. ISBN 1-56006-476-5. BE57680.
*active euthanasia; *allowing to die; artificial feeding; *assisted suicide; attitudes; *autonomy; biomedical technologies; coercion; competence; constitutional law; *decision making; due process; economics; equal protection; food; freedom; judicial action; *legal aspects; legal rights; legislation; pain; persistent vegetative state; physically disabled; physician patient relationship; physician's role; *physicians; prolongation of life; quality of life; *right to die; state government; state interest; suffering; Supreme Court decisions; terminal care; terminally ill; third party consent; treatment refusal; trust; value of life; ventilators; vulnerable populations; *wedge argument; withholding treatment; Bouvia, Elizabeth; Cruzan, Nancy; Death with Dignity Act (OR); Netherlands; New York; Oregon; Patient Self–Determination Act 1990; Quinlan, Karen; *United States; Washington

Murder charge against Dutch nursing home dropped. [News]. *BMJ (British Medical Journal).* 1997 Sep 13; 315(7109): 624. BE57364.
*allowing to die; *artificial feeding; criminal law; *dementia; intention; killing; *legal liability; *nursing homes; *withholding treatment; dehydration; *Netherlands

ALLOWING TO DIE/RELIGIOUS ASPECTS

Cozby, Dimitri. Prolonging life: an Orthodox Christian perspective. *Christian Bioethics.* 1997 Dec; 3(3): 204–221. 21 refs. 18 fn. BE58487.
*allowing to die; *attitudes to death; decision making; *Eastern Orthodox ethics; family members; human body; pain; pastoral care; personhood; physicians; *prolongation of life; psychological stress; *suffering; terminal care; *terminally ill; *theology; treatment refusal; uncertainty; withholding treatment
While Orthodox Christianity does not find explicit statements about the morality of prolonging life in the usual doctrinal sources, the Scriptures and the Fathers of the Church, there are elements in Tradition which bear upon the issue. These include Orthodox spirituality's emphasis on the "wholeness" of the human person, its liturgical and synergistic view of human life, and its understanding of our moral ambiguity as fallen human beings in a fallen world. This last point, in particular, means that we do not usually have a clear choice between right and wrong, and that we cannot always trust ourselves to know which choice is the right, or even the better one. Therefore, we must always approach decisions about death and dying with humility and in a spirit of repentance, aware of the imperfection of all we do and trusting in the mercy of God.

Donovan, G. Kevin. Decisions at the end of life: Catholic

---

tradition. *Christian Bioethics.* 1997 Dec; 3(3): 188–203. 22 refs. 4 fn. BE58488.

> *active euthanasia; *allowing to die; artificial feeding; *assisted suicide; *attitudes to death; *brain death; cardiac death; costs and benefits; decision making; *determination of death; drugs; family members; informed consent; intention; organ donation; *pain; *palliative care; persistent vegetative state; prolongation of life; resuscitation; risks and benefits; *Roman Catholic ethics; *suffering; suicide; terminal care; *terminally ill; theology; third party consent; treatment outcome; treatment refusal; value of life; *withholding treatment; Congregation for the Doctrine of the Faith; National Conference of Catholic Bishops; United States

Medical decisions regarding end-of-life care have undergone significant changes in recent decades, driven by changes in both medicine and society. Catholic tradition in medical ethics offers clear guidance in many issues, and a moral framework accessible to those who do not share the same faith as well as to members of its faith community. In some areas, a Catholic perspective can be seen clearly and confidently, such as in teachings on the permissibility of suicide and euthanasia. In others, such as withdrawal of nutrition and hydration, the Church does not yet speak with one voice and has not closed out the discussion. Yet, it is not in the teaching on individual issues that a Catholic moral tradition offers the most help and comfort, but in its account of what it means to lead a life in Christ, and to prepare for a Christian death. As in the problem of pain and suffering, it is the spiritual support more than the ethical guidance that helps both patients and physicians bear the unbearable and fathom the unfathomable.

Eber, George. End-of-life decision making: an authentic Christian death. *Christian Bioethics.* 1997 Dec; 3(3): 183–187. 6 refs. BE58489.

> *allowing to die; assisted suicide; *attitudes to death; *Christian ethics; costs and benefits; decision making; pastoral care; prolongation of life; psychological stress; risks and benefits; secularism; *suffering; terminal care; *terminally ill; theology; treatment refusal; value of life; withholding treatment

Fournier, Keith A.; Watkins, William D. In Defense of Life. Colorado Springs, CO: NavPress; 1996. 159 p. 352 fn. ISBN 08910–98801. BE56728.

> aborted fetuses; *abortion, induced; *active euthanasia; aged; *allowing to die; *assisted suicide; beginning of life; body parts and fluids; brain death; *Christian ethics; commodification; congenital disorders; death; determination of death; disabled; economics; eugenics; fetal tissue donation; fetuses; government regulation; health personnel; historical aspects; human experimentation; infanticide; international aspects; judicial action; *killing; legal aspects; love; *morality; *newborns; organ donation; *political activity; population control; pregnant women; psychological stress; public policy; quality of life; rights; *value of life; *values; violence; hope; Humphry, Derek; Kevorkian, Jack; *Right to Life Movement; Roe v. Wade; Smith, Susan; United States

Geis, Sally B.; Messer, Donald E., eds. How Shall We Die?: Helping Christians Debate Assisted Suicide. Nashville, TN: Abingdon Press; 1997. 201 p. Annotated bibliography: p. 183–189. Appendices include generic forms for advance directives and for organ/tissue donation. ISBN 0-687-06140-7. BE57384.

> *active euthanasia; advance directives; *allowing to die; *assisted suicide; attitudes to death; autonomy; beneficence; case studies; *Christian ethics; clergy; *decision making; diagnosis; drugs; ethics consultation; family members; forms; freedom; informed consent; killing; legal aspects; love; pain; palliative care; pastoral care; patients; physicians; prognosis;

Protestant ethics; quality of life; resource allocation; right to die; Roman Catholic ethics; suffering; *suicide; terminally ill; *theology; treatment refusal; truth disclosure; value of life; voluntary euthanasia; wedge argument; withholding treatment; Compassion in Dying v. State of Washington; Death with Dignity Act (OR); New York; Quill v. Vacco; United States; Washington

Guroian, Vigen. Life's Living toward Dying: A Theological and Medical-Ethical Study. Grand Rapids, MI: W.B. Eerdmans; 1996. 108 p. 130 fn. ISBN 0-8028-4190-2. BE55682.

> *active euthanasia; *allowing to die; *assisted suicide; *attitudes to death; autonomy; *Christian ethics; Eastern Orthodox ethics; human experimentation; infants; killing; *literature; medicine; morality; physician's role; prolongation of life; religion; right to die; secularism; social impact; suffering; *terminal care; terminally ill; *theology; trends; values; Baby Rena; Kevorkian, Jack

McGann, John R. To care for the dying. *Origins.* 1997 Mar 20; 26(39): 640–648. 99 fn. Text of a pastoral letter, "Comfort my people: finding peace as life ends," by Bishop John R. McGann of Rockville Centre, NY, 19 Feb 1997. BE56596.

> active euthanasia; *allowing to die; *assisted suicide; attitudes to death; biomedical technologies; clergy; coercion; compassion; depressive disorder; double effect; drugs; economics; emotions; family members; government regulation; health care; health personnel; hospices; intention; love; pain; *palliative care; pastoral care; patients; physician patient relationship; physician's role; physicians; prolongation of life; psychological stress; *Roman Catholic ethics; social interaction; suffering; *terminal care; terminally ill; trust; vulnerable populations; withholding treatment; dignity; United States

Morrison, Mary F.; DeMichele, Sarah Gelbach. How culture and religion affect attitudes toward medical futility. *In:* Zucker, Marjorie B.; Zucker Howard D., eds. Medical Futility and the Evaluation of Life-Sustaining Interventions. New York, NY: Cambridge University Press; 1997: 71–84. 36 refs. ISBN 0-521-56877-3. BE55981.

> active euthanasia; advance directives; *allowing to die; alternative therapies; American Indians; Asian Americans; *attitudes to death; autonomy; blacks; Buddhist ethics; communication; *cultural pluralism; *decision making; *determination of death; family members; females; *futility; Hindu ethics; Hispanic Americans; Islamic ethics; Jewish ethics; males; *minority groups; pain; physician's role; *prolongation of life; Protestant ethics; quality of life; *religion; Roman Catholic ethics; socioeconomic factors; suffering; suicide; *terminally ill; treatment refusal; trust; truth disclosure; value of life; *values; withholding treatment; United States

O'Rourke, Kevin. Euthanasia and assisted suicide: a response to Edmund Pellegrino. *In:* Wildes, Kevin Wm.; Mitchell, Alan C., eds. Choosing Life: A Dialogue on *Evangelium Vitae.* Washington, DC: Georgetown University Press; 1997: 259–261. ISBN 0-87840-646-8. BE56693.

> *allowing to die; artificial feeding; assisted suicide; persistent vegetative state; prolongation of life; quality of life; risks and benefits; *Roman Catholic ethics; terminally ill; treatment refusal; voluntary euthanasia; withholding treatment; Evangelium Vitae

O'Rourke, Kevin D. Withdrawal of life support: mistaken assumptions. *Health Progress.* 1996 Nov–Dec; 77(6): 60–61, 65. 14 fn. BE56324.

> advance directives; *allowing to die; artificial feeding; family members; love; moral obligations; persistent vegetative state; prolongation of life; risks and benefits; *Roman Catholic

---

BE = bioethics accession number   fn. = footnotes   refs. = references

ethics; terminally ill; third party consent; withholding treatment

Paris, John J.; Poorman, Mark. When religious beliefs and medical judgments conflict: civic polity and the social good. *In:* Zucker, Marjorie B.; Zucker, Howard D., eds. Medical Futility and the Evaluation of Life-Sustaining Interventions. New York, NY: Cambridge University Press; 1997: 85–97. 54 refs. ISBN 0-521-56877-3. BE55982.
    *allowing to die; autonomy; *common good; conscience; constitutional law; *cultural pluralism; *decision making; democracy; determination of death; *dissent; *family members; *futility; justice; legal aspects; medicine; *patients; *physician's role; *physicians; professional autonomy; *prolongation of life; *public policy; *refusal to treat; *religion; secularism; *terminally ill; value of life; integrity; First Amendment; In re Baby K; In re Wanglie; United States

Rosin, Arnold J.; Sonnenblick, Moshe. Autonomy and paternalism in geriatric medicine: the Jewish ethical approach to issues of feeding terminally ill patients, and to cardiopulmonary resuscitation. *Journal of Medical Ethics.* 1998 Feb; 24(1): 44–48. 45 refs. BE57409.
    *aged; *allowing to die; *artificial feeding; attitudes; *autonomy; decision making; *dementia; family members; futility; *Jewish ethics; palliative care; *paternalism; physicians; prognosis; *prolongation of life; religious hospitals; resuscitation; *resuscitation orders; risks and benefits; suffering; *terminal care; *terminally ill; treatment outcome; treatment refusal; *value of life; withholding treatment; *Israel; Orthodox Judaism; Shaare Zedek Medical Center (Jerusalem)
Respecting and encouraging autonomy in the elderly is basic to the practice of geriatrics. In this paper, we examine the practice of cardiopulmonary resuscitation (CPR) and "artificial" feeding in a geriatric unit in a general hospital subscribing to Jewish orthodox religious principles, in which the sanctity of life is a fundamental ethical guideline. The literature on the administration of food and water in terminal stages of illness, including dementia, still shows division of opinion on the morality of withdrawing nutrition. We uphold the principle that as long as feeding by naso-gastric (N–G) or percutaneous endoscopic gastrostomy (PEG) does not constitute undue danger or arouse serious opposition it should be given, without causing suffering to the patient. This is part of basic care, and the doctor has no mandate to withdraw this. The question of CPR still shows much discrepancy regarding elderly patients' wishes, and doctors' opinions about its worthwhileness, although up to 10 percent survive. Our geriatric patients rarely discuss the subject, but it is openly ventilated with families who ask about it, who are then involved in the decision-making, and the decision about CPR or "do-not-resuscitate" (DNR) is based on clinical and prognostic considerations.

Rosner, Fred. Euthanasia. *In:* Dorff, Elliot N.; Newman, Louis E., eds. Contemporary Jewish Ethics and Morality: A Reader. New York, NY: Oxford University Press; 1995: 350–362. 76 fn. Reprinted from Rosner, Fred; Bleich, J. David, eds., *Jewish Bioethics*, New York, NY: Hebrew Publishing Co., 1979: 253–265. ISBN 0-19-509066-7. BE58528.
    *active euthanasia; *allowing to die; assisted suicide; Christian ethics; eugenics; *euthanasia; international aspects; involuntary euthanasia; *Jewish ethics; killing; legal aspects; physicians; suffering; terminally ill; terminology; *theology; voluntary euthanasia; withholding treatment; Orthodox Judaism

Rushton, Cindy Hylton; Russell, Kathleen. The language of miracles: ethical challenges. *Pediatric Nursing.* 1996 Jan–Feb; 22(1): 64–67. 1 ref. BE55579.
    *allowing to die; attitudes; case studies; children; communication; *decision making; dissent; emotions; futility; *health personnel; leukemia; *parents; professional family relationship; *prolongation of life; *religion; resuscitation orders; terminal care; *terminally ill; withholding treatment; *hope

Shatz, David. Concepts of autonomy in Jewish medical ethics. *In:* Jewish Law Annual. Volume Twelve. Amsterdam, Netherlands: Harwood Academic Publishers; 1997: 3–43. 84 fn. ISBN 90-5702-551-5. BE58346.
    *allowing to die; altruism; *autonomy; *beneficence; bioethics; coercion; comparative studies; *decision making; disclosure; historical aspects; *informed consent; *Jewish ethics; medical ethics; moral obligations; *moral policy; pain; paternalism; patient compliance; prolongation of life; risks and benefits; secularism; *theology; treatment refusal; uncertainty; values; withholding treatment

Stempsey, William E. End-of-life decisions: Christian perspectives. *Christian Bioethics.* 1997 Dec; 3(3): 249–261. 21 refs. 3 fn. BE58490.
    *active euthanasia; *allowing to die; *assisted suicide; *attitudes to death; autonomy; *Christian ethics; conscience; constitutional law; costs and benefits; decision making; *Eastern Orthodox ethics; human body; legal rights; libertarianism; moral obligations; morality; *natural law; personhood; physicians; prolongation of life; *Protestant ethics; risks and benefits; *Roman Catholic ethics; *secularism; suffering; Supreme Court decisions; *terminally ill; *theology; value of life; values; withholding treatment; *Methodist Church; United States; Vacco v. Quill; Washington v. Glucksberg
While legal rights to make medical treatment decisions at the end of one's life have been recognized by the courts, particular religious traditions put axiological and metaphysical meat on the bare bones of legal rights. Mere legal rights do not capture the full reality, meaning and importance of death. End-of-life decisions reflect not only the meaning we find in dying, but also the meaning we have found in living. The Christian religions bring particular understandings of the vision of life as a gift from God, human responsibility for stewardship of that life, the wholeness of the person, and the importance of the dying process in preparing spiritually for life beyond earthly life, to bear on end-of-life decisions.

Thobaben, James R. A United Methodist approach to end-of-life decisions: intentional ambiguity or ambiguous intentions. *Christian Bioethics.* 1997 Dec; 3(3): 222–248. 40 refs. 22 fn. BE58491.
    *active euthanasia; advance directives; *allowing to die; *assisted suicide; autonomy; *clergy; competence; *decision making; *dissent; family members; historical aspects; hospices; *organizational policies; pain; pastoral care; personhood; physicians; *Protestant ethics; quality of life; suffering; suicide; terminal care; *terminally ill; terminology; theology; third party consent; treatment refusal; uncertainty; vulnerable populations; withholding treatment; *Methodist Church; *Wesley, John
The position of the United Methodist Church on end-of-life decisions is best described as intentional ambiguity or ambiguous intentions or both. The paper analyzes the official position of the denomination and then considers the actions of a U.M.C. bishop who served as a foreman for a trial of Dr. Jack Kevorkian. In an effort to find some common ground within an increasingly divided denomination, the work concludes with a consideration of the work of John Wesley and his approach to human death.

BE = bioethics accession number   fn. = footnotes   refs. = references

Werber, Stephen J. Ancient answers to modern questions: death, dying, and organ transplants -- a Jewish law perspective. *Journal of Law and Health.* 1996–1997; 11(1–2): 13–44. 139 fn. BE57589.
  *active euthanasia; *allowing to die; *assisted suicide; brain death; cadavers; chronically ill; *determination of death; hearts; *Jewish ethics; killing; *organ donation; organ donors; organ transplantation; physicians; *resuscitation orders; right to die; *suicide; terminally ill; tissue donation; treatment refusal; value of life; withholding treatment; Orthodox Judaism

Wildes, Kevin Wm. Sanctity of life: a study in ambiguity and confusion. *In:* Hoshino, Kazumasa, ed. Japanese and Western Bioethics: Studies in Moral Diversity. Boston, MA: Kluwer Academic; 1997: 89–101. 33 refs. 5 fn. ISBN 0–7923–4112–0. BE57085.
  abortion, induced; *allowing to die; *bioethics; *Buddhist ethics; *Christian ethics; compassion; euthanasia; killing; legal aspects; personhood; *prolongation of life; religion; Roman Catholic ethics; *secularism; state interest; suicide; *terminology; theology; *value of life; withholding treatment; Cruzan v. Director, Missouri Department of Health; Cruzan v. Harmon; United States

ANIMAL EXPERIMENTATION

Balls, Michael; Goldberg, Alan M.; Fentem, Julia H., et al. The three Rs: the way forward: the report and recommendations of ECVAM [European Centre for the Validation of Alternative Methods] Workshop 11. *ATLA: Alternatives to Laboratory Animals.* 1995 Nov–Dec; 23(6): 838–866. 112 refs. BE56085.
  animal care committees; *animal experimentation; *animal testing alternatives; drugs; education; ethical review; financial support; government regulation; guidelines; historical aspects; information dissemination; *international aspects; investigators; primates; public policy; research design; risks and benefits; suffering; transgenic animals; Europe; *European Union; Great Britain; Twentieth Century; United States

Beauchamp, Tom L. Opposing views on animal experimentation: do animals have rights? *Ethics and Behavior.* 1997; 7(2): 113–121. 13 refs. 4 fn. BE56400.
  *animal experimentation; *animal rights; autonomy; dementia; emotions; *moral obligations; *moral policy; pain; personhood; quality of life; rights; *speciesism; standards; suffering; value of life
Animals have moral standing; that is, they have properties (including the ability to feel pain) that qualify them for the protections of morality. It follows from this that humans have moral obligations toward animals, and because rights are logically correlative to obligations, animals have rights.

Brestrup, Craig. Experimenting on animals. *In:* his Disposable Animals: Ending the Tragedy of Throwaway Pets. Leander, TX: Camino Bay Books; 1997: 115–128. 3 refs. ISBN 0–9657285–9–5. BE57227.
  *animal experimentation; animal testing alternatives; human characteristics; investigators; moral obligations; organizational policies; risks and benefits; self concept; *speciesism; value of life; Animals (Scientific Procedures) Act 1986; Great Britain; Institute of Medical Ethics (Great Britain)

Brody, Baruch A., comp. Appendixes: international research ethics policies; European transnational research ethics policies; U.S. research ethics policies; research ethics policies from other countries. *In:* his The Ethics of Biomedical Research: An International Perspective. New York, NY: Oxford University Press; 1998: 213–358. ISBN 0–19–509007–1. BE57677.
  *animal experimentation; *biomedical research; codes of ethics; embryo research; federal government; fetal research; gene therapy; genetic research; genetic screening; genome mapping; government regulation; *guidelines; *human experimentation; *international aspects; patents; professional organizations; *research ethics; Australia; Canada; Council for International Organizations of Medical Sciences (CIOMS); Council of Europe; Declaration of Helsinki; Department of Health and Human Services; Europe; Food and Drug Administration; Great Britain; Japan; National Institutes of Health; Nuremberg Code; Public Health Service; United States; World Medical Association

Brody, Baruch A. Research ethics: international perspectives. *Cambridge Quarterly of Healthcare Ethics.* 1997 Fall; 6(4): 376–384. 22 fn. BE56458.
  adults; *animal experimentation; animal rights; bioethics; comparative studies; *consensus; *cultural pluralism; *dissent; *embryo research; embryos; ethical review; guidelines; *human experimentation; in vitro fertilization; informed consent; *international aspects; moral obligations; moral policy; regulation; research embryo creation; research subjects; speciesism; value of life; Asia; Australia; Europe; North America

Brody, Baruch A. The use of animals in research. *In:* his The Ethics of Biomedical Research: An International Perspective. New York, NY: Oxford University Press; 1998: 11–30, 361–362. 37 fn. ISBN 0–19–509007–1. BE57668.
  animal care committees; *animal experimentation; animal organs; animal rights; animal testing alternatives; comparative studies; ethical review; government regulation; historical aspects; *international aspects; *moral policy; organ transplantation; patents; *public policy; review; risks and benefits; speciesism; statistics; suffering; transgenic animals; utilitarianism; Australia; Europe; United States

Burch, Rex L. The progress of humane experimental technique since 1959: a personal view. *ATLA: Alternatives to Laboratory Animals.* 1995 Nov–Dec; 23(6): 776–783. 37 refs. BE55739.
  *animal experimentation; animal testing alternatives; historical aspects; trends; Great Britain; Twentieth Century

Coghlan, Andy. Silent slaughter. [News]. *New Scientist.* 1997 Oct 25; 156(2105): 25. BE59088.
  *animal experimentation; body parts and fluids; investigators; killing; political activity; statistics; *Great Britain

Cohen, Carl. Do animals have rights? *Ethics and Behavior.* 1997; 7(2): 91–102. 3 refs. BE56404.
  *animal experimentation; *animal rights; biomedical research; human rights; killing; *moral obligations; *moral policy; philosophy; rights; risks and benefits; *speciesism; rodents; Regan, Tom
A right, unlike an interest, is a valid claim, or potential claim, made by a moral agent, under principles that govern both the claimant and the target of the claim. Animals cannot be the bearers of rights because the concept of rights is essentially human; it is rooted in and has force within a human moral world.

Cohen, Carl. Ethical aspects of animal research. *In:* Eder, G.; Kaiser, E.; King, F.A., eds. The Role of the Chimpanzee in Research. Symposium, Vienna, Austria, May 22–24, 1992. New York, NY: Karger; 1994: 18–25. 3 refs. ISBN 3–8055–5850–3. BE58158.
  *animal experimentation; *animal rights; drugs; human experimentation; human rights; *moral obligations; *moral policy; pain; *primates; *risks and benefits; *speciesism; utilitarianism

---

BE = bioethics accession number   fn. = footnotes   refs. = references

Cooper, J.E. Ethics and laboratory animals. *Veterinary Record.* 1985 Jun 1; 116(22): 594–595. 6 refs. BE56955.
accountability; administrators; anesthesia; animal care committees; *animal experimentation; animal testing alternatives; euthanasia; *guidelines; *international aspects; moral obligations; pain; professional competence; public policy; speciesism; suffering; surgery; analgesia; Biological Council (Great Britain); *Council for International Organizations of Medical Sciences; Great Britain

Dombrowski, Daniel A. Babies and Beasts: The Argument from Marginal Cases. Urbana, IL: University of Illinois Press; 1997. 221 p. Bibliography: p. 211–218. ISBN 0-252-06638-3. BE56144.
animal experimentation; *animal rights; infants; killing; mentally retarded; *moral policy; persistent vegetative state; personhood; philosophy; primates; review; rights; *speciesism; suffering; slavery; Becker, Lawrence; Carruthers, Peter; Frey, R.G.; Leahy, Michael; McCloskey, H.J.; Narveson, Jan; Nozick, Robert; Rachels, James; Rawls, John; Regan, Tom; Singer, Peter; Watson, Richard

Dresser, Rebecca. Scientists in the sunshine. *Hastings Center Report.* 1997 Nov–Dec; 27(6): 26–28. 11 refs. BE57857.
*advisory committees; animal experimentation; *biomedical research; *committee membership; conflict of interest; *decision making; federal government; government financing; government regulation; guidelines; information dissemination; investigators; *legal aspects; legislation; private sector; *public participation; public policy; public sector; *science; *standards; Supreme Court decisions; technical expertise; values; *Animal Legal Defense Fund v. Shalala; *Federal Advisory Committee Act 1994; Guide for the Care and Use of Laboratory Animals (National Research Council); *National Academy of Sciences; Public Citizen v. U.S. Department of Justice; *United States

Feldmann, Bruce Max. The immorality of nonhuman animal research. *Journal of the American Veterinary Medical Association.* 1996 Jun 1; 208(11): 1798–1801. 10 refs. BE57412.
alternatives; *animal experimentation; animal rights; biomedical research; epidemiology; health services research; human rights; intelligence; moral obligations; *moral policy; pain; preventive medicine; speciesism; suffering

Frey, R.G. Moral community and animal research in medicine. *Ethics and Behavior.* 1997; 7(2): 123–136. 8 refs. 6 fn. BE56849.
allowing to die; anencephaly; *animal experimentation; *animal rights; assisted suicide; biomedical research; mentally disabled; *moral obligations; *moral policy; pain; personhood; quality of life; religion; rights; *speciesism; suffering; utilitarianism; *value of life; wedge argument
The invocation of moral rights in moral/social debate today is a recipe for deadlock in our consideration of substantive issues. How we treat animals and humans in part should derive from the value of their lives, which is a function of the quality of their lives, which in turn is a function of the richness of their lives. Consistency in argument requires that humans with a low quality of life should be chosen as experimental subjects over animals with a higher quality of life.

Gluck, John P.; Shapiro, Kenneth J. Behavioral research and animal welfare. [Case study and commentaries]. *Ethics and Behavior.* 1997; 7(2): 185–192. 20 refs. BE56409.
*animal care committees; *animal experimentation; animal testing alternatives; behavioral research; case studies; committee membership; conflict of interest; dissent; ethical review; investigators; psychological stress; *research design; suffering; technical expertise; utilitarianism

Gluck, John P. Harry F. Harlow and animal research: reflection on the ethical paradox. *Ethics and Behavior.* 1997; 7(2): 149–161. 24 refs. 1 fn. BE56410.
*animal experimentation; attitudes; behavior disorders; behavioral research; brain pathology; emotions; *evaluation; famous persons; interprofessional relations; *investigators; motivation; peer review; *primates; professional ethics; psychological stress; psychology; *research design; *scientific misconduct; self regulation; social interaction; suffering; *Harlow, Harry
With respect to the ethical debate about the treatment of animals in biomedical and behavioral research, Harry F. Harlow represents a paradox. On the one hand, his work on monkey cognition and social development fostered a view of the animals as having rich subjective lives filled with intention and emotion. On the other, he has been criticized for the conduct of research that seemed to ignore the ethical implications of his own discoveries. The basis of this contradiction is discussed and propositions for current research practice are presented.

Gluck, John P.; Orlans, F. Barbara. Institutional animal care and use committees: a flawed paradigm or work in progress? *Ethics and Behavior.* 1997; 7(4): 329–336. 6 refs. BE58664.
*animal care committees; *animal experimentation; committee membership; conflict of interest; ethical review; evaluation; federal government; government regulation; investigators; legislation; public participation; scientific misconduct; self regulation; standards; technical expertise; universities; Animal Welfare Act; United States
In his challenging article, Steneck (1997) criticized the creation of the Institutional Animal Care and Use Committee (IACUC) system established by the 1985 amendments to the Animal Welfare Act. He saw the IACUC review and approval of biomedical and behavioral research with animals as an unnecessary "reassignment" of duties from existing animal care programs to IACUC committees. He argued that the committees are unable to do the work expected of them for basically three reasons: (a) the membership lacks the expertise in matters relevant to animal research and care, (b) there exists an inherent and disabling conflict of interest, and (c) the committee's operational base of authority is alien to academic culture and violates essential aspects of academic freedom. In addition, he found that the system is burdensome, requiring enormous expenditures of time and money that inappropriately diverts resources away from the business of scientific discovery. We dispute several aspects of Steneck's historical account and the coherence of his proposals. We believe his proposals, if followed, would be a step back into a failed past.

Golden, Frederic. Cock-a-doodle quail. [News]. *Time.* 1997 Mar 17; 149(11): 60. BE58042.
*animal experimentation; *brain; embryo research; *embryos; *tissue transplantation; *animal behavior; Balaban, Evan; Neurosciences Institute (San Diego, CA)

Great Britain. Parliamentary Office of Science and Technology. The Use of Animals in Research, Development and Testing. London: Parliamentary Office of Science and Technology; 1992 Sep. 92 p. 94 refs. 11 fn. ISBN 1-897941-05-6. BE56242.
accountability; *animal experimentation; animal testing alternatives; government regulation; international aspects; investigators; legislation; political activity; primates; public policy; research institutes; risks and benefits; statistics; toxicity; transgenic animals; Animals (Scientific Procedures) Act 1986; Europe; European Community; *Great Britain

---

BE = bioethics accession number   fn. = footnotes   refs. = references

Griffin, Gilly. Alternatives in Canada. *ATLA: Alternatives to Laboratory Animals.* 1995 Nov–Dec; 23(6): 824–826. 12 refs. BE55552.
animal care committees; *animal experimentation; *animal testing alternatives; *Canada; Canadian Council on Animal Care

Groves, Julian McAllister. Hearts and Minds: The Controversy over Laboratory Animals. Philadelphia, PA: Temple University Press; 1997. 230 p. (Animals, culture, and society). Bibliography: p. 213–221. ISBN 1–56639–476–7. BE58944.
animal care committees; *animal experimentation; animal rights; *attitudes; emotions; females; historical aspects; *investigators; males; motivation; *political activity; regulation; risks and benefits; ethnographic studies; United States

Hart, C.B. Legal control of use of animals for scientific purposes. *In:* Tuffery, A.A., ed. Laboratory Animals: An Introduction for Experimenters. Second Edition. New York, NY: Wiley; 1995: 37–65. 19 refs. ISBN 0–471–95257–5. BE56089.
anesthesia; animal care committees; *animal experimentation; *government regulation; killing; *legal aspects; legislation; records; risks and benefits; suffering; *Animals (Scientific Procedures) Act 1986; Council of Europe; *Cruelty to Animals Act 1876 (Great Britain); Europe; European Union; *Great Britain

Häyry, Matti. Ethics committees, principles and consequences. *Journal of Medical Ethics.* 1998 Apr; 24(2): 81–85. 8 refs. BE58079.
*animal care committees; *animal experimentation; autonomy; beneficence; *human experimentation; infants; justice; *moral policy; pain; personhood; principle–based ethics; prisoners; *research ethics committees; research subjects; risks and benefits; speciesism; suffering; value of life
When ethics committees evaluate the research proposals submitted to them by biomedical scientists, they can seek guidance from laws and regulations, their own beliefs, values and experiences, and from the theories of philosophers. The starting point of this paper is that philosophers can only be helpful to the members of ethics committees if they take into account in their models both the basic moral intuitions that most of us share and the consequences of people's choices. A moral view which can be labelled as a consequentialist interpretation of mid–level principlism is developed, defended and applied to some real–life and hypothetical research proposals.

Horton, Larry. Changing cultural and political attitudes toward research with animals. *In:* Eder, G.; Kaiser, E.; King, F.A., eds. The Role of the Chimpanzee in Research. Symposium, Vienna, Austria, May 22–24, 1992. New York, NY: Karger; 1994: 7–17. 7 refs. 3 fn. ISBN 3–8055–5850–3. BE58157.
adults; *animal experimentation; animal rights; attitudes; children; empirical research; government regulation; guidelines; human experimentation; informed consent; international aspects; investigators; mass media; *political activity; *politics; *public opinion; violence; Europe; Nuremberg Code; United States

James, Barbara. Animals in experiments. *In:* her Animal Rights. Hove, East Sussex, Eng.: Wayland; 1990: 20–26. (Points of view). ISBN 1–85210–842–8. BE56243.
*animal experimentation; animal rights; animal testing alternatives; attitudes; drugs; education; investigators; political activity; suffering; toxicity; cosmetics

Jamieson, Dale. Experimenting on animals: a

reconsideration. *Between the Species.* 1985 Summer; 1(3): 4–11. 12 fn. BE57061.
*animal experimentation; *animal rights; attitudes; biomedical research; freedom; humanism; investigators; *morality; pain; political activity; privacy; regulation; scientific misconduct; suffering; universities; violence

Jennings, Maggy; Silcock, Sheila. Benefits, necessity and justification in animal research. *ATLA: Alternatives to Laboratory Animals.* 1995 Nov–Dec; 23(6): 828–836. 40 refs. BE55585.
*animal experimentation; animal testing alternatives; biomedical research; costs and benefits; *decision making; drug industry; drugs; ethical review; government regulation; legislation; motivation; primates; research design; *risks and benefits; suffering; Animals (Scientific Procedures) Act 1986; *Great Britain

Jones, Bidda. Current Standards in Europe for the Care of Non–Human Primates in Laboratories. West Sussex, England: Royal Society for the Prevention of Cruelty to Animals; 1996 Mar. 25 p. 12 refs. ISBN 0–901098–05–1. BE57743.
*animal experimentation; animal testing alternatives; *evaluation; *guidelines; international aspects; legislation; organizational policies; *primates; *standards; statistics; *Europe; *European Convention for the Protection of Animals in Experimental Procedures; *European Primate Resources Network; *European Union

Kestenbaum, David. Groups vie for space chimp colony. [News]. *Science.* 1998 May 22; 280(5367): 1186. BE58269.
*animal experimentation; animal rights; federal government; political activity; *primates; U.S. Air Force; *United States

Kolata, Gina. Tough tactics are used over animals in the lab. [News]. *New York Times.* 1998 Mar 24: E1, E6. BE57731.
*animal experimentation; *animal rights; deception; industry; laboratories; *political activity; suffering; violence; Boys Town National Research Hospital; Colgate–Palmolive; *Huntingdon Life Sciences; *People for the Ethical Treatment of Animals (PETA); Proctor and Gamble; United States; Walsh, Edward

LaFollette, Hugh; Shanks, Niall. The origin of speciesism. *Philosophy.* 1996 Jan; 71(275): 41–61. 35 fn. BE57249.
*animal experimentation; behavioral research; deontological ethics; human characteristics; *moral policy; morality; philosophy; social discrimination; *speciesism; utilitarianism

Lewin, David I. Animal welfare group seeks ban on MAbs from mouse ascites. [News]. *Journal of NIH Research.* 1997 Jul; 9(7): 22–23. BE55587.
*animal experimentation; *animal testing alternatives; biomedical research; federal government; *government regulation; legal aspects; methods; *political activity; *rodents; American Anti–Vivisection Society; National Institutes of Health; *United States

McCarthy, Charles R. The rights of human research subjects and the necessity of conducting animal research as illuminated by the Nuremberg Code and the Declaration of Helsinki. *In:* Eder, G.; Kaiser, E.; King, F.A., eds. The Role of the Chimpanzee in Research. Symposium, Vienna, Austria, May 22–24, 1992. New York, NY: Karger; 1994: 1–6. 5 refs. ISBN 3–8055–5850–3. BE58156.
*animal experimentation; autonomy; codes of ethics; deontological ethics; *guidelines; *human experimentation; human rights; informed consent; international aspects; nontherapeutic research; primates; research subjects; utilitarianism; *Declaration of Helsinki; *Nuremberg Code

---

BE = bioethics accession number   fn. = footnotes   refs. = references

Macilwain, Colin. NIH urged to address chimp care 'crisis'. [News]. *Nature.* 1997 Jul 17; 388(6639): 218. BE56311.
     AIDS; *animal experimentation; federal government; government financing; political activity; *primates; research institutes; resource allocation; Chimpanzee Management Program (ChiMP); National Academy of Sciences; *National Institutes of Health; United States

Masood, Ehsan. Pressure grows for inquiry into welfare of transgenic animals. [News]. *Nature.* 1997 Jul 24; 388(6640): 311–312. BE56579.
     advisory committees; animal experimentation; animal organs; animal rights; genetic research; organ transplantation; political activity; politics; public opinion; *public policy; risks and benefits; *transgenic animals; Europe; *Great Britain

Masood, Ehsan. UK tightens regime for animal research. [News]. *Nature.* 1997 Oct 30; 389(6654): 896. BE56164.
     *animal experimentation; animal testing alternatives; economics; education; government financing; *government regulation; industry; information dissemination; public opinion; public policy; *Great Britain

Miller, Barbara. Germany remains split on animal testing. [News]. *Nature.* 1998 Feb 12; 391(6668): 624. BE58023.
     *animal experimentation; animal rights; *government regulation; international aspects; legal aspects; political activity; politics; European Union; *Germany

Morton, David. A comparison of the controls regarding the ethical judgements on animal and human research. *In:* Close, Bryony; Combes, Robert; Hubbard, Anthony; Illingworth, John, eds. Volunteers in Research and Testing. Bristol, PA: Taylor and Francis; 1997: 109–116. 7 refs. ISBN 0-7484-0397-3. BE57035.
     accountability; animal care committees; *animal experimentation; animal testing alternatives; committee membership; government regulation; guidelines; human experimentation; public participation; *regulation; suffering; *Great Britain

Morton, David B. Advances in refinement in animal experimentation over the past 25 years. *ATLA: Alternatives to Laboratory Animals.* 1995 Nov–Dec; 23(6): 812–822. 73 refs. BE55590.
     *animal experimentation; animal testing alternatives; education; government regulation; guidelines; historical aspects; investigators; primates; public opinion; *standards; suffering; *Great Britain; Twentieth Century

National Science Teachers Association. Code of Practice on Use of Animals in Schools. [Position statement]. Issued by the National Science Teachers Association, 1742 Connecticut Avenue, N.W., Washington, DC 20009; 1985 Jul. 2 p. Adopted by the NSTA Board of Directors, Jul 1985. BE57149.
     *animal experimentation; *education; faculty; *guidelines; *organizational policies; professional organizations; *schools; *science; primary schools; secondary schools; *National Science Teachers Association; United States

Noble, Denis; Vincent, Jean–Didier. The Ethics of Life. Paris: Unesco; 1997. 238 p. Bibliography: p. 221–230. Papers presented at a seminar "Physiology and the Respect for Life," held under the joint auspices of the International Union of Physical Scientists and Unesco in Paris, Sep 1995. ISBN 92-3-103422-7. BE58647.
     *animal experimentation; *animal rights; attitudes to death; beginning of life; behavioral research; *bioethical issues; bioethics; *biomedical research; brain death; Buddhist ethics; competence; determination of death; education; embryo research; females; fetal research; genetic determinism;

homosexuals; human experimentation; *human rights; humanism; informed consent; international aspects; legal aspects; moral obligations; *moral policy; nontherapeutic research; organ donation; personhood; philosophy; political activity; prisoners; regulation; research ethics committees; research subjects; risks and benefits; science; speciesism; suffering; therapeutic research; *value of life; vulnerable populations; Europe; Japan

Orlans, F. Barbara. Ethical decision making about animal experiments. *Ethics and Behavior.* 1997; 7(2): 163–171. 8 refs. BE56416.
     *animal care committees; *animal experimentation; committee membership; decision making; *ethical review; international aspects; pain; public participation; public policy; risks and benefits; standards; suffering; Guide for the Care and Use of Laboratory Animals (National Research Council); United States
Laboratory animals, being vulnerable subjects, need the protection provided by adequate ethical review. This review falls primarily to Institutional Animal Care and Use Committees. A review committee's first duty is to identify which procedures ethically are unacceptable irrespective of any knowledge that might be derived. Examples are provided. These projects should be disapproved. Then, "on balance" judgments are assessed that weigh the animal harms against the potential benefits to humans. Several countries (but not the United States) use a classification system for ranking the degree of animal pain and distress. This type of assessment is essential for careful ethical analysis. Another way to enhance ethical discussion is to strive for a more balanced perspective of different viewpoints among members of decision making committees. Inclusion of representatives of animal welfare organizations and a greater proportion of nonanimal researchers would likely achieve this objective.

Orlans, F. Barbara; Beauchamp, Tom L.; Dresser, Rebecca, et al. The Human Use of Animals: Case Studies in Ethical Choice. New York, NY: Oxford University Press; 1998. 330 p. 669 fn. ISBN 0-19-511907-X. BE57045.
     aggression; animal care committees; *animal experimentation; animal organs; animal rights; animal testing alternatives; behavioral research; brain; case studies; deontological ethics; drugs; ecology; education; emotions; *ethical analysis; ethical review; evolution; food; force feeding; government regulation; historical aspects; injuries; investigators; killing; *moral policy; morality; mothers; organ donation; organ transplantation; pain; patents; personhood; primates; professional ethics; quality of life; religion; review; rights; speciesism; suffering; toxicity; transgenic animals; utilitarianism; cosmetics

Parascandola, Mark. Animal research. *In:* Chadwick, Ruth, ed. Encyclopedia of Applied Ethics, Volume 1. San Diego, CA: Academic Press; 1998: 151–160. 9 refs. ISBN 0-12-227066-5. BE56368.
     *animal experimentation; animal rights; animal testing alternatives; attitudes; biomedical research; decision making; drugs; education; government regulation; guidelines; historical aspects; international aspects; investigators; legislation; pain; political activity; public participation; risks and benefits; self regulation; speciesism; standards; statistics; suffering; toxicity; cosmetics; United States

Parnham, Michael J. Animal experimentation. *In: his* Ethical Issues in Drug Research: Through a Glass Darkly. Washington, DC: IOS Press; 1996: 97–114. 46 fn. ISBN 90-5199-279-3. BE55678.
     *animal experimentation; animal rights; animal testing alternatives; attitudes; biomedical research; conscience; drugs; emotions; evolution; guidelines; historical aspects;

BE = bioethics accession number   fn. = footnotes   refs. = references

investigators; killing; moral policy; philosophy; political activity; regulation; religious ethics; research design; *risks and benefits; science; speciesism; utilitarianism

Regan, Tom. The rights of humans and other animals. *Ethics and Behavior.* 1997; 7(2): 103–111. 2 refs. 1 fn. BE56417.
> *animal experimentation; *animal rights; autonomy; biomedical research; emotions; *human rights; infants; mentally disabled; moral policy; morality; pain; personhood; *speciesism; utilitarianism; rationality

Human moral rights place justified limits on what people are free to do to one another. Animals also have moral rights, and arguments to support the use of animals in scientific research based on the benefits allegedly derived from animal model research are thus invalid. Animals do not belong in laboratories because placing them there, in the hope of benefits for others, violates their rights.

Rollin, Bernard E. Laws relevant to animal research in the United States. *In:* Tuffery, A.A., ed. Laboratory Animals: An Introduction for Experimenters. Second Edition. New York, NY: Wiley; 1995: 67–86. 24 refs. ISBN 0-471-95257-5. BE56090.
> accountability; animal care committees; *animal experimentation; animal testing alternatives; federal government; *government regulation; historical aspects; *legal aspects; legislation; pain; public policy; standards; suffering; Animal Enterprise Protection Act 1992; Animal Welfare Act 1966; Department of Agriculture; Health Research Extension Act 1985; National Institutes of Health; NIH Revitalization Act 1993; Twentieth Century; *United States

Rose, John C. Animals in research: an investigator's perspective. *Pharos.* 1985 Fall; 48(4): 19–22. 10 refs. BE57072.
> *animal experimentation; animal rights; biomedical research; biomedical technologies; historical aspects; investigators; pain; *risks and benefits; suffering

Ross, Michael W. The ethics of experiments on higher animals. *Social Science and Medicine.* 1981; 15F: 51–60. 30 refs. BE56496.
> animal care committees; *animal experimentation; animal rights; behavioral research; communication; historical aspects; intelligence; pain; *primates; psychological stress; psychology; recall; research design; self concept; *speciesism; *suffering

It has been demonstrated over the last decade that some higher animals can learn sign language and communicate with humans. This finding radically alters some earlier conceptions of animals as being non–sentient, and forces a re–evaluation of the use of higher animals in research. The ethics of using animals are examined in this paper in relation to postulated levels of consciousness, and in relation to experimental design and experimental goals. In particular, an attempt is made to classify experimental situations with regard to potential psychological trauma, and to examine in detail the ethics of using higher animals in psychological research and situations in which such use can be justified. Analysis concentrates on the scientific ramifications of ethical use of animals, and concludes that in the majority of cases, ethical treatment and scientific approach are synonymous.

Roush, Wade. Chimp retirement plan proposed. [News]. *Science.* 1997 Jul 25; 277(5325): 471. BE56315.
> AIDS; *animal experimentation; federal government; government financing; political activity; *primates; research institutes; Chimpanzee Management Program (ChiMP); National Academy of Sciences; *National Institutes of Health; United States

Rozmiarek, Harry. Animal welfare regulations and accreditation by the American Association for Accreditation of Laboratory Animal Care: impact on chimpanzees in research. *In:* Eder, G.; Kaiser, E.; King, F.A., eds. The Role of the Chimpanzee in Research. Symposium, Vienna, Austria, May 22–24, 1992. New York, NY: Karger; 1994: 26–33. 19 refs. ISBN 3-8055-5850-3. BE58159.
> animal care committees; *animal experimentation; ethical review; federal government; government regulation; guidelines; international aspects; peer review; primates; professional organizations; public policy; *regulation; self regulation; *standards; American Association for Accreditation of Laboratory Animal Care; Animal Welfare Act; Guide for the Care and Use of Laboratory Animals; Public Health Service; *United States

Runkle, Deborah; Granger, Ellen. Animal rights: teaching or deceiving kids. [Editorial]. *Science.* 1997 Sep 5; 277(5331): 1419. 2 refs. BE56052.
> *animal experimentation; animal rights; attitudes; biomedical research; *education; information dissemination; political activity; professional organizations; risks and benefits; schools; science; students; teaching methods; *primary schools; *secondary schools; United States

Saegusa, Asako. Storm in Japan over sale of zoo monkeys for research. [News]. *Nature.* 1998 Jun 4; 393(6684): 404. BE58826.
> *animal experimentation; primates; scarcity; *zoo animals; *Japan

Service, Robert F., ed. Research to continue on infected chimps. [News]. *Science.* 1998 Aug 14; 281(5379): 909. BE58838.
> age factors; *animal experimentation; federal government; *primates; public policy; *U.S. Air Force; United States

Smith, David H. Religion and the use of animals in research: some first thoughts. *Ethics and Behavior.* 1997; 7(2): 137–147. 14 refs. BE56419.
> *animal experimentation; animal rights; biomedical research; Christian ethics; health; investigators; killing; love; medicine; moral obligations; pain; *religion; speciesism; suffering; theology; value of life; values; United States

Religious traditions can be drawn on in a number of ways to illuminate discussions of the moral standing of animals and the ethical use of animals in scientific research. I begin with some general comments about relevant points in the history of major religions. I then briefly describe American civil religion, including the cult of health, and its relation to scientific research. Finally, I offer a critique of American civil religion from a Christian perspective.

Smith, Jane A.; Boyd, Kenneth M. Ethics and laboratory animals: can the use of animals in experiments be justified? *In:* Tuffery, A.A., ed. Laboratory Animals: An Introduction for Experimenters. Second Edition. New York, NY: Wiley; 1995: 1–13. 38 refs. 2 fn. ISBN 0-471-95257-5. BE56247.
> *animal experimentation; animal rights; animal testing alternatives; communication; deontological ethics; investigators; moral obligations; *moral policy; pain; philosophy; risks and benefits; *speciesism; suffering; utilitarianism

Steneck, Nicholas H. Role of the institutional animal care and use committee in monitoring research. *Ethics and Behavior.* 1997; 7(2): 173–184. 17 refs. 10 fn. BE56420.
> advisory committees; *animal care committees; *animal experimentation; committee membership; conflict of interest; federal government; freedom; *government regulation;

BE = bioethics accession number   fn. = footnotes   refs. = references

guidelines; historical aspects; investigators; political activity; research institutes; resource allocation; *self regulation; technical expertise; time factors; universities; United States; University of Michigan

During the 1980s, federal regulations transferred significant portions of the responsibility for monitoring the care and use of research animals from animal care programs to Institutional Animal Care and Use Committees (IACUCs). After a brief review of the history of the regulation of the use of animals in research preceding and during the 4 decades following World War II, this article raises 4 problems associated with the role IACUCs currently play in monitoring the use of animals in research: (a) lack of expertise, (b) diverted resources, (c) conflict of interest, and (d) restrictions of academic freedom. It is concluded that the care and treatment of animals used in research would be served better and organized more rationally if the day-to-day responsibilities for approving projects and caring for animals were separated more clearly from broader, oversight functions, with the former being assigned to animal care programs and the latter to IACUCs.

Swiss Academy of Medical Sciences; Swiss Academy of Sciences. Ethical principles and guidelines for scientific experiments on animals [revised edition]. *ATLA: Alternatives to Laboratory Animals.* 1997 May–Jun; 25(3): 379–384. Approved 7 May 1994 by the Senate of the Swiss Academy of Sciences and on 24 Feb 1995 by the Senate of the Swiss Academy of Medical Sciences. BE55543.
　　*animal experimentation; animal rights; animal testing alternatives; genetic diversity; *guidelines; institutional ethics; investigators; legislation; moral obligations; pain; research institutes; risks and benefits; self regulation; suffering; *Swiss Academy of Medical Sciences; *Swiss Academy of Sciences; *Switzerland

U.S. Congress. House. A bill to amend the Animal Welfare Act to strengthen the annual reporting requirements of research facilities conducting animal experimentation or testing and to improve the accountability of animal experimentation programs of the Department of Defense [Animal Experimentation Right to Know Act]. H.R. 4971, 103d Cong., 2d Sess. Introduced by Robert G. Torricelli; 1994 Aug 16. 6 p. Referred jointly to the Committees on Agriculture and Armed Services. BE56778.
　　*accountability; *animal experimentation; federal government; government financing; *government regulation; *legal aspects; legislation; records; research institutes; *Animal Experimentation Right to Know Act (1994 bill); Animal Welfare Act; *Department of Defense; *United States

Wacks, Raymond. Sacrificed for science: are animal experiments morally defensible? *In:* Becker, Gerhold K., ed. Changing Nature's Course: The Ethical Challenge of Biotechnology. Hong Kong: Hong Kong University Press; 1996: 37–57. 73 fn. ISBN 962–209–403–1. BE56714.
　　animal care committees; *animal experimentation; *animal rights; animal testing alternatives; autonomy; ethical theory; government regulation; international aspects; moral obligations; *moral policy; pain; personhood; rights; speciesism; suffering; utilitarianism; value of life

Wadman, Meredith. Bid to give legal protection to laboratory mice in US. [News]. *Nature.* 1998 May 7; 393(6680): 6. BE58026.
　　*animal experimentation; attitudes; federal government; *government regulation; investigators; political activity; *rodents; Animal Welfare Act; Department of Agriculture;

*United States

Wadman, Meredith. Population explosion raises alarm over lab animal health. [News]. *Nature.* 1998 Feb 12; 391(6668): 623. BE58027.
　　*animal experimentation; communicable diseases; federal government; government financing; government regulation; research institutes; *standards; Biomedical Models and Resources (National Research Council); National Center for Research Resources; National Institutes of Health; United States

Yount, Lisa. Should animals be used in medical research and testing? [Juvenile literature]. *In:* her Issues in Biomedical Ethics. San Diego, CA: Lucent Books; 1998: 56–74, 102–104. 34 fn. ISBN 1–56006–476–5. BE57681.
　　animal care committees; *animal experimentation; animal organs; animal rights; animal testing alternatives; drugs; government financing; government regulation; guidelines; hormones; human rights; moral obligations; morbidity; mortality; organ transplantation; pain; *political activity; primates; public health; recombinant DNA research; *risks and benefits; speciesism; suffering; toxicity; value of life; violence; Animal Liberation Front; Animal Welfare Act; People for the Ethical Treatment of Animals (PETA); United States

Publication of experimental animal research: ethical aspects. [Editorial]. *Veterinary Quarterly.* 1985 Apr; 7(2): 81–83. BE57780.
　　*animal experimentation; *editorial policies; ethical review; international aspects; research design; scientific misconduct; *standards; Netherlands; United States; *Veterinary Quarterly

The means to an end. [Editorial]. *New Scientist.* 1997 Oct 25; 156(2105): 3. BE59086.
　　*animal experimentation; *animal testing alternatives; government financing; political activity; Europe

ANIMAL ORGANS *See* ORGAN AND TISSUE TRANSPLANTATION, ORGAN AND TISSUE DONATION

ANIMALS, TRANSGENIC *See* GENETIC INTERVENTION, PATENTING LIFE FORMS, RECOMBINANT DNA RESEARCH

ARTIFICIAL INSEMINATION

See also REPRODUCTIVE TECHNOLOGIES

Black, Douglas. Corporate tyranny. [Editorial]. *Journal of Medical Ethics.* 1997 Oct; 23(5): 269–270. 4 refs. BE56903.
　　*advisory committees; *artificial insemination; beneficence; *bioethical issues; *confidentiality; *consensus; death; *decision making; famous persons; *informed consent; married persons; *posthumous reproduction; regulation; *semen donors; suicide; *General Medical Council (Great Britain); Great Britain; *Human Fertilisation and Embryology Authority; Wingate, Orde

Bleich, J. David. Sperm banking in anticipation of infertility. *In:* Feldman, Emanuel; Wolowelsky, Joel B., eds. Jewish Law and the New Reproductive Technologies. Hoboken, NJ: Ktav; 1997: 139–154. 27 fn. ISBN 0–88125–586–6. BE57460.
　　artificial insemination; cryopreservation; infertility; *Jewish ethics; *males; married persons; moral obligations; reproduction; single persons; *sperm; theology; *tissue

---

BE = bioethics accession number　　　fn. = footnotes　　　refs. = references

banks; Orthodox Judaism

Brazier, Margaret. Hard cases make bad law? [Editorial]. *Journal of Medical Ethics.* 1997 Dec; 23(6): 341–343. 3 refs. BE57656.

*artificial insemination; cesarean section; *coercion; compensation; *competence; cryopreservation; death; *decision making; *fetuses; government regulation; guidelines; informed consent; *judicial action; *legal aspects; legal rights; married persons; physicians; *posthumous reproduction; *pregnant women; professional organizations; remuneration; semen donors; sperm; *surrogate mothers; *treatment refusal; Blood, Diane; European Union; *Great Britain; Human Fertilisation and Embryology Act 1990; Human Fertilisation and Embryology Authority; In re MB (Caesarean Section); R v. Human Fertilisation and Embryology Authority (ex parte Blood); Re S (Adult: Medical Treatment); Royal College of Obstetricians and Gynaecologists

California. Court of Appeal, Second District, Division 7. Hecht v. Superior Court (Kane). *California Reporter, 2d Series.* 1996 Nov 13 (date of decision; modified Nov 19). 59: 222–229. BE57349.

adults; advance directives; *artificial insemination; children; *cryopreservation; death; intention; *legal aspects; *posthumous reproduction; *property rights; reproduction; *semen donors; single persons; *sperm; suicide; tissue banks; adult offspring; *California; *Hecht v. Superior Court (Kane)

The Superior Court of Los Angeles County reversed the probate court and allowed Deborah Hecht, as the girlfriend of decedent William Kane, access to all vials of cryobanked sperm left to her under Kane's will. Kane's adult children argued that the sperm were property or assets of the estate; as such, under terms of a property settlement between the heirs, Hecht was entitled to 20% of the property or only three vials of sperm. The court based this decision on its first opinion in the case that "the fate of the sperm must be decided by the person from whom it is drawn," because genetic material is a unique form of property and sperm is tied to the fundamental liberty right of procreation. The decedent's clear intent was to leave the sperm to his girlfriend for future insemination if she chose. According to the court, only she had a right to the sperm and the decision concerning insemination was hers, though she could not contract, sell, or otherwise negotiate about the sperm. (KIE abstract)

Cook, Rachel; Golombok, Susan; Bish, Alison, et al. Disclosure of donor insemination: parental attitudes. *American Journal of Orthopsychiatry.* 1995 Oct; 65(4): 549–559. 50 refs. BE55711.

adoption; *artificial insemination; *attitudes; *children; comparative studies; *confidentiality; *disclosure; family members; fathers; genetic information; in vitro fertilization; infertility; mothers; motivation; parent child relationship; *parents; psychological stress; *reproductive technologies; semen donors; survey; Great Britain

Daniels, Ken; Lalos, Othon. The Swedish insemination act and the availability of donors. *Human Reproduction.* 1995 Jul; 10(7): 1871–1874. 17 refs. BE55763.

*artificial insemination; children; *confidentiality; *disclosure; health facilities; institutional policies; *legal aspects; *legislation; motivation; *public policy; records; *semen donors; social impact; New Zealand; *Sweden

Delany, Linda. Bending the statutory rules: the case of Mrs. Blood. *Health Care Analysis.* 1997 Sep; 5(3): 238–240, 243. 4 fn. BE55821.

*artificial insemination; *cryopreservation; death; government regulation; informed consent; international

aspects; *legal aspects; married persons; *posthumous reproduction; semen donors; *sperm; tissue banks; Belgium; European Union; *Great Britain; Human Fertilisation and Embryology Act 1990; *R v. Human Fertilisation and Embryology Authority (ex parte Blood)

Durna, Eva M.; Bebe, Judy; Steigrad, Stephen J., et al. Donor insemination: attitudes of parents towards disclosure. *Medical Journal of Australia.* 1997 Sep 1; 167(5): 256–259. 15 refs. BE58971.

age factors; *artificial insemination; *attitudes; *children; *confidentiality; counseling; *disclosure; *parents; psychological stress; semen donors; survey; New South Wales

Dyer, Clare. Government reviews law on "posthumous conceptions." [News]. *BMJ (British Medical Journal).* 1997 Oct 4; 315(7112): 834. BE56058.

*artificial insemination; competence; cryopreservation; *death; informed consent; *legal aspects; married persons; *posthumous reproduction; semen donors; sperm; coma; *Great Britain; *R v. Human Fertilisation and Embryology Authority (ex parte Blood)

Great Britain. England. Court of Appeal, Civil Division. R v. Human Fertilisation and Embryology Authority, ex parte Blood. *All England Law Reports.* 1997 Feb 6 (date of decision). [1997] 2: 687–704. BE57097.

*artificial insemination; *cryopreservation; *death; informed consent; international aspects; *legal aspects; *married persons; *posthumous reproduction; semen donors; *sperm; coma; European Community; *Great Britain; *R v. Human Fertilisation and Embryology Authority, ex parte Blood

England's Court of Appeal, Civil Division, upheld the lower court decision that, without the necessary written consent of the deceased husband, the 1990 Human Fertilisation and Embryology Act prohibits the storage of his cryopreserved sperm and its use in artificial insemination by the widow. When doctors retrieved sperm from Stephen Blood, he was already comatose from meningitis and would die soon thereafter. His widow sought release of the sperm to her for posthumous conception. Without the actual existence of a written consent for cryopreservation and also for disposition upon death, both storage of the sperm and its later use are prohibited under the licensing statute. The court did not address common law issues concerning consent to the retrieval of sperm from an unconscious man because those issues were not argued. In dicta (nonbinding opinion), the court noted that written consent is not required under the statute in a case involving fresh, i.e., nonpreserved, sperm where the donor later dies. The court did uphold the right to appeal the licensing authority's refusal to authorize the widow's export of the sperm for insemination at a medical clinic in another state of the European Community, such as Belgium, as infringing on her right to treatment under Community law. (KIE abstract)

Humphrey, Michael; Humphrey, Heather. Parenthood by donor insemination. *In: their* Families with a Difference: Varieties of Surrogate Parenthood. New York, NY: Routledge; 1988: 131–148, 181–182. 9 fn. ISBN 0-415-00690-2. BE56733.

adoption; *artificial insemination; attitudes; children; deception; females; infertility; males; marital relationship; married persons; parent child relationship; psychological stress; selection for treatment; semen donors

Iserson, Kenneth V.; Klepper, Howard; Andereck, William S. Sperm donation from a comatose, dying man. [Case study and commentaries]. *Cambridge*

BE = bioethics accession number   fn. = footnotes   refs. = references

Quarterly of Healthcare Ethics. 1998 Spring; 7(2): 209–217. 12 refs. 1 fn. BE57559.
  *artificial insemination; case studies; clinical ethics committees; cryopreservation; death; *decision making; directed donation; family members; legal aspects; minors; mothers; motivation; parent child relationship; parental consent; *posthumous reproduction; *semen donors; single persons; sperm; *terminally ill; *third party consent; *coma

Njikam Savage, Olayinka Margaret. Secrecy still the best policy: donor insemination in Cameroon. *Politics and the Life Sciences.* 1995 Feb; 14(1): 87–88. 5 refs. BE55701.
  *artificial insemination; *attitudes; *confidentiality; developing countries; family relationship; females; *infertility; males; parent child relationship; psychological stress; *semen donors; stigmatization; values; *Cameroon

Pozda, Richard; Miedema, Felicia; Matthews, Mary. Sperm collection in the brain–dead patient. [Case study and commentaries]. *Dimensions of Critical Care Nursing.* 1996 Mar–Apr; 15(2): 98–104. 25 refs. BE56881.
  *artificial insemination; autonomy; *brain death; cadavers; case studies; *cryopreservation; *decision making; directed donation; ethics consultation; informed consent; legal aspects; *married persons; organ donation; *posthumous reproduction; religion; reproductive technologies; *semen donors; *sperm; spousal consent; state government; withholding treatment; United States

Reichman, Edward. The rabbinic conception of conception: an exercise in fertility. *In:* Feldman, Emanuel; Wolowelsky, Joel B., eds. Jewish Law and the New Reproductive Technologies. Hoboken, NJ: Ktav; 1997: 1–35. 120 fn. ISBN 0–88125–586–6. BE57454.
  *artificial insemination; embryos; females; germ cells; *historical aspects; *Jewish ethics; males; *reproduction; reproductive technologies; theology; Orthodox Judaism

Diane Blood and the HFEA. *Bulletin of Medical Ethics.* 1997 Jan; No. 124: 2. BE55741.
  *artificial insemination; children; cryopreservation; *death; government regulation; informed consent; *legal aspects; *married persons; *posthumous reproduction; sperm; state interest; *Blood, Diane; *Great Britain; *Human Fertilisation and Embryology Authority

Widow allowed to export husband's sperm. [News]. *BMJ (British Medical Journal).* 1997 Mar 8; 314(7082): 696. BE58622.
  *artificial insemination; cryopreservation; *death; international aspects; *legal aspects; *married persons; *posthumous reproduction; sperm; Belgium; *Blood, Diane; *Great Britain; Human Fertilisation and Embryology Authority

ASSISTED SUICIDE *See* SUICIDE

ATTITUDES
  See under
  ABORTION/ATTITUDES
  ALLOWING TO DIE/ATTITUDES
  EUTHANASIA/ATTITUDES

BEHAVIOR CONTROL

See also PSYCHOSURGERY

Agich, George J.; May, Thomas. Alcoholism, moral agency, and paternalism: a theoretical framework. *In:* Shelton, Wayne N.; Edwards, Rem B., eds. Advances

in Bioethics. Volume 3: Values, Ethics, and Alcoholism. Greenwich, CT: JAI Press; 1997: 103–118. 20 refs. ISBN 0–7623–0219–4. BE57634.
  *accountability; *alcohol abuse; *autonomy; *behavior control; *behavior disorders; beneficence; coercion; competence; dangerousness; disabled; *disease; freedom; goals; government regulation; *injuries; morality; *paternalism; *patient care; patient compliance; patients; *physicians; psychological stress; risk; *self induced illness; social interaction; traffic accidents; values; dependency; liberalism; rationality; Mills, John Stuart; Raz, Joseph

Berghmans, Ron L.P. Coercive treatment in psychiatry. *In:* Chadwick, Ruth, ed. Encyclopedia of Applied Ethics, Volume 1. San Diego, CA: Academic Press; 1998: 535–542. 12 refs. ISBN 0–12–227066–5. BE56374.
  *autonomy; *behavior control; beneficence; *coercion; *competence; dangerousness; decision making; deinstitutionalized persons; incentives; institutionalized persons; international aspects; involuntary commitment; mental institutions; *mentally ill; *moral policy; outpatient commitment; *paternalism; *patient care; psychiatric diagnosis; psychiatric wills; *psychiatry; psychosurgery; review; risks and benefits; standards; suffering; *treatment refusal

Crenshaw, Wesley B.; Cain, Kimberly A.; Francis, Paul S. An updated national survey on seclusion and restraint. *Psychiatric Services.* 1997 Mar; 48(3): 395–397. 2 refs. BE56861.
  *behavior control; *institutionalized persons; *mental institutions; *mentally ill; *patient care; *physical restraint; statistics; survey; time factors; United States

Davis, Anne J.; Aroskar, Mila A.; Liaschenko, Joan, et al. Behavior control. *In: their* Ethical Dilemmas and Nursing Practice. Fourth Edition. Stamford, CT: Appleton and Lange; 1997: 185–211. 85 fn. ISBN 0–8385–2283–1. BE58598.
  *behavior control; case studies; coercion; dangerousness; drug abuse; females; involuntary commitment; mentally disabled; *mentally ill; normality; *nurses; operant conditioning; paternalism; patients' rights; psychoactive drugs; psychosurgery; psychotherapy; public policy; risks and benefits; social control; treatment refusal; homeless persons; United States

Evans, Lois K.; Strumpf, Neville E.; Allen–Taylor, S. Lynne, et al. A clinical trial to reduce restraints in nursing homes. *Journal of the American Geriatrics Society.* 1997 Jun; 45(6): 675–681. 43 refs. BE55720.
  *aged; *behavior control; comparative studies; *control groups; dementia; depressive disorder; *education; evaluation studies; *health personnel; injuries; nurses; *nursing homes; *patient care; *physical restraint; psychoactive drugs; *referral and consultation; time factors; continuing education; dependency; follow–up studies; Pennsylvania

Hantikainen, Virpi. Physical restraint: a descriptive study in Swiss nursing homes. *Nursing Ethics.* 1998 Jul; 5(4): 330–346. 30 refs. BE58872.
  *aged; allied health personnel; alternatives; *behavior control; competence; decision making; disclosure; *institutional policies; institutionalized persons; *knowledge, attitudes, practice; motivation; *nurses; *nursing homes; nursing research; *patient care; patient participation; *physical restraint; risks and benefits; statistics; survey; qualitative research; *Switzerland

Harris, Cathleen M.; Mahowald, Mary B. Women and alcohol abuse. *In:* Shelton, Wayne N.; Edwards, Rem B., eds. Advances in Bioethics. Volume 3: Values, Ethics, and Alcoholism. Greenwich, CT: JAI Press; 1997:

BE = bioethics accession number   fn. = footnotes   refs. = references

153–170. 69 refs. ISBN 0–7623–0219–4. BE57637.
accountability; *alcohol abuse; autonomy; *behavior control; *coercion; congenital disorders; criminal law; decision making; disease; *females; *fetuses; indigents; legal aspects; mandatory programs; minority groups; moral obligations; newborns; *patient care; *pregnant women; *prenatal injuries; privacy; psychological stress; public policy; reproduction; rights; self concept; sexuality; social discrimination; socioeconomic factors; state interest; *stigmatization; value of life; women's health services; women's rights; United States

Hsu, Irene; DuChane, Janeen; Veatch, Robert M. Recommendation of treatment that would allow parole -- Scenario; Position 1: pharmacist should recommend the hormonal treatment; Position 2: pharmacist should not recommend the hormonal treatment; Analysis and commentary. *American Journal of Health–System Pharmacy.* 1995 Apr 15; 52(8): 829–833. 5 refs. BE58105.
*behavior control; case studies; codes of ethics; competence; freedom; government financing; health insurance reimbursement; HIV seropositivity; *hormones; legal aspects; mental institutions; mentally ill; obligations to society; patient compliance; patients' rights; *pharmacists; *prisoners; professional ethics; *selection for treatment; *sex offenses; sexuality; technical expertise; withholding treatment; professional role

Illingworth, Patricia. Warning: AIDS health promotion programs may be hazardous to your autonomy. *In:* Overall, Christine and Zion, William P., eds. Perspectives on AIDS: Ethical and Social Issues. New York, NY: Oxford University Press; 1991: 138–154. 39 fn. ISBN 0–19–540749–0. BE58292.
*AIDS; attitudes; *autonomy; *behavior control; *coercion; common good; drug abuse; *health education; *health promotion; HIV seropositivity; *information dissemination; methods; motivation; operant conditioning; preventive medicine; *public health; public policy; self concept; sexuality; social discrimination; social impact; Canada

Kapp, Marshall B. Persons with dementia as "liability magnets": ethical implications. *Journal of Clinical Ethics.* 1998 Spring; 9(1): 66–70. 18 fn. BE57715.
allowing to die; *attitudes; *autonomy; *behavior control; dangerousness; decision making; *dementia; *family members; *health facilities; *health personnel; hospices; human experimentation; injuries; legal guardians; *legal liability; motivation; *paternalism; *patient care; prolongation of life; quality of health care; refusal to treat; residential facilities; risk; selection of subjects; terminal care; *risk management

Kellett, John M.; Curtis, David. Suspension of nurse who gave drug on consultant's instructions. [Letters]. *BMJ (British Medical Journal).* 1997 Apr 5; 314(7086): 1043–1044. 2 refs. BE55897.
*administrators; *behavior control; behavior disorders; *deception; *misconduct; *nurse's role; *nurses; patient care; *patient care team; physician nurse relationship; *physicians; *psychoactive drugs; *punishment; treatment refusal; *Great Britain; National Health Service

Lupton, Deborah. The Imperative of Health: Public Health and the Regulated Body. Thousand Oaks, CA: Sage Publications; 1995. 181 p. Bibliography: p. 162–175. ISBN 0–8039–7936–3. BE56130.
advertising; autonomy; *behavior control; diagnosis; freedom; health; health education; *health promotion; HIV seropositivity; mass media; mass screening; *public health; public policy; risk; self induced illness; *social control; social dominance; social sciences; uncertainty

Phillips, Charles D.; Hawes, Catherine; Mor, Vince,
et al. Facility and area variation affecting the use of physical restraints in nursing homes. *Medical Care.* 1996 Nov; 34(11): 1149–1162. 36 refs. BE59072.
*aged; *behavior control; evaluation studies; health personnel; institutional policies; *nursing homes; nursing research; *patient care; *physical restraint; resource allocation; selection for treatment; statistics; cognition disorders; *geographic factors; California; Connecticut; Iowa; Maryland; Minnesota; Ohio; Oregon; Tennessee; Texas; *United States; Virginia

Shuttleworth, John Sterling. Ethical issues of cost in long–term care. *Journal of the Medical Association of Georgia.* 1990 Nov; 79(11): 843–845. 5 refs. BE55642.
administrators; *aged; *behavior control; communication; *economics; family members; government financing; *long–term care; *nursing homes; physicians; psychoactive drugs; *psychological stress; quality of life; personal financing; Medicare; United States

Westall, Jessica. Shackling of prisoners denounced. [News]. *BMJ (British Medical Journal).* 1997 Feb 8; 314(7078): 393. BE58603.
guidelines; *hospitals; institutional policies; patient care; *physical restraint; *prisoners; terminally ill; *Great Britain; Thomas, Geoffrey

Williams, Carter Catlett; Finch, Caleb E. Physical restraint: not fit for woman, man, or beast. [Editorial]. *Journal of the American Geriatrics Society.* 1997 Jun; 45(6): 773–775. 27 refs. BE55735.
administrators; *aged; alternatives; *behavior control; brain pathology; dementia; education; empirical research; health personnel; injuries; *morbidity; *nursing homes; *patient care; *physical restraint; psychoactive drugs; psychological stress; referral and consultation; United States

Wisconsin. Supreme Court. State v. Kruzicki. *North Western Reporter, 2d Series.* 1997 Apr 22 (date of decision). 561: 729–749. BE56745.
*behavior control; coercion; *criminal law; *drug abuse; *fetuses; government regulation; *legal aspects; *personhood; *pregnant women; *prenatal injuries; state government; treatment refusal; *viability; *Angela M.W.; *State v. Kruzicki; Wisconsin
The Wisconsin Supreme Court reversed the appellate court's denial of review of writs under which a pregnant woman sought release from the court's detention and protective custody of her viable fetus. Although she had given birth, the court considered the now moot issue of a child in need of protection or services. When Angela M.W. was thirty–six weeks pregnant, blood tests confirmed drug use in each of the preceding three months and it was decided that her continued use of drugs would cause the fetus serious harm. The county took protective custody of the fetus by a court order requiring that the woman be confined to an inpatient drug treatment facility. After considering the meanings of "child" and "person", the court concluded that under state law a child is a human being born alive, not a fetus. The dissenting judge argued that the meanings of "child" and "person" include a viable fetus. (KIE abstract)

BEHAVIORAL GENETICS

Allen, Garland E. Genetics and behavior. *In:* Chadwick, Ruth, ed. Encyclopedia of Applied Ethics, Volume 2. San Diego, CA: Academic Press; 1998: 435–443. 6 refs. ISBN 0–12–227067–3. BE56390.
behavior disorders; *behavioral genetics; eugenics; genetic research; genetics; historical aspects; homosexuals; intelligence; investigators; mass media; moral policy; public

---

policy; research design; resource allocation; social control; social problems; stigmatization

Carey, Gregory; Gottesman, Irving I. Genetics and antisocial behavior: substance versus sound bytes. *Politics and the Life Sciences.* 1996 Mar; 15(1): 88–90. 11 refs. BE55646.
adoption; behavior disorders; *behavioral genetics; *behavioral research; genetic disorders; *genetic predisposition; genetic research; public policy; socioeconomic factors; twins; *violence; XYY karyotype

Daniels, Jo; McGuffin, Peter; Owen, Mike. Molecular genetic research on IQ: can it be done? Should it be done? *Journal of Biosocial Science.* 1996 Oct; 28(4): 491–507. 37 refs. BE55762.
*behavioral genetics; genes; *genetic research; genetic screening; genetics; genome mapping; *intelligence; Great Britain; United States

Duster, Troy. Persistence and continuity in human genetics and social stratification. *In:* Peters, Ted, ed. Genetics: Issues of Social Justice. Cleveland, OH: Pilgrim Press; 1998: 218–238. 57 fn. ISBN 0-8298-1251-2. BE57481.
aliens; anthropology; behavior control; *behavioral genetics; blacks; *eugenics; *evolution; *genetics; genome mapping; historical aspects; intelligence; involuntary sterilization; legal aspects; *public policy; social problems; violence; emigration and immigration; Social Darwinism; United States

Fishbein, Diana H. Prospects for the application of genetic findings to crime and violence prevention. *Politics and the Life Sciences.* 1996 Mar; 15(1): 91–94. 22 refs. BE55633.
*behavioral genetics; *behavioral research; drug abuse; *genetic predisposition; *genetic research; goals; health care; law enforcement; legal aspects; mental health; preventive medicine; public health; rehabilitation; social control; social discrimination; socioeconomic factors; *violence

Goldman, David. Interdisciplinary perceptions of genetics and behavior. *Politics and the Life Sciences.* 1996 Mar; 15(1): 97–98. BE55634.
*behavioral genetics; eugenics; *genetic predisposition; *genetic research; genetics; goals; interdisciplinary communication; social control; social discrimination; violence

Goodey, Chris. Genes that are all in the mind. *New Scientist.* 1997 Jun 7; 154(2085): 49. BE56411.
*behavioral genetics; genetic research; *intelligence; mental health; normality; *psychiatric diagnosis; *public policy; *Great Britain; Medical Research Council (Great Britain)

Goodey, Chris. Genetic markers for intelligence. *Bulletin of Medical Ethics.* 1996 Aug; No. 120: 13–16. 2 refs. BE55865.
*behavioral genetics; eugenics; *genetic research; *intelligence; mentally retarded; prenatal diagnosis; selective abortion; stigmatization; suffering; wedge argument; Great Britain

Hamer, Dean; Copeland, Peter. Engineering temperament: cloning and the future politics of personality. *In: their* Living with Our Genes: Why They Matter More Than You Think. New York, NY: Doubleday; 1998: 295–316, 344. 11 refs. ISBN 0-385-48583-2. BE57647.
*behavioral genetics; brain; *cloning; gene therapy; *genetic determinism; genetic enhancement; *genetic intervention; genetic predisposition; genetic screening; germ cells; industry; psychoactive drugs; risks and benefits; uncertainty; *personality

Hefner, Philip. Determinism, freedom, and moral failure. *Dialog: A Journal of Theology.* 1994 Winter; 33(1): 23–29. 10 fn. BE57534.
*behavioral genetics; *Christian ethics; evolution; *freedom; *genetic determinism; *genetic intervention; genetics; *genome mapping; *human characteristics; *theology; ELSI-funded publication

Herbert, Wray. How the nature vs. nurture debate shapes public policy -- and our view of ourselves. *U.S. News and World Report.* 1997 Apr 21; 122(15): 72–74, 77–80. BE58045.
accountability; alcohol abuse; attitudes; *behavioral genetics; eugenics; federal government; genetic determinism; *genetic predisposition; genetic research; government financing; health care; homosexuals; mentally ill; public policy; resource allocation; schizophrenia; self concept; sexuality; social discrimination; social impact; *social problems; stigmatization; violence; United States

Jones, Owen D. Genes, behavior, and law. *Politics and the Life Sciences.* 1996 Mar; 15(1): 101–103. BE55631.
*behavioral genetics; evolution; *genetics; interdisciplinary communication; *law; social control; social discrimination; terminology; United States; University of Maryland

Masters, Roger D. Neuroscience, genetics, and society: is the biology of human social behavior too controversial to study? *Politics and the Life Sciences.* 1996 Mar; 15(1): 103–104. 4 refs. BE55626.
behavior control; *behavioral genetics; *behavioral research; education; eugenics; genetic predisposition; genetic research; mass media; *political activity; psychoactive drugs; social discrimination; *socioeconomic factors; *violence; United States; University of Maryland

Murphy, Timothy F. Gay Science: The Ethics of Sexual Orientation Research. New York, NY: Columbia University Press; 1997. 268 p. 416 fn. ISBN 0-231-10848-6. BE58226.
*behavioral genetics; *behavioral research; brain; children; females; fetal therapy; genetic determinism; genetic predisposition; genetic screening; historical aspects; *homosexuals; hormones; legal aspects; males; military personnel; moral obligations; normality; parent child relationship; prenatal diagnosis; psychology; psychotherapy; religion; science; selective abortion; sexuality; siblings; social discrimination; stigmatization

Nelkin, Dorothy; Lindee, M. Susan. "Genes made me do it": the appeal of biological explanations. *Politics and the Life Sciences.* 1996 Mar; 15(1): 95–97. 12 refs. BE55624.
*behavioral genetics; behavioral research; *genetic predisposition; justice; mass media; moral obligations; obligations of society; public policy; social problems; socioeconomic factors; *violence; United States

Paul, Diane B. Culpability and compassion: lessons from the history of eugenics. *Politics and the Life Sciences.* 1996 Mar; 15(1): 99–100. 7 refs. BE55623.
accountability; *behavioral genetics; *eugenics; *genetic predisposition; punishment; sexuality; social control; *social discrimination; social problems; stigmatization; *violence; culpability

Peters, Ted F. On the gay gene: back to original sin again? *Dialog: A Journal of Theology.* 1994 Winter; 33(1): 30–38. 15 fn. BE57535.
*behavioral genetics; behavioral research; *Christian ethics; freedom; gene therapy; *genetic determinism; genetic intervention; *genetic predisposition; genetic research; *homosexuals; males; selective abortion; social discrimination; *stigmatization; *theology; ELSI-funded

---

BE = bioethics accession number   fn. = footnotes   refs. = references

publication

Rafter, Nicole Hahn. Creating Born Criminals. Urbana, IL: University of Illinois Press; 1997. 284 p. Bibliography: p. 241–270. ISBN 0–252–06741–X. BE57201.
    anthropology; *behavioral genetics; dangerousness; *eugenics; females; government regulation; *historical aspects; indigents; institutionalized persons; intelligence; mental institutions; *mentally ill; *mentally retarded; *prisoners; *public policy; social impact; state government; sterilization (sexual); *violence; *Nineteenth Century; *Twentieth Century; *United States

Sherman, Stephanie L.; DeFries, John C.; Gottesman, Irving I., et al. Behavioral genetics '97 -- ASHG statement: recent developments in human behavioral genetics: past accomplishments and future directions. *American Journal of Human Genetics.* 1997 Jun; 60(6): 1265–1275. 54 refs. BE56013.
    adoption; *behavioral genetics; *behavioral research; emotions; eugenics; family relationship; genetic counseling; *genetic research; research design; review; schizophrenia; twins; population genetics; American Society of Human Genetics

Walters, LeRoy B. Behavioural and germ–line genetic research. *In:* Kilner, John F.; Pentz, Rebecca D.; Young, Frank E., eds. Genetic Ethics: Do the Ends Justify the Genes? Grand Rapids, MI: W.B. Eerdmans; 1997: 104–112. 15 fn. ISBN 0–8028–4428–6. BE56718.
    aggression; *behavioral genetics; *Christian ethics; embryos; empirical research; family members; freedom; future generations; *gene therapy; genetic determinism; genetic enhancement; *genetic intervention; genetic research; genome mapping; *germ cells; intelligence; methods; moral obligations; parents; preimplantation diagnosis; prenatal diagnosis; quality of life; *risks and benefits; twins; personality

Wasserman, David. Research into genetics and crime: consensus and controversy. *Politics and the Life Sciences.* 1996 Mar; 15(1): 107–109. BE55637.
    *behavioral genetics; behavioral research; consensus; dissent; *genetic predisposition; *genetic research; *interdisciplinary communication; investigators; mass media; *political activity; social control; social discrimination; *socioeconomic factors; *violence; United States; University of Maryland

Zimring, Franklin E. The genetics of crime: a skeptic's vision of the future. *Politics and the Life Sciences.* 1996 Mar; 15(1): 105–106. BE55636.
    adolescents; *behavioral genetics; behavioral research; children; genetic research; motivation; normality; preventive medicine; psychoactive drugs; resource allocation; selection for treatment; social control; social discrimination; social problems; *socioeconomic factors; *violence; wedge argument; United States

BEHAVIORAL RESEARCH

See also BIOMEDICAL RESEARCH, HUMAN EXPERIMENTATION

Aitkenhead, Marilyn; Dordoy, Jackie. What the subjects have to say. *British Journal of Social Psychology.* 1985 Nov; 24(Pt. 4): 293–305. 17 refs. BE56650.
    *attitudes; *behavioral research; codes of ethics; *deception; *empirical research; evaluation studies; investigator subject relationship; investigators; *psychological stress; *psychology; research design; *research subjects; *students; universities; volunteers; Great Britain

Badaway, Abdulla A.-B. Ethics in alcohol research and publishing. [Editorial]. *Alcohol and Alcoholism.* 1996 Jan; 31(1): 7–9. 10 refs. BE55753.
    *alcohol abuse; *behavioral research; *biomedical research; codes of ethics; conflict of interest; disclosure; *editorial policies; financial support; *investigators; peer review; *professional ethics; scientific misconduct; *self regulation; universities; *journalism

Butler, Declan. Advances in neuroscience 'may threaten human rights.' [News]. *Nature.* 1998 Jan 22; 391(6665): 316. BE57764.
    advisory committees; behavioral genetics; *behavioral research; biomedical technologies; *brain; human rights; privacy; *neurology; France; National Ethics Advisory Committee (France)

Carey, Gregory; Gottesman, Irving I. Genetics and antisocial behavior: substance versus sound bytes. *Politics and the Life Sciences.* 1996 Mar; 15(1): 88–90. 11 refs. BE55646.
    adoption; behavior disorders; *behavioral genetics; *behavioral research; genetic disorders; *genetic predisposition; genetic research; public policy; socioeconomic factors; twins; *violence; XYY karyotype

Childress, Craig A.; Asamen, Joy K. The emerging relationship of psychology and the Internet: proposed guidelines for conducting Internet intervention research. *Ethics and Behavior.* 1998; 8(1): 19–35. 30 refs. BE58915.
    *behavioral research; communication; *computer communication networks; computers; confidentiality; counseling; disclosure; emergency care; empirical research; *guidelines; health personnel; *health services research; investigator subject relationship; investigators; legal aspects; mentally ill; methods; professional ethics; professional patient relationship; psychiatric diagnosis; psychology; *psychotherapy; referral and consultation; research design; risks and benefits; socioeconomic factors; standards; suicide; *Internet
The Internet is rapidly developing into an important medium of communication in modern society, and both psychological research and therapeutic interventions are being increasingly conducted using this new communication medium. As therapeutic interventions using the Internet are becoming more prevalent, it is becoming increasingly important to conduct research on psychotherapeutic Internet interventions to assist in the development of an appropriate standard of practice regarding interventions using this new medium. In this article, we examine the Internet and the current psychological uses which are being initiated using this medium. Ethical concerns related to the psychological use of the Internet are discussed, and guidelines are proposed for the conduct of Internet intervention research.

Fishbein, Diana H. Prospects for the application of genetic findings to crime and violence prevention. *Politics and the Life Sciences.* 1996 Mar; 15(1): 91–94. 22 refs. BE55633.
    *behavioral genetics; *behavioral research; drug abuse; *genetic predisposition; *genetic research; goals; health care; law enforcement; legal aspects; mental health; preventive medicine; public health; rehabilitation; social control; social discrimination; socioeconomic factors; *violence

Gallagher, Bernard; Creighton, Susan; Gibbons, Jane. Ethical dilemmas in social research: no easy solutions. *British Journal of Social Work.* 1995 Jun; 25(3): 295–311. 49 refs. BE56911.
    *behavioral research; child abuse; children; confidentiality; deception; family members; guidelines; informed consent;

BE = bioethics accession number   fn. = footnotes   refs. = references

methods; professional organizations; psychological stress; records; registries; research design; research ethics committees; risks and benefits; social workers; time factors; vulnerable populations; Great Britain

Kemp, Martin. Hyde's horrors. *Nature.* 1998 May 21; 393(6682): 219. BE58037.
*behavioral research; eugenics; historical aspects; literature; violence; *medical illustration; Darwin, Charles; Nineteenth Century; The Strange Case of Dr. Jekyll and Mr. Hyde (Stevenson, R.L.)

McHaffie, Hazel. Researching sensitive issues. *In:* Frith, Lucy, ed. Ethics and Midwifery: Issues in Contemporary Pratice. Boston, MA: Butterworth–Heinemann; 1996: 258–273. 14 refs. ISBN 0–7506–3056–6. BE58642.
accountability; AIDS; *behavioral research; case studies; child abuse; confidentiality; deception; drug abuse; interprofessional relations; *investigator subject relationship; investigators; moral obligations; newborns; *nurse midwives; nurses; nursing ethics; *nursing research; physicians; privacy; psychological stress; research subjects; risks and benefits; sexuality; withholding treatment; *research ethics

Masters, Roger D. Neuroscience, genetics, and society: is the biology of human social behavior too controversial to study? *Politics and the Life Sciences.* 1996 Mar; 15(1): 103–104. 4 refs. BE55626.
behavior control; *behavioral genetics; *behavioral research; education; eugenics; genetic predisposition; genetic research; mass media; *political activity; psychoactive drugs; social discrimination; *socioeconomic factors; *violence; United States; University of Maryland

Paavilainen, Eija; Astedt–Kurki, Päivi; Paunonen, Marita. Ethical problems in research on families who are abusing children. *Nursing Ethics.* 1998 May; 5(3): 200–205. 15 refs. BE58719.
*behavioral research; *child abuse; confidentiality; *domestic violence; *family members; informed consent; investigator subject relationship; *nursing research; research design; qualitative research; *Finland

Plant, Martin; Plant, Moira; Vernon, Bryan. Ethics, funding and alcohol research. *Alcohol and Alcoholism.* 1996 Jan; 31(1): 17–25. 36 refs. BE55770.
*alcohol abuse; *behavioral research; *biomedical research; codes of ethics; *conflict of interest; disclosure; economics; editorial policies; *financial support; government financing; guidelines; industry; information dissemination; *investigators; peer review; *professional ethics; science; scientific misconduct; *self regulation; social sciences; universities; values; whistleblowing

Rose, Mary R.; Fischer, Karla. Do authorship policies impact students' judgments of perceived wrongdoing? *Ethics and Behavior.* 1998; 8(1): 59–79. 18 refs. 4 fn. BE58918.
*authorship; *behavioral research; codes of ethics; *faculty; females; institutional policies; interprofessional relations; males; professional organizations; *scientific misconduct; *students; survey; universities; whistleblowing; American Psychological Association
Although authorship policies exist, researchers understand little about their impact on perceptions of authorship scenarios. Graduate students (N=277) at a large university read 1 of 3 vignettes about a graduate student–faculty collaboration. One half of the surveys included the American Psychological Association's statement on authorship. Participants rated (a) the ethics of the professor as first author and (b) the likelihood of a dissatisfied student reporting the authorship result, as well as the effectiveness and negative consequences of reporting. Work arrangements on the project had a consistent main effect. Also, an authorship policy impacted women's ratings of first authorship when the student contributed the idea for a project. For men, a policy impacted only ratings of the likelihood of reporting when a professor was first author on a student's dissertation. Apart from sex, no other demographic variables on participants were predictive. Discussion focuses on the policy's potential for making only some specific issues salient.

Ross, Michael W. The ethics of experiments on higher animals. *Social Science and Medicine.* 1981; 15F: 51–60. 30 refs. BE56496.
animal care committees; *animal experimentation; animal rights; behavioral research; communication; historical aspects; intelligence; pain; *primates; psychological stress; psychology; recall; research design; self concept; *speciesism; *suffering
It has been demonstrated over the last decade that some higher animals can learn sign language and communicate with humans. This finding radically alters some earlier conceptions of animals as being non-sentient, and forces a re-evaluation of the use of higher animals in research. The ethics of using animals are examined in this paper in relation to postulated levels of consciousness, and in relation to experimental design and experimental goals. In particular, an attempt is made to classify experimental situations with regard to potential psychological trauma, and to examine in detail the ethics of using higher animals in psychological research and situations in which such use can be justified. Analysis concentrates on the scientific ramifications of ethical use of animals, and concludes that in the majority of cases, ethical treatment and scientific approach are synonymous.

Sherman, Stephanie L.; DeFries, John C.; Gottesman, Irving I., et al. Behavioral genetics '97 -- ASHG statement: recent developments in human behavioral genetics: past accomplishments and future directions. *American Journal of Human Genetics.* 1997 Jun; 60(6): 1265–1275. 54 refs. BE56013.
adoption; *behavioral genetics; *behavioral research; emotions; eugenics; family relationship; genetic counseling; *genetic research; research design; review; schizophrenia; twins; population genetics; American Society of Human Genetics

BEHAVIORAL RESEARCH/ETHICS COMMITTEES

Kallgren, Carl A.; Tauber, Robert T. Undergraduate research and the institutional review board: a mismatch or happy marriage? *Teaching of Psychology.* 1996 Feb; 23(1): 20–25. 23 refs. 3 fn. BE55785.
*attitudes; *behavioral research; education; ethical review; evaluation; *investigators; *psychology; *research ethics committees; *students; survey; *universities; Pennsylvania State University

BEHAVIORAL RESEARCH/FOREIGN COUNTRIES

Kondro, Wayne. New rules on human subjects could end debate in Canada. [News]. *Science.* 1998 Jun 5; 280(5369): 1521. BE58875.
advisory committees; *behavioral research; biomedical research; committee membership; consensus; deception; dissent; ethical review; genetic research; *guidelines; *human experimentation; humanities; informed consent; interdisciplinary communication; lawyers; minority groups; *regulation; research ethics committees; research institutes;

BE = bioethics accession number   fn. = footnotes   refs. = references

research subjects; science; social sciences; universities; community consent; *Canada; *Code of Conduct for Research Involving Humans; *Medical Research Council of Canada; *Natural Sciences and Engineering Research Council (Canada); *Social Sciences and Humanities Research Council (Canada)

BEHAVIORAL RESEARCH/INFORMED CONSENT

Adair, John G.; Dushenko, Terrance W.; Lindsay, R.C.L. Ethical regulations and their impact on research practice. *American Psychologist.* 1985 Jan; 40(1): 59–72. 82 refs. 5 fn. BE57821.
> *behavioral research; codes of ethics; consent forms; *deception; editorial policies; empirical research; *ethical review; evaluation studies; *informed consent; literature; methods; *psychology; *regulation; research design; risks and benefits; social impact; statistics; survey; qualitative research; Journal of Personality and Social Psychology

Brody, Janet L.; Gluck, John P.; Aragon, Alfredo S. Participants' understanding of the process of psychological research: informed consent. *Ethics and Behavior.* 1997; 7(4): 285–298. 22 refs. BE58661.
> attitudes; autonomy; *behavioral research; coercion; communication; comprehension; consent forms; deception; disclosure; evaluation studies; historical aspects; *informed consent; *psychology; *research subjects; risks and benefits; scientific misconduct; *students; survey; *universities; University of New Mexico

Sixty-five undergraduates participating in a wide range of psychological research experiments were interviewed in depth about their research experiences and their views on the process of informed consent. Overall, 32% of research experiences were characterized positively and 41% were characterized negatively. One major theme of the negative experiences was that experiments were perceived as too invasive, suggesting incomplete explication of negative aspects of research during the informed consent process. Informed consent experiences were viewed positively 80% of the time. However, most of the participants had a limited view of the purpose of informed consent: less than 20% viewed the process as a decision point. Results suggest a number of common pitfalls to standard informed consent practices that have not generally been recognized. Results are discussed in terms of both ethical and methodological implications. Suggestions for improving the informed consent process are also provided.

Gutscher, Heinz. Informed consent in the social sciences: agreeing to being deceived. *In:* Berthoud, Gérald; Sitter-Liver, Beat, eds. The Responsible Scholar: Ethical Considerations in the Humanities and Social Sciences. Canton, MA: Watson Publishing International; 1996: 255–269. 40 refs. ISBN 0-88135-165-2. BE57225.
> *alternatives; *behavioral research; *deception; *disclosure; guidelines; *informed consent; investigator subject relationship; investigators; professional ethics; psychological stress; *research subjects; risks and benefits; social impact; social sciences; trust; debriefing; American Psychological Association

Kirsch, Irving; Rosadino, Michael J. Do double-blind studies with informed consent yield externally valid results? An empirical test. *Psychopharmacology (Berlin).* 1993; 110(4): 437–442. 13 refs. BE55567.
> adolescents; *behavioral research; control groups; disclosure; *drugs; *evaluation; evaluation studies; human experimentation; *informed consent; *placebos; psychology; *random selection; *research design; research subjects;

students

Sigmon, Sandra T.; Rohan, Kelly J.; Dorhofer, Diana, et al. Effects of consent form information on self–disclosure. *Ethics and Behavior.* 1997; 7(4): 299–310. 17 refs. BE58662.
> autonomy; *behavioral research; beneficence; communication; comparative studies; comprehension; *consent forms; *depressive disorder; *disclosure; females; informed consent; investigators; *males; *psychological stress; psychology; psychotherapy; recall; referral and consultation; *research subjects; students; suicide; survey; universities; United States

When researchers encounter preexisting psychological distress in participants, ethical codes provide little guidance on how to balance issues of beneficence and autonomy. Although researchers may inform participants what will occur given responses indicating distress, this information may lead to biased self-reports. This important issue was addressed in this study by manipulating consent form information regarding the type of psychopathology to be assessed and various levels of possible follow-up. In comparing responses on self-report measures of anxiety, depression, and general psychological distress, men who believed depression was the focus of the study reported fewer symptoms of depression and less trait anxiety as intrusiveness of experimenter follow-up increased. These results are discussed within the framework of socialization theory. Given that half of the sample did not correctly answer questions regarding information contained in the consent form, guidelines to improve consent form comprehension are offered.

Singer, Eleanor. Public reactions to some ethical issues of social research: attitudes and behavior. *Journal of Consumer Research.* 1984 Jun; 11: 501–509. 26 refs. 4 fn. BE57838.
> *attitudes; *behavioral research; confidentiality; disclosure; *informed consent; investigator subject relationship; *public opinion; research subjects; social sciences; socioeconomic factors; survey; trust; United States

BEHAVIORAL RESEARCH/MINORS

Wadman, Meredith. Row erupts over child aggression study. [News]. *Nature.* 1998 Apr 23; 392(6678): 747. BE58075.
> *aggression; *behavioral research; blacks; *children; *drugs; ethical review; federal government; government regulation; Hispanic Americans; *human experimentation; indigents; males; *minority groups; *nontherapeutic research; research ethics committees; research subjects; scientific misconduct; selection of subjects; *fenfluramine; New York City; *New York State Psychiatric Institute (NYC); Office for Protection from Research Risks; United States

BEHAVIORAL RESEARCH/REGULATION

Adair, John G.; Dushenko, Terrance W.; Lindsay, R.C.L. Ethical regulations and their impact on research practice. *American Psychologist.* 1985 Jan; 40(1): 59–72. 82 refs. 5 fn. BE57821.
> *behavioral research; codes of ethics; consent forms; *deception; editorial policies; empirical research; *ethical review; evaluation studies; *informed consent; literature; methods; *psychology; *regulation; research design; risks and benefits; social impact; statistics; survey; qualitative research; Journal of Personality and Social Psychology

Kondro, Wayne. New rules on human subjects could end

debate in Canada. [News]. *Science.* 1998 Jun 5; 280(5369): 1521. BE58875.

> advisory committees; *behavioral research; biomedical research; committee membership; consensus; deception; dissent; ethical review; genetic research; *guidelines; *human experimentation; humanities; informed consent; interdisciplinary communication; lawyers; minority groups; *regulation; research ethics committees; research institutes; research subjects; science; social sciences; universities; community consent; *Canada; *Code of Conduct for Research Involving Humans; *Medical Research Council of Canada; *Natural Sciences and Engineering Research Council (Canada); *Social Sciences and Humanities Research Council (Canada)

Pattullo, Edward L. Governmental regulation of the investigation of human subjects in social research. *Minerva.* 1985 Winter; 23(4): 521–533. 34 fn. BE56677.

> *behavioral research; ethical review; faculty; federal government; freedom; *government regulation; historical aspects; human experimentation; injuries; investigators; psychoactive drugs; research ethics committees; research subjects; scientific misconduct; *self regulation; *social sciences; students; *universities; Alpert, Richard; Department of Health and Human Services; Department of Health, Education, and Welfare; Harvard University; Leary, Timothy; LSD; Twentieth Century; *United States

BEHAVIORAL RESEARCH/RESEARCH DESIGN

Beeson, Diane. Nuance, complexity, and context: qualitative methods in genetic counseling research. *Journal of Genetic Counseling.* 1997 Mar; 6(1): 21–43. 66 refs. BE57337.

> *behavioral research; confidentiality; evaluation; *genetic counseling; methods; *research design; ethnographic studies; *qualitative research

Kirsch, Irving; Rosadino, Michael J. Do double–blind studies with informed consent yield externally valid results? An empirical test. *Psychopharmacology (Berlin).* 1993; 110(4): 437–442. 13 refs. BE55567.

> adolescents; *behavioral research; control groups; disclosure; *drugs; *evaluation; evaluation studies; human experimentation; *informed consent; *placebos; psychology; *random selection; *research design; research subjects; students

Swartz, Marvin S.; Burns, Barbara J.; George, Linda K., et al. The ethical challenges of a randomized controlled trial of involuntary outpatient commitment. *Journal of Mental Health Administration.* 1997 Winter; 24(1): 35–43. 27 refs. BE57762.

> *behavioral research; coercion; informed consent; legal aspects; *mentally ill; *outpatient commitment; patient compliance; *random selection; *research design; research subjects; selection of subjects; treatment outcome; North Carolina

BEHAVIORAL RESEARCH/SPECIAL POPULATIONS

Latvala, Eila; Janhonen, Sirpa; Moring, Juha. Ethical dilemmas in a psychiatric nursing study. *Nursing Ethics.* 1998 Jan; 5(1): 27–35. 33 refs. BE58714.

> autonomy; *behavioral research; coercion; competence; confidentiality; informed consent; *institutionalized persons; investigators; *mental institutions; *mentally ill; nurses; nursing ethics; *nursing research; privacy; research design; research subjects; third party consent; qualitative research; Finland

Murphy, Timothy F. Gay Science: The Ethics of Sexual

Orientation Research. New York, NY: Columbia University Press; 1997. 268 p. 416 fn. ISBN 0–231–10848–6. BE58226.

> *behavioral genetics; *behavioral research; brain; children; females; fetal therapy; genetic determinism; genetic predisposition; genetic screening; historical aspects; *homosexuals; hormones; legal aspects; males; military personnel; moral obligations; normality; parent child relationship; prenatal diagnosis; psychology; psychotherapy; religion; science; selective abortion; sexuality; siblings; social discrimination; stigmatization

Sigmon, Sandra T.; Rohan, Kelly J.; Dorhofer, Diana, et al. Effects of consent form information on self–disclosure. *Ethics and Behavior.* 1997; 7(4): 299–310. 17 refs. BE58662.

> autonomy; *behavioral research; beneficence; communication; comparative studies; comprehension; *consent forms; *depressive disorder; *disclosure; females; informed consent; investigators; *males; *psychological stress; psychology; psychotherapy; recall; referral and consultation; *research subjects; students; suicide; survey; universities; United States

When researchers encounter preexisting psychological distress in participants, ethical codes provide little guidance on how to balance issues of beneficence and autonomy. Although researchers may inform participants what will occur given responses indicating distress, this information may lead to biased self–reports. This important issue was addressed in this study by manipulating consent form information regarding the type of psychopathology to be assessed and various levels of possible follow–up. In comparing responses on self–report measures of anxiety, depression, and general psychological distress, men who believed depression was the focus of the study reported fewer symptoms of depression and less trait anxiety as intrusiveness of experimenter follow–up increased. These results are discussed within the framework of socialization theory. Given that half of the sample did not correctly answer questions regarding information contained in the consent form, guidelines to improve consent form comprehension are offered.

Swartz, Marvin S.; Burns, Barbara J.; George, Linda K., et al. The ethical challenges of a randomized controlled trial of involuntary outpatient commitment. *Journal of Mental Health Administration.* 1997 Winter; 24(1): 35–43. 27 refs. BE57762.

> *behavioral research; coercion; informed consent; legal aspects; *mentally ill; *outpatient commitment; patient compliance; *random selection; *research design; research subjects; selection of subjects; treatment outcome; North Carolina

Wadman, Meredith. Row erupts over child aggression study. [News]. *Nature.* 1998 Apr 23; 392(6678): 747. BE58075.

> *aggression; *behavioral research; blacks; *children; *drugs; ethical review; federal government; government regulation; Hispanic Americans; *human experimentation; indigents; males; *minority groups; *nontherapeutic research; research ethics committees; research subjects; scientific misconduct; selection of subjects; *fenfluramine; New York City; *New York State Psychiatric Institute (NYC); Office for Protection from Research Risks; United States

BIOETHICS

See also MEDICAL ETHICS, NURSING ETHICS, PROFESSIONAL ETHICS

Abbott, Alison. Germany's past still casts a long shadow. [News]. *Nature.* 1997 Oct 16; 389(6652): 660. BE55958.
advisory committees; *bioethical issues; bioethics; cloning; embryo research; genetic intervention; historical aspects; human experimentation; international aspects; misconduct; National Socialism; physicians; politics; *public policy; regulation; religion; Europe; European Convention on Human Rights and Biomedicine; German Chamber of Physicians; *Germany

Agich, George J.; Spielman, Bethany. Ethics expert testimony: against the skeptics. *Journal of Medicine and Philosophy.* 1997 Aug; 22(4): 381–403. 53 refs. 14 fn. BE55811.
advisory committees; bioethical issues; bioethics; case studies; *clinical ethics; conscience; cultural pluralism; democracy; ethical analysis; ethical theory; *ethicist's role; *ethicists; *ethics; *expert testimony; human experimentation; *judicial action; *law; metaethics; physicians; professional competence; public policy; *technical expertise; values; withholding treatment; United States

There is great skepticism about the admittance of expert normative ethics testimony into evidence. However, a practical analysis of the way ethics testimony has been used in courts of law reveals that the skeptical position is itself based on assumptions that are controversial. We argue for an alternative way to understand such expert testimony. This alternative understanding is based on the practice of clinical ethics.

Akabayashi, Akira. The concept of happiness in Oriental thought and its significance in clinical medicine. *In:* Hoshino, Kazumasa, ed. Japanese and Western Bioethics: Studies in Moral Diversity. Boston, MA: Kluwer Academic; 1997: 161–164. 5 refs. 1 fn. ISBN 0–7923–4112–0. BE57092.
altruism; *Buddhist ethics; *clinical ethics; compassion; *emotions; *goals; patients; *physicians; *quality of life; suffering; virtues; Asia; *Japan

American Nurses Association. Compendium of American Nurses Association Position Statements. Washington, DC: American Nurses Publishing; 1996. 232 p. Includes references. Pub. No. PR26–.75M–2/96. ISBN 1–55810–123–3. BE57450.
active euthanasia; advance directives; aged; AIDS; AIDS serodiagnosis; alcohol abuse; allowing to die; artificial feeding; assisted suicide; *bioethical issues; capital punishment; *clinical ethics; communicable diseases; computers; confidentiality; counseling; cultural pluralism; drug abuse; drugs; employment; financial support; health care delivery; health personnel; HIV seropositivity; human rights; iatrogenic disease; mass screening; medical records; *nurses; nursing education; *nursing ethics; nursing research; occupational exposure; *organizational policies; palliative care; patient care; pregnant women; prenatal injuries; primary health care; *professional organizations; resuscitation orders; *standards; terminal care; voluntary programs; women's health services; infection control; needle–exchange programs; tuberculosis; *American Nurses Association; United States

Andre, Judith. The week of November seventh: bioethics as a practice. [Personal narrative]. *In:* Carson, Ronald A.; Burns, Chester R., eds. Philosophy of Medicine and Bioethics: A Twenty–Year Retrospective and Critical Appraisal. Boston, MA: Kluwer Academic; 1997: 153–172. 18 refs. 6 fn. ISBN 0–7923–3545–7. BE56532.
bioethical issues; bioethics; clinical ethics; education; emotions; *ethicist's role; *ethicists; ethics consultation; goals; health care; indigents; interdisciplinary communication; justice; medicine; *obligations to society; philosophy; professional competence

Ashley, Benedict M.; O'Rourke, Kevin D. Health Care Ethics: A Theological Analysis. Fourth Edition. Washington, DC: Georgetown University Press; 1997. 530 p. Bibliography: p. 463–518. ISBN 0–87840–644–1. BE56501.
abortion, induced; assisted suicide; beginning of life; *bioethical issues; Christian ethics; conscience; contraception; death; decision making; determination of death; electroconvulsive therapy; ethical theory; euthanasia; family planning; fetuses; genetic counseling; genetic intervention; genetic screening; health; health care; health personnel; human experimentation; informed consent; interprofessional relations; mental health; organ transplantation; pastoral care; patients' rights; personhood; prenatal diagnosis; preventive medicine; professional ethics; professional patient relationship; psychoactive drugs; psychosurgery; psychotherapy; reproductive technologies; *Roman Catholic ethics; sexuality; terminal care; *theology; transsexualism; truth disclosure; value of life; virtues; Humanae Vitae; Instruction on Respect for Human Life

Benatar, Solomon R. Just healthcare beyond individualism: challenges for North American bioethics. *Cambridge Quarterly of Healthcare Ethics.* 1997 Fall; 6(4): 397–415. 208 fn. Appendix: proposed World Medical Association statement on health and human rights, p. 414–415. Article based on a presentation at the World Medical Association Symposium, "Medical Ethics, Humanities' Needs: Formulating a Future Ethical Program for the WMA," held in Stockholm, Sep 1994, and on the Rosenstadt Lecture, University of Toronto, Mar 1995. BE56455.
autonomy; beneficence; *bioethics; *common good; communitarianism; cultural pluralism; democracy; developing countries; disadvantaged; *economics; ethicist's role; freedom; health; *health care; *health care delivery; health care reform; health promotion; *human rights; industry; institutional ethics; *international aspects; *justice; medical ethics; medicine; moral complicity; moral obligations; *obligations to society; organizational policies; physician patient relationship; *physician's role; political systems; professional organizations; public health; resource allocation; review; science; *socioeconomic factors; trends; values; non–Western World; Western World; United States; World Medical Organization

Black, Douglas. Corporate tyranny. [Editorial]. *Journal of Medical Ethics.* 1997 Oct; 23(5): 269–270. 4 refs. BE56903.
*advisory committees; *artificial insemination; beneficence; *bioethical issues; *confidentiality; *consensus; death; *decision making; famous persons; *informed consent; married persons; *posthumous reproduction; regulation; *semen donors; suicide; *General Medical Council (Great Britain); Great Britain; *Human Fertilisation and Embryology Authority; Wingate, Orde

Blacksher, Erika. Desperately seeking difference. *Cambridge Quarterly of Healthcare Ethics.* 1998 Winter; 7(1): 11–16. 17 fn. BE58504.
bioethical issues; *clinical ethics; communication; consensus; *cultural pluralism; decision making; dissent; empirical research; ethical analysis; health care delivery; managed care programs; *minority groups; patient care; *professional patient relationship; self concept; stigmatization; terminal care; trust; truth disclosure; *values; United States

Blustein, Jeffrey. What bioethics needs to learn about families: The Worth of a Child, by Thomas Murray; The Patient in the Family: An Ethics of Medicine and Families, by Hilde Lindemann Nelson and James Lindemann Nelson. [Book review essay]. *Theoretical Medicine and Bioethics.* 1998 Apr; 19(2): 101–115. 5 fn. BE57573.
adults; aged; bioethical issues; *bioethics; caring; children;

---

decision making; *ethical analysis; ethical theory; family members; *family relationship; friends; love; *methods; models, theoretical; *moral obligations; moral policy; morality; *parent child relationship; parents; principle-based ethics; values; adult offspring; *The Patient in the Family: An Ethics of Medicine and Families (Nelson, H.L.; Nelson, J.L.); *The Worth of a Child (Murray, T.)

Boyd, Kenneth M.; Higgs, Roger; Pinching, Anthony J., eds. The New Dictionary of Medical Ethics. London: BMJ Publishing Group; 1997. 285 p. 16 refs. ISBN 0-7279-1001-9. BE58160.
*bioethical issues; *bioethics; ethics; medical ethics; professional ethics; *terminology

Boyle, Joseph. The Roman Catholic tradition and bioethics. *In:* Lustig, B. Andrew, ed.; Center for Medical Ethics and Health Policy (Houston, TX). Bioethics Yearbook, Volume 5: Theological Developments in Bioethics, 1992-1994. Boston, MA: Kluwer Academic; 1997: 11-32. 33 refs. ISBN 0-7923-4428-6. BE58379.
aborted fetuses; active euthanasia; advance directives; artificial feeding; assisted suicide; beginning of life; *bioethical issues; *bioethics; casuistry; double effect; embryos; fetal tissue donation; fetuses; health facilities; institutional policies; intention; killing; moral complicity; moral policy; morality; natural law; persistent vegetative state; personhood; public policy; religious hospitals; *Roman Catholic ethics; sterilization (sexual); *theology; value of life; withholding treatment; craniotomy; ectopic pregnancy; hysterectomy; uterine isolation; Ethical and Religious Directives for Catholic Health Care Services; National Conference of Catholic Bishops; United States; Veritatis Splendor

Bradley, Peter M.; Shenkin, Henry A.; Rivlin, Michael M., et al. The ethics industry. [Letters]. *Lancet.* 1997 Nov 22; 350(9090): 1547-1549. 9 refs. BE58150.
*bioethical issues; decision making; *ethicist's role; *ethicists; medical ethics; *physicians; professional autonomy; technical expertise

Brody, Howard. Who gets to tell the story? Narrative in postmodern bioethics. *In:* Nelson, Hilde Lindemann, ed. Stories and Their Limits: Narrative Approaches to Bioethics. New York, NY: Routledge; 1997: 18-30. 13 fn. ISBN 0-415-91910-X. BE57464.
*bioethics; clinical ethics; communication; emotions; empathy; ethicist's role; evaluation; medicine; *narrative ethics; patients; physician patient relationship; physicians; self concept; suffering; technical expertise; *postmodernism; sick role; The Wounded Storyteller (Frank, A.W.)

Butler, Declan. 'Bioethics needs better input from public.' [News]. *Nature.* 1997 Oct 23; 389(6653): 775. BE56203.
*advisory committees; *bioethical issues; committee membership; common good; *decision making; *ethics committees; eugenics; human rights; interdisciplinary communication; *international aspects; preimplantation diagnosis; *public participation; public policy; values; national ethics committees; European Union; *France; *Great Britain

Butler, Declan. France reaps benefits and costs of going by the book. [News]. *Nature.* 1997 Oct 16; 389(6652): 661-662. BE55957.
advisory committees; *bioethical issues; bioethics; cloning; *embryo research; genetic research; *government regulation; international aspects; *public policy; *France; National Ethics Advisory Committee (France)

Butler, Declan. Unesco board set to agree on compromise on bioethics committee. [News]. *Nature.* 1998 Apr 30; 392(6679): 854. BE58407.

*advisory committees; *bioethical issues; ecology; genetic research; *international aspects; science; *International Bioethics Committee (Unesco); *Unesco; *World Commission on the Ethics of Scientific Knowledge and Technology

Callahan, Daniel. Cloning: then and now. *Cambridge Quarterly of Healthcare Ethics.* 1998 Spring; 7(2): 141-144. BE58006.
advisory committees; attitudes; *bioethics; biomedical research; *cloning; economics; genetic intervention; government regulation; historical aspects; reproduction; reproductive technologies; rights; risks and benefits; National Bioethics Advisory Commission; United States

Callahan, Daniel. Communitarian bioethics: a pious hope? *Responsive Community.* 1996 Fall; 6(4): 26-33. BE55845.
*autonomy; bioethical issues; *bioethics; biomedical technologies; common good; *communitarianism; freedom; goals; health care; historical aspects; *libertarianism; medicine; moral obligations; obligations to society; physician patient relationship; public health; rights; trends; values; *Twentieth Century; *United States

Callahan, Daniel. International perspectives. *Hastings Center Report.* 1998 Jan-Feb; 28(1): 45-46. BE57298.
attitudes to death; bioethical issues; *bioethics; biomedical technologies; *cultural pluralism; health care; *international aspects; medicine; values; Hastings Center; United States

Campbell, Courtney S. Ecclesiology and ethics: an LDS response. *In:* Lustig, B. Andrew, ed.; Center for Medical Ethics and Health Policy (Houston, TX). Bioethics Yearbook, Volume 5: Theological Developments in Bioethics, 1992-1994. Boston, MA: Kluwer Academic; 1997: 33-53. 16 refs. ISBN 0-7923-4428-6. BE58380.
accountability; active euthanasia; allowing to die; alternative therapies; assisted suicide; *bioethical issues; biomedical technologies; conscience; cultural pluralism; decision making; family relationship; health personnel; historical aspects; killing; marital relationship; medical ethics; moral obligations; morality; physicians; political activity; *Protestant ethics; public policy; sexuality; suicide; *theology; uncertainty; faith; integrity; rationality; Death with Dignity Act (OR); *Mormonism; Nineteenth Century; Oregon; Twentieth Century; United States

Campbell, Courtney S. The crumbling foundations of medical ethics: Rethinking Life and Death: The Collapse of Our Traditional Ethics, by Peter Singer; The Foundations of Bioethics, by H. Tristram Engelhardt; Deciding Together: Bioethics and Moral Consensus, by Jonathan D. Moreno. [Book review essay]. *Theoretical Medicine and Bioethics.* 1998 Apr; 19(2): 143-152. BE57574.
bioethical issues; *bioethics; consensus; cultural pluralism; *decision making; dissent; ethical relativism; *goals; medical ethics; *medicine; morality; religious ethics; secularism; value of life; values; *Deciding Together: Bioethics and Moral Consensus (Moreno, J.D.); *Rethinking Life and Death: The Collapse of Our Traditional Ethics (Singer, P.); *The Foundations of Bioethics (Engelhardt, H.T.)

Caplan, Arthur L. Am I My Brother's Keeper? The Ethical Frontiers of Biomedicine. Bloomington, IN: Indiana University Press; 1997. 241 p. (Medical ethics series). Bibliography: p. 221-235. ISBN 0-253-33358-X. BE56949.
active euthanasia; allowing to die; animal organs; artificial organs; assisted suicide; autonomy; *bioethical issues; bioethics; cloning; determination of death; disease; donors; economics; eugenics; federal government; fetal tissue donation; futility; gatekeeping; gene therapy; government financing; health; health care delivery; hearts; hospices; human experimentation; informed consent; legal aspects;

misconduct; moral complicity; National Socialism; newborns; organ transplantation; physician patient relationship; physicians; public policy; regulation; remuneration; reproductive technologies; resource allocation; risk; self induced illness; suffering; tissue donation; trust; withholding treatment; Baby Jane Doe; Germany; In re Treatment and Care of Infant Doe; Tuskegee Syphilis Study; United States

Carse, Alisa L. Impartial principle and moral context: securing a place for the particular in ethical theory. *Journal of Medicine and Philosophy.* 1998 Apr; 23(2): 153–169. 44 refs. 10 fn. BE58652.
  *caring; *ethical analysis; *ethical theory; justice; moral development; personhood; principle–based ethics
This essay critically assesses two strategies of accommodation used by defenders of impartialism in ethics to argue that the care orientation represents no genuine challenge to impartialist theoretical paradigms. One strategy focuses on impartiality as a constraint on moral deliberation, the other as a constraint on moral justification. While highlighting respects in which the commitment to impartiality is more consonant with the care orientation than many advocates of care have acknowledged, this essay attempts to clarify crucial ways in which each accommodationist strategy fails, thus locating some of the more important contributions and challenges the care orientation offers to moral theory.

Carson, Ronald A. Medical ethics as reflective practice. *In:* Carson, Ronald A.; Burns, Chester R., eds. Philosophy of Medicine and Bioethics: A Twenty–Year Retrospective and Critical Appraisal. Boston, MA: Kluwer Academic; 1997: 181–191. 20 refs. 2 fn. ISBN 0–7923–3545–7. BE56534.
  *bioethics; casuistry; historical aspects; medical ethics; medicine; metaphor; methods; narrative ethics; principle–based ethics; theology

Carson, Ronald A.; Burns, Chester R., eds. Philosophy of Medicine and Bioethics: A Twenty–Year Retrospective and Critical Appraisal. Boston, MA: Kluwer Academic; 1997. 341 p. (Philosophy and medicine; v. 50). 553 refs. 84 fn. ISBN 0–7923–3545–7. BE56522.
  *bioethical issues; *bioethics; circumcision; cultural pluralism; economics; ethical relativism; ethicist's role; ethicists; females; health care delivery; humanism; humanities; interdisciplinary communication; legal obligations; medical education; *medicine; moral obligations; morality; normality; pain; palliative care; patient advocacy; patient care; *philosophy; physician patient relationship; resource allocation; secularism; self concept; standards; suffering; values; women's health; postmodernism; research ethics

Cassell, Jackie. Against medical ethics: opening the can of worms. *Journal of Medical Ethics.* 1998 Feb; 24(1): 8–12. 13 fn. BE57404.
  *bioethics; deontological ethics; ethical theory; *ethics; medical education; *medical ethics; medical specialties; *medicine; morality; *philosophy; utilitarianism
In a controversial paper, David Seedhouse argues that medical ethics is not and cannot be a distinct discipline with it own field of study. He derives this claim from a characterization of ethics, which he states but does not defend. He claims further that the project of medical ethics as it exists and of moral philosophy do not overlap. I show that Seedhouse's views on ethics have wide implications which he does not declare, and in the light of this argue that Seedhouse owes us a defence of his characterization of ethics. Further, I show that his characterization of ethics, which he uses to attack

medical ethics, is a committed position within moral philosophy. As a consequence of this, it does not allow the relation between moral philosophy and medical ethics to be discussed without prejudice to its outcome. Finally, I explore the relation between Seedhouse's position and naturalism, and its implications for medical epistemology. I argue that this shows us that Seedhouse's position, if it can be defended, is likely to lead to a fruitful and important line of inquiry which reconnects philosophy and medical ethics.

Chambers, Tod. What to expect from an ethics case (and what it expects from you). *In:* Nelson, Hilde Lindemann, ed. Stories and Their Limits: Narrative Approaches to Bioethics. New York, NY: Routledge; 1997: 171–184. 32 refs. 2 fn. ISBN 0–415–91910–X. BE57469.
  *bioethics; *case studies; clinical ethics; *narrative ethics

Cherry, Mark J. Moral strangers: a humanity that does not bind. *In:* Hoshino, Kazumasa, ed. Japanese and Western Bioethics: Studies in Moral Diversity. Boston, MA: Kluwer Academic; 1997: 201–223. 42 refs. 6 fn. ISBN 0–7923–4112–0. BE57096.
  attitudes to death; autonomy; beneficence; *bioethical issues; biomedical technologies; caring; Christian ethics; coercion; communitarianism; comparative studies; consensus; *cultural pluralism; decision making; dissent; emotions; *ethical relativism; ethical theory; family members; gene therapy; genetic enhancement; genetic intervention; germ cells; health care; informed consent; legal aspects; *morality; nursing ethics; organ donation; paternalism; patients; physician patient relationship; public policy; reproductive technologies; resource allocation; secularism; terminology; treatment refusal; truth disclosure; value of life; *values; postmodernism; rationality; *Western World; *Japan

Childress, James F. Narrative(s) versus norm(s): a misplaced debate in bioethics. *In:* Nelson, Hilde Lindemann, ed. Stories and Their Limits: Narrative Approaches to Bioethics. New York, NY: Routledge; 1997: 252–271. 57 fn. ISBN 0–415–91910–X. BE57472.
  autonomy; beneficence; *bioethics; case studies; casuistry; *ethical analysis; ethical theory; ethics; killing; *methods; *moral policy; *narrative ethics; nuclear warfare; paternalism; principle–based ethics; treatment refusal; war; Cowart, Dax; Hiroshima

Churchill, Larry R. Bioethics in social context. *In:* Carson, Ronald A.; Burns, Chester R., eds. Philosophy of Medicine and Bioethics: A Twenty–Year Retrospective and Critical Appraisal. Boston, MA: Kluwer Academic; 1997: 137–151. 20 refs. 7 fn. ISBN 0–7923–3545–7. BE56531.
  autonomy; *bioethics; clinical ethics; clinical ethics committees; decision making; empathy; ethical theory; ethics; ethics consultation; humanities; interdisciplinary communication; methods; narrative ethics; paternalism; patient participation; patients; professional patient relationship; social dominance; social sciences

Clouser, K. Danner. Biomedical ethics. *In:* Borchert, Donald M., ed. The Encyclopedia of Philosophy. Supplement. New York, NY: Simon and Schuster Macmillan; 1996: 61–67. 21 refs. ISBN 0–02–864629–0. BE57220.
  abortion, induced; allowing to die; bioethical issues; *bioethics; ethical relativism; ethical theory; ethics; genetic intervention; health care; historical aspects; human experimentation; interdisciplinary communication; methods; moral policy; *philosophy; physician patient relationship; professional organizations; reproductive technologies; resource allocation; terminology

---

BE = bioethics accession number   fn. = footnotes   refs. = references

Cole, Thomas R. Toward a humanist bioethics: commentary on Churchill and Andre. *In:* Carson, Ronald A.; Burns, Chester R., eds. Philosophy of Medicine and Bioethics: A Twenty-Year Retrospective and Critical Appraisal. Boston, MA: Kluwer Academic; 1997: 173–179. 18 refs. 2 fn. ISBN 0–7923–3545–7. BE56533.
*bioethics; communication; emotions; ethical theory; ethicist's role; *humanism

Crawford, Cromwell. Hindu developments in bioethics. *In:* Lustig, B. Andrew, ed.; Center for Medical Ethics and Health Policy (Houston, TX). Bioethics Yearbook, Volume 5: Theological Developments in Bioethics, 1992–1994. Boston, MA: Kluwer Academic; 1997: 55–74. 15 refs. ISBN 0–7923–4428–6. BE58381.
allowing to die; assisted suicide; attitudes to death; autonomy; beginning of life; *bioethical issues; compassion; females; fetal development; health; health care; *Hindu ethics; human body; involuntary euthanasia; justice; medicine; mother fetus relationship; newborns; obligations of society; personhood; philosophy; pregnant women; quality of life; religion; science; selective abortion; self concept; sex determination; sexuality; suicide; therapeutic abortion; value of life; voluntary euthanasia; rationality; Ayurveda; India

Crigger, Bette–Jane. As time goes by: an intellectual ethnography of bioethics. *In:* DeVries, Raymond: Subedi, Janardan, eds. Bioethics and Society: Constructing the Ethical Enterprise. Upper Saddle River, NJ: Prentice Hall; 1998: 192–215. 5 refs. 20 fn. ISBN 0–13–531252–3. BE58736.
abortion, induced; AIDS; allowing to die; behavior control; *bioethical issues; *bioethics; clinical ethics; genetic intervention; genetic research; health care delivery; historical aspects; interdisciplinary communication; *literature; methods; organ donation; organ transplantation; population control; pregnant women; prolongation of life; public policy; reproduction; reproductive technologies; review; terminal care; *trends; Hastings Center Report; Twentieth Century

Crigger, Bette–Jane. Bioethnography: fieldwork in the lands of medical ethics. [Book review essay]. *Medical Anthropology Quarterly.* 1995 Sep; 9(3): 400–417. 26 refs. 11 fn. BE56559.
*anthropology; artificial organs; autonomy; *bioethics; biomedical technologies; chronically ill; commodification; cultural pluralism; decision making; ethical theory; ethics consultation; genetic counseling; gifts; health personnel; hearts; human experimentation; intensive care units; *interdisciplinary communication; interprofessional relations; medical ethics; medicine; organ donation; organ transplantation; patient participation; professional patient relationship; resource allocation; resuscitation orders; selection for treatment; self concept; *social sciences; *sociology of medicine; values; sick role; *All God's Mistakes: Genetic Counseling in a Pediatric Hospital (Bosk, C.L.); *Good Days, Bad Days: The Self and Time in Chronic Illness (Charmaz, K.); *Intensive Care: Medical Ethics and the Medical Profession (Zussman, R.); *Social Science Perspectives on Medical Ethics (Weisz, G., ed.); *Spare Parts: Organ Replacement in American Society (Fox, R.C.; Swazey, J.P.); United States

Curran, William J.; Hall, Mark A.; Bobinski, Mary Anne, et al. Health Care Law and Ethics. Fifth Edition. New York, NY: Aspen Law and Business; 1998. 1,463 p. Includes references. ISBN 1–56706–809–X. BE57442.
abortion, induced; adults; advance directives; AIDS serodiagnosis; allowing to die; alternative therapies; assisted suicide; *bioethical issues; brain death; communicable diseases; competence; confidentiality; conflict of interest; contact tracing; contraception; decision making; determination of death; drugs; economics; futility;

government regulation; *health care delivery; health facilities; health personnel; HIV seropositivity; informed consent; *legal aspects; malpractice; managed care programs; mandatory programs; mentally ill; minors; organ donation; organ transplantation; *patient care; pregnant women; prenatal injuries; professional patient relationship; public health; reproduction; reproductive technologies; right to die; standards; third party consent; treatment refusal; *United States

Davis, Anne J.; Aroskar, Mila A.; Liaschenko, Joan, et al. Health care ethics and ethical dilemmas. *In: their* Ethical Dilemmas and Nursing Practice. Fourth Edition. Stamford, CT: Appleton and Lange; 1997: 1–15. 12 refs. ISBN 0–8385–2283–1. BE58589.
bioethical issues; *bioethics; codes of ethics; ethicists; ethics; health care; justice; legal aspects; medical ethics; morality; nursing ethics; professional organizations; American Medical Association; American Nurses Association; Hippocratic Oath; International Council of Nurses

Davis, Dena S. Legal trends in bioethics. *Journal of Clinical Ethics.* 1997 Summer; 8(2): 204–207. 14 fn. BE55950.
abortion, induced; AIDS serodiagnosis; assisted suicide; *bioethical issues; brain death; cadavers; cloning; contraception; drug abuse; fetuses; government regulation; health insurance reimbursement; hospitals; human experimentation; informed consent; international aspects; law enforcement; *legal aspects; legal liability; methods; personhood; posthumous reproduction; pregnant women; psychoactive drugs; reproductive technologies; resuscitation orders; semen donors; Australia; Blood, Diane; Great Britain; In re Baby K; Japan; Tarbuck, Joanne; United States

Davis, Dena S. Legal trends in bioethics. *Journal of Clinical Ethics.* 1997 Fall; 8(3): 313–319. 19 fn. BE57588.
abortion, induced; AIDS; allowing to die; assisted suicide; *bioethical issues; brain death; children; circumcision; cloning; drugs; females; government regulation; HIV seropositivity; human experimentation; international aspects; *legal aspects; managed care programs; organ transplantation; parents; persistent vegetative state; physicians; religion; selection for treatment; state government; Supreme Court decisions; treatment refusal; withholding treatment; Egypt; Japan; RU–486; *United States

Davis, Dena S. Legal trends in bioethics. *Journal of Clinical Ethics.* 1997 Winter; 8(4): 405–410. 17 fn. BE57606.
abortion, induced; accountability; assisted suicide; *bioethical issues; child abuse; cloning; compensation; contraception; cryopreservation; disabled; drugs; federal government; fetal development; genetic disorders; government financing; government regulation; health insurance reimbursement; HIV seropositivity; human experimentation; *legal aspects; legal liability; managed care programs; mental health; mentally retarded; minors; negligence; occupational exposure; ovum; parental consent; patients' rights; physicians; pregnant women; prenatal injuries; semen donors; state government; sterilization (sexual); surrogate mothers; tissue banks; torts; voluntary euthanasia; Australia; California; Colombia; Kevorkian, Jack; Oregon; Poland; *United States

Davis, Dena S. Legal trends in bioethics. *Journal of Clinical Ethics.* 1998 Spring; 9(1): 92–96. 14 fn. BE57718.
abortion, induced; AIDS; animal organs; assisted suicide; *bioethical issues; cloning; disabled; employment; fetuses; genetic screening; HIV seropositivity; human experimentation; incentives; *legal aspects; managed care programs; organ transplantation; physicians; pregnant women; privacy; psychoactive drugs; refusal to treat; terminally ill; treatment refusal; marijuana; Council of Europe; *United States

---

BE = bioethics accession number   fn. = footnotes   refs. = references

Davis, Dena S. Legal trends in bioethics. *Journal of Clinical Ethics.* 1998 Summer; 9(2): 209–211. 5 fn. BE58969.
> abortion, induced; assisted suicide; *bioethical issues; disclosure; informed consent; *legal aspects; managed care programs; minors; nontherapeutic research; organ transplantation; patient care; physicians; professional competence; reproductive technologies; resource allocation; scientific misconduct; *United States

Dell'Oro, Roberto; Viafora, Corrado, eds. History of Bioethics: International Perspectives. San Francisco, CA: International Scholars Publications; 1996. 313 p. 428 fn. English translation from the Italian, by R. Dell'Oro, of *Vent'Anni di Bioetica Idee Protagonisti Istituzioni*, C. Viafora, ed. (Padua, Italy: Lanza Foundation; 1990). ISBN 1-57309-048-4. BE56240.
> abortion, induced; animal experimentation; attitudes to death; *bioethical issues; *bioethics; biomedical technologies; clinical ethics; *cultural pluralism; education; ethical analysis; ethical theory; ethics; ethics committees; euthanasia; future generations; genetic intervention; *historical aspects; human experimentation; *international aspects; justice; law; moral obligations; *moral policy; morality; organ donation; physician patient relationship; prenatal diagnosis; principle-based ethics; public policy; religion; reproductive technologies; research institutes; review; Roman Catholic ethics; science; secularism; sociology of medicine; terminology; trends; values; virtues; France; Germany; Italy; Latin America; Netherlands; Spain; United States

DeRenzo, Evan G.; Strauss, Michelle. A feminist model for clinical ethics consultation: increasing attention to context and narrative. *HEC (HealthCare Ethics Committee) Forum.* 1997 Sep; 9(3): 212–227. 42 refs. BE56180.
> *clinical ethics; clinical ethics committees; communication; consensus; *decision making; emotions; ethical analysis; *ethicists; *ethics consultation; *feminist ethics; models, theoretical; narrative ethics; social dominance

DeVries, Raymond; Subedi, Janardan, eds. Bioethics and Society: Constructing the Ethical Enterprise. Upper Saddle River, NJ: Prentice Hall; 1998. 276 p. 463 refs. 4 fn. ISBN 0-13-531252-3. BE58726.
> attitudes; attitudes to death; autonomy; *bioethical issues; *bioethics; clinical ethics committees; cultural pluralism; decision making; economics; empirical research; ethical analysis; ethicists; ethics consultation; euthanasia; evaluation; federal government; genetic counseling; health care delivery; historical aspects; human experimentation; informed consent; interdisciplinary communication; international aspects; literature; managed care programs; medical ethics; medicine; methods; minority groups; patient care; physician patient relationship; physicians; public policy; radiation; review; right to die; social sciences; sociology of medicine; standards; trends; Atomic Energy Commission; Twentieth Century; United States

DeVries, Raymond; Conrad, Peter. Why bioethics needs sociology. *In:* DeVries, Raymond; Subedi, Janardan, eds. Bioethics and Society: Constructing the Ethical Enterprise. Upper Saddle River, NJ: Prentice Hall; 1998: 233–257. 41 refs. 13 fn. ISBN 0-13-531252-3. BE58738.
> adults; bioethical issues; *bioethics; clinical ethics; clinical ethics committees; cultural pluralism; decision making; education; empirical research; ethicist's role; *ethicists; evaluation; goals; historical aspects; intensive care units; *interdisciplinary communication; international aspects; interprofessional relations; newborns; nursing ethics; physicians; professional competence; professional organizations; *social sciences; social workers; sociology of medicine; standards; technical expertise; values; withholding

treatment; Twentieth Century; *United States

Dickens, B. Canadian developments [bioethics and the law]. [News]. *International Journal of Bioethics.* 1997 Mar–Jun; 8(1–2): 131–134. BE59101.
> artificial insemination; *bioethical issues; compensation; HIV seropositivity; involuntary sterilization; judicial action; *legal aspects; legal liability; medical devices; physicians; pregnant women; prenatal injuries; refusal to treat; sperm; wrongful life; *Canada

Dickson, David. UK takes pride in 'principled pragmatism'. [News]. *Nature.* 1997 Oct 16; 389(6652): 663. BE55847.
> advisory committees; *bioethical issues; cloning; genetic intervention; government regulation; public opinion; *public policy; self regulation; social impact; *Great Britain; Human Genetics Advisory Commission (Great Britain); Nuffield Council on Bioethics

Di Noia, J. Augustine. The virtues of the Good Samaritan: health care ethics in the perspective of a renewed moral theology. *Dolentium Hominum: Church and Health in the World.* 1996; 31(11th Yr., No. 1): 211–214. 13 fn. BE57368.
> *bioethics; ethical theory; health care; *health personnel; patient advocacy; patient care; principle-based ethics; professional ethics; professional patient relationship; *Roman Catholic ethics; *theology; *virtues; Good Samaritanism; Veritatis Splendor

Dorff, Elliot N. A methodology for Jewish medical ethics. *In:* Dorff, Elliot N.; Newman, Louis E., eds. Contemporary Jewish Ethics and Morality: A Reader. New York, NY: Oxford University Press; 1995: 161–176. 22 fn. Reprinted from *Jewish Law Association Studies*, 1991; 7: 35–57. ISBN 0-19-509066-7. BE58526.
> autonomy; *bioethical issues; *bioethics; clergy; conscience; covenant; *decision making; dissent; ethical analysis; historical aspects; *Jewish ethics; law; medicine; *methods; morality; quality of life; *theology; value of life; *Conservative Judaism; *Orthodox Judaism; *Reform Judaism; United States

Dorff, Elliot N. Review of recent work in Jewish bioethics. *In:* Lustig, B. Andrew, ed.; Center for Medical Ethics and Health Policy (Houston, TX). Bioethics Yearbook, Volume 5: Theological Developments in Bioethics, 1992–1994. Boston, MA: Kluwer Academic; 1997: 75–91. 41 refs. ISBN 0-7923-4428-6. BE58382.
> AIDS serodiagnosis; allowing to die; animal experimentation; artificial feeding; autonomy; *bioethical issues; brain death; cadavers; decision making; disclosure; double effect; drugs; fetuses; gene therapy; germ cells; HIV seropositivity; iatrogenic disease; *Jewish ethics; medical education; mothers; multiple pregnancy; newborns; organ donation; persistent vegetative state; physicians; privacy; reproductive technologies; selective abortion; terminally ill; *theology; therapeutic abortion; truth disclosure; viability; voluntary euthanasia; withholding treatment; Conservative Judaism; Israel; North America; Orthodox Judaism; Reconstructionist Judaism; Reform Judaism

Dossetor, John B. Human values in health care: trying to get it right. *Canadian Medical Association Journal.* 1997 Dec 15; 157(12): 1689–1690. 4 refs. BE59051.
> *bioethical issues; *bioethics; ethical theory; health care delivery; trends; values; *Canada

Dyson, Anthony O. Reflections on method in theology and genetics: from suspicion to critical cooperation. *In:* Becker, Gerhold K., ed. Changing Nature's Course: The Ethical Challenge of Biotechnology. Hong Kong: Hong Kong University Press; 1996: 159–169. 40 fn. ISBN

962-209-403-1. BE56711.
autonomy; *bioethics; *Christian ethics; freedom; future generations; *genetic intervention; genetics; germ cells; historical aspects; philosophy; *Protestant ethics; Roman Catholic ethics; secularism; *theology; Twentieth Century; United States

Elliott, Carl. Hedgehogs and hermaphrodites: toward a more anthropological bioethics. *In:* Carson, Ronald A.; Burns, Chester R., eds. Philosophy of Medicine and Bioethics: A Twenty-Year Retrospective and Critical Appraisal. Boston, MA: Kluwer Academic; 1997: 197-211. 19 refs. 2 fn. ISBN 0-7923-3545-7. BE56536.
anthropology; autonomy; *bioethics; biomedical technologies; children; cosmetic surgery; *cultural pluralism; disease; futility; gene therapy; genetic disorders; genetic enhancement; goals; growth disorders; health; homosexuals; hormones; justice; medicine; mental health; metaphor; methods; morality; *normality; psychoactive drugs; psychotherapy; quality of life; *self concept; sexuality; transsexualism; *values; dignity; *personal identity; Prozac

Elliott, Carl. On being unprincipled: Principles of Health Care Ethics, edited by Raanan Gillon and Ann Lloyd; A Matter of Principles? Ferment in U.S. Bioethics, by Edwin R. DuBose, Ron Hamel, and Laurence J. O'Connell. [Book review essay]. *Theoretical Medicine and Bioethics.* 1998 Apr; 19(2): 153-159. 13 fn. BE57575.
alternatives; *bioethics; ethical theory; ethicists; *methods; *principle-based ethics; *A Matter of Principles? Ferment in U.S. Bioethics (DuBose, E.R.; Hamel, R.; O'Connell, L.J.); *Principles of Health Care Ethics (Gillon, R.; Lloyd, A., eds.)

Elliott, Deni; Blanford, Patricia; Watson, Marci, comps. Scientific research ethics videography. *Professional Ethics.* 1995 Spring-Summer; 4(3-4): 199-204. List of video titles with short summaries. BE55684.
animal experimentation; *audiovisual aids; *bioethical issues; *biomedical research; education; genetic research; human experimentation; mass media; prenatal diagnosis; professional ethics; resource allocation; science; *scientific misconduct; teaching methods; United States

Ellos, William J. Some narrative methodologies for clinical ethics. *Cambridge Quarterly of Healthcare Ethics.* 1998 Summer; 7(3): 315-322. 21 fn. BE58559.
case studies; *clinical ethics; ethicist's role; *ethics consultation; *narrative ethics; philosophy; Barthes, Roland; Foucault, Michel

Engelhardt, H. Tristram. Bioethics and the philosophy of medicine reconsidered. *In:* Carson, Ronald A.; Burns, Chester R., eds. Philosophy of Medicine and Bioethics: A Twenty-Year Retrospective and Critical Appraisal. Boston, MA: Kluwer Academic; 1997: 85-103. 65 refs. 8 fn. ISBN 0-7923-3545-7. BE56528.
advisory committees; bioethical issues; *bioethics; caring; consensus; *cultural pluralism; decision making; historical aspects; humanism; humanities; interdisciplinary communication; medical ethics; *medicine; *morality; *philosophy; political systems; principle-based ethics; public policy; religious ethics; *secularism; theology; values; postmodernism

Engelhardt, H. Tristram. Japanese and Western bioethics: studies in moral diversity. *In:* Hoshino, Kazumasa, ed. Japanese and Western Bioethics: Studies in Moral Diversity. Boston, MA: Kluwer Academic; 1997: 1-10. 6 refs. ISBN 0-7923-4112-0. BE57079.
attitudes to death; *bioethical issues; *bioethics; Christian ethics; common good; communitarianism; comparative studies; *cultural pluralism; *ethical relativism; ethics; family

relationship; health care; historical aspects; *international aspects; *morality; public policy; religion; secularism; *values; virtues; *non-Western World; rationality; *Western World; *Japan; United States

Engelhardt, H. Tristram. Moral puzzles concerning the human genome: Western taboos, intuitions, and beliefs at the end of the Christian era. *In:* Hoshino, Kazumasa, ed. Japanese and Western Bioethics: Studies in Moral Diversity. Boston, MA: Kluwer Academic; 1997: 181-186. 6 refs. ISBN 0-7923-4112-0. BE57094.
*bioethics; *Christian ethics; ethical relativism; future generations; gene therapy; genetic enhancement; genetic identity; *genetic intervention; germ cells; *morality; risks and benefits; *secularism; *values; *rationality; Western World; *Europe; Germany; *Japan

Fan, Ruiping. Three levels of problems in cross-cultural explorations of bioethics: a methodological approach. *In:* Hoshino, Kazumasa, ed. Japanese and Western Bioethics: Studies in Moral Diversity. Boston, MA: Kluwer Academic; 1997: 189-199. 15 refs. 3 fn. ISBN 0-7923-4112-0. BE57095.
*autonomy; *beneficence; *bioethics; communitarianism; comparative studies; *cultural pluralism; decision making; disclosure; *ethical relativism; family members; family relationship; informed consent; international aspects; *moral policy; *morality; patient participation; patients; physicians; religion; secularism; third party consent; *values; Confucian ethics; *non-Western World; *Western World; *China; Japan

Fineschi, Vittorio; Turillazzi, Emanuela; Cateni, Cecilia. The new Italian code of medical ethics. *Journal of Medical Ethics.* 1997 Aug; 23(4): 239-244. 14 refs. BE55905.
advance directives; advisory committees; autonomy; *bioethical issues; bioethics; *codes of ethics; competence; confidentiality; conscience; cultural pluralism; decision making; democracy; disclosure; government regulation; historical aspects; informed consent; legal aspects; *medical ethics; physician patient relationship; physicians; professional autonomy; professional organizations; reproductive technologies; selection for treatment; self regulation; *Italy; National Committee for Bioethics (Italy); Twentieth Century
In June 1995, the Italian code of medical ethics was revised in order that its principles should reflect the ever-changing relationship between the medical profession and society and between physicians and patients. The updated code is also a response to new ethical problems created by scientific progress; the discussion of such problems often shows up a need for better understanding on the part of the medical profession itself. Medical deontology is defined as the discipline for the study of norms of conduct for the health care professions, including moral and legal norms as well as those pertaining more strictly to professional performance. The aim of deontology is therefore, the in-depth investigation and revision of the code of medical ethics. It is in the light of this conceptual definition that one should interpret a review of the different codes which have attempted, throughout the various periods of Italy's recent history, to adapt ethical norms to particular social and health care climates.

Fins, Joseph J. Approximation and negotiation: clinical pragmatism and difference. *Cambridge Quarterly of Healthcare Ethics.* 1998 Winter; 7(1): 68-76. 17 fn. BE58453.
attitudes to death; *blacks; *brain death; case studies; children; *clinical ethics; *communication; *consensus; *cultural pluralism; *decision making; *determination of

---

BE = bioethics accession number   fn. = footnotes   refs. = references

death; diagnosis; *dissent; Jewish ethics; *Jews; *knowledge, attitudes, practice; legal aspects; *minority groups; parents; *patient care; *physicians; *professional family relationship; religion; secularism; terminal care; trust; *values; *pragmatism; New York; Orthodox Judaism; United States

Fletcher, John C. Bioethics in a legal forum: confessions of an "expert" witness. *Journal of Medicine and Philosophy.* 1997 Aug; 22(4): 297–324. 55 refs. 18 fn. BE55855.

allowing to die; anencephaly; *bioethical issues; bioethics; case studies; clinical ethics; deception; decision making; dissent; emergency care; ethical analysis; *ethicist's role; *ethicists; *ethics; ethics consultation; *expert testimony; futility; hospitals; infants; informed consent; interprofessional relations; *judicial action; *law; legal aspects; misconduct; mothers; patient care; physicians; prolongation of life; public policy; refusal to treat; remuneration; *technical expertise; ventilators; Americans with Disabilities Act 1990; Child Abuse Amendments 1984; Emergency Medical Treatment and Active Labor Act 1986; Fairfax Hospital (Falls Church, VA); In re Baby K; Osheroff v. Greenspan; *United States; Veatch, Robert

This article reflects on the author's modest experience as an expert witness in two trials: Osheroff vs. Greenspan (1983), and In the Matter of Baby K (1994). Bioethicists' expertise as scholar-teachers and consultants on particular issues merits qualification by judges as expert witnesses. The article argues that a different kind of expertise — strong moral advocacy — is required to be an effective expert witness. The major lessons of expert witnessing for the author concern the demands and strains on the bioethicist's role as scholar, teacher, and consultant. The Baby K case is analyzed in some detail, due to its importance for bioethics, ethics consultation, and the testimony of bioethicists on either side of the case. Rules of thumb are offered to guide decisions as to choices regarding expert witnessing, as well as a discussion of the interaction of law and bioethics.

Fletcher, John C.; Miller, Franklin G. The promise and perils of public bioethics. *In:* Vanderpool, Harold Y., ed. The Ethics of Research Involving Human Subjects: Facing the 21st Century. Frederick, MD: University Publishing Group; 1996: 155–184. 74 fn. ISBN 1-55572-036-6. BE56986.

abortion, induced; accountability; *advisory committees; AIDS; *bioethical issues; *bioethics; biomedical research; embryo research; federal government; fetal research; fetal tissue donation; government financing; government regulation; health care delivery; historical aspects; *human experimentation; morality; politics; *public policy; *regulation; research institutes; scientific misconduct; Department of Health and Human Services; Ethics Advisory Board; National Bioethics Advisory Commission; National Commission for the Protection of Human Subjects; President's Commission for the Study of Ethical Problems; *United States

Fox, Mark D.; McGee, Glenn; Caplan, Arthur. Paradigms for clinical ethics consultation practice. *Cambridge Quarterly of Healthcare Ethics.* 1998 Summer; 7(3): 308–314. 27 fn. BE58558.

accountability; *clinical ethics; conflict of interest; *ethicist's role; *ethicists; *ethics consultation; evaluation; health personnel; *hospitals; interprofessional relations; *models, theoretical; organization and administration; patient care team; professional family relationship; referral and consultation; technical expertise; community hospitals; preventive ethics; teaching hospitals

Fox, Renée C.; DeVries, Raymond. Afterword: the sociology of bioethics. *In:* DeVries, Raymond; Subedi, Janardan, eds. Bioethics and Society: Constructing the

Ethical Enterprise. Upper Saddle River, NJ: Prentice Hall; 1998: 270–276. 4 fn. ISBN 0-13-531252-3. BE58740.

autonomy; *bioethics; evaluation; *social sciences; sociology of medicine; United States

Frank, Arthur W. Enacting illness stories: when, what, and why. *In:* Nelson, Hilde Lindemann, ed. Stories and Their Limits: Narrative Approaches to Bioethics. New York, NY: Routledge; 1997: 31–49. 31 refs. 17 fn. ISBN 0-415-91910-X. BE57465.

autonomy; *communication; emotions; medicine; *narrative ethics; *patients; physician patient relationship; self concept; social dominance; sick role

Frith, Lucy, ed. Ethics and Midwifery: Issues in Contemporary Practice. Boston, MA: Butterworth–Heinemann; 1996. 282 p. Includes references. ISBN 0-7506-3056-6. BE58631.

aborted fetuses; allowing to die; autonomy; behavioral research; *bioethical issues; childbirth; conflict of interest; congenital disorders; decision making; drugs; fetal tissue donation; human experimentation; informed consent; intensive care units; moral policy; newborns; *nurse midwives; nurse patient relationship; *nursing ethics; nursing research; pain; patient advocacy; *patient care; physician nurse relationship; *pregnant women; prematurity; prenatal diagnosis; professional autonomy; public policy; regulation; reproductive technologies; risk; risks and benefits; selection for treatment; selective abortion; sexuality; standards; analgesia; ultrasonography; *Great Britain; United Kingdom Central Council for Nursing, Midwifery and Health Visiting

Gallagher, Eugene B.; Schlomann, Pamela; Sloan, Rebecca S., et al. To enrich bioethics, add one part social to one part clinical. *In:* DeVries, Raymond; Subedi, Janardan, eds. Bioethics and Society: Constructing the Ethical Enterprise. Upper Saddle River, NJ: Prentice Hall; 1998: 166–191. 24 refs. 9 fn. ISBN 0-13-531252-3. BE58735.

allowing to die; attitudes; autonomy; *bioethical issues; *bioethics; case studies; clinical ethics; congenital disorders; decision making; disadvantaged; emotions; health personnel; historical aspects; human experimentation; incentives; informed consent; intensive care units; *interdisciplinary communication; interprofessional relations; kidney diseases; kidneys; newborns; nontherapeutic research; nursing research; organ transplantation; pain; parents; patient care; patient compliance; patients; prematurity; quality of life; remuneration; renal dialysis; research subjects; resource allocation; social sciences; socioeconomic factors; *sociology of medicine; stigmatization; therapeutic research; treatment refusal; Twentieth Century; United States

Garrett, Thomas M.; Baillie, Harold W.; Garrett, Rosellen M. Health Care Ethics: Principles and Problems. Third Edition. Upper Saddle River, NJ: Prentice Hall; 1998. 344 p. Bibliography: p. 323–338. ISBN 0-13-856634-8. BE56097.

abortion, induced; active euthanasia; advance directives; allowing to die; assisted suicide; autonomy; beneficence; *bioethical issues; brain death; case studies; clinical ethics committees; cloning; confidentiality; determination of death; disclosure; fetal research; fetuses; gene therapy; genetic research; health care; *health personnel; hospitals; human experimentation; informed consent; institutional ethics; legal aspects; mass screening; moral obligations; organ donation; organ transplantation; paternalism; pregnant women; *professional ethics; professional organizations; quality of health care; reproductive technologies; resource allocation; resuscitation orders; selection for treatment; suicide; third party consent; treatment refusal; truth disclosure; withholding treatment

Gillett, Grant. "We be of one blood, you and I":

---

commentary on Kopelman. *In:* Carson, Ronald A.; Burns, Chester R., eds. Philosophy of Medicine and Bioethics: A Twenty-Year Retrospective and Critical Appraisal. Boston, MA: Kluwer Academic; 1997: 239–245. 9 refs. 2 fn. ISBN 0-7923-3545-7. BE56539.
circumcision; *cultural pluralism; dissent; *ethical relativism; females; goals; international aspects; medicine; *morality; suffering; values; women's health; non-Western World; Western World

Gillon, Raanan. Bioethics, overview. *In:* Chadwick, Ruth, ed. Encyclopedia of Applied Ethics, Volume 1. San Diego, CA: Academic Press; 1998: 305–317. 41 refs. ISBN 0-12-227066-5. BE56369.
autonomy; beneficence; *bioethical issues; *bioethics; biomedical research; biomedical technologies; casuistry; clinical ethics; cultural pluralism; ecology; education; ethical theory; feminist ethics; health care; health personnel; historical aspects; *interdisciplinary communication; international aspects; investigators; justice; law; medical ethics; medicine; methods; moral obligations; narrative ethics; patient care; patients' rights; personhood; philosophy; political activity; political systems; principle-based ethics; professional ethics; professional patient relationship; religious ethics; research institutes; resource allocation; review; social problems; social sciences; terminology; utilitarianism; virtues

Goodman, Kenneth W. Bioethics and health informatics: an introduction. *In:* Goodman, Kenneth W., ed. Ethics, Computing, and Medicine: Informatics and the Transformation of Health Care. New York, NY: Cambridge University Press; 1998: 1–31. 117 refs. 1 fn. ISBN 0-521-46905-8. BE57001.
advance directives; *bioethics; *computer communication networks; *computers; confidentiality; decision making; DNA data banks; epidemiology; ethical theory; genetic information; *health care; information dissemination; informed consent; medical education; *medicine; moral obligations; organ transplantation; patient education; professional competence; professional ethics; professional patient relationship; psychiatry; psychology; quality of health care; referral and consultation; registries; risks and benefits; standards; surgery; trends; values; *informatics; *telemedicine

Goold, Susan Dorr. Is distance critical for clinical ethicists? A reply to Glenn McGee. *HEC (HealthCare Ethics Committee) Forum.* 1997 Sep; 9(3): 280–283. 1 ref. BE56172.
accountability; *clinical ethics; education; *ethicist's role; *ethicists; professional competence; technical expertise

Graber, Glenn C. Basic theories in medical ethics. [Revised]. *In:* Monagle, John F.; Thomasma, David C., eds. Health Care Ethics: Critical Issues for the 21st Century. Gaithersburg, MD: Aspen Publishers; 1998: 515–526. 31 refs. 20 fn. ISBN 0-8342-0911-X. BE56296.
*bioethics; covenant; deontological ethics; *ethical theory; evaluation; moral obligations; narrative ethics; principle-based ethics; review; rights; teleological ethics; utilitarianism; values; virtues

Granbois, Judith A.; Smith, David H. The Anglican Communion and bioethics. *In:* Lustig, B. Andrew, ed.; Center for Medical Ethics and Health Policy (Houston, TX). Bioethics Yearbook, Volume 5: Theological Developments in Bioethics, 1992–1994. Boston, MA: Kluwer Academic; 1997: 93–122. 26 refs. 2 fn. ISBN 0-7923-4428-6. BE58383.
aborted fetuses; active euthanasia; advance directives; AIDS; allowing to die; artificial feeding; assisted suicide; *bioethical issues; double effect; drugs; embryo research; fetal development; fetal tissue donation; gene therapy; genetic

screening; germ cells; health care delivery; HIV seropositivity; homosexuals; hospices; international aspects; obligations of society; ovum donors; pain; personhood; physicians; preimplantation diagnosis; *Protestant ethics; public policy; reproductive technologies; research embryo creation; selective abortion; semen donors; sex preselection; social discrimination; surrogate mothers; *theology; therapeutic abortion; value of life; ovaries; *Anglican Church; Australia; Canada; England; *Episcopal Church; New Zealand; Scotland; United States; Wales

Grey, William. Playing God. *In:* Chadwick, Ruth, ed. Encyclopedia of Applied Ethics, Volume 3. San Diego, CA: Academic Press; 1998: 525–530. 7 refs. ISBN 0-12-227068-1. BE56261.
abortion, induced; *bioethical issues; bioethics; biomedical technologies; decision making; euthanasia; *genetic intervention; killing; *metaphor; *morality; natural law; *terminology; theology; value of life

Groenhout, Ruth. Care theory and the ideal of neutrality in public moral discourse. *Journal of Medicine and Philosophy.* 1998 Apr; 23(2): 170–189. 32 refs. 8 fn. BE58653.
altruism; bioethics; *caring; common good; consensus; cultural pluralism; democracy; empathy; ethical analysis; *ethical theory; feminist ethics; moral development; moral obligations; mothers; parent child relationship; *public policy; social interaction; *virtues
In this paper I argue that Care theory has the resources to offer an insightful and original theoretical perspective on issues in medical ethics. The paper begins with a discussion of the sort of theory Care is, and argues that it closely resembles virtue theory. After a discussion of common features of Care theories, I respond to a few of the criticisms that have been levied against the theory. The final section of the paper is a discussion of the question of neutrality in public moral discourse. Care theory is not a neutral theory with regard to questions of the nature of the good life for humans, but I argue that this should not preclude Care from playing a part in the public debate over policy decisions.

Guillemin, Jeanne. Bioethics and the coming of the corporation to medicine. *In:* DeVries, Raymond; Subedi, Janardan, eds. Bioethics and Society: Constructing the Ethical Enterprise. Upper Saddle River, NJ: Prentice Hall; 1998: 60–77. 32 refs. ISBN 0-13-531252-3. BE58730.
*bioethics; biomedical technologies; clinical ethics; dehumanization; *economics; emotions; entrepreneurship; ethicists; government financing; government regulation; *health care delivery; historical aspects; hospitals; managed care programs; medical education; organization and administration; physician patient relationship; physicians; professional autonomy; secularism; *sociology of medicine; terminal care; trends; values; rationality; Twentieth Century; United States

Gustafson, James M. Ethics: an American growth industry. *Perspectives in Biology and Medicine.* 1998 Winter; 41(2): 191–199. Reprinted from *The Key Reporter,* 1991 Spring; 36(3). BE59027.
attitudes; *bioethical issues; bioethics; common good; ecology; ethicists; *ethics; expert testimony; historical aspects; literature; *morality; religious ethics; technical expertise; *trends; values; war; business ethics; Twentieth Century; United States

Hanson, Mark J. The religious difference in clinical healthcare. *Cambridge Quarterly of Healthcare Ethics.* 1998 Winter; 7(1): 57–67. 24 fn. BE58454.
attitudes to death; autonomy; beneficence; bioethical issues; bioethics; Christian Scientists; *clinical ethics;

BE = bioethics accession number   fn. = footnotes   refs. = references

communication; *cultural pluralism; *decision making; goals; health; health care; health care delivery; *knowledge, attitudes, practice; medicine; morality; *patient care; *patients; physician patient relationship; *religion; religious ethics; secularism; self concept; suffering; terminal care; *values; faith healing

Hawkins, Anne Hunsaker. Medical ethics and the epiphanic dimension of narrative. *In:* Nelson, Hilde Lindemann, ed. Stories and Their Limits: Narrative Approaches to Bioethics. New York, NY: Routledge; 1997: 153–170. 29 refs. 2 fn. ISBN 0–415–91910–X. BE57468.
> bioethics; *comprehension; *decision making; empathy; *literature; medical education; *medical ethics; *medicine; *narrative ethics; physician patient relationship; *physicians; self concept; suffering; sick role; Joyce, James

Hill, T. Patrick. A religious voice for bioethics? *NCCE News (Veterans Health Administration National Center for Clinical Ethics).* 1997 Winter–Spring; 5(1): 1–2, 9–10. 11 fn. BE56616.
> autonomy; beneficence; *bioethics; cultural pluralism; *interdisciplinary communication; justice; morality; physician patient relationship; principle-based ethics; public policy; *religion; secularism; theology; values; United States

Holden, Constance, ed. All quiet on the bioethics front. [News]. *Science.* 1998 Jul 10; 281(5374): 169. BE58441.
> *advisory committees; *bioethical issues; federal government; government financing; time factors; *National Bioethics Advisory Commission; United States

Holm, Søren. Ethical Problems in Clinical Practice -- A Study of the Ethical Reasoning of Health Care Professionals. Copenhagen: University of Copenhagen; 1996. 258 p. Includes references. Dissertation, Ph.D., University of Copenhagen, Dept. of Medical Philosophy and Clinical Theory. BE57888.
> *bioethics; caring; case studies; *clinical ethics; *decision making; disclosure; education; empirical research; ethical analysis; ethical theory; health care delivery; *health personnel; hospitals; interprofessional relations; medical ethics; models, theoretical; *moral development; negligence; nurses; nursing ethics; philosophy; physicians; *professional ethics; science; sociology of medicine; survey; whistleblowing; medical errors; *qualitative research; *Denmark

Hoshino, Kazumasa. Japanese and Western Bioethics: Studies in Moral Diversity. Boston, MA: Kluwer Academic; 1997. 243 p. (Philosophy and medicine; v. 54). Proceedings of the United States–Japan Bioethics Congress held 2–4 Sep 1994 in Tokyo. ISBN 0–7923–4112–0. BE57078.
> allowing to die; attitudes to death; autonomy; beneficence; *bioethical issues; *bioethics; Buddhist ethics; Christian ethics; common good; communitarianism; comparative studies; *cultural pluralism; decision making; ethical relativism; family relationship; genetic identity; genetic information; genetic intervention; historical aspects; informed consent; international aspects; *morality; nursing ethics; organ donation; paternalism; physician patient relationship; quality of life; religion; secularism; suffering; terminal care; truth disclosure; value of life; values; non-Western World; rationality; *Western World; China; Europe; Germany; *Japan; United States

Houtepen, Rob. The social construction of euthanasia and medical ethics in the Netherlands. *In:* DeVries, Raymond; Subedi, Janardan, eds. Bioethics and Society: Constructing the Ethical Enterprise. Upper Saddle River, NJ: Prentice Hall; 1998: 117–144. 76 refs. 1 fn. ISBN 0–13–531252–3. BE58733.
> accountability; active euthanasia; allowing to die; assisted suicide; attitudes; autonomy; bioethical issues; *bioethics; codes of ethics; *decision making; ethicists; *euthanasia; goals; guidelines; *historical aspects; *interdisciplinary communication; lawyers; *medical ethics; medicine; patients' rights; physician patient relationship; *physicians; professional autonomy; professional organizations; quality of life; *right to die; social control; *social sciences; *sociology of medicine; terminal care; terminology; treatment refusal; trends; value of life; *Netherlands; Royal Dutch Society of Physicians; *Twentieth Century

Howe, Edmund G. Resisting the siren: commentary. *Journal of Clinical Ethics.* 1998 Summer; 9(2): 207–208. 4 fn. Commentary on Spudis, E.V., p. 286. BE58968.
> abortion, induced; death; decision making; *dehumanization; *emotions; ethical analysis; *health personnel; law; literature; medicine; public policy; schizophrenia; values

Imber, Jonathan B. Medical publicity before bioethics: nineteenth-century illustrations of twentieth-century dilemmas. *In:* DeVries, Raymond; Subedi, Janardan, eds. Bioethics and Society: Constructing the Ethical Enterprise. Upper Saddle River, NJ: Prentice Hall; 1998: 16–37. 61 refs. 16 fn. ISBN 0–13–531252–3. BE58728.
> abortion, induced; accountability; animal experimentation; assisted suicide; *attitudes to death; *autopsies; *bioethical issues; *bioethics; *cadavers; death; emotions; entrepreneurship; *ethicist's role; *ethicists; famous persons; goals; *historical aspects; human body; human experimentation; law; legal aspects; mass media; *medical education; medical ethics; *medicine; organ donation; personhood; *physicians; public opinion; scientific misconduct; *sociology of medicine; theology; *trust; twins; conjoined twins; Garfield, James; *Nineteenth Century; *Twentieth Century; United States

Jennings, Bruce. Autonomy and difference: the travails of liberalism in bioethics. *In:* DeVries, Raymond; Subedi, Janardan, eds. Bioethics and Society: Constructing the Ethical Enterprise. Upper Saddle River, NJ: Prentice Hall; 1998: 258–269. 14 refs. ISBN 0–13–531252–3. BE58739.
> *autonomy; *bioethics; clinical ethics; *cultural pluralism; democracy; freedom; historical aspects; minority groups; physician patient relationship; *social sciences; socioeconomic factors; *liberalism; Twentieth Century; United States

Johnstone, Megan–Jane. Bioethics: A Nursing Perspective. Second Edition. Philadelphia, PA: W.B. Saunders; 1994. 574 p. Includes references and ten appendices of codes of ethics and patients' bills of rights. ISBN 0–7295–1421–8. BE56507.
> abortion, induced; active euthanasia; allowing to die; *bioethical issues; *bioethics; clinical ethics committees; codes of ethics; confidentiality; conscience; cultural pluralism; decision making; ethical analysis; ethical relativism; ethical theory; feminist ethics; fetuses; informed consent; international aspects; legal aspects; misconduct; moral complicity; moral development; *moral policy; National Socialism; nurse patient relationship; *nurse's role; nursing education; *nursing ethics; organ donation; organ transplantation; patient advocacy; patients' rights; physician nurse relationship; political activity; pregnant women; professional organizations; quality of life; religious ethics; resuscitation orders; strikes; suicide; truth disclosure; Australia; New Zealand

Jones, Anne Hudson. From principles to reflective practice or narrative ethics? Commentary on Carson. *In:* Carson, Ronald A.; Burns, Chester R., eds. Philosophy of Medicine and Bioethics: A Twenty-Year Retrospective and Critical Appraisal. Boston, MA:

Kluwer Academic; 1997: 193–195. 6 refs. ISBN 0-7923-3545-7. BE56535.
*bioethics; *narrative ethics; principle-based ethics

Jonsen, Albert R.; Siegler, Mark; Winslade, William J. Clinical Ethics: A Practical Approach to Ethical Decisions in Clinical Medicine. Fourth Edition. New York, NY: McGraw-Hill, Health Professions Division; 1998. 206 p. ISBN 0-07-033120-0. BE59103.
active euthanasia; adults; advance directives; AIDS; allowing to die; assisted suicide; *bioethical issues; brain death; case studies; *clinical ethics; competence; confidentiality; cultural pluralism; decision making; disclosure; economics; emergency care; ethical analysis; ethics consultation; family members; futility; goals; health care; human experimentation; informed consent; legal aspects; *medical ethics; medicine; minors; pain; patient care; patient participation; physician patient relationship; *physicians; quality of life; resource allocation; resuscitation orders; review; selection for treatment; suicide; third party consent; treatment refusal; truth disclosure; withholding treatment

Jonsen, Albert R.; Veatch, Robert M.; Walters, LeRoy, eds. Source Book in Bioethics: A Documentary History. Washington, DC: Georgetown University Press; 1998. 510 p. 65 refs. 55 fn. ISBN 0-87840-683-2. BE57889.
advisory committees; allowing to die; *bioethical issues; bioethics; confidentiality; decision making; determination of death; duty to warn; embryo research; federal government; fetal research; gene therapy; genetic intervention; genetic screening; genome mapping; government regulation; guidelines; historical aspects; human experimentation; informed consent; international aspects; legal aspects; organ donation; organ transplantation; reproductive technologies; third party consent; Belmont Report; Canterbury v. Spence; Committee for the Study of Inborn Errors of Metabolism; Cruzan v. Director, Missouri Department of Health; Declaration of Helsinki; DHEW Guidelines; DHHS Guidelines; Human Fetal Tissue Transplantation Research Panel; In re Baby K; In re Conroy; In re Quinlan; National Commission for the Protection of Human Subjects; Nuremberg Code; Office of Technology Assessment; President's Commission for the Study of Ethical Problems; Royal Commission on New Reproductive Technologies (Canada); Superintendent v. Saikewicz; Tarasoff v. Regents of the University of California; Task Force on Organ Transplantation; Tuskegee Syphilis Study; *Twentieth Century; Uniform Anatomical Gift Act; *United States; Waller Committee; Warnock Committee

Jonsen, Albert R. The Birth of Bioethics. New York, NY: Oxford University Press; 1998. 431 p. 1,173 fn. ISBN 0-19-510325-4. BE58983.
abortion, induced; advisory committees; allowing to die; *bioethical issues; *bioethics; biomedical technologies; brain death; clinical ethics committees; education; ethical theory; ethicists; federal government; genetic intervention; genome mapping; government regulation; *historical aspects; human experimentation; interdisciplinary communication; international aspects; legal aspects; medical ethics; medicine; misconduct; National Socialism; organ transplantation; philosophy; professional organizations; public policy; reproductive technologies; research institutes; review; theology; National Institutes of Health; Tuskegee Syphilis Study; Twentieth Century; United States

Junkerman, Charles; Schiedermayer, David. Practical Ethics for Students, Interns, and Residents: A Short Reference Manual. Second Edition. Frederick, MD: University Publishing Group; 1998. 73 p. Includes references. ISBN 1-55572-054-4. BE57923.
active euthanasia; advance directives; AIDS; allowing to die; assisted suicide; autopsies; *bioethical issues; brain death; clinical ethics committees; competence; confidentiality; determination of death; ethics consultation; futility; informed consent; legal aspects; managed care programs; *medical ethics; organ donation; palliative care; patient care; patient compliance; pediatrics; persistent vegetative state; physician patient relationship; physician's role; refusal to treat; resource allocation; resuscitation orders; terminal care; third party consent; withholding treatment; United States

Kennedy Institute of Ethics (Georgetown University). Bioethics Information Retrieval Project. Bioethics Thesaurus. 1998 Edition. Washington, DC: The Institute; 1998. 91 p. Also available at Web address http://bioethics.georgetown.edu. BE58583.
*bioethics; data banks; *terminology; *BIOETHICSLINE

Khushf, George. Bioethics and the Pentecostal traditions: Christianity as an alternative healing system. *In:* Lustig, B. Andrew, ed.; Center for Medical Ethics and Health Policy (Houston, TX). Bioethics Yearbook, Volume 5: Theological Developments in Bioethics, 1992–1994. Boston, MA: Kluwer Academic; 1997: 123–141. 44 refs. 22 fn. ISBN 0-7923-4428-6. BE58384.
allowing to die; *alternative therapies; attitudes; *bioethical issues; *bioethics; disease; literature; *medicine; patient compliance; professional patient relationship; *Protestant ethics; secularism; stigmatization; *theology; treatment refusal; *values; withholding treatment; faith; *faith healing; Evangelical Christians; *Pentecostal Christians; Right to Life Movement; United States

Kipnis, Kenneth. Confessions of an expert ethics witness. *Journal of Medicine and Philosophy.* 1997 Aug; 22(4): 325–343. 6 refs. 6 fn. BE55913.
adults; allowing to die; artificial feeding; *bioethical issues; blood transfusions; cancer; case studies; clinical ethics; competence; conflict of interest; consensus; decision making; DNA data banks; DNA fingerprinting; education; ethical theory; *ethicist's role; *ethicists; *ethics consultation; *expert testimony; family members; federal government; infants; Jehovah's Witnesses; *judicial action; mandatory programs; military personnel; parents; privacy; professional competence; professional ethics; public policy; remuneration; *standards; *technical expertise; therapeutic research; third party consent; treatment refusal; withholding treatment; Department of Defense; Hawaii; The Health Care Ethics Consultant (F.E. Baylis, ed.); United States
The aim of this essay is to describe and reflect upon the concrete particulars of one academician's work as an expert ethics witness. The commentary on my practices and the narrative descriptions of three cases are offered as evidence for the thesis that it is possible to act honorably within a role that some have considered to be inherently illicit. Practical measures are described for avoiding some of the best known pitfalls. The discussion concludes with a listing of the distinctive competencies and understandings that are useful in serving as an expert ethics witness.

Kleinman, Arthur. Anthropology of bioethics. *In: his* Writing at the Margin: Discourse Between Anthropology and Medicine. Berkeley, CA: University of California Press; 1995: 41–67, 268–269. 9 fn. An earlier version of this article appeared under the title "Anthropology of medicine" in Reich, Warren T., ed. *Encyclopedia of Bioethics*, Revised Edition (New York, NY: Simon and Schuster Macmillan, 1995). ISBN 0-520-20965-6. BE57749.
*anthropology; autonomy; beneficence; *bioethics; biomedical technologies; clinical ethics; *cultural pluralism; developing countries; disease; *ethical relativism; ethicists; health; health care; *interdisciplinary communication; *international aspects; justice; medicine; metaphor; minority groups; morality; patient care; *social sciences; *sociology of medicine; suffering; *values; folk medicine; non-Western World; Western World

---

BE = bioethics accession number   fn. = footnotes   refs. = references

Koch, Tom; Ridgley, Mark. Distanced perspectives: AIDS, anencephaly, and AHP [Analytic Hierarchy Process]. *Theoretical Medicine and Bioethics.* 1998 Jan; 19(1): 47–58. 26 fn. BE57311.

AIDS; *allowing to die; *anencephaly; *bioethical issues; brain pathology; *decision analysis; *decision making; equal protection; *futility; infants; *law; legal aspects; medicine; models, theoretical; *newborns; *personhood; prolongation of life; *quality of life; self concept; social interaction; speciesism; *standards; value of life; ventilators; withholding treatment; In re Baby K; In re T.A.C.P.; United States

Kopelman, Loretta M. Medicine's challenge to relativism: the case of female genital mutilation. *In:* Carson, Ronald A.; Burns, Chester R., eds. Philosophy of Medicine and Bioethics: A Twenty-Year Retrospective and Critical Appraisal. Boston, MA: Kluwer Academic; 1997: 221–237. 32 refs. 9 fn. ISBN 0–7923–3545–7. BE56538.

bioethics; case studies; children; *circumcision; *cultural pluralism; dissent; *ethical relativism; *females; goals; health; health personnel; *international aspects; medicine; methods; minority groups; *morality; morbidity; mortality; pain; physicians; refusal to treat; religion; risks and benefits; suffering; surgery; *values; *women's health; non–Western World; Western World; Africa; Middle East

Kuczewski, Mark. Bioethics' consensus on method: *who could ask for anything more?* *In:* Nelson, Hilde Lindemann, ed. Stories and Their Limits: Narrative Approaches to Bioethics. New York, NY: Routledge; 1997: 134–149. 46 fn. ISBN 0–415–91910–X. BE57467.

autonomy; beneficence; *bioethics; casuistry; communitarianism; *consensus; cultural pluralism; *decision making; dissent; ethical analysis; ethical theory; ethicists; evaluation; informed consent; interdisciplinary communication; *methods; *narrative ethics; physician patient relationship; principle–based ethics; rights; virtues

Kuczewski, Mark G. Fragmentation and Consensus: Communitarian and Casuist Bioethics. Washington, DC: Georgetown University Press; 1997. 177 p. Bibliography: p. 163–168. ISBN 0–87840–648–4. BE56503.

advance directives; autonomy; beneficence; *bioethics; blood transfusions; case studies; *casuistry; common good; *communitarianism; consensus; decision making; *ethical analysis; ethical relativism; ethical theory; family members; informed consent; Jehovah's Witnesses; medical ethics; medicine; narrative ethics; natural law; personhood; philosophy; physician patient relationship; principle–based ethics; rights; treatment refusal; virtues; wedge argument; liberalism; rationality; Aristotle

Lammers, Stephen E.; Verhey, Allen, eds. On Moral Medicine: Theological Perspectives in Medical Ethics. Second Edition. Grand Rapids, MI: Eerdmans; 1998. 1,004 p. Includes references. ISBN 0–8028–4249–6. BE58318.

abortion, induced; active euthanasia; aged; AIDS; allowing to die; animal experimentation; assisted suicide; attitudes to death; *bioethical issues; *bioethics; biomedical technologies; *Christian ethics; codes of ethics; contraception; feminist ethics; fetuses; genetic intervention; health; human experimentation; indigents; informed consent; interdisciplinary communication; justice; love; managed care programs; medical ethics; medicine; mentally ill; newborns; patient care; personhood; physician patient relationship; prolongation of life; Protestant ethics; religion; *religious ethics; reproductive technologies; resource allocation; Roman Catholic ethics; suffering; technology assessment; terminal care; *theology; value of life; sick role; United States

Lebacqz, Karen. Difficult difference. *Cambridge Quarterly of Healthcare Ethics.* 1998 Winter; 7(1): 17–26. 58 fn.

BE58457.

autonomy; bioethics; *cultural pluralism; *females; *feminist ethics; homosexuals; *justice; males; *minority groups; *politics; self concept; *sexuality; *social control; *social dominance; socioeconomic factors; postmodernism

Levin, Betty Wolder; Schiller, Nina Glick. Social class and medical decisionmaking: a neglected topic in bioethics. *Cambridge Quarterly of Healthcare Ethics.* 1998 Winter; 7(1): 41–56. 23 fn. BE58458.

AIDS; allowing to die; attitudes; autonomy; *bioethics; case studies; *clinical ethics; *cultural pluralism; *decision making; ethicists; family relationship; females; health; health care delivery; health personnel; heart diseases; hearts; *indigents; justice; *knowledge, attitudes, practice; literature; minority groups; organ transplantation; *patient care; *patients; self concept; *social discrimination; social dominance; *socioeconomic factors; terminal care; treatment refusal; trust; values; *vulnerable populations; withholding treatment; United States

Lewins, Frank. Bioethics for Health Professionals: An Introduction and Critical Approach. South Melbourne, VIC: MacMillan Education Australia; 1996. 154 p. Bibliography: p. 144–151. ISBN 0–7329–3046–4. BE57151.

abortion, induced; active euthanasia; allowing to die; attitudes; autonomy; beneficence; *bioethical issues; *bioethics; blood transfusions; brain death; confidentiality; decision making; determination of death; empirical research; ethical analysis; ethical theory; ethics; *evaluation; health care; health personnel; informed consent; interdisciplinary communication; legal aspects; methods; organ donation; organ transplantation; public opinion; public policy; regulation; resource allocation; *social sciences; sociology of medicine; surgery; transsexualism; *values; voluntary euthanasia; Australia; United States

Lewis, Marcia A.; Tamparo, Carol D. Medical Law, Ethics, and Bioethics for Ambulatory Care. Fourth Edition. Philadelphia, PA: F.A. Davis; 1998. 295 p. Includes references and discussion questions. Appendix 1: Codes of ethics; Appendix 2: Sample documents for choices about health care, life, and death. ISBN 0–8036–0348–7. BE57279.

abortion, induced; advance directives; AIDS; *allied health personnel; assisted suicide; *bioethical issues; case studies; codes of ethics; confidentiality; cultural pluralism; decision making; drugs; *employment; euthanasia; fetuses; genetic services; government regulation; health care delivery; health facilities; informed consent; interprofessional relations; law; *legal aspects; *legal liability; *legal obligations; malpractice; mandatory reporting; medical fees; medical records; negligence; *organization and administration; *patient care; *professional ethics; professional patient relationship; reproductive technologies; resource allocation; standards; terminal care; third party consent; *ambulatory care; United States

Light, Donald W.; McGee, Glenn. On the social embeddedness of bioethics. *In:* DeVries, Raymond; Subedi, Janardan, eds. Bioethics and Society: Constructing the Ethical Enterprise. Upper Saddle River, NJ: Prentice Hall; 1998: 1–15. 31 refs. ISBN 0–13–531252–3. BE58727.

autonomy; behavior control; bioethical issues; *bioethics; clinical ethics; cultural pluralism; emotions; empirical research; *ethical analysis; ethical theory; health insurance; incentives; *interdisciplinary communication; *methods; moral policy; paternalism; resource allocation; risk; self induced illness; smoking; *social sciences; sociology of medicine

Little, Margaret Olivia. Care: from theory to orientation and back. *Journal of Medicine and Philosophy.* 1998 Apr;

23(2): 190–209. 26 refs. 10 fn. BE58654.
*caring; *ethical analysis; *ethical theory; females; feminist ethics; *justice; males; *moral development; moral obligations; philosophy; psychology; rights; self concept; social interaction; virtues; *Gilligan, Carol

In this paper, I urge that the very real lessons Carol Gilligan's work in moral psychology offer to moral philosophy can best be appreciated if we take seriously the gap between the two disciplines. The care and justice perspectives Gilligan explores are psychological orientations, and orientations are defined as much by matters of emphasis, selectivity of interpretation, and gestalt as they are by propositional commitment. As such, I argue, their contribution to moral theory is best seen as stances from which to do theory, rather than as constituting ready-made theories themselves. In pursuing this train of thought, I examine how Gilligan's work has developed over time and how, in the end, we should understand the juxtaposition between the two orientations.

Little, Margaret Olivia. Introduction [to a set of articles on care theory]. *Journal of Medicine and Philosophy.* 1998 Apr; 23(2): 127–130. 4 refs. BE58669.
*caring; *ethical theory; females; justice; males; moral development; principle-based ethics; virtues; Gilligan, Carol

Löw, Reinhard. Anthropology as the basis of bioethics. *In:* Becker, Gerhold K., ed. Changing Nature's Course: The Ethical Challenge of Biotechnology. Hong Kong: Hong Kong University Press; 1996: 147–157. 13 fn. ISBN 962-209-403-1. BE56710.
*anthropology; beginning of life; *bioethics; Christian ethics; eugenics; *evolution; genetics; human rights; philosophy; *sociobiology; value of life

Lustig, B. Andrew, ed.; Center for Medical Ethics and Health Policy (Houston, TX). Bioethics Yearbook, Volume 5: Theological Developments in Bioethics, 1992-1994. Boston, MA: Kluwer Academic; 1997. 301 p. (Bioethics yearbook; v. 5). 452 refs. 24 fn. ISBN 0-7923-4428-6. BE58377.
abortion, induced; active euthanasia; advance directives; allowing to die; animal rights; assisted suicide; attitudes to death; beginning of life; *bioethical issues; bioethics; confidentiality; contraception; cultural pluralism; determination of death; developing countries; ecology; embryo research; fetal research; fetal tissue donation; genetic information; genetic intervention; health care; Hindu ethics; human body; informed consent; international aspects; Islamic ethics; Jehovah's Witnesses; Jewish ethics; newborns; organ donation; personhood; political activity; Protestant ethics; public policy; *religious ethics; reproductive technologies; resource allocation; review; rights; Roman Catholic ethics; terminal care; *theology; value of life; African Methodist Episcopal Church; African Methodist Episcopal Zion Church; Anglican Church; Australia; Baptist Church; Christian Methodist Episcopal Church; Church of Scotland; Church of the Nazarene; Episcopal Church; Europe; Evangelical Christians; Free Methodist Church; Great Britain; India; Israel; Lutheran Church; Methodist Church; Mormonism; New Zealand; Pentecostal Christians; Presbyterian Church; Reformed Church; United Methodist Church; United States; Wesleyan Church

Lustig, B. Andrew. Recent trends in theological bioethics. *In:* Lustig, B. Andrew, ed.; Center for Medical Ethics and Health Policy (Houston, TX). Bioethics Yearbook, Volume 5: Theological Developments in Bioethics, 1992-1994. Boston, MA: Kluwer Academic; 1997: 1–9. 23 refs. ISBN 0-7923-4428-6. BE58378.
abortion, induced; assisted suicide; autonomy; *bioethical issues; Christian ethics; Eastern Orthodox ethics; health care; Hindu ethics; Islamic ethics; Jewish ethics; morality;

Protestant ethics; *religious ethics; reproductive technologies; rights; Roman Catholic ethics; *theology; *trends; values; voluntary euthanasia; Europe; United States

McCullough, Laurence B. Molecular medicine, managed care, and the moral responsibilities of patients and physicians. *Journal of Medicine and Philosophy.* 1998 Feb; 23(1): 3–9. 11 refs. BE57517.
alcohol abuse; bioethics; biomedical technologies; *clinical ethics; disease; entrepreneurship; genetic information; genetic predisposition; genetic screening; goals; health; historical aspects; justice; *managed care programs; *medical ethics; *medicine; models, theoretical; *moral obligations; obligations to society; organ transplantation; patents; *patients; patients' rights; physician patient relationship; physician's role; *physicians; resource allocation; selection for treatment; self induced illness; social impact

Macer, Darryl. What can bioethics offer to Japanese culture? *Nichibunken Newsletter.* 1993 Aug; No. 15: 3–6. 8 fn. Commented on by C. Becker and D. Macer, "What can Japan offer to bioethics? A response to Dr. Macer," *Nichibunken Newsletter,* 1994 Jun; No. 18, p. 1–12. BE57778.
attitudes; autonomy; bioethical issues; *bioethics; brain death; *cultural pluralism; decision making; informed consent; *international aspects; organ donation; paternalism; physician patient relationship; public opinion; public policy; religion; trust; non-Western World; Western World; *Japan

McGee, Glenn. Therapeutic clinical ethics. *HEC (HealthCare Ethics Committee) Forum.* 1997 Sep; 9(3): 276–279. BE56173.
accountability; bioethics; *clinical ethics; education; *ethicist's role; *ethicists; *ethics consultation; hospitals; professional competence; technical expertise

McKenny, Gerald P. An anthropological bioethics: hermeneutical or critical? Commentary on Elliott. *In:* Carson, Ronald A.; Burns, Chester R., eds. Philosophy of Medicine and Bioethics: A Twenty-Year Retrospective and Critical Appraisal. Boston, MA: Kluwer Academic; 1997: 213–220. 5 refs. 3 fn. ISBN 0-7923-3545-7. BE56537.
anthropology; *bioethics; biomedical technologies; casuistry; *cultural pluralism; ethicist's role; medicine; methods; mortality; *normality; principle-based ethics; *self concept; *values; dignity; *personal identity

McKenny, Gerald P. Technology, authority and the loss of tradition: the roots of American bioethics in comparison with Japanese bioethics. *In:* Hoshino, Kazumasa, ed. Japanese and Western Bioethics: Studies in Moral Diversity. Boston, MA: Kluwer Academic; 1997: 73–87. 20 refs. 2 fn. ISBN 0-7923-4112-0. BE57084.
autonomy; bioethical issues; *bioethics; biomedical technologies; comparative studies; *cultural pluralism; decision making; ethicists; goals; health; historical aspects; human body; *international aspects; medical ethics; medicine; *morality; philosophy; physicians; Protestant ethics; religion; rights; secularism; suffering; values; rationality; Western World; *Japan; *United States

McKenny, Gerald P. To Relieve the Human Condition: Bioethics, Technology, and the Body. Albany, NY: State University of New York Press; 1997. 279 p. Bibliography: p. 261-272. ISBN 0-7914-3474-5. BE58646.
active euthanasia; allowing to die; assisted suicide; autonomy; beneficence; bioethical issues; *bioethics; biomedical research; biomedical technologies; casuistry; dehumanization; *ethics; gene therapy; genetic enhancement;

BE = bioethics accession number   fn. = footnotes   refs. = references

germ cells; *goals; health; *human body; killing; medical ethics; *medicine; mentally retarded; methods; moral obligations; moral policy; obligations of society; *philosophy; physicians; religious ethics; reproductive technologies; secularism; social control; suffering; suicide; withholding treatment; liberalism; Bacon, Francis; Gustafson, James; Hauerwas, Stanley; Jonas, Hans; Kass, Leon

Mackler, Aaron L. Cases and principles in Jewish bioethics: toward a holistic model. *In:* Dorff, Elliot N.; Newman, Louis E., eds. Contemporary Jewish Ethics and Morality: A Reader. New York, NY: Oxford University Press; 1995: 177–193. 49 fn. ISBN 0-19-509066-7. BE58527.
autonomy; *bioethical issues; *bioethics; casuistry; conscience; consensus; cultural pluralism; *decision making; dissent; *ethical analysis; ethical theory; health care; historical aspects; indigents; *Jewish ethics; justice; law; *methods; *models, theoretical; moral policy; morality; *theology; value of life; Conservative Judaism; Orthodox Judaism; Reform Judaism; United States

McLean, Sheila A.M., ed. Contemporary Issues in Law, Medicine and Ethics. Brookfield, VT: Dartmouth; 1996. 277 p. (Medico–legal series). 963 fn. ISBN 1-85521-586-1. BE57786.
advance directives; anencephaly; animal organs; *bioethical issues; biomedical research; brain death; cardiac death; cesarean section; coercion; confidentiality; decision making; fetal tissue donation; fetuses; genetic information; genetic screening; health care; health care delivery; human rights; informed consent; international aspects; *legal aspects; legal liability; medical ethics; mentally retarded; minors; moral policy; negligence; organ donation; patents; patients' rights; physician patient relationship; physicians; pregnant women; prenatal diagnosis; prenatal injuries; professional ethics; prolongation of life; *public policy; recombinant DNA research; resource allocation; rights; sterilization (sexual); treatment refusal; ventilators; wrongful life; business ethics; Australia; Europe; *Great Britain; National Health Service; United States

Mason, John Kenyon; McCall Smith, R.A. Law and Medical Ethics. Fourth Edition. London: Butterworths; 1994. 451 p. Includes references. Appendixes include the Hippocratic Oath, international codes and declarations, and a specimen living will. ISBN 0-406-02478-2. BE55694.
abortion, induced; active euthanasia; aged; AIDS; allowing to die; *bioethical issues; brain death; codes of ethics; competence; confidentiality; contraception; determination of death; embryo research; fetal research; fetuses; forensic psychiatry; gene therapy; genetic counseling; homosexuals; human experimentation; informed consent; international aspects; involuntary commitment; *legal aspects; legal liability; *medical ethics; mentally ill; minors; negligence; newborns; nontherapeutic research; organ donation; organ transplantation; prenatal diagnosis; reproductive technologies; resource allocation; scientific misconduct; sex offenses; sexuality; sexually transmitted diseases; sterilization (sexual); transsexualism; wrongful life; *Great Britain

Miller, Franklin G.; Fins, Joseph J.; Bacchetta, Matthew D. Clinical pragmatism: John Dewey and clinical ethics. *Journal of Contemporary Health Law and Policy.* 1996 Fall; 13(1): 27–51. 58 fn. BE55789.
autonomy; bioethical issues; *bioethics; casuistry; *clinical ethics; common good; communication; cultural pluralism; *decision making; democracy; emotions; *ethical analysis; *ethical theory; ethicists; family members; health personnel; interprofessional relations; *morality; paternalism; patient care; patient participation; *philosophy; physician patient relationship; principle–based ethics; science; technical expertise; values; *pragmatism; *Dewey, John

Miller, Franklin G. Dedicatory essay on John C. Fletcher [and] Bibliography of publications by John C. Fletcher. *Journal of Contemporary Health Law and Policy.* 1996 Fall; 13(1): ix–xxxii. BE55790.
*bioethical issues; bioethics; ethicist's role; ethicists; ethics consultation; research institutes; *Fletcher, John C.; National Institutes of Health; University of Virginia

Minogue, Brendan P.; Palmer–Fernández, Gabriel; Reagan, James E., eds. Reading Engelhardt: Essays on the Thought of H. Tristram Engelhardt, Jr. Boston, MA: Kluwer Academic; 1997. 312 p. 547 fn. Papers presented at the conference, "Ethics, Medicine and Health Care: An Appraisal of the Thought of H. Tristram Engelhardt, Jr.," held at Youngstown State University, 30 Sep 1995. Includes list of publications by Engelhardt, p. 293–305. ISBN 0-7923-4572-X. BE56546.
autonomy; beneficence; bioethical issues; *bioethics; children; Christian ethics; coercion; common good; communitarianism; consensus; cultural pluralism; disease; economics; *ethical analysis; *ethical theory; ethicists; females; feminist ethics; fetuses; freedom; health; health care delivery; humanism; justice; libertarianism; medicine; moral obligations; *moral policy; *morality; personhood; *philosophy; physician's role; property rights; public policy; resource allocation; rights; secularism; social discrimination; values; postmodernism; rationality; sick role; *Engelhardt, H. Tristram; The Foundations of Bioethics (Engelhardt, H.T.)

Monagle, John F.; Thomasma, David C., eds. Health Care Ethics: Critical Issues for the 21st Century. Gaithersburg, MD: Aspen Publishers; 1998. 614 p. Includes references. Contains original and previously published material. ISBN 0-8342-0911-X. BE56274.
abortion, induced; active euthanasia; aged; AIDS; allowing to die; assisted suicide; autonomy; *bioethical issues; biomedical technologies; brain death; casuistry; clinical ethics committees; cloning; competence; cultural pluralism; decision making; dementia; domestic violence; emergency care; ethical theory; ethics consultation; family members; fetuses; futility; gatekeeping; genetic predisposition; genetic screening; health insurance; home care; human experimentation; informed consent; justice; long–term care; managed care programs; mentally ill; moral obligations; organ donation; physician patient relationship; pregnant women; preimplantation diagnosis; prenatal diagnosis; reproductive technologies; research ethics committees; resource allocation; selective abortion; Patient Self-Determination Act 1990; United States

Montello, Martha. Narrative competence. *In:* Nelson, Hilde Lindemann, ed. Stories and Their Limits: Narrative Approaches to Bioethics. New York, NY: Routledge; 1997: 185–197. 51 refs. 2 fn. ISBN 0-415-91910-X. BE57470.
clinical ethics; empathy; *literature; medical education; *medical ethics; medicine; *moral development; *narrative ethics; physician patient relationship; *physicians; *professional competence

Morreim, E. Haavi. Bioethics, expertise, and the courts: an overview and an argument for inevitability. *Journal of Medicine and Philosophy.* 1997 Aug; 22(4): 291–295. 8 refs. Introduction to a set of six articles, on the ethicist's role as expert witness in legal proceedings, by J.C. Fletcher, p. 298–324; by K. Kipnis, p. 325–343; by M. Yarborough, p. 345–365; by K. Wm. Wildes, p. 365–371; by V.A. Sharpe and E.D. Pellegrino, p. 378–379; and by G.F. Agich and B.J. Spielman, p. 381–403. BE55827.
*bioethical issues; bioethics; clinical ethics; cultural pluralism; decision making; ethical analysis; *ethicist's role; *ethicists; *ethics; *expert testimony; *judicial action; *law; morality; secularism; technical expertise; values; United

States

Murray, Thomas H. What do we mean by "narrative ethics"? *In:* Nelson, Hilde Lindemann, ed. Stories and Their Limits: Narrative Approaches to Bioethics. New York, NY: Routledge; 1997: 3–17. 13 refs. 1 fn. ISBN 0–415–91910–X. BE57463.
bioethics; casuistry; cultural pluralism; ethical theory; *ethics; literature; methods; moral development; moral policy; *morality; *narrative ethics; philosophy

Nelson, Hilde Lindemann, ed. Stories and Their Limits: Narrative Approaches to Bioethics. New York, NY: Routledge; 1997. 284 p. 184 refs. 328 fn. ISBN 0–415–91910–X. BE57462.
audiovisual aids; autonomy; *bioethics; case studies; communication; consensus; decision making; empathy; ethical theory; ethicists; ethics; informed consent; literature; medical ethics; methods; moral development; moral policy; morality; *narrative ethics; patients; physician patient relationship; physicians; self concept; suffering; sick role; James, Henry; Joyce, James

Nelson, Paul. Bioethics and the Lutheran Communion. *In:* Lustig, B. Andrew, ed.; Center for Medical Ethics and Health Policy (Houston, TX). Bioethics Yearbook, Volume 5: Theological Developments in Bioethics, 1992–1994. Boston, MA: Kluwer Academic; 1997: 143–169. 38 refs. ISBN 0–7923–4428–6. BE58385.
aborted fetuses; advance directives; advisory committees; allowing to die; beneficence; *bioethical issues; disclosure; ecology; embryo research; employment; fetal tissue donation; genetic information; genetic intervention; genetic screening; human rights; international aspects; justice; love; national health insurance; natural law; ovum donors; parent child relationship; privacy; *Protestant ethics; public participation; public policy; reproductive technologies; resource allocation; selective abortion; semen donors; sex determination; sex preselection; surrogate mothers; *theology; therapeutic abortion; transgenic animals; value of life; voluntary euthanasia; Denmark; Europe; Finland; Golden Rule; Iceland; *Lutheran Church; Norway; United States

Noble, Denis; Vincent, Jean–Didier. The Ethics of Life. Paris: Unesco; 1997. 238 p. Bibliography: p. 221–230. Papers presented at a seminar "Physiology and the Respect for Life," held under the joint auspices of the International Union of Physical Scientists and Unesco in Paris, Sep 1995. ISBN 92–3–103422–7. BE58647.
*animal experimentation; *animal rights; attitudes to death; beginning of life; behavioral research; *bioethical issues; bioethics; *biomedical research; brain death; Buddhist ethics; competence; determination of death; education; embryo research; females; fetal research; genetic determinism; homosexuals; human experimentation; *human rights; humanism; informed consent; international aspects; legal aspects; moral obligations; *moral policy; nontherapeutic research; organ donation; personhood; philosophy; political activity; prisoners; regulation; research ethics committees; research subjects; risks and benefits; science; speciesism; suffering; therapeutic research; *value of life; vulnerable populations; Europe; Japan

Nordgren, Anders. Ethics and imagination: implications of cognitive semantics for medical ethics. *Theoretical Medicine and Bioethics.* 1998 Apr; 19(2): 117–141. 42 fn. BE57576.
*autonomy; beneficence; *bioethics; *casuistry; consensus; empirical research; *ethical analysis; *ethical theory; *justice; medicine; metaethics; *metaphor; *methods; moral obligations; morality; narrative ethics; personhood; philosophy; *principle–based ethics; psychology; resource allocation; utilitarianism; virtues; integrity; Brody, Baruch; Johnson, Mark; Jonsen, Albert; Toulmin, Stephen

Parens, Erik. What differences make a difference? [Editorial]. *Cambridge Quarterly of Healthcare Ethics.* 1998 Winter; 7(1): 1–6. BE58486.
advance directives; bioethical issues; *clinical ethics; consensus; *cultural pluralism; decision making; *disabled; dissent; empirical research; health care delivery; health personnel; justice; *minority groups; patient care; *professional patient relationship; religion; self concept; sexuality; *socioeconomic factors; stigmatization; terminal care; *values

Payne–James, Jason; Dean, Peter; Wall, Ian. Medicolegal Essentials in Healthcare. New York, NY: Churchill Livingstone; 1996. 177 p. Includes references. ISBN 0–443–05240–9. BE58648.
abortion, induced; active euthanasia; AIDS; AIDS serodiagnosis; *bioethical issues; blood donation; confidentiality; determination of death; disclosure; drug industry; drugs; emergency care; guidelines; health personnel; HIV seropositivity; human experimentation; infertility; informed consent; judicial action; *legal aspects; legal liability; legislation; living wills; mentally disabled; minors; negligence; organ donation; patient care; physicians; property rights; reproductive technologies; self regulation; third party consent; treatment refusal; withholding treatment; Children Act 1989 (Great Britain); General Medical Council (Great Britain); *Great Britain; Medicines Act 1968 (Great Britain); Mental Health Act 1983 (Great Britain); National Health Service; United Kingdom Central Council for Nursing, Midwifery and Health Visiting

Pellegrino, Edmund D. Bioethics as an interdisciplinary enterprise: where does ethics fit in the mosaic of disciplines? *In:* Carson, Ronald A.; Burns, Chester R., eds. Philosophy of Medicine and Bioethics: A Twenty–Year Retrospective and Critical Appraisal. Boston, MA: Kluwer Academic; 1997: 1–23. 75 refs. ISBN 0–7923–3545–7. BE56523.
*bioethics; biology; ethical theory; ethics; historical aspects; humanism; humanities; *interdisciplinary communication; law; literature; medical ethics; medicine; methods; models, theoretical; *philosophy; principle–based ethics; review; social sciences; terminology; theology; Twentieth Century

Pellegrino, Edmund D.; Thomasma, David C. Edmund D. Pellegrino on the future of bioethics. [Interview]. *Cambridge Quarterly of Healthcare Ethics.* 1997 Fall; 6(4): 373–375. BE56480.
*bioethical issues; *bioethics; cultural pluralism; decision making; family members; managed care programs; physician patient relationship; *trends

Pence, Gregory E., ed. Classic Works in Medical Ethics: Core Philosophical Readings. Boston, MA: McGraw–Hill; 1998. 399 p. Includes references. ISBN 0–07–038115–1. BE56190.
abortion, induced; active euthanasia; AIDS; alcohol abuse; allowing to die; animal experimentation; autonomy; beneficence; *bioethical issues; biomedical technologies; congenital disorders; embryos; ethical theory; genetic counseling; genetic intervention; genome mapping; health care; health care delivery; infanticide; involuntary commitment; justice; medical ethics; mentally ill; newborns; organ transplantation; persistent vegetative state; personhood; public policy; quality of life; reproductive technologies; resource allocation; retreatment; review; selection for treatment; suicide; surrogate mothers; value of life

Petersen, Kerry, ed. Intersections: Women on Law, Medicine and Technology. Brookfield, VT: Ashgate; 1997. 246 p. (Medico–legal series). 438 refs. 174 fn. ISBN 1–85521–882–8. BE57483.
allowing to die; attitudes; autonomy; *bioethical issues; brain death; codes of ethics; decision making; disabled; family

---

planning; females; fetuses; government regulation; guidelines; historical aspects; human experimentation; human rights; infertility; international aspects; *legal aspects; medical ethics; mentally retarded; patient care; persistent vegetative state; physicians; population control; pregnant women; public policy; reproductive technologies; selection of subjects; sexuality; sociology of medicine; sterilization (sexual); stigmatization; third party consent; withholding treatment; women's rights; Hippocratic Oath

Phelps, Ruth-Ann. VHA policy-related clinical ethical issues. *HEC (HealthCare Ethics Committee) Forum.* 1997 Jun; 9(2): 159–168. 8 refs. 1 fn. BE55962.
advance directives; allowing to die; assisted suicide; autonomy; *bioethical issues; *clinical ethics; clinical ethics committees; competence; *federal government; guidelines; health care delivery; health facilities; human experimentation; informed consent; institutional ethics; institutional policies; medical education; *public hospitals; *public policy; research ethics committees; research subjects; resuscitation orders; third party consent; withholding treatment; United States; Veterans Affairs National Center for Clinical Ethics (White River Junction, VT); *Veterans Health Administration

Rachels, James. The principle of agency. *Bioethics.* 1998 Apr; 12(2): 150–161. 15 fn. BE58625.
active euthanasia; *bioethical issues; *bioethics; biomedical technologies; cloning; genetic intervention; in vitro fertilization; *intention; preimplantation diagnosis; religion; reproductive technologies; rights; teleological ethics; *agency; nature
The Principle of Agency says that if it would be good for a state of affairs to occur "naturally," then it is permissable to take action to bring it about. This contradicts the views of some bioethicists, who object to euthanasia, in vitro fertilization, and cloning, even though they acknowledge that the states of affairs produced are good. But the principle, or some form of it, seems inescapable. The opposite view -- that we may not, by our action, reproduce "natural" goods -- may owe its appeal to an implicitly religious view of nature.

Reagan, James E.; Lomax, Karen J.; Nelson, William A. Clinical ethics in the Veterans Health Administration. *HEC (HealthCare Ethics Committee) Forum.* 1997 Jun; 9(2): 120–128. 2 refs. 2 fn. BE55961.
advisory committees; bioethics; *clinical ethics; *clinical ethics committees; committee membership; education; ethics consultation; *federal government; health care delivery; health facilities; *organization and administration; primary health care; *program descriptions; *public hospitals; public policy; research institutes; United States; *Veterans Health Administration

Reitemeier, Paul J. Musings on medical mistakes: a four-piece ensemble in search of an orchestra. *Journal of Clinical Ethics.* 1997 Winter; 8(4): 353–358. 5 fn. BE57612.
attitudes; bioethics; *clinical ethics; clinical ethics committees; communication; conscience; *disclosure; emotions; empirical research; *ethicist's role; ethics consultation; family members; *iatrogenic disease; legal liability; malpractice; moral obligations; moral policy; negligence; patient care; patients' rights; physician patient relationship; physicians; professional competence; quality of health care; standards; terminal care; *truth disclosure; virtues; whistleblowing; *medical errors

Rich, Ben A. A legacy of silence: bioethics and the culture of pain. *Journal of Medical Humanities.* 1997 Winter; 18(4): 233–259. 47 refs. BE57245.
assisted suicide; attitudes; bioethical issues; *bioethics; cancer; chronically ill; clinical ethics; drug abuse; drugs; ethical analysis; ethicists; goals; government regulation;

historical aspects; hospices; legal aspects; medical education; medical ethics; medicine; moral obligations; morality; *pain; *palliative care; *patient care; physicians; quality of health care; review; self regulation; standards; state government; *suffering; technical expertise; *terminal care; terminally ill; Study to Understand Prognoses and Preferences for Outcomes and Risks of Treatments (SUPPORT); United States
For over 20 years the medical literature has carefully documented the undertreatment of all types of pain by physicians. During this same period, as the field of bioethics came of age, the phenomenon of undertreated pain received almost no attention from the bioethics literature. This article takes bioethicists to task for failing to recognize the undertreatment of pain as a major ethical, and not merely a clinical, failing of the medical profession. The nature and extent of the problem of undertreated pain is examined, as well as possible reasons for its disregard by bioethicists. The factors contributing to undertreated pain in the clinical setting are considered, as well as the hazards posed by recent failures to address ethically questionable clinical practices. Finally, suggestions are offered for refocusing the attention of bioethicists to this significant problem.

Roleff, Tamara L., ed. Biomedical Ethics: Opposing Viewpoints. San Diego, CA: Greenhaven Press; 1998. 252 p. (Opposing viewpoints series). Includes references. ISBN 1-56510-792-6. BE59107.
age factors; animal organs; autonomy; beneficence; *bioethical issues; body parts and fluids; brain death; cadavers; capital punishment; childbirth; *cloning; eugenics; females; genes; *genetic intervention; *genetic research; genetic screening; genome mapping; government regulation; indigents; moral policy; *organ donation; organ transplantation; patents; personhood; posthumous reproduction; pregnant women; presumed consent; prisoners; public policy; remuneration; *reproductive technologies; risks and benefits; selection for treatment; surrogate mothers; transgenic animals

Saegusa, Asako. Japan's bioethics debate lags behind thinking in the West. [News]. *Nature.* 1997 Oct 16; 389(6652): 661. BE55953.
*bioethical issues; brain death; cloning; eugenics; genetic research; genetic services; information dissemination; organ donation; organ transplantation; paternalism; public opinion; *public policy; *Japan

Seedhouse, David. What's the difference between health care ethics, medical ethics and nursing ethics? [Editorial]. *Health Care Analysis.* 1997 Dec; 5(4): 267–274. 16 refs. BE57543.
*bioethics; caring; cultural pluralism; ethical theory; ethics; *goals; health; health care; health personnel; interdisciplinary communication; *medical ethics; medicine; nurses; *nursing ethics; philosophy; physicians; professional ethics; values

Serour, Gamal I. Islamic developments in bioethics. *In:* Lustig, B. Andrew, ed.; Center for Medical Ethics and Health Policy (Houston, TX). Bioethics Yearbook, Volume 5: Theological Developments in Bioethics, 1992-1994. Boston, MA: Kluwer Academic; 1997: 171–188. 47 refs. ISBN 0-7923-4428-6. BE58386.
aborted fetuses; active euthanasia; allowing to die; autonomy; beneficence; *bioethical issues; biomedical technologies; carriers; confidentiality; congenital disorders; cryopreservation; cultural pluralism; determination of death; developing countries; embryo research; embryos; fetal research; fetal tissue donation; gene therapy; genetic enhancement; genetic identity; genetic information; genetic screening; health care; human experimentation; informed consent; *Islamic ethics; justice; married persons; medical

ethics; multiple pregnancy; newborns; organ donors; parent child relationship; pregnant women; property rights; reproductive technologies; resource allocation; selective abortion; sex preselection; *theology; therapeutic abortion; tissue transplantation

Shelton, Robert L. Biomedical ethics in Methodist traditions. *In:* Lustig, B. Andrew, ed.; Center for Medical Ethics and Health Policy (Houston, TX). Bioethics Yearbook, Volume 5: Theological Developments in Bioethics, 1992–1994. Boston, MA: Kluwer Academic; 1997: 189–220. 63 refs. ISBN 0-7923-4428-6. BE58387.
   active euthanasia; advance directives; AIDS; allowing to die; artificial feeding; assisted suicide; beginning of life; *bioethical issues; confidentiality; cultural pluralism; determination of death; developing countries; ecology; embryo disposition; gene therapy; genetic materials; genetic research; health care; health hazards; human body; human experimentation; informed consent; justice; marital relationship; newborns; nuclear energy; organ donation; organ transplantation; patents; patient care; persistent vegetative state; political activity; *Protestant ethics; reproductive technologies; resource allocation; rights; selective abortion; semen donors; terminally ill; *theology; therapeutic abortion; value of life; withholding treatment; African Methodist Episcopal Church; African Methodist Episcopal Zion Church; Christian Methodist Episcopal Church; Church of the Nazarene; Free Methodist Church; Kazakhstan; *Methodist Church; United Methodist Church; United States; Wesleyan Church

Shi, Da-pu; Yu, Lin. The conflict between the advancement of medical science and technology and traditional Chinese medical ethics. *In:* Becker, Gerhold K., ed. Changing Nature's Course: The Ethical Challenge of Biotechnology. Hong Kong: Hong Kong University Press; 1996: 111–118. ISBN 962-209-403-1. BE56708.
   *bioethical issues; *biomedical technologies; communication; economics; goals; informed consent; justice; life extension; medical ethics; *medicine; moral obligations; physician patient relationship; physician's role; quality of life; reproductive technologies; resource allocation; social impact; transsexualism; trust; *China

Shildrick, Margrit. Leaky Bodies and Boundaries: Feminism, Postmodernism and (Bio)ethics. New York, NY: Routledge; 1997. 252 p. Bibliography: p. 231–244. ISBN 0-415-14617-8. BE56731.
   autonomy; *bioethics; body parts and fluids; caring; cultural pluralism; *ethical theory; *females; *feminist ethics; health care; historical aspects; homosexuals; *human body; humanism; infertility; informed consent; males; moral development; mother fetus relationship; paternalism; *philosophy; physician patient relationship; pregnant women; reproduction; *reproductive technologies; risks and benefits; selection for treatment; *self concept; sexuality; social dominance; stigmatization; *postmodernism; rationality; Derrida, Jacques; Foucault, Michel; Irigaray, Luce

Simini, Bruno. New ethical guidelines issued by the Vatican. [News]. *Lancet.* 1997 Sep 20; 350(9081): 874. BE56337.
   abortion, induced; active euthanasia; allowing to die; animal experimentation; *bioethical issues; capital punishment; contraception; morality; organ donation; *Roman Catholic ethics; sexuality; *Catechism of the Catholic Church

Simmons, Paul D. Baptist-Evangelical medical ethics. *In:* Lustig, B. Andrew, ed.; Center for Medical Ethics and Health Policy (Houston, TX). Bioethics Yearbook, Volume 5: Theological Developments in Bioethics, 1992–1994. Boston, MA: Kluwer Academic; 1997: 221–257. 70 refs. ISBN 0-7923-4428-6. BE58388.
   aborted fetuses; abortion, induced; active euthanasia; advance directives; AIDS; allowing to die; animal rights; artificial feeding; assisted suicide; attitudes to death; *bioethical issues; capital punishment; contraception; embryo research; fetal research; fetal tissue donation; genetic screening; genome mapping; health care reform; health facilities; health personnel; killing; moral complicity; morality; patents; physicians; *political activity; preimplantation diagnosis; *Protestant ethics; public policy; recombinant DNA research; sex determination; suffering; terminal care; *theology; *value of life; violence; war; withholding treatment; *Baptist Church; *Evangelical Christians; Right to Life Movement; United States

Sinclair, Daniel B. Jewish law in the state of Israel. *In:* Jewish Law Annual. Volume Twelve. Amsterdam, Netherlands: Harwood Academic Publishers; 1997: 253–266. 57 fn. ISBN 90-5702-551-5. BE58348.
   adults; allowing to die; *bioethical issues; brain death; cesarean section; cryopreservation; death; dissent; embryo transfer; embryos; family members; fathers; fetuses; in vitro fertilization; *Jewish ethics; *legal aspects; minors; pregnant women; reproductive technologies; resuscitation orders; surrogate mothers; Tay Sachs disease; terminally ill; third party consent; treatment refusal; value of life; Attorney General v. B; Eyal v. Willenski; *Israel; Nahmani v. Nahmani; Yael Sheffer v. State of Israel; Zadok v. Beth Haelah

Smalley, M. Gene. Jehovah's Witnesses: help with bioethical issues. *In:* Lustig, B. Andrew, ed.; Center for Medical Ethics and Health Policy (Houston, TX). Bioethics Yearbook, Volume 5: Theological Developments in Bioethics, 1992–1994. Boston, MA: Kluwer Academic; 1997: 259–267. 25 refs. ISBN 0-7923-4428-6. BE58389.
   abortion, induced; active euthanasia; advance directives; allowing to die; alternatives; beginning of life; *bioethical issues; blood transfusions; contraception; embryo disposition; *Jehovah's Witnesses; married persons; methods; personhood; *Protestant ethics; reproductive technologies; *theology; treatment refusal; *value of life

Spicker, Stuart F. The philosophy of medicine and bioethics: commentary on ten Have and Engelhardt. *In:* Carson, Ronald A.; Burns, Chester R., eds. Philosophy of Medicine and Bioethics: A Twenty-Year Retrospective and Critical Appraisal. Boston, MA: Kluwer Academic; 1997: 125–133. 2 refs. ISBN 0-7923-3545-7. BE56530.
   *bioethics; consensus; cultural pluralism; *medicine; *philosophy; religious ethics; secularism; postmodernism

Spudis, Edward V. Non-simultaneous deaths of parallel personhoods crashing through a Denver S & L. [Poetry]. *Journal of Clinical Ethics.* 1998 Summer; 9(2): 206. Commented on by E.G. Howe, p. 207–208. BE58967.
   *death; *dehumanization; determination of death; emotions; law; literature; medicine; personhood

ten Have, Henk. From synthesis and system to morals and procedure: the development of philosophy of medicine. *In:* Carson, Ronald A.; Burns, Chester R., eds. Philosophy of Medicine and Bioethics: A Twenty-Year Retrospective and Critical Appraisal. Boston, MA: Kluwer Academic; 1997: 105–123. 37 refs. ISBN 0-7923-3545-7. BE56529.
   *bioethics; cultural pluralism; historical aspects; international aspects; *medicine; *philosophy; trends; postmodernism

Thomasma, David C., ed. The Influence of Edmund D. Pellegrino's Philosophy of Medicine. Boston, MA: Kluwer Academic; 1997. 215 p. 561 fn. Reprinted from *Theoretical Medicine,* 18(1-2); 1997. ISBN

BE = bioethics accession number   fn. = footnotes   refs. = references

0–7923–4412–X. BE57642.
    allowing to die; assisted suicide; *bioethical issues; *bioethics; caring; clinical ethics; communitarianism; conflict of interest; covenant; cultural pluralism; decision making; disease; economics; *ethical theory; ethicists; health; international aspects; managed care programs; medical education; *medical ethics; *medicine; nursing ethics; patient advocacy; patient care; patient participation; *philosophy; *physician patient relationship; *physician's role; primary health care; principle–based ethics; psychiatry; public policy; quality of health care; religious ethics; resource allocation; secularism; sociology of medicine; trust; values; *virtues; voluntary euthanasia; *Pellegrino, Edmund; United States

Tong, Rosemarie. The ethics of care: a feminist virtue ethics of care for healthcare practitioners. *Journal of Medicine and Philosophy.* 1998 Apr; 23(2): 131–152. 28 refs. 1 fn. BE58651.
    *caring; *ethical analysis; *ethical theory; *females; *feminist ethics; historical aspects; *justice; *males; moral development; moral obligations; morality; *narrative ethics; philosophy; social dominance; values; *virtues; Eighteenth Century; Nineteenth Century
In this paper I seek to distinguish a feminist virtue ethics of care from (1) justice ethics, (2) narrative ethics, (3) care ethics and (4) virtue ethics. I also connect this contemporary discussion of what makes a virtue ethics of care feminist to eighteenth and nineteenth century debates about male, female, and human virtue. I conclude that by focusing on issues related to gender -- primarily those related to the systems, structures, and ideologies that create and sustain patterns of male domination and female subordination -- we can begin to appreciate that true care and bona–fide virtue can flourish only in societies that treat all persons with equal respect and consideration.

Toombs, S. Kay. Taking the body seriously. [Book review essay]. *Hastings Center Report.* 1997 Sep–Oct; 27(5): 39–43. 4 fn. BE56126.
    *bioethical issues; *bioethics; clinical ethics; cultural pluralism; disabled; feminist ethics; health; *human body; literature; medicine; narrative ethics; normality; religious ethics; sociology of medicine; stigmatization; suffering; postmodernism; sick role; Embodiment, Morality, and Medicine (Cahill, L.S.; Farley, M.A., eds.); Enforcing Normalcy: Disability, Deafness and the Body (Davis, L.J.); The Wounded Storyteller: Body, Illness and Ethics (Frank, A.W.); Troubled Bodies: Critical Perspectives (Komesaroff, P.A., ed.)

Turner, Leigh. An anthropological exploration of contemporary bioethics: the varieties of common sense. *Journal of Medical Ethics.* 1998 Apr; 24(2): 127–133. 17 fn. BE58071.
    active euthanasia; anthropology; assisted suicide; autonomy; *bioethical issues; *bioethics; brain death; cancer; casuistry; *cultural pluralism; deception; decision making; determination of death; developing countries; diagnosis; ethical relativism; ethicist's role; ethics consultation; family members; informed consent; international aspects; minority groups; *morality; organ donation; organ transplantation; patients; principle–based ethics; prognosis; public policy; religious ethics; socioeconomic factors; suffering; truth disclosure; value of life; community consent; postmodernism; *Canada; *United States
Patients and physicians can inhabit distinctive social worlds where they are guided by diverse understandings of moral practice. Despite the contemporary presence of multiple moral traditions, religious communities and ethnic backgrounds, two of the major methodological approaches in bioethics, casuistry and principlism, rely upon the notion of a common morality. However, the heterogeneity of ethnic, moral, and religious traditions

raises questions concerning the singularity of common sense. Indeed, it might be more appropriate to consider plural traditions of moral reasoning. This poses a considerable challenge for bioethicists because the existence of plural moral traditions can lead to difficulties regarding "closure" in moral reasoning. The topics of truth–telling, informed consent, euthanasia, and brain death and organ transplantation reveal the presence of different understandings of common sense. With regard to these subjects, plural accounts of "common sense" moral reasoning exist.

Turner, Leigh. The greening of bioethics: corporate funding of bioethics research. *Cambridge Quarterly of Healthcare Ethics.* 1998 Summer; 7(3): 326–328. BE58561.
    *bioethics; *conflict of interest; education; *ethicists; federal government; *financial support; government financing; *industry; *research institutes; scarcity

U.S. Congress. Senate. A bill to provide for the establishment of a Commission to Promote a National Dialogue on Bioethics. S. 1595, 105th Cong., 2d Sess. Introduced by Bill Frist; 1998 Feb 2. 9 p. Referred to the Committee on Labor and Human Resources. BE58438.
    *advisory committees; *bioethical issues; cloning; committee membership; legal aspects; *organization and administration; *public participation; *public policy; *Commission to Promote a National Dialogue on Bioethics; Institute of Medicine; *United States

van der Burg, Wibren. Slippery slope arguments. *In:* Chadwick, Ruth, ed. Encyclopedia of Applied Ethics, Volume 4. San Diego, CA: Academic Press; 1998: 129–142. 5 refs. ISBN 0–12–227069–X. BE56345.
    *bioethical issues; case studies; emotions; involuntary euthanasia; moral policy; morality; philosophy; public policy; social impact; trends; *voluntary euthanasia; *wedge argument; Netherlands

Veatch, Robert M. The place of care in ethical theory. *Journal of Medicine and Philosophy.* 1998 Apr; 23(2): 210–224. 53 refs. 1 fn. BE58655.
    autonomy; beneficence; bioethics; *caring; *ethical analysis; *ethical theory; justice; principle–based ethics; social interaction; *virtues
The concept of care and a related ethical theory of care have emerged as increasingly important in biomedical ethics. This essay outlines a series of questions about the conceptualization of care and its place in ethical theory. First, it considers the possibility that care should be conceptualized as an alternative principle of right action; then as a virtue, a cluster of virtues, or as a synonym for virtue theory. The implications for various interpretations of the debate of the relation of care and justice are then explored, suggesting three possible meanings for that contrast. Next, the possibility that care theorists are taking up the debate over the relation between principles and cases is considered. Finally, it is suggested that care theorists may be pressing for consideration of an entirely new question in moral theory: the assessment of the normative appropriateness of relationships. Issues needing to be addressed in an ethic of relationships are suggested.

Verhey, Allen. Bioethics in the Reformed tradition. *In:* Lustig, B. Andrew, ed.; Center for Medical Ethics and Health Policy (Houston, TX). Bioethics Yearbook, Volume 5: Theological Developments in Bioethics, 1992–1994. Boston, MA: Kluwer Academic; 1997: 269–282. 11 refs. ISBN 0–7923–4428–6. BE58390.
    active euthanasia; adults; AIDS; allowing to die; assisted

---

BE = bioethics accession number   fn. = footnotes   refs. = references

suicide; autonomy; *bioethical issues; confidentiality; disabled; dissent; genetic disorders; genetic information; genetic screening; health care reform; HIV seropositivity; human body; international aspects; national health insurance; newborns; obligations of society; pastoral care; patient advocacy; personhood; physicians; *Protestant ethics; quality of life; stigmatization; suffering; *theology; treatment refusal; viability; Church of Scotland; Lindeboom Institute (Netherlands); Netherlands; *Presbyterian Church; *Reformed Church; Royal Dutch Medical Society; United States

Wadman, Meredith. Business booms for guides to biology's moral maze. [News]. *Nature.* 1997 Oct 16; 389(6652): 658–659. BE55951.
   advisory committees; *bioethics; cloning; education; ethicist's role; *ethicists; genome mapping; government regulation; human experimentation; literature; politics; private sector; public policy; public sector; research institutes; science; social impact; statistics; *trends; National Bioethics Advisory Commission; NCHGR Program on Ethical, Legal, and Social Implications (ELSI); President's Commission for the Study of Ethical Problems; *United States

Wadman, Meredith. National Institutes of Health sets up its own bioethics panel. [News]. *Nature.* 1997 Dec 18–25; 390(6661): 651. BE57320.
   *advisory committees; *bioethical issues; *federal government; organization and administration; *public policy; *National Institutes of Health; *Trans–NIH Bioethics Committee; *United States

Warren, Mary Anne. Moral Status: Obligations to Persons and Other Living Things. New York, NY: Oxford University Press; 1997. 265 p. (Issues in biomedical ethics). Bibliography: p. 243–253. ISBN 0-19-823668-9. BE56996.
   abortion, induced; allowing to die; animal experimentation; *animal rights; assisted suicide; *bioethical issues; cultural pluralism; ecology; embryos; emotions; ethical relativism; ethical theory; euthanasia; fetal development; fetuses; food; freedom; genetic intervention; historical aspects; *human rights; infants; mentally disabled; *moral obligations; *moral policy; morality; pain; *personhood; religion; *rights; self concept; social interaction; speciesism; utilitarianism; *value of life; viability; women's rights; potentiality; rationality; Callicott, J. Baird; Kant, Immanuel; Regan, Tom

Watson, Rory. European bioethics convention signed. [News]. *BMJ (British Medical Journal).* 1997 Apr 12; 314(7087): 1066. BE56442.
   *bioethical issues; embryo research; gene therapy; government regulation; human experimentation; human rights; informed consent; *international aspects; organ donation; Council of Europe; *Europe; *European Convention on Human Rights and Biomedicine

Weijer, Charles. Film and narrative in bioethics: Akira Kurosawa's *Ikiru. In:* Nelson, Hilde Lindemann, ed. Stories and Their Limits: Narrative Approaches to Bioethics. New York, NY: Routledge; 1997: 113–122. 26 fn. ISBN 0-415-91910-X. BE57466.
   *audiovisual aids; *bioethics; cancer; competence; empathy; ethicist's role; family members; health personnel; mass media; *narrative ethics; *patients; self concept; terminally ill; truth disclosure; postmodernism; *Ikiru (Kurosawa, A.); Japan

Wheeler, Sondra Ely. Stewards of Life: Bioethics and Pastoral Care. Nashville, TN: Abingdon Press; 1996. 126 p. Includes references. ISBN 0-687-02087-5. BE57203.
   aged; artificial feeding; autonomy; beneficence; *bioethical issues; *bioethics; case studies; *Christian ethics; chronically ill; *clergy; critically ill; decision making; family members;

food; futility; justice; newborns; *pastoral care; patient care; physicians; prematurity; quality of life; resource allocation; risks and benefits; suffering; suicide; *theology; treatment refusal; virtues; United States

Whitehouse, Peter J. Readdressing our moral relationship to nonhuman creatures: commentary on "A dialogue on species–specific rights: humans and animals in bioethics." *Cambridge Quarterly of Healthcare Ethics.* 1997 Fall; 6(4): 445–448. 13 fn. BE56499.
   *animal rights; *bioethics; *ecology; *human rights; moral obligations; *moral policy; *personhood; religion; rights; *speciesism; rationality; Potter, Van Rensselear

Wildes, Keven Wm. Institutional identity, integrity, and conscience. *Kennedy Institute of Ethics Journal.* 1997 Dec; 7(4): 413–419. 9 refs. BE59024.
   accountability; *bioethics; *conscience; economics; *goals; guidelines; health care delivery; historical aspects; *institutional ethics; *institutional policies; justice; *managed care programs; medicine; models, theoretical; religious hospitals; Roman Catholic ethics; science; postmodernism; United States
Bioethics has focused on the areas of individual ethical choices — patient care — or public policy and law. There are however, important arenas for ethical choices that have been overlooked. Health care is populated with intermediate arenas such as hospitals, nursing homes, hospices, and health care systems. This essay argues that bioethics needs to develop a language and concepts for institutional ethics. A first step in this direction is to think about institutional conscience.

Wildes, Kevin Wm. Healthy skepticism: the emperor has very few clothes. *Journal of Medicine and Philosophy.* 1997 Aug; 22(4): 365–371. 16 refs. BE55927.
   autonomy; *bioethics; consensus; *cultural pluralism; democracy; ethical relativism; *ethicist's role; *ethicists; *ethics; *expert testimony; *judicial action; *morality; *secularism; *technical expertise
The role of an expert witness in ethics, as part of a legal proceeding, is examined in this essay. The essay argues that the use of such expertise rests on confusions about normative and non–normative ethics compounded by misunderstandings about the challenges of moral argument in secular, morally pluralistic societies.

Wildes, Kevin Wm. *In vitro* fertilization: secular moral authority, biomedicine, and the role of the state. *In:* Wildes, Kevin Wm., ed. Infertility: A Crossroad of Faith, Medicine, and Technology. Boston, MA: Kluwer Academic; 1997: 181–194. 13 refs. 1 fn. ISBN 0-7923-4061-2. BE55998.
   *bioethics; casuistry; *cultural pluralism; ethical analysis; ethical theory; in vitro fertilization; libertarianism; *morality; *natural law; principle–based ethics; *public policy; Roman Catholic ethics; *secularism; values; Instruction on Respect for Human Life

Wildes, Kevin Wm. Redesigning the human genome: are there constraints from nature? *In:* Agius, Emmanuel; Busuttil, Salvino, eds. Germ–Line Intervention and Our Responsibilities to Future Generations. Boston, MA: Kluwer Academic; 1998: 35–49. 21 refs. 2 fn. ISBN 0-7923-4828-1. BE57878.
   bioethics; casuistry; *cultural pluralism; *decision making; democracy; deontological ethics; *ethical analysis; ethical theory; future generations; *gene therapy; *germ cells; human characteristics; informed consent; methods; *morality; *natural law; principle–based ethics; privacy; *secularism; teleological ethics; theology; values; *nature; rationality

---

BE = bioethics accession number   fn. = footnotes   refs. = references

Wildes, Kevin Wm. Sanctity of life: a study in ambiguity and confusion. *In:* Hoshino, Kazumasa, ed. Japanese and Western Bioethics: Studies in Moral Diversity. Boston, MA: Kluwer Academic; 1997: 89–101. 33 refs. 5 fn. ISBN 0–7923–4112–0. BE57085.
  abortion, induced; *allowing to die; *bioethics; *Buddhist ethics; *Christian ethics; compassion; euthanasia; killing; legal aspects; personhood; *prolongation of life; religion; Roman Catholic ethics; *secularism; state interest; suicide; *terminology; theology; *value of life; withholding treatment; Cruzan v. Director, Missouri Department of Health; Cruzan v. Harmon; United States

Wolpe, Paul Root. The triumph of autonomy in American bioethics: a sociological view. *In:* DeVries, Raymond; Subedi, Janardan, eds. Bioethics and Society: Constructing the Ethical Enterprise. Upper Saddle River, NJ: Prentice Hall; 1998: 38–59. 51 refs. 20 fn. ISBN 0–13–531252–3. BE58729.
  *autonomy; beneficence; bioethical issues; *bioethics; common good; cultural pluralism; ethicists; government regulation; health care delivery; historical aspects; human experimentation; iatrogenic disease; informed consent; justice; law; medical ethics; medicine; patient care; physician patient relationship; physicians; principle–based ethics; professional autonomy; public policy; rights; secularism; *sociology of medicine; trends; trust; values; Twentieth Century; United States

Wreen, Michael. Nihilism, relativism, and Engelhardt. *Theoretical Medicine and Bioethics.* 1998 Jan; 19(1): 73–88. 7 fn. BE57322.
  *bioethics; cultural pluralism; *ethical relativism; ethical theory; methods; *morality; philosophy; *religious ethics; *secularism; *Engelhardt, H. Tristram; The Foundations of Bioethics (Engelhardt, H.T.)

Yount, Lisa. Issues in Biomedical Ethics. [Juvenile literature]. San Diego, CA: Lucent Books; 1998. 128 p. (Contemporary issues). Bibliography: p. 113–119. ISBN 1–56006–476–5. BE57678.
  active euthanasia; allowing to die; animal experimentation; animal rights; assisted suicide; attitudes; *bioethical issues; biomedical technologies; cloning; competence; decision making; economics; eugenics; future generations; gene therapy; genetic enhancement; genetic intervention; genetic screening; germ cells; health care; international aspects; legal aspects; moral policy; persistent vegetative state; physicians; public participation; public policy; resource allocation; risks and benefits; selection for treatment; speciesism; terminal care; terminally ill; treatment refusal; wedge argument; withholding treatment; United States

Zohar, Noam J. Alternatives in Jewish Bioethics. Albany, NY: State University of New York Press; 1997. 165 p. (SUNY series in Jewish philosophy). Bibliography: p. 153–160. ISBN 0–7914–3274–2. BE57041.
  active euthanasia; allowing to die; assisted suicide; *bioethical issues; *bioethics; cadavers; cultural pluralism; ethical relativism; ethics; human body; humanism; *Jewish ethics; medicine; morality; natural law; random selection; religious ethics; reproductive technologies; resource allocation; secularism; teleological ethics; *theology; voluntary euthanasia

Zoloth–Dorfman, Laurie; Rubin, Susan B. Navigators and captains: expertise in clinical ethics consultation. [Book review essay]. *Theoretical Medicine.* 1997 Dec; 18(4): 421–432. 5 fn. BE56341.
  bioethics; *clinical ethics; clinical ethics committees; education; employment; *ethicist's role; *ethicists; *ethics consultation; goals; health personnel; *interdisciplinary communication; interprofessional relations; metaphor; professional competence; professional patient relationship; review; standards; *technical expertise; *Ethics

Consultation: A Practical Guide (La Puma, J.; Schiedermayer, D.); *The Health Care Ethics Consultant (Baylis, F.E., ed.)

Zribi, Ahmed. Medical ethics and Islam. *Dolentium Hominum: Church and Health in the World.* 1996; 31(11th Yr., No. 1): 82–85. 7 refs. BE57377.
  abortion, induced; active euthanasia; beneficence; *bioethical issues; cadavers; confidentiality; contraception; fetal development; freedom; gene therapy; genetic identity; genetic intervention; human experimentation; *Islamic ethics; justice; *medical ethics; organ donation; organ donors; organ transplantation; parent child relationship; reproductive technologies; *theology; Hippocrates

European Directory of Bioethics, 1996. Second Edition. Secaucus, NJ: Lavoisier; distributed by Springer Verlag; 1996. 703 p. Produced under the direction of Gérard Huber. French title: *Annuaire Europeen de Bioethique 1996*; text in French with English translation. Includes the bilingual *Thesaurus d'ethique biomedicale/Thesaurus of Biomedical Ethics*, p. 566–599. ISBN 2–7430–0094–5. BE56506.
  advisory committees; bioethical issues; *bioethics; education; *ethicists; ethics committees; *international aspects; literature; *research institutes; terminology; national ethics committees; *Europe

From the editors [the future of bioethics]. *Cambridge Quarterly of Healthcare Ethics.* 1997 Fall; 6(4): 365–369. 12 fn. BE56490.
  *bioethical issues; *bioethics; cultural pluralism; international aspects; *trends; Twenty–First Century

Light in dark places. [Editorial]. *Nature.* 1997 Oct 23; 389(6653): 767. BE56875.
  *bioethical issues; *international aspects; investigators; public participation; public policy; regulation; social impact; *France; *Great Britain

Trust and the bioethics industry. [Editorial]. *Nature.* 1997 Oct 16; 389(6652): 647. BE56576.
  attitudes; bioethical issues; *bioethics; cloning; ethicist's role; genetic research; politics; public opinion; public policy; risk; *science; trust

BIOETHICS/EDUCATION

Armstrong, Kerri; Weber, Kurt. Genetic engineering: a lesson on bioethics for the classroom. *American Biology Teacher.* 1991 May; 53(5): 294–297. BE58115.
  bioethics; *education; *genetic intervention; schools; *teaching methods; *secondary schools; United States

Ashcroft, Richard; Baron, Dennis; Benatar, Solomon, et al. Teaching medical ethics and law within medical education: a model for the UK core curriculum. [Consensus statement by teachers of medical ethics and law in UK medical schools]. *Journal of Medical Ethics.* 1998 Jun; 24(3): 188–192. 1 ref. This consensus statement is also available at the *British Medical Journal* website: www.bmj.com. Additional authors: Jackson, Jennifer; Jessiman, Ian; Johnson, Alan; King, Jennifer; Lutrell, Steven; Matthews, Eric; Meakin, Richard; Parker, Michael; Portsmouth, O.; Schwartz, Lisa; Shenfield, Francoise; Snashall, David; Somerville, Ann; Steiner, Timothy; Vernon, Bryan; Ward, Christopher; Zander, Luke; de Zulueta, Paquita. BE59121.
  *bioethical issues; bioethics; children; confidentiality; *consensus; *curriculum; *faculty; genetics; goals; human experimentation; informed consent; interprofessional relations; law; *medical education; *medical ethics; *medical schools; mentally disabled; physician patient relationship;

BE = bioethics accession number   fn. = footnotes   refs. = references

reproduction; resource allocation; *standards; teaching methods; terminal care; treatment refusal; General Medical Council (Great Britain); *Great Britain

Biermann, Carol A. What's a nice biology teacher like you doing teaching humanities? *American Biology Teacher.* 1990 Nov–Dec; 52(8): 487–490. 11 refs. BE58116.
    *bioethics; biology; curriculum; *education; humanities; interdisciplinary communication; *teaching methods; Kingsborough Community College (Brooklyn, NY)

Doyal, Len; Gillon, Raanan. Medical ethics and law as a core subject in medical education: a core curriculum offers flexibility in how it is taught -- but not that it is taught. [Editorial]. *BMJ (British Medical Journal).* 1998 May 30; 316(7145): 1623–1624. 2 refs. BE58252.
    *bioethical issues; consensus; *curriculum; law; *medical education; *medical ethics; *standards; *Great Britain

Fielder, John. Ethical experts and *Dr. Ethics. IEEE Engineering in Medicine and Biology Magazine.* 1993 Dec; 12(4): 116–119. 3 fn. BE56030.
    advance directives; allowing to die; assisted suicide; *audiovisual aids; bioethical issues; case studies; casuistry; codes of ethics; *computers; decision making; ethical analysis; ethical theory; ethicists; *ethics; evaluation; feminist ethics; informed consent; medical ethics; methods; professional ethics; *teaching methods; technical expertise; *software; *Dr. Ethics (software program)

Gastmans, Chris. Contemporary challenges in health care ethics. *Nursing Ethics.* 1998 Jan; 5(1): 81–83. 1 ref. BE58717.
    *bioethics; curriculum; *education; program descriptions; research institutes; *Kennedy Institute of Ethics

Homenko, Donna F. Overview of ethical issues perceived by allied health professionals in the workplace. *Journal of Allied Health.* 1997 Summer; 26(3): 97–103. 15 refs. BE58466.
    *allied health personnel; *bioethical issues; *bioethics; *education; hospitals; *knowledge, attitudes, practice; *professional ethics; survey; questionnaires; Midwestern United States

Hope, Tony. Ethics and law for medical students: the core curriculum. [Editorial]. *Journal of Medical Ethics.* 1998 Jun; 24(3): 147–148. 2 refs. BE59115.
    attitudes; *bioethical issues; bioethics; consensus; *curriculum; faculty; goals; law; *medical education; *medical ethics; physicians; teaching methods; General Medical Council (Great Britain); *Great Britain

Kane, Gregory C.; Leone, Frank T.; Rowane, Joseph, et al. Nationwide perspective on the use of a formal ethics curriculum during critical care fellowship training. [Letter]. *Academic Medicine.* 1998 Jan; 73(1): 103. 1 ref. BE56627.
    administrators; advance directives; allowing to die; attitudes; *bioethical issues; bioethics; biomedical technologies; critically ill; *curriculum; human experimentation; intensive care units; *medical education; *medical ethics; patient care; survey; withholding treatment; United States

Kent, Heather. Medical, health–science students bring different perspectives to interdisciplinary ethics course. *Canadian Medical Association Journal.* 1997 May 1; 156(9): 1317–1318. BE56155.
    bioethical issues; *clinical ethics; curriculum; *education; faculty; *health personnel; *interdisciplinary communication; professional ethics; program descriptions; teaching methods; British Columbia; *University of British Columbia

Lewthwaite, Barbara; Erickson–Nesmith, Sharon. Needs assessment for healthcare ethics education. *HEC (HealthCare Ethics Committee) Forum.* 1998 Mar; 10(1): 86–101. 6 refs. BE59061.
    *attitudes; *bioethical issues; *clinical ethics committees; *education; evaluation; *health personnel; hospitals; nurses; physicians; survey; teaching methods; time factors; questionnaires; teaching hospitals; *Canada

Neff–Smith, Martha; Giles, Scott; Spencer, Edward M., et al. Ethics program evaluation: the Virginia Hospital Ethics Fellows example. *HEC (HealthCare Ethics Committee) Forum.* 1997 Dec; 9(4): 375–388. 3 refs. BE58088.
    administrators; attitudes; *clinical ethics; clinical ethics committees; *education; *ethics consultation; *evaluation; *evaluation studies; health personnel; *hospitals; organization and administration; program descriptions; standards; *community hospitals; *Center for Biomedical Ethics, University of Virginia; Virginia; West Virginia

Price, John; Price, David; Williams, Gail, et al. Changes in medical student attitudes as they progress through a medical course. *Journal of Medical Ethics.* 1998 Apr; 24(2): 110–117. 30 refs. BE58064.
    aged; *attitudes; autonomy; beneficence; *bioethical issues; comparative studies; confidentiality; duty to warn; females; informed consent; justice; law enforcement; males; *medical education; *medical ethics; minority groups; misconduct; moral development; moral obligations; obligations to society; patient compliance; patients' rights; physicians; political activity; professional autonomy; resource allocation; self induced illness; social discrimination; *students; survey; *time factors; truth disclosure; value of life; *Australia; Queensland
    OBJECTIVES: To explore the way ethical principles develop during a medical education course for three groups of medical students -- in their first year, at the beginning of their penultimate (fifth) year and towards the end of their final (sixth) year. DESIGN: Survey questionnaire administered to medical students in their first, fifth and final (sixth) year. SETTING: A large medical school in Queensland, Australia. SURVEY SAMPLE: Approximately half the students in each of three years (first, fifth and sixth) provided data on a voluntary basis, a total of 385 students. RESULTS: At the point of entry, minor differences were found between medical students and first year law and psychology students. More striking were differences between male and female medical students, suggesting early socialization had a substantial impact here. CONCLUSIONS: Results indicate that substantial changes in attitude have developed by the beginning of fifth year with little change thereafter. Gender difference persisted. Some difference in ethical attitudes were found when groups of different ethnic backgrounds were compared. The impact of a move to a graduate medical course, which gives high priority to ethics within a professional development domain, can now be evaluated.

Seedhouse, David. Against medical ethics: a response to Cassell. *Journal of Medical Ethics.* 1998 Feb; 24(1): 13–17. 12 refs. BE57435.
    *bioethics; curriculum; ethical theory; ethicists; *ethics; health personnel; *medical education; *medical ethics; medical specialties; medicine; morality; philosophy; physicians; Great Britain

BIOLOGICAL WARFARE *See* WAR

Columbia

BIOMEDICAL RESEARCH

See also BEHAVIORAL RESEARCH, EMBRYO
AND FETAL RESEARCH, GENETIC
RESEARCH, HUMAN EXPERIMENTATION

Abbott, Alison. Germany tightens grip on misconduct.
[News]. *Nature.* 1997 Dec 4; 390(6659): 430. BE56850.
  biomedical research; financial support; *fraud; investigators;
  research institutes; *scientific misconduct; *self regulation;
  universities; Brach, Marion; *Deutsche
  Forschungsgemeinschaft; *Germany; Herrmann, Friedhelm;
  *Max Planck Society

Abbott, Alison. Researcher sues over 'fraud' sanction.
[News]. *Nature.* 1997 Dec 18–25; 390(6661): 652.
BE57300.
  authorship; biomedical research; due process; editorial
  policies; faculty; *fraud; *investigators; *legal aspects;
  punishment; *scientific misconduct; self regulation;
  *universities; orthopedics; *Germany; *Goertzen, Meinolf;
  Journal of Bone and Joint Surgery; *University of
  Düsseldorf

**Angell, Marcia; Kassirer, Jerome; Manson, JoAnn E.,
et al.** Conflict of interest. [Letter and responses].
Epidemiology. 1997 Nov; 8(6): 686–687. 10 refs. BE58351.
  authorship; *biomedical research; *conflict of interest;
  *disclosure; *drug industry; drugs; *editorial policies;
  *financial support; investigators; referral and consultation;
  time factors; obesity; *New England Journal of Medicine

Atterstam, Inger. Karolinska Institute rocked by research
misconduct. [News]. *Lancet.* 1997 Aug 30; 350(9078):
643. BE56082.
  biomedical research; cancer; fraud; genetic research;
  investigators; research institutes; *scientific misconduct; self
  regulation; *Karolinska Institute (Sweden); *Lönn, Ulf;
  *Sweden

Badaway, Abdulla A.-B. Ethics in alcohol research and
publishing. [Editorial]. *Alcohol and Alcoholism.* 1996 Jan;
31(1): 7–9. 10 refs. BE55753.
  *alcohol abuse; *behavioral research; *biomedical research;
  codes of ethics; conflict of interest; disclosure; *editorial
  policies; financial support; investigators; peer review;
  *professional ethics; scientific misconduct; *self regulation;
  universities; *journalism

Beach, Doré. The Responsible Conduct of Research.
Weinheim, Germany; New York, NY: VCH Publishers;
1996. 161 p. Includes references and discussion
questions. Designed as a textbook for "pre- and
postdoctoral students planning careers in scientific
research." ISBN 3-527-29333-7. BE56145.
  authorship; *biomedical research; biomedical technologies;
  confidentiality; conflict of interest; education; embryo
  research; ethical analysis; ethical theory; ethics; faculty;
  federal government; fraud; genetic research; genetic
  screening; genome mapping; government regulation;
  guidelines; human experimentation; information
  dissemination; informed consent; interprofessional relations;
  *investigators; laboratories; legal aspects; misconduct; moral
  obligations; obligations to society; patents; peer review;
  professional ethics; property rights; records; research ethics
  committees; *science; scientific misconduct; self regulation;
  standards; students; terminology; whistleblowing;
  technology transfer; Nuremberg Code; United States

Bebeau, M.J.; Holt, S.C. Proceedings of a symposium,
"Toward Responsible Research Conduct: The Role of
Scientific Societies." [Introduction to a set of five papers
and a consensus statement]. *Journal of Dental Research.*
1996 Feb; 75(2): 823–824. 2 refs. Paper presented at the

symposium at the annual meeting of the American
Association for Dental Research, held in San Antonio,
TX, Mar 1995. BE56453.
  biomedical research; codes of ethics; *dentistry;
  *investigators; organizational policies; *professional ethics;
  *professional organizations; *scientific misconduct; *self
  regulation; standards; *dental research; professional role;
  American Association for Dental Research

Bebeau, M.J.; Davis, E.L. Survey of ethical issues in
dental research. *Journal of Dental Research.* 1996 Feb;
75(2): 845–855. 10 refs. Paper presented at the
symposium, "Toward Responsible Research Conduct:
The Role of Scientific Societies," during the annual
meeting of the American Association for Dental
Research, held in San Antonio, TX, Mar 1995. BE56452.
  administrators; *attitudes; authorship; biomedical research;
  codes of ethics; *dentistry; education; ethics committees;
  *investigators; *professional ethics; professional
  organizations; *scientific misconduct; self regulation;
  standards; survey; *dental research; professional role;
  *American Association for Dental Research; International
  Association for Dental Research

**Bebeau, Muriel J.; Holt, Stanley C.; American
Association for Dental Research. Ethics Committee.**
The role of the AADR in promoting research integrity:
perspectives and consensus statements. *Journal of Dental
Research.* 1996 Feb; 75(2): 856–860. 9 refs. BE56454.
  biomedical research; *codes of ethics; *dentistry; due
  process; education; ethics committees; goals; guidelines;
  *investigators; professional autonomy; *professional ethics;
  *professional organizations; *scientific misconduct; *self
  regulation; *standards; *dental research; professional role;
  *American Association for Dental Research; International
  Association for Dental Research

Benatar, Solomon R. Editorial ethics. [Personal view].
BMJ (British Medical Journal). 1998 Jan 10; 316(7125):
155–156. BE57772.
  accountability; biomedical research; communication;
  *editorial policies; guidelines; investigators; peer review;
  *professional ethics; time factors; *journalism

Berger, Edward M.; Gert, Bernard. The institutional
context for research. *Professional Ethics.* 1995
Spring–Summer; 4(3–4): 17–46. 2 fn. References
embedded in back–of–issue bibliography. BE55693.
  administrators; authorship; biomedical research;
  confidentiality; education; federal government; fraud;
  government financing; government regulation; *guidelines;
  *institutional ethics; *institutional policies; interprofessional
  relations; investigators; legal aspects; misconduct; moral
  obligations; organization and administration; professional
  ethics; *research institutes; *science; *scientific misconduct;
  *self regulation; terminology; universities; whistleblowing;
  Breuning, Stephen; California Institute of Technology;
  Department of Justice; National Academy of Sciences;
  Ninnemann, John; Responsible Science: Ensuring the
  Integrity of the Research Process (NAS); United States;
  University of California, San Diego; University of Illinois;
  University of Pittsburgh; University of Utah

Bero, Lisa A. Disclosure policies for gifts from industry
to academic faculty. [Editorial]. *JAMA.* 1998 Apr 1;
279(13): 1031–1032. 10 refs. BE57331.
  *biomedical research; *conflict of interest; contracts;
  *disclosure; education; *faculty; federal government;
  *financial support; gifts; government regulation; *guidelines;
  human experimentation; *industry; information
  dissemination; *institutional policies; *investigators; patents;
  property rights; records; self regulation; *universities;
  California; United States; *University of California, San
  Francisco

BE = bioethics accession number   fn. = footnotes   refs. = references

Bersoff, D.N. Process and procedures for dealing with misconduct: a necessity or a nightmare? *Journal of Dental Research.* 1996 Feb; 75(2): 836–840. 14 refs. Paper presented at the symposium, "Toward Responsible Research Conduct: The Role of Scientific Societies," during the annual meeting of the American Association for Dental Research, held in San Antonio, TX, Mar 1995. BE56457.
> biomedical research; codes of ethics; dentistry; *due process; economics; ethics committees; *investigators; *legal aspects; legal liability; *organizational policies; *professional ethics; *professional organizations; psychology; punishment; *science; *scientific misconduct; *self regulation; dental research; professional role; American Association for Dental Research; American Psychological Association

Bird, Stephanie J.; Housman, David E. Conducting and reporting research. *Professional Ethics.* 1995 Spring–Summer; 4(3–4): 127–154. 4 fn. References embedded in back-of-issue bibliography. BE55692.
> administrators; authorship; *biomedical research; contracts; financial support; information dissemination; interprofessional relations; *investigators; mass media; methods; obligations to society; peer review; *professional ethics; property rights; research design; *science; scientific misconduct; standards; students; United States

Böttiger, Lars Erik. Scientific misconduct -- does it exist? [Editorial]. *Journal of Internal Medicine.* 1994 Feb; 235(2): 103–105. 6 refs. BE55610.
> biomedical research; editorial policies; fraud; human experimentation; investigators; medical education; peer review; physicians; public participation; *regulation; *scientific misconduct; Denmark; Great Britain; United States

Bowie, Cameron. Was the paper I wrote a fraud? [Personal view]. *BMJ (British Medical Journal).* 1998 Jun 6; 316(7146): 1755–1756. BE58234.
> authorship; biomedical research; community services; fraud; interprofessional relations; investigators; physically disabled; *scientific misconduct; trust; Great Britain

Breyer, Stephen. The interdependence of science and law. *Science.* 1998 Apr 24; 280(5363): 537–538. 9 refs. Revised text of an address given by Justice Breyer at the 150th Annual Meeting of the American Association for the Advancement of Science, 16 Feb 1998. BE58202.
> biomedical research; compensation; *expert testimony; genetics; health hazards; *interdisciplinary communication; *investigators; judicial action; justice; *law; psychiatry; right to die; *science; Supreme Court decisions; *technical expertise; toxicity; uncertainty; judges; *United States

Brody, Baruch A., comp. Appendixes: international research ethics policies; European transnational research ethics policies; U.S. research ethics policies; research ethics policies from other countries. *In: his* The Ethics of Biomedical Research: An International Perspective. New York, NY: Oxford University Press; 1998: 213–358. ISBN 0-19-509007-1. BE57677.
> *animal experimentation; *biomedical research; codes of ethics; embryo research; federal government; fetal research; gene therapy; genetic research; genetic screening; genome mapping; government regulation; *guidelines; *human experimentation; *international aspects; patents; professional organizations; *research ethics; Australia; Canada; Council for International Organizations of Medical Sciences (CIOMS); Council of Europe; Declaration of Helsinki; Department of Health and Human Services; Europe; Food and Drug Administration; Great Britain; Japan; National Institutes of Health; Nuremberg Code; Public Health Service; United States; World Medical Association

Brody, Baruch A. Epidemiological research. *In: his* The Ethics of Biomedical Research: An International Perspective. New York, NY: Oxford University Press; 1998: 55–75, 364–366. 43 fn. ISBN 0-19-509007-1. BE57670.
> anonymous testing; behavioral research; confidentiality; conflict of interest; consensus; cultural pluralism; data banks; developing countries; disclosure; DNA data banks; *epidemiology; ethical relativism; ethical review; financial support; genetic research; government regulation; guidelines; historical aspects; HIV seropositivity; information dissemination; informed consent; *international aspects; investigators; medical records; moral obligations; moral policy; nontherapeutic research; political activity; prevalence; privacy; public health; public policy; random selection; research design; research subjects; review; risks and benefits; smoking; tissue banks; community consent; multicenter studies; Canada; Europe; United States

Brody, Baruch A. The Ethics of Biomedical Research: An International Perspective. New York, NY: Oxford University Press; 1998. 386 p. 393 fn. ISBN 0-19-509007-1. BE57667.
> animal experimentation; *biomedical research; control groups; drugs; embryo research; epidemiology; females; fetal research; genetic research; guidelines; *human experimentation; *international aspects; medical devices; mentally disabled; minority groups; minors; pregnant women; prisoners; public policy; random selection; regulation; research design; review; vulnerable populations; *research ethics; United States

Burd, Larry; Gregory, Jennifer M.; Kerbeshian, Jacob. The brain–mind quiddity: ethical issues in the use of human brain tissue for therapeutic and scientific purposes. *Journal of Medical Ethics.* 1998 Apr; 24(2): 118–122. 13 refs. BE58051.
> animal experimentation; *biomedical research; *brain; brain death; computers; electrical stimulation of the brain; *emotions; ethical review; human body; human experimentation; informed consent; laboratories; models, theoretical; *organ donation; *organ transplantation; *personhood; regulation; *tissue donation; *tissue transplantation; cell lines; personal identity
The use of human brain tissue in neuroscience research is increasing. Recent developments include transplanting neural tissue, growing or maintaining neural tissue in laboratories and using surgically removed tissue for experimentation. Also, it is likely that in the future there will be attempts at partial or complete brain transplants. A discussion of the ethical issues of using human brain tissue for research and brain transplantation has been organized around nine broadly defined topic areas. Criteria for human brain tissue transplantation and laboratory use of brain tissue are proposed.

Burrows, Beth. Second thoughts about U.S. Patent #4,438,032. *Bulletin of Medical Ethics.* 1997 Jan; No. 124: 11–14. 3 refs. BE55740.
> *biomedical research; *body parts and fluids; conflict of interest; deception; disclosure; drug industry; informed consent; *investigators; *legal aspects; *patents; *patients; *property rights; remuneration; *tissue donation; universities; *cell lines; California; Golde, David; *Moore v. Regents of the University of California; United States

Butler, Declan. European grants to face ethics scrutiny. [News]. *Nature.* 1997 Dec 4; 390(6659): 433. BE57255.
> advisory committees; bioethics; *biomedical research; *ethical review; financial support; genetic intervention; *international aspects; public policy; national ethics committees; *Europe; *European Commission; European Union; Group of Advisers on the Ethical Implications of Biotechnology (European Commission)

BE = bioethics accession number   fn. = footnotes   refs. = references

Butler, Declan; DeGandt, Olivier. French ministry reopens inquiry into conduct of INSERM unit. [News]. *Nature.* 1998 Feb 5; 391(6667): 519–520. BE58020.
> administrators; *biomedical research; government regulation; industry; patents; *research institutes; *scientific misconduct; universities; whistleblowing; Bihain, Bernard; *France; Genset; *INSERM

Butler, Declan. Karolinska Institute disowns work of cancer researcher. [News]. *Nature.* 1997 Aug 28; 388(6645): 816. BE56071.
> biomedical research; cancer; fraud; investigators; research institutes; *scientific misconduct; self regulation; *Karolinska Institute (Sweden); *Lönn, Ulf; *Sweden

Callahan, Daniel. Cloning: the work not done. *Hastings Center Report.* 1997 Sep–Oct; 27(5): 18–20. 2 fn. BE56116.
> advisory committees; bioethical issues; bioethics; *biomedical research; children; *cloning; common good; future generations; government regulation; human experimentation; informed consent; *moral policy; *public policy; reproduction; reproductive technologies; research subjects; rights; *risks and benefits; science; standards; *values; *Cloning Human Beings (NBAC); *National Bioethics Advisory Commission; United States

Camenisch, P.F. The moral foundations of scientific ethics and responsibility. *Journal of Dental Research.* 1996 Feb; 75(2): 825–831. 16 refs. Paper presented at the symposium, "Toward Responsible Research Conduct: The Role of Scientific Societies," during the annual meeting of the American Association for Dental Research, held in San Antonio, TX, Mar 1995. BE56459.
> biomedical research; codes of ethics; common good; conflict of interest; *dentistry; disclosure; goals; information dissemination; *investigators; moral obligations; obligations to society; organizational policies; professional autonomy; professional competence; *professional ethics; *professional organizations; science; *scientific misconduct; *self regulation; trust; values; *dental research; professional role; *American Association for Dental Research; *International Association for Dental Research

Campbell, Eric G.; Louis, Karen Seashore; Blumenthal, David. Looking a gift horse in the mouth: corporate gifts supporting life sciences research. *JAMA.* 1998 Apr 1; 279(13): 995–999. 12 fn. BE57332.
> attitudes; *biomedical research; conflict of interest; contracts; disclosure; education; evaluation studies; *faculty; federal government; females; *financial support; *gifts; government financing; guidelines; human experimentation; *industry; information dissemination; institutional policies; *investigators; males; medical schools; patents; property rights; self regulation; statistics; survey; *universities; NCHGR–funded publication; *United States
> CONTEXT: Throughout the last decade a number of studies have been conducted to examine academic–industry research relationships. However, to our knowledge, no studies to date have empirically examined academic scientists' experience with research-related gifts from companies. OBJECTIVE: To examine the frequency, importance, and potential implications of research-related gifts from companies to academic life scientists. DESIGN: A mailed survey conducted in 1994 and 1995 of 3394 faculty who conduct life science research at the 50 universities that received the most research funding from the National Institutes of Health in 1993. SETTING: Research-intensive universities. PARTICIPANTS: A total of 2167 of the 3394 faculty responded to the survey (response rate, 64%). MAIN OUTCOME MEASURES: The percentage of faculty who received a research-related

gift from a company in the last 3 years, the perceived importance of gifts to respondents' research, and what, if anything, the recipient thought the donor(s) expected in return for the gift. RESULTS: Forty-three percent of respondents received a research-related gift in the last 3 years independent of a grant or contract. The most frequently received gifts were biomaterials (24%), discretionary funds (15%), research equipment and trips to meetings (11% each), support for students (9%), and other research-related gifts (3%). Of those who received a gift, 66% reported the gift was important to their research. More than half of the recipients reported that donors expected the following in return for the gift: acknowledgment in publications (63%), that the gift not be passed on to a third party (60%), and that the gift be used only for the agreed-on purposes (59%). A total of 32% of recipients reported that the donor wanted prepublication review of any articles or reports stemming from the use of the gift, 30% indicated the company expected testing of their products, and 19% indicated that a donor expected ownership of all patentable results from the research in which a gift was used. However, what recipients thought donors expected differed by the type of gift received. CONCLUSIONS: Research-related gifts are a common and important form of research support for academic life scientists. However, recipients frequently think that donors place restrictions and expect returns that may be problematic for recipients as well as institutions.

Canada. Medical Research Council of Canada; Canada. Natural Sciences and Engineering Research Council of Canada; Canada. Social Sciences and Humanities Research Council of Canada. Integrity in Research and Scholarship: A Tri–Council Policy Statement. Ottawa, ON: Medical Research Council of Canada; 1994 Jan. 4 p. BE56727.
> accountability; biomedical research; government financing; government regulation; institutional policies; investigators; peer review; *regulation; research institutes; science; *scientific misconduct; self regulation; *Canada

Carlson, John W. On the justification and limits of medical research: a response to Kevin Wildes. *In:* Wildes, Kevin Wm.; Mitchell, Alan C., eds. Choosing Life: A Dialogue on *Evangelium Vitae.* Washington, DC: Georgetown University Press; 1997: 199–205. 18 fn. ISBN 0–87840–646–8. BE56689.
> beginning of life; *biomedical research; *embryo research; fetal research; genetic enhancement; *genetic research; germ cells; nontherapeutic research; *Roman Catholic ethics; theology; *therapeutic research; value of life; dignity; Evangelium Vitae

Chantler, Cyril; Chantler, Shireen. Dealing with research misconduct in the United Kingdom: deception: difficulties and initiatives. *BMJ (British Medical Journal).* 1998 Jun 6; 316(7146): 1731–1732. 8 refs. BE58204.
> biomedical research; due process; editorial policies; fraud; guidelines; institutional policies; investigators; medical education; medical schools; physicians; professional organizations; *regulation; *scientific misconduct; self regulation; whistleblowing; General Medical Council (Great Britain); Great Britain; Royal College of Physicians

Cho, Mildred. Disclosing conflicts of interest. [Letter]. *Lancet.* 1997 Jul 5; 350(9070): 72–73. 5 refs. BE56565.
> *biomedical research; *conflict of interest; *disclosure; *financial support; government financing; investigators; moral obligations; trust; universities

Coghlan, Andy. Organs for research are on the cards.

[News]. *New Scientist.* 1997 Apr 5; 154(2076): 5. BE56220.
    *biomedical research; cadavers; *donor cards; drug industry; *organ donation; presumed consent; *public policy; *tissue donation; Department of Health (Great Britain); *Great Britain

Cooper–Mahkorn, Déirdre. Many journals have not retracted "fraudulent" research. [News]. *BMJ (British Medical Journal).* 1998 Jun 20; 316(7148): 1850. BE58276.
    authorship; biomedical research; *editorial policies; *fraud; investigators; *scientific misconduct; *retraction of publication; Brach, Marion; *Germany; *Herrmann, Friedhelm; University of Ulm

Coughlin, Steven S. Advancing professional ethics in epidemiology. *Journal of Epidemiology and Biostatistics.* 1996; 1(2): 71–77. 41 refs. BE58494.
    bioethics; biomedical research; conflict of interest; curriculum; *education; *epidemiology; ethical review; ethics committees; financial support; guidelines; historical aspects; international aspects; *investigators; *professional ethics; professional organizations; public health; schools; self regulation; American College of Epidemiology; International Epidemiological Association; Society for Epidemiologic Research; Twentieth Century; United States

Coughlin, Steven S. Ethics in Epidemiology and Public Health Practice: Collected Works. Columbus, GA: Quill Publications; 1997. 232 p. Includes references. ISBN 0–9661520–0–X. BE58542.
    American Indians; autonomy; beneficence; biomedical research; cancer; case studies; confidentiality; control groups; curriculum; ecology; education; *epidemiology; ethical theory; ethics committees; federal government; females; government regulation; health hazards; health personnel; HIV seropositivity; human experimentation; informed consent; international aspects; investigators; justice; *preventive medicine; *professional ethics; professional organizations; *public health; random selection; research design; research ethics committees; risks and benefits; scientific misconduct; selection of subjects; self regulation; socioeconomic factors; violence; vulnerable populations; professional role; Tuskegee Syphilis Study; United States

Coughlin, Steven S. Implementing breast and cervical cancer prevention programs among the Houma Indians of southern Louisiana: cultural and ethical considerations. *Journal of Health Care for the Poor and Underserved.* 1998 Feb; 9(1): 30–41. 44 refs. BE58493.
    *American Indians; attitudes; autonomy; beneficence; *breast cancer; *cancer; confidentiality; *cultural pluralism; epidemiology; *females; health; *health services research; informed consent; *mass screening; *preventive medicine; public participation; research design; research subjects; risks and benefits; socioeconomic factors; vulnerable populations; ethnographic studies; qualitative research; Louisiana

Dalton, Rex. Collins' student sanctioned over 'most severe' case of fraud. [News]. *Nature.* 1997 Jul 24; 388(6640): 313. BE56069.
    biomedical research; federal government; genetic research; government regulation; *investigators; *scientific misconduct; *students; universities; Collins, Francis; *Hajra, Amitov; National Center for Human Genome Research; Office of Research Integrity; United States; University of Michigan

Dalton, Rex. Neuroscientist accused of misconduct turns on his accusers. [News]. *Nature.* 1998 Apr 2; 392(6675): 424. BE58021.
    *administrators; *biomedical research; federal government; fraud; government regulation; *investigators; *legal aspects; *legal liability; *medical schools; *scientific misconduct;

torts; universities; *Angelides, Kimon; *Baylor College of Medicine; National Institutes of Health; Office of Research Integrity

DeGroot, Leslie J.; St. Germain, Donald L.; Ridgway, E. Chester, et al. Bioequivalence of levothyroxine preparations: issues of science, publication, and advertising. [Letters and responses]. *JAMA.* 1997 Sep 17; 278(11): 895–900. 21 refs. BE55903.
    *advertising; alternatives; *biomedical research; coercion; conflict of interest; contracts; *drug industry; *drugs; *editorial policies; evaluation studies; *financial support; health services research; industry; *information dissemination; *investigators; legal aspects; managed care programs; organizational policies; peer review; proprietary health facilities; research design; scientific misconduct; self regulation; *Dong, Betty; *JAMA; Jones Medical Industries; *Knoll Pharmaceutical Co.; *Levoxyl; *Synthroid

Deichmann, Ute; Müller–Hill, Benno. The fraud of Abderhalden's enzymes. *Nature.* 1998 May 14; 393(6681): 109–111. 19 refs. BE58302.
    *biomedical research; cancer; communicable diseases; *diagnosis; eugenics; *fraud; genetics; historical aspects; human experimentation; investigators; moral complicity; National Socialism; pregnant women; prisoners; schizophrenia; *scientific misconduct; *sociology of medicine; whistleblowing; *Abderhalden, Emil; *Germany; Twentieth Century

Dresser, Rebecca. Scientists in the sunshine. *Hastings Center Report.* 1997 Nov–Dec; 27(6): 26–28. 11 refs. BE57857.
    *advisory committees; animal experimentation; *biomedical research; *committee membership; conflict of interest; *decision making; federal government; government financing; government regulation; guidelines; information dissemination; investigators; *legal aspects; legislation; private sector; *public participation; public policy; public sector; *science; *standards; Supreme Court decisions; technical expertise; values; *Animal Legal Defense Fund v. Shalala; *Federal Advisory Committee Act 1994; Guide for the Care and Use of Laboratory Animals (National Research Council); *National Academy of Sciences; Public Citizen v. U.S. Department of Justice; *United States

Dresser, Rebecca. Setting priorities for science support. *Hastings Center Report.* 1998 May–Jun; 28(3): 21–23. 7 fn. BE58609.
    accountability; administrators; *biomedical research; *decision making; *federal government; *government financing; investigators; justice; politics; professional autonomy; public participation; public policy; *resource allocation; science; *National Institutes of Health; *U.S. Congress; *United States

Dyer, Clare. Tobacco company set up network of sympathetic scientists. [News]. *BMJ (British Medical Journal).* 1998 May 23; 316(7144): 1555. BE58277.
    *biomedical research; *conflict of interest; editorial policies; *financial support; *industry; *international aspects; *investigators; legal aspects; research institutes; scientific misconduct; *smoking; Europe; Great Britain; *Philip Morris; United States

Edwards, Griffith. Should industry sponsor research? If the drinks industry does not clean up its act, pariah status is inevitable. *BMJ (British Medical Journal).* 1998 Aug 1; 317(7154): 336. 4 refs. BE58754.
    *alcohol abuse; *biomedical research; conflict of interest; *financial support; health hazards; *industry; investigators; Great Britain

Eisenberg, Rebecca S. Proprietary rights and the norms of science in biotechnology research. *Yale Law Journal.*

1987 Dec; 97(2): 177–231. 261 fn. BE56488.
 AIDS; *biomedical research; confidentiality; disclosure; editorial policies; federal government; financial support; government financing; incentives; industry; *information dissemination; investigators; *legal aspects; methods; microbiology; *patents; *property rights; *recombinant DNA research; *science; state government; Supreme Court decisions; transgenic organisms; universities; *values; Diamond v. Chakrabarty; Uniform Trade Secrets Act; *United States

Elliott, Deni. Case studies for teaching research ethics. *Professional Ethics.* 1995 Spring–Summer; 4(3–4): 179–198. 26 fn. References embedded in back-of-issue bibliography. BE55685.
 accountability; authorship; *biomedical research; *case studies; conflict of interest; *education; ethical analysis; financial support; fraud; industry; interprofessional relations; misconduct; *professional ethics; property rights; *science; *scientific misconduct; self regulation; students; *teaching methods; universities; whistleblowing

Elliott, Deni. Researchers as professionals, professionals as researchers: a context for laboratory research ethics. *Professional Ethics.* 1995 Spring–Summer; 4(3–4): 5–16. 8 fn. References embedded in back-of-issue bibliography. BE55686.
 biomedical research; common good; conflict of interest; consensus; deception; goals; health hazards; injuries; *investigators; *laboratories; moral obligations; *morality; obligations to society; *professional ethics; research subjects; *science; self regulation; values; community consent; journalism; rationality

Elliott, Deni; Blanford, Patricia; Watson, Marci, comps. Scientific research ethics videography. *Professional Ethics.* 1995 Spring–Summer; 4(3–4): 199–204. List of video titles with short summaries. BE55684.
 animal experimentation; *audiovisual aids; *bioethical issues; *biomedical research; education; genetic research; human experimentation; mass media; prenatal diagnosis; professional ethics; resource allocation; science; *scientific misconduct; teaching methods; United States

Endocrine Society. Ethical guidelines for publications of research. *Journal of Clinical Endocrinology and Metabolism.* 1996 Jan; 81(1): R1–R2. Guidelines prepared by the Publications Committee of the Endocrine Society and approved for publication and distribution by the Society's Council. BE57688.
 *authorship; biomedical research; due process; *editorial policies; *guidelines; information dissemination; investigators; peer review; professional organizations; *scientific misconduct; *publishing; *Endocrine Society

Evans, Imogen. Dealing with research misconduct in the United Kingdom: conduct unbecoming -- the MRC's approach. *BMJ (British Medical Journal).* 1998 Jun 6; 316(7146): 1728–1729. 1 ref. BE58206.
 biomedical research; confidentiality; deception; education; fraud; investigators; negligence; *regulation; *scientific misconduct; standards; *Great Britain; *Medical Research Council (Great Britain)

Farthing, Michael J.G. Dealing with research misconduct in the United Kingdom: an editor's response to fraudsters. *BMJ (British Medical Journal).* 1998 Jun 6; 316(7146): 1729–1731. 9 refs. BE58207.
 biomedical research; *editorial policies; fraud; international aspects; investigators; public health; *regulation; *scientific misconduct; self regulation; uncertainty; whistleblowing; Committee on Publication Ethics (Great Britain); Great Britain

Ferguson, James R. Biomedical research and insider trading. *New England Journal of Medicine.* 1997 Aug 28; 337(9): 631–634. 21 refs. BE59003.
 *biomedical research; *confidentiality; *conflict of interest; criminal law; *disclosure; *drug industry; drugs; *economics; fraud; human experimentation; *investigators; *legal aspects; *legal liability; *legal obligations; Supreme Court decisions; torts; Securities and Exchange Commission; *Securities Exchange Act 1934; *United States

Fischer, Beth A.; Zigmond, Michael J. Scientific publishing. *In:* Chadwick, Ruth, ed. Encyclopedia of Applied Ethics, Volume 4. San Diego, CA: Academic Press; 1998: 29–38. 7 refs. ISBN 0-12-227069-X. BE56344.
 authorship; biomedical research; confidentiality; *editorial policies; fraud; information dissemination; interprofessional relations; investigators; *peer review; *science; *scientific misconduct

Flanagin, Annette; Carey, Lisa A.; Fontanarosa, Phil B.; et al. Prevalence of articles with honorary authors and ghost authors in peer-reviewed medical journals. *JAMA.* 1998 Jul 15; 280(3): 222–224. 17 refs. BE58412.
 accountability; *authorship; *biomedical research; editorial policies; guidelines; *investigators; peer review; scientific misconduct; *standards; statistics; survey; guideline adherence; *publishing; *American Journal of Cardiology; *American Journal of Medicine; *American Journal of Obstetrics and Gynecology; *Annals of Internal Medicine; *JAMA; *New England Journal of Medicine; United States
 CONTEXT: Authorship in biomedical publications establishes accountability, responsibility, and credit. Misappropriation of authorship undermines the integrity of the authorship system, but accurate data on its prevalence are limited. OBJECTIVES: To determine the prevalence of articles with honorary authors (named authors who have not met authorship criteria) and ghost authors (individuals not named as authors but who contributed substantially to the work) in peer-reviewed medical journals and to identify journal characteristics and article types associated with such authorship misappropriation. DESIGN: Mailed, self-administered, confidential survey. PARTICIPANTS: A total of 809 corresponding authors (1179 surveyed, 69% response rate) of articles published in 1996 in 3 peer-reviewed, large-circulation general medical journals (Annals of Internal Medicine, JAMA, and The New England Journal of Medicine) and 3 peer-reviewed, smaller-circulation journals that publish supplements (American Journal of Cardiology, American Journal of Medicine, and American Journal of Obstetrics and Gynecology). MAIN OUTCOME MEASURES: Prevalence of articles with honorary authors and ghost authors, as reported by corresponding authors. RESULTS: Of the 809 articles, 492 were original research reports, 240 were reviews and articles not reporting original data, and 77 were editorials. A total of 156 articles (1 9%) had evidence of honorary authors (range, 11%–25% among journals); 93 articles (11%) had evidence of ghost authors (range, 7%–16% among journals); and 13 articles (2%) had evidence of both. The prevalence of articles with honorary authors was greater among review articles than research articles (odds ratio [OR], 1.8; 95% confidence interval [CI], 1.2–2.6) but did not differ significantly between large-circulation and smaller-circulation journals (OR, 1.4; 95% CI, 0.96–2.03). Compared with similar-type articles in large-circulation journals, articles with ghost authors in smaller-circulation journals were more likely to be reviews (OR, 4.2; 95% CI, 1.5–13.5) and less likely to be research articles (OR, 0.49; 95% CI, 0.27–0.88).

BE = bioethics accession number   fn. = footnotes   refs. = references

CONCLUSION: A substantial proportion of articles in peer-reviewed medical journals demonstrate evidence of honorary authors or ghost authors.

Frankel, M.S. Developing ethical standards for responsible research: why? form? functions? process? outcomes? *Journal of Dental Research.* 1996 Feb; 75(2): 832–835. 6 refs. Paper presented at the symposium, "Toward Responsible Research Conduct: The Role of Scientific Societies," during the annual meeting of the American Association for Dental Research, held in San Antonio, TX, Mar 1995. BE56461.
> accountability; biomedical research; *codes of ethics; decision making; *dentistry; education; *investigators; professional autonomy; *professional ethics; *professional organizations; *science; *scientific misconduct; *self regulation; *standards; dental research; American Association for Dental Research

Freedman, Monroe H.; Hoenig, Leonard J.; Spiro, Howard M., et al. Nazi research: too evil to cite. [Letters]. *Hastings Center Report.* 1985 Aug; 15(4): 31–32. BE57827.
> animal experimentation; *biomedical research; *editorial policies; historical aspects; *human experimentation; killing; moral complicity; *National Socialism; research subjects; *scientific misconduct; torture; utilitarianism; Germany; Twentieth Century

Goldbeck–Wood, Sandra. Scientists call for whistleblowers' charter. [News]. *BMJ (British Medical Journal).* 1997 Nov 15; 315(7118): 1252. BE56914.
> biomedical research; *editorial policies; fraud; investigators; regulation; *scientific misconduct; *whistleblowing; *Committee on Publication Ethics (Great Britain); *Great Britain

Green, Charles R.; Barnes, Deborah E.; Bero, Lisa A. Industry-funded research and conflict of interest: funding by the Center for Indoor Air Research [title supplied]. [Letter and response]. *Journal of Health Politics, Policy and Law.* 1997 Oct; 22(5): 1279–1293. 21 refs. BE58260.
> *biomedical research; *conflict of interest; *financial support; *health hazards; *industry; *investigators; peer review; research design; research institutes; *smoking; *Center for Indoor Air Research; R.J. Reynolds Tobacco Co.; United States

Grinnell, Frederick. Truth, fairness, and the definition of scientific misconduct. *Journal of Laboratory and Clinical Medicine.* 1997 Feb; 129(2): 189–192. 18 refs. BE57515.
> advisory committees; biomedical research; deception; fraud; *investigators; methods; *science; *scientific misconduct; self regulation; terminology; Commission on Research Integrity; United States

Hannum, Hurst. Should industry sponsor research? Condemning the drinks industry rules out potentially useful research. *BMJ (British Medical Journal).* 1998 Aug 1; 317(7154): 335–336. BE58753.
> *alcohol abuse; *biomedical research; conflict of interest; disclosure; *financial support; government financing; health hazards; *industry; investigators; public health; regulation; Great Britain; United States

Hedley, A.J.; Whidden, Phillip. The tobacco industry and scientific publications. [Letters]. *BMJ (British Medical Journal).* 1997 May 3; 314(7090): 1350–1351. 7 refs. BE55910.
> *biomedical research; *conflict of interest; disclosure; epidemiology; *financial support; *health hazards; *industry; *investigators; morbidity; mortality; *smoking

Heller, Michael A.; Eisenberg, Rebecca S. Can patents deter innovation? The anticommons in biomedical research. *Science.* 1998 May 1; 280(5364): 698–701. 40 fn. BE58036.
> *biomedical research; DNA sequences; drug industry; economics; *genome mapping; industry; legal aspects; *patents; private sector; *property rights; public sector; *social impact; United States

The "tragedy of the commons" metaphor helps explain why people overuse shared resources. However, the recent proliferation of intellectual property rights in biomedical research suggests a different tragedy, an "anticommons" in which people underuse scarce resources because too many owners can block each other. Privatization of biomedical research must be more carefully deployed to sustain both upstream research and downstream product development. Otherwise, more intellectual property rights may lead paradoxically to fewer useful products for improving human health.

Holden, Constance. Tricky ethics of tissue samples. [News]. *Science.* 1998 Mar 13; 279(5357): 1621. BE57779.
> advisory committees; *biomedical research; blood donation; body parts and fluids; *donors; guidelines; informed consent; legal rights; *public policy; stigmatization; *tissue donation; *community consent; *National Bioethics Advisory Commission; United States

Horton, Richard. ICRF: from mayhem to meltdown. *Lancet.* 1997 Oct 11; 350(9084): 1043–1044. BE56927.
> *biomedical research; *breast cancer; *conflict of interest; editorial policies; epidemiology; females; *financial support; *hormones; *human experimentation; *information dissemination; investigators; mass media; organizational policies; *risk; women's health; *estrogen replacement therapy; *Great Britain; *Imperial Cancer Research Fund; Lancet

Horton, Richard. Sponsorship, authorship, and a tale of two media. *Lancet.* 1997 May 17; 349(9063): 1411–1412. 4 refs. BE56307.
> advertising; authorship; *biomedical research; computer communication networks; *conflict of interest; disclosure; drug industry; *editorial policies; financial support; *guidelines; investigators; professional organizations; *standards; *journalism; *International Committee of Medical Journal Editors; Internet; Lancet

Horton, Richard. The unmasked carnival of science. [Commentary]. *Lancet.* 1998 Mar 7; 351(9104): 688–689. 15 refs. BE58852.
> *authorship; *biomedical research; disclosure; *editorial policies; guidelines; institutional policies; international aspects; investigators; public participation; scientific misconduct; universities; guideline adherence

Horton, Richard. Will the UK COPE? [Letter]. *Lancet.* 1997 Jul 26; 350(9073): 234. 9 refs. BE56154.
> advisory committees; biomedical research; *editorial policies; *scientific misconduct; *self regulation; *Committee on Publication Ethics (Great Britain); *Great Britain

Jacobsen, Geir; Hals, Arild. Medical investigators' views about ethics and fraud in medical research. *Journal of the Royal College of Physicians of London.* 1995 Sep–Oct; 29(5): 405–409. 20 refs. BE55562.
> advisory committees; age factors; *attitudes; *biomedical research; *ethical review; evaluation; females; *fraud; freedom; historical aspects; human experimentation; information dissemination; *investigators; *knowledge, attitudes, practice; males; medical ethics; physicians; professional autonomy; professional ethics; regional ethics committees; *regulation; *research design; *research ethics committees; retrospective moral judgment; science;

BE = bioethics accession number   fn. = footnotes   refs. = references

*scientific misconduct; *self regulation; statistics; survey; trends; *Norway; Twentieth Century

Johnson, Timothy. Shattuck lecture -- medicine and the media. *New England Journal of Medicine.* 1998 Jul 9; 339(2): 87–92. 12 refs. Presented as the 108th Shattuck Lecture to the Annual Meeting of the Massachusetts Medical Society, Boston, 9 May 1998. BE58613.
advertising; *biomedical research; biomedical technologies; conflict of interest; disclosure; economics; *editorial policies; entrepreneurship; famous persons; health; health care; *information dissemination; *mass media; *medicine; peer review; physician's role; physicians; professional competence; technical expertise; time factors; publishing; New England Journal of Medicine; United States

Jones, R. Scott; Fletcher, John C. Self-regulation of surgical practice and research. *In:* McCullough, Laurence B.; Jones, James W.; Brody, Baruch A., eds. Surgical Ethics. New York, NY: Oxford University Press; 1998: 255–279. 63 refs. ISBN 0-19-510347-5. BE58328.
*accountability; animal experimentation; authorship; beneficence; *biomedical research; conflict of interest; continuing education; economics; *goals; government regulation; guidelines; historical aspects; human experimentation; incentives; interprofessional relations; managed care programs; medical ethics; *medicine; *moral obligations; patient advocacy; peer review; physician patient relationship; *physicians; professional autonomy; professional competence; professional organizations; review; scientific misconduct; *self regulation; *surgery; whistleblowing; integrity; medical errors; physician impairment; United States

Jones, Roger; Murphy, Elizabeth; Crosland, Ann. Primary care research ethics. *British Journal of General Practice.* 1995 Nov; 45(400): 623–626. 16 refs. BE56868.
confidentiality; data banks; *epidemiology; *family practice; *health services research; information dissemination; informed consent; investigator subject relationship; patients; physician patient relationship; *primary health care; research design; selection of subjects; qualitative research; questionnaires; Great Britain

Kaiser, Jocelyn. British editors form misconduct panel. [News]. *Science.* 1997 Aug 1; 277(5326): 627. BE56330.
biomedical research; *editorial policies; government regulation; information dissemination; *scientific misconduct; *self regulation; *journalism; *Committee on Publication Ethics (Great Britain); Great Britain

Kaiser, Jocelyn. Fisher wins $2.75 million settlement. [News]. *Science.* 1997 Sep 5; 277(5331): 1425. BE56077.
biomedical research; cancer; *compensation; due process; federal government; fraud; *investigators; legal aspects; *scientific misconduct; universities; *Fisher, Bernard; National Cancer Institute; National Surgical Adjuvant Breast and Bowel Project; United States; University of Pittsburgh

Kaiser, Jocelyn. Privacy rules set no new research curbs. [News]. *Science.* 1997 Sep 19; 277(5333): 1757. BE56210.
*biomedical research; *confidentiality; drug industry; epidemiology; federal government; *government regulation; guidelines; informed consent; *medical records; *privacy; research subjects; state government; *United States

Kaiser, Jocelyn. Tobacco consultants find letters lucrative. [News]. *Science.* 1998 Aug 14; 281(5379): 895, 897. BE58877.
*biomedical research; *conflict of interest; *disclosure; *editorial policies; *financial support; health hazards; *industry; *investigators; physicians; *smoking; United States

Kiernan, Vincent. Truth is no longer its own reward. [News]. *New Scientist.* 1997 Mar 1; 153(2071): 11. BE55536.
*biomedical research; *conflict of interest; disclosure; editorial policies; *entrepreneurship; faculty; *financial support; industry; *investigators; patents; universities; Massachusetts; United States

Koenig, Robert. Panel calls falsification in German case 'unprecedented.' [News]. *Science.* 1997 Aug 15; 277(5328): 894. BE56065.
authorship; biomedical research; *fraud; gene therapy; genetic research; investigators; peer review; *scientific misconduct; self regulation; standards; universities; *Brach, Marion; *Germany; *Herrmann, Friedhelm; University of Ulm

Koenig, Robert. Panel proposes ways to combat fraud. [News]. *Science.* 1997 Dec 19; 278(5346): 2049–2050. BE56872.
biomedical research; financial support; *fraud; investigators; research institutes; *scientific misconduct; *self regulation; standards; universities; Brach, Marion; *Deutsche Forschungsgemeinschaft; *Germany; Herrmann, Friedhelm; *Max Planck Society

Korenman, Stanley G.; Berk, Richard; Wenger, Neil S., et al. Evaluation of the research norms of scientists and administrators responsible for academic research integrity. *JAMA.* 1998 Jan 7; 279(1): 41–47. 28 refs. BE57816.
*administrators; *attitudes; authorship; biomedical research; comparative studies; *conflict of interest; financial support; fraud; industry; *information dissemination; interprofessional relations; *investigators; *professional ethics; punishment; *scientific misconduct; survey; universities; *research ethics; United States

CONTEXT: The professional integrity of scientists is important to society as a whole and particularly to disciplines such as medicine that depend heavily on scientific advances for their progress. OBJECTIVE: To characterize the professional norms of active scientists and compare them with those of individuals with institutional responsibility for the conduct of research. DESIGN: A mailed survey consisting of 12 scenarios in 4 domains of research ethics. Respondents were asked whether an act was unethical and, if so, the degree to which they considered it unethical and to select responses and punishments for the act. PARTICIPANTS: A total of 924 National Science Foundation research grantees in 1993 or 1994 in molecular or cellular biology and 140 representatives from the researchers' institutions to the US Department of Health and Human Services Office of Research Integrity. MAIN OUTCOME MEASURES: Percentage of respondents considering an act unethical and the mean malfeasance rating on a scale of 1 to 10. RESULTS: A total of 606 research grantees and 91 institutional representatives responded to the survey (response rate of 69% of those who could be contacted). Respondents reported a hierarchy of unethical research behaviors. The mean malfeasance rating was unrelated to the characteristics of the investigator performing the hypothetical act or to its consequences. Fabrication, falsification, and plagiarism received malfeasance ratings higher than 8.6, and virtually all thought they were unethical. Deliberately misleading statements about a paper or failure to give proper attribution received ratings between 7 and 8. Sloppiness, oversights, conflicts of interest, and failure to share were less serious still, receiving malfeasance ratings between 5 and 6. Institutional representatives proposed more and different

---

BE = bioethics accession number   fn. = footnotes   refs. = references

interventions and punishments than the scientists. CONCLUSIONS: Surveyed scientists and institutional representatives had strong and similar norms of professional behavior, but differed in their approaches to an unethical act.

Krimsky, Sheldon; Rothenberg, L.S. Financial interest and its disclosure in scientific publications. *JAMA.* 1998 Jul 15; 280(3): 225–226. 18 refs. BE58418.
    *biomedical research; *conflict of interest; *disclosure; *economics; *editorial policies; entrepreneurship; *financial support; industry; *investigators
Journal policies and requirements of funding agencies on financial disclosure of authors and grant applicants have divided editors and scientists who disagree on whether such policies can improve the integrity of science or manage conflicts of interest. Those opposed to such disclosure policies argue that financial interest is one of many interests held by scientists, is the least scientifically dangerous, and should not be singled out. Those who favor open reporting of financial interests argue that full disclosure removes the suspicion that something of relevance to objectivity is being hidden and allows readers to form their own opinions on whether a conflict of interest exists and what relevance that has to the study. The authors believe that the scientific community and the public will be best served by open publication of financial disclosures for readers and reviewers to evaluate.

LaFollette, Marcel C. The pathology of research fraud: the history and politics of the US experience. *Journal of Internal Medicine.* 1994 Feb; 235(2): 129–135. 29 refs. BE55603.
    biomedical research; federal government; *fraud; government financing; *government regulation; historical aspects; institutional policies; investigators; *politics; research institutes; science; *scientific misconduct; self regulation; universities; whistleblowing; National Institutes of Health; U.S. Congress; *United States

Laurie, Graeme T. Biotechnology and intellectual property: a marriage of inconvenience? *In:* McLean, Sheila A.M., ed. Contemporary Issues in Law, Medicine and Ethics. Brookfield, VT: Dartmouth; 1996: 237–267. 151 fn. ISBN 1-85521-586-1. BE57798.
    *biomedical research; biomedical technologies; body parts and fluids; DNA sequences; donors; genome mapping; guidelines; human body; *industry; informed consent; international aspects; investigators; *legal aspects; *morality; *patents; property rights; *recombinant DNA research; standards; Supreme Court decisions; tissue donation; transgenic animals; cell lines; Diamond v. Chakrabarty; *Europe; European Patent Convention; European Patent Office; *Great Britain; Moore v. Regents of the University of California; National Institutes of Health; Patent and Trademark Office; *United States

Lock, Stephen. Research misconduct: a brief history and a comparison. *Journal of Internal Medicine.* 1994 Feb; 235(2): 123–127. 16 refs. BE55602.
    authorship; biomedical research; editorial policies; *fraud; historical aspects; human experimentation; institutional policies; international aspects; investigators; physicians; regulation; research ethics committees; research institutes; science; *scientific misconduct; universities; Great Britain; United States

Lowrance, William W. Privacy and Health Research: A Report to the U.S. Secretary of Health and Human Services. Washington, DC: U.S. Department of Health and Human Services, Office of the Assistant Secretary for Planning and Evaluation; 1997 May. 80 p. 125 fn.

BE58644.
    biomedical research; communicable diseases; computers; *confidentiality; data banks; disclosure; economics; *epidemiology; genetic research; government regulation; guidelines; *health services research; human experimentation; informed consent; *international aspects; legal aspects; legislation; mandatory reporting; medical records; organization and administration; *privacy; private sector; public health; public policy; *records; registries; research ethics committees; research subjects; computer security; *Council of Europe; *Europe; *United States

Lucas, Alan. Should industry sponsor research? Collaborative research with infant formula companies should not always be censored. *BMJ (British Medical Journal).* 1998 Aug 1; 317(7154): 337–338. 12 refs. BE58755.
    *biomedical research; developing countries; *financial support; *food; *industry; *infants; international aspects; nutrition; risks and benefits

McCarthy, Michael. Conflict of interest highlighted in debate on calcium–channel blockers. [News]. *Lancet.* 1998 Jan 17; 351(9097): 191. BE57776.
    *biomedical research; *conflict of interest; disclosure; *drug industry; *drugs; economics; *financial support; *investigators

Macilwain, Colin. Scientists defy their ethics codes and take gifts from industry. [News]. *Nature.* 1998 Apr 2; 392(6675): 427. BE58022.
    *biomedical research; *conflict of interest; *gifts; *industry; information dissemination; institutional policies; *investigators; misconduct; property rights; survey; universities; United States

Mandel, I.D. On being a scientist in a rapidly changing world. *Journal of Dental Research.* 1996 Feb; 75(2): 841–844. 18 refs. Paper presented at the symposium, "Toward Responsible Research Conduct: The Role of Scientific Societies," during the annual meeting of the American Association for Dental Research, held in San Antonio, TX, Mar 1995. BE56471.
    animal experimentation; biological warfare; *biomedical research; dentistry; economics; entrepreneurship; federal government; goals; government regulation; health hazards; *historical aspects; industry; *investigators; microbiology; political activity; *professional ethics; recombinant DNA research; research ethics committees; *science; scientific misconduct; self regulation; trends; universities; values; dental research; Twentieth Century; United States

Marshall, Eliot. Medline searches turn up cases of suspected plagiarism. [News]. *Science.* 1998 Jan 23; 279(5350): 473–474. Includes inset article, "The Internet: a powerful tool for plagiarism sleuths," p. 474. BE56877.
    authorship; biomedical research; computer communication networks; data banks; *fraud; international aspects; investigators; literature; regulation; *scientific misconduct; Denmark; Internet; *Jendryczko, Andrzej; MEDLINE; *Poland

Marshall, Eliot. Need a reagent? Just sign here. [News]. *Science.* 1997 Oct 10; 278(5336): 212–213. Includes inset article by E. Marshall, "Devilish details," p. 213. BE56312.
    *biomedical research; *contracts; DNA sequences; drugs; guidelines; *industry; *information dissemination; institutional policies; international aspects; interprofessional relations; investigators; patents; *property rights; regulation; *universities; *biological materials; National Institutes of Health; United States; University of California, San Francisco

---

BE = bioethics accession number   fn. = footnotes   refs. = references

Martin, Judith; Stent, Gunther S. Bioetiquette. *Perspectives in Biology and Medicine.* 1998 Winter; 41(2): 267–281. 11 refs. BE59029.

> *authorship; *biomedical research; ethics; guidelines; historical aspects; *information dissemination; *interprofessional relations; *investigators; law; *medical etiquette; morality; *peer review; *professional ethics; regulation; *science; scientific misconduct; smoking; *social interaction

Melton, L. Joseph. The threat to medical–records research. *New England Journal of Medicine.* 1997 Nov 13; 337(20): 1466–1470. 38 refs. BE56431.

> autonomy; *biomedical research; common good; *confidentiality; *disclosure; *epidemiology; *government regulation; health services research; hospitals; informed consent; legislation; *medical records; privacy; quality of health care; regulation; research design; research subjects; *risks and benefits; social impact; state government; treatment outcome; Mayo Clinic; Minnesota

Mitchell, Peter. Drug industry lobbies against European research–data directive. [News]. *Lancet.* 1997 May 10; 349(9062): 1378. BE56414.

> *biomedical research; *confidentiality; drug industry; epidemiology; human experimentation; informed consent; *international aspects; *medical records; *regulation; self regulation; *Europe; European Federation of Pharmaceutical Industries' Associations; *European Union

Noble, Denis; Vincent, Jean–Didier. The Ethics of Life. Paris: Unesco; 1997. 238 p. Bibliography: p. 221–230. Papers presented at a seminar "Physiology and the Respect for Life," held under the joint auspices of the International Union of Physical Scientists and Unesco in Paris, Sep 1995. ISBN 92-3-103422-7. BE58647.

> *animal experimentation; *animal rights; attitudes to death; beginning of life; behavioral research; *bioethical issues; bioethics; *biomedical research; brain death; Buddhist ethics; competence; determination of death; education; embryo research; females; fetal research; genetic determinism; homosexuals; human experimentation; *human rights; humanism; informed consent; international aspects; legal aspects; moral obligations; *moral policy; nontherapeutic research; organ donation; personhood; philosophy; political activity; prisoners; regulation; research ethics committees; research subjects; risks and benefits; science; speciesism; suffering; therapeutic research; *value of life; vulnerable populations; Europe; Japan

Olson, Carin M.; Glass, Richard M.; Thacker, Stephen B., et al. Ethical issues in studying submissions to a medical journal. *JAMA.* 1998 Jul 15; 280(3): 290–291. 4 refs. BE58423.

> *authorship; *biomedical research; confidentiality; *editorial policies; informed consent; *investigators; *peer review; *publishing; *JAMA

A protocol to prospectively study characteristics of meta-analyses submitted to a weekly medical journal raised several ethical issues. In submitting a manuscript for publication, authors do not implicitly consent to have their work used for research. Authors must be free to refuse to consent, without it affecting their chances for publication. Systematically analyzing data on manuscript characteristics might influence the decision to publish. Having investigators who are not on the editorial staff or peer reviewers extract the manuscripts' characteristics breaks the confidentiality of the author–editor–reviewer relationship. In response to these issues, we added a statement to our journal's instructions for authors that submitted manuscripts may be systematically analyzed to improve the quality of the editorial or peer review process. Authors had to actively consent to participate, but editors and external reviewers were unaware of which authors were participating. The manuscript characteristics were not shared with authors, editors, or external reviewers. The investigators were blinded to each manuscript's author and institution. After we addressed ethical issues encountered in studying manuscripts submitted to a medical journal, 99 of 105 authors submitting a meta-analysis during the study's first 24 months agreed to participate.

Parnham, Michael J. Ethical Issues in Drug Research: Through a Glass Darkly. Washington, DC: IOS Press; 1996. 155 p. Includes references. ISBN 90-5199-279-3. BE55677.

> advertising; animal experimentation; attitudes; *biomedical research; conscience; deception; developing countries; drug industry; *drugs; freedom; genetic research; government regulation; health; hormones; human experimentation; human rights; information dissemination; international aspects; investigators; pain; patents; patient care; psychoactive drugs; quality of life; research design; *risks and benefits; science; toxicity; universities; utilitarianism

Plant, Martin; Plant, Moira; Vernon, Bryan. Ethics, funding and alcohol research. *Alcohol and Alcoholism.* 1996 Jan; 31(1): 17–25. 36 refs. BE55770.

> *alcohol abuse; *behavioral research; *biomedical research; codes of ethics; *conflict of interest; disclosure; economics; editorial policies; *financial support; government financing; guidelines; industry; information dissemination; *investigators; peer review; *professional ethics; science; scientific misconduct; *self regulation; social sciences; universities; values; whistleblowing

Poste, George; Roberts, David; Gentry, Simon. Patents, ethics and improving healthcare. *Bulletin of Medical Ethics.* 1997 Jan; No. 124: 29–31. BE55745.

> *biomedical research; *drug industry; drugs; economics; genes; *genetic materials; health care; hormones; international aspects; legal aspects; *patents; risks and benefits

Powers, Madison. Theories of justice in the context of research. *In:* Kahn, Jeffrey P.; Mastroianni, Anna C.; Sugarman, Jeremy, eds. Beyond Consent: Seeking Justice in Research. New York, NY: Oxford University Press; 1998: 147–165. 26 fn. ISBN 0-19-511353-5. BE58848.

> age factors; AIDS; autonomy; *biomedical research; critically ill; decision making; developing countries; disadvantaged; ecology; economics; emergency care; females; freedom; health care delivery; *human experimentation; informed consent; *justice; libertarianism; military personnel; *moral policy; nontherapeutic research; occupational medicine; political activity; prisoners; *public policy; research design; research ethics committees; research subjects; *resource allocation; *risks and benefits; selection of subjects; social discrimination; vulnerable populations; United States

Proctor, Christopher J. Should industry sponsor research? Tobacco industry research: collaboration, not confrontation, is the best approach. *BMJ (British Medical Journal).* 1998 Aug 1; 317(7154): 333–334. 2 refs. BE58751.

> *biomedical research; *financial support; health hazards; *industry; peer review; public health; *smoking; BAT Industries [British American Tobacco]; Great Britain

Rennie, Drummond. Dealing with research misconduct in the United Kingdom: an American perspective on research integrity. *BMJ (British Medical Journal).* 1998 Jun 6; 316(7146): 1726–1728. 9 refs. BE58217.

> biomedical research; federal government; fraud; government financing; government regulation; institutional policies; international aspects; investigators; motivation; *regulation;

BE = bioethics accession number   fn. = footnotes   refs. = references

*scientific misconduct; self regulation; whistleblowing; *Great Britain; Office of Research Integrity; *United States

Riis, Povl. Dealing with research misconduct in the United Kingdom: honest advice from Denmark. *BMJ (British Medical Journal).* 1998 Jun 6; 316(7146): 1733. BE58218.
advisory committees; authorship; biomedical research; committee membership; fraud; international aspects; investigators; organization and administration; *regulation; *scientific misconduct; whistleblowing; *national ethics committees; Denmark; *Great Britain

Riis, Povl. Prevention and management of fraud -- in theory. *Journal of Internal Medicine.* 1994 Feb; 235(2): 107–113. 3 refs. BE55608.
advisory committees; biomedical research; editorial policies; *fraud; international aspects; investigators; public participation; public policy; punishment; *regulation; research ethics committees; research institutes; science; *scientific misconduct; self regulation; standards; universities; whistleblowing; national ethics committees; Denmark

Rossignol, Annette MacKay; Goodmonson, Sharon. Are ethical topics in epidemiology included in the graduate epidemiology curricula? *American Journal of Epidemiology.* 1995 Dec 15; 142(12): 1265–1268. 38 refs. BE55523.
*attitudes; *curriculum; *education; *epidemiology; *faculty; human experimentation; investigators; *professional ethics; public health; schools; survey; teaching methods; United States

Rundall, Patti. Should industry sponsor research? How much research in infant feeding comes from unethical marketing? *BMJ (British Medical Journal).* 1998 Aug 1; 317(7154): 338–339. 3 refs. BE58756.
advertising; *biomedical research; conflict of interest; *financial support; *food; *industry; *infants; international aspects; investigators; nutrition; public health

Schiermeier, Quirin. Gene therapist accused of fraud to seek redress in German court. [News]. *Nature.* 1997 Sep 11; 389(6647): 105. BE56062.
biomedical research; *fraud; gene therapy; genetic research; interprofessional relations; investigators; *legal aspects; *scientific misconduct; universities; Brach, Marion; *Germany; *Herrmann, Friedhelm; University of Freiburg; University of Ulm

Silvestrini, Bruno. Respect for life and biomedical research. *Dolentium Hominum: Church and Health in the World.* 1996; 31(11th Yr., No. 1): 159–162. 6 refs. BE57375.
advisory committees; beginning of life; bioethical issues; biology; *biomedical research; education; evaluation; evolution; human characteristics; human rights; prolongation of life; public health; public policy; quality of life; religion; risks and benefits; Roman Catholic ethics; *value of life; values; Council of Europe

Smith, Richard. Beyond conflict of interest: transparency is the key. [Editorial]. *BMJ (British Medical Journal).* 1998 Aug 1; 317(7154): 291–292. 18 refs. BE58818.
accountability; *biomedical research; *conflict of interest; *disclosure; economics; *editorial policies; *financial support; *industry; *investigators; *physicians; *BMJ (British Medical Journal)

Smith, Richard. Conflict of interest in clinical research: opprobrium or obsession? [Letter]. *Lancet.* 1997 Jun 7; 349(9066): 1703. 2 refs. BE56564.
*biomedical research; *conflict of interest; *disclosure; economics; *editorial policies; financial support;

investigators; terminology; BMJ (British Medical Journal)

Smith, Richard. Informed consent: edging forwards (and backwards). [Editorial]. *BMJ (British Medical Journal).* 1998 Mar 28; 316(7136): 949–951. 17 refs. Includes the text of the *BMJ*'s guidelines for "Publishing information that emerges from the doctor–patient relationship." BE58067.
attitudes; *biomedical research; case studies; *confidentiality; death; *editorial policies; *guidelines; human experimentation; *informed consent; patient care; patients; physician patient relationship; privacy; research subjects; time factors; pedigree studies; photography; *BMJ (British Medical Journal); General Medical Council (Great Britain); International Committee of Medical Journal Editors

Smith, Richard. Misconduct in research: editors respond -- the Committee on Publication Ethics (COPE) is formed. [Editorial]. *BMJ (British Medical Journal).* 1997 Jul 26; 315(7102): 201–202. 8 refs. BE58501.
biomedical research; *editorial policies; fraud; investigators; *scientific misconduct; *self regulation; *Committee on Publication Ethics (Great Britain); Great Britain

Smith, Richard. The need for a national body for research misconduct: nothing less will reassure the public. [Editorial]. *BMJ (British Medical Journal).* 1998 Jun 6; 316(7146): 1686–1687. 12 refs. BE58221.
advisory committees; biomedical research; editorial policies; fraud; international aspects; *regulation; *scientific misconduct; self regulation; national ethics committees; Committee on Publication Ethics (Great Britain); *Great Britain

Sorell, Tom. Should industry sponsor research? Tobacco company sponsorship discredits medical but not all research. *BMJ (British Medical Journal).* 1998 Aug 1; 317(7154): 334. BE58752.
*biomedical research; conflict of interest; deception; *financial support; health hazards; *industry; investigators; risk; *smoking; BAT Industries [British American Tobacco]; Europe; United States

Spurgeon, David. Trials sponsored by drug companies: review ordered. [News]. *BMJ (British Medical Journal).* 1998 Sep 5; 317(7159): 618. BE59078.
*biomedical research; confidentiality; contracts; *disclosure; *drug industry; *drugs; *financial support; *hospitals; *human experimentation; *institutional policies; *investigators; livers; minors; *regulation; *thalassemia; therapeutic research; *toxicity; *Apotex; Canada; *deferiprone; *Hospital for Sick Children (Toronto); *Olivieri, Nancy

Stern, Jerome M.; Simes, R. John. Publication bias: evidence of delayed publication in a cohort study of clinical research projects. *BMJ (British Medical Journal).* 1997 Sep 13; 315(7109): 640–645. 27 refs. BE57251.
*biomedical research; *editorial policies; human experimentation; *information dissemination; investigators; registries; research design; statistics; survey; *time factors; *publication bias; qualitative research; quantitative research; Australia
OBJECTIVES: To determine the extent to which publication is influenced by study outcome. DESIGN: A cohort of studies submitted to a hospital ethics committee over 10 years were examined retrospectively by reviewing the protocols and by questionnaire. The primary method of analysis was Cox's proportional hazards model. SETTING: University hospital, Sydney, Australia. STUDIES: 748 eligible studies submitted to Royal Prince Alfred Hospital Ethics Committee between 1979 and 1988. MAIN OUTCOME MEASURES: Time

to publication. RESULTS: Response to the questionnaire was received for 520 (70%) of the eligible studies. Of the 218 studies analysed with tests of significance, those with positive results (P less than 0.05) were much more likely to be published than those with negative results (P greater than or = 0.10) (hazard ratio 2.32 (95% confidence interval 1.47 to 3.66), P = 0.0003), with a significantly shorter time to publication (median 4.8 v 8.0 years). This finding was even stronger for the group of 130 clinical trials (hazard ratio 3.13 (1.76 to 5.58), P = 0.0001), with median times to publication of 4.7 and 8.0 years respectively. These results were not materially changed after adjusting for other significant predictors of publication. Studies with indefinite conclusions (0.05 less than/= P less than 0.10) tended to have an even lower publication rate and longer time to publication than studies with negative results (hazard ratio 0.39 (0.13 to 1.12), P = 0.08). For the 103 studies in which outcome was rated qualitatively, there was no clear cut evidence of publication bias, although the number of studies in this group was not large. CONCLUSIONS: This study confirms the evidence of publication bias found in other studies and identifies delay in publication as an additional important factor. The study results support the need for prospective registration of trials to avoid publication bias and also support restricting the selection of trials to those started before a common date in undertaking systematic reviews.

Sternberg, S. Release of study ends drug fracas. [News]. *Science News.* 1997 Apr 19; 151(16): 236. BE56149.
*biomedical research; conflict of interest; contracts; *drug industry; *drugs; *financial support; *information dissemination; *investigators; peer review; universities; *Boots Pharmaceutical Ltd.; Dong, Betty; *Knoll Pharmaceutical Co.; *Synthroid; University of California, San Francisco

Strauss, Evelyn. The tissue issue: losing oneself to science? *Science News.* 1997 Sep 20; 152(12): 190–191. BE56635.
*biomedical research; cadavers; confidentiality; consent forms; federal government; genetic research; government financing; government regulation; human experimentation; *informed consent; property rights; research ethics committees; time factors; *tissue banks; *tissue donation; United States

Swazey, Judith P.; Bird, Stephanie J. Teaching and learning research ethics. *Professional Ethics.* 1995 Spring–Summer; 4(3–4): 155–178. 3 fn. References embedded in back–of–issue bibliography. BE55674.
adults; *biomedical research; *case studies; communication; *education; ethical analysis; ethics; faculty; goals; interprofessional relations; moral development; *professional ethics; science; scientific misconduct; students; *teaching methods; universities; values

U.S. Congress. Senate. Committee on Labor and Human Resources. Women's Health: Ensuring Quality and Equity in Biomedical Research. Hearing, 29 Jun 1992. Washington, DC: U.S. Government Printing Office; 1992. 48 p. S. Hrg. 102–1180. BE58949.
*biomedical research; cancer; diagnosis; drugs; federal government; *females; government financing; heart diseases; *human experimentation; males; morbidity; mortality; patient care; *public policy; research subjects; selection of subjects; social discrimination; *women's health; ovaries; National Institutes of Health; Office of Research on Women's Health; *United States; Women's Health Initiative

U.S. Department of Health and Human Services. Departmental Appeals Board. Research Integrity

Adjudications Panel. Mikulas Popovic, M.D., Ph.D. [Docket No. A–93–100; Decision No. 1446. 1993 Nov 3 (date of decision)]. Washington, DC: U.S. Department of Health and Human Services; 1993 Nov 3. 79+ p. Includes an additional 18 p. of appendices. BE57697.
AIDS; biomedical research; *due process; expert testimony; *federal government; government regulation; investigators; *legal aspects; *scientific misconduct; standards; Department of Health and Human Services; Departmental Appeals Board (DHHS); *Office of Research Integrity; *Popovic, Mikulas; Research Integrity Adjudications Panel (DHHS); Science; *United States

Vandenbroucke, Jan P. Maintaining privacy and the health of the public should not be seen as in opposition. [Editorial]. *BMJ (British Medical Journal).* 1998 May 2; 316(7141): 1331–1332. 12 refs. BE58602.
biomedical research; *confidentiality; editorial policies; *epidemiology; *government regulation; informed consent; international aspects; *medical records; *privacy; public health; risks and benefits; state government; retrospective studies; Europe; United States

Vanderpool, Harold Y. What's happening in research ethics? Commentary on Brody. *In:* Carson, Ronald A.; Burns, Chester R., eds. Philosophy of Medicine and Bioethics: A Twenty–Year Retrospective and Critical Appraisal. Boston, MA: Kluwer Academic; 1997: 287–297. 35 refs. 9 fn. ISBN 0–7923–3545–7. BE56543.
advisory committees; bioethical issues; bioethics; *biomedical research; drugs; education; *ethicist's role; ethicists; government regulation; *human experimentation; *literature; research design; research ethics committees; risks and benefits; scientific misconduct; *trends; *research ethics

Wadman, Meredith. Cancer 'cure' article stirs up hot debate. [News]. *Nature.* 1998 May 14; 393(6681): 104–105. Includes inset article, "Reporter backs away from lucrative book deal," p. 104. BE58431.
animal experimentation; *biomedical research; *cancer; *conflict of interest; *drugs; economics; *industry; investigators; *mass media; Folkman, Judah; Kolata, Gina; *New York Times; United States

Wadman, Meredith. $100m payout after drug data withheld. [News]. *Nature.* 1997 Aug 21; 388(6644): 703. BE56353.
*biomedical research; *compensation; contracts; costs and benefits; *drug industry; *drugs; economics; *financial support; human experimentation; *information dissemination; investigators; legal liability; *misconduct; patients; universities; Dong, Betty; *Knoll Pharmaceutical Co.; *Synthroid; United States; University of California, San Francisco

Walters, LeRoy. Research and experimentation: a response to Kevin Wildes's essay. *In:* Wildes, Kevin Wm.; Mitchell, Alan C., eds. Choosing Life: A Dialogue on *Evangelium Vitae*. Washington, DC: Georgetown University Press; 1997: 206–209. 1 fn. ISBN 0–87840–646–8. BE56690.
aborted fetuses; abortion, induced; *biomedical research; contraception; *embryo research; *fetal research; fetal tissue donation; gene therapy; killing; nontherapeutic research; research embryo creation; *Roman Catholic ethics; therapeutic research; tissue transplantation; value of life; Evangelium Vitae

Waters, W.E. Ethics and epidemiological research. *International Journal of Epidemiology.* 1985 Mar; 14(1): 48–51. 10 refs. BE56679.
*attitudes; *biomedical research; confidentiality; *epidemiology; *ethical review; health services research; *human experimentation; informed consent; *international

aspects; *investigators; random selection; research design; research ethics committees; research subjects; survey

Weil, Vivian; Arzbaecher, Robert. Ethics and relationships in laboratories and research communities. *Professional Ethics.* 1995 Spring–Summer; 4(3–4): 83–125. 17 fn. BE55673.
accountability; administrators; authorship; *biomedical research; *case studies; communication; confidentiality; conflict of interest; deception; *faculty; females; financial support; goals; *interprofessional relations; *investigators; *laboratories; minority groups; organization and administration; peer review; professional autonomy; *professional ethics; property rights; *science; *scientific misconduct; self regulation; social control; social dominance; standards; *students; trust; values; Gallo, Robert; National Institutes of Health; Popovic, Mikulas; United States

Wells, Frank O. Management of research misconduct -- in practice. *Journal of Internal Medicine.* 1994 Feb; 235(2): 115–121. 10 refs. BE55606.
biomedical research; *drug industry; financial support; *fraud; guidelines; human experimentation; investigators; medical education; motivation; *organizational policies; *physicians; punishment; *regulation; review committees; *scientific misconduct; Association of the British Pharmaceutical Industry; General Medical Council (Great Britain); *Great Britain; WHO Guidelines for Good Clinical Practice (GCP) for Trials on Pharmaceutical Products

Werhane, Patricia; Doering, Jeffrey. Conflicts of interest and conflicts of commitment. *Professional Ethics.* 1995 Spring–Summer; 4(3–4): 47–81. 4 fn. BE55672.
accountability; administrators; *biomedical research; case studies; codes of ethics; *conflict of interest; disclosure; editorial policies; financial support; genome mapping; industry; information dissemination; institutional policies; interprofessional relations; *investigators; patents; *professional ethics; professional organizations; property rights; research subjects; *scientific misconduct; *self regulation; standards; trust; universities

Whitbeck, Caroline. Research ethics. *In:* Chadwick, Ruth, ed. Encyclopedia of Applied Ethics, Volume 3. San Diego, CA: Academic Press; 1998: 835–843. 13 refs. ISBN 0–12–227068–1. BE56270.
authorship; *biomedical research; editorial policies; faculty; federal government; fraud; government regulation; information dissemination; interprofessional relations; investigators; peer review; professional ethics; professional organizations; *scientific misconduct; self regulation; students; universities; United States

White, Caroline. Call for research misconduct agency. [News]. *BMJ (British Medical Journal).* 1998 Jun 6; 316(7146): 1695. BE58247.
biomedical research; editorial policies; fraud; guidelines; human experimentation; investigators; *regulation; *scientific misconduct; standards; whistleblowing; Committee on Publication Ethics (Great Britain); *Great Britain

Wigzell, Hans; Pontén, Jan. Refutation of investigation commissioned by Karolinska Institute. [Letter]. *Lancet.* 1998 May 16; 351(9114): 1510–1511. 3 refs. BE58856.
biomedical research; fraud; investigators; peer review; research institutes; *scientific misconduct; self regulation; *Karolinska Institute; Lönn, Ulf; *Sweden

Wildes, Kevin Wm. In the service of life: Evangelium Vitae and medical research. *In:* Wildes, Kevin Wm.; Mitchell, Alan C., eds. Choosing Life: A Dialogue on *Evangelium Vitae.* Washington, DC: Georgetown University Press; 1997: 186–198. 26 fn. ISBN

0–87840–646–8. BE56688.
autonomy; beginning of life; beneficence; *biomedical research; coercion; common good; deontological ethics; *embryo research; embryos; fetuses; human rights; informed consent; killing; moral obligations; nontherapeutic research; personhood; *Roman Catholic ethics; *theology; therapeutic research; *value of life; dignity; *Evangelium Vitae; Instruction on Respect for Human Life

Williams, Nigel. Editors call for misconduct watchdog. [News]. *Science.* 1998 Jun 12; 280(5370): 1685–1686. BE58272.
biomedical research; editorial policies; ethical review; fraud; investigators; *regulation; *scientific misconduct; Committee on Publication Ethics (Great Britain); General Medical Council (Great Britain); *Great Britain

Williams, Nigel. Editors seek ways to cope with fraud. [News]. *Science.* 1997 Nov 14; 278(5341): 1221. BE56893.
biomedical research; *editorial policies; fraud; *international aspects; investigators; *scientific misconduct; whistleblowing; *Committee on Publication Ethics (Great Britain); Deutsche Forschungsgemeinschaft; *Europe; Max Planck Society

Wise, Jacqui. Research suppressed for seven years by drug company. [News]. *BMJ (British Medical Journal).* 1997 Apr 19; 314(7088): 1145. BE56774.
*biomedical research; contracts; *drug industry; *drugs; editorial policies; federal government; *financial support; government regulation; *information dissemination; *investigators; legal aspects; research design; universities; *Boots Pharmaceuticals Ltd.; *Dong, Betty; Food and Drug Administration; JAMA; Knoll Pharmaceutical Co.; *Synthroid; United States

Youngner, Julius S. The scientific misconduct process: a scientist's view from the inside. *JAMA.* 1998 Jan 7; 279(1): 62–64. 7 refs. BE57815.
biomedical research; *due process; federal government; *government regulation; investigators; lawyers; legal aspects; *peer review; science; *scientific misconduct; Department of Health and Human Services; *Office of Research Integrity; *Research Integrity Adjudications Panel (DHHS); *United States

A time for responsibility. [Editorial]. *Nature.* 1997 Dec 4; 390(6659): 427. BE57271.
accountability; bioethics; *biomedical research; *ethical review; financial support; freedom; *international aspects; investigators; public policy; science; social impact; *Europe; *European Commission

Integrity in Scientific Research. [Videorecording].American Association for the Advancement of Science; available for sale from Science Integrity Videos, AAAS Directorate for Science and Policy Programs, 1200 New York Ave., NW, Washington, DC 20005, 202–326–6600; 1996. 5 videocassettes; 44 min. (8–10 min. each); sd.; color; 1/2 in.; VHS. Produced by Amram Nowak Associates, Inc. for the AAAS in cooperation with the Medical College of Georgia's Division of Health Communication; directed by Stuart Hersh; written and produced by Manya Starr. Accompanied by a 50–page Discussion and Resource Guide. BE57897.
animal experimentation; *authorship; *biomedical research; case studies; *conflict of interest; contracts; disclosure; *financial support; *industry; *information dissemination; *investigators; peer review; professional ethics; psychological stress; *scientific misconduct; universities; whistleblowing; publication bias; *research ethics

---

BE = bioethics accession number   fn. = footnotes   refs. = references

BIOMEDICAL TECHNOLOGIES

See also HEALTH CARE, ORGAN AND TISSUE
TRANSPLANTATION, REPRODUCTIVE
TECHNOLOGIES
See also under
RESOURCE ALLOCATION/BIOMEDICAL
TECHNOLOGIES

Alpert, Sheri A. Health care information: access,
confidentiality, and good practice. *In:* Goodman,
Kenneth W., ed. Ethics, Computing, and Medicine:
Informatics and the Transformation of Health Care.
New York, NY: Cambridge University Press; 1998:
75–101. 64 refs. ISBN 0–521–46905–8. BE57005.
*computer communication networks; *computers;
*confidentiality; data banks; *disclosure; drug industry;
economics; employment; genetic information; government
regulation; *health care; health insurance; health services
research; information dissemination; informed consent; legal
aspects; *medical records; moral obligations; physician
patient relationship; privacy; privileged communication; self
regulation; social discrimination; standards; computer
security; health data cards; United States

Anderson, James G.; Aydin, Carolyn E. Evaluating
medical information systems: social contexts and ethical
challenges. *In:* Goodman, Kenneth W., ed. Ethics,
Computing, and Medicine: Informatics and the
Transformation of Health Care. New York, NY:
Cambridge University Press; 1998: 57–74. 99 refs. ISBN
0–521–46905–8. BE57004.
accountability; administrators; attitudes; computer
communication networks; *computers; decision making;
economics; evaluation; *health care delivery;
interprofessional relations; *medical records; organization
and administration; patient care; patient participation;
physicians; professional autonomy; quality of health care;
social impact; values; *informatics; physician's practice
patterns; professional role

Balsamo, Anne. On the cutting edge: cosmetic surgery
and new imaging technologies. *In: her:* Technologies of
the Gendered Body: Reading Cyborg Women. Durham,
NC: Duke University Press; 1996: 56–79, 177–184. 71
fn. ISBN 0–8223–1698–6. BE58521.
*advertising; age factors; *audiovisual aids; *biomedical
technologies; *commodification; *cosmetic surgery;
counseling; *females; feminist ethics; human body; informed
consent; males; motivation; normality; patient care; physician
patient relationship; physicians; self concept; social control;
standards; beauty; video recording

Boyle, Philip J., ed. Getting Doctors to Listen: Ethics
and Outcomes Data in Context. Washington, DC:
Georgetown University Press; 1998. 234 p. (Hastings
Center studies in ethics). 479 fn. ISBN 0–87840–654–9.
BE57925.
accountability; *biomedical technologies; bone marrow;
cancer; communication; consensus; *decision making; drugs;
economics; *evaluation; federal government; females; goals;
*guidelines; health care; health insurance reimbursement;
hormones; international aspects; knowledge, attitudes,
practice; legal liability; medicine; moral obligations; *patient
care; patient compliance; physician patient relationship;
*physicians; political activity; *practice guidelines;
professional autonomy; professional organizations; public
participation; public policy; risks and benefits; science;
*standards; surgery; technical expertise; *technology
assessment; tissue transplantation; *treatment outcome;
uncertainty; values; *guideline adherence; *investigational
therapies; menopause; France; Great Britain; National
Institutes of Health; Netherlands; *United States

**Burt, R.A.P.; Goldschmidt, Peter G.; Monaco, Grace
Powers, et al.** Investigational treatments: process,
payment, and priorities. [Letters and response]. *JAMA.*
1997 Nov 5; 278(17): 1402–1404. 13 refs. BE57252.
*biomedical technologies; decision making; *evaluation;
*health insurance reimbursement; health maintenance
organizations; human experimentation; patient care; random
selection; *research design; review committees; risks and
benefits; standards; *technology assessment; terminology;
*therapeutic research; *evidence-based medicine;
*investigational therapies; United States

Bynum, Terrell Ward; Fodor, John L. Medical
informatics and human values. *In:* Goodman, Kenneth
W., ed. Ethics, Computing, and Medicine: Informatics
and the Transformation of Health Care. New York,
NY: Cambridge University Press; 1998: 32–42. 21 refs.
ISBN 0–521–46905–8. BE57002.
*computers; economics; *health care; health personnel;
information dissemination; patient care; patient education;
professional ethics; quality of health care; *risks and benefits;
values; *informatics; professional role

Chelala, César. German dialysis firm quits Chinese
interest. [News]. *Lancet.* 1998 Mar 14; 351(9105): 812.
BE58443.
aliens; *cadavers; capital punishment; health facilities;
industry; *international aspects; kidneys; *misconduct; moral
complicity; *organ donation; organ transplantation;
*prisoners; *renal dialysis; *China; *Fresenius Medical Care
AG; Germany

Cher, Daniel J.; Lenert, Leslie A. Method of Medicare
reimbursement and the rate of potentially ineffective care
of critically ill patients. *JAMA.* 1997 Sep 24; 278(12):
1001–1007. 29 refs. Correction appears in *JAMA*, 1998
Jun 17; 279(23): 1876. BE55815.
aged; allowing to die; biomedical technologies; comparative
studies; *critically ill; *economics; *futility; *health
maintenance organizations; hospitals; *intensive care units;
*managed care programs; *mortality; *patient care;
physicians; prolongation of life; quality of health care;
remuneration; resource allocation; selection for treatment;
*terminal care; time factors; *treatment outcome;
withholding treatment; *fee-for-service plans; severity of
illness index; *California; *Medicare
CONTEXT: The worst outcome of critical care may
not be death itself; rather, the worst may be an extended
death process in which a patient's and his or her family's
suffering has been prolonged by services that are
ultimately impotent. We have previously used potentially
ineffective care (PIC) as a proxy measure for this type
of care. OBJECTIVE: To determine if PIC is delivered
less often to Medicare patients enrolled in health
maintenance organizations (HMOs) than those in
traditional fee-for-service health plans. PATIENTS: All
Medicare patients hospitalized in intensive care units in
California during fiscal year 1994. OUTCOME:
Potentially ineffective care was defined as the
concurrence of in-hospital death or death within 100
days of hospital discharge and resource use (total hospital
costs) above the 90th percentile. METHODS: Hospital
costs were adjusted for institution-specific
cost-to-charge ratios and local wage indices derived
from Health Care Financing Administration cost reports.
A multivariate regression model adjusted PIC rates for
age, sex, race, elective admission to the hospital,
Charlson index diseases, the 15 most common diagnosis
related groups for death by 100 days, intensive care unit
size, and number of residents at the hospital. RESULTS:
A total of 3914 (4.8%) of 81,494 patients experienced
PIC and used 21.6% of total intensive care unit
resources. The occurrence of PIC was less common

BE = bioethics accession number   fn. = footnotes   refs. = references

among HMO members (adjusted odds ratio, 0.75; 95% confidence interval, 0.65–0.87). However, HMO members were not more likely to experience in–hospital death (adjusted odds ratio, 0.99; 95% confidence interval, 0.91–1.07) and only slightly more likely to experience death by 100 days after hospital discharge (adjusted odds ratio, 1.08; 95% confidence interval, 1.01–1.15). CONCLUSIONS: Patients who experience PIC outcomes are not uncommon in the Medicare population, and patients experiencing this outcome consume a disproportionate amount of medical resources. Medicare beneficiaries in HMO practice settings had a lower risk of experiencing PIC outcomes after adjusting for age, sex, diagnosis, comorbid conditions, and characteristics of the treating hospital. This suggests that HMO practices may be better at limiting or avoiding injudicious use of critical care near the end of life.

Curtis, J. Randall; Rubenfeld, Gordon D. Aggressive medical care at the end of life; does capitated reimbursement encourage the right care for the wrong reason? [Editorial]. *JAMA.* 1997 Sep 24; 278(12): 1025–1026. 12 refs. BE55814.
  biomedical technologies; *critically ill; decision making; *economics; *health maintenance organizations; hospitals; *intensive care units; *managed care programs; mortality; *patient care; physicians; prolongation of life; quality of health care; remuneration; *terminal care; time factors; treatment outcome; withholding treatment; capitation fee; *fee–for–service plans; *Medicare; *United States

Daniels, Norman; Sabin, James E. Last chance therapies and managed care: pluralism, fair procedures, and legitimacy. *Hastings Center Report.* 1998 Mar–Apr; 28(2): 27–41. 19 fn. BE57541.
  accountability; autonomy; *biomedical technologies; *bone marrow; *breast cancer; cancer; case studies; communication; comparative studies; cultural pluralism; *decision making; democracy; *due process; females; government regulation; guidelines; health insurance; *health insurance reimbursement; historical aspects; industry; institutional policies; *justice; legal aspects; *managed care programs; *moral policy; paternalism; patient care; patients; physicians; policy analysis; political activity; *public participation; resource allocation; risks and benefits; state government; technology assessment; terminally ill; therapeutic research; *tissue transplantation; *investigational therapies; seriously ill; Aetna; Blue Cross–Blue Shield; Northern California Kaiser Permanente; Twentieth Century; United States

Flax, Robert A. Silicone breast implants: two stories of informed consent. *In:* BioLaw: A Legal and Ethical Reporter on Medicine, Health Care, and Bioengineering. Special Sections, 2(9). Frederick, MD: University Publications of America; 1997 Sep: S311–S330. 58 refs. BE56646.
  autonomy; breast cancer; coercion; communication; comprehension; *cosmetic surgery; *disclosure; *federal government; *females; *government regulation; human experimentation; *industry; *information dissemination; *informed consent; legal liability; *medical devices; paternalism; patient care; *patient education; physicians; *risk; risks and benefits; standards; uncertainty; women's health; *breast implants; *Dow Corning; *Food and Drug Administration; United States

Goldberg, Allen I.; Faure, Eveline A.M.; O'Callaghan, John J. High–technology home care: critical issues and ethical choices. *In:* Monagle, John F.; Thomasma, David C., eds. Health Care Ethics: Critical Issues for the 21st Century. Gaithersburg, MD: Aspen Publishers; 1998: 146–163. 30 fn. ISBN 0–8342–0911–X. BE56282.
  adults; autonomy; beneficence; *biomedical technologies;

*children; *chronically ill; community services; *economics; family members; federal government; goals; government financing; *health care delivery; health care reform; health insurance reimbursement; health maintenance organizations; health personnel; historical aspects; *home care; justice; models, theoretical; moral policy; patient care team; private sector; public policy; resource allocation; state government; trends; values; ventilators; case managers; poliomyelitis; Medicaid; Twentieth Century; United States

Goodman, Kenneth W. Bioethics and health informatics: an introduction. *In:* Goodman, Kenneth W., ed. Ethics, Computing, and Medicine: Informatics and the Transformation of Health Care. New York, NY: Cambridge University Press; 1998: 1–31. 117 refs. 1 fn. ISBN 0–521–46905–8. BE57001.
  advance directives; *bioethics; *computer communication networks; *computers; confidentiality; decision making; DNA data banks; epidemiology; ethical theory; genetic information; *health care; information dissemination; informed consent; medical education; *medicine; moral obligations; organ transplantation; patient education; professional competence; professional ethics; professional patient relationship; psychiatry; psychology; quality of health care; referral and consultation; registries; risks and benefits; standards; surgery; trends; values; *informatics; *telemedicine

Goodman, Kenneth W., ed. Ethics, Computing, and Medicine: Informatics and the Transformation of Health Care. New York, NY: Cambridge University Press; 1998. 180 p. Includes references. ISBN 0–521–46905–8. BE57000.
  accountability; bioethics; *computer communication networks; *computers; confidentiality; data banks; decision making; disclosure; economics; evaluation; futility; *health care; health care delivery; information dissemination; informed consent; legal aspects; managed care programs; medical records; medicine; patient care; physician patient relationship; practice guidelines; professional autonomy; professional competence; quality of health care; resource allocation; risks and benefits; selection for treatment; standards; technical expertise; uncertainty; values; withholding treatment; evidence–based medicine; *informatics; professional role; telemedicine; United States

Goodman, Kenneth W. Outcomes, futility, and health policy research. *In:* Goodman, Kenneth W., ed. Ethics, Computing, and Medicine: Informatics and the Transformation of Health Care. New York, NY: Cambridge University Press; 1998: 116–138. 61 refs. ISBN 0–521–46905–8. BE57007.
  allowing to die; *computers; *critically ill; *decision making; disclosure; economics; epidemiology; evaluation; family members; futility; human experimentation; informed consent; patient care; patients; practice guidelines; *prognosis; resource allocation; *selection for treatment; social discrimination; *treatment outcome; *uncertainty; withholding treatment; evidence–based medicine; severity of illness index

Lantos, John D. Was the UK collaborative ECMO trial ethical? *Paediatric and Perinatal Epidemiology.* 1997 Jul; 11(3): 264–268. 7 refs. BE58033.
  alternatives; *biomedical technologies; coercion; congenital disorders; critically ill; *human experimentation; international aspects; mortality; *newborns; parental consent; *patient care; *random selection; *research design; risks and benefits; *technology assessment; *therapeutic research; time factors; *treatment outcome; uncertainty; *extracorporeal membrane oxygenation; *Great Britain

Maiorca, Rosario; Maggiore, Quirino; Mordacci, Roberto, et al. Ethical problems in dialysis and transplantation. *Nephrology, Dialysis, Transplantation.*

BE = bioethics accession number   fn. = footnotes   refs. = references

1996; 11(Suppl. 9): 100–112. BE57965.
   age factors; aliens; allowing to die; cultural pluralism; decision making; developing countries; directed donation; economics; health care delivery; international aspects; *kidneys; organ donation; organ donors; *organ transplantation; physicians; professional autonomy; prolongation of life; quality of life; *renal dialysis; resource allocation; selection for treatment; treatment refusal; withholding treatment; Europe; Great Britain; India; *Italy; United States

Mazen, Noël–Jean. Human DNA on trial in French law. *In:* Knoppers, Bartha Maria, ed. Human DNA: Law and Policy: International and Comparative Perspectives. Proceedings of the First International Conference on DNA Sampling and Human Genetic Research: Ethical, Legal, and Policy Aspects, held in Montreal, Canada, 6–8 Sep 1996. Boston, MA: Kluwer Law International; 1997: 43–54. 45 fn. ISBN 90–411–0361–9. BE58168.
   *biomedical technologies; body parts and fluids; DNA sequences; drugs; gene therapy; genetic intervention; *genetic materials; genetic research; gifts; *government regulation; informed consent; *legal aspects; legislation; *patents; *remuneration; *tissue donation; Europe; European Community; *France

Mead, Gillian E.; Pendleton, Neil; Pendleton, Deborah E., et al. High technology medical interventions: what do older people want? [Letter]. *Journal of the American Geriatrics Society.* 1997 Nov; 45(11): 1409–1411. 12 refs. BE56552.
   *aged; allowing to die; *attitudes; *biomedical technologies; *cancer; critically ill; diagnosis; drugs; *heart diseases; *patient care; radiology; referral and consultation; surgery; survey; truth disclosure; *withholding treatment; Great Britain

Melzer, David. Patent protection for medical technologies: why some and not others? *Lancet.* 1998 Feb 14; 351(9101): 518–519. 21 refs. BE58470.
   biomedical research; *biomedical technologies; drug industry; drugs; *financial support; government regulation; human experimentation; incentives; *industry; international aspects; medical devices; methods; organizational policies; *patents; *physicians; professional organizations; *public policy; surgery; technology assessment; transgenic animals; British Medical Association; *Great Britain; National Health Service

Miller, Pam. Ethical issues in neonatal intensive care. *In:* Frith, Lucy, ed. Ethics and Midwifery: Issues in Contemporary Practice. Boston, MA: Butterworth–Heinemann; 1996: 123–139. 24 refs. ISBN 0–7506–3056–6. BE58636.
   *allowing to die; artificial feeding; biomedical technologies; case studies; communication; *congenital disorders; *decision making; *intensive care units; moral policy; mothers; *newborns; *nurse midwives; *nurse's role; nurses; parents; patient advocacy; patient care; personhood; physicians; *prematurity; professional family relationship; prognosis; quality of life; resource allocation; risks and benefits; *selection for treatment; suffering; terminal care; treatment outcome; value of life; withholding treatment; Great Britain

Miller, Randolph A.; Goodman, Kenneth W. Ethical challenges in the use of decision-support software in clinical practice. *In:* Goodman, Kenneth W., ed. Ethics, Computing, and Medicine: Informatics and the Transformation of Health Care. New York, NY: Cambridge University Press; 1998: 102–115. 32 refs. ISBN 0–521–46905–8. BE57006.
   *computers; *decision making; guidelines; informed consent; medical education; *patient care; physician patient relationship; professional competence; referral and consultation; standards; technical expertise

Morain, William D. Patently unethical. [Editorial]. *Annals of Plastic Surgery.* 1996 Mar; 36(3): 334. BE56213.
   *biomedical technologies; cosmetic surgery; economics; entrepreneurship; federal government; government regulation; health care; medical ethics; *methods; *patents; physicians; *surgery; United States

Napper, Stan A.; Hale, Paul N. Teaching of ethics in biomedical engineering. *IEEE Engineering in Medicine and Biology Magazine.* 1993 Dec; 12(4): 100–105. 26 refs. BE56038.
   animal experimentation; artificial organs; bioethical issues; biomedical research; *biomedical technologies; body parts and fluids; computers; costs and benefits; economics; *education; federal government; government regulation; hearts; human experimentation; industry; medical devices; organ donation; organ transplantation; professional ethics; resource allocation; selection for treatment; teaching methods; transplant recipients; *engineering; Louisiana Tech University; United States

Nyman, Deborah J.; Sprung, Charles L. International perspectives on ethics in critical care. *Critical Care Clinics.* 1997 Apr; 13(2): 409–415. 36 refs. BE58360.
   allowing to die; *critically ill; decision making; euthanasia; informed consent; *intensive care units; *international aspects; medical ethics; patient admission; *patient care; physicians; prognosis; quality of life; resource allocation; resuscitation orders; selection for treatment; values; withholding treatment

Ong, Bie Nio. The lay perspective in health technology assessment. *International Journal of Technology Assessment in Health Care.* 1996 Summer; 12(3): 511–517. 24 refs. BE55573.
   *biomedical technologies; health services research; *patient participation; physicians; *public participation; quality of life; resource allocation; technical expertise; *technology assessment; treatment outcome; *health planning

Parens, Erik. Is better always good? The enhancement project. [Project on the Prospect of Technologies Aimed at the Enhancement of Human Capacities and Traits]. *Hastings Center Report.* 1998 Jan–Feb; 28(1): S1–S17. 35 fn. BE57294.
   behavior control; *biomedical technologies; *cosmetic surgery; disabled; entrepreneurship; ethical analysis; females; *genetic enhancement; *goals; *health; *health care; health insurance reimbursement; *human characteristics; *justice; *medicine; moral complicity; *moral policy; motivation; *normality; preventive medicine; *psychoactive drugs; *public policy; resource allocation; *self concept; social control; social impact; social problems; socioeconomic factors; suffering; terminology; *values; authenticity; beauty; *enhancement technologies; life style; Hastings Center; *Project on the Prospect of Technologies Aimed at the Enhancement of Human Capabilities and Traits; Prozac
The following essay begins to say why and when it will sometimes make sense to worry about the prospect of aiming new biotechnologies at the enhancement of human capacities and traits. It grows out of a two–year, Hastings Center project, generously funded by the National Endowment for the Humanities.

Paris, John J.; Muir, J. Cameron; Reardon, Frank E. Ethical and legal issues in intensive care. *Journal of Intensive Care Medicine.* 1997 Nov–Dec; 12(6): 298–309. 98 refs. BE58495.
   allowing to die; anencephaly; assisted suicide; autonomy; brain death; clinical ethics committees; *critically ill; *decision making; determination of death; dissent; family

---

BE = bioethics accession number   fn. = footnotes   refs. = references

members; futility; guidelines; hospitals; infants; institutional policies; *intensive care units; judicial action; managed care programs; pain; patient care; physicians; prognosis; prolongation of life; quality of health care; quality of life; resuscitation orders; risks and benefits; surgery; *terminal care; terminally ill; treatment refusal; withholding treatment; seriously ill; Study to Understand Prognoses and Preferences for Outcomes and Risks of Treatments (SUPPORT); United States

Parker, Lisa S. Beauty and breast implantation: how candidate selection affects autonomy and informed consent. *In:* DiQuinzio, Patrice; Young, Iris Marion, eds. Feminist Ethics and Social Policy. Bloomington, IN: Indiana University Press; 1997: 255–273. 47 refs. 9 fn. ISBN 0-253-21125-5. BE57287.
*autonomy; breast cancer; competence; *cosmetic surgery; *decision making; *females; *feminist ethics; *informed consent; *medical devices; motivation; risks and benefits; *selection for treatment; self concept; *values; beauty; *breast implants; United States

Prokes, Mary Timothy. Technology and the lived body. *In: her* Toward a Theology of the Body. Grand Rapids, MI: W.B. Eerdmans; 1996: 104–117. 10 fn. Includes references embedded in list at back of book. ISBN 0-8028-4339-5. BE56246.
*biomedical technologies; conscience; contraception; embryos; eugenics; *human body; human characteristics; intention; marital relationship; mass media; moral obligations; morality; *personhood; reproduction; reproductive technologies; *Roman Catholic ethics; *theology; value of life; Humanae Vitae; Instruction on Respect for Human Life; Veritatis Splendor

Reisman, Joseph M. Physicians and surgeons as inventors: reconciling medical process patents and medical ethics. [Comment]. *High Technology Law Journal.* 1995; 10(2): 355–403. 228 fn. BE56920.
*biomedical technologies; conflict of interest; entrepreneurship; information dissemination; interprofessional relations; *legal aspects; legislation; moral obligations; ophthalmology; organizational policies; *patents; patient care; *physicians; professional organizations; surgery; American Medical Association; Medical Procedures Innovation and Affordability Act (1995 bill); Moore v. Regents of the University of California; Pallin, Samuel; *United States

Reiss, Michael. Biotechnology. *In:* Chadwick, Ruth, ed. Encyclopedia of Applied Ethics, Volume 1. San Diego, CA: Academic Press; 1998: 319–333. 10 refs. ISBN 0-12-227066-5. BE56370.
animal experimentation; animal rights; *biomedical technologies; drugs; ecology; food; *gene therapy; genetic enhancement; *genetic intervention; genetic materials; germ cells; growth disorders; historical aspects; hormones; international aspects; methods; moral policy; patents; *recombinant DNA research; reproductive technologies; risk; *risks and benefits; suffering; terminology; *transgenic animals; *transgenic organisms; agriculture

Shi, Da-pu; Yu, Lin. The conflict between the advancement of medical science and technology and traditional Chinese medical ethics. *In:* Becker, Gerhold K., ed. Changing Nature's Course: The Ethical Challenge of Biotechnology. Hong Kong: Hong Kong University Press; 1996: 111–118. ISBN 962-209-403-1. BE56708.
*bioethical issues; *biomedical technologies; communication; economics; goals; informed consent; justice; life extension; medical ethics; *medicine; moral obligations; physician patient relationship; physician's role; quality of life; reproductive technologies; resource allocation; social impact; transsexualism; trust; *China

Sirmon, Maryella D. The combative patient: ethical issues in patient selection for chronic dialysis. *Seminars in Dialysis.* 1996 Jan–Feb; 9(1): 56–60. 38 refs. BE55798.
adolescents; adults; allowing to die; attitudes; case studies; chronically ill; costs and benefits; critically ill; *decision making; dementia; family members; guidelines; mentally retarded; palliative care; *patient compliance; persistent vegetative state; physicians; practice guidelines; professional organizations; *renal dialysis; resource allocation; risks and benefits; *selection for treatment; terminally ill; treatment refusal; *withholding treatment; United States

Slifkin, Robert F.; Charytan, Chaim. Ethical issues related to the provision or denial of renal services to non-citizens. [Case commentaries on ethical issues in dialysis]. *Seminars in Dialysis.* 1997 May–Jun; 10(3): 173–175. 5 refs. BE57921.
*aliens; emergency care; federal government; government financing; government regulation; *kidney diseases; obligations of society; *public policy; *refusal to treat; *renal dialysis; *selection for treatment; state government; Medicaid; *United States

Snapper, John W. Responsibility for computer-based decisions in health care. *In:* Goodman, Kenneth W., ed. Ethics, Computing, and Medicine: Informatics and the Transformation of Health Care. New York, NY: Cambridge University Press; 1998: 43–56. 28 refs. ISBN 0-521-46905-8. BE57003.
*accountability; *computers; *decision making; diagnosis; *health care; legal aspects; *legal liability; patient care; physician's role; *physicians; professional competence; referral and consultation; standards; informatics; *medical errors; professional role; United States

Stewart, F.E. *JAMA* 100 years ago: is it ethical for medical men to patent medical inventions? [Reprint]. *JAMA.* 1997 Sep 10; 278(10): 816. BE55942.
*biomedical technologies; conflict of interest; drugs; *economics; *historical aspects; medical etiquette; *patents; patient care; *pharmacists; *physicians; *Nineteenth Century; United States

Tulsky, James A.; Cassileth, Barrie R.; Bennett, Charles L. The effect of ethnicity on ICU use and DNR orders in hospitalized AIDS patients. *Journal of Clinical Ethics.* 1997 Summer; 8(2): 150–157. 18 fn. BE55777.
advance care planning; *AIDS; allowing to die; attitudes; *blacks; comparative studies; *Hispanic Americans; hospitals; *intensive care units; males; medical records; *minority groups; mortality; *patient admission; *patient care; patients; prolongation of life; *resuscitation orders; statistics; *terminal care; *time factors; treatment outcome; *whites; multicenter studies; retrospective studies; severity of illness index; Chicago; Los Angeles; Miami

Veatch, Robert M. Technology assessment: inevitably a value judgment. *In:* Boyle, Philip J., ed. Getting Doctors to Listen: Ethics and Outcomes Data in Context. Washington, DC: Georgetown University Press; 1998: 180–195. 29 fn. ISBN 0-87840-654-9. BE57926.
*biomedical technologies; consensus; costs and benefits; *decision making; empirical research; goals; guidelines; investigators; patients; physicians; practice guidelines; public policy; risks and benefits; science; selection for treatment; technical expertise; *technology assessment; therapeutic research; treatment outcome; *values; National Institutes of Health; United States

Wear, Stephen E.; Coles, William H.; Szczygiel, Anthony H., et al. Patenting medical and surgical techniques: an ethical-legal analysis. *Journal of Medicine and Philosophy.* 1998 Feb; 23(1): 75–97. 34 refs. 30 fn. BE57521.

biomedical research; *biomedical technologies; conflict of interest; diagnosis; entrepreneurship; ethical analysis; financial support; incentives; investigators; *legal aspects; medical ethics; medicine; methods; ophthalmology; organizational policies; *patents; patient care; *physicians; policy analysis; professional organizations; *public policy; risks and benefits; social impact; *surgery; American Medical Association; Pallin, Samuel; *United States

Considerable controversy has recently arisen regarding the patenting of medical and surgical processes in the United States. One such patent, viz. for a "chevron" incision used in ophthalmologic surgery, has especially occasioned heated response including a major, condemnatory ethics policy statement from the American Medical Association as well as federal legislation denying patent protection for most uses of a patented medical or surgical procedure. This article identifies and discusses the major legal, ethical and public policy considerations offered by proponents and opponents of such patents. The existing literature divides up into those who favor such patents essentially without qualification, and those who condemn and wish to outlaw them. We advance a compromise position where administrative and legislative action is called for to provide more specific guidelines regarding the patentability of such processes by the Patent and Trademark Office. Our position, in sum, will be that too much is at stake in this complicated area for either the blanket prohibition, or wholesale, uncritical acceptance, of the patenting of medical and surgical processes or techniques.

Wilson, Donna. A report of an investigation of end–of–life care practices in health care facilities and the influences on those practices. *Journal of Palliative Care.* 1997 Winter; 13(4): 34–40. 63 refs. BE58824.
   age factors; artificial feeding; *biomedical technologies; death; decision making; family members; females; *health facilities; hospitals; intensive care units; males; palliative care; resuscitation; resuscitation orders; statistics; survey; *terminal care; terminally ill; ventilators; retrospective studies; *Alberta; Canada

BLOOD DONATION

See also ORGAN AND TISSUE DONATION

American College of Obstetricians and Gynecologists. Committee on Obstetric Practice. Routine storage of umbilical cord blood for potential future transplantation. ACOG Committee Opinion No. 183, April 1997. *International Journal of Gynaecology and Obstetrics.* 1997 Aug; 58(2): 257–259. 8 refs. BE57952.
   advertising; alternatives; *blood banks; *blood donation; bone marrow; confidentiality; costs and benefits; cryopreservation; *directed donation; disclosure; donors; genetic screening; industry; *newborns; *obstetrics and gynecology; *organizational policies; parental consent; parents; *physicians; professional organizations; property rights; *risks and benefits; *stem cells; time factors; tissue transplantation; *cord blood; *American College of Obstetricians and Gynecologists; United States

Emanuel, Ezekiel J. Is health care a commodity? [Book review essay]. *Lancet.* 1997 Dec 6; 350(9092): 1713–1714. BE56925.
   AIDS; *altruism; *blood donation; blood transfusions; commodification; comparative studies; *economics; freedom; gifts; *health care delivery; hemophilia; *international aspects; quality of health care; values; Great Britain; *The Gift Relationship: From Human Blood to Social Policy (Titmuss, R.); *United States

Goldfinger, Dennis. Controversies in transfusion medicine: directed blood donations -- pro. *Transfusion.* 1989 Jan–Feb; 29(1): 70–74. 9 refs. BE56781.
   AIDS; *blood banks; *blood donation; *blood transfusions; costs and benefits; *directed donation; hepatitis; HIV seropositivity; institutional policies; *risks and benefits; standards

Kaplan, Edward H. Israel's ban on use of Ethiopians' blood: how many infectious donations were prevented? *Lancet.* 1998 Apr 11; 351(9109): 1127–1128. 15 refs. BE58309.
   aliens; blood banks; *blood donation; *deception; *HIV seropositivity; prevalence; *preventive medicine; *public policy; risk; statistics; *stigmatization; *emigration and immigration; Ethiopia; *Israel

McMillan, Margaret P. Banking on cord blood. [Editorial]. *Journal of Obstetric, Gynecologic and Neonatal Nursing.* 1996 Feb; 25(2): 115. 1 ref. BE55880.
   advertising; *blood banks; blood donation; costs and benefits; cryopreservation; deception; *economics; health insurance reimbursement; hospitals; *industry; institutional policies; legal liability; newborns; nurses; parents; property rights; proprietary health facilities; stem cells; *cord blood; United States

Mudur, Ganapati. Ban on payment to donors causes blood shortage in India. [News]. *BMJ (British Medical Journal).* 1998 Jan 17; 316(7126): 172. BE57913.
   blood banks; *blood donation; *donors; *government regulation; hepatitis; HIV seropositivity; *remuneration; scarcity; *India

Rogers, Arthur. Europe–wide blood–donor system debated. [News]. *Lancet.* 1998 Apr 11; 351(9109): 1112. BE58243.
   blood banks; *blood donation; data banks; *donors; *international aspects; registries; *standards; questionnaires; *Europe; European Commission

Sazama, Kathleen; Lind, Stuart E. Cord blood stem cells belong to the infant, not to the mother. [Letter and response]. *Transfusion.* 1995 Nov–Dec; 35(11): 967. 2 refs. BE55773.
   *blood donation; fetal tissue donation; legal rights; *mothers; *newborns; parental consent; property rights; risks and benefits; standards; *stem cells; *cord blood; placentas

Titmuss, Richard M. The Gift Relationship: From Human Blood to Social Policy. Original Edition with New Chapters Edited by Ann Oakley and John Ashton. New York, NY: New Press; 1997. 360 p. Bibliography: p. 340–345. Originally published by Allen and Unwin, 1970. ISBN 1–56584–403–3. BE57204.
   AIDS; AIDS serodiagnosis; *altruism; attitudes; *blood donation; blood transfusions; comparative studies; *donors; *economics; *gifts; health care delivery; hemophilia; homosexuals; industry; *international aspects; legal aspects; moral obligations; motivation; obligations to society; *public policy; remuneration; socioeconomic factors; values; voluntary programs; *Great Britain; National Health Service; South Africa; *United States; USSR

Warwick, Ruth. Collections of cord blood. [Letter]. *Lancet.* 1997 Jul 26; 350(9073): 297. 3 refs. BE56890.
   *blood banks; *blood donation; bone marrow; costs and benefits; *directed donation; gene therapy; genetic disorders; genetic screening; prenatal diagnosis; risks and benefits; selective abortion; *siblings; tissue donation; tissue transplantation; *cord blood

Wise, Jacqui. Doctors fight US company patent on umbilical cord blood. [News]. *BMJ (British Medical*

BE = bioethics accession number   fn. = footnotes   refs. = references

Journal). 1997 Apr 19; 314(7088): 1146. BE56895.
> biomedical technologies; *blood banks; blood donation; blood transfusions; cryopreservation; *industry; *international aspects; *patents; *cord blood; *Biocyte; *Europe; *United States

Young, Ian F. Medical ethics in relation to transfusion medicine. *Transfusion Medicine Reviews.* 1996 Jan; 10(1): 23–30. 43 refs. BE55548.
> advance directives; AIDS serodiagnosis; autonomy; beneficence; blood banks; *blood donation; *blood transfusions; competence; confidentiality; developing countries; directed donation; disclosure; donors; economics; family members; fetuses; health hazards; HIV seropositivity; informed consent; institutional policies; international aspects; justice; organ donation; organ transplantation; paternalism; patients; pregnant women; property rights; religion; remuneration; resource allocation; risk; selection for treatment; self induced illness; standards; third party consent; treatment refusal; cord blood

Trading trust for blood money. [Editorial]. *Lancet.* 1995 Sep 30; 346(8979): 855. BE56102.
> *blood banks; *blood donation; *confidentiality; conflict of interest; disclosure; *donors; economics; industry; organization and administration; organizational policies; records; *Great Britain; *National Blood Authority (Great Britain); *National Health Service

BRAIN DEATH
See under
DETERMINATION OF DEATH/BRAIN DEATH

CAPITAL PUNISHMENT

Chelala, César. Prospect of discussions on prisoners' organs for sale in China. [News]. *Lancet.* 1997 Nov 1; 350(9087): 1307. BE57268.
> body parts and fluids; cadavers; *capital punishment; disclosure; family members; human rights; informed consent; misconduct; *organ donation; *prisoners; public policy; *remuneration; Amnesty International; *China; Human Rights Watch/Asia; Singapore; Taiwan; United Nations

Curriden, Mark. Inmate's last wish is to donate kidney. [News]. *ABA Journal: The Lawyer's Magazine.* 1996 Jun; 82: 26. BE57625.
> autonomy; *capital punishment; kidneys; *legal aspects; *organ donation; *prisoners; *Georgia; *Lonchar, Larry

Dunea, George. Death by Injection. *BMJ (British Medical Journal).* 1998 May 2; 316(7141): 1394. BE58834.
> allied health personnel; *capital punishment; drugs; federal government; legal aspects; nurses; organizational policies; *physician's role; physicians; professional organizations; public opinion; state government; *United States

Egbert, Lawrence D. Physicians and the death penalty. *America.* 1998 Mar 7; 178(7): 15–16. BE58565.
> anesthesia; *capital punishment; drugs; *physician's role

Gorman, Christine. Body parts for sale. [News]. *Time.* 1998 Mar 9; 151(9): 76. BE58043.
> *body parts and fluids; cadavers; *capital punishment; federal government; human rights; informed consent; *international aspects; legal aspects; *organ donation; *prisoners; *remuneration; *China; United States

Josefson, Deborah. Two arrested in US for selling organs for transplantation. [News]. *BMJ (British Medical Journal).* 1998 Mar 7; 316(7133): 725. BE57705.
> *body parts and fluids; *capital punishment; international

aspects; *law enforcement; legal aspects; *organ donation; *prisoners; *remuneration; *tissue donation; China; United States

Loewy, Erich H. Harming, healing, and euthanasia. *In:* Emanuel, Linda L., ed. Regulating How We Die: The Ethical, Medical, and Legal Issues Surrounding Physician–Assisted Suicide. Cambridge, MA: Harvard University Press; 1998: 48–67, 267–269. 18 fn. ISBN 0–674–66654–2. BE58533.
> *active euthanasia; allowing to die; assisted suicide; autonomy; *capital punishment; health personnel; *killing; moral obligations; *moral policy; morality; National Socialism; physician patient relationship; *physician's role; physicians; prolongation of life; public policy; risks and benefits; *suffering; *suicide; terminal care; terminally ill; value of life; voluntary euthanasia; wedge argument; withholding treatment; Netherlands; United States

White, Caroline. Lethal injection is medicalising execution. [News]. *BMJ (British Medical Journal).* 1998 Jan 31; 316(7128): 328. BE58125.
> *capital punishment; *drugs; forensic medicine; *international aspects; *physicians; political activity; trends; *Amnesty International; Lethal Injection: The Medical Technology of Execution (Amnesty International)

Doctors' involvement in death penalty is morally wrong. [BMA Annual Meeting, July 1998]. *BMJ (British Medical Journal).* 1998 Jul 18; 317 (7152): 215–216. BE58511.
> *capital punishment; international aspects; organizational policies; *physician's role; physicians; professional organizations; *British Medical Association; Great Britain

CIVIL COMMITMENT *See* INVOLUNTARY COMMITMENT

CLINICAL ETHICISTS *See* ETHICISTS AND ETHICS COMMITTEES

CLINICAL ETHICS *See* BIOETHICS, ETHICISTS AND ETHICS COMMITTEES, MEDICAL ETHICS, NURSING ETHICS, PROFESSIONAL ETHICS

CLINICAL ETHICS COMMITTEES *See* ETHICISTS AND ETHICS COMMITTEES

CLINICAL RESEARCH *See* HUMAN EXPERIMENTATION

CLONING

See also REPRODUCTIVE TECHNOLOGIES, GENETIC INTERVENTION

Allmers, Henning; Kenwright, Simon. Ethics of cloning. [Letters]. *Lancet.* 1997 May 10; 349(9062): 1401. 1 ref. BE56851.
> bone marrow; cadavers; *cloning; cryopreservation; decision making; *directed donation; leukemia; motivation; *organ donation; parents; regulation; *reproduction; siblings; time factors; *tissue donation; transplant recipients; Ayala, Anissa; Ayala, Marissa; Great Britain; United States

Andrews, Lori B. Mom, Dad, clone: implications for reproductive privacy. *Cambridge Quarterly of Healthcare Ethics.* 1998 Spring; 7(2): 176–186. 71 fn. BE58004.
> children; *cloning; constitutional law; genetic determinism;

genetic identity; genetic information; genetic screening; *government regulation; *legal rights; parent child relationship; privacy; *reproduction; risks and benefits; social discrimination; social impact; United States

Andrews, Lori B.; Rothstein, Mark A.; Latham, Stephen R., et al. The clone age. *ABA Journal: The Lawyer's Magazine.* 1997 Jul; 83: 68–73. BE57526.
*cloning; embryo transfer; genetic enhancement; genetic information; genetic research; government regulation; international aspects; *legal aspects; parent child relationship; property rights; reproductive technologies; United States

Annas, George J.; Robertson, John A. Human cloning: should the United States legislate against it? Yes: individual dignity demands nothing less [Annas]; No: the potential for good is too compelling [Robertson]. *ABA Journal: The Lawyer's Magazine.* 1997 May; 83: 80–81. BE57624.
*cloning; commodification; dehumanization; genetic identity; *government regulation; human experimentation; *public policy; *risks and benefits; dignity; United States

Annas, George J. Why we should ban human cloning. *New England Journal of Medicine.* 1998 Jul 9; 339(2): 122–125. 25 refs. BE58657.
children; *cloning; death; dehumanization; federal government; *government regulation; human experimentation; human rights; infertility; investigators; literature; moral obligations; parent child relationship; personhood; *public policy; reproduction; reproductive technologies; *risks and benefits; social control; *United States

Bailey, Ronald. What exactly is wrong with cloning people? *In:* McGee, Glenn, ed. The Human Cloning Debate. Berkeley, CA: Berkeley Hills Books; 1998: 181–188. ISBN 0–9653774–8–2. BE58991.
advisory committees; *cloning; government regulation; moral policy; reproductive technologies; risks and benefits; *social control; United States

Blacksher, Erika. Cloning human beings: responding to the National Bioethics Advisory Commission's Report [Introduction to a set of articles by J.F. Childress; S.M. Wolf, C.S. Campbell, D. Callahan, and E. Parens; includes excerpts from the Executive Summary of the Commission's report]. *Hastings Center Report.* 1997 Sep–Oct; 27(5): 6–9. BE56112.
advisory committees; animal experimentation; biomedical research; children; *cloning; cultural pluralism; embryo research; embryo transfer; federal government; freedom; government financing; government regulation; human experimentation; industry; methods; moral policy; private sector; *public policy; public sector; religious ethics; reproductive technologies; research embryo creation; *risks and benefits; social impact; nuclear transplantation; *Cloning Human Beings (NBAC); *National Bioethics Advisory Commission; *United States

In February of this year two figures were added to our daily life. Dolly, a cloned sheep, and her maker, Scottish scientist Ian Wilmut, could be found in our newspapers, on our televisions, across the Internet, and in our conversations. What Wilmut had done was indeed new, if not fantastic. By transferring the nucleus of a somatic cell from an adult animal into an egg from which the nucleus had been removed, Wilmut successfully cloned a mammal—a technique that had never before succeeded.

Bower, Hilary. Public consultation on human cloning launched. [News]. *BMJ (British Medical Journal).* 1998 Feb 7; 316(7129): 411. BE58092.

advisory committees; *cloning; *embryo research; government regulation; public participation; *public policy; research embryo creation; nuclear transplantation; *Great Britain; Human Fertilisation and Embryology Authority; Human Genetics Advisory Commission (Great Britain)

Boyd, Kenneth M. Little lamb, who made thee? A letter from Edinburgh. *Cambridge Quarterly of Healthcare Ethics.* 1998 Spring; 7(2): 199–202. 7 fn. BE58005.
animal experimentation; *cloning; embryo research; *government regulation; international aspects; public opinion; public participation; *public policy; risks and benefits; self regulation; transgenic animals; *Great Britain; Roslin Institute (Scotland); Scotland

Broyde, Michael J. Cloning people and Jewish law: a preliminary analysis. *Journal of Halacha and Contemporary Society.* 1997 Fall; No. 34: 27–65. 64 fn. BE57177.
childbirth; *cloning; dehumanization; embryo transfer; *family relationship; fathers; genetic materials; human experimentation; in vitro fertilization; *Jewish ethics; moral obligations; mothers; organ donation; ovum donors; *parent child relationship; property rights; reproduction; reproductive technologies; semen donors; sexuality; siblings; stigmatization; surrogate mothers; twins; nuclear transplantation; Orthodox Judaism

Bruce, Donald M. A view from Edinburgh. *In:* Cole–Turner, Ronald, ed. Human Cloning: Religious Responses. Louisville, KY: Westminster John Knox Press; 1997: 1–11. 10 fn. ISBN 0–664–25771–2. BE58138.
animal experimentation; *Christian ethics; *cloning; embryo research; genetic diversity; intention; investigators; Protestant ethics; public participation; regulation; reproductive technologies; risks and benefits; nuclear transplantation; Church of Scotland; Europe; Roslin Institute (Scotland); Scotland

Buck, Gene. An open letter to Dr. Seed. [Satire]. *JAMA.* 1998 Apr 1; 279(10): 977. BE57339.
*cloning; volunteers; Seed, Richard

Byers, David M. An absence of love. *In:* Cole–Turner, Ronald, ed. Human Cloning: Religious Responses. Louisville, KY: Westminster John Knox Press; 1997: 66–77. 4 fn. ISBN 0–664–25771–2. BE58145.
*cloning; embryo disposition; embryo research; embryos; love; parent child relationship; personhood; reproduction; *Roman Catholic ethics; *social discrimination; social impact; theology; value of life

California. Human cloning. *California Health and Safety Code (West).* 1997 Oct 4 (date enacted). Sects. 24185, 24187, 24189. 2 p. In effect 1 Jan 1998 until 1 Jan 2003. BE58573.
*cloning; *government regulation; *legal aspects; state government; nuclear transplantation; *California

Callahan, Daniel. Cloning: the work not done. *Hastings Center Report.* 1997 Sep–Oct; 27(5): 18–20. 2 fn. BE56116.
advisory committees; bioethical issues; bioethics; *biomedical research; children; *cloning; common good; future generations; government regulation; human experimentation; informed consent; *moral policy; *public policy; reproduction; reproductive technologies; research subjects; rights; *risks and benefits; science; standards; *values; *Cloning Human Beings (NBAC); *National Bioethics Advisory Commission; United States

Callahan, Daniel. Cloning: then and now. *Cambridge Quarterly of Healthcare Ethics.* 1998 Spring; 7(2): 141–144. BE58006.

BE = bioethics accession number   fn. = footnotes   refs. = references

advisory committees; attitudes; *bioethics; biomedical research; *cloning; economics; genetic intervention; government regulation; historical aspects; reproduction; reproductive technologies; rights; risks and benefits; National Bioethics Advisory Commission; United States

Campbell, Courtney S. Prophecy and policy. *Hastings Center Report.* 1997 Sep–Oct; 27(5): 15–17. 1 fn. BE56115.
 advisory committees; bioethics; *cloning; common good; *cultural pluralism; dehumanization; family relationship; federal government; morality; public participation; *public policy; *religion; *religious ethics; science; *values; liberalism; National Bioethics Advisory Commission; United States

Childress, James F. The challenges of public ethics: reflections on NBAC's report. *Hastings Center Report.* 1997 Sep–Oct; 27(5): 9–11. BE56113.
 *advisory committees; autonomy; beneficence; casuistry; children; *cloning; consensus; cultural pluralism; *ethical analysis; federal government; government regulation; *moral policy; *morality; organizational policies; principle-based ethics; public participation; *public policy; religious ethics; *risks and benefits; secularism; social impact; *Cloning Human Beings (NBAC); *National Bioethics Advisory Commission; United States

Cohen, Philip. Cult's bizarre vision rekindles cloning debate. [News]. *New Scientist.* 1997 May 31; 154(2084): 12. BE56403.
 *cloning; federal government; government financing; *government regulation; human experimentation; industry; legislation; private sector; universities; *Canada; Raëlians; *United States

Cole–Turner, Ronald. At the beginning. *In:* Cole–Turner, Ronald, ed. Human Cloning: Religious Responses. Louisville, KY: Westminister John Knox Press; 1997: 119–130. 11 fn. ISBN 0–664–25771–2. BE58149.
 *Christian ethics; *cloning; embryo research; embryos; genetic determinism; genetic identity; parent child relationship; public participation; public policy; reproduction; nature

Cole–Turner, Ronald, ed. Human Cloning: Religious Responses. Louisville, KY: Westminister John Knox Press; 1997. 151 p. 123 fn. Appendix I: Recommendations of the National Bioethics Advisory Commission [Chapter 6 of the 1997 NBAC report *Cloning Human Beings*]; Appendix II: Denominational statements on cloning. ISBN 0–664–25771–2. BE58137.
 animal experimentation; *Christian ethics; *cloning; embryo research; embryos; eugenics; family relationship; genetic determinism; genetic identity; human rights; love; motivation; parent child relationship; personhood; Protestant ethics; public policy; regulation; reproduction; reproductive technologies; risks and benefits; Roman Catholic ethics; social impact; theology; twins; value of life

Council for Responsible Genetics. Position statement on cloning. *Bulletin of Medical Ethics.* 1997 Sep; No. 131: 10–11. BE57628.
 animal experimentation; *cloning; genetic diversity; genetic enhancement; genetic materials; human experimentation; international aspects; *organizational policies; public opinion; *public policy; value of life; agriculture; *Council for Responsible Genetics; United States

Dickson, David. UK consults public on clones for research. [News]. *Nature.* 1998 Feb 5; 391(6667): 523. Includes an inset article by M. Wadman, "US sees flurry of bills in bids to legislate." BE58054.
 advisory committees; *cloning; *embryo research;

government regulation; public participation; *public policy; nuclear transplantation; *Great Britain; Human Fertilisation and Embryology Authority; Human Genetics Advisory Commission (Great Britain)

Elshtain, Jean Bethke. Bad Seed: the hard questions. *New Republic.* 1998 Feb 9; 218(6): 9. BE58439.
 *cloning; freedom; investigators; morality; motivation; theology; *Seed, Richard

Enserink, Martin. Dutch pull the plug on cow cloning. [News]. *Science.* 1998 Mar 6; 279(5356): 1444. BE57304.
 animal experimentation; *cloning; *drug industry; *government regulation; *transgenic animals; *Netherlands; Pharming Holding N.V.

European Commission. Group of Advisers on the Ethical Implications of Biotechnology. Ethical aspects of cloning techniques. *Journal of Medical Ethics.* 1997 Dec; 23(6): 349–352. Advisers: Anne McLaren; Margareta Mikkelsen; Luis Archer; Octavi Quintana; Stefano Rodota; Egbert Schroten; Dietmar Mieth; Gilbert Hottois; Chairman, Noëlle Lenoir. BE57661.
 advisory committees; animal experimentation; *cloning; embryo research; *ethical review; eugenics; genetic diversity; goals; guidelines; human experimentation; information dissemination; international aspects; methods; nontherapeutic research; *organizational policies; public participation; public policy; *regulation; *risks and benefits; twinning; embryo splitting; nuclear transplantation; Europe; *European Commission; *Group of Advisers on the Ethical Implications of Biotechnology (European Commission)

European Parliament. Cloning animals and human beings. [Resolution of 12 March 1997]. *Bulletin of Medical Ethics.* 1997 May; No. 128: 10–11. Includes extracts from the European Parliament's resolution on the cloning of the human embryo of 28 Oct 1993. BE55687.
 animal experimentation; *cloning; embryo research; embryos; ethics committees; genetic identity; genetic research; government regulation; human experimentation; human rights; *international aspects; investigators; *regulation; self regulation; Europe; *European Union

Evans, Abigail Rian. Saying no to human cloning. *In:* Cole–Turner, Ronald, ed. Human Cloning: Religious Responses. Louisville, KY: Westminister John Knox Press; 1997: 25–34. 11 fn. ISBN 0–664–25771–2. BE58140.
 biomedical technologies; *cloning; common good; eugenics; freedom; parent child relationship; personhood; *Protestant ethics; regulation; reproduction; reproductive technologies; risks and benefits; Reformed Church

Fielding, Ellen Wilson. Fear of cloning. *Human Life Review.* 1997 Spring; 23(2): 15–22. BE57428.
 abortion, induced; attitudes; beneficence; *cloning; common good; compassion; euthanasia; marital relationship; reproductive technologies; sexuality; social impact; value of life; United States

FitzGerald, Kevin T. Human cloning: analysis and evaluation. *Cambridge Quarterly of Healthcare Ethics.* 1998 Spring; 7(2): 218–222. 3 refs. BE58007.
 animal experimentation; *cloning; gene therapy; genetic identity; motivation; organ donation; reproductive technologies; *risks and benefits; nuclear transplantation; Roslin Institute (Scotland)

FitzGerald, Kevin T. Proposals for human cloning: a review and ethical evaluation. *In:* Monagle, John F.; Thomasma, David C., eds. Health Care Ethics: Critical Issues for the 21st Century. Gaithersburg, MD: Aspen

---

BE = bioethics accession number   fn. = footnotes   refs. = references

Publishers; 1998: 3–7. 10 fn. ISBN 0–8342–0911–X. BE56275.
> *cloning; embryos; family members; gene therapy; genetic disorders; organ donation; reproduction; reproductive technologies; rights; risks and benefits

France. National Ethics Advisory Committee for the Biological and Health Sciences (Comité Consultatif National d'Éthique pour les Sciences de la Vie et de la Santé). Reply to the President of the French Republic on the Subject of Reproductive Cloning [Report No. 54]. [English translation]. Internet Web Site: http://www.ccne–ethique.org/ccne—uk/avis/a—054.htm; 1997 Apr 22 [online]. 25 p. 35 refs. Downloaded 2 Jun 1997. BE57396.
> advisory committees; animal experimentation; *cloning; embryos; genetic identity; genetics; *government regulation; human experimentation; human rights; infertility; information dissemination; international aspects; legal aspects; mass media; motivation; *public policy; reproduction; reproductive technologies; risks and benefits; terminology; transgenic animals; twins; *nuclear transplantation; European Union; *France; *National Ethics Advisory Committee (France)

Franklin, Sarah. Dolly: a new form of transgenic breedwealth. *Environmental Values.* 1997 Nov; 6(4): 427–437. 11 refs. BE58569.
> *cloning; commodification; historical aspects; mass media; patents; property rights; public opinion; reproductive technologies; *speciesism; *transgenic animals; *agriculture; nuclear transplantation; Great Britain

Gorman, Christine. To ban or not to ban? [News]. *Time.* 1997 Jun 16; 149(24): 66. BE57991.
> advisory committees; *cloning; embryo research; federal government; *government regulation; legal aspects; political activity; private sector; public sector; reproductive technologies; Cloning Human Beings (NBAC); *National Bioethics Advisory Commission; *United States

Haglund, Keith. Ninety–day wonder. [Editorial]. *Journal of NIH Research.* 1997 Jul; 9(7): 10. BE55553.
> abortion, induced; advisory committees; *cloning; embryo research; federal government; freedom; *government regulation; legislation; reproductive technologies; science; National Bioethics Advisory Commission; U.S. Congress; *United States

Hamer, Dean; Copeland, Peter. Engineering temperament: cloning and the future politics of personality. *In: their* Living with Our Genes: Why They Matter More Than You Think. New York, NY: Doubleday; 1998: 295–316, 344. 11 refs. ISBN 0–385–48583–2. BE57647.
> *behavioral genetics; brain; *cloning; gene therapy; *genetic determinism; genetic enhancement; *genetic intervention; genetic predisposition; genetic screening; germ cells; industry; psychoactive drugs; risks and benefits; uncertainty; *personality

Harris, John. Cloning and bioethical thinking. [Letter]. *Nature.* 1997 Oct 2; 389(6650): 433. BE57157.
> *cloning; embryo research; embryos; ethical theory; moral obligations; motivation

Harris, John. Cloning and human dignity. *Cambridge Quarterly of Healthcare Ethics.* 1998 Spring; 7(2): 163–167. 11 fn. BE58008.
> attitudes; autonomy; *cloning; embryos; human rights; moral obligations; morality; motivation; public policy; reproductive technologies; risks and benefits; social impact; twins; *dignity; Kant, Immanuel

...Appeals to human dignity are, of course, universally attractive; they are also comprehensively vague. A first question to ask when the idea of human dignity is invoked is: whose dignity is attacked and how? If it is the duplication of a large part of the human genome that is supposed to constitute the attack on human dignity, or where the issue of "genetic identity" is invoked, we might legitimately ask whether and how the dignity of a natural twin is threatened by the existence of her sister and what follows as to the permissibility of natural monozygotic twinning? However, the notion of human dignity is often linked to Kantian ethics and it is this link I wish to examine more closely here.

Harris, John. "Goodbye Dolly?" The ethics of human cloning. *Journal of Medical Ethics.* 1997 Dec; 23(6): 353–360. 34 fn. BE57662.
> attitudes; autonomy; *cloning; deontological ethics; embryo research; embryo transfer; eugenics; gene therapy; genetic diversity; genetic identity; germ cells; human experimentation; human rights; international aspects; preimplantation diagnosis; public policy; reproduction; *risks and benefits; twinning; cell lines; dignity; embryo splitting; nuclear transplantation; European Parliament; Unesco; World Health Organization

The ethical implications of human clones have been much alluded to, but have seldom been examined with any rigour. This paper examines the possible uses and abuses of human cloning and draws out the principal ethical dimensions, both of what might be done and its meaning. The paper examines some of the major public and official responses to cloning by authorities such as President Clinton, the World Health Organisation, the European parliament, UNESCO, and others and reveals their inadequacies as foundations for a coherent public policy on human cloning. The paper ends by defending a conception of reproductive rights of "procreative autonomy" which shows human cloning to be not inconsistent with human rights and dignity.

Hauerwas, Stanley; Shuman, Joel. Cloning the human body. *In:* Cole–Turner, Ronald, ed. Human Cloning: Religious Responses. Louisville, KY: Westminster John Knox Press; 1997: 58–65. 4 fn. ISBN 0–644–25771–2. BE58144.
> animal experimentation; *Christian ethics; *cloning; *human body; reproduction; self concept; suffering; *theology

Herbert, Wray; Sheler, Jeffery L.; Watson, Traci. The world after cloning. *U.S. News and World Report.* 1997 Mar 10; 122(9): 59–63. BE56227.
> *cloning; human experimentation; industry; methods; motivation; religious ethics; risks and benefits; social impact

Hodgson, John. Dolly opens a farm full of possibilities. [News]. *Nature Biotechnology.* 1997 Apr; 15(4): 306. BE55966.
> animal experimentation; *cloning; drug industry; economics; methods; *risks and benefits; transgenic animals; nuclear transplantation; PPL Therapeutics; Scotland

Holden, Constance. UN weighs in on cloning. [News]. *Science.* 1997 Nov 21; 278(5342): 1407. BE57341.
> *cloning; genetic information; genetic intervention; genetic research; genome mapping; guidelines; human rights; *international aspects; Declaration on the Human Genome (Unesco); *Unesco

Holm, Søren. A life in the shadow: one reason why we should not clone humans. *Cambridge Quarterly of Healthcare Ethics.* 1998 Spring; 7(2): 160–162. 1 ref.

BE = bioethics accession number   fn. = footnotes   refs. = references

BE58009.
    *cloning; *genetic determinism; *genetic identity; twins
Introduction: One of the arguments that is often put forward in the discussion of human cloning is that it is in itself wrong to create a copy of a human being. This argument is usually dismissed by pointing out that a) we do not find anything wrong in the existence of monozygotic twins even though they are genetically identical, and b) the clone would not be an exact copy of the original even in those cases where it is an exact genetic copy, since it would have experienced a different environment that would have modified its biological and psychological development. In my view both these counterarguments are valid, but nevertheless I think that there is some core of truth in the assertion that it is wrong deliberately to try to create a copy of an already existing human being. It is this idea that I will briefly try to explicate here.

Hopkins, Patrick D. Bad copies: how popular media represent cloning as an ethical problem. *Hastings Center Report.* 1998 Mar–Apr; 28(2): 6–13. 4 fn. BE57538.
    attitudes; *cloning; genetic determinism; genetic identity; human experimentation; *mass media; morality; motivation; public opinion; science; United States

Johnson, Dirk. Eccentric's hubris set off global frenzy over cloning. [News]. *New York Times.* 1998 Jan 24: A1, A11. BE58128.
    *cloning; embryo research; financial support; government regulation; *investigators; *mass media; reproductive technologies; technical expertise; *Seed, Richard

Jones, Steve. Arguing ethics, forfeiting progress. *New York Times.* 1998 Mar 14: A17. BE57987.
    *cloning; emotions; genetic identity; organ transplantation; public policy; regulation; reproductive technologies; risks and benefits; *social control; United States

Josefson, Deborah. US scientist plans human cloning clinic. [News]. *BMJ (British Medical Journal).* 1998 Jan 17; 316(7126): 167. BE57910.
    *cloning; health facilities; human experimentation; international aspects; investigators; private sector; public policy; reproductive technologies; risks and benefits; Europe; *Seed, Richard; United States

Kahn, Axel. Cloning, dignity and ethical revisionism. [Letter]. *Nature.* 1997 Jul 24; 388(6640): 320. BE56592.
    *cloning; dehumanization; embryos; reproductive technologies; research embryo creation; dignity

Kassirer, Jerome P.; Rosenthal, Nadia A. Should human cloning research be off limits? [Editorial]. *New England Journal of Medicine.* 1998 Mar 26; 338(13): 905–906. 8 refs. BE57414.
    *cloning; embryo research; federal government; genetic research; government regulation; human experimentation; public policy; risks and benefits; United States

Keeler, William. The problem with human cloning. *Origins.* 1998 Feb 26; 27(36): 597, 599–601. 8 fn. Testimony before the House Commerce Committee's Subcommittee on Health and the Environment on behalf of the National Conference of Catholic Bishops' Pro-Life Activities Committee, 12 Feb 1998. BE58775.
    advisory committees; *cloning; dehumanization; embryo research; moral policy; parent child relationship; public policy; reproduction; risks and benefits; *Roman Catholic ethics; National Bioethics Advisory Commission; United States

Kestenbaum, David. Cloning plan spawns ethics debate. [News]. *Science.* 1998 Jan 16; 279(5349): 315. BE57420.
    *cloning; human experimentation; investigators; mass media; public policy; Seed, Richard; United States

Klotzko, Arlene Judith. Dolly, cloning, and the public misunderstanding of science: a challenge for us all. [Editorial]. *Cambridge Quarterly of Healthcare Ethics.* 1998 Spring; 7(2): 115–116. 1 ref. BE58010.
    *cloning; comprehension; decision making; education; *information dissemination; investigators; mass media; public opinion; science

Klotzko, Arlene Judith. Science fictions: cloning is bad and septuplets are good. *Washington Post.* 1997 Dec 14: C3. BE58498.
    *cloning; mass media; *multiple pregnancy; *reproductive technologies; *risks and benefits

Klotzko, Arlene Judith. The debate about Dolly. *Bioethics.* 1997 Oct; 11(5): 427–438. 27 fn. BE56332.
    abortion, induced; advisory committees; animal experimentation; attitudes; *cloning; embryo research; ethical theory; federal government; government financing; government regulation; human experimentation; legislation; mass media; political activity; politics; public opinion; *public policy; religion; state government; nuclear transplantation; Great Britain; Human Embryo Research Panel; National Bioethics Advisory Commission; *United States

Klotzko, Arlene Judith; Bulfield, Grahame; Campbell, Keith, et al. Voices from Roslin: the creators of Dolly discuss science, ethics, and social responsibility. [Interview]. *Cambridge Quarterly of Healthcare Ethics.* 1998 Spring; 7(2): 121–140. 8 fn. BE58011.
    animal experimentation; biomedical research; *cloning; embryos; expert testimony; *genetic intervention; goals; *investigators; methods; obligations to society; regulation; reproductive technologies; research institutes; risks and benefits; science; *transgenic animals; nuclear transplantation; PPL Therapeutics; *Roslin Institute (Scotland); Scotland; U.S. Congress; United States

Kolata, Gina. Clone: The Road to Dolly, and the Path Ahead. New York, NY: William Morrow; 1998. 276 p. Includes references. ISBN 0–688–15692–4. BE56508.
    animal experimentation; *cloning; genetic intervention; genetic materials; historical aspects; industry; infertility; investigators; mass media; methods; reproductive technologies; risks and benefits; science; scientific misconduct; social impact; trends; agriculture; *nuclear transplantation; Illmensee, Karl; PPL Therapeutics; Scotland; Wilmut, Ian

Kuhse, Helga; Singer, Peter. Cloning our way to Armageddon? [Editorial]. *Bioethics.* 1997 Oct; 11(5): iii–v. 1 fn. BE56333.
    *attitudes; *cloning; human experimentation; international aspects; mass media; *risks and benefits

Kuhse, Helga; Singer, Peter. On the ethics of bringing people into existence. [Editorial]. *Bioethics.* 1998 Apr; 12(2): iii–v. 2 fn. BE58623.
    bioethical issues; *cloning; *future generations; genetic intervention; genome mapping; moral obligations; population control; *quality of life; *reproduction; theology; *value of life

Labib, Karim. Don't leave dignity out of the cloning debate. [Letter]. *Nature.* 1997 Jul 3; 388(6637): 15. BE56575.
    *cloning; *dehumanization; embryo research; *dignity

BE = bioethics accession number   fn. = footnotes   refs. = references

Lebacqz, Karen. Genes, justice, and clones. *In:* Cole–Turner, Ronald, ed. Human Cloning: Religious Responses. Louisville, KY: Westminister John Knox Press; 1997: 49–57. 21 fn. ISBN 0–664–25771–2. BE58143.
*cloning; disadvantaged; females; genetic identity; genetics; homosexuals; infertility; *justice; males; parent child relationship; *reproduction; reproductive technologies; resource allocation; *rights; social discrimination; socioeconomic factors

McGee, Glenn; Wilmut, Ian. Cloning and the adoption model. *In:* McGee, Glenn, ed. The Human Cloning Debate. Berkeley, CA: Berkeley Hills Books; 1998: 93–105. 7 fn. ISBN 0–9653774–8–2. BE58990.
*adoption; beneficence; children; *cloning; freedom; *government regulation; infertility; models, theoretical; obligations of society; parent child relationship; public policy; reproduction; reproductive technologies; rights; risks and benefits; United States

McGee, Glenn, ed. The Human Cloning Debate. Berkeley, CA: Berkeley Hills Books; 1998. 270 p. 73 fn. ISBN 0–9653774–8–2. BE58988.
adoption; advisory committees; Buddhist ethics; children; Christian ethics; *cloning; eugenics; genetic identity; government regulation; Islamic ethics; Jewish ethics; methods; moral policy; motivation; parent child relationship; personhood; philosophy; public policy; religious ethics; reproduction; reproductive technologies; rights; *risks and benefits; Roman Catholic ethics; *social control; social impact; value of life; National Bioethics Advisory Commission; United States

Macklin, Ruth. Human cloning? Don't just say no. *U.S. News and World Report.* 1997 Mar 10; 122(9): 64. BE56233.
*cloning; genetic enhancement; genetic identity; government regulation; human experimentation; risks and benefits

McLaren, Anne; European Commission. Group of Advisers on the Ethical Implications of Biotechnology. Ethical aspects of cloning techniques: opinion of the Group of Advisers on the Ethical Implications of Biotechnology of the European Commission. [Statement and commentary]. *Cambridge Quarterly of Healthcare Ethics.* 1998 Spring; 7(2): 187–193. BE58012.
advisory committees; animal experimentation; *cloning; embryo research; embryos; international aspects; *public policy; regulation; reproductive technologies; risks and benefits; terminology; twins; embryo splitting; nuclear transplantation; Europe; *European Commission; Group of Advisers on the Ethical Implications of Biotechnology (European Commission)

MacQuitty, Jonathan J. The real implications of Dolly. *Nature Biotechnology.* 1997 Apr; 15(4): 294. BE55956.
animal experimentation; *cloning; embryo research; federal government; genetic research; goals; government regulation; human experimentation; mass media; methods; transgenic animals; nuclear transplantation; Great Britain; United States

Marshall, Eliot. Biomedical groups derail fast–track anticloning bill. [News]. *Science.* 1998 Feb 20; 279(5354): 1123–1124. BE58108.
biomedical research; *cloning; drug industry; embryo research; federal government; *government regulation; *investigators; legislation; *political activity; politics; *U.S. Congress; *United States

Marwick, Charles. Put human cloning on hold, say bioethicists. [News]. *JAMA.* 1997 Jul 2; 278(1): 13–14.

BE56313.
advisory committees; *cloning; federal government; genetic research; government financing; *government regulation; human experimentation; morality; *public policy; reproductive technologies; self regulation; *National Bioethics Advisory Commission; *United States

Miller, Franklin G.; Caplan, Arthur L.; Fletcher, John C. Dealing with Dolly: inside the National Bioethics Advisory Commission. *Health Affairs.* 1998 May–Jun; 17(3): 264–267. 6 fn. BE58758.
*advisory committees; bioethical issues; *cloning; embryo research; federal government; genetic information; genetic research; government financing; government regulation; human experimentation; mentally ill; moral policy; politics; *public policy; religion; risks and benefits; *National Bioethics Advisory Commission; *United States

Mohler, R. Albert. The brave new world of cloning: a Christian worldview perspective. *In:* Cole–Turner, Ronald, ed. Human Cloning: Religious Responses. Louisville, KY: Westminister John Knox Press; 1997: 91–105. 27 fn. ISBN 0–664–25771–2. BE58147.
animal experimentation; *Christian ethics; *cloning; coercion; *eugenics; family relationship; genetic screening; parent child relationship; reproduction; reproductive technologies; secularism; social impact; theology; value of life

Morton, Oliver; Williams, Nigel. First Dolly, now headless tadpoles. [News]. *Science.* 1997 Oct 31; 278(5339): 798. BE58063.
animal experimentation; animal organs; *cloning; editorial policies; embryo research; industry; *mass media; organ donation; *Great Britain

Nelkin, Dorothy; Lindee, M. Susan. Cloning in the popular imagination. *Cambridge Quarterly of Healthcare Ethics.* 1998 Spring; 7(2): 145–149. 20 fn. BE58013.
animal experimentation; *attitudes; *cloning; genetic determinism; genetics; mass media; regulation; religion; reproductive technologies; risks and benefits; science; *social impact; Roslin Institute (Scotland)

Newman, Stephen A. Human cloning and the family: reflections on cloning existing children. *New York Law School Journal of Human Rights.* 1997 Spring; 13(3): 523–530. 1 fn. BE57777.
*children; *cloning; *family relationship; genetic identity; human experimentation; motivation; parents; psychological stress; risks and benefits; *self concept; siblings; terminally ill; twins

Parens, Erik. Tools from and for democratic deliberations. *Hastings Center Report.* 1997 Sep–Oct; 27(5): 20–22. 1 ref. BE56117.
advisory committees; *cloning; consensus; cultural pluralism; *decision making; democracy; embryo research; genetic intervention; methods; moral policy; *public policy; religion; reproductive technologies; risks and benefits; secularism; social impact; nuclear transplantation; *Cloning Human Beings (NBAC); *National Bioethics Advisory Commission; United States

Paris, Peter J. A view from the underside. *In:* Cole–Turner, Ronald, ed. Human Cloning: Religious Responses. Louisville, KY: Westminister John Knox Press; 1997: 43–48. ISBN 0–664–25771–2. BE58142.
*cloning; dehumanization; eugenics; genetic diversity; human experimentation; investigators; minority groups; misconduct; motivation; public participation; public policy; regulation; religion; *risks and benefits; *social discrimination; utilitarianism; slavery

---

BE = bioethics accession number   fn. = footnotes   refs. = references

Pence, Gregory E., ed. Flesh of My Flesh: The Ethics of Cloning Humans: A Reader. Lanham, MD: Rowman and Littlefield; 1998. 154 p. Includes references. ISBN 0-8476-8982-4. BE57848.
advisory committees; autonomy; bioethics; brain; *cloning; dehumanization; embryo research; emotions; eugenics; genetic identity; government regulation; historical aspects; homosexuals; human experimentation; informed consent; libertarianism; marital relationship; methods; *moral policy; parent child relationship; Protestant ethics; public opinion; *public policy; reproductive technologies; research embryo creation; rights; risks and benefits; self concept; sexuality; social control; *social impact; twins; values; wedge argument; nuclear transplantation; National Bioethics Advisory Commission; United States

Pence, Gregory E. Who's Afraid of Human Cloning? Lanham, MD: Rowman and Littlefield; 1998. 181 p. Includes references. ISBN 0-8476-8782-1. BE56784.
advisory committees; attitudes; *cloning; embryo research; embryos; emotions; ethicists; eugenics; evolution; freedom; gene therapy; genetic determinism; genetic diversity; genetic identity; government regulation; homosexuals; human experimentation; industry; infertility; investigators; *moral policy; morality; personhood; policy analysis; preimplantation diagnosis; *public policy; religious ethics; reproductive technologies; rights; *risks and benefits; sexuality; social discrimination; twins; wedge argument; Human Embryo Research Panel; National Bioethics Advisory Commission; United States

Pennisi, Elizabeth. After Dolly, a pharming frenzy. [News]. *Science.* 1998 Jan 30; 279(5351): 646-648. BE57421.
animal experimentation; animal organs; *cloning; drug industry; genetic research; *industry; international aspects; *methods; *transgenic animals; nuclear transplantation; Netherlands; Pharming Holding N.V.; United States

Pennisi, Elizabeth. The lamb that roared. [News]. *Science.* 1997 Dec 19; 278(5346): 2038-2039. BE57316.
animal experimentation; *cloning; genetic intervention; risks and benefits; *social impact; transgenic animals; nuclear transplantation; Roslin Institute (Scotland)

Peters, Ted. Cloning shock: a theological reaction. *In:* Cole-Turner, Ronald, ed. Human Cloning: Religious Responses. Louisville, KY: Westminister John Knox Press; 1997: 12-24. 12 fn. ISBN 0-664-25771-2. BE58139.
animal experimentation; *children; *Christian ethics; *cloning; *commodification; embryo research; genetic identity; *human rights; love; regulation; reproduction; reproductive technologies; social worth; *theology; twins; dignity; quality assurance; Roslin Institute (Scotland)

Polkinghorne, John. Cloning and the moral imperative. *In:* Cole-Turner, Ronald, ed. Human Cloning: Religious Responses. Louisville, KY: Westminister John Knox Press; 1997: 35-42. 1 fn. ISBN 0-664-25771-2. BE58141.
*Christian ethics; *cloning; embryo research; embryos; personhood; regulation; risks and benefits; theology; value of life; Great Britain

Ramsay, Sarah. UK public consulted on ethics of human cloning. [News]. *Lancet.* 1998 Feb 7; 351(9100): 427. BE59082.
advisory committees; *cloning; decision making; embryo research; government regulation; morality; *public participation; *public policy; *Great Britain; *Human Fertilisation and Embryology Authority; *Human Genetics Advisory Commission (Great Britain)

Ravindra, Ravi; Roach, Geshe Michael; LaFleur,

William, et al. Buddhists on cloning. *In:* McGee, Glenn, ed. The Human Cloning Debate. Berkeley, CA: Berkeley Hills Books; 1998: 227-230. ISBN 0-9653774-8-2. BE58992.
*Buddhist ethics; *cloning; conscience; genetic identity; investigators; motivation; reproductive technologies

Robertson, John A. Human cloning and the challenge of regulation. *New England Journal of Medicine.* 1998 Jul 9; 339(2): 119-122. 24 refs. BE58656.
children; *cloning; federal government; financial support; genetic intervention; *government regulation; investigators; motivation; parent child relationship; parents; private sector; *public policy; reproduction; reproductive technologies; rights; *risks and benefits; tissue donation; twins; *United States

Robertson, John A. Liberty, identity, and human cloning. *Texas Law Review.* 1998 May; 76(6): 1371-1456. 298 fn. BE57440.
adults; advisory committees; animal experimentation; autonomy; children; *cloning; disclosure; donors; embryo research; embryos; eugenics; family relationship; federal government; *freedom; genetic determinism; genetic enhancement; genetic identity; genetic intervention; genetic materials; *government regulation; guidelines; human experimentation; infertility; informed consent; intention; mandatory programs; methods; *moral policy; motivation; organ donation; parents; policy analysis; *public policy; remuneration; *reproduction; reproductive technologies; review; *rights; *risks and benefits; transgenic animals; twins; wrongful life; embryo donation; embryo splitting; nuclear transplantation; National Bioethics Advisory Commission; United States

Rogers, Arthur. Britain denies prevarication over human-cloning ban. [News]. *Lancet.* 1997 Oct 18; 350(9085): 1151. BE56236.
*cloning; genetic research; guidelines; human experimentation; *international aspects; politics; *public policy; Council of Europe; European Convention on Bioethics; Germany; *Great Britain

Rogers, Arthur. Europe takes steps to outlaw human cloning. [News]. *Lancet.* 1997 Oct 4; 350(9083): 1012. BE57344.
*cloning; genetic intervention; *government regulation; human experimentation; *international aspects; *Council of Europe; Europe; European Bioethics Convention; Germany

Rovner, Julie. USA to think again about ban on human cloning. [News]. *Lancet.* 1998 Feb 21; 351(9102): 578. BE58515.
*cloning; government regulation; *politics; *public policy; research embryo creation; U.S. Congress; *United States

Roy, Ina. Philosophical perspectives. *In:* McGee, Glenn, ed. The Human Cloning Debate. Berkeley, CA: Berkeley Hills Books; 1998: 41-66. 7 fn. ISBN 0-9653774-8-2. BE58989.
children; *cloning; eugenics; feminist ethics; genetic identity; life extension; moral policy; motivation; organ donation; personhood; philosophy; reproduction; risks and benefits; surrogate mothers; theology

Sachedina, Abdulaziz. Human clones: an Islamic view. *In:* McGee, Glenn, ed. The Human Cloning Debate. Berkeley, CA: Berkeley Hills Books; 1998: 231-244. 19 fn. ISBN 0-9653774-8-2. BE58993.
*cloning; embryo research; family relationship; *Islamic ethics; personhood; reproductive technologies; resource allocation; risks and benefits; social impact; theology

Saegusa, Asako. Japan gears up to debate brake on human

BE = bioethics accession number   fn. = footnotes   refs. = references

cloning. [News]. *Nature*. 1998 Jan 22; 391(6665): 313. BE57361.
  advisory committees; *cloning; embryo research; government regulation; human experimentation; *public policy; *Japan

Shapiro, David. Cloning, dignity and ethical reasoning. [Letter]. *Nature*. 1997 Aug 7; 388(6642): 511. BE56436.
  animal experimentation; autonomy; *cloning; dehumanization; family relationship; genetic determinism; reproductive technologies; dignity

Shinn, Roger L. Between Eden and Babel. *In:* Cole-Turner, Ronald, ed. Human Cloning: Religious Responses. Louisville, KY: Westminister John Knox Press; 1997: 106–118. 8 fn. ISBN 0-664-25771-2. BE58148.
  animal experimentation; Christian ethics; *cloning; eugenics; genetic intervention; historical aspects; motivation; regulation; reproduction; rights; risks and benefits; science

Silberner, Joanne. Seeding the cloning debate. *Hastings Center Report*. 1998 Mar–Apr; 28(2): 5. BE57537.
  *cloning; investigators; mass media; politics; Seed, Richard; United States

Silver, Lee M. Cloning, ethics, and religion. *Cambridge Quarterly of Healthcare Ethics*. 1998 Spring; 7(2): 168–172. 14 fn. This article is based on material extracted from L.M. Silver, *Remaking Eden: Cloning and Beyond in a Brave New World*, Avon Books, 1997. BE58015.
  *cloning; genetic identity; regulation; *religion; reproductive technologies; risks and benefits; social impact

Silver, Lee M. Remaking Eden: Cloning and Beyond in a Brave New World. New York, NY: Avon Books; 1997. 317 p. Includes references. ISBN 0-380-97494-0. BE56517.
  artificial insemination; beginning of life; *cloning; cryopreservation; embryos; eugenics; family relationship; fathers; females; fetal development; freedom; future generations; genetic enhancement; genetics; germ cells; government regulation; homosexuals; in vitro fertilization; infertility; males; mothers; motivation; ovum donors; parent child relationship; preimplantation diagnosis; religion; reproduction; *reproductive technologies; rights; semen donors; single persons; *social impact; socioeconomic factors; surrogate mothers; transgenic animals; *trends; United States

Stolberg, Sheryl Gay. F.D.A. stand on cloning raises even more questions. [News]. *New York Times*. 1998 Jan 21: A14. BE58047.
  biomedical research; *cloning; embryo research; federal government; gene therapy; *government regulation; industry; investigators; political activity; reproductive technologies; *Food and Drug Administration; U.S. Congress; *United States

Strong, Carson. Cloning and infertility. *Cambridge Quarterly of Healthcare Ethics*. 1998 Summer; 7(3): 279-293. 40 fn. BE58556.
  autonomy; children; *cloning; confidentiality; counseling; disclosure; freedom; genetic disorders; genetic enhancement; genetic identity; government regulation; *infertility; injuries; *moral policy; motivation; parent child relationship; privacy; psychological stress; public policy; reproduction; reproductive technologies; research embryo creation; risks and benefits; self concept; wrongful life

Turner, Leigh. A sheep named Dolly. [Editorial]. *Canadian Medical Association Journal*. 1997 Apr 15; 156(8): 1149-1150. 2 refs. BE57357.
  animal experimentation; *cloning; embryos; moral policy;

personhood; risks and benefits; Roslin Institute (Scotland); Wilmut, Ian

U.S. Congress. House. Committee on Science. Subcommittee on Technology. Biotechnology and the Ethics of Cloning: How Far Should We Go? Hearing, 5 Mar 1997. Washington, DC: U.S. Government Printing Office; 1997. 59 p. No. 3. ISBN 0-16-055267-2. BE56349.
  animal experimentation; *cloning; embryo research; federal government; genetic research; government financing; government regulation; human experimentation; industry; morality; public policy; reproductive technologies; risks and benefits; transgenic organisms; agriculture; nuclear transplantation; United States

U.S. Congress. House. Committee on Science. Subcommittee on Technology. Review of the President's Commission's Recommendations on Cloning. Hearing, 12 Jun 1997. Washington, DC: U.S. Government Printing Office; 1997. 227 p. No. 19. Includes text of the National Bioethics Advisory Commission's *Cloning Human Beings: Report and Recommendations*, Jun 1997. ISBN 0-16-055881-6. BE58987.
  *advisory committees; animal experimentation; *cloning; embryo research; federal government; *government regulation; private sector; *public policy; public sector; reproductive technologies; *risks and benefits; national ethics committees; nuclear transplantation; *National Bioethics Advisory Commission; *United States

U.S. Congress. Senate. Committee on Labor and Human Resources. Subcommittee on Public Health and Safety. Ethics and Theology: A Continuation of the National Discussion on Human Cloning. Hearing, 17 Jun 1997. Washington, DC: U.S. Government Printing Office; 1997. 69 p. S. Hrg. 105-123. ISBN 0-16-055475-6. BE58698.
  advisory committees; autonomy; children; *cloning; embryo research; family relationship; federal government; Islamic ethics; Jewish ethics; Protestant ethics; public policy; *religious ethics; reproductive technologies; rights; *risks and benefits; Roman Catholic ethics; science; social impact; theology; nuclear transplantation; National Bioethics Advisory Commission; United States

U.S. Congress. Senate. Committee on Labor and Human Resources. Subcommittee on Public Health and Safety. Scientific Discoveries in Cloning: Challenges for Public Policy. Hearing, 12 Mar 1997. Washington, DC: U.S. Government Printing Office; 1997. 87 p. S. Hrg. 105-22. ISBN 0-16-054938-8. BE56519.
  advisory committees; animal experimentation; biomedical research; *cloning; embryo research; embryos; federal government; genetic disorders; government financing; government regulation; human experimentation; industry; investigators; organ transplantation; *public policy; reproductive technologies; *risks and benefits; social impact; transgenic animals; nuclear transplantation; Great Britain; National Bioethics Advisory Commission; United States; Wilmut, Ian

Verhey, Allen. Theology after Dolly. *Christian Century*. 1997 Mar 19-26; 114(10): 285-286. BE56046.
  autonomy; children; *cloning; *dehumanization; family relationship; freedom; human body; motivation; parent child relationship; *reproduction; rights; risks and benefits; self concept; *theology; utilitarianism; personal identity; Lederberg, Joshua; *Ramsey, Paul

Wachbroit, Robert. Genetic encores: the ethics of human

BE = bioethics accession number   fn. = footnotes   refs. = references

cloning. *Philosophy and Public Policy.* 1997 Fall; 17(4): 1–7. 7 fn. BE58776.
    advisory committees; *cloning; genetic determinism; genetic intervention; moral policy; motivation; parent child relationship; public policy; reproductive technologies; *risks and benefits; social impact; National Bioethics Advisory Commission; United States

Wadman, Meredith. Backing for anti–cloning bill reopens embryo debate. [News]. *Nature.* 1997 Aug 7; 388(6642): 505. BE56318.
    biomedical research; *cloning; *embryo research; embryos; federal government; government financing; *government regulation; legislation; private sector; research embryo creation; *U.S. Congress; *United States

Wadman, Meredith. Cloning for research 'should be allowed.' [News]. *Nature.* 1997 Jul 3; 388(6637): 6. BE56319.
    attitudes; *cloning; federal government; freedom; genetic research; *government regulation; human experimentation; international aspects; investigators; regulation; research embryo creation; nuclear transplantation; United States; Wilmut, Ian

Wadman, Meredith. Seed sows further doubts on cloning. [News]. *Nature.* 1998 Jan 15; 391(6664): 218–219. Includes inset articles by M. Wadman, "US ban 'would resist challenges in court'," p. 218; by M. Wadman and D. Butler, "Unesco declaration lacks legal teeth," p. 219; and by D. Butler, "Europe brings in first international ban," p. 219. BE58024.
    *cloning; embryo research; federal government; government regulation; international aspects; investigators; legal aspects; reproductive technologies; Europe; Seed, Richard; U.S. Congress; United States

Wadman, Meredith. Unesco text will target gene techniques. [News]. *Nature.* 1997 Aug 7; 388(6642): 508. BE56218.
    advisory committees; *cloning; embryo research; *gene therapy; genetic research; *germ cells; government regulation; guidelines; human rights; *international aspects; public policy; Canada; Germany; International Bioethics Committee (Unesco); *Unesco

Wadman, Meredith. US Senate bills on cloning under fire from researchers. [News]. *Nature.* 1998 Feb 12; 391(6668): 623. BE58073.
    *cloning; dissent; embryo research; embryo transfer; *government regulation; investigators; legislation; politics; professional organizations; American Association for Cancer Research; Association of American Medical Colleges; Federation of American Societies for Experimental Biology; *U.S. Congress; *United States

Warnock, Mary. The regulation of technology. *Cambridge Quarterly of Healthcare Ethics.* 1998 Spring; 7(2): 173–175. BE58016.
    biomedical research; *cloning; embryos; freedom; government regulation; investigators; *regulation; risks and benefits; self regulation; social control
Everybody recognizes that most of the problems in medical ethics arise, these days, from innovations in medical technology. We would not have had to lay down laws or ethical guidelines about assisted reproduction had it not been for the new technology of in vitro fertilization, which produced the first IVF baby in 1978. We would not be currently anxious about the ethics of possible human cloning, had it not been for the production in Edinburgh of Dolly, the lamb whose birth resulted from the removal of a mammary gland cell from an adult sheep. So the question is whether there is some

research into developing technology that is too dangerous, that will lead to consequences too dramatic for humanity, for the research itself to be permitted. Should there be control over what technological innovation should be permitted?

Water, Brent. One flesh? Cloning, procreation, and the family. *In:* Cole-Turner, Ronald, ed. Human Cloning: Religious Responses. Louisville, KY: Westminister John Knox Press; 1997: 78–90. 10 fn. ISBN 0-664-25771-2. BE58146.
    *cloning; *family relationship; freedom; love; motivation; parent child relationship; *reproduction; reproductive technologies; *rights; social impact

Watson, Rory. European parliament wants world ban on human cloning. [News]. *BMJ (British Medical Journal).* 1997 Mar 22; 314(7084): 847. BE58502.
    advisory committees; animal experimentation; *cloning; human experimentation; *international aspects; *public policy; regulation; risks and benefits; national ethics committees; *Europe; European Parliament; European Union

Watson, Rory. The [European] Union gets interested in ethics. [News]. *BMJ (British Medical Journal).* 1997 Jun 28; 314(7098): 1854. BE56443.
    advisory committees; animal experimentation; *cloning; embryos; ethics committees; *genetic intervention; human experimentation; *international aspects; patents; public participation; *regulation; *Europe; *European Union

Wilkie, Tom; Graham, Elizabeth. Power without responsibility: media portrayals of Dolly and science. *Cambridge Quarterly of Healthcare Ethics.* 1998 Spring; 7(2): 150–159. 33 fn. BE58017.
    animal experimentation; *cloning; comparative studies; editorial policies; eugenics; government regulation; *information dissemination; international aspects; investigators; *mass media; risks and benefits; *science; social impact; technical expertise; *Great Britain; *Roslin Institute (Scotland); United States
...In this article, we will analyze principally the British broadsheet newspaper coverage of the Dolly story. We also look at some of the corresponding U.S. newspaper coverage and find striking contrasts, relating not just to journalistic practices but also to the public status and position of science in the two countries. For reasons of space and difficulty of obtaining archive material, we do not address the role of the broadcast media.

Winston, Robert. The promise of cloning for human medicine: not a moral threat but an exciting challenge. [Editorial]. *BMJ (British Medical Journal).* 1997 Mar 29; 314(7085): 913–914. 9 refs. BE58604.
    *cloning; genetic research; regulation; reproductive technologies; *risks and benefits

Wise, Jacqui. Bills on human cloning are full of loopholes. [News]. *BMJ (British Medical Journal).* 1998 Feb 21; 316(7131): 573. BE57365.
    *cloning; federal government; *government regulation; *legislation; state government; *United States

Wolf, Susan M. Ban cloning? Why NBAC is wrong. *Hastings Center Report.* 1997 Sep–Oct; 27(5): 12–15. 21 fn. BE56114.
    *advisory committees; biomedical research; children; *cloning; constitutional law; cultural pluralism; embryo research; embryo transfer; federal government; freedom; genetic intervention; *government regulation; human experimentation; industry; legal aspects; methods; models, theoretical; morality; politics; private sector; *public policy;

BE = bioethics accession number   fn. = footnotes   refs. = references

reproductive technologies; risks and benefits; self regulation; social impact; embryo splitting; nuclear transplantation; Cloning Human Beings (NBAC); *National Bioethics Advisory Commission; Recombinant DNA Advisory Committee; U.S. Congress; *United States

Yount, Lisa. Should human genes be altered? [Juvenile literature]. *In: her* Issues in Biomedical Ethics. San Diego, CA: Lucent Books; 1998: 75–93, 104–105. 30 fn. ISBN 1-56006-476-5. BE57682.
*cloning; coercion; employment; eugenics; future generations; gene pool; *gene therapy; genetic disorders; *genetic enhancement; genetic information; *genetic intervention; genetic screening; *germ cells; health insurance; informed consent; insurance selection bias; involuntary sterilization; killing; prenatal diagnosis; regulation; *risks and benefits; selective abortion; *social discrimination; wedge argument

A force of nature? Human need could prove too strong for any ban on cloning. [Editorial]. *New Scientist.* 1998 Jan 17; 156(2117): 3. BE59089.
attitudes; *cloning; infertility; *regulation; reproductive technologies; social control

A triumph of hope.... [Editorial]. *New Scientist.* 1997 May 31; 154(2084): 3. BE56421.
advisory committees; *cloning; *government regulation; human experimentation; industry; international aspects; private sector; *public policy; risks and benefits; Canada; Great Britain; National Bioethics Advisory Commission; *United States

Cooling down over cloning. [Editorial]. *Lancet.* 1998 Jan 17; 351(9097): 151. BE57413.
*cloning; genetic research; human experimentation; *international aspects; *public policy; regulation; *risks and benefits; Europe; Great Britain; Seed, Richard; United States

Crossing the line: Richard Seed may not win a place in history for cloning humans, but someone probably will. [News]. *New Scientist.* 1998 Jan 17; 156(2117): 4. BE59090.
animal experimentation; *cloning; industry; investigators; primates; regulation; reproductive technologies; risks and benefits; technical expertise; nuclear transplantation; Seed, Richard

Dolly clone institute wins research funding reprieve. [News]. *Nature.* 1998 Jan 1; 391(6662): 10. BE58091.
*cloning; *government financing; *research institutes; nuclear transplantation; *Great Britain; *Roslin Institute (Scotland)

Double trouble: Unesco should think again before endorsing an outright condemnation of human cloning. [Editorial]. *Nature.* 1997 Aug 7; 388(6642): 501. BE56057.
*cloning; guidelines; *international aspects; *public policy; reproduction; *Unesco

French Academy split on cloning policy. [News]. *Nature.* 1997 Jul 3; 388(6637): 11. BE56327.
*cloning; dissent; human experimentation; investigators; *organizational policies; professional organizations; regulation; *Academy of Sciences (France); *France

Hubris, benefits and minefields of human cloning. [Editorial]. *Nature.* 1998 Jan 15; 391(6664): 211. BE58031.
biomedical research; *cloning; government regulation; international aspects; reproductive technologies; risks and benefits; Seed, Richard

Thinking about cloning. [Editorial]. *Nature Biotechnology.* 1997 Apr.; 15(4): 293. BE55969.

*cloning; human experimentation; public policy; reproductive technologies; social impact

To clone or not to clone? [News]. *Christian Century.* 1997 Mar 19–26; 114(10): 286–288. BE56045.
*cloning; eugenics; gene therapy; genetic intervention; germ cells; government regulation; public policy; *religious ethics; reproductive technologies; risks and benefits; social impact; United States; Wilmut, Ian; World Health Organization

CODES OF ETHICS
See under
MEDICAL ETHICS/CODES OF ETHICS
NURSING ETHICS/CODES OF ETHICS
PROFESSIONAL ETHICS/CODES OF ETHICS

CONFIDENTIALITY

See also PATIENT ACCESS TO RECORDS
See also under
AIDS/CONFIDENTIALITY

Allen, Anita L. Genetic privacy: emerging concepts and values. *In:* Rothstein, Mark A., ed. Genetic Secrets: Protecting Privacy and Confidentiality in the Genetic Era. New Haven, CT: Yale University Press; 1997: 31–59. 141 fn. ISBN 0-300-07251-1. BE58674.
autonomy; beneficence; *confidentiality; democracy; disclosure; DNA data banks; family members; *genetic information; genetic intervention; genetic materials; genetic research; *genetic screening; genetic services; historical aspects; informed consent; legal rights; mandatory testing; mass screening; morality; *privacy; property rights; public policy; reproduction; review; social discrimination; stigmatization; terminology; values; biological specimen banks; Nineteenth Century; Twentieth Century; United States

Allison, Althea; Ewens, Ann. Tensions in sharing client confidences while respecting autonomy: implications for interprofessional practice. *Nursing Ethics.* 1998 Sep; 5(5): 441–450. 19 refs. BE58906.
autonomy; case studies; communication; *confidentiality; disclosure; health personnel; intention; *interprofessional relations; *patient care team; privacy; *professional patient relationship; referral and consultation; social workers

Alpert, Sheri A. Health care information: access, confidentiality, and good practice. *In:* Goodman, Kenneth W., ed. Ethics, Computing, and Medicine: Informatics and the Transformation of Health Care. New York, NY: Cambridge University Press; 1998: 75–101. 64 refs. ISBN 0-521-46905-8. BE57005.
*computer communication networks; *computers; *confidentiality; data banks; *disclosure; drug industry; economics; employment; genetic information; government regulation; *health care; health insurance; health services research; information dissemination; informed consent; legal aspects; *medical records; moral obligations; physician patient relationship; privacy; privileged communication; self regulation; social discrimination; standards; computer security; health data cards; United States

American Medical Record Association. Confidentiality of Patient Health Information. *American Medical Record Association Journal.* 1985 Dec; 56(12): 4–14. BE57866.
*confidentiality; *disclosure; forms; *health facilities; *institutional policies; *medical records; *organization and administration; *organizational policies; *patient access to records; professional organizations; *American Medical Record Association

---

BE = bioethics accession number   fn. = footnotes   refs. = references

American Society of Human Genetics. Social Issues Subcommittee on Familial Disclosure. ASHG statement: professional disclosure of familial genetic information. *American Journal of Human Genetics.* 1998 Feb; 62(2): 474–483. 46 refs. 32 fn. BE57550.
*confidentiality; *disclosure; *duty to warn; *family members; genetic counseling; genetic disorders; *genetic information; *genetic screening; *guidelines; *health personnel; informed consent; international aspects; legal obligations; moral obligations; *organizational policies; privacy; professional family relationship; professional organizations; professional patient relationship; risk; risks and benefits; *American Society of Human Genetics; United States

Andrews, Lori B. Gen-etiquette: genetic information, family relationships, and adoption. *In:* Rothstein, Mark A., ed. Genetic Secrets: Protecting Privacy and Confidentiality in the Genetic Era. New Haven, CT: Yale University Press; 1997: 255–280. 86 fn. ISBN 0-300-07251-1. BE58686.
*adoption; anthropology; children; *confidentiality; *disclosure; duty to warn; *family members; *family relationship; *genetic information; *genetic screening; health personnel; legal obligations; moral obligations; parent child relationship; parents; privacy; professional family relationship; rights; pedigree studies; United States

Andrews, Lori B. Genetic fallout: new technologies are changing the legal landscape. *Trial.* 1995 Dec; 31(12): 20–23, 25–27. 30 fn. BE57273.
carriers; *confidentiality; *disclosure; duty to warn; employment; family members; federal government; genetic disorders; *genetic information; genetic predisposition; *genetic screening; government regulation; health insurance; *legal aspects; legal liability; mandatory testing; mass screening; newborns; physicians; pregnant women; prenatal diagnosis; risk; *social discrimination; state government; stigmatization; treatment refusal; wrongful life; ELSI-funded publication; Americans with Disabilities Act 1990; Equal Employment Opportunity Commission; *United States

Armstrong, Mary Beth. Confidentiality, general issues of. *In:* Chadwick, Ruth, ed. Encyclopedia of Applied Ethics, Volume 1. San Diego, CA: Academic Press; 1998: 579–582. 5 refs. ISBN 0-12-227066-5. BE56375.
*confidentiality; deontological ethics; disclosure; moral obligations; professional ethics; risks and benefits; standards; utilitarianism; whistleblowing

Auguste, Valérie; Guérin, Corinne; Hervé, Christian, et al. Professional secret in hospitals: study conducted in a pharmacy department. *International Journal of Bioethics.* 1997 Dec; 8(4): 89–99. 12 refs. BE58366.
*attitudes; *confidentiality; disclosure; *drugs; *hospitals; *patient care; *patients; *pharmacists; *privacy; professional patient relationship; survey; *outpatients; *France

Baird, Patricia A. Registries, record linkage, and research in genetics: protecting privacy. *In:* Knoppers, Bartha Maria, ed. Human DNA: Law and Policy: International and Comparative Perspectives. Proceedings of the First International Conference on DNA Sampling and Human Genetic Research: Ethical, Legal, and Policy Aspects, held in Montreal, Canada, 6–8 Sep 1996. Boston, MA: Kluwer Law International; 1997: 165–175. 12 fn. ISBN 90-411-0361-9. BE58176.
computers; *confidentiality; *data banks; *DNA data banks; epidemiology; genetic disorders; *genetic information; genetic materials; *genetic research; genetic screening; informed consent; *medical records; privacy; *registries; tissue donation; *biological specimen banks; Canada

Barrett, Nicholas A. The medical student and the suicidal patient. *Journal of Medical Ethics.* 1997 Oct; 23(5): 277–281. 32 fn. BE57102.
*autonomy; communication; *confidentiality; dangerousness; decision making; *disclosure; legal aspects; legal liability; *medical education; *moral obligations; negligence; patient advocacy; patient care; *patients; professional competence; *students; *suicide; rationality; Australia; Bolan v. Friern Hospital Management Committee; Great Britain; Tarasoff v. Regents of the University of California; United States
Today's medical students are being confronted with ethical situations of far greater complexity than were their predecessors and yet the medical education system does little to prepare students for the ethical dilemmas which they inevitably face when entering the hospital environment. The following article addresses the issues surrounding a case where a patient has told a student in confidence of his plans to commit suicide. What should the student do? The only way for the student to prevent death is by breaking confidentiality because the student has insufficient clinical experience to provide adequate guidance. However, this requires ignoring the patient's right to autonomy, a right enshrined in both case law and medical ethics. Clearly the student's ethical, moral and legal position must be carefully evaluated.

Biesecker, Barbara Bowles. Privacy in genetic counseling. *In:* Rothstein, Mark A., ed. Genetic Secrets: Protecting Privacy and Confidentiality in the Genetic Era. New Haven, CT: Yale University Press; 1997: 108–125. 21 fn. ISBN 0-300-07251-1. BE58678.
adoption; autonomy; *confidentiality; deception; directive counseling; disclosure; family members; *genetic counseling; genetic information; genetic screening; health personnel; prenatal diagnosis; *privacy; professional family relationship; professional patient relationship; incidental findings; paternity

Black, Douglas. Corporate tyranny. [Editorial]. *Journal of Medical Ethics.* 1997 Oct; 23(5): 269–270. 4 refs. BE56903.
*advisory committees; *artificial insemination; beneficence; *bioethical issues; *confidentiality; *consensus; death; *decision making; famous persons; *informed consent; married persons; *posthumous reproduction; regulation; *semen donors; suicide; *General Medical Council (Great Britain); Great Britain; *Human Fertilisation and Embryology Authority; Wingate, Orde

Bloche, M. Gregg. Managed care, medical privacy, and the paradigm of consent. *Kennedy Institute of Ethics Journal.* 1997 Dec; 7(4): 381–386. 2 refs. BE59020.
advertising; *computer communication networks; computers; *confidentiality; contracts; disclosure; *informed consent; *managed care programs; *medical records; patient care; patients; *privacy; United States
The market success of managed health plans in the 1990s is bringing to medicine the easy availability of electronically stored information that is characteristic of the securities and consumer credit industries. Protection for medical confidentiality, however, has not kept pace with this information revolution. Employers, the managed care industry, and legal and ethics commentators frequently look to the concept of informed consent to justify particular uses of health information, but the elastic use of informed consent as a way of responding to managed care health plans' disclosure of information to third parties fails to address underlying questions involving substantive value choices.

Block, Marian R.; Schaffner, Kenneth F.; Coulehan, John L. Ethical problems of recording physician-patient interactions in family practice settings.

Journal of Family Practice. 1985; 21(6): 467–472. 14 refs. BE57823.
 *audiovisual aids; autonomy; coercion; competence; *confidentiality; *family practice; guidelines; *informed consent; *medical education; physician patient relationship; privacy; teaching methods; outpatients; *video recording

Botkin, Jeffrey R.; McMahon, William M.; Smith, Ken R., et al. Privacy and confidentiality in the publication of pedigrees: a survey of investigators and biomedical journals. *JAMA.* 1998 Jun 10; 279(22): 1808–1812. 11 refs. BE58763.
 *attitudes; *confidentiality; *disclosure; *editorial policies; evaluation studies; *family members; *genetic information; *genetic research; genetic screening; guidelines; *informed consent; international aspects; *investigators; *knowledge, attitudes, practice; *privacy; *research subjects; survey; guideline adherence; medical illustration; *pedigree studies; publishing; International Committee of Medical Journal Editors
CONTEXT: Pedigree diagrams efficiently communicate family information to genetics investigators; however, the publication of pedigrees poses a risk to the privacy and confidentiality of individuals depicted in the diagrams. Two sets of authoritative guidelines have been published to protect the privacy and confidentiality of subjects, but the influence of these guidelines on publication practices for pedigrees is unknown. OBJECTIVE: To determine the attitudes, practices, and experiences of investigators and journals with respect to privacy and confidentiality concerns in the publication of pedigrees. DESIGN: Investigators who have published pedigrees and editors of 26 biomedical journals were surveyed. Journals were reviewed for content in their "information for authors" sections and for documentation of informed consent in articles containing pedigrees. OUTCOME MEASURES: Practices regarding confidentiality and privacy reported by investigators and editors. RESULTS: Of 226 surveys sent to investigators, 177 were returned (78% response rate). Sixty-one investigators (36%) stated that family members were not informed that their pedigree would be published; 131 (78%) do not obtain informed consent specifically for pedigree publication and only 12 (28%) of the 43 who obtained consent obtained consent from all family members depicted. Thirty-two individuals (19%) reported having altered published pedigrees and 14 (45%) of 31 who had altered pedigrees stated that alterations were not disclosed to journals. Of the 14 journals that responded (54% response rate), only 3 reported written policies for managing potentially identifying information. Two journals reported having asked authors to alter pedigrees and 3 stated they had permitted alterations. A review of 5 genetics journals over a 2–year period revealed no documentation of consent for pedigree publication. CONCLUSIONS: Current practices in the publication of pedigrees do not conform with established recommendations and risk the privacy and confidentiality of subjects, often without informed consent. Attempts to address this problem through the alteration of data are being used, although this practice impairs the integrity of scientific communication.

Cain, Paul. The limits of confidentiality. *Nursing Ethics.* 1998 Mar; 5(2): 158–165. 12 refs. BE58473.
 autonomy; *confidentiality; *disclosure; health personnel; models, theoretical; moral obligations; nurse patient relationship; patient care team; *privacy; professional ethics; *standards; trust; professional role

Carnall, Douglas. Report urges widespread reform of

handling of NHS data. [News]. *BMJ (British Medical Journal).* 1997 Dec 13; 315(7122): 1562. BE58117.
 advisory committees; *computer communication networks; *confidentiality; health care reform; *medical records; *Great Britain; *National Health Service

Cook–Deegan, Robert Mullan. Confidentiality, collective resources, and commercial genomics. *In:* Rothstein, Mark A., ed. Genetic Secrets: Protecting Privacy and Confidentiality in the Genetic Era. New Haven, CT: Yale University Press; 1997: 161–183. 32 fn. ISBN 0–300–07251–1. BE58681.
 *confidentiality; conflict of interest; dementia; disclosure; DNA data banks; donors; *drug industry; family members; *financial support; genes; *genetic information; *genetic research; *genome mapping; government financing; government regulation; *industry; information dissemination; informed consent; investigators; legal aspects; patents; private sector; *property rights; public sector; regulation; *research subjects; tissue donation; universities; biological specimen banks; pedigree studies; United States

Cook, Rachel; Golombok, Susan; Bish, Alison, et al. Disclosure of donor insemination: parental attitudes. *American Journal of Orthopsychiatry.* 1995 Oct; 65(4): 549–559. 50 refs. BE55711.
 adoption; *artificial insemination; *attitudes; *children; comparative studies; *confidentiality; *disclosure; family members; fathers; genetic information; in vitro fertilization; infertility; mothers; motivation; parent child relationship; *parents; psychological stress; *reproductive technologies; semen donors; survey; Great Britain

Daniels, Ken; Lalos, Othon. The Swedish insemination act and the availability of donors. *Human Reproduction.* 1995 Jul; 10(7): 1871–1874. 17 refs. BE55763.
 *artificial insemination; children; *confidentiality; *disclosure; health facilities; institutional policies; *legal aspects; *legislation; motivation; *public policy; records; *semen donors; social impact; New Zealand; *Sweden

David, T.J.; Wynne, Jane; Kessel, Anthony S., et al. Child sexual abuse: when a doctor's duty to report abuse conflicts with a duty of confidentiality to the victim. *BMJ (British Medical Journal).* 1998 Jan 3; 316(7124): 55–57. 12 refs. BE57702.
 adults; *child abuse; *confidentiality; *disclosure; *duty to warn; females; guidelines; legal aspects; males; medical records; moral obligations; obligations to society; patient access to records; patient advocacy; pediatrics; physician patient relationship; *physicians; privacy; referral and consultation; *sex offenses; social workers; time factors; Access to Health Records Act 1990 (Great Britain); General Medical Council (Great Britain); *Great Britain

Ford, Carol A.; Millstein, Susan G.; Halpern–Felsher, Bonnie L., et al. Influence of physician confidentiality assurances on adolescents' willingness to disclose information and seek future health care: a randomized controlled trial. *JAMA.* 1997 Sep 24; 278(12): 1029–1034. 20 refs. BE56303.
 *adolescents; alcohol abuse; *attitudes; communication; *confidentiality; contraception; depressive disorder; *disclosure; evaluation studies; females; males; mental health; *patient care; physician patient relationship; physicians; recall; sexuality; smoking; socioeconomic factors; suicide; survey; California
CONTEXT: Adolescents' concerns about privacy in clinical settings decrease their willingness to seek health care for sensitive problems and may inhibit their communication with physicians. OBJECTIVE: To investigate the influence of physicians' assurances of confidentiality on adolescents' willingness to disclose information and seek future health care. DESIGN:

BE = bioethics accession number   fn. = footnotes   refs. = references

Randomized controlled trial. SETTING: Three suburban public high schools in California. PARTICIPANTS: The 562 participating adolescents represented 92% of students in mandatory classes. INTERVENTION: After random assignment to 1 of 3 groups, the adolescents listened to a standardized audiotape depiction of an office visit during which they heard a physician who assured unconditional confidentiality, a physician who assured conditional confidentiality, or a physician who did not mention confidentiality. MAIN OUTCOME MEASURES: Adolescents' willingness to disclose general information, willingness to disclose information about sensitive topics, intended honesty, and likelihood of return visits to the physician depicted in the scenario were assessed by anonymous written questionnaire. RESULTS: Assurances of confidentiality increased the number of adolescents willing to disclose sensitive information about sexuality, substance use, and mental health from 39% (68/175) to 46.5% (178/383) (beta = .10, P = .02) and increased the number willing to seek future health care from 53% (93/175) to 67% (259/386) (beta = .17, P less than .001). When comparing the unconditional with the conditional groups, assurances of unconditional confidentiality increased the number of adolescents willing to return for a future visit by 10 percentage points, from 62% (122/196) to 72% (137/190) (beta = .14, P = .001). CONCLUSIONS: Adolescents are more willing to communicate with and seek health care from physicians who assure confidentiality. Further investigation is needed to identify a confidentiality assurance statement that explains the legal and ethical limitations of confidentiality without decreasing adolescents' likelihood of seeking future health care for routine and nonreportable sensitive health concerns.

Gallagher, Hugh Gregory. FDR's Splendid Deception: The Moving Story of Roosevelt's Massive Disability -- and the Intense Efforts to Conceal It from the Public. Revised Edition. Arlington, VA: Vandamere Press; 1994. 242 p. Bibliography: p. 230–236. First edition published in 1985 by Dodd, Mead. ISBN 0–918339–33–2. BE56098.

attitudes; *confidentiality; *deception; disclosure; emotions; *famous persons; *health; historical aspects; mass media; *physically disabled; physicians; *politics; rehabilitation; *Roosevelt, Franklin; Twentieth Century; United States

General Medical Council (Great Britain). Duties of a Doctor: Guidance from the General Medical Council. [Booklets]. London: The Council; 1995. portfolio of 4 booklets. BE57156.

advertising; AIDS serodiagnosis; biomedical research; *confidentiality; conflict of interest; disclosure; duty to warn; family practice; gifts; *guidelines; *HIV seropositivity; iatrogenic disease; informed consent; *interprofessional relations; *medical ethics; medical fees; medical specialties; occupational exposure; patient care; *physician patient relationship; *physicians; professional competence; referral and consultation; refusal to treat; self regulation; traffic accidents; *General Medical Council (Great Britain); *Great Britain

Gevers, Sjef; Olsthoorn–Heim, Els. DNA sampling: Dutch and other European approaches to the issues of informed consent and confidentiality. In: Knoppers, Bartha Maria, ed. Human DNA: Law and Policy: International and Comparative Perspectives. Proceedings of the First International Conference on DNA Sampling and Human Genetic Research: Ethical, Legal, and Policy Aspects, held in Montreal, Canada, 6–8 Sep 1996. Boston, MA: Kluwer Law International; 1997: 109–120. 18 fn. ISBN 90–411–0361–9. BE58171.

advisory committees; *confidentiality; *DNA data banks; *genetic information; *genetic materials; genetic research; *genetic screening; government regulation; guidelines; *informed consent; *international aspects; privacy; *public policy; *regulation; *tissue donation; *biological specimen banks; Council of Europe; *Europe; National Ethics Advisory Committee (France); *Netherlands; Nuffield Council on Bioethics

Glen, Sally. Confidentiality: a critique of the traditional view. Nursing Ethics. 1997 Sep; 4(5): 403–406. 5 refs. BE56904.

*confidentiality; nurse patient relationship; *nurses; paternalism; patient access to records; social dominance; Great Britain

Gostin, Lawrence O. Personal privacy in the health care system: employer–sponsored insurance, managed care, and integrated delivery systems. Kennedy Institute of Ethics Journal. 1997 Dec; 7(4): 361–376. 27 refs. 3 fn. BE59018.

biomedical research; computer communication networks; computers; *confidentiality; data banks; *disclosure; *employment; *health care delivery; health facilities; *health insurance; health personnel; *informed consent; law; *managed care programs; *medical records; patient care; *privacy; public health; quality assurance; *United States Widespread collection and use of identifiable information can promote social goods while, at the same time, infringing on personal privacy. Information systems are developing within the context of a fundamental transformation in the organization, delivery, and financing of health care. Changes in the health care system include rapid development of employer–sponsored health coverage, managed care organizations, and integrated delivery systems. These complex, multifaceted arrangements for delivering and paying for health care require ever–more–sophisticated information systems that facilitate extensive sharing of personal data. Systemic flows of sensitive health information occur both vertically and horizontally among employers, hospitals, insurers, laboratories, and suppliers. Beyond this complex web of vertical and horizontal sharing are the multiple demands for information management, quality assurance, research, governmental regulation, and public health. Theoretical problems exist with the law and ethics of informational privacy. The traditional method of exercising control over personal health information is through informed consent. Informed consent, however, within a modern health information infrastructure becomes highly complex. In this kind of environment, the doctrine of informed consent is flawed and does not provide sufficient control over personal information to assure adequate protection of privacy.

Hood, Catherine A.; Hope, Tony; Dove, Phillip. Videos, photographs, and patient consent. BMJ (British Medical Journal). 1998 Mar 28; 316(7136): 1009–1011. 13 refs. BE57555.

*audiovisual aids; *computer communication networks; *confidentiality; consent forms; editorial policies; *information dissemination; *informed consent; *patients; physicians; professional organizations; property rights; *medical illustration; *photography; Great Britain; Internet

Hook, C. Christopher. Genetic testing and confidentiality. In: Kilner, John F.; Pentz, Rebecca D.; Young, Frank E., eds. Genetic Ethics: Do the Ends Justify the Genes? Grand Rapids, MI: W.B. Eerdmans; 1997: 124–135. 28 fn. ISBN 0–8028–4428–6. BE56720.

carriers; children; *Christian ethics; *confidentiality; *disclosure; employment; family members; genetic

---

BE = bioethics accession number   fn. = footnotes   refs. = references

counseling; genetic disorders; *genetic information; genetic predisposition; *genetic screening; informed consent; insurance; legislation; medical records; preimplantation diagnosis; prenatal diagnosis; psychological stress; reproduction; risk; *risks and benefits; selective abortion; social discrimination; state government; United States

Juengst, Eric T. Respecting human subjects in genome research: a preliminary policy agenda. *In:* Vanderpool, Harold Y., ed. The Ethics of Research Involving Human Subjects: Facing the 21st Century. Frederick, MD: University Publishing Group; 1996: 401–429. 74 fn. ISBN 1-55572-036-6. BE56995.
children; *confidentiality; *disclosure; employment; *family members; genetic information; genetic materials; genetic predisposition; *genetic research; *genome mapping; *informed consent; insurance; international aspects; mentally ill; minority groups; privacy; property rights; public policy; research subjects; *risks and benefits; *selection of subjects; stigmatization; truth disclosure; *pedigree studies; Human Genome Project; United States

Kaiser, Jocelyn. Archive available for genetic studies. [News]. *Science.* 1997 Nov 21; 278(5342): 1389. BE57439.
*confidentiality; *DNA data banks; donors; federal government; *genetic information; *genetic research; government regulation; *Centers for Disease Control and Prevention; United States

Kelly, Grant. Patient data, confidentiality, and electronics: identifiable data should no longer be freely available within the NHS. [Editorial]. *BMJ (British Medical Journal).* 1998 Mar 7; 316(7133): 718–719. 6 refs. BE57352.
administrators; *computer communication networks; *computers; *confidentiality; hospitals; informed consent; *medical records; physicians; *public policy; British Medical Association; Department of Health (Great Britain); *Great Britain; *National Health Service

Kuhse, Helga. Confidentiality and the AMA's [Australian Medical Association] new code of ethics: an imprudent formulation? *Medical Journal of Australia.* 1996 Sep 16; 165(6): 327–329. 11 refs. BE58972.
*codes of ethics; *confidentiality; dangerousness; disclosure; duty to warn; guidelines; *medical ethics; *physicians; *professional organizations; *Australia; *Australian Medical Association

Lebacqz, Karen. Genetic privacy: no deal for the poor. *In:* Peters, Ted, ed. Genetics: Issues of Social Justice. Cleveland, OH: Pilgrim Press; 1998: 239–254. 60 fn. Reprinted from *Dialog,* Winter 1994, 33:1, 39–48. ISBN 0-8298-1251-2. BE57482.
computers; *confidentiality; directive counseling; *disadvantaged; disclosure; employment; genetic counseling; *genetic information; genetic predisposition; *genetic screening; *health insurance; indigents; informed consent; insurance selection bias; justice; medical records; minority groups; prenatal diagnosis; *privacy; risk; selective abortion; *social discrimination; socioeconomic factors; truth disclosure; United States

Lehrman, Sally. Clinton backs congressional efforts on genetic discrimination. [News]. *Nature.* 1997 Jul 17; 388(6639): 216. BE56167.
*confidentiality; federal government; *genetic information; genetic research; *government regulation; *health insurance; industry; insurance selection bias; political activity; *social discrimination; Department of Health and Human Services; *United States

Lowrance, William W. Privacy and Health Research: A Report to the U.S. Secretary of Health and Human Services. Washington, DC: U.S. Department of Health and Human Services, Office of the Assistant Secretary for Planning and Evaluation; 1997 May. 80 p. 125 fn. BE58644.
biomedical research; communicable diseases; computers; *confidentiality; data banks; disclosure; economics; *epidemiology; genetic research; government regulation; guidelines; *health services research; human experimentation; informed consent; *international aspects; legal aspects; legislation; mandatory reporting; medical records; organization and administration; *privacy; private sector; public health; public policy; *records; registries; research ethics committees; research subjects; computer security; *Council of Europe; *Europe; *United States

Marshall, Mary Faith; Smith, C.D. Confidentiality in surgical practice. *In:* McCullough, Laurence B.; Jones, James W.; Brody, Baruch A., eds. Surgical Ethics. New York, NY: Oxford University Press; 1998: 38–56. 33 refs. ISBN 0-19-510347-5. BE58332.
audiovisual aids; competence; computer communication networks; computers; *confidentiality; dangerousness; decision making; disclosure; domestic violence; duty to warn; emergency care; employment; family members; famous persons; health insurance; HIV seropositivity; hospitals; iatrogenic disease; information dissemination; informed consent; institutional policies; law enforcement; legal aspects; legal liability; legal obligations; *medical records; *moral obligations; occupational exposure; patient access to records; patients; physician patient relationship; physicians; privacy; privileged communication; public health; risk; *surgery; third party consent; trust; computer security; United States

Melton, L. Joseph. The threat to medical-records research. *New England Journal of Medicine.* 1997 Nov 13; 337(20): 1466–1470. 38 refs. BE56431.
autonomy; *biomedical research; common good; *confidentiality; *disclosure; *epidemiology; *government regulation; health services research; hospitals; informed consent; legislation; *medical records; privacy; quality of health care; regulation; research design; research subjects; *risks and benefits; social impact; state government; treatment outcome; Mayo Clinic; Minnesota

Mendelson, Danuta. The concept of medical confidentiality in Australian and Jewish law. *In:* Jewish Law Annual. Volume Twelve. Amsterdam, Netherlands: Harwood Academic Publishers; 1997: 217–249. 99 fn. ISBN 90-5702-551-5. BE58344.
Christian ethics; codes of ethics; *confidentiality; disclosure; duty to warn; health personnel; historical aspects; international aspects; interprofessional relations; *Jewish ethics; law enforcement; *legal aspects; legal liability; legal obligations; married persons; medical education; medical ethics; medical records; medical schools; moral obligations; physician patient relationship; *physicians; privileged communication; professional organizations; public health; *Australia; Australian Medical Association; Declaration of Geneva; Great Britain; Hippocratic Oath; International Code of Ethics; World Medical Association

Miller, Hugh. DNA blueprints, personhood, and genetic privacy. *Health Matrix.* 1998 Summer; 8(2): 179–221. 105 fn. BE58953.
*autonomy; confidentiality; constitutional law; disclosure; *genetic determinism; *genetic identity; *genetic information; genetic research; genetic screening; legal aspects; *legal rights; *personhood; philosophy; *privacy; *personal identity; United States

Mitchell, Peter. Drug industry lobbies against European research-data directive. [News]. *Lancet.* 1997 May 10; 349(9062): 1378. BE56414.
*biomedical research; *confidentiality; drug industry;

epidemiology; human experimentation; informed consent; *international aspects; *medical records; *regulation; self regulation; *Europe; European Federation of Pharmaceutical Industries' Associations; *European Union

Mitchell, Peter. France gets smart with health à la carte. [News]. *Lancet.* 1998 Mar 7; 351(9104): 736. BE58854.
*computer communication networks; *computers; *confidentiality; *data banks; *economics; health insurance; international aspects; *medical records; national health insurance; patient access to records; *public policy; computer security; *France; Internet

National Research Council. Committee on Maintaining Privacy and Security in Health Care Applications of the National Information Infrastructure. For the Record: Protecting Electronic Health Information. Washington, DC: National Academy Press; 1997. 264 p. Bibliography: p. 197–207. ISBN 0–309–05697–7. BE56132.
*computer communication networks; *confidentiality; federal government; government regulation; health care delivery; *information dissemination; *medical records; *methods; organization and administration; *privacy; *public policy; state government; *computer security; *United States

Njikam Savage, Olayinka Margaret. Secrecy still the best policy: donor insemination in Cameroon. *Politics and the Life Sciences.* 1995 Feb; 14(1): 87–88. 5 refs. BE55701.
*artificial insemination; *attitudes; *confidentiality; developing countries; family relationship; females; *infertility; males; parent child relationship; psychological stress; *semen donors; stigmatization; values; *Cameroon

Nowakowski, Loretta H. Confidentiality and customary practices. *Journal of Professional Nursing.* 1985 Mar–Apr; 1(2): 86–89. 11 refs. BE57832.
audiovisual aids; communication; *confidentiality; contracts; disclosure; family members; guidelines; health personnel; informed consent; interprofessional relations; professional patient relationship; students

Odenbach, Erwin. Respect for the patient's privacy. *Dolentium Hominum: Church and Health in the World.* 1996; 31(11th Yr., No. 1): 119–123. BE57372.
communication; computer communication networks; *confidentiality; cultural pluralism; emergency care; health facilities; health personnel; medical education; medical records; pastoral care; patient care; patients; patients' rights; *privacy; socioeconomic factors; computer security; dignity; Hippocratic Oath; World Medical Association

O'Flynn, Norma; Spencer, John; Jones, Roger. Consent and confidentiality in teaching in general practice: survey of patients' views on presence of students. *BMJ (British Medical Journal).* 1997 Nov 1; 315(7116): 1142. 5 refs. BE56225.
*attitudes; *confidentiality; *disclosure; *family practice; informed consent; *medical education; medical records; *patient care; *patient satisfaction; *patients; physicians; *privacy; referral and consultation; sexuality; *students; survey; group practice; outpatients; Great Britain

Orentlicher, David. Genetic privacy in the physician–patient relationship. *In:* Rothstein, Mark A., ed. Genetic Secrets: Protecting Privacy and Confidentiality in the Genetic Era. New Haven, CT: Yale University Press; 1997: 77–91. 40 fn. ISBN 0–300–07251–1. BE58676.
computers; *confidentiality; data banks; *genetic information; genetic screening; health; health insurance; managed care programs; medical ethics; medical records; patient care; physician patient relationship; *privacy; social discrimination; stigmatization; trust

Pergament, Eugene. A clinical geneticist perspective of the patient–physician relationship. *In:* Rothstein, Mark A., ed. Genetic Secrets: Protecting Privacy and Confidentiality in the Genetic Era. New Haven, CT: Yale University Press; 1997: 92–107. 21 fn. ISBN 0–300–07251–1. BE58677.
autonomy; behavioral genetics; computer communication networks; *confidentiality; data banks; directive counseling; disclosure; family members; *genetic counseling; *genetic information; genetic predisposition; genetic screening; genome mapping; insurance; legal obligations; managed care programs; medical records; moral obligations; patient advocacy; physician patient relationship; privacy; professional family relationship; United States

Pokorski, Robert J. A test for the insurance industry. *Nature.* 1998 Feb 26; 391(6670): 835–836. 11 refs. BE57970.
*confidentiality; dementia; disclosure; *economics; *genetic information; genetic predisposition; *genetic screening; *industry; insurance selection bias; *justice; *life insurance; public policy; rights; risk; United States

Powers, Madison. Justice and genetics: privacy protection and the moral basis of public policy. *In:* Rothstein, Mark A., ed. Genetic Secrets: Protecting Privacy and Confidentiality in the Genetic Era. New Haven, CT: Yale University Press; 1997: 355–368. 15 fn. ISBN 0–300–07251–1. BE58691.
autonomy; common good; *confidentiality; data banks; *disclosure; economics; employment; epidemiology; family members; *genetic information; genetic predisposition; *genetic research; *genetic screening; government regulation; health care delivery; health hazards; health insurance; incentives; informed consent; *justice; legal rights; mass screening; medical records; moral policy; policy analysis; *privacy; public health; *public policy; registries; risks and benefits; social discrimination; stigmatization; *pragmatism; United States

Rankine, James J. Most patients don't read the BMJ. [Personal view]. *BMJ (British Medical Journal).* 1998 Mar 28; 316(7136): 1026–1027. BE57581.
biomedical research; *confidentiality; *editorial policies; *informed consent; *patients; physicians; *medical illustration; *publishing; *BMJ (British Medical Journal); Great Britain

Reilly, Philip R. Laws to regulate the use of genetic information. *In:* Rothstein, Mark A., ed. Genetic Secrets: Protecting Privacy and Confidentiality in the Genetic Era. New Haven, CT: Yale University Press; 1997: 369–391. 76 fn. ISBN 0–300–07251–1. BE58692.
blacks; *confidentiality; *disclosure; DNA data banks; DNA fingerprinting; *employment; *federal government; *genetic information; genetic materials; genetic research; *genetic screening; *government regulation; *health insurance; historical aspects; informed consent; *legislation; mandatory testing; mass screening; medical records; model legislation; newborns; phenylketonuria; privacy; *public policy; sickle cell anemia; *social discrimination; *state government; *trends; biological specimen banks; Twentieth Century; *United States

Rosner, Fred. Medical confidentiality in Judaism. *Journal of Halacha and Contemporary Society.* 1997 Spring; No. 33: 5–15. 8 fn. BE55592.
altruism; *confidentiality; dangerousness; *disclosure; *duty to warn; health; injuries; *Jewish ethics; marital relationship; mental health; moral obligations; motivation; physicians; privileged communication

Rothstein, Mark A. Genetic secrets: a policy framework. *In:* Rothstein, Mark A., ed. Genetic Secrets: Protecting

---

BE = bioethics accession number   fn. = footnotes   refs. = references

Privacy and Confidentiality in the Genetic Era. New Haven, CT: Yale University Press; 1997: 451–495. 90 fn. ISBN 0–300–07251–1. BE58694.

adoption; anonymous testing; autonomy; *confidentiality; criminal law; *disclosure; DNA data banks; DNA fingerprinting; duty to warn; economics; employment; family members; federal government; genetic counseling; *genetic information; genetic predisposition; genetic research; *genetic screening; *government regulation; health care delivery; health insurance; health personnel; industry; informed consent; international aspects; legal liability; *legislation; mandatory testing; medical records; military personnel; parent child relationship; *privacy; professional competence; public health; *public policy; schools; self regulation; social discrimination; standards; state government; trends; biological specimen banks; United States

Rothstein, Mark A., ed. Genetic Secrets: Protecting Privacy and Confidentiality in the Genetic Era. New Haven, CT: Yale University Press; 1997. 511 p. 1,175 fn. ISBN 0–300–07251–1. BE58672.

adoption; *confidentiality; disclosure; DNA data banks; DNA fingerprinting; employment; epidemiology; family members; family relationship; financial support; genetic counseling; genetic determinism; *genetic information; genetic predisposition; genetic research; *genetic screening; genome mapping; government regulation; health hazards; health insurance; industry; informed consent; international aspects; legal aspects; legislation; life insurance; occupational exposure; *privacy; property rights; public health; public policy; research subjects; review; schools; biological specimen banks; Europe; United States

Rothstein, Mark A. The law of medical and genetic privacy in the workplace. *In:* Rothstein, Mark A., ed. Genetic Secrets: Protecting Privacy and Confidentiality in the Genetic Era. New Haven, CT: Yale University Press; 1997: 281–298. 54 fn. ISBN 0–300–07251–1. BE58687.

*confidentiality; *disclosure; *employment; genetic information; *genetic screening; health; health insurance; *legal aspects; legislation; medical records; privacy; social discrimination; state government; Americans with Disabilities Act 1990; *United States

Rushton, Cindy Hylton; Infante, Marie C. Keeping secrets: the ethical and legal challenges. *Pediatric Nursing.* 1995 Sep–Oct; 21(5): 479–482. 7 refs. BE55526.

accountability; *adolescents; case studies; communication; *confidentiality; diagnosis; *disclosure; legal aspects; minors; *nurses; nursing ethics; *parents; patient advocacy; pediatrics; privacy; sexuality; sexually transmitted diseases

Samet, Jonathan M.; Bailey, Linda A. Environmental population screening. *In:* Rothstein, Mark A., ed. Genetic Secrets: Protecting Privacy and Confidentiality in the Genetic Era. New Haven, CT: Yale University Press; 1997: 197–211. 20 fn. ISBN 0–300–07251–1. BE58683.

*confidentiality; disclosure; *epidemiology; *genetic information; genetic predisposition; *genetic research; genetic screening; health; informed consent; mass screening; occupational exposure; privacy; research subjects; genetic markers; recontact

Schwartz, Paul M. European data protection law and medical privacy. *In:* Rothstein, Mark A., ed. Genetic Secrets: Protecting Privacy and Confidentiality in the Genetic Era. New Haven, CT: Yale University Press; 1997: 392–417. 91 fn. ISBN 0–300–07251–1. BE58693.

comparative studies; *confidentiality; *disclosure; DNA fingerprinting; federal government; *genetic information; genetic research; *genetic screening; *government regulation; insurance; *international aspects; *legislation;

*medical records; privacy; public policy; state government; Austria; *Europe; European Union; France; Germany; Switzerland; United States

Shalala, Donna E. Health care information and privacy. *Health Matrix.* 1998 Summer; 8(2): 223–232. BE58954.

accountability; computers; *confidentiality; disclosure; federal government; health care delivery; informed consent; *medical records; *privacy; *public policy; *United States

Sheldon, Tony. Dutch face disclosure of medical records. [News]. *BMJ (British Medical Journal).* 1998 Feb 21; 316(7131): 572. BE57250.

*confidentiality; *disclosure; fraud; government regulation; industry; *life insurance; *medical records; organizational policies; physicians; professional organizations; *Netherlands; Royal Dutch Medical Association

Shickle, Darren. Privacy versus public right to know. *In:* Chadwick, Ruth, ed. Encyclopedia of Applied Ethics, Volume 3. San Diego, CA: Academic Press; 1998: 661–669. 9 refs. ISBN 0–12–227068–1. BE56263.

autonomy; codes of ethics; common good; *confidentiality; dangerousness; deception; disclosure; duty to warn; forensic psychiatry; legal aspects; physician patient relationship; *privacy; professional ethics; rights; risks and benefits; social interaction

Smith, Richard. Informed consent: edging forwards (and backwards). [Editorial]. *BMJ (British Medical Journal).* 1998 Mar 28; 316(7136): 949–951. 17 refs. Includes the text of the *BMJ*'s guidelines for "Publishing information that emerges from the doctor–patient relationship." BE58067.

attitudes; *biomedical research; case studies; *confidentiality; death; *editorial policies; *guidelines; human experimentation; *informed consent; patient care; patients; physician patient relationship; privacy; research subjects; time factors; pedigree studies; photography; *BMJ (British Medical Journal); General Medical Council (Great Britain); International Committee of Medical Journal Editors

Stephenson, Joan. Ethics group drafts guidelines for control of genetic material and information. [News]. *JAMA.* 1998 Jan 21; 279(3): 184. BE58069.

advisory committees; *confidentiality; disclosure; *DNA data banks; family members; *genetic information; *genetic materials; *genetic research; *guidelines; *international aspects; property rights; *tissue banks; *tissue donation; *biological specimen banks; *Ethical, Legal, and Social Issues Committee (HUGO-ELSI); *Human Genome Organization

Veatch, Robert M., ed. Ethical issues in the changing health care system. *In:* Jonsen, Albert R.; Veatch, Robert M.; Walters, LeRoy, eds. Source Book in Bioethics: A Documentary History. Washington, DC: Georgetown University Press; 1998: 407–504. 8 fn. ISBN 0–87840–683–2. BE57894.

advance directives; advisory committees; aliens; autonomy; body parts and fluids; cadavers; competence; *confidentiality; dangerousness; disclosure; *duty to warn; federal government; historical aspects; *informed consent; legal aspects; mentally ill; model legislation; *organ donation; organ donors; *organ transplantation; patient care; patients' rights; physician patient relationship; remuneration; selection for treatment; *third party consent; tissue donation; transplant recipients; *Canterbury v. Spence; National Organ Transplant Act 1984; President's Commission for the Study of Ethical Problems; *Tarasoff v. Regents of the University of California; *Task Force on Organ Transplantation; *Twentieth Century; *Uniform Anatomical Gift Act; *United States

Wadman, Meredith. Genome panel defends researchers'

BE = bioethics accession number   fn. = footnotes   refs. = references

-- and families' -- interests. [News]. *Nature.* 1998 Feb 26; 391(6670): 826. BE58072.
  advisory committees; *confidentiality; *disclosure; DNA data banks; family members; *genetic information; *genetic research; *genome mapping; informed consent; *international aspects; investigators; medical records; *privacy; tissue banks; *Human Genome Organization (HUGO)

Wainwright, Paul; Cain, Paul. Using clients: a response to Paul Cain. [Commentary and response]. *Nursing Ethics.* 1998 Jul; 5(4): 363-369. 3 refs. BE58881.
  autonomy; case studies; *confidentiality; *disclosure; hospitals; *informed consent; *moral obligations; nurse patient relationship; *nursing education; *nursing ethics; nursing research; paternalism; *patient care; *patients; privacy; research subjects; *students; teaching methods

Warwick, Ruth. Anonymity for unrelated bone marrow donors should remain. [Letter]. *BMJ (British Medical Journal).* 1997 Aug 30; 315(7107): 548-549. 3 refs. BE58224.
  *bone marrow; coercion; *confidentiality; directed donation; *donors; *privacy; retreatment; risks and benefits; siblings; *tissue donation; *unrelated donors; Great Britain

Wertz, Dorothy C. Society and the not-so-new genetics: what are we afraid of? Some future predictions from a social scientist. *Journal of Contemporary Health Law and Policy.* 1997 Spring; 13(2): 299-346. 130 fn. BE56015.
  *attitudes; autonomy; codes of ethics; common good; *confidentiality; directive counseling; disabled; *disclosure; DNA fingerprinting; employment; eugenics; family members; *genetic counseling; genetic determinism; genetic disorders; *genetic enhancement; *genetic information; genetic intervention; genetic predisposition; genetic screening; *genetic services; *genetics; genome mapping; guidelines; *health personnel; indigents; industry; insurance; *international aspects; *knowledge, attitudes, practice; late-onset disorders; *physicians; prenatal diagnosis; *privacy; *public opinion; reproduction; resource allocation; *rights; risk; selective abortion; sex determination; social discrimination; *social impact; survey; *values; Human Genome Project; *United States; WHO Guidelines on Ethical Issues in Genetics

Williamson, Charlotte; Wilkie, Patricia. Teaching medical students in general practice: respecting patients' rights. [Editorial]. *BMJ (British Medical Journal).* 1997 Nov 1; 315(7116): 1108-1109. 11 refs. BE56894.
  attitudes; communication; *confidentiality; disclosure; family practice; *informed consent; *medical education; medical ethics; medical records; *patient care; patients; *students; Great Britain; National Health Service

Woodrow, Philip. Exploring confidentiality in nursing practice. *Nursing Standard.* 1996 May 1; 10(32): 38-42. 22 refs. BE55929.
  common good; *confidentiality; disclosure; duty to warn; ethical theory; guidelines; HIV seropositivity; legal aspects; legislation; nurse patient relationship; *nurses; professional organizations; psychiatry; rights; utilitarianism; Great Britain; United Kingdom Central Council for Nursing, Midwifery and Health Visiting

Zuger, Abigail. Ever elusive, privacy slips from grasp of patients. *New York Times.* 1998 Nov 3: F7. BE58939.
  computers; *confidentiality; hospitals; *medical records; *privacy

Zweig, Franklin M.; Walsh, Joseph T.; Freeman, Daniel M. Courts and the challenges of adjudicating genetic testing's secrets. *In:* Rothstein, Mark A., ed. Genetic Secrets: Protecting Privacy and Confidentiality

in the Genetic Era. New Haven, CT: Yale University Press; 1997: 332-351. 23 fn. ISBN 0-300-07251-1. BE58690.
  *adoption; aggression; behavioral genetics; capital punishment; competence; *confidentiality; criminal law; disclosure; *genetic information; *genetic predisposition; *genetic screening; judicial action; *legal aspects; legal liability; mentally ill; privacy; violence; *United States

Human Genetics Advisory Commission meets. [News; title supplied]. *Gene Therapy.* 1997 Apr; 4(4): 271. BE56184.
  advisory committees; *confidentiality; disclosure; *genetic information; *genetic screening; *industry; insurance selection bias; *life insurance; *organizational policies; professional organizations; social discrimination; *Association of British Insurers; Great Britain; *Human Genetics Advisory Commission (Great Britain)

Trading trust for blood money. [Editorial]. *Lancet.* 1995 Sep 30; 346(8979): 855. BE56102.
  *blood banks; *blood donation; *confidentiality; conflict of interest; disclosure; *donors; economics; industry; organization and administration; organizational policies; records; *Great Britain; *National Blood Authority (Great Britain); *National Health Service

CONFIDENTIALITY/LEGAL ASPECTS

Abbasi, Kamran. BMJ to act on media abuse. [News]. *BMJ (British Medical Journal).* 1998 Jan 17; 316(7126): 170. BE58113.
  *computer communication networks; *confidentiality; *editorial policies; informed consent; *legal aspects; *mass media; organizational policies; patients; *medical illustration; *photography; *BMJ (British Medical Journal); Great Britain; *Internet

Andrews, Lori B.; Elster, Nanette. Adoption, reproductive technologies, and genetic information. *Health Matrix.* 1998 Summer; 8(2): 125-151. 125 fn. BE58951.
  *adoption; artificial insemination; behavioral genetics; children; *confidentiality; *disclosure; *genetic information; *genetic screening; government regulation; informed consent; *legal aspects; ovum donors; parents; records; registries; *reproductive technologies; semen donors; state government; *United States

Andrews, Lori B. The genetic information superhighway: rules of the road for contacting relatives and recontacting former patients. *In:* Knoppers, Bartha Maria, ed. Human DNA: Law and Policy: International and Comparative Perspectives. Proceedings of the First International Conference on DNA Sampling and Human Genetic Research: Ethical, Legal, and Policy Aspects, held in Montreal, Canada, 6-8 Sep 1996. Boston, MA: Kluwer Law International; 1997: 133-143. 42 fn. ISBN 90-411-0361-9. BE58173.
  *confidentiality; *disclosure; duty to warn; *family members; *genetic counseling; genetic disorders; *genetic information; genetic predisposition; *genetic screening; guidelines; *legal aspects; *patients; physicians; professional organizations; risks and benefits; wrongful life; *recontact; United States

Appelbaum, Paul S. A "health information infrastructure" and the threat to confidentiality of health records. *Psychiatric Services.* 1998 Jan; 49(1): 27-28, 33. 8 refs. BE58201.
  computers; *confidentiality; data banks; *disclosure; federal government; health personnel; informed consent; investigators; *legal aspects; managed care programs; *medical records; mentally ill; *psychiatry; *public policy; Department of Health and Human Services; Health Insurance Portability and Accountability Act 1996; U.S.

Congress; *United States

Baird, Rachel. Gene tests pose challenge for privacy guardian. [News]. *New Scientist.* 1997 Jun 28; 154(2088): 4. BE59084.
*confidentiality; genetic information; *genetic screening; *government regulation; industry; *insurance; Data Protection Act 1984 (Great Britain); *Great Britain; Human Genetics Advisory Commission (Great Britain)

Berger, John. Patient confidentiality in a high tech world. *Journal of Pharmacy and Law.* 1996; 5(1): 139–145. BE57591.
codes of ethics; computers; *confidentiality; disclosure; *drugs; federal government; government regulation; *legal aspects; legal liability; medical records; *patient care; *pharmacists; privacy; professional organizations; American Pharmaceutical Association; United States

Berry, Roberta M. The genetic revolution and the physician's duty of confidentiality: the role of the old Hippocratic virtues in the regulation of the new genetic intimacy. *Journal of Legal Medicine.* 1997 Dec; 18(4): 401–441. 110 fn. BE58650.
autonomy; *caring; codes of ethics; *confidentiality; decision making; *disclosure; dissent; duty to warn; employment; *family members; genetic determinism; *genetic information; genetic predisposition; genetic screening; government regulation; historical aspects; insurance; law; *legal aspects; legal liability; *legal obligations; medical ethics; *medicine; *moral obligations; obligations to society; patients; physician patient relationship; *physicians; policy analysis; privacy; professional family relationship; *public policy; risks and benefits; schools; *virtues; Hippocratic Oath

Brown, Iona Jane; Gannon, Philippa. Confidentiality and the Human Genome Project: a prophecy for conflict. *In:* McLean, Sheila A.M., ed. Contemporary Issues in Law, Medicine and Ethics. Brookfield, VT: Dartmouth; 1996: 215–236. 88 fn. ISBN 1–85521–586–1. BE57797.
carriers; common good; *confidentiality; disabled; *disclosure; duty to warn; eugenics; family members; genetic counseling; genetic disorders; *genetic information; genetic predisposition; *genetic screening; genome mapping; *legal aspects; legal obligations; medical ethics; moral obligations; physician patient relationship; physicians; prenatal diagnosis; preventive medicine; risk; selective abortion; social discrimination; stigmatization; *Great Britain; Human Genome Project

Chan, Kevin W. Jaffee v. Redmond: making the courts a tool of injustice? *Journal of the American Academy of Psychiatry and the Law.* 1997; 25(3): 383–389. 10 refs. 3 fn. BE57303.
*confidentiality; disclosure; federal government; justice; law enforcement; *legal aspects; *privileged communication; *psychotherapy; social workers; state government; Supreme Court decisions; *Jaffee v. Redmond; United States

Dale, Ruth; Barton, Roger; Shepherd, Jonathan, et al. Why are doctors ambivalent about patients who misuse alcohol? [Case study and commentaries]. *BMJ (British Medical Journal).* 1997 Nov 15; 315(7118): 1297–1300. 14 refs. BE57242.
*alcohol abuse; *attitudes; case studies; common good; *confidentiality; *disclosure; employment; family practice; guidelines; hospitals; *legal aspects; legal liability; legal obligations; *mandatory reporting; *obligations to society; patient compliance; *patients; physician patient relationship; *physicians; preventive medicine; *risk; survey; *traffic accidents; Driver and Vehicle Licensing Agency (Great Britain); General Medical Council (Great Britain); *Great Britain

Davis, Helen R.; Mitrius, Janice V. Recent legislation on genetics and insurance. [Note]. *Jurimetrics Journal.* 1996 Fall; 37(1): 69–82. 50 fn. BE57689.
*confidentiality; *disclosure; family members; federal government; genetic disorders; *genetic information; genetic predisposition; *genetic screening; *government regulation; hospitals; informed consent; *insurance; insurance selection bias; *legislation; physicians; privacy; social discrimination; *state government; Americans with Disabilities Act 1990; Employment Retirement Income Security Act (ERISA) 1974; *United States

Dickens, Bernard M. Choices, control, access -- the Canadian position. *In:* Knoppers, Bartha Maria, ed. Human DNA: Law and Policy: International and Comparative Perspectives. Proceedings of the First International Conference on DNA Sampling and Human Genetic Research: Ethical, Legal, and Policy Aspects, held in Montreal, Canada, 6–8 Sep 1996. Boston, MA: Kluwer Law International; 1997: 71–89. 59 fn. ISBN 90–411–0361–9. BE58169.
*confidentiality; criminal law; *disclosure; *DNA data banks; DNA fingerprinting; employment; federal government; *genetic information; *genetic materials; *genetic research; *genetic screening; government regulation; health personnel; *informed consent; law enforcement; *legal aspects; legislation; mandatory testing; privacy; private sector; public sector; state government; tissue donation; *biological specimen banks; *Canada; *Privacy Act 1983 (Canada); Quebec

Ferguson, James R. Biomedical research and insider trading. *New England Journal of Medicine.* 1997 Aug 28; 337(9): 631–634. 21 refs. BE59003.
*biomedical research; *confidentiality; *conflict of interest; criminal law; *disclosure; *drug industry; drugs; *economics; fraud; human experimentation; *investigators; *legal aspects; *legal liability; *legal obligations; Supreme Court decisions; torts; Securities and Exchange Commission; *Securities Exchange Act 1934; *United States

Ferris, Lorraine E. Protecting the public from risk of harm: Ontario's forthcoming regulatory law protects doctors, public, and the patient. [Editorial]. *BMJ (British Medical Journal).* 1998 Apr 4; 316(7137): 1033–1034. 4 refs. BE58253.
*confidentiality; *dangerousness; *duty to warn; *legal aspects; legal liability; *mandatory reporting; *physicians; violence; *Ontario

Gostin, Lawrence. Health care information and the protection of personal privacy: ethical and legal considerations. *Annals of Internal Medicine.* 1997 Oct 15; 127(8, Pt. 2): 683–690. 33 refs. BE55862.
autonomy; *computer communication networks; *confidentiality; *data banks; disclosure; employment; evaluation; federal government; *government regulation; guidelines; health care delivery; *information dissemination; insurance; *legal aspects; legislation; managed care programs; *medical records; mental health; physician patient relationship; physicians; *privacy; *public policy; quality of health care; standards; state government; values; Health Insurance Portability and Accountability Act 1996; *United States
During the early 1990s, the U.S. government addressed the issue of providing universal health care to all its citizens. Although this issue has not been completely resolved, centralization of electronic data and sharing of health care information among insurers and providers have been pursued. The emergence of electronic data banks in health care has raised another issue: each citizen's right to privacy compared with the collective benefit to society when critical data on quality assurance and scientific research are shared by an array of network

---

BE = bioethics accession number   fn. = footnotes   refs. = references

users. The choices we face are difficult, and the solution may necessarily reflect a compromise that alters traditional beliefs in the right to personal privacy. However, Congress can take the initiative by enacting statutes to ensure that sensitive information contained in electronic patient records is not divulged without a patient's consent and is protected against fraudulent access and abuse.

Great Britain. Department of Health. Protection and Use of Patient Information: Guidance from the Department of Health. London: The Department; 1996 Mar. 24 p. 36 fn. BE58132.

adults; biomedical research; computers; *confidentiality; *disclosure; *government regulation; *guidelines; health care delivery; health personnel; informed consent; international aspects; law enforcement; *legal aspects; mass media; *medical records; minors; patient access to records; public health; Data Protection Act 1984 (Great Britain); *Department of Health (Great Britain); European Union; *Great Britain; *National Health Service; Patient's Charter (Great Britain)

Kaiser, Jocelyn. Privacy rules set no new research curbs. [News]. *Science.* 1997 Sep 19; 277(5333): 1757. BE56210.

*biomedical research; *confidentiality; drug industry; epidemiology; federal government; *government regulation; guidelines; informed consent; *medical records; *privacy; research subjects; state government; *United States

Kondro, Wayne. Canada's privacy legislation warning. [News]. *Lancet.* 1997 Oct 11; 350(9084): 1085. BE56929.

*computer communication networks; *confidentiality; *legislation; *medical records; privacy; *public policy; *Canada; *Canadian Health Information Network

Leong, Gregory B.; Silva, J. Arturo; Weinstock, Robert. Another courtroom assault on the confidentiality of the psychotherapist–patient relationship. *Journal of Forensic Sciences.* 1995 Sep; 40(5): 862–864. 19 refs. BE55878.

competence; *confidentiality; *criminal law; dangerousness; disclosure; *legal aspects; medical records; physician patient relationship; *privileged communication; *psychotherapy; *California; *People v. Webb

Litman, Moe M. The legal status of genetic material. *In:* Knoppers, Bartha Maria, ed. Human DNA: Law and Policy: International and Comparative Perspectives. Proceedings of the First International Conference on DNA Sampling and Human Genetic Research: Ethical, Legal, and Policy Aspects, held in Montreal, Canada, 6–8 Sep 1996. Boston, MA: Kluwer Law International; 1997: 17–32. 76 fn. ISBN 90–411–0361–9. BE58165.

biomedical research; *body parts and fluids; commodification; *confidentiality; DNA data banks; economics; *genetic information; *genetic materials; *genetic research; international aspects; *legal aspects; patents; privacy; *property rights; public policy; *tissue donation; *Canada; Moore v. Regents of the University of California; *United States

Mendelson, Danuta. The concept of medical confidentiality in Australian and Jewish law. *In:* Jewish Law Annual. Volume Twelve. Amsterdam, Netherlands: Harwood Academic Publishers; 1997: 217–249. 99 fn. ISBN 90–5702–551–5. BE58344.

Christian ethics; codes of ethics; *confidentiality; disclosure; duty to warn; health personnel; historical aspects; international aspects; interprofessional relations; *Jewish ethics; law enforcement; *legal aspects; legal liability; legal obligations; married persons; medical education; medical ethics; medical records; medical schools; moral obligations; physician patient relationship; *physicians; privileged

communication; professional organizations; public health; *Australia; Australian Medical Association; Declaration of Geneva; Great Britain; Hippocratic Oath; International Code of Ethics; World Medical Association

Montgomery, Jonathan. The position of the patient: consent to treatment; confidentiality and access to health care records; care for children; mental health; research. *In: his* Health Care Law. New York, NY: Oxford University Press; 1997: 225–356. 701 fn. ISBN 0–19–876260–7. BE56244.

*adults; AIDS serodiagnosis; animal experimentation; coercion; compensation; competence; computers; *confidentiality; dangerousness; disclosure; dissent; duty to warn; genetic information; government regulation; *human experimentation; *informed consent; injuries; involuntary commitment; *legal aspects; legal guardians; legal liability; legislation; medical records; *mentally ill; *minors; parental consent; patient access to records; *patient care; patient discharge; patients' rights; research ethics committees; treatment refusal; *Great Britain; National Health Service

Pear, Robert. States pass laws to regulate uses of genetic testing. [News]. *New York Times.* 1997 Oct 18: A1, A9. BE58094.

attitudes; *confidentiality; disclosure; drug industry; employment; genetic disorders; *genetic information; genetic materials; genetic predisposition; genetic research; *genetic screening; *government regulation; health insurance; investigators; life insurance; patients; privacy; property rights; *social discrimination; *state government; *United States

Roche, Patricia (Winnie). Caveat venditor: protecting privacy and ownership interests in DNA. *In:* Knoppers, Bartha Maria, ed. Human DNA: Law and Policy: International and Comparative Perspectives. Proceedings of the First International Conference on DNA Sampling and Human Genetic Research: Ethical, Legal, and Policy Aspects, held in Montreal, Canada, 6–8 Sep 1996. Boston, MA: Kluwer Law International; 1997: 33–41. 30 fn. ISBN 90–411–0361–9. BE58166.

*confidentiality; disclosure; *DNA data banks; DNA fingerprinting; federal government; *genetic information; *genetic materials; *genetic research; *genetic screening; *government regulation; informed consent; *legal aspects; model legislation; privacy; *property rights; tissue donation; *Genetic Privacy Act; Moore v. Regents of the University of California; *United States

Schwartz, Paul M. Protection of privacy in health care reform. *Vanderbilt Law Review.* 1995 Mar; 48(2): 295–347. 264 fn. BE57192.

computers; *confidentiality; *disclosure; drug industry; economics; federal government; *government regulation; health care delivery; *health care reform; industry; informed consent; international aspects; legal rights; *medical records; preventive medicine; *privacy; private sector; social control; social discrimination; state government; Europe; *United States

Sfikas, Peter M. Does the dentist have an ethical duty to report child abuse? *Journal of the American Dental Association.* 1996 Apr; 127(4): 521–523. 9 refs. BE55581.

*child abuse; codes of ethics; confidentiality; *dentistry; government regulation; *health personnel; *legal aspects; legal liability; *mandatory reporting; moral obligations; professional organizations; state government; American Dental Association; United States

Shuman, Daniel W. The origins of the physician–patient privilege and professional secret. *Southwestern Law Journal.* 1985 Jun; 39(2): 661–687. 160 fn. BE56968.

clergy; comparative studies; *confidentiality; deontological ethics; disclosure; *historical aspects; *international aspects;

BE = bioethics accession number   fn. = footnotes   refs. = references

law; law enforcement; lawyers; *legal aspects; physician patient relationship; physicians; *privacy; *privileged communication; risks and benefits; state government; utilitarianism; England; France; Rome; United States

Silberner, Joanne. Keeping confidence. *Hastings Center Report.* 1997 Nov–Dec; 27(6): 8. BE57853.
accountability; *confidentiality; disclosure; epidemiology; federal government; genetic information; *government regulation; health insurance; law enforcement; *medical records; patient access to records; politics; privacy; standards; *Department of Health and Human Services; *United States

Skolnick, Andrew A. Opposition to law officers having unfettered access to medical records. *JAMA.* 1998 Jan 28; 279(4): 257–259. Includes an inset article, "Protecting research as well as patient privacy," p. 258. BE58066.
computer communication networks; *confidentiality; *disclosure; dissent; drug abuse; *epidemiology; federal government; HIV seropositivity; informed consent; investigators; *law enforcement; *legal aspects; legislation; managed care programs; *medical records; mental health; patients; privacy; psychotherapy; *public policy; state government; Supreme Court decisions; *Department of Health and Human Services; U.S. Congress; *United States

U.S. Congress. House. A bill to amend the Fair Labor Standards Act of 1938 to restrict employers in obtaining, disclosing, and using of genetic information. H.R. 3477, 104th Cong., 2d Sess. Introduced by Joseph P. Kennedy; 1996 May 16. 3 p. Referred to Committee on Economic and Educational Opportunities. BE56944.
*confidentiality; *disclosure; *employment; *genetic information; genetic screening; informed consent; *legal aspects; legislation; Americans with Disabilities Act 1990; *Fair Labor Standards Act 1938 (1996 Amendment); *United States

U.S. Congress. House. A bill to protect the privacy of health information in the age of genetic and other new technologies, and for other purposes [Medical Privacy in the Age of New Technologies Act of 1996]. H.R. 3482, 104th Cong., 2d Sess. Introduced by Jim McDermott; 1996 May 16. 73 p. Referred to the Committee on Commerce, and in addition to the Committee on Government Reform and Oversight. BE56779.
advisory committees; biomedical research; computers; *confidentiality; criminal law; *disclosure; emergency care; family members; federal government; genetic information; government regulation; health; health insurance; information dissemination; informed consent; law enforcement; *legal aspects; legislation; *medical records; *privacy; public health; state government; torts; *Medical Privacy in the Age of New Technologies Act (1996 bill); *United States

U.S. Congress. Senate. A bill to establish limitation with respect to the disclosure and use of genetic information, and for other purposes [Genetic Privacy and Nondiscrimination Act of 1995]. S. 1416, 104th Cong., 1st Sess. Introduced by Mark O. Hatfield; 1995 Nov 15. 7 p. Referred to the Committee on Labor and Human Resources. BE56946.
advisory committees; *confidentiality; *disclosure; DNA data banks; employment; federal government; *genetic information; genetic screening; government regulation; health insurance; informed consent; law enforcement; *legal aspects; legislation; *privacy; social discrimination; state government; *Genetic Privacy and Nondiscrimination Act (1995 bill); National Bioethics Advisory Commission; *United States

U.S. Department of Health and Human Services.

Confidentiality of Individually Identifiable Health Information: Recommendations of the Secretary of Health and Human Services, Pursuant to Section 264 of the Health Insurance Portability and Accountability Act of 1996. U.S. Government Printing Office; downloaded from Web site: http://aspe.os.hhs.gov/admnsimp/index.htm; 1997 Sep 11. 50 p. 10 fn. Downloaded 10 Dec 1997. Submitted to the Committee on Labor and Human Resources and the Committee on Finance of the U.S. Senate, and to the Committee on Commerce and the Committee on Ways and Means of the U.S. House of Representatives, 11 Sep 1997. BE56249.
accountability; biomedical research; computers; *confidentiality; *disclosure; *federal government; *guidelines; health care delivery; health facilities; health insurance; health personnel; information dissemination; informed consent; law enforcement; *legislation; medical records; patient access to records; *privacy; public health; *public policy; computer security; quality assurance; *Department of Health and Human Services; Health Insurance Portability and Accountability Act 1996; U.S. Congress; *United States

Vandenbroucke, Jan P. Maintaining privacy and the health of the public should not be seen as in opposition. [Editorial]. *BMJ (British Medical Journal).* 1998 May 2; 316(7141): 1331–1332. 12 refs. BE58602.
biomedical research; *confidentiality; editorial policies; *epidemiology; *government regulation; informed consent; international aspects; *medical records; *privacy; public health; risks and benefits; state government; retrospective studies; Europe; United States

Wadman, Meredith. Privacy bill under fire from researchers. [News]. *Nature.* 1998 Mar 5; 392(6671): 6. BE57258.
biomedical research; *confidentiality; disclosure; *ethical review; federal government; *government regulation; *human experimentation; industry; informed consent; investigators; *legislation; *medical records; privacy; *private sector; research ethics committees; research subjects; expedited review; *Medical Information Protection Act 1998; *United States

Wadman, Meredith. US to tighten protection of medical data. [News]. *Nature.* 1997 Aug 14; 388(6643): 611. BE56557.
*biomedical research; *confidentiality; criminal law; drugs; federal government; government regulation; health personnel; human experimentation; industry; informed consent; insurance; investigators; *legal liability; legislation; *medical records; patients; *privacy; research ethics committees; Department of Health and Human Services; U.S. Congress; *United States

Yee, Yale H. Criminal DNA data banks: revolution for law enforcement or threat to individual privacy? [Note]. *American Journal of Criminal Law.* 1995 Winter; 22(2): 461–490. 212 fn. BE56910.
computers; *confidentiality; constitutional law; *criminal law; *DNA data banks; *DNA fingerprinting; expert testimony; *genetic information; genetic screening; government regulation; *law enforcement; *legal aspects; legal rights; mandatory testing; minority groups; *prisoners; *privacy; public policy; records; social discrimination; standards; state government; state interest; DNA Identification Act 1994; *United States

Flawed US proposals on patients' privacy. [Editorial]. *Lancet.* 1997 Sep 20; 350(9081): 823. BE56170.
computers; *confidentiality; federal government; *government regulation; law enforcement; *medical records; privacy; standards; Department of Health and Human Services; *United States

---

BE = bioethics accession number   fn. = footnotes   refs. = references

CONFIDENTIALITY/MENTAL HEALTH

Appelbaum, Paul S. A "health information infrastructure" and the threat to confidentiality of health records. *Psychiatric Services.* 1998 Jan; 49(1): 27–28, 33. 8 refs. BE58201.
computers; *confidentiality; data banks; *disclosure; federal government; health personnel; informed consent; investigators; *legal aspects; managed care programs; *medical records; mentally ill; *psychiatry; *public policy; Department of Health and Human Services; Health Insurance Portability and Accountability Act 1996; U.S. Congress; *United States

Appelbaum, Paul S.; Bourne, Richard; Candilis, Philip J., et al. Case vignette: unanticipated propinquity. [Case study and commentaries]. *Ethics and Behavior.* 1997; 7(4): 377–388. 5 refs. BE58667.
beneficence; case studies; *confidentiality; *conflict of interest; *disclosure; *expert testimony; *forensic psychiatry; *health personnel; informed consent; justice; lawyers; malpractice; medical records; privileged communication; professional patient relationship; psychology; *psychotherapy; referral and consultation; *professional role
CASE VIGNETTE: UNANTICIPATED PROPINQUITY. Dr. Marge N. O'Vera has a reputation in the community as a thoughtful, caring, and highly ethical psychotherapist. For more than a year she has been treating Greta Grievance, helping her to cope with emotional and financial insecurities in the aftermath of a highly contentious divorce. During a therapy session, Ms. Grievance tells Dr. O'Vera that she has decided to sue the attorney who represented her during the divorce. Ms. Grievance believes that he did not represent her interests effectively and that she foolishly took his advice in accepting a very inferior settlement. She has retained another attorney who, she tells O'Vera, will soon be calling to request information on the stress of the divorce and Ms. Grievance's continuing need for therapy. Dr. O'Vera will be asked to testify as to the harm caused to her client and resulting treatment expenses. As Ms. Grievance gets up to leave, she tells Dr. O'Vera, "I'm so glad you'll help me teach that awful Tom Tort a lesson." As she hears the name of Attorney Tort for the first time, Dr. O'Vera begins to sweat. Thomas Tort, attorney at law, is also a client of hers. She had no idea that he had been Ms. Grievance's divorce lawyer. She has treated him for recurring major depression over several years and knows that he probably was sufficiently depressed so as to compromise his professional work at the time he represented Ms. Grievance. When she is named as an expert witness for the plaintiff, Attorney Tort will learn that his therapist was also treating Ms. Grievance. At the same time, her duty of confidentiality precludes her informing others that Tort is also her client. What is Dr. O'Vera to do?

Artnak, Kathryn E.; Dimmitt, Jane H. Choosing a framework for ethical analysis in advanced practice settings: the case for casuistry. *Archives of Psychiatric Nursing.* 1996 Feb; 10(1): 16–23. 12 refs. BE55660.
adolescents; blacks; case studies; *casuistry; *clinical ethics; *confidentiality; *dangerousness; decision making; *disadvantaged; *domestic violence; *duty to warn; ethical analysis; family relationship; fathers; females; law enforcement; mentally ill; mothers; *nurses; *nursing ethics; patient care; patient participation; principle-based ethics; privacy; *psychotherapy; quality of life; sex offenses; *social problems; trust; values; *violence

Chan, Kevin W. Jaffee v. Redmond: making the courts a tool of injustice? *Journal of the American Academy of Psychiatry and the Law.* 1997; 25(3): 383–389. 10 refs. 3 fn. BE57303.
*confidentiality; disclosure; federal government; justice; law enforcement; *legal aspects; *privileged communication; *psychotherapy; social workers; state government; Supreme Court decisions; *Jaffee v. Redmond; United States

Furlong, Mark; Leggatt, Margaret. Reconciling the patient's right to confidentiality and the family's need to know. *Australian and New Zealand Journal of Psychiatry.* 1996 Oct; 30(5): 614–622. 27 refs. BE56002.
communication; *confidentiality; *disclosure; *family members; home care; legal aspects; *mentally ill; patient care team; physician patient relationship; *professional family relationship; psychiatry; Australia

Great Britain. England. Court of Appeal, Civil Division. W v. Egdell. *All England Law Reports.* 1989 Nov 9 (date of decision). [1990] 1: 835–853. BE56783.
*confidentiality; *dangerousness; *disclosure; *duty to warn; *institutionalized persons; *legal aspects; mental institutions; *mentally ill; physicians; psychiatry; schizophrenia; violence; *Great Britain; *W v. Egdell
The English Court of Appeal, Civil Division, affirmed the lower court's dismissal of a mental patient's claim of breach of confidentiality by his psychiatrist, who released information to the patient's hospital and prompted the later release of such information by the hospital to a mental health review tribunal. W, a paranoid schizophrenic, was detained in a secure hospital because he had shot seven people, killing five and wounding two. Ten years later his attorneys requested Dr. Henry George Egdell, a psychiatrist, to evaluate W's mental condition in order to prepare an application for eventual release or transfer to a less secure facility. Upon receipt of Egdell's negative report, which pointed out that W's interest in guns and homemade bombs predated his schizophrenia, the attorneys withdrew W's application. When Egdell learned that neither W's hospital nor review tribunal had seen the report, in the interest of further treatment, he sent a copy to the hospital and asked the hospital to send a copy to the tribunal. W claimed Egdell had breached his duty of confidentiality. Balancing the public interests in confidence and in disclosure, the court held in favor of the restricted disclosure of vital information about W's dangerousness because of the grave concern for public safety. As in *Tarasoff,* circumstances dictated the breadth of the psychiatrist's duty of confidentiality, which was liable to be overridden by public interest in disclosure. (KIE abstract)

Leong, Gregory B.; Silva, J. Arturo; Weinstock, Robert. Another courtroom assault on the confidentiality of the psychotherapist–patient relationship. *Journal of Forensic Sciences.* 1995 Sep; 40(5): 862–864. 19 refs. BE55878.
competence; *confidentiality; *criminal law; dangerousness; disclosure; *legal aspects; medical records; physician patient relationship; *privileged communication; *psychotherapy; *California; *People v. Webb

Muehleman, Thomas; Pickens, Bruce K.; Robinson, Franklin. Informing clients about the limits to confidentiality, risks, and their rights: is self-disclosure inhibited? *Professional Psychology: Research and Practice.* 1985 Jun; 16(3): 385–397. 17 refs. BE56950.
*confidentiality; consent forms; depressive disorder; *disclosure; evaluation studies; *informed consent; *psychotherapy; risks and benefits; students; universities

Schlossberger, Eugene; Hecker, Lorna. HIV and family

therapists' duty to warn: a legal and ethical analysis. *Journal of Marital and Family Therapy.* 1996 Jan; 22(1): 27–40. 63 refs. BE57065.
     autonomy; *confidentiality; disclosure; *duty to warn; government regulation; health personnel; *HIV seropositivity; informed consent; *legal aspects; legal liability; *psychotherapy; sexuality; state government; *family therapy; Tarasoff v. Regents of the University of California; United States

Wedding, Danny; Topolski, James; McGaha, Annette. Maintaining the confidentiality of computerized mental health outcome data. *Journal Of Mental Health Administration.* 1995 Summer; 22(3): 237–244. 31 refs. BE55926.
     administrators; *computers; *confidentiality; *data banks; evaluation; federal government; *information dissemination; managed care programs; *medical records; mental health; privacy; *psychotherapy; public policy; quality of health care; treatment outcome; trends; *computer communication networks; *computer security; United States

Weiner, Myron F.; Shuman, Daniel W. The privilege study. *Archives of General Psychiatry.* 1983 Sep; 40(9): 1027–1030. 9 refs. BE57231.
     *attitudes; *confidentiality; disclosure; evaluation studies; *knowledge, attitudes, practice; law; legal aspects; legislation; patients; physicians; *privileged communication; psychiatry; *psychotherapy; public opinion; judges; questionnaires; *Texas

CONTRACEPTION

See also POPULATION CONTROL, STERILIZATION

Callahan, Joan C. Birth control ethics. *In:* Chadwick, Ruth, ed. Encyclopedia of Applied Ethics, Volume 1. San Diego, CA: Academic Press; 1998: 335–351. 17 refs. ISBN 0-12-227066-5. BE56371.
     abortion on demand; *abortion, induced; attitudes; autonomy; beginning of life; coercion; congenital disorders; *contraception; drug abuse; eugenics; family planning; females; fetuses; government regulation; hormones; infanticide; international aspects; involuntary sterilization; males; medical devices; *methods; *moral policy; *morality; multiple pregnancy; personhood; physicians; politics; *population control; pregnant women; prenatal diagnosis; prenatal injuries; *public policy; religion; *reproduction; selective abortion; sex determination; sexuality; *social control; socioeconomic factors; voluntary sterilization; wedge argument; women's rights

Charo, R. Alta. The interaction between family planning policies and the introduction of new reproductive technologies. *In:* Petersen, Kerry, ed. Intersections: Women on Law, Medicine and Technology. Brookfield, VT: Ashgate; 1997: 73–97. 55 refs. 10 fn. ISBN 1-85521-882-8. BE57487.
     abortion, induced; autonomy; *contraception; decision making; drugs; eugenics; *family planning; *females; historical aspects; international aspects; legal aspects; physician's role; political activity; *population control; public health; public policy; *reproductive technologies; social dominance; women's health services; *women's rights; Nineteenth Century; RU-486; Twentieth Century; United States

Grisez, Germain. Difficult moral questions: may a physician remain in a group that provides immoral services? *Linacre Quarterly.* 1997 May; 64(2): 21–25. BE55616.
     *abortion, induced; *conscience; *contraception; drugs; employment; family planning; family practice; health

maintenance organizations; intention; interprofessional relations; *moral complicity; obstetrics and gynecology; *physicians; *referral and consultation; *Roman Catholic ethics; *Roman Catholics; voluntary sterilization; group practice

International Federation of Gynecology and Obstetrics. Recommendations on ethical issues in obstetrics and gynecology. [Official statement]. *Bulletin of Medical Ethics.* 1997 Nov; No. 133: 8–9. BE57629.
     circumcision; *contraception; disclosure; *females; government regulation; human rights; informed consent; international aspects; obstetrics and gynecology; *organizational policies; ovum donors; physicians; professional competence; professional organizations; remuneration; *reproduction; semen donors; sexuality; embryo donation; *International Federation of Gynecology and Obstetrics

King, Leslie; Meyer, Madonna Harrington. The politics of reproductive benefits: U.S. insurance coverage of contraceptive and infertility treatments. *Gender and Society.* 1997 Feb; 11(1): 8–30. 83 refs. 3 fn. BE57686.
     age factors; *contraception; employment; eugenics; federal government; females; *government financing; health insurance; *health insurance reimbursement; indigents; infertility; political activity; politics; *public policy; *reproductive technologies; *socioeconomic factors; state government; survey; *women's health services; Illinois; Medicaid; *United States

Ollila, Eeva; Hemminki, Elina. Does licensing of drugs in industrialized countries guarantee drug quality and safety for Third World countries? The case of Norplant licensing in Finland. *International Journal of Health Services.* 1997; 27(2): 309–328. 35 refs. BE56009.
     *contraception; *developing countries; drug industry; *drugs; *evaluation; *evaluation studies; females; government regulation; hormones; *human experimentation; information dissemination; *international aspects; patient care; patient education; *records; research design; research subjects; risks and benefits; *standards; *Finland; *Norplant; Sweden

Riddle, John M. Eve's Herbs: A History of Contraception and Abortion in the West. Cambridge, MA: Harvard University Press; 1997. 341 p. 1,330 fn. ISBN 0-674-27024-X. BE56628.
     *abortion, induced; *alternative therapies; ancient history; attitudes; *contraception; drugs; *females; fetuses; health personnel; *historical aspects; infanticide; information dissemination; international aspects; legal aspects; literature; nurse midwives; population control; religion; reproduction; technical expertise; *folk medicine; *plants; *Western World; Eighteenth Century; Europe; Middle Ages; Nineteenth Century; Seventeenth Century; Sixteenth Century; Twentieth Century; United States

Roberts, Dorothy. Killing the Black Body: Race, Reproduction, and the Meaning of Liberty. New York, NY: Pantheon Books; 1997. 373 p. 1,073 fn. ISBN 0-679-44226-X. BE57998.
     abortion, induced; adolescents; autonomy; *blacks; *coercion; *contraception; criminal law; deception; dehumanization; *drug abuse; eugenics; family relationship; *females; genetic identity; government financing; historical aspects; indigents; *involuntary sterilization; justice; legal aspects; misconduct; morality; parent child relationship; physicians; *pregnant women; *prenatal injuries; property rights; public policy; rape; *reproduction; *reproductive technologies; risks and benefits; sexuality; *social control; *social discrimination; socioeconomic factors; stigmatization; surrogate mothers; personal identity; slavery; Depo-provera; Medicaid; Nineteenth Century; Norplant; Twentieth Century; United States

---

BE = bioethics accession number   fn. = footnotes   refs. = references

Savage, Wendy. Taking liberties with women: abortion, sterilization, and contraception. *International Journal of Health Services.* 1982; 12(2): 293–308. 27 refs. BE57235.
    abortion, induced; coercion; *contraception; drug industry; informed consent; international aspects; involuntary sterilization; medical devices; methods; misconduct; morbidity; physicians; risks and benefits; socioeconomic factors; *sterilization (sexual); *women's health services; *women's rights; hysterectomy; intrauterine devices; Dalkon Shield; Depo-provera; Great Britain; National Health Service

Stubblefield, Phillip. Self-administered emergency contraception -- a second chance. [Editorial]. *New England Journal of Medicine.* 1998 Jul 2; 339(1): 41–42. 8 refs. BE58507.
    abortion, induced; *contraception; drugs; females; international aspects; statistics; *postcoital contraceptives; self care; United States

Tanne, Janice Hopkins. US hospital mergers threaten reproductive services. [News]. *BMJ (British Medical Journal).* 1997 Nov 22; 315(7119): 1330. BE56886.
    abortion, induced; contraception; *family planning; *hospitals; indigents; institutional policies; managed care programs; organization and administration; refusal to treat; religion; *religious hospitals; Roman Catholic ethics; *Roman Catholics; secularism; social impact; trends; voluntary sterilization; *women's health services; *health facility mergers; United States

World Medical Association. Family planning and the right of a woman to contraception. [Official statement]. *Bulletin of Medical Ethics.* 1997 Nov; No. 133: 9–10. BE57630.
    conscience; *contraception; *family planning; females; health education; international aspects; males; medical education; *organizational policies; physicians; professional organizations; referral and consultation; women's health; *women's rights; *World Medical Association

CONTRACEPTION/MINORS

Williams, Glanville. The Gillick saga [and] The Gillick saga -- II. *New Law Journal.* 1985 Nov 22, Nov 29; 135(6230 and 6231): 1156–1158, 1179–1182. 13 fn. BE57066.
    adolescents; confidentiality; *contraception; females; informed consent; judicial action; *legal aspects; *minors; parental consent; parental notification; physicians; public policy; sexuality; Department of Health and Social Security; *Gillick v. West Norfolk and Wisbech AHA; *Great Britain

COST OF HEALTH CARE *See* HEALTH CARE/ECONOMICS

DANGEROUSNESS *See* CONFIDENTIALITY/MENTAL HEALTH

DEATH *See* DETERMINATION OF DEATH

DEATH WITH DIGNITY *See* ALLOWING TO DIE, EUTHANASIA, SUICIDE, TERMINAL CARE

DELIVERY OF HEALTH CARE *See* HEALTH CARE

DETERMINATION OF DEATH

Al, Joop. Comparative observations on some current medico–legal issues in Dutch law. *In:* Jewish Law Annual. Volume Twelve. Amsterdam, Netherlands: Harwood Academic Publishers; 1997: 167–215. 127 fn. ISBN 90–5702–551–5. BE58341.
    *active euthanasia; *allowing to die; assisted suicide; body parts and fluids; brain death; cadavers; cardiac death; competence; congenital disorders; criminal law; decision making; depressive disorder; *determination of death; donor cards; family members; futility; guidelines; involuntary euthanasia; *Jewish ethics; *legal aspects; newborns; *organ donation; *organ donors; organ transplantation; persistent vegetative state; physicians; professional organizations; *public policy; quality of life; referral and consultation; resource allocation; self regulation; suffering; voluntary euthanasia; withholding treatment; Austria; Belgium; Denmark; France; Germany; *Netherlands; Norway; Sweden

Capron, Alexander Morgan. Death, definition of. *In:* Chadwick, Ruth, ed. Encyclopedia of Applied Ethics, Volume 1. San Diego, CA: Academic Press; 1998: 717–725. 6 refs. ISBN 0–12–227066–5. BE56376.
    anencephaly; brain death; *determination of death; legal aspects; model legislation; organ donation; *standards; withholding treatment; Uniform Determination of Death Act; United States

Dorff, Elliot N. Jewish law and lore: the case of organ transplantation. *In:* Jewish Law Annual. Volume Twelve. Amsterdam, Netherlands: Harwood Academic Publishers; 1997: 65–114. 86 fn. ISBN 90–5702–551–5. BE58343.
    abortion, induced; advance directives; attitudes to death; beginning of life; brain death; cadavers; cardiac death; Christian ethics; communitarianism; compassion; *determination of death; donor cards; family members; fetal development; *human body; *Jewish ethics; justice; moral obligations; *organ donation; *organ donors; organ transplantation; philosophy; religion; risks and benefits; secularism; terminally ill; theology; third party consent; transplant recipients; *value of life; *values; United States

Hoffenberg, R.; Lock, M.; Tilney, N., et al. Should organs from patients in permanent vegetative state be used for transplantation? [For the International Forum for Transplant Ethics]. *Lancet.* 1997 Nov 1; 350(9087): 1320–1321. 7 refs. BE56463.
    allowing to die; anencephaly; body parts and fluids; brain; conscience; *determination of death; futility; health personnel; involuntary euthanasia; *killing; legal aspects; newborns; *organ donation; organizational policies; *persistent vegetative state; professional organizations; prolongation of life; withholding treatment; Airedale NHS Trust v. Bland; American Neurological Association; British Medical Association; Great Britain; United States

Lamb, David. Death, medical aspects of. *In:* Chadwick, Ruth, ed. Encyclopedia of Applied Ethics, Volume 1. San Diego, CA: Academic Press; 1998: 727–734. 5 refs. ISBN 0–12–227066–5. BE56377.
    brain death; *determination of death; diagnosis; historical aspects; organ donation; standards; uncertainty; withholding treatment

Morrison, Mary F.; DeMichele, Sarah Gelbach. How culture and religion affect attitudes toward medical futility. *In:* Zucker, Marjorie B.; Zucker Howard D., eds. Medical Futility and the Evaluation of Life–Sustaining Interventions. New York, NY: Cambridge University Press; 1997: 71–84. 36 refs. ISBN 0–521–56877–3. BE55981.

BE = bioethics accession number   fn. = footnotes   refs. = references

active euthanasia; advance directives; *allowing to die; alternative therapies; American Indians; Asian Americans; *attitudes to death; autonomy; blacks; Buddhist ethics; communication; *cultural pluralism; *decision making; *determination of death; family members; females; *futility; Hindu ethics; Hispanic Americans; Islamic ethics; Jewish ethics; males; *minority groups; pain; physician's role; *prolongation of life; Protestant ethics; quality of life; *religion; Roman Catholic ethics; socioeconomic factors; suffering; suicide; *terminally ill; treatment refusal; trust; truth disclosure; value of life; *values; withholding treatment; United States

Veatch, Robert M., ed. The ethics of death and dying. *In:* Jonsen, Albert R.; Veatch, Robert M.; Walters, LeRoy, eds. Source Book in Bioethics: A Documentary History. Washington, DC: Georgetown University Press; 1998: 111–252. 14 fn. ISBN 0–87840–683–2. BE57891.
adults; advisory committees; age factors; *allowing to die; anencephaly; artificial feeding; attitudes to death; brain death; competence; *determination of death; family members; federal government; futility; government regulation; guidelines; historical aspects; *legal aspects; mentally disabled; model legislation; moral policy; newborns; persistent vegetative state; prolongation of life; public policy; standards; state government; third party consent; ventilators; withholding treatment; *Cruzan v. Director, Missouri Department of Health; *In re Baby K; *In re Conroy; *In re Quinlan; Natural Death Act (CA); *President's Commission for the Study of Ethical Problems; *Superintendent v. Saikewicz; *Twentieth Century; *United States

Werber, Stephen J. Ancient answers to modern questions: death, dying, and organ transplants -- a Jewish law perspective. *Journal of Law and Health.* 1996–1997; 11(1–2): 13–44. 139 fn. BE57589.
*active euthanasia; *allowing to die; *assisted suicide; brain death; cadavers; chronically ill; *determination of death; hearts; *Jewish ethics; killing; *organ donation; organ donors; organ transplantation; physicians; *resuscitation orders; right to die; *suicide; terminally ill; tissue donation; treatment refusal; value of life; withholding treatment; Orthodox Judaism

Youngner, Stuart J.; Shuck, Jerry M. Advance directives and the determination of death. *In:* McCullough, Laurence B.; Jones, James W.; Brody, Baruch A., eds. Surgical Ethics. New York, NY: Oxford University Press; 1998: 57–77. 49 refs. ISBN 0–19–510347–5. BE58340.
advance care planning; *advance directives; brain death; cardiac death; *communication; decision making; *determination of death; family members; goals; guidelines; living wills; organ donation; palliative care; *physicians; professional autonomy; prolongation of life; quality of life; *resuscitation orders; *surgery; terminally ill; third party consent; treatment refusal; values; withholding treatment; Patient Self-Determination Act 1990; United States

DETERMINATION OF DEATH/BRAIN DEATH

Abbott, Alison. German law could boost prospects for organ transplants. [News]. *Nature.* 1997 Jul 3; 388(6637): 4. BE56072.
body parts and fluids; *brain death; cadavers; *determination of death; *legal aspects; *organ donation; organ donors; remuneration; standards; Europe; Eurotransplant; *Germany

Bernat, James L. A defense of the whole-brain concept of death. *Hastings Center Report.* 1998 Mar–Apr; 28(2): 14–23. 36 fn. BE57539.
*brain; *brain death; cardiac death; consensus;

*determination of death; model legislation; organ donation; public policy; religion; *standards; Uniform Determination of Death Act; United States

Brannigan, Michael. On asking the right questions: personal death vs. brain death in Japan. *Death Studies.* 1998 Mar–Apr; 22(2): 157–169. 2 refs. 10 fn. BE58049.
*attitudes; *attitudes to death; *brain death; *determination of death; hearts; organ donation; organ transplantation; personhood; self concept; survey; *ethnographic studies; non-Western World; *Japan

Brooks, Chandler McC. A consideration of the ethics of brain death. *Sangyo Ika Daigaku Zasshi/Journal of University of Occupational and Environmental Health.* 1985 Jun 1; 7(2): 139–150. 14 refs. BE57826.
allowing to die; *brain death; death; *determination of death; ethics; organ donation; physicians; standards; values

Defanti, C.A. Brain death. *In:* Chadwick, Ruth, ed. Encyclopedia of Applied Ethics, Volume 1. San Diego, CA: Academic Press; 1998: 369–376. 9 refs. ISBN 0–12–227066–5. BE56372.
advisory committees; anencephaly; attitudes; bioethics; brain; *brain death; committee membership; consensus; *determination of death; diagnosis; dissent; evaluation; fetal development; historical aspects; international aspects; organ donation; persistent vegetative state; personhood; review; *standards; terminology; withholding treatment; Harvard Committee on Brain Death; President's Commission for the Study of Ethical Problems

Donovan, G. Kevin. Decisions at the end of life: Catholic tradition. *Christian Bioethics.* 1997 Dec; 3(3): 188–203. 22 refs. 4 fn. BE58488.
*active euthanasia; *allowing to die; artificial feeding; *assisted suicide; *attitudes to death; *brain death; cardiac death; costs and benefits; decision making; *determination of death; drugs; family members; informed consent; intention; organ donation; *pain; *palliative care; persistent vegetative state; prolongation of life; resuscitation; risks and benefits; *Roman Catholic ethics; *suffering; suicide; terminal care; *terminally ill; theology; third party consent; treatment outcome; treatment refusal; value of life; *withholding treatment; Congregation for the Doctrine of the Faith; National Conference of Catholic Bishops; United States

Medical decisions regarding end-of-life care have undergone significant changes in recent decades, driven by changes in both medicine and society. Catholic tradition in medical ethics offers clear guidance in many issues, and a moral framework accessible to those who do not share the same faith as well as to members of its faith community. In some areas, a Catholic perspective can be seen clearly and confidently, such as in teachings on the permissibility of suicide and euthanasia. In others, such as withdrawal of nutrition and hydration, the Church does not yet speak with one voice and has not closed out the discussion. Yet, it is not in the teaching on individual issues that a Catholic moral tradition offers the most help and comfort, but in its account of what it means to lead a life in Christ, and to prepare for a Christian death. As in the problem of pain and suffering, it is the spiritual support more than the ethical guidance that helps both patients and physicians bear the unbearable and fathom the unfathomable.

Fins, Joseph J. Approximation and negotiation: clinical pragmatism and difference. *Cambridge Quarterly of Healthcare Ethics.* 1998 Winter; 7(1): 68–76. 17 fn. BE58453.
attitudes to death; *blacks; *brain death; case studies;

BE = bioethics accession number   fn. = footnotes   refs. = references

children; *clinical ethics; *communication; *consensus; *cultural pluralism; *decision making; *determination of death; diagnosis; *dissent; Jewish ethics; *Jews; *knowledge, attitudes, practice; legal aspects; *minority groups; parents; *patient care; *physicians; *professional family relationship; religion; secularism; terminal care; trust; *values; *pragmatism; New York; Orthodox Judaism; United States

Goldworth, Amnon; White, Robert J.; Truog, Robert. On brain death. [Letters and response]. *Hastings Center Report.* 1997 Sep–Oct; 27(5): 4–5. BE56124.
   *brain death; cardiac death; children; *determination of death; organ donation; *standards

Gutierrez, Ed. Japan's House of Representatives passes brain-death bill. [News]. *Lancet.* 1997 May 3; 349(9061): 1304. BE56078.
   *brain death; *determination of death; guidelines; *legal aspects; legislation; organ donation; organ transplantation; professional organizations; standards; *Japan; Society for Transplantation (Japan)

Korein, Julius. Ontogenesis of the brain in the human organism: definitions of life and death of the human being and person. *In:* Edwards, Rem B., ed. Advances in Bioethics. Volume 2: New Essays on Abortion and Bioethics. Greenwich, CT: JAI Press; 1997: 1–74. 298 refs. ISBN 0-7623-0194-5. BE56789.
   abortion, induced; adults; *anencephaly; *beginning of life; *brain; *brain death; children; *determination of death; diagnosis; embryos; *fetal development; *fetuses; infants; newborns; organ transplantation; persistent vegetative state; *personhood; prognosis; tissue transplantation

New York. Supreme Court, Queens County. In re Long Island Jewish Medical Center. *New York Supplement, 2d Series.* 1996 Feb 28 (date of decision). 641: 989–992. BE56740.
   *allowing to die; *brain death; *decision making; *determination of death; dissent; *hospitals; *infants; institutional policies; *legal aspects; *parents; physicians; religion; ventilators; withholding treatment; *In re Long Island Jewish Medical Center; New York
The New York Supreme Court for Queens County authorized hospital withdrawal of a respirator from a brain dead infant. Three experts, two board certified pediatric specialists, retained by the hospital and another medical expert retained by the parents, certified the brain death of the five-month-old infant. Although hospital policy did not provide in writing for "reasonable accommodation" of religious or moral objections to determinations of death by the patient or the patient's family, the court found that the hospital did provide reasonable accommodation by keeping the parents informed, having its doctors available for consultation, encouraging a second opinion, and seeking judicial intervention. (KIE abstract)

Paris, John J.; Bell, Anthony J.; Murphy, James J. Pediatric brain death: dead is dead. *Journal of Perinatology.* 1995 Jan–Feb; 15(1): 67–70. 17 refs. BE55886.
   *adolescents; *brain death; children; *communication; *decision making; *determination of death; dissent; infants; legal aspects; parents; physician family relationship; physicians; ventilators; withholding treatment; Florida; New York

Patterson, Elizabeth G. Human rights and human life: an uneven fit. *Tulane Law Review.* 1994 Jun; 68(6): 1527–1561. 168 fn. BE55539.
   abortion, induced; adults; allowing to die; *anencephaly; autonomy; beginning of life; *brain death; cadavers;

*competence; determination of death; equal protection; *fetuses; human rights; informed consent; *legal aspects; *legal rights; mentally disabled; *minors; newborns; *persistent vegetative state; *personhood; quality of life; Supreme Court decisions; third party consent; treatment refusal; *value of life; withholding treatment; *United States

Provisional Commission for the Study on Brain Death and Organ Transplantation (Japan). Important Considerations with Respect to Brain Death and Organ Transplants, January 22, 1992. Tokyo: the Commission; translation issued by the Osaka Kidney Foundation; 1994 Jun. 39 p. English version of a report submitted to the Prime Minister. BE58449.
   advisory committees; *brain death; *cadavers; consensus; *determination of death; dissent; informed consent; *organ donation; *organ transplantation; personhood; physicians; public policy; resource allocation; *standards; transplant recipients; trust; *Japan; *Provisional Commission for the Study on Brain Death and Organ Transplantation (Japan)

Stevens, M.L. Tina. Redefining death in America, 1968. *Caduceus.* 1995 Winter; 11(3): 207–219. 41 fn. BE55530.
   allowing to die; *brain death; cadavers; *cardiac death; conflict of interest; *determination of death; hearts; historical aspects; human experimentation; killing; legal liability; motivation; *organ donation; organ transplantation; physicians; prolongation of life; public opinion; public policy; resuscitation; Roman Catholic ethics; standards; ventilators; withholding treatment; coma; Harvard Committee on Brain Death; Twentieth Century; United States

Tonti–Filippini, Nicholas. Revising brain death: cultural imperialism? *Linacre Quarterly.* 1998 May; 65(2): 51–72. 47 fn. BE58934.
   *brain death; comprehension; *determination of death; family members; legal aspects; organ donation; psychological stress; Roman Catholic ethics; *standards; third party consent; time factors

Wise, Jacqui. Japan to allow organ transplants. [News]. *BMJ (British Medical Journal).* 1997 May 3; 314(7090): 1298. BE55928.
   attitudes; *brain death; *determination of death; *legal aspects; legislation; *organ donation; organ transplantation; *Japan

DISCLOSURE *See* CONFIDENTIALITY,
   INFORMED CONSENT, PATIENT ACCESS TO
   RECORDS, TRUTH DISCLOSURE

DISTRIBUTIVE JUSTICE *See* RESOURCE
   ALLOCATION

DNA FINGERPRINTING

See also GENETIC SCREENING

de Bousingen, Denis Durand. Exhumation angers French ethicists. [News]. *Lancet.* 1997 Nov 15; 350(9089): 1458. BE56924.
   *cadavers; death; *DNA fingerprinting; *famous persons; fathers; informed consent; parent child relationship; paternity; *France; *Montand, Yves

Dorozynski, Alexander. Yves Montand to be exhumed to test paternity. [News]. *BMJ (British Medical Journal).* 1997 Nov 29; 315(7120): 1398. BE56913.
   *cadavers; death; *DNA fingerprinting; *famous persons; fathers; informed consent; *legal aspects; parent child relationship; *paternity; *France; *Montand, Yves

---

BE = bioethics accession number   fn. = footnotes   refs. = references

Humphreys, Martin; Brockman, Bea. DNA profiling of detained patients. [Letter]. *Lancet.* 1998 Mar 7; 351(9104): 760. 2 refs. BE58855.
> blood specimen collection; *DNA fingerprinting; informed consent; *law enforcement; *mentally ill; prisoners; Great Britain

McEwen, Jean E. DNA data banks. *In:* Rothstein, Mark A., ed. Genetic Secrets: Protecting Privacy and Confidentiality in the Genetic Era. New Haven, CT: Yale University Press; 1997: 231–251. 71 fn. ISBN 0–300–07251–1. BE58685.
> *DNA data banks; *DNA fingerprinting; donors; family members; genetic counseling; genetic information; genetic materials; *genetic research; government regulation; industry; informed consent; legal aspects; military personnel; prisoners; privacy; public policy; standards; state government; universities; *biological specimen banks; Department of Defense; United States

McEwen, Jean E. DNA sampling and banking: practices and procedures in the United States. *In:* Knoppers, Bartha Maria, ed. Human DNA: Law and Policy: International and Comparative Perspectives. Proceedings of the First International Conference on DNA Sampling and Human Genetic Research: Ethical, Legal, and Policy Aspects, held in Montreal, Canada, 6–8 Sep 1996. Boston, MA: Kluwer Law International; 1997: 407–421. 76 fn. ISBN 90–411–0361–9. BE58197.
> blood specimen collection; confidentiality; *DNA data banks; *DNA fingerprinting; family members; federal government; genetic research; genetic screening; government regulation; guidelines; informed consent; institutional policies; *law enforcement; legal aspects; mandatory programs; *military personnel; newborns; organization and administration; prisoners; privacy; professional organizations; public policy; regulation; state government; statistics; *tissue banks; *biological specimen banks; DNA Identification Act 1994; Human Genome Privacy Act; *United States

Mnookin, Seth. Department of Defense DNA registry raises legal, ethical issues. *GeneWATCH.* 1996 Aug; 10(1): 1, 3, 11. BE56919.
> *DNA data banks; *DNA fingerprinting; employment; federal government; genetic information; genetic predisposition; health insurance; informed consent; legal aspects; *mandatory testing; *military personnel; *public policy; *registries; *social discrimination; time factors; *Department of Defense; *United States

Murch, Randall S.; Budowle, Bruce. Are developments in forensic applications of DNA technology consistent with privacy protections? *In:* Rothstein, Mark A., ed. Genetic Secrets: Protecting Privacy and Confidentiality in the Genetic Era. New Haven, CT: Yale University Press; 1997: 212–230. 27 fn. ISBN 0–300–07251–1. BE58684.
> *DNA data banks; *DNA fingerprinting; forensic medicine; law enforcement; methods; privacy; regulation; genetic markers

Roeper, Burkhardt. Germany approves DNA tests for visas. [News]. *Nature.* 1998 Feb 19; 391(6669): 723. BE58065.
> *aliens; confidentiality; *DNA fingerprinting; *family members; *genetic screening; *public policy; *emigration and immigration; *Germany

Smith, J. Clay. The precarious implications of DNA profiling. *University of Pittsburgh Law Review.* 1994 Spring; 55(3): 865–888. 137 fn. BE55940.
> behavioral genetics; blacks; criminal law; DNA data banks; *DNA fingerprinting; federal government; forensic

medicine; genetic screening; genetics; law enforcement; *legal aspects; *legal rights; methods; *privacy; risks and benefits; *social discrimination; standards; state government; violence; Daubert v. Merrell Dow Pharmaceuticals; Fourth Amendment; *United States

U.S. Congress. House. A bill to amend title 10, United States Code, to limit the collection and use by the Department of Defense of individual genetic identifying information for the purpose of identification of remains, other than when the consent of the individual concerned is obtained. H.R. 2873, 104th Cong., 2d Sess. Introduced by Joseph P. Kennedy; 1996 Jan 24. 2 p. Referred to the Committee on National Security. BE57198.
> blood specimen collection; *DNA fingerprinting; federal government; *genetic information; *genetic screening; informed consent; *legal aspects; legislation; *military personnel; *Department of Defense; *United States

U.S. Court of Appeals, Ninth Circuit. Mayfield v. Dalton. *Federal Reporter, 3d Series.* 1997 Mar 27 (date of decision). 109: 1423–1427. BE56741.
> alternatives; blood specimen collection; *DNA data banks; *DNA fingerprinting; federal government; *legal aspects; *mandatory programs; *military personnel; *public policy; *Department of Defense; Fourth Amendment; *Mayfield v. Dalton; *United States

The U.S. Court of Appeals for the Ninth Circuit vacated a case in which the Department of Defense's compulsory taking of blood and tissue specimens from armed services members was claimed to be an unreasonable search and seizure under the Fourth Amendment. Mayfield and Vlacovsky were on active duty in the U.S. Marines when they challenged the military's order to give up blood and tissue samples for its DNA Registry, a repository for identification of remains of soldiers killed on duty. Mayfield and Vlacovsky also feared the possibility of discrimination from genetic information concerning propensity for disease. Between the decision of the federal district court and oral argument in this case, Mayfield and Vlacovsky had gone off active duty and joined the reserves. The court found the issue to be moot because Mayfield and Vlacovsky were not subject to the DNA collection program except in the remote possibility that they returned to active duty in an emergency situation. Also, between the two cases, the Department of Defense had shortened its specimen storage policy from 75 to 50 years and added the option of destroying the specimens at the donor's request upon separation from the service. (KIE abstract)

U.S. District Court, D. Hawaii. Mayfield v. Dalton. *Federal Supplement.* 1995 Sep 8 (date of decision). 901: 300–306. BE56743.
> blood specimen collection; *DNA data banks; *DNA fingerprinting; *federal government; genetic materials; *legal aspects; legal rights; *mandatory programs; *military personnel; privacy; *public policy; *Department of Defense; Fourth Amendment; *Mayfield v. Dalton; *United States

The U.S. District Court for the District of Hawaii denied motions for summary judgment and certification of a class action suit by two members of the armed services who refused to give blood and tissue samples for DNA identification of bodies in wartime. Mayfield and Vlacovsky were U.S. Marines on active duty at the time they refused to obey an order to supply specimens for the Department of Defense DNA Registry. That repository was set up following Operation Desert Storm for DNA analysis of soldiers' remains. Specimens were to be stored for 75 years before being destroyed. Mayfield and Vlacovsky alledged violation of the Fourth Amendment's prohibition against unreasonable search

---

and seizure. The court found the identification use of the samples to be far less intrusive than an evidentiary one for criminal or disciplinary purposes. Furthermore, use of the samples to diagnose hereditary disease and the possible discrimination by employers or insurers was too hypothetical. The court also found that the DNA Registry did not meet the definition of "research" under the Code of Federal Regulations on Protection of Human Subjects, because the sample was not to be used unless a service member was believed to be killed in action. (KIE abstract)

U.S. Federal Bureau of Investigation. Legislative Guidelines for DNA Databases [and] Text of the DNA Identification Act (1994), as Enacted: Subtitle C -- DNA Identification [and] Statutes and Legislation Regarding Mandatory Submission of Blood Samples for DNA Identification Purposes, July 1996. Quantico, VA: Federal Bureau of Investigation; 1991. 51 p. BE58041.
> blood specimen collection; *DNA data banks; *DNA fingerprinting; federal government; *government regulation; guidelines; *law enforcement; *legal aspects; legal rights; legislation; mandatory programs; privacy; standards; state government; DNA Identification Act (1991 bill); *Federal Bureau of Investigation; United States

Wade, Nicholas. F.B.I. set to open its DNA database for fighting crime: some fear for privacy. [News]. *New York Times.* 1998 Oct 12: A1, A15. BE58938.
> confidentiality; criminal law; *DNA data banks; *DNA fingerprinting; federal government; *law enforcement; mass screening; *prisoners; *privacy; state government; Federal Bureau of Investigation; *Great Britain; *United States

Washington. Supreme Court. State v. Olivas. *Pacific Reporter, 2d Series.* 1993 Aug 12 (date of decision). 856: 1076-1094. BE57099.
> blood specimen collection; *constitutional law; criminal law; DNA data banks; *DNA fingerprinting; due process; equal protection; law enforcement; *legal aspects; *legal rights; *mandatory testing; *prisoners; privacy; state government; state interest; *Fourth Amendment; *State v. Olivas; *Washington

The Supreme Court of Washington upheld the constitutionality of a state law requiring DNA testing of persons convicted of violent crimes or sex offenses in order to establish a DNA data bank for use in future prosecution of recidivist acts. The court allowed "the drawing of blood without a search warrant, probable cause or individualized suspicion." The court reasoned that it was preferable "to balance the general privacy right of persons to be free from unjustified governmental intrusion against the 'special needs beyond normal law enforcement' of the government" rather than "to balance the limited privacy rights of convicted persons against a compelling governmental interest." (KIE abstract)

Yee, Yale H. Criminal DNA data banks: revolution for law enforcement or threat to individual privacy? [Note]. *American Journal of Criminal Law.* 1995 Winter; 22(2): 461-490. 212 fn. BE56910.
> computers; *confidentiality; constitutional law; *criminal law; *DNA data banks; *DNA fingerprinting; expert testimony; *genetic information; genetic screening; government regulation; *law enforcement; *legal aspects; legal rights; mandatory testing; minority groups; *prisoners; *privacy; public policy; records; social discrimination; standards; state government; state interest; DNA Identification Act 1994; *United States

Banking Our Genes. [Videorecording].Eunice Kennedy Shriver Center; available for sale from Fanlight Productions, 47 Halifax St., Boston, MA 02130,

800-937-4113; 1995. 1 videocassette; 33 min.; sd.; color; 1/2 in.; VHS. Executive producer: Philip Reilly. BE57896.
> behavioral genetics; computers; *DNA data banks; *DNA fingerprinting; family members; federal government; genetic information; genetic predisposition; *genetic research; genetic screening; insurance; law enforcement; legal aspects; mass screening; military personnel; newborns; *privacy; public policy; *risks and benefits; stigmatization; violence; *biological specimen banks; ELSI-funded publication; pedigree studies; Department of Defense; Federal Bureau of Investigation; United States

Convict DNA bank unconstitutional? [News]. *Science.* 1998 Aug 21; 281(5380): 1121. BE59093.
> blood specimen collection; *DNA data banks; DNA fingerprinting; *legal aspects; legal rights; *prisoners; privacy; *biological specimen banks; *Massachusetts

DRUGS
See under
    PATIENT CARE/DRUGS

DURABLE POWERS OF ATTORNEY *See*
    ADVANCE DIRECTIVES

ECONOMICS
See under
    HEALTH CARE/ECONOMICS

EDUCATION
See under
    BIOETHICS/EDUCATION
    MEDICAL ETHICS/EDUCATION
    NURSING ETHICS/EDUCATION
    PROFESSIONAL ETHICS/EDUCATION

ELECTROCONVULSIVE THERAPY

Heitman, Elizabeth. The public's role in the evaluation of health care technology: the conflict over ECT. *International Journal of Technology Assessment in Health Care.* 1996 Fall; 12(4): 657-672. 89 refs. 2 fn. BE55556.
> brain pathology; *electroconvulsive therapy; evaluation; *government regulation; human experimentation; informed consent; mentally ill; municipal government; patient care; *patient participation; patients' rights; physicians; *political activity; psychiatry; public opinion; *public participation; *risks and benefits; selection for treatment; state government; technical expertise; *technology assessment; treatment outcome; treatment refusal; Berkeley; California; United States

Illinois. Appellate Court, Fourth District. In re Branning. *North Eastern Reporter, 2d Series.* 1996 Dec 18 (date of decision). 674: 463-472. BE58897.
> *decision making; *due process; *electroconvulsive therapy; institutionalized persons; judicial action; *legal aspects; *legal guardians; *mentally ill; psychosurgery; *third party consent; treatment refusal; *Illinois; *In re Branning

The Appellate Court of Illinois, Fourth District, invalidated a law permitting a guardian, with court approval, to provide consent for a ward's participation in any medical procedure which the guardian deems to be in the best interests of the ward. Branning, age 70, had received electroconvulsive therapy (ECT) throughout her life, beginning at age 14 or 15, until two years earlier. Her guardian petitioned the court for approval of the guardian's consent to ECT. The court held that the law facially violated the due process rights

---

of the patient. The court held that due process required, at a minimum, that the ward receive a hearing at which she be allowed to appear, present witnesses on her behalf, and cross-examine witnesses against her. She must also receive competent assistance at the hearing and she is entitled to an independent psychiatric examination. The ward must also be shown to be unable to make a reasoned decision about the treatment, and the treatment must be shown to be in her best interest and to be the least restrictive alternative. (KIE abstract)

Wisconsin. Court of Appeals. In re Guardianship of Ruth E.J. *North Western Reporter, 2d Series.* 1995 Sep 6 (date of decision). 540: 213–217. BE56744.
    *competence; constitutional law; critically ill; depressive disorder; *electroconvulsive therapy; equal protection; *informed consent; *legal aspects; legal guardians; legal rights; *legislation; *mentally ill; state government; *third party consent; *In re Guardianship of Ruth E.J.; *Wisconsin
The Wisconsin Court of Appeals allowed the guardian of an incompetent ward to consent to electroconvulsive therapy (ECT) because a state statute which required the patient's consent prior to treatment in effect denied the right to treatment to a patient who is incapable of consent. Ruth E.J. suffered from severe depression and was in danger of starvation and dehydration. Her doctor had decided that she would likely die without ECT, yet she was so ill that she could not make a decision concerning treatment. The court concluded that the state statute requiring "express and informed consent" for ECT and other drastic treatment violated equal protection under the federal and state constitutions because it applied to all patients, including those unable to express consent. (KIE abstract)

Electroconvulsive therapy. *Medical Journal of Australia.* 1985 Sep 2; 143(5): 190–191. 13 refs. BE56957.
    competence; depressive disorder; disclosure; *electroconvulsive therapy; *guidelines; informed consent; *mentally ill; methods; morbidity; mortality; *organizational policies; patient care; patient care team; physicians; professional organizations; psychiatry; referral and consultation; risks and benefits; selection for treatment; *standards; third party consent; Australia; *Royal Australian and New Zealand College of Psychiatrists

EMBRYO AND FETAL RESEARCH

See also FETUSES

Anleu, Sharyn L. Roach. Regulating new reproductive technologies: an examination of the emergence of legislation in two Australian states. *In:* Holstein, J.A.; Miller, G., eds. Perspectives on Social Problems: A Research Annual. Volume 8. Greenwich, CT: JAI Press; 1996: 175–197. 60 refs. 2 fn. ISBN 0–7623–0035–3. BE57747.
    advisory committees; artificial insemination; cryopreservation; embryo disposition; *embryo research; embryo transfer; embryos; *family relationship; feminist ethics; government financing; *government regulation; health insurance reimbursement; human experimentation; in vitro fertilization; infertility; *investigators; law; *legislation; married persons; mass media; medicine; national health insurance; personhood; political activity; professional autonomy; public policy; reproduction; *reproductive technologies; rights; selection for treatment; social dominance; social impact; surrogate mothers; *women's rights; Australia; Council on Reproductive Technology (South Australia); Medical Procedures (Infertility) Act 1984 (Victoria); Reproductive Technology Act 1988 (South Australia); *South Australia; *Victoria; Waller Committee

Blank, Robert H. Fetal research. *In:* Chadwick, Ruth, ed. Encyclopedia of Applied Ethics, Volume 2. San Diego, CA: Academic Press; 1998: 279–288. 7 refs. ISBN 0–12–227067–3. BE56384.
    aborted fetuses; abortion, induced; advisory committees; cadavers; *embryo research; embryos; federal government; *fetal research; fetal tissue donation; fetuses; goals; government financing; government regulation; in vitro fertilization; informed consent; motivation; pregnant women; public policy; risks and benefits; state government; viability; United States

Bower, Hilary. Public consultation on human cloning launched. [News]. *BMJ (British Medical Journal).* 1998 Feb 7; 316(7129): 411. BE58092.
    advisory committees; *cloning; *embryo research; government regulation; public participation; *public policy; research embryo creation; nuclear transplantation; *Great Britain; Human Fertilisation and Embryology Authority; Human Genetics Advisory Commission (Great Britain)

Brody, Baruch A. Reproductive and fetal research. *In: his* The Ethics of Biomedical Research: An International Perspective. New York, NY: Oxford University Press; 1998: 99–118, 368–370. 49 fn. ISBN 0–19–509007–1. BE57672.
    aborted fetuses; abortion, induced; comparative studies; consensus; *embryo research; embryos; ethical review; fathers; federal government; *fetal research; fetal tissue donation; genetic intervention; government regulation; guidelines; human experimentation; in vitro fertilization; informed consent; *international aspects; methods; nontherapeutic research; pregnant women; *public policy; research embryo creation; review; therapeutic research; value of life; Australia; Canada; Europe; United States

Brody, Baruch A. Research ethics: international perspectives. *Cambridge Quarterly of Healthcare Ethics.* 1997 Fall; 6(4): 376–384. 22 fn. BE56458.
    adults; *animal experimentation; animal rights; bioethics; comparative studies; *consensus; *cultural pluralism; *dissent; *embryo research; embryos; ethical review; guidelines; *human experimentation; in vitro fertilization; informed consent; *international aspects; moral obligations; moral policy; regulation; research embryo creation; research subjects; speciesism; value of life; Asia; Australia; Europe; North America

Butler, Declan. France reaps benefits and costs of going by the book. [News]. *Nature.* 1997 Oct 16; 389(6652): 661–662. BE55957.
    advisory committees; *bioethical issues; bioethics; cloning; *embryo research; genetic research; *government regulation; international aspects; *public policy; *France; National Ethics Advisory Committee (France)

Cahill, Lisa Sowle. The status of the embryo and policy discourse. *Journal of Medicine and Philosophy.* 1997 Oct; 22(5): 407–414. 9 refs. 3 fn. BE56618.
    advisory committees; beginning of life; cloning; *consensus; dissent; *embryo research; *embryos; federal government; fetal development; government financing; government regulation; *moral obligations; personhood; private sector; public opinion; *public policy; research embryo creation; value of life; values; Ethics Advisory Board; Human Embryo Research Panel; National Bioethics Advisory Commission; National Institutes of Health; United States

Carlson, John W. On the justification and limits of medical research: a response to Kevin Wildes. *In:* Wildes, Kevin Wm.; Mitchell, Alan C., eds. Choosing Life: A Dialogue on *Evangelium Vitae.* Washington, DC: Georgetown University Press; 1997: 199–205. 18 fn. ISBN 0–87840–646–8. BE56689.

BE = bioethics accession number   fn. = footnotes   refs. = references

beginning of life; *biomedical research; *embryo research; fetal research; genetic enhancement; *genetic research; germ cells; nontherapeutic research; *Roman Catholic ethics; theology; *therapeutic research; value of life; dignity; Evangelium Vitae

Diamond, Eugene F. Reflections on the 50th anniversary of the Nuremberg doctors' trials. *Linacre Quarterly.* 1997 May; 64(2): 17–20. 12 refs. BE55618.

aborted fetuses; abortion, induced; advisory committees; codes of ethics; eugenics; euthanasia; federal government; *fetal research; government regulation; historical aspects; human rights; international aspects; involuntary sterilization; killing; misconduct; National Socialism; nontherapeutic research; parental consent; *value of life; vulnerable populations; genocide; Declaration of Helsinki; Germany; Nuremberg Code; Twentieth Century; *United States

Dickson, David. UK consults public on clones for research. [News]. *Nature.* 1998 Feb 5; 391(6667): 523. Includes an inset article by M. Wadman, "US sees flurry of bills in bids to legislate." BE58054.

advisory committees; *cloning; *embryo research; government regulation; public participation; *public policy; nuclear transplantation; *Great Britain; Human Fertilisation and Embryology Authority; Human Genetics Advisory Commission (Great Britain)

Fletcher, John C. Ethical considerations in and beyond experimental fetal therapy. *Seminars in Perinatology.* 1985 Jul; 9(2): 130–135. 20 refs. BE56960.

abortion, induced; cesarean section; coercion; costs and benefits; federal government; *fetal development; *fetal research; *fetal therapy; *fetuses; financial support; government regulation; guidelines; legal aspects; moral obligations; mortality; parental consent; patient care team; pregnant women; prenatal diagnosis; private sector; research ethics committees; risks and benefits; selection for treatment; state interest; surgery; therapeutic research; treatment outcome; treatment refusal; trends; twins; viability; United States

Jonsen, Albert R., ed. The ethics of research with human subjects. *In:* Jonsen, Albert R.; Veatch, Robert M.; Walters, LeRoy, eds. Source Book in Bioethics: A Documentary History. Washington, DC: Georgetown University Press; 1998: 3–110. 3 refs. 31 fn. ISBN 0–87840–683–2. BE57890.

aborted fetuses; advisory committees; children; *embryo research; ethical review; federal government; *fetal research; fetal tissue donation; government regulation; *guidelines; historical aspects; *human experimentation; in vitro fertilization; informed consent; international aspects; investigators; legal aspects; literature; nontherapeutic research; patients; physicians; professional organizations; research design; research ethics committees; research subjects; risks and benefits; scientific misconduct; self regulation; therapeutic research; volunteers; vulnerable populations; *Belmont Report; *Declaration of Helsinki; *DHEW Guidelines; *DHHS Guidelines; *Ethics Advisory Board; Germany; *Human Fetal Tissue Transplantation Research Panel; *National Commission for the Protection of Human Subjects; National Institutes of Health; Nineteenth Century; *Nuremberg Code; *Tuskegee Syphilis Study; *Twentieth Century; *United States

Khushf, George. Embryo research: the ethical geography of the debate. *Journal of Medicine and Philosophy.* 1997 Oct; 22(5): 495–519. 36 refs. 9 fn. BE56624.

abortion, induced; advisory committees; *beginning of life; consensus; *embryo research; *embryos; federal government; fetal development; *government financing; *government regulation; human experimentation; in vitro fertilization; informed consent; libertarianism; *moral obligations; *moral policy; nontherapeutic research; *personhood; *policy analysis; *politics; private sector;

*public policy; reproductive technologies; research design; research embryo creation; risks and benefits; science; twinning; value of life; *Human Embryo Research Panel; United States

Three basic political positions on embryo research will be identified as libertarian, conservative, and social–democratic. The Human Embryo Research Panel will be regarded as an expression of the social–democratic position. A taxonomy of the ethical issues addressed by the Panel will then be developed at the juncture of political and ethical modes of reflection. Among the arguments considered will be those for the separability of the abortion and embryo research debates; arguments against the possibility of the preembryo being a person, especially arguments associated with totipotency and the significance of the primitive streak; and the various reasons for regulating embryo research, including those associated with respect for the preembryo, the protection of traditional views of human procreation, and the prevention of commercialization.

King, Patricia A. Embryo research: the challenge for public policy. *Journal of Medicine and Philosophy.* 1997 Oct; 22(5): 441–455. 27 refs. 6 fn. BE56621.

abortion, induced; advisory committees; attitudes; beginning of life; bioethical issues; *consensus; cultural pluralism; democracy; *embryo research; *embryos; fetal development; fetal tissue donation; fetuses; genetic identity; government financing; government regulation; *moral obligations; *moral policy; personhood; private sector; *public policy; research embryo creation; risks and benefits; standards; value of life; Human Fetal Tissue Transplantation Research Panel; United States

Complete moral consensus on the status of the human embryo is neither feasible nor necessary for the formulation of ethically acceptable public policy for human embryo research. Significant consensus on permissible human embryo research can rest upon diverse but overlapping moral traditions. Thus, human embryo research policy should do more than reflect mere abstract assertions about the moral status of human embryos. Rather, the moral underpinnings of human embryo research should be derived from a range of values, including the facilitation of human procreation, the advancement of applied scientific knowledge, the reduction of human suffering, and the protection of vulnerable persons from coercion and exploitation.

Kolata, Gina. Scientists face new ethical quandaries in baby-making. [News]. *New York Times.* 1997 Aug 19: C1, C8. BE55537.

*embryo research; *methods; *ovum; physicians; *reproductive technologies; risks and benefits; trends; United States

Krebs, D. Rules and ethics concerning assisted procreation established by the government in Germany. *Journal of Assisted Reproduction and Genetics.* 1996 Mar; 13(3): 193–195. 3 refs. BE55876.

beginning of life; cloning; criminal law; *embryo research; embryo transfer; genetic disorders; genetic intervention; germ cells; *government regulation; hybrids; in vitro fertilization; informed consent; *legal aspects; multiple pregnancy; ovum donors; physicians; posthumous reproduction; preimplantation diagnosis; *reproductive technologies; semen donors; sex preselection; surrogate mothers; Embryo Protection Act 1990 (Germany); *Germany

Langston, J. William; Palfreman, Jon. The Case of the Frozen Addicts: Working at the Edge of the Mysteries of the Human Brain. New York, NY: Vintage Books;

1996. 309 p. ISBN 0–678–74708–7. BE56698.
*aborted fetuses; animal experimentation; biomedical research; *brain; *brain pathology; diagnosis; disadvantaged; *drug abuse; federal government; *fetal research; *fetal tissue donation; government financing; *heroin; human experimentation; international aspects; interprofessional relations; *investigators; moral complicity; *paralysis; patients; primates; research institutes; research subjects; risks and benefits; selection of subjects; therapeutic research; *tissue transplantation; *toxicity; *Parkinson disease; Human Fetal Tissue Transplantation Research Panel; *Langston, J. William; Lindvall, Olle; National Institutes of Health; Sweden; United States

Merchant, Jennifer. Biogenetics, artificial procreation, and public policy in the United States and France. *Technology in Society.* 1996; 18(1): 1–15. 26 fn. BE56595.
abortion, induced; advisory committees; biomedical research; cesarean section; coercion; comparative studies; criminal law; cryopreservation; drug abuse; embryo disposition; *embryo research; federal government; *fetal research; fetal therapy; *fetuses; *genetic research; genetic screening; genetic services; *government financing; in vitro fertilization; indigents; industry; international aspects; judicial action; *legal aspects; legal liability; legal rights; personhood; physicians; *pregnant women; preimplantation diagnosis; prenatal diagnosis; *prenatal injuries; private sector; *public policy; *reproductive technologies; state government; state interest; Supreme Court decisions; torts; treatment refusal; women's health services; women's rights; *wrongful life; Bonbrest v. Kotz; France; Roe v. Wade; *United States

Mulkay, Michael. The Embryo Research Debate: Science and the Politics of Reproduction. New York, NY: Cambridge University Press; 1997. 212 p. (Cambridge cultural social studies). 556 fn. ISBN 0–521–57683–0. BE56513.
abortion, induced; beginning of life; *embryo research; embryos; females; genetic intervention; genetic screening; *government regulation; historical aspects; males; mass media; political activity; *politics; preimplantation diagnosis; *public policy; religion; reproductive technologies; *risks and benefits; Roman Catholic ethics; science; sex preselection; value of life; wedge argument; *Great Britain; Human Fertilisation and Embryology Act 1990; Human Fertilisation and Embryology Authority; Twentieth Century; Warnock Committee

Pechura, Constance M. Fetal and embryo research: a changing scientific, political, and ethical landscape. *In:* Vanderpool, Harold Y., ed. The Ethics of Research Involving Human Subjects: Facing the 21st Century. Frederick, MD: University Publishing Group; 1996: 371–400. 74 fn. ISBN 1–55572–036–6. BE56994.
aborted fetuses; advisory committees; body parts and fluids; *embryo research; federal government; *fetal research; *fetal tissue donation; government financing; *government regulation; historical aspects; parental consent; pregnant women; prenatal diagnosis; professional organizations; *public policy; reproductive technologies; research embryo creation; risks and benefits; stem cells; tissue banks; trends; cord blood; American College of Obstetricians and Gynecologists; American Fertility Society; Biomedical Ethics Advisory Committee; Department of Health and Human Services; Ethics Advisory Board; Human Fetal Tissue Transplantation Research Panel; National Advisory Board on Ethics in Reproduction (NABER); National Institutes of Health; Office of Technology Assessment; United States

Peel, John. After the embryo, the fetus? *Ethics and Medicine.* 1986; 2(2): 19–22. BE57494.
aborted fetuses; Christian ethics; *embryo research; embryos; fetal research; in vitro fertilization; infertility; personhood; public policy; regulation; Great Britain;

Warnock Committee

Pyers, Greg; Gott, Robert. Fertility Rights: The IVF Debate. Carlton, VIC, Australia: CIS Publishers; 1993. 49 p. (Australian issues series). ISBN 1–86391–102–2. BE57445.
beginning of life; children; cryopreservation; economics; *embryo research; *embryo transfer; embryos; feminist ethics; *in vitro fertilization; infertility; legal aspects; *methods; *public policy; *reproductive technologies; *risks and benefits; social impact; terminology; treatment outcome; *Australia

Shanner, Laura. Teaching women's health issues in a government committee: the story of a successful policy group. *Women's Health Issues.* 1997 Nov–Dec; 7(6): 393–399. 2 refs. BE57577.
*advisory committees; committee membership; *embryo research; embryos; *females; genetic intervention; government regulation; guidelines; human experimentation; infertility; informed consent; moral obligations; organization and administration; ovum donors; preimplantation diagnosis; program descriptions; *public policy; reproductive technologies; *women's health; embryo donation; *Canada; *Discussion Group on Embryo Research (Health Canada)

Shenfield, F.; Sureau, C. Ethics of embryo research. *In:* Shenfield, F.; Sureau, C., eds. Ethical Dilemmas in Assisted Reproduction. New York, NY: Parthenon Pub. Group; 1997: 15–21. 23 refs. ISBN 1–85070–916–5. BE57942.
cloning; cryopreservation; donors; *embryo research; embryos; government regulation; in vitro fertilization; informed consent; *international aspects; legislation; moral policy; personhood; research embryo creation; value of life; Council of Europe; *Europe; European Convention on Bioethics; France; Great Britain; Human Fertilisation and Embryology Act 1990; Human Fertilisation and Embryology Authority; United States

Tauer, Carol A. Embryo research and public policy: a philosopher's appraisal. *Journal of Medicine and Philosophy.* 1997 Oct; 22(5): 423–439. 20 refs. 1 fn. BE56620.
advisory committees; beginning of life; committee membership; *embryo research; *embryos; federal government; fetal development; government financing; government regulation; *guidelines; human experimentation; *in vitro fertilization; *moral obligations; *moral policy; nontherapeutic research; ovum donors; parent child relationship; personhood; policy analysis; public opinion; *public policy; reproductive technologies; research embryo creation; risks and benefits; semen donors; twinning; value of life; values; Ethics Advisory Board; *Human Embryo Research Panel; National Institutes of Health; United States
The development of public policy on bioethical issues can be approached through substantive moral and philosophic reasoning, or through balancing perceived societal views as to what is ethically acceptable. The Human Embryo Research Panel had to apply the first approach to the question of the moral status of the preimplantation embryo. Only after concluding that the preimplantation embryo was not a full human subject could the panel consider the conditions under which embryo research was ethically acceptable, given a range of societal views, concerns, and interests.

Tedeschi, Christopher M. Foetal tissue transplantation research: scientific progress and the role of special interest groups. *Minerva.* 1995 Spring; 33(1): 45–66. 88 fn. BE57270.
*aborted fetuses; abortion, induced; advisory committees; attitudes; federal government; *fetal research; *fetal tissue donation; *government financing; *government regulation;

---

informed consent; investigators; legal aspects; mass media; moral policy; organizational policies; patient advocacy; *political activity; politics; pregnant women; professional organizations; *public policy; tissue transplantation; *Parkinson disease; American College of Obstetricians and Gynecologists; American Medical Association; *Department of Health and Human Services; Human Fetal Tissue Transplantation Research Panel; *National Institutes of Health; *United States

U.S. General Accounting Office. NIH–Funded Research: Therapeutic Human Fetal Tissue Transplantation Projects Meet Federal Requirements. Report to the Chairmen and Ranking Minority Members, Committee on Labor and Human Resources, U.S. Senate, and Committee on Commerce, House of Representatives. Washington, DC: U.S. General Accounting Office; 1997 Mar. 8 p. 6 fn. GAO/HEHS–97–61. BE58135.
*aborted fetuses; abortion, induced; donors; federal government; *fetal research; *fetal tissue donation; *government financing; *government regulation; guidelines; human experimentation; informed consent; investigators; research institutes; therapeutic research; tissue transplantation; transplant recipients; *guideline adherence; NIH Guidelines; NIH Revitalization Act 1993; *United States

Wade, Nicholas. Scientists cultivate cells at root of human life: hope for transplants and gene therapy -- ethics at issue. [News]. *New York Times.* 1998 Nov 6: A1, A24. BE59031.
aborted fetuses; cloning; embryo disposition; *embryo research; federal government; *fetal tissue donation; gene therapy; government financing; government regulation; industry; investigators; private sector; risks and benefits; *stem cells; tissue transplantation; United States

Wadman, Meredith. Backing for anti–cloning bill reopens embryo debate. [News]. *Nature.* 1997 Aug 7; 388(6642): 505. BE56318.
biomedical research; *cloning; *embryo research; embryos; federal government; government financing; *government regulation; legislation; private sector; research embryo creation; *U.S. Congress; *United States

Walters, LeRoy. Research and experimentation: a response to Kevin Wildes's essay. *In:* Wildes, Kevin Wm.; Mitchell, Alan C., eds. Choosing Life: A Dialogue on *Evangelium Vitae.* Washington, DC: Georgetown University Press; 1997: 206–209. 1 fn. ISBN 0–87840–646–8. BE56690.
aborted fetuses; abortion, induced; *biomedical research; contraception; *embryo research; *fetal research; fetal tissue donation; gene therapy; killing; nontherapeutic research; research embryo creation; *Roman Catholic ethics; therapeutic research; tissue transplantation; value of life; Evangelium Vitae

Wildes, Kevin Wm. In the service of life: Evangelium Vitae and medical research. *In:* Wildes, Kevin Wm.; Mitchell, Alan C., eds. Choosing Life: A Dialogue on *Evangelium Vitae.* Washington, DC: Georgetown University Press; 1997: 186–198. 26 fn. ISBN 0–87840–646–8. BE56688.
autonomy; beginning of life; beneficence; *biomedical research; coercion; common good; deontological ethics; *embryo research; embryos; fetuses; human rights; informed consent; killing; moral obligations; nontherapeutic research; personhood; *Roman Catholic ethics; *theology; therapeutic research; *value of life; dignity; *Evangelium Vitae; Instruction on Respect for Human Life

A ban on cells that could heal. [Editorial]. *New York Times.* 1998 Nov 7: 14. BE59094.

aborted fetuses; embryo disposition; *embryo research; federal government; fetal tissue donation; government financing; *government regulation; industry; private sector; *stem cells; *tissue donation; tissue transplantation; *United States

EMBRYOS *See* EMBRYO AND FETAL RESEARCH, FETUSES

EPIDEMIOLOGY *See* BIOMEDICAL RESEARCH

ETHICISTS AND ETHICS COMMITTEES

Agich, George J.; Spielman, Bethany. Ethics expert testimony: against the skeptics. *Journal of Medicine and Philosophy.* 1997 Aug; 22(4): 381–403. 53 refs. 14 fn. BE55811.
advisory committees; bioethical issues; bioethics; case studies; *clinical ethics; conscience; cultural pluralism; democracy; ethical analysis; ethical theory; *ethicist's role; *ethicists; *ethics; *expert testimony; human experimentation; *judicial action; *law; metaethics; physicians; professional competence; public policy; *technical expertise; values; withholding treatment; United States
There is great skepticism about the admittance of expert normative ethics testimony into evidence. However, a practical analysis of the way ethics testimony has been used in courts of law reveals that the skeptical position is itself based on assumptions that are controversial. We argue for an alternative way to understand such expert testimony. This alternative understanding is based on the practice of clinical ethics.

American College of Obstetricians and Gynecologists. Committee on Ethics. Endorsement of institutional ethics committees. ACOG Committee Opinion No. 46. *ACOG Committee Opinions.* 1985 Oct; No. 46: 3 p. 12 refs. BE56907.
*clinical ethics committees; decision making; hospitals; obstetrics and gynecology; *organizational policies; physicians; professional organizations; *American College of Obstetricians and Gynecologists

Andre, Judith. Goals of ethics consultation: toward clarity, utility, and fidelity. *Journal of Clinical Ethics.* 1997 Summer; 8(2): 193–198. 5 fn. BE55752.
clinical ethics; *clinical ethics committees; communication; comparative studies; consensus; decision making; education; ethicists; *ethics consultation; evaluation; family members; *goals; health personnel; hospitals; institutional policies; patients; standards; Sparrow Hospital (Lansing, MI)

Andre, Judith. Speaking truth to employers. *Journal of Clinical Ethics.* 1997 Summer; 8(2): 199–203. 10 fn. BE56354.
clinical ethics committees; communication; *conflict of interest; *conscience; *dissent; *employment; *ethicist's role; *ethicists; ethics consultation; expert testimony; institutional policies; interprofessional relations; mass media; *moral obligations; patient advocacy; physicians; *professional ethics; truth disclosure; *virtues; whistleblowing; courage; *integrity

Andre, Judith. The week of November seventh: bioethics as a practice. [Personal narrative]. *In:* Carson, Ronald A.; Burns, Chester R., eds. Philosophy of Medicine and Bioethics: A Twenty-Year Retrospective and Critical Appraisal. Boston, MA: Kluwer Academic; 1997: 153–172. 18 refs. 6 fn. ISBN 0–7923–3545–7. BE56532.
bioethical issues; *bioethics; clinical ethics; education;

emotions; *ethicist's role; *ethicists; ethics consultation; goals; health care; indigents; interdisciplinary communication; justice; medicine; *obligations to society; philosophy; professional competence

Aulisio, Mark P.; Arnold, Robert M.; Youngner, Stuart J. Can there be educational and training standards for those conducting health care ethics consultation? *In:* Monagle, John F.; Thomasma, David C., eds. Health Care Ethics: Critical Issues for the 21st Century. Gaithersburg, MD: Aspen Publishers; 1998: 484–496. 27 fn. ISBN 0-8342-0911-X. BE56295.
    accountability; *clinical ethics committees; communication; *education; ethical analysis; ethicist's role; *ethicists; *ethics consultation; goals; interdisciplinary communication; legal aspects; models, theoretical; professional competence; self regulation; social dominance; *standards; technical expertise; virtues; quality assurance; Bouvia v. Superior Court (Glenchur); United States

Bacchetta, Matthew D.; Fins, Joseph J. The economics of clinical ethics programs: a quantitative justification. *Cambridge Quarterly of Healthcare Ethics.* 1997 Fall; 6(4): 451–460. 20 fn. BE56451.
    administrators; clinical ethics; *clinical ethics committees; communication; *costs and benefits; *economics; *education; *ethicists; *ethics consultation; *evaluation; health personnel; *hospitals; institutional policies; models, theoretical; referral and consultation; remuneration; resource allocation; social impact; *standards

Bateman, Randall B. Attorneys on bioethics committees: unwelcome menace or valuable asset? *Journal of Law and Health.* 1994–1995; 9(2): 247–272. 133 fn. BE57178.
    case studies; *clinical ethics committees; *committee membership; conflict of interest; education; ethical review; ethics consultation; historical aspects; hospitals; institutional policies; interdisciplinary communication; interprofessional relations; *lawyers; legal aspects; methods; social dominance; *professional role; United States

Black, Douglas. Corporate tyranny. [Editorial]. *Journal of Medical Ethics.* 1997 Oct; 23(5): 269–270. 4 refs. BE56903.
    *advisory committees; *artificial insemination; beneficence; *bioethical issues; *confidentiality; *consensus; death; *decision making; famous persons; *informed consent; married persons; *posthumous reproduction; regulation; *semen donors; suicide; *General Medical Council (Great Britain); Great Britain; *Human Fertilisation and Embryology Authority; Wingate, Orde

Bosk, Charles L.; Frader, Joel. Institutional ethics committees: sociological oxymoron, empirical black box. *In:* DeVries, Raymond; Subedi, Janardan, eds. Bioethics and Society: Constructing the Ethical Enterprise. Upper Saddle River, NJ: Prentice Hall; 1998: 94–116. 61 refs. 17 fn. ISBN 0-13-531252-3. BE58732.
    accountability; bioethical issues; *clinical ethics committees; committee membership; conflict of interest; decision making; empirical research; ethicist's role; ethicists; *ethics consultation; *evaluation; historical aspects; hospitals; legal aspects; organization and administration; professional competence; research ethics committees; review; social sciences; *standards; professional role; Twentieth Century; United States

Bradley, Peter M.; Shenkin, Henry A.; Rivlin, Michael M., et al. The ethics industry. [Letters]. *Lancet.* 1997 Nov 22; 350(9090): 1547–1549. 9 refs. BE58150.
    *bioethical issues; decision making; *ethicist's role; *ethicists; medical ethics; *physicians; professional autonomy; technical expertise

Brody, Baruch. Whatever happened to research ethics? *In:* Carson, Ronald A.; Burns, Chester R., eds. Philosophy of Medicine and Bioethics: A Twenty-Year Retrospective and Critical Appraisal. Boston, MA: Kluwer Academic; 1997: 275–286. 25 refs. ISBN 0-7923-3545-7. BE56542.
    advisory committees; bioethical issues; bioethics; biomedical research; clinical ethics; control groups; drugs; education; *ethicist's role; ethicists; federal government; freedom; *government regulation; historical aspects; *human experimentation; international aspects; literature; moral policy; public policy; random selection; *research design; research ethics committees; risks and benefits; selection of subjects; time factors; *trends; values; *research ethics; Europe; Twentieth Century; United States

Burdick, James F.; Turcotte, Jeremiah G.; Veatch, Robert M. Principles of organ and tissue allocation and donation by living donors. [Foreword]. *Transplantation Proceedings.* 1992 Oct; 24(5): 2226. Foreword to the Report on Organ Allocation (p. 2227–2235) and Living Donors (p. 2236–2237) by the 1991 Ethics Committee of the United Network for Organ Sharing, Richmond, VA. BE56844.
    committee membership; *ethics committees; *organ donation; *organ transplantation; organizational policies; *United Network for Organ Sharing; *United States

Butler, Declan. 'Bioethics needs better input from public.' [News]. *Nature.* 1997 Oct 23; 389(6653): 775. BE56203.
    *advisory committees; *bioethical issues; committee membership; common good; *decision making; *ethics committees; eugenics; human rights; interdisciplinary communication; *international aspects; preimplantation diagnosis; *public participation; public policy; values; national ethics committees; European Union; *France; *Great Britain

Butler, Declan. European biotech industry plans ethics panel. [News]. *Nature.* 1997 Jul 3; 388(6637): 6. BE56151.
    advisory committees; cloning; codes of ethics; embryo research; *ethics committees; *genetic intervention; *genetic research; germ cells; *industry; institutional ethics; professional ethics; *self regulation; *EuropaBio; *Europe

Butler, Declan. Unesco board set to agree on compromise on bioethics committee. [News]. *Nature.* 1998 Apr 30; 392(6679): 854. BE58407.
    *advisory committees; *bioethical issues; ecology; genetic research; *international aspects; science; *International Bioethics Committee (Unesco); *Unesco; *World Commission on the Ethics of Scientific Knowledge and Technology

Childress, James F. The challenges of public ethics: reflections on NBAC's report. *Hastings Center Report.* 1997 Sep–Oct; 27(5): 9–11. BE56113.
    *advisory committees; autonomy; beneficence; casuistry; children; *cloning; consensus; cultural pluralism; *ethical analysis; federal government; government regulation; *moral policy; *morality; organizational policies; principle-based ethics; public participation; *public policy; religious ethics; *risks and benefits; secularism; social impact; *Cloning Human Beings (NBAC); *National Bioethics Advisory Commission; United States

Collier, Joe. The future of ethics committees. *In:* Close, Bryony; Combes, Robert; Hubbard, Anthony; Illingworth, John, eds. Volunteers in Research and Testing. Bristol, PA: Taylor and Francis; 1997: 177–183. ISBN 0-7484-0397-3. BE57040.
    clinical ethics committees; committee membership; ethicists; *ethics committees; hospitals; human experimentation; organization and administration; *research ethics

---

BE = bioethics accession number   fn. = footnotes   refs. = references

committees; Europe; *Great Britain

Coughlin, Steven S. Invited commentary: on the role of ethics committees in epidemiology professional societies. *American Journal of Epidemiology.* 1997 Aug 1; 146(3): 209–213. 28 refs. BE57501.
    bioethics; continuing education; *epidemiology; *ethics committees; guidelines; human experimentation; interdisciplinary communication; international aspects; investigators; law; legal aspects; professional ethics; *professional organizations; public health; scientific misconduct; self regulation

Csikai, Ellen L. The status of hospital ethics committees in Pennsylvania. *Cambridge Quarterly of Healthcare Ethics.* 1998 Winter; 7(1): 104–107. 4 fn. BE58451.
    administrators; bioethical issues; clergy; *clinical ethics committees; *committee membership; ethics consultation; females; *hospitals; males; medical specialties; nurses; *organization and administration; physicians; *social workers; statistics; survey; *Pennsylvania

Degnin, Francis Dominic. Max Weber on ethics case consultation: a methodological critique of the Conference on Evaluation of Ethics Consultation. *Journal of Clinical Ethics.* 1997 Summer; 8(2): 181–192. 38 fn. BE55764.
    case studies; communication; *consensus; education; *empirical research; *ethical analysis; *ethicist's role; ethicists; *ethics; *ethics consultation; *evaluation; *goals; institutional policies; *methods; politics; principle–based ethics; social sciences; values; dispute resolution; *Conference on Evaluation of Ethics Consultation; *Weber, Max

DeRenzo, Evan G.; Strauss, Michelle. A feminist model for clinical ethics consultation: increasing attention to context and narrative. *HEC (HealthCare Ethics Committee) Forum.* 1997 Sep; 9(3): 212–227. 42 refs. BE56180.
    *clinical ethics; clinical ethics committees; communication; consensus; *decision making; emotions; ethical analysis; *ethicists; *ethics consultation; *feminist ethics; models, theoretical; narrative ethics; social dominance

DeVries, Raymond; Conrad, Peter. Why bioethics needs sociology. *In:* DeVries, Raymond; Subedi, Janardan, eds. Bioethics and Society: Constructing the Ethical Enterprise. Upper Saddle River, NJ: Prentice Hall; 1998: 233–257. 41 refs. 13 fn. ISBN 0–13–531252–3. BE58738.
    adults; bioethical issues; *bioethics; clinical ethics; clinical ethics committees; cultural pluralism; decision making; education; empirical research; ethicist's role; *ethicists; evaluation; goals; historical aspects; intensive care units; *interdisciplinary communication; international aspects; interprofessional relations; newborns; nursing ethics; physicians; professional competence; professional organizations; *social sciences; social workers; sociology of medicine; standards; technical expertise; values; withholding treatment; Twentieth Century; *United States

de Wachter, Maurice A.M.; Knoppers, Bartha M.; Monti, Chantal LeGris. Ethical decision–making by hospital committees. [Letter]. *Canadian Medical Association Journal.* 1984 Oct 1; 131(7): 713–714. BE57425.
    *clinical ethics committees; decision making; *ethics committees; evaluation; *hospitals; *research ethics committees; survey; *Canada; *Quebec

Dresser, Rebecca. Scientists in the sunshine. *Hastings Center Report.* 1997 Nov–Dec; 27(6): 26–28. 11 refs. BE57857.

*advisory committees; animal experimentation; *biomedical research; *committee membership; conflict of interest; *decision making; federal government; government financing; government regulation; guidelines; information dissemination; investigators; *legal aspects; legislation; private sector; *public participation; public policy; public sector; *science; *standards; Supreme Court decisions; technical expertise; values; *Animal Legal Defense Fund v. Shalala; *Federal Advisory Committee Act 1994; Guide for the Care and Use of Laboratory Animals (National Research Council); *National Academy of Sciences; Public Citizen v. U.S. Department of Justice; *United States

Ehleben, Carole M.; Childs, Brian H.; Saltzman, Steven L. HEC self assessment: what is it exactly that you do? A "snapshot" of an ethicist at work. *HEC (HealthCare Ethics Committee) Forum.* 1998 Mar; 10(1): 71–74. 4 refs. BE59059.
    clinical ethics; communication; employment; *ethicist's role; *ethicists; *ethics consultation; evaluation studies; family members; hospitals; medical education; patients; physicians; statistics; time factors

Ellos, William J. Some narrative methodologies for clinical ethics. *Cambridge Quarterly of Healthcare Ethics.* 1998 Summer; 7(3): 315–322. 21 fn. BE58559.
    case studies; *clinical ethics; ethicist's role; *ethics consultation; *narrative ethics; philosophy; Barthes, Roland; Foucault, Michel

Felder, Michael. Bioethics and the HMO. *HEC (HealthCare Ethics Committee) Forum.* 1997 Dec; 9(4): 355–364. 5 refs. BE58084.
    *clinical ethics committees; committee membership; economics; financial support; *health maintenance organizations; institutional policies; organization and administration; program descriptions; public participation; regional ethics committees; *Community Health Plan
The expanded role of managed healthcare has raised numerous ethical questions for which there has been no previous appropriate or convenient venue for discussion. Contrary to what many think, the relevant ethical questions are not the same as those raised by healthcare reform. To serve as a forum for dialogue and recommendations, in 1991 Community Health Plan (CHP) established a unique health maintenance organization (HMO) planwide ethics committee to address sub–acute and out–patient oriented issues. It is called the CHP Ethical Issues Committee (CHPEIC).

Ferrell, Betty R. The role of ethics committees in responding to the moral outrage of unrelieved pain. *Bioethics Forum.* 1997 Fall; 13(3): 11–16. 20 refs. BE57528.
    accountability; *clinical ethics committees; drugs; government regulation; institutional ethics; interdisciplinary communication; *pain; *palliative care; patient care; patient education; placebos; *quality of health care; quality of life; standards; technical expertise; vulnerable populations

Fletcher, John C. Bioethics in a legal forum: confessions of an "expert" witness. *Journal of Medicine and Philosophy.* 1997 Aug; 22(4): 297–324. 55 refs. 18 fn. BE55855.
    allowing to die; anencephaly; *bioethical issues; bioethics; case studies; clinical ethics; deception; decision making; dissent; emergency care; ethical analysis; *ethicist's role; *ethicists; *ethics; ethics consultation; *expert testimony; futility; hospitals; infants; informed consent; interprofessional relations; *judicial action; *law; legal aspects; misconduct; mothers; patient care; physicians; prolongation of life; public policy; refusal to treat; remuneration; *technical expertise; ventilators; Americans with Disabilities Act 1990; Child Abuse Amendments 1984; Emergency Medical Treatment and Active Labor Act 1986; Fairfax Hospital (Falls Church,

---

VA); In re Baby K; Osheroff v. Greenspan; *United States; Veatch, Robert

This article reflects on the author's modest experience as an expert witness in two trials: Osheroff vs. Greenspan (1983), and In the Matter of Baby K (1994). Bioethicists' expertise as scholar-teachers and consultants on particular issues merits qualification by judges as expert witnesses. The article argues that a different kind of expertise -- strong moral advocacy -- is required to be an effective expert witness. The major lessons of expert witnessing for the author concern the demands and strains on the bioethicist's role as scholar, teacher, and consultant. The Baby K case is analyzed in some detail, due to its importance for bioethics, ethics consultation, and the testimony of bioethicists on either side of the case. Rules of thumb are offered to guide decisions as to choices regarding expert witnessing, as well as a discussion of the interaction of law and bioethics.

Fletcher, John C.; Miller, Franklin G. The promise and perils of public bioethics. *In:* Vanderpool, Harold Y., ed. The Ethics of Research Involving Human Subjects: Facing the 21st Century. Frederick, MD: University Publishing Group; 1996: 155-184. 74 fn. ISBN 1-55572-036-6. BE56986.

abortion, induced; accountability; *advisory committees; AIDS; *bioethical issues; *bioethics; biomedical research; embryo research; federal government; fetal research; fetal tissue donation; government financing; government regulation; health care delivery; historical aspects; *human experimentation; morality; politics; *public policy; *regulation; research institutes; scientific misconduct; Department of Health and Human Services; Ethics Advisory Board; National Bioethics Advisory Commission; National Commission for the Protection of Human Subjects; President's Commission for the Study of Ethical Problems; *United States

Fox, Mark D.; McGee, Glenn; Caplan, Arthur. Paradigms for clinical ethics consultation practice. *Cambridge Quarterly of Healthcare Ethics.* 1998 Summer; 7(3): 308-314. 27 fn. BE58558.

accountability; *clinical ethics; conflict of interest; *ethicist's role; *ethicists; *ethics consultation; evaluation; health personnel; *hospitals; interprofessional relations; *models, theoretical; organization and administration; patient care team; professional family relationship; referral and consultation; technical expertise; community hospitals; preventive ethics; teaching hospitals

Gillon, Raanan. Clinical ethics committees -- pros and cons. [Editorial]. *Journal of Medical Ethics.* 1997 Aug; 23(4): 203-204. 14 fn. BE55906.

clinical ethics; *clinical ethics committees; ethics consultation; *goals; hospitals; interdisciplinary communication; *risks and benefits; Great Britain

Goold, Susan Dorr. Is distance critical for clinical ethicists? A reply to Glenn McGee. *HEC (HealthCare Ethics Committee) Forum.* 1997 Sep; 9(3): 280-283. 1 ref. BE56172.

accountability; *clinical ethics; education; *ethicist's role; *ethicists; professional competence; technical expertise

Great Britain. England. High Court of Justice, Queen's Bench Division. R v. Ethical Committee of St. Mary's Hospital (Manchester) ex parte H. *Family Law Reports.* 1987 Oct 26 (date of decision). [1988] 1: 512-520. BE58576.

adoption; *clinical ethics committees; *decision making; hospitals; in vitro fertilization; infertility; judicial action; *legal aspects; *physicians; referral and consultation; *refusal

to treat; *reproductive technologies; *selection for treatment; sex offenses; standards; prostitution; *Great Britain; *National Health Service; *R v. Ethical Committee of St. Mary's Hospital (Manchester) ex parte H.

The Queen's Bench Division of England's High Court of Justice refused judicial review of a hospital ethics committee's decision that the medical team rather than the committee should determine denial of IVF services, in effect, refusal of treatment, to a patient and her husband. Because the patient, who was unable to conceive, had a past history of prostitution and poor understanding of the parental role, she and her husband were refused adoption and foster children by social services. They then sought IVF treatment and were put on a waiting list for services. After learning of the reasons for the adoption refusal, the consultant in obstetrics and gynecology decided that IVF should not be given and that the patient's name should be taken off the wait list. An ethics committee, which had been set up to provide advice and guidance on infertility services, as recommended by the Warnock Report, concluded that the decision on IVF services should be made by the medical consultant. Seeking judicial review, the patient claimed that once any matter is brought to the committee's attention, it was under a charge first to investigate and then to advise. The court found that the committtee with its "wide range of expertise" was intended to be advisory, not decision-making. In the court's opinion, the committee served as an informal forum for professionals. (KIE abstract)

Guyer, Ruth Levy. When decisions are life-and-death: patients and their families are increasingly turning to hospital ethicists to help them make tough calls on treatments. *USA Weekend.* 1998 Feb 6-8: 26. BE59105.

bioethical issues; bioethics; decision making; education; *ethicists; *ethics consultation; family members; health personnel; *hospitals; patients; United States

Hauerwas, Stanley M. How Christian ethics became medical ethics: the case of Paul Ramsey. *In: his:* Wilderness Wanderings: Probing Twentieth-Century Theology and Philosophy. Boulder, CO: Westview Press; 1997: 124-140. 22 refs. 11 fn. ISBN 0-8133-3349-0. BE58529.

bioethics; *Christian ethics; covenant; ethicists; interdisciplinary communication; love; medical ethics; medicine; natural law; *Protestant ethics; *theology; *Ramsey, Paul; The Patient as Person (Ramsey, P.)

Heilig, Steve; Brody, Robert V. Physician-hastened death and end-of-life care: development of a community-wide consensus statement and guidelines. *Cambridge Quarterly of Healthcare Ethics.* 1998 Spring; 7(2): 223-225. 7 refs. BE57558.

*assisted suicide; *clinical ethics committees; committee membership; consensus; guidelines; physicians; *practice guidelines; program descriptions; public participation; regional ethics committees; *terminal care; *Bay Area Network of Ethics Committees; San Francisco

Heitman, Elizabeth; Bulger, Ruth Ellen. The healthcare ethics committee in the structural transformation of health care: administrative and organization ethics in changing times. *HEC (HealthCare Ethics Committee) Forum.* 1998 Jun; 10(2): 152-176. 40 refs. BE59064.

clinical ethics; *clinical ethics committees; committee membership; *economics; education; ethics consultation; federal government; government financing; health care delivery; health insurance; health maintenance organizations; hospitals; incentives; *institutional ethics; institutional policies; *managed care programs; *organization and administration; patients' rights; physicians; standards;

business ethics; utilization review; Joint Commission on the Accreditation of Healthcare Organizations; Medicare; United States

Herb, Alice; Lazar, Eliot J. Ethics committees and end-of-life decision making. *In:* Zucker, Marjorie B.; Zucker, Howard D., eds. Medical Futility and the Evaluation of Life-Sustaining Interventions. New York, NY: Cambridge University Press; 1997: 110–122. 13 refs. ISBN 0-521-56877-3. BE55984.
  advance directives; *allowing to die; case studies; *clinical ethics committees; committee membership; *decision making; *dissent; education; ethicist's role; *family members; hospitals; institutional policies; interdisciplinary communication; legal aspects; *mediation; organization and administration; patient care; *physicians; prognosis; prolongation of life; *referral and consultation; resuscitation orders; uncertainty; withholding treatment; Joint Commission on the Accreditation of Healthcare Organizations; United States

Holden, Constance, ed. All quiet on the bioethics front. [News]. *Science.* 1998 Jul 10; 281(5374): 169. BE58441.
  *advisory committees; *bioethical issues; federal government; government financing; time factors; *National Bioethics Advisory Commission; United States

Howe, Edmund G. Everyday heroes, part 2: should careproviders ever be Quintilian? *Journal of Clinical Ethics.* 1997 Summer; 8(2): 115–123. 27 fn. BE56355.
  bioethical issues; *clinical ethics committees; coercion; communication; decision making; *dissent; *emotions; *ethicists; females; health personnel; *interprofessional relations; males; professional ethics; self concept; sexuality; social dominance; truth disclosure; virtues

Imber, Jonathan B. Medical publicity before bioethics: nineteenth-century illustrations of twentieth-century dilemmas. *In:* DeVries, Raymond; Subedi, Janardan, eds. Bioethics and Society: Constructing the Ethical Enterprise. Upper Saddle River, NJ: Prentice Hall; 1998: 16–37. 61 refs. 16 fn. ISBN 0-13-531252-3. BE58728.
  abortion, induced; accountability; animal experimentation; assisted suicide; *attitudes to death; *autopsies; *bioethical issues; *bioethics; *cadavers; death; emotions; entrepreneurship; *ethicist's role; *ethicists; famous persons; goals; *historical aspects; human body; human experimentation; law; legal aspects; mass media; *medical education; medical ethics; *medicine; organ donation; personhood; *physicians; public opinion; scientific misconduct; *sociology of medicine; theology; *trust; twins; conjoined twins; Garfield, James; *Nineteenth Century; *Twentieth Century; United States

Jacobson, Jay A.; Francis, L.P.; Battin, Margaret P., et al. Dialogue to action: lessons learned from some family members of deceased patients at an interactive program in seven Utah hospitals. *Journal of Clinical Ethics.* 1997 Winter; 8(4): 359–371. 12 fn. BE57609.
  advance directives; allowing to die; *attitudes; autopsies; *clinical ethics committees; *communication; death; decision making; diagnosis; education; ethicist's role; *evaluation; *family members; health personnel; *hospitals; information dissemination; *institutional policies; pain; palliative care; *professional family relationship; prognosis; program descriptions; prolongation of life; *public participation; quality of health care; resuscitation; survey; *terminal care; truth disclosure; *Dialogue to Action (LDS Hospital, Salt Lake City, UT); Utah
Dialogue to Action is a program we developed to establish a link between hospital ethics committees (HECs) and the public. We began Dialogue to Action in 1995 as a pilot program to consider how ethics committees should define their role. We described the

format of this program and the results from the first Dialogue to Action in another publication. Now, the program has been completed at seven Utah hospitals, which has enabled us to validate the findings from the first program and learn substantially more information. In this article, we make our findings and methods available to others in the hope that they will benefit by using Dialogue to Action as a model for other programs.

Jurchak, Martha. Clinical ethics consultants: survey and practice. *In:* Monagle, John F.; Thomasma, David C., eds. Health Care Ethics: Critical Issues for the 21st Century. Gaithersburg, MD: Aspen Publishers; 1998: 471–483. 36 fn. ISBN 0-8342-0911-X. BE56294.
  allowing to die; clinical ethics committees; committee membership; consensus; education; employment; ethical analysis; *ethicist's role; *ethicists; *ethics consultation; health facilities; knowledge, attitudes, practice; mediation; models, theoretical; patient participation; survey; retrospective studies; Society for Bioethics Consultation; United States

Kelly, Susan E.; Marshall, Patricia A.; Sanders, Lee M., et al. Understanding the practice of ethics consultation: results of an ethnographic multi-site study. *Journal of Clinical Ethics.* 1997 Summer; 8(2): 136–149. 35 fn. BE55765.
  allowing to die; case studies; *clinical ethics committees; committee membership; communication; comparative studies; consensus; decision making; *dissent; empirical research; *ethicists; *ethics consultation; *evaluation; evaluation studies; family members; gatekeeping; health maintenance organizations; *hospitals; institutional policies; minority groups; nurses; organization and administration; patient care; patient care team; patients; physician nurse relationship; physician patient relationship; physicians; public hospitals; social dominance; sociology of medicine; standards; survey; community hospitals; *ethnographic studies; multicenter studies; teaching hospitals; Pacific States

Khushf, George. Administrative and organizational ethics. *HEC (HealthCare Ethics Committee) Forum.* 1997 Dec; 9(4): 299–309. 35 refs. BE58087.
  accountability; *administrators; bioethics; *clinical ethics committees; decision making; goals; guidelines; *health facilities; *hospitals; *institutional ethics; institutional policies; managed care programs; *organization and administration; *professional ethics; regulation; religious hospitals; values; *institutional ethics; professional role; United States

Kipnis, Kenneth. Confessions of an expert ethics witness. *Journal of Medicine and Philosophy.* 1997 Aug; 22(4): 325–343. 6 refs. 6 fn. BE55913.
  adults; allowing to die; artificial feeding; *bioethical issues; blood transfusions; cancer; case studies; clinical ethics; competence; conflict of interest; consensus; decision making; DNA data banks; DNA fingerprinting; education; ethical theory; *ethicist's role; *ethicists; *ethics consultation; *expert testimony; family members; federal government; infants; Jehovah's Witnesses; *judicial action; mandatory programs; military personnel; parents; privacy; professional competence; professional ethics; public policy; remuneration; *standards; *technical expertise; therapeutic research; third party consent; treatment refusal; withholding treatment; Department of Defense; Hawaii; The Health Care Ethics Consultant (F.E. Baylis, ed.); United States
The aim of this essay is to describe and reflect upon the concrete particulars of one academician's work as an expert ethics witness. The commentary on my practices and the narrative descriptions of three cases are offered as evidence for the thesis that it is possible to act honorably within a role that some have considered to be inherently illicit. Practical measures are described

---

BE = bioethics accession number   fn. = footnotes   refs. = references

for avoiding some of the best known pitfalls. The discussion concludes with a listing of the distinctive competencies and understandings that are useful in serving as an expert ethics witness.

Lagnado, Lucette. Columbia urges ethics officers at its hospitals. [News]. *Wall Street Journal.* 1997 Dec 12: B6. BE58240.
> *administrators; *ethicists; fraud; *industry; private sector; *proprietary hospitals; *self regulation; business ethics; *Columbia/HCA Healthcare Corp.; Medicare

Larcher, Victor F.; Lask, Bryan; McCarthy, Jean M. Paediatrics at the cutting edge: do we need clinical ethics committees? *Journal of Medical Ethics.* 1997 Aug; 23(4): 245-249. 22 refs. BE55915.
> accountability; attitudes; children; clinical ethics; *clinical ethics committees; committee membership; education; ethicists; ethics consultation; evaluation studies; *goals; guidelines; health personnel; hospitals; human experimentation; informed consent; interdisciplinary communication; legal aspects; organization and administration; parental consent; patient care; patient care team; *pediatrics; research ethics committees; survey; withholding treatment; national ethics committees; *Great Britain; Great Ormond Street Hospital for Children (London); United States

OBJECTIVES: To investigate the need for hospital clinical ethics committees by studying the frequency with which ethical dilemmas arose, the perceived adequacy of the process of their resolution, and the teaching and training of staff in medical ethics. DESIGN: Interviews with individuals and three multidisciplinary teams; questionnaire to randomly selected individuals. SETTING: Two major London children's hospitals. RESULTS: Ethical dilemmas arose frequently but were resolved in a relatively unstructured fashion. Ethical concerns included: the validity of consent for investigations and treatment; lack of children's involvement in consent; initiation of heroic or futile treatments; resource allocation. Staff expressed the need for a forum which would provide consultation on ethical issues, develop guidelines for good ethical practice, undertake teaching and training, and provide ethical reflection outside the acute clinical setting. CONCLUSION: Multidisciplinary, accountable and audited clinical ethics committees with predominantly advisory, practice development and educational roles could provide a valuable contribution to UK clinical practice and perhaps in other countries that have not developed hospital clinical ethics committees.

Le Bris, Sonia. National Ethics Bodies: Report. Strasbourg, France: Council of Europe Press; 1993. 77 p. 73 fn. Study commissioned by the Council of Europe's Ad Hoc Committee of Experts on Bioethics (CAHBI). ISBN 92-871-2225-3. BE56509.
> *advisory committees; bioethical issues; committee membership; *ethics committees; financial support; international aspects; *organization and administration; public policy; statistics; survey; questionnaires; *Europe; Holy See; Turkey; United States

Lewthwaite, Barbara; Erickson-Nesmith, Sharon. Needs assessment for healthcare ethics education. *HEC (HealthCare Ethics Committee) Forum.* 1998 Mar; 10(1): 86-101. 6 refs. BE59061.
> *attitudes; *bioethical issues; *clinical ethics committees; *education; evaluation; *health personnel; hospitals; nurses; physicians; survey; teaching methods; time factors; questionnaires; teaching hospitals; *Canada

Lowenthal, Barbara; Getz, Marjorie; Kaye, Celia. The

special educator and the hospital ethics committee. Available from the ERIC Document Reproduction Service, DYNCORP I&ET, 7420 Fullerton Rd., Suite 110, Springfield, VA 22153-2852; Document No. ED320338; EC231146; 1990 Feb. 40 p. 34 refs. Paper presented at the Conference of the Learning Disabilities Association, Anaheim, CA, 1990 February 21-24. BE57693.
> *allowing to die; biomedical technologies; brain death; case studies; child abuse; children; *clinical ethics committees; committee membership; *congenital disorders; *decision making; determination of death; disabled; dissent; education; *ethics consultation; federal government; government regulation; hospitals; *infants; *institutional policies; legislation; low birth weight; mentally retarded; *newborns; organ donation; parents; *patient care; persistent vegetative state; *prolongation of life; psychological stress; *quality of life; suffering; surgery; treatment refusal; *value of life; ventilators; *withholding treatment; Department of Health and Human Services; Education of the Handicapped Act Amendments 1986; *Lutheran General Hospital (Park Ridge, IL); United States

McCullough, Laurence B. Preventive ethics, managed practice, and the hospital ethics committee as a resource for physician executives. *HEC (HealthCare Ethics Committee) Forum.* 1998 Jun; 10(2): 136-151. 16 refs. BE59063.
> accountability; *administrators; *clinical ethics committees; conflict of interest; costs and benefits; decision making; disclosure; *economics; health facilities; informed consent; *institutional ethics; institutional policies; *managed care programs; medicine; moral obligations; organization and administration; patient care; patients' rights; *physicians; private sector; public sector; quality of health care; remuneration; resource allocation; treatment outcome; *business ethics; *preventive ethics; United States

McGee, Glenn. Therapeutic clinical ethics. *HEC (HealthCare Ethics Committee) Forum.* 1997 Sep; 9(3): 276-279. BE56173.
> accountability; bioethics; *clinical ethics; education; *ethicist's role; *ethicists; *ethics consultation; hospitals; professional competence; technical expertise

McGurn, William. Princeton defends its philosopher of infanticide. *Wall Street Journal.* 1998 Nov 13: W17. BE58995.
> *attitudes; bioethics; dissent; *ethicists; *faculty; infanticide; morality; quality of life; speciesism; universities; value of life; *values; *Princeton University; *Singer, Peter

Marshall, Patricia A. Boundary crossings: gender and power in clinical ethics consultations. *In:* Sargent, Carolyn F.; Brettell; Caroline B., eds. Gender and Health: An International Perspective. Upper Saddle River, NJ: Prentice Hall; 1996: 205-226. 88 refs. 5 fn. ISBN 0-13-079427-9. BE58097.
> case studies; clinical ethics; *communication; *critically ill; *decision making; dissent; *ethicist's role; *ethics consultation; family members; family relationship; *females; *feminist ethics; futility; *narrative ethics; *organ transplantation; patient care team; patient transfer; *professional patient relationship; prognosis; psychological stress; *retreatment; self concept; social dominance; time factors; *uncertainty; values; sick role; Loyola University of Chicago Medical Center

Meslin, Eric M. Oxford Radcliffe Hospital Clinical Ethics Project 1994-1995: final report and recommendations. Oxford Radcliffe Hospital, Clinical Ethics Project, Stable Block, Manor House, Headley Way, Headington, Oxford, England OX3 9DZ; 1995 Jun 12. 53 p. 8 fn. BE57694.

---

*clinical ethics committees; committee membership;
*ethicists; *ethics consultation; *evaluation; hospitals;
interdisciplinary communication; *organization and
administration; program descriptions; standards; England;
*Oxford Radcliffe Hospital

Miller, Franklin G.; Caplan, Arthur L.; Fletcher, John C. Dealing with Dolly: inside the National Bioethics Advisory Commission. *Health Affairs.* 1998 May–Jun; 17(3): 264–267. 6 fn. BE58758.
*advisory committees; bioethical issues; *cloning; embryo research; federal government; genetic information; genetic research; government financing; government regulation; human experimentation; mentally ill; moral policy; politics; *public policy; religion; risks and benefits; *National Bioethics Advisory Commission; *United States

Miller, Franklin G. Dedicatory essay on John C. Fletcher [and] Bibliography of publications by John C. Fletcher. *Journal of Contemporary Health Law and Policy.* 1996 Fall; 13(1): ix–xxxii. BE55790.
*bioethical issues; ethicist's role; ethicists; ethics consultation; research institutes; *Fletcher, John C.; National Institutes of Health; University of Virginia

Miller, Tracy E.; Coleman, Carl H.; Cugliari, Anna Maria. Treatment decisions for patients without surrogates: rethinking policies for a vulnerable population. *Journal of the American Geriatrics Society.* 1997 Mar; 45(3): 369–374. 35 refs. BE56473.
advisory committees; aged; allowing to die; *alternatives; biomedical technologies; *clinical ethics committees; committee membership; *competence; *decision making; dementia; *ethics committees; guidelines; hospitals; indigents; *institutional policies; institutionalized persons; judicial action; legal aspects; legal guardians; managed care programs; mentally disabled; models, theoretical; *nursing homes; *patient advocacy; *patient care; patient care team; physician's role; physicians; referral and consultation; review committees; risks and benefits; single persons; standards; *third party consent; treatment refusal; *vulnerable populations; withholding treatment; *absence of proxy; New York State Task Force on Life and the Law; United States

Morreim, E. Haavi. Bioethics, expertise, and the courts: an overview and an argument for inevitability. *Journal of Medicine and Philosophy.* 1997 Aug; 22(4): 291–295. 8 refs. Introduction to a set of six articles, on the ethicist's role as expert witness in legal proceedings, by J.C. Fletcher, p. 298–324; by K. Kipnis, p. 325–343; by M. Yarborough, p. 345–365; by K. Wm. Wildes, p. 365–371; by V.A. Sharpe and E.D. Pellegrino, p. 378–379; and by G.F. Agich and B.J. Spielman, p. 381–403. BE55827.
*bioethical issues; bioethics; clinical ethics; cultural pluralism; decision making; ethical analysis; *ethicist's role; *ethicists; *ethics; *expert testimony; *judicial action; *law; morality; secularism; technical expertise; values; United States

Neff-Smith, Martha; Giles, Scott; Spencer, Edward M., et al. Ethics program evaluation: the Virginia Hospital Ethics Fellows example. *HEC (HealthCare Ethics Committee) Forum.* 1997 Dec; 9(4): 375–388. 3 refs. BE58088.
administrators; attitudes; *clinical ethics; clinical ethics committees; *education; *ethics consultation; *evaluation; *evaluation studies; health personnel; *hospitals; organization and administration; program descriptions; standards; *community hospitals; *Center for Biomedical Ethics, University of Virginia; Virginia; West Virginia

Nelson, Lawrence J. Editor's introduction [conscience]. *HEC (HealthCare Ethics Committee) Forum.* 1998 Mar; 10(1): 2–8. 2 refs. 1 fn. BE59079.

accountability; beneficence; blood transfusions; *clinical ethics committees; committee membership; *conscience; *decision making; *ethicists; ethics consultation; *health personnel; informed consent; institutional policies; minors; moral development; moral obligations; physicians; religion; treatment refusal; values

Nelson, William A.; Wlody, Ginger Schafer. The evolving role of ethics advisory committees in VHA. *HEC (HealthCare Ethics Committee) Forum.* 1997 Jun; 9(2): 129–146. 31 refs. BE55963.
advisory committees; *clinical ethics committees; committee membership; disadvantaged; education; ethics consultation; evaluation; *federal government; goals; government financing; health care delivery; *health facilities; health services research; institutional ethics; institutional policies; males; organization and administration; patients; primary health care; *public hospitals; resource allocation; standards; technical expertise; ambulatory care; Department of Veterans Affairs; United States; Veterans Affairs National Center for Clinical Ethics (White River Junction, VT); *Veterans Health Administration

Orr, Robert D.; Morton, Kelly R.; deLeon, Dennis M., et al. Evaluation of an ethics consultation service: patient and family perspective. *American Journal of Medicine.* 1996 Aug; 101(2): 135–141. 18 refs. BE55574.
*attitudes; decision making; *ethicists; *ethics consultation; *evaluation; evaluation studies; *family members; minority groups; patient care; *patient satisfaction; *patients; prognosis; survey; California; Loma Linda Community Medical Center; Loma Linda University Medical Center

Pentz, Rebecca D. Expanding into organizational ethics: the experience of one clinical ethics committee. *HEC (HealthCare Ethics Committee) Forum.* 1998 Jun; 10(2): 213–219. 5 fn. BE59068.
bone marrow; cancer; case studies; *clinical ethics committees; costs and benefits; decision making; *economics; *ethics consultation; guidelines; hospitals; *institutional ethics; *institutional policies; justice; moral obligations; physicians; *resource allocation; tissue transplantation; treatment outcome; M.D. Anderson Cancer Center; Texas

Rayner, Claire. A new ethics committee. *Bulletin of Medical Ethics.* 1997 May; No. 128: 20–21. 4 refs. BE55675.
*clinical ethics committees; health personnel; hospitals; interprofessional relations; organization and administration; professional competence; whistleblowing; *Great Britain; National Health Service

Reagan, James E.; Lomax, Karen J.; Nelson, William A. Clinical ethics in the Veterans Health Administration. *HEC (HealthCare Ethics Committee) Forum.* 1997 Jun; 9(2): 120–128. 2 refs. 2 fn. BE55961.
advisory committees; bioethics; *clinical ethics; *clinical ethics committees; committee membership; education; ethics consultation; *federal government; health care delivery; health facilities; *organization and administration; primary health care; *program descriptions; *public hospitals; public policy; research institutes; United States; *Veterans Health Administration

Reitemeier, Paul J. Musings on medical mistakes: a four-piece ensemble in search of an orchestra. *Journal of Clinical Ethics.* 1997 Winter; 8(4): 353–358. 5 fn. BE57612.
attitudes; bioethics; *clinical ethics; clinical ethics committees; communication; conscience; *disclosure; emotions; empirical research; *ethicist's role; ethics consultation; family members; *iatrogenic disease; legal liability; malpractice; moral obligations; moral policy; negligence; patient care; patients' rights; physician patient relationship; physicians; professional competence; quality of

---

BE = bioethics accession number   fn. = footnotes   refs. = references

health care; standards; terminal care; *truth disclosure; virtues; whistleblowing; *medical errors

Rothrock, Jane C. Nurses belong at the table of the ethics committee. *AORN Journal (Association of Operating Room Nurses).* 1985 Mar; 41(3): 527–528. 3 refs. BE57835.
    allowing to die; *clinical ethics committees; decision making; newborns; *nurse's role; patient advocacy

Sanfilippo, Alfred. Optimizing the quality of health care through better communication: case conferences. *HEC (HealthCare Ethics Committee) Forum.* 1997 Sep; 9(3): 256–263. 1 ref. BE56176.
    *clinical ethics committees; *communication; *ethics consultation; family members; goals; guidelines; health personnel; hospitals; patient participation; records; standards

Schenkenberg, Tom. Salt Lake City VA Medical Center's first 150 ethics committee case consultations: what we have learned (so far). *HEC (HealthCare Ethics Committee) Forum.* 1997 Jun; 9(2): 147–158. 6 refs. BE55960.
    bioethical issues; *clinical ethics committees; education; ethicists; *ethics consultation; evaluation; institutional policies; *public hospitals; survey; *Salt Lake City Veterans Affairs Medical Center; Utah

Schick, Ida Critelli; Moore, Sally. Ethics committees identify four key factors for success. *HEC (HealthCare Ethics Committee) Forum.* 1998 Mar; 10(1): 75–85. 14 refs. BE59060.
    administrators; aged; attitudes; *clinical ethics committees; committee membership; *evaluation; financial support; home care; hospices; hospitals; organization and administration; physicians; residential facilities; survey; focus groups; qualitative research; Indiana; Kentucky; Ohio

Self, Donnie J.; Skeel, Joy D. The moral reasoning of HEC members. *HEC (HealthCare Ethics Committee) Forum.* 1998 Mar; 10(1): 43–54. 41 refs. BE59057.
    age factors; *clinical ethics committees; *committee membership; comparative studies; control groups; evaluation studies; females; hospitals; males; *moral development; morality; United States

Shalit, Ruth. When we were philosopher kings: the rise of the medical ethicist. *New Republic.* 1997 Apr 28; 216(17): 24–28. BE57837.
    *accountability; *clinical ethics; clinical ethics committees; conflict of interest; decision making; economics; education; employment; *ethicist's role; *ethicists; *ethics consultation; *evaluation; family members; hospitals; legal liability; malpractice; managed care programs; patient care; physicians; *professional competence; standards; *technical expertise; proprietary organizations; Society for Bioethics Consultation; United States

Shanner, Laura. Teaching women's health issues in a government committee: the story of a successful policy group. *Women's Health Issues.* 1997 Nov–Dec; 7(6): 393–399. 2 refs. BE57577.
    *advisory committees; committee membership; *embryo research; embryos; *females; genetic intervention; government regulation; guidelines; human experimentation; infertility; informed consent; moral obligations; organization and administration; ovum donors; preimplantation diagnosis; program descriptions; *public policy; reproductive technologies; *women's health; embryo donation; *Canada; *Discussion Group on Embryo Research (Health Canada)

Sharpe, Virginia A.; Pellegrino, Edmund D. Medical ethics in the courtroom: a reappraisal. *Journal of Medicine and Philosophy.* 1997 Aug; 22(4): 373–379. 3

refs. BE55923.
    assisted suicide; bioethical issues; conflict of interest; cultural pluralism; due process; education; ethical analysis; *ethicist's role; *ethicists; ethics; ethics consultation; *expert testimony; *judicial action; law; legal aspects; morality; remuneration; state interest; *technical expertise; values; Compassion in Dying v. State of Washington; Quill v. Vacco
Following up on a 1989 paper on the subject, this essay revisits the question of ethical expertise in the court room. Informed by recent developments in the use of ethics experts, the authors argue 1) that the adversarial nature of court proceedings challenges the integrity of the ethicist's pedagogical role; 2) that the use of ethics experts as normative authorities remains dubious; 3) that clarification of the State's interest in "protecting the ethical integrity of the medical profession" is urgently required; and 4) that the expertise of the ethicist may be more appropriately used in advising the legislature that in influencing the court.

Silverman, Henry. The role of emotions in decisional competence, standards of competency, and altruistic acts. *Journal of Clinical Ethics.* 1997 Summer; 8(2): 171–175. 10 fn. Commentary on J. Spike, "What's love got to do with it? The altruistic giving of organs," p. 165–170. BE55954.
    *altruism; case studies; clinical ethics committees; *competence; comprehension; decision making; *directed donation; *emotions; *ethics consultation; family relationship; *informed consent; kidneys; love; *mentally retarded; motivation; *organ donation; *organ donors; risks and benefits; standards; *unrelated donors

Slowther, Anne; Underwood, Martin. Is there a demand for a clinical ethics advisory service in the UK? [Letter]. *Journal of Medical Ethics.* 1998 Jun; 24(3): 207. 5 refs. BE59118.
    *attitudes; *clinical ethics committees; ethicists; *ethics consultation; hospitals; *physicians; survey; *Great Britain

Spencer, Edward M. A new role for institutional ethics committees: organizational ethics. *Journal of Clinical Ethics.* 1997 Winter; 8(4): 372–376. 12 fn. BE57614.
    administrators; *clinical ethics committees; codes of ethics; committee membership; economics; ethicist's role; *health facilities; *institutional ethics; managed care programs; moral obligations; *organization and administration; *professional ethics; proprietary health facilities; regulation; *standards; business ethics; *institutional ethics; *Joint Commission for Accreditation of Healthcare Organizations
New methods for financing and managing healthcare organizations have caused concerns regarding how these changes will affect the ethics of the care of patients. To address these concerns, the JCAHO has, for the first time, promulgated a standard requiring that each HCO develop and operate under a code of organizational ethics. This standard is now a part of the requirements that JCAHO will consider in its accreditation of HCOs. Development of the required code is mandatory for JCAHO subscribers and will, by necessity, need to be addressed by each institution. An IEC is the proper forum for undertaking this work.

Spencer, Edward M. Physician's conscience and HECs: friends or foes? *HEC (HealthCare Ethics Committee) Forum.* 1998 Mar; 10(1): 34–42. 7 refs. BE59056.
    *clinical ethics committees; committee membership; communication; *conscience; consensus; decision making; dissent; institutional policies; managed care programs; physician's role; *physicians; public participation; terminology; institutional ethics
No matter the future of healthcare financing and management, physicians of conscience and integrity must

---

BE = bioethics accession number   fn. = footnotes   refs. = references

still be an important force in the consideration of ethical issues. The traditional role for the conscientious physician -- being the only or even the major determinant of the morality of specific clinical decisions -- is, for better or worse, no longer in effect. Much of this authority now belongs to patients and HECs are the mechanism within HCOs to help maintain this authority and to observe, comment on, recommend, and occasionally "regulate" the ethics of the healthcare arena. It is natural that these mechanisms for addressing areas of moral uncertainty create a certain tension. This tension should be acknowledged by conscientious physicians and HEC members. Total agreement on all moral issues in the clinical setting is impossible and should not be a goal. However, the respectful recognition of the importance of each perspective by both HEC members and conscientious physicians, and cooperation in developing effective mechanisms to address real differences, are possible and desirable. All who are interested in the ethics of healthcare now and in the future should support these endeavors.

Spicker, Stuart F., ed. The Healthcare Ethics Committee Experience: Selected Readings from HEC Forum. Malabar, FL: Krieger; 1998. 452 p. Includes references. ISBN 1-57524-024-6. BE57076.
  accountability; caring; clergy; *clinical ethics committees; committee membership; competence; conflict of interest; cultural pluralism; decision making; due process; economics; education; ethical review; ethicists; ethics consultation; family members; gatekeeping; health personnel; hospitals; institutional policies; lawyers; legal aspects; legal liability; nursing homes; *organization and administration; patient participation; psychiatry; public participation; remuneration; United States

Spike, Jeffrey. What's love got to do with it? The altruistic giving of organs. *Journal of Clinical Ethics.* 1997 Summer; 8(2): 165-170. 4 fn. Commented on by H. Silverman, p. 171-175. BE55955.
  *altruism; case studies; clinical ethics committees; *competence; comprehension; decision making; *directed donation; disclosure; *ethics consultation; family members; family relationship; *informed consent; kidneys; love; *mentally retarded; *organ donation; *organ donors; risks and benefits; self concept; *unrelated donors

ten Have, Henk A.M.J.; Janssens, Rien M.J.P.A. Regulating euthanasia in the Netherlands: ethics committees for review of euthanasia? *HEC (HealthCare Ethics Committee) Forum.* 1997 Dec; 9(4): 393-399. 7 refs. BE58089.
  *active euthanasia; *clinical ethics committees; *decision making; disclosure; *ethics consultation; government regulation; legal aspects; *palliative care; physicians; *public policy; quality of health care; *regional ethics committees; technical expertise; *Netherlands
In this essay we critically review recent regulations with regard to euthanasia policy in The Netherlands. Euthanasia in Holland is formally structured under the penal code. However, because of court cases in which, from the beginning of the 1970s, conditions were formulated wherein euthanizing physicians would not be prosecuted, euthanasia could easily become part of the future standard of medical practice. Recently, new rules concerning the practice of euthanasia have been proposed by the Dutch government in order to adequately control euthanasia practice. These proposals mainly focus on retrospective review. Until now, relatively little attention was paid to preventability of euthanasia. In order to prevent euthanasia, prospective consultation with physicians considering to commit

euthanasia would have to receive more attention. In the United States, ample experience has been acquired providing prospective consultative services in neonatalogy. In the aftermath of the "Baby Doe" case, infant care review committees (ICRCs) were established to enhance decisionmaking with regard to severely compromised newborns. These experiences provide interesting points of departure for the development of prospective consultative services in The Netherlands, particularly for physicians who are considering to euthanize patients.

Tripp, Glenn; McCotter, Patricia I. Ethics committee consultation: a case. *HEC (HealthCare Ethics Committee) Forum.* 1997 Dec; 9(4): 389-392. BE58090.
  *allowing to die; brain pathology; cancer; case studies; *clinical ethics committees; competence; *critically ill; *decision making; *ethicist's role; hospitals; legal aspects; legal guardians; palliative care; prognosis; resuscitation orders; third party consent; time factors
Our hospital's Medical Ethics Committee (HEC) is routinely asked by attending physicians for advice regarding the ethical approach to difficult treatment decisions in patient care. As a result of several recent cases, the HEC is reevaluating its role during *ad hoc* consultations. At issue is whether the HEC should function in an advisory capacity only, or upon request, as a surrogate decisionmaker when urgent medical treatment decisions are needed.

Tuffs, Annette. Central ethics committee formed in Germany. [News]. *Lancet.* 1995 Aug 12; 346(8972): 433. BE56133.
  advisory committees; committee membership; *ethics committees; guidelines; human experimentation; medical ethics; preimplantation diagnosis; research ethics committees; *national ethics committees; Federal Medical Council (Germany); *Germany

Tunisia. Decree No. 94-1939 of 19 September 1994 laying down the functions, composition, and working procedures of the National Committee on Medical Ethics. *International Digest of Health Legislation.* 1995; 46(2): 201. BE57181.
  *advisory committees; bioethical issues; public policy; *National Committee on Medical Ethics (Tunisia); *Tunisia

Turner, Leigh. The greening of bioethics: corporate funding of bioethics research. *Cambridge Quarterly of Healthcare Ethics.* 1998 Summer; 7(3): 326-328. BE58561.
  *bioethics; *conflict of interest; education; *ethicists; federal government; *financial support; government financing; *industry; *research institutes; scarcity

U.S. Congress. House. Committee on Government Reform and Oversight. Subcommittee on Human Resources. Oversight of NIH and FDA: Bioethics and the Adequacy of Informed Consent. Hearing, 8 May 1997. Washington, DC: U.S. Government Printing Office; 1997. Serial No. 105-49. ISBN 0-16-055827-1. BE58891.
  *advisory committees; bioethics; children; cloning; control groups; developing countries; disclosure; drugs; emergency care; *ethical review; evaluation; federal government; genetic research; government financing; *government regulation; hepatitis; HIV seropositivity; *human experimentation; immunization; *informed consent; international aspects; mentally ill; military personnel; parental consent; placebos; pregnant women; public policy; research design; research ethics committees; research subjects; scientific misconduct; *vulnerable populations; war; Africa; AZT; Centers for Disease Control and Prevention; Department of Defense; Food and Drug Administration;

---

*National Bioethics Advisory Commission; National Institutes of Health; *United States

U.S. Congress. Senate. A bill to provide for the establishment of a Commission to Promote a National Dialogue on Bioethics. S. 1595, 105th Cong., 2d Sess. Introduced by Bill Frist; 1998 Feb 2. 9 p. Referred to the Committee on Labor and Human Resources. BE58438.
  *advisory committees; *bioethical issues; cloning; committee membership; legal aspects; *organization and administration; *public participation; *public policy; *Commission to Promote a National Dialogue on Bioethics; Institute of Medicine; *United States

Ubel, Peter A.; Asch, David A. Semantic and moral debates about hastening death: a survey of bioethicists. *Journal of Clinical Ethics.* 1997 Fall; 8(3): 242–249. 24 fn. BE57617.
  *active euthanasia; *allowing to die; artificial feeding; *assisted suicide; *attitudes; case studies; competence; *consensus; *dissent; *double effect; *drugs; *ethicists; family members; intention; involuntary euthanasia; killing; *moral policy; *morality; pain; palliative care; physicians; survey; *terminology; third party consent; treatment refusal; ventilators; *voluntary euthanasia; *withholding treatment; American Association of Bioethics; United States

Vanderpool, Harold Y. What's happening in research ethics? Commentary on Brody. *In:* Carson, Ronald A.; Burns, Chester R., eds. Philosophy of Medicine and Bioethics: A Twenty-Year Retrospective and Critical Appraisal. Boston, MA: Kluwer Academic; 1997: 287–297. 35 refs. 9 fn. ISBN 0-7923-3545-7. BE56543.
  advisory committees; bioethical issues; bioethics; *biomedical research; drugs; education; *ethicist's role; ethicists; government regulation; *human experimentation; *literature; research design; research ethics committees; risks and benefits; scientific misconduct; *trends; *research ethics

Veterans Affairs National Headquarters. Bioethics Committee. Ethics Advisory Committees: Committee Report. Issued by the VA National Center for Clinical Ethics, White River Junction, VT 05009; 1996 May. 8 p. 16 refs. BE56736.
  *clinical ethics committees; committee membership; education; ethics consultation; federal government; health facilities; institutional policies; organization and administration; public hospitals; standards; *United States; *Veterans Health Administration

Wadman, Meredith. Business booms for guides to biology's moral maze. [News]. *Nature.* 1997 Oct 16; 389(6652): 658–659. BE55951.
  advisory committees; *bioethics; cloning; education; ethicist's role; *ethicists; genome mapping; government regulation; human experimentation; literature; politics; private sector; public policy; public sector; research institutes; science; social impact; statistics; *trends; National Bioethics Advisory Commission; NCHGR Program on Ethical, Legal, and Social Implications (ELSI); President's Commission for the Study of Ethical Problems; *United States

Wadman, Meredith. National Institutes of Health sets up its own bioethics panel. [News]. *Nature.* 1997 Dec 18–25; 390(6661): 651. BE57320.
  *advisory committees; *bioethical issues; *federal government; organization and administration; *public policy; *National Institutes of Health; *Trans–NIH Bioethics Committee; *United States

Webb, Sally L.; Marshall, Mary Faith; Boettcher, Flint, et al. Refusal of treatment by an adolescent: the deliverances of different consciences. *HEC (HealthCare Ethics Committee) Forum.* 1998 Mar; 10(1): 9–23. 15 refs. 3 fn. BE59054.
  *adolescents; advance directives; allowing to die; *blood transfusions; case studies; competence; *conscience; *decision making; dissent; *ethicists; ethics consultation; informed consent; *Jehovah's Witnesses; legal aspects; *parents; *physicians; religion; risks and benefits; surgery; third party consent; *treatment refusal; uncertainty; values

White, Jocelyn C.; Dunn, Patrick M.; Homer, Lou. A practical instrument to evaluate ethics consultations. *HEC (HealthCare Ethics Committee) Forum.* 1997 Sep; 9(3): 228–246. 14 refs. BE56178.
  bioethical issues; clinical ethics; *clinical ethics committees; *ethicists; *ethics consultation; *evaluation; evaluation studies; forms; goals; hospitals; professional competence; community hospitals; Oregon

Wildes, Kevin Wm. Healthy skepticism: the emperor has very few clothes. *Journal of Medicine and Philosophy.* 1997 Aug; 22(4): 365–371. 16 refs. BE55927.
  autonomy; *bioethics; consensus; *cultural pluralism; democracy; ethical relativism; *ethicist's role; *ethicists; *ethics; *expert testimony; *judicial action; *morality; *secularism; *technical expertise
The role of an expert witness in ethics, as part of a legal proceeding, is examined in this essay. The essay argues that the use of such expertise rests on confusions about normative and non–normative ethics compounded by misunderstandings about the challenges of moral argument in secular, morally pluralistic societies.

Wolf, Susan M. Ban cloning? Why NBAC is wrong. *Hastings Center Report.* 1997 Sep–Oct; 27(5): 12–15. 21 fn. BE56114.
  *advisory committees; biomedical research; children; *cloning; constitutional law; cultural pluralism; embryo research; embryo transfer; federal government; freedom; genetic intervention; *government regulation; human experimentation; industry; legal aspects; methods; models, theoretical; morality; politics; private sector; *public policy; reproductive technologies; risks and benefits; self regulation; social impact; embryo splitting; nuclear transplantation; Cloning Human Beings (NBAC); *National Bioethics Advisory Commission; Recombinant DNA Advisory Committee; U.S. Congress; *United States

Woods, David. AMA launches institute for ethics. [News]. *BMJ (British Medical Journal).* 1997 Mar 29; 314(7085): 920. BE58446.
  bioethical issues; *ethics committees; medical ethics; physicians; professional organizations; *American Medical Association

Yarborough, Mark. The reluctant retained witness: alleged sexual misconduct in the doctor/patient relationship. *Journal of Medicine and Philosophy.* 1997 Aug; 22(4): 345–364. 10 refs. BE55930.
  bioethical issues; case studies; conflict of interest; *decision making; *ethicist's role; *ethicists; *expert testimony; faculty; interprofessional relations; judicial action; *legal aspects; *misconduct; *physician patient relationship; *physicians; professional ethics; remuneration; *sexuality; *technical expertise; uncertainty; universities; Colorado
Testifying as an expert ethics witness raises a number of important issues. These include: the prospect of generating adverse publicity for oneself and one's institution, avoiding bias, giving testimony that is at odds with testimony given by colleagues, potential conflicts of interest introduced by reimbursement, the need of those who hear the testimony of bioethicists to appreciate the nature of moral expertise, the difficulty of assessing the quality of legal evidence which emerges from

---

BE = bioethics accession number   fn. = footnotes   refs. = references

adversarial legal proceedings, and the need to consider what weight should be assigned to expert ethics testimony. Along with these issues, what might constitute sexual misconduct is addressed in the essay so that readers can review the decision-making of the author in two cases.

Zoloth-Dorfman, Laurie; Rubin, Susan B. Insider trading: conscience and critique in bioethics. *HEC (HealthCare Ethics Committee) Forum.* 1998 Mar; 10(1): 24–33. 6 refs. BE59055.
*clinical ethics committees; *conscience; dissent; economics; ethicist's role; *ethicists; *ethics consultation; health care delivery; managed care programs; professional ethics

Zoloth-Dorfman, Laurie; Rubin, Susan B. Navigators and captains: expertise in clinical ethics consultation. [Book review essay]. *Theoretical Medicine.* 1997 Dec; 18(4): 421–432. 5 fn. BE56341.
bioethics; *clinical ethics; clinical ethics committees; education; employment; *ethicist's role; *ethicists; *ethics consultation; goals; health personnel; *interdisciplinary communication; interprofessional relations; metaphor; professional competence; professional patient relationship; review; standards; *technical expertise; *Ethics Consultation: A Practical Guide (La Puma, J.; Schiedermayer, D.); *The Health Care Ethics Consultant (Baylis, F.E., ed.)

European Directory of Bioethics, 1996. Second Edition. Secaucus, NJ: Lavoisier; distributed by Springer Verlag; 1996. 703 p. Produced under the direction of Gérard Huber. French title: *Annuaire Europeen de Bioethique 1996*; text in French with English translation. Includes the bilingual *Thesaurus d'ethique biomedicale/Thesaurus of Biomedical Ethics*, p. 566–599. ISBN 2-7430-0094-5. BE56506.
advisory committees; bioethical issues; *bioethics; education; *ethicists; ethics committees; *international aspects; literature; *research institutes; terminology; national ethics committees; *Europe

New US regulatory framework emerges for genetics. [News]. *Nature Biotechnology.* 1997 Apr; 15(4): 300. BE55967.
*advisory committees; federal government; *genome mapping; government regulation; *public policy; *Advisory Committee on Genetics and Public Policy; National Human Genome Research Institute; NIH-DOE Working Group on Ethical, Legal, and Social Implications (ELSI); *United States

Thanks for the advice. [Editorial]. *Nature Biotechnology.* 1997 Apr; 15(4): 293. BE55970.
*advisory committees; bioethical issues; gene therapy; *genetic intervention; genetic screening; international aspects; prenatal diagnosis; *public policy; Great Britain; Japan; United States

ETHICS COMMITTEES *See* ETHICISTS AND ETHICS COMMITTEES
See under
BEHAVIORAL RESEARCH/ETHICS COMMITTEES
HUMAN EXPERIMENTATION/ETHICS COMMITTEES

EUGENICS

See also GENETIC INTERVENTION

Armstrong, Claire. Thousands of women sterilised in

Sweden without consent. [News]. *BMJ (British Medical Journal).* 1997 Sep 6; 315(7108): 563. BE57302.
*eugenics; *females; historical aspects; institutionalized persons; *involuntary sterilization; legal aspects; mentally disabled; public policy; social problems; standards; sterilization (sexual); *Sweden; Twentieth Century

Beardsley, Tim. China syndrome: China's eugenics law makes trouble for science and business. *Scientific American.* 1997 Mar; 276(3): 33–34. BE56853.
*eugenics; *genetic disorders; genetic research; government regulation; human rights; industry; international aspects; investigators; legislation; *mandatory programs; political activity; *public policy; *reproduction; *China

Boisaubin, Eugene V. Nazi medicine: In the Shadow of the Reich: Nazi Medicine [videorecording], by John Michalczyk. [Audiovisual review essay]. *JAMA.* 1998 May 13; 279(18): 1496. BE57824.
audiovisual aids; *eugenics; *historical aspects; human experimentation; involuntary euthanasia; involuntary sterilization; mandatory programs; *medicine; *misconduct; *National Socialism; *physicians; *Germany; *In the Shadow of the Reich: Nazi Medicine (Michalczyk, J.); *Twentieth Century; United States

Broberg, Gunnar; Roll-Hansen, Nils, eds. Eugenics and the Welfare State: Sterilization Policy in Denmark, Sweden, Norway, and Finland. East Lansing, MI: Michigan State University Press; 1996. 294 p. (Uppsala studies in history of science; v. 21). Bibliography: p. 273–280. ISBN 0-87013-413-2. BE57995.
alcohol abuse; anthropology; coercion; consensus; democracy; *eugenics; family planning; females; *genetic disorders; genetic predisposition; *genetics; *historical aspects; informed consent; institutionalized persons; international aspects; investigators; *involuntary sterilization; *legal aspects; legislation; mentally ill; mentally retarded; minority groups; minors; National Socialism; physically disabled; physicians; *public policy; research institutes; secularism; sex offenses; sexuality; social control; social discrimination; social problems; social worth; socialism; *socioeconomic factors; *sterilization (sexual); third party consent; *voluntary sterilization; *Denmark; *Finland; Germany; Nineteenth Century; *Norway; *Scandinavia; *Sweden; *Twentieth Century; World War II

Bucur, Maria. Disciplining the Future: Eugenics and Modernization in Interwar Romania. Ann Arbor, MI: University Microfilms International; 1996. 315 p. Bibliography: p. 280–312. Dissertation, Ph.D. in History, University of Illinois at Urbana-Champaign, 1996. UMI No. 9712209. BE58499.
autonomy; biology; common good; education; *eugenics; females; *genetic determinism; *goals; government regulation; *historical aspects; law; minority groups; obligations of society; obligations to society; *physician's role; political systems; politics; public health; *public policy; reproduction; secularism; *social control; social dominance; social sciences; socioeconomic factors; values; rationality; *Romania; *Twentieth Century

Burleigh, Michael. Ethics and Extermination: Reflections on Nazi Genocide. New York, NY: Cambridge University Press; 1997. 261 p. 538 fn. ISBN 0-521-58816-2. BE57155.
clergy; *eugenics; *historical aspects; homosexuals; *involuntary euthanasia; involuntary sterilization; Jews; *killing; literature; *mentally disabled; minority groups; *misconduct; *National Socialism; *physically disabled; physicians; Protestants; psychiatry; Roman Catholics; war; *Germany; Nineteenth Century; *Twentieth Century

Burleigh, Michael. Psychiatry, German society, and the

Nazi "euthanasia" programme. *Social History of Medicine.* 1994 Aug; 7(2): 213–228. 61 fn. BE57594.

adults; children; coercion; deinstitutionalized persons; *eugenics; *health personnel; *historical aspects; *involuntary euthanasia; involuntary sterilization; Jews; *killing; mental institutions; *mentally ill; mentally retarded; *National Socialism; nurses; parental consent; physically disabled; *physicians; *psychiatry; *public policy; socioeconomic factors; sociology of medicine; utilitarianism; war; *Germany; *Twentieth Century

Burleigh, Michael. Saving money, spending lives: psychiatry, society and the 'euthanasia' programme. *In:* Burleigh, Michael, ed. Confronting the Nazi Past: New Debates on Modern German History. New York, NY: St. Martin's Press; 1996: 98–111. 3 refs. ISBN 0–312–16353–3. BE57395.

administrators; adults; children; chronically ill; deinstitutionalized persons; *economics; employment; *eugenics; genetic disorders; health care; health personnel; *historical aspects; institutionalized persons; *involuntary euthanasia; involuntary sterilization; *killing; legislation; *mass media; mental institutions; *mentally ill; *mentally retarded; *misconduct; motivation; *National Socialism; parental consent; *physically disabled; physician's role; *psychiatry; public opinion; *public policy; stigmatization; volunteers; starvation; *Germany; Twentieth Century

Butler, Declan. Eugenics scandal reveals silence of Swedish scientists. [News]. *Nature.* 1997 Sep 4; 389(6646): 9. BE55806.

attitudes; disadvantaged; *eugenics; females; historical aspects; investigators; *involuntary sterilization; legal aspects; mentally disabled; misconduct; physicians; *public policy; *socioeconomic factors; statistics; *sterilization (sexual); *Sweden; *Twentieth Century

Canadian College of Medical Geneticists. China's eugenics law: position statement of the Canadian College of Medical Geneticists. *Journal of Medical Genetics.* 1997 Nov; 34(11): 960. Statement prepared by the CCMG's Ethics and Public Policy Committee and endorsed by its Board of Directors, June 1997. BE58367.

*eugenics; genetic disorders; genetic screening; government regulation; *international aspects; *organizational policies; physicians; prenatal diagnosis; professional organizations; *public policy; selective abortion; voluntary programs; *Canadian College of Medical Geneticists; *China

Dowbiggin, Ian Robert. Keeping America Sane: Psychiatry and Eugenics in the United States and Canada, 1880–1940. Ithaca, NY: Cornell University Press; 1997. 245 p. (Cornell studies in the history of psychiatry). 638 fn. ISBN 0–8014–3356–8. BE56505.

administrators; aliens; attitudes; behavior control; disadvantaged; *eugenics; females; government financing; health care reform; *historical aspects; institutionalized persons; international aspects; interprofessional relations; involuntary commitment; involuntary sterilization; legislation; males; mental institutions; *mentally ill; *mentally retarded; National Socialism; patient care; *physician's role; *physicians; political activity; population control; professional organizations; *psychiatry; public health; public hospitals; public policy; reproduction; resource allocation; sexuality; social discrimination; socioeconomic factors; state government; emigration and immigration; American Medico–Psychological Association; Blumer, George; *Canada; Clarke, Charles; Nineteenth Century; Twentieth Century; *United States

Duster, Troy. Persistence and continuity in human genetics and social stratification. *In:* Peters, Ted, ed. Genetics: Issues of Social Justice. Cleveland, OH: Pilgrim Press; 1998: 218–238. 57 fn. ISBN 0–8298–1251–2. BE57481.

aliens; anthropology; behavior control; *behavioral genetics;

blacks; *eugenics; *evolution; *genetics; genome mapping; historical aspects; intelligence; involuntary sterilization; legal aspects; *public policy; social problems; violence; emigration and immigration; Social Darwinism; United States

Dyck, Arthur J. Eugenics in historical and ethical perspective. *In:* Kilner, John F.; Pentz, Rebecca D.; Young, Frank E., eds. Genetic Ethics: Do the Ends Justify the Genes? Grand Rapids, MI: W.B. Eerdmans; 1997: 25–39. 31 fn. ISBN 0–8028–4428–6. BE56716.

*Christian ethics; coercion; disabled; *eugenics; evolution; genetic counseling; genetic determinism; genetic screening; health personnel; historical aspects; Huntington's disease; international aspects; involuntary euthanasia; involuntary sterilization; killing; mentally disabled; minority groups; National Socialism; prenatal diagnosis; public policy; reproduction; social discrimination; social worth; sociobiology; stigmatization; *value of life; Germany; Great Britain; Nineteenth Century; Twentieth Century; United States

Ernst, Edzard. Killing in the name of healing: the active role of the German medical profession during the Third Reich. *American Journal of Medicine.* 1996 May; 100(5): 579–581. 18 refs. BE55719.

disabled; employment; *eugenics; genetic disorders; *historical aspects; human experimentation; involuntary euthanasia; involuntary sterilization; Jews; *killing; legal aspects; mentally disabled; metaphor; *misconduct; *National Socialism; *physician's role; *physicians; prisoners; social discrimination; sociology of medicine; technical expertise; *Germany; Social Darwinism; Twentieth Century

Galton, David J.; Galton, Clare J. Francis Galton and eugenics today. *Journal of Medical Ethics.* 1998 Apr; 24(2): 99–105. 25 refs. BE58077.

employment; *eugenics; evolution; gene therapy; genetic disorders; genetic enhancement; genetic intervention; *genetic predisposition; *genetic screening; genome mapping; germ cells; government regulation; *historical aspects; insurance selection bias; international aspects; mentally disabled; prenatal diagnosis; public policy; reproduction; risk; selective abortion; *social discrimination; social worth; socioeconomic factors; sterilization (sexual); values; virtues; pedigree studies; Darwin, Charles; *Galton, Francis; Germany; *Great Britain; *Nineteenth Century; *Twentieth Century; United States

Eugenics can be defined as the use of science applied to the qualitative and quantitative improvement of the human genome. The subject was initiated by Francis Galton with considerable support from Charles Darwin in the latter half of the 19th century. Its scope has increased enormously since the recent revolution in molecular genetics. Genetic files can be easily obtained for individuals either antenatally or at birth; somatic gene therapy has been introduced for some rare inborn errors of metabolism; and gene manipulation of human germ–line cells will no doubt occur in the near future to generate organs for transplantation. The past history of eugenics has been appalling, with gross abuses in the USA between 1931 and 1945 when compulsory sterilization was practised; and in Germany between 1933 and 1945 when mass extermination and compulsory sterilization were performed. To prevent such abuses in the future statutory bodies, such as a genetics commission, should be established to provide guidance and rules of conduct for use of the new information and technologies as applied to the human genome.

Glass, James M. "Life Unworthy of Life": Racial Phobia and Mass Murder in Hitler's Germany. New York, NY: Basic Books; 1997. 252 p. Bibliography: p. 227–240. ISBN 0–465–09844–4. BE57385.

BE = bioethics accession number   fn. = footnotes   refs. = references

adults; children; communicable diseases; consensus; *dehumanization; disabled; *disease; *eugenics; genetic disorders; *genetics; health; historical aspects; human body; human experimentation; investigators; involuntary euthanasia; involuntary sterilization; *Jews; *killing; medicine; mentally ill; minority groups; moral complicity; *National Socialism; physician's role; prisoners; *psychology; public health; *public policy; quarantine; *social discrimination; stigmatization; Europe; *Germany; Twentieth Century; United States

Kerr, Anne; Cunningham-Burley, Sarah; Amos, Amanda. Eugenics and the new genetics in Britain: examining contemporary professionals' accounts. *Science, Technology, and Human Values.* 1998 Spring; 23(2): 175-198. 41 refs. 11 fn. BE57723.
    *attitudes; autonomy; behavioral genetics; coercion; democracy; directive counseling; disabled; *eugenics; gene pool; gene therapy; genetic counseling; genetic determinism; genetic disorders; genetic intervention; genetic predisposition; *genetic research; genetic screening; genetic services; *genetics; homosexuals; intelligence; *investigators; mass media; *physicians; political systems; prenatal diagnosis; resource allocation; schizophrenia; selective abortion; *social impact; socioeconomic factors; survey; *Great Britain; National Health Service

Kevles, Daniel J. In the Name of Eugenics: Genetics and the Uses of Human Heredity. With a New Preface by the Author. Cambridge, MA: Harvard University Press; 1995. 426 p. 918 fn. ISBN 0-674-44557-0. BE57444.
    attitudes; behavioral genetics; behavioral research; disadvantaged; *eugenics; genetic counseling; genetic disorders; genetic screening; *genetics; government regulation; *historical aspects; intelligence; international aspects; investigators; involuntary sterilization; legal aspects; literature; mandatory programs; mentally disabled; minority groups; National Socialism; political activity; prenatal diagnosis; public policy; reproduction; selective abortion; sexuality; social discrimination; social impact; sociobiology; socioeconomic factors; voluntary sterilization; women's rights; emigration and immigration; American Eugenics Society; Davenport, Charles; Galton, Francis; Germany; Great Britain; Nineteenth Century; Pearson, Karl; Penrose, Lionel; Twentieth Century; United States

King, David. Eugenic tendencies in modern genetics. *In:* Doherty, Peter; Sutton, Agneta, eds. Man-Made Man: Ethical and Legal Issues in Genetics. Dublin, Ireland: Open Air; 1997: 71-82. 2 refs. ISBN 1-85182-278-X. BE58297.
    autonomy; disabled; *eugenics; genetic determinism; genetic predisposition; genetic screening; genetics; moral obligations; obligations to society; preimplantation diagnosis; prenatal diagnosis; reproduction; reproductive technologies; science; selective abortion; social control; social discrimination; socioeconomic factors; stigmatization; trends; values; liberalism; rationality

Larson, Edward J. "In the finest, most womanly way": women in the Southern eugenics movement. *American Journal of Legal History.* 1995 Apr; 39(2): 119-147. 124 fn. BE56032.
    blacks; *eugenics; *females; *historical aspects; investigators; involuntary sterilization; males; mentally disabled; physicians; *political activity; *politics; public policy; social discrimination; state government; whites; women's rights; *Southeastern United States; *Twentieth Century

Lombardo, Paul A. Medicine, eugenics, and the Supreme Court: from coercive sterilization to reproductive freedom. *Journal of Contemporary Health Law and Policy.* 1996 Fall; 13(1): 1-25. 180 fn. BE55766.
    aliens; behavioral genetics; blacks; *constitutional law; criminal law; *eugenics; federal government; *genetic

determinism; *genetic predisposition; historical aspects; *human rights; *involuntary sterilization; *legal aspects; legal rights; legislation; marital relationship; *mentally retarded; *prisoners; privacy; public health; *public policy; *reproduction; social discrimination; social problems; state government; *Supreme Court decisions; whites; *Buck v. Bell; Immigration Restriction Act 1924; Loving v. Commonwealth; *Skinner v. Oklahoma; *Twentieth Century; *United States; Virginia

Maranto, Gina. Quest for Perfection: The Drive to Breed Better Human Beings. New York, NY: Scribner; 1996. 335 p. Bibliography: p. 303-315. ISBN 0-684-80029-2. BE56131.
    age factors; ancient history; anthropology; artificial insemination; attitudes; children; cloning; confidentiality; congenital disorders; cryopreservation; death; disabled; disclosure; embryo research; embryo transfer; embryos; *eugenics; females; gene therapy; genetic disorders; genetic enhancement; genetic intervention; genetic research; *historical aspects; in vitro fertilization; infanticide; infertility; international aspects; involuntary sterilization; legal aspects; males; medical specialties; minority groups; ovum donors; physicians; posthumous reproduction; preimplantation diagnosis; psychological stress; reproduction; *reproductive technologies; selection for treatment; semen donors; sex preselection; sociology of medicine; sperm; Eighteenth Century; Europe; Middle Ages; Nineteenth Century; Renaissance; Twentieth Century; United States

Miller, Marvin D. Terminating the "Socially Inadequate": The American Eugenicists and the German Race Hygienists, California to Cold Spring Harbor, Long Island to Germany. Commack, NY: Malamud-Rose; 1996. 289 p. Bibliography: p. 245-280. ISBN 0-9610466-1-9. BE57153.
    active euthanasia; attitudes; blacks; contraception; *eugenics; financial support; genetic research; government regulation; *historical aspects; indigents; *international aspects; *interprofessional relations; investigators; *involuntary sterilization; Jews; legislation; mentally ill; mentally retarded; misconduct; National Socialism; physically disabled; political activity; professional organizations; reproduction; Roman Catholics; social discrimination; state government; *vulnerable populations; whites; pedigree studies; California; *Germany; Great Britain; *Twentieth Century; *United States

Milliez, J.; Sureau, C. Pre-implantation diagnosis and the eugenics debate: our responsibility to future generations. *In:* Shenfield, F.; Sureau, C., eds. Ethical Dilemmas in Assisted Reproduction. New York, NY: Parthenon Pub. Group; 1997: 57-66. 26 refs. ISBN 1-85070-916-5. BE57947.
    confidentiality; data banks; embryos; epidemiology; *eugenics; fetal therapy; future generations; gene therapy; genetic disorders; germ cells; informed consent; mandatory reporting; methods; *preimplantation diagnosis; risks and benefits; stem cells

Mohler, R. Albert. The brave new world of cloning: a Christian worldview perspective. *In:* Cole-Turner, Ronald, ed. Human Cloning: Religious Responses. Louisville, KY: Westminister John Knox Press; 1997: 91-105. 27 fn. ISBN 0-664-25771-2. BE58147.
    animal experimentation; *Christian ethics; *cloning; coercion; *eugenics; family relationship; genetic screening; parent child relationship; reproduction; reproductive technologies; secularism; social impact; theology; value of life

Neri, Demetrio. Eugenics. *In:* Chadwick, Ruth, ed. Encyclopedia of Applied Ethics, Volume 2. San Diego, CA: Academic Press; 1998: 161-173. 9 refs. ISBN

BE = bioethics accession number   fn. = footnotes   refs. = references

0-12-227067-3. BE56381.
    ancient history; beneficence; *eugenics; future generations;
    gene therapy; genetic counseling; genetic disorders; genetic
    diversity; genetic enhancement; *genetic intervention;
    genetic screening; germ cells; historical aspects; international
    aspects; justice; mandatory programs; moral obligations;
    moral policy; normality; preventive medicine; reproduction;
    reproductive technologies; review; risks and benefits; social
    control; social discrimination; terminology; voluntary
    programs; Galton, Francis; Nineteenth Century; Plato;
    Twentieth Century

Paul, Diane. From eugenics to medical genetics. *In:*
Marcus, Alan I.; Cravens, Hamilton, eds. Health Care
Policy in Contemporary America. University Park, PA:
Pennsylvania State University Press; 1997: 96-116. 79
fn. Published also in a special issue of *Journal of Policy
History*, 1997; 9(1). ISBN 0-271-01740-6. BE56799.
    attitudes; coercion; contraception; directive counseling;
    *eugenics; gene pool; *genetic counseling; genetic disorders;
    genetic screening; genetic services; genetics; historical
    aspects; intelligence; investigators; mass screening; mentally
    disabled; minority groups; newborns; physically disabled;
    prenatal diagnosis; public opinion; public policy;
    reproduction; selective abortion; socioeconomic factors;
    sterilization (sexual); Great Britain; Twentieth Century;
    United States

Paul, Diane B. Culpability and compassion: lessons from
the history of eugenics. *Politics and the Life Sciences.* 1996
Mar; 15(1): 99-100. 7 refs. BE55623.
    accountability; *behavioral genetics; *eugenics; *genetic
    predisposition; punishment; sexuality; social control; *social
    discrimination; social problems; stigmatization; *violence;
    culpability

Pearson, Roger. Heredity and Humanity: Race, Eugenics
and Modern Science. Washington, DC:
Scott-Townsend; 1996. 162 p. Bibliography: p. 146-156.
ISBN 1-878365-15-5. BE57200.
    altruism; ancient history; anthropology; behavioral genetics;
    communism; developing countries; DNA fingerprinting;
    *eugenics; evolution; genetic determinism; *genetic research;
    *genetics; genome mapping; historical aspects; legislation;
    mass media; medicine; minority groups; psychology; public
    policy; reproduction; science; social sciences; socialism;
    sociobiology; twins; *population genetics; Western World;
    Great Britain; Nineteenth Century; Twentieth Century;
    United States

Qiu, Ren-Zong. Germ-line engineering as the eugenics
of the future. *In:* Agius, Emmanuel; Busuttil, Salvino,
eds. Germ-Line Intervention and Our Responsibilities
to Future Generations. Boston, MA: Kluwer Academic;
1998: 105-116. 22 refs. ISBN 0-7923-4828-1. BE57882.
    contracts; developing countries; *eugenics; *future
    generations; *gene therapy; genetic determinism; *genetic
    enhancement; genetic intervention; *germ cells; international
    aspects; *moral obligations; morality; *rights; values;
    Confucian ethics; non-Western World; Western World;
    Parfit, Derek

Rafter, Nicole Hahn. Creating Born Criminals. Urbana,
IL: University of Illinois Press; 1997. 284 p.
Bibliography: p. 241-270. ISBN 0-252-06741-X.
BE57201.
    anthropology; *behavioral genetics; dangerousness;
    *eugenics; females; government regulation; *historical
    aspects; indigents; institutionalized persons; intelligence;
    mental institutions; *mentally ill; *mentally retarded;
    *prisoners; *public policy; social impact; state government;
    sterilization (sexual); *violence; *Nineteenth Century;
    *Twentieth Century; *United States

Resta, Robert G. Eugenics and nondirectiveness in genetic

counseling. *Journal of Genetic Counseling.* 1997 Jun; 6(2):
255-258. 15 refs. BE55668.
    attitudes; directive counseling; *eugenics; *genetic
    counseling; historical aspects; physicians; Twentieth
    Century; United States

Rifkin, Jeremy. The Biotech Century: Harnessing the
Gene and Remaking the World. New York, NY: Jeremy
P. Tarcher/Putnam; 1998. 271 p. 486 fn. ISBN
0-87477-909-X. BE57152.
    animal experimentation; animal organs; animal rights;
    biological warfare; biomedical research; cloning;
    commodification; computers; developing countries;
    *ecology; *economics; *eugenics; future generations; gene
    pool; gene therapy; genes; genetic disorders; genetic
    diversity; genetic enhancement; *genetic information;
    *genetic intervention; genetic predisposition; *genetic
    research; genetics; genome mapping; *industry; international
    aspects; legal aspects; patents; property rights; regulation;
    reproduction; reproductive technologies; review; *risks and
    benefits; *social impact; social problems; stigmatization;
    transgenic animals; *transgenic organisms; *trends; wedge
    argument; agriculture; transgenic plants; Europe; Human
    Genome Diversity Project; Human Genome Project;
    Twenty-First Century; United States

Rodriguez, Eduardo. The Human Genome Project and
eugenics. *Linacre Quarterly.* 1998 May; 65(2): 73-82. 24
fn. BE58935.
    economics; *eugenics; genetic disorders; *genetic screening;
    genome mapping; historical aspects; prenatal diagnosis;
    reproduction; reproductive technologies; selective abortion;
    social discrimination; Human Genome Project; United States

Suzuki, David. A personal journey through genetics and
civil rights. *Science.* 1998 Sep 18; 281(5384): 1796-1797.
BE59030.
    *eugenics; genetic research; *genetics; historical aspects;
    *investigators; minority groups; moral obligations;
    obligations to society; science; social discrimination; social
    impact; values; Canada

Tännsjö, Torbjörn. Compulsory sterilisation in Sweden.
Bioethics. 1998 Jul; 12(3): 236-249. 1 fn. BE58892.
    *autonomy; children; *coercion; *competence; congenital
    disorders; *disabled; *eugenics; genetic disorders;
    government regulation; historical aspects; informed consent;
    involuntary euthanasia; *involuntary sterilization; mandatory
    programs; mass media; mentally retarded; *moral policy;
    paternalism; politics; prenatal diagnosis; *public policy;
    quality of life; *reproduction; reproductive technologies;
    *rights; selective abortion; social discrimination; sterilization
    (sexual); suffering; third party consent; value of life; wedge
    argument; *Sweden; Twentieth Century
In the Fall of 1997 the leading Swedish newspaper,
Dagens Nyheter, created a media hype over the Swedish
policy of compulsory sterilisation that had been in
operation between 1935 and 1975. In the discussion that
followed, the moral condemnation of our medical past
was unanimous. However, the reasons for rejecting what
had gone on were varied and mutually inconsistent.
Three strands of criticism were common: the argument
from autonomy, the argument from caution, and the
argument from biological scepticism. In the paper it is
argued that what point of departure you choose in your
criticism of the past should be of consequence also for
your ideas about present and future medical practice.
In particular, if you rely on the argument from
autonomy, you should be prepared to accept a liberal
(present and future) use of reproductive techniques.

Thielman, Samuel B. Psychiatry and social values: the
American Psychiatric Association and immigration
restriction, 1880-1930. *Psychiatry.* 1985 Nov; 48(4):

BE = bioethics accession number   fn. = footnotes   refs. = references

299–310. 45 refs. 3 fn. BE56965.
*aliens; *attitudes; *eugenics; genetic determinism; *historical aspects; intelligence; mental health; *mentally disabled; minority groups; *organizational policies; *physicians; political activity; professional organizations; *psychiatry; *public policy; *emigration and immigration; geographic factors; *American Psychiatric Association; *Nineteenth Century; *Twentieth Century; *United States

Veglia, Geremia; Shmaefsky, Brian R.; Johnson, Walter. Public Attitudes Toward Human Genetic Manipulation: A Revitalization of Eugenics? Available from ERIC Document Reproduction Service, DYNCORP I&ET, 7420 Fullerton Rd., Suite 110, Springfield, VA 22153–2852; Document No. ED327408; SE051655; 1990. 26 p. Paper presented at the Fifth National Technological Literacy Conference of the National Association of Science, Technology and Society, Arlington, VA, 2–4 Feb 1990. BE57782.
*attitudes; behavioral genetics; *eugenics; females; genetic disorders; *genetic enhancement; *genetic intervention; health; intelligence; involuntary sterilization; law; males; prenatal diagnosis; *public policy; reproduction; *risks and benefits; science; selective abortion; *social impact; *students; survey; *universities; *United States

Watson, James D. Genes and politics. *Journal Of Molecular Medicine.* 1997 Sep; 75(9): 624–636. Keynote address to the Congress of Molecular Medicine, Berlin, May 1997. BE57981.
active euthanasia; aliens; behavioral genetics; blacks; dissent; *eugenics; gene therapy; genes; genetic determinism; genetic disorders; genetic intervention; *genetic research; genetic screening; *genetics; genome mapping; *historical aspects; intelligence; international aspects; investigators; involuntary sterilization; Jews; killing; mentally disabled; military personnel; physically disabled; physician's role; political activity; prenatal diagnosis; *public policy; recombinant DNA research; social discrimination; social problems; war; emigration and immigration; Eugenics Record Station (Cold Spring Harbor, NY); Germany; Human Genome Project; Lysenkoism; NCHGR Program on Ethical, Legal, and Social Implications (ELSI); Nineteenth Century; Social Darwinism; Twentieth Century; United States; USSR; World War I; World War II

Weindling, Paul. Weimar eugenics: the Kaiser Wilhelm Institute for Anthropology, Human Heredity and Eugenics in social context. *Annals of Science.* 1985 May; 42(3): 303–318. 45 fn. BE56782.
anthropology; attitudes; biology; disabled; *eugenics; genetic research; genetics; government financing; *historical aspects; *investigators; involuntary sterilization; medicine; National Socialism; physicians; *political activity; public health; *public policy; research institutes; social problems; *Germany; *Kaiser Wilhelm Institute for Anthropology, Human Heredity and Eugenics; *Twentieth Century

Zoloth-Dorfman, Laurie. Mapping the normal human self: the Jew and the mark of otherness. *In:* Peters, Ted, ed. Genetics: Issues of Social Justice. Cleveland, OH: Pilgrim Press; 1998: 180–202. 60 fn. ISBN 0-8298-1251-2. BE57479.
aliens; blacks; cosmetic surgery; *disease; *eugenics; genetic disorders; genetic diversity; genetic intervention; genetic research; genetic screening; *genome mapping; historical aspects; *human body; intelligence; *Jewish ethics; *Jews; justice; medicine; *normality; public policy; *risks and benefits; science; sexuality; social discrimination; *stigmatization; theology; emigration and immigration; population genetics; Europe; Human Genome Project; Nineteenth Century; Twentieth Century; United States

Opportunity for depth in Chinese eugenics debate. [Editorial]. *Nature.* 1998 Mar 12; 392(6672): 109.

BE57256.
communication; cultural pluralism; disabled; *eugenics; *international aspects; investigators; legislation; political activity; professional organizations; *public policy; social problems; *socioeconomic factors; *China; *International Congress on Genetics; Law on Maternal and Infant Health Care (China)

EUTHANASIA

See also ALLOWING TO DIE, INFANTICIDE, SUICIDE

Admiraal, Pieter. Voluntary euthanasia: the Dutch way. *In:* McLean, Sheila A.M., ed. Death, Dying and the Law. Brookfield, VT: Dartmouth; 1996: 113–127. 35 fn. ISBN 1-85521-657-4. BE57216.
allowing to die; autonomy; criminal law; futility; guidelines; hospices; hospitals; international aspects; involuntary euthanasia; legal aspects; mandatory reporting; pain; palliative care; physicians; professional organizations; psychological stress; public opinion; *public policy; suffering; terminally ill; *voluntary euthanasia; wedge argument; Great Britain; *Netherlands; Royal Dutch Medical Association

Admiraal, Pieter V. Euthanasia in the Netherlands. *Free Inquiry.* 1996–1997 Winter; 17(1): 5–8. 1 ref. BE55781.
allowing to die; assisted suicide; autonomy; cancer; criminal law; decision making; depressive disorder; guidelines; involuntary euthanasia; legal aspects; organizational policies; pain; physicians; professional organizations; psychological stress; public opinion; suffering; terminal care; terminally ill; *voluntary euthanasia; wedge argument; dignity; *Netherlands; Royal Dutch Medical Association

Angell, Marcia. Helping desperately ill people to die. *In:* Emanuel, Linda L., ed. Regulating How We Die: The Ethical, Medical, and Legal Issues Surrounding Physician-Assisted Suicide. Cambridge, MA: Harvard University Press; 1998: 3–20, 263–264. 19 fn. ISBN 0-674-66654-2. BE58531.
*active euthanasia; *allowing to die; *assisted suicide; attitudes; autonomy; competence; critically ill; decision making; family members; government regulation; legal aspects; persistent vegetative state; physician's role; *physicians; public opinion; public policy; right to die; standards; state government; suffering; terminally ill; third party consent; treatment refusal; *voluntary euthanasia; wedge argument; withholding treatment; Brophy v. New England Sinai Hospital; In re Quinlan; Lane v. Candura; Netherlands; *United States

Arras, John D. Physician-assisted suicide: a tragic view. *In:* Battin, Margaret P.; Rhodes, Rosamond; Silvers, Anita, eds. Physician Assisted Suicide: Expanding the Debate. New York, NY: Routledge; 1998: 279–300. 88 fn. ISBN 0-415-92003-5. BE58794.
*active euthanasia; advance directives; allowing to die; *assisted suicide; autonomy; chronically ill; compassion; competence; constitutional law; cultural pluralism; depressive disorder; disabled; equal protection; government regulation; killing; legal aspects; legal rights; legislation; moral policy; pain; *palliative care; *physicians; policy analysis; professional family relationship; *public policy; quality of health care; risks and benefits; social impact; state government; suffering; Supreme Court decisions; terminally ill; theology; third party consent; treatment refusal; trust; *voluntary euthanasia; vulnerable populations; *wedge argument; withholding treatment; Compassion in Dying v. State of Washington; Quill v. Vacco; United States

Battin, Margaret P. Euthanasia: the way we do it, the way they do it. [Revised]. *In:* Monagle, John F.;

Thomasma, David C., eds. Health Care Ethics: Critical Issues for the 21st Century. Gaithersburg, MD: Aspen Publishers; 1998: 311–322. 15 fn. ISBN 0-8342-0911-X. BE56288.
active euthanasia; advance directives; *allowing to die; *assisted suicide; autonomy; *international aspects; involuntary euthanasia; legal aspects; national health insurance; physician patient relationship; physicians; policy analysis; *public policy; resource allocation; risks and benefits; *socioeconomic factors; standards; suffering; *terminally ill; third party consent; treatment refusal; *voluntary euthanasia; wedge argument; withholding treatment; German Society for Humane Dying; *Germany; *Netherlands; *United States

Beauchamp, Tom L. Physician–assisted suicide: a response to Edmund Pellegrino. In: Wildes, Kevin Wm.; Mitchell, Alan C., eds. Choosing Life: A Dialogue on Evangelium Vitae. Washington, DC: Georgetown University Press; 1997: 254–258. 3 fn. ISBN 0-87840-646-8. BE56692.
*allowing to die; *assisted suicide; autonomy; intention; *killing; moral obligations; *moral policy; physician patient relationship; physicians; Protestant ethics; risks and benefits; Roman Catholic ethics; treatment refusal; *voluntary euthanasia; withholding treatment; Evangelium Vitae

Beecham, Linda. BMA opposes legalisation of euthanasia. [News]. BMJ (British Medical Journal). 1997 Jul 12; 315(7100): 80. BE55808.
*active euthanasia; *assisted suicide; legal aspects; *organizational policies; physician's role; *physicians; professional organizations; public policy; terminal care; *British Medical Association; Great Britain

Begley, Ann–Marie. Beneficent voluntary active euthanasia: a challenge to professionals caring for terminally ill patients. Nursing Ethics. 1998 Jul; 5(4): 294–306. 33 refs. BE58869.
active euthanasia; attitudes; autonomy; beneficence; Christian ethics; coercion; compassion; family members; killing; morality; nurses; palliative care; physicians; quality of life; right to die; terminal care; *terminally ill; trust; value of life; *voluntary euthanasia; Great Britain

Bernardin, Joseph. Euthanasia: ethical and legal challenge. In: Langan, John P., ed. Joseph Cardinal Bernardin: A Moral Vision for America. Washington, DC: Georgetown University Press; 1998: 59–69, 170. 1 fn. Reference embedded in list at back of book. Address at the Center for Clinical Medical Ethics, University of Chicago Hospital, 26 May 1988. ISBN 0-87840-675-1. BE58523.
*active euthanasia; aged; allowing to die; artificial feeding; *assisted suicide; autonomy; biomedical technologies; common good; cultural pluralism; economics; hospices; indigents; legal aspects; *moral policy; obligations of society; privacy; prolongation of life; *public policy; resource allocation; Roman Catholic ethics; state interest; terminally ill; *value of life; *United States

Bradley, Peter; Przygoda, Pablo; Saimovici, Javier, et al. Physician assisted suicide, euthanasia, and withdrawal of treatment. [Letters]. BMJ (British Medical Journal). 1998 Jan 3; 316(7124): 71–72. 9 refs. BE57955.
*active euthanasia; *allowing to die; *assisted suicide; attitudes; double effect; intention; moral policy; *physicians; survey; terminal care; terminology; wedge argument; withholding treatment; Argentina; Great Britain

Budziszewski, J. Why we kill the weak. Human Life Review. 1997 Fall; 23(4): 67–74. BE57427.
*abortion, induced; *active euthanasia; *allowing to die; compassion; conscience; family relationship; justice; *killing; love; moral development; moral obligations; motivation;

*vulnerable populations; withholding treatment; duty to die

Burleigh, Michael. Ethics and Extermination: Reflections on Nazi Genocide. New York, NY: Cambridge University Press; 1997. 261 p. 538 fn. ISBN 0-521-58816-2. BE57155.
clergy; *eugenics; *historical aspects; homosexuals; *involuntary euthanasia; involuntary sterilization; Jews; *killing; literature; *mentally disabled; minority groups; *misconduct; *National Socialism; *physically disabled; physicians; Protestants; psychiatry; Roman Catholics; war; *Germany; Nineteenth Century; *Twentieth Century

Burleigh, Michael. Psychiatry, German society, and the Nazi "euthanasia" programme. Social History of Medicine. 1994 Aug; 7(2): 213–228. 61 fn. BE57594.
adults; children; coercion; deinstitutionalized persons; *eugenics; *health personnel; *historical aspects; *involuntary euthanasia; involuntary sterilization; Jews; *killing; mental institutions; *mentally ill; mentally retarded; *National Socialism; nurses; parental consent; physically disabled; *physicians; *psychiatry; *public policy; socioeconomic factors; sociology of medicine; utilitarianism; war; *Germany; *Twentieth Century

Burleigh, Michael. Saving money, spending lives: psychiatry, society and the 'euthanasia' programme. In: Burleigh, Michael, ed. Confronting the Nazi Past: New Debates on Modern German History. New York, NY: St. Martin's Press; 1996: 98–111. 3 refs. ISBN 0-312-16353-3. BE57395.
administrators; adults; children; chronically ill; deinstitutionalized persons; *economics; employment; *eugenics; genetic disorders; health care; health personnel; *historical aspects; institutionalized persons; *involuntary euthanasia; involuntary sterilization; *killing; legislation; *mass media; mental institutions; *mentally ill; *mentally retarded; *misconduct; motivation; *National Socialism; parental consent; *physically disabled; physician's role; *psychiatry; public opinion; *public policy; stigmatization; volunteers; starvation; *Germany; Twentieth Century

Callahan, Sydney. A feminist case against euthanasia. Health Progress. 1996 Nov–Dec; 77(6): 21–27, 29. 11 fn. BE56323.
aged; *assisted suicide; autonomy; coercion; communication; decision making; family relationship; females; *feminist ethics; informed consent; involuntary euthanasia; killing; palliative care; physicians; quality of life; *right to die; self concept; social discrimination; social impact; social interaction; suffering; suicide; third party consent; *value of life; *voluntary euthanasia; vulnerable populations; *wedge argument; women's rights; dependency; United States

Coatney, Caryn. Outback's assisted–suicide law: Australia delivers world's first dose of legal euthanasia. [News]. Christian Science Monitor. 1997 Jan 8: 1, 18. BE55736.
*active euthanasia; adults; *assisted suicide; attitudes; cultural pluralism; international aspects; *legislation; minority groups; physicians; public opinion; terminally ill; *voluntary euthanasia; *Australia; *Northern Territory

Cooke, Molly; Gourlay, Linda; Collette, Linda, et al. Informal caregivers and the intention to hasten AIDS–related death. Archives of Internal Medicine. 1998 Jan 12; 158(1): 69–75. 35 refs. BE56300.
*active euthanasia; *AIDS; assisted suicide; *drugs; evaluation studies; family members; friends; HIV seropositivity; home care; homosexuals; hospices; hospitals; *intention; males; motivation; *palliative care; physician's role; psychological stress; survey; *terminal care; terminally ill; voluntary euthanasia; *caregivers; narcotics; prospective studies; sedatives; San Francisco
OBJECTIVES: To determine the extent to which

BE = bioethics accession number   fn. = footnotes   refs. = references

homosexual men dying of the acquired immunodeficiency syndrome (AIDS) receive medication intended to hasten death. To assess the impact on caregivers of administering medications intended to hasten death. METHODS: In a prospective study of caregiving partners of men with AIDS (n = 140), characteristics of the ill partner, the caregiver, and the relationship were assessed at baseline and 1 month before the ill partner's death. Three months after the death, caregivers were asked if they had increased their partner's narcotic and/or sedative–hypnotic medication dose and if so, what had been the objective of the increase, and their comfort with their medication decisions. RESULTS: Of 140 ill partners who died of AIDS, 17 (12.1%) received an increase in the use of medications immediately before death intended to hasten death. Diagnoses and care needs of ill partners who received increases in the use of medications to hasten death did not differ from those of ill partners receiving medication for symptoms. Fourteen increases (10%) in use of medications were administered by caregivers. These caregivers did not differ from those administering medication for symptom control in level of distress, caregiving burden, relationship characteristics, or comfort with the medication decision, but they reported more social support and positive meaning in caregiving. CONCLUSION: The decision to hasten death is not a rare event in this group of men. There is no evidence that it is the result of caregiver distress, poor relationship quality, or intolerable caregiving burden; and it does not cause excessive discomfort in the surviving partner. This study, although small, has implications for the policy debate on assisted suicide.

Corner, Jessica. More openness needed in palliative care. [Medicine and the media]. *BMJ (British Medical Journal).* 1997 Nov 8; 315(7117): 1242. BE56780.
*double effect; drugs; *mass media; *palliative care; *paralysis; *physically disabled; physicians; right to die; suffering; *terminal care; *voluntary euthanasia; *Great Britain; *Lindsell, Annie

Davis, Anne J.; Aroskar, Mila A.; Liaschenko, Joan, et al. Dying and death. *In: their* Ethical Dilemmas and Nursing Practice. Fourth Edition. Stamford, CT: Appleton and Lange; 1997: 159–183. 58 fn. ISBN 0-8385-2283-1. BE58597.
*active euthanasia; adults; advance directives; *allowing to die; assisted suicide; caring; case studies; decision making; determination of death; hospices; legal aspects; newborns; *nurses; nursing ethics; resuscitation orders; right to die; suffering; suicide; *terminal care; third party consent; treatment refusal; withholding treatment; United States

Devine, Philip E. Homicide, criminal versus justifiable. *In:* Chadwick, Ruth, ed. Encyclopedia of Applied Ethics, Volume 2. San Diego, CA: Academic Press; 1998: 587–595. 14 refs. ISBN 0-12-227067-3. BE56396.
*abortion, induced; *active euthanasia; assisted suicide; Christian ethics; criminal law; double effect; intention; involuntary euthanasia; *killing; moral policy; personhood; philosophy; public policy; secularism; speciesism; *suicide; theology; utilitarianism; voluntary euthanasia; wedge argument

Docker, Christopher. The way forward? *In:* McLean, Sheila A.M., ed. Death, Dying and the Law. Brookfield, VT: Dartmouth; 1996: 129–160. 99 fn. ISBN 1-85521-657-4. BE57217.
*active euthanasia; *advance directives; aged; *allowing to die; *assisted suicide; decision making; double effect; economics; hospices; legal aspects; living wills; pain;

*palliative care; *persistent vegetative state; physicians; public policy; *resource allocation; selection for treatment; terminal care; withholding treatment; *Great Britain; National Health Service; Netherlands; United States

Draper, Heather. Euthanasia. *In:* Chadwick, Ruth, ed. Encyclopedia of Applied Ethics, Volume 2. San Diego, CA: Academic Press; 1998: 175–187. 5 refs. ISBN 0-12-227067-3. BE56382.
*active euthanasia; *allowing to die; artificial feeding; autonomy; beneficence; competence; deontological ethics; double effect; drugs; *euthanasia; futility; informed consent; intention; involuntary euthanasia; killing; *moral policy; motivation; pain; palliative care; persistent vegetative state; physicians; public policy; quality of life; resource allocation; resuscitation; review; right to die; risks and benefits; suffering; suicide; terminology; third party consent; treatment refusal; utilitarianism; value of life; voluntary euthanasia; wedge argument; withholding treatment; culpability

Dyer, Clare. Two doctors confess to helping patients to die. [News]. *BMJ (British Medical Journal).* 1997 Jul 26; 315(7102): 206. BE58514.
*active euthanasia; attitudes; double effect; legal liability; organizational policies; palliative care; *physicians; professional organizations; terminally ill; voluntary euthanasia; British Medical Association; *Great Britain; *Irwin, Michael; *Moor, David

Emanuel, Ezekiel. Whose right to die? *Atlantic Monthly.* 1997 Mar; 279(3): 73–79. BE57684.
accountability; allowing to die; *assisted suicide; attitudes; biomedical technologies; coercion; decision making; depressive disorder; economics; guidelines; historical aspects; international aspects; involuntary euthanasia; legal aspects; motivation; newborns; pain; physicians; psychological stress; public opinion; *public policy; *right to die; suffering; *voluntary euthanasia; vulnerable populations; wedge argument; dependency; dignity; duty to die; guideline adherence; Hippocratic Oath; *Netherlands; Nineteenth Century; Remmelink Commission; Twentieth Century; *United States

Emanuel, Ezekiel J. Why now? *In:* Emanuel, Linda L., ed. Regulating How We Die: The Ethical, Medical, and Legal Issues Surrounding Physician–Assisted Suicide. Cambridge, MA: Harvard University Press; 1998: 175–202, 307–312. 48 fn. ISBN 0-674-66654-2. BE58538.
*active euthanasia; allowing to die; ancient history; *assisted suicide; attitudes; autonomy; economics; eugenics; *historical aspects; killing; legal aspects; moral obligations; pain; philosophy; physician patient relationship; *physicians; *public policy; social dominance; social worth; terminal care; terminally ill; values; voluntary euthanasia; wedge argument; Canada; Eighteenth Century; Europe; Nineteenth Century; Seventeenth Century; Sixteenth Century; Twentieth Century; United States

Emanuel, Linda L. A question of balance. *In:* Emanuel, Linda L., ed. Regulating How We Die: The Ethical, Medical, and Legal Issues Surrounding Physician–Assisted Suicide. Cambridge, MA: Harvard University Press; 1998: 234–260. ISBN 0-674-66654-2. BE58540.
*active euthanasia; *advance care planning; allowing to die; *assisted suicide; autonomy; compassion; cultural pluralism; decision making; health care delivery; intention; killing; legal rights; medical education; moral obligations; motivation; palliative care; physician's role; physicians; privacy; public policy; religious ethics; suffering; *terminal care; values; wedge argument; withholding treatment; dignity; Netherlands; United States

Emanuel, Linda L., ed. Regulating How We Die: The

BE = bioethics accession number   fn. = footnotes   refs. = references

Ethical, Medical, and Legal Issues Surrounding Physician–Assisted Suicide. Cambridge, MA: Harvard University Press; 1998. 325 p. 401 fn. ISBN 0–674–66654–2. BE58530.
*active euthanasia; adolescents; advance care planning; allowing to die; *assisted suicide; beneficence; capital punishment; children; critically ill; government regulation; historical aspects; Jewish ethics; *killing; legal aspects; legal rights; moral obligations; moral policy; physician's role; *physicians; Protestant ethics; public policy; religious ethics; right to die; Roman Catholic ethics; state government; *suffering; suicide; *terminally ill; Netherlands; United States

Farsides, Bobbie. Palliative care -- a euthanasia–free zone? [Editorial]. *Journal of Medical Ethics.* 1998 Jun; 24(3): 149–150. BE59110.
*active euthanasia; communication; dissent; goals; health personnel; hospices; legal aspects; moral policy; *palliative care; patients; philosophy; quality of life; *terminal care

Fenigsen, Richard. Dutch euthanasia revisited. *Issues in Law and Medicine.* 1997 Winter; 13(3): 301–311. 68 fn. BE58706.
*active euthanasia; adults; age factors; allowing to die; *assisted suicide; cancer; comparative studies; drugs; empirical research; guidelines; infants; *involuntary euthanasia; knowledge, attitudes, practice; legal liability; mandatory reporting; mentally ill; mortality; motivation; newborns; *physicians; referral and consultation; statistics; *trends; *voluntary euthanasia; wedge argument; withholding treatment; *guideline adherence; *Netherlands

Fenigsen, Richard. Physician–assisted death in the Netherlands: impact on long–term care. *Issues in Law and Medicine.* 1995 Winter; 11(3): 283–297. 59 fn. BE58820.
*active euthanasia; adults; age factors; *aged; *allowing to die; assisted suicide; attitudes; children; congenital disorders; decision making; *disabled; Down syndrome; hospitals; infants; *involuntary euthanasia; *long–term care; mentally retarded; newborns; nurses; nursing homes; physicians; public opinion; *public policy; quality of health care; *social impact; *voluntary euthanasia; *withholding treatment; *Netherlands

Gert, Bernard; Culver, Charles M.; Clouser, K. Danner. An alternative to physician–assisted suicide: a conceptual and moral analysis. *In:* Battin, Margaret P.; Rhodes, Rosamond; Silvers, Anita, eds. Physician Assisted Suicide: Expanding the Debate. New York, NY: Routledge; 1998: 182–202. 25 fn. ISBN 0–415–92003–5. BE58789.
*active euthanasia; *allowing to die; alternatives; artificial feeding; *assisted suicide; competence; double effect; drugs; food; freedom; government regulation; informed consent; intention; *killing; legal aspects; model legislation; *moral obligations; *moral policy; pain; *palliative care; *physicians; policy analysis; prolongation of life; public policy; right to die; state government; suffering; suicide; Supreme Court decisions; terminal care; terminally ill; time factors; treatment refusal; *voluntary euthanasia; withholding treatment; analgesia; dehydration; rationality; United States; Vacco v. Quill; Washington v. Glucksberg

Gert, Bernard. Euthanasia. *In:* Borchert, Donald M., ed. The Encyclopedia of Philosophy. Supplement. New York, NY: Simon and Schuster Macmillan; 1996: 155–158. 12 refs. ISBN 0–02–864629–0. BE57221.
*active euthanasia; advance directives; *allowing to die; competence; killing; moral policy; patient participation; physicians; public policy; suffering; treatment refusal; withholding treatment

Gibson, Susanne. Acts and omissions. *In:* Chadwick, Ruth,

ed. Encyclopedia of Applied Ethics, Volume 1. San Diego, CA: Academic Press; 1998: 23–28. 8 refs. ISBN 0–12–227066–5. BE56363.
*active euthanasia; *allowing to die; deontological ethics; *ethical analysis; ethical theory; *killing; moral obligations; moral policy; rights; teleological ethics; virtues; culpability

Greenberg, Samuel I. Euthanasia and Assisted Suicide: Psychosocial Issues. Springfield, IL: Charles C. Thomas; 1997. 164 p. (American series in behavioral science and law). 113 refs. ISBN 0–398–06785–6. BE58317.
*active euthanasia; adults; advance directives; aged; allowing to die; *assisted suicide; attitudes; case studies; decision making; economics; ethicists; hospices; international aspects; judicial action; lawyers; legal rights; managed care programs; minors; newborns; nursing homes; organizational policies; pain; palliative care; physician patient relationship; physician's role; physicians; professional organizations; public policy; resuscitation orders; right to die; spina bifida; suffering; Supreme Court decisions; terminal care; treatment refusal; wedge argument; Germany; Great Britain; Kevorkian, Jack; Netherlands; *United States

Gunning, K.F.; Crowther, C.A. End of life decisions. [Letters]. *BMJ (British Medical Journal).* 1997 Nov 1; 315(7116): 1164–1165. 6 refs. BE58153.
*active euthanasia; allowing to die; attitudes; competence; *decision making; editorial policies; legal aspects; *mentally retarded; palliative care; physicians; suffering; terminal care; *vulnerable populations; BMJ (British Medical Journal); *Great Britain; *Netherlands

Hecht, Barbara K.; Hecht, Frederick. Murder of son with a genital malformation. [Letter]. *American Journal of Medical Genetics.* 1995 Sep 25; 58(4): 381. BE56169.
adults; congenital disorders; depressive disorder; family members; *genetic disorders; *killing; legal liability; *mothers; sexuality; *suffering; *voluntary euthanasia; adult offspring; *France; *Féron, Anne; *Féron, Marc

Hendin, Herbert. Assisted suicide and euthanasia. *In:* his Suicide in America. New and Expanded Edition. New York, NY: W.W. Norton; 1995: 236–277, 294–297. 43 fn. ISBN 0–393–31368–9. BE56135.
*active euthanasia; aged; *assisted suicide; attitudes to death; autonomy; behavior control; chronically ill; coercion; competence; depressive disorder; freedom; guidelines; involuntary euthanasia; legal aspects; motivation; paternalism; physicians; psychiatric diagnosis; psychotherapy; public policy; right to die; statistics; suffering; suicide; terminally ill; voluntary euthanasia; vulnerable populations; wedge argument; Chabot, Boudewijn; Netherlands; United States

Hendin, Herbert; Goold, Susan Dorr; Meier, Diane E., et al. Physician–assisted suicide and euthanasia in the United States. [Letters and response]. *New England Journal of Medicine.* 1998 Sep 10; 339(11): 775–776. 8 refs. BE59075.
*active euthanasia; *assisted suicide; drugs; females; government regulation; guidelines; *knowledge, attitudes, practice; legal aspects; males; *physicians; state government; voluntary euthanasia; guideline adherence; *Oregon; United States

Houtepen, Rob. The social construction of euthanasia and medical ethics in the Netherlands. *In:* DeVries, Raymond; Subedi, Janardan, eds. Bioethics and Society: Constructing the Ethical Enterprise. Upper Saddle River, NJ: Prentice Hall; 1998: 117–144. 76 refs. 1 fn. ISBN 0–13–531252–3. BE58733.
accountability; active euthanasia; allowing to die; assisted suicide; attitudes; autonomy; bioethical issues; *bioethics; codes of ethics; *decision making; ethicists; *euthanasia;

BE = bioethics accession number   fn. = footnotes   refs. = references

goals; guidelines; *historical aspects; *interdisciplinary communication; lawyers; *medical ethics; medicine; patients' rights; physician patient relationship; *physicians; professional autonomy; professional organizations; quality of life; *right to die; social control; *social sciences; *sociology of medicine; terminal care; terminology; treatment refusal; trends; value of life; *Netherlands; Royal Dutch Society of Physicians; *Twentieth Century

Howard, Philip J.; Cole, A.P.; Grassin, Marc, et al. End–of–life decisions in Dutch paediatric practice. [Letters]. *Lancet.* 1997 Sep 13; 350(9080): 816–817. 5 refs. BE57165.
    *active euthanasia; *allowing to die; artificial feeding; *decision making; drugs; *infants; *intention; killing; *knowledge, attitudes, practice; legal aspects; legal liability; mandatory reporting; *newborns; parental consent; parents; *paternalism; *pediatrics; peer review; *physicians; *professional autonomy; psychological stress; referral and consultation; regulation; wedge argument; *withholding treatment; neonatology; France; Great Britain; *Netherlands; United States

Humphry, Derek. Final Exit: The Practicalities of Self–Deliverance and Assisted Suicide for the Dying. Second Edition. New York, NY: Dell Trade Paperback; 1996. 206 p. 25 refs. ISBN 0–440–50785–5. BE58643.
    advance directives; allowing to die; *assisted suicide; autonomy; autopsies; dementia; depressive disorder; *drugs; family members; food; hospices; international aspects; legal liability; life insurance; *methods; model legislation; pain; physically disabled; physicians; privacy; quality of life; *right to die; suffering; *suicide; terminal care; terminally ill; terminology; toxicity; treatment refusal; *voluntary euthanasia; support groups; United States

Kamm, Frances M. Physician–assisted suicide, euthanasia, and intending death. *In:* Battin, Margaret P.; Rhodes, Rosamond; Silvers, Anita, eds. Physician Assisted Suicide: Expanding the Debate. New York, NY: Routledge; 1998: 28–62. 53 fn. ISBN 0–415–92003–5. BE58779.
    accountability; *active euthanasia; *allowing to die; *assisted suicide; beneficence; *death; deontological ethics; *double effect; *drugs; *ethical analysis; *euthanasia; *intention; involuntary euthanasia; *killing; *moral obligations; *moral policy; morality; *pain; *palliative care; paralysis; personhood; *physicians; psychological stress; quality of life; right to die; suffering; suicide; terminal care; terminally ill; terminology; treatment refusal; value of life; *voluntary euthanasia; withholding treatment

Kelly, Brian J.; Varghese, Francis T. Assisted suicide and euthanasia: what about the clinical issues? *Australian and New Zealand Journal of Psychiatry.* 1996 Feb; 30(1): 3–8. 34 refs. BE56870.
    *active euthanasia; AIDS; *assisted suicide; autonomy; depressive disorder; medical education; mentally ill; palliative care; physician patient relationship; psychiatric diagnosis; psychiatry; quality of life; suffering; suicide; *terminal care; terminally ill; grief

Kowalski, Susan D. Assisted suicide: is there a future? Ethical and nursing considerations. *Critical Care Nursing Quarterly.* 1996 May; 19(1): 45–54. 10 refs. BE55723.
    *active euthanasia; *allowing to die; artificial feeding; *assisted suicide; autonomy; case studies; chronically ill; common good; competence; double effect; economics; guidelines; *nurses; organizational policies; pain; palliative care; persistent vegetative state; physicians; professional organizations; professional patient relationship; quality of life; *right to die; suffering; terminal care; terminally ill; terminology; third party consent; treatment refusal; ventilators; *voluntary euthanasia; wedge argument; withholding treatment; American Nurses Association; Netherlands; United States

Kuhse, Helga. From intention to consent: learning from experience with euthanasia. *In:* Battin, Margaret P.; Rhodes, Rosamond; Silvers, Anita, eds. Physician Assisted Suicide: Expanding the Debate. New York, NY: Routledge; 1998: 252–266. 38 fn. ISBN 0–415–92003–5. BE58792.
    *allowing to die; *assisted suicide; autonomy; comparative studies; *double effect; drugs; empirical research; informed consent; *intention; international aspects; involuntary euthanasia; killing; *knowledge, attitudes, practice; legal aspects; *moral policy; *palliative care; *physicians; policy analysis; *public policy; statistics; terminal care; *terminally ill; treatment refusal; *voluntary euthanasia; wedge argument; *withholding treatment; sedatives; *Australia; *Euthanasia Laws Act 1996 (Australia); *Netherlands; New York State Task Force on Life and the Law; United States

Loewy, Erich H. Harming, healing, and euthanasia. *In:* Emanuel, Linda L., ed. Regulating How We Die: The Ethical, Medical, and Legal Issues Surrounding Physician–Assisted Suicide. Cambridge, MA: Harvard University Press; 1998: 48–67, 267–269. 18 fn. ISBN 0–674–66654–2. BE58533.
    *active euthanasia; allowing to die; assisted suicide; autonomy; *capital punishment; health personnel; *killing; moral obligations; *moral policy; morality; National Socialism; physician patient relationship; *physician's role; physicians; prolongation of life; public policy; risks and benefits; *suffering; *suicide; terminal care; terminally ill; value of life; voluntary euthanasia; wedge argument; withholding treatment; Netherlands; United States

Logue, Barbara J. Physician–assisted suicide: a social science perspective on international trends. *In:* McLean, Sheila A.M., ed. Death, Dying and the Law. Brookfield, VT: Dartmouth; 1996: 95–112. 56 fn. ISBN 1–85521–657–4. BE57215.
    *active euthanasia; aged; anthropology; assisted suicide; attitudes; competence; dementia; disabled; economics; family members; health personnel; historical aspects; humanities; international aspects; killing; legal aspects; long–term care; physicians; professional patient relationship; psychological stress; psychology; quality of life; resource allocation; *social sciences; suffering; vulnerable populations

Lusthaus, Evelyn W. Involuntary euthanasia and current attempts to define persons with mental retardation as less than human. *Mental Retardation.* 1985 Jun; 23(3): 148–154. 46 refs. BE56962.
    *allowing to die; children; congenital disorders; *dehumanization; human characteristics; *involuntary euthanasia; legal aspects; *mentally retarded; *newborns; parents; *personhood; *quality of life; selection for treatment; treatment refusal; *value of life; withholding treatment; United States

Macer, Darryl R.J. Views of euthanasia for sufferers of genetic disease: comments on the Felon [Féron] case. [Letter]. *American Journal of Medical Genetics.* 1995 Sep 25; 58(4): 379–380. BE56165.
    adults; *congenital disorders; depressive disorder; family members; *genetic disorders; *killing; legal liability; *mothers; sexuality; *suffering; *voluntary euthanasia; adult offspring; *France; Féron, Anne; Féron, Marc

McLean, Sheila A.M., ed. Death, Dying and the Law. Brookfield, VT: Dartmouth; 1996. 185 p. (Medico–legal series). 531 fn. ISBN 1–85521–657–4. BE57209.
    *active euthanasia; *advance directives; *allowing to die; *assisted suicide; competence; decision making; disabled; futility; international aspects; legal aspects; palliative care; persistent vegetative state; *physicians; prognosis; public policy; resource allocation; suffering; *terminal care; treatment refusal; *voluntary euthanasia; withholding treatment; Airedale NHS Trust v. Bland; Death with

---

BE = bioethics accession number   fn. = footnotes   refs. = references

Dignity Act (OR); *Great Britain; Netherlands; United States

Mason, J.K. Death and dying: one step at a time? *In:* McLean, Sheila A.M., ed. Death, Dying and the Law. Brookfield, VT: Dartmouth; 1996: 161–178. 62 fn. ISBN 1–85521–657–4. BE57218.
> *active euthanasia; advance directives; allowing to die; artificial feeding; attitudes; autonomy; double effect; drugs; futility; intention; involuntary euthanasia; legal aspects; pain; paternalism; patients; persistent vegetative state; physician patient relationship; physician's role; *physicians; professional autonomy; psychological stress; quality of life; suffering; treatment refusal; *voluntary euthanasia; withholding treatment; Great Britain; Netherlands

Moreno, Jonathan D., ed. Arguing Euthanasia: The Controversy Over Mercy Killing, Assisted Suicide, and the "Right to Die." New York, NY: Simon and Schuster; 1995. 251 p. ISBN 0–684–80760–2. BE55810.
> *active euthanasia; allowing to die; *assisted suicide; attitudes; autonomy; cultural pluralism; economics; family members; involuntary euthanasia; killing; legal aspects; moral policy; morality; pain; palliative care; physician's role; physicians; public opinion; public policy; religion; resource allocation; right to die; secularism; suffering; terminally ill; value of life; voluntary euthanasia; wedge argument; Death with Dignity Act (OR); Netherlands; United States

Mount, Balfour. Morphine drips, terminal sedation, and slow euthanasia: definitions and facts, not anecdotes. [Commentary]. *Journal of Palliative Care.* 1996 Winter; 12(4): 31–37. 27 refs. Commentary on J.A. Billings and S.D. Block, p. 21–30. BE55729.
> *active euthanasia; attitudes; case studies; *double effect; *drugs; empirical research; hospices; *intention; killing; pain; *palliative care; physicians; psychological stress; suffering; *terminal care; *terminally ill; time factors; *morphine; *sedatives

Muller, Martien T.; van der Wal, Gerrit; van Eijk, Jacques Th.M., et al. Active euthanasia and physician–assisted suicide in Dutch nursing homes: patients' characteristics. *Age and Ageing.* 1995 Sep; 24(5): 429–433. 6 refs. BE56606.
> age factors; *aged; *assisted suicide; cancer; central nervous system diseases; comparative studies; diagnosis; females; males; *nursing homes; *patients; *physicians; religion; socioeconomic factors; statistics; survey; time factors; *voluntary euthanasia; *Netherlands

National Council for Hospice and Specialist Palliative Care Services. Voluntary euthanasia: the Council's view. *Nursing Ethics.* 1998 Jul; 5(4): 371–374. 3 refs. 2 fn. Approved by the Council 17 Jul 1997. BE58874.
> advance directives; allowing to die; double effect; drugs; hospices; *organizational policies; *palliative care; public policy; *terminal care; treatment refusal; *voluntary euthanasia; Great Britain; House of Lords Select Committee on Medical Ethics; *National Council for Hospice and Specialist Palliative Care Services (Great Britain)

Norris, Patrick F. Palliative care and killing: understanding ethical distinctions. *Bioethics Forum.* 1997 Fall; 13(3): 25–30. 6 refs. 1 fn. BE57529.
> *active euthanasia; *allowing to die; *assisted suicide; *double effect; drugs; *intention; *killing; moral policy; pain; *palliative care; suicide; *terminal care; terminally ill; withholding treatment; sedatives

O'Connor, Nancy K.; Cheng, Tsung O.; Hendin, Herbert, et al. Physician–assisted suicide and euthanasia in the Netherlands: lessons from the Dutch. [Letters and response]. *JAMA.* 1997 Sep 10; 278(10):

817–818. 12 refs. BE57253.
> assisted suicide; *drugs; evaluation; *intention; *involuntary euthanasia; *killing; palliative care; *physicians; quality of life; self regulation; social worth; statistics; survey; terminally ill; terminology; value of life; voluntary euthanasia; *vulnerable populations; *Netherlands

Onwuteaka–Philipsen, B.D.; van der Wal, G. Cases of euthanasia and physician assisted suicide among AIDS patients reported to the Public Prosecutor in North Holland. *Public Health.* 1998 Jan; 112(1): 53–56. 17 refs. BE58216.
> *AIDS; *assisted suicide; evaluation studies; females; males; mandatory reporting; medical specialties; mortality; *patients; physicians; referral and consultation; statistics; trends; *voluntary euthanasia; retrospective studies; *Netherlands

Onwuteaka–Philipsen, Bregje D.; Muller, Martien T.; van der Wal, Gerrit. Euthanasia and old age. *Age and Ageing.* 1997 Nov; 26(6): 487–492. 10 refs. BE57967.
> *age factors; *aged; AIDS; *assisted suicide; cancer; *diagnosis; family practice; females; home care; hospitals; males; mandatory reporting; medical specialties; nursing homes; *physicians; *statistics; time factors; *voluntary euthanasia; cerebrovascular disorders; multiple sclerosis; retrospective studies; *Netherlands; North Holland

Orentlicher, David. The Supreme Court and terminal sedation: an ethically inferior alternative to physician–assisted suicide. *In:* Battin, Margaret P.; Rhodes, Rosamond; Silvers, Anita, eds. Physician Assisted Suicide: Expanding the Debate. New York, NY: Routledge; 1998: 301–311. 29 fn. ISBN 0–415–92003–5. BE58795.
> active euthanasia; *allowing to die; *artificial feeding; *assisted suicide; competence; double effect; drugs; food; *intention; involuntary euthanasia; *legal aspects; moral policy; *palliative care; *physicians; right to die; suffering; *Supreme Court decisions; terminally ill; vulnerable populations; wedge argument; *withholding treatment; *sedatives; United States; *Vacco v. Quill; *Washington v. Glucksberg

Orlowski, James P.; Smith, Martin L.; Van Zwienen, Jan. Medical decisions concerning the end of life in children in the Netherlands. [Letter]. *American Journal of Diseases of Children.* 1993 Jun; 147(6): 613–614. 8 refs. BE57873.
> accountability; *active euthanasia; *children; drugs; *infants; intention; palliative care; quality of life; suffering; voluntary euthanasia; *wedge argument; guideline adherence; *Netherlands; Remmelink Commission

Pellegrino, Edmund D. The false promise of beneficent killing. *In:* Emanuel, Linda L., ed. Regulating How We Die: The Ethical, Medical, and Legal Issues Surrounding Physician–Assisted Suicide. Cambridge, MA: Harvard University Press; 1998: 71–91, 269–274. 48 fn. ISBN 0–674–66654–2. BE58534.
> *active euthanasia; advance directives; aged; *assisted suicide; autonomy; *beneficence; coercion; compassion; decision making; depressive disorder; freedom; infants; informed consent; *killing; legal aspects; medical ethics; moral obligations; *moral policy; pain; palliative care; patients; physician's role; *physicians; privacy; prolongation of life; public policy; right to die; *suffering; terminal care; value of life; voluntary euthanasia; wedge argument; dignity; Netherlands; United States

Portenoy, Russell K. Morphine infusions at the end of life: the pitfalls in reasoning from anecdote. [Commentary]. *Journal of Palliative Care.* 1996 Winter; 12(4): 44–46. 12 refs. Commentary on J.A. Billings and

---

BE = bioethics accession number   fn. = footnotes   refs. = references

S.D. Block, p. 21–30. BE55731.
*active euthanasia; assisted suicide; attitudes; *double effect; *drugs; empirical research; intention; killing; *palliative care; physicians; suffering; *terminal care; terminally ill; *morphine; sedatives

Quill, Timothy E.; Kimsma, Gerrit. End–of–life care in the Netherlands and the United States: a comparison of values, justifications, and practices. *Cambridge Quarterly of Healthcare Ethics.* 1997 Spring; 6(2): 189–204. 127 fn. BE56476.
*allowing to die; *assisted suicide; autonomy; case studies; common good; comparative studies; competence; consensus; decision making; dissent; double effect; drugs; freedom; government regulation; guidelines; health care delivery; hospices; intention; *international aspects; *knowledge, attitudes, practice; legal aspects; mass media; obligations of society; *palliative care; physician patient relationship; *physicians; policy analysis; public opinion; *public policy; social control; socioeconomic factors; statistics; *suffering; *terminal care; *values; *voluntary euthanasia; *Netherlands; *United States
Voluntary active euthanasia (VAE) and physician–assisted suicide (PAS) remain technically illegal in the Netherlands, but the practices are openly tolerated provided that physicians adhere to carefully constructed guidelines. Harsh criticism of the Dutch practice by authors in the United States and Great Britain has made achieving a balanced understanding of its clinical, moral, and policy implications very difficult. Similar practice patterns probably exist in the United States, but they are conducted in secret because of a more uncertain legal and ethical climate. In this manuscript, we plan to compare end–of–life care in the United States and the Netherlands with regard to underlying values, justifications, and practices. We will explore the risks and benefits of each system for a real patient who was faced with a common end–of–life clinical dilemma, and close with challenges for public policies in both countries.

Quill, Timothy E.; Lo, Bernard; Brock, Dan W. Palliative options of last resort: a comparison of voluntarily stopping eating and drinking, terminal sedation, physician–assisted suicide, and voluntary active euthanasia. *JAMA.* 1997 Dec 17; 278(23): 2099–2104. 70 refs. BE56434.
*active euthanasia; *allowing to die; artificial feeding; *assisted suicide; autonomy; beneficence; chronically ill; comparative studies; competence; conscience; diagnosis; double effect; *drugs; ethical analysis; family members; food; guidelines; informed consent; intention; legal aspects; *moral policy; pain; *palliative care; physician's role; physicians; prognosis; *public policy; suffering; *terminal care; terminally ill; treatment refusal; *voluntary euthanasia; *sedatives; United States
Palliative care is generally agreed to be the standard of care for the dying, but there remain some patients for whom intolerable suffering persists. In the face of ethical and legal controversy about the acceptability of physician–assisted suicide and voluntary active euthanasia, voluntarily stopping eating and drinking and terminal sedation have been proposed as ethically superior responses of last resort that do not require changes in professional standards or the law. The clinical and ethical differences and similarities between these 4 practices are critically compared in light of the doctrine of double effect, the active/passive distinction, patient voluntariness, proportionality between risks and benefits, and the physician's potential conflict of duties. Terminal sedation and voluntarily stopping eating and drinking would allow clinicians to remain responsive to a wide range of patient suffering, but they are ethically and

clinically more complex and closer to physician–assisted suicide and voluntary active euthanasia than is ordinarily acknowledged. Safeguards are presented for any medical action that may hasten death, including determining that palliative care is ineffective, obtaining informed consent, ensuring diagnostic and prognostic clarity, obtaining an independent second opinion, and implementing reporting and monitoring processes. Explicit public policy about which of these practices are permissible would reassure the many patients who fear a bad death in their future and allow for a predictable response for the few whose suffering becomes intolerable in spite of optimal palliative care.

Reiman, Jeffrey. On euthanasia and health care. *In: his* Critical Moral Liberalism: Theory and Practice. Lanham, MD: Rowman and Littlefield; 1997: 211–219. 8 fn. ISBN 0–8476–8314–1. BE57649.
*active euthanasia; age factors; aged; allowing to die; autonomy; *health care; *moral policy; personhood; public policy; quality of life; *resource allocation; *right to die; self concept; suffering; value of life; *voluntary euthanasia; wedge argument

Rhodes, Rosamond. Physicians, assisted suicide, and the right to live or die. *In:* Battin, Margaret P.; Rhodes, Rosamond; Silvers, Anita, eds. Physician Assisted Suicide: Expanding the Debate. New York, NY: Routledge; 1998: 165–176. 20 fn. ISBN 0–415–92003–5. BE58787.
advance directives; allowing to die; *assisted suicide; autonomy; *beneficence; caring; killing; medical ethics; *moral obligations; *moral policy; palliative care; physician patient relationship; *physician's role; *physicians; public policy; *right to die; *rights; suffering; suicide; third party consent; treatment refusal; trust; value of life; *voluntary euthanasia; withholding treatment; rationality

Roy, David J. On the ethics of euthanasia discourse. [Editorial]. *Journal of Palliative Care.* 1996 Winter; 12(4): 3–5. 3 fn. BE55733.
*active euthanasia; *communication; palliative care; public participation; terminal care; values

Schotsman, Paul. Debating euthanasia in Belgium. [News]. *Hastings Center Report.* 1997 Sep–Oct; 27(5): 46–47. BE56122.
advisory committees; bioethical issues; decision making; guidelines; palliative care; physicians; *public policy; regulation; *voluntary euthanasia; *Belgium; *Federal Advisory Committee on Bioethics (Belgium)

Shanahan, Timothy; Wang, Robin. Suicide and euthanasia. *In: their* Reason and Insight: Western and Eastern Perspectives on the Pursuit of Moral Wisdom. Belmont, CA: Wadsworth; 1996: 396–425. Includes references, readings, and discussion questions. Designed as a textbook for college students. ISBN 0–534–23167–5. BE56142.
*active euthanasia; *allowing to die; attitudes; attitudes to death; brain death; Buddhist ethics; determination of death; Hindu ethics; international aspects; *moral policy; *morality; physician's role; *suicide; non–Western World; rationality; Western World; India; Japan

Smith, Anthony M.; Edmonds, Polly; Davies, Andrew, et al. More openness needed in palliative care. [Letters]. *BMJ (British Medical Journal).* 1998 Jan 31; 316(7128): 390–391. 6 refs. BE57801.
*active euthanasia; *double effect; drugs; *intention; *palliative care; physicians; quality of life; *terminal care; Great Britain

---

BE = bioethics accession number   fn. = footnotes   refs. = references

Smith, Wesley J. "Inevitable" assisted suicide?: don't bet your life. *Human Life Review.* 1997 Spring; 23(2): 61–74. 37 fn. BE57431.
*active euthanasia; alternatives; *assisted suicide; autonomy; chronically ill; conflict of interest; congenital disorders; depressive disorder; disabled; economics; emotions; gatekeeping; guidelines; health maintenance organizations; hospices; involuntary euthanasia; legal aspects; managed care programs; mandatory reporting; mass media; newborns; palliative care; physicians; prolongation of life; proprietary health facilities; public opinion; *public policy; quality of life; referral and consultation; right to die; social impact; suffering; terminally ill; voluntary euthanasia; wedge argument; capitation fee; Compassion in Dying v. State of Washington; Death with Dignity Act (OR); *Netherlands; Oregon; Remmelink Commission; *United States

Supanich, Barbara; Brody, Howard. Ethical issues concerning physician–assisted death. *In:* Monagle, John F.; Thomasma, David C., eds. Health Care Ethics: Critical Issues for the 21st Century. Gaithersburg, MD: Aspen Publishers; 1998: 302–310. 29 fn. ISBN 0–8342–0911–X. BE56287.
*assisted suicide; autonomy; communication; compassion; competence; comprehension; decision making; disclosure; palliative care; patients; physician patient relationship; physician's role; public policy; quality of health care; referral and consultation; right to die; suffering; values; *voluntary euthanasia; wedge argument; United States

ten Have, Henk A.M.J.; Janssens, Rien M.J.P.A. Regulating euthanasia in the Netherlands: ethics committees for review of euthanasia? *HEC (HealthCare Ethics Committee) Forum.* 1997 Dec; 9(4): 393–399. 7 refs. BE58089.
*active euthanasia; *clinical ethics committees; *decision making; disclosure; *ethics consultation; government regulation; legal aspects; *palliative care; physicians; *public policy; quality of health care; *regional ethics committees; technical expertise; *Netherlands
In this essay we critically review recent regulations with regard to euthanasia policy in The Netherlands. Euthanasia in Holland is formally structured under the penal code. However, because of court cases in which, from the beginning of the 1970s, conditions were formulated wherein euthanizing physicians would not be prosecuted, euthanasia could easily become part of the future standard of medical practice. Recently, new rules concerning the practice of euthanasia have been proposed by the Dutch government in order to adequately control euthanasia practice. These proposals mainly focus on retrospective review. Until now, relatively little attention was paid to preventability of euthanasia. In order to prevent euthanasia, prospective consultation with physicians considering to commit euthanasia would have to receive more attention. In the United States, ample experience has been acquired providing prospective consultative services in neonatalogy. In the aftermath of the "Baby Doe" case, infant care review committees (ICRCs) were established to enhance decisionmaking with regard to severely compromised newborns. These experiences provide interesting points of departure for the development of prospective consultative services in The Netherlands, particularly for physicians who are considering to euthanize patients.

Ubel, Peter A.; Asch, David A. Semantic and moral debates about hastening death: a survey of bioethicists. *Journal of Clinical Ethics.* 1997 Fall; 8(3): 242–249. 24 fn. BE57617.
*active euthanasia; *allowing to die; artificial feeding; *assisted suicide; *attitudes; case studies; competence;

*consensus; *dissent; *double effect; *drugs; *ethicists; family members; intention; involuntary euthanasia; killing; *moral policy; *morality; pain; palliative care; physicians; survey; *terminology; third party consent; treatment refusal; ventilators; *voluntary euthanasia; *withholding treatment; American Association of Bioethics; United States

Uhlmann, Michael M., ed. Last Rights? Assisted Suicide and Euthanasia Debated. Washington, DC: Ethics and Public Policy Center; Grand Rapids, MI: W.B. Eerdmans; 1998. 667 p. 511 fn. ISBN 0–8028–4199–6. BE57202.
*active euthanasia; *allowing to die; *assisted suicide; attitudes to death; autonomy; Christian ethics; coercion; compassion; competence; double effect; drugs; freedom; government regulation; historical aspects; intention; Jewish ethics; killing; legal aspects; medical ethics; model legislation; *moral policy; morality; natural law; pain; personhood; philosophy; physician's role; physicians; quality of life; review; *right to die; Roman Catholic ethics; state interest; suffering; *suicide; Supreme Court decisions; theology; treatment refusal; utilitarianism; value of life; vulnerable populations; wedge argument; withholding treatment; rationality; Western World; American Medical Association; Netherlands; United States; Vacco v. Quill; Washington v. Glucksberg

van der Arend, Arie J.G. An ethical perspective on euthanasia and assisted suicide in the Netherlands from a nursing point of view. *Nursing Ethics.* 1998 Jul; 5(4): 307–318. 16 refs. BE58870.
active euthanasia; *assisted suicide; communication; *decision making; drugs; *empirical research; government regulation; guidelines; *knowledge, attitudes, practice; legal aspects; *nurse's role; nursing ethics; patient advocacy; physician nurse relationship; *physicians; professional organizations; referral and consultation; statistics; terminal care; *voluntary euthanasia; *Netherlands

van der Burg, Wibren. Slippery slope arguments. *In:* Chadwick, Ruth, ed. Encyclopedia of Applied Ethics, Volume 4. San Diego, CA: Academic Press; 1998: 129–142. 5 refs. ISBN 0–12–227069–X. BE56345.
*bioethical issues; case studies; emotions; involuntary euthanasia; moral policy; morality; philosophy; public policy; social impact; trends; *voluntary euthanasia; *wedge argument; Netherlands

van der Heide, A.; van der Maas, P.J.; Kollée, L.A.A. End–of–life decisions in Dutch paediatric practice. [Letter]. *Lancet.* 1997 Dec 6; 350(9092): 1711. 2 refs. BE58154.
*active euthanasia; *allowing to die; attitudes; *decision making; drugs; *infants; legal aspects; *newborns; parents; *pediatrics; peer review; *physicians; *Netherlands

van der Maas, Paul J. End of life decisions in mentally disabled people: protecting vulnerable life does not mean prolonging it regardless of suffering. [Editorial]. *BMJ (British Medical Journal).* 1997 Jul 12; 315(7100): 73. 10 refs. BE55597.
*active euthanasia; *allowing to die; *decision making; drugs; *mentally retarded; patient care team; *physicians; statistics; *terminally ill; withholding treatment; *Netherlands

van der Maas, Paul J.; Emanuel, Linda L. Factual findings. *In:* Emanuel, Linda L., ed. Regulating How We Die: The Ethical, Medical, and Legal Issues Surrounding Physician–Assisted Suicide. Cambridge, MA: Harvard University Press; 1998: 151–174, 300–307. 28 fn. ISBN 0–674–66654–2. BE58537.
*active euthanasia; *assisted suicide; *attitudes; autonomy; cancer; coercion; cultural pluralism; decision making;

BE = bioethics accession number   fn. = footnotes   refs. = references

depressive disorder; *empirical research; intention; international aspects; involuntary euthanasia; legal aspects; moral obligations; *motivation; organizational policies; pain; palliative care; physicians; professional organizations; *public opinion; public policy; suffering; terminally ill; value of life; voluntary euthanasia; wedge argument; withholding treatment; dignity; Netherlands; United States

van Thiel, G.J.M.W.; van Delden, J.J.M.; de Haan, K., et al. Retrospective study of doctors' "end of life decisions" in caring for mentally handicapped people in institutions in the Netherlands. *BMJ (British Medical Journal).* 1997 Jul 12; 315(7100): 88–91. 8 refs. BE55583.
*active euthanasia; *allowing to die; communication; competence; *decision making; drugs; family members; *institutionalized persons; *mentally retarded; mortality; motivation; nurses; *palliative care; *physicians; referral and consultation; statistics; suffering; survey; *terminal care; *terminally ill; withholding treatment; retrospective studies; *Netherlands
OBJECTIVES: To gain insight into the reasons behind and the prevalence of doctors' decisions at the end of life that might hasten a patient's death ("end of life decisions") in institutions caring for mentally handicapped people in the Netherlands, and to describe important aspects of the decisions making process. DESIGN: Survey of random sample of doctors caring for mentally handicapped people by means of self completed questionnaires and structured interviews. SUBJECTS: 89 of the 101 selected doctors completed the questionnaire. 67 doctors had taken an end of life decision and were interviewed about their most recent case. MAIN OUTCOME MEASURES: Prevalence of end of life decisions; types of decisions; characteristics of patients; reasons why the decision was taken; and the decision making process. RESULTS: The 89 doctors reported 222 deaths for 1995. An end of life decision was taken in 97 cases (44%); in 75 the decision was to withdraw or withhold treatment, and in 22 it was to relieve pain or symptoms with opiates in dosages that may have shortened life. In the 67 most recent cases with an end of life decision the patients were mostly incompetent (63) and under 65 years old (51). Only two patients explicitly asked to die, but in 23 cases there had been some communication with the patient. In 60 cases the doctors discussed the decision with nursing staff and in 46 with a colleague. CONCLUSIONS: End of life decisions are an important aspect of the institutionalised care of mentally handicapped people. The proportion of such decisions in the total number of deaths is similar to that in other specialties. However, the discussion of such decisions is less open in the care of mental handicap than in other specialties. Because of distinctive features of care in this specialty an open debate about end of life decisions should not be postponed.

Warren, Mary Anne. Euthanasia and the moral status of human beings. *In: her:* Moral Status: Obligations to Persons and Other Living Things. New York, NY: Oxford University Press; 1997: 185–200. 13 fn. ISBN 0-19-823668-9. BE56997.
*active euthanasia; adults; advance directives; *allowing to die; anencephaly; *assisted suicide; brain death; children; coercion; competence; *euthanasia; *human rights; *involuntary euthanasia; killing; legal aspects; *moral obligations; *moral policy; newborns; persistent vegetative state; prolongation of life; public policy; quality of life; suffering; suicide; terminally ill; terminology; third party consent; treatment refusal; *value of life; *voluntary euthanasia; Netherlands; United States

Wolf, Susan. Facing assisted suicide and euthanasia in children and adolescents. *In:* Emanuel, Linda L., ed.

Regulating How We Die: The Ethical, Medical, and Legal Issues Surrounding Physician–Assisted Suicide. Cambridge, MA: Harvard University Press; 1998: 92–119, 274–294. 154 fn. ISBN 0-674-66654-2. BE58535.
abortion, induced; *active euthanasia; *adolescents; adults; age factors; allowing to die; *assisted suicide; autonomy; beneficence; *children; coercion; competence; congenital disorders; decision making; infanticide; infants; international aspects; involuntary euthanasia; killing; legal aspects; legal rights; National Socialism; newborns; palliative care; parental consent; physicians; public policy; quality of life; socioeconomic factors; state interest; treatment refusal; voluntary euthanasia; withholding treatment; Netherlands; United States

Zwart, Frédérique. A very special day. [Personal narrative on voluntary euthanasia]. *BMJ (British Medical Journal).* 1997 Jul 26; 315(7102): 260. BE58572.
aged; attitudes; physicians; suffering; terminally ill; *voluntary euthanasia; Netherlands

Dutch GPs to be offered advice on euthanasia. [News]. *BMJ (British Medical Journal).* 1997 Jun 21; 314(7097): 1782. BE55819.
family practice; interprofessional relations; medical education; *organizational policies; *physicians; professional organizations; referral and consultation; *voluntary euthanasia; *Amsterdam; *Netherlands; *Royal Dutch Medical Association

EUTHANASIA/ATTITUDES

Berger, Douglas; Fukunishi, Isao; O'Dowd, Mary Alice, et al. A comparison of Japanese and American psychiatrists' attitudes towards patients wishing to die in the general hospital. *Psychotherapy and Psychosomatics.* 1997; 66(6): 319–328. 27 refs. BE59010.
*active euthanasia; *allowing to die; *assisted suicide; *attitudes; comparative studies; competence; depressive disorder; hospitals; international aspects; mental health; motivation; *physicians; *psychiatry; quality of life; referral and consultation; right to die; suicide; survey; terminally ill; treatment refusal; truth disclosure; values; *voluntary euthanasia; rationality; *Japan; *United States

Berger, Douglas; Takahashi, Yoshitomo; Fukunishi, Isao, et al. Japanese psychiatrists' attitudes toward patients wishing to die in the general hospital: a cultural perspective. *Cambridge Quarterly of Healthcare Ethics.* 1997 Fall; 6(4): 470–479. 44 fn. BE56456.
active euthanasia; *allowing to die; *assisted suicide; *attitudes; competence; *depressive disorder; *euthanasia; family members; family relationship; hospitals; patients; persistent vegetative state; *physicians; prolongation of life; *psychiatric diagnosis; *psychiatry; *quality of life; resuscitation orders; *right to die; suffering; *suicide; survey; terminally ill; third party consent; treatment refusal; voluntary euthanasia; withholding treatment; rationality; *Japan

Billings, J. Andrew; Block, Susan D. Slow euthanasia. *Journal of Palliative Care.* 1996 Winter; 12(4): 21–30. 80 refs. Commented on by B. Mount, p. 31–37; by H. Brody, p. 38–41; by B.M. Dickens, p. 42–43; and by R.K. Portenoy, p. 44–46. BE55706.
*active euthanasia; allowing to die; *attitudes; beneficence; case studies; decision making; *double effect; *drugs; family members; hospices; informed consent; *intention; involuntary euthanasia; killing; pain; *palliative care; paternalism; patients; physicians; psychological stress; suffering; *terminal care; *terminally ill; time factors; voluntary euthanasia; withholding treatment; analgesia; *morphine; sedatives

Chochinov, Harvey Max; Wilson, Keith G. The euthanasia debate: attitudes, practices and psychiatric considerations. *Canadian Journal of Psychiatry.* 1995 Dec; 40(10): 593–602. 69 refs. BE56325.

*assisted suicide; *attitudes; cancer; competence; criminal law; depressive disorder; empirical research; family relationship; international aspects; *knowledge, attitudes, practice; legal aspects; mental health; mentally ill; palliative care; patients; *physician's role; *physicians; psychiatric diagnosis; *psychiatry; *public opinion; public policy; referral and consultation; suicide; terminal care; terminally ill; *voluntary euthanasia; wedge argument; Canada; Netherlands; United States

de Boer, Anthonius; Lau, Hong Sang; Porsius, Arijan. Physician–assisted death and pharmacy practice in the Netherlands. [Letter]. *New England Journal of Medicine.* 1997 Oct 9; 337(15): 1091–1092. 5 refs. BE57169.

*active euthanasia; *assisted suicide; *attitudes; *drugs; guidelines; hospitals; *knowledge, attitudes, practice; legal aspects; *pharmacists; physicians; practice guidelines; professional organizations; statistics; survey; *Netherlands; Royal Dutch Pharmaceutical Association

Domino, George; Kempton, Susan; Cavender, Jim. Physician assisted suicide: a scale and some empirical findings. *Omega: A Journal of Death and Dying.* 1996–1997; 34(3): 247–257. 15 refs. BE56487.

aged; *assisted suicide; *attitudes; comparative studies; competence; *evaluation; family members; legal aspects; morality; *physicians; public policy; right to die; students; survey; terminally ill; universities; *voluntary euthanasia; *questionnaires; United States

Emanuel, Ezekiel J.; Daniels, Elisabeth R.; Fairclough, Diane L., et al. The practice of euthanasia and physician–assisted suicide in the United States: adherence to proposed safeguards and effects on physicians. *JAMA.* 1998 Aug 12; 280(6): 507–513. 34 refs. BE58766.

*active euthanasia; *assisted suicide; *attitudes; *cancer; competence; decision making; drugs; empirical research; evaluation studies; family members; guidelines; hospices; involuntary euthanasia; *knowledge, attitudes, practice; medical specialties; motivation; pain; palliative care; physician patient relationship; *physicians; psychological stress; public policy; referral and consultation; religion; suffering; survey; terminal care; *terminally ill; *voluntary euthanasia; *guideline adherence; *oncology; *United States

CONTEXT: Despite intense debates about legalization, there are few data examining the details of actual euthanasia and physician–assisted suicide (PAS) cases in the United States. OBJECTIVE: To determine whether the practices of euthanasia and PAS are consistent with proposed safeguards and the effect on physicians of having performed euthanasia or PAS. DESIGN: Structured in–depth telephone interviews. SETTING AND PARTICIPANTS: Randomly selected oncologists in the United States. OUTCOME MEASURES: Adherence to primary and secondary safeguards for the practice of euthanasia and PAS; regret, comfort, and fear of prosecution from performing euthanasia or PAS. RESULTS: A total of 355 oncologists (72.6% response rate) were interviewed on euthanasia and PAS. On 2 screening questions, 56 oncologists (15.8%) reported participating in euthanasia or PAS; 53 oncologists (94.6% response rate) participated in in–depth interviews. Thirty–eight of 53 oncologists described clearly defined cases of euthanasia or PAS. Twenty–three patients (60.5%) both initiated and repeated their request for euthanasia or PAS, but 6 patients (15.8%) did not participate in the decision for euthanasia or PAS. Thirty–seven patients (97.4%) were experiencing unremitting pain or such poor physical

functioning they could not perform self–care. Physicians sought consultation in 15 cases (39.5%). Overall, oncologists adhered to all 3 main safeguards in 13 cases (34.2%): (1) having the patient initiate and repeat the request for euthanasia or PAS, (2) ensuring the patient was experiencing extreme physical pain or suffering, and (3) consulting with a colleague. Those who adhered to the safeguards had known their patients longer and tended to be more religious. In 28 cases (73.7%), the family supported the decision. In all cases of pain, patients were receiving narcotic analgesia. Fifteen patients (39.5%) were enrolled in a hospice. While 19 oncologists (52.6%) received comfort from having helped a patient with euthanasia or PAS, 9 (23.7%) regretted having performed euthanasia or PAS, and 15 (39.5%) feared prosecution. CONCLUSIONS: Intractable pain or poor physical functioning seem to be nearly absolute requirements for physicians to perform euthanasia or PAS. Only one third of cases are performed consistently with proposed safeguards. For some patients, end–of–life care that includes opioid analgesia and hospice care does not obviate their desire for euthanasia or PAS. While the majority of physicians seem comforted by their actions, some experience adverse consequences from having performed euthanasia or PAS.

Hassan, Riaz. Euthanasia and the medical profession: an Australian study. *Australian Journal of Social Issues.* 1996 Aug; 31(3): 239–252. 12 refs. BE58274.

*active euthanasia; *allowing to die; *assisted suicide; *attitudes; family members; *knowledge, attitudes, practice; legal aspects; motivation; patients; *physicians; survey; *voluntary euthanasia; *Australia; Netherlands; *South Australia

Hooper, S.C.; Vaughan, K.J.; Tennant, C.C., et al. Preferences for voluntary euthanasia during major depression and following improvement in an elderly population. *Australian Journal on Ageing.* 1997 Feb; 16(1): 3–7. 18 refs. BE57685.

*aged; *attitudes; *competence; *depressive disorder; morbidity; *motivation; patient care; prognosis; suicide; survey; *voluntary euthanasia; severity of illness index; *Australia

Kinsella, T. Douglas; Verhoef, Marja J. Assisted suicide: opinions of Alberta physicians. *Clinical and Investigative Medicine.* 1995 Oct; 18(5): 406–412. 13 refs. BE55511.

age factors; *assisted suicide; *attitudes; criminal law; *legal aspects; *physicians; public policy; religion; statistics; survey; uncertainty; *voluntary euthanasia; *Alberta; Canada

Meier, Diane E.; Emmons, Carol–Ann; Wallenstein, Sylvan, et al. A national survey of physician–assisted suicide and euthanasia in the United States. *New England Journal of Medicine.* 1998 Apr 23; 338(17): 1193–1201. 23 refs. BE57820.

*active euthanasia; *assisted suicide; *attitudes; family members; *knowledge, attitudes, practice; legal aspects; medical specialties; motivation; patients; *physicians; prognosis; survey; terminally ill; *voluntary euthanasia; *United States

BACKGROUND: Although there have been many studies of physician–assisted suicide and euthanasia in the United States, national data are lacking. METHODS: In 1996, we mailed questionnaires to a stratified probability sample of 3102 physicians in the 10 specialties in which doctors are most likely to receive requests from patients for assistance with suicide or euthanasia. We weighted the results to obtain nationally representative

---

BE = bioethics accession number   fn. = footnotes   refs. = references

data. RESULTS: We received 1902 completed questionnaires (response rate, 61 percent). Eleven percent of the physicians said that under current legal constraints, there were circumstances in which they would be willing to hasten a patient's death by prescribing medication, and 7 percent said that they would provide a lethal injection; 36 percent and 24 percent, respectively, said that they would do so if it were legal. Since entering practice, 18.3 percent of the physicians (unweighted number, 320) reported having received a request from a patient for assistance with suicide and 11.1 percent (unweighted number, 196) had received a request for a lethal injection. Sixteen percent of the physicians receiving such requests (unweighted number, 42), or 3.3 percent of the entire sample, reported that they had written at least one prescription to be used to hasten death, and 4.7 percent (unweighted number, 59), said that they had administered at least one lethal injection. CONCLUSIONS: A substantial proportion of physicians in the United States report that they receive requests for physician-assisted suicide and euthanasia, and about 7 percent of those who responded to our survey have complied with such requests at least once.

Morrow, Elizabeth. Attitudes of women from vulnerable populations toward physician-assisted death: a qualitative approach. *Journal of Clinical Ethics.* 1997 Fall; 8(3): 279-289. 22 fn. BE57610.
> aged; allowing to die; *assisted suicide; *attitudes; *autonomy; coercion; comparative studies; conflict of interest; *decision making; *disadvantaged; domestic violence; economics; family members; family relationship; *females; Hispanic Americans; indigents; physician patient relationship; physicians; public opinion; *public policy; referral and consultation; religion; social discrimination; social dominance; students; survey; terminally ill; third party consent; *trust; universities; *voluntary euthanasia; *vulnerable populations; empowerment; homeless persons; qualitative research; California; United States

Muller, M.T.; Onwuteaka-Philipsen, B.D.; Kriegsman, D.M.W., et al. Voluntary active euthanasia and doctor-assisted suicide: knowledge and attitudes of Dutch medical students. *Medical Education.* 1996 Nov; 30(6): 428-433. 9 refs. BE57056.
> *assisted suicide; *attitudes; females; guidelines; *knowledge, attitudes, practice; males; *medical education; *physicians; religion; *students; survey; *voluntary euthanasia; *Netherlands

NOP Consumer Market Research. Euthanasia (Fieldwork: 31 March-5 April 1993): A Report Produced for [the] Voluntary Euthanasia Society. Issued by NOP [National Opinion Poll] Consumer Market Research, London; 1993 Apr. 13 p. NOP/41341. BE57398.
> active euthanasia; legal aspects; *public opinion; *public policy; religion; statistics; suffering; survey; *voluntary euthanasia; *Great Britain; *Voluntary Euthanasia Society (Great Britain)

Oliver, John. Voluntary euthanasia commands majority support. [Letter]. *BMJ (British Medical Journal).* 1995 Aug 19; 311(7003): 510. 3 refs. BE56104.
> *public opinion; terminal care; *voluntary euthanasia; *Great Britain

Onwuteaka-Philipsen, Bregje D.; Muller, Martien T.; van der Wal, Gerrit, et al. Active voluntary euthanasia or physician-assisted suicide? *Journal of the American Geriatrics Society.* 1997 Oct; 45(10): 1208-1213. 18 refs. BE56474.
> *assisted suicide; *attitudes; comparative studies; *family practice; *knowledge, attitudes, practice; morality; morbidity; *motivation; *nursing homes; *patients; *physicians; survey; *voluntary euthanasia; retrospective studies; *Netherlands

Suarez-Almazor, Maria E.; Belzile, Michelle; Bruera, Eduardo. Euthanasia and physician-assisted suicide: a comparative study of physicians, terminally ill cancer patients, and the general population. *Journal of Clinical Oncology.* 1997 Feb; 15(2): 418-427. 37 refs. BE58258.
> *active euthanasia; *assisted suicide; *attitudes; *cancer; comparative studies; family practice; medical specialties; *patients; *physicians; *public opinion; public policy; religion; socioeconomic factors; suffering; survey; *terminally ill; *Alberta

Sullivan, Mark; Rapp, Suzanne; Fitzgibbon, Dermot, et al. Pain and the choice to hasten death in patients with painful metastatic cancer. *Journal of Palliative Care.* 1997 Autumn; 13(3): 18-28. 34 refs. BE58070.
> *active euthanasia; *allowing to die; artificial feeding; *assisted suicide; *attitudes; *cancer; depressive disorder; double effect; drugs; hospitals; living wills; *pain; *palliative care; *patients; physicians; *quality of life; resuscitation orders; right to die; suicide; *terminal care; *terminally ill; treatment refusal; values; voluntary euthanasia; withholding treatment; analgesia; outpatients; United States; University of Washington Medical Center

Walker, Gail C. The right to die: healthcare workers' attitudes compared with a national public poll. *Omega: A Journal of Death and Dying.* 1997; 35(4): 339-345. 4 refs. BE57722.
> *active euthanasia; advance directives; *allowing to die; *attitudes; autonomy; clinical ethics committees; comparative studies; competence; congenital disorders; *decision making; drugs; family members; hospitals; newborns; *nurses; pain; palliative care; parents; patients; *public opinion; quality of life; *right to die; suffering; *suicide; survey; terminally ill; third party consent; treatment refusal; withholding treatment; dependency; New York; Times Mirror Center; United States

Dutch GPs often fail to honor euthanasia requests. [News]. *BMJ (British Medical Journal).* 1997 Jan 18; 314(7075): 166. BE58616.
> family practice; *knowledge, attitudes, practice; *physicians; survey; time factors; *voluntary euthanasia; *directive adherence; *Netherlands

EUTHANASIA/LEGAL ASPECTS

Al, Joop. Comparative observations on some current medico-legal issues in Dutch law. *In:* Jewish Law Annual. Volume Twelve. Amsterdam, Netherlands: Harwood Academic Publishers; 1997: 167-215. 127 fn. ISBN 90-5702-551-5. BE58341.
> *active euthanasia; *allowing to die; assisted suicide; body parts and fluids; brain death; cadavers; cardiac death; competence; congenital disorders; criminal law; decision making; depressive disorder; *determination of death; donor cards; family members; futility; guidelines; involuntary euthanasia; *Jewish ethics; *legal aspects; newborns; *organ donation; *organ donors; organ transplantation; persistent vegetative state; physicians; professional organizations; *public policy; quality of life; referral and consultation; resource allocation; self regulation; suffering; voluntary euthanasia; withholding treatment; Austria; Belgium; Denmark; France; Germany; *Netherlands; Norway; Sweden

Arras, John D. Physician-assisted suicide: a tragic view. *Journal of Contemporary Health Law and Policy.* 1997

Spring; 13(2): 361–389. 94 fn. BE56000.

advance directives; *allowing to die; *assisted suicide; autonomy; chronically ill; coercion; competence; constitutional law; cultural pluralism; decision making; depressive disorder; due process; economics; equal protection; freedom; government regulation; intention; judicial action; killing; *legal aspects; legal rights; legislation; managed care programs; *moral policy; pain; *palliative care; physically disabled; physician patient relationship; *physicians; *public policy; religion; review; *right to die; secularism; *social impact; state government; suffering; terminally ill; third party consent; *voluntary euthanasia; vulnerable populations; *wedge argument; withholding treatment; Compassion in Dying v. State of Washington; Quill v. Vacco; *United States

Brody, Howard. Commentary on Billings and Block's "Slow euthanasia." *Journal of Palliative Care.* 1996 Winter; 12(4): 38–41. 11 refs. Commentary on J.A. Billings and S.D. Block, p. 21–30. BE55709.

*active euthanasia; allowing to die; *assisted suicide; decision making; double effect; drugs; *government regulation; intention; justice; killing; *legal aspects; *palliative care; physicians; resource allocation; suffering; *terminal care; *terminally ill; wedge argument; withholding treatment; morphine; Compassion in Dying v. State of Washington; Netherlands; United States

Brooks, Timothy Paul. State v. Forrest: mercy killing and malice in North Carolina. [Note]. *North Carolina Law Review.* 1988 Sep; 66(6): 1160–1176. 113 fn. BE56655.

*active euthanasia; *criminal law; *family members; *killing; *legal aspects; *legal liability; motivation; right to die; state government; suffering; *North Carolina; *State v. Forrest

Churchill, Larry R.; King, Nancy M.P. Physician assisted suicide, euthanasia, or withdrawal of treatment. [Editorial]. *BMJ (British Medical Journal).* 1997 Jul 19; 315(7101): 137–138. 16 refs. BE58500.

*active euthanasia; *assisted suicide; government regulation; international aspects; *legal aspects; physicians; public policy; right to die; state government; Supreme Court decisions; treatment refusal; wedge argument; withholding treatment; Death with Dignity Act (OR); Great Britain; Netherlands; Northern Territory; Rights of the Terminally Ill Act (NT); *United States; Vacco v. Quill; Washington v. Glucksberg

DePalma, Anthony. Canadian gets light term in child's death. [News]. *New York Times.* 1997 Dec 2: A8. BE58126.

*active euthanasia; attitudes; children; compassion; constitutional law; criminal law; disabled; *family members; fathers; *killing; *legal liability; legal rights; motivation; pain; *physically disabled; *punishment; social worth; value of life; Canada; Canadian Charter of Rights and Freedom; *Latimer, Robert; *Latimer, Tracy; *Saskatchewan

DePalma, Anthony. Father's killing of Canadian girl: mercy or murder? [News]. *New York Times.* 1997 Dec 1: A3. BE58127.

*active euthanasia; attitudes; autonomy; children; criminal law; decision making; disabled; *family members; fathers; *killing; *legal aspects; *legal liability; pain; patient advocacy; *physically disabled; public opinion; *punishment; quality of life; social worth; value of life; Canada; *Latimer, Robert; *Latimer, Tracy; *Saskatchewan

Dickens, Bernard M. Commentary on "Slow euthanasia." *Journal of Palliative Care.* 1996 Winter; 12(4): 42–43. 4 refs. Commentary on J.A. Billings and S.D. Block, p. 21–30. BE55716.

*active euthanasia; assisted suicide; criminal law; double effect; *drugs; intention; *legal aspects; motivation;

*palliative care; physicians; suffering; *terminal care; terminally ill; withholding treatment; *morphine; Canada; Criminal Code of Canada

Dyer, Clare. Newcastle GP charged with murder. [News]. *BMJ (British Medical Journal).* 1998 Jun 20; 316(7148): 1849. BE58237.

*active euthanasia; cancer; drugs; intention; killing; *legal aspects; *legal liability; pain; *physicians; terminally ill; *Great Britain; Liddell, George; *Moore, David

Ferguson, Pamela R. Causing death or allowing to die? Developments in the law. *Journal of Medical Ethics.* 1997 Dec; 23(6): 368–372. 19 fn. Commented on by F. Randall, p. 373–376. BE57658.

*active euthanasia; *allowing to die; artificial feeding; *criminal law; decision making; *double effect; drugs; futility; *intention; *killing; law; *legal aspects; *legal liability; moral obligations; moral policy; *morality; motivation; pain; patients; *persistent vegetative state; *physicians; public policy; quality of life; *terminally ill; voluntary euthanasia; *withholding treatment; *Airedale NHS Trust v. Bland; *Great Britain; *Law Hospital NHS Trust v. Lord Advocate; *R v. Cox

Several cases which have been considered by the courts in recent years have highlighted the legal dilemmas facing doctors whose decisions result in the ending of a patient's life. This paper considers the case of Dr Cox, who was convicted of attempting to murder one of his patients, and explores the roles of motive, diminished responsibility and consent in cases of "mercy killing". The Cox decision is compared to that of Tony Bland and Janet Johnstone, in which the patients were in a persistent vegetative state. In all three cases, the doctors believed that their patients' quality of life was so poor that their continued existence was of no benefit to them, and decided that their lives should not be unduly prolonged, yet the doctor who was prosecuted was the one whose dying patient had requested that her death be hastened. The paper examines the law's seemingly contradictory approaches to such cases.

Hanafin, Patrick. Last Rights: Death, Dying and the Law in Ireland. Cork, Ireland: Cork University Press; 1997. 114 p. (Undercurrents; 12). 255 fn. ISBN 1-85918-156-2. BE57047.

advance directives; *allowing to die; artificial feeding; assisted suicide; attitudes; attitudes to death; *autonomy; beneficence; brain pathology; clergy; constitutional law; criminal law; *decision making; dissent; family members; *international aspects; judicial action; killing; legal rights; legislation; natural law; persistent vegetative state; physicians; privacy; *right to die; Roman Catholic ethics; Supreme Court decisions; terminally ill; third party consent; treatment refusal; trends; *value of life; *voluntary euthanasia; withholding treatment; Australia; Canada; Great Britain; In re a Ward of Court; *Ireland; *Medical Council (Ireland); Netherlands; Northern Territory; Right to Life Movement; United States

Hemlock Society. Mercy killing: a position statement regarding David Rodriguez. *Issues in Law and Medicine.* 1997 Winter; 13(3): 341–342. BE58711.

*active euthanasia; chronically ill; compassion; competence; family members; killing; *legal aspects; *legal liability; motivation; *organizational policies; right to die; suffering; terminally ill; *Hemlock Society; *Rodriguez, David; United States

Hodgson, John. Rights of the terminally ill patient. *Annals of Health Law.* 1996; 5: 169–191. 93 fn. BE58364.

*active euthanasia; adults; advance directives; *allowing to die; artificial feeding; assisted suicide; competence; *decision making; family members; informed consent; judicial action;

BE = bioethics accession number   fn. = footnotes   refs. = references

*legal aspects; legal liability; *legal rights; minors; palliative care; *persistent vegetative state; physicians; quality of life; right to die; standards; *terminally ill; *third party consent; *treatment refusal; withholding treatment; Airedale NHS Trust v. Bland; *Great Britain; House of Lords Select Committee on Medical Ethics; Law Commission (Great Britain)

Keown, John. The euthanasia debate in Britain. *International Journal of Bioethics.* 1997 Mar–Jun; 8(1–2): 55–63. 23 fn. BE59095.
    *active euthanasia; advisory committees; allowing to die; assisted suicide; autonomy; criminal law; decision making; double effect; drugs; intention; involuntary euthanasia; killing; *legal aspects; legal rights; palliative care; physicians; *public policy; regulation; treatment refusal; *voluntary euthanasia; vulnerable populations; wedge argument; *Great Britain; *House of Lords Select Committee on Medical Ethics; Netherlands

Kimura, Rihito. Death, dying, and advance directives in Japan: sociocultural and legal points of view. *In:* Sass, Hans-Martin; Veatch, Robert M.; Kimura, Rihito, eds. Advance Directives and Surrogate Decision Making in Health Care: United States, Germany, and Japan. Baltimore, MD: Johns Hopkins University Press; 1998: 187–208. 29 refs. ISBN 0-8018-5831-3. BE59042.
    *active euthanasia; *advance directives; *allowing to die; assisted suicide; attitudes; *attitudes to death; cancer; common good; criminal law; decision making; diagnosis; drugs; family members; *family relationship; historical aspects; *legal aspects; living wills; model legislation; national health insurance; organ donation; organizational policies; pain; palliative care; paternalism; patient advocacy; physician patient relationship; physicians; professional organizations; prognosis; prolongation of life; public opinion; *public policy; resuscitation orders; social dominance; *terminal care; terminally ill; third party consent; trends; trust; truth disclosure; *values; voluntary euthanasia; withholding treatment; oral directives; *Japan; Japan Medical Association; Japan Science Council; Japanese Society for Dying with Dignity

Kondro, Wayne. "Mercy killing" takes centre stage in Canada. [News]. *Lancet.* 1997 Nov 15; 350(9089): 1458. BE57174.
    *active euthanasia; advisory committees; assisted suicide; cancer; *criminal law; *killing; *legal aspects; *legal liability; *legislation; parents; patients; physically disabled; physicians; *Canada; Halifax (NS); Latimer, Robert; Morrison, Nancy; Nova Scotia; Saskatchewan

Kondro, Wayne. Murder-or-mercy case tested in Canada. [News]. *Lancet.* 1997 May 17; 349(9063): 1458. BE55824.
    *active euthanasia; cancer; *criminal law; family members; hospitals; intensive care units; *killing; *legal liability; patients; *physicians; right to die; third party consent; *withholding treatment; *Canada; Mills, Paul; *Morrison, Nancy; Nova Scotia; Victoria General Hospital (Halifax, NS)

Küng, Hans; Jens, Walter. A dignified dying: a plea for personal responsiblity. London: SCM Press; 1995. 132 p. 101 fn. Contributions by Dietrich Niethammer and Albin Eser. Translated from the 1995 German publication *Menschenw4rdig Sterben: Ein Pl1doyer f4r Selbstverantwortung.* ISBN 0-334-02609-1. BE55842.
    *active euthanasia; advance directives; allowing to die; *assisted suicide; *attitudes to death; *autonomy; biomedical technologies; *Christian ethics; conscience; criminal law; *death; decision making; double effect; drugs; *freedom; guidelines; intention; international aspects; killing; *legal aspects; *literature; moral policy; physician patient relationship; *physicians; prolongation of life; public policy; quality of life; *right to die; Roman Catholic ethics; *suffering; suicide; terminal care; terminally ill; theology;

treatment refusal; value of life; *voluntary euthanasia; withholding treatment; *dignity; patient abandonment; Evangelium Vitae; Germany; Netherlands

Legemaate, Johan; Gevers, J.K.M. Physician-assisted suicide in psychiatry: developments in the Netherlands. *Cambridge Quarterly of Healthcare Ethics.* 1997 Spring; 6(2): 175–188. 45 fn. BE56430.
    *active euthanasia; advisory committees; *assisted suicide; behavior disorders; competence; criminal law; depressive disorder; expert testimony; guidelines; judicial action; *legal aspects; legal liability; *mentally ill; *physicians; professional organizations; *psychiatry; *psychological stress; public policy; right to die; self regulation; *suffering; treatment refusal; *voluntary euthanasia; wedge argument; anorexia nervosa; Chabot, Boudewijn; *Netherlands
    In this paper we give an overview of the legal developments in this area [physician-assisted suicide in psychiatry]. First, we will briefly outline the general legal situation in the Netherlands regarding euthanasia and assisted suicide. Second, we will analyze the case law on physician-assisted suicide in psychiatry. Third, we would like to give an impression of the debate outside the courtroom on physician-assisted suicide in psychiatry. That debate started even before publication of the first court ruling on this issue (by the Central Medical Disciplinary Board in 1990) and has not only continued but intensified as a result of subsequent decisions of criminal courts over the last four years. We sketch a general picture of the positions taken by different actors, mainly by referring to reports and statements of the most important organizations and advisory committees.

McLean, Sheila A.M. Law at the end of life: what next? *In:* McLean, Sheila A.M., ed. Death, Dying and the Law. Brookfield, VT: Dartmouth; 1996: 49–66. 56 fn. ISBN 1-85521-657-4. BE57213.
    *active euthanasia; advance directives; advisory committees; *allowing to die; assisted suicide; autonomy; congenital disorders; decision making; double effect; *legal aspects; newborns; palliative care; persistent vegetative state; *public policy; quality of life; state interest; terminal care; treatment refusal; value of life; withholding treatment; Airedale NHS Trust v. Bland; *Great Britain; *House of Lords Select Committee on Medical Ethics

NOP Consumer Market Research. Euthanasia (Fieldwork: 31 March–5 April 1993): A Report Produced for [the] Voluntary Euthanasia Society. Issued by NOP [National Opinion Poll] Consumer Market Research, London; 1993 Apr. 13 p. NOP/41341. BE57398.
    active euthanasia; legal aspects; *public opinion; *public policy; religion; statistics; suffering; survey; *voluntary euthanasia; *Great Britain; *Voluntary Euthanasia Society (Great Britain)

Ogilvie, Alan D. Colombia is confused over legalisation of euthanasia. [News]. *BMJ (British Medical Journal).* 1997 Jun 28; 314(7098): 1852. BE55829.
    *legal aspects; palliative care; physicians; value of life; *voluntary euthanasia; *Colombia

Orentlicher, David. The Supreme Court and physician-assisted suicide -- rejecting assisted suicide but embracing euthanasia. *New England Journal of Medicine.* 1997 Oct 23; 337(17): 1236–1239. 19 refs. BE55800.
    *active euthanasia; artificial feeding; *assisted suicide; constitutional law; double effect; *drugs; intention; involuntary euthanasia; *legal aspects; *legal rights; pain; *palliative care; *physicians; right to die; suffering;

BE = bioethics accession number   fn. = footnotes   refs. = references

*Supreme Court decisions; *terminal care; *terminally ill; wedge argument; withholding treatment; coma; *sedatives; *United States; *Vacco v. Quill; *Washington v. Glucksberg

Otlowski, Margaret. Voluntary Euthanasia and the Common Law. New York, NY: Oxford University Press; 1997. 564 p. Bibliography: p. 520–552. ISBN 0–19–825996–4. BE57847.
    active euthanasia; advisory committees; allowing to die; *assisted suicide; autonomy; constitutional law; *criminal law; double effect; drugs; *government regulation; informed consent; intention; *international aspects; knowledge, attitudes, practice; *legal aspects; legal liability; legislation; libertarianism; moral policy; morality; motivation; organizational policies; palliative care; physicians; policy analysis; professional organizations; public opinion; *public policy; terminally ill; treatment refusal; *voluntary euthanasia; withholding treatment; Appleton Consensus; *Australia; *Canada; Council of Europe; European Parliament; *Great Britain; *Netherlands; Netherlands State Commission on Euthanasia; Northern Territory; Remmelink Commission; Rights of the Terminally Ill Act (NT); Royal Dutch Medical Association; *United States

Randall, Fiona. Why causing death is not necessarily morally equivalent to allowing to die -- a response to Ferguson. *Journal of Medical Ethics.* 1997 Dec; 23(6): 373–376. 1 ref. Commentary on P.R. Ferguson, "Causing death or allowing to die? Developments in the law," p. 368–372. BE57665.
    *active euthanasia; *allowing to die; artificial feeding; *criminal law; futility; *intention; involuntary euthanasia; *killing; law; *legal aspects; legal liability; moral obligations; *moral policy; *morality; pain; patients; *persistent vegetative state; *physicians; public policy; quality of life; terminally ill; *withholding treatment; Airedale NHS Trust v. Bland; *Great Britain; Law Hospital NHS Trust v. Lord Advocate; R v. Cox

Schneider, Carl E. Hard cases. *Hastings Center Report.* 1998 Mar–Apr; 28(2): 24–26. 2 refs. BE57540.
    *active euthanasia; *children; *congenital disorders; *disabled; *fathers; justice; *killing; law; *legal aspects; *legal liability; pain; paralysis; punishment; quality of life; suffering; value of life; quadriplegia; *Canada; *Latimer v. the Queen; *Latimer, Robert; Latimer, Tracy; *R. v. Latimer; Saskatchewan

Sheldon, Tony. Dutch GP in euthanasia case will not go to prison. [News]. *BMJ (British Medical Journal).* 1997 Apr 19; 314(7088): 1148. BE57173.
    breast cancer; criminal law; drugs; guidelines; killing; *legal liability; mandatory reporting; *physicians; punishment; referral and consultation; terminally ill; *voluntary euthanasia; *Netherlands; Royal Dutch Medical Association; *Schat, Sippe

Sneiderman, Barney; Verhoef, Marja. Patient autonomy and the defence of medical necessity: five Dutch euthanasia cases. *Alberta Law Review.* 1996; 34(2): 374–415. 74 fn. BE59012.
    *active euthanasia; *assisted suicide; autonomy; *beneficence; case studies; chronically ill; criminal law; depressive disorder; drugs; guidelines; killing; *legal aspects; *legal liability; mentally ill; motivation; physically disabled; physician patient relationship; *physicians; professional organizations; public policy; quality of life; *suffering; treatment refusal; *voluntary euthanasia; *Netherlands; Royal Dutch Medical Association

Wallerstein, Claire. Philippines considers euthanasia bill. [News]. *BMJ (British Medical Journal).* 1997 Jun 7; 314(7095): 1644. BE55836.
    allowing to die; *euthanasia; *legal aspects; legislation; patients' rights; political activity; right to die; Roman

Catholics; *Philippines

Yount, Lisa. Should doctors ever hasten patients' deaths? [Juvenile literature]. *In: her* Issues in Biomedical Ethics. San Diego, CA: Lucent Books; 1998: 36–55, 101–102. 29 fn. ISBN 1–56006–476–5. BE57680.
    *active euthanasia; *allowing to die; artificial feeding; *assisted suicide; attitudes; *autonomy; biomedical technologies; coercion; competence; constitutional law; *decision making; due process; economics; equal protection; food; freedom; judicial action; *legal aspects; legal rights; legislation; pain; persistent vegetative state; physically disabled; physician patient relationship; physician's role; *physicians; prolongation of life; quality of life; *right to die; state government; state interest; suffering; Supreme Court decisions; terminal care; terminally ill; third party consent; treatment refusal; trust; value of life; ventilators; vulnerable populations; *wedge argument; withholding treatment; Bouvia, Elizabeth; Cruzan, Nancy; Death with Dignity Act (OR); Netherlands; New York; Oregon; Patient Self-Determination Act 1990; Quinlan, Karen; *United States; Washington

Zinn, Christopher. Australian doctors renew battle over euthanasia. [News]. *BMJ (British Medical Journal).* 1996 Jun 8; 312(7044): 1437. BE57347.
    *assisted suicide; attitudes; *decision making; *guidelines; *legal aspects; *organizational policies; *physicians; professional organizations; right to die; uncertainty; *voluntary euthanasia; *Australia; *Australian Medical Association; *Northern Territory; *Rights of the Terminally Ill Act (NT)

Zinn, Christopher. Australian voluntary euthanasia law is overturned. [News]. *BMJ (British Medical Journal).* 1997 Apr 5; 314(7086): 994. BE55838.
    *assisted suicide; attitudes; federal government; government financing; *legislation; organizational policies; *palliative care; physicians; professional organizations; terminal care; *voluntary euthanasia; *Australia; Australian Medical Association; *Northern Territory; *Rights of the Terminally Ill Act (NT)

EUTHANASIA/RELIGIOUS ASPECTS

Bernardin, Joseph. Euthanasia in the Catholic tradition. *In:* Langan, John P., ed. Joseph Cardinal Bernardin: A Moral Vision for America. Washington, DC: Georgetown University Press; 1998: 119–128. Visiting scholar lecture at Rockhurst College, Kansas City, MO, 1 Feb 1995. ISBN 0–87840–675–1. BE58525.
    *active euthanasia; *assisted suicide; attitudes; autonomy; biomedical technologies; international aspects; judicial action; legal aspects; legislation; *moral policy; physicians; *public policy; quality of life; *Roman Catholic ethics; state government; terminal care; *value of life; Europe; Kevorkian, Jack; Netherlands; *United States

Childress, James F. Religious viewpoints. *In:* Emanuel, Linda L., ed. Regulating How We Die: The Ethical, Medical, and Legal Issues Surrounding Physician–Assisted Suicide. Cambridge, MA: Harvard University Press; 1998: 120–147, 294–300. 54 fn. ISBN 0–674–66654–2. BE58536.
    active euthanasia; allowing to die; *assisted suicide; autonomy; covenant; dissent; double effect; extraordinary treatment; gifts; *Jewish ethics; killing; palliative care; *Protestant ethics; public policy; quality of life; *religious ethics; *Roman Catholic ethics; suffering; suicide; theology; value of life; voluntary euthanasia; wedge argument; withholding treatment; Evangelium Vitae; United States

Cook, E. David. The Medical Maze: A Christian Approach to Healthcare Ethics. London: Christian

---

BE = bioethics accession number   fn. = footnotes   refs. = references

Medical Fellowship; 1991. 22 p. ISBN 0–906747–24–4. BE58130.

*active euthanasia; attitudes to death; *Christian ethics; compassion; conscience; cultural pluralism; decision making; *medical ethics; moral policy; *physicians; suffering; *theology; value of life

Donovan, G. Kevin. Decisions at the end of life: Catholic tradition. *Christian Bioethics.* 1997 Dec; 3(3): 188–203. 22 refs. 4 fn. BE58488.

*active euthanasia; *allowing to die; artificial feeding; *assisted suicide; *attitudes to death; *brain death; cardiac death; costs and benefits; decision making; *determination of death; drugs; family members; informed consent; intention; organ donation; *pain; *palliative care; persistent vegetative state; prolongation of life; resuscitation; risks and benefits; *Roman Catholic ethics; *suffering; suicide; terminal care; *terminally ill; theology; third party consent; treatment outcome; treatment refusal; value of life; *withholding treatment; Congregation for the Doctrine of the Faith; National Conference of Catholic Bishops; United States

Medical decisions regarding end–of–life care have undergone significant changes in recent decades, driven by changes in both medicine and society. Catholic tradition in medical ethics offers clear guidance in many issues, and a moral framework accessible to those who do not share the same faith as well as to members of its faith community. In some areas, a Catholic perspective can be seen clearly and confidently, such as in teachings on the permissibility of suicide and euthanasia. In others, such as withdrawal of nutrition and hydration, the Church does not yet speak with one voice and has not closed out the discussion. Yet, it is not in the teaching on individual issues that a Catholic moral tradition offers the most help and comfort, but in its account of what it means to lead a life in Christ, and to prepare for a Christian death. As in the problem of pain and suffering, it is the spiritual support more than the ethical guidance that helps both patients and physicians bear the unbearable and fathom the unfathomable.

Fournier, Keith A.; Watkins, William D. In Defense of Life. Colorado Springs, CO: NavPress; 1996. 159 p. 352 fn. ISBN 08910–98801. BE56728.

aborted fetuses; *abortion, induced; *active euthanasia; aged; *allowing to die; *assisted suicide; beginning of life; body parts and fluids; brain death; *Christian ethics; commodification; congenital disorders; death; determination of death; disabled; economics; eugenics; fetal tissue donation; fetuses; government regulation; health personnel; historical aspects; human experimentation; infanticide; international aspects; judicial action; *killing; legal aspects; love; *morality; *newborns; organ donation; *political activity; population control; pregnant women; psychological stress; public policy; quality of life; rights; *value of life; *values; violence; hope; Humphry, Derek; Kevorkian, Jack; *Right to Life Movement; Roe v. Wade; Smith, Susan; United States

Geis, Sally B.; Messer, Donald E., eds. How Shall We Die?: Helping Christians Debate Assisted Suicide. Nashville, TN: Abingdon Press; 1997. 201 p. Annotated bibliography: p. 183–189. Appendices include generic forms for advance directives and for organ/tissue donation. ISBN 0–687–06140–7. BE57384.

*active euthanasia; advance directives; *allowing to die; *assisted suicide; attitudes to death; autonomy; beneficence; case studies; *Christian ethics; clergy; *decision making; diagnosis; drugs; ethics consultation; family members; forms; freedom; informed consent; killing; legal aspects; love; pain; palliative care; pastoral care; patients; physicians; prognosis; Protestant ethics; quality of life; resource allocation; right to die; Roman Catholic ethics; suffering; *suicide; terminally

ill; *theology; treatment refusal; truth disclosure; value of life; voluntary euthanasia; wedge argument; withholding treatment; Compassion in Dying v. State of Washington; Death with Dignity Act (OR); New York; Quill v. Vacco; United States; Washington

Guroian, Vigen. Life's Living toward Dying: A Theological and Medical–Ethical Study. Grand Rapids, MI: W.B. Eerdmans; 1996. 108 p. 130 fn. ISBN 0–8028–4190–2. BE55682.

*active euthanasia; *allowing to die; *assisted suicide; *attitudes to death; autonomy; *Christian ethics; Eastern Orthodox ethics; human experimentation; infants; killing; *literature; medicine; morality; physician's role; prolongation of life; religion; right to die; secularism; social impact; suffering; *terminal care; terminally ill; *theology; trends; values; Baby Rena; Kevorkian, Jack

Küng, Hans; Jens, Walter. A dignified dying: a plea for personal responsiblity. London: SCM Press; 1995. 132 p. 101 fn. Contributions by Dietrich Niethammer and Albin Eser. Translated from the 1995 German publication *Menschenw4rdig Sterben: Ein Pl1doyer f4r Selbstverantwortung.* ISBN 0–334–02609–1. BE55842.

*active euthanasia; advance directives; allowing to die; *assisted suicide; *attitudes to death; *autonomy; biomedical technologies; *Christian ethics; conscience; criminal law; *death; decision making; double effect; drugs; *freedom; guidelines; intention; international aspects; killing; *legal aspects; *literature; moral policy; physician patient relationship; *physicians; prolongation of life; public policy; quality of life; *right to die; Roman Catholic ethics; *suffering; suicide; terminal care; terminally ill; theology; treatment refusal; value of life; *voluntary euthanasia; withholding treatment; *dignity; patient abandonment; Evangelium Vitae; Germany; Netherlands

Larson, Edward J.; Amundsen, Darrel W. A Different Death: Euthanasia and the Christian Tradition. Downers Grove, IL: InterVarsity Press; 1998. 288 p. 587 fn. ISBN 0–8308–1518–X. BE58946.

*active euthanasia; advance directives; allowing to die; ancient history; artificial feeding; *assisted suicide; attitudes to death; biomedical technologies; caring; *Christian ethics; due process; equal protection; freedom; *historical aspects; hospices; involuntary euthanasia; Jewish ethics; killing; legal aspects; palliative care; physicians; privacy; public opinion; public policy; *right to die; selection for treatment; state interest; suffering; *suicide; terminally ill; *theology; third party consent; treatment refusal; value of life; voluntary euthanasia; war; wedge argument; withholding treatment; Eighteenth Century; Europe; Middle Ages; Netherlands; Nineteenth Century; Seventeenth Century; Sixteenth Century; Twentieth Century; United States

Paris, John J. Autonomy and physician–assisted suicide. *America.* 1997 May 17; 176(17): 11–14. BE55792.

*active euthanasia; *allowing to die; *assisted suicide; attitudes to death; *autonomy; biomedical technologies; *killing; *morality; patients' rights; *physicians; prolongation of life; public opinion; quality of life; *right to die; *Roman Catholic ethics; sociology of medicine; suffering; treatment refusal; withholding treatment; United States

Pellegrino, Edmund D. Evangelium Vitae, euthanasia, and physician–assisted suicide: John Paul II's dialogue with the culture and ethics of contemporary medicine. *In:* Wildes, Kevin Wm.; Mitchell, Alan C., eds. Choosing Life: A Dialogue on *Evangelium Vitae.* Washington, DC: Georgetown University Press; 1997: 236–253. 35 fn. ISBN 0–87840–646–8. BE56691.

allowing to die; artificial feeding; *assisted suicide; autonomy; bioethics; compassion; determination of death; double effect; freedom; intention; killing; moral obligations; morality; natural law; organ donation; pain; palliative care;

BE = bioethics accession number   fn. = footnotes   refs. = references

physician's role; *physicians; quality of life; *Roman
Catholic ethics; suffering; *theology; value of life;
*voluntary euthanasia; withholding treatment; dignity;
*Evangelium Vitae; John Paul II, Pope

Previn, Matthew P. Assisted suicide and religion:
conflicting conceptions of the sanctity of human life.
[Note]. *Georgetown Law Journal.* 1995 Feb; 84(3):
589–616. 163 fn. BE56701.
active euthanasia; ancient history; *assisted suicide;
autonomy; Christian ethics; compassion; competence;
*constitutional law; freedom; government regulation;
historical aspects; *humanism; *legal aspects; *legal rights;
love; philosophy; physicians; *religion; *religious ethics;
right to die; secularism; state government; state interest;
suffering; suicide; terminally ill; theology; *value of life;
*voluntary euthanasia; *United States

Rosner, Fred. Euthanasia. *In:* Dorff, Elliot N.; Newman,
Louis E., eds. Contemporary Jewish Ethics and
Morality: A Reader. New York, NY: Oxford University
Press; 1995: 350–362. 76 fn. Reprinted from Rosner,
Fred; Bleich, J. David, eds., *Jewish Bioethics*, New
York, NY: Hebrew Publishing Co., 1979: 253–265. ISBN
0-19-509066-7. BE58528.
*active euthanasia; *allowing to die; assisted suicide;
Christian ethics; eugenics; *euthanasia; international aspects;
involuntary euthanasia; *Jewish ethics; killing; legal aspects;
physicians; suffering; terminally ill; terminology; *theology;
voluntary euthanasia; withholding treatment; Orthodox
Judaism

Stempsey, William E. End-of-life decisions: Christian
perspectives. *Christian Bioethics.* 1997 Dec; 3(3): 249–261.
21 refs. 3 fn. BE58490.
*active euthanasia; *allowing to die; *assisted suicide;
*attitudes to death; autonomy; *Christian ethics; conscience;
constitutional law; costs and benefits; decision making;
*Eastern Orthodox ethics; human body; legal rights;
libertarianism; moral obligations; morality; *natural law;
personhood; physicians; prolongation of life; *Protestant
ethics; risks and benefits; *Roman Catholic ethics;
*secularism; suffering; Supreme Court decisions; *terminally
ill; *theology; value of life; values; withholding treatment;
*Methodist Church; United States; Vacco v. Quill;
Washington v. Glucksberg
While legal rights to make medical treatment decisions
at the end of one's life have been recognized by the
courts, particular religious traditions put axiological and
metaphysical meat on the bare bones of legal rights. Mere
legal rights do not capture the full reality, meaning and
importance of death. End-of-life decisions reflect not
only the meaning we find in dying, but also the meaning
we have found in living. The Christian religions bring
particular understandings of the vision of life as a gift
from God, human responsibility for stewardship of that
life, the wholeness of the person, and the importance
of the dying process in preparing spiritually for life
beyond earthly life, to bear on end-of-life decisions.

Thobaben, James R. A United Methodist approach to
end-of-life decisions: intentional ambiguity or ambiguous
intentions. *Christian Bioethics.* 1997 Dec; 3(3): 222–248.
40 refs. 22 fn. BE58491.
*active euthanasia; advance directives; *allowing to die;
*assisted suicide; autonomy; *clergy; competence; *decision
making; *dissent; family members; historical aspects;
hospices; *organizational policies; pain; pastoral care;
personhood; physicians; *Protestant ethics; quality of life;
suffering; suicide; terminal care; *terminally ill; terminology;
theology; third party consent; treatment refusal; uncertainty;
vulnerable populations; withholding treatment; *Methodist
Church; *Wesley, John
The position of the United Methodist Church on

end-of-life decisions is best described as intentional
ambiguity or ambiguous intentions or both. The paper
analyzes the official position of the denomination and
then considers the actions of a U.M.C. bishop who
served as a foreman for a trial of Dr. Jack Kevorkian.
In an effort to find some common ground within an
increasingly divided denomination, the work concludes
with a consideration of the work of John Wesley and
his approach to human death.

Werber, Stephen J. Ancient answers to modern questions:
death, dying, and organ transplants -- a Jewish law
perspective. *Journal of Law and Health.* 1996–1997;
11(1–2): 13–44. 139 fn. BE57589.
*active euthanasia; *allowing to die; *assisted suicide; brain
death; cadavers; chronically ill; *determination of death;
hearts; *Jewish ethics; killing; *organ donation; organ
donors; organ transplantation; physicians; *resuscitation
orders; right to die; *suicide; terminally ill; tissue donation;
treatment refusal; value of life; withholding treatment;
Orthodox Judaism

Zohar, Noam J. Death: natural process and human
intervention. *In: his* Alternatives in Jewish Bioethics.
Albany, NY: State University of New York Press; 1997:
37–68. 42 fn. ISBN 0-7914-3274-2. BE57042.
*active euthanasia; allowing to die; *assisted suicide; death;
deontological ethics; hospices; *Jewish ethics; killing;
medicine; palliative care; prolongation of life; suffering;
suicide; terminally ill; *theology; value of life; *voluntary
euthanasia

FAMILY PLANNING *See* CONTRACEPTION, POPULATION CONTROL

FETUSES

See also ABORTION, EMBRYO AND FETAL
RESEARCH, PRENATAL INJURIES

**Andersen, C. Yding; Westergaard, L.G.; Grinsted, J.,
et al.** Frozen embryos: too cold to touch? Frozen
pre-embryos in Denmark. *Human Reproduction.* 1996
Apr; 11(4): 703. 3 refs. BE56852.
*cryopreservation; *embryo disposition; embryo transfer;
*embryos; *government regulation; *in vitro fertilization;
legal aspects; statistics; time factors; *Denmark

Annas, George J. The shadowlands -- secrets, lies, and
assisted reproduction. *New England Journal of Medicine.*
1998 Sep 24; 339(13): 935–939. 28 refs. BE59074.
advisory committees; *children; confidentiality; contracts;
cryopreservation; *embryo disposition; embryo research;
embryo transfer; *embryos; federal government; government
regulation; in vitro fertilization; informed consent; judicial
action; *legal aspects; mothers; ovum donors; *parent child
relationship; *public policy; records; *reproductive
technologies; semen donors; standards; surrogate mothers;
divorce; *Buzzanca v. Buzzanca; California; *Kass v. Kass;
New York; *New York State Task Force on Life and the
Law; *United States

Barlow, Bicka A. Severe penalties for the destruction of
"potential life" -- cruel and unusual punishment?
[Comment]. *University of San Francisco Law Review.* 1995
Winter; 29(2): 463–508. 401 fn. Appendix: [model] Fetal
Homicide Statute. BE57274.
abortion, induced; beginning of life; constitutional law;
*criminal law; fetal development; *fetuses; intention;
*killing; *legal liability; model legislation; *personhood;
pregnant women; punishment; standards; state government;
state interest; viability; violence; wrongful death;

---

miscarriage; *Eighth Amendment; United States

Bermúdez, José Luis. The moral significance of birth. *Ethics.* 1996 Jan; 106(2): 378–403. 31 fn. BE55688.
   abortion, induced; beginning of life; *childbirth; *ethical analysis; fetal development; *fetuses; infanticide; killing; *moral policy; *newborns; *personhood; philosophy; prematurity; primates; psychology; *self concept; speciesism; *value of life

Brazier, Margaret. Hard cases make bad law? [Editorial]. *Journal of Medical Ethics.* 1997 Dec; 23(6): 341–343. 3 refs. BE57656.
   *artificial insemination; cesarean section; *coercion; compensation; *competence; cryopreservation; death; *decision making; *fetuses; government regulation; guidelines; informed consent; *judicial action; *legal aspects; legal rights; married persons; physicians; *posthumous reproduction; *pregnant women; professional organizations; remuneration; semen donors; sperm; *surrogate mothers; *treatment refusal; Blood, Diane; European Union; *Great Britain; Human Fertilisation and Embryology Act 1990; Human Fertilisation and Embryology Authority; In re MB (Caesarean Section); R v. Human Fertilisation and Embryology Authority (ex parte Blood); Re S (Adult: Medical Treatment); Royal College of Obstetricians and Gynaecologists

Breitowitz, Yitzchok A. Halakhic approaches to the resolution of disputes concerning the disposition of preembryos. *In:* Feldman, Emanuel; Wolowelsky, Joel B., eds. Jewish Law and the New Reproductive Technologies. Hoboken, NJ: Ktav; 1997: 155–186. 95 fn. ISBN 0–88125–586–6. BE57461.
   cryopreservation; death; *decision making; dissent; *embryo disposition; embryo research; embryo transfer; *embryos; fathers; *in vitro fertilization; *Jewish ethics; marital relationship; mothers; parent child relationship; property rights; reproductive technologies; surrogate mothers; theology; divorce; Orthodox Judaism

Brown, Barry. Reconciling property law with advances in reproductive science. *Stanford Law and Policy Review.* 1995; 6(2): 73–88. 113 fn. BE56485.
   artificial insemination; body parts and fluids; confidentiality; *cryopreservation; death; decision making; dissent; *embryo disposition; *embryos; eugenics; females; future generations; gene therapy; genetic enhancement; genetic information; *genetic intervention; genetic screening; *germ cells; government regulation; in vitro fertilization; international aspects; *legal aspects; males; mandatory testing; parents; preimplantation diagnosis; privacy; *property rights; *public policy; reproduction; *reproductive technologies; state interest; divorce; Davis v. Davis; Hecht v. Superior Court (Kane); *United States

Chervenak, Frank A.; McCullough, Laurence B.; Kurjak, Asim. An essential clinical ethical concept. *In:* Chervenak, Frank A.; Kurjak, Asim, eds. Current Perspectives on the Fetus as a Patient. New York, NY: Parthenon Publishing Group; 1996: 1–9. 27 refs. ISBN 1–85070–742–1. BE57644.
   autonomy; beginning of life; beneficence; congenital disorders; *counseling; cultural pluralism; *directive counseling; *ethical analysis; ethics; *fetal therapy; *fetuses; informed consent; law; medical ethics; *moral obligations; morality; mother fetus relationship; *obstetrics and gynecology; patient care; personhood; physician patient relationship; *physicians; *pregnant women; prematurity; prenatal diagnosis; selective abortion; treatment refusal; value of life; *viability; virtues

Chervenak, Frank A.; McCullough, Laurence B. What is obstetric ethics? *Journal of Perinatal Medicine.* 1995; 23(5): 331–341. 52 refs. BE57763.
   autonomy; beneficence; clinical ethics; consensus; directive counseling; embryos; ethical analysis; ethical theory; fetal development; fetal therapy; *fetuses; informed consent; law; *medical ethics; moral obligations; *obstetrics and gynecology; *patient care; physicians; *pregnant women; prenatal diagnosis; religion; value of life; viability

Csordas, Thomas J. A handmaid's tale: the rhetoric of personhood in American and Japanese healing of abortions. *In:* Sargent, Carolyn F.; Brettell, Caroline B., eds. Gender and Health: An International Perspective. Upper Saddle River, NJ: Prentice Hall; 1996: 227–241. 23 refs. 5 fn. ISBN 0–13–079427–9. BE58095.
   *aborted fetuses; *abortion, induced; *Buddhist ethics; comparative studies; emotions; *females; international aspects; mother fetus relationship; *personhood; *psychological stress; psychology; *religion; *Roman Catholics; grief; guilt; *Japan; *Pentecostal Christians; *United States

Delany, Linda. Court-authorised caesareans: new guidance. *Health Care Analysis.* 1997 Sep; 5(3): 240–241, 243. 10 fn. BE55820.
   autonomy; *cesarean section; coercion; *competence; *fetuses; guidelines; *judicial action; *legal aspects; legal rights; *pregnant women; *treatment refusal; *Great Britain; *Re MB (Caesarean Section)

Demartis, Francesco. Mass pre-embryo adoption. *Cambridge Quarterly of Healthcare Ethics.* 1998 Winter; 7(1): 101–103. 15 fn. BE58452.
   *adoption; *beginning of life; *cryopreservation; dissent; *embryo disposition; embryo transfer; *embryos; international aspects; personhood; *Roman Catholics; *value of life; Great Britain; *Italy

Elkins, Thomas E.; Brown, Douglas. Ethical issues in the utilization of cesarean section. *In:* Flamm, B.L.; Quilligan, E.J., eds. Cesarean Section: Guidelines for Appropriate Utilization. New York, NY: Springer-Verlag; 1995: 191–205. 69 refs. ISBN 0387–94238–6. BE56682.
   autonomy; blood transfusions; *cesarean section; childbirth; *coercion; *decision making; developing countries; fetal therapy; *fetuses; informed consent; *judicial action; *legal aspects; maternal health; minority groups; *moral obligations; newborns; *obstetrics and gynecology; *organizational policies; *patient care; patient compliance; patient participation; physician patient relationship; *physicians; *pregnant women; privacy; professional organizations; prognosis; *risks and benefits; selection for treatment; socioeconomic factors; state interest; terminally ill; *treatment refusal; viability; *American Academy of Pediatrics; *American College of Obstetricians and Gynecologists; *American Medical Association; District of Columbia; *In re A.C.; *United States

Elliston, Sarah. Life after death? Legal and ethical considerations of maintaining pregnancy in brain dead women. *In:* Petersen, Kerry, ed. Intersections: Women on Law, Medicine and Technology. Brookfield, VT: Ashgate; 1997: 145–164. 23 refs. 7 fn. ISBN 1–85521–882–8. BE57490.
   advance directives; *autonomy; *brain death; cadavers; childbirth; *decision making; determination of death; *fetuses; informed consent; *legal aspects; models, theoretical; mother fetus relationship; *patient care; *pregnant women; *prolongation of life; treatment refusal; *withholding treatment; women's rights; *Great Britain

Espinoza, Leslie G. Dissecting women, dissecting law: the court-ordering of caesarean section operations and the failure of informed consent to protect women of color. *National Black Law Journal.* 1994; 13: 211–237.

---

211 fn. BE58974.

    Asian Americans; autonomy; blacks; *cesarean section;
*coercion; communication; competence; cultural pluralism;
decision making; *fetuses; Hispanic Americans; hospitals;
indigents; *informed consent; judicial action; *legal aspects;
legal rights; *minority groups; mother fetus relationship;
physicians; *pregnant women; social discrimination; *state
interest; terminally ill; *treatment refusal; *viability; District
of Columbia; George Washington University Hospital; *In
re A.C.; In re Madyun

Flagler, Elizabeth; Baylis, Françoise; Rodgers, Sanda.
Bioethics for clinicians: 12. Ethical dilemmas that arise
in the care of pregnant women: rethinking
"maternal–fetal conflicts." *Canadian Medical Association
Journal.* 1997 Jun 15; 156(12): 1729–1732. 34 refs.
BE57354.

    AIDS serodiagnosis; autonomy; case studies; cesarean
section; coercion; *fetuses; *legal aspects; legal rights; moral
obligations; mother fetus relationship; obstetrics and
gynecology; patient care; personhood; physicians; *pregnant
women; *treatment refusal; *Canada

Fletcher, John C. Ethical considerations in and beyond
experimental fetal therapy. *Seminars in Perinatology.* 1985
Jul; 9(2): 130–135. 20 refs. BE56960.

    abortion, induced; cesarean section; coercion; costs and
benefits; federal government; *fetal development; *fetal
research; *fetal therapy; *fetuses; financial support;
government regulation; guidelines; legal aspects; moral
obligations; mortality; parental consent; patient care team;
pregnant women; prenatal diagnosis; private sector; research
ethics committees; risks and benefits; selection for treatment;
state interest; surgery; therapeutic research; treatment
outcome; treatment refusal; trends; twins; viability; United
States

Folscheid, Dominique. The status of the embryo from a
Christian perspective. *Studies in Christian Ethics.* 1996;
9(2): 16–21. BE55683.

    beginning of life; *embryos; moral obligations; personhood;
*Roman Catholic ethics; science; *value of life

Ford, Norman. Fetus. *In:* Chadwick, Ruth, ed.
Encyclopedia of Applied Ethics, Volume 2. San Diego,
CA: Academic Press; 1998: 289–298. 11 refs. ISBN
0–12–227067–3. BE56385.

    aborted fetuses; abortion, induced; *beginning of life;
*embryos; fetal development; fetal research; fetal therapy;
fetal tissue donation; *fetuses; gene therapy; *moral policy;
mother fetus relationship; nontherapeutic research;
personhood; pregnant women; rights; risks and benefits;
surgery; theology; therapeutic research; treatment refusal;
twinning; value of life

German, L.G. The beginning of individual human life.
Linacre Quarterly. 1997 May; 64(2): 94–95. 8 fn. BE55617.
    *beginning of life; *embryos; genetic identity

Gillam, Lynn. Arguing by analogy in the fetal tissue
debate. *Bioethics.* 1997 Oct; 11(5): 397–412. 18 fn.
BE56328.

    *aborted fetuses; *abortion, induced; adults; attitudes;
cadavers; *ethical analysis; ethical theory; *fetal tissue
donation; government regulation; incentives; *killing; *moral
complicity; *moral policy; organ donation; physicians;
pregnant women; prisoners; public policy; social impact;
tissue transplantation

In the debate over fetal tissue use, an analogy is often
drawn between removing organs from the body of a
person who has been murdered to use for transplantation,
and collecting tissue from an aborted fetus to use for
the same purpose. The murder victim analogy is taken
by its proponents to show that even if abortion is the

moral equivalent of murder, there is still no good reason
to refrain from using the fetal tissue, since as a society
we do not see any problem about using organs from
murder victims. However, I argue that the analogy
between murder victims and aborted fetuses does not
hold -- the two situations are not the same in all morally
relevant respects. Thus the murder victim analogy does
not provide an argument in favour of fetal tissue
transplant. In conclusion, I point to some of the potential
pitfalls of using analogies in ethical argument.

Graber, Glenn C. The moral status of gametes and
embryos: storage and surrogacy. *In:* Monagle, John F.;
Thomasma, David C., eds. Health Care Ethics: Critical
Issues for the 21st Century. Gaithersburg, MD: Aspen
Publishers; 1998: 8–14. 10 refs. ISBN 0–8342–0911–X.
BE56276.

    cryopreservation; *embryos; moral obligations; *moral
policy; parent child relationship; personhood; reproductive
technologies; surrogate mothers

Grubb, Andrew. The Human Fertilisation and
Embryology (Statutory Storage Period for Embryos)
Regulations 1996 (S.I. 1996 No. 375). [Comment].
Medical Law Review. 1996 Summer; 4(2): 211–215.
BE56591.

    *cryopreservation; donors; *embryo disposition; embryo
research; embryo transfer; *embryos; genetic disorders;
*government regulation; guidelines; *in vitro fertilization;
infertility; informed consent; legislation; patients; surrogate
mothers; *time factors; *Great Britain; Human Fertilisation
and Embryology Act 1990; *Human Fertilisation and
Embryology Authority

Harris, Cathleen M.; Mahowald, Mary B. Women and
alcohol abuse. *In:* Shelton, Wayne N.; Edwards, Rem
B., eds. Advances in Bioethics. Volume 3: Values, Ethics,
and Alcoholism. Greenwich, CT: JAI Press; 1997:
153–170. 69 refs. ISBN 0–7623–0219–4. BE57637.

    accountability; *alcohol abuse; autonomy; *behavior control;
*coercion; congenital disorders; criminal law; decision
making; disease; *females; *fetuses; indigents; legal aspects;
mandatory programs; minority groups; moral obligations;
newborns; *patient care; *pregnant women; *prenatal
injuries; privacy; psychological stress; public policy;
reproduction; rights; self concept; sexuality; social
discrimination; socioeconomic factors; state interest;
*stigmatization; value of life; women's health services;
women's rights; United States

Hersey, Jonathan. Enigma of the unborn mother: legal
and ethical considerations of aborted fetal ovarian tissue
and ova transplantations. *UCLA Law Review.* 1995 Oct;
43(1): 159–207. 228 fn. BE57196.

    *aborted fetuses; abortion, induced; advisory committees;
conflict of interest; decision making; directed donation;
federal government; females; fetal research; *fetal tissue
donation; *government regulation; in vitro fertilization;
infertility; informed consent; *legal aspects; legal rights;
*organ donation; *ovum donors; property rights; *public
policy; risks and benefits; scarcity; social impact; state
government; *ovaries; Great Britain; National Organ
Transplant Act 1984; Uniform Anatomical Gift Act; *United
States

Holm, Søren. Embryology, ethics of. *In:* Chadwick, Ruth,
ed. Encyclopedia of Applied Ethics, Volume 2. San
Diego, CA: Academic Press; 1998: 39–45. 7 refs. ISBN
0–12–227067–3. BE56380.

    abortion, induced; *beginning of life; embryo research;
*embryos; fetal development; *fetuses; in vitro fertilization;
killing; *moral policy; philosophy; reproductive
technologies; research embryo creation; rights; theology;
twinning; viability; personal identity

Inciardi, James A.; Surratt, Hilary L.; Saum, Christine A. Prenatal cocaine use and the prosecution of pregnant addicts. *In: their* Cocaine-Exposed Infants: Social, Legal, and Public Health Issues. Thousand Oaks, CA: Sage Publications; 1997: 62–85. References embedded in list at back of book. ISBN 0-8039-7087-0. BE57226.

alcohol abuse; child abuse; constitutional law; criminal law; death; *drug abuse; due process; equal protection; *fetuses; health facilities; involuntary commitment; killing; *legal aspects; *legal liability; *legal rights; newborns; parents; personhood; *pregnant women; *prenatal injuries; privacy; punishment; state government; state interest; torts; viability; Alaska v. Grubbs; California; Eighth Amendment; Florida; Florida v. Johnson; Fourteenth Amendment; In re Ruiz; Ohio; People v. Stewart; Roe v. Wade; *United States; Webster v. Reproductive Health Services

Johnston, S.R.D.; Broadley, K.; Henson, G., et al. Management of metastatic melanoma during pregnancy. [Case study and commentaries]. *BMJ (British Medical Journal).* 1998 Mar 14; 316(7134): 848–851. 13 refs. BE57757.

altruism; *cancer; case studies; cesarean section; *childbirth; *decision making; drugs; fetal development; *fetuses; maternal health; morbidity; mortality; parents; *patient care; *pregnant women; *prognosis; radiology; *risks and benefits; terminally ill; *therapeutic abortion; viability

Khushf, George. Embryo research: the ethical geography of the debate. *Journal of Medicine and Philosophy.* 1997 Oct; 22(5): 495–519. 36 refs. 9 fn. BE56624.

abortion, induced; advisory committees; *beginning of life; consensus; *embryo research; *embryos; federal government; fetal development; *government financing; *government regulation; human experimentation; in vitro fertilization; informed consent; libertarianism; *moral obligations; *moral policy; nontherapeutic research; *personhood; *policy analysis; *politics; private sector; *public policy; reproductive technologies; research design; research embryo creation; risks and benefits; science; twinning; value of life; *Human Embryo Research Panel; United States

Three basic political positions on embryo research will be identified as libertarian, conservative, and social-democratic. The Human Embryo Research Panel will be regarded as an expression of the social-democratic position. A taxonomy of the ethical issues addressed by the Panel will then be developed at the juncture of political and ethical modes of reflection. Among the arguments considered will be those for the separability of the abortion and embryo research debates; arguments against the possibility of the preembryo being a person, especially arguments associated with totipotency and the significance of the primitive streak; and the various reasons for regulating embryo research, including those associated with respect for the preembryo, the protection of traditional views of human procreation, and the prevention of commercialization.

Kinney, Joanna H. Restricting donative choice: fetal tissue transplantation and respect for human life. *Journal of Law and Health.* 1995-1996; 10(2): 259–285. 121 fn. BE57145.

*aborted fetuses; abortion, induced; casuistry; diabetes; *directed donation; fetal research; *fetal tissue donation; fetuses; government regulation; intention; *legal aspects; legal rights; moral obligations; motivation; pregnant women; state government; tissue transplantation; war; *United States

Kischer, C. Ward. The media and human embryology. *Linacre Quarterly.* 1998 May; 65(2): 33–42. 12 refs. BE58932.

abortion, induced; anencephaly; *beginning of life; embryo research; *embryos; *fetal development; fetal tissue donation; *fetuses; *mass media; organ donation; prenatal injuries; technical expertise; United States

Klasing, Murphy S. Death of an unborn child: jurisprudential inconsistencies in wrongful death, criminal homicide, and abortion cases. *Pepperdine Law Review.* 1995; 22(3): 933–979. 385 fn. BE56670.

*abortion, induced; *beginning of life; criminal law; fetal development; *fetuses; judicial action; killing; *legal aspects; *legal liability; negligence; newborns; *personhood; prenatal injuries; *state government; Supreme Court decisions; torts; *viability; *wrongful death; *United States

Korein, Julius. Ontogenesis of the brain in the human organism: definitions of life and death of the human being and person. *In:* Edwards, Rem B., ed. Advances in Bioethics. Volume 2: New Essays on Abortion and Bioethics. Greenwich, CT: JAI Press; 1997: 1–74. 298 refs. ISBN 0-7623-0194-5. BE56789.

abortion, induced; adults; *anencephaly; *beginning of life; *brain; *brain death; children; *determination of death; diagnosis; embryos; *fetal development; *fetuses; infants; newborns; organ transplantation; persistent vegetative state; *personhood; prognosis; tissue transplantation

Lamb, David. Ethics of fetal tissue transplants. *In:* Frith, Lucy, ed. Ethics and Midwifery: Issues in Contemporary Practice. Boston, MA: Butterworth-Heinemann; 1996: 156–169. 14 refs. ISBN 0-7506-3056-6. BE58638.

*aborted fetuses; abortion, induced; advisory committees; commodification; *fetal tissue donation; guidelines; incentives; informed consent; *moral policy; pregnant women; public policy; risks and benefits; *Great Britain; Polkinghorne Report

Langston, J. William; Palfreman, Jon. The Case of the Frozen Addicts: Working at the Edge of the Mysteries of the Human Brain. New York, NY: Vintage Books; 1996. 309 p. ISBN 0-678-74708-7. BE56698.

*aborted fetuses; animal experimentation; biomedical research; *brain; *brain pathology; diagnosis; disadvantaged; *drug abuse; federal government; *fetal research; *fetal tissue donation; government financing; *heroin; human experimentation; international aspects; interprofessional relations; *investigators; moral complicity; *paralysis; patients; primates; research institutes; research subjects; risks and benefits; selection of subjects; therapeutic research; *tissue transplantation; *toxicity; *Parkinson disease; Human Fetal Tissue Transplantation Research Panel; *Langston, J. William; Lindvall, Olle; National Institutes of Health; Sweden; United States

Leavine, Barbara Ann. Court-ordered cesareans: can a pregnant woman refuse? *Houston Law Review.* 1992 Spring; 29(1): 185–218. 276 fn. BE56978.

abortion, induced; autonomy; *cesarean section; coercion; decision making; *fetuses; *judicial action; *legal aspects; *legal rights; physicians; *pregnant women; privacy; *state interest; Supreme Court decisions; *treatment refusal; value of life; viability; *women's rights; District of Columbia; In re A.C.; Roe v. Wade; *United States

Macready, Norra. US state rules that a viable fetus is a person. [News]. *BMJ (British Medical Journal).* 1997 Dec 6; 315(7121): 1488. BE57262.

child abuse; *drug abuse; *fetuses; *legal aspects; legal liability; *personhood; *pregnant women; *prenatal injuries; state government; *viability; *South Carolina; *Whitner, Cornelia

Mair, Jane. Maternal/foetal conflict: defined or defused? *In:* McLean, Sheila A.M., ed. Contemporary Issues in

---

Law, Medicine and Ethics. Brookfield, VT: Dartmouth; 1996: 79–97. 45 fn. ISBN 1-85521-586-1. BE57791.
autonomy; cesarean section; *coercion; communication; compensation; *drug abuse; *fetuses; freedom; guidelines; health; informed consent; international aspects; judicial action; *legal aspects; *legal liability; legal obligations; *legal rights; moral obligations; newborns; personhood; physicians; *pregnant women; *prenatal injuries; privacy; religion; state interest; torts; *treatment refusal; viability; women's rights; *Great Britain; United States

Patterson, Elizabeth G. Human rights and human life: an uneven fit. *Tulane Law Review.* 1994 Jun; 68(6): 1527–1561. 168 fn. BE55539.
abortion, induced; adults; allowing to die; *anencephaly; autonomy; beginning of life; *brain death; cadavers; *competence; determination of death; equal protection; *fetuses; human rights; informed consent; *legal aspects; *legal rights; mentally disabled; *minors; newborns; *persistent vegetative state; *personhood; quality of life; Supreme Court decisions; third party consent; treatment refusal; *value of life; withholding treatment; *United States

Peters, Ted. Designer genes and selective abortion. *In: his* For the Love of Children: Genetic Technology and the Future of the Family. Louisville, KY: Westminster John Knox Press; 1996: 85–118, 193–199. 63 fn. ISBN 0-664-25468-3. BE55697.
adoption; beginning of life; coercion; confidentiality; decision making; disabled; employment; eugenics; fetal development; *fetuses; genetic counseling; *genetic disorders; genetic information; *genetic predisposition; *genetic screening; government regulation; insurance; killing; legal rights; *personhood; pregnant women; prenatal diagnosis; privacy; Protestant ethics; public policy; risk; *Roman Catholic ethics; *selective abortion; *social discrimination; value of life; viability; dignity; Genetic Privacy Act 1994; United States

Pinkerton, JoAnn V.; Finnerty, James J.; Sosnowski, J. Richard. Resolving the clinical and ethical dilemma involved in fetal-maternal conflicts. [Article and discussion]. *American Journal of Obstetrics and Gynecology.* 1996 Aug; 175(2): 289–295. 28 refs. Presented at the Fifty-Eighth Annual Meeting of the South Atlantic Association of Obstetricians and Gynecologists, 27–30 Jan 1996. BE57969.
allowing to die; *autonomy; *beneficence; *cesarean section; clinical ethics committees; *coercion; competence; counseling; *decision making; ethics consultation; fetal therapy; *fetuses; guidelines; informed consent; *hospitals; *institutional policies; *judicial action; moral obligations; moral policy; patient care team; patient transfer; *practice guidelines; *pregnant women; prolongation of life; religion; rights; risks and benefits; state interest; terminally ill; third party consent; *treatment refusal; viability; In re A.C.; In re Baby Boy Doe v. Mother Doe; In re Madgun; Jefferson v. Griffin Spalding Co. Hospital Authority; United States; *University of Virginia Health Services Center

Ramsay, Sarah. UK woman wins right to refuse caesarean section. [News]. *Lancet.* 1998 May 16; 351(9114): 1499. BE58888.
*cesarean section; *fetuses; *legal aspects; *legal rights; *pregnant women; *treatment refusal; *Great Britain; *Re S; St. George's Hospital

Robertson, John A. Meaning what you sign. *Hastings Center Report.* 1998 Jul–Aug; 28(4): 22–23. 4 refs. BE58924.
advance directives; autonomy; contracts; *cryopreservation; decision making; *embryo disposition; embryo research; *embryos; *in vitro fertilization; informed consent; *legal aspects; marital relationship; married persons; *property rights; *divorce; Davis v. Davis; *Kass v. Kass; *New York;

Tennessee

Rossiter, Graham P. Contemporary transatlantic developments concerning compelled medical treatment of pregnant women. *Australian and New Zealand Journal of Obstetrics and Gynaecology.* 1995 May; 35(2): 132–138. 28 fn. BE55889.
*autonomy; blood transfusions; cesarean section; *coercion; competence; decision making; emergency care; *fetuses; hospitals; informed consent; *international aspects; Jehovah's Witnesses; judicial action; *legal aspects; legal liability; legal rights; obstetrics and gynecology; physicians; *pregnant women; prognosis; religion; state interest; *treatment refusal; viability; women's rights; *Great Britain; In re A.C.; Jefferson v. Griffin Spalding Co. Hospital Authority; New Zealand; Re S (Adult: Refusal of Medical Treatment); Re T (Adult: Refusal of Medical Treatment); State of Illinois v. Bricci; *United States

Sapin, Emmanuel. The horizons of fetal medicine and its ethical consequences. *Dolentium Hominum: Church and Health in the World.* 1996; 31(11th Yr., No. 1): 155–158. BE57374.
aborted fetuses; beginning of life; blood transfusions; congenital disorders; counseling; diabetes; drugs; eugenics; *fetal therapy; fetal tissue donation; fetuses; genetic disorders; neural tube defects; parents; pregnant women; prematurity; *prenatal diagnosis; preventive medicine; quality of life; selective abortion; value of life; vitamins

Schwartz, Lewis M. An essay on the moral status question. *In:* Edwards, Rem B., ed. Advances in Bioethics. Volume 2: New Essays on Abortion and Bioethics. Greenwich, CT: JAI Press; 1997: 267–301. 11 refs. ISBN 0-7623-0194-5. BE56797.
*abortion, induced; adults; *fetal development; *fetuses; *killing; *moral obligations; *moral policy; pain; persistent vegetative state; *personhood; philosophy

Shannon, Thomas A. Fetal status: sources and implications. *Journal of Medicine and Philosophy.* 1997 Oct; 22(5): 415–422. 2 refs. BE56619.
abortion, induced; *attitudes; beginning of life; biomedical technologies; cesarean section; coercion; drug abuse; embryo research; *embryos; fetal development; fetal therapy; fetal tissue donation; *fetuses; intensive care units; *moral obligations; newborns; *personhood; pregnant women; preimplantation diagnosis; prematurity; prenatal diagnosis; prenatal injuries; public policy; reproductive technologies; treatment refusal; utilitarianism; *value of life; viability; United States
This essay considers the ways in which the various contexts — abortion, prenatal diagnosis, fetal research, and the use of fetuses in transplantation — shape the American debate on the moral standing of the fetus. This discussion gives rise to several philosophical debates on the status of the preimplantation embryo, particularly the debate over when the preimplantation embryo becomes individuated. How that questions is resolved has critical ethical and policy implications.

Shannon, Thomas A. Response to Khushf. *Journal of Medicine and Philosophy.* 1997 Oct; 22(5): 525–527. 4 refs. BE56626.
*beginning of life; embryo research; *embryos; fetal development; moral obligations; *personhood; twinning

Strasser, Mark. Dependence, reliance and abortion. *Philosophical Quarterly.* 1985 Jan; 35(138): 73–82. 6 fn. Commentary on M. Davis, "Foetuses, famous violinists, and the right to continued aid," *PQ* 1983 Jul; 33(132): 259–278. BE57840.
*abortion, induced; altruism; *fetuses; justice; killing; *moral obligations; *moral policy; *mother fetus relationship;

BE = bioethics accession number   fn. = footnotes   refs. = references

personhood; *pregnant women; rights; viability

Strong, Carson. Response to Khushf. *Journal of Medicine and Philosophy.* 1997 Oct; 22(5): 521–523. 5 refs. BE56625.
   *beginning of life; embryo research; *embryos; *fetal development; moral obligations; *personhood; research embryo creation; value of life

Strong, Carson. The moral status of preembryos, embryos, fetuses, and infants. *Journal of Medicine and Philosophy.* 1997 Oct; 22(5): 457–478. 32 refs. 4 fn. BE56622.
   *beginning of life; embryo disposition; embryo research; *embryos; *fetal development; *fetuses; *human characteristics; legal aspects; *moral obligations; *moral policy; *newborns; *personhood; property rights; research embryo creation; risks and benefits; self concept; social interaction; teleological ethics; value of life; viability
Some have argued that embryos and fetuses have the moral status of personhood because of certain criteria that are satisfied during gestation. However, these attempts to base personhood during gestation on intrinsic characteristics have uniformly been unsuccessful. Within a secular framework, another approach to establishing a moral standing for embryos and fetuses is to argue that we ought to confer some moral status upon them. There appear to be two main approaches to defending conferred moral standing; namely, consequentialist and contractarian arguments. This article puts forward a consequentialist argument for the conferred moral standing of preembryos, embryos, fetuses, and infants. It states and defends an original version of the commonly-held view that moral standing increases during gestation. It also explores the implications of this viewpoint for several issues: what is involved in showing 'respect' for preembryos; and whether it is permissible to create preembryos solely for research.

Sweden. Ministry of Health and Social Affairs. The Swedish Transplant Act. [Pamphlet]. Stockholm: Ministry of Health and Social Affairs; 1997. 52 p. Appendix: text of the Swedish Transplant Act 1995. BE57746.
   aborted fetuses; cadavers; economics; family members; *fetal tissue donation; informed consent; *legal aspects; legislation; mentally disabled; minors; *organ donation; organ donors; presumed consent; third party consent; tissue donation; *Sweden; *Transplant Act 1995 (Sweden)

Wallace, Ruth; Wiegand, Frances; Warren, Connie. Beneficence toward whom? Ethical decision-making in a maternal-fetal conflict. *AACN Clinical Issues in Critical Care Nursing.* 1997 Nov; 8(4): 586–594. 22 refs. BE58362.
   *beneficence; case studies; childbirth; critically ill; *decision making; drugs; ethical analysis; fetal development; *fetuses; informed consent; *leukemia; nurse's role; *patient care; patient participation; *pregnant women; prematurity; prenatal injuries; *prognosis; quality of life; *risks and benefits; time factors; toxicity; values; withholding treatment; *chemotherapy

Werpehowski, William. Persons, practices, and the conception argument. *Journal of Medicine and Philosophy.* 1997 Oct; 22(5): 479–494. 18 refs. 6 fn. BE56623.
   *beginning of life; embryo research; *embryos; fetal development; genetic identity; justice; *moral obligations; moral policy; parent child relationship; *personhood; *Roman Catholic ethics; theology; twinning; value of life; Declaration on Procured Abortion; Instruction on Respect for Human Life
The argument that human life should be fully protected once conception is complete has been challenged by the claim that at that time such life is not genuinely individuated in the morally required sense. This essay analyzes the "conception versus individuation" exchange and directs attention to the communal contexts within which the relevant arguments and counter-arguments arise.

Wisconsin. Supreme Court. State v. Kruzicki. *North Western Reporter, 2d Series.* 1997 Apr 22 (date of decision). 561: 729–749. BE56745.
   *behavior control; coercion; *criminal law; *drug abuse; *fetuses; government regulation; *legal aspects; *personhood; *pregnant women; *prenatal injuries; state government; treatment refusal; *viability; *Angela M.W.; *State v. Kruzicki; Wisconsin
The Wisconsin Supreme Court reversed the appellate court's denial of review of writs under which a pregnant woman sought release from the court's detention and protective custody of her viable fetus. Although she had given birth, the court considered the now moot issue of a child in need of protection or services. When Angela M.W. was thirty-six weeks pregnant, blood tests confirmed drug use in each of the preceding three months and it was decided that her continued use of drugs would cause the fetus serious harm. The county took protective custody of the fetus by a court order requiring that the woman be confined to an inpatient drug treatment facility. After considering the meanings of "child" and "person", the court concluded that under state law a child is a human being born alive, not a fetus. The dissenting judge argued that the meanings of "child" and "person" include a viable fetus. (KIE abstract)

FINANCIAL SUPPORT See BIOMEDICAL
   RESEARCH, HEALTH CARE/ECONOMICS
See under
   ABORTION/FINANCIAL SUPPORT

FORCE FEEDING

Draper, Heather. Treating anorexics without consent: some reservations. [Editorial]. *Journal of Medical Ethics.* 1998 Feb; 24(1): 5–7. 9 fn. BE57405.
   *behavior disorders; competence; decision making; food; *force feeding; informed consent; legal aspects; prolongation of life; *treatment refusal; *anorexia nervosa; Great Britain

Great Britain. England. Court of Appeal, Civil Division. B v. Croydon Health Authority. *All England Law Reports.* 1994 Nov 29 (date of decision). [1995] 1: 683–690. BE57784.
   *artificial feeding; behavior disorders; coercion; emergency care; *food; *force feeding; informed consent; involuntary commitment; *legal aspects; *mentally ill; patient care; *treatment refusal; *B v. Croydon Health Authority; *Great Britain; *Mental Health Act 1983 (Great Britain)
England's Court of Appeal, Civil Division, dismissed the appeal of B, a mentally ill patient, and upheld the lower court's order allowing force feeding by a nasogastric tube. In an attempt to harm herself, B had refused to eat while she was involuntarily hospitalized. Under threat of tubal feeding, she accepted food. B argued that she could not be fed without her consent because, although the Mental Health Act did not require her consent for "any medical treatment" given for her mental illness, force feeding was not medical treatment in the sense of psychotherapy. The court interpreted "medical treatment" to include ancillary acts such as "nursing and care concurrent with the core treatment or as a necessary prerequisite to such treatment or to prevent the patient from causing harm to himself or to alleviate the

consequences of the disorder." A concurring judge agreed that "any medical treatment" included treatment to alleviate symptoms of the disorder as well as treatment to remedy the underlying cause of the disorder. (KIE abstract)

Johannes Wier Foundation. Assistance in Hunger Strikes: A Manual for Physicians and Other Health Personnel Dealing with Hunger Strikers. Amersfoort, the Netherlands: Johannes Wier Foundation for Health and Human Rights; 1995. 44 p. Includes references. Published in cooperation with the Royal Dutch Medical Association and the Pharos Foundation for Refugee Health Care. BE57785.

   aliens; allowing to die; artificial feeding; competence; *dissent; *force feeding; *guidelines; human rights; *international aspects; legal aspects; organizational policies; *physician's role; physicians; *political activity; *prisoners; professional organizations; public policy; torture; treatment refusal; British Medical Association; Declaration of Malta; Declaration of Tokyo; Great Britain; Royal Dutch Medical Association; World Medical Association

FOREIGN COUNTRIES
See under
   ABORTION/FOREIGN COUNTRIES
   BEHAVIORAL RESEARCH/FOREIGN
       COUNTRIES
   HEALTH CARE/FOREIGN COUNTRIES
   HUMAN EXPERIMENTATION/FOREIGN
       COUNTRIES
   INVOLUNTARY COMMITMENT/FOREIGN
       COUNTRIES

FRAUD AND MISCONDUCT

Abbott, Alison. Germany tightens grip on misconduct. [News]. *Nature.* 1997 Dec 4; 390(6659): 430. BE56850.
   biomedical research; financial support; *fraud; investigators; research institutes; *scientific misconduct; *self regulation; universities; Brach, Marion; *Deutsche Forschungsgemeinschaft; *Germany; Herrmann, Friedhelm; *Max Planck Society

Abbott, Alison. Researcher sues over 'fraud' sanction. [News]. *Nature.* 1997 Dec 18–25; 390(6661): 652. BE57300.
   authorship; biomedical research; due process; editorial policies; faculty; *fraud; *investigators; *legal aspects; punishment; *scientific misconduct; self regulation; *universities; orthopedics; *Germany; *Goertzen, Meinolf; Journal of Bone and Joint Surgery; *University of Düsseldorf

Advisory Committee on Human Radiation Experiments. The Human Radiation Experiments: Final Report of the Advisory Committee. New York, NY: Oxford University Press; 1996. 620 p. 2,134 fn. "The Advisory Committee submitted its final report to the President in late 1995, and this book contains the entire text of the report issued by the U.S. Government Printing Office in October 1995. It also includes the full text of the President's remarks in acceptance of the report and a complete index." ISBN 0-19-510792-6. BE56500.
   *advisory committees; attitudes; blacks; children; codes of ethics; compensation; consent forms; deception; disclosure; ecology; ethical relativism; ethical review; *evaluation; evaluation studies; *federal government; government regulation; *guidelines; health hazards; *historical aspects; *human experimentation; information dissemination; informed consent; injuries; institutional policies; military

personnel; nontherapeutic research; nuclear warfare; occupational exposure; organization and administration; patients; policy analysis; prisoners; *public policy; *radiation; records; research institutes; research subjects; retrospective moral judgment; risks and benefits; *scientific misconduct; selection of subjects; *standards; survey; universities; volunteers; *Advisory Committee on Human Radiation Experiments; Atomic Energy Commission; Central Intelligence Agency; Cold War; Department of Defense; Department of Energy; Department of Health and Human Services; Department of Health, Education, and Welfare; National Aeronautics and Space Administration; Nuremberg Code; *Twentieth Century; *United States; Veterans Administration

Aller, Robert; Aller, Gregory. An institutional response to patient/family complaints. *In:* Shamoo, Adil E., ed. Ethics in Neurobiological Research with Human Subjects: The Baltimore Conference on Ethics. Amsterdam: Gordon and Breach; 1997: 155–172. 32 fn. This paper provides the viewpoints of a father and of his son, who was a research subject at the UCLA Clinical Research Center. ISBN 2-88449-161-9. BE57013.
   administrators; case studies; consent forms; *deception; *disclosure; family members; *human experimentation; iatrogenic disease; *informed consent; medical records; *mentally ill; patients; physician patient relationship; placebos; professional family relationship; *psychoactive drugs; *research design; research subjects; risks and benefits; *schizophrenia; *scientific misconduct; suicide; treatment outcome; universities; *withholding treatment; patient abandonment; *UCLA Neuropsychiatric Institute; United States; *University of California, Los Angeles

American College of Obstetricians and Gynecologists. Committee on Ethics. Sexual misconduct in the practice of obstetrics and gynecology: ethical considerations. ACOG Committee Opinion No. 144. *ACOG Committee Opinions.* 1994 Nov; No. 144: 3 p. 12 refs. BE56909.
   females; *guidelines; *misconduct; *obstetrics and gynecology; *organizational policies; patient care; *physician patient relationship; *physicians; professional organizations; *sexuality; *American College of Obstetricians and Gynecologists; American Medical Association; Society of Obstetricians and Gynecologists of Canada

Angell, Marcia; Kassirer, Jerome; Manson, JoAnn E., et al. Conflict of interest. [Letter and responses]. *Epidemiology.* 1997 Nov; 8(6): 686–687. 10 refs. BE58351.
   authorship; *biomedical research; *conflict of interest; *disclosure; *drug industry; drugs; *editorial policies; *financial support; investigators; referral and consultation; time factors; obesity; *New England Journal of Medicine

Atterstam, Inger. Karolinska Institute rocked by research misconduct. [News]. *Lancet.* 1997 Aug 30; 350(9078): 643. BE56082.
   biomedical research; cancer; fraud; genetic research; investigators; research institutes; *scientific misconduct; self regulation; *Karolinska Institute (Sweden); *Lönn, Ulf; *Sweden

Bass, Larry J.; DeMers, Stephen T.; Ogloff, James R.P., et al. Professional Conduct and Discipline in Psychology. Washington, DC; Montgomery, AL: American Psychological Association; Association of State and Provincial Psychology Boards; 1996. 330 p. Includes references. Appendixes include ASPPB and APA codes of conduct and Canadian Code of Ethics for Psychologists. ISBN 1-55798-372-0. BE57075.
   *codes of ethics; confidentiality; economics; education; federal government; government regulation; health

---

BE = bioethics accession number   fn. = footnotes   refs. = references

personnel; human experimentation; informed consent; legal aspects; legal liability; malpractice; *misconduct; professional competence; *professional ethics; professional organizations; professional patient relationship; *psychology; *regulation; self regulation; sexuality; *standards; state government; trends; American Psychological Association; Association of State and Provincial Psychology Boards; Canada; Canadian Psychological Association; United States

Bebeau, M.J.; Holt, S.C. Proceedings of a symposium, "Toward Responsible Research Conduct: The Role of Scientific Societies." [Introduction to a set of five papers and a consensus statement]. *Journal of Dental Research.* 1996 Feb; 75(2): 823–824. 2 refs. Paper presented at the symposium at the annual meeting of the American Association for Dental Research, held in San Antonio, TX, Mar 1995. BE56453.
biomedical research; codes of ethics; *dentistry; *investigators; organizational policies; *professional ethics; *professional organizations; *scientific misconduct; *self regulation; standards; *dental research; professional role; American Association for Dental Research

Bebeau, M.J.; Davis, E.L. Survey of ethical issues in dental research. *Journal of Dental Research.* 1996 Feb; 75(2): 845–855. 10 refs. Paper presented at the symposium, "Toward Responsible Research Conduct: The Role of Scientific Societies," during the annual meeting of the American Association for Dental Research, held in San Antonio, TX, Mar 1995. BE56452.
administrators; *attitudes; authorship; biomedical research; codes of ethics; *dentistry; education; ethics committees; *investigators; *professional ethics; professional organizations; *scientific misconduct; self regulation; standards; survey; *dental research; professional role; *American Association for Dental Research; International Association for Dental Research

Bebeau, Muriel J.; Holt, Stanley C.; American Association for Dental Research. Ethics Committee. The role of the AADR in promoting research integrity: perspectives and consensus statements. *Journal of Dental Research.* 1996 Feb; 75(2): 856–860. 9 refs. BE56454.
biomedical research; *codes of ethics; *dentistry; due process; education; ethics committees; goals; guidelines; *investigators; professional autonomy; *professional ethics; *professional organizations; *scientific misconduct; *self regulation; *standards; *dental research; professional role; *American Association for Dental Research; International Association for Dental Research

Berger, Edward M.; Gert, Bernard. The institutional context for research. *Professional Ethics.* 1995 Spring–Summer; 4(3–4): 17–46. 2 fn. References embedded in back–of–issue bibliography. BE55693.
administrators; authorship; biomedical research; confidentiality; education; federal government; fraud; government financing; government regulation; *guidelines; *institutional ethics; *institutional policies; interprofessional relations; investigators; legal aspects; misconduct; moral obligations; organization and administration; professional ethics; *research institutes; *science; *scientific misconduct; *self regulation; terminology; universities; whistleblowing; Breuning, Stephen; California Institute of Technology; Department of Justice; National Academy of Sciences; Ninnemann, John; Responsible Science: Ensuring the Integrity of the Research Process (NAS); United States; University of California, San Diego; University of Illinois; University of Pittsburgh; University of Utah

Bersoff, D.N. Process and procedures for dealing with misconduct: a necessity or a nightmare? *Journal of Dental Research.* 1996 Feb; 75(2): 836–840. 14 refs. Paper presented at the symposium, "Toward Responsible

Research Conduct: The Role of Scientific Societies," during the annual meeting of the American Association for Dental Research, held in San Antonio, TX, Mar 1995. BE56457.
biomedical research; codes of ethics; dentistry; *due process; economics; ethics committees; *investigators; *legal aspects; legal liability; *organizational policies; *professional ethics; *professional organizations; psychology; punishment; *science; *scientific misconduct; *self regulation; dental research; professional role; American Association for Dental Research; American Psychological Association

Blakely, Robert L.; Harrington, Judith M., eds. Bones in the Basement: Postmortem Racism in Nineteenth–Century Medical Training. Washington, DC: Smithsonian Institution Press; 1997. 380 p. Includes references. ISBN 1–56098–750–2. BE57441.
attitudes; autopsies; *blacks; *body parts and fluids; *cadavers; drugs; health; health care; *historical aspects; *human body; indigents; injuries; legal aspects; *medical education; medical ethics; medical schools; *misconduct; morbidity; nutrition; *physicians; social control; *social discrimination; sociology of medicine; students; *teaching methods; whites; ethnographic studies; slavery; Georgia; Harris, Grandison; *Medical College of Georgia (Augusta); *Nineteenth Century; Twentieth Century; United States

Bloche, M. Gregg. Cutting waste and keeping faith. [Editorial]. *Annals of Internal Medicine.* 1998 Apr 15; 128(8): 688–689. 11 refs. BE57901.
conflict of interest; *economics; entrepreneurship; *fraud; *government regulation; incentives; managed care programs; physician patient relationship; physician self–referral; *physicians; self regulation; trust; Health Care Financing Administration; *United States

Boisaubin, Eugene V. Nazi medicine: In the Shadow of the Reich: Nazi Medicine [videorecording], by John Michalczyk. [Audiovisual review essay]. *JAMA.* 1998 May 13; 279(18): 1496. BE57824.
audiovisual aids; *eugenics; *historical aspects; human experimentation; involuntary euthanasia; involuntary sterilization; mandatory programs; *medicine; *misconduct; *National Socialism; *physicians; *Germany; *In the Shadow of the Reich: Nazi Medicine (Michalczyk, J.); *Twentieth Century; United States

Böttiger, Lars Erik. Scientific misconduct –– does it exist? [Editorial]. *Journal of Internal Medicine.* 1994 Feb; 235(2): 103–105. 6 refs. BE55610.
biomedical research; editorial policies; fraud; human experimentation; investigators; medical education; peer review; physicians; public participation; *regulation; *scientific misconduct; Denmark; Great Britain; United States

Bowie, Cameron. Was the paper I wrote a fraud? [Personal view]. *BMJ (British Medical Journal).* 1998 Jun 6; 316(7146): 1755–1756. BE58234.
authorship; biomedical research; community services; fraud; interprofessional relations; investigators; physically disabled; *scientific misconduct; trust; Great Britain

Bradby, Hannah; Gabe, Jonathan; Bury, Michael. 'Sexy docs' and 'busty blondes': press coverage of professional misconduct cases brought before the General Medical Council. *Sociology of Health and Illness.* 1995 Sep; 17(4): 458–476. 59 refs. 2 fn. BE55691.
*females; *males; marital relationship; *mass media; *misconduct; *patients; *physician patient relationship; *physicians; self regulation; *sex offenses; *sexuality; social discrimination; sociology of medicine; stigmatization; General Medical Council (Great Britain); *Great Britain

---

BE = bioethics accession number   fn. = footnotes   refs. = references

Brahams, Diana. UK gynaecologist found guilty of serious professional misconduct. [News]. *Lancet.* 1997 Oct 4; 350(9083): 1014. BE56923.

females; *informed consent; *misconduct; *obstetrics and gynecology; *physicians; punishment; regulation; *surgery; *hysterectomy; *ovaries; General Medical Council (Great Britain); *Great Britain; *Studd, John

Bunce, Christina. Doctors involved in human rights' abuses in Kenya. [News]. *BMJ (British Medical Journal).* 1997 Jan 18; 314(7075): 166. BE58741.

death; deception; health care; human rights; medical records; *misconduct; physician's role; *physicians; *prisoners; *torture; Amnesty International; *Kenya

Burleigh, Michael. Ethics and Extermination: Reflections on Nazi Genocide. New York, NY: Cambridge University Press; 1997. 261 p. 538 fn. ISBN 0-521-58816-2. BE57155.

clergy; *eugenics; *historical aspects; homosexuals; *involuntary euthanasia; involuntary sterilization; Jews; *killing; literature; *mentally disabled; minority groups; *misconduct; *National Socialism; *physically disabled; physicians; Protestants; psychiatry; Roman Catholics; war; *Germany; Nineteenth Century; *Twentieth Century

Burleigh, Michael. Saving money, spending lives: psychiatry, society and the 'euthanasia' programme. *In:* Burleigh, Michael, ed. Confronting the Nazi Past: New Debates on Modern German History. New York, NY: St. Martin's Press; 1996: 98-111. 3 refs. ISBN 0-312-16353-3. BE57395.

administrators; adults; children; chronically ill; deinstitutionalized persons; *economics; employment; *eugenics; genetic disorders; health care; health personnel; *historical aspects; institutionalized persons; *involuntary euthanasia; involuntary sterilization; *killing; legislation; *mass media; mental institutions; *mentally ill; *mentally retarded; *misconduct; motivation; *National Socialism; parental consent; *physically disabled; physician's role; *psychiatry; public opinion; *public policy; stigmatization; volunteers; starvation; *Germany; Twentieth Century

Butler, Declan; DeGandt, Olivier. French ministry reopens inquiry into conduct of INSERM unit. [News]. *Nature.* 1998 Feb 5; 391(6667): 519-520. BE58020.

administrators; *biomedical research; government regulation; industry; patents; *research institutes; *scientific misconduct; universities; whistleblowing; Bihain, Bernard; *France; Genset; *INSERM

Butler, Declan. Karolinska Institute disowns work of cancer researcher. [News]. *Nature.* 1997 Aug 28; 388(6645): 816. BE56071.

biomedical research; cancer; fraud; investigators; research institutes; *scientific misconduct; self regulation; *Karolinska Institute (Sweden); *Lönn, Ulf; *Sweden

Camenisch, P.F. The moral foundations of scientific ethics and responsibility. *Journal of Dental Research.* 1996 Feb; 75(2): 825-831. 16 refs. Paper presented at the symposium, "Toward Responsible Research Conduct: The Role of Scientific Societies," during the annual meeting of the American Association for Dental Research, held in San Antonio, TX, Mar 1995. BE56459.

biomedical research; codes of ethics; common good; conflict of interest; *dentistry; disclosure; goals; information dissemination; *investigators; moral obligations; obligations to society; organizational policies; professional autonomy; professional competence; *professional ethics; *professional organizations; science; *scientific misconduct; *self regulation; trust; values; *dental research; professional role; *American Association for Dental Research; *International Association for Dental Research

Campbell, Duncan. Medicine needs its MI5. *BMJ (British Medical Journal).* 1997 Dec 20-27; 315(7123): 1677-1680. 2 refs. BE57651.

biomedical research; fraud; *human experimentation; *investigators; mass media; *misconduct; *patient care; *physicians; professional competence; *scientific misconduct; *self regulation; stigmatization; whistleblowing; medical audit; *General Medical Council (Great Britain); *Great Britain

Canada. Medical Research Council of Canada; Canada. Natural Sciences and Engineering Research Council of Canada; Canada. Social Sciences and Humanities Research Council of Canada. Integrity in Research and Scholarship: A Tri-Council Policy Statement. Ottawa, ON: Medical Research Council of Canada; 1994 Jan. 4 p. BE56727.

accountability; biomedical research; government financing; government regulation; institutional policies; investigators; peer review; *regulation; research institutes; science; *scientific misconduct; self regulation; *Canada

Caplan, Arthur L. Time to get down and dirty in defining misconduct. [Editorial]. *Journal of Laboratory and Clinical Medicine.* 1997 Feb; 129(2): 172-173. 8 refs. BE57514.

science; *scientific misconduct; self regulation; standards; terminology

Castledine, George. Whistleblowing guidelines for nursing colleagues. *British Journal of Nursing.* 1997 Jun 12-25; 6(11): 654. 3 refs. BE58254.

communication; *guidelines; interprofessional relations; *misconduct; *nurses; regulation; *whistleblowing; *professional impairment; *Great Britain; *United Kingdom Central Council for Nursing, Midwifery and Health Visiting

Chambers, Timothy. Questionable ethics — whistle-blowing or tale-telling? *Journal of Medical Ethics.* 1997 Dec; 23(6): 382-383. 2 refs. BE57657.

case studies; disclosure; *editorial policies; informed consent; *kidney diseases; *nontherapeutic research; parental consent; patient care; peer review; physicians; prognosis; *scientific misconduct; *surgery; *whistleblowing; medical audit

Renal biopsy is a potentially hazardous procedure, generally performed for therapeutic reasons. An open renal biopsy was performed when there appeared to be no accepted clinical indication and its results published in a specialty journal, whose editors declined publication of subsequent correspondence, questioning the ethical propriety of such a procedure. The implications for clinical practice, authors, editors and readers are discussed.

Chantler, Cyril; Chantler, Shireen. Dealing with research misconduct in the United Kingdom: deception: difficulties and initiatives. *BMJ (British Medical Journal).* 1998 Jun 6; 316(7146): 1731-1732. 8 refs. BE58204.

biomedical research; due process; editorial policies; fraud; guidelines; institutional policies; investigators; medical education; medical schools; physicians; professional organizations; *regulation; *scientific misconduct; self regulation; whistleblowing; General Medical Council (Great Britain); Great Britain; Royal College of Physicians

Chelala, César. German dialysis firm quits Chinese interest. [News]. *Lancet.* 1998 Mar 14; 351(9105): 812. BE58443.

aliens; *cadavers; capital punishment; health facilities; industry; *international aspects; kidneys; *misconduct; moral complicity; *organ donation; organ transplantation; *prisoners; *renal dialysis; *China; *Fresenius Medical Care AG; Germany

---

BE = bioethics accession number   fn. = footnotes   refs. = references

Chen, Yuan–Fang. Japanese death factories and the American cover–up. *Cambridge Quarterly of Healthcare Ethics.* 1997 Spring; 6(2): 240–242. BE56425.
    accountability; aliens; *biological warfare; communicable diseases; *historical aspects; *human experimentation; human rights; international aspects; investigators; killing; medical ethics; military personnel; moral complicity; National Socialism; physicians; *prisoners; *public policy; *research subjects; *scientific misconduct; torture; *war; China; Factories of Death (Harris, S.); Germany; Ishii, Shiro; *Japan; Twentieth Century; *United States; *World War II

Clinton, William J. Remarks by the president in apology for study done in Tuskegee. Washington, DC: The White House, Office of the Press Secretary, [Online]. Available: http://www1.whitehouse.gov/New/Remarks/Fri/199 70516-898.html; 1997 May 16. 3 p. Downloaded 22 Aug 1997. BE57692.
    advisory committees; bioethics; *blacks; compensation; education; ethical review; federal government; *human experimentation; indigents; informed consent; *nontherapeutic research; *public policy; *research subjects; *scientific misconduct; selection of subjects; syphilis; trust; *withholding treatment; National Bioethics Advisory Commission; *Tuskegee Syphilis Study; *United States

College of Physicians and Surgeons of British Columbia. Committee on Physician Sexual Misconduct. Crossing the Boundaries. The Report of the Committee on Physician Sexual Misconduct. Issued by the College of Physicians and Surgeons of British Columbia, Vancouver, BC; 1992 Nov. 28 p. BE57276.
    attitudes; mandatory reporting; medical education; *misconduct; *organizational policies; patient advocacy; *patients; *physician patient relationship; *physicians; professional organizations; public opinion; public participation; *self regulation; *sexuality; social dominance; statistics; survey; *College of Physicians and Surgeons of British Columbia

Cooper–Mahkorn, Déirdre. Many journals have not retracted "fraudulent" research. [News]. *BMJ (British Medical Journal).* 1998 Jun 20; 316(7148): 1850. BE58276.
    authorship; biomedical research; *editorial policies; *fraud; investigators; *scientific misconduct; *retraction of publication; Brach, Marion; *Germany; *Herrmann, Friedhelm; University of Ulm

Coverdale, John H.; Thomson, Alex N.; White, Gillian E. Social and sexual contact between general practitioners and patients in New Zealand: attitudes and prevalence. *British Journal of General Practice.* 1995 May; 45(394): 245–247. 16 refs. BE56554.
    *attitudes; family practice; *knowledge, attitudes, practice; *misconduct; *physician patient relationship; *physicians; risks and benefits; *sexuality; *social interaction; statistics; survey; *New Zealand

Dalton, Rex. Collins' student sanctioned over 'most severe' case of fraud. [News]. *Nature.* 1997 Jul 24; 388(6640): 313. BE56069.
    biomedical research; federal government; genetic research; government regulation; *investigators; *scientific misconduct; *students; universities; Collins, Francis; *Hajra, Amitov; National Center for Human Genome Research; Office of Research Integrity; United States; University of Michigan

Dalton, Rex. Neuroscientist accused of misconduct turns on his accusers. [News]. *Nature.* 1998 Apr 2; 392(6675): 424. BE58021.
    *administrators; *biomedical research; federal government; fraud; government regulation; *investigators; *legal aspects;

*legal liability; *medical schools; *scientific misconduct; torts; universities; *Angelides, Kimon; *Baylor College of Medicine; National Institutes of Health; Office of Research Integrity

de Bousingen, Denis Durand. French Medical Association apologises to Jews. [News]. *Lancet.* 1997 Oct 18; 350(9085): 1153. BE56221.
    eugenics; *historical aspects; *Jews; *misconduct; *National Socialism; *organizational policies; *physicians; professional organizations; *social discrimination; *France; *French Medical Association; Twentieth Century; World War II

Dehlendorf, Christine E.; Wolfe, Sidney M. Physicians disciplined for sex-related offenses. *JAMA.* 1998 Jun 17; 279(23): 1883–1888. 25 refs. BE58410.
    age factors; family practice; federal government; *government regulation; medical specialties; *misconduct; obstetrics and gynecology; *physician patient relationship; *physicians; psychiatry; *punishment; *self regulation; *sex offenses; *sexuality; state government; statistics; *United States
CONTEXT: Physicians who abuse their patients sexually cause immense harm, and, therefore, the discipline of physicians who commit any sex-related offenses is an important public health issue that should be examined. OBJECTIVES: To determine the frequency and severity of discipline against physicians who commit sex-related offenses and to describe the characteristics of these physicians. DESIGN AND SETTING: Analysis of sex-related orders from a national database of disciplinary orders taken by state medical boards and federal agencies. SUBJECTS: A total of 761 physicians disciplined for sex-related offenses from 1981 through 1996. MAIN OUTCOME MEASURES: Rate and severity of discipline over time for sex-related offenses and specialty, age, and board certification status of disciplined physicians. RESULTS: The number of physicians disciplined per year for sex-related offenses increased from 42 in 1989 to 147 in 1996, and the proportion of all disciplinary orders that were sex related increased from 2.1% in 1989 to 4.4% in 1996 (P less than .001 for trend). Discipline for sex-related offenses was significantly more severe (P less than .001) than for non-sex-related offenses, with 71.9% of sex-related orders involving revocation, surrender, or suspension of medical license. Of 761 physicians disciplined, the offenses committed by 567 (75%) involved patients, including sexual intercourse, rape, sexual molestation, and sexual favors for drugs. As of March 1997, 216 physicians (39.9%) disciplined for sex-related offenses between 1981 and 1994 were licensed to practice. Compared with all physicians, physicians disciplined for sex-related offenses were more likely to practice in the specialties of psychiatry, child psychiatry, obstetrics and gynecology, and family and general practice (all P less than .001) than in other specialties and were older than the national physician population, but were no different in terms of board certification status. CONCLUSIONS: Discipline against physicians for sex-related offenses is increasing over time and is relatively severe, although few physicians are disciplined for sexual offenses each year. In addition, a substantial proportion of physicians disciplined for these offenses are allowed to either continue to practice or return to practice.

Deichmann, Ute; Müller–Hill, Benno. The fraud of Abderhalden's enzymes. *Nature.* 1998 May 14; 393(6681): 109–111. 19 refs. BE58302.
    *biomedical research; cancer; communicable diseases; *diagnosis; eugenics; *fraud; genetics; historical aspects;

BE = bioethics accession number   fn. = footnotes   refs. = references

human experimentation; investigators; moral complicity; National Socialism; pregnant women; prisoners; schizophrenia; *scientific misconduct; *sociology of medicine; whistleblowing; *Aberhalden, Emil; *Germany; Twentieth Century

Dorozynski, Alexander. French doctors apologise for wartime antisemitism. [News]. *BMJ (British Medical Journal)*. 1997 Nov 1; 315(7116): 1116. BE56912.
 *historical aspects; *Jews; *misconduct; *National Socialism; *organizational policies; *physicians; professional organizations; *social discrimination; *France; *Ordre National des Médecins; Twentieth Century

Dorozynski, Alexander. Scandal unfolds over blood donation in French prisons. [News]. *BMJ (British Medical Journal)*. 1998 Jan 17; 316(7126): 171. BE57958.
 *administrators; blood donation; *blood transfusions; disclosure; *HIV seropositivity; legal liability; *misconduct; *physicians; prisoners; risk; *France

Dracy, David L.; Yutrzenka, Barbara A. Responses of direct-care paraprofessional mental health staff to hypothetical ethics violations. *Psychiatric Services*. 1997 Sep; 48(9): 1160–1163. 8 refs. BE55717.
 *allied health personnel; decision making; education; institutionalized persons; *interprofessional relations; *knowledge, attitudes, practice; *mental institutions; mentally ill; mentally retarded; *misconduct; patient care; *professional ethics; survey; *whistleblowing; Midwestern United States

Dyer, Clare. Cardiologist admits research misconduct. [News]. *BMJ (British Medical Journal)*. 1997 May 24; 314(7093): 1501. BE56070.
 human experimentation; informed consent; *legal aspects; mass media; *physicians; research design; *scientific misconduct; cardiology; journalism; *Great Britain; *Nixon, Peter

Dyer, Clare. Consultant struck off over research fraud. [News]. *BMJ (British Medical Journal)*. 1997 Jul 26; 315(7102): 205. BE58744.
 consent forms; deception; drug industry; drugs; *fraud; *human experimentation; investigators; *physicians; punishment; records; regulation; *scientific misconduct; *Anderton, George; *General Medical Council (Great Britain); *Great Britain

Dyer, Clare. Consultant suspended for not getting consent for cardiac procedure. [News]. *BMJ (British Medical Journal)*. 1998 Mar 28; 316(7136): 955. BE58056.
 children; death; deception; hearts; *malpractice; *misconduct; *parental consent; *patient care; *physicians; punishment; surgery; General Medical Council (Great Britain); Jenkins, Debbie; London; *Taylor, James

Dyer, Clare. Gynaecologist admonished for removing ovaries without consent. [News]. *BMJ (British Medical Journal)*. 1997 Oct 4; 315(7112): 832. BE56080.
 females; *informed consent; *misconduct; *obstetrics and gynecology; *physicians; punishment; self regulation; *surgery; *hysterectomy; *ovaries; Bartley, Jacqueline; General Medical Council (Great Britain); Great Britain; *Studd, John

Elliott, Deni. Case studies for teaching research ethics. *Professional Ethics*. 1995 Spring–Summer; 4(3–4): 179–198. 26 fn. References embedded in back-of-issue bibliography. BE55685.
 accountability; authorship; *biomedical research; *case studies; conflict of interest; *education; ethical analysis; financial support; fraud; industry; interprofessional relations; misconduct; *professional ethics; property rights; *science;

*scientific misconduct; self regulation; students; *teaching methods; universities; whistleblowing

Elliott, Deni; Blanford, Patricia; Watson, Marci, comps. Scientific research ethics videography. *Professional Ethics*. 1995 Spring–Summer; 4(3–4): 199–204. List of video titles with short summaries. BE55684.
 animal experimentation; *audiovisual aids; *bioethical issues; *biomedical research; education; genetic research; human experimentation; mass media; prenatal diagnosis; professional ethics; resource allocation; science; *scientific misconduct; teaching methods; United States

Endocrine Society. Ethical guidelines for publications of research. *Journal of Clinical Endocrinology and Metabolism*. 1996 Jan; 81(1): R1–R2. Guidelines prepared by the Publications Committee of the Endocrine Society and approved for publication and distribution by the Society's Council. BE57688.
 *authorship; biomedical research; due process; *editorial policies; *guidelines; information dissemination; investigators; peer review; professional organizations; *scientific misconduct; *publishing; *Endocrine Society

Ernst, Edzard. Killing in the name of healing: the active role of the German medical profession during the Third Reich. *American Journal of Medicine*. 1996 May; 100(5): 579–581. 18 refs. BE55719.
 disabled; employment; *eugenics; genetic disorders; *historical aspects; human experimentation; involuntary euthanasia; involuntary sterilization; Jews; *killing; legal aspects; mentally disabled; metaphor; *misconduct; *National Socialism; *physician's role; *physicians; prisoners; social discrimination; sociology of medicine; technical expertise; *Germany; Social Darwinism; Twentieth Century

Evans, Imogen. Dealing with research misconduct in the United Kingdom: conduct unbecoming -- the MRC's approach. *BMJ (British Medical Journal)*. 1998 Jun 6; 316(7146): 1728–1729. 1 ref. BE58206.
 biomedical research; confidentiality; deception; education; fraud; investigators; negligence; *regulation; *scientific misconduct; standards; *Great Britain; *Medical Research Council (Great Britain)

Farthing, Michael J.G. Dealing with research misconduct in the United Kingdom: an editor's response to fraudsters. *BMJ (British Medical Journal)*. 1998 Jun 6; 316(7146): 1729–1731. 9 refs. BE58207.
 biomedical research; *editorial policies; fraud; international aspects; investigators; public health; *regulation; *scientific misconduct; self regulation; uncertainty; whistleblowing; Committee on Publication Ethics (Great Britain); Great Britain

Finetti, Marco. Second careers of the Nazis' doctors. [Book review essay]. *Nature*. 1997 Dec 4; 390(6659): 457–458. BE56933.
 accountability; attitudes; employment; *faculty; historical aspects; interprofessional relations; medical education; medicine; *misconduct; *National Socialism; *physicians; time factors; *universities; *Germany; *Kontinuität und Neuanfang in der Hochschulmedizin nach 1945 (Aumüller, G., et al., eds.); Twentieth Century

Fischer, Beth A.; Zigmond, Michael J. Scientific publishing. *In:* Chadwick, Ruth, ed. Encyclopedia of Applied Ethics, Volume 4. San Diego, CA: Academic Press; 1998: 29–38. 7 refs. ISBN 0-12-227069-X. BE56344.
 authorship; biomedical research; confidentiality; *editorial policies; fraud; information dissemination; interprofessional

---

BE = bioethics accession number   fn. = footnotes   refs. = references

relations; investigators; *peer review; *science; *scientific misconduct

Fishman, Rachelle H.B. Israeli surgeon questioned over transplantation ethics. [News]. *Lancet.* 1998 Mar 14; 351(9105): 812. BE58440.
   international aspects; *kidneys; *misconduct; *organ donation; organ donors; organ transplantation; *physicians; *remuneration; *Israel; Romania; *Shapiro, Zaki

Frankel, M.S. Developing ethical standards for responsible research: why? form? functions? process? outcomes? *Journal of Dental Research.* 1996 Feb; 75(2): 832–835. 6 refs. Paper presented at the symposium, "Toward Responsible Research Conduct: The Role of Scientific Societies," during the annual meeting of the American Association for Dental Research, held in San Antonio, TX, Mar 1995. BE56461.
   accountability; biomedical research; *codes of ethics; decision making; *dentistry; education; *investigators; professional autonomy; *professional ethics; *professional organizations; *science; *scientific misconduct; *self regulation; *standards; dental research; American Association for Dental Research

Freedman, Monroe H.; Hoenig, Leonard J.; Spiro, Howard M., et al. Nazi research: too evil to cite. [Letters]. *Hastings Center Report.* 1985 Aug; 15(4): 31–32. BE57827.
   animal experimentation; *biomedical research; *editorial policies; historical aspects; *human experimentation; killing; moral complicity; *National Socialism; research subjects; *scientific misconduct; torture; utilitarianism; Germany; Twentieth Century

Geltman, Paul. Rwanda: physician complicity and rebuilding the medical community. *Lancet.* 1997 Jul 5; 350(9070): 64. 2 refs. BE56571.
   *human rights; *killing; *misconduct; moral complicity; *physician's role; physicians; *torture; *genocide; *Rwanda

Gitanjali, B.; Shashindran, C.H.; Tripathi, K.D., et al. Are drug advertisements in Indian edition of BMJ unethical? [Article and commentary]. *BMJ (British Medical Journal).* 1997 Aug 23; 315(7106): 459–460. 12 refs. BE56649.
   *advertising; alternative therapies; comparative studies; *deception; *drug industry; *drugs; *editorial policies; financial support; health personnel; *international aspects; *misconduct; *standards; survey; technical expertise; *BMJ (British Medical Journal); Great Britain; *India; World Health Organization

Glass, Nigel. Austrian medicine encouraged to confront its Nazi past. [News]. *Lancet.* 1998 Feb 7; 351(9100): 427. BE58884.
   historical aspects; killing; *misconduct; *National Socialism; *physicians; psychiatry; *Austria; Twentieth Century

Gluck, John P. Harry F. Harlow and animal research: reflection on the ethical paradox. *Ethics and Behavior.* 1997; 7(2): 149–161. 24 refs. 1 fn. BE56410.
   *animal experimentation; attitudes; behavior disorders; behavioral research; brain pathology; emotions; *evaluation; famous persons; interprofessional relations; *investigators; motivation; peer review; *primates; professional ethics; psychological stress; psychology; *research design; *scientific misconduct; self regulation; social interaction; suffering; *Harlow, Harry
With respect to the ethical debate about the treatment of animals in biomedical and behavioral research, Harry F. Harlow represents a paradox. On the one hand, his work on monkey cognition and social development

fostered a view of the animals as having rich subjective lives filled with intention and emotion. On the other, he has been criticized for the conduct of research that seemed to ignore the ethical implications of his own discoveries. The basis of this contradiction is discussed and propositions for current research practice are presented.

Godfrey, Nelda S.; Kuehne, Dale S.; Wildes, Kevin Wm. In the care of a nurse. [Case study and commentaries]. *Hastings Center Report.* 1997 Sep–Oct; 27(5): 23–24. BE56125.
   active euthanasia; advance directives; *allowing to die; autonomy; case studies; *conscience; *deception; *decision making; *dissent; drugs; family members; hospitals; institutional ethics; institutional policies; intensive care units; *misconduct; moral obligations; *nurses; *nursing ethics; patient advocacy; *patient care team; *prolongation of life; terminally ill; treatment refusal; withholding treatment

Gold, Hal. Unit 731: Testimony –– Japan's Wartime Human Experimentation Program. Tokyo: Yenbooks; 1996. 256 p. Bibliography: p. 251–256. ISBN 4–900737–39–9. BE57996.
   *biological warfare; children; confidentiality; dehumanization; disclosure; federal government; females; historical aspects; *human experimentation; international aspects; investigators; killing; military personnel; *moral complicity; *prisoners; public policy; *scientific misconduct; torture; China; Cold War; Ishii, Shiro; *Japan; Manchuria; *Twentieth Century; *United States; USSR; *World War II

Goldbeck–Wood, Sandra. Scientists call for whistleblowers' charter. [News]. *BMJ (British Medical Journal).* 1997 Nov 15; 315(7118): 1252. BE56914.
   biomedical research; *editorial policies; fraud; investigators; regulation; *scientific misconduct; *whistleblowing; *Committee on Publication Ethics (Great Britain); *Great Britain

Gorton, Gregg E.; Samuel, Steven E. A national survey of training directors about education for prevention of psychiatrist–patient sexual exploitation. *Academic Psychiatry.* 1996 Summer; 20(2): 92–98. 15 refs. BE58119.
   administrators; curriculum; faculty; *internship and residency; *medical education; medical ethics; *misconduct; *physician patient relationship; *psychiatry; *sexuality; survey; teaching methods; United States

Grayson, Lesley. Scientific Deception: An Overview and Guide to the Literature of Misconduct and Fraud in Scientific Research. London: British Library, Science Reference and Information Service; 1995. 107 p. (Science policy series). 230 refs. ISBN 0–7123–0831–8. BE55702.
   biomedical research; *deception; financial support; *fraud; government financing; government regulation; industry; *international aspects; investigators; motivation; peer review; professional organizations; *public policy; *regulation; *science; *scientific misconduct; self regulation; statistics; universities; whistleblowing; Australia; Europe; Great Britain; United States

Greenberg, Daniel S. Hidden data and abuse in research come to light in the USA. [News]. *Lancet.* 1997 Oct 11; 350(9084): 1083. BE56926.
   cancer; compensation; *disclosure; federal government; government regulation; *health hazards; historical aspects; *human experimentation; industry; informed consent; mentally ill; *nuclear warfare; public health; *public policy; *radiation; research ethics committees; *scientific misconduct; Cold War; Twentieth Century; *United States

---

BE = bioethics accession number   fn. = footnotes   refs. = references

Grinnell, Frederick. Truth, fairness, and the definition of scientific misconduct. *Journal of Laboratory and Clinical Medicine.* 1997 Feb; 129(2): 189–192. 18 refs. BE57515.
advisory committees; biomedical research; deception; fraud; *investigators; methods; *science; *scientific misconduct; self regulation; terminology; Commission on Research Integrity; United States

Hornblum, Allen M. Acres of Skin: Human Experiments at Holmesburg Prison –– A True Story of Abuse and Exploitation in the Name of Medical Science. New York, NY: Routledge; 1998. 297 p. Bibliography: p. 271–284. ISBN 0-415-91990-8. BE58697.
administrators; blacks; disclosure; drug industry; federal government; government regulation; *historical aspects; *human experimentation; *incentives; informed consent; institutionalized persons; *investigators; mass media; methods; National Socialism; *nontherapeutic research; *prisoners; psychoactive drugs; radiation; remuneration; research design; research subjects; risks and benefits; *scientific misconduct; state government; toxicity; volunteers; chemical warfare; dermatology; Atomic Energy Commission; Department of the Army; Environmental Protection Agency; Food and Drug Administration; *Holmesburg Prison (Philadelphia, PA); *Kligman, Albert; *Twentieth Century; *United States; University of Pennsylvania

Hornblum, Allen M. They were cheap and available: prisoners as research subjects in twentieth century America. *BMJ (British Medical Journal).* 1997 Nov 29; 315(7120): 1437–1441. 49 refs. BE57051.
attitudes; coercion; death; disclosure; drug industry; federal government; government regulation; guidelines; *historical aspects; *human experimentation; incentives; injuries; investigators; *nontherapeutic research; physicians; *prisoners; *public policy; research subjects; risk; *scientific misconduct; selection of subjects; trends; utilitarianism; volunteers; war; guideline adherence; Cold War; Nuremberg Code; *Twentieth Century; *United States; World War II

Horton, Richard. Doctors, the General Medical Council, and Bristol. *Lancet.* 1998 May 23; 351(9115): 1525–1526. 5 refs. BE58239.
administrators; biomedical research; disclosure; fraud; informed consent; mass media; *misconduct; mortality; *patient care; *physicians; *professional competence; quality of health care; risks and benefits; *self regulation; surgery; technical expertise; medical audit; *General Medical Council (Great Britain); Good Medical Practice (General Medical Council); *Great Britain

Horton, Richard. Will the UK COPE? [Letter]. *Lancet.* 1997 Jul 26; 350(9073): 234. 9 refs. BE56154.
advisory committees; biomedical research; *editorial policies; *scientific misconduct; *self regulation; *Committee on Publication Ethics (Great Britain); *Great Britain

Hunt, Geoffrey. The human condition of the professional: discretion and accountability. *Nursing Ethics.* 1997 Nov; 4(6): 519–526. 6 refs. BE57416.
*accountability; *conscience; *decision making; *misconduct; nursing ethics; *professional ethics; punishment; resuscitation

Hunt, Geoffrey, ed. Whistleblowing in the Health Service: Accountability, Law and Professional Practice. London: Edward Arnold; 1995. 170 p. Includes references. ISBN 0-340-59234-6. BE55681.
*accountability; *administrators; confidentiality; democracy; employment; *government regulation; health care delivery; *health personnel; hospitals; information dissemination; international aspects; *legal aspects; malpractice; *misconduct; nurses; organization and administration; patient care; physicians; professional autonomy; *professional

competence; *quality of health care; *self regulation; standards; values; *whistleblowing; *Great Britain; *National Health Service; United States

Hutchens, Michael P. Grave robbing and ethics in the 19th century. *JAMA.* 1997 Oct 1; 278(13): 1115. 7 refs. BE55868.
*cadavers; confidentiality; health insurance; *historical aspects; legal aspects; *medical education; medical ethics; *misconduct; *physicians; Great Britain; *Nineteenth Century

Irving, Miles; Berwick, Donald M.; Rubin, Peter, et al. Five times: coincidence or something more serious? [Article and commentaries]. *BMJ (British Medical Journal).* 1998 Jun 6; 316(7146): 1736–1740. 8 refs. BE58368.
interprofessional relations; *misconduct; mortality; *physicians; *professional competence; self regulation; *surgery; treatment outcome; *whistleblowing; medical audit; General Medical Council (Great Britain); Great Britain

Jacobsen, Geir; Hals, Arild. Medical investigators' views about ethics and fraud in medical research. *Journal of the Royal College of Physicians of London.* 1995 Sep–Oct; 29(5): 405–409. 20 refs. BE55562.
advisory committees; age factors; *attitudes; *biomedical research; *ethical review; evaluation; females; *fraud; freedom; historical aspects; human experimentation; information dissemination; *investigators; *knowledge, attitudes, practice; males; medical ethics; physicians; professional autonomy; professional ethics; regional ethics committees; *regulation; *research design; *research ethics committees; retrospective moral judgment; science; *scientific misconduct; *self regulation; statistics; survey; trends; *Norway; Twentieth Century

Jayaraman, K.S. Inquiry looks into Indian cancer deaths. [News]. *Nature.* 1997 Dec 18–25; 390(6661): 653. BE57309.
attitudes; *cancer; *disadvantaged; disclosure; *females; historical aspects; *human experimentation; *informed consent; investigators; retrospective moral judgment; *scientific misconduct; *withholding treatment; *India; Indian Council of Medical Research

Jehu, Derek. Patients as Victims: Sexual Abuse in Psychotherapy and Counselling. New York, NY: Wiley; 1994. 241 p. (Wiley series in psychotherapy and counselling). Bibliography: p. 225–238. ISBN 0-471-94398-3. BE55680.
age factors; attitudes; *counseling; females; *health personnel; legal aspects; males; mentally ill; *misconduct; patient care; prevalence; professional ethics; *professional patient relationship; *psychotherapy; regulation; *sex offenses; *sexuality; statistics; Great Britain; United States

Josefson, Deborah. US journal embroiled in another conflict of interest scandal. [News]. *BMJ (British Medical Journal).* 1998 Jan 24; 316(7127): 251. BE58120.
authorship; cancer; *conflict of interest; *disclosure; *ecology; *editorial policies; employment; epidemiology; *health hazards; *industry; misconduct; *physicians; public health; *Berke, Jerry; Living Downstream: An Ecologist Looks at Cancer and the Environment (Steingraber, S.); *New England Journal of Medicine

Kaiser, Jocelyn. British editors form misconduct panel. [News]. *Science.* 1997 Aug 1; 277(5326): 627. BE56330.
biomedical research; *editorial policies; government regulation; information dissemination; *scientific misconduct; *self regulation; *journalism; *Committee on Publication Ethics (Great Britain); Great Britain

Kaiser, Jocelyn. Fisher wins $2.75 million settlement. [News]. *Science.* 1997 Sep 5; 277(5331): 1425. BE56077.
  biomedical research; cancer; *compensation; due process; federal government; fraud; *investigators; legal aspects; *scientific misconduct; universities; *Fisher, Bernard; National Cancer Institute; National Surgical Adjuvant Breast and Bowel Project; United States; University of Pittsburgh

Kellett, John M.; Curtis, David. Suspension of nurse who gave drug on consultant's instructions. [Letters]. *BMJ (British Medical Journal).* 1997 Apr 5; 314(7086): 1043-1044. 2 refs. BE55897.
  *administrators; *behavior control; behavior disorders; *deception; *misconduct; *nurse's role; *nurses; patient care; *patient care team; physician nurse relationship; *physicians; *psychoactive drugs; *punishment; treatment refusal; *Great Britain; National Health Service

King, Patricia A. Race, justice, and research. *In:* Kahn, Jeffrey P.; Mastroianni, Anna C.; Sugarman, Jeremy, eds. Beyond Consent: Seeking Justice in Research. New York, NY: Oxford University Press; 1998: 88-110. 82 fn. ISBN 0-19-511353-5. BE58845.
  *blacks; females; genetic screening; health care delivery; historical aspects; *human experimentation; informed consent; *justice; males; medical education; medicine; minority groups; public participation; public policy; research subjects; *scientific misconduct; selection of subjects; sickle cell anemia; *social discrimination; stigmatization; surgery; syphilis; trends; trust; vulnerable populations; whites; withholding treatment; slavery; Tuskegee Syphilis Study; United States

Klein, Rudolf. Competence, professional self regulation, and the public interest. *BMJ (British Medical Journal).* 1998 Jun 6; 316(7146): 1740-1742. 6 refs. BE58213.
  children; heart diseases; hospitals; interprofessional relations; *misconduct; mortality; *pediatrics; *physicians; *professional competence; quality of health care; *self regulation; standards; *surgery; technical expertise; whistleblowing; medical audit; Bristol Royal Infirmary; *General Medical Council (Great Britain); *Great Britain; National Health Service

Kmietowicz, Zosia. MRC cleared of unethical research practices. [News]. *BMJ (British Medical Journal).* 1998 May 30; 316(7145): 1628. BE58278.
  financial support; *historical aspects; *human experimentation; informed consent; *radiation; research subjects; retrospective moral judgment; review committees; *scientific misconduct; standards; *Great Britain; *Medical Research Council (Great Britain); *Twentieth Century

Koenig, Robert. Panel calls falsification in German case 'unprecedented.' [News]. *Science.* 1997 Aug 15; 277(5328): 894. BE56065.
  authorship; biomedical research; *fraud; gene therapy; genetic research; investigators; peer review; *scientific misconduct; self regulation; standards; universities; *Brach, Marion; *Germany; *Herrmann, Friedhelm; University of Ulm

Koenig, Robert. Panel proposes ways to combat fraud. [News]. *Science.* 1997 Dec 19; 278(5346): 2049-2050. BE56872.
  biomedical research; financial support; *fraud; investigators; research institutes; *scientific misconduct; *self regulation; standards; universities; Brach, Marion; *Deutsche Forschungsgemeinschaft; *Germany; Herrmann, Friedhelm; *Max Planck Society

Korenman, Stanley G.; Berk, Richard; Wenger, Neil S., et al. Evaluation of the research norms of scientists and administrators responsible for academic research integrity. *JAMA.* 1998 Jan 7; 279(1): 41-47. 28 refs. BE57816.
  *administrators; *attitudes; authorship; biomedical research; comparative studies; *conflict of interest; financial support; fraud; industry; *information dissemination; interprofessional relations; *investigators; *professional ethics; punishment; *scientific misconduct; survey; universities; *research ethics; United States
  CONTEXT: The professional integrity of scientists is important to society as a whole and particularly to disciplines such as medicine that depend heavily on scientific advances for their progress. OBJECTIVE: To characterize the professional norms of active scientists and compare them with those of individuals with institutional responsibility for the conduct of research. DESIGN: A mailed survey consisting of 12 scenarios in 4 domains of research ethics. Respondents were asked whether an act was unethical and, if so, the degree to which they considered it unethical and to select responses and punishments for the act. PARTICIPANTS: A total of 924 National Science Foundation research grantees in 1993 or 1994 in molecular or cellular biology and 140 representatives from the researchers' institutions to the US Department of Health and Human Services Office of Research Integrity. MAIN OUTCOME MEASURES: Percentage of respondents considering an act unethical and the mean malfeasance rating on a scale of 1 to 10. RESULTS: A total of 606 research grantees and 91 institutional representatives responded to the survey (response rate of 69% of those who could be contacted). Respondents reported a hierarchy of unethical research behaviors. The mean malfeasance rating was unrelated to the characteristics of the investigator performing the hypothetical act or to its consequences. Fabrication, falsification, and plagiarism received malfeasance ratings higher than 8.6, and virtually all thought they were unethical. Deliberately misleading statements about a paper or failure to give proper attribution received ratings between 7 and 8. Sloppiness, oversights, conflicts of interest, and failure to share were less serious still, receiving malfeasance ratings between 5 and 6. Institutional representatives proposed more and different interventions and punishments than the scientists. CONCLUSIONS: Surveyed scientists and institutional representatives had strong and similar norms of professional behavior, but differed in their approaches to an unethical act.

LaFollette, Marcel C. The pathology of research fraud: the history and politics of the US experience. *Journal of Internal Medicine.* 1994 Feb; 235(2): 129-135. 29 refs. BE55603.
  biomedical research; federal government; *fraud; government financing; *government regulation; historical aspects; institutional policies; investigators; *politics; research institutes; science; *scientific misconduct; self regulation; universities; whistleblowing; National Institutes of Health; U.S. Congress; *United States

Lazarus, Jeremy A. Ethical issues in doctor-patient sexual relationships. *Psychiatric Clinics of North America.* 1995 Mar; 18(1): 55-70. 37 refs. BE55512.
  codes of ethics; emotions; ethics committees; family members; females; health personnel; injuries; internship and residency; interprofessional relations; males; malpractice; medical ethics; mentally ill; *misconduct; patients; *physician patient relationship; *physicians; professional family relationship; professional organizations; *psychiatry; *psychotherapy; punishment; self regulation; sex offenses; *sexuality; time factors; American Medical Association; *American Psychiatric Association; United States

---

BE = bioethics accession number   fn. = footnotes   refs. = references

Lee, Nick. Spotlight on South African medical profession. [News]. *Lancet.* 1997 Jul 5; 350(9070): 39. BE56593.
blacks; historical aspects; *human rights; *misconduct; organizational policies; *physician's role; physicians; politics; prisoners; *professional organizations; social discrimination; *torture; Biko, Steve; *Medical Association of South Africa; *South Africa; Twentieth Century

Lehrman, Sally. University settles with patients over trade in 'stolen' embryos. [News]. *Nature.* 1997 Jul 31; 388(6641): 411. BE56064.
*embryo transfer; human experimentation; *in vitro fertilization; informed consent; investigational drugs; investigators; *legal liability; *misconduct; physicians; *scientific misconduct; *universities; Asch, Ricardo; Balmaceda, Jose; California; Center for Reproductive Health (Irvine, CA); Stone, Sergio; *University of California, Irvine; *University of California, San Diego

Lock, Stephen. Research misconduct: a brief history and a comparison. *Journal of Internal Medicine.* 1994 Feb; 235(2): 123–127. 16 refs. BE55602.
authorship; biomedical research; editorial policies; *fraud; historical aspects; human experimentation; institutional policies; international aspects; investigators; physicians; regulation; research ethics committees; research institutes; science; *scientific misconduct; universities; Great Britain; United States

Macready, Norra. US doctors lie to help patients. [News]. *BMJ (British Medical Journal).* 1997 Jul 19; 315(7101): 148. BE58620.
*attitudes; *deception; diagnosis; health care delivery; *health insurance; *misconduct; moral obligations; *patient advocacy; *physicians; remuneration; survey; United States

Mansour, Paul. Turkish doctors collude in torture. [News]. *BMJ (British Medical Journal).* 1997 Mar 8; 314(7082): 699. 1 ref. BE58747.
dissent; fraud; human rights; medical records; *misconduct; organizational policies; physician's role; *physicians; *prisoners; professional organizations; *torture; Amnesty International; *Turkey; Turkish Medical Association

Marshall, Eliot. Medline searches turn up cases of suspected plagiarism. [News]. *Science.* 1998 Jan 23; 279(5350): 473–474. Includes inset article, "The Internet: a powerful tool for plagiarism sleuths," p. 474. BE56877.
authorship; biomedical research; computer communication networks; data banks; *fraud; international aspects; investigators; literature; regulation; *scientific misconduct; Denmark; Internet; *Jendryczko, Andrzej; MEDLINE; *Poland

Mitchell, Peter. Edinburgh doctor struck off because of clinical–trial fraud. [News]. *Lancet.* 1997 Jul 26; 350(9073): 273. BE56075.
consent forms; human experimentation; investigational drugs; *physicians; *punishment; *scientific misconduct; self regulation; *Anderton, John; General Medical Council (Great Britain); *Scotland

Mollica, Richard F. Human rights reflections in daily medical practice. [Editorial]. *Medical Journal of Australia.* 1996 Dec 2–16; 165(11–12): 594–595. 9 refs. BE58973.
*disadvantaged; *human rights; *misconduct; *obligations to society; *patient care; *physician's role; prisoners; public policy; *social problems; torture; violence; war

Morris, Kelly. UK GMC finds lack of consent merits serious–misconduct judgment. [News]. *Lancet.* 1998 Mar 28; 351(9107): 966. BE58748.
death; *minors; *misconduct; *parental consent; patient care;

*physicians; punishment; *regulation; heart catheterization; *General Medical Council (Great Britain); *Great Britain; Jenkins, Deborah; *Taylor, James

Morris, Kelly. UK misconduct case raises informed–consent issues. [News]. *Lancet.* 1998 Mar 21; 351(9106): 885. BE58857.
children; death; heart diseases; informed consent; *misconduct; *parental consent; *physicians; surgery; *angioplasty; directive adherence; *Great Britain

Morrison, James; Wickersham, Peter. Physicians disciplined by a state medical board. *JAMA.* 1998 Jun 17; 279(23): 1889–1893. 33 refs. BE58422.
alcohol abuse; drug abuse; females; fraud; *government regulation; males; medical specialties; *misconduct; negligence; patient care; physician patient relationship; *physicians; professional competence; *punishment; *self regulation; sex offenses; sexuality; state government; statistics; professional impairment; *California; *Medical Board of California
CONTEXT: State medical boards discipline several thousand physicians each year. Although certain subgroups, such as those disciplined for malpractice, substance use, or sexual abuse, have been studied, little is known about disciplined physicians as a group. OBJECTIVE: To assess the offenses, contributing factors, and type of discipline of a consecutive series of disciplined physicians. DESIGN: Case–control study on publicly available data matching 375 disciplined physicians with 2 groups of control physicians, one matched solely by locale, and a second matched for sex, type of practice, and locale. SUBJECTS: All disciplined physicians publicly reported by the Medical Board of California from October 1995 through April 1997. MAIN OUTCOME MEASURES: Characteristics of disciplined physicians, offenses leading to discipline, and type of discipline. RESULTS: A total of 375 physicians licensed by the Medical Board of California (approximately 0.24% per year) were disciplined for 465 offenses. The most frequent causes for discipline were negligence or incompetence (34%), abuse of alcohol or other drugs (14%), inappropriate prescribing practices (11%), inappropriate contact with patients (10%), and fraud (9%). Discipline imposed was revocation of medical license (21%), actual suspension of license (13%), stayed suspension of license (45%), and reprimand (21%). Type of offense was significantly associated with severity of discipline (P=.03). In logistic regression models comparing disciplined physicians with controls matched by locale, board discipline was significantly associated with physicians' sex (odds ratio [OR] for women, 0.44; 95% confidence interval [CI], 0.28–0.70) and involvement in direct patient care (OR, 2.56; 95% CI, 1.75–3.75). In the regression model with additional matching criteria, disciplinary action was negatively associated with specialty board certification (OR, 0.42; 95% CI, 0.29–0.60) and positively associated with being in practice more than 20 years (OR, 2.02; 95% CI, 1.39–2.92). CONCLUSIONS: A small but substantial proportion of physicians is disciplined each year for a variety of offenses. Further study of disciplined physicians is necessary to identify physicians at high risk for offenses leading to disciplinary action and to develop effective interventions to prevent these offenses.

Mudur, Ganapati. Indian study of women with cervical lesions called unethical. [News]. *BMJ (British Medical Journal).* 1997 Apr 12; 314(7087): 1065. BE56063.
attitudes; *cancer; developing countries; *disadvantaged; disclosure; *females; historical aspects; *human

---

BE = bioethics accession number   fn. = footnotes   refs. = references

experimentation; *informed consent; investigators; retrospective moral judgment; *scientific misconduct; withholding treatment; *India; Institute of Cytology and Preventive Oncology (New Delhi)

Pasztor, Andy; Lagnado, Lucette. Ethics czar aims to heal Columbia. [News]. *Wall Street Journal.* 1997 Nov 26: B1, B6. BE56343.
administrators; disclosure; federal government; *fraud; government regulation; *health care delivery; *industry; institutional policies; *private sector; *proprietary hospitals; *self regulation; voluntary programs; business ethics; *Columbia/HCA Healthcare Corporation; Medicare

RAGE (Radiotherapy Action Group Exposure) National [Great Britain]. All treatment and trials must have informed consent. [Personal view]. *BMJ (British Medical Journal).* 1997 Apr 12; 314(7087): 1134–1135. BE55676.
cancer; disclosure; *females; *human experimentation; *informed consent; *injuries; morbidity; patient participation; *patients; physicians; *political activity; *radiology; research ethics committees; risks and benefits; *scientific misconduct; trust; *Great Britain; *RAGE (Radiotherapy Action Group Exposure)

Rennie, Drummond. Dealing with research misconduct in the United Kingdom: an American perspective on research integrity. *BMJ (British Medical Journal).* 1998 Jun 6; 316(7146): 1726–1728. 9 refs. BE58217.
biomedical research; federal government; fraud; government financing; government regulation; institutional policies; international aspects; investigators; motivation; *regulation; *scientific misconduct; self regulation; whistleblowing; *Great Britain; Office of Research Integrity; *United States

Riis, Povl. Dealing with research misconduct in the United Kingdom: honest advice from Denmark. *BMJ (British Medical Journal).* 1998 Jun 6; 316(7146): 1733. BE58218.
advisory committees; authorship; biomedical research; committee membership; fraud; international aspects; investigators; organization and administration; *regulation; *scientific misconduct; whistleblowing; *national ethics committees; Denmark; *Great Britain

Riis, Povl. Prevention and management of fraud -- in theory. *Journal of Internal Medicine.* 1994 Feb; 235(2): 107–113. 3 refs. BE55608.
advisory committees; biomedical research; editorial policies; *fraud; international aspects; investigators; public participation; public policy; punishment; *regulation; research ethics committees; research institutes; science; *scientific misconduct; self regulation; standards; universities; whistleblowing; national ethics committees; Denmark

Rinchuse, Daniel J.; Rinchuse, Donald J.; Deluzio, Charles. Ethical checklist for dental practice. *Journal of the American College of Dentists.* 1995 Fall; 62(3): 45–48. 5 refs. BE55771.
advertising; deception; *dentistry; economics; *gifts; *health personnel; *interprofessional relations; legal aspects; medical specialties; *misconduct; professional ethics; *referral and consultation; business ethics; health services misuse; United States

Roman, Brenda; Kay, Jerald. Residency education on the prevention of physician–patient sexual misconduct. *Academic Psychiatry.* 1997 Spring; 21(1): 26–34. 34 refs. BE58123.
curriculum; *internship and residency; *medical education; *misconduct; *physician patient relationship; *psychiatry; *psychotherapy; *sexuality; teaching methods

Rose, Mary R.; Fischer, Karla. Do authorship policies impact students' judgments of perceived wrongdoing? *Ethics and Behavior.* 1998; 8(1): 59–79. 18 refs. 4 fn. BE58918.
*authorship; *behavioral research; codes of ethics; *faculty; females; institutional policies; interprofessional relations; males; professional organizations; *scientific misconduct; *students; survey; universities; whistleblowing; American Psychological Association
Although authorship policies exist, researchers understand little about their impact on perceptions of authorship scenarios. Graduate students (N=277) at a large university read 1 of 3 vignettes about a graduate student–faculty collaboration. One half of the surveys included the American Psychological Association's statement on authorship. Participants rated (a) the ethics of the professor as first author and (b) the likelihood of a dissatisfied student reporting the authorship result, as well as the effectiveness and negative consequences of reporting. Work arrangements on the project had a consistent main effect. Also, an authorship policy impacted women's ratings of first authorship when the student contributed the idea for a project. For men, a policy impacted only ratings of the likelihood of reporting when a professor was first author on a student's dissertation. Apart from sex, no other demographic variables on participants were predictive. Discussion focuses on the policy's potential for making only some specific issues salient.

Rosen, Linda. Reporting incompetent or unethical behavior: an ethical and legal dilemma. *Today's OR Nurse.* 1985 Oct; 7(10): 36–37. 4 refs. BE56966.
codes of ethics; *health personnel; interprofessional relations; *legal aspects; *misconduct; *nurses; nursing ethics; *professional competence; *whistleblowing; *professional impairment

Ross, Lena B.; Roy, Manisha, eds. Cast the First Stone: Ethics in Analytic Practice. Wilmette, IL: Chiron Publications; 1995. 146 p. Includes references. ISBN 0-933029-89-6. BE58319.
emotions; females; *health personnel; love; males; *misconduct; morality; *professional ethics; *professional patient relationship; psychology; *psychotherapy; self concept; self regulation; *sexuality; values; Jung, Carl

Schiermeier, Quirin. Gene therapist accused of fraud to seek redress in German court. [News]. *Nature.* 1997 Sep 11; 389(6647): 105. BE56062.
biomedical research; *fraud; gene therapy; genetic research; interprofessional relations; investigators; *legal aspects; *scientific misconduct; universities; Brach, Marion; *Germany; *Herrmann, Friedhelm; University of Freiburg; University of Ulm

Scutchfield, F. Douglas; Benjamin, Regina. The role of the medical profession in physician discipline. [Editorial]. *JAMA.* 1998 Jun 17; 279(23): 1915–1916. 5 refs. BE58425.
*government regulation; medical education; medical ethics; *misconduct; physician patient relationship; *physicians; punishment; *self regulation; sex offenses; sexuality; state government; United States

Shapiro, Joseph P. Death be not swift enough: fraud fighters begin to probe the expense of hospice care. [News]. *U.S. News and World Report.* 1997 Mar 24; 122(11): 34–35. BE55794.
diagnosis; *economics; federal government; *fraud; *government financing; *hospices; prognosis; proprietary health facilities; selection for treatment; *terminal care; terminally ill; time factors; Florida; *Medicare; *United

---

BE = bioethics accession number   fn. = footnotes   refs. = references

States

Sharav, Vera Hassner. Independent family advocates challenge the fraternity of silence. *In:* Shamoo, Adil E., ed. Ethics in Neurobiological Research with Human Subjects: The Baltimore Conference on Ethics. Amsterdam: Gordon and Breach; 1997: 175–181. ISBN 2-88449-161-9. BE57015.

attitudes; *conflict of interest; deception; disclosure; drug industry; drugs; family members; federal government; financial support; government regulation; *human experimentation; iatrogenic disease; informed consent; institutionalized persons; *investigators; *mentally ill; *nontherapeutic research; *patient advocacy; physician's role; placebos; professional organizations; psychiatry; psychoactive drugs; research design; research ethics committees; research subjects; risks and benefits; schizophrenia; *scientific misconduct; state government; withholding treatment; *Alliance for the Mentally Ill of New York State; Bronx VA Medical Center (NY); National Institute of Mental Health; New York; Office for Protection from Research Risks; United States

Sidley, Pat. AIDS drug scandal in South Africa continues. [News]. *BMJ (British Medical Journal).* 1998 Mar 14; 316(7134): 800. BE57761.

administrators; *AIDS; conflict of interest; drug industry; *drugs; economics; ethical review; government financing; government regulation; *human experimentation; investigators; legal aspects; *politics; *scientific misconduct; *South Africa; *Virodene; Zuma, Nkosazana

Sidley, Pat. Doctors involved in South Africa's biological warfare programme. [News]. *BMJ (British Medical Journal).* 1998 Jun 20; 316(7148): 1852. BE58124.

*biological warfare; criminal law; historical aspects; investigators; *misconduct; *physicians; psychoactive drugs; public policy; *chemical warfare; Basson, Wouter; *South Africa; Twentieth Century

Sidley, Pat. South Africa Truth Commission calls doctors to account for their actions during the apartheid era. [News]. *BMJ (British Medical Journal).* 1997 Jun 28; 314(7098): 1850. BE56594.

blacks; *human rights; *misconduct; *physicians; political activity; prisoners; *social discrimination; *torture; *South Africa

Sidley, Pat. South Africa's doctors apologise for apartheid years. [News]. *BMJ (British Medical Journal).* 1995 Jul 15; 311(6998): 148. BE56667.

*blacks; human rights; minority groups; *misconduct; *moral complicity; obligations to society; *organizational policies; patient care; *physicians; political activity; prisoners; *professional organizations; public policy; *social discrimination; torture; wrongful death; Biko, Steve; *Medical Association of South Africa; *South Africa

Skolnick, Andrew A. Advisory committee report recommends that US make amends for human radiation experiments. [News]. *JAMA.* 1995 Sep 27; 274(12): 933. BE56668.

*advisory committees; compensation; *federal government; historical aspects; *human experimentation; *public policy; *radiation; research subjects; *scientific misconduct; *Advisory Committee on Human Radiation Experiments; Twentieth Century; *United States

Smith, Richard. All doctors are problem doctors: doctors worldwide must do better with managing problem colleagues. [Editorial]. *BMJ (British Medical Journal).* 1997 Mar 22; 314(7084): 841–842. 3 refs. BE58601.

international aspects; interprofessional relations; malpractice; medical education; *misconduct; *physicians; professional competence; psychological stress; *self regulation; *sociology of medicine; uncertainty; medical errors; *physician impairment; Great Britain

Smith, Richard. Beyond conflict of interest: transparency is the key. [Editorial]. *BMJ (British Medical Journal).* 1998 Aug 1; 317(7154): 291–292. 18 refs. BE58818.

accountability; *biomedical research; *conflict of interest; *disclosure; economics; *editorial policies; *financial support; *industry; *investigators; *physicians; *BMJ (British Medical Journal)

Smith, Richard. Misconduct in research: editors respond -- the Committee on Publication Ethics (COPE) is formed. [Editorial]. *BMJ (British Medical Journal).* 1997 Jul 26; 315(7102): 201–202. 8 refs. BE58501.

biomedical research; *editorial policies; fraud; investigators; *scientific misconduct; *self regulation; *Committee on Publication Ethics (Great Britain); Great Britain

Smith, Richard. The need for a national body for research misconduct: nothing less will reassure the public. [Editorial]. *BMJ (British Medical Journal).* 1998 Jun 6; 316(7146): 1686–1687. 12 refs. BE58221.

advisory committees; biomedical research; editorial policies; fraud; international aspects; *regulation; *scientific misconduct; self regulation; national ethics committees; Committee on Publication Ethics (Great Britain); *Great Britain

Stecklow, Steve; Johannes, Laura. Drug makers relied on clinical researchers who now await trial. [News]. *Wall Street Journal.* 1997 Aug 15: A1, A6. BE55547.

competence; contracts; dementia; *drug industry; entrepreneurship; faculty; financial support; *fraud; government regulation; health personnel; human experimentation; *incentives; informed consent; *investigators; medical schools; physicians; psychoactive drugs; research subjects; schizophrenia; *scientific misconduct; *selection of subjects; *self regulation; technical expertise; guideline adherence; *Borison, Richard; *Diamond, Bruce; Food and Drug Administration; Georgia; Medical College of Georgia

U.S. Congress. Senate. Committee on Labor and Human Resources. Human Subjects Research: Radiation Experimentation. Hearing, 13 Jan 1994 (Waltham, MA). Washington, DC: U.S. Government Printing Office; 1994. 61 p. S. Hrg. 103–511. ISBN 0-16-044800-X. BE58699.

children; consent forms; deception; disclosure; *federal government; food; health hazards; *historical aspects; *human experimentation; informed consent; *institutionalized persons; *mentally retarded; nontherapeutic research; *radiation; records; research subjects; risks and benefits; *scientific misconduct; universities; vulnerable populations; Advisory Committee on Human Radiation Experiments; Fernald State School (MA); Massachusetts; Massachusetts Institute of Technology; *Twentieth Century; *United States

U.S. Department of Health and Human Services. Departmental Appeals Board. Research Integrity Adjudications Panel. Mikulas Popovic, M.D., Ph.D. [Docket No. A–93–100; Decision No. 1446. 1993 Nov 3 (date of decision)]. Washington, DC: U.S. Department of Health and Human Services; 1993 Nov 3. 79+ p. Includes an additional 18 p. of appendices. BE57697.

AIDS; biomedical research; *due process; expert testimony; *federal government; government regulation; investigators; *legal aspects; *scientific misconduct; standards; Department of Health and Human Services; Departmental Appeals Board (DHHS); *Office of Research Integrity; *Popovic, Mikulas; Research Integrity Adjudications Panel (DHHS);

BE = bioethics accession number   fn. = footnotes   refs. = references

Science; *United States

Wadman, Meredith. Mentally disabled research subjects 'need protection.' [News]. *Nature.* 1997 Oct 16; 389(6652): 652. BE56161.
advisory committees; federal government; government regulation; *human experimentation; informed consent; *mentally disabled; psychoactive drugs; *public policy; research subjects; *scientific misconduct; withholding treatment; National Bioethics Advisory Commission; National Institute of Mental Health; United States

Wadman, Meredith. $100m payout after drug data withheld. [News]. *Nature.* 1997 Aug 21; 388(6644): 703. BE56353.
*biomedical research; *compensation; contracts; costs and benefits; *drug industry; *drugs; economics; *financial support; human experimentation; legal liability; *misconduct; patients; universities; Dong, Betty; *Knoll Pharmaceutical Co.; *Synthroid; United States; University of California, San Francisco

Watts, Jonathan. Japan taken to court over germ-warfare allegations. [News]. *Lancet.* 1998 Feb 28; 351(9103): 657. BE58264.
*biological warfare; *historical aspects; *human experimentation; international aspects; legal aspects; *scientific misconduct; war; China; *Japan; Twentieth Century; *World War II

Weil, Vivian; Arzbaecher, Robert. Ethics and relationships in laboratories and research communities. *Professional Ethics.* 1995 Spring–Summer; 4(3-4): 83–125. 17 fn. BE55673.
accountability; administrators; authorship; *biomedical research; *case studies; communication; confidentiality; conflict of interest; deception; *faculty; females; financial support; goals; *interprofessional relations; *investigators; *laboratories; minority groups; organization and administration; peer review; professional autonomy; *professional ethics; property rights; *science; *scientific misconduct; self regulation; social control; social dominance; standards; *students; trust; values; Gallo, Robert; National Institutes of Health; Popovic, Mikulas; United States

Wells, Frank O. Management of research misconduct -- in practice. *Journal of Internal Medicine.* 1994 Feb; 235(2): 115–121. 10 refs. BE55606.
biomedical research; *drug industry; financial support; *fraud; guidelines; human experimentation; investigators; medical education; motivation; *organizational policies; *physicians; punishment; *regulation; review committees; *scientific misconduct; Association of the British Pharmaceutical Industry; General Medical Council (Great Britain); *Great Britain; WHO Guidelines for Good Clinical Practice (GCP) for Trials on Pharmaceutical Products

Werhane, Patricia; Doering, Jeffrey. Conflicts of interest and conflicts of commitment. *Professional Ethics.* 1995 Spring–Summer; 4(3-4): 47–81. 4 fn. BE55672.
accountability; administrators; *biomedical research; case studies; codes of ethics; *conflict of interest; disclosure; editorial policies; financial support; genome mapping; industry; information dissemination; institutional policies; interprofessional relations; *investigators; patents; *professional ethics; professional organizations; property rights; research subjects; *scientific misconduct; *self regulation; standards; trust; universities

Werner, Michael J.; American College of Physicians. Understanding the fraud and abuse laws: guidance for internists. *Annals of Internal Medicine.* 1998 Apr 15; 128(8): 678–684. Paper developed by the ACP Health and Public Policy Committee and approved by the ACP

Board of Regents on 11 Jan 1998. BE58001.
*conflict of interest; *economics; entrepreneurship; federal government; *fraud; government financing; *government regulation; guidelines; internal medicine; managed care programs; *physician self-referral; *physicians; professional organizations; proprietary health facilities; punishment; referral and consultation; remuneration; group practice; *American College of Physicians; Department of Health and Human Services; Ethics in Patient Referrals Act 1989; False Claims Act; Health Care Financing Administration; Medicare; *United States

Whitbeck, Caroline. Research ethics. *In:* Chadwick, Ruth, ed. Encyclopedia of Applied Ethics, Volume 3. San Diego, CA: Academic Press; 1998: 835–843. 13 refs. ISBN 0-12-227068-1. BE56270.
authorship; *biomedical research; editorial policies; faculty; federal government; fraud; government regulation; information dissemination; interprofessional relations; investigators; peer review; professional ethics; professional organizations; *scientific misconduct; self regulation; students; universities; United States

White, Caroline. Call for research misconduct agency. [News]. *BMJ (British Medical Journal).* 1998 Jun 6; 316(7146): 1695. BE58247.
biomedical research; editorial policies; fraud; guidelines; human experimentation; investigators; *regulation; *scientific misconduct; standards; whistleblowing; Committee on Publication Ethics (Great Britain); *Great Britain

Wigzell, Hans; Pontén, Jan. Refutation of investigation commissioned by Karolinska Institute. [Letter]. *Lancet.* 1998 May 16; 351(9114): 1510–1511. 3 refs. BE58856.
biomedical research; fraud; investigators; peer review; research institutes; *scientific misconduct; self regulation; *Karolinska Institute; Lönn, Ulf; *Sweden

Wilbers, Doaitse; Willibrord, C.M.; Schultz, Weijmar, et al. Sexual contact between doctors and patients. *In:* Lens, Peter; van der Wal, Gerrit, eds. Problem Doctors: A Conspiracy of Silence. Washington, DC: IOS Press; 1997: 75–85. 47 refs. ISBN 90-5199-287-4. BE56999.
continuing education; criminal law; emotions; international aspects; mass media; medical education; medical specialties; *misconduct; organizational policies; patients; *physician patient relationship; *physicians; prevalence; professional organizations; psychotherapy; risk; self regulation; *sexuality; social dominance; time factors; American Medical Association; Canada; Europe; Great Britain; United States

Williams, Nigel. Editors call for misconduct watchdog. [News]. *Science.* 1998 Jun 12; 280(5370): 1685–1686. BE58272.
biomedical research; editorial policies; ethical review; fraud; investigators; *regulation; *scientific misconduct; Committee on Publication Ethics (Great Britain); General Medical Council (Great Britain); *Great Britain

Williams, Nigel. Editors seek ways to cope with fraud. [News]. *Science.* 1997 Nov 14; 278(5341): 1221. BE56893.
biomedical research; *editorial policies; fraud; *international aspects; investigators; *scientific misconduct; whistleblowing; *Committee on Publication Ethics (Great Britain); Deutsche Forschungsgemeinschaft; *Europe; Max Planck Society

Williams, Peter; Wallace, David. Unit 731: The Japanese Army's Secret of Secrets. London: Hodder and Stoughton; 1989. 366 p. 596 fn. ISBN 0-340-39463-3. BE57390.
*biological warfare; confidentiality; dehumanization;

---

disclosure; federal government; *historical aspects; *human experimentation; international aspects; *investigators; killing; military personnel; *moral complicity; *prisoners; public policy; *scientific misconduct; technical expertise; torture; war; chemical warfare; Canada; China; France; Germany; Great Britain; Ishii, Shiro; *Japan; Korean War; Netherlands; Twentieth Century; *United States; USSR; *World War II

Wise, Jacqui. Karolinska professor broke research rules. [News]. *BMJ (British Medical Journal).* 1997 Sep 6; 315(7108): 563. BE56896.
> biomedical research; cancer; fraud; investigators; research institutes; *scientific misconduct; *Karolinska Institute; *Lönn, Ulf; *Sweden

Wolinsky, Howard. Steps still being taken to undo damage of "America's Nuremberg." [News]. *Annals of Internal Medicine.* 1997 Aug 15; 127(4): I43–I44. BE56100.
> attitudes; *blacks; codes of ethics; compensation; drugs; federal government; historical aspects; *human experimentation; informed consent; males; National Socialism; organ donation; physicians; *research subjects; *scientific misconduct; social impact; *syphilis; trust; withholding treatment; Germany; *Nuremberg Code; Public Health Service; *Tuskegee Syphilis Study; Twentieth Century; *United States

Woody, Robert Henley. Dubious and bogus credentials in mental health practice. *Ethics and Behavior.* 1997; 7(4): 337–345. 13 refs. BE58665.
> counseling; education; *health personnel; mental health; *misconduct; *professional competence; professional ethics; *professional organizations; psychology; *psychotherapy; *self regulation; social workers; *standards; quality assurance

Within an ethics framework, this article explores mental health practitioners' use of credentials that lack acceptable accreditation or authority. Increased competition among mental health care providers has elevated the importance of credentials for marketing professional services. Practitioners worried about economic survival, along with certain personality characteristics (e.g., sheer ego), are tempted to rely on credentials that lack proof of quality, thereby potentially jeopardizing professionalism. Specific assertions and recommendations are set forth in the interest of safeguarding consumers and promoting professionalism.

Yarborough, Mark. The reluctant retained witness: alleged sexual misconduct in the doctor/patient relationship. *Journal of Medicine and Philosophy.* 1997 Aug; 22(4): 345–364. 10 refs. BE55930.
> bioethical issues; case studies; conflict of interest; *decision making; *ethicist's role; *ethicists; *expert testimony; faculty; interprofessional relations; judicial action; *legal aspects; *misconduct; *physician patient relationship; *physicians; professional ethics; remuneration; *sexuality; *technical expertise; uncertainty; universities; Colorado

Testifying as an expert ethics witness raises a number of important issues. These include: the prospect of generating adverse publicity for oneself and one's institution, avoiding bias, giving testimony that is at odds with testimony given by colleagues, potential conflicts of interest introduced by reimbursement, the need of those who hear the testimony of bioethicists to appreciate the nature of moral expertise, the difficulty of assessing the quality of legal evidence which emerges from adversarial legal proceedings, and the need to consider what weight should be assigned to expert ethics testimony. Along with these issues, what might constitute sexual misconduct is addressed in the essay so that readers can review the decision-making of the

author in two cases.

Youngner, Julius S. The scientific misconduct process: a scientist's view from the inside. *JAMA.* 1998 Jan 7; 279(1): 62–64. 7 refs. BE57815.
> biomedical research; *due process; federal government; *government regulation; investigators; lawyers; legal aspects; *peer review; science; *scientific misconduct; Department of Health and Human Services; *Office of Research Integrity; *Research Integrity Adjudications Panel (DHHS); *United States

Zinn, Christopher. Australian orphans were used as guinea pigs. [News]. *BMJ (British Medical Journal).* 1997 Jun 21; 314(7097): 1783. BE56129.
> *children; historical aspects; *human experimentation; *immunization; *infants; institutionalized persons; research subjects; retrospective moral judgment; *scientific misconduct; vulnerable populations; *Australia; Commonwealth Serum Laboratories (Australia); Twentieth Century

Human rights begin at home. [Editorial]. *BMJ (British Medical Journal).* 1997 Nov 29; 315(7120): 1387. BE56915.
> health personnel; *human experimentation; *human rights; investigators; mentally ill; *misconduct; patient care; *prisoners; *scientific misconduct; *torture; Great Britain; United Nations; United States; Universal Declaration of Human Rights

Integrity in Scientific Research. [Videorecording].American Association for the Advancement of Science; available for sale from Science Integrity Videos, AAAS Directorate for Science and Policy Programs, 1200 New York Ave., NW, Washington, DC 20005, 202–326–6600; 1996. 5 videocassettes; 44 min. (8–10 min. each); sd.; color; 1/2 in.; VHS. Produced by Amram Nowak Associates, Inc. for the AAAS in cooperation with the Medical College of Georgia's Division of Health Communication; directed by Stuart Hersh; written and produced by Manya Starr. Accompanied by a 50–page Discussion and Resource Guide. BE57897.
> animal experimentation; *authorship; *biomedical research; case studies; *conflict of interest; contracts; disclosure; *financial support; *industry; *information dissemination; *investigators; peer review; professional ethics; psychological stress; *scientific misconduct; universities; whistleblowing; publication bias; *research ethics

Research without consent in South Africa. [News; title supplied]. *BMJ (British Medical Journal).* 1997 Jun 28; 314(7098): 1850. BE56128.
> *blacks; *human experimentation; *industry; informed consent; *occupational exposure; *occupational medicine; *scientific misconduct; *South Africa

GENE THERAPY

See also GENETIC INTERVENTION, RECOMBINANT DNA RESEARCH, GENETIC SERVICES

Archer, Luis. Genetic testing and gene therapy: the scientific and ethical background. *In:* Doherty, Peter; Sutton, Agneta, eds. Man–Made Man: Ethical and Legal Issues in Genetics. Dublin, Ireland: Open Air; 1997: 29–45. 18 fn. ISBN 1-85182-278-X. BE58294.
> advisory committees; autonomy; confidentiality; embryos; employment; eugenics; family members; *gene therapy; genetic enhancement; genetic predisposition; *genetic screening; germ cells; informed consent; insurance; justice; legal aspects; occupational exposure; parental consent; public

---

policy; rights; *risks and benefits; social discrimination; Europe

Areen, Judith. Regulating human gene therapy. *West Virginia Law Review.* 1985 Fall; 88(2): 153–171. 90 fn. BE56608.
advisory committees; decision making; federal government; *gene therapy; *government regulation; historical aspects; human experimentation; investigators; public policy; recombinant DNA research; research ethics committees; risks and benefits; science; scientific misconduct; self regulation; Biotechnology Science Board; Department of Health and Human Services; Recombinant DNA Advisory Committee; Twentieth Century; *United States

Bailey, Keith; Ridgway, Anthony. A rational approach to regulation of gene therapy in Canada. *Transfusion Science.* 1996 Mar; 17(1): 197–202. 1 ref. BE55667.
advisory committees; drugs; *gene therapy; *government regulation; guidelines; human experimentation; industry; investigational drugs; public policy; risks and benefits; voluntary programs; *Canada; United States

Bayertz, Kurt. Ethical aspects of gene therapy and molecular genetic diagnostics. *Cytokines and Molecular Therapy.* 1996 Sep; 2(3): 207–211. 13 refs. BE58352.
coercion; *gene therapy; genetic disorders; genetic predisposition; *genetic screening; health insurance; late-onset disorders; mass screening; preventive medicine; public opinion; *risks and benefits; social control; social discrimination; social impact; Europe; Germany

Boyce, Nell. In sickness and in health. [News]. *New Scientist.* 1997 Oct 25; 156(2105): 20–21. BE59087.
advisory committees; federal government; *gene therapy; *genetic enhancement; germ cells; *government regulation; human characteristics; nontherapeutic research; normality; therapeutic research; Recombinant DNA Advisory Committee; United States

Deepandung, Attajinda; Noonpakdee, Wilai T. The moral status of the human genome. *In:* Agius, Emmanuel; Busuttil, Salvino, eds. Germ–Line Intervention and Our Responsibilities to Future Generations. Boston, MA: Kluwer Academic; 1998: 13–18. 9 refs. ISBN 0–7923–4828–1. BE57876.
confidentiality; future generations; *gene therapy; genetic counseling; genetic information; genetic research; *genetic screening; *genome mapping; human experimentation; moral obligations; obligations of society; privacy; public policy; resource allocation; risks and benefits; Thailand

Dickens, Bernard M. Legal and ethical challenges in gene therapy. *Transfusion Science.* 1996 Mar; 17(1): 191–196. 10 refs. BE55671.
advisory committees; age factors; children; conflict of interest; cosmetic surgery; critically ill; disclosure; emergency care; ethical review; freedom; *gene therapy; genetic disorders; genetic enhancement; genetic research; germ cells; government regulation; health insurance reimbursement; human experimentation; industry; informed consent; investigators; *justice; paternalism; patient care; peer review; private sector; property rights; resource allocation; selection for treatment; *therapeutic research; withholding treatment; investigational therapies; seriously ill; Clothier Committee; Great Britain

Doherty, Peter; Sutton, Agneta, eds. Man–Made Man: Ethical and Legal Issues in Genetics. Dublin, Ireland: Open Air; 1997. 116 p. Includes references. ISBN 1–85182–278–X. BE58293.
autonomy; children; confidentiality; disabled; embryos; eugenics; fetuses; *gene therapy; genetic counseling; genetic determinism; *genetic intervention; genetic predisposition; genetic research; *genetic screening; genetics; genome

mapping; informed consent; international aspects; personhood; preimplantation diagnosis; prenatal diagnosis; public policy; regulation; reproduction; rights; risks and benefits; selective abortion; social control; social discrimination; trends; values; Europe; Great Britain

Engelhardt, H. Tristram. Human nature genetically re-engineered: moral responsibilities to future generations. *In:* Agius, Emmanuel; Busuttil, Salvino, eds. Germ–Line Intervention and Our Responsibilities to Future Generations. Boston, MA: Kluwer Academic; 1998: 51–63. 2 refs. 1 fn. ISBN 0–7923–4828–1. BE57879.
beneficence; contraception; *cultural pluralism; decision making; ecology; *ethical analysis; *freedom; *future generations; *gene therapy; *genetic enhancement; *genetic intervention; *germ cells; goals; guidelines; international aspects; *moral obligations; morality; regulation; reproduction; *risks and benefits; *secularism

Feinberg, John S. A theological basis for genetic intervention. *In:* Kilner, John F.; Pentz, Rebecca D.; Young, Frank E., eds. Genetic Ethics: Do the Ends Justify the Genes? Grand Rapids, MI: W.B. Eerdmans; 1997: 183–192. 12 fn. ISBN 0–8028–4428–6. BE56724.
*Christian ethics; eugenics; *gene therapy; *genetic enhancement; *genetic intervention; germ cells; morality; recombinant DNA research; risks and benefits; secularism; theology

Fox, Jeffrey L. Green light for gene therapy in healthy volunteers. [News]. *Nature Biotechnology.* 1997 Apr; 15(4): 314. BE55858.
advisory committees; federal government; *gene therapy; genetic research; *government regulation; *human experimentation; investigators; *nontherapeutic research; *volunteers; Crystal, Ron; Food and Drug Administration; National Institutes of Health; *Recombinant DNA Advisory Committee; United States

Gillott, John. Germ line gene therapy –– why not? *GenEthics News.* 1995 Nov–Dec; No. 9: 6. BE56224.
attitudes; disabled; eugenics; *gene therapy; genetic counseling; genetic intervention; *germ cells; *risks and benefits; Genetic Interest Group (Great Britain); Great Britain

Glannon, Walter. Genes, embryos, and future people. *Bioethics.* 1998 Jul; 12(3): 187–211. 36 fn. BE58893.
beginning of life; *beneficence; children; *cryopreservation; *embryo disposition; *embryos; *eugenics; fetal therapy; fetuses; future generations; *gene therapy; *genetic disorders; genetic enhancement; *genetic intervention; *genetic screening; germ cells; *injuries; justice; late-onset disorders; mentally disabled; *moral obligations; *moral policy; pain; parents; personhood; physically disabled; posthumous reproduction; *preimplantation diagnosis; *quality of life; reproduction; reproductive technologies; risks and benefits; self concept; suffering; time factors; value of life; *wrongful life

Testing embryonic cells for genetic abnormalities gives us the capacity to predict whether and to what extent people will exist with disease and disability. Moreover, the freezing of embryos for long periods of time enables us to alter the length of a normal human lifespan. After highlighting the shortcomings of somatic-cell gene therapy and germ-line genetic alteration, I argue that the testing and selective termination of genetically defective embryos is the only medically and morally defensible way to prevent the existence of people with severe disability, pain and suffering that make their lives not worth living for them on the whole. In addition, I consider the possible harmful effects on children born from frozen embryos after the deaths of their biological parents, or when their parents are at an advanced age.

BE = bioethics accession number   fn. = footnotes   refs. = references

I also explore whether embryos have moral status and whether the prospects for disease-preventing genetic alteration can justify long-term cryopreservation of embryos.

Hedgecoe, Adam M. Gene therapy. *In:* Chadwick, Ruth, ed. Encyclopedia of Applied Ethics, Volume 2. San Diego, CA: Academic Press; 1998: 383–390. 4 refs. ISBN 0–12–227067–3. BE56386.
    beneficence; eugenics; future generations; *gene therapy; genetic enhancement; germ cells; *moral policy; risks and benefits; dignity

Holtug, Nils. Altering humans -- the case for and against human gene therapy. *Cambridge Quarterly of Healthcare Ethics.* 1997 Spring; 6(2): 157–174. 68 fn. BE56427.
    aggression; altruism; autonomy; behavioral genetics; beneficence; deontological ethics; disabled; embryos; eugenics; evolution; future generations; gene pool; *gene therapy; genetic disorders; *genetic enhancement; genetic identity; *germ cells; justice; *moral policy; preimplantation diagnosis; prenatal diagnosis; religious ethics; reproduction; review; *risks and benefits; selective abortion; social control; social discrimination; teleological ethics
In this paper, I shall consider how deontological and consequentialist objections apply to somatic, germ-line, and enhancement gene therapy, and whether they provide overall reasons not to perform one or several of these kinds of therapy.

Juengst, Eric T. Should we treat the human germ-line as a global human resource? *In:* Agius, Emmanuel; Busuttil, Salvino, eds. Germ-Line Intervention and Our Responsibilities to Future Generations. Boston, MA: Kluwer Academic; 1998: 85–102. 13 refs. 8 fn. ISBN 0–7923–4828–1. BE57881.
    disabled; eugenics; *future generations; *gene pool; *gene therapy; *genes; genetic disorders; genetic enhancement; genetic intervention; genetic research; genome mapping; *germ cells; human rights; international aspects; justice; metaphor; moral obligations; preventive medicine; privacy; public health; social discrimination; stigmatization

Qiu, Ren–Zong. Germ-line engineering as the eugenics of the future. *In:* Agius, Emmanuel; Busuttil, Salvino, eds. Germ-Line Intervention and Our Responsibilities to Future Generations. Boston, MA: Kluwer Academic; 1998: 105–116. 22 refs. ISBN 0–7923–4828–1. BE57882.
    contracts; developing countries; *eugenics; *future generations; *gene therapy; genetic determinism; *genetic enhancement; genetic intervention; *germ cells; international aspects; *moral obligations; morality; *rights; values; Confucian ethics; non–Western World; Western World; Parfit, Derek

Reiss, Michael. Biotechnology. *In:* Chadwick, Ruth, ed. Encyclopedia of Applied Ethics, Volume 1. San Diego, CA: Academic Press; 1998: 319–333. 10 refs. ISBN 0–12–227066–5. BE56370.
    animal experimentation; animal rights; *biomedical technologies; drugs; ecology; food; *gene therapy; genetic enhancement; *genetic intervention; genetic materials; germ cells; growth disorders; historical aspects; hormones; international aspects; methods; moral policy; patents; *recombinant DNA research; reproductive technologies; risk; *risks and benefits; suffering; terminology; *transgenic animals; *transgenic organisms; agriculture

Rubenstein, Donald S. Response to "Dimensions and classification of genetic interventions in the human genome," by Matthew D. Bacchetta and Gerd Richter (*CQ* Vol. 5, No. 3): misinterpretations and misrepresentations. *Cambridge Quarterly of Healthcare*

Ethics. 1998 Winter; 7(1): 90–93. BE58460.
    cloning; *gene therapy; genetic enhancement; *germ cells; *methods; ovum; reproductive technologies; research design; nuclear transplantation

Shinn, Roger L. Genetics, ethics, and theology: the ecumenical discussion. *In:* Peters, Ted, ed. Genetics: Issues of Social Justice. Cleveland, OH: Pilgrim Press; 1998: 122–143. 43 fn. ISBN 0–8298–1251–2. BE57477.
    advisory committees; *Christian ethics; eugenics; future generations; *gene therapy; genetic counseling; genetic enhancement; *genetic intervention; genetic research; *genetics; genome mapping; *germ cells; historical aspects; organizational policies; political activity; Protestant ethics; public policy; Roman Catholic ethics; science; Catechism of the Catholic Church; *National Council of Churches; President's Commission for the Study of Ethical Problems; Rifkin, Jeremy; Twentieth Century; United Methodist Church; United States; *World Council of Churches

Shinn, Roger Lincoln. The New Genetics: Challenges for Science, Faith, and Politics. Wakefield, RI: Moyer Bell; distributed in North America by Publishers Group West, Emeryville, CA; 1996. 175 p. Bibliography: p. 159–170. ISBN 1–55921–171–7. BE56094.
    behavioral genetics; cultural pluralism; decision making; ethics; eugenics; freedom; future generations; *gene therapy; genetic determinism; genetic diversity; *genetic intervention; genetic screening; *genetics; *genome mapping; *germ cells; health; intelligence; investigators; morality; normality; political activity; politics; prenatal diagnosis; *public policy; religion; risks and benefits; science; *social impact; theology; *values; *Human Genome Project; NIH-DOE Working Group on Ethical, Legal, and Social Implications (ELSI); United States

Sutton, Agneta. The new genetics and traditional Hippocratic medicine. *In:* Doherty, Peter; Sutton, Agneta, eds. Man–Made Man: Ethical and Legal Issues in Genetics. Dublin, Ireland: Open Air; 1997: 58–70. 13 refs. ISBN 1–85182–278–X. BE58296.
    adults; carriers; children; confidentiality; eugenics; family members; *gene therapy; genetic enhancement; genetic predisposition; *genetic screening; germ cells; goals; informed consent; mass screening; medical ethics; medicine; obligations to society; physicians; pregnant women; prenatal diagnosis; risks and benefits; virtues; voluntary programs

U.S. National Institutes of Health. Recombinant DNA research: proposed actions under the guidelines; notice. *Federal Register.* 1996 Nov 22; 61(227): 59726–59742. BE57536.
    *advisory committees; committee membership; data banks; *ethical review; *federal government; *gene therapy; *government regulation; guidelines; *human experimentation; organization and administration; *public policy; recombinant DNA research; review committees; Food and Drug Administration; *Gene Therapy Policy Conferences; *National Institutes of Health; NIH Guidelines; Office of Recombinant DNA Activities; Points to Consider: Transfer of Recombinant DNA into Human Subjects; *Recombinant DNA Advisory Committee; *United States

van Berkel, Dymphie; Klinge, Ineke. Gene technology: also a gender issue: views of Dutch informed women on genetic screening and gene therapy. *Patient Education and Counseling.* 1997 May; 31(1): 49–55. 6 refs. BE57525.
    *attitudes; autonomy; decision making; *females; fetal research; fetal therapy; *gene therapy; *genetic screening; genetic services; genome mapping; *knowledge, attitudes, practice; males; prenatal diagnosis; social discrimination; social impact; *Netherlands

Vogel, Gretchen. Genetic enhancement: from science fiction to ethics quandary. [News]. *Science.* 1997 Sep 19;

BE = bioethics accession number   fn. = footnotes   refs. = references

277(5333): 1753–1754. BE56160.

advisory committees; federal government; *gene therapy; *genetic enhancement; *genetic research; government regulation; human experimentation; mass media; trends; wedge argument; Recombinant DNA Advisory Committee; United States

Wadman, Meredith. Germline gene therapy 'must be spared excessive regulation.' [News]. *Nature.* 1998 Mar 26; 392(6674): 317. Includes inset article, "European states outlaw permanent changes." BE57918.

advisory committees; federal government; *gene therapy; genetic enhancement; *germ cells; government regulation; international aspects; *regulation; Europe; Recombinant DNA Advisory Committee; *United States

Wadman, Meredith. Unesco text will target gene techniques. [News]. *Nature.* 1997 Aug 7; 388(6642): 508. BE56218.

advisory committees; *cloning; embryo research; *gene therapy; genetic research; *germ cells; government regulation; guidelines; human rights; *international aspects; public policy; Canada; Germany; International Bioethics Committee (Unesco); *Unesco

Walters, LeRoy, ed. Ethical issues in human genetics. *In:* Jonsen, Albert R.; Veatch, Robert M.; Walters, LeRoy, eds. Source Book in Bioethics: A Documentary History. Washington, DC: Georgetown University Press; 1998: 253–333. 40 refs. ISBN 0-87840-683-2. BE57892.

advisory committees; carriers; federal government; *gene therapy; genetic counseling; genetic disorders; *genetic intervention; genetic research; *genetic screening; genetic services; *genome mapping; germ cells; guidelines; historical aspects; industry; international aspects; legal aspects; mass screening; moral policy; newborns; prenatal diagnosis; public policy; recombinant DNA research; resource allocation; universities; *Committee for the Study of Inborn Errors of Metabolism; Council of Europe; Declaration of Inuyama; European Medical Research Councils; *NIH Guidelines; *Office of Technology Assessment; *President's Commission for the Study of Ethical Problems; Recombinant DNA Advisory Committee; *Twentieth Century; *United States

Walters, LeRoy B. Behavioural and germ-line genetic research. *In:* Kilner, John F.; Pentz, Rebecca D.; Young, Frank E., eds. Genetic Ethics: Do the Ends Justify the Genes? Grand Rapids, MI: W.B. Eerdmans; 1997: 104–112. 15 fn. ISBN 0-8028-4428-6. BE56718.

aggression; *behavioral genetics; *Christian ethics; embryos; empirical research; family members; freedom; future generations; *gene therapy; genetic determinism; genetic enhancement; *genetic intervention; genetic research; genome mapping; *germ cells; intelligence; methods; moral obligations; parents; preimplantation diagnosis; prenatal diagnosis; quality of life; *risks and benefits; twins; personality

Wildes, Kevin Wm. Redesigning the human genome: are there constraints from nature? *In:* Agius, Emmanuel; Busuttil, Salvino, eds. Germ-Line Intervention and Our Responsibilities to Future Generations. Boston, MA: Kluwer Academic; 1998: 35–49. 21 refs. 2 fn. ISBN 0-7923-4828-1. BE57878.

bioethics; casuistry; *cultural pluralism; *decision making; democracy; deontological ethics; *ethical analysis; ethical theory; future generations; *gene therapy; *germ cells; human characteristics; informed consent; methods; *morality; *natural law; principle-based ethics; privacy; *secularism; teleological ethics; theology; values; *nature; rationality

Williams, Janet K.; Lessick, Mira. Genome research: implications for children. *Pediatric Nursing.* 1996 Jan-Feb; 22(1): 40–46. 46 refs. BE55584.

carriers; *children; chromosome abnormalities; cystic fibrosis; *gene therapy; genetic counseling; genetic determinism; genetic disorders; genetic information; genetic predisposition; *genetic research; *genetic screening; genome mapping; germ cells; nurses; parent child relationship; patient advocacy; pediatrics; *risks and benefits; social discrimination; social impact; adenosine deaminase deficiency; fragile X syndrome

Young, Frank E. Genetic therapy. *In:* Kilner, John F.; Pentz, Rebecca D.; Young, Frank E., eds. Genetic Ethics: Do the Ends Justify the Genes? Grand Rapids, MI: W.B. Eerdmans; 1997: 171–182. 35 fn. ISBN 0-8028-4428-6. BE56723.

*Christian ethics; embryos; evolution; federal government; *gene therapy; genetic identity; genetic research; genome mapping; germ cells; human rights; recombinant DNA research; regulation; risks and benefits; theology; transgenic organisms; United States

Yount, Lisa. Should human genes be altered? [Juvenile literature]. *In: her* Issues in Biomedical Ethics. San Diego, CA: Lucent Books; 1998: 75–93, 104–105. 30 fn. ISBN 1-56006-476-5. BE57682.

*cloning; coercion; employment; eugenics; future generations; gene pool; *gene therapy; genetic disorders; *genetic enhancement; genetic information; *genetic intervention; genetic screening; *germ cells; health insurance; informed consent; insurance selection bias; involuntary sterilization; killing; prenatal diagnosis; regulation; *risks and benefits; selective abortion; *social discrimination; wedge argument

Perils in free market genomics. [Editorial]. *Nature.* 1998 Mar 26; 392(6674): 315. BE57318.

*gene therapy; genetic enhancement; *genetic research; *germ cells; *regulation; risks and benefits

GENETIC COUNSELING

See also GENETIC INTERVENTION, GENETIC SCREENING, PRENATAL DIAGNOSIS, GENETIC SERVICES

Allen, Jill S. Fonda; Mulhauser, Lynda C. Genetic counseling after abnormal prenatal diagnosis: facilitating coping in families who continue their pregnancies. *Journal of Genetic Counseling.* 1995 Dec; 4(4): 251–265. 43 refs. BE56020.

allowing to die; *attitudes; case studies; *childbirth; decision making; disabled; fetuses; *genetic counseling; *genetic disorders; guidelines; marital relationship; motivation; newborns; parents; patient care; pregnant women; *prenatal diagnosis; prognosis; *psychological stress; risk; selective abortion; uncertainty; *values

Andrews, Lori B. The genetic information superhighway: rules of the road for contacting relatives and recontacting former patients. *In:* Knoppers, Bartha Maria, ed. Human DNA: Law and Policy: International and Comparative Perspectives. Proceedings of the First International Conference on DNA Sampling and Human Genetic Research: Ethical, Legal, and Policy Aspects, held in Montreal, Canada, 6–8 Sep 1996. Boston, MA: Kluwer Law International; 1997: 133–143. 42 fn. ISBN 90-411-0361-9. BE58173.

*confidentiality; *disclosure; duty to warn; *family members; *genetic counseling; genetic disorders; *genetic information; genetic predisposition; *genetic screening; guidelines; *legal aspects; *patients; physicians; professional organizations; risks and benefits; wrongful life; *recontact; United States

Beeson, Diane. Nuance, complexity, and context:

qualitative methods in genetic counseling research. *Journal of Genetic Counseling.* 1997 Mar; 6(1): 21–43. 66 refs. BE57337.
> *behavioral research; confidentiality; evaluation; *genetic counseling; methods; *research design; ethnographic studies; *qualitative research

Begleiter, Michael L.; Rogers, Jill Cellars. Genetic counseling for a family with two distinct anomalies: a case report of a neural tube defect and 5p– syndrome in a fetus. *Journal of Genetic Counseling.* 1994 Jun; 3(2): 87–93. 14 refs. BE57378.
> amniocentesis; *autonomy; *beneficence; caring; *chromosome abnormalities; communication; *decision making; *directive counseling; *genetic counseling; *neural tube defects; parents; prenatal diagnosis; professional patient relationship; *psychological stress; time factors; treatment refusal; grief; ultrasonography

Bernhardt, Barbara A.; Geller, Gail; Strauss, Misha, et al. Toward a model informed consent process for BRCA1 testing: a qualitative assessment of women's attitudes. *Journal of Genetic Counseling.* 1997 Jun; 6(2): 207–222. 16 refs. BE55666.
> adults; *breast cancer; children; comprehension; decision making; directive counseling; *disclosure; *females; *genetic counseling; *genetic screening; *genetic predisposition; *informed consent; insurance; *knowledge, attitudes, practice; models, theoretical; patient participation; physician patient relationship; physicians; public opinion; risk; *risks and benefits; social discrimination; socioeconomic factors; survey; trust; uncertainty; qualitative research; urban population; Baltimore

Biesecker, Barbara Bowles. Future directions in genetic counseling: practical and ethical considerations. *Kennedy Institute of Ethics Journal.* 1998 Jun; 8(2): 145–160. 45 refs. Commented on by S.M. Suter, p. 161–163. BE58373.
> autonomy; communication; confidentiality; decision making; directive counseling; disclosure; education; empirical research; eugenics; family members; *genetic counseling; genetic screening; genetic services; *health personnel; mass screening; moral obligations; patients; professional patient relationship; referral and consultation; reproduction; technical expertise; *trends; truth disclosure; values; *professional role

The accelerated discovery of gene mutations that lead to increased risk of disease has led to the rapid development of predictive genetic tests. These tests improve the accuracy of assigning risk, but at a time when intervention or prevention strategies are largely unproved. In coming years, however, data will become increasingly available to guide treatment of genetic diseases. Eventually genetic testing will be performed for common diseases as well as for rare genetic conditions. This will challenge genetic counseling practice. The ethical principles that now guide this practice take into account the personal nature of test decision making, the need to respect individual self-determination, and the importance of client confidentiality. Certain of these principles may have to be modified as genetic testing becomes more widespread in order to meet the changing needs of clients and society. This paper offers recommendations to ensure that genetic counselors will take a leading role in the future delivery of ethical genetic services.

Biesecker, Barbara Bowles. Privacy in genetic counseling. *In:* Rothstein, Mark A., ed. Genetic Secrets: Protecting Privacy and Confidentiality in the Genetic Era. New Haven, CT: Yale University Press; 1997: 108–125. 21 fn. ISBN 0–300–07251–1. BE58678.
> adoption; autonomy; *confidentiality; deception; directive

counseling; disclosure; family members; *genetic counseling; genetic information; genetic screening; health personnel; prenatal diagnosis; *privacy; professional family relationship; professional patient relationship; incidental findings; paternity

Burgess, M.M.; Hayden, M.R. Patients' rights to laboratory data: trinucleotide repeat length in Huntington disease. [Editorial]. *American Journal of Medical Genetics.* 1996 Mar 1; 62(1): 6–9. 25 refs. BE55662.
> autonomy; beneficence; decision making; *diagnosis; ethical analysis; *genetic counseling; *genetic information; genetic screening; *Huntington's disease; institutional policies; laboratories; late-onset disorders; paternalism; patient participation; professional patient relationship; risks and benefits; trust; *truth disclosure

Chapple, Alison; May, Carl; Campion, Peter. Lay understanding of genetic disease: a British study of families attending a genetic counseling service. *Journal of Genetic Counseling.* 1995 Dec; 4(4): 281–300. 37 refs. 9 fn. BE56024.
> *attitudes; children; communication; *comprehension; disclosure; females; *genetic counseling; *genetic disorders; genetics; knowledge, attitudes, practice; males; parents; *patients; physicians; *stigmatization; guilt; qualitative research; Great Britain; National Health Service

Clarke, Angus. Genetic counseling. *In:* Chadwick, Ruth, ed. Encyclopedia of Applied Ethics, Volume 2. San Diego, CA: Academic Press; 1998: 391–405. 32 refs. ISBN 0–12–227067–3. BE56387.
> adults; autonomy; carriers; children; confidentiality; directive counseling; disclosure; economics; employment; eugenics; family members; *genetic counseling; genetic disorders; genetic predisposition; genetic screening; goals; informed consent; insurance; late-onset disorders; mass screening; newborns; prenatal diagnosis; privacy; psychological stress; risks and benefits

Clarke, Joe T.R.; Ray, Peter N. Look-back: the duty to update genetic counselling. *In:* Knoppers, Bartha Maria, ed. Human DNA: Law and Policy: International and Comparative Perspectives. Proceedings of the First International Conference on DNA Sampling and Human Genetic Research: Ethical, Legal, and Policy Aspects, held in Montreal, Canada, 6–8 Sep 1996. Boston, MA: Kluwer Law International; 1997: 121–132. 13 fn. ISBN 90–411–0361–9. BE58172.
> confidentiality; DNA data banks; family members; *genetic counseling; genetic information; *genetic screening; *guidelines; health personnel; informed consent; laboratories; legal obligations; physicians; primary health care; professional organizations; biological specimen banks; *recontact

Cohen, Cynthia B.; McCloskey, Elizabeth Leibold. Introduction [to a set of five articles and one commentary on genetic information]. *Kennedy Institute of Ethics Journal.* 1998 Jun; 8(2): vii–x. Introduction to articles by C.B. Cohen, R. Wachbroit, B.B. Biesecker, J.L. Nelson, and E.T. Juengst, and a commentary on Biesecker by S.M. Suter. BE58370.
> adults; children; decision making; directive counseling; *disclosure; *genetic counseling; *genetic information; genetic predisposition; genetic research; *genetic screening; informed consent; late-onset disorders; moral obligations; patients; prenatal diagnosis; risks and benefits; truth disclosure; vulnerable populations; population genetics

Cohen, Pamela E.; Wertz, Dorothy C.; Nippert, Irmgard, et al. Genetic counseling practices in Germany: a comparison between East German and West

German geneticists. *Journal of Genetic Counseling*. 1997 Mar; 6(1): 61–80. 40 refs. BE56326.

*attitudes; comparative studies; confidentiality; congenital disorders; *directive counseling; disabled; eugenics; *genetic counseling; genetic disorders; genetic information; genetic predisposition; genetic screening; *health personnel; *knowledge, attitudes, practice; National Socialism; political systems; prenatal diagnosis; rape; reproduction; selective abortion; sex determination; socioeconomic factors; survey; therapeutic abortion; *East Germany; *Germany; *West Germany

Eng, Christine M.; Schechter, Clyde; Robinowitz, Jane, et al. Prenatal genetic carrier testing using triple disease screening. *JAMA*. 1997 Oct 15; 278(15): 1268–1272. 30 refs. BE56056.

*carriers; *cystic fibrosis; decision making; disclosure; evaluation studies; females; *genetic counseling; genetic disorders; *genetic screening; informed consent; Jews; *knowledge, attitudes, practice; males; married persons; patient education; pregnant women; prenatal diagnosis; privacy; prognosis; program descriptions; selective abortion; *Tay Sachs disease; *Gaucher's disease; NCHGR-funded publication; severity of illness index; Mount Sinai Medical Center (New York City); United States

CONTEXT: Rapid progress in gene discovery has dramatically increased diagnostic capabilities for carrier screening and prenatal testing for genetic diseases. However, simultaneous prenatal carrier screening for prevalent genetic disease has not been evaluated, and patient acceptance and attitudes toward this testing strategy remain undefined. OBJECTIVE: To evaluate an educational, counseling, and carrier testing program for 3 genetic disorders: Tay–Sachs disease (TSD), type 1 Gaucher disease (GD), and cystic fibrosis (CF) that differ in detectability, severity, and availability of therapy. DESIGN: Potential participants received education and genetic counseling, gave informed consent, chose screening tests, and completed pre–education and posteducation questionnaires that assessed knowledge, attitudes toward genetic testing, and disease testing preferences. SETTING: Medical genetics referral center. PATIENTS: Volunteer sample of 2824 Ashkenazi Jewish individuals enrolled as couples who were referred for TSD testing. INTERVENTION: Genetic counseling, education, and if chosen, genetic testing for any or all 3 disorders. MAIN OUTCOME MEASURE: Acceptance of screening for each of the 3 disorders. Secondary outcomes include attitudes toward genetic testing and reproductive considerations. RESULTS: Of the 2824 individuals tested for TSD, 97% and 95% also chose testing for CF and GD, respectively. The frequency of detected carriers was 1:21 for TSD, 1:25 for CF, and 1:18 for GD. Twenty-one carriercoupleswere identified, counseled, and all postconception couples opted for prenatal diagnosis. Pre–education and posteducation questionnaires revealed that patients initially knew little about the diseases, but acquired disease information and increased knowledge of genetic concepts. Education and genetic counseling increased understanding and retention of genetic concepts and disease–related information, and minimized test–related anxiety. Although individuals sought screening for all 3 diseases, reproductive attitudes and decisions varied directly with disease severity and treatability. CONCLUSIONS: These findings emphasize the importance of genetic counseling for prenatal carrier testing and may improve understanding, acceptance, and informed decision making for prenatal carrier screening for multiple genetic diseases.

Fine, Beth A. Genetic counseling and women. *Women's*

Health Issues. 1997 Jul–Aug; 7(4): 220–224. 15 refs. BE55722.

caring; eugenics; *females; *genetic counseling; genetic research; *goals; health personnel; justice; prenatal diagnosis; terminology; women's health; ELSI–funded publication

Geller, Gail; Botkin, Jeffrey R.; Green, Michael J., et al. Genetic testing for susceptibility to adult–onset cancer: the process and content of informed consent. *JAMA*. 1997 May 14; 277(18): 1467–1474. 122 refs. BE55859.

adults; advisory committees; alternatives; audiovisual aids; *cancer; communication; comprehension; confidentiality; consent forms; decision making; *disclosure; DNA data banks; employment; *genetic counseling; genetic information; *genetic predisposition; *genetic screening; *guidelines; information dissemination; *informed consent; insurance; *late-onset disorders; minority groups; *patient education; privacy; professional patient relationship; psychology; *public policy; risks and benefits; social discrimination; teaching methods; time factors; NHGRI–funded publication; Cancer Genetics Studies Consortium; *Task Force on Informed Consent

OBJECTIVE: To provide guidance on informed consent to clinicians offering cancer susceptibility testing. PARTICIPANTS: The Task Force on Informed Consent is part of the Cancer Genetics Studies Consortium (CGSC), whose members were recipients of National Institutes of Health grants to assess the implications of cancer susceptibility testing. The 10 task force members represent a range of relevant backgrounds, including various medical specialties, social science, genetic counseling, and consumer advocacy. EVIDENCE: The CGSC held 3 public meetings from 1994 to 1996. At its first meeting, the task force jointly established a list of topics. The cochairs (G.G. and J.R.B) then developed an outline and assigned each topic to an appropriate writer and reviewer. Writers summarized the literature on their topics and drafted recommendations, which were then revised by the reviewers. The cochairs compiled and edited the entire manuscript. All members were involved in writing this report. CONSENSUS PROCESS: The first draft was distributed to task force members, after which a meeting was held to discuss its content and organization. Consensus was reached by voting. A subsequent draft was presented to the entire CGSC at its third meeting, and comments were incorporated. CONCLUSIONS: The task force recommends that informed consent for cancer susceptibility testing be an ongoing process of education and counseling in which (1) providers elicit participant, family, and community values and disclose their own, (2) decision making is shared, (3) the style of information disclosure is individualized, and (4) specific content areas are discussed.

Hallowell, N.; Murton, F.; Statham, H., et al. Women's need for information before attending genetic counselling for familial breast or ovarian cancer: a questionnaire, interview, and observational study. *BMJ (British Medical Journal)*. 1997 Jan 25; 314(7076): 281–283. 8 refs. BE58810.

*attitudes; *breast cancer; *cancer; *comprehension; *females; *genetic counseling; *genetic predisposition; *patient education; *patient satisfaction; *patients; survey; Great Britain

OBJECTIVES: To describe women's information needs prior to genetic counselling for familial breast or ovarian cancer. DESIGN: Prospective study including semistructured telephone interviews before genetic counselling, observations of consultations, completion of postal questionnaires, and face–to face interviews within

---

BE = bioethics accession number   fn. = footnotes   refs. = references

two months of counselling. SUBJECTS: 46 women attending genetic counselling for familial breast or ovarian cancer. MAIN OUTCOME MEASURES: Subjects' understanding of process and content of genetic counselling before attending and attitudes about their preparation for the counselling session. RESULTS: Although all women interviewed before the clinic expected to discuss their risk of developing cancer and risk management options, there was evidence of a lack of knowledge about the process and content of genetic counselling, 17 (37%) women said they did not know what else would happen. Most women interviewed after counselling viewed it positively, but 26 (65%) felt they had been inadequately prepared and 11 (28%) felt that their lack of preparation meant that they could not be given an accurate estimation of their risk of cancer. CONCLUSIONS: Some women felt that they did not obtain optimum benefit from genetic counselling because they were inadequately prepared for it. We suggest that cancer family history clinics should provide women with written information about the process and content of genetic counselling before their clinic attendance.

Harper, Peter S.; Clarke, Angus J. Genetics, Society, and Clinical Practice. Herndon, VA: BIOS Scientific Publishers; 1997. 253 p. 564 refs. ISBN 1-85996-206-8. BE59033.
  carriers; children; confidentiality; cystic fibrosis; decision making; directive counseling; Down syndrome; economics; eugenics; family members; *genetic counseling; genetic disorders; genetic diversity; genetic information; genetic predisposition; genetic research; *genetic screening; *genetic services; goals; health care delivery; Huntington's disease; informed consent; insurance; intelligence; late-onset disorders; mass screening; newborns; prenatal diagnosis; privacy; public health; public policy; registries; reproduction; selective abortion; social discrimination; terminology; population genetics; China; Great Britain

Heimler, Audrey; Zanko, Andrea. Huntington disease: a case study describing the complexities and nuances of predictive testing of monozygotic twins. *Journal of Genetic Counseling.* 1995 Jun; 4(2): 125-137. 13 refs. 1 fn. BE56031.
  adults; autonomy; case studies; communication; confidentiality; disclosure; DNA data banks; family members; *genetic counseling; *genetic screening; *Huntington's disease; informed consent; late-onset disorders; psychological stress; *twins; geographic factors; United States

Henn, Wolfram. Predictive diagnosis and genetic screening: manipulation of fate? *Perspectives in Biology and Medicine.* 1998 Winter; 41(2): 282-289. 18 refs. BE59009.
  carriers; diagnosis; directive counseling; eugenics; family members; *genetic counseling; genetic disorders; genetic predisposition; *genetic screening; insurance; late-onset disorders; motivation; preventive medicine; *risks and benefits; uncertainty; right not to know

Jan, Sheau-Wen; Chen, Chih-Ping; Huang, Lian-Hua, et al. Attitudes toward maternal serum screening in Chinese women with positive results. *Journal of Genetic Counseling.* 1996 Dec; 5(4): 169-180. 33 refs. BE56329.
  amniocentesis; *attitudes; decision making; *Down syndrome; females; *genetic counseling; *genetic screening; knowledge, attitudes, practice; *pregnant women; *prenatal diagnosis; survey; *alpha fetoproteins; *Taiwan

Juengst, Eric T. Ethics of prediction: genetic risk and the physician-patient relationship. *Genome Science and Technology.* 1995; 1(1): 21-36. 72 refs. BE57993.

autonomy; carriers; confidentiality; decision making; directive counseling; disabled; disclosure; DNA data banks; duty to warn; eugenics; family members; fathers; *genetic counseling; genetic determinism; *genetic disorders; genetic identity; *genetic information; genetic materials; *genetic predisposition; genetic research; *genetic screening; genetic services; genome mapping; health insurance; informed consent; late-onset disorders; medical ethics; minors; parent child relationship; parents; prenatal diagnosis; property rights; public policy; reproduction; *risk; *risks and benefits; sex determination; social discrimination; stigmatization; tissue banks; uncertainty; ELSI-funded publication; National Center for Human Genome Research; Office for Protection from Research Risks; United States

Kielstein, Rita. Clinical and ethical challenges of genetic markers for severe human hereditary disorders. *In:* Becker, Gerhold K., ed. Changing Nature's Course: The Ethical Challenge of Biotechnology. Hong Kong: Hong Kong University Press; 1996: 61-70. 10 refs. 9 fn. ISBN 962-209-403-1. BE56705.
  autonomy; case studies; children; decision making; directive counseling; family planning; *genetic counseling; *genetic disorders; genetic screening; *kidney diseases; *late-onset disorders; moral obligations; patients; preimplantation diagnosis; prenatal diagnosis; reproduction; risk; selective abortion; suffering; truth disclosure; value of life; values

McGee, Glenn; Arruda, Monica. A crossroads in genetic counseling and ethics. *Cambridge Quarterly of Healthcare Ethics.* 1998 Winter; 7(1): 97-100. 2 fn. BE58459.
  bioethics; curriculum; *directive counseling; *education; evaluation; *genetic counseling; genetic screening; genetic services; *health personnel; mass screening; schools; statistics; survey; United States

McKinnon, Wendy C.; Baty, Bonnie J.; Bennett, Robin L., et al. Predisposition genetic testing for late-onset disorders in adults: a position paper of the National Society of Genetic Counselors. [Policy statement]. *JAMA.* 1997 Oct 15; 278(15): 1217-1220. 58 refs. BE56054.
  *adults; confidentiality; disclosure; *genetic counseling; genetic information; genetic materials; *genetic predisposition; *genetic screening; *guidelines; informed consent; laboratories; *late-onset disorders; *organizational policies; patient education; professional organizations; risks and benefits; social discrimination; uncertainty; NCHGR-funded publication; *National Society of Genetic Counselors; United States

Mao, Xin; Wertz, Dorothy C. China's genetic services providers' attitudes towards several ethical issues: a cross-cultural survey. *Clinical Genetics.* 1997 Aug; 52(2): 100-109. 38 refs. BE57506.
  *attitudes; common good; confidentiality; congenital disorders; developing countries; *directive counseling; *disclosure; *DNA data banks; DNA fingerprinting; duty to warn; eugenics; *genetic counseling; *genetic disorders; *genetic information; genetic materials; genetic predisposition; genetic services; genome mapping; government regulation; *health personnel; informed consent; law enforcement; minority groups; population control; public policy; reproductive technologies; *selective abortion; *sex determination; socioeconomic factors; survey; *China

Marteau, Theresa M.; Croyle, Robert T. The new genetics: psychological responses to genetic testing. *BMJ (British Medical Journal).* 1998 Feb 28; 316(7132): 693-696. 34 refs. BE57756.
  breast cancer; carriers; cystic fibrosis; family members; females; *genetic counseling; genetic disorders; genetic predisposition; *genetic screening; Huntington's disease; late-onset disorders; males; patient care; prenatal diagnosis;

preventive medicine; *psychological stress; risk; selective abortion; social impact; uncertainty; Great Britain

Michie, Susan; Marteau, Theresa M.; Bobrow, Martin. Genetic counselling: the psychological impact of meeting patients' expectations. *Journal of Medical Genetics.* 1997 Mar; 34(3): 237–241. 22 refs. BE56158.
> *attitudes; directive counseling; emotions; evaluation; *genetic counseling; *patient satisfaction; *patients; psychological stress; survey; treatment outcome; Great Britain

New Jersey. Superior Court, Appellate Division. Safer v. Estate of Pack. *Atlantic Reporter, 2d Series.* 1996 Jul 11 (date of decision). 677: 1188–1193. BE58828.
> cancer; confidentiality; *duty to warn; *family members; *genetic counseling; *genetic predisposition; *legal liability; *legal obligations; negligence; patient care; physician patient relationship; *physicians; standards; New Jersey; *Safer v. Estate of Pack

The Superior Court of New Jersey, Appellate Division, recognized "a physician's duty to warn those known to be at risk of avoidable harm from a genetically transmissible condition." During the 1950s, Dr. George Pack treated Donna Shafer's father for a cancerous blockage of the colon and multiple polyposis. In 1990, Safer was diagnosed with the same condition, which she claims is inherited, and, if not diagnosed and treated, invariably will lead to metastic colorectal cancer. Safer alleged that Dr. Pack knew the hereditary nature of the disease, yet failed to warn the immediate family, thus breaching his professional duty to warn. The court did not follow the analysis of the trial court, that a physician has no legal duty to warn the child of a patient of the genetic risk of disease because no physician and patient relationship exists between the doctor and the child. (KIE abstract)

Paul, Diane. From eugenics to medical genetics. *In:* Marcus, Alan I.; Cravens, Hamilton, eds. Health Care Policy in Contemporary America. University Park, PA: Pennsylvania State University Press; 1997: 96–116. 79 fn. Published also in a special issue of *Journal of Policy History,* 1997; 9(1). ISBN 0–271–01740–6. BE56799.
> attitudes; coercion; contraception; directive counseling; *eugenics; gene pool; *genetic counseling; genetic disorders; genetic screening; genetic services; genetics; historical aspects; intelligence; investigators; mass screening; mentally disabled; minority groups; newborns; physically disabled; prenatal diagnosis; public opinion; public policy; reproduction; selective abortion; socioeconomic factors; sterilization (sexual); Great Britain; Twentieth Century; United States

Pergament, Eugene. A clinical geneticist perspective of the patient–physician relationship. *In:* Rothstein, Mark A., ed. Genetic Secrets: Protecting Privacy and Confidentiality in the Genetic Era. New Haven, CT: Yale University Press; 1997: 92–107. 21 fn. ISBN 0–300–07251–1. BE58677.
> autonomy; behavioral genetics; computer communication networks; *confidentiality; data banks; directive counseling; disclosure; family members; *genetic counseling; *genetic information; genetic predisposition; genetic screening; genome mapping; insurance; legal obligations; managed care programs; medical records; moral obligations; patient advocacy; physician patient relationship; privacy; professional family relationship; United States

Räikkä, Juha. Freedom and a right (not) to know. *Bioethics.* 1998 Jan; 12(1): 49–63. 21 fn. BE58482.
> *autonomy; coercion; competence; *decision making; freedom; *genetic counseling; *genetic information; *moral

obligations; *moral policy; *patient participation; *rights; *truth disclosure; *right not to know

Reich, Elsa; Zanko, Andrea; Heimler, Audrey. Testing for HD in twins. [Letter and response]. *Journal of Genetic Counseling.* 1996 Mar; 5(1): 47–51. BE56495.
> autonomy; coercion; confidentiality; family members; *genetic counseling; genetic information; *genetic screening; *Huntington's disease; privacy; truth disclosure; *twins

Resta, Robert G. Eugenics and nondirectiveness in genetic counseling. *Journal of Genetic Counseling.* 1997 Jun; 6(2): 255–258. 15 refs. BE55668.
> attitudes; directive counseling; *eugenics; *genetic counseling; historical aspects; physicians; Twentieth Century; United States

Rhodes, Rosamond. Genetic links, family ties, and social bonds: rights and responsibilities in the face of genetic knowledge. *Journal of Medicine and Philosophy.* 1998 Feb; 23(1): 10–30. 42 refs. 19 fn. BE57518.
> *autonomy; beneficence; case studies; confidentiality; decision making; directive counseling; disclosure; *family members; family relationship; friends; *genetic counseling; genetic disorders; *genetic information; genetic research; *genetic screening; Huntington's disease; *moral obligations; *moral policy; *obligations to society; patient participation; *patients; privacy; rights; social interaction; Tay Sachs disease; *truth disclosure; volunteers; pedigree studies; population genetics; *right not to know

Currently, some of the most significant moral issues involving genetic links relate to genetic knowledge. In this paper, instead of looking at the frequently addressed issues of responsibilities professionals or institutions have to individuals, I take up the question of what responsibilities individuals have to one another with respect to genetic knowledge. I address the questions of whether individuals have a moral right to pursue their own goals without contributing to society's knowledge of population genetics, without adding to their family's knowledge of its genetic history, and without discovering genetic information about themselves and their offspring. These questions lead to an examination of the presumed right to genetic ignorance and an exploration of a variety of social bonds. Analyzing cases in light of these considerations leads to a surprising conclusion about a widely accepted precept of genetic counseling, to some ethical insights into typical problems, and to some further unanswered questions about personal responsibility in the face of genetic knowledge.

Salihu, Hamisu Mohammed. Genetic counselling among Muslims: questions remain unanswered. [Letter]. *Lancet.* 1997 Oct 4; 350(9083): 1035–1036. 2 refs. BE57359.
> clergy; fetal development; *genetic counseling; genetic disorders; *genetic screening; *Islamic ethics; *preimplantation diagnosis; *prenatal diagnosis; *selective abortion; socioeconomic factors; Cameroon; Great Britain

Saxton, Marsha; Anderson, Betsy; Blatt, Robin J.R., et al. Prenatal diagnosis and pregnancy options. *Genetic Resource.* 1991; 6(1): 31–42. 14 refs. Includes a list of resources for pregnant women who receive an abnormal prenatal test result. BE56042.
> adoption; *alternatives; childbirth; community services; *congenital disorders; *counseling; *decision making; disabled; Down syndrome; *genetic counseling; genetic disorders; *guidelines; health personnel; parents; patient care; pregnant women; *prenatal diagnosis; psychological stress; referral and consultation; selective abortion; self-help groups; United States

Silvers, Anita; Miller, Franklin G.; Davis, Dena. An open future. [Letters and response]. *Hastings Center Report.* 1997 Sep–Oct; 27(5): 5. BE56111.
   *autonomy; *children; congenital disorders; directive counseling; *genetic counseling; health personnel; normality; parents; *physically disabled; professional ethics; reproduction; sex determination; *hearing disorders

Suter, Sonia M. Value neutrality and nondirectiveness: comments on "Future directions in genetic counseling." *Kennedy Institute of Ethics Journal.* 1998 Jun; 8(2): 161–163. 1 ref. Commentary on B.B. Biesecker, p. 146–160. BE58374.
   decision making; *directive counseling; *genetic counseling; goals; *health personnel; patients; professional patient relationship; technical expertise; values; *professional role
Common wisdom in genetic counseling, which is supported by Biesecker, holds that counselors should strive not to influence their clients' decision making. Such a presumption of nondirectiveness is challenged in this commentary.

Thomson, Elizabeth J. Genetic counselling. *In:* Kilner, John F.; Pentz, Rebecca D.; Young, Frank E., eds. Genetic Ethics: Do the Ends Justify the Genes? Grand Rapids, MI: W.B. Eerdmans; 1997: 146–155. 10 refs. ISBN 0-8028-4428-6. BE56722.
   education; family members; family relationship; *genetic counseling; genetic disorders; goals; health personnel; patient education; psychological stress; professional role; support groups

Tibben, A.; Stevens, M.; de Wert, G.M.W.R., et al. Preparing for presymptomatic DNA testing for early onset Alzheimer's disease/cerebral haemorrhage and hereditary Pick disease. *Journal of Medical Genetics.* 1997 Jan; 34(1): 63–72. 22 refs. BE56014.
   *attitudes; autonomy; *brain pathology; competence; dementia; disclosure; family members; *genetic counseling; genetic information; *genetic predisposition; genetic research; *genetic screening; genetic services; informed consent; *late–onset disorders; minors; motivation; preimplantation diagnosis; prenatal diagnosis; psychological stress; reproduction; risk; selective abortion; social discrimination; suicide; survey; third party consent; Netherlands

Wertz, Dorothy C. International research in bioethics: the challenges of cross–cultural interpretation. *In:* DeVries, Raymond; Subedi, Janardan, eds. Bioethics and Society: Constructing the Ethical Enterprise. Upper Saddle River, NJ: Prentice Hall; 1998: 145–165. 17 refs. 1 fn. ISBN 0-13-531252-3. BE58734.
   *attitudes; autonomy; bioethics; confidentiality; *cultural pluralism; disabled; *empirical research; *genetic counseling; genetic screening; health personnel; *international aspects; methods; paternalism; prenatal diagnosis; privacy; professional patient relationship; research design; *survey; ELSI–funded publication; non–Western World; Western World

Wertz, Dorothy C. Provider gender and moral reasoning: the politics of an "ethics of care." *Journal of Genetic Counseling.* 1994 Jun; 3(2): 95–112. 49 refs. BE57380.
   *attitudes; autonomy; caring; chromosome abnormalities; comparative studies; confidentiality; decision making; *directive counseling; disclosure; family members; *females; *genetic counseling; genetic disorders; *health personnel; international aspects; justice; knowledge, attitudes, practice; *males; *moral development; neural tube defects; paternalism; patients; pregnant women; prenatal diagnosis; professional patient relationship; psychological stress; reproductive technologies; sex determination; social dominance; surrogate mothers; survey; ELSI–funded

publication; United States

Wertz, Dorothy C. Society and the not–so–new genetics: what are we afraid of? Some future predictions from a social scientist. *Journal of Contemporary Health Law and Policy.* 1997 Spring; 13(2): 299–346. 130 fn. BE56015.
   *attitudes; autonomy; codes of ethics; common good; *confidentiality; directive counseling; disabled; *disclosure; DNA fingerprinting; employment; eugenics; family members; *genetic counseling; genetic determinism; genetic disorders; *genetic enhancement; *genetic information; genetic intervention; genetic predisposition; genetic screening; *genetic services; *genetics; genome mapping; guidelines; *health personnel; indigents; industry; insurance; *international aspects; *knowledge, attitudes, practice; late–onset disorders; *physicians; prenatal diagnosis; *privacy; *public opinion; reproduction; resource allocation; *rights; risk; selective abortion; sex determination; social discrimination; *social impact; survey; *values; Human Genome Project; *United States; WHO Guidelines on Ethical Issues in Genetics

White, Mary Terrell. Decision–making through dialogue: reconfiguring autonomy in genetic counseling. *Theoretical Medicine and Bioethics.* 1998 Jan; 19(1): 5–19. 24 refs. BE57321.
   accountability; *autonomy; coercion; *communication; competence; comprehension; cultural pluralism; *decision making; *directive counseling; *genetic counseling; genetic information; genetic screening; *goals; *health personnel; models, theoretical; patient participation; patients; prenatal diagnosis; professional ethics; professional patient relationship; reproduction; technical expertise; values; *professional role

White, Mary Terrell. "Respect for autonomy" in genetic counseling: an analysis and a proposal. *Journal of Genetic Counseling.* 1997 Sep; 6(3): 297–313. 45 refs. BE57266.
   *autonomy; coercion; communication; decision making; *directive counseling; disclosure; *genetic counseling; genetic information; goals; health personnel; patients; professional patient relationship; psychological stress; rights; risk; uncertainty; values

Wilcke, Jon Torgny R. Late onset genetic disease: where ignorance is bliss, is it folly to inform relatives? *BMJ (British Medical Journal).* 1998 Sep 12; 317(7160): 744–747. 17 refs. BE58837.
   advisory committees; autonomy; *disclosure; *duty to warn; *family members; *genetic counseling; *genetic predisposition; health personnel; *late–onset disorders; moral obligations; *moral policy; paternalism; patients; preventive medicine; privacy; professional family relationship; *risks and benefits; smoking; right not to know; Danish Ethics Council; Denmark

Wolff, Gerhard; Jung, Christine. Nondirectiveness and genetic counseling. *Journal of Genetic Counseling.* 1995 Mar; 4(1): 3–25. 42 refs. 5 fn. BE56048.
   communication; *decision making; *directive counseling; *genetic counseling; goals; health personnel; parents; prenatal diagnosis; preventive medicine; professional patient relationship; review; selective abortion; social dominance; standards; *professional role

World Health Organization. Genetic counselling. *In:* Control of Hereditary Diseases: Report of a WHO Scientific Group. Geneva: World Health Organization; 1996: 50–58. References embedded in list at back of book. ISBN 92-4-120865-1. BE58940.
   carriers; decision making; directive counseling; family members; *genetic counseling; genetic disorders; genetic screening; genetic services; Huntington's disease; marital relationship; prenatal diagnosis; primary health care; prognosis; psychological stress; reproduction; risk; selection

---

BE = bioethics accession number   fn. = footnotes   refs. = references

for treatment; selective abortion; social discrimination

GENETIC ENGINEERING *See* GENE THERAPY, GENETIC INTERVENTION, RECOMBINANT DNA RESEARCH

GENETIC INTERVENTION

See also EUGENICS, CLONING, GENE THERAPY, GENETIC COUNSELING, GENETIC SCREENING, GENOME MAPPING, GENETIC RESEARCH, RECOMBINANT DNA RESEARCH

Abbott, Alison. Euro–vote lifts block on biotech patents ... but Parliament wants closer scrutiny. [News]. *Nature.* 1997 Jul 24; 388(6640): 314–315. BE56422.
  biomedical technologies; ethical review; ethics committees; genes; *genetic intervention; *international aspects; legal aspects; *patents; political activity; *regulation; risks and benefits; transgenic animals; *transgenic organisms; agriculture; *Europe; *European Parliament; European Patent Office

Agius, Emmanuel; Busuttil, Salvino, eds. Germ–Line Intervention and Our Responsibilities to Future Generations. Boston, MA: Kluwer Academic; 1998. 174 p. (Philosophy and medicine; v. 55). 148 refs. 33 fn. ISBN 0-7923-4828-1. BE57875.
  accountability; Buddhist ethics; cultural pluralism; decision making; democracy; deontological ethics; ethical analysis; freedom; *future generations; gene pool; gene therapy; genes; genetic diversity; genetic enhancement; *genetic intervention; genetic research; genetic screening; genome mapping; germ cells; international aspects; moral obligations; morality; natural law; patents; peer review; property rights; regulation; review; rights; risks and benefits; secularism; teleological ethics; transgenic organisms; values

Armstrong, Kerri; Weber, Kurt. Genetic engineering: a lesson on bioethics for the classroom. *American Biology Teacher.* 1991 May; 53(5): 294–297. BE58115.
  bioethics; *education; *genetic intervention; schools; *teaching methods; *secondary schools; United States

Badoux, John C.; Hunkeler, David; Waldner, Rosmarie, et al. Swiss democracy has its advantages. [Letters]. *Nature.* 1998 May 21; 393(6682): 205. BE58029.
  animal experimentation; decision making; democracy; *genetic intervention; *government regulation; information dissemination; political activity; *public participation; public policy; quality of life; *transgenic animals; *Switzerland

Bayertz, Kurt. The normative status of the human genome: a European perspective. *In:* Hoshino, Kazumasa, ed. Japanese and Western Bioethics: Studies in Moral Diversity. Boston, MA: Kluwer Academic; 1997: 167–180. 17 refs. 2 fn. ISBN 0-7923-4112-0. BE57093.
  autonomy; body parts and fluids; cultural pluralism; freedom; gene therapy; genetic enhancement; *genetic identity; *genetic information; *genetic intervention; *genetic materials; *human body; infertility; informed consent; legal aspects; *morality; personhood; property rights; remuneration; reproductive technologies; *values; *dignity; integrity; personality; Council of Europe; Embryo Protection Act 1990 (Germany); *Europe; *European Convention on Bioethics; *Germany; Switzerland

Becker, Evelyn S. Ethical issues arising in biotechnology. *In:* Haddad, Amy Marie, ed. Teaching and Learning Strategies in Pharmacy Ethics. Second Edition. New York, NY: Pharmaceutical Products Press; 1997: 33–47.

25 refs. Co–published simultaneously in *Journal of Pharmacy Teaching*, 1997; 6(1/2): 33–47. ISBN 0-7890-0378-3. BE57931.
  case studies; confidentiality; economics; gene therapy; genetic disorders; genetic information; *genetic intervention; genetic research; genetic screening; genome mapping; justice; pharmacists; prenatal diagnosis; professional ethics; resource allocation; selection for treatment; professional role

Becker, Gerhold K., ed. Changing Nature's Course: The Ethical Challenge of Biotechnology. Hong Kong: Hong Kong University Press; 1996. 208 p. Includes references. Articles based on a November 1993 symposium, "Biotechnology and Ethics: Scientific Liberty and Moral Responsibility," organized and sponsored by the Centre for Applied Ethics at Hong Kong Baptist University in cooperation with the Hong Kong University of Science and Technology and the Goethe Institut. ISBN 962-209-403-1. BE56704.
  animal experimentation; anthropology; bioethics; biomedical technologies; Christian ethics; ecology; economics; food; gene therapy; genetic counseling; genetic disorders; *genetic intervention; genetic screening; genome mapping; international aspects; philosophy; public policy; recombinant DNA research; reproductive technologies; risk; *risks and benefits; technology assessment; theology; transgenic organisms; agriculture; transgenic plants

Brown, Barry. Reconciling property law with advances in reproductive science. *Stanford Law and Policy Review.* 1995; 6(2): 73–88. 113 fn. BE56485.
  artificial insemination; body parts and fluids; confidentiality; *cryopreservation; death; decision making; dissent; *embryo disposition; *embryos; eugenics; females; future generations; gene therapy; genetic enhancement; genetic information; *genetic intervention; genetic screening; *germ cells; government regulation; in vitro fertilization; international aspects; *legal aspects; males; mandatory testing; parents; preimplantation diagnosis; privacy; *property rights; *public policy; reproduction; *reproductive technologies; state interest; divorce; Davis v. Davis; Hecht v. Superior Court (Kane); *United States

Buchanan, James P. Future-perfect? Biotechnology and the ethics of the unknown: an afterword. *In:* Becker, Gerhold K., ed. Changing Nature's Course: The Ethical Challenge of Biotechnology. Hong Kong: Hong Kong University Press; 1996: 185–201. 28 fn. ISBN 962-209-403-1. BE56713.
  body parts and fluids; common good; ecology; economics; eugenics; genetic diversity; genetic enhancement; genetic information; *genetic intervention; genetic materials; genome mapping; health hazards; industry; minority groups; normality; patents; property rights; recombinant DNA research; *risks and benefits; science; social impact; transgenic animals; uncertainty; cybernetics

Butler, Declan. European biotech industry plans ethics panel. [News]. *Nature.* 1997 Jul 3; 388(6637): 6. BE56151.
  advisory committees; cloning; codes of ethics; embryo research; *ethics committees; *genetic intervention; *genetic research; germ cells; *industry; institutional ethics; professional ethics; *self regulation; *EuropaBio; *Europe

Byk, Christian. The ambiguous intent of genetics law: to ease the social fear or safeguard the human condition? *In:* Doherty, Peter; Sutton, Agneta, eds. Man-Made Man: Ethical and Legal Issues in Genetics. Dublin, Ireland: Open Air; 1997: 83–97. 19 fn. ISBN 1-85182-278-X. BE58298.
  advisory committees; confidentiality; directive counseling; ecology; food; gene therapy; genetic counseling; genetic information; *genetic intervention; genetic screening; germ cells; government regulation; human experimentation;

BE = bioethics accession number   fn. = footnotes   refs. = references

*international aspects; preimplantation diagnosis; prenatal diagnosis; public policy; recombinant DNA research; *regulation; risks and benefits; selective abortion; social discrimination; transgenic organisms; Denmark; European Union; France; Germany; Great Britain; Netherlands; United States

Canada. Minister of Health. New Reproductive and Genetic Technologies: Setting Boundaries, Enhancing Health. Ottawa, ON: Minister of Supply and Services Canada; 1996 Jun. 48 p. Cat.H21-127/1996E. ISBN 0-662-24101-0. BE59032.
accountability; advisory committees; children; cloning; disabled; embryo research; embryos; federal government; gene therapy; *genetic intervention; genetic screening; *government regulation; hybrids; industry; infertility; informed consent; moral policy; ovum donors; prenatal diagnosis; *public policy; registries; remuneration; *reproductive technologies; research embryo creation; selective abortion; semen donors; sex determination; standards; surrogate mothers; ectogenesis; Advisory Committee on the Interim Moratorium on Reproductive and Genetic Technologies (Canada); *Canada; *Human Reproductive and Genetic Technologies Act 1996 (Canada); *Royal Commission on New Reproductive and Genetic Technologies (Canada)

Cuschieri, Alfred. Screening for genetic diseases: what are the moral constraints? *In:* Agius, Emmanuel; Busuttil, Salvino, eds. Germ-Line Intervention and Our Responsibilities to Future Generations. Boston, MA: Kluwer Academic; 1998: 3-11. ISBN 0-7923-4828-1. BE57886.
confidentiality; disclosure; eugenics; fetal therapy; *future generations; gene pool; gene therapy; genetic counseling; genetic disorders; genetic enhancement; genetic information; *genetic intervention; genetic research; *genetic screening; genome mapping; germ cells; late-onset disorders; mandatory testing; mass screening; moral obligations; preimplantation diagnosis; prenatal diagnosis; privacy; *risks and benefits; selective abortion; voluntary programs

Dickson, David. Biosafety code gathers pace through bilateral agreements. [News]. *Nature.* 1995 Sep 14; 377(6545): 94. BE56107.
developing countries; *ecology; *genetic intervention; guidelines; industry; *international aspects; regulation; risk; *transgenic organisms; voluntary programs; Argentina; Europe; Great Britain; Netherlands; United Nations

Dobson, Andrew. Genetic engineering and environmental ethics. *Cambridge Quarterly of Healthcare Ethics.* 1997 Spring; 6(2): 205-221. 69 fn. BE56426.
animal rights; communitarianism; *ecology; economics; genetic identity; *genetic intervention; industry; justice; microbiology; moral obligations; *moral policy; patents; public participation; public policy; *recombinant DNA research; regulation; review; rights; risks and benefits; *speciesism; *transgenic animals; *transgenic organisms; utilitarianism; *values; agriculture; *environmental ethics; transgenic plants
I shall be saying something about the ethical dilemmas raised by genetic engineering in both these contexts -- that is to say, human and animal. But the bulk of what I have to say refers to a field that covers both humans and animals but extends beyond them -- the field of environmental ethics....

Doherty, Peter; Sutton, Agneta, eds. Man-Made Man: Ethical and Legal Issues in Genetics. Dublin, Ireland: Open Air; 1997. 116 p. Includes references. ISBN 1-85182-278-X. BE58293.
autonomy; children; confidentiality; disabled; embryos; eugenics; fetuses; *gene therapy; genetic counseling; genetic determinism; *genetic intervention; genetic predisposition;

genetic research; *genetic screening; genetics; genome mapping; informed consent; international aspects; personhood; preimplantation diagnosis; prenatal diagnosis; public policy; regulation; reproduction; rights; risks and benefits; selective abortion; social control; social discrimination; trends; values; Europe; Great Britain

Durant, John, ed. Biotechnology in Public: A Review of Recent Research. London: Science Museum for the European Federation of Biotechnology; 1992. 201 p. 353 refs. 109 fn. ISBN 0-901805-52-1. BE56194.
animal experimentation; animal rights; ecology; food; gene therapy; *genetic intervention; genetic research; genetics; industry; information dissemination; international aspects; investigators; knowledge, attitudes, practice; mass media; political activity; *public opinion; public participation; public policy; recombinant DNA research; regulation; risk; *risks and benefits; science; social control; *social impact; socioeconomic factors; statistics; survey; technology assessment; transgenic animals; trust; journalism; *Europe; European Community; Great Britain

Dyson, Anthony O. Reflections on method in theology and genetics: from suspicion to critical cooperation. *In:* Becker, Gerhold K., ed. Changing Nature's Course: The Ethical Challenge of Biotechnology. Hong Kong: Hong Kong University Press; 1996: 159-169. 40 fn. ISBN 962-209-403-1. BE56711.
autonomy; *bioethics; *Christian ethics; freedom; future generations; *genetic intervention; genetics; germ cells; historical aspects; philosophy; *Protestant ethics; Roman Catholic ethics; secularism; *theology; Twentieth Century; United States

Engelhardt, H. Tristram. Human nature genetically re-engineered: moral responsibilities to future generations. *In:* Agius, Emmanuel; Busuttil, Salvino, eds. Germ-Line Intervention and Our Responsibilities to Future Generations. Boston, MA: Kluwer Academic; 1998: 51-63. 2 refs. 1 fn. ISBN 0-7923-4828-1. BE57879.
beneficence; contraception; *cultural pluralism; decision making; ecology; *ethical analysis; *freedom; *future generations; *gene therapy; *genetic enhancement; *genetic intervention; *germ cells; goals; guidelines; international aspects; *moral obligations; morality; regulation; reproduction; *risks and benefits; *secularism

Engelhardt, H. Tristram. Moral puzzles concerning the human genome: Western taboos, intuitions, and beliefs at the end of the Christian era. *In:* Hoshino, Kazumasa, ed. Japanese and Western Bioethics: Studies in Moral Diversity. Boston, MA: Kluwer Academic; 1997: 181-186. 6 refs. ISBN 0-7923-4112-0. BE57094.
*bioethics; *Christian ethics; ethical relativism; future generations; gene therapy; genetic enhancement; genetic identity; *genetic intervention; germ cells; *morality; risks and benefits; *secularism; *values; *rationality; Western World; *Europe; Germany; *Japan

Enserink, Martin. Dutch pull the plug on cow cloning. [News]. *Science.* 1998 Mar 6; 279(5356): 1444. BE57304.
animal experimentation; *cloning; *drug industry; *government regulation; *transgenic animals; *Netherlands; Pharming Holding N.V.

Feinberg, John S. A theological basis for genetic intervention. *In:* Kilner, John F.; Pentz, Rebecca D.; Young, Frank E., eds. Genetic Ethics: Do the Ends Justify the Genes? Grand Rapids, MI: W.B. Eerdmans; 1997: 183-192. 12 fn. ISBN 0-8028-4428-6. BE56724.
*Christian ethics; eugenics; *gene therapy; genetic enhancement; *genetic intervention; germ cells; morality; recombinant DNA research; risks and benefits; secularism; theology

---

BE = bioethics accession number   fn. = footnotes   refs. = references

Felice, Alex E. Guardianship by peer review in genetic engineering and biotechnology. *In:* Agius, Emmanuel; Busuttil, Salvino, eds. Germ–Line Intervention and Our Responsibilities to Future Generations. Boston, MA: Kluwer Academic; 1998: 117–129. 20 refs. 1 fn. ISBN 0-7923-4828-1. BE57883.
   developing countries; future generations; gene therapy; *genetic intervention; *genetic research; genome mapping; international aspects; investigators; *peer review; public participation; regulation; resource allocation; risks and benefits; self regulation; time factors

Fielder, John H. Patenting biotechnology: ethical and philosophical issues. *IEEE Engineering in Medicine and Biology Magazine.* 1997 Nov–Dec; 16(6): 118–120. 13 refs. BE58411.
   animal rights; commodification; ecology; eugenics; food; *genetic intervention; industry; *patents; risk; social impact; *transgenic organisms; values

Fox, Michael W. Genetic engineering and biomedical research. *In: his* Eating with Conscience: The Bioethics of Food. Troutdale, OR: NewSage Press; 1997: 85–103, 185. 9 fn. ISBN 0-939165-30-9. BE56512.
   animal experimentation; cloning; disclosure; drug industry; ecology; federal government; food; *genetic intervention; government regulation; health hazards; industry; recombinant DNA research; *risks and benefits; *transgenic animals; transgenic organisms; agriculture; transgenic plants; Food and Drug Administration; United States

Franklin, Sarah. Dolly: a new form of transgenic breedwealth. *Environmental Values.* 1997 Nov; 6(4): 427–437. 11 refs. BE58569.
   *cloning; commodification; historical aspects; mass media; patents; property rights; public opinion; reproductive technologies; *speciesism; *transgenic animals; *agriculture; nuclear transplantation; Great Britain

Glannon, Walter. Genes, embryos, and future people. *Bioethics.* 1998 Jul; 12(3): 187–211. 36 fn. BE58893.
   beginning of life; *beneficence; children; *cryopreservation; *embryo disposition; *embryos; *eugenics; fetal therapy; fetuses; future generations; *gene therapy; *genetic disorders; genetic enhancement; *genetic intervention; *genetic screening; germ cells; *injuries; justice; late–onset disorders; mentally disabled; *moral obligations; *moral policy; pain; parents; personhood; physically disabled; posthumous reproduction; *preimplantation diagnosis; *quality of life; reproduction; reproductive technologies; risks and benefits; self concept; suffering; time factors; value of life; *wrongful life

Testing embryonic cells for genetic abnormalities gives us the capacity to predict whether and to what extent people will exist with disease and disability. Moreover, the freezing of embryos for long periods of time enables us to alter the length of a normal human lifespan. After highlighting the shortcomings of somatic–cell gene therapy and germ–line genetic alteration, I argue that the testing and selective termination of genetically defective embryos is the only medically and morally defensible way to prevent the existence of people with severe disability, pain and suffering that make their lives not worth living for them on the whole. In addition, I consider the possible harmful effects on children born from frozen embryos after the deaths of their biological parents, or when their parents are at an advanced age. I also explore whether embryos have moral status and whether the prospects for disease–preventing genetic alteration can justify long–term cryopreservation of embryos.

Gore, Albert; Owens, Steve. The challenge of biotechnology. *Yale Law and Policy Review.* 1985 Spring; 3(2): 336–357. 88 fn. BE56491.
   advisory committees; ecology; federal government; gene therapy; *genetic intervention; germ cells; *government regulation; guidelines; historical aspects; industry; investigators; *public policy; *recombinant DNA research; *risks and benefits; self regulation; transgenic organisms; Asilomar Conference; Department of Agriculture; Environmental Protection Agency; National Institutes of Health; NIH Guidelines; Recombinant DNA Advisory Committee; Twentieth Century; U.S. Congress; *United States

Grace, Eric S. Ethical issues. *In: his* Biotechnology Unzipped: Promises and Realities. Washington, DC: Joseph Henry Press; 1997: 191–224, 237. 8 refs. ISBN 0-309-05777-9. BE56684.
   developing countries; ecology; economics; federal government; food; gene therapy; genetic diversity; *genetic intervention; genetic materials; genetic research; genetic screening; industry; information dissemination; international aspects; legal aspects; mass media; patents; public opinion; recombinant DNA research; *risks and benefits; social discrimination; transgenic organisms; universities; agriculture; Europe; Human Genome Diversity Project; National Institutes of Health; United States

Great Britain. Department of Health. Advisory Group on the Ethics of Xenotransplantation (Chair: Ian Kennedy). Animal Tissue into Humans: A Report by the Advisory Group on the Ethics of Xenotransplantation, 1996. London: Her Majesty's Stationery Office; 1997. 258 p. 92 fn. Appendixes include Glossary of terms; The consultation exercise; Report of the Workshop on Xenotransplantation and Infectious Disease; and Development of transgenic pigs. ISBN 0-11-321866-4. BE55999.
   advisory committees; alternatives; animal experimentation; *animal organs; animal rights; artificial organs; body parts and fluids; communicable diseases; ethical review; *evaluation; gene therapy; genetic intervention; *government regulation; *guidelines; health promotion; *human experimentation; informed consent; international aspects; legal aspects; organ donation; *organ transplantation; preventive medicine; primates; private sector; public health; *public policy; public sector; research ethics committees; resource allocation; *risks and benefits; scarcity; selection of subjects; suffering; therapeutic research; *tissue transplantation; *transgenic animals; swine; Advisory Group on the Ethics of Xenotransplantation (Great Britain); Animals (Scientific Procedures) Act 1986; Department of Health (Great Britain); *Great Britain

Grey, William. Playing God. *In:* Chadwick, Ruth, ed. Encyclopedia of Applied Ethics, Volume 3. San Diego, CA: Academic Press; 1998: 525–530. 7 refs. ISBN 0-12-227068-1. BE56261.
   abortion, induced; *bioethical issues; bioethics; biomedical technologies; decision making; euthanasia; *genetic intervention; killing; *metaphor; *morality; natural law; *terminology; theology; value of life

Gustafson, James M. Where theologians and geneticists meet. *Dialog: A Journal of Theology.* 1994 Winter; 33(1): 7–16. 31 fn. BE57533.
   attitudes; biology; *Christian ethics; clergy; ethicists; freedom; genetic enhancement; *genetic intervention; genetic research; *genetics; *human characteristics; interdisciplinary communication; investigators; morality; natural law; personhood; *theology; value of life; ELSI-funded publication; nature; Barth, Karl; Ramsey, Paul

Hamer, Dean; Copeland, Peter. Engineering temperament: cloning and the future politics of personality. *In: their* Living with Our Genes: Why They

Matter More Than You Think. New York, NY: Doubleday; 1998: 295–316, 344. 11 refs. ISBN 0–385–48583–2. BE57647.
*behavioral genetics; brain; *cloning; gene therapy; *genetic determinism; genetic enhancement; *genetic intervention; genetic predisposition; genetic screening; germ cells; industry; psychoactive drugs; risks and benefits; uncertainty; *personality

Harris, John. Clones, Genes, and Immortality: Ethics and the Genetic Revolution. New York, NY: Oxford University Press; 1998. 328 p. Bibliography: p. 305–321. ISBN 0–19–288080–2. BE58945.
aborted fetuses; anencephaly; beginning of life; body parts and fluids; cadavers; cloning; confidentiality; DNA fingerprinting; embryo research; embryos; employment; eugenics; fetal tissue donation; future generations; gene therapy; genes; genetic diversity; genetic information; *genetic intervention; genetic screening; germ cells; hybrids; informed consent; injuries; insurance; justice; moral obligations; moral policy; morality; personhood; prenatal diagnosis; property rights; remuneration; reproduction; *reproductive technologies; risks and benefits; selective abortion; social discrimination; tissue banks; tissue donation; transgenic organisms; wrongful life

Häyry, Matti; Häyry, Heta. Genetic engineering. *In:* Chadwick, Ruth, ed. Encyclopedia of Applied Ethics, Volume 2. San Diego, CA: Academic Press; 1998: 407–417. 4 refs. ISBN 0–12–227067–3. BE56388.
advisory committees; biomedical technologies; costs and benefits; deontological ethics; developing countries; ecology; eugenics; freedom; gene therapy; *genetic intervention; genome mapping; international aspects; justice; moral obligations; *moral policy; public participation; recombinant DNA research; resource allocation; rights; risk; *risks and benefits; teleological ethics; transgenic organisms; utilitarianism; dignity

Hefner, Philip. Determinism, freedom, and moral failure. *Dialog: A Journal of Theology.* 1994 Winter; 33(1): 23–29. 10 fn. BE57534.
*behavioral genetics; *Christian ethics; evolution; *freedom; *genetic determinism; *genetic intervention; genetics; *genome mapping; *human characteristics; *theology; ELSI-funded publication

Hettinger, Ned. Patenting life: biotechnology, intellectual property, and environmental ethics. *Boston College Environmental Affairs Law Review.* 1995 Winter; 22(2): 267–305. 184 fn. BE57193.
developing countries; *ecology; economics; financial support; genes; *genetic intervention; *genetic materials; genetic research; goals; government regulation; incentives; industry; investigators; legal aspects; *patents; private sector; property rights; public sector; rights; *risks and benefits; social impact; transgenic animals; *transgenic organisms; value of life; agriculture; transgenic plants; United States

Heyd, David. Are we our descendants' keepers? *In:* Agius, Emmanuel; Busuttil, Salvino, eds. Germ-Line Intervention and Our Responsibilities to Future Generations. Boston, MA: Kluwer Academic; 1998: 131–145. 9 refs. 10 fn. ISBN 0–7923–4828–1. BE57884.
autonomy; beneficence; *decision making; ecology; eugenics; *future generations; *gene pool; genetic diversity; genetic identity; *genetic intervention; goals; justice; legal guardians; metaethics; metaphor; *moral obligations; philosophy; regulation; rights; theology; values; vulnerable populations

Heyd, David. *Human Genome Research and the Challenge of Contingent Future Persons: Toward an Impersonal Theocentric Approach to Value,* by Jan Christian Heller. [Book review essay]. *Bioethics.* 1998 Apr; 12(2): 173–176.

BE58627.
Christian ethics; decision making; economics; *future generations; *genetic intervention; *genome mapping; moral policy; reproduction; social impact; teleological ethics; *theology; *values; Human Genome Project; *Human Genome Research and the Challenge of Contingent Future Persons (Heller, J.C.)

Holtzman, Neil A. The gene: harnessing the gene and remaking the world, by Jeremy Rifkin. [Book review essay]. *JAMA.* 1998 Aug 12; 280(6): 575. BE58774.
gene therapy; *genetic intervention; *genetic research; genetic screening; genetics; patents; *The Biotech Century: Harnessing the Gene and Remaking the World (Rifkin, J.)

Kaiser, Jocelyn. UNESCO drafts bioethics declaration. [News]. *Science.* 1997 Oct 3; 278(5335): 23. BE56412.
cloning; *genetic intervention; genetic research; *genome mapping; *human rights; *international aspects; patents; *Unesco; United States; Universal Declaration of Human Rights; *Universal Declaration on the Human Genome and Human Rights

Kilner, John F.; Pentz, Rebecca D.; Young, Frank E., eds. Genetic Ethics: Do the Ends Justify the Genes? Grand Rapids, MI: W.B. Eerdmans; 1997. 291 p. (Horizon in bioethics series). 14 refs. 489 fn. Presented by the Center for Bioethics and Human Dignity, Bannockburn, IL. ISBN 0–8028–4428–6. BE56715.
behavioral genetics; *Christian ethics; confidentiality; disclosure; eugenics; gene therapy; genetic counseling; genetic determinism; genetic disorders; genetic enhancement; *genetic identity; *genetic information; *genetic intervention; genetic research; genetic screening; genetics; genome mapping; germ cells; growth disorders; health education; historical aspects; hormones; patents; preimplantation diagnosis; prenatal diagnosis; reproduction; selective abortion; suffering; *theology; value of life

King, David. No to genetic engineering of humans! *GenEthics News.* 1995 Nov–Dec; No. 9: 7. BE56230.
gene therapy; genetic disorders; genetic enhancement; *genetic intervention; germ cells; prenatal diagnosis; *risks and benefits; transgenic animals

Klotzko, Arlene Judith; Bulfield, Grahame; Campbell, Keith, et al. Voices from Roslin: the creators of Dolly discuss science, ethics, and social responsibility. [Interview]. *Cambridge Quarterly of Healthcare Ethics.* 1998 Spring; 7(2): 121–140. 8 fn. BE58011.
animal experimentation; biomedical research; *cloning; embryos; expert testimony; *genetic intervention; goals; *investigators; methods; obligations to society; regulation; reproductive technologies; research institutes; risks and benefits; science; *transgenic animals; nuclear transplantation; PPL Therapeutics; *Roslin Institute (Scotland); Scotland; U.S. Congress; United States

Koenig, Robert. Switzerland: voters reject antigenetics initiative. [News]. *Science.* 1998 Jun 12; 280(5370): 1685. BE58415.
drug industry; *government regulation; investigators; patents; *political activity; public opinion; public participation; *transgenic organisms; *Switzerland

Lenoir, Noëlle, et al.; European Commission. Group of Advisers on the Ethical Implications of Biotechnology. Ethical aspects of the labelling of foods derived from modern biotechnology. [Report]. *Politics and the Life Sciences.* 1996 Mar; 15(1): 117–119. BE55628.
disclosure; education; *food; *information dissemination; *international aspects; rights; technology assessment; *transgenic organisms; *Europe; Group of Advisers on the Ethical Implications of Biotechnology (European

Commission)

Levitin, Carl. Russia warned: act now or regret it later. [News]. *Nature.* 1997 Oct 16; 389(6652): 659. BE55959.
  *genetic intervention; *government regulation; industry; transgenic organisms; *Russia

Macer, Darryl. Bioethics and genetics in Asia and the Pacific: is universal bioethics possible? *In:* Becker, Gerhold K., ed. Changing Nature's Course: The Ethical Challenge of Biotechnology. Hong Kong: Hong Kong University Press; 1996: 171–184. 23 fn. ISBN 962-209-403-1. BE56712.
  *attitudes; bioethics; biomedical technologies; comparative studies; confidentiality; *cultural pluralism; economics; empirical research; ethical relativism; eugenics; gene therapy; genetic diversity; genetic enhancement; *genetic intervention; genetic screening; germ cells; human rights; *international aspects; prenatal diagnosis; *public opinion; *risks and benefits; trust; values; *Asia

McGleenan, Tony. Genetic technology, legal regulation of. *In:* Chadwick, Ruth, ed. Encyclopedia of Applied Ethics, Volume 2. San Diego, CA: Academic Press; 1998: 451–462. 17 refs. ISBN 0-12-227067-3. BE56392.
  ecology; eugenics; gene therapy; *genetic intervention; genetic research; genetic screening; *government regulation; guidelines; human experimentation; *international aspects; legislation; recombinant DNA research; *regulation; reproductive technologies; research ethics committees; risks and benefits; transgenic organisms; Australia; Canada; Europe; European Community; Great Britain; United States

Macklin, Ruth. Genetics and reproductive technologies. *In:* Borchert, Donald M., ed. The Encyclopedia of Philosophy. Supplement. New York, NY: Simon and Schuster and Macmillan; 1996: 217–220. 13 refs. ISBN 0-02-864629-0. BE57222.
  embryo disposition; eugenics; genetic counseling; genetic enhancement; genetic information; *genetic intervention; genetic predisposition; genetic screening; parent child relationship; *reproductive technologies

Marteau, Theresa; Michie, Susan; Drake, Harriet, et al. Public attitudes towards the selection of desirable characteristics in children. *Journal of Medical Genetics.* 1995 Oct; 32(10): 796–798. 9 refs. BE57760.
  congenital disorders; drugs; gene therapy; genetic disorders; *genetic enhancement; *genetic intervention; genetic predisposition; *human characteristics; prenatal diagnosis; *public opinion; selective abortion; statistics; survey; *Great Britain

Masood, Ehsan. Pressure grows for inquiry into welfare of transgenic animals. [News]. *Nature.* 1997 Jul 24; 388(6640): 311–312. BE56579.
  advisory committees; animal experimentation; animal organs; animal rights; genetic research; organ transplantation; political activity; politics; public opinion; *public policy; risks and benefits; *transgenic animals; Europe; *Great Britain

Mehlman, Maxwell J.; Botkin, Jeffrey R. Access to the Genome: The Challenge to Equality. Washington, DC: Georgetown University Press; 1998. 152 p. 231 fn. ISBN 0-87840-678-6. BE57386.
  carriers; communitarianism; disclosure; economics; employment; eugenics; gene pool; gene therapy; genetic counseling; genetic disorders; genetic enhancement; genetic information; *genetic intervention; genetic predisposition; genetic screening; *genetic services; *genome mapping; germ cells; health insurance reimbursement; insurance; *justice; late-onset disorders; libertarianism; managed care programs; mandatory testing; moral policy; newborns;

policy analysis; prenatal diagnosis; *public policy; *resource allocation; rights; *risks and benefits; scarcity; selection for treatment; selective abortion; social discrimination; *social impact; social worth; stigmatization; utilitarianism; ELSI-funded publication; personal financing; *Human Genome Project; Medicaid; Medicare; National Center for Human Genome Research; United States

Nelkin, Dorothy. Genetics, God, and sacred DNA. *Society.* 1996 May–Jun; 33(4): 22–25. BE57171.
  behavioral genetics; clergy; genes; genetic diversity; *genetic intervention; genetic materials; genetic research; genetics; genome mapping; investigators; patents; political activity; *religion; *science; *terminology; transgenic animals; Human Genome Diversity Project

Neri, Demetrio. Eugenics. *In:* Chadwick, Ruth, ed. Encyclopedia of Applied Ethics, Volume 2. San Diego, CA: Academic Press; 1998: 161–173. 9 refs. ISBN 0-12-227067-3. BE56381.
  ancient history; beneficence; *eugenics; future generations; gene therapy; genetic counseling; genetic disorders; genetic diversity; genetic enhancement; *genetic intervention; genetic screening; germ cells; historical aspects; international aspects; justice; mandatory programs; moral obligations; moral policy; normality; preventive medicine; reproduction; reproductive technologies; review; risks and benefits; social control; social discrimination; terminology; voluntary programs; Galton, Francis; Nineteenth Century; Plato; Twentieth Century

O'Mathúna, Dónal P. The case of human growth hormone. *In:* Kilner, John F.; Pentz, Rebecca D.; Young, Frank E., eds. Genetic Ethics: Do the Ends Justify the Genes? Grand Rapids, MI: W.B. Eerdmans; 1997: 203–217. 62 fn. ISBN 0-8028-4428-6. BE56726.
  *children; *Christian ethics; costs and benefits; *genetic enhancement; *genetic intervention; goals; *growth disorders; *hormones; justice; medicine; *normality; psychological stress; resource allocation; *risks and benefits; selection for treatment; self concept; social discrimination; social worth; stigmatization; suffering; theology; treatment outcome

Palazzani, Laura. Genetic engineering and human nature. *In:* Doherty, Peter; Sutton, Agneta, eds. Man–Made Man: Ethical and Legal Issues in Genetics. Dublin, Ireland: Open Air; 1997: 46–57. 17 fn. ISBN 1-85182-278-X. BE58295.
  autonomy; economics; embryo research; eugenics; fetal therapy; gene therapy; *genetic intervention; genetic screening; germ cells; natural law; nontherapeutic research; personhood; prenatal diagnosis; therapeutic research; utilitarianism; value of life

Parens, Erik. Is better always good? The enhancement project. [Project on the Prospect of Technologies Aimed at the Enhancement of Human Capacities and Traits]. *Hastings Center Report.* 1998 Jan–Feb; 28(1): S1–S17. 35 fn. BE57294.
  behavior control; *biomedical technologies; *cosmetic surgery; disabled; entrepreneurship; ethical analysis; females; *genetic enhancement; *goals; *health; *health care; health insurance reimbursement; *human characteristics; *justice; *medicine; moral complicity; *moral policy; motivation; *normality; preventive medicine; *psychoactive drugs; *public policy; resource allocation; *self concept; social control; social impact; social problems; socioeconomic factors; suffering; terminology; *values; authenticity; beauty; *enhancement technologies; life style; Hastings Center; *Project on the Prospect of Technologies Aimed at the Enhancement of Human Capabilities and Traits; Prozac
  The following essay begins to say why and when it will sometimes make sense to worry about the prospect of aiming new biotechnologies at the enhancement of

human capacities and traits. It grows out of a two–year, Hastings Center project, generously funded by the National Endowment for the Humanities.

Parrott, Robert H., et al.; American Academy of Pediatrics. Council on Research. Proposed guidelines on genetic engineering. *Pediatrics.* 1985 Jun; 75(6): 1159. BE56676.
> federal government; genetic disorders; *genetic intervention; genetic research; germ cells; *government regulation; *guidelines; *organizational policies; pediatrics; physicians; professional organizations; public policy; *recombinant DNA research; risks and benefits; *American Academy of Pediatrics; National Institutes of Health; United States

Pennisi, Elizabeth. After Dolly, a pharming frenzy. [News]. *Science.* 1998 Jan 30; 279(5351): 646–648. BE57421.
> animal experimentation; animal organs; *cloning; drug industry; genetic research; *industry; international aspects; *methods; *transgenic animals; nuclear transplantation; Netherlands; Pharming Holding N.V.; United States

Peters, Ted, ed. Genetics: Issues of Social Justice. Cleveland, OH: Pilgrim Press; 1998. 262 p. (The pilgrim library of ethics). 659 fn. ISBN 0–8298–1251–2. BE57474.
> behavioral genetics; Christian ethics; cloning; confidentiality; disadvantaged; eugenics; evolution; gene therapy; genetic determinism; genetic diversity; genetic information; *genetic intervention; genetic materials; genetic research; genetic screening; *genetics; *genome mapping; germ cells; health insurance; international aspects; Jewish ethics; *justice; normality; patents; privacy; religious ethics; review; risks and benefits; selective abortion; social discrimination; *social impact; stigmatization; Human Genome Diversity Project; Human Genome Project; United States

Peterson, James C. Ethical standards for genetic intervention. *In:* Kilner, John F.; Pentz, Rebecca D.; Young, Frank E., eds. Genetic Ethics: Do the Ends Justify the Genes? Grand Rapids, MI: W.B. Eerdmans; 1997: 193–202. 23 fn. ISBN 0–8028–4428–6. BE56725.
> accountability; *Christian ethics; decision making; future generations; gene therapy; genetic enhancement; *genetic intervention; germ cells; normality; parents; public policy; risks and benefits; standards; *theology

Pharmaceutical Research and Manufacturers of America. Ethical Principles on GENOMICS. [Statement]. Washington, DC: Pharmaceutical Research and Manufacturers of America; 1996 May 16. 1 p. BE57399.
> *drug industry; genetic information; *genetic intervention; genetic research; genetic screening; health care; *organizational policies; public participation; standards; *Pharmaceutical Research and Manufacturers of America (PhRMA)

Pluhar, Evelyn. On the genetic manipulation of animals. *Between the Species.* 1985 Summer; 1(3): 13–18. 23 fn. BE57062.
> animal experimentation; ecology; *genetic intervention; human experimentation; *morality; paternalism; *risks and benefits; *speciesism; *transgenic animals; transgenic plants

Privitera, Salvatore. Moral reasoning in bioethics and posterity. *In:* Agius, Emmanuel; Busuttil, Salvino, eds. Germ–Line Intervention and Our Responsibilities to Future Generations. Boston, MA: Kluwer Academic; 1998: 27–33. 1 fn. ISBN 0–7923–4828–1. BE57877.
> bioethics; *deontological ethics; ethical theory; future generations; gene therapy; *genetic intervention; germ cells; *teleological ethics

Reiss, Michael. Biotechnology. *In:* Chadwick, Ruth, ed. Encyclopedia of Applied Ethics, Volume 1. San Diego, CA: Academic Press; 1998: 319–333. 10 refs. ISBN 0–12–227066–5. BE56370.
> animal experimentation; animal rights; *biomedical technologies; drugs; ecology; food; *gene therapy; genetic enhancement; *genetic intervention; genetic materials; germ cells; growth disorders; historical aspects; hormones; international aspects; methods; moral policy; patents; *recombinant DNA research; reproductive technologies; risk; *risks and benefits; suffering; terminology; *transgenic animals; *transgenic organisms; agriculture

Rifkin, Jeremy. The Biotech Century: Harnessing the Gene and Remaking the World. New York, NY: Jeremy P. Tarcher/Putnam; 1998. 271 p. 486 fn. ISBN 0–87477–909–X. BE57152.
> animal experimentation; animal organs; animal rights; biological warfare; biomedical research; cloning; commodification; computers; developing countries; *ecology; *economics; *eugenics; future generations; gene pool; gene therapy; genes; genetic disorders; genetic diversity; genetic enhancement; *genetic information; *genetic intervention; genetic predisposition; *genetic research; genetics; genome mapping; *industry; international aspects; legal aspects; patents; property rights; regulation; reproduction; reproductive technologies; review; *risks and benefits; *social impact; social problems; stigmatization; transgenic animals; *transgenic organisms; wedge argument; agriculture; transgenic plants; Europe; Human Genome Diversity Project; Human Genome Project; Twenty–First Century; United States

Rogers, Arthur. European Parliament approves intellectual property rights directive. [News]. *Lancet.* 1997 Jul 26; 350(9073): 272. BE56418.
> developing countries; *genetic intervention; *international aspects; *patents; property rights; *regulation; *transgenic organisms; *Europe; *European Parliament

Roleff, Tamara L., ed. Biomedical Ethics: Opposing Viewpoints. San Diego, CA: Greenhaven Press; 1998. 252 p. (Opposing viewpoints series). Includes references. ISBN 1–56510–792–6. BE59107.
> age factors; animal organs; autonomy; beneficence; *bioethical issues; body parts and fluids; brain death; cadavers; capital punishment; childbirth; *cloning; eugenics; females; genes; *genetic intervention; *genetic research; genetic screening; genome mapping; government regulation; indigents; moral policy; *organ donation; organ transplantation; patents; personhood; posthumous reproduction; pregnant women; presumed consent; prisoners; public policy; remuneration; *reproductive technologies; risks and benefits; selection for treatment; surrogate mothers; transgenic animals

Sass, Hans–Martin. Moral risk assessment in biotechnology. *In:* Becker, Gerhold K., ed. Changing Nature's Course: The Ethical Challenge of Biotechnology. Hong Kong: Hong Kong University Press; 1996: 127–144. 27 refs. 27 fn. ISBN 962–209–403–1. BE56709.
> autonomy; carriers; cultural pluralism; gene therapy; genetic information; *genetic intervention; genetic predisposition; germ cells; *guidelines; *moral obligations; moral policy; preventive medicine; public policy; recombinant DNA research; regulation; *risk; *risks and benefits; self induced illness; truth disclosure; values; agriculture

Schenker, Joseph G.; International Federation of Gynecology and Obstetrics. Committee for the Study of Ethical Aspects of Human Reproduction. Report of the FIGO Committee for the Study of Ethical Aspects of Human Reproduction. *International Journal of*

BE = bioethics accession number   fn. = footnotes   refs. = references

Gynaecology and Obstetrics. 1997 Jun; 57(3): 333–337. 1 fn. BE57508.

> *allowing to die; confidentiality; *congenital disorders; contraception; gene therapy; genetic enhancement; *genetic intervention; genetic materials; germ cells; guidelines; HIV seropositivity; informed consent; *newborns; organizational policies; quality of health care; remuneration; *reproduction; sexuality; withholding treatment; women's health services; women's rights; International Federation of Gynecology and Obstetrics

Schiermeier, Quirin. Swiss researchers facing 'anti-transgenics' vote. [News]. *Nature.* 1997 Jul 24; 388(6640): 315. BE56580.

> animal experimentation; drug industry; *genetic intervention; genetic research; *government regulation; patents; *public participation; *transgenic animals; *transgenic organisms; universities; *transgenic plants; *Switzerland

Schiermeier, Quirin. Switzerland seeks to head off ban on use of transgenic animals. [News]. *Nature.* 1998 Jan 22; 391(6665): 312. BE57257.

> animal experimentation; attitudes; *genetic intervention; *government regulation; investigators; political activity; public opinion; *transgenic animals; *Switzerland

Schroten, Egbert; European Commission. Group of Advisers on the Ethical Implications of Biotechnology. Ethical aspects of genetic modification of animals: opinion of the Group of Advisers on the Ethical Implications of Biotechnology of the European Commission. [Statement and commentary]. *Cambridge Quarterly of Healthcare Ethics.* 1998 Spring; 7(2): 194–198. BE58014.

> advisory committees; animal experimentation; ecology; economics; genetic intervention; *international aspects; public opinion; public participation; *public policy; regulation; risks and benefits; *transgenic animals; Europe; *European Commission; Group of Advisers on the Ethical Implications of Biotechnology (European Commission); United States

Seifert, Franz; Torgersen, Helge. How to keep out what we don't want: an assessment of 'Sozialverträglichkeit' under the Austrian Genetic Engineering Act. *Public Understanding of Science.* 1997 Oct; 6(4): 301–327. 101 fn. BE59104.

> *decision making; democracy; ecology; *genetic intervention; *government regulation; industry; international aspects; legislation; politics; *public participation; *public policy; *risk; risks and benefits; social impact; technology assessment; transgenic organisms; agriculture; *transgenic plants; *Austria; European Union; *Genetic Engineering Act 1994 (Austria)

Shannon, Thomas A. Genetics, ethics, and theology: the Roman Catholic discussion. *In:* Peters, Ted, ed. Genetics: Issues of Social Justice. Cleveland, OH: Pilgrim Press; 1998: 144–179. 174 fn. ISBN 0-8298-1251-2. BE57478.

> abortion, induced; autonomy; embryo research; embryos; eugenics; fetal research; gene therapy; genetic counseling; *genetic intervention; genetic research; genetic screening; *genetics; genome mapping; human characteristics; marital relationship; moral obligations; morality; natural law; prenatal diagnosis; *reproduction; reproductive technologies; *Roman Catholic ethics; sexuality; sociobiology; *theology; value of life; Ashley, Benedict; Catholic Health Association; Curran, Charles; Haring, Bernard; Humanae Vitae; Instruction on Respect for Human Life; John Paul II, Pope; May, William; McCormick, Richard; O'Rourke, Kevin; Rahner, Karl; Vatican II

Shinn, Roger L. Genetics, ethics, and theology: the

ecumenical discussion. *In:* Peters, Ted, ed. Genetics: Issues of Social Justice. Cleveland, OH: Pilgrim Press; 1998: 122–143. 43 fn. ISBN 0-8298-1251-2. BE57477.

> advisory committees; *Christian ethics; eugenics; future generations; *gene therapy; genetic counseling; genetic enhancement; *genetic intervention; genetic research; *genetics; genome mapping; *germ cells; historical aspects; organizational policies; political activity; Protestant ethics; public policy; Roman Catholic ethics; science; Catechism of the Catholic Church; *National Council of Churches; President's Commission for the Study of Ethical Problems; Rifkin, Jeremy; Twentieth Century; United Methodist Church; United States; *World Council of Churches

Shinn, Roger Lincoln. The New Genetics: Challenges for Science, Faith, and Politics. Wakefield, RI: Moyer Bell; distributed in North America by Publishers Group West, Emeryville, CA; 1996. 175 p. Bibliography: p. 159–170. ISBN 1-55921-171-7. BE56094.

> behavioral genetics; cultural pluralism; decision making; ethics; eugenics; freedom; future generations; *gene therapy; genetic determinism; genetic diversity; *genetic intervention; genetic screening; *genetics; *genome mapping; *germ cells; health; intelligence; investigators; morality; normality; political activity; politics; prenatal diagnosis; *public policy; religion; risks and benefits; science; *social impact; theology; *values; *Human Genome Project; NIH–DOE Working Group on Ethical, Legal, and Social Implications (ELSI); United States

Singer, Maxine F. Genetics and the law: a scientist's view. *Yale Law and Policy Review.* 1985 Spring; 3(2): 315–335. 44 fn. BE56497.

> biological warfare; clergy; education; evolution; federal government; *genetic intervention; *genetic research; *genetics; germ cells; government regulation; *interdisciplinary communication; investigators; *law; *lawyers; legal aspects; *political activity; political systems; professional competence; public policy; *recombinant DNA research; *risks and benefits; *science; self regulation; technical expertise; transgenic organisms; agriculture; Lysenko, T.D.; Rifkin, Jeremy; *United States; USSR

Spicker, Stuart F. The unknowable effects of genetic interventions on future generations (or, who guards the genetic engineers in democratic republics?). *In:* Agius, Emmanuel; Busuttil, Salvino, eds. Germ-Line Intervention and Our Responsibilities to Future Generations. Boston, MA: Kluwer Academic; 1998: 147–163. 41 refs. 8 fn. ISBN 0-7923-4828-1. BE57885.

> *accountability; consensus; *decision making; *democracy; eugenics; *future generations; gene therapy; genetic enhancement; *genetic intervention; *genetic research; germ cells; investigators; moral obligations; public participation; public policy; regulation; risks and benefits; social control; uncertainty

United Methodist Church. Faithful Witness on Today's Issues: Genetic Science. [Pamphlet]. Washington, DC: General Board of Church and Society; 1992. 23 p. Includes General Conference resolutions on genetic science adopted 1992, and on organ and tissue donation adopted 1984. BE57388.

> Christian ethics; clergy; confidentiality; ecology; education; gene therapy; genes; genetic information; *genetic intervention; genetic research; genetic screening; genetic services; genome mapping; *organ donation; *organizational policies; patents; property rights; *Protestant ethics; public participation; public policy; resource allocation; risks and benefits; social impact; *tissue donation; agriculture; *Methodist Church; United States

Veglia, Geremia; Shmaefsky, Brian R.; Johnson, Walter. Public Attitudes Toward Human Genetic Manipulation: A Revitalization of Eugenics? Available

from ERIC Document Reproduction Service, DYNCORP I&ET, 7420 Fullerton Rd., Suite 110, Springfield, VA 22153-2852; Document No. ED327408; SE051655; 1990. 26 p. Paper presented at the Fifth National Technological Literacy Conference of the National Association of Science, Technology and Society, Arlington, VA, 2–4 Feb 1990. BE57782.
  *attitudes; behavioral genetics; *eugenics; females; genetic disorders; *genetic enhancement; *genetic intervention; health; intelligence; involuntary sterilization; law; males; prenatal diagnosis; *public policy; reproduction; *risks and benefits; science; selective abortion; *social impact; *students; survey; *universities; *United States

Vines, Gail. Genetics: let the public decide. [News]. *BMJ (British Medical Journal).* 1997 Apr 5; 314(7086): 1055. BE56338.
  behavioral genetics; *decision making; eugenics; *genetic intervention; genetic materials; *genetic research; genetic screening; *genetics; industry; *knowledge, attitudes, practice; mass media; *public opinion; *public participation; Great Britain

Walters, LeRoy, ed. Ethical issues in human genetics. *In:* Jonsen, Albert R.; Veatch, Robert M.; Walters, LeRoy, eds. Source Book in Bioethics: A Documentary History. Washington, DC: Georgetown University Press; 1998: 253–333. 40 refs. ISBN 0-87840-683-2. BE57892.
  advisory committees; carriers; federal government; *gene therapy; genetic counseling; genetic disorders; *genetic intervention; genetic research; *genetic screening; genetic services; *genome mapping; germ cells; guidelines; historical aspects; industry; international aspects; legal aspects; mass screening; moral policy; newborns; prenatal diagnosis; public policy; recombinant DNA research; resource allocation; universities; *Committee for the Study of Inborn Errors of Metabolism; Council of Europe; Declaration of Inuyama; European Medical Research Councils; *NIH Guidelines; *Office of Technology Assessment; *President's Commission for the Study of Ethical Problems; Recombinant DNA Advisory Committee; *Twentieth Century; *United States

Walters, LeRoy B. Behavioural and germ-line genetic research. *In:* Kilner, John F.; Pentz, Rebecca D.; Young, Frank E., eds. Genetic Ethics: Do the Ends Justify the Genes? Grand Rapids, MI: W.B. Eerdmans; 1997: 104–112. 15 fn. ISBN 0-8028-4428-6. BE56718.
  aggression; *behavioral genetics; *Christian ethics; embryos; empirical research; family members; freedom; future generations; *gene therapy; genetic determinism; genetic enhancement; *genetic intervention; genetic research; genome mapping; *germ cells; intelligence; methods; moral obligations; parents; preimplantation diagnosis; prenatal diagnosis; quality of life; *risks and benefits; twins; personality

Watson, Rory. EU approves rights to genetic material. [News]. *BMJ (British Medical Journal).* 1997 Dec 6; 315(7121): 1487. BE57346.
  biomedical technologies; cloning; embryo research; genetic intervention; *genetic materials; *genetic research; *international aspects; legislation; *patents; political activity; *regulation; *transgenic organisms; *Europe; *European Union

Watson, Rory. The [European] Union gets interested in ethics. [News]. *BMJ (British Medical Journal).* 1997 Jun 28; 314(7098): 1854. BE56443.
  advisory committees; animal experimentation; *cloning; embryos; ethics committees; *genetic intervention; human experimentation; *international aspects; patents; public participation; *regulation; *Europe; *European Union

Weiss, Rick. Patent sought on making of part–human

creatures: scientist seeks to touch off ethics debate. [News]. *Washington Post.* 1998 Apr 2: A12. BE58048.
  *genetic intervention; government regulation; human experimentation; *hybrids; investigators; *legal aspects; *patents; primates; public policy; *Newman, Stuart; Patent and Trademark Office; United States

Williams, Nigel. European Parliament backs new biopatent guidelines. [News]. *Science.* 1997 Jul 25; 277(5325): 472. BE56444.
  genes; *genetic intervention; industry; *international aspects; legal aspects; *patents; political activity; *regulation; risks and benefits; transgenic animals; *transgenic organisms; *Europe; *European Parliament

Yount, Lisa. Should human genes be altered? [Juvenile literature]. *In: her* Issues in Biomedical Ethics. San Diego, CA: Lucent Books; 1998: 75–93, 104–105. 30 fn. ISBN 1-56006-476-5. BE57682.
  *cloning; coercion; employment; eugenics; future generations; gene pool; *gene therapy; genetic disorders; *genetic enhancement; genetic information; *genetic intervention; genetic screening; *germ cells; health insurance; informed consent; insurance selection bias; involuntary sterilization; killing; prenatal diagnosis; regulation; *risks and benefits; selective abortion; *social discrimination; wedge argument

Zinkernagel, Rolf M. Gene technology and democracy. [Editorial]. *Science.* 1997 Nov 14; 278(5341): 1207. BE57423.
  attitudes; biomedical research; ecology; education; *genetic intervention; *government regulation; industry; patents; *political activity; public opinion; *public participation; science; social control; *transgenic organisms; *Switzerland

Genethics in the mid–1990s. [News]. *GenEthics News.* 1996 Jul/Aug; 13: 6–7. BE56408.
  behavioral genetics; ecology; economics; food; *genetic intervention; genetic screening; genome mapping; government regulation; industry; information dissemination; international aspects; patents; political activity; risks and benefits; social discrimination; social impact; transgenic organisms; agriculture; transgenic plants; European Union; Great Britain; United States

How not to run a scientifically successful country. [Editorial]. *Nature.* 1998 Apr 23; 392(6678): 741. BE58025.
  attitudes; *genetic intervention; *government regulation; investigators; patents; political activity; *public participation; *transgenic animals; transgenic organisms; *Switzerland

MPs call for tough controls on human genetics. [News]. *GenEthics News.* 1995 Jul–Aug; No. 7: 1, 3. BE56335.
  advisory committees; employment; gene therapy; genes; genetic information; *genetic intervention; genetic predisposition; *genetic screening; germ cells; *government regulation; insurance; patents; privacy; *public policy; *social discrimination; *Great Britain; House of Commons; Human Genetics Commission (Great Britain)

Referendum's challenge to transgenic research [Switzerland]. [Editorial]. *Nature.* 1997 Sep 11; 389(6647): 103. BE56477.
  *government regulation; industry; information dissemination; investigators; *legislation; mass media; morality; public opinion; *public participation; *recombinant DNA research; risks and benefits; social control; *transgenic animals; *Switzerland

Swiss to vote on genetic engineering. [News]. *ATLA: Alternatives to Laboratory Animals.* 1997 May–Jun; 25(3): 220–221. BE55596.
  biomedical research; ecology; government regulation;

BE = bioethics accession number   fn. = footnotes   refs. = references

industry; patents; *political activity; public opinion; public participation; transgenic animals; *transgenic organisms; *Switzerland

Thanks for the advice. [Editorial]. *Nature Biotechnology.* 1997 Apr; 15(4): 293. BE55970.
   *advisory committees; bioethical issues; gene therapy; *genetic intervention; genetic screening; international aspects; prenatal diagnosis; *public policy; Great Britain; Japan; United States

GENETIC RESEARCH

See also BIOMEDICAL RESEARCH, GENOME MAPPING, HUMAN EXPERIMENTATION, PATENTING LIFE FORMS, RECOMBINANT DNA RESEARCH

Agius, Emmanuel. Patenting life: our responsibilities to present and future generations. *In:* Agius, Emmanuel; Busuttil, Salvino, eds. Germ–Line Intervention and Our Responsibilities to Future Generations. Boston, MA: Kluwer Academic; 1998: 67–83. 10 refs. 2 fn. ISBN 0–7923–4828–1. BE57880.
   common good; *developing countries; ecology; evolution; freedom; *future generations; gene pool; gene therapy; genes; *genetic diversity; genetic enhancement; genetic intervention; *genetic research; germ cells; guidelines; human rights; industry; *international aspects; legal aspects; *moral obligations; *patents; *property rights; recombinant DNA research; *regulation; risks and benefits; *transgenic organisms; war; agriculture; *World Patent Convention on Biotechnological Inventions

Andrews, Lori; Nelkin, Dorothy. Whose body is it anyway? Disputes over body tissue in a biotechnology age. *Lancet.* 1998 Jan 3; 351(9095): 53–57. 43 refs. BE57900.
   *attitudes; biomedical research; *body parts and fluids; *cultural pluralism; deception; economics; gene therapy; *genetic materials; *genetic research; genetic screening; *human body; industry; informed consent; international aspects; investigators; legal aspects; patents; *property rights; psychology; public policy; *self concept; tissue banks; *values; vulnerable populations; integrity; Human Genome Diversity Project; United States

Baird, Patricia A. Registries, record linkage, and research in genetics: protecting privacy. *In:* Knoppers, Bartha Maria, ed. Human DNA: Law and Policy: International and Comparative Perspectives. Proceedings of the First International Conference on DNA Sampling and Human Genetic Research: Ethical, Legal, and Policy Aspects, held in Montreal, Canada, 6–8 Sep 1996. Boston, MA: Kluwer Law International; 1997: 165–175. 12 fn. ISBN 90–411–0361–9. BE58176.
   computers; *confidentiality; *data banks; *DNA data banks; epidemiology; genetic disorders; *genetic information; genetic materials; *genetic research; genetic screening; informed consent; *medical records; privacy; *registries; tissue donation; *biological specimen banks; Canada

Bankowski, Zbigniew. International ethics guidelines and genetic epidemiology. *In:* Knoppers, Bartha Maria, ed. Human DNA: Law and Policy: International and Comparative Perspectives. Proceedings of the First International Conference on DNA Sampling and Human Genetic Research: Ethical, Legal, and Policy Aspects, held in Montreal, Cananda, 6–8 Sep 1996. Boston, MA: Kluwer Law International; 1997: 9–13. 5 refs. ISBN 90–411–0361–9. BE58164.
   bioethics; developing countries; *epidemiology; ethical relativism; *genetic research; *genetic screening;

*guidelines; human rights; informed consent; *international aspects; tissue donation; Council for International Organizations of Medical Sciences

Botkin, Jeffrey R.; McMahon, William M.; Smith, Ken R., et al. Privacy and confidentiality in the publication of pedigrees: a survey of investigators and biomedical journals. *JAMA.* 1998 Jun 10; 279(22): 1808–1812. 11 refs. BE58763.
   *attitudes; *confidentiality; *disclosure; *editorial policies; evaluation studies; *family members; *genetic information; *genetic research; genetic screening; guidelines; *informed consent; international aspects; *investigators; *knowledge, attitudes, practice; *privacy; *research subjects; survey; guideline adherence; medical illustration; *pedigree studies; publishing; International Committee of Medical Journal Editors
   CONTEXT: Pedigree diagrams efficiently communicate family information to genetics investigators; however, the publication of pedigrees poses a risk to the privacy and confidentiality of individuals depicted in the diagrams. Two sets of authoritative guidelines have been published to protect the privacy and confidentiality of subjects, but the influence of these guidelines on publication practices for pedigrees is unknown. OBJECTIVE: To determine the attitudes, practices, and experiences of investigators and journals with respect to privacy and confidentiality concerns in the publication of pedigrees. DESIGN: Investigators who have published pedigrees and editors of 26 biomedical journals were surveyed. Journals were reviewed for content in their "information for authors" sections and for documentation of informed consent in articles containing pedigrees. OUTCOME MEASURES: Practices regarding confidentiality and privacy reported by investigators and editors. RESULTS: Of 226 surveys sent to investigators, 177 were returned (78% response rate). Sixty-one investigators (36%) stated that family members were not informed that their pedigree would be published; 131 (78%) do not obtain informed consent specifically for pedigree publication and only 12 (28%) of the 43 who obtained consent obtained consent from all family members depicted. Thirty-two individuals (19%) reported having altered published pedigrees and 14 (45%) of 31 who had altered pedigrees stated that alterations were not disclosed to journals. Of the 14 journals that responded (54% response rate), only 3 reported written policies for managing potentially identifying information. Two journals reported having asked authors to alter pedigrees and 3 stated they had permitted alterations. A review of 5 genetics journals over a 2-year period revealed no documentation of consent for pedigree publication. CONCLUSIONS: Current practices in the publication of pedigrees do not conform with established recommendations and risk the privacy and confidentiality of subjects, often without informed consent. Attempts to address this problem through the alteration of data are being used, although this practice impairs the integrity of scientific communication.

Brandt-Rauf, Paul W.; Brandt-Rauf, Sherry I. Biomarkers -- scientific advances and societal implications. *In:* Rothstein, Mark A., ed. Genetic Secrets: Protecting Privacy and Confidentiality in the Genetic Era. New Haven, CT: Yale University Press; 1997: 184–196. 30 fn. ISBN 0–300–07251–1. BE58682.
   biomedical research; compensation; confidentiality; ecology; employment; *genetic predisposition; *genetic research; *genetic screening; *health hazards; *occupational exposure; toxicity; *genetic markers

---

Brody, Baruch A. Genetic research. *In: his* The Ethics of Biomedical Research: An International Perspective. New York, NY: Oxford University Press; 1998: 77–97, 366–368. 53 fn. ISBN 0–19–509007–1. BE57671.
advisory committees; consensus; containment; ecology; ethical review; federal government; gene therapy; genes; genetic enhancement; genetic information; *genetic research; genetic screening; genetic services; genome mapping; germ cells; government regulation; guidelines; human experimentation; industry; insurance; international aspects; mass screening; patents; public policy; recombinant DNA research; *regulation; review; transgenic organisms; Europe; United States

Brunner, E.J.; Sheppard, J.; Ravetz, J. Public is concerned about gene testing. [Letter]. *BMJ (British Medical Journal).* 1997 May 24; 314(7093): 1552–1553. 2 refs. BE56856.
*attitudes; confidentiality; *disclosure; drug industry; economics; *genetic information; *genetic materials; *genetic research; *genetic screening; informed consent; life insurance; *public opinion; survey; tissue donation; *Great Britain

Butler, Declan. European biotech industry plans ethics panel. [News]. *Nature.* 1997 Jul 3; 388(6637): 6. BE56151.
advisory committees; cloning; codes of ethics; embryo research; *ethics committees; *genetic intervention; *genetic research; germ cells; *industry; institutional ethics; professional ethics; *self regulation; *EuropaBio; *Europe

Butler, Declan. Tensions grow over access to DNA bank. [News]. *Nature.* 1998 Feb 19; 391(6669): 727. BE58028.
*aged; confidentiality; contracts; disclosure; *DNA data banks; financial support; genetic information; *genetic research; *industry; *information dissemination; investigators; legal aspects; patents; research institutes; *tissue banks; *Centre d'Etude du Polymorphisme Humain (CEPH); *France; *Genset; *Schächter, François

Carlson, John W. On the justification and limits of medical research: a response to Kevin Wildes. *In:* Wildes, Kevin Wm.; Mitchell, Alan C., eds. Choosing Life: A Dialogue on *Evangelium Vitae.* Washington, DC: Georgetown University Press; 1997: 199–205. 18 fn. ISBN 0–87840–646–8. BE56689.
beginning of life; *biomedical research; *embryo research; fetal research; genetic enhancement; *genetic research; germ cells; nontherapeutic research; *Roman Catholic ethics; theology; *therapeutic research; value of life; dignity; Evangelium Vitae

Chadwick, Ruth. The status of human genetic material -- European approaches. *In:* Knoppers, Bartha Maria, ed. Human DNA: Law and Policy: International and Comparative Perspectives. Proceedings of the First International Conference on DNA Sampling and Human Genetic Research: Ethical, Legal, and Policy Aspects, held in Montreal, Canada, 6–8 Sep 1996. Boston, MA: Kluwer Law International; 1997: 55–62. 20 fn. ISBN 90–411–0361–9. BE58167.
body parts and fluids; confidentiality; genes; *genetic information; *genetic materials; genetic screening; *international aspects; legal aspects; *property rights; tissue donation; *Europe

Clayton, Ellen Wright. Informed consent and genetic research. *In:* Rothstein, Mark A., ed. Genetic Secrets: Protecting Privacy and Confidentiality in the Genetic Era. New Haven, CT: Yale University Press; 1997: 126–136. 13 fn. ISBN 0–300–07251–1. BE58679.
anonymous testing; confidentiality; disclosure; DNA data banks; family members; genetic information; *genetic research; genetic screening; *informed consent; insurance;

mass screening; newborns; parental consent; records; *research subjects; risks and benefits; social discrimination; stigmatization; biological specimen banks; pedigree studies

Clayton, Ellen Wright. Prospective uses of DNA samples for research. *In:* Knoppers, Bartha Maria, ed. Human DNA: Law and Policy: International and Comparative Perspectives. Proceedings of the First International Conference on DNA Sampling and Human Genetic Research: Ethical, Legal, and Policy Aspects, held in Montreal, Canada, 6–8 Sep 1996. Boston, MA: Kluwer Law International; 1997: 291–301. 34 fn. ISBN 90–411–0361–9. BE58186.
advisory committees; comparative studies; confidentiality; consent forms; decision making; disclosure; *DNA data banks; federal government; genetic information; *genetic materials; *genetic research; genetic screening; *government regulation; guidelines; *informed consent; *international aspects; model legislation; professional organizations; *public policy; research subjects; risk; tissue donation; *biological specimen banks; *Canada; Genetic Privacy Act; *Great Britain; Nuffield Council on Bioethics; *United States

Cook–Deegan, Robert Mullan. Confidentiality, collective resources, and commercial genomics. *In:* Rothstein, Mark A., ed. Genetic Secrets: Protecting Privacy and Confidentiality in the Genetic Era. New Haven, CT: Yale University Press; 1997: 161–183. 32 fn. ISBN 0–300–07251–1. BE58681.
*confidentiality; conflict of interest; dementia; disclosure; DNA data banks; donors; *drug industry; family members; *financial support; genes; *genetic information; *genetic research; *genome mapping; government financing; government regulation; *industry; information dissemination; informed consent; investigators; legal aspects; patents; private sector; *property rights; public sector; regulation; *research subjects; tissue donation; universities; biological specimen banks; pedigree studies; United States

Cunningham, Brian C. Impact of the Human Genome Project at the interface between patent and FDA laws. *Risk: Health, Safety and Environment.* 1996 Summer; 7(3): 253–266. 56 fn. BE55932.
advisory committees; decision making; federal government; gene therapy; *genetic research; genome mapping; *government regulation; *industry; *legal aspects; *patents; *public policy; recombinant DNA research; transgenic organisms; Diamond v. Chakrabarty; Food and Drug Administration; Patent and Trademark Office; Recombinant DNA Advisory Committee; *United States

Daniels, Jo; McGuffin, Peter; Owen, Mike. Molecular genetic research on IQ: can it be done? Should it be done? *Journal of Biosocial Science.* 1996 Oct; 28(4): 491–507. 37 refs. BE55762.
*behavioral genetics; genes; *genetic research; genetic screening; genetics; genome mapping; *intelligence; Great Britain; United States

Dickens, Bernard M. Choices, control, access -- the Canadian position. *In:* Knoppers, Bartha Maria, ed. Human DNA: Law and Policy: International and Comparative Perspectives. Proceedings of the First International Conference on DNA Sampling and Human Genetic Research: Ethical, Legal, and Policy Aspects, held in Montreal, Canada, 6–8 Sep 1996. Boston, MA: Kluwer Law International; 1997: 71–89. 59 fn. ISBN 90–411–0361–9. BE58169.
*confidentiality; criminal law; *disclosure; *DNA data banks; DNA fingerprinting; employment; federal government; *genetic information; *genetic materials; *genetic research; *genetic screening; government regulation; health personnel; *informed consent; law enforcement; *legal aspects; legislation; mandatory testing;

BE = bioethics accession number   fn. = footnotes   refs. = references

privacy; private sector; public sector; state government; tissue donation; *biological specimen banks; *Canada; *Privacy Act 1983 (Canada); Quebec

Enríquez, Juan. Genomics and the world's economy. [News]. *Science.* 1998 Aug 14; 281(5379): 925–926. 26 refs. BE58878.
*drug industry; *economics; genetic intervention; *genetic research; *industry; *international aspects; patients; regulation; social impact; transgenic organisms; *trends

Enserink, Martin. Physicians wary of scheme to pool Icelanders' genetic data. [News]. *Science.* 1998 Aug 14; 281(5379): 890–891. BE58876.
attitudes; computer communication networks; confidentiality; *DNA data banks; epidemiology; *genetic information; *genetic research; *industry; legislation; *medical records; physicians; privacy; public opinion; public policy; *population genetics; *deCODE Genetics; *Iceland; Icelandic Health Ministry

Felice, Alex E. Guardianship by peer review in genetic engineering and biotechnology. *In:* Agius, Emmanuel; Busuttil, Salvino, eds. Germ-Line Intervention and Our Responsibilities to Future Generations. Boston, MA: Kluwer Academic; 1998: 117–129. 20 refs. 1 fn. ISBN 0-7923-4828-1. BE57883.
developing countries; future generations; gene therapy; *genetic intervention; *genetic research; genome mapping; international aspects; investigators; *peer review; public participation; regulation; resource allocation; risks and benefits; self regulation; time factors

Fishbein, Diana H. Prospects for the application of genetic findings to crime and violence prevention. *Politics and the Life Sciences.* 1996 Mar; 15(1): 91–94. 22 refs. BE55633.
*behavioral genetics; *behavioral research; drug abuse; *genetic predisposition; *genetic research; goals; health care; law enforcement; legal aspects; mental health; preventive medicine; public health; rehabilitation; social control; social discrimination; socioeconomic factors; *violence

Fishman, Rachelle H.B. Jerusalem: flourishing legal environment nurtures protected genetic inquiry. [News]. *Lancet.* 1998 Jun 27; 351(9120): 1939. BE58496.
breast cancer; confidentiality; disclosure; economics; *genetic research; *genetic screening; informed consent; international aspects; Jews; legal aspects; *Israel

Godard, Béatrice; Kinsella, T. Douglas. DNA sampling and banking: practices and procedures. *In:* Knoppers, Bartha Maria, ed. Human DNA: Law and Policy: International and Comparative Perspectives. Proceedings of the First International Conference on DNA Sampling and Human Genetic Research: Ethical, Legal, and Policy Aspects, held in Montreal, Canada, 6–8 Sep 1996. Boston, MA: Kluwer Law International; 1997: 429–434. ISBN 90-411-0361-9. BE58199.
confidentiality; *DNA data banks; DNA fingerprinting; donors; genetic information; genetic materials; genetic research; genetic screening; informed consent; institutional policies; international aspects; law enforcement; tissue donation; *biological specimen banks; Canada; Europe; United States

Goldman, David. Interdisciplinary perceptions of genetics and behavior. *Politics and the Life Sciences.* 1996 Mar; 15(1): 97–98. BE55634.
*behavioral genetics; eugenics; *genetic predisposition; *genetic research; genetics; goals; interdisciplinary communication; social control; social discrimination; violence

Goodey, Chris. Genetic markers for intelligence. *Bulletin of Medical Ethics.* 1996 Aug; No. 120: 13–16. 2 refs. BE55865.
*behavioral genetics; eugenics; *genetic research; *intelligence; mentally retarded; prenatal diagnosis; selective abortion; stigmatization; suffering; wedge argument; Great Britain

Greely, Henry T. The ethics of the Human Genome Diversity Project: the North American Regional Committee's proposed model ethical protocol. *In:* Knoppers, Bartha Maria, ed. Human DNA: Law and Policy: International and Comparative Perspectives. Proceedings of the First International Conference on DNA Sampling and Human Genetic Research: Ethical, Legal, and Policy Aspects, held in Montreal, Canada, 6–8 Sep 1996. Boston, MA: Kluwer Law International; 1997: 239–256. 33 fn. ISBN 90-411-0361-9. BE58181.
anthropology; developing countries; ethical review; *genetic diversity; genetic materials; *genetic research; *genome mapping; *guidelines; industry; informed consent; *international aspects; investigators; legal aspects; minority groups; patents; property rights; public participation; remuneration; *population genetics; *Human Genome Diversity Project; Human Genome Organization (HUGO); North America

Greely, Henry T. The Human Genome Diversity Project: ethical, legal, and social issues. *In:* Peters, Ted, ed. Genetics: Issues of Social Justice. Cleveland, OH: Pilgrim Press; 1998: 71–81. 9 fn. ISBN 0-8298-1251-2. BE57475.
confidentiality; costs and benefits; developing countries; DNA data banks; *genetic diversity; genetic information; *genetic research; *genome mapping; informed consent; *international aspects; minority groups; property rights; public participation; risks and benefits; social discrimination; community consent; *population genetics; *Human Genome Diversity Project

Guo, Sun-Wei; Zheng, Chang-Jiang; Li, C.C. "Gene war of the century?" [Letter]. *Science.* 1997 Dec 5; 278(5344): 1693–1694. 3 refs. BE57704.
advisory committees; blood specimen collection; drug industry; *economics; *genetic materials; *genetic research; government regulation; *international aspects; patents; *public policy; *population genetics; *China

Hirtle, Marie. Genetic screening and research revisited. *In:* Knoppers, Bartha Maria, ed. Human DNA: Law and Policy: International and Comparative Perspectives. Proceedings of the First International Conference on DNA Sampling and Human Genetic Research: Ethical, Legal, and Policy Aspects, held in Montreal, Canada, 6–8 Sep 1996. Boston, MA: Kluwer Law International; 1997: 333–340. 7 fn. ISBN 90-411-0361-9. BE58190.
cancer; *carriers; cystic fibrosis; DNA data banks; federal government; genetic materials; *genetic research; *genetic screening; *informed consent; legal aspects; *newborns; *parental consent; prenatal diagnosis; presumed consent; thalassemia; biological specimen banks; Europe; National Center for Human Genome Research; United States

Holtzman, Neil A. The gene: harnessing the gene and remaking the world, by Jeremy Rifkin. [Book review essay]. *JAMA.* 1998 Aug 12; 280(6): 575. BE58774.
gene therapy; *genetic intervention; *genetic research; genetic screening; genetics; patents; *The Biotech Century: Harnessing the Gene and Remaking the World (Rifkin, J.)

Juengst, Eric T. Groups as gatekeepers to genomic research: conceptually confusing, morally hazardous, and practically useless. *Kennedy Institute of Ethics*

Journal. 1998 June; 8(2): 183–200. 31 refs. BE58376.
autonomy; *cultural pluralism; *decision making; epidemiology; eugenics; *genetic diversity; *genetic research; genetic screening; genome mapping; *informed consent; international aspects; minority groups; research design; research subjects; self concept; social discrimination; *vulnerable populations; *community consent; *population genetics; Human Genome Diversity Project

Some argue that human groups have a stake in the outcome of population-genomics research and that the decision to participate in such research should therefore be subject to group permission. It is not possible, however, to obtain prior group permission, because the actual human groups under study, human demes, are unidentifiable before research begins. Moreover, they lack moral standing. If identifiable social groups with moral standing are used as proxies for demes, group approval could be sought, but at the expense of unfairly exposing these surrogates to risks from which prior group approval is powerless to protect them. Unless population genomics can proceed without targeting socially defined groups, or can find other ways of protecting them, it may fall to individuals to protect the interests of the groups they care about, and to scientists to warn their subjects of the need to do so.

Juengst, Eric T. Respecting human subjects in genome research: a preliminary policy agenda. *In:* Vanderpool, Harold Y., ed. The Ethics of Research Involving Human Subjects: Facing the 21st Century. Frederick, MD: University Publishing Group; 1996: 401–429. 74 fn. ISBN 1-55572-036-6. BE56995.
children; *confidentiality; *disclosure; employment; *family members; genetic information; genetic materials; genetic predisposition; *genetic research; *genome mapping; *informed consent; insurance; international aspects; mentally ill; minority groups; privacy; property rights; public policy; research subjects; *risks and benefits; *selection of subjects; stigmatization; truth disclosure; *pedigree studies; Human Genome Project; United States

Kääriäinen, Helena. Genetic studies in populations. *In:* Knoppers, Bartha Maria, ed. Human DNA: Law and Policy: International and Comparative Perspectives. Proceedings of the First International Conference on DNA Sampling and Human Genetic Research: Ethical, Legal, and Policy Aspects, held in Montreal, Canada, 6–8 Sep 1996. Boston, MA: Kluwer Law International; 1997: 177–188. 9 fn. ISBN 90-411-0361-9. BE58177.
cancer; DNA data banks; family members; *genetic predisposition; *genetic research; *genetic screening; human experimentation; *informed consent; mass screening; patients; asthma; biological specimen banks; *population genetics; *Finland

Kahn, Mary Jo Ellis; Jamison, Kay Redfield; Collins, Francis S. Protecting our 'family secrets'. *Washington Post.* 1997 Jul 31: A15. BE55546.
employment; family members; federal government; *genetic information; genetic predisposition; *genetic research; *genetic screening; government regulation; *health insurance; insurance selection bias; legislation; preventive medicine; *risks and benefits; social discrimination; state government; United States

Kaiser, Jocelyn. Archive available for genetic studies. [News]. *Science.* 1997 Nov 21; 278(5342): 1389. BE57439.
*confidentiality; *DNA data banks; donors; federal government; *genetic information; *genetic research; government regulation; *Centers for Disease Control and Prevention; United States

Kerr, Anne; Cunningham-Burley, Sarah; Amos,

Amanda. Eugenics and the new genetics in Britain: examining contemporary professionals' accounts. *Science, Technology, and Human Values.* 1998 Spring; 23(2): 175–198. 41 refs. 11 fn. BE57723.
*attitudes; autonomy; behavioral genetics; coercion; democracy; directive counseling; disabled; *eugenics; gene pool; gene therapy; genetic counseling; genetic determinism; genetic disorders; genetic intervention; genetic predisposition; *genetic research; genetic screening; genetic services; *genetics; homosexuals; intelligence; *investigators; mass media; *physicians; political systems; prenatal diagnosis; resource allocation; schizophrenia; selective abortion; *social impact; socioeconomic factors; survey; *Great Britain; National Health Service

Knoppers, Bartha Maria, ed. Human DNA: Law and Policy: International and Comparative Perspectives. Proceedings of the First International Conference on DNA Sampling and Human Genetic Research: Ethical, Legal, and Policy Aspects, held in Montreal, Canada, 6–8 Sep 1996. Boston, MA: Kluwer Law International; 1997. 455 p. 898 fn. ISBN 90-411-0361-9. BE58163.
body parts and fluids; carriers; confidentiality; disclosure; *DNA data banks; DNA fingerprinting; DNA sequences; epidemiology; *genetic diversity; genetic information; genetic intervention; *genetic materials; *genetic research; *genetic screening; genome mapping; government regulation; guidelines; incentives; industry; informed consent; *international aspects; legal aspects; mass screening; minority groups; newborns; patents; prenatal diagnosis; property rights; *public policy; registries; review; tissue donation; *biological specimen banks; population genetics; recontact; Canada; Europe; Human Genome Diversity Project; Human Genome Project; United States

Lehrman, Sally. Coalition to pursue ethnic concerns over gene research. [News]. *Nature.* 1998 Apr 2; 392(6675): 428. BE58058.
*genetic research; genome mapping; *minority groups; *public policy; United States

Litman, Moe M. The legal status of genetic material. *In:* Knoppers, Bartha Maria, ed. Human DNA: Law and Policy: International and Comparative Perspectives. Proceedings of the First International Conference on DNA Sampling and Human Genetic Research: Ethical, Legal, and Policy Aspects, held in Montreal, Canada, 6–8 Sep 1996. Boston, MA: Kluwer Law International; 1997: 17–32. 76 fn. ISBN 90-411-0361-9. BE58165.
biomedical research; *body parts and fluids; commodification; *confidentiality; DNA data banks; economics; *genetic information; *genetic materials; *genetic research; international aspects; *legal aspects; patents; privacy; *property rights; public policy; *tissue donation; *Canada; Moore v. Regents of the University of California; *United States

Lock, Margaret. The Human Genome Diversity Project: a perspective from cultural anthropolgy. *In:* Knoppers, Bartha Maria, ed. Human DNA: Law and Policy: International and Comparative Perspectives. Proceedings of the First International Conference on DNA Sampling and Human Genetic Research: Ethical, Legal, and Policy Aspects, held in Montreal, Canada, 6–8 Sep 1996. Boston, MA: Kluwer Law International; 1997: 229–237. 16 fn. ISBN 90-411-0361-9. BE58180.
*anthropology; blood specimen collection; cultural pluralism; *genetic diversity; genetic materials; genetic predisposition; *genetic research; *genome mapping; goals; informed consent; *international aspects; *minority groups; patents; politics; property rights; social discrimination; social impact; *population genetics; *Human Genome Diversity Project

---

BE = bioethics accession number   fn. = footnotes   refs. = references

Luther, Lori; Hirtle, Marie. Genetic diversity -- a clash of world views? *In:* Knoppers, Bartha Maria, ed. Human DNA: Law and Policy: International and Comparative Perspectives. Proceedings of the First International Conference on DNA Sampling and Human Genetic Research: Ethical, Legal, and Policy Aspects, held in Montreal, Canada, 6–8 Sep 1996. Boston, MA: Kluwer Law International; 1997: 275–280. 11 fn. ISBN 90–411–0361–9. BE58184.
    blood specimen collection; economics; *genetic diversity; *genetic research; *genome mapping; informed consent; *international aspects; minority groups; public participation; selection of subjects; social discrimination; values; *population genetics; *Human Genome Diversity Project

Macer, Darryl R.J. Bioethics and genetic diversity from the perspective of UNESCO and non–governmental organizations. *In:* Knoppers, Bartha Maria, ed. Human DNA: Law and Policy: International and Comparative Perspectives. Proceedings of the First International Conference on DNA Sampling and Human Genetic Research: Ethical, Legal, and Policy Aspects, held in Montreal, Canada, 6–8 Sep 1996. Boston, MA: Kluwer Law International; 1997: 265–273. 15 fn. ISBN 90–411–0361–9. BE58183.
    advisory committees; bioethics; confidentiality; DNA data banks; eugenics; *genetic diversity; genetic materials; *genetic research; genetic screening; *genome mapping; guidelines; informed consent; *international aspects; investigators; minority groups; *population genetics; *Human Genome Diversity Project; Human Genome Organization; International Bioethics Committee (Unesco); *Unesco

McEwen, Jean E. DNA data banks. *In:* Rothstein, Mark A., ed. Genetic Secrets: Protecting Privacy and Confidentiality in the Genetic Era. New Haven, CT: Yale University Press; 1997: 231–251. 71 fn. ISBN 0–300–07251–1. BE58685.
    *DNA data banks; *DNA fingerprinting; donors; family members; genetic counseling; genetic information; genetic materials; *genetic research; government regulation; industry; informed consent; legal aspects; military personnel; prisoners; privacy; public policy; standards; state government; universities; *biological specimen banks; Department of Defense; United States

McEwen, Jean E. DNA sampling and banking: practices and procedures in the United States. *In:* Knoppers, Bartha Maria, ed. Human DNA: Law and Policy: International and Comparative Perspectives. Proceedings of the First International Conference on DNA Sampling and Human Genetic Research: Ethical, Legal, and Policy Aspects, held in Montreal, Canada, 6–8 Sep 1996. Boston, MA: Kluwer Law International; 1997: 407–421. 76 fn. ISBN 90–411–0361–9. BE58197.
    blood specimen collection; confidentiality; *DNA data banks; *DNA fingerprinting; family members; federal government; genetic research; genetic screening; government regulation; guidelines; informed consent; institutional policies; *law enforcement; legal aspects; mandatory programs; *military personnel; newborns; organization and administration; prisoners; privacy; professional organizations; public policy; regulation; state government; statistics; *tissue banks; *biological specimen banks; DNA Identification Act 1994; Human Genome Privacy Act; *United States

Marshall, Eliot. Whose DNA is it, anyway? [News]. *Science.* 1997 Oct 24; 278(5338): 564–567. Includes two inset articles by E. Marshall, "Gene prospecting in remote populations," p. 565, and "Tapping Iceland's DNA," p. 566. Correction appears in *Science* 1997 Nov

28; 278(5343): 1551. BE57314.
    attitudes; confidentiality; *DNA data banks; *DNA sequences; federal government; financial support; genes; genetic disorders; genetic information; *genetic materials; *genetic research; *genome mapping; industry; *information dissemination; international aspects; investigators; patents; private sector; property rights; public sector; time factors; cell lines; deCode Genetics, Inc.; Iceland; National Institutes of Health; Stefansson, Kari; United States

Mason R.O.; Tomlinson, G.E. Genetic research. *In:* Chadwick, Ruth, ed. Encyclopedia of Applied Ethics, Volume 2. San Diego, CA: Academic Press; 1998: 419–434. 14 refs. ISBN 0–12–227067–3. BE56389.
    behavioral genetics; confidentiality; containment; disclosure; DNA data banks; DNA fingerprinting; eugenics; financial support; gene therapy; genetic disorders; genetic enhancement; genetic materials; *genetic research; genetic screening; genetics; genome mapping; guidelines; historical aspects; human experimentation; industry; information dissemination; informed consent; investigators; moral policy; patents; privacy; public policy; recombinant DNA research; research design; research ethics committees; research subjects; resource allocation; review; risks and benefits; science; scientific misconduct; selection of subjects; terminology; Twentieth Century

Merchant, Jennifer. Biogenetics, artificial procreation, and public policy in the United States and France. *Technology in Society.* 1996; 18(1): 1–15. 26 fn. BE56595.
    abortion, induced; advisory committees; biomedical research; cesarean section; coercion; comparative studies; criminal law; cryopreservation; drug abuse; embryo disposition; *embryo research; federal government; *fetal research; fetal therapy; *fetuses; *genetic research; genetic screening; genetic services; *government financing; in vitro fertilization; indigents; industry; international aspects; judicial action; *legal aspects; legal liability; legal rights; personhood; physicians; *pregnant women; preimplantation diagnosis; prenatal diagnosis; *prenatal injuries; private sector; *public policy; *reproductive technologies; state government; state interest; Supreme Court decisions; torts; treatment refusal; women's health services; women's rights; *wrongful life; Bonbrest v. Kotz; France; Roe v. Wade; *United States

Murashige, Kate H. Genome research and traditional intellectual property protection -- a bad fit? *Risk: Health, Safety and Environment.* 1996 Summer; 7(3): 231–238. 16 fn. BE55938.
    DNA sequences; genes; *genetic research; industry; *legal aspects; *patents; recombinant DNA research; transgenic animals; United States

National Research Council. Committee on Human Genome Diversity. Human rights and human genetic–variation research. *In: its* Evaluating Human Genetic Diversity. Washington, DC: National Academy Press; 1997: 55–68. ISBN 0–309–05931–3. BE57648.
    confidentiality; cultural pluralism; *DNA data banks; DNA sequences; genes; *genetic diversity; *genetic research; genome mapping; guidelines; *human rights; informed consent; international aspects; minority groups; patents; property rights; public participation; *research design; research subjects; risks and benefits; social discrimination; *biological specimen banks; community consent; *population genetics

Neel, James V. Looking ahead: some genetic issues of the future. *Perspectives in Biology and Medicine.* 1997 Spring; 40(3): 328–347. 77 refs. Based on a presentation at the Ninth International Congress of Human Genetics in Rio de Janeiro, 23 Aug 1996. BE59007.
    drug industry; ecology; eugenics; financial support; food; future generations; *gene pool; gene therapy; genetic

---

disorders; genetic diversity; genetic predisposition; *genetic research; genetic screening; *genetics; health hazards; international aspects; investigators; *moral obligations; morbidity; nutrition; *population control; psychoactive drugs; public policy; radiation; social problems; trends; *population genetics; China

Nørgaard–Pederson, Bent. Use of stored samples from the Danish PKU register. *In:* Knoppers, Bartha Maria, ed. Human DNA: Law and Policy: International and Comparative Perspectives. Proceedings of the First International Conference on DNA Sampling and Human Genetic Research: Ethical, Legal, and Policy Aspects, held in Montreal, Canada, 6–8 Sep 1996. Boston, MA: Kluwer Law International; 1997: 303–311. 24 fn. ISBN 90–411–0361–9. BE58187.
  congenital disorders; *DNA data banks; genetic disorders; genetic information; genetic materials; *genetic research; *genetic screening; guidelines; *newborns; *phenylketonuria; pregnant women; *registries; *biological specimen banks; *Denmark

Page, David L.; Jensen, Roy A.; Geller, Gail, et al. Genetic testing and informed consent. [Letter and response]. *JAMA.* 1997 Sep 10; 278(10): 821–822. 2 refs. BE57315.
  biomedical research; *cancer; confidentiality; disclosure; DNA data banks; epidemiology; federal government; genetic information; *genetic predisposition; *genetic research; *genetic screening; government regulation; guidelines; health insurance; *informed consent; patients; research ethics committees; research subjects; risks and benefits; social discrimination; tissue banks; Office for Protection from Research Risks; United States

Pearson, Roger. Heredity and Humanity: Race, Eugenics and Modern Science. Washington, DC: Scott–Townsend; 1996. 162 p. Bibliography: p. 146–156. ISBN 1–878365–15–5. BE57200.
  altruism; ancient history; anthropology; behavioral genetics; communism; developing countries; DNA fingerprinting; *eugenics; evolution; genetic determinism; *genetic research; *genetics; genome mapping; historical aspects; legislation; mass media; medicine; minority groups; psychology; public policy; reproduction; science; social sciences; socialism; sociobiology; twins; *population genetics; Western World; Great Britain; Nineteenth Century; Twentieth Century; United States

Powers, Madison. Justice and genetics: privacy protection and the moral basis of public policy. *In:* Rothstein, Mark A., ed. Genetic Secrets: Protecting Privacy and Confidentiality in the Genetic Era. New Haven, CT: Yale University Press; 1997: 355–368. 15 fn. ISBN 0–300–07251–1. BE58691.
  autonomy; common good; *confidentiality; data banks; *disclosure; economics; employment; epidemiology; family members; *genetic information; genetic predisposition; *genetic research; *genetic screening; government regulation; health care delivery; health hazards; health insurance; incentives; informed consent; *justice; legal rights; mass screening; medical records; moral policy; policy analysis; *privacy; public health; *public policy; registries; risks and benefits; social discrimination; stigmatization; *pragmatism; United States

Quintana, Octavi. Human tissue banks in Europe. *In:* Knoppers, Bartha Maria, ed. Human DNA: Law and Policy: International and Comparative Perspectives. Proceedings of the First International Conference on DNA Sampling and Human Genetic Research: Ethical, Legal, and Policy Aspects, held in Montreal, Canada, 6–8 Sep 1996. Boston, MA: Kluwer Law International; 1997: 423–427. 11 fn. ISBN 90–411–0361–9. BE58198.

confidentiality; *DNA data banks; genetic research; informed consent; international aspects; medical devices; organization and administration; *regulation; *tissue banks; tissue donation; *biological specimen banks; *Europe; European Union; Group of Advisers on the Ethical Implications of Biotechnology (European Commission)

Rifkin, Jeremy. The Biotech Century: Harnessing the Gene and Remaking the World. New York, NY: Jeremy P. Tarcher/Putnam; 1998. 271 p. 486 fn. ISBN 0–87477–909–X. BE57152.
  animal experimentation; animal organs; animal rights; biological warfare; biomedical research; cloning; commodification; computers; developing countries; *ecology; *economics; *eugenics; future generations; gene pool; gene therapy; genes; genetic disorders; genetic diversity; genetic enhancement; *genetic information; *genetic intervention; genetic predisposition; *genetic research; genetics; genome mapping; *industry; international aspects; legal aspects; patents; property rights; regulation; reproduction; reproductive technologies; review; *risks and benefits; *social impact; social problems; stigmatization; transgenic animals; *transgenic organisms; *trends; wedge argument; agriculture; transgenic plants; Europe; Human Genome Diversity Project; Human Genome Project; Twenty–First Century; United States

Roche, Patricia (Winnie). Caveat venditor: protecting privacy and ownership interests in DNA. *In:* Knoppers, Bartha Maria, ed. Human DNA: Law and Policy: International and Comparative Perspectives. Proceedings of the First International Conference on DNA Sampling and Human Genetic Research: Ethical, Legal, and Policy Aspects, held in Montreal, Canada, 6–8 Sep 1996. Boston, MA: Kluwer Law International; 1997: 33–41. 30 fn. ISBN 90–411–0361–9. BE58166.
  *confidentiality; disclosure; *DNA data banks; DNA fingerprinting; federal government; *genetic information; *genetic materials; *genetic research; *genetic screening; *government regulation; informed consent; *legal aspects; model legislation; privacy; *property rights; tissue donation; *Genetic Privacy Act; Moore v. Regents of the University of California; *United States

Roleff, Tamara L., ed. Biomedical Ethics: Opposing Viewpoints. San Diego, CA: Greenhaven Press; 1998. 252 p. (Opposing viewpoints series). Includes references. ISBN 1–56510–792–6. BE59107.
  age factors; animal organs; autonomy; beneficence; *bioethical issues; body parts and fluids; brain death; cadavers; capital punishment; childbirth; *cloning; eugenics; females; genes; *genetic intervention; *genetic research; genetic screening; genome mapping; government regulation; indigents; moral policy; *organ donation; organ transplantation; patents; personhood; posthumous reproduction; pregnant women; presumed consent; prisoners; public policy; remuneration; *reproductive technologies; risks and benefits; selection for treatment; surrogate mothers; transgenic animals

Roy, David J.; Kramar, Giulia; de Langavant, Ghislaine Cleret. Ethics for complexity. *In:* Knoppers, Bartha Maria, ed. Human DNA: Law and Policy: International and Comparative Perspectives. Proceedings of the First International Conference on DNA Sampling and Human Genetic Research: Ethical, Legal, and Policy Aspects, held in Montreal, Canada, 6–8 Sep 1996. Boston, MA: Kluwer Law International; 1997: 189–209. 60 fn. ISBN 90–411–0361–9. BE58178.
  confidentiality; *DNA data banks; *epidemiology; ethical theory; *ethics; evolution; genetic counseling; genetic disorders; *genetic diversity; genetic materials; genetic predisposition; *genetic research; *genetic screening; *genetics; informed consent; international aspects; mass screening; public health; risks and benefits; *biological

specimen banks; *population genetics

Samet, Jonathan M.; Bailey, Linda A. Environmental population screening. *In:* Rothstein, Mark A., ed. Genetic Secrets: Protecting Privacy and Confidentiality in the Genetic Era. New Haven, CT: Yale University Press; 1997: 197–211. 20 fn. ISBN 0–300–07251–1. BE58683.
*confidentiality; disclosure; *epidemiology; *genetic information; genetic predisposition; *genetic research; genetic screening; health; informed consent; mass screening; occupational exposure; privacy; research subjects; genetic markers; recontact

Sherman, Stephanie L.; DeFries, John C.; Gottesman, Irving I., et al. Behavioral genetics '97 — ASHG statement: recent developments in human behavioral genetics: past accomplishments and future directions. *American Journal of Human Genetics.* 1997 Jun; 60(6): 1265–1275. 54 refs. BE56013.
adoption; *behavioral genetics; *behavioral research; emotions; eugenics; family relationship; genetic counseling; *genetic research; research design; review; schizophrenia; twins; population genetics; American Society of Human Genetics

Singer, Maxine F. Genetics and the law: a scientist's view. *Yale Law and Policy Review.* 1985 Spring; 3(2): 315–335. 44 fn. BE56497.
biological warfare; clergy; education; evolution; federal government; *genetic intervention; *genetic research; *genetics; germ cells; government regulation; *interdisciplinary communication; investigators; *law; *lawyers; legal aspects; *political activity; political systems; professional competence; public policy; *recombinant DNA research; *risks and benefits; *science; self regulation; technical expertise; transgenic organisms; agriculture; Lysenko, T.D.; Rifkin, Jeremy; *United States; USSR

Spicker, Stuart F. The unknowable effects of genetic interventions on future generations (or, who guards the genetic engineers in democratic republics?). *In:* Agius, Emmanuel; Busuttil, Salvino, eds. Germ-Line Intervention and Our Responsibilities to Future Generations. Boston, MA: Kluwer Academic; 1998: 147–163. 41 refs. 8 fn. ISBN 0–7923–4828–1. BE57885.
*accountability; consensus; *decision making; *democracy; eugenics; *future generations; gene therapy; genetic enhancement; *genetic intervention; *genetic research; germ cells; investigators; moral obligations; public participation; public policy; regulation; risks and benefits; social control; uncertainty

Sprunger, Suzanne A.; Julian-Arnold, Gianna. Promoting and managing genome innovation. *Risk: Health, Safety and Environment.* 1996 Summer; 7(3): 197–200. 12 fn. BE55941.
DNA sequences; *genetic research; genetic screening; genome mapping; industry; patents; regulation; social impact; United States

Stephenson, Joan. Ethics group drafts guidelines for control of genetic material and information. [News]. *JAMA.* 1998 Jan 21; 279(3): 184. BE58069.
advisory committees; *confidentiality; disclosure; *DNA data banks; family members; *genetic information; *genetic materials; *genetic research; *guidelines; *international aspects; property rights; *tissue banks; *tissue donation; *biological specimen banks; *Ethical, Legal, and Social Issues Committee (HUGO-ELSI); *Human Genome Organization

Thomson, Elizabeth J. Sampling issues in clinical impact of genetic testing and counselling studies. *In:* Knoppers,

Bartha Maria, ed. Human DNA: Law and Policy: International and Comparative Perspectives. Proceedings of the First International Conference on DNA Sampling and Human Genetic Research: Ethical, Legal, and Policy Aspects, held in Montreal, Canada, 6–8 Sep 1996. Boston, MA: Kluwer Law International; 1997: 313–317. 9 fn. ISBN 90–411–0361–9. BE58188.
cancer; confidentiality; cystic fibrosis; DNA data banks; federal government; genetic counseling; genetic materials; genetic predisposition; *genetic research; *genetic screening; genetic services; government financing; informed consent; risks and benefits; social impact; National Center for Human Genome Research; NCHGR Program on Ethical, Legal, and Social Implications (ELSI); United States

Verhoef, Marja J.; Lewkonia, Raymond M.; Kinsella, T. Douglas. Ethical issues concerning current human DNA banking practices in Canada: three perspectives. *In:* Knoppers, Bartha Maria, ed. Human DNA: Law and Policy: International and Comparative Perspectives. Proceedings of the First International Conference on DNA Sampling and Human Genetic Research: Ethical, Legal, and Policy Aspects, held in Montreal, Canada, 6–8 Sep 1996. Boston, MA: Kluwer Law International; 1997: 393–405. 17 fn. ISBN 90–411–0361–9. BE58196.
*administrators; comparative studies; confidentiality; consent forms; disclosure; *DNA data banks; donors; ethical review; evaluation; *genetic research; informed consent; *institutional policies; *investigators; *knowledge, attitudes, practice; organization and administration; organizational policies; professional organizations; property rights; *research ethics committees; research institutes; survey; tissue donation; *biological specimen banks; *Canada; Canadian College of Medical Genetics

Verma, Ishwar C. Ethical concerns in genome diversity studies in developing countries. *In:* Knoppers, Bartha Maria, ed. Human DNA: Law and Policy: International and Comparative Perspectives. Proceedings of the First International Conference on DNA Sampling and Human Genetic Research: Ethical, Legal, and Policy Aspects, held in Montreal, Canada, 6–8 Sep 1996. Boston, MA: Kluwer Law International; 1997: 257–263. 14 fn. ISBN 90–411–0361–9. BE58182.
blood specimen collection; confidentiality; consent forms; *developing countries; *genetic diversity; *genetic research; *genome mapping; incentives; informed consent; *international aspects; investigators; minority groups; moral obligations; remuneration; research ethics committees; social impact; population genetics; *Human Genome Diversity Project; *India

Vines, Gail. Genetics: let the public decide. [News]. *BMJ (British Medical Journal).* 1997 Apr 5; 314(7086): 1055. BE56338.
behavioral genetics; *decision making; eugenics; *genetic intervention; genetic materials; *genetic research; genetic screening; *genetics; industry; *knowledge, attitudes, practice; mass media; *public opinion; *public participation; Great Britain

Vogel, Gretchen. Genetic enhancement: from science fiction to ethics quandary. [News]. *Science.* 1997 Sep 19; 277(5333): 1753–1754. BE56160.
advisory committees; federal government; *gene therapy; *genetic enhancement; *genetic research; government regulation; human experimentation; mass media; trends; wedge argument; Recombinant DNA Advisory Committee; United States

Wadman, Meredith. Genome panel defends researchers' — and families' — interests. [News]. *Nature.* 1998 Feb 26; 391(6670): 826. BE58072.
advisory committees; *confidentiality; *disclosure; DNA

---

data banks; family members; *genetic information; *genetic research; *genome mapping; informed consent; *international aspects; investigators; medical records; *privacy; tissue banks; *Human Genome Organization (HUGO)

Wadman, Meredith. 'Group debate' urged for gene studies. [News]. *Nature.* 1998 Jan 22; 391(6665): 314. BE57319.
advisory committees; attitudes; *genetic research; *human experimentation; *informed consent; investigators; Jews; minority groups; *public participation; *public policy; risks and benefits; *tissue banks; *tissue donation; *population genetics; *National Bioethics Advisory Commission; United States

Wadman, Meredith. Jewish leaders meet NIH chiefs on genetic stigmatization fears. [News]. *Nature.* 1998 Apr 30; 392(6679): 851. BE58432.
genetic predisposition; *genetic research; *genetic screening; *Jews; social discrimination; *stigmatization; National Institutes of Health; United States

Wasserman, David. Research into genetics and crime: consensus and controversy. *Politics and the Life Sciences.* 1996 Mar; 15(1): 107–109. BE55637.
*behavioral genetics; behavioral research; consensus; dissent; *genetic predisposition; *genetic research; *interdisciplinary communication; investigators; mass media; *political activity; social control; social discrimination; *socioeconomic factors; *violence; United States; University of Maryland

Watson, James D. Genes and politics. *Journal Of Molecular Medicine.* 1997 Sep; 75(9): 624–636. Keynote address to the Congress of Molecular Medicine, Berlin, May 1997. BE57981.
active euthanasia; aliens; behavioral genetics; blacks; dissent; *eugenics; gene therapy; genes; genetic determinism; genetic disorders; genetic intervention; *genetic research; genetic screening; *genetics; genome mapping; *historical aspects; intelligence; international aspects; investigators; involuntary sterilization; Jews; killing; mentally disabled; military personnel; physically disabled; physician's role; political activity; prenatal diagnosis; *public policy; recombinant DNA research; social discrimination; social problems; war; emigration and immigration; Eugenics Record Station (Cold Spring Harbor, NY); Germany; Human Genome Project; Lysenkoism; NCHGR Program on Ethical, Legal, and Social Implications (ELSI); Nineteenth Century; Social Darwinism; Twentieth Century; United States; USSR; World War I; World War II

Watson, Rory. EU approves rights to genetic material. [News]. *BMJ (British Medical Journal).* 1997 Dec 6; 315(7121): 1487. BE57346.
biomedical technologies; cloning; embryo research; genetic intervention; *genetic materials; *genetic research; *international aspects; legislation; *patents; political activity; *regulation; *transgenic organisms; *Europe; *European Union

Weir, Robert F. Differing perspectives on consent, choice and control. *In:* Knoppers, Bartha Maria, ed. Human DNA: Law and Policy: International and Comparative Perspectives. Proceedings of the First International Conference on DNA Sampling and Human Genetic Research: Ethical, Legal, and Policy Aspects, held in Montreal, Canada, 6–8 Sep 1996. Boston, MA: Kluwer Law International; 1997: 91–107. 31 fn. ISBN 90-411-0361-9. BE58170.
attitudes; confidentiality; consent forms; *disclosure; *DNA data banks; donors; federal government; *genetic information; *genetic materials; *genetic research; genetic screening; government regulation; guidelines; *informed

consent; model legislation; privacy; professional organizations; research ethics committees; *tissue banks; *tissue donation; *biological specimen banks; American College of Medical Genetics; American Society of Human Genetics; Centers for Disease Control and Prevention; Genetic Privacy Act; National Center for Human Genome Research; *United States

Williams, Janet K.; Lessick, Mira. Genome research: implications for children. *Pediatric Nursing.* 1996 Jan–Feb; 22(1): 40–46. 46 refs. BE55584.
carriers; *children; chromosome abnormalities; cystic fibrosis; *gene therapy; genetic counseling; genetic determinism; genetic disorders; genetic information; genetic predisposition; *genetic research; *genetic screening; genome mapping; germ cells; nurses; parent child relationship; patient advocacy; pediatrics; *risks and benefits; social discrimination; social impact; adenosine deaminase deficiency; fragile X syndrome

Banking Our Genes. [Videorecording].Eunice Kennedy Shriver Center; available for sale from Fanlight Productions, 47 Halifax St., Boston, MA 02130, 800-937-4113; 1995. 1 videocassette; 33 min.; sd.; color; 1/2 in.; VHS. Executive producer: Philip Reilly. BE57896.
behavioral genetics; computers; *DNA data banks; *DNA fingerprinting; family members; federal government; genetic information; genetic predisposition; *genetic research; genetic screening; insurance; law enforcement; legal aspects; mass screening; military personnel; newborns; *privacy; public policy; *risks and benefits; stigmatization; violence; *biological specimen banks; ELSI-funded publication; pedigree studies; Department of Defense; Federal Bureau of Investigation; United States

Perils in free market genomics. [Editorial]. *Nature.* 1998 Mar 26; 392(6674): 315. BE57318.
*gene therapy; genetic enhancement; *genetic research; *germ cells; *regulation; risks and benefits

GENETIC SCREENING

See also DNA FINGERPRINTING, GENETIC COUNSELING, GENETIC INTERVENTION, GENETIC SERVICES, GENOME MAPPING, MASS SCREENING, PRENATAL DIAGNOSIS

Allen, Anita L. Genetic privacy: emerging concepts and values. *In:* Rothstein, Mark A., ed. Genetic Secrets: Protecting Privacy and Confidentiality in the Genetic Era. New Haven, CT: Yale University Press; 1997: 31–59. 141 fn. ISBN 0-300-07251-1. BE58674.
autonomy; beneficence; *confidentiality; democracy; disclosure; DNA data banks; family members; *genetic information; genetic intervention; genetic materials; genetic research; *genetic screening; genetic services; historical aspects; informed consent; legal rights; mandatory testing; mass screening; morality; *privacy; property rights; public policy; reproduction; review; social discrimination; stigmatization; terminology; values; biological specimen banks; Nineteenth Century; Twentieth Century; United States

American Medical Association. Council on Ethical and Judicial Affairs. Multiplex genetic testing. [Policy statement]. *Hastings Center Report.* 1998 Jul–Aug; 28(4): 15–21. 14 fn. Report adopted by the House of Delegates of the American Medical Association Dec 1996 and subsequently revised in response to comments from peer reviewers. BE58923.
breast cancer; carriers; disclosure; genetic counseling; genetic disorders; genetic information; genetic predisposition; *genetic screening; guidelines; informed

---

BE = bioethics accession number   fn. = footnotes   refs. = references

consent; late-onset disorders; methods; minority groups; *organizational policies; physician's role; physicians; professional organizations; risk; risks and benefits; social discrimination; technical expertise; uncertainty; population genetics; *American Medical Association

As panels of multiple genetic tests become increasingly available, clinicians face new challenges in helping patients understand the nature of these tests. Diagnostic tests for conditions that inevitably lead to disease, "susceptibility" tests that reveal heightened risk of disease, and tests for carrier status raise different concerns about informed consent and pose different needs for counseling. Clinicians must understand the implications of different kinds of tests, and of different arrays of tests in multiple panels, if multiplex tests are to be used wisely in clinical practice.

American Society of Human Genetics. Social Issues Subcommittee on Familial Disclosure. ASHG statement: professional disclosure of familial genetic information. *American Journal of Human Genetics.* 1998 Feb; 62(2): 474-483. 46 refs. 32 fn. BE57550.
> *confidentiality; *disclosure; *duty to warn; *family members; genetic counseling; genetic disorders; *genetic information; *genetic screening; *guidelines; *health personnel; informed consent; international aspects; legal obligations; moral obligations; *organizational policies; privacy; professional family relationship; professional organizations; professional patient relationship; risk; risks and benefits; *American Society of Human Genetics; United States

Andrews, Lori B.; Elster, Nanette. Adoption, reproductive technologies, and genetic information. *Health Matrix.* 1998 Summer; 8(2): 125-151. 125 fn. BE58951.
> *adoption; artificial insemination; behavioral genetics; children; *confidentiality; *disclosure; *genetic information; *genetic screening; government regulation; informed consent; *legal aspects; ovum donors; parents; records; registries; *reproductive technologies; semen donors; state government; *United States

Andrews, Lori B. Gen-etiquette: genetic information, family relationships, and adoption. *In:* Rothstein, Mark A., ed. Genetic Secrets: Protecting Privacy and Confidentiality in the Genetic Era. New Haven, CT: Yale University Press; 1997: 255-280. 86 fn. ISBN 0-300-07251-1. BE58686.
> *adoption; anthropology; children; *confidentiality; *disclosure; duty to warn; *family members; *family relationship; *genetic information; *genetic screening; health personnel; legal obligations; moral obligations; parent child relationship; parents; privacy; professional family relationship; rights; pedigree studies; United States

Andrews, Lori B. Genetic fallout: new technologies are changing the legal landscape. *Trial.* 1995 Dec; 31(12): 20-23, 25-27. 30 fn. BE57273.
> carriers; *confidentiality; *disclosure; duty to warn; employment; family members; federal government; genetic disorders; *genetic information; genetic predisposition; *genetic screening; government regulation; health insurance; *legal aspects; legal liability; mandatory testing; mass screening; newborns; physicians; pregnant women; prenatal diagnosis; risk; *social discrimination; state government; stigmatization; treatment refusal; wrongful life; ELSI-funded publication; Americans with Disabilities Act 1990; Equal Employment Opportunity Commission; *United States

Andrews, Lori B. The genetic information superhighway: rules of the road for contacting relatives and recontacting former patients. *In:* Knoppers, Bartha

Maria, ed. Human DNA: Law and Policy: International and Comparative Perspectives. Proceedings of the First International Conference on DNA Sampling and Human Genetic Research: Ethical, Legal, and Policy Aspects, held in Montreal, Canada, 6-8 Sep 1996. Boston, MA: Kluwer Law International; 1997: 133-143. 42 fn. ISBN 90-411-0361-9. BE58173.
> *confidentiality; *disclosure; duty to warn; *family members; *genetic counseling; genetic disorders; *genetic information; genetic predisposition; *genetic screening; guidelines; *legal aspects; *patients; physicians; professional organizations; risks and benefits; wrongful life; *recontact; United States

Archer, Luis. Genetic testing and gene therapy: the scientific and ethical background. *In:* Doherty, Peter; Sutton, Agneta, eds. Man-Made Man: Ethical and Legal Issues in Genetics. Dublin, Ireland: Open Air; 1997: 29-45. 18 fn. ISBN 1-85182-278-X. BE58294.
> advisory committees; autonomy; confidentiality; embryos; employment; eugenics; family members; *gene therapy; genetic enhancement; genetic predisposition; *genetic screening; germ cells; informed consent; insurance; justice; legal aspects; occupational exposure; parental consent; public policy; rights; *risks and benefits; social discrimination; Europe

Association of British Insurers. Genetic Testing: ABI Code of Practice. London: Association of British Insurers [online]. Internet Web Site: http://www.abi.org.uk/Industry/abikey/genetics/gentest97 [1998 April 29]; 1997 Dec. 23 p. BE57074.
> administrators; confidentiality; due process; genetic information; *genetic screening; *guidelines; *industry; *institutional ethics; *insurance; medical records; *Association of British Insurers; Great Britain

Baird, Rachel. Gene tests pose challenge for privacy guardian. [News]. *New Scientist.* 1997 Jun 28; 154(2088): 4. BE59084.
> *confidentiality; genetic information; *genetic screening; *government regulation; industry; *insurance; Data Protection Act 1984 (Great Britain); *Great Britain; Human Genetics Advisory Commission (Great Britain)

Bankowski, Zbigniew. International ethics guidelines and genetic epidemiology. *In:* Knoppers, Bartha Maria, ed. Human DNA: Law and Policy: International and Comparative Perspectives. Proceedings of the First International Conference on DNA Sampling and Human Genetic Research: Ethical, Legal, and Policy Aspects, held in Montreal, Cananda, 6-8 Sep 1996. Boston, MA: Kluwer Law International; 1997: 9-13. 5 refs. ISBN 90-411-0361-9. BE58164.
> bioethics; developing countries; *epidemiology; ethical relativism; *genetic research; *genetic screening; *guidelines; human rights; informed consent; *international aspects; tissue donation; Council for International Organizations of Medical Sciences

Barnes, Frank L. Ethical considerations of preimplantation genetic diagnosis and embryo selection. *In:* Monagle, John F.; Thomasma, David C., eds. Health Care Ethics: Critical Issues for the 21st Century. Gaithersburg, MD: Aspen Publishers; 1998: 56-59. 10 fn. ISBN 0-8342-0911-X. BE56279.
> embryo transfer; embryos; gene therapy; *genetic disorders; genetic predisposition; *genetic screening; in vitro fertilization; methods; parents; *preimplantation diagnosis; selection for treatment

Bayertz, Kurt. Ethical aspects of gene therapy and molecular genetic diagnostics. *Cytokines and Molecular Therapy.* 1996 Sep; 2(3): 207-211. 13 refs. BE58352.

BE = bioethics accession number   fn. = footnotes   refs. = references

coercion; *gene therapy; genetic disorders; genetic predisposition; *genetic screening; health insurance; late-onset disorders; mass screening; preventive medicine; public opinion; *risks and benefits; social control; social discrimination; social impact; Europe; Germany

Bernhardt, Barbara A.; Geller, Gail; Strauss, Misha, et al. Toward a model informed consent process for BRCA1 testing: a qualitative assessment of women's attitudes. *Journal of Genetic Counseling.* 1997 Jun; 6(2): 207–222. 16 refs. BE55666.
  adults; *breast cancer; children; comprehension; decision making; directive counseling; *disclosure; *females; *genetic counseling; *genetic predisposition; *genetic screening; guidelines; health education; *informed consent; insurance; *knowledge, attitudes, practice; models, theoretical; patient participation; physician patient relationship; physicians; public opinion; risk; *risks and benefits; social discrimination; socioeconomic factors; survey; trust; uncertainty; qualitative research; urban population; Baltimore

Berry, Roberta M. The genetic revolution and the physician's duty of confidentiality: the role of the old Hippocratic virtues in the regulation of the new genetic intimacy. *Journal of Legal Medicine.* 1997 Dec; 18(4): 401–441. 110 fn. BE58650.
  autonomy; *caring; codes of ethics; *confidentiality; decision making; *disclosure; dissent; duty to warn; employment; *family members; genetic determinism; *genetic information; genetic predisposition; genetic screening; government regulation; historical aspects; insurance; law; *legal aspects; legal liability; *legal obligations; medical ethics; *medicine; *moral obligations; obligations to society; patients; physician patient relationship; *physicians; policy analysis; privacy; professional family relationship; *public policy; risks and benefits; schools; *virtues; Hippocratic Oath

Bove, Catherine M.; Fry, Sara T.; MacDonald, Deborah J. Presymptomatic and predisposition genetic testing: ethical and social considerations. *Seminars in Oncology Nursing.* 1997 May; 13(2): 135–140. 30 refs. BE58977.
  autonomy; cancer; children; disclosure; employment; genetic counseling; genetic information; *genetic predisposition; *genetic screening; informed consent; insurance; late-onset disorders; nurses; prenatal diagnosis; privacy; psychological stress; social discrimination

Brandt–Rauf, Paul W.; Brandt–Rauf, Sherry I. Biomarkers -- scientific advances and societal implications. *In:* Rothstein, Mark A., ed. Genetic Secrets: Protecting Privacy and Confidentiality in the Genetic Era. New Haven, CT: Yale University Press; 1997: 184–196. 30 fn. ISBN 0–300–07251–1. BE58682.
  biomedical research; compensation; confidentiality; ecology; employment; *genetic predisposition; *genetic research; *genetic screening; *health hazards; *occupational exposure; toxicity; *genetic markers

Brockett, Patrick L.; Tankersley, E. Susan. The genetics revolution, economics, ethics, and insurance. *Journal of Business Ethics.* 1997 Nov; 16(15): 1661–1676. 13 refs. 6 fn. BE58890.
  age factors; confidentiality; disclosure; *economics; employment; federal government; *genetic information; *genetic screening; *genome mapping; government regulation; health insurance; industry; *insurance; *insurance selection bias; justice; legal rights; legislation; life insurance; medical records; privacy; *public policy; *risk; risks and benefits; *social discrimination; social impact; state government; traffic accidents; Americans with Disabilities Act 1990; Human Genome Privacy Act (1991 bill); *United States

Brodaty, Henry; Alzheimer's Disease International. Medical and Scientific Advisory Committee. Consensus statement on predictive testing for Alzheimer disease. *Alzheimer Disease and Associated Disorders.* 1995 Winter; 9(4): 182–187. 15 refs. BE55708.
  confidentiality; *dementia; disclosure; family members; genetic counseling; *genetic predisposition; *genetic screening; informed consent; methods; *organizational policies; professional organizations; rights; risk; risks and benefits; *Alzheimer's Disease International

Brown, Iona Jane; Gannon, Philippa. Confidentiality and the Human Genome Project: a prophecy for conflict. *In:* McLean, Sheila A.M., ed. Contemporary Issues in Law, Medicine and Ethics. Brookfield, VT: Dartmouth; 1996: 215–236. 88 fn. ISBN 1–85521–586–1. BE57797.
  carriers; common good; *confidentiality; disabled; *disclosure; duty to warn; eugenics; family members; genetic counseling; genetic disorders; *genetic information; genetic predisposition; *genetic screening; genome mapping; *legal aspects; legal obligations; medical ethics; moral obligations; physician patient relationship; physicians; prenatal diagnosis; preventive medicine; risk; selective abortion; social discrimination; stigmatization; *Great Britain; Human Genome Project

Brunner, E.J.; Sheppard, J.; Ravetz, J. Public is concerned about gene testing. [Letter]. *BMJ (British Medical Journal).* 1997 May 24; 314(7093): 1552–1553. 2 refs. BE56856.
  *attitudes; confidentiality; *disclosure; drug industry; economics; *genetic information; *genetic materials; *genetic research; *genetic screening; informed consent; life insurance; *public opinion; survey; tissue donation; *Great Britain

Burris, Scott; Gostin, Lawrence O. Genetic screening from a public health perspective: some lessons from the HIV experience. *In:* Rothstein, Mark A., ed. Genetic Secrets: Protecting Privacy and Confidentiality in the Genetic Era. New Haven, CT: Yale University Press; 1997: 137–158. 57 fn. ISBN 0–300–07251–1. BE58680.
  adults; AIDS serodiagnosis; costs and benefits; DNA data banks; epidemiology; *genetic information; genetic research; *genetic screening; *government regulation; guidelines; HIV seropositivity; informed consent; justice; legal aspects; mandatory reporting; mandatory testing; mass screening; moral policy; newborns; *privacy; *public health; *public policy; resource allocation; risks and benefits; social discrimination; socioeconomic factors; stigmatization; biological specimen banks; United States

Cao, Antonio. Technical and social aspects of beta-thalassemia screening in Europe and developing countries. *In:* Knoppers, Bartha Maria, ed. Human DNA: Law and Policy: International and Comparative Perspectives. Proceedings of the First International Conference on DNA Sampling and Human Genetic Research: Ethical, Legal, and Policy Aspects, held in Montreal, Canada, 6–8 Sep 1996. Boston, MA: Kluwer Law International; 1997: 319–332. 36 refs. ISBN 90–411–0361–9. BE58189.
  *carriers; communication; *developing countries; directive counseling; evaluation; genetic counseling; *genetic screening; health education; mass media; mass screening; *prenatal diagnosis; *preventive medicine; program descriptions; *thalassemia; *Europe; *Mediterranean Region; Middle East

Chadwick, Ruth. Genetic screening. *In:* Chadwick, Ruth, ed. Encyclopedia of Applied Ethics, Volume 2. San Diego, CA: Academic Press; 1998: 445–449. 8 refs. ISBN 0–12–227067–3. BE56391.
  advisory committees; autonomy; communitarianism;

---

confidentiality; decision making; disclosure; eugenics; family members; genetic counseling; genetic disorders; genetic information; genetic predisposition; *genetic screening; genetic services; guidelines; informed consent; international aspects; justice; mandatory programs; *mass screening; moral policy; normality; public health; risks and benefits; stigmatization; voluntary programs; incidental findings; Council of Europe; Danish Council of Ethics; Nuffield Council on Bioethics

Chadwick, Ruth. The status of human genetic material -- European approaches. *In:* Knoppers, Bartha Maria, ed. Human DNA: Law and Policy: International and Comparative Perspectives. Proceedings of the First International Conference on DNA Sampling and Human Genetic Research: Ethical, Legal, and Policy Aspects, held in Montreal, Canada, 6-8 Sep 1996. Boston, MA: Kluwer Law International; 1997: 55-62. 20 fn. ISBN 90-411-0361-9. BE58167.
> body parts and fluids; confidentiality; genes; *genetic information; *genetic materials; genetic screening; *international aspects; legal aspects; *property rights; tissue donation; *Europe

Clarke, Joe T.R.; Ray, Peter N. Look-back: the duty to update genetic counselling. *In:* Knoppers, Bartha Maria, ed. Human DNA: Law and Policy: International and Comparative Perspectives. Proceedings of the First International Conference on DNA Sampling and Human Genetic Research: Ethical, Legal, and Policy Aspects, held in Montreal, Canada, 6-8 Sep 1996. Boston, MA: Kluwer Law International; 1997: 121-132. 13 fn. ISBN 90-411-0361-9. BE58172.
> confidentiality; DNA data banks; family members; *genetic counseling; genetic information; *genetic screening; *guidelines; health personnel; informed consent; laboratories; legal obligations; physicians; primary health care; professional organizations; biological specimen banks; *recontact

Clayton, Ellen Wright. Screening and treatment of newborns. *Houston Law Review.* 1992 Spring; 29(1): 85-148. 263 fn. BE56567.
> carriers; congenital disorders; disclosure; empirical research; *family relationship; genetic counseling; genetic disorders; genetic information; *genetic screening; health insurance; insurance selection bias; late-onset disorders; *legal aspects; *mandatory testing; *mass screening; *newborns; *parents; privacy; psychological stress; public health; *public policy; reproduction; *risks and benefits; state government; *state interest; stigmatization; *voluntary programs; United States

Cohen, Cynthia B.; McCloskey, Elizabeth Leibold. Introduction [to a set of five articles and one commentary on genetic information]. *Kennedy Institute of Ethics Journal.* 1998 Jun; 8(2): vii-x. Introduction to articles by C.B. Cohen, R. Wachbroit, B.B. Biesecker, J.L. Nelson, and E.T. Juengst, and a commentary on Biesecker by S.M. Suter. BE58370.
> adults; children; decision making; directive counseling; *disclosure; *genetic counseling; *genetic information; genetic predisposition; genetic research; *genetic screening; informed consent; late-onset disorders; moral obligations; patients; prenatal diagnosis; risks and benefits; truth disclosure; vulnerable populations; population genetics

Cohen, Cynthia B. Wrestling with the future: should we test children for adult-onset genetic conditions? *Kennedy Institute of Ethics Journal.* 1998 Jun; 8(2): 111-130. 40 refs. BE58371.
> *adolescents; advance care planning; age factors; autonomy; beneficence; *children; competence; *decision making; family relationship; genetic counseling; *genetic screening; health insurance; health personnel; informed consent;

*late-onset disorders; moral policy; parental consent; *parents; policy analysis; prognosis; psychological stress; risk; *risks and benefits; social discrimination; stigmatization; time factors; uncertainty

Genetics professionals have been reluctant to test children for adult-onset conditions because they believe this would create psychosocial harm to children not counterbalanced by significant benefits. An additional concern they express is that such testing would violate the autonomy of these children as adults. Yet weighing the harms and benefits of such testing results in a draw, with no substantial harms proven. Moreover, such testing can enhance, rather than violate the adult autonomy of these children. In deciding whether to proceed with predictive testing of children, parents, mature children, and health care professionals should consider a complex of factors relevant to the particular child. The importance of these factors will vary depending on the condition at issue, the age and stage of development of the child, family dynamics, and the concerns, values, and objectives of the parents and mature child. The final decision whether to test a child for an adult-onset condition should rest with the parents and the mature child.

Cuschieri, Alfred. Screening for genetic diseases: what are the moral constraints? *In:* Agius, Emmanuel; Busuttil, Salvino, eds. Germ-Line Intervention and Our Responsibilities to Future Generations. Boston, MA: Kluwer Academic; 1998: 3-11. ISBN 0-7923-4828-1. BE57886.
> confidentiality; disclosure; eugenics; fetal therapy; *future generations; gene pool; gene therapy; genetic counseling; genetic disorders; genetic enhancement; genetic information; *genetic intervention; genetic research; *genetic screening; genome mapping; germ cells; late-onset disorders; mandatory testing; mass screening; moral obligations; preimplantation diagnosis; prenatal diagnosis; privacy; *risks and benefits; selective abortion; voluntary programs

Dankert-Roelse, Jeannette E.; te Meerman, Gerard J. Screening for cystic fibrosis -- time to change our position? [Editorial]. *New England Journal of Medicine.* 1997 Oct 2; 337(14): 997-999. 10 refs. BE56407.
> carriers; *costs and benefits; *cystic fibrosis; diagnosis; genetic counseling; *genetic screening; *mass screening; methods; *newborns; patient care; prognosis; public policy; reproduction; *risks and benefits; treatment outcome

Davis, Helen R.; Mitrius, Janice V. Recent legislation on genetics and insurance. [Note]. *Jurimetrics Journal.* 1996 Fall; 37(1): 69-82. 50 fn. BE57689.
> *confidentiality; *disclosure; family members; federal government; genetic disorders; *genetic information; genetic predisposition; *genetic screening; *government regulation; hospitals; informed consent; *insurance; insurance selection bias; *legislation; physicians; privacy; social discrimination; *state government; Americans with Disabilities Act 1990; Employment Retirement Income Security Act (ERISA) 1974; *United States

Deepandung, Attajinda; Noonpakdee, Wilai T. The moral status of the human genome. *In:* Agius, Emmanuel; Busuttil, Salvino, eds. Germ-Line Intervention and Our Responsibilities to Future Generations. Boston, MA: Kluwer Academic; 1998: 13-18. 9 refs. ISBN 0-7923-4828-1. BE57876.
> confidentiality; future generations; *gene therapy; genetic counseling; genetic information; genetic research; *genetic screening; *genome mapping; human experimentation; moral obligations; obligations of society; privacy; public policy; resource allocation; risks and benefits; Thailand

---

BE = bioethics accession number   fn. = footnotes   refs. = references

de Wachter, Maurice A.M. DNA sampling and duties to relatives -- looking back: European approaches. *In:* Knoppers, Bartha Maria, ed. Human DNA: Law and Policy: International and Comparative Perspectives. Proceedings of the First International Conference on DNA Sampling and Human Genetic Research: Ethical, Legal, and Policy Aspects, held in Montreal, Canada, 6–8 Sep 1996. Boston, MA: Kluwer Law International; 1997: 145–156. 30 fn. ISBN 90–411–0361–9. BE58174.
　　carriers; confidentiality; *disclosure; DNA data banks; *family members; family planning; genetic counseling; genetic disorders; *genetic information; genetic predisposition; *genetic screening; informed consent; international aspects; patients; psychological stress; *Europe

Dhondt, Jean–Louis; Farriaux, Jean–Pierre. Impact of French legislation on neonatal screening. *In:* Knoppers, Bartha Maria, ed. Human DNA: Law and Policy: International and Comparative Perspectives. Proceedings of the First International Conference on DNA Sampling and Human Genetic Research: Ethical, Legal, and Policy Aspects, held in Montreal, Canada, 6–8 Sep 1996. Boston, MA: Kluwer Law International; 1997: 285–289. 5 fn. ISBN 90–411–0361–9. BE58185.
　　costs and benefits; disclosure; DNA data banks; genetic disorders; genetic research; *genetic screening; guidelines; *legal aspects; legislation; *mass screening; *newborns; parental consent; professional organizations; biological specimen banks; Association for Neonatal Screening (France); *France

Dickens, Bernard M. Choices, control, access -- the Canadian position. *In:* Knoppers, Bartha Maria, ed. Human DNA: Law and Policy: International and Comparative Perspectives. Proceedings of the First International Conference on DNA Sampling and Human Genetic Research: Ethical, Legal, and Policy Aspects, held in Montreal, Canada, 6–8 Sep 1996. Boston, MA: Kluwer Law International; 1997: 71–89. 59 fn. ISBN 90–411–0361–9. BE58169.
　　*confidentiality; criminal law; *disclosure; *DNA data banks; DNA fingerprinting; employment; federal government; *genetic information; *genetic materials; *genetic research; *genetic screening; government regulation; health personnel; *informed consent; law enforcement; *legal aspects; legislation; mandatory testing; privacy; private sector; public sector; state government; tissue donation; *biological specimen banks; *Canada; *Privacy Act 1983 (Canada); Quebec

Dickson, David. Physicians prepare guidelines on use of human genome data. [News]. *Nature.* 1995 Sep 28; 377(6547): 279. BE56109.
　　genetic predisposition; *genetic screening; genome mapping; *guidelines; *international aspects; *organizational policies; physicians; professional organizations; *World Medical Association

Doherty, Peter; Sutton, Agneta, eds. Man–Made Man: Ethical and Legal Issues in Genetics. Dublin, Ireland: Open Air; 1997. 116 p. Includes references. ISBN 1–85182–278–X. BE58293.
　　autonomy; children; confidentiality; disabled; embryos; eugenics; fetuses; *gene therapy; genetic counseling; genetic determinism; *genetic intervention; genetic predisposition; genetic research; *genetic screening; genetics; genome mapping; informed consent; international aspects; personhood; preimplantation diagnosis; prenatal diagnosis; public policy; regulation; reproduction; rights; risks and benefits; selective abortion; social control; social discrimination; trends; values; Europe; Great Britain

Donahue, James. Patenting of human DNA sequences -- implications for prenatal genetic testing. [Note]. *Journal*

of Family Law. 1997–1998 Spring; 36(2): 267–283. 127 fn. BE58773.
　　*DNA sequences; eugenics; genetic counseling; genetic predisposition; genetic research; *genetic screening; genome mapping; indigents; industry; *legal aspects; negligence; *patents; physicians; *prenatal diagnosis; selective abortion; social impact; wrongful life; Patent and Trademark Office; *United States

Draper, Elaine Alma. Social issues of genome innovation and intellectual property. *Risk: Health, Safety and Environment.* 1996 Summer; 7(3): 201–229. 37 fn. BE55934.
　　coercion; confidentiality; data banks; DNA data banks; drug abuse; *employment; females; genetic disorders; *genetic information; genetic predisposition; genetic research; *genetic screening; genome mapping; health hazards; industry; insurance; legislation; medical records; minority groups; occupational exposure; preconception injuries; prenatal injuries; privacy; *social discrimination; Americans with Disabilities Act 1990; United States

DudokdeWit, A.C.; Tibben, A.; Duivenvoorden, H.J., et al. Psychological distress in applicants for predictive DNA testing for autosomal dominant, heritable, late onset disorders. [For the Rotterdam/Leiden Genetics Workgroup]. *Journal of Medical Genetics.* 1997 May; 34(5): 382–390. 61 refs. BE56001.
　　attitudes; *brain pathology; breast cancer; *cancer; comparative studies; decision making; emotions; family members; genetic counseling; *genetic predisposition; *genetic screening; Huntington's disease; *late–onset disorders; motivation; patients; *psychological stress; risk; stigmatization; Netherlands

Durfy, Sharon J.; Page, Andrea; Eng, Barry, et al. Attitudes of high school students toward carrier screening and prenatal diagnosis of cystic fibrosis. *Journal of Genetic Counseling.* 1994 Jun; 3(2): 141–155. 23 refs. BE57379.
　　*adolescents; *attitudes; *carriers; *cystic fibrosis; disclosure; females; *genetic screening; males; *mass screening; *prenatal diagnosis; reproduction; self concept; social discrimination; *students; survey; uncertainty; voluntary programs; NCHGR–funded publication; *secondary schools; Ontario

Eng, Christine M.; Schechter, Clyde; Robinowitz, Jane, et al. Prenatal genetic carrier testing using triple disease screening. *JAMA.* 1997 Oct 15; 278(15): 1268–1272. 30 refs. BE56056.
　　*carriers; *cystic fibrosis; decision making; disclosure; evaluation studies; females; *genetic counseling; genetic disorders; *genetic screening; informed consent; Jews; *knowledge, attitudes, practice; males; married persons; patient education; pregnant women; prenatal diagnosis; privacy; prognosis; program descriptions; selective abortion; *Tay Sachs disease; *Gaucher's disease; NCHGR–funded publication; severity of illness index; Mount Sinai Medical Center (New York City); United States
　　CONTEXT: Rapid progress in gene discovery has dramatically increased diagnostic capabilities for carrier screening and prenatal testing for genetic diseases. However, simultaneous prenatal carrier screening for prevalent genetic disease has not been evaluated, and patient acceptance and attitudes toward this testing strategy remain undefined. OBJECTIVE: To evaluate an educational, counseling, and carrier testing program for 3 genetic disorders: Tay–Sachs disease (TSD), type 1 Gaucher disease (GD), and cystic fibrosis (CF) that differ in detectability, severity, and availability of therapy. DESIGN: Potential participants received education and genetic counseling, gave informed consent, chose screening tests, and completed

---

BE = bioethics accession number　　　　fn. = footnotes　　　　refs. = references

pre-education and posteducation questionnaires that assessed knowledge, attitudes toward genetic testing, and disease testing preferences. SETTING: Medical genetics referral center. PATIENTS: Volunteer sample of 2824 Ashkenazi Jewish individuals enrolled as couples who were referred for TSD testing. INTERVENTION: Genetic counseling, education, and if chosen, genetic testing for any or all 3 disorders. MAIN OUTCOME MEASURE: Acceptance of screening for each of the 3 disorders. Secondary outcomes include attitudes toward genetic testing and reproductive considerations. RESULTS: Of the 2824 individuals tested for TSD, 97% and 95% also chose testing for CF and GD, respectively. The frequency of detected carriers was 1:21 for TSD, 1:25 for CF, and 1:18 for GD. Twenty-one carriercoupleswere identified, counseled, and all postconception couples opted for prenatal diagnosis. Pre-education and posteducation questionnaires revealed that patients initially knew little about the diseases, but acquired disease information and increased knowledge of genetic concepts. Education and genetic counseling increased understanding and retention of genetic concepts and disease-related information, and minimized test-related anxiety. Although individuals sought screening for all 3 diseases, reproductive attitudes and decisions varied directly with disease severity and treatability. CONCLUSIONS: These findings emphasize the importance of genetic counseling for prenatal carrier testing and may improve understanding, acceptance, and informed decision making for prenatal carrier screening for multiple genetic diseases.

Fanos, Joanna H.; Johnson, John P. Barriers to carrier testing for adult cystic fibrosis sibs: the importance of not knowing. *American Journal of Medical Genetics.* 1995 Oct 23; 59(1): 85–91. 50 refs. ELSI: R01 HG00639; NIH/CFSC BE58000.

    *adults; *carriers; communication; *cystic fibrosis; family relationship; females; genetic counseling; *genetic screening; insurance; *knowledge, attitudes, practice; males; married persons; motivation; parents; psychology; reproduction; selective abortion; *siblings; value of life; ELSI–funded publication; California

Fishman, Rachelle H.B. Jerusalem: flourishing legal environment nurtures protected genetic inquiry. [News]. *Lancet.* 1998 Jun 27; 351(9120): 1939. BE58496.

    breast cancer; confidentiality; disclosure; economics; *genetic research; *genetic screening; informed consent; international aspects; Jews; legal aspects; *Israel

Galton, David J.; Galton, Clare J. Francis Galton and eugenics today. *Journal of Medical Ethics.* 1998 Apr; 24(2): 99–105. 25 refs. BE58077.

    employment; *eugenics; evolution; gene therapy; genetic disorders; genetic enhancement; genetic intervention; *genetic predisposition; *genetic screening; genome mapping; germ cells; government regulation; *historical aspects; insurance selection bias; international aspects; mentally disabled; prenatal diagnosis; public policy; reproduction; risk; selective abortion; *social discrimination; social worth; socioeconomic factors; sterilization (sexual); values; virtues; pedigree studies; Darwin, Charles; *Galton, Francis; Germany; *Great Britain; *Nineteenth Century; *Twentieth Century; United States

Eugenics can be defined as the use of science applied to the qualitative and quantitative improvement of the human genome. The subject was initiated by Francis Galton with considerable support from Charles Darwin in the latter half of the 19th century. Its scope has increased enormously since the recent revolution in molecular genetics. Genetic files can be easily obtained for individuals either antenatally or at birth; somatic gene therapy has been introduced for some rare inborn errors of metabolism; and gene manipulation of human germ-line cells will no doubt occur in the near future to generate organs for transplantation. The past history of eugenics has been appalling, with gross abuses in the USA between 1931 and 1945 when compulsory sterilization was practised; and in Germany between 1933 and 1945 when mass extermination and compulsory sterilization were performed. To prevent such abuses in the future statutory bodies, such as a genetics commission, should be established to provide guidance and rules of conduct for use of the new information and technologies as applied to the human genome.

Geller, Gail; Botkin, Jeffrey R.; Green, Michael J., et al. Genetic testing for susceptibility to adult-onset cancer: the process and content of informed consent. *JAMA.* 1997 May 14; 277(18): 1467–1474. 122 refs. BE55859.

    adults; advisory committees; alternatives; audiovisual aids; *cancer; communication; comprehension; confidentiality; consent forms; decision making; *disclosure; DNA data banks; employment; *genetic counseling; genetic information; *genetic predisposition; *genetic screening; *guidelines; information dissemination; *informed consent; insurance; *late–onset disorders; minority groups; *patient education; privacy; professional patient relationship; psychology; *public policy; risks and benefits; social discrimination; teaching methods; time factors; NHGRI–funded publication; Cancer Genetics Studies Consortium; *Task Force on Informed Consent

OBJECTIVE: To provide guidance on informed consent to clinicians offering cancer susceptibility testing. PARTICIPANTS: The Task Force on Informed Consent is part of the Cancer Genetics Studies Consortium (CGSC), whose members were recipients of National Institutes of Health grants to assess the implications of cancer susceptibility testing. The 10 task force members represent a range of relevant backgrounds, including various medical specialties, social science, genetic counseling, and consumer advocacy. EVIDENCE: The CGSC held 3 public meetings from 1994 to 1996. At its first meeting, the task force jointly established a list of topics. The cochairs (G.G. and J.R.B) then developed an outline and assigned each topic to an appropriate writer and reviewer. Writers summarized the literature on their topics and drafted recommendations, which were then revised by the reviewers. The cochairs compiled and edited the entire manuscript. All members were involved in writing this report. CONSENSUS PROCESS: The first draft was distributed to task force members, after which a meeting was held to discuss its content and organization. Consensus was reached by voting. A subsequent draft was presented to the entire CGSC at its third meeting, and comments were incorporated. CONCLUSIONS: The task force recommends that informed consent for cancer susceptibility testing be an ongoing process of education and counseling in which (1) providers elicit participant, family, and community values and disclose their own, (2) decision making is shared, (3) the style of information disclosure is individualized, and (4) specific content areas are discussed.

Gevers, Sjef; Olsthoorn-Heim, Els. DNA sampling: Dutch and other European approaches to the issues of informed consent and confidentiality. *In:* Knoppers, Bartha Maria, ed. Human DNA: Law and Policy: International and Comparative Perspectives. Proceedings of the First International Conference on DNA Sampling and Human Genetic Research: Ethical,

---

BE = bioethics accession number   fn. = footnotes   refs. = references

Legal, and Policy Aspects, held in Montreal, Canada, 6–8 Sep 1996. Boston, MA: Kluwer Law International; 1997: 109–120. 18 fn. ISBN 90–411–0361–9. BE58171.
advisory committees; *confidentiality; *DNA data banks; *genetic information; *genetic materials; genetic research; *genetic screening; government regulation; guidelines; *informed consent; *international aspects; privacy; *public policy; *regulation; *tissue donation; *biological specimen banks; Council of Europe; *Europe; National Ethics Advisory Committee (France); *Netherlands; Nuffield Council on Bioethics

Glannon, Walter. Genes, embryos, and future people. *Bioethics.* 1998 Jul; 12(3): 187–211. 36 fn. BE58893.
beginning of life; *beneficence; children; *cryopreservation; *embryo disposition; *embryos; *eugenics; fetal therapy; fetuses; future generations; *gene therapy; *genetic disorders; genetic enhancement; *genetic intervention; *genetic screening; germ cells; *injuries; justice; late–onset disorders; mentally disabled; *moral obligations; *moral policy; pain; parents; personhood; physically disabled; posthumous reproduction; *preimplantation diagnosis; *quality of life; reproduction; reproductive technologies; risks and benefits; self concept; suffering; time factors; value of life; *wrongful life
Testing embryonic cells for genetic abnormalities gives us the capacity to predict whether and to what extent people will exist with disease and disability. Moreover, the freezing of embryos for long periods of time enables us to alter the length of a normal human lifespan. After highlighting the shortcomings of somatic–cell gene therapy and germ–line genetic alteration, I argue that the testing and selective termination of genetically defective embryos is the only medically and morally defensible way to prevent the existence of people with severe disability, pain and suffering that make their lives not worth living for them on the whole. In addition, I consider the possible harmful effects on children born from frozen embryos after the deaths of their biological parents, or when their parents are at an advanced age. I also explore whether embryos have moral status and whether the prospects for disease-preventing genetic alteration can justify long-term cryopreservation of embryos.

Glass, Kathleen Cranley. Challenging the paradigm: stored tissue samples and access to genetic information. *In:* Knoppers, Bartha Maria, ed. Human DNA: Law and Policy: International and Comparative Perspectives. Proceedings of the First International Conference on DNA Sampling and Human Genetic Research: Ethical, Legal, and Policy Aspects, held in Montreal, Canada, 6–8 Sep 1996. Boston, MA: Kluwer Law International; 1997: 157–162. 16 fn. ISBN 90–411–0361–9. BE58175.
confidentiality; *disclosure; *DNA data banks; family members; *genetic information; *genetic materials; genetic predisposition; genetic research; *genetic screening; informed consent; international aspects; regulation; tissue donation; *biological specimen banks; Canada; Europe; United States

Godard, Béatrice; Kinsella, T. Douglas. DNA sampling and banking: practices and procedures. *In:* Knoppers, Bartha Maria, ed. Human DNA: Law and Policy: International and Comparative Perspectives. Proceedings of the First International Conference on DNA Sampling and Human Genetic Research: Ethical, Legal, and Policy Aspects, held in Montreal, Canada, 6–8 Sep 1996. Boston, MA: Kluwer Law International; 1997: 429–434. ISBN 90–411–0361–9. BE58199.
confidentiality; *DNA data banks; DNA fingerprinting; donors; genetic information; genetic materials; genetic research; genetic screening; informed consent; institutional

policies; international aspects; law enforcement; tissue donation; *biological specimen banks; Canada; Europe; United States

Golub, Edward S. Ethical considerations arising from economic aspects of human genetics. *In:* Becker, Gerhold K., ed. Changing Nature's Course: The Ethical Challenge of Biotechnology. Hong Kong: Hong Kong University Press; 1996: 71–83. 21 refs. 21 fn. ISBN 962–209–403–1. BE56706.
behavioral genetics; biomedical technologies; disease; drug industry; drugs; *economics; genetic disorders; genetic predisposition; *genetic screening; genome mapping; government financing; kidney diseases; legal aspects; organ transplantation; renal dialysis; science; End Stage Renal Disease Program; Great Britain; United States

Grandjean, P. Ethical aspects of genetic predisposition to disease. *In:* Grandjean, Phillippe, ed. Ecogenetics: Genetic Predisposition to the Toxic Effects of Chemicals. New York, NY: Chapman and Hall on behalf of the World Health Organization, Regional Office for Europe; 1991: 237–251. 18 refs. BE57646.
confidentiality; costs and benefits; disabled; *employment; freedom; *genetic predisposition; *genetic screening; *health hazards; justice; moral policy; *occupational exposure; paternalism; privacy; rights; risks and benefits; social discrimination; utilitarianism

Green, Ronald M.; Thomas, A. Mathew. Whose gene is it? A case discussion about familial conflict over genetic testing for breast cancer. *Journal of Genetic Counseling.* 1997 Jun; 6(2): 245–254. 14 refs. BE55669.
*breast cancer; case studies; confidentiality; death; decision making; *disclosure; *dissent; DNA data banks; *family members; family relationship; females; genetic counseling; genetic disorders; *genetic information; *genetic predisposition; genetic research; *genetic screening; mothers; property rights; risks and benefits; *siblings; *twins; uncertainty

Harper, Peter S.; Clarke, Angus J. Genetics, Society, and Clinical Practice. Herndon, VA: BIOS Scientific Publishers; 1997. 253 p. 564 refs. ISBN 1-85996-206-8. BE59033.
carriers; children; confidentiality; cystic fibrosis; decision making; directive counseling; Down syndrome; economics; eugenics; family members; *genetic counseling; genetic disorders; genetic diversity; genetic information; genetic predisposition; genetic research; *genetic screening; *genetic services; goals; health care delivery; Huntington's disease; informed consent; insurance; intelligence; late–onset disorders; mass screening; newborns; prenatal diagnosis; privacy; public health; public policy; registries; reproduction; selective abortion; social discrimination; terminology; population genetics; China; Great Britain

Hartley, N.E.; Scotcher, D.; Harris, H., et al. The uptake and acceptability to patients of cystic fibrosis carrier testing offered in pregnancy by the GP. *Journal of Medical Genetics.* 1997 Jun; 34(6): 459–464. 16 refs. BE56153.
*attitudes; *carriers; *cystic fibrosis; *decision making; disclosure; *genetic screening; informed consent; mass screening; motivation; *patient satisfaction; physicians; *pregnant women; psychological stress; survey; truth disclosure; Great Britain

Healy, Bernadine. BRCA genes -- bookmaking, fortunetelling, and medical care. [Editorial]. *New England Journal of Medicine.* 1997 May 15; 336(20): 1448–1449. 12 refs. BE55909.
*breast cancer; females; *genetic predisposition; *genetic screening; preventive medicine; *risk; risks and benefits;

BE = bioethics accession number   fn. = footnotes   refs. = references

surgery; ovarian cancer

Hedgecoe, Adam. Genetic Catch–22: testing, risk and private health insurance. *Business and Professional Ethics Journal.* 1996 Summer; 15(2): 69–86. 26 refs. 4 fn. BE58570.
> carriers; employment; genetic determinism; genetic disorders; genetic information; genetic predisposition; *genetic screening; health care delivery; *health insurance; industry; *insurance; *insurance selection bias; *justice; national health insurance; *risk; social discrimination; United States

Heimler, Audrey; Zanko, Andrea. Huntington disease: a case study describing the complexities and nuances of predictive testing of monozygotic twins. *Journal of Genetic Counseling.* 1995 Jun; 4(2): 125–137. 13 refs. 1 fn. BE56031.
> adults; autonomy; case studies; communication; confidentiality; disclosure; DNA data banks; family members; *genetic counseling; *genetic screening; *Huntington's disease; informed consent; late–onset disorders; psychological stress; *twins; geographic factors; United States

Henn, Wolfram. Predictive diagnosis and genetic screening: manipulation of fate? *Perspectives in Biology and Medicine.* 1998 Winter; 41(2): 282–289. 18 refs. BE59009.
> carriers; diagnosis; directive counseling; eugenics; family members; *genetic counseling; genetic disorders; genetic predisposition; *genetic screening; insurance; late–onset disorders; motivation; preventive medicine; *risks and benefits; uncertainty; right not to know

Hirtle, Marie. Genetic screening and research revisited. *In:* Knoppers, Bartha Maria, ed. Human DNA: Law and Policy: International and Comparative Perspectives. Proceedings of the First International Conference on DNA Sampling and Human Genetic Research: Ethical, Legal, and Policy Aspects, held in Montreal, Canada, 6–8 Sep 1996. Boston, MA: Kluwer Law International; 1997: 333–340. 7 fn. ISBN 90–411–0361–9. BE58190.
> cancer; *carriers; cystic fibrosis; DNA data banks; federal government; genetic materials; *genetic research; *genetic screening; *informed consent; legal aspects; *newborns; *parental consent; prenatal diagnosis; presumed consent; thalassemia; biological specimen banks; Europe; National Center for Human Genome Research; United States

Holmes–Farley, S. Rebecca. CRG files amicus brief in workplace privacy and discrimination case. [News]. *GeneWATCH.* 1997 Feb; 10(4–5): 1, 4. 1 fn. BE58492.
> blacks; confidentiality; constitutional law; *deception; *employment; females; *genetic screening; informed consent; *legal aspects; males; mandatory programs; occupational medicine; privacy; social discrimination; California; *Council for Responsible Genetics; *Lawrence Berkeley National Laboratory

Holtzman, Neil A.; Murphy, Patricia D.; Watson, Michael S., et al. Predictive genetic testing: from basic research to clinical practice. *Science.* 1997 Oct 24; 278(5338): 602–605. 26 fn. BE57334.
> advisory committees; confidentiality; DNA data banks; *evaluation; federal government; genetic disorders; *genetic predisposition; genetic research; *genetic screening; *genetic services; goals; government regulation; industry; informed consent; investigators; public policy; research ethics committees; risks and benefits; self regulation; uncertainty; diagnostic kits; NHGRI–funded publication; Department of Health and Human Services; *Task Force on Genetic Testing; United States

Holtzman, Neil A.; Shapiro, David. The new genetics: genetic testing and public policy. *BMJ (British Medical Journal).* 1998 Mar 14; 316(7134): 852–856. 46 refs. BE57754.
> advisory committees; comparative studies; confidentiality; cystic fibrosis; disclosure; Duchenne muscular dystrophy; duty to warn; employment; family members; genetic counseling; genetic disorders; genetic information; genetic predisposition; *genetic screening; health insurance; Huntington's disease; informed consent; insurance selection bias; *international aspects; *laboratories; legal aspects; life insurance; medical records; prenatal diagnosis; *privacy; private sector; psychological stress; *public policy; risk; *risks and benefits; selective abortion; *social discrimination; diagnostic kits; *quality assurance; *quality control; Advisory Committee on Genetic Testing (Great Britain); British Insurers Code of Practice; *Great Britain; Health Insurance Portability and Accountability Act 1996; Human Genetics Advisory Commission (Great Britain); National Health Service; Task Force on Genetic Testing; *United States

Hook, C. Christopher. Genetic testing and confidentiality. *In:* Kilner, John F.; Pentz, Rebecca D.; Young, Frank E., eds. Genetic Ethics: Do the Ends Justify the Genes? Grand Rapids, MI: W.B. Eerdmans; 1997: 124–135. 28 fn. ISBN 0–8028–4428–6. BE56720.
> carriers; children; *Christian ethics; *confidentiality; *disclosure; employment; family members; genetic counseling; genetic disorders; *genetic information; genetic predisposition; *genetic screening; informed consent; insurance; legislation; medical records; preimplantation diagnosis; prenatal diagnosis; psychological stress; reproduction; risk; *risks and benefits; selective abortion; social discrimination; state government; United States

Jacobs, R. Genetic screening –– uses, potential abuses and ethical issues. *Occupational Medicine.* 1997 Aug; 47(6): 367–370. 7 refs. BE59006.
> advisory committees; *employment; genetic counseling; *genetic predisposition; *genetic screening; health hazards; informed consent; legal aspects; mass screening; occupational exposure; public policy; social discrimination; *Great Britain

Jan, Sheau–Wen; Chen, Chih–Ping; Huang, Lian–Hua, et al. Attitudes toward maternal serum screening in Chinese women with positive results. *Journal of Genetic Counseling.* 1996 Dec; 5(4): 169–180. 33 refs. BE56329.
> amniocentesis; *attitudes; decision making; *Down syndrome; females; *genetic counseling; *genetic screening; knowledge, attitudes, practice; *pregnant women; *prenatal diagnosis; survey; *alpha fetoproteins; *Taiwan

Jayaraman, K.S. Indian guidelines allow limited gene screening. [News]. *Nature.* 1998 Jan 8; 391(6663): 115. BE58057.
> aborted fetuses; disclosure; embryo research; employment; family members; fetal tissue donation; genetic research; *genetic screening; government regulation; *guidelines; international aspects; life insurance; prenatal diagnosis; *India; *Indian Council of Medical Research

Juengst, Eric T. Ethics of prediction: genetic risk and the physician–patient relationship. *Genome Science and Technology.* 1995; 1(1): 21–36. 72 refs. BE57993.
> autonomy; carriers; confidentiality; decision making; directive counseling; disabled; disclosure; DNA data banks; duty to warn; eugenics; family members; fathers; *genetic counseling; genetic determinism; *genetic disorders; genetic identity; *genetic information; genetic materials; *genetic predisposition; genetic research; *genetic screening; genetic services; genome mapping; health insurance; informed consent; late–onset disorders; medical ethics; minors; parent child relationship; parents; prenatal diagnosis; property

---

BE = bioethics accession number   fn. = footnotes   refs. = references

rights; public policy; reproduction; *risk; *risks and benefits; sex determination; social discrimination; stigmatization; tissue banks; uncertainty; ELSI-funded publication; National Center for Human Genome Research; Office for Protection from Research Risks; United States

Kääriäinen, Helena. Genetic studies in populations. *In:* Knoppers, Bartha Maria, ed. Human DNA: Law and Policy: International and Comparative Perspectives. Proceedings of the First International Conference on DNA Sampling and Human Genetic Research: Ethical, Legal, and Policy Aspects, held in Montreal, Canada, 6–8 Sep 1996. Boston, MA: Kluwer Law International; 1997: 177–188. 9 fn. ISBN 90–411–0361–9. BE58177.
  cancer; DNA data banks; family members; *genetic predisposition; *genetic research; *genetic screening; human experimentation; *informed consent; mass screening; patients; asthma; biological specimen banks; *population genetics; *Finland

Kadlec, Josef V.; McPherson, Richard A. Ethical issues in screening and testing for genetic diseases. *Clinics in Laboratory Medicine.* 1995 Dec; 15(4): 989–999. 3 refs. BE55564.
  cancer; coercion; confidentiality; dementia; disclosure; family members; financial support; genetic counseling; genetic disorders; genetic information; genetic predisposition; *genetic screening; heart diseases; obligations of society; privacy; risks and benefits; social discrimination

Kahn, Mary Jo Ellis; Jamison, Kay Redfield; Collins, Francis S. Protecting our 'family secrets'. *Washington Post.* 1997 Jul 31: A15. BE55546.
  employment; family members; federal government; *genetic information; genetic predisposition; *genetic research; *genetic screening; government regulation; *health insurance; insurance selection bias; legislation; preventive medicine; *risks and benefits; social discrimination; state government; United States

Kapp, Marshall B. Medicolegal, employment, and insurance issues in APOE genotyping and Alzheimer's disease. *Annals of the New York Academy of Sciences.* 1996 Dec 16; 802: 139–148. 22 refs. BE57911.
  competence; confidentiality; *dementia; disclosure; *employment; genetic information; genetic research; *genetic screening; government regulation; health personnel; informed consent; *insurance; *legal aspects; legal obligations; risks and benefits; social discrimination; standards; United States

Kass, Nancy E. The implications of genetic testing for health and life insurance. *In:* Rothstein, Mark A., ed. Genetic Secrets: Protecting Privacy and Confidentiality in the Genetic Era. New Haven, CT: Yale University Press; 1997: 299–316. 46 fn. ISBN 0–300–07251–1. BE58688.
  employment; *genetic information; genetic predisposition; genetic research; *genetic screening; *health insurance; international aspects; *legal aspects; legal rights; *life insurance; medical records; records; risk; social discrimination; Americans with Disabilities Act 1990; Employee Retirement Income Security Act 1974 (ERISA); Health Insurance Portability and Accountability Act 1996; United States

King, David. Is knowledge always good? *GenEthics News.* 1996 May–Jun; No. 12: 6–7. BE56331.
  adults; attitudes; autonomy; children; decision making; federal government; genetic counseling; genetic disorders; *genetic information; genetic predisposition; *genetic screening; genetic services; government regulation; health personnel; industry; international aspects; parents; paternalism; prenatal diagnosis; public opinion; rights; Great

Britain; United States

Kirk, Maggie. Commercial gene testing: the need for professional and public debate. *British Journal of Nursing.* 1997 Oct 9–22; 6(18): 1043–1047. 22 refs. BE58255.
  carriers; cystic fibrosis; genetic counseling; genetic predisposition; *genetic screening; *genetic services; industry; informed consent; mass screening; nurses; *risks and benefits; uncertainty; *diagnostic kits; *Great Britain

Knoppers, Bartha Maria, ed. Human DNA: Law and Policy: International and Comparative Perspectives. Proceedings of the First International Conference on DNA Sampling and Human Genetic Research: Ethical, Legal, and Policy Aspects, held in Montreal, Canada, 6–8 Sep 1996. Boston, MA: Kluwer Law International; 1997. 455 p. 898 fn. ISBN 90–411–0361–9. BE58163.
  body parts and fluids; carriers; confidentiality; disclosure; *DNA data banks; DNA fingerprinting; DNA sequences; epidemiology; *genetic diversity; genetic information; genetic intervention; *genetic materials; *genetic research; *genetic screening; genome mapping; government regulation; guidelines; incentives; industry; informed consent; *international aspects; legal aspects; mass screening; minority groups; newborns; patents; prenatal diagnosis; property rights; *public policy; registries; review; tissue donation; *biological specimen banks; population genetics; recontact; Canada; Europe; Human Genome Diversity Project; Human Genome Project; United States

Kodish, Eric; Wiesner, Georgia L.; Mehlman, Maxwell, et al. Genetic testing for cancer risk: how to reconcile the conflicts. *JAMA.* 1998 Jan 21; 279(3): 179–181. 26 refs. BE57811.
  *breast cancer; *cancer; decision making; dissent; federal government; genetic counseling; *genetic predisposition; genetic research; *genetic screening; guidelines; informed consent; mass screening; *organizational policies; patient advocacy; *practice guidelines; professional organizations; public policy; risk; *risks and benefits; American Society of Clinical Oncology; National Advisory Council for Human Genome Research; National Breast Cancer Coalition; United States

Koh, D.; Jeyaratnam, J. Biomarkers, screening and ethics. *Occupational Medicine.* 1998 Jan; 48(1): 27–30. 10 refs. BE59077.
  *employment; *genetic predisposition; *genetic screening; guidelines; *health hazards; informed consent; medical ethics; *occupational exposure; *occupational medicine; preventive medicine; social discrimination

Kolata, Gina. Genetic testing falls short of public embrace. [News]. *New York Times.* 1998 Mar 27: A16. BE57727.
  attitudes; breast cancer; cancer; employment; genetic information; genetic predisposition; *genetic screening; genetic services; health insurance; industry; preventive medicine; psychological stress; social discrimination; colon cancer; United States

Lebacqz, Karen. Genetic privacy: no deal for the poor. *In:* Peters, Ted, ed. Genetics: Issues of Social Justice. Cleveland, OH: Pilgrim Press; 1998: 239–254. 60 fn. Reprinted from *Dialog,* Winter 1994, 33:1, 39–48. ISBN 0–8298–1251–2. BE57482.
  computers; *confidentiality; directive counseling; *disadvantaged; disclosure; employment; genetic counseling; *genetic information; genetic predisposition; *genetic screening; *health insurance; indigents; informed consent; insurance selection bias; justice; medical records; minority groups; prenatal diagnosis; *privacy; risk; selective abortion; *social discrimination; socioeconomic factors; truth disclosure; United States

---

BE = bioethics accession number   fn. = footnotes   refs. = references

Lehrman, Sally. Genetic testing for Alzheimer's disease 'not appropriate.' [News]. *Nature.* 1997 Oct 30; 389(6654): 898. BE56168.
advisory committees; *dementia; diagnosis; disclosure; economics; genetic predisposition; *genetic screening; psychological stress; public policy; risks and benefits; Program in Genomics, Ethics and Society (Stanford University); United States

Lippman, Abby. The politics of health: geneticization versus health promotion. *In:* Sherwin, Susan, et al. The Politics of Women's Health: Exploring Agency and Autonomy. Philadelphia, PA: Temple University Press; 1998: 64–82. 30 fn. ISBN 1-56639-633-6. BE58394.
accountability; behavioral genetics; ecology; *females; *feminist ethics; *genetic determinism; genetic diversity; *genetic predisposition; *genetic screening; genetics; health; *health promotion; normality; obligations of society; *politics; prenatal diagnosis; public policy; self induced illness; social control; social discrimination; socioeconomic factors; stigmatization; *women's health; Canada

Lock, Margaret. Perfecting society: reproductive technologies, genetic testing, and the planned family in Japan. *In:* Lock, Margaret; Kaufert, Patricia A., eds. Pragmatic Women and Body Politics. New York, NY: Cambridge University Press; 1998: 206–239. 57 refs. ISBN 0-521-62929-2. BE58695.
abortion, induced; adoption; anthropology; *attitudes; autonomy; coercion; contraception; disabled; eugenics; family planning; family relationship; *females; feminist ethics; genetic disorders; *genetic screening; historical aspects; infanticide; married persons; paternalism; prenatal diagnosis; religion; *reproduction; *reproductive technologies; selective abortion; self concept; sex determination; single persons; social discrimination; *social dominance; social impact; stigmatization; women's rights; non-Western World; *Japan

Lucassen, Emy. Prenatal genetic testing: the need for legislation. *In:* Doherty, Peter; Sutton, Agneta, eds. Man-Made Man: Ethical and Legal Issues in Genetics. Dublin, Ireland: Open Air; 1997: 98–112. 23 refs. ISBN 1-85182-278-X. BE58299.
amniocentesis; chorionic villi sampling; competence; disclosure; fetuses; genetic disorders; *genetic screening; government regulation; informed consent; *legal aspects; legal liability; physicians; pregnant women; *prenatal diagnosis; risks and benefits; selective abortion; torts; wrongful life; *Great Britain

McKinnon, Wendy C.; Baty, Bonnie J.; Bennett, Robin L., et al. Predisposition genetic testing for late-onset disorders in adults: a position paper of the National Society of Genetic Counselors. [Policy statement]. *JAMA.* 1997 Oct 15; 278(15): 1217–1220. 58 refs. BE56054.
*adults; confidentiality; disclosure; *genetic counseling; genetic information; genetic materials; *genetic predisposition; *genetic screening; *guidelines; informed consent; laboratories; *late-onset disorders; *organizational policies; patient education; professional organizations; risks and benefits; social discrimination; uncertainty; NCHGR-funded publication; *National Society of Genetic Counselors; United States

Marteau, Theresa M.; Croyle, Robert T. The new genetics: psychological responses to genetic testing. *BMJ (British Medical Journal).* 1998 Feb 28; 316(7132): 693–696. 34 refs. BE57756.
breast cancer; carriers; cystic fibrosis; family members; females; *genetic counseling; genetic disorders; genetic predisposition; *genetic screening; Huntington's disease; late-onset disorders; males; patient care; prenatal diagnosis;

preventive medicine; *psychological stress; risk; selective abortion; social impact; uncertainty; Great Britain

Masood, Ehsan. UK insurers oppose moratorium plea on use of genetic data. [News]. *Nature.* 1998 Jan 1; 391(6662): 3. BE58061.
advisory committees; confidentiality; *disclosure; *genetic information; *genetic screening; *industry; *life insurance; *organizational policies; public policy; *Association of British Insurers; *Great Britain; Human Genetics Advisory Commission (Great Britain)

Michie, Susan; McDonald, Valerie; Bobrow, Martin, et al. Parents' responses to predictive genetic testing in their children: report of a single case study. *Journal of Medical Genetics.* 1996 Apr; 33(4): 313–318. 14 refs. BE56007.
age factors; *attitudes; autonomy; case studies; *children; confidentiality; *decision making; emotions; genetic counseling; *genetic predisposition; *genetic screening; health personnel; *late-onset disorders; motivation; parent child relationship; *parents; preventive medicine; risk; truth disclosure; professional role; Great Britain

Miller, Hugh. DNA blueprints, personhood, and genetic privacy. *Health Matrix.* 1998 Summer; 8(2): 179–221. 105 fn. BE58953.
*autonomy; confidentiality; constitutional law; disclosure; *genetic determinism; *genetic identity; *genetic information; genetic research; genetic screening; legal aspects; *legal rights; *personhood; philosophy; *privacy; *personal identity; United States

Mosenkis, Ari. Genetic screening for breast cancer susceptibility: a Torah perspective. *Journal of Halacha and Contemporary Society.* 1997 Fall; No. 34: 5–26. 66 fn. BE57176.
adolescents; age factors; *breast cancer; carriers; confidentiality; disclosure; employment; females; genetic information; *genetic predisposition; *genetic screening; insurance; *Jewish ethics; *Jews; *mass screening; moral obligations; prevalence; preventive medicine; *psychological stress; reproduction; risk; *risks and benefits; self concept; single persons; social discrimination; stigmatization; Tay Sachs disease; uncertainty; Orthodox Judaism

Murray, Thomas H. Genetic exceptionalism and "future diaries": is genetic information different from other medical information? *In:* Rothstein, Mark A., ed. Genetic Secrets: Protecting Privacy and Confidentiality in the Genetic Era. New Haven, CT: Yale University Press; 1997: 60–73. 20 fn. ISBN 0-300-07251-1. BE58675.
confidentiality; DNA data banks; DNA fingerprinting; family members; *genetic determinism; *genetic information; genetic materials; *genetic predisposition; genetic screening; health; health insurance; insurance selection bias; medical records; metaphor; minority groups; *privacy; risk; social discrimination; stigmatization; biological specimen banks

Murray, Thomas H. Genetic screening in the workplace: ethical issues. *Journal of Occupational Medicine.* 1983 Jun; 25(6): 451–454. BE57631.
*employment; genetic predisposition; genetic research; *genetic screening; goals; health hazards; informed consent; *occupational exposure; social discrimination

Natowicz, Marvin R.; Ard, Catherine. The commercialization of clinical genetics: an analysis of interrelations between academic centers and for-profit clinical genetics diagnostics companies. *Journal of Genetic Counseling.* 1997 Sep; 6(3): 337–355. 60 refs. BE57247.
administrators; conflict of interest; faculty; financial support; genetic counseling; genetic research; *genetic screening;

BE = bioethics accession number   fn. = footnotes   refs. = references

*genetic services; health personnel; *industry; investigators; professional organizations; *proprietary health facilities; social impact; statistics; survey; *trends; *universities; American Society of Human Genetics; National Academy of Sciences; United States

NIH–DOE Working Group on Ethical, Legal, and Social Implications of Human Genome Research. Task Force on Genetic Testing. Interim Principles. Issued by the Task Force, 550 N. Broadway, Suite 511, Baltimore, MD 21205; 1997 Mar 11. 42 p. 17 fn. Interim document for public comment; not to be construed as final. BE57695.

adults; advisory committees; carriers; confidentiality; conflict of interest; directive counseling; education; ethical review; evaluation; federal government; genetic counseling; genetic disorders; genetic predisposition; *genetic screening; *genetic services; health personnel; health insurance; human experimentation; industry; informed consent; laboratories; newborns; pregnant women; *public policy; quality of health care; research design; risks and benefits; selection of subjects; *standards; technical expertise; terminology; truth disclosure; diagnostic kits; quality control; *NIH–DOE Working Group on Ethical, Legal, and Social Implications (ELSI); *Task Force on Genetic Testing; United States

Nørgaard–Pederson, Bent. Use of stored samples from the Danish PKU register. *In:* Knoppers, Bartha Maria, ed. Human DNA: Law and Policy: International and Comparative Perspectives. Proceedings of the First International Conference on DNA Sampling and Human Genetic Research: Ethical, Legal, and Policy Aspects, held in Montreal, Canada, 6–8 Sep 1996. Boston, MA: Kluwer Law International; 1997: 303–311. 24 fn. ISBN 90–411–0361–9. BE58187.

congenital disorders; *DNA data banks; genetic disorders; genetic information; genetic materials; *genetic research; *genetic screening; guidelines; *newborns; *phenylketonuria; pregnant women; *registries; *biological specimen banks; *Denmark

Page, David L.; Jensen, Roy A.; Geller, Gail, et al. Genetic testing and informed consent. [Letter and response]. *JAMA.* 1997 Sep 10; 278(10): 821–822. 2 refs. BE57315.

biomedical research; *cancer; confidentiality; disclosure; DNA data banks; epidemiology; federal government; genetic information; *genetic predisposition; *genetic research; *genetic screening; government regulation; guidelines; health insurance; *informed consent; patients; research ethics committees; research subjects; risks and benefits; social discrimination; tissue banks; Office for Protection from Research Risks; United States

Parsons, Evelyn; Bradley, Don; Clarke, Angus. Disclosure of Duchenne muscular dystrophy after newborn screening. *Archives of Disease in Childhood.* 1996 Jun; 74(6): 550–553. 13 refs. BE56314.

attitudes; communication; *diagnosis; *Duchenne muscular dystrophy; evaluation; *genetic screening; informed consent; interdisciplinary communication; mass screening; *newborns; parents; patient care team; *patient satisfaction; professional patient relationship; program descriptions; time factors; *truth disclosure; voluntary programs; Wales

Patenaude, Andrea Farkas; Basili, Laura; Fairclough, Diane L., et al. Attitudes of 47 mothers of pediatric oncology patients toward genetic testing for cancer predisposition. *Journal of Clinical Oncology.* 1996 Feb; 14(2): 415–421. 17 refs. BE55519.

adults; age factors; *attitudes; *cancer; *children; decision making; disclosure; family planning; genetic counseling; *genetic predisposition; *genetic screening; *knowledge, attitudes, practice; *mothers; parental consent; psychological

stress; risks and benefits; survey; Massachusetts

Pear, Robert. States pass laws to regulate uses of genetic testing. [News]. *New York Times.* 1997 Oct 18: A1, A9. BE58094.

attitudes; *confidentiality; disclosure; drug industry; employment; genetic disorders; *genetic information; genetic materials; genetic predisposition; genetic research; *genetic screening; *government regulation; health insurance; investigators; life insurance; patients; privacy; property rights; *social discrimination; *state government; *United States

Peters, David A. Risk classification, genetic testing, and health care: a conflict between libertarian and egalitarian values? *In:* Peters, Ted, ed. Genetics: Issues of Social Justice. Cleveland, OH: Pilgrim Press; 1998: 205–217. 17 fn. ISBN 0–8298–1251–2. BE57480.

economics; ethical analysis; freedom; genes; genetic disorders; genetic information; genetic predisposition; *genetic screening; health care delivery; *health insurance; industry; insurance selection bias; *justice; *libertarianism; moral policy; property rights; *risk; social impact; United States

Peters, Ted. Designer genes and selective abortion. *In: his* For the Love of Children: Genetic Technology and the Future of the Family. Louisville, KY: Westminster John Knox Press; 1996: 85–118, 193–199. 63 fn. ISBN 0–664–25468–3. BE55697.

adoption; beginning of life; coercion; confidentiality; decision making; disabled; employment; eugenics; fetal development; *fetuses; genetic counseling; *genetic disorders; genetic information; *genetic predisposition; *genetic screening; government regulation; insurance; killing; legal rights; *personhood; pregnant women; prenatal diagnosis; privacy; Protestant ethics; public policy; risk; *Roman Catholic ethics; *selective abortion; *social discrimination; value of life; viability; dignity; Genetic Privacy Act 1994; United States

Pokorski, Robert J. A test for the insurance industry. *Nature.* 1998 Feb 26; 391(6670): 835–836. 11 refs. BE57970.

*confidentiality; dementia; disclosure; *economics; *genetic information; genetic predisposition; *genetic screening; *industry; insurance selection bias; *justice; *life insurance; public policy; rights; risk; United States

Ponder, Bruce. Genetic testing for cancer risk. *Science.* 1997 Nov 7; 278(5340): 1050–1054. 36 fn. BE57335.

*breast cancer; *cancer; confidentiality; decision making; education; employment; genetic counseling; *genetic predisposition; *genetic screening; genetic services; guidelines; informed consent; insurance; resource allocation; risk; risks and benefits; social discrimination; uncertainty; Great Britain; United States

Genetic testing for cancer susceptibility is already part of the clinical management of families with some of the well-defined (but uncommon) inherited cancer syndromes. In cases where the risks associated with a predisposing mutation are less certain, or where there is no clearly effective intervention to offer those with a positive result, its use is more controversial. Careful evaluation of costs and benefits, and of the efficacy of interventions in those found to be at risk, is essential and is only just beginning. An immediate challenge is to ensure that both health professionals and the public understand clearly the issues involved.

Powers, Madison. Justice and genetics: privacy protection and the moral basis of public policy. *In:* Rothstein, Mark A., ed. Genetic Secrets: Protecting Privacy and Confidentiality in the Genetic Era. New Haven, CT:

BE = bioethics accession number   fn. = footnotes   refs. = references

Yale University Press; 1997: 355–368. 15 fn. ISBN 0–300–07251–1. BE58691.

autonomy; common good; *confidentiality; data banks; *disclosure; economics; employment; epidemiology; family members; *genetic information; genetic predisposition; *genetic research; *genetic screening; government regulation; health care delivery; health hazards; health insurance; incentives; informed consent; *justice; legal rights; mass screening; medical records; moral policy; policy analysis; *privacy; public health; *public policy; registries; risks and benefits; social discrimination; stigmatization; *pragmatism; United States

Rae, Scott B. Prenatal genetic testing, abortion, and beyond. *In:* Kilner, John F.; Pentz, Rebecca D.; Young, Frank E., eds. Genetic Ethics: Do the Ends Justify the Genes? Grand Rapids, MI: W.B. Eerdmans; 1997: 136–145. 12 fn. ISBN 0–8028–4428–6. BE56721.

*Christian ethics; disabled; embryos; fetal therapy; fetuses; genetic counseling; *genetic disorders; *genetic screening; genome mapping; late–onset disorders; personhood; *preimplantation diagnosis; *prenatal diagnosis; quality of life; *selective abortion; sex determination; uncertainty; value of life; United States

Reich, Elsa; Zanko, Andrea; Heimler, Audrey. Testing for HD in twins. [Letter and response]. *Journal of Genetic Counseling.* 1996 Mar; 5(1): 47–51. BE56495.

autonomy; coercion; confidentiality; family members; *genetic counseling; genetic information; *genetic screening; *Huntington's disease; privacy; truth disclosure; *twins

Reilly, Philip R. Laws to regulate the use of genetic information. *In:* Rothstein, Mark A., ed. Genetic Secrets: Protecting Privacy and Confidentiality in the Genetic Era. New Haven, CT: Yale University Press; 1997: 369–391. 76 fn. ISBN 0–300–07251–1. BE58692.

blacks; *confidentiality; *disclosure; DNA data banks; DNA fingerprinting; *employment; *federal government; *genetic information; genetic materials; genetic research; *genetic screening; *government regulation; *health insurance; historical aspects; informed consent; *legislation; mandatory testing; mass screening; medical records; model legislation; newborns; phenylketonuria; privacy; *public policy; sickle cell anemia; *social discrimination; *state government; *trends; biological specimen banks; Twentieth Century; *United States

Rhodes, Rosamond. Genetic links, family ties, and social bonds: rights and responsibilities in the face of genetic knowledge. *Journal of Medicine and Philosophy.* 1998 Feb; 23(1): 10–30. 42 refs. 19 fn. BE57518.

*autonomy; beneficence; case studies; confidentiality; decision making; directive counseling; disclosure; *family members; family relationship; friends; *genetic counseling; genetic disorders; *genetic information; genetic research; *genetic screening; Huntington's disease; *moral obligations; *moral policy; *obligations to society; patient participation; *patients; privacy; rights; social interaction; Tay Sachs disease; *truth disclosure; volunteers; pedigree studies; population genetics; *right not to know

Currently, some of the most significant moral issues involving genetic links relate to genetic knowledge. In this paper, instead of looking at the frequently addressed issues of responsibilities professionals or institutions have to individuals, I take up the question of what responsibilities individuals have to one another with respect to genetic knowledge. I address the questions of whether individuals have a moral right to pursue their own goals without contributing to society's knowledge of population genetics, without adding to their family's knowledge of its genetic history, and without discovering genetic information about themselves and their offspring. These questions lead to an examination of the presumed right to genetic ignorance and an exploration of a variety of social bonds. Analyzing cases in light of these considerations leads to a surprising conclusion about a widely accepted precept of genetic counseling, to some ethical insights into typical problems, and to some further unanswered questions about personal responsibility in the face of genetic knowledge.

Roche, Patricia (Winnie). Caveat venditor: protecting privacy and ownership interests in DNA. *In:* Knoppers, Bartha Maria, ed. Human DNA: Law and Policy: International and Comparative Perspectives. Proceedings of the First International Conference on DNA Sampling and Human Genetic Research: Ethical, Legal, and Policy Aspects, held in Montreal, Canada, 6–8 Sep 1996. Boston, MA: Kluwer Law International; 1997: 33–41. 30 fn. ISBN 90–411–0361–9. BE58166.

*confidentiality; disclosure; *DNA data banks; DNA fingerprinting; federal government; *genetic information; *genetic materials; *genetic research; *genetic screening; *government regulation; informed consent; *legal aspects; model legislation; privacy; *property rights; tissue donation; *Genetic Privacy Act; Moore v. Regents of the University of California; *United States

Rodriguez, Eduardo. The Human Genome Project and eugenics. *Linacre Quarterly.* 1998 May; 65(2): 73–82. 24 fn. BE58935.

economics; *eugenics; genetic disorders; *genetic screening; genome mapping; historical aspects; prenatal diagnosis; reproduction; reproductive technologies; selective abortion; social discrimination; Human Genome Project; United States

Roeper, Burkhardt. Germany approves DNA tests for visas. [News]. *Nature.* 1998 Feb 19; 391(6669): 723. BE58065.

*aliens; confidentiality; *DNA fingerprinting; *family members; *genetic screening; *public policy; *emigration and immigration; *Germany

Rothenberg, Karen H. Genetic accountability and pregnant women. *Women's Health Issues.* 1997 Jul–Aug; 7(4): 215–219. 12 refs. BE55732.

*accountability; autonomy; coercion; conflict of interest; contraception; decision making; disabled; economics; eugenics; females; genetic counseling; genetic disorders; *genetic screening; genetic services; government financing; health education; health personnel; incentives; legal aspects; mandatory testing; medical education; obligations to society; *pregnant women; *prenatal diagnosis; public policy; *reproduction; selective abortion; state interest; *voluntary programs; wrongful life; ELSI–funded publication; United States

Rothstein, Laura F. Genetic information in schools. *In:* Rothstein, Mark A., ed. Genetic Secrets: Protecting Privacy and Confidentiality in the Genetic Era. New Haven, CT: Yale University Press; 1997: 317–331. 38 fn. ISBN 0–300–07251–1. BE58689.

children; confidentiality; education; *genetic information; *genetic screening; informed consent; legal aspects; privacy; *schools; social discrimination; students; United States

Rothstein, Mark A. Genetic discrimination in employment and the Americans with Disabilities Act. *Houston Law Review.* 1992 Spring; 29(1): 23–84. 386 fn. BE56975.

carriers; confidentiality; disabled; *disclosure; economics; *employment; *federal government; genetic disorders; *genetic information; genetic predisposition; *genetic screening; *government regulation; health insurance; insurance selection bias; late–onset disorders; *legal aspects; *legislation; *social discrimination; *Americans with

---

BE = bioethics accession number   fn. = footnotes   refs. = references

Disabilities Act 1990; Equal Employment Opportunity Commission; *United States

Rothstein, Mark A. Genetic secrets: a policy framework. *In:* Rothstein, Mark A., ed. Genetic Secrets: Protecting Privacy and Confidentiality in the Genetic Era. New Haven, CT: Yale University Press; 1997: 451–495. 90 fn. ISBN 0–300–07251–1. BE58694.
adoption; anonymous testing; autonomy; *confidentiality; criminal law; *disclosure; DNA data banks; DNA fingerprinting; duty to warn; economics; employment; family members; federal government; genetic counseling; *genetic information; genetic predisposition; genetic research; *genetic screening; *government regulation; health care delivery; health insurance; health personnel; industry; informed consent; international aspects; legal liability; *legislation; mandatory testing; medical records; military personnel; parent child relationship; *privacy; professional competence; public health; *public policy; schools; self regulation; social discrimination; standards; state government; trends; biological specimen banks; United States

Rothstein, Mark A., ed. Genetic Secrets: Protecting Privacy and Confidentiality in the Genetic Era. New Haven, CT: Yale University Press; 1997. 511 p. 1,175 fn. ISBN 0–300–07251–1. BE58672.
adoption; *confidentiality; disclosure; DNA data banks; DNA fingerprinting; employment; epidemiology; family members; family relationship; financial support; genetic counseling; genetic determinism; *genetic information; genetic predisposition; genetic research; *genetic screening; genome mapping; government regulation; health hazards; health insurance; industry; informed consent; international aspects; legal aspects; legislation; life insurance; occupational exposure; *privacy; property rights; public health; public policy; research subjects; review; schools; biological specimen banks; Europe; United States

Rothstein, Mark A. The law of medical and genetic privacy in the workplace. *In:* Rothstein, Mark A., ed. Genetic Secrets: Protecting Privacy and Confidentiality in the Genetic Era. New Haven, CT: Yale University Press; 1997: 281–298. 54 fn. ISBN 0–300–07251–1. BE58687.
*confidentiality; *disclosure; *employment; genetic information; *genetic screening; health; health insurance; *legal aspects; legislation; medical records; privacy; social discrimination; state government; Americans with Disabilities Act 1990; *United States

Roy, David J.; Kramar, Giulia; de Langavant, Ghislaine Cleret. Ethics for complexity. *In:* Knoppers, Bartha Maria, ed. Human DNA: Law and Policy: International and Comparative Perspectives. Proceedings of the First International Conference on DNA Sampling and Human Genetic Research: Ethical, Legal, and Policy Aspects, held in Montreal, Canada, 6–8 Sep 1996. Boston, MA: Kluwer Law International; 1997: 189–209. 60 fn. ISBN 90–411–0361–9. BE58178.
confidentiality; *DNA data banks; *epidemiology; ethical theory; *ethics; evolution; genetic counseling; genetic disorders; *genetic diversity; genetic materials; genetic predisposition; *genetic research; *genetic screening; *genetics; informed consent; international aspects; mass screening; public health; risks and benefits; *biological specimen banks; *population genetics

Saegusa, Asako. Japan okays test–tube baby gene tests. [News]. *Nature.* 1998 Jul 9; 394(6689): 110. BE58865.
*genetic screening; guidelines; in vitro fertilization; *organizational policies; physicians; *preimplantation diagnosis; professional organizations; *Japan; *Japan Society of Obstetrics and Gynecology

Salihu, Hamisu Mohammed. Genetic counselling among Muslims: questions remain unanswered. [Letter]. *Lancet.* 1997 Oct 4; 350(9083): 1035–1036. 2 refs. BE57359.
clergy; fetal development; *genetic counseling; genetic disorders; *genetic screening; *Islamic ethics; *preimplantation diagnosis; *prenatal diagnosis; *selective abortion; socioeconomic factors; Cameroon; Great Britain

Schwartz, Paul M. European data protection law and medical privacy. *In:* Rothstein, Mark A., ed. Genetic Secrets: Protecting Privacy and Confidentiality in the Genetic Era. New Haven, CT: Yale University Press; 1997: 392–417. 91 fn. ISBN 0–300–07251–1. BE58693.
comparative studies; *confidentiality; *disclosure; DNA fingerprinting; federal government; *genetic information; genetic research; *genetic screening; *government regulation; insurance; *international aspects; *legislation; *medical records; privacy; public policy; state government; Austria; *Europe; European Union; France; Germany; Switzerland; United States

Sharp, David. Gene tests offered to UK public. [News]. *Lancet.* 1997 Oct 4; 350(9083): 1013. BE57345.
advisory committees; *genetic screening; *genetic services; guidelines; *home care; *industry; regulation; *diagnostic kits; *Advisory Committee on Genetic Testing (Great Britain); *Great Britain

Sharpe, Neil F. Presymptomatic testing for Huntington disease: is there a duty to test those under the age of eighteen years? [Letter]. *American Journal of Medical Genetics.* 1993 Apr 15; 46(2): 250–253. 54 refs. BE57994.
age factors; *disclosure; genetic counseling; *genetic screening; health personnel; *Huntington's disease; informed consent; late–onset disorders; legal liability; *minors; parents; *risks and benefits; uncertainty; Canada; United States

Spiegler, Gerard E.; Motulsky, Arno G. Genetic screening of adolescents. [Letter and response]. *New England Journal of Medicine.* 1997 Aug 28; 337(9): 639–640. 7 refs. BE59004.
*adolescents; carriers; confidentiality; genetic counseling; genetic disorders; *genetic information; *genetic screening; health insurance; *mass screening; national health insurance; patient compliance; risks and benefits; social discrimination; Montreal; United States

Sutton, Agneta. The new genetics and traditional Hippocratic medicine. *In:* Doherty, Peter; Sutton, Agneta, eds. Man–Made Man: Ethical and Legal Issues in Genetics. Dublin, Ireland: Open Air; 1997: 58–70. 13 refs. ISBN 1–85182–278–X. BE58296.
adults; carriers; children; confidentiality; eugenics; family members; *gene therapy; genetic enhancement; genetic predisposition; *genetic screening; germ cells; goals; informed consent; mass screening; medical ethics; medicine; obligations to society; physicians; pregnant women; prenatal diagnosis; risks and benefits; virtues; voluntary programs

Thomas, A. Mathew; Cohen, Gene; Cook–Deegan, Robert M., et al. Alzheimer testing at Silver Years. *Cambridge Quarterly of Healthcare Ethics.* 1998 Summer; 7(3): 294–307. 38 fn. BE58557.
*aged; autonomy; beneficence; community services; contracts; *dementia; diagnosis; *economics; *genetic predisposition; *genetic screening; informed consent; *institutional policies; insurance selection bias; justice; late–onset disorders; legal aspects; *mandatory testing; *moral policy; nursing homes; *patient admission; *patient care; *residential facilities; *social discrimination; standards; Americans with Disabilities Act 1990; United States

Thomson, Elizabeth J. Sampling issues in clinical impact of genetic testing and counselling studies. *In:* Knoppers,

---

BE = bioethics accession number   fn. = footnotes   refs. = references

Bartha Maria, ed. Human DNA: Law and Policy: International and Comparative Perspectives. Proceedings of the First International Conference on DNA Sampling and Human Genetic Research: Ethical, Legal, and Policy Aspects, held in Montreal, Canada, 6–8 Sep 1996. Boston, MA: Kluwer Law International; 1997: 313–317. 9 fn. ISBN 90–411–0361–9. BE58188.
cancer; confidentiality; cystic fibrosis; DNA data banks; federal government; genetic counseling; genetic materials; genetic predisposition; *genetic research; *genetic screening; genetic services; government financing; informed consent; risks and benefits; social impact; National Center for Human Genome Research; NCHGR Program on Ethical, Legal, and Social Implications (ELSI); United States

Tibben, A.; Stevens, M.; de Wert, G.M.W.R., et al. Preparing for presymptomatic DNA testing for early onset Alzheimer's disease/cerebral haemorrhage and hereditary Pick disease. *Journal of Medical Genetics.* 1997 Jan; 34(1): 63–72. 22 refs. BE56014.
*attitudes; autonomy; *brain pathology; competence; dementia; disclosure; family members; *genetic counseling; genetic information; *genetic predisposition; genetic research; *genetic screening; genetic services; informed consent; *late-onset disorders; minors; motivation; preimplantation diagnosis; prenatal diagnosis; psychological stress; reproduction; risk; selective abortion; social discrimination; suicide; survey; third party consent; Netherlands

Tracy, Kathryn Bayard; Post, Stephen G.; Whitehouse, Peter J. Genetic testing for Alzheimer disease. [Letter and response]. *JAMA.* 1997 Sep 24; 278(12): 978–979. 8 refs. BE57166.
breast cancer; comprehension; confidentiality; *dementia; family members; *genetic predisposition; *genetic screening; genetics; human experimentation; Huntington's disease; *preventive medicine; professional organizations; psychological stress; risk; *risks and benefits; social discrimination; time factors; United States

Tyler, Audrey; Ball, David; Clarke, Angus. Genetic testing in the classroom. [Letter]. *BMJ (British Medical Journal).* 1995 Jul 29; 311(7000): 330. 1 ref. BE56103.
anonymous testing; confidentiality; genetic counseling; genetic disorders; *genetic screening; informed consent; *medical education; medical schools; *students; teaching methods; Great Britain

U.S. Congress. House. A bill to amend the Fair Labor Standards Act of 1938 to restrict employers in obtaining, disclosing, and using of genetic information. H.R. 3477, 104th Cong., 2d Sess. Introduced by Joseph P. Kennedy; 1996 May 16. 3 p. Referred to Committee on Economic and Educational Opportunities. BE56944.
*confidentiality; *disclosure; *employment; *genetic information; genetic screening; informed consent; *legal aspects; legislation; Americans with Disabilities Act 1990; *Fair Labor Standards Act 1938 (1996 Amendment); *United States

U.S. Congress. House. A bill to amend title 10, United States Code, to limit the collection and use by the Department of Defense of individual genetic identifying information for the purpose of identification of remains, other than when the consent of the individual concerned is obtained. H.R. 2873, 104th Cong., 2d Sess. Introduced by Joseph P. Kennedy; 1996 Jan 24. 2 p. Referred to the Committee on National Security. BE57198.
blood specimen collection; *DNA fingerprinting; federal government; *genetic information; *genetic screening; informed consent; *legal aspects; legislation; *military personnel; *Department of Defense; *United States

U.S. Congress. House. A bill to prohibit insurance providers from denying or canceling health insurance coverage, or varying the premiums, terms, or conditions for health insurance coverage on the basis of genetic information or a request for genetic services, and for other purposes [Genetic Information Nondiscrimination in Health Insurance Act of 1995]. H.R. 2748, 104th Cong., 1st Sess. Introduced by Louise McIntosh Slaughter; 1995 Dec 7. 8 p. Referred to the Committee on Commerce and to the Committee on Economic and Educational Opportunities. BE56948.
*genetic information; *genetic screening; genetic services; government regulation; *health insurance; *insurance selection bias; *legal aspects; legislation; *social discrimination; state government; *Genetic Information Nondiscrimination in Health Insurance Act (1995 bill); *United States

U.S. Congress. House. Committee on Science. Subcommittee on Technology. Technological Advances in Genetics Testing: Implications for the Future. Hearing, 17 Sep 1996. Washington, DC: U.S. Government Printing Office; 1996. 191 p. No. 68. ISBN 0–16–053777–0. BE57641.
confidentiality; federal government; genetic information; genetic predisposition; genetic research; *genetic screening; genetic services; government regulation; health insurance; industry; laboratories; legislation; privacy; public policy; social discrimination; standards; Food and Drug Administration; Genetic Privacy and Nondiscrimination Act 1996 (1996 bill); *United States

U.S. Congress. Senate. A bill to establish limitation with respect to the disclosure and use of genetic information, and for other purposes [Genetic Privacy and Nondiscrimination Act of 1995]. S. 1416, 104th Cong., 1st Sess. Introduced by Mark O. Hatfield; 1995 Nov 15. 7 p. Referred to the Committee on Labor and Human Resources. BE56946.
advisory committees; *confidentiality; *disclosure; DNA data banks; employment; federal government; *genetic information; genetic screening; government regulation; health insurance; informed consent; law enforcement; *legal aspects; legislation; *privacy; social discrimination; state government; *Genetic Privacy and Nondiscrimination Act (1995 bill); National Bioethics Advisory Commission; *United States

U.S. Congress. Senate. A bill to establish limitations on health plans with respect to genetic information, and for other purposes [Genetic Fairness Act of 1996]. S. 1600, 104th Cong., 2d Sess. Introduced by Diane Feinstein; 1996 Mar 7. 7 p. Referred to the Committee on Labor and Human Resources. BE56945.
family members; *genetic information; *genetic screening; genetic services; government regulation; *health insurance; *insurance selection bias; *legal aspects; legislation; *social discrimination; state government; *Genetic Fairness Act (1996 bill); *United States

U.S. Congress. Senate. A bill to prohibit discrimination against individuals and their family members on the basis of genetic information, or a request for genetic services [Genetic Information Nondiscrimination in Health Insurance Act of 1997]. S. 89, 105th Cong., 1st Sess. Introduced by Olympia Snowe; 1997 Jan 21. 15 p. Referred to the Committee on Labor and Human Resources. BE56947.
confidentiality; disclosure; family members; *genetic information; *genetic screening; genetic services; *health insurance; informed consent; *insurance selection bias; *legal aspects; legislation; *social discrimination; Employee Retirement Income Security Act 1974 (ERISA); *Genetic

---

BE = bioethics accession number   fn. = footnotes   refs. = references

Information Nondiscrimination in Health Insurance Act (1997 bill); Medicare; Public Health Service Act; Social Security Act; *United States

U.S. Department of Health and Human Services. Health Insurance in the Age of Genetics. Report: Executive Summary. *In:* BioLaw: A Legal and Ethical Reporter on Medicine, Health Care, and Bioengineering. Special Sections, 2(9). Frederick, MD: University Publications of America; 1997 Sep: S265–S277. 7 refs. Appended: Statement of Francis Collins on President Clinton's announcement to end genetic discrimination in health insurance, 14 July 1997. BE56647.

confidentiality; *federal government; genetic information; genetic research; *genetic screening; genome mapping; *government regulation; *health insurance; insurance selection bias; legislation; privacy; risks and benefits; *social discrimination; state government; Health Insurance Portability and Accountability Act 1996; U.S. Congress; *United States

U.S. National Center for Human Genome Research. ELSI 1990–1995: A Review of the Ethical, Legal, and Social Implications Research Program and Related Activities. Bethesda, MD: U.S. National Center for Human Genome Research; 1996 Apr 12. 17 p. 10 refs. BE59047.

cancer; cystic fibrosis; education; ethical review; federal government; genetic disorders; genetic information; genetic predisposition; *genetic screening; genetic services; *genome mapping; goals; government financing; government regulation; health insurance; health personnel; information dissemination; informed consent; law enforcement; minority groups; privacy; *program descriptions; *public policy; social discrimination; ELSI-funded publication; Human Genome Project; *NCHGR Program on Ethical, Legal, and Social Implications (ELSI); *United States

van Berkel, Dymphie; Klinge, Ineke. Gene technology: also a gender issue: views of Dutch informed women on genetic screening and gene therapy. *Patient Education and Counseling.* 1997 May; 31(1): 49–55. 6 refs. BE57525.

*attitudes; autonomy; decision making; *females; fetal research; fetal therapy; *gene therapy; *genetic screening; genetic services; genome mapping; *knowledge, attitudes, practice; males; prenatal diagnosis; social discrimination; social impact; *Netherlands

Wachbroit, Robert. The question not asked: the challenge of pleiotropic genetic tests. *Kennedy Institute of Ethics Journal.* 1998 Jun; 8(2): 131–144. 10 refs. BE58372.

*dementia; *disclosure; double effect; genetic counseling; *genetic disorders; *genetic information; genetic predisposition; *genetic screening; *heart diseases; informed consent; moral obligations; moral policy; obligations to society; patients; physicians; policy analysis; psychological stress; risks and benefits; social discrimination; time factors; *truth disclosure; *incidental findings

Nearly all of the literature on the ethical, legal, or social issues surrounding genetic tests has proceeded on the assumption that any particular test for a gene mutation yields information about only one disease condition. Even though the phenomenon of pleiotropy, where a single gene has multiple, apparently unrelated phenotypic effects, is widely recognized in genetics, it has not had much significance for genetic testing until recently. In this article, I examine a moral dilemma created by one sort of pleiotropic testing, APOE genotyping, which can yield information about the risk of two different conditions -- coronary heart disease and Alzheimer's disease. A physician administering APOE testing for the beneficial purpose of assessing the risk of heart disease may discover medically useless and socially harmful information about the patient's risk of

Alzheimer's disease. I explore how much providers should disclose to patients about pleiotropic test results and whether patients are obligated to know as much about their genetic condition as possible.

Wadman, Meredith. Ethical terms set for breast cancer test. [News]. *Nature.* 1997 Nov 27; 390(6658): 324. BE57336.

*breast cancer; genes; genetic counseling; *genetic screening; genetic services; *industry; patents; *self regulation; Cancer Research Campaign Technology (London); Duke University; Great Britain; National Health Service; Oncormed; United States

Wadman, Meredith. Jewish leaders meet NIH chiefs on genetic stigmatization fears. [News]. *Nature.* 1998 Apr 30; 392(6679): 851. BE58432.

genetic predisposition; *genetic research; *genetic screening; *Jews; social discrimination; *stigmatization; National Institutes of Health; United States

Walters, LeRoy, ed. Ethical issues in human genetics. *In:* Jonsen, Albert R.; Veatch, Robert M.; Walters, LeRoy, eds. Source Book in Bioethics: A Documentary History. Washington, DC: Georgetown University Press; 1998: 253–333. 40 refs. ISBN 0-87840-683-2. BE57892.

advisory committees; carriers; federal government; *gene therapy; genetic counseling; genetic disorders; *genetic intervention; genetic research; *genetic screening; genetic services; *genome mapping; germ cells; guidelines; historical aspects; industry; international aspects; legal aspects; mass screening; moral policy; newborns; prenatal diagnosis; public policy; recombinant DNA research; resource allocation; universities; *Committee for the Study of Inborn Errors of Metabolism; Council of Europe; Declaration of Inuyama; European Medical Research Councils; *NIH Guidelines; *Office of Technology Assessment; *President's Commission for the Study of Ethical Problems; Recombinant DNA Advisory Committee; *Twentieth Century; *United States

Watzman, Haim. Israel split on rights to genetic privacy. [News]. *Nature.* 1998 Jul 16; 394(6690): 214. BE58866.

confidentiality; *disclosure; *genetic information; genetic materials; genetic research; *genetic screening; *government regulation; insurance; *legislation; privacy; property rights; *Israel

Weaver, Kirke D. Genetic screening and the right not to know. *Issues in Law and Medicine.* 1997 Winter; 13(3): 243–281. 192 fn. BE58704.

coercion; dementia; disabled; *employment; federal government; genetic counseling; genetic disorders; genetic predisposition; *genetic screening; government regulation; health hazards; Huntington's disease; industry; *insurance; *legal aspects; *legal rights; legislation; *mandatory testing; occupational exposure; privacy; private sector; psychological stress; public sector; *risks and benefits; social discrimination; state interest; stigmatization; treatment refusal; *truth disclosure; voluntary programs; *right not to know; Americans with Disabilities Act 1990; Fourth Amendment; United States

Wertz, Dorothy C.; Reilly, Philip R. Laboratory policies and practices for the genetic testing of children: a survey of the Helix network. *American Journal of Human Genetics.* 1997 Nov; 61(5): 1163–1168. 19 refs. BE58850.

*adolescents; *age factors; autonomy; carriers; *children; cystic fibrosis; Duchenne muscular dystrophy; genetic counseling; genetic disorders; *genetic screening; *genetic services; guidelines; Huntington's disease; informed consent; *institutional policies; *laboratories; late-onset disorders; organizational policies; parental consent; physicians; primary health care; professional organizations; regulation; risks and benefits; statistics; survey; ELSI-funded publication; United States

---

BE = bioethics accession number   fn. = footnotes   refs. = references

Wilke, Joanne. From a survivor: the emotional experience of genetic testing. [Personal narrative]. *Journal of Psychosocial Nursing and Mental Health Services.* 1995 Apr; 33(4): 28–37. BE55779.
emotions; family members; genetic counseling; *genetic screening; *Huntington's disease; *patients; prenatal diagnosis; *psychological stress

Willer, Roger A., ed. Genetic Testing and Screening: Critical Engagement at the Intersection of Faith and Science. Minneapolis, MN: Kirk House Publishers; 1998. 210 p. 184 fn. ISBN 1–886513–11–2. BE59048.
behavioral genetics; carriers; children; *Christian ethics; commodification; eugenics; genetic counseling; genetic disorders; genetic predisposition; *genetic screening; genetic services; genetics; genome mapping; industry; late–onset disorders; normality; pastoral care; prenatal diagnosis; *Protestant ethics; selective abortion; theology; value of life; Evangelical Lutheran Church

Williams, Janet K.; Lessick, Mira. Genome research: implications for children. *Pediatric Nursing.* 1996 Jan–Feb; 22(1): 40–46. 46 refs. BE55584.
carriers; *children; chromosome abnormalities; cystic fibrosis; *gene therapy; genetic counseling; genetic determinism; genetic disorders; genetic information; genetic predisposition; *genetic research; *genetic screening; genome mapping; germ cells; nurses; parent child relationship; patient advocacy; pediatrics; *risks and benefits; social discrimination; social impact; adenosine deaminase deficiency; fragile X syndrome

World Health Organization. Ethical, social and legal aspects of genetic technology in medicine [and] Conclusions and recommendations. *In:* Control of Hereditary Diseases: Report of a WHO Scientific Group. Geneva: World Health Organization; 1996: 73–81. References embedded in list at back of book. ISBN 92–4–120865–1. BE58941.
autonomy; carriers; confidentiality; consensus; data banks; decision making; directive counseling; disclosure; family members; genetic counseling; *genetic information; genetic predisposition; *genetic screening; genetic services; genome mapping; guidelines; human rights; informed consent; international aspects; late–onset disorders; newborns; patents; prenatal diagnosis; privacy; public health; selective abortion; stigmatization; voluntary programs; right not to know

Yesley, Michael S. Genetic privacy, discrimination, and social policy: challenges and dilemmas. *Microbial and Comparative Genomics.* 1997; 2(1): 19–35. 81 refs. Remarks delivered at a workshop on genetics and public policy sponsored by the Institute for Genomic Research Science Education Foundation and held as part of the Third World Conference on Bioethics, San Francisco, CA, 22 Nov 1996. BE58447.
blacks; confidentiality; *employment; *federal government; genetic disorders; *genetic information; genetic predisposition; *genetic screening; genome mapping; *government regulation; *health insurance; *legal aspects; legislation; *life insurance; mass screening; occupational exposure; *privacy; risks and benefits; sickle cell anemia; *social discrimination; *state government; ELSI–funded publication; Americans with Disabilities Act 1990; Genetic Privacy Act; U.S. Congress; *United States

Zweig, Franklin M.; Walsh, Joseph T.; Freeman, Daniel M. Courts and the challenges of adjudicating genetic testing's secrets. *In:* Rothstein, Mark A., ed. Genetic Secrets: Protecting Privacy and Confidentiality in the Genetic Era. New Haven, CT: Yale University Press; 1997: 332–351. 23 fn. ISBN 0–300–07251–1. BE58690.
*adoption; aggression; behavioral genetics; capital punishment; competence; *confidentiality; criminal law; disclosure; *genetic information; *genetic predisposition; *genetic screening; judicial action; *legal aspects; legal liability; mentally ill; privacy; violence; *United States

British guidelines set out standards for genetic tests. [News]. *Nature.* 1997 Oct 2; 389(6650): 427. BE55807.
advisory committees; confidentiality; cystic fibrosis; genetic counseling; *genetic screening; *genetic services; *guidelines; *industry; public policy; *standards; voluntary programs; *Advisory Committee on Genetic Testing (Great Britain); *Great Britain

Human Genetics Advisory Commission meets. [News; title supplied]. *Gene Therapy.* 1997 Apr; 4(4): 271. BE56184.
advisory committees; *confidentiality; disclosure; *genetic information; *genetic screening; *industry; insurance selection bias; *life insurance; *organizational policies; professional organizations; social discrimination; *Association of British Insurers; Great Britain; *Human Genetics Advisory Commission (Great Britain)

Knowing your genes. [Editorial]. *Lancet.* 1997 Oct 4; 350(9083): 969. BE57310.
advisory committees; genetic information; *genetic screening; *genetic services; guidelines; *home care; *industry; regulation; *diagnostic kits; Advisory Committee on Genetic Testing (Great Britain); *Great Britain

MPs call for tough controls on human genetics. [News]. *GenEthics News.* 1995 Jul–Aug; No. 7: 1, 3. BE56335.
advisory committees; employment; gene therapy; genes; genetic information; *genetic intervention; genetic predisposition; *genetic screening; germ cells; *government regulation; insurance; patents; privacy; *public policy; *social discrimination; *Great Britain; House of Commons; Human Genetics Commission (Great Britain)

National Ethical Consultative Committee for the Life and Health Sciences in France issues opinion entitled "Genetics and medicine: from prediction to prevention." *International Digest of Health Legislation.* 1996; 47(2): 263–265. BE57188.
adults; advisory committees; confidentiality; disclosure; DNA data banks; family members; genetic counseling; genetic information; genetic research; *genetic screening; *guidelines; health personnel; informed consent; minors; occupational exposure; professional competence; social discrimination; *standards; *France; *National Ethics Advisory Committee (France)

Task force finalizes genetic testing recommendations. [News]. *Nature Biotechnology.* 1997 Apr; 15(4): 300. BE55968.
advisory committees; federal government; *genetic screening; government regulation; laboratories; *public policy; technical expertise; Food and Drug Administration; National Genetics Board; *Task Force on Genetic Testing; *United States

GENETIC SERVICES

See also GENE THERAPY, GENETIC COUNSELING, GENETIC SCREENING

Andrews, Lori B. Torts and the double helix: malpractice liability for failure to warn of genetic risks. *Houston Law Review.* 1992 Spring; 29(1): 149–184. 189 fn. BE56977.
age factors; carriers; children; compensation; confidentiality; congenital disorders; disabled; *disclosure; *family members; *genetic counseling; *genetic disorders; *genetic information; *genetic predisposition; *genetic screening; *genetic services; health education; late–onset disorders; *legal aspects; *legal liability; legislation; mass media;

BE = bioethics accession number   fn. = footnotes   refs. = references

minority groups; negligence; parents; *patients; *physicians; prenatal diagnosis; privacy; reproduction; risk; selective abortion; state government; torts; trends; *wrongful life; *recontact; *United States

Cassel, Christine K. Policy implications of the Human Genome Project for women. *Women's Health Issues.* 1997 Jul–Aug; 7(4): 225–229. 10 refs. BE55710.

confidentiality; disabled; *females; genetic counseling; genetic disorders; genetic research; genetic screening; *genetic services; genome mapping; government financing; health care reform; health insurance; indigents; insurance selection bias; minority groups; patient care; pregnant women; prenatal diagnosis; public policy; risks and benefits; selective abortion; sex determination; social impact; stigmatization; *women's health; *women's health services; ELSI-funded publication; Medicaid; United States

Harper, Peter S.; Clarke, Angus J. Genetics, Society, and Clinical Practice. Herndon, VA: BIOS Scientific Publishers; 1997. 253 p. 564 refs. ISBN 1–85996–206–8. BE59033.

carriers; children; confidentiality; cystic fibrosis; decision making; directive counseling; Down syndrome; economics; eugenics; family members; *genetic counseling; genetic disorders; genetic diversity; genetic information; genetic predisposition; genetic research; *genetic screening; *genetic services; goals; health care delivery; Huntington's disease; informed consent; insurance; intelligence; late-onset disorders; mass screening; newborns; prenatal diagnosis; privacy; public health; public policy; registries; reproduction; selective abortion; social discrimination; terminology; population genetics; China; Great Britain

Holtzman, Neil A.; Murphy, Patricia D.; Watson, Michael S., et al. Predictive genetic testing: from basic research to clinical practice. *Science.* 1997 Oct 24; 278(5338): 602–605. 26 fn. BE57334.

advisory committees; confidentiality; DNA data banks; *evaluation; federal government; genetic disorders; *genetic predisposition; genetic research; *genetic screening; *genetic services; goals; government regulation; industry; informed consent; investigators; public policy; research ethics committees; risks and benefits; self regulation; uncertainty; diagnostic kits; NHGRI-funded publication; Department of Health and Human Services; *Task Force on Genetic Testing; United States

Kinmonth, Ann Louise; Reinhard, John; Bobrow, Martin, et al. The new genetics: implications for clinical services in Britain and the United States. *BMJ (British Medical Journal).* 1998 Mar 7; 316(7133): 767–770. 34 refs. BE57755.

comparative studies; computer communication networks; continuing education; data banks; genetic counseling; genetic disorders; genetic information; genetic predisposition; genetic research; genetic screening; *genetic services; genetics; guidelines; health care delivery; interdisciplinary communication; *international aspects; medical specialties; patient care team; patient education; physicians; *primary health care; private sector; public sector; referral and consultation; registries; risk; support groups; *Great Britain; Internet; National Health Service; *United States

Kirk, Maggie. Commercial gene testing: the need for professional and public debate. *British Journal of Nursing.* 1997 Oct 9–22; 6(18): 1043–1047. 22 refs. BE58255.

carriers; cystic fibrosis; genetic counseling; genetic predisposition; *genetic screening; *genetic services; industry; informed consent; mass screening; nurses; *risks and benefits; uncertainty; *diagnostic kits; *Great Britain

Mahowald, Mary B. Gender justice in genetics. *Women's Health Issues.* 1997 Jul–Aug; 7(4): 230–233. 4 refs. BE55725.

biology; blacks; carriers; confidentiality; cystic fibrosis; disclosure; dissent; fathers; *females; genetic counseling; genetic disorders; genetic screening; *genetic services; *genetics; genome mapping; *justice; males; minority groups; mothers; obligations of society; pregnant women; prenatal diagnosis; sickle cell anemia; single persons; spousal consent; *women's rights; ELSI-funded publication; incidental findings

Mehlman, Maxwell J.; Botkin, Jeffrey R. Access to the Genome: The Challenge to Equality. Washington, DC: Georgetown University Press; 1998. 152 p. 231 fn. ISBN 0–87840–678–6. BE57386.

carriers; communitarianism; disclosure; economics; employment; eugenics; gene pool; gene therapy; genetic counseling; genetic disorders; genetic enhancement; genetic information; *genetic intervention; genetic predisposition; genetic screening; *genetic services; *genome mapping; germ cells; health insurance reimbursement; insurance; *justice; late-onset disorders; libertarianism; managed care programs; mandatory testing; moral policy; newborns; policy analysis; prenatal diagnosis; *public policy; *resource allocation; rights; *risks and benefits; scarcity; selection for treatment; selective abortion; social discrimination; *social impact; social worth; stigmatization; utilitarianism; ELSI-funded publication; personal financing; *Human Genome Project; Medicaid; Medicare; National Center for Human Genome Research; United States

Natowicz, Marvin R.; Ard, Catherine. The commercialization of clinical genetics: an analysis of interrelations between academic centers and for-profit clinical genetics diagnostics companies. *Journal of Genetic Counseling.* 1997 Sep; 6(3): 337–355. 60 refs. BE57247.

administrators; conflict of interest; faculty; financial support; genetic counseling; genetic research; *genetic screening; *genetic services; health personnel; *industry; investigators; professional organizations; *proprietary health facilities; social impact; statistics; survey; *trends; *universities; American Society of Human Genetics; National Academy of Sciences; United States

NIH–DOE Working Group on Ethical, Legal, and Social Implications of Human Genome Research. Task Force on Genetic Testing. Interim Principles. Issued by the Task Force, 550 N. Broadway, Suite 511, Baltimore, MD 21205; 1997 Mar 11. 42 p. 17 fn. Interim document for public comment; not to be construed as final. BE57695.

adults; advisory committees; carriers; confidentiality; conflict of interest; directive counseling; education; ethical review; evaluation; federal government; genetic counseling; genetic disorders; genetic predisposition; *genetic screening; *genetic services; health personnel; health insurance; human experimentation; industry; informed consent; laboratories; newborns; pregnant women; *public policy; quality of health care; research design; risks and benefits; selection of subjects; *standards; technical expertise; terminology; truth disclosure; diagnostic kits; quality control; *NIH–DOE Working Group on Ethical, Legal, and Social Implications (ELSI); *Task Force on Genetic Testing; United States

Sharp, David. Gene tests offered to UK public. [News]. *Lancet.* 1997 Oct 4; 350(9083): 1013. BE57345.

advisory committees; *genetic screening; *genetic services; guidelines; *home care; *industry; regulation; *diagnostic kits; *Advisory Committee on Genetic Testing (Great Britain); *Great Britain

Wertz, Dorothy C.; Reilly, Philip R. Laboratory policies and practices for the genetic testing of children: a survey of the Helix network. *American Journal of Human Genetics.* 1997 Nov; 61(5): 1163–1168. 19 refs. BE58850.

*adolescents; *age factors; autonomy; carriers; *children;

BE = bioethics accession number   fn. = footnotes   refs. = references

cystic fibrosis; Duchenne muscular dystrophy; *genetic counseling*; genetic disorders; *genetic screening; *genetic services*; guidelines; Huntington's disease; informed consent; *institutional policies; *laboratories; late-onset disorders; organizational policies; parental consent; physicians; primary health care; professional organizations; regulation; risks and benefits; statistics; survey; ELSI-funded publication; United States

Wertz, Dorothy C. Society and the not-so-new genetics: what are we afraid of? Some future predictions from a social scientist. *Journal of Contemporary Health Law and Policy.* 1997 Spring; 13(2): 299–346. 130 fn. BE56015.
 *attitudes; autonomy; codes of ethics; common good; *confidentiality; directive counseling; disabled; *disclosure; DNA fingerprinting; employment; eugenics; family members; *genetic counseling; genetic determinism; genetic disorders; *genetic enhancement; *genetic information; genetic intervention; genetic predisposition; genetic screening; *genetic services; *genetics; genome mapping; guidelines; *health personnel; indigents; industry; insurance; *international aspects; *knowledge, attitudes, practice; late-onset disorders; *physicians; prenatal diagnosis; *privacy; *public opinion; reproduction; resource allocation; *rights; risk; selective abortion; sex determination; social discrimination; *social impact; survey; *values; Human Genome Project; *United States; WHO Guidelines on Ethical Issues in Genetics

British guidelines set out standards for genetic tests. [News]. *Nature.* 1997 Oct 2; 389(6650): 427. BE55807.
 advisory committees; confidentiality; cystic fibrosis; genetic counseling; *genetic screening; *genetic services; *guidelines; *industry; public policy; *standards; voluntary programs; *Advisory Committee on Genetic Testing (Great Britain); *Great Britain

Knowing your genes. [Editorial]. *Lancet.* 1997 Oct 4; 350(9083): 969. BE57310.
 advisory committees; genetic information; *genetic screening; *genetic services; guidelines; *home care; *industry; regulation; *diagnostic kits; Advisory Committee on Genetic Testing (Great Britain); *Great Britain

GENOME MAPPING

See also GENETIC INTERVENTION, GENETIC RESEARCH, GENETIC SCREENING

Austin, Christopher P.; Tribble, Jack L. Gene patents and drug development: the perspective from Merck. *In:* Knoppers, Bartha Maria, ed. Human DNA: Law and Policy: International and Comparative Perspectives. Proceedings of the First International Conference on DNA Sampling and Human Genetic Research: Ethical, Legal, and Policy Aspects, held in Montreal, Canada, 6–8 Sep 1996. Boston, MA: Kluwer Law International; 1997: 379–383. 13 fn. ISBN 90–411–0361–9. BE58194.
 *DNA sequences; *drug industry; drugs; federal government; financial support; *genes; genetic research; genome mapping; information dissemination; *patents; private sector; public sector; risks and benefits; Merck Gene Index; *Merck Inc.; *United States

Bonn, Dorothy. Genome directory causes controversy. [News]. *Lancet.* 1995 Sep 30; 346(8979): 893. BE56136.
 *DNA data banks; *DNA sequences; *drug industry; *editorial policies; *genome mapping; *information dissemination; international aspects; interprofessional relations; investigators; private sector; property rights; Human Genome Sciences Inc.; *Institute for Genomic Research; Maddox, John; *Nature; SmithKline Beecham; United States; Venter, Craig

Brockett, Patrick L.; Tankersley, E. Susan. The genetics revolution, economics, ethics, and insurance. *Journal of Business Ethics.* 1997 Nov; 16(15): 1661–1676. 13 refs. 6 fn. BE58890.
 age factors; confidentiality; disclosure; *economics; employment; federal government; *genetic information; *genetic screening; *genome mapping; government regulation; health insurance; industry; *insurance; *insurance selection bias; justice; legal rights; legislation; life insurance; medical records; privacy; *public policy; *risk; risks and benefits; *social discrimination; social impact; state government; traffic accidents; Americans with Disabilities Act 1990; Human Genome Privacy Act (1991 bill); *United States

Caplan, Arthur L. The Human Genome Project and the future of health care. [Book review essay]. *Journal of Legal Medicine.* 1997 Dec; 18(4): 547–551. BE58668.
 cloning; employment; genetic information; genetic intervention; genetic screening; *genome mapping; *health care delivery; health insurance; insurance selection bias; justice; risks and benefits; social discrimination; *social impact; Human Genome Project; *The Human Genome Project and the Future of Health Care (Murray, T.H.; Rothstein, M.A.; Murray, R.F. *United States

Cavalli–Sforza, L. Luca. Human genome diversity: where is the project now? *In:* Knoppers, Bartha Maria, ed. Human DNA: Law and Policy: International and Comparative Perspectives. Proceedings of the First International Conference on DNA Sampling and Human Genetic Research: Ethical, Legal, and Policy Aspects, held in Montreal, Canada, 6–8 Sep 1996. Boston, MA: Kluwer Law International; 1997: 219–227. 14 fn. ISBN 90–411–0361–9. BE58179.
 anthropology; DNA data banks; eugenics; evolution; *genetic diversity; genetic screening; *genome mapping; *international aspects; *population genetics; *Human Genome Diversity Project; Human Genome Project

Cho, Mildred K.; Merz, Jon F. Patients and patents. [Letter]. *Nature.* 1997 Nov 20; 390(6657): 221. BE58265.
 *DNA sequences; economics; genetic services; *genome mapping; government financing; industry; *patents; public sector; universities; United States

Collins, Francis S. The Human Genome Project. *In:* Kilner, John F.; Pentz, Rebecca D.; Young, Frank E., eds. Genetic Ethics: Do the Ends Justify the Genes? Grand Rapids, MI: W.B. Eerdmans; 1997: 95–103. 23 fn. ISBN 0–8028–4428–6. BE56717.
 breast cancer; *Christian ethics; cystic fibrosis; disclosure; genetic information; genetic predisposition; genetic screening; *genome mapping; *risks and benefits; social discrimination

Cook–Deegan, Robert Mullan. Confidentiality, collective resources, and commercial genomics. *In:* Rothstein, Mark A., ed. Genetic Secrets: Protecting Privacy and Confidentiality in the Genetic Era. New Haven, CT: Yale University Press; 1997: 161–183. 32 fn. ISBN 0–300–07251–1. BE58681.
 *confidentiality; conflict of interest; dementia; disclosure; DNA data banks; donors; *drug industry; family members; *financial support; genes; *genetic information; *genetic research; *genome mapping; government financing; government regulation; *industry; information dissemination; informed consent; investigators; legal aspects; patents; private sector; public sector; regulation; *research subjects; tissue donation; universities; biological specimen banks; pedigree studies; United States

Deepandung, Attajinda; Noonpakdee, Wilai T. The moral status of the human genome. *In:* Agius, Emmanuel;

Busuttil, Salvino, eds. Germ–Line Intervention and Our Responsibilities to Future Generations. Boston, MA: Kluwer Academic; 1998: 13–18. 9 refs. ISBN 0–7923–4828–1. BE57876.

> confidentiality; future generations; *gene therapy; genetic counseling; genetic information; genetic research; *genetic screening; *genome mapping; human experimentation; moral obligations; obligations of society; privacy; public policy; resource allocation; risks and benefits; Thailand

de Witte, Joke I.; ten Have, Henk. Ownership of genetic material and information. *Social Science and Medicine.* 1997 Jul; 45(1): 51–60. 32 refs. BE58152.

> *autonomy; body parts and fluids; common good; DNA sequences; *donors; family members; genes; genetic counseling; *genetic information; *genetic materials; genetic screening; genome mapping; gifts; *human body; organ donation; patents; privacy; *property rights; remuneration; tissue donation; Bentham, Jeremy; Human Genome Project; Kant, Immanuel; Locke, John; Nozick, Robert

As a result of the International Human Genome Project genetic information is rapidly multiplying. To avoid some of the problems regarding the availability and use of genetic information, it is sometimes suggested to apply the concept of ownership. This article focuses on the clarification of the status of genetic material and genetic information, obtained as a result of screening and counseling of individual patients. First, some philosophical theories of ownership are examined for a justification of the use of the concept of ownership with regard to the human body. Next, arguments with regard to ownership of the human body are examined. The results of this analysis are applied to genetic material and genetic information.

Dickson, David; Wadman, Meredith. Genome effort 'still in need of support.' [News]. *Nature.* 1998 May 21; 393(6682): 201. Includes inset article by D. Dickson, "British finding boost is Wellcome news." BE58205.

> DNA sequences; federal government; *financial support; *genome mapping; *government financing; industry; *private sector; *public sector; Great Britain; *Human Genome Project; Institute for Genomic Research; Perkin–Elmer Corp.; *United States; Venter, Craig; Wellcome Trust

Doll, John J. The patenting of DNA. *Science.* 1998 May 1; 280(5364): 689–690. 9 refs. BE58035.

> *DNA sequences; federal government; genetic research; *genome mapping; industry; legal aspects; *patents; Patent and Trademark Office; United States

Eisenberg, Rebecca S. Genomic patents and product development incentives. *In:* Knoppers, Bartha Maria, ed. Human DNA: Law and Policy: International and Comparative Perspectives. Proceedings of the First International Conference on DNA Sampling and Human Genetic Research: Ethical, Legal, and Policy Aspects, held in Montreal, Canada, 6–8 Sep 1996. Boston, MA: Kluwer Law International; 1997: 373–378. 5 fn. ISBN 90–411–0361–9. BE58193.

> *DNA sequences; federal government; *genome mapping; government financing; *incentives; *industry; *patents; private sector; *public policy; public sector; National Center for Human Genome Research; *United States

Galloux, Jean–Christophe. The patentability of the human genome: a European perspective. *In:* Knoppers, Bartha Maria, ed. Human DNA: Law and Policy: International and Comparative Perspectives. Proceedings of the First International Conference on DNA Sampling and Human Genetic Research: Ethical, Legal, and Policy Aspects, held in Montreal, Canada,

6–8 Sep 1996. Boston, MA: Kluwer Law International; 1997: 361–371. 20 fn. ISBN 90–411–0361–9. BE58192.

> advisory committees; *DNA sequences; genes; *genome mapping; international aspects; *legal aspects; *patents; property rights; transgenic animals; *Europe; European Patent Convention; European Patent Office

Gibbons, Ann. Which of our genes makes us human? [News]. *Science.* 1998 Sep 4; 281(5382): 1432–1434. BE58976.

> DNA sequences; *genes; *genome mapping; *human characteristics; *primates

Greely, Henry T. The ethics of the Human Genome Diversity Project: the North American Regional Committee's proposed model ethical protocol. *In:* Knoppers, Bartha Maria, ed. Human DNA: Law and Policy: International and Comparative Perspectives. Proceedings of the First International Conference on DNA Sampling and Human Genetic Research: Ethical, Legal, and Policy Aspects, held in Montreal, Canada, 6–8 Sep 1996. Boston, MA: Kluwer Law International; 1997: 239–256. 33 fn. ISBN 90–411–0361–9. BE58181.

> anthropology; developing countries; ethical review; *genetic diversity; genetic materials; *genetic research; *genome mapping; *guidelines; industry; informed consent; *international aspects; investigators; legal aspects; minority groups; patents; property rights; public participation; remuneration; *population genetics; *Human Genome Diversity Project; Human Genome Organization (HUGO); North America

Greely, Henry T. The Human Genome Diversity Project: ethical, legal, and social issues. *In:* Peters, Ted, ed. Genetics: Issues of Social Justice. Cleveland, OH: Pilgrim Press; 1998: 71–81. 9 fn. ISBN 0–8298–1251–2. BE57475.

> confidentiality; costs and benefits; developing countries; DNA data banks; *genetic diversity; genetic information; *genetic research; *genome mapping; informed consent; *international aspects; minority groups; property rights; public participation; risks and benefits; social discrimination; community consent; *population genetics; *Human Genome Diversity Project

Hedgecoe, Adam M. Genome analysis. *In:* Chadwick, Ruth, ed. Encyclopedia of Applied Ethics, Volume 2. San Diego, CA: Academic Press; 1998: 463–470. 6 refs. ISBN 0–12–227067–3. BE56393.

> developing countries; DNA sequences; economics; financial support; genetic diversity; genetic materials; genetic research; *genome mapping; guidelines; industry; information dissemination; informed consent; *international aspects; investigators; metaphor; minority groups; patents; property rights; public policy; resource allocation; risks and benefits; science; social discrimination; terminology; population genetics; Declaration on the Protection of the Human Genome and Human Rights; Human Genome Diversity Project; Human Genome Project; Unesco

Hefner, Philip. Determinism, freedom, and moral failure. *Dialog: A Journal of Theology.* 1994 Winter; 33(1): 23–29. 10 fn. BE57534.

> *behavioral genetics; *Christian ethics; evolution; *freedom; *genetic determinism; *genetic intervention; genetics; *genome mapping; *human characteristics; *theology; ELSI–funded publication

Heller, Michael A.; Eisenberg, Rebecca S. Can patents deter innovation? The anticommons in biomedical research. *Science.* 1998 May 1; 280(5364): 698–701. 40 fn. BE58036.

> *biomedical research; DNA sequences; drug industry; economics; *genome mapping; industry; legal aspects;

BE = bioethics accession number   fn. = footnotes   refs. = references

*patents; private sector; *property rights; public sector; *social impact; United States

The "tragedy of the commons" metaphor helps explain why people overuse shared resources. However, the recent proliferation of intellectual property rights in biomedical research suggests a different tragedy, an "anticommons" in which people underuse scarce resources because too many owners can block each other. Privatization of biomedical research must be more carefully deployed to sustain both upstream research and downstream product development. Otherwise, more intellectual property rights may lead paradoxically to fewer useful products for improving human health.

Heyd, David. *Human Genome Research and the Challenge of Contingent Future Persons: Toward an Impersonal Theocentric Approach to Value*, by Jan Christian Heller. [Book review essay]. *Bioethics.* 1998 Apr; 12(2): 173–176. BE58627.
> Christian ethics; decision making; economics; *future generations; *genetic intervention; *genome mapping; moral policy; reproduction; social impact; teleological ethics; *theology; *values; Human Genome Project; *Human Genome Research and the Challenge of Contingent Future Persons (Heller, J.C.)

Hood, Leroy; Rowen, Lee. Genes, genomes, and society. *In:* Rothstein, Mark A., ed. Genetic Secrets: Protecting Privacy and Confidentiality in the Genetic Era. New Haven, CT: Yale University Press; 1997: 3–30. 19 fn. ISBN 0-300-07251-1. BE58673.
> biology; confidentiality; genetic determinism; genetic information; genetic intervention; genetic screening; genetics; *genome mapping; information dissemination; medicine; privacy; science; social impact; values; Human Genome Project

Human Genome Organization. HUGO Statement on Patenting Issues Related to Early Release of Raw Sequence Data. London: HUGO; 1997 May. 2 p. Statement prepared by the Intellectual Property Rights Committee and approved by the Council of HUGO, 1997 May. BE58133.
> *DNA sequences; *genes; *genome mapping; information dissemination; *international aspects; legal aspects; *organizational policies; *patents; property rights; public policy; Europe; *Human Genome Organization (HUGO); United States

Juengst, Eric T. Respecting human subjects in genome research: a preliminary policy agenda. *In:* Vanderpool, Harold Y., ed. The Ethics of Research Involving Human Subjects: Facing the 21st Century. Frederick, MD: University Publishing Group; 1996: 401–429. 74 fn. ISBN 1-55572-036-6. BE56995.
> children; *confidentiality; *disclosure; employment; *family members; genetic information; genetic materials; genetic predisposition; *genetic research; *genome mapping; *informed consent; insurance; international aspects; mentally ill; minority groups; privacy; property rights; public policy; research subjects; *risks and benefits; *selection of subjects; stigmatization; truth disclosure; *pedigree studies; Human Genome Project; United States

Kaiser, Jocelyn. UNESCO drafts bioethics declaration. [News]. *Science.* 1997 Oct 3; 278(5335): 23. BE56412.
> cloning; *genetic intervention; genetic research; *genome mapping; *human rights; *international aspects; patents; *Unesco; United States; Universal Declaration of Human Rights; *Universal Declaration on the Human Genome and Human Rights

Lebacqz, Karen. Fair shares: is the genome project just?

In: Peters, Ted, ed. Genetics: Issues of Social Justice. Cleveland, OH: Pilgrim Press; 1998: 82–107. 86 fn. ISBN 0-8298-1251-2. BE57476.
> costs and benefits; developing countries; economics; *financial support; genetic intervention; genetic research; *genome mapping; government financing; *industry; information dissemination; *international aspects; *justice; patents; philosophy; *risks and benefits; universities; *Human Genome Project; Japan; *United States

Lock, Margaret. The Human Genome Diversity Project: a perspective from cultural anthropolgy. *In:* Knoppers, Bartha Maria, ed. Human DNA: Law and Policy: International and Comparative Perspectives. Proceedings of the First International Conference on DNA Sampling and Human Genetic Research: Ethical, Legal, and Policy Aspects, held in Montreal, Canada, 6–8 Sep 1996. Boston, MA: Kluwer Law International; 1997: 229–237. 16 fn. ISBN 90-411-0361-9. BE58180.
> *anthropology; blood specimen collection; cultural pluralism; *genetic diversity; genetic materials; genetic predisposition; *genetic research; *genome mapping; goals; informed consent; *international aspects; *minority groups; patents; politics; property rights; social discrimination; social impact; *population genetics; *Human Genome Diversity Project

Luther, Lori; Hirtle, Marie. Genetic diversity -- a clash of world views? *In:* Knoppers, Bartha Maria, ed. Human DNA: Law and Policy: International and Comparative Perspectives. Proceedings of the First International Conference on DNA Sampling and Human Genetic Research: Ethical, Legal, and Policy Aspects, held in Montreal, Canada, 6–8 Sep 1996. Boston, MA: Kluwer Law International; 1997: 275–280. 11 fn. ISBN 90-411-0361-9. BE58184.
> blood specimen collection; economics; *genetic diversity; *genetic research; *genome mapping; informed consent; *international aspects; minority groups; public participation; selection of subjects; social discrimination; values; *population genetics; *Human Genome Diversity Project

McCarthy, Michael. US panel urges caution in study of human genetic differences. [News]. *Lancet.* 1997 Nov 1; 350(9087): 1306. BE57343.
> confidentiality; DNA data banks; donors; evolution; *genetic diversity; genetic research; *genome mapping; informed consent; *international aspects; Evaluating Human Genetic Diversity (National Research Council); *Human Genome Diversity Project; National Research Council; United States

Macer, Darryl R.J. Bioethics and genetic diversity from the perspective of UNESCO and non-governmental organizations. *In:* Knoppers, Bartha Maria, ed. Human DNA: Law and Policy: International and Comparative Perspectives. Proceedings of the First International Conference on DNA Sampling and Human Genetic Research: Ethical, Legal, and Policy Aspects, held in Montreal, Canada, 6–8 Sep 1996. Boston, MA: Kluwer Law International; 1997: 265–273. 15 fn. ISBN 90-411-0361-9. BE58183.
> advisory committees; bioethics; confidentiality; DNA data banks; eugenics; *genetic diversity; genetic materials; *genetic research; genetic screening; *genome mapping; guidelines; informed consent; *international aspects; investigators; minority groups; *population genetics; *Human Genome Diversity Project; Human Genome Organization; International Bioethics Committee (Unesco); *Unesco

Mahowald, Mary B. An overview of the Human Genome Project and its implications for women. *Women's Health Issues.* 1997 Jul-Aug; 7(4): 206–208. 5 refs. BE55726.
> females; genetic disorders; *genome mapping; males; social

BE = bioethics accession number   fn. = footnotes   refs. = references

impact; *women's health; ELSI–funded publication

Marshall, Eliot; Pennisi, Elizabeth. Hubris and the human genome. [News]. *Science.* 1998 May 15; 280(5366): 994–995. Includes inset article by R.F. Service, "Picking up the pace of sequencing," p. 995. BE58059.
> attitudes; *DNA sequences; federal government; *genome mapping; *industry; investigators; methods; patents; time factors; Human Genome Project; *Perkin–Elmer Corp.; United States; *Venter, Craig

Marshall, Eliot. 'Playing chicken' over gene markers. [News]. *Science.* 1997 Dec 19; 278(5346): 2046–2048. BE57313.
> blood specimen collection; confidentiality; *DNA data banks; *DNA sequences; donors; federal government; *genetic diversity; genetic information; *genetic research; *genome mapping; government financing; industry; *information dissemination; informed consent; patents; private sector; property rights; *public sector; time factors; *National Institutes of Health; *United States

Marshall, Eliot. Whose DNA is it, anyway? [News]. *Science.* 1997 Oct 24; 278(5338): 564–567. Includes two inset articles by E. Marshall, "Gene prospecting in remote populations," p. 565, and "Tapping Iceland's DNA," p. 566. Correction appears in *Science* 1997 Nov 28; 278(5343): 1551. BE57314.
> attitudes; confidentiality; *DNA data banks; *DNA sequences; federal government; financial support; genes; genetic disorders; genetic information; *genetic materials; *genetic research; *genome mapping; industry; *information dissemination; international aspects; investigators; patents; private sector; property rights; public sector; time factors; cell lines; deCode Genetics, Inc.; Iceland; National Institutes of Health; Stefansson, Kari; United States

Mehlman, Maxwell J.; Botkin, Jeffrey R. Access to the Genome: The Challenge to Equality. Washington, DC: Georgetown University Press; 1998. 152 p. 231 fn. ISBN 0–87840–678–6. BE57386.
> carriers; communitarianism; disclosure; economics; employment; eugenics; gene pool; gene therapy; genetic counseling; genetic disorders; genetic enhancement; genetic information; *genetic intervention; genetic predisposition; genetic screening; *genetic services; *genome mapping; germ cells; health insurance reimbursement; insurance; *justice; late–onset disorders; libertarianism; managed care programs; mandatory testing; moral policy; newborns; policy analysis; prenatal diagnosis; *public policy; *resource allocation; rights; *risks and benefits; scarcity; selection for treatment; selective abortion; social discrimination; *social impact; social worth; stigmatization; utilitarianism; ELSI–funded publication; personal financing; *Human Genome Project; Medicaid; Medicare; National Center for Human Genome Research; United States

Pennisi, Elizabeth. NRC OKs long–delayed survey of human genome diversity. [News]. *Science.* 1997 Oct 24; 278(5338): 568. BE57317.
> anthropology; confidentiality; DNA data banks; donors; ethical review; evolution; financial support; *genetic diversity; genetic research; *genome mapping; goals; *international aspects; privacy; risks and benefits; Evaluating Human Genetic Diversity (National Research Council); *Human Genome Diversity Project; National Institutes of Health; National Research Council; National Science Foundation; United States

Peters, Ted, ed. Genetics: Issues of Social Justice. Cleveland, OH: Pilgrim Press; 1998. 262 p. (The pilgrim library of ethics). 659 fn. ISBN 0–8298–1251–2. BE57474.
> behavioral genetics; Christian ethics; cloning; confidentiality; disadvantaged; eugenics; evolution; gene therapy; genetic determinism; genetic diversity; genetic information; *genetic

intervention; genetic materials; genetic research; genetic screening; *genetics; *genome mapping; germ cells; health insurance; international aspects; Jewish ethics; *justice; normality; patents; privacy; religious ethics; review; risks and benefits; selective abortion; social discrimination; *social impact; stigmatization; Human Genome Diversity Project; Human Genome Project; United States

Salgo, Reinhold C. Patenting the human genome. *Bulletin of Medical Ethics.* 1997 Jan; No. 124: 15–16. BE55747.
> DNA sequences; *genetic materials; *genome mapping; legal aspects; *patents; transgenic organisms; Europe; European Patent Convention; European Patent Office

Shinn, Roger Lincoln. The New Genetics: Challenges for Science, Faith, and Politics. Wakefield, RI: Moyer Bell; distributed in North America by Publishers Group West, Emeryville, CA; 1996. 175 p. Bibliography: p. 159–170. ISBN 1–55921–171–7. BE56094.
> behavioral genetics; cultural pluralism; decision making; ethics; eugenics; freedom; future generations; *gene therapy; genetic determinism; genetic diversity; *genetic intervention; genetic screening; *genetics; *genome mapping; *germ cells; health; intelligence; investigators; morality; normality; political activity; politics; prenatal diagnosis; *public policy; religion; risks and benefits; science; *social impact; theology; *values; *Human Genome Project; NIH–DOE Working Group on Ethical, Legal, and Social Implications (ELSI); United States

Stephenson, Joan. Private venture galvanizes public effort on Human Genome Project. [News]. *JAMA.* 1998 Jun 24; 279(24): 1933, 1935. BE58430.
> DNA sequences; genetic research; *genome mapping; government financing; *industry; information dissemination; international aspects; methods; *private sector; *public policy; *public sector; time factors; *Human Genome Project; Perkin–Elmer Corp.; United States; Venter, Craig

U.S. National Center for Human Genome Research. ELSI 1990–1995: A Review of the Ethical, Legal, and Social Implications Research Program and Related Activities. Bethesda, MD: U.S. National Center for Human Genome Research; 1996 Apr 12. 17 p. 10 refs. BE59047.
> cancer; cystic fibrosis; education; ethical review; federal government; genetic disorders; genetic information; genetic predisposition; *genetic screening; genetic services; *genome mapping; goals; government financing; government regulation; health insurance; health personnel; information dissemination; informed consent; law enforcement; minority groups; privacy; *program descriptions; *public policy; social discrimination; ELSI–funded publication; Human Genome Project; *NCHGR Program on Ethical, Legal, and Social Implications (ELSI); *United States

Verma, Ishwar C. Ethical concerns in genome diversity studies in developing countries. *In:* Knoppers, Bartha Maria, ed. Human DNA: Law and Policy: International and Comparative Perspectives. Proceedings of the First International Conference on DNA Sampling and Human Genetic Research: Ethical, Legal, and Policy Aspects, held in Montreal, Canada, 6–8 Sep 1996. Boston, MA: Kluwer Law International; 1997: 257–263. 14 fn. ISBN 90–411–0361–9. BE58182.
> blood specimen collection; confidentiality; consent forms; *developing countries; *genetic diversity; *genetic research; *genome mapping; incentives; informed consent; *international aspects; investigators; minority groups; moral obligations; remuneration; research ethics committees; social impact; population genetics; *Human Genome Diversity Project; *India

Wadman, Meredith. Company aims to beat NIH human genome efforts. [News]. *Nature.* 1998 May 14; 393(6681):

BE = bioethics accession number   fn. = footnotes   refs. = references

101. BE58266.
    DNA data banks; economics; federal government; financial support; *genome mapping; *industry; *private sector; public sector; time factors; Human Genome Project; National Institutes of Health; United States; Venter, Craig

Wadman, Meredith. Gene marker database stirs up debate. [News]. *Nature.* 1998 Feb 19; 391(6669): 726. BE58074.
    cancer; *DNA data banks; *genetic diversity; *genome mapping; international aspects; *minority groups; research institutes; *genetic markers; *Centre d'Etude du Polymorphisme Humain (CEPH); France; *National Cancer Institute; National Human Genome Research Institute; United States

Wadman, Meredith. Genome panel defends researchers' -- and families' -- interests. [News]. *Nature.* 1998 Feb 26; 391(6670): 826. BE58072.
    advisory committees; *confidentiality; *disclosure; DNA data banks; family members; *genetic information; *genetic research; *genome mapping; informed consent; *international aspects; investigators; medical records; *privacy; tissue banks; *Human Genome Organization (HUGO)

Walters, LeRoy, ed. Ethical issues in human genetics. *In:* Jonsen, Albert R.; Veatch, Robert M.; Walters, LeRoy, eds. Source Book in Bioethics: A Documentary History. Washington, DC: Georgetown University Press; 1998: 253–333. 40 refs. ISBN 0–87840–683–2. BE57892.
    advisory committees; carriers; federal government; *gene therapy; genetic counseling; genetic disorders; *genetic intervention; genetic research; *genetic screening; genetic services; *genome mapping; germ cells; guidelines; historical aspects; industry; international aspects; legal aspects; mass screening; moral policy; newborns; prenatal diagnosis; public policy; recombinant DNA research; resource allocation; universities; *Committee for the Study of Inborn Errors of Metabolism; Council of Europe; Declaration of Inuyama; European Medical Research Councils; *NIH Guidelines; *Office of Technology Assessment; *President's Commission for the Study of Ethical Problems; Recombinant DNA Advisory Committee; *Twentieth Century; *United States

Zimbelman, Joel. Technology assessment, ethics and public policy in biotechnology: the case of the Human Genome Project. *In:* Becker, Gerhold K., ed. Changing Nature's Course: The Ethical Challenge of Biotechnology. Hong Kong: Hong Kong University Press; 1996: 85–108. 97 refs. 51 fn. ISBN 962–209–403–1. BE56707.
    common good; confidentiality; education; freedom; genetic information; genetic screening; *genome mapping; government regulation; justice; private sector; *public policy; risks and benefits; social impact; *technology assessment; *Human Genome Project; United States

Zoloth–Dorfman, Laurie. Mapping the normal human self: the Jew and the mark of otherness. *In:* Peters, Ted, ed. Genetics: Issues of Social Justice. Cleveland, OH: Pilgrim Press; 1998: 180–202. 60 fn. ISBN 0–8298–1251–2. BE57479.
    aliens; blacks; cosmetic surgery; *disease; *eugenics; genetic disorders; genetic diversity; genetic intervention; genetic research; genetic screening; *genome mapping; historical aspects; *human body; intelligence; *Jewish ethics; *Jews; justice; medicine; *normality; public policy; *risks and benefits; science; sexuality; social discrimination; *stigmatization; theology; emigration and immigration; population genetics; Europe; Human Genome Project; Nineteenth Century; Twentieth Century; United States

A challenge to genetic transparency. [Editorial]. *Nature.* 1998 May 21; 393(6682): 195. BE58032.
    financial support; *genome mapping; government financing;

*industry; *private sector; *public sector; time factors; *Human Genome Project; United States

New US regulatory framework emerges for genetics. [News]. *Nature Biotechnology.* 1997 Apr; 15(4): 300. BE55967.
    *advisory committees; federal government; *genome mapping; government regulation; *public policy; *Advisory Committee on Genetics and Public Policy; National Human Genome Research Institute; NIH–DOE Working Group on Ethical, Legal, and Social Implications (ELSI); *United States

HEALTH

See also MENTAL HEALTH, OCCUPATIONAL HEALTH, PUBLIC HEALTH

Alcalá, Maria José; Family Care International. Commitments to Sexual and Reproductive Health and Rights for All: Framework for Action. New York, NY: Family Care International; 1995. 64 p. 3 fn. Based on relevant international agreements and conventions, including the Beijing, Copenhagen, Cairo, and Vienna conferences. BE56148.
    abortion, induced; adolescents; AIDS; autonomy; biomedical research; children; family planning; females; goals; *health; health care; health education; health services research; *human rights; indigents; *international aspects; justice; legal aspects; males; pregnant women; *public policy; quality of health care; regulation; *reproduction; resource allocation; *sexuality; sexually transmitted diseases; social discrimination; socioeconomic factors; standards; violence; voluntary programs; *women's health; *women's health services; *women's rights; *health planning; United Nations

Bhopal, Raj. Spectre of racism in health and health care: lessons from history and the United States. *BMJ (British Medical Journal).* 1998 Jun 27; 316(7149): 1970–1973. 62 refs. BE58812.
    biomedical technologies; *blacks; comparative studies; diagnosis; eugenics; *health; *health care; health education; health services research; heart diseases; historical aspects; investigators; *minority groups; morbidity; paternalism; patient care; physician patient relationship; physicians; preventive medicine; public policy; quality of health care; selection for treatment; *social discrimination; *social dominance; socioeconomic factors; surgery; trust; values; *whites; Europe; Great Britain; Nineteenth Century; Twentieth Century; *United States

Bram, Anthony D. The physically ill or dying psychotherapist: a review of ethical and clinical considerations. *Psychotherapy.* 1995 Winter; 32(4): 568–580. 34 refs. BE56023.
    attitudes to death; beneficence; codes of ethics; confidentiality; *disclosure; emotions; empirical research; guidelines; *health; *health personnel; patient care; patient transfer; patients; professional competence; *professional ethics; professional organizations; *professional patient relationship; psychology; *psychotherapy; referral and consultation; risks and benefits; *terminally ill; patient abandonment; patient care planning; professional impairment; *seriously ill; American Psychological Association

Brandt, Allan M.; Rozin, Paul. Morality and Health. New York, NY: Routledge; 1997. 416 p. Includes references. ISBN 0–415–91582–1. BE55841.
    adolescents; advertising; alcohol abuse; attitudes; behavior control; childbirth; communicable diseases; cultural pluralism; disadvantaged; disease; drug abuse; food; freedom; government regulation; *health; *health promotion; historical aspects; international aspects; mass media;

metaphor; *morality; nutrition; *public health; public policy; religion; secularism; *self induced illness; sexuality; single persons; smoking; social problems; socioeconomic factors; stigmatization; suffering; life style; tuberculosis; China; Great Britain; India; Nineteenth Century; Twentieth Century; United States

Calman, Kenneth C. Equity, poverty and health for all. *BMJ (British Medical Journal).* 1997 Apr 19; 314(7088): 1187–1191. 8 refs. BE56859.
  *economics; *health; health care; *health care delivery; *indigents; international aspects; justice; public health; public policy; quality of life; *resource allocation; socioeconomic factors; Great Britain; National Health Service; World Health Organization

Cassel, Christine K. Policy implications of the Human Genome Project for women. *Women's Health Issues.* 1997 Jul–Aug; 7(4): 225–229. 10 refs. BE55710.
  confidentiality; disabled; *females; genetic counseling; genetic disorders; genetic research; genetic screening; *genetic services; genome mapping; government financing; health care reform; health insurance; indigents; insurance selection bias; minority groups; patient care; pregnant women; prenatal diagnosis; public policy; risks and benefits; selective abortion; sex determination; social impact; stigmatization; *women's health; *women's health services; ELSI-funded publication; Medicaid; United States

De Koninck, Maria. Reflections on the transfer of "progress": the case of reproduction. *In:* Sherwin, Susan, et al. The Politics of Women's Health: Exploring Agency and Autonomy. Philadelphia, PA: Temple University Press; 1998: 150–177. 14 fn. ISBN 1–56639–633–6. BE58397.
  attitudes to death; cesarean section; childbirth; *developing countries; emergency care; family planning; *females; health personnel; indigents; international aspects; *mortality; nurse midwives; obstetrics and gynecology; patient care; physicians; *pregnant women; professional patient relationship; *reproduction; risk; *socioeconomic factors; *women's health; *women's health services; technology transfer; *Benin

Edgar, A. Health care allocation, public consultation and the concept of 'health'. *Health Care Analysis.* 1998 Sep; 6(3): 193–198. 10 refs. BE58980.
  autonomy; commodification; democracy; economics; *health; *health care; *health care delivery; health insurance; health promotion; humanism; justice; libertarianism; managed care programs; *moral policy; obligations of society; public participation; *public policy; *resource allocation; self induced illness; state medicine; values; Great Britain; National Health Service; Oregon; United States

Edgar, Andrew. Quality of life indicators. *In:* Chadwick, Ruth, ed. Encyclopedia of Applied Ethics, Volume 3. San Diego, CA: Academic Press; 1998: 759–776. 16 refs. ISBN 0–12–227068–1. BE56268.
  aged; contracts; costs and benefits; decision making; disabled; *evaluation; *health; health care; health services research; patient participation; physicians; prognosis; public participation; public policy; *quality adjusted life years; *quality of life; *resource allocation; social discrimination; *treatment outcome; utilitarianism; values; severity of illness index; Great Britain

Gallagher, Hugh Gregory. FDR's Splendid Deception: The Moving Story of Roosevelt's Massive Disability –– and the Intense Efforts to Conceal It from the Public. Revised Edition. Arlington, VA: Vandamere Press; 1994. 242 p. Bibliography: p. 230–236. First edition published in 1985 by Dodd, Mead. ISBN 0–918339–33–2. BE56098.
  attitudes; *confidentiality; *deception; disclosure; emotions; *famous persons; *health; historical aspects; mass media;

*physically disabled; physicians; *politics; rehabilitation; *Roosevelt, Franklin; Twentieth Century; United States

Hagihara, Akihito; Murakami, Masayoshi; Miller, Alan S., et al. Association between attitudes toward health promotion and opinions regarding organ transplants in Japan. *Health Policy.* 1997 Nov; 42(2): 157–170. 30 refs. BE57982.
  *attitudes; *health promotion; *organ transplantation; preventive medicine; *public opinion; resource allocation; *self induced illness; survey; transplant recipients; *Japan

Keville, Terri D. The invisible woman: gender bias in medical research. *Women's Rights Law Reporter.* 1994; 15: 123–142. 209 fn. BE56661.
  biomedical research; biomedical technologies; cancer; coercion; contraception; diagnosis; employment; federal government; *females; fetuses; government regulation; health hazards; health insurance; heart diseases; historical aspects; *human experimentation; *investigators; justice; *legal aspects; males; obstetrics and gynecology; occupational exposure; patient care; pregnant women; prenatal injuries; *public policy; research design; *research subjects; *selection of subjects; *social discrimination; treatment refusal; *women's health; International Union, UAW v. Johnson Controls, Inc.; National Institutes of Health; Office of Research on Women's Health; *United States; Women's Health Equity Act 1991

Kopelman, Loretta M. Female circumcision and genital mutilation. *In:* Chadwick, Ruth, ed. Encyclopedia of Applied Ethics, Volume 2. San Diego, CA: Academic Press; 1998: 249–259. 16 refs. ISBN 0–12–227067–3. BE56383.
  anthropology; *circumcision; *cultural pluralism; *ethical relativism; *females; health hazards; human rights; international aspects; morality; risks and benefits; values; women's health

Kopelman, Loretta M. Medicine's challenge to relativism: the case of female genital mutilation. *In:* Carson, Ronald A.; Burns, Chester R., eds. Philosophy of Medicine and Bioethics: A Twenty-Year Retrospective and Critical Appraisal. Boston, MA: Kluwer Academic; 1997: 221–237. 32 refs. 9 fn. ISBN 0–7923–3545–7. BE56538.
  bioethics; case studies; children; *circumcision; *cultural pluralism; dissent; *ethical relativism; *females; goals; health; health personnel; *international aspects; medicine; methods; minority groups; *morality; morbidity; mortality; pain; physicians; refusal to treat; religion; risks and benefits; suffering; surgery; *values; *women's health; non-Western World; Western World; Africa; Middle East

Lippman, Abby. The politics of health: geneticization versus health promotion. *In:* Sherwin, Susan, et al. The Politics of Women's Health: Exploring Agency and Autonomy. Philadelphia, PA: Temple University Press; 1998: 64–82. 30 fn. ISBN 1–56639–633–6. BE58394.
  accountability; behavioral genetics; ecology; *females; *feminist ethics; *genetic determinism; genetic diversity; *genetic predisposition; *genetic screening; genetics; health; *health promotion; normality; obligations of society; *politics; prenatal diagnosis; public policy; self induced illness; social control; social discrimination; socioeconomic factors; stigmatization; *women's health; Canada

Lock, Margaret. Anomalous women and political strategies for aging societies. *In:* Sherwin, Susan, et al. The Politics of Women's Health: Exploring Agency and Autonomy. Philadelphia, PA: Temple University Press; 1998: 178–204. 3 fn. ISBN 1–56639–633–6. BE58398.
  *age factors; aged; attitudes; comparative studies; disclosure; drug industry; drugs; economics; family relationship; *females; *feminist ethics; home care; human body;

*international aspects; medicine; patient care; public policy; risks and benefits; *women's health; women's health services; estrogen replacement therapy; *menopause; *Japan; *North America

Lock, Margaret. Situating women in the politics of health. *In:* Sherwin, Susan, et al. The Politics of Women's Health: Exploring Agency and Autonomy. Philadelphia, PA: Temple University Press; 1998: 48–63. 7 fn. ISBN 1–56639–633–6. BE58393.
> American Indians; autonomy; behavior control; cultural pluralism; disease; economics; *females; *feminist ethics; *health; health care delivery; health promotion; historical aspects; males; medicine; moral obligations; obligations of society; *politics; public policy; self induced illness; social discrimination; social problems; *women's health; Confucian ethics; holistic health; self-help groups; Europe; North America

Mitchinson, Wendy. 'It's not society that's the problem, it's women's bodies': a historical view of medical treatment of women. *In:* Petersen, Kerry, ed. Intersections: Women on Law, Medicine and Technology. Brookfield, VT: Ashgate; 1997: 25–48. 84 fn. ISBN 1–85521–882–8. BE57485.
> adolescents; *attitudes; disease; *females; historical aspects; *human body; males; marital relationship; normality; *physicians; *sexuality; socioeconomic factors; *sociology of medicine; stigmatization; *women's health; menopause; Canada; Western World

Mordacci, Roberto; Sobel, Richard. Health: a comprehensive concept. *Hastings Center Report.* 1998 Jan-Feb; 28(1): 34–37. 21 fn. BE57297.
> disease; *goals; *health; *medicine; narrative ethics; physician's role; *quality of life; *self concept; socioeconomic factors; *value of life; *values; postmodernism

Health is one of those everyday words that only seems self-evident in its meaning. Physiological measurements alone fail to capture the subjective dimension of health. "Health" is an end and a means — it is a foundation for achievement, a first achievement itself, and a precondition for further achievement.

Morgan, Kathryn Pauly. Contested bodies, contested knowledges: women, health, and the politics of medicalization. *In:* Sherwin, Susan, et al. The Politics of Women's Health: Exploring Agency and Autonomy. Philadelphia, PA: Temple University Press; 1998: 83–121. 44 fn. ISBN 1–56639–633–6. BE58395.
> biomedical technologies; childbirth; disadvantaged; *females; *feminist ethics; health care; *human body; informal social control; *medicine; moral obligations; patient care; physician patient relationship; *political activity; politics; pregnant women; preventive medicine; reproduction; social dominance; technical expertise; *women's health; *women's health services; women's rights; estrogen replacement therapy; menopause

Parens, Erik. Is better always good? The enhancement project. [Project on the Prospect of Technologies Aimed at the Enhancement of Human Capacities and Traits]. *Hastings Center Report.* 1998 Jan-Feb; 28(1): S1–S17. 35 fn. BE57294.
> behavior control; *biomedical technologies; *cosmetic surgery; disabled; entrepreneurship; ethical analysis; females; *genetic enhancement; *goals; *health; *health care; health insurance reimbursement; *human characteristics; *justice; *medicine; moral complicity; *moral policy; motivation; *normality; preventive medicine; *psychoactive drugs; *public policy; resource allocation; *self concept; social control; social impact; social problems; socioeconomic factors; suffering; terminology; *values; authenticity; beauty;

*enhancement technologies; life style; Hastings Center; *Project on the Prospect of Technologies Aimed at the Enhancement of Human Capabilities and Traits; Prozac

The following essay begins to say why and when it will sometimes make sense to worry about the prospect of aiming new biotechnologies at the enhancement of human capacities and traits. It grows out of a two–year, Hastings Center project, generously funded by the National Endowment for the Humanities.

Sargent, Carolyn F.; Brettell, Caroline B., eds. Gender and Health: An International Perspective. Upper Saddle River, NJ: Prentice Hall; 1996. 370 p. Includes references. ISBN 0–13–079427–9. BE58098.
> aborted fetuses; abortion, induced; age factors; AIDS; bioethics; biomedical technologies; blacks; breast cancer; cancer; cesarean section; childbirth; cultural pluralism; developing countries; economics; ethics consultation; *females; *feminist ethics; *health; *health care; health hazards; Hispanic Americans; human body; human experimentation; *international aspects; males; medicine; occupational exposure; politics; preventive medicine; psychological stress; religion; reproduction; risk; self concept; sexuality; *socioeconomic factors; terminology; violence; *women's health; ethnographic studies; menopause; premenstrual syndrome; Africa; Japan; United States

Seedhouse, David. Health Promotion: Philosophy, Prejudice and Practice. New York, NY: Wiley; 1997. 202 p. Includes references. An accompanying handbook for teachers and lecturers is available on request. ISBN 0–471–93910–2. BE58320.
> alcohol abuse; case studies; decision making; dissent; fluoridation; goals; *health; health personnel; *health promotion; informed consent; models, theoretical; paternalism; patient compliance; philosophy; public health; public policy; quality of life; risks and benefits; self induced illness; smoking; *values

Shanner, Laura. Teaching women's health issues in a government committee: the story of a successful policy group. *Women's Health Issues.* 1997 Nov-Dec; 7(6): 393–399. 2 refs. BE57577.
> *advisory committees; committee membership; *embryo research; embryos; *females; genetic intervention; government regulation; guidelines; human experimentation; infertility; informed consent; moral obligations; organization and administration; ovum donors; preimplantation diagnosis; program descriptions; *public policy; reproductive technologies; *women's health; embryo donation; *Canada; *Discussion Group on Embryo Research (Health Canada)

Sherwin, Susan, et al. The Politics of Women's Health: Exploring Agency and Autonomy. Philadelphia, PA: Temple University Press; 1998. 321 p. 216 fn. ISBN 1–56639–633–6. BE58391.
> age factors; *autonomy; cultural pluralism; decision making; domestic violence; *females; *feminist ethics; genetic determinism; genetic predisposition; genetic screening; genetics; health care delivery; health promotion; historical aspects; human body; human experimentation; international aspects; medicine; mortality; obligations of society; patient care; physician patient relationship; political activity; politics; pregnant women; reproduction; selection of subjects; socioeconomic factors; *women's health; *women's health services; menopause; Feminist Health Care Ethics Research Network (Canada); North America

Silvers, Anita. Disability rights. *In:* Chadwick, Ruth, ed. Encyclopedia of Applied Ethics, Volume 1. San Diego, CA: Academic Press; 1998: 781–796. 20 refs. ISBN 0–12–227066–5. BE56378.
> *disabled; education; employment; health; health care; human rights; legal rights; legislation; normality; patients'

---

rights; rehabilitation; right to die; social discrimination; stigmatization; terminology; Americans with Disabilities Act 1990; Disability Discrimination Act 1995 (Great Britain); Great Britain; United States

Tsevat, Joel; Dawson, Neal V.; Wu, Albert W., et al. Health values of hospitalized patients 80 years or older. [For the HELP Investigators]. *JAMA.* 1998 Feb 4; 279(5): 371–375. 42 refs. BE57814.
*aged; *attitudes; comparative studies; depressive disorder; evaluation studies; family members; *health; hospitals; institutionalized persons; pain; palliative care; patient care; *patients; prognosis; prolongation of life; quality adjusted life years; *quality of life; resuscitation; survey; time factors; *value of life; *values; severity of illness index; Hospitalized Elderly Longitudinal Project (HELP)
CONTEXT: Health values (utilities or preferences for health states) are often incorporated into clinical decisions and health care policy when issues of quality vs length of life arise, but little is known about health values of the very old. OBJECTIVE: To assess health values of older hospitalized patients, compare their values with those of their surrogate decision makers, investigate possible determinants of health values, and determine whether health values change over time. DESIGN: A prospective, longitudinal, multicenter cohort study. SETTING: Four academic medical centers. PARTICIPANTS: Four hundred fourteen hospitalized patients aged 80 years or older and their surrogate decision makers who were interviewed and understood the task. MAIN OUTCOME MEASURES: Time–trade–off utilities, reflecting preferences for current health relative to a shorter but healthy life. RESULTS: On average, patients equated living 1 year in their current state of health with living 9.7 months in excellent health (mean [SD] utility, 0.81 [0.28]). Although only 126 patients (30.7%) rated their current quality of life as excellent or very good, 284 (68.6%) were willing to give up at most 1 month of 12 in exchange for excellent health (utility greater than or =0.92). At the other extreme, 25 (6.0%) were willing to live 2 weeks or less in excellent health rather than 1 year in their current state of health (utility less than or =0.04). Patients were willing to trade significantly less time for a healthy life than their surrogates assumed they would (mean difference, 0.05; P=.007); 61 surrogates (20.3%) underestimated the patient's time–trade–off score by 0.25 (3 months of 12) or more. Patients willing to trade less time for better health were more likely to want resuscitation and other measures to extend life. Time–trade–off score correlated only modestly with quality–of–life rating (r=0.28) and inversely with depression score (r=-0.27), but there were few other clinical or demographic predictors of health values. When patients who survived were asked the time–trade–off question again at 1 year, they were willing to trade less time for better health than at baseline (mean difference, 0.04; P=.04). CONCLUSION: Very old hospitalized patients who could be interviewed were able, in most cases, to have their health values assessed using the time–trade–off technique. Most patients were unwilling to trade much time for excellent health, but preferences varied greatly. Because proxies and multivariable analyses cannot gauge health values of elderly hospitalized patients accurately, health values of the very old should be elicited directly from the patient.

U.S. Congress. Senate. Committee on Labor and Human Resources. Women's Health: Ensuring Quality and Equity in Biomedical Research. Hearing, 29 Jun 1992. Washington, DC: U.S. Government Printing Office; 1992. 48 p. S. Hrg. 102–1180. BE58949.
*biomedical research; cancer; diagnosis; drugs; federal government; *females; government financing; heart diseases; *human experimentation; males; morbidity; mortality; patient care; *public policy; research subjects; selection of subjects; social discrimination; *women's health; ovaries; National Institutes of Health; Office of Research on Women's Health; *United States; Women's Health Initiative

Wachbroit, Robert. Health and disease, concepts of. *In:* Chadwick, Ruth, ed. Encyclopedia of Applied Ethics, Volume 2. San Diego, CA: Academic Press; 1998: 533–538. 13 refs. ISBN 0-12-227067-3. BE56394.
disabled; *disease; eugenics; genetic disorders; genetic enhancement; genetic predisposition; goals; *health; medicine; normality; paternalism; philosophy; review; terminology; values

Younger–Lewis, Catherine. Genital mutilation may raise awkward issues for MDs after birth. [News]. *Canadian Medical Association Journal.* 1997 Oct 15; 157(8): 1013. BE56583.
*childbirth; *circumcision; *cultural pluralism; decision making; ethical relativism; *females; minority groups; *patient care; *physicians; *refusal to treat; sexuality; surgery; *women's health; emigration and immigration; *Canada

HEALTH CARE

See also BIOMEDICAL TECHNOLOGIES, PATIENT CARE

Alcalá, Maria José; Family Care International. Commitments to Sexual and Reproductive Health and Rights for All: Framework for Action. New York, NY: Family Care International; 1995. 64 p. 3 fn. Based on relevant international agreements and conventions, including the Beijing, Copenhagen, Cairo, and Vienna conferences. BE56148.
abortion, induced; adolescents; AIDS; autonomy; biomedical research; children; family planning; females; goals; *health; health care; health education; health services research; *human rights; indigents; *international aspects; justice; legal aspects; males; pregnant women; *public policy; quality of health care; regulation; *reproduction; resource allocation; *sexuality; sexually transmitted diseases; social discrimination; socioeconomic factors; standards; violence; voluntary programs; *women's health; *women's health services; *women's rights; *health planning; United Nations

Alpert, Sheri A. Health care information: access, confidentiality, and good practice. *In:* Goodman, Kenneth W., ed. Ethics, Computing, and Medicine: Informatics and the Transformation of Health Care. New York, NY: Cambridge University Press; 1998: 75–101. 64 refs. ISBN 0-521-46905-8. BE57005.
*computer communication networks; *computers; *confidentiality; data banks; *disclosure; drug industry; economics; employment; genetic information; government regulation; *health care; health insurance; health services research; information dissemination; informed consent; legal aspects; *medical records; moral obligations; physician patient relationship; privacy; privileged communication; self regulation; social discrimination; standards; computer security; health data cards; United States

Anderson, James G.; Aydin, Carolyn E. Evaluating medical information systems: social contexts and ethical challenges. *In:* Goodman, Kenneth W., ed. Ethics, Computing, and Medicine: Informatics and the Transformation of Health Care. New York, NY: Cambridge University Press; 1998: 57–74. 99 refs. ISBN

0–521–46905–8. BE57004.
accountability; administrators; attitudes; computer communication networks; *computers; decision making; economics; evaluation; *health care delivery; interprofessional relations; *medical records; organization and administration; patient care; patient participation; physicians; professional autonomy; quality of health care; social impact; values; *informatics; physician's practice patterns; professional role

Asch, Adrienne. Distracted by disability. *Cambridge Quarterly of Healthcare Ethics.* 1998 Winter; 7(1): 77–87. 22 fn. BE58450.
assisted suicide; *attitudes; autonomy; bioethics; chronically ill; communication; cultural pluralism; *decision making; depressive disorder; *disabled; goals; *health care; health facilities; *health personnel; medicine; minority groups; *moral obligations; motivation; *obligations of society; *patient care; *physically disabled; physician patient relationship; physicians; quality of life; rehabilitation; *resource allocation; social discrimination; *stigmatization; treatment refusal; withholding treatment; dependency

Benatar, Solomon R. What makes a just healthcare system? Broader professional ethics, including consideration of the public interest and the common good. [Editorial]. *BMJ (British Medical Journal).* 1996 Dec 21–28; 313(7072): 1567–1568. 13 refs. BE58404.
biomedical research; common good; developing countries; federal government; freedom; *health care delivery; international aspects; *justice; managed care programs; national health insurance; private sector; professional ethics; public sector; resource allocation; retrospective moral judgment; *standards; Buchanan, Allen; *United States

Berwick, Donald; Hiatt, Howard; Janeway, Penny, et al. An ethical code for everybody in health care. [Editorial]. *BMJ (British Medical Journal).* 1997 Dec 20–27; 315(7123): 1633–1634. 1 ref. BE57554.
administrators; *codes of ethics; confidentiality; economics; *health care; health care delivery; health facilities; health personnel; information dissemination; institutional ethics; interdisciplinary communication; international aspects; managed care programs; moral obligations; physicians; *professional ethics; rights; Great Britain; National Health Service

Bhopal, Raj. Spectre of racism in health and health care: lessons from history and the United States. *BMJ (British Medical Journal).* 1998 Jun 27; 316(7149): 1970–1973. 62 refs. BE58812.
biomedical technologies; *blacks; comparative studies; diagnosis; eugenics; *health; *health care; health education; health services research; heart diseases; historical aspects; investigators; *minority groups; morbidity; paternalism; patient care; physician patient relationship; physicians; preventive medicine; public policy; quality of health care; selection for treatment; *social discrimination; *social dominance; socioeconomic factors; surgery; trust; values; *whites; Europe; Great Britain; Nineteenth Century; Twentieth Century; *United States

Boozang, Kathleen M. Deciding the fate of religious hospitals in the emerging health care market. *Houston Law Review.* 1995; 31: 1429–1516. 403 fn. BE57195.
abortion, induced; allowing to die; artificial feeding; assisted suicide; autonomy; bioethical issues; *conscience; contraception; counseling; cultural pluralism; disclosure; economics; emergency care; freedom; *government regulation; *health care delivery; health care reform; HIV seropositivity; institutional ethics; *institutional policies; *legal aspects; legal liability; moral policy; patient transfer; quality of health care; referral and consultation; *refusal to treat; religion; *religious hospitals; right to die; *Roman Catholic ethics; secularism; Supreme Court decisions; *health facility mergers; Ethical and Religious Directives

for Catholic Health Care Services; First Amendment; Religious Freedom Restoration Act 1994; *United States

Borowsky, Steven J.; Davis, Margaret K.; Goertz, Christine, et al. Are all health plans created equal? The physician's view. *JAMA.* 1997 Sep 17; 278(11): 917–921. 13 refs. BE55653.
*attitudes; comparative studies; continuing education; emergency care; *evaluation; evaluation studies; health care delivery; health education; health maintenance organizations; home care; *managed care programs; medical specialties; mental health; patient education; physician patient relationship; *physicians; preventive medicine; primary health care; *quality of health care; referral and consultation; survey; physician's practice patterns; utilization review; Minneapolis-St. Paul; Minnesota
CONTEXT: The health care market is demanding increasing amounts of information regarding quality of care in health plans. Physicians are a potentially important but infrequently used source of such information. OBJECTIVE: To assess physicians' views on health plan practices that promote or impede delivery of high-quality care in health plans and to compare ratings between plans. SETTING: Minneapolis-St Paul, Minn. PARTICIPANTS: One hundred physicians in each of 3 health plans. Each physician rated 1 health plan. MAIN OUTCOME MEASURES: Likert-type items that assessed health plan practices that promote or impede delivery of high-quality care. RESULTS: A total of 249 physicians (84%) completed the survey. Fewer than 20% of all physicians gave plans the highest rating (excellent or strongly agree) for health plan practices that promote delivery of high-quality care (such as providing continuing medical education for physicians, identifying patients needing preventive care, and providing physicians feedback about practice patterns). Barriers to delivering high-quality care related to sufficiency of time to spend with patients, covered benefits and copayment structure, and utilization management practices. Ratings differed across health plans. For example, the percentage of physicians indicating that they would recommend the plan they rated to their own family was 64% for plan 1, 92% for plan 2, and 24% for plan 3 (P less than .001 for all comparisons). CONCLUSIONS: Physician surveys can highlight strengths and weaknesses in health plans, and their ratings differ across plans. Physician ratings of health plan practices that promote or impede delivery of high-quality care may be useful to consumers and purchasers of health care as a tool to evaluate health plans and promote quality improvement.

Brett, Allan S.; Raymond, James I.; Saunders, Donald E., et al. An ethics discussion series for hospital administrators. *HEC (HealthCare Ethics Committee) Forum.* 1998 Jun; 10(2): 177–185. 13 refs. BE59065.
*administrators; *communication; ethicists; evaluation; *hospitals; *institutional ethics; *institutional policies; *interprofessional relations; *professional ethics; *program descriptions; Richland Memorial Hospital (Columbia, SC); South Carolina; University of South Carolina

Brodeur, Dennis. Redefining long-term care, personal choices and "futile care." *Journal of Long-Term Care Administration.* 1993 Fall; 21(3): 78–80. BE56018.
aged; allowing to die; autonomy; community services; disabled; financial support; food; futility; home care; *long-term care; nursing homes; patient care; patients' rights; rehabilitation; resource allocation; risk

Brody, Howard. Is there a treatment for cynicism? Expanding moral conversation from health care to the

---

BE = bioethics accession number   fn. = footnotes   refs. = references

public sphere. *Medical Humanities Review.* 1996 Fall; 10(2): 9–19. 15 fn. Paper originally presented as the Annual Faculty Oration at the Society for Health and Human Values annual meeting held in San Diego, CA, 15 Oct 1995. BE56654.
  *attitudes; clinical ethics committees; common good; *communication; communitarianism; cultural pluralism; federal government; government financing; government regulation; *health care delivery; *health care reform; justice; *politics; public opinion; public participation; public policy; trust; *values; *United States

Bynum, Terrell Ward; Fodor, John L. Medical informatics and human values. *In:* Goodman, Kenneth W., ed. Ethics, Computing, and Medicine: Informatics and the Transformation of Health Care. New York, NY: Cambridge University Press; 1998: 32–42. 21 refs. ISBN 0–521–46905–8. BE57002.
  *computers; economics; *health care; health personnel; information dissemination; patient care; patient education; professional ethics; quality of health care; *risks and benefits; values; *informatics; professional role

Callahan, Daniel. False Hopes: Why America's Quest for Perfect Health Is a Recipe for Failure. New York, NY: Simon and Schuster; 1998. 330 p. 235 fn. ISBN 0–684–81109–X. BE58541.
  aged; attitudes to death; biomedical technologies; chronically ill; common good; ecology; economics; *goals; health; *health care; *health care delivery; health care reform; health promotion; international aspects; *medicine; models, theoretical; obligations of society; obligations to society; primary health care; public health; public policy; quality of life; resource allocation; self induced illness; standards; suffering; *United States

Caplan, Arthur L. The Human Genome Project and the future of health care. [Book review essay]. *Journal of Legal Medicine.* 1997 Dec; 18(4): 547–551. BE58668.
  cloning; employment; genetic information; genetic intervention; genetic screening; *genome mapping; *health care delivery; health insurance; insurance selection bias; justice; risks and benefits; social discrimination; *social impact; Human Genome Project; *The Human Genome Project and the Future of Health Care (Murray, T.H.; Rothstein, M.A.; Murray, R.F. *United States

Cassel, Christine K. Policy implications of the Human Genome Project for women. *Women's Health Issues.* 1997 Jul–Aug; 7(4): 225–229. 10 refs. BE55710.
  confidentiality; disabled; *females; genetic counseling; genetic disorders; genetic research; genetic screening; *genetic services; genome mapping; government financing; health care reform; health insurance; indigents; insurance selection bias; minority groups; patient care; pregnant women; prenatal diagnosis; public policy; risks and benefits; selective abortion; sex determination; social impact; stigmatization; *women's health; *women's health services; ELSI-funded publication; Medicaid; United States

Chafey, Kathleen. "Caring" is not enough: ethical paradigms for community-based care. *N and HC Perspectives on Community.* 1996 Jan–Feb; 17(1): 10–15. 26 refs. BE58300.
  caring; children; community services; feminist ethics; *health care; health promotion; historical aspects; indigents; *justice; minority groups; nurse's role; nurses; *nursing ethics; *obligations of society; political activity; public health; public policy; resource allocation; social impact; social problems; socioeconomic factors; values; women's health; Nineteenth Century; Twentieth Century; *United States; Wald, Lillian

Cherry, Christopher. Health care, human worth and the limits of the particular. *Journal of Medical Ethics.* 1997

Oct; 23(5): 310–314. 10 fn. BE57103.
  common good; costs and benefits; disabled; *health care; human characteristics; *managed care programs; physician patient relationship; quality adjusted life years; quality of life; *resource allocation; social worth; speciesism; *value of life
An ethics concerned with health care developments and systems must be historically continuous, especially as it concerns the application to managed structures of key moral–epistemic concepts such as care, love and empathy. These concepts are traditionally most at home in the personal, individual domain. Human beings have non–instrumental worth just because they are human beings and not by virtue of their capacities. Managed health care systems tend to abstract from this worth in respect of both individuals' distinctness and individual identity. The first, a common feature of quantitative approaches to health care assessment and delivery, is avoidable. The second, by contrast, is necessarily sacrificed in impersonally managed structures. Failure to distinguish the two encourages confusion and distress, and the demand for impossible medico–moral relationships.

Curran, William J.; Hall, Mark A.; Bobinski, Mary Anne, et al. Health Care Law and Ethics. Fifth Edition. New York, NY: Aspen Law and Business; 1998. 1,463 p. Includes references. ISBN 1–56706–809–X. BE57442.
  abortion, induced; adults; advance directives; AIDS serodiagnosis; allowing to die; alternative therapies; assisted suicide; *bioethical issues; brain death; communicable diseases; competence; confidentiality; conflict of interest; contact tracing; contraception; decision making; determination of death; drugs; economics; futility; government regulation; *health care delivery; health facilities; health personnel; HIV seropositivity; informed consent; *legal aspects; malpractice; managed care programs; mandatory programs; mentally ill; minors; organ donation; organ transplantation; *patient care; pregnant women; prenatal injuries; professional patient relationship; public health; reproduction; reproductive technologies; right to die; standards; third party consent; treatment refusal; *United States

Davis, Anne J.; Aroskar, Mila A.; Liaschenko, Joan, et al. Policy, ethics, and health care. *In: their* Ethical Dilemmas and Nursing Practice. Fourth Edition. Stamford, CT: Appleton and Lange; 1997: 245–263. 41 fn. ISBN 0–8385–2283–1. BE58600.
  aged; biomedical research; case studies; federal government; goals; *health care; health care reform; historical aspects; indigents; justice; managed care programs; moral obligations; *nurses; obligations of society; *public policy; resource allocation; United States

Dougherty, Charles J. How to avoid flying blind: to truly improve U.S. healthcare, leaders must consider seven moral values. *Health Progress.* 1997 Mar–Apr; 78(2): 20–22. BE56448.
  caring; common good; disadvantaged; economics; *health care delivery; *health care reform; moral obligations; obligations of society; quality of health care; resource allocation; *values; dignity; United States

Dougherty, Charles J. Tradition, mission, and the market: faith in ultimate purposefulness makes Catholic healthcare different. *Health Progress.* 1997 Jul–Aug; 78(4): 44–51. BE56447.
  autonomy; commodification; cultural pluralism; disadvantaged; economics; employment; goals; health care; health care delivery; health care reform; human rights; *institutional ethics; institutional policies; public policy; *religious hospitals; *Roman Catholic ethics; standards; United States

---

Doyal, Len. Need for moral audit in evaluating quality in health care. *Quality in Health Care.* 1992 Sep; 1(3): 178–183. 25 refs. BE56406.
> autonomy; confidentiality; guidelines; health; *health care delivery; informed consent; justice; patients' rights; *quality of health care; resource allocation; selection for treatment; truth disclosure; medical audit; Great Britain; National Health Service

Edgar, A. Health care allocation, public consultation and the concept of 'health'. *Health Care Analysis.* 1998 Sep; 6(3): 193–198. 10 refs. BE58980.
> autonomy; commodification; democracy; economics; *health; *health care; *health care delivery; health insurance; health promotion; humanism; justice; libertarianism; managed care programs; *moral policy; obligations of society; public participation; *public policy; *resource allocation; self induced illness; state medicine; values; Great Britain; National Health Service; Oregon; United States

Engelhardt, H. Tristram. Holiness, virtue, and social justice: contrasting understandings of the moral life. *Christian Bioethics.* 1997 Mar; 3(1): 3–19. 25 refs. 18 fn. BE56357.
> abortion, induced; bioethical issues; bioethics; *Christian ethics; clergy; communication; *conscience; cultural pluralism; euthanasia; *health care delivery; *health personnel; historical aspects; indigents; interprofessional relations; justice; love; managed care programs; *moral obligations; morality; *religious hospitals; remuneration; *Roman Catholics; secularism; *theology; virtues; ecumenism

Being a Christian involves metaphysical, epistemological, and social commitments that set Christians at variance with the dominant secular culture. Because Christianity is not syncretical, but proclaims the unique truth of its revelations, Christians will inevitably be placed in some degree of conflict with secular health care institutions. Because being Christian involves a life of holiness, not merely living justly or morally, Christians will also be in conflict with the ethos of many contemporary Christian health care institutions which have abandoned a commitment to Christian spirituality. In this regard, managed care raises the special question of how Christian institutions can act morally under financial constraints and maintain their character while under the control of secular managers. This question itself raises the further question as to why health care institutions need even pose this query when there are Christian physicians and nurses who could work for less, or Christian men and women who could become sisters and brothers and work for nothing. Contemporary challenges to Christians to maintain their integrity in a post-Christian world have much of their force because Christians have failed to maintain traditional Christian sprituality. In the face of that failure, Christian physicians and nurses will find themselves in greater conflict with health care institutions, because few will any longer understand the requirements of traditional Christianity. In its place, they will have put a generic spirituality, a value–neutral understanding of the role of the health professional, and an anonymous commitment to social justice.

Entwistle, Vikki A.; Renfrew, Mary J.; Yearley, Steven, et al. Lay perspectives: advantages for health research. *BMJ (British Medical Journal).* 1998 Feb 7; 316(7129): 463–466. 26 refs. BE57959.
> evaluation; health care; *health services research; patient participation; politics; *public participation; research design; risks and benefits

Franks, Peter; Clancy, Carolyn M.; Naumburg,

Elizabeth H. Sex, access, and excess. [Editorial]. *Annals of Internal Medicine.* 1995 Oct 1; 123(7): 548–549. 20 refs. BE56106.
> biomedical technologies; diagnosis; *females; *health care; health services research; heart diseases; *males; *patient care; *patient satisfaction; preventive medicine; primary health care; quality of health care; referral and consultation; *selection for treatment; social discrimination; surgery; treatment outcome; women's health; continuity of patient care; United States

Goodman, Kenneth W. Bioethics and health informatics: an introduction. *In:* Goodman, Kenneth W., ed. Ethics, Computing, and Medicine: Informatics and the Transformation of Health Care. New York, NY: Cambridge University Press; 1998: 1–31. 117 refs. 1 fn. ISBN 0–521–46905–8. BE57001.
> advance directives; *bioethics; *computer communication networks; *computers; confidentiality; decision making; DNA data banks; epidemiology; ethical theory; genetic information; *health care; information dissemination; informed consent; medical education; *medicine; moral obligations; organ transplantation; patient education; professional competence; professional ethics; professional patient relationship; psychiatry; psychology; quality of health care; referral and consultation; registries; risks and benefits; standards; surgery; trends; values; *informatics; *telemedicine

Goodman, Kenneth W., ed. Ethics, Computing, and Medicine: Informatics and the Transformation of Health Care. New York, NY: Cambridge University Press; 1998. 180 p. Includes references. ISBN 0–521–46905–8. BE57000.
> accountability; bioethics; *computer communication networks; *computers; confidentiality; data banks; decision making; disclosure; economics; evaluation; futility; *health care; health care delivery; information dissemination; informed consent; legal aspects; managed care programs; medical records; medicine; patient care; physician patient relationship; practice guidelines; professional autonomy; professional competence; quality of health care; resource allocation; risks and benefits; selection for treatment; standards; technical expertise; uncertainty; values; withholding treatment; evidence–based medicine; *informatics; professional role; telemedicine; United States

Jamison, Tena. Should God be practicing medicine? *Human Rights.* 1995 Summer; 22(3): 10–13. BE55875.
> abortion, induced; clergy; contraception; females; government regulation; guidelines; *hospitals; legal aspects; prenatal diagnosis; public opinion; refusal to treat; *religious hospitals; *reproduction; *Roman Catholic ethics; state government; sterilization (sexual); *women's health services; *community hospitals; *health facility mergers; Amelia E. v. Public Health Council; California; Leonard Hospital (Troy, NY); Massachusetts; New York; Seton Health Systems (NY); St. Mary's Hospital (NY)

Kerridge, Ian; Lowe, Michael; Henry, David. Ethics and evidence based medicine. *BMJ (British Medical Journal).* 1998 Apr 11; 316(7138): 1151–1153. 29 refs. BE58212.
> *decision making; empirical research; evaluation; *health services research; human experimentation; *medicine; morality; patient participation; quality of health care; random selection; research design; resource allocation; teleological ethics; treatment outcome; *values; *evidence–based medicine

Khushf, George. The scope of organizational ethics: editor's introduction. *HEC (HealthCare Ethics Committee) Forum.* 1998 Jun; 10(2): 127–135. 13 refs. 4 fn. BE59080.
> clinical ethics; conflict of interest; economics; ethical theory;

BE = bioethics accession number   fn. = footnotes   refs. = references

ethics consultation; health care delivery; *health facilities; incentives; *institutional ethics; organization and administration; professional ethics; professional organizations; standards; business ethics; evidence-based medicine; quality assurance; utilization review; American Society for Bioethics and Humanities; United States

King, Patricia A.; Wolf, Leslie E. Lessons for physician-assisted suicide from the African-American experience. *In:* Battin, Margaret P.; Rhodes, Rosamond; Silvers, Anita, eds. Physician Assisted Suicide: Expanding the Debate. New York, NY: Routledge; 1998: 91-112. 80 fn. A version of this paper, "Empowering and protecting patients: lessons for physician assisted suicide from the African-American experience," was published in the *Minnesota Law Review* 82(1998): 1015-1043. ISBN 0-415-92003-5. BE58782.
　　*assisted suicide; *attitudes; autonomy; autopsies; *blacks; coercion; *communication; cultural pluralism; eugenics; health; *health care delivery; historical aspects; human experimentation; medical education; medicine; morbidity; mortality; paternalism; physician patient relationship; *physicians; public policy; quality of health care; research subjects; scientific misconduct; selection for treatment; self concept; *social discrimination; social dominance; social worth; socioeconomic factors; *stigmatization; trust; voluntary euthanasia; vulnerable populations; whites; empowerment; Nineteenth Century; Tuskegee Syphilis Study; Twentieth Century; United States

Kinn, Sue. The relationship between clinical audit and ethics. *Journal of Medical Ethics.* 1997 Aug; 23(4): 250-253. 20 refs. BE55912.
　　administrators; confidentiality; disclosure; ethical review; health personnel; *health services research; information dissemination; medical records; patient care; patient participation; privacy; *quality of health care; research design; research ethics committees; standards; *medical audit; quality assurance; Scotland
The aim of this paper is to start a debate about ethical issues associated with the practice of clinical audit. This is an area that has not received much consideration. The role of clinical audit is to raise general clinical standards. The ethical issues of clinical audit may have far-reaching consequences for clinicians, patients, health care providers and purchasers. Guidance is required to provide consistency in approach so that those involved in clinical audit, at whatever level, can be confident that they are following good practice. Clinicians and managers often think of good practice as being a technical matter. The main point of this paper is to bring out important ethical dimensions to good practice.

Kopaczynski, Germain. Catholic identity in health care and the relevance of the 1994 Ethical and Religious Directives for Catholic Health Care Services. *Linacre Quarterly.* 1997 May; 64(2): 26-35. Address to the 1996 meeting of the National Association of Catholic Nurses. BE55615.
　　economics; *health care delivery; *institutional policies; moral obligations; nurses; organization and administration; religion; *religious hospitals; *Roman Catholic ethics; *health facility mergers; *Ethical and Religious Directives for Catholic Health Care Services; United States

La Puma, John. Should medical ethics be part of public relations? *Managed Care.* 1997 Sep; 6(9): 111-112. BE58469.
　　clinical ethics; ethicist's role; *managed care programs; organization and administration; terminal care; United States

Laney, James T. Ethics in health care: what do we have

to do? What should we do? *Journal of the Medical Association of Georgia.* 1990 Nov; 79(11): 829-833. Article based on a speech delivered to the Georgia Hospital Association in Atlanta, GA, 11 Jan 1990. BE55629.
　　age factors; common good; economics; *health care; historical aspects; medical education; *obligations of society; preventive medicine; public health; public policy; quality of life; resource allocation; socioeconomic factors; terminal care; Georgia; Woodruff, Robert

Lipton, Eric. In houses of healing, an uneasy alliance: worried by church rules, hospital may end union with Catholic facility. [News]. *Washington Post.* 1998 Apr 3: B1, B8. BE58046.
　　abortion, induced; allowing to die; bioethical issues; contraception; economics; *health care delivery; *hospitals; *institutional policies; legal rights; municipal government; political activity; professional autonomy; *religious hospitals; *Roman Catholic ethics; selective abortion; sterilization (sexual); treatment refusal; *health facility mergers; Ethical and Religious Directives for Catholic Health Care Services; Memorial Hospital (Cumberland, MD); Sacred Heart Hospital (Cumberland, MD)

Loewy, Erich H. Justice and health care systems: what would an ideal health care system look like? *Health Care Analysis.* 1998 Sep; 6(3): 185-192. 15 fn. BE58979.
　　capitalism; *common good; decision making; democracy; disadvantaged; economics; employment; goals; health care; *health care delivery; health insurance; *justice; models, theoretical; *obligations of society; public participation; resource allocation; socioeconomic factors; standards; *values; United States

Lomax, Karen J.; Garthwaite, Thomas L. VHA's mission: institutional integrity, non-abandonment and VHA special emphasis programs. *HEC (HealthCare Ethics Committee) Forum.* 1997 Jun; 9(2): 182-193. 11 refs. BE55964.
　　economics; federal government; government regulation; *health care delivery; *health facilities; *institutional ethics; military personnel; moral obligations; program descriptions; public hospitals; *public policy; resource allocation; trust; values; vulnerable populations; patient abandonment; United States; *Veterans Health Administration

Mehuron, Kate. "Undemocratic afflictions": a feminist response to the AIDS epidemic. *In:* DiQuinzio, Patrice; Young, Iris Marion, eds. Feminist Ethics and Social Policy. Bloomington, IN: Indiana University Press; 1997: 208-225. 83 refs. 12 fn. ISBN 0-253-21125-5. BE57286.
　　*AIDS; attitudes; biological warfare; *blacks; community services; drug abuse; federal government; *females; *feminist ethics; guidelines; *health care delivery; historical aspects; HIV seropositivity; *homosexuals; human experimentation; *indigents; males; mass media; metaphor; minority groups; morality; *political activity; preventive medicine; *public policy; resource allocation; selection of subjects; sexuality; social control; *social discrimination; *socioeconomic factors; *stigmatization; trust; values; women's health; women's health services; empowerment; *genocide; Centers for Disease Control and Prevention; The Social Impact of AIDS in the United States (National Research Council); *United States

Millard, Charles E.; McManus, Robert. The enigma of today's physician. *Linacre Quarterly.* 1997 May; 64(2): 89-93. BE55613.
　　bioethical issues; economics; education; *health care delivery; intention; *moral complicity; *physicians; *religious hospitals; Roman Catholic ethics; *Roman Catholics; *health facility mergers; United States

Morgan, Kathryn Pauly. Contested bodies, contested

---

knowledges: women, health, and the politics of medicalization. *In:* Sherwin, Susan, et al. The Politics of Women's Health: Exploring Agency and Autonomy. Philadelphia, PA: Temple University Press; 1998: 83–121. 44 fn. ISBN 1–56639–633–6. BE58395.

biomedical technologies; childbirth; disadvantaged; *females; *feminist ethics; health care; *human body; informal social control; *medicine; moral obligations; patient care; physician patient relationship; *political activity; politics; pregnant women; preventive medicine; reproduction; social dominance; technical expertise; *women's health; *women's health services; women's rights; estrogen replacement therapy; menopause

Nikku, Nina; Eriksson, Bengt Erik. Preventive medicine. *In:* Chadwick, Ruth, ed. Encyclopedia of Applied Ethics, Volume 3. San Diego, CA: Academic Press; 1998: 643–648. 7 refs. ISBN 0–12–227068–1. BE56262.

autonomy; behavior control; genetic information; health education; *health promotion; informed consent; mass screening; paternalism; *preventive medicine; *public health; risks and benefits; selection for treatment; self induced illness; social control; socioeconomic factors

Nilstun, Tore; Ohlsson, Rolf. Should health care be rationed by age? *Scandinavian Journal of Social Medicine.* 1995 Jun; 23(2): 81–84. 18 refs. BE55518.

*age factors; autonomy; biomedical technologies; costs and benefits; *health care; justice; *moral policy; organ transplantation; *resource allocation; *scarcity; *selection for treatment; utilitarianism; Sweden

O'Rourke, Kevin D. Catholic healthcare as "leaven": to penetrate and renew society, Catholic healthcare must meet five requirements. *Health Progress.* 1997 Mar–Apr; 78(2): 34–38, 43. 54 refs. 12 fn. BE56449.

common good; employment; *health care delivery; health facilities; health personnel; indigents; moral obligations; pain; quality of health care; *Roman Catholic ethics; suffering; terminal care; theology; values; United States

Parens, Erik. Is better always good? The enhancement project. [Project on the Prospect of Technologies Aimed at the Enhancement of Human Capacities and Traits]. *Hastings Center Report.* 1998 Jan–Feb; 28(1): S1–S17. 35 fn. BE57294.

behavior control; *biomedical technologies; *cosmetic surgery; disabled; entrepreneurship; ethical analysis; females; *genetic enhancement; *goals; *health; *health care; health insurance reimbursement; *human characteristics; *justice; *medicine; moral complicity; *moral policy; motivation; *normality; preventive medicine; *psychoactive drugs; *public policy; resource allocation; *self concept; social control; social impact; social problems; socioeconomic factors; suffering; terminology; *values; authenticity; beauty; *enhancement technologies; life style; Hastings Center; *Project on the Prospect of Technologies Aimed at the Enhancement of Human Capabilities and Traits; Prozac

The following essay begins to say why and when it will sometimes make sense to worry about the prospect of aiming new biotechnologies at the enhancement of human capacities and traits. It grows out of a two-year, Hastings Center project, generously funded by the National Endowment for the Humanities.

Presbyterian Church (U.S.A.). General Assembly. Life Abundant: Values, Choices and Health Care -- The Responsibility and Role of the Presbyterian Church (U.S.A.). [Policy statement]. Louisville, KY: Office of the General Assembly, the Presbyterian Church (U.S.A.); 1988. 83 p. 9 refs. A policy statement adopted by the 200th General Assembly (1988), Presbyterian Church (U.S.A.) BE56195.

biomedical technologies; economics; health; health care delivery; *health care reform; health insurance; health promotion; indigents; justice; moral obligations; obligations of society; *organizational policies; preventive medicine; *Protestant ethics; public policy; resource allocation; theology; life style; *Presbyterian Church; United States

Reiman, Jeffrey. On euthanasia and health care. *In: his* Critical Moral Liberalism: Theory and Practice. Lanham, MD: Rowman and Littlefield; 1997: 211–219. 8 fn. ISBN 0–8476–8314–1. BE57649.

*active euthanasia; age factors; aged; allowing to die; autonomy; *health care; *moral policy; personhood; public policy; quality of life; *resource allocation; *right to die; self concept; suffering; value of life; *voluntary euthanasia; wedge argument

Sargent, Carolyn F.; Brettell, Caroline B., eds. Gender and Health: An International Perspective. Upper Saddle River, NJ: Prentice Hall; 1996. 370 p. Includes references. ISBN 0–13–079427–9. BE58098.

aborted fetuses; abortion, induced; age factors; AIDS; bioethics; biomedical technologies; blacks; breast cancer; cancer; cesarean section; childbirth; cultural pluralism; developing countries; economics; ethics consultation; *females; *feminist ethics; *health; *health care; health hazards; Hispanic Americans; human body; human experimentation; *international aspects; males; medicine; occupational exposure; politics; preventive medicine; psychological stress; religion; reproduction; risk; self concept; sexuality; *socioeconomic factors; terminology; violence; *women's health; ethnographic studies; menopause; premenstrual syndrome; Africa; Japan; United States

Savulescu, Julian. Consequentialism, reasons, value and justice. *Bioethics.* 1998 Jul; 12(3): 212–235. 61 fn. BE58894.

age factors; autonomy; *health care; *justice; *moral policy; philosophy; *prognosis; *resource allocation; rights; *selection for treatment; *teleological ethics; *utilitarianism; values; rationality; *Harris, John

Over the past 10 years, John Harris has made important contributions to thinking about distributive justice in health care. In his latest work, Harris controversially argues that clinicians should stop prioritising patients according to prognosis. He argues that the good or benefit of health care is providing each individual with an opportunity to live the best and longest life possible for him or her. I call this thesis, opportunism. For the purpose of distribution of resources in health care, Harris rejects welfarism (the thesis that the good of health care is well–being) and argues that utilitarianism in general may lead to de facto discrimination against groups of people needing health care. I argue that well–being is a superior theory of the good of health care to Harris' opportunism. Harris' concerns about utilitarianism can be better addressed by: (i) relating justice more closely to reasons for action; (ii) by conceptualising the relationship between reasons for action and the value of the consequences of those actions as a plateau rather than scalar relationship. Justice can be understood as satisfying as many equally rational claims on resources as possible. The rationality of a person's claim on health resources turns on the strength of that person's reasons to promote certain health–related states of affairs. I argue that the strength of that reason does not track the expected value of that state of affairs in a fully scalar fashion. Rather a person can have most reason to promote some state of affairs, even though he or she could promote other more valuable states of affairs. Thus there can be equal reason for a distributor of public resources to save either of two people, even though one

---

BE = bioethics accession number   fn. = footnotes   refs. = references

will have a better and more valuable life. This approach, while addressing many of Harris' concerns about utilitarianism, does not imply that doctors should give up prioritising patients according to prognosis altogether, but it does allow that patients with lower but reasonable prognosis should have a share of public resources.

Sherwin, Susan. A relational approach to autonomy in health care. *In:* Sherwin, Susan, et al. The Politics of Women's Health: Exploring Agency and Autonomy. Philadelphia, PA: Temple University Press; 1998: 19–47. 30 fn. ISBN 1–56639–633–6. BE58392.
　　*autonomy; bioethics; coercion; competence; *decision making; disadvantaged; disclosure; females; *feminist ethics; *health care; health care delivery; informed consent; paternalism; *patient care; physician patient relationship; public policy; self concept; social discrimination; social dominance; social interaction; values; women's health; women's health services

Sherwin, Susan, et al. The Politics of Women's Health: Exploring Agency and Autonomy. Philadelphia, PA: Temple University Press; 1998. 321 p. 216 fn. ISBN 1–56639–633–6. BE58391.
　　age factors; *autonomy; cultural pluralism; decision making; domestic violence; *females; *feminist ethics; genetic determinism; genetic predisposition; genetic screening; genetics; health care delivery; health promotion; historical aspects; human body; human experimentation; international aspects; medicine; mortality; obligations of society; patient care; physician patient relationship; political activity; politics; pregnant women; reproduction; selection of subjects; socioeconomic factors; *women's health; *women's health services; menopause; Feminist Health Care Ethics Research Network (Canada); North America

Smith, Allyne L. In the world but not of it: managing the conflict between Christian and institution. *Christian Bioethics.* 1997 Mar; 3(1): 74–84. 20 refs. 7 fn. Commentary on H.T. Engelhardt, p. 3–19; on S.A. Salladay and J.A. Shelly, p. 20–38; on J.F. Peppin, p. 39–54; and on E.D. Pellegrino, p. 55–73. BE56361.
　　*Christian ethics; conscience; cultural pluralism; Eastern Orthodox ethics; goals; *health care delivery; health facilities; *health personnel; justice; managed care programs; nurse patient relationship; nurses; patient care; physician patient relationship; religion; Roman Catholic ethics; secularism; terminology; values; virtues
Christian physicians, nurses and other health care workers must manage a daily conflict of conscience between their Christian faith and predominantly secular health care institutions. This essay examines various efforts for managing these conflicts: a turn towards social justice or a seeking of holiness. Seeking social justice, however, is theologically empty. Traditionally, the Christian requirement that we be "in this world but not of it" requires a journey along a narrow path to holiness. Christian medical morality must, therefore, be understood within this light. However, just as there cannot be generic health care, but rather health care for a particular person's needs and problems there cannot be generic holiness, but only a holiness grounded in worshiping God rightly. In so worshiping the Christian will be assisted in negotiating the inescapable and perilous vocation of being in the world but not of it.

Snapper, John W. Responsibility for computer-based decisions in health care. *In:* Goodman, Kenneth W., ed. Ethics, Computing, and Medicine: Informatics and the Transformation of Health Care. New York, NY: Cambridge University Press; 1998: 43–56. 28 refs. ISBN 0–521–46905–8. BE57003.
　　*accountability; *computers; *decision making; diagnosis;

*health care; legal aspects; *legal liability; patient care; physician's role; *physicians; professional competence; referral and consultation; standards; informatics; *medical errors; professional role; United States

Tanne, Janice Hopkins. US hospital mergers threaten reproductive services. [News]. *BMJ (British Medical Journal).* 1997 Nov 22; 315(7119): 1330. BE56886.
　　abortion, induced; contraception; *family planning; *hospitals; indigents; institutional policies; managed care programs; organization and administration; refusal to treat; religion; *religious hospitals; Roman Catholic ethics; *Roman Catholics; secularism; social impact; trends; voluntary sterilization; *women's health services; *health facility mergers; United States

Torrey, E. Fuller. Out of the Shadows: Confronting America's Mental Illness Crisis. New York, NY: Wiley; 1997. 244 p. Includes references. ISBN 0–471–24532–1. BE58948.
　　accountability; biomedical research; brain pathology; dangerousness; *deinstitutionalized persons; economics; family members; federal government; government financing; *health care delivery; involuntary commitment; legal aspects; managed care programs; mental health; mental institutions; *mentally ill; patient care; politics; prisoners; proprietary health facilities; psychiatry; psychoactive drugs; public policy; schizophrenia; state government; stigmatization; treatment outcome; violence; homeless persons; nonprofit organizations; Medicaid; Medicare; Twentieth Century; *United States

Ubel, Peter A.; Goold, Susan Dorr. 'Rationing' health care: not all definitions are created equal. *Archives of Internal Medicine.* 1998 Feb 9; 158(3): 209–214. 24 refs. BE57980.
　　costs and benefits; decision making; *health care; health insurance; justice; physicians; *resource allocation; review; scarcity; *terminology; values; *withholding treatment; United States

Weiss, Lawrence D. Private Medicine and Public Health: Profit, Politics, and Prejudice in the American Health Care Enterprise. Boulder, CO: Westview Press; 1997. 220 p. Includes references. ISBN 0–8133–3351–2. BE56786.
　　alternative therapies; capitalism; children; diagnosis; drug industry; economics; entrepreneurship; federal government; females; government financing; government regulation; *health care delivery; health care reform; health insurance; health maintenance organizations; historical aspects; hospitals; indigents; industry; laboratories; managed care programs; medical fees; medicine; minority groups; misconduct; nurses; physician self-referral; physicians; politics; professional organizations; public health; renal dialysis; social discrimination; trends; Canada; Medicaid; Medicare; *United States

Worthley, John Abbott. The Ethics of the Ordinary in Healthcare: Concepts and Cases. Chicago, IL: Health Administration Press; 1997. 332 p. Includes references. ISBN 1–56793–056–5. BE57077.
　　*accountability; *administrators; bioethical issues; bioethics; case studies; codes of ethics; decision making; ethical analysis; *health care delivery; *health facilities; health insurance; *health personnel; hospitals; institutional ethics; interprofessional relations; misconduct; moral obligations; patient admission; *professional ethics; professional organizations; regulation; resource allocation; social dominance; standards; values; whistleblowing; microethics; American College of Healthcare Executives; American Hospital Association; United States

---

BE = bioethics accession number　　　　fn. = footnotes　　　refs. = references

HEALTH CARE/ECONOMICS

Ad Hoc Committee to Defend Health Care (Cambridge, MA). For our patients, not for profits: a Call to Action. *JAMA.* 1997 Dec 3; 278(21): 1733-1738. 4 refs. Drafters of the Call to Action: Joan Agretelis, Jerry Avorn, Charles M. Blatt, Susanna E. Bedell, Susan E. Bennett, David H. Bor, Emil Frei, Ernesto Gonzalez, Suzanne Gordon, Thomas Graboys, Charles Hatern, David U. Himmelstein, Timothy H. Holtz, Barry S. Levy, Bernard Lown, Robert J. Master, Timothy B. McCall, Mitchell T. Rabkin, Jeffrey Scavron, John D. Stoeckle, Lee Swislow, John Walsh, Steffie Woolhandler. Includes a 5-page list of persons endorsing the statement. BE56306.
　　attitudes; caring; *economics; entrepreneurship; goals; *health care delivery; *health care reform; incentives; *industry; managed care programs; medicine; *nurses; *patient advocacy; physician patient relationship; *physicians; *political activity; private sector; *proprietary health facilities; public policy; social impact; time factors; *trends; *values; vulnerable populations; withholding treatment; *Massachusetts; *United States

Ader, Mary. Investigational treatments: coverage, controversy, and consensus. *Annals of Health Law.* 1996; 5: 45-60. 20 fn. BE58363.
　　biomedical technologies; contracts; financial support; *health insurance reimbursement; *legal aspects; public policy; risks and benefits; standards; technology assessment; terminally ill; *therapeutic research; evidence-based medicine; *investigational therapies; United States

Altman, Stuart H.; Reinhardt, Uwe E.; Shields, Alexandra E., eds. The Future U.S. Healthcare System: Who Will Care for the Poor and Uninsured? Chicago, IL: Health Administration Press; Waltham, MA: Council on the Economic Impact of Health System Change; 1998. 426 p. Includes references. ISBN 1-56793-067-0. BE58579.
　　aged; children; common good; *economics; employment; federal government; financial support; government financing; government regulation; health; *health care delivery; *health care reform; *health insurance; *indigents; industry; justice; managed care programs; medical education; national health insurance; obligations of society; *policy analysis; proprietary hospitals; public hospitals; public opinion; *public policy; remuneration; resource allocation; social impact; state government; trends; utilitarianism; teaching hospitals; Health Insurance Portability and Accountability Act 1996; Medicaid; Medicare; *United States

American College of Obstetricians and Gynecologists. Committee on Ethics. Guidelines for relationships with industry. ACOG Committee Opinion No. 182, April 1997 (replaces No. 45, October 1985). *International Journal of Gynaecology and Obstetrics.* 1997 Aug; 58(2): 255-256. 2 refs. BE57951.
　　advertising; biomedical research; conflict of interest; continuing education; *drug industry; *financial support; gifts; *guidelines; hospitals; *industry; medical education; medical schools; *obstetrics and gynecology; *organizational policies; patient care; *physicians; professional organizations; referral and consultation; remuneration; *American College of Obstetricians and Gynecologists; United States

American Medical Association. Council on Ethical and Judicial Affairs. Sale of non-health-related goods from physicians' offices. *JAMA.* 1998 Aug 12; 280(6): 563. 2 refs. BE58767.
　　community services; *conflict of interest; *economics; *entrepreneurship; *guidelines; medical ethics; *organizational policies; physician patient relationship; *physicians; professional organizations; *American Medical Association; United States

Appleby, Chuck. True values: while ethical decisionmaking and managed care aren't mutually exclusive, executives are struggling to find a common denominator. *Hospitals and Health Networks.* 1996 Jul 5; 70(13): 20-22, 26. BE55611.
　　community services; *contracts; employment; *guidelines; health care delivery; health maintenance organizations; *hospitals; indigents; industry; *institutional ethics; *managed care programs; primary health care; religious hospitals; social discrimination; business ethics; rural population; United States

Arno, Peter S.; Bonuck, Karen. The economics and financing of HIV disease. *In:* Cohen, P.T.; Sande, Merle A.; Volberding, Paul A., eds. The AIDS Knowledge Base: A Textbook on HIV Disease from the University of California, San Francisco, and the San Francisco General Hospital. Second Edition. Boston, MA: Little, Brown; 1994: 9.3-1 to 9.3-12. 79 refs. ISBN 0-316-77067-1. BE56645.
　　*AIDS; children; chronically ill; community services; critically ill; drugs; *economics; females; government financing; health care; *HIV seropositivity; home care; hospitals; long-term care; males; patient care; social impact; terminally ill; trends; outpatients; undertreatment; Medicaid; Orphan Drug Act 1983; United States

Austad, Carol Shaw. Is Long-Term Psychotherapy Unethical? Toward a Social Ethic in an Era of Managed Care. San Francisco, CA: Jossey-Bass; 1996. 283 p. Includes references. ISBN 0-7879-0218-7. BE56093.
　　accountability; alternatives; behavior disorders; beneficence; case studies; confidentiality; conflict of interest; costs and benefits; *economics; empirical research; evaluation; health care delivery; health care reform; health insurance; health personnel; justice; long-term care; *managed care programs; mental health; mentally ill; *patient care; practice guidelines; professional competence; professional ethics; professional patient relationship; psychoactive drugs; *psychotherapy; quality of health care; remuneration; *resource allocation; selection for treatment; standards; *time factors; treatment outcome; health services misuse; United States

Bailit, Howard. When the benefit is in doubt, who decides? *Journal of the American Geriatrics Society.* 1998 Mar; 46(3): 342-345. 5 refs. Paper presented at the 1996 Congress of Clinical Societies. BE56751.
　　accountability; contracts; *decision making; financial support; government regulation; guidelines; *health insurance reimbursement; *health maintenance organizations; industry; legal aspects; *managed care programs; organization and administration; *organizational policies; patient care; physicians; practice guidelines; quality of health care; risk; standards; therapeutic research; utilization review; *United States

Bernat, James L.; Ringel, Steven P.; Vickrey, Barbara G., et al. Attitudes of US neurologists concerning the ethical dimensions of managed care. *Neurology.* 1997 Jul; 49(1): 4-13. 40 refs. BE58867.
　　*attitudes; conflict of interest; costs and benefits; deception; diagnosis; disclosure; drugs; economics; health insurance reimbursement; hospitals; incentives; legal liability; *managed care programs; patient admission; patient advocacy; *physicians; practice guidelines; professional autonomy; professional organizations; quality of health care; resource allocation; survey; guideline adherence; investigational therapies; *neurology; United States

Bernat, James L. Quality of neurological care: balancing cost control and ethics. *Archives of Neurology.* 1997 Nov;

54(11): 1341–1345. 52 refs. BE58353.
> conflict of interest; *costs and benefits; *economics; government regulation; guidelines; *health care delivery; incentives; institutional ethics; justice; managed care programs; medical ethics; obligations to society; patient advocacy; patients; *physicians; practice guidelines; public policy; *quality of health care; resource allocation; withholding treatment; health planning; neurology; United States

Bickell, Nina A. Drug companies and continuing medical education. *Journal of General Internal Medicine.* 1995 Jul; 10(7): 392–394. 9 refs. BE56600.
> *continuing education; disclosure; *drug industry; *financial support; guidelines; *medical education; misconduct; professional organizations; regulation; guideline adherence; United States

Bleich, J. David. Medical and life insurance: a halakhic mandate. *Tradition: A Journal of Orthodox Jewish Thought.* 1997 Spring; 31(3): 52–70. 33 fn. BE58771.
> economics; *health insurance; historical aspects; *insurance; *Jewish ethics; *life insurance; managed care programs; mandatory programs; risk; *theology; voluntary programs; personal financing

Bloche, M. Gregg. Cutting waste and keeping faith. [Editorial]. *Annals of Internal Medicine.* 1998 Apr 15; 128(8): 688–689. 11 refs. BE57901.
> conflict of interest; *economics; entrepreneurship; *fraud; *government regulation; incentives; managed care programs; physician patient relationship; physician self-referral; *physicians; self regulation; trust; Health Care Financing Administration; *United States

Bloche, M. Gregg. Managed care, medical privacy, and the paradigm of consent. *Kennedy Institute of Ethics Journal.* 1997 Dec; 7(4): 381–386. 2 refs. BE59020.
> advertising; *computer communication networks; computers; *confidentiality; contracts; *disclosure; *informed consent; *managed care programs; *medical records; patient care; patients; *privacy; United States

The market success of managed health plans in the 1990s is bringing to medicine the easy availability of electronically stored information that is characteristic of the securities and consumer credit industries. Protection for medical confidentiality, however, has not kept pace with this information revolution. Employers, the managed care industry, and legal and ethics commentators frequently look to the concept of informed consent to justify particular uses of health information, but the elastic use of informed consent as a way of responding to managed care health plans' disclosure of information to third parties fails to address underlying questions involving substantive value choices.

Bodenheimer, Thomas. The Oregon Health Plan — lessons for the nation. [First of two parts]. *New England Journal of Medicine.* 1997 Aug 28; 337(9): 651–655. 20 refs. BE59005.
> decision making; disabled; *economics; employment; federal government; *government financing; government regulation; *health care delivery; health insurance; *indigents; *managed care programs; public participation; *public policy; quality of life; *resource allocation; social discrimination; state government; treatment outcome; capitation fee; *Medicaid; *Oregon; *Oregon Health Plan; Oregon Health Services Commission

Bodenheimer, Thomas S.; Grumbach, Kevin. Medical ethics and the rationing of health care. *In: their* Understanding Health Policy: A Clinical Approach. Stamford, CT: Appleton and Lange; 1995: 173–194. 45 refs. ISBN 0–8385–3678–6. BE56193.

allowing to die; autonomy; beneficence; case studies; costs and benefits; decision making; *economics; futility; gatekeeping; *health care; health insurance; indigents; intensive care units; *justice; medical ethics; organ transplantation; physician patient relationship; physicians; prolongation of life; public policy; *resource allocation; scarcity; selection for treatment; self induced illness; terminally ill; withholding treatment; Oregon; United States

Brecher, Bob. What would a socialist health service look like? *Health Care Analysis.* 1997 Sep; 5(3): 217–225. 29 fn. BE55812.
> accountability; capitalism; democracy; economics; freedom; health; *health care delivery; health care reform; justice; obligations of society; paternalism; politics; private sector; public participation; public sector; resource allocation; *socialism; socioeconomic factors; standards; state medicine; values; liberalism; *Great Britain; Kant, Immanuel; *National Health Service; Rawls, John

A socialist health service cannot be a socialist island in a sea of capitalism, as the record of the British National Health Service shows. Nonetheless, since health is a basic need, it can be a key component of the advocacy of socialism. I propose two central socialist principles. On the basis of these I suggest that a socialist health system would emphasise care rather than service; insist on democratic structures and control of resources; and require the prohibition of private medicine.

Brodell, Robert T. Ethics and micromanaged care. *Archives of Dermatology.* 1996 Sep; 132(9): 1013–1015. 22 refs. BE55902.
> *alternatives; case studies; *costs and benefits; decision making; disclosure; *drugs; *health insurance reimbursement; informed consent; *managed care programs; patient advocacy; *patient care; physicians; professional autonomy; quality of health care; *risks and benefits; dermatology; *formularies; *undertreatment; United States

Brody, Howard; Bonham, Vence L. Gag rules and trade secrets in managed care contracts: ethical and legal concerns. *Archives of Internal Medicine.* 1997 Oct 13; 157(18): 2037–2043. 34 refs. BE55809.
> alternatives; confidentiality; conscience; *contracts; *disclosure; economics; federal government; guidelines; *health maintenance organizations; incentives; industry; *information dissemination; legal aspects; *managed care programs; medical ethics; organizational policies; patient advocacy; patient education; peer review; physician patient relationship; *physicians; practice guidelines; professional organizations; quality of health care; standards; state government; withholding treatment; business ethics; guideline adherence; *proprietary information; utilization review; American Medical Association; United States

Gag rules–clauses in managed care contracts that prevent physicians from disclosing information that the plan may find disparaging, but that could relate directly to the patient's health–have recently been the subject of ethical condemnation and legislative prohibition. Another serious problem in managed care contracts, trade secrets, or guidelines and quality assurance mechanisms that are imposed on physicians while their origins are shrouded in proprietary secrecy, have by contrast received little attention. Responses to these ethical challenges to the physician's integrity must involve individual physicians, managed care organizations, professional organizations, and public policymakers.

Brown, Lawrence D. Health reform in America: the mystery of the missing moral momentum. *Cambridge Quarterly of Healthcare Ethics.* 1998 Summer; 7(3): 239–246. BE58551.
> communication; cultural pluralism; democracy; government financing; *health care reform; indigents; national health

---

BE = bioethics accession number   fn. = footnotes   refs. = references

insurance; political activity; *politics; public opinion; public participation; *public policy; religion; resource allocation; *socioeconomic factors; values; *United States

Burgoyne, Carole B. Distributive justice and rationing in the NHS: framing effects in press coverage of a controversial decision. *Journal of Community and Applied Social Psychology*. 1997 Apr; 7(2): 119–136. 28 refs. BE57544.
   administrators; bone marrow; *children; costs and benefits; *decision making; *government financing; *health care delivery; justice; leukemia; *mass media; parents; physicians; prognosis; public opinion; *public sector; quality of life; *refusal to treat; *resource allocation; social worth; tissue transplantation; value of life; values; *withholding treatment; *Bowen, Jaymee; *Great Britain; *National Health Service; R v. Cambridge Health Authority

Callahan, Daniel. Managed care and the goals of medicine. *Journal of the American Geriatrics Society*. 1998 Mar; 46(3): 385–388. 1 ref. Paper presented at the 1996 Congress of Clinical Societies. BE56753.
   administrators; *conflict of interest; *economics; entrepreneurship; *goals; health care delivery; health care reform; incentives; industry; *managed care programs; *medicine; physicians; professional autonomy; values; withholding treatment; integrity; nonprofit organizations; United States

Calman, Kenneth C. Equity, poverty and health for all. *BMJ (British Medical Journal)*. 1997 Apr 19; 314(7088): 1187–1191. 8 refs. BE56859.
   *economics; *health; health care; *health care delivery; *indigents; international aspects; justice; public health; public policy; quality of life; *resource allocation; socioeconomic factors; Great Britain; National Health Service; World Health Organization

Cassell, Eric J. The future of the doctor-payer-patient relationship. *Journal of the American Geriatrics Society*. 1998 Mar; 46(3): 318–321. 5 refs. Paper presented at the 1996 Congress of Clinical Societies. BE56754.
   biomedical technologies; *chronically ill; commodification; diagnosis; disabled; disease; informed consent; *managed care programs; *medicine; patient care; *physician patient relationship; *physician's role; trends; self care; United States

Chambers, Tod. Letting the patient backstage: informed consent for HMO enrollees. *Journal of the American Geriatrics Society*. 1998 Mar; 46(3): 355–358. 10 refs. Paper presented at the 1996 Congress of Clinical Societies. BE56755.
   administrators; alternatives; conflict of interest; contracts; decision making; *disclosure; economics; gatekeeping; *health maintenance organizations; incentives; *informed consent; *organizational policies; patient care; physician's role; physicians; referral and consultation; remuneration; risks and benefits; gag clauses; United States

Cher, Daniel J.; Lenert, Leslie A. Method of Medicare reimbursement and the rate of potentially ineffective care of critically ill patients. *JAMA*. 1997 Sep 24; 278(12): 1001–1007. 29 refs. Correction appears in *JAMA*, 1998 Jun 17; 279(23): 1876. BE55815.
   aged; allowing to die; biomedical technologies; comparative studies; *critically ill; *economics; *futility; *health maintenance organizations; hospitals; *intensive care units; *managed care programs; *mortality; *patient care; physicians; prolongation of life; quality of health care; remuneration; resource allocation; selection for treatment; *terminal care; time factors; *treatment outcome; withholding treatment; *fee-for-service plans; severity of illness index; *California; *Medicare
   CONTEXT: The worst outcome of critical care may

not be death itself; rather, the worst may be an extended death process in which a patient's and his or her family's suffering has been prolonged by services that are ultimately impotent. We have previously used potentially ineffective care (PIC) as a proxy measure for this type of care. OBJECTIVE: To determine if PIC is delivered less often to Medicare patients enrolled in health maintenance organizations (HMOs) than those in traditional fee-for-service health plans. PATIENTS: All Medicare patients hospitalized in intensive care units in California during fiscal year 1994. OUTCOME: Potentially ineffective care was defined as the concurrence of in-hospital death or death within 100 days of hospital discharge and resource use (total hospital costs) above the 90th percentile. METHODS: Hospital costs were adjusted for institution-specific cost-to-charge ratios and local wage indices derived from Health Care Financing Administration cost reports. A multivariate regression model adjusted PIC rates for age, sex, race, elective admission to the hospital, Charlson index diseases, the 15 most common diagnosis related groups for death by 100 days, intensive care unit size, and number of residents at the hospital. RESULTS: A total of 3914 (4.8%) of 81,494 patients experienced PIC and used 21.6% of total intensive care unit resources. The occurrence of PIC was less common among HMO members (adjusted odds ratio, 0.75; 95% confidence interval, 0.65–0.87). However, HMO members were not more likely to experience in-hospital death (adjusted odds ratio, 0.99; 95% confidence interval, 0.91–1.07) and only slightly more likely to experience death by 100 days after hospital discharge (adjusted odds ratio, 1.08; 95% confidence interval, 1.01–1.15). CONCLUSIONS: Patients who experience PIC outcomes are not uncommon in the Medicare population, and patients experiencing this outcome consume a disproportionate amount of medical resources. Medicare beneficiaries in HMO practice settings had a lower risk of experiencing PIC outcomes after adjusting for age, sex, diagnosis, comorbid conditions, and characteristics of the treating hospital. This suggests that HMO practices may be better at limiting or avoiding injudicious use of critical care near the end of life.

Childress, James F. Conscience and conscientious actions in the context of MCOs. *Kennedy Institute of Ethics Journal*. 1997 Dec; 7(4): 403–411. 12 refs. BE59023.
   *conflict of interest; *conscience; contracts; deception; disclosure; dissent; employment; gatekeeping; government regulation; health care; health maintenance organizations; *incentives; legal obligations; *managed care programs; moral complicity; *moral obligations; patients; *physicians; public policy; referral and consultation; remuneration; resource allocation; whistleblowing; withholding treatment; gag clauses; utilization review
   Managed care organizations can produce conflicts of obligation and conflicts of interest that may lead to problems of conscience for health care professionals. This paper provides a basis for understanding the notions of conscience and conscientious objection and offers a framework for clinicians to stake out positions grounded in personal conscience as a way for them to respond to unacceptable pressures from managers to limit services.

Christensen, Kate; Miles, Steven H. The ethical importance of differences between managed care systems. *HEC (HealthCare Ethics Committee) Forum*. 1997 Dec; 9(4): 313–322. 38 refs. BE58082.
   administrators; comparative studies; conflict of interest; economics; goals; incentives; *managed care programs; *organization and administration; physician patient

relationship; physician's role; physicians; professional autonomy; *proprietary health facilities; quality of health care; remuneration; withholding treatment; capitation fee; *nonprofit organizations; United States

Though many articles have been written on the "ethics of managed care", few distinguish between how differences between various managed care systems may affect medical professionalism. We will focus on four important differences between managed care organizations: [1] the differences between for-profit and non-profit systems; [2] the various incentives used to control costs; [3] the degreee of integration of the various parts of the organization; and [4] the degree of involvement of physicians in administering the quality of care. Understanding these distinctions is the key to a productive debate because differences between managed care organizations (MCOs) mitigate or accentuate the threat to medical professionalism and patient care.

Cohen, Jordan J. Remembering the real questions. *Annals of Internal Medicine.* 1998 Apr 1; 128(7): 563–566. 3 refs. BE57324.
>   communication; cultural pluralism; *economics; genetic information; internal medicine; *managed care programs; medicine; organizational policies; *patient advocacy; patient care; patient education; *physician patient relationship; *physician's role; physicians; practice guidelines; prognosis; treatment outcome; evidence-based medicine; United States

Coney, Sandra. To the uninformed: managed care means damaged ethics. [Letter]. *Health Care Analysis.* 1997 Sep; 5(3): 252–258. 6 refs. BE55816.
>   accountability; administrators; conflict of interest; decision making; disclosure; *economics; gatekeeping; government financing; guidelines; health care delivery; *health care reform; health promotion; hospitals; incentives; industry; insurance selection bias; international aspects; *managed care programs; physician patient relationship; physicians; primary health care; private sector; public participation; public policy; public sector; quality of health care; referral and consultation; resource allocation; *social impact; withholding treatment; capitation fee; personal financing; *New Zealand

Cotler, Miriam P. Dimensions of time in managed care: metaphor or measure? *HEC (HealthCare Ethics Committee) Forum.* 1997 Dec; 9(4): 323–332. 6 refs. BE58083.
>   allied health personnel; communication; costs and benefits; economics; goals; health care delivery; indigents; institutional ethics; *managed care programs; metaphor; moral obligations; patient care; patients; physician patient relationship; quality of health care; resource allocation; *time factors; values

This article poses questions about time -- how much and whose? We have time pieces, but we do not measure the true costs of time. Time management is one example of our confusion about the nature of the problems in trying to control financial costs of medical care. The imposition of time constraints on benefit packages and/or medical practice is an oversimplified, misleading mode of external control. Providers are expected to "produce" x number of patients, tests, or procedures per day. Treatment costs and benefits are judged by short-term results and prejudices. Patients and plans change affiliations in rapid order. These adjustments may be impractical; some are unwise and a source of serious dissatisfaction to patients and providers. We often do not acknowledge other associated costs and benefits. Time and knowledge are the physician's primary tools.

Culyer, Anthony. Need: is a consensus possible? [Editorial]. *Journal of Medical Ethics.* 1998 Apr; 24(2): 77–80. 7 refs. BE58053.
>   biomedical research; biomedical technologies; consensus; costs and benefits; decision making; goals; health; *health care; health care delivery; health promotion; justice; *resource allocation; rights; terminology; *needs; Great Britain; National Health Service

Curtis, J. Randall; Rubenfeld, Gordon D. Aggressive medical care at the end of life; does capitated reimbursement encourage the right care for the wrong reason? [Editorial]. *JAMA.* 1997 Sep 24; 278(12): 1025–1026. 12 refs. BE55814.
>   biomedical technologies; *critically ill; decision making; *economics; *health maintenance organizations; hospitals; *intensive care units; *managed care programs; mortality; *patient care; physicians; prolongation of life; quality of health care; remuneration; *terminal care; time factors; treatment outcome; withholding treatment; capitation fee; *fee-for-service plans; *Medicare; *United States

Daniels, Norman; Sabin, James. Closure, fair procedures, and setting limits within managed care organizations. *Journal of the American Geriatrics Society.* 1998 Mar; 46(3): 351–354. 16 refs. Paper presented at the 1996 Congress of Clinical Societies. BE56756.
>   accountability; *biomedical technologies; costs and benefits; *decision making; democracy; disclosure; *economics; goals; health care delivery; health care reform; *health insurance reimbursement; industry; international aspects; justice; *managed care programs; medicine; organization and administration; *organizational policies; physicians; *resource allocation; risks and benefits; technology assessment; therapeutic research; withholding treatment; *United States

Daniels, Norman. Family responsibility initiatives and justice between age groups. *Law, Medicine and Health Care.* 1985 Sep; 13(4): 153–159. 25 fn. BE56702.
>   adults; *age factors; *aged; beneficence; biomedical technologies; children; *community services; disabled; economics; *family members; *family relationship; *financial support; *health care; health care delivery; home care; *justice; legal obligations; *long-term care; love; *moral obligations; *obligations of society; parents; patient care; private sector; *public policy; public sector; quality of life; *resource allocation; selection for treatment; socioeconomic factors; trends; prudence; United States

Daniels, Norman; Sabin, James E. Last chance therapies and managed care: pluralism, fair procedures, and legitimacy. *Hastings Center Report.* 1998 Mar–Apr; 28(2): 27–41. 19 fn. BE57541.
>   accountability; autonomy; *biomedical technologies; *bone marrow; *breast cancer; cancer; case studies; communication; comparative studies; cultural pluralism; *decision making; democracy; *due process; females; government regulation; guidelines; health insurance; *health insurance reimbursement; historical aspects; industry; institutional policies; *justice; legal aspects; *managed care programs; *moral policy; paternalism; patient care; patients; physicians; policy analysis; political activity; *public participation; resource allocation; risks and benefits; state government; technology assessment; terminally ill; therapeutic research; *tissue transplantation; *investigational therapies; seriously ill; Aetna; Blue Cross-Blue Shield; Northern California Kaiser Permanente; Twentieth Century; United States

Daniels, Norman; Sabin, James. Limits to health care: fair procedures, democratic deliberation, and the legitimacy problem for insurers. *Philosophy and Public Affairs.* 1997 Fall; 26(4): 303–350. 32 fn. BE57340.
>   *accountability; alternatives; *biomedical technologies; bone marrow; breast cancer; common good; costs and benefits;

BE = bioethics accession number   fn. = footnotes   refs. = references

*decision making; *democracy; disclosure; due process; economics; growth disorders; guidelines; health care; health care delivery; health insurance; *health insurance reimbursement; hormones; industry; *institutional ethics; *justice; law; *managed care programs; mediation; *moral policy; national health insurance; obligations of society; *private sector; *public participation; public policy; public sector; regulation; *resource allocation; risks and benefits; selection for treatment; technology assessment; therapeutic research; tissue transplantation; *investigational therapies; United States

Darragh, Martina, comp. Ethical issues in managed care: selected bibliography. *Kennedy Institute of Ethics Journal.* 1997 Dec; 7(4): 421–426. This selected bibliography supplements and updates Scope Note 31, "Managed Health Care: New Ethical Issues for All," *KIE Journal*, 1996 Jun; 6(2): 189–207. BE59025.
  accountability; conflict of interest; decision making; economics; health care delivery; health facilities; health insurance; industry; institutional ethics; *managed care programs; medical ethics; moral obligations; obligations to society; patient advocacy; patient care; physician patient relationship; physicians; quality of health care; resource allocation; social impact; United States

Davidoff, Frank. Medicine and commerce. 1: Is managed care a "monstrous hybrid"? [Editorial]. *Annals of Internal Medicine.* 1998 Mar 15; 128(6): 496–499. 20 refs. BE57325.
  codes of ethics; conflict of interest; *economics; fraud; health care delivery; *managed care programs; *medicine; morality; physician patient relationship; regulation; sociology of medicine; United States

Davidoff, Frank. Medicine and commerce. 2: The gift. [Editorial]. *Annals of Internal Medicine.* 1998 Apr 1; 128(7): 572–575. 13 refs. BE57326.
  *commodification; covenant; *economics; *gifts; information dissemination; interprofessional relations; *managed care programs; medical education; *medicine; organ donation; patient care; physician patient relationship; physicians; remuneration; research subjects; social interaction; volunteers; United States

Davis, Fran; Post, Edward R.; Rogers, Connie S., et al. What could have saved John Worthy? *Hastings Center Report.* 1998 Jul–Aug; 28(4): S1–S17. 34 refs. BE58928.
  accountability; administrators; case studies; contracts; decision making; economics; *emergency care; gatekeeping; guidelines; health care delivery; health insurance reimbursement; health maintenance organizations; hospitals; incentives; institutional ethics; *managed care programs; patients; physicians; primary health care; proprietary health facilities; public policy; quality of health care; referral and consultation; capitation fee; case managers; utilization review; United States

Davis, Kenneth M.; Clark, Doug; Koch, Karen E., et al. Physician marketing of nutritional supplements. [Letter and response]. *JAMA.* 1998 Sep 16; 280(11): 967–968. 9 refs. BE58768.
  advertising; conflict of interest; counseling; *drug industry; *economics; *entrepreneurship; federal government; financial support; government regulation; medical ethics; *nutrition; patient care; *physicians; *vitamins; Food and Drug Administration; Rexall Showcase International; United States

DeGroot, Leslie J.; St. Germain, Donald L.; Ridgway, E. Chester, et al. Bioequivalence of levothyroxine preparations: issues of science, publication, and advertising. [Letters and responses]. *JAMA.* 1997 Sep

17; 278(11): 895–900. 21 refs. BE55903.
  *advertising; alternatives; *biomedical research; coercion; conflict of interest; contracts; *drug industry; *drugs; *editorial policies; evaluation studies; *financial support; health services research; industry; *information dissemination; *investigators; legal aspects; managed care programs; organizational policies; peer review; proprietary health facilities; research design; scientific misconduct; self regulation; *Dong, Betty; *JAMA; Jones Medical Industries; *Knoll Pharmaceutical Co.; *Levoxyl; *Synthroid

Downie, R.S. Professional ethics and business ethics. *In:* McLean, Sheila A.M., ed. Contemporary Issues in Law, Medicine and Ethics. Brookfield, VT: Dartmouth; 1996: 1–14. 14 fn. ISBN 1-85521-586-1. BE57787.
  administrators; beneficence; confidentiality; decision making; disadvantaged; *economics; health care; *health care delivery; justice; *medical ethics; paternalism; patient advocacy; peer review; physician patient relationship; *professional ethics; *public policy; quality of health care; social dominance; trust; *business ethics; integrity; quality control; Great Britain; National Health Service

Dubler, Nancy Neveloff. Mediation and managed care. *Journal of the American Geriatrics Society.* 1998 Mar; 46(3): 359–364. 56 refs. Paper presented at the 1996 Congress of Clinical Societies. BE56758.
  communication; conflict of interest; *decision making; disclosure; *dissent; *due process; economics; ethics consultation; health insurance reimbursement; informed consent; *managed care programs; *mediation; moral obligations; *organizational policies; patient advocacy; *patient participation; physician patient relationship; physicians; regulation; social dominance; standards

Dworkin, Ronald. Justice in the distribution of health care. *McGill Law Journal.* 1993; 38(4): 883–898. 3 fn. The McGill Lecture in Jurisprudence and Public Policy, delivered at the Faculty of Law, McGill University, 17 Mar 1993. BE59026.
  *economics; *health care; health care reform; health insurance; *justice; models, theoretical; obligations of society; public participation; public policy; *resource allocation; Canada; United States

Dyer, Allen R. Ethics, advertising, and assisted reproduction: the goals and methods of advertising. *Women's Health Issues.* 1997 May–Jun; 7(3): 143–148. 11 refs. Paper presented at a workshop on "Assisted Reproductive Technologies, Ads, and Ethics: Philosophical, Ethical, and Clinical Perspectives on the Use of Advertising in Reproductive Medicine," held by the National Advisory Board on Ethics in Reproduction in Washington, DC on 19 Oct 1996. BE55850.
  *advertising; autonomy; codes of ethics; commodification; decision making; *economics; government regulation; *health care; medical ethics; organizational policies; personhood; physicians; professional organizations; reproductive technologies; postmodernism; American Medical Association; United States

Emanuel, Ezekiel J. Is health care a commodity? [Book review essay]. *Lancet.* 1997 Dec 6; 350(9092): 1713–1714. BE56925.
  AIDS; *altruism; *blood donation; blood transfusions; commodification; comparative studies; *economics; freedom; gifts; *health care delivery; hemophilia; *international aspects; quality of health care; values; Great Britain; *The Gift Relationship: From Human Blood to Social Policy (Titmuss, R.); *United States

Emanuel, Ezekiel J.; Battin, Margaret P. What are the potential cost savings from legalizing physician–assisted suicide? *New England Journal of Medicine.* 1998 Jul 16;

339(3): 167–172. 45 refs. BE58612.
*assisted suicide; cancer; costs and benefits; *economics; *evaluation; government financing; health care; home care; hospices; hospitals; legal aspects; managed care programs; nursing homes; physicians; *public policy; *social impact; statistics; *terminal care; time factors; personal financing; Medicare; Netherlands; *United States

Engelhardt, H. Tristram. Freedom and moral diversity: the moral failures of health care in the welfare state. *Social Philosophy and Policy.* 1997 Summer; 14(2): 180–196. 32 fn. BE55549.
age factors; coercion; costs and benefits; democracy; *economics; ethical relativism; females; *freedom; government financing; *health care delivery; health insurance; indigents; international aspects; *justice; males; moral obligations; *moral policy; morality; morbidity; mortality; obligations of society; *public policy; religion; resource allocation; *rights; risk; secularism; self induced illness; socioeconomic factors; standards; suffering; values; personal financing; postmodernism; rationality; Medicare; United States

Evans, Roger W. Limits of chronological age as a basis for rationing health care. *Dialysis and Transplantation.* 1994 Sep; 23(9): 506–507, 510–512+. 42 refs. BE57063.
*age factors; *aged; *economics; government financing; health; *health care; kidneys; morbidity; mortality; organ transplantation; patient care; *quality of life; rehabilitation; *renal dialysis; *resource allocation; *selection for treatment; statistics; *treatment outcome; Medicare; *United States

Faden, Ruth. Managed care and informed consent. *Kennedy Institute of Ethics Journal.* 1997 Dec; 7(4): 377–379. 7 refs. BE59019.
alternatives; contracts; *costs and benefits; *disclosure; economics; incentives; *informed consent; institutional policies; *managed care programs; medical specialties; patient care; physicians; withholding treatment; gag clauses; United States
Arguments for efficiency in health care delivery have been used to support some level of withholding of information about available treatment options from patients in managed care systems. To the extent that such arguments prevail, they may necessitate changes in the established understanding of and commitment to informed consent and the disclosure of information to patients.

Farmer, Paul. Listening for prophetic voices in medicine. *America.* 1997 Jul 5; 177(1): 8–10, 12–13. BE55935.
AIDS; biomedical technologies; children; Christian ethics; communicable diseases; developing countries; drugs; *economics; females; *health care delivery; *indigents; industry; international aspects; *justice; obligations of society; patient compliance; prognosis; *resource allocation; selection of subjects; *social discrimination; *socioeconomic factors; suffering; therapeutic research; value of life; withholding treatment; tuberculosis; Haiti; Peru; United States

Felder, Stefan. Costs of dying: alternatives to rationing. *Health Policy.* 1997 Feb; 39(2): 167–176. 21 refs. 3 fn. Published erratum appears in *Health Policy* 1997 Jun; 40(3): 269. BE55605.
age factors; *aged; biomedical technologies; death; decision making; economic value of life; *economics; family members; *health care; *health insurance; health maintenance organizations; health personnel; incentives; justice; motivation; organ transplantation; prolongation of life; public policy; *resource allocation; risk; *terminal care; terminally ill; *personal financing

Feldstein, Bruce D.; Ogle, Richard D. Satisfaction, managed ethics, and the duty to design. *HEC*

(HealthCare Ethics Committee) Forum. 1997 Dec; 9(4): 333–354. 10 refs. BE58085.
administrators; clinical ethics committees; decision making; economics; emergency care; goals; *health care delivery; *institutional ethics; institutional policies; interprofessional relations; *managed care programs; moral obligations; *organization and administration; *patient care team; *professional ethics; professional patient relationship; *quality of health care; time factors; *institutional ethics; myocardial infarction; thrombolytic therapy; Kaiser–Permanente Medical Center (Santa Clara, CA)
Healthcare ethics committee (HEC) members and healthcare professionals at all levels are facing a crisis in ethics as a result of the pervasive organizational, economic, scientific, and technological changes in medicine and healthcare. Our current approach to medical ethics does not effectively address the fundamental challenge this crisis poses: to provide ethically principled care to the satisfaction of all stakeholders. In this paper we present a new approach that extends the scope and understanding of ethics by building links between the disciplines of ethics, management, and design. We call such an approach "Managed Ethics and Design." After outlining the main tenets of this approach, we illustrate its application with a design-based quality improvement project at the Kaiser–Permanente Medical Center at Santa Clara, California, that successfully enhanced delivery of thrombolytic drugs to treat patients arriving with acute MI. We conclude that in order to provide and ensure ethically principled care to the satisfaction of all stakeholders, we have a "duty to design," a duty to improve, create and innovate new practices, processes, standards, and understandings of healthcare. Good design can lead to new possibilities that will enable us to achieve higher, rather than lower, ethical standards. In the current era of organizational medicine and managed care, the duty to design is an inescapable moral imperative.

Finkelstein, Beth S.; Silvers, J.B.; Marrero, Ursula, et al. Insurance coverage, physician recommendations, and access to emerging treatments: growth hormone therapy for childhood short stature. *JAMA.* 1998 Mar 4; 279(9): 663–668. 37 refs. BE57809.
*children; costs and benefits; *decision making; *drugs; economics; family practice; *government financing; *growth disorders; health care delivery; *health insurance reimbursement; *health maintenance organizations; *hormones; medical specialties; *patient care; pediatrics; primary health care; *referral and consultation; selection for treatment; state government; survey; *physician's practice patterns; *Medicaid; United States
CONTEXT: There is concern in both the medical community and the general public about mechanisms of medical decision making and the interplay of physician and insurer decisions in determining access to care. OBJECTIVE: To examine the medical process influencing access to growth hormone (GH) therapy for childhood short stature by comparing coverage policies of US insurers with the treatment recommendations of US physicians. DESIGN AND PARTICIPANTS: Independent national representative surveys were mailed to insurers (private, Blue Cross/Blue Shield, health maintenance organizations, programs for Children with Special Health Care Needs, and Medicaid programs, n=113), primary care physicians (n=1504), and pediatric endocrinologists (n=534) with response rates of 75%, 60%, and 81%, respectively. Each survey included identical case scenarios. Primary care physicians were asked decisions about referrals to pediatric endocrinologists. Endocrinologists were asked

---

BE = bioethics accession number   fn. = footnotes   refs. = references

GH treatment recommendations. Insurers were asked coverage decisions for GH therapy. MAIN OUTCOME MEASURES: Insurer coverage decisions for GH in specific case scenarios were compared with the recommendations of primary care physicians and pediatric endocrinologists. RESULTS: Physician recommendations and insurance coverage decisions differed strikingly. For example, while 96% of pediatric endocrinologists recommended GH therapy for children with Turner syndrome, insurer policies covered GH therapy for only 52% of these children. Overall, referral and treatment decisions by physicians resulted in recommendations for GH therapy in 78% of children with GH deficiency, Turner syndrome, or renal failure; of those recommended for treatment, 28% were denied coverage by insurers. Similarly, GH therapy would be recommended by physicians for only 9% of children with idiopathic short stature, but insurers would not cover GH for the vast majority of these children. Furthermore, the data indicated considerable variation among insurers regarding coverage policies for GH (P less than .01). CONCLUSIONS: Access to GH therapy differs depending on the type of insurance coverage. The deep discord between physician recommendations and insurance coverage decisions, exemplified by these findings, represents a major challenge to mechanisms of health care decision making, access, and costs.

Fins, Joseph J. A medical trust fund for managed care: the legacy of Hughley *vs* Rocky Mountain Health Care Maintenance Organization. *Journal of the American Geriatrics Society.* 1998 Mar; 46(3): 365–368. 30 refs. Paper presented at the 1996 Congress of Clinical Societies. BE56761.
  bone marrow; breast cancer; *decision making; *dissent; due process; *health insurance reimbursement; *health maintenance organizations; judicial action; *legal aspects; *managed care programs; mediation; tissue transplantation; Colorado; *Hughley v. Rocky Mountain Health Maintenance Organization; United States

Fins, Joseph J. Drug benefits in managed care: seeking ethical guidance from the formulary? *Journal of the American Geriatrics Society.* 1998 Mar; 46(3): 346–350. 27 refs. Paper presented at the 1996 Congress of Clinical Societies. BE56759.
  conflict of interest; costs and benefits; decision making; disclosure; drug industry; *drugs; *economics; guidelines; health insurance reimbursement; hospitals; informed consent; *managed care programs; organization and administration; *organizational policies; patient advocacy; patient care; physicians; professional autonomy; resource allocation; review committees; *standards; *formularies; *pharmacy and therapeutics committees; quality assurance; United States

Fins, Joseph J.; Blacksher, Erika. The ethics of managed care: report on a Congress of Clinical Societies. *Journal of the American Geriatrics Society.* 1998 Mar; 46(3): 309–313. 5 refs. BE56760.
  accountability; conflict of interest; disclosure; drugs; *economics; government financing; health care delivery; incentives; legal liability; *managed care programs; mediation; medicine; palliative care; patient advocacy; physician patient relationship; physicians; practice guidelines; public policy; resource allocation; terminal care; trends; formularies; United States

Foglio, John; Gauthier, Candace; Mengel, Norma, et al. What ethicists talk about when they talk about managed care. *Hospitals and Health Networks.* 1996 Jul 5; 70(13): 24–25. BE55604.
  economics; ethicist's role; health care reform; *managed care

programs; medical education; religious hospitals; values; capitation fee; health facility mergers; United States

Fox, Daniel M. Managed care: the third reorganization of health care. *Journal of the American Geriatrics Society.* 1998 Mar; 46(3): 314–317. 1 fn. Paper presented at the 1996 Congress of Clinical Societies. BE56762.
  *economics; federal government; government financing; government regulation; *health care delivery; health insurance; historical aspects; hospitals; *managed care programs; medical education; organization and administration; physician patient relationship; private sector; *public policy; public sector; state government; *trends; Medicaid; Medicare; Nineteenth Century; *Twentieth Century; *United States

Fry, Sara T. Rationing health care: the ethics of cost containment. *Nursing Economics.* 1983 Nov–Dec; 1(3): 165–169. 11 refs. BE57495.
  alternatives; decision making; *economics; federal government; government financing; *health care; health care delivery; health care reform; health insurance; justice; nurses; *public policy; *resource allocation; personal financing; Medicaid; Securing Access to Health Care (President's Commission for the Study of Ethical Problems); *United States

Gervais, Karen G. Changing society, changing medicine, changing bioethics. *In:* DeVries, Raymond; Subedi, Janardan, eds. Bioethics and Society: Constructing the Ethical Enterprise. Upper Saddle River, NJ: Prentice Hall; 1998: 216–232. 5 refs. 1 fn. ISBN 0–13–531252–3. BE58737.
  autonomy; bioethics; *communication; conflict of interest; *cultural pluralism; *health care delivery; historical aspects; justice; *managed care programs; methods; *minority groups; patient care; *physician patient relationship; physicians; professional patient relationship; resource allocation; sociology of medicine; trends; trust; values; non–Western World; Western World; *Hmong; Twentieth Century; United States

Gitanjali, B.; Shashindran, C.H.; Tripathi, K.D., et al. Are drug advertisements in Indian edition of BMJ unethical? [Article and commentary]. *BMJ (British Medical Journal).* 1997 Aug 23; 315(7106): 459–460. 12 refs. BE56649.
  *advertising; alternative therapies; comparative studies; *deception; *drug industry; *drugs; *editorial policies; financial support; health personnel; *international aspects; *misconduct; *standards; survey; technical expertise; *BMJ (British Medical Journal); Great Britain; *India; World Health Organization

Giuffrida, Antonio; Torgerson, David J. Should we pay the patient? Review of financial incentives to enhance patient compliance. *BMJ (British Medical Journal).* 1997 Sep 20; 315(7110): 703–707. 64 refs. BE57308.
  *costs and benefits; *empirical research; health services research; *incentives; *patient care; *patient compliance; *remuneration; treatment outcome; United States
  OBJECTIVE: To determine whether financial incentives increase patients' compliance with healthcare treatments. DATA SOURCES: Systematic literature review of computer databases––Medline, Embase, PsychLit, EconLit, and the Cochrane Database of Clinical Trials. In addition, the reference list of each retrieved article was reviewed and relevant citations retrieved. STUDY SELECTION: Only randomised trials with quantitative data concerning the effect, of financial incentives (cash, vouchers, lottery tickets, or gifts) on compliance with medication, medical advice, or medical appointments were included in the review. Eleven papers were identified as meeting the selection

BE = bioethics accession number   fn. = footnotes   refs. = references

criteria. DATA EXTRACTION: Data on study populations, interventions, and outcomes were extracted and analysed using odds ratios and the number of patients needed to be treated to improve compliance by one patient. RESULTS: 10 of the 11 studies showed improvements in patient compliance with the use of financial incentives. CONCLUSIONS: Financial incentives can improve patient compliance.

Goldberg, Allen I.; Faure, Eveline A.M.; O'Callaghan, John J. High-technology home care: critical issues and ethical choices. *In:* Monagle, John F.; Thomasma, David C., eds. Health Care Ethics: Critical Issues for the 21st Century. Gaithersburg, MD: Aspen Publishers; 1998: 146–163. 30 fn. ISBN 0-8342-0911-X. BE56282.
    adults; autonomy; beneficence; *biomedical technologies; *children; *chronically ill; community services; *economics; family members; federal government; goals; government financing; *health care delivery; health care reform; health insurance reimbursement; health maintenance organizations; health personnel; historical aspects; *home care; justice; models, theoretical; moral policy; patient care team; private sector; public policy; resource allocation; state government; trends; values; ventilators; case managers; poliomyelitis; Medicaid; Twentieth Century; United States

Gonsoulin, Thomas P. Ethical issues raised by managed care. *Laryngoscope.* 1997 Nov; 107(11, Part 1): 1425–1428. 9 refs. Presented at the Meeting of the Southern Section of the American Laryngoical, Rhinological and Otological Society, Captiva Island, FL, 18 Jan 1997. BE58864.
    autonomy; conflict of interest; disclosure; economics; health care reform; incentives; interprofessional relations; *managed care programs; physician patient relationship; physicians; quality of health care; remuneration; resource allocation; capitation fee; United States

Gostin, Lawrence O. Personal privacy in the health care system: employer-sponsored insurance, managed care, and integrated delivery systems. *Kennedy Institute of Ethics Journal.* 1997 Dec; 7(4): 361–376. 27 refs. 3 fn. BE59018.
    biomedical research; computer communication networks; computers; *confidentiality; data banks; *disclosure; *employment; *health care delivery; health facilities; *health insurance; health personnel; *informed consent; law; *managed care programs; *medical records; patient care; *privacy; public health; quality assurance; *United States Widespread collection and use of identifiable information can promote social goods while, at the same time, infringing on personal privacy. Information systems are developing within the context of a fundamental transformation in the organization, delivery, and financing of health care. Changes in the health care system include rapid development of employer-sponsored health coverage, managed care organizations, and integrated delivery systems. These complex, multifaceted arrangements for delivering and paying for health care require ever-more-sophisticated information systems that facilitate extensive sharing of personal data. Systemic flows of sensitive health information occur both vertically and horizontally among employers, hospitals, insurers, laboratories, and suppliers. Beyond this complex web of vertical and horizontal sharing are the multiple demands for information management, quality assurance, research, governmental regulation, and public health. Theoretical problems exist with the law and ethics of informational privacy. The traditional method of exercising control over personal health information is through informed consent. Informed consent, however, within a modern

health information infrastructure becomes highly complex. In this kind of environment, the doctrine of informed consent is flawed and does not provide sufficient control over personal information to assure adequate protection of privacy.

Greenberg, Henry M. American medicine is on the right track. *JAMA.* 1998 Feb 11; 279(6): 426–428. 12 refs. BE57810.
    *economics; government regulation; health care delivery; *health care reform; health maintenance organizations; industry; *managed care programs; medical education; medicine; physician's role; politics; professional autonomy; proprietary health facilities; *public policy; *United States

Grim, Pamela. The price of life. *Discover.* 1997 Sep; 18(9): 39, 41–43. BE57264.
    brain pathology; case studies; decision making; drugs; *emergency care; *health insurance; *hospitals; patient care; patient transfer; physicians; *time factors; *cerebrovascular disorders

Guillemin, Jeanne. Bioethics and the coming of the corporation to medicine. *In:* DeVries, Raymond; Subedi, Janardan, eds. Bioethics and Society: Constructing the Ethical Enterprise. Upper Saddle River, NJ: Prentice Hall; 1998: 60–77. 32 refs. ISBN 0-13-531252-3. BE58730.
    *bioethics; biomedical technologies; clinical ethics; dehumanization; *economics; emotions; entrepreneurship; ethicists; government financing; government regulation; *health care delivery; historical aspects; hospitals; managed care programs; medical education; organization and administration; physician patient relationship; physicians; professional autonomy; secularism; *sociology of medicine; terminal care; trends; values; rationality; Twentieth Century; United States

Gunderman, Richard. Medicine and the pursuit of wealth. *Hastings Center Report.* 1998 Jan–Feb; 28(1): 8–13. 3 refs. BE57291.
    *altruism; *economics; *entrepreneurship; *goals; humanism; love; managed care programs; medical education; *medical ethics; *medicine; *motivation; physician patient relationship; *physicians; self concept; sociology of medicine; students; trends; trust; *values; virtues; *greed; Smith, Adam; United States

Gurewich, Victor; Johnson, James R.; Sobieraj, Jerry, et al. Truth or consequences. [Letters and response]. *New England Journal of Medicine.* 1998 Aug 6; 339(6): 410–412. 4 refs. BE58975.
    alternatives; communication; costs and benefits; *disclosure; *economics; health insurance reimbursement; health maintenance organizations; incentives; patient care; *physician's role; *resource allocation; time factors; withholding treatment

Haas, Jennifer. The cost of being a woman. *New England Journal of Medicine.* 1998 Jun 4; 338(23): 1694–1695. 12 refs. BE58104.
    age factors; attitudes; biomedical technologies; chronically ill; *economics; *females; *health care; indigents; *males; morbidity; mortality; patient care; physicians; *selection for treatment; women's health; longevity; Canada; United States

Hackler, Chris. Is rationing of health care ethically defensible? *In:* Monagle, John F.; Thomasma, David C., eds. Health Care Ethics: Critical Issues for the 21st Century. Gaithersburg, MD: Aspen Publishers; 1998: 371–377. 12 fn. ISBN 0-8342-0911-X. BE56291.
    *decision making; *economics; *health care; justice; public participation; public policy; *resource allocation; standards; terminology; values; United States

---

BE = bioethics accession number   fn. = footnotes   refs. = references

Hall, Mark A.; Berenson, Robert A. Ethical practice in managed care: a dose of realism. *Annals of Internal Medicine.* 1998 Mar 1; 128(5): 395–402. 72 refs. BE57850.

administrators; common good; conflict of interest; *decision making; disclosure; *economics; ethical analysis; *guidelines; health; health care delivery; health insurance reimbursement; *incentives; *managed care programs; *medical ethics; moral obligations; moral policy; patient advocacy; patient care; *physician patient relationship; physician's role; *physicians; practice guidelines; public policy; remuneration; *resource allocation; *trust; withholding treatment; capitation fee; United States

This article examines the ethics of medical practice under managed care from a pragmatic perspective that gives physicians more useful guidance than do existing ethical statements. The article begins with a framework for constructing a realistic set of ethical principles, namely, that medical ethics derives from physicians' role as healers; that ethical statements are primarily aspirational, not regulatory; and that preserving patient trust is the primary objective. The following concrete ethical guidelines are presented: Financial incentives should influence physicians to maximize the health of the group of patients under their care; physicians should not enter into incentive arrangements that they are embarrassed to describe accurately to their patients; physicians should treat each patient impartially without regard to source of payment, consistent with the physician's own treatment style; if physicians depart from this ideal, they should inform their patients honestly; and it is desirable, although not mandatory, to differentiate medical treatment recommendations from insurance coverage decisions by clearly assigning authority over these different roles and by physicians advocating for recommended treatment that is not covered.

Halm, Ethan A.; Causino, Nancyanne; Blumenthal, David. Is gatekeeping better than traditional care? A survey of physicians' attitudes. *JAMA.* 1997 Nov 26; 278(20): 1677–1681. 23 refs. BE56305.

*attitudes; comparative studies; *economics; *evaluation; *gatekeeping; health insurance; knowledge, attitudes, practice; *managed care programs; organization and administration; patient care; physician patient relationship; *physicians; preventive medicine; primary health care; professional autonomy; *quality of health care; *referral and consultation; *resource allocation; *risks and benefits; *social impact; survey; time factors; continuity of patient care; outpatients; Boston; Massachusetts General Hospital

CONTEXT: Nearly all managed care plans rely on a physician "gatekeeper" to control use of specialty, hospital, and other expensive services. Gatekeeping is intended to reduce costs while maintaining or improving quality of care by increasing coordination and prevention and reducing duplicative or inappropriate care. Whether gatekeeping achieves these goals remains largely unproven. OBJECTIVE: To assess physicians' attitudes about the effects of gatekeeping compared with traditional care on administrative work, quality of patient care, appropriateness of resource use, and cost. DESIGN: Cross-sectional survey of primary care physicians. SETTING: Outpatient facilities in metropolitan Boston, Mass. PARTICIPANTS: All physicians who served as both primary care gatekeepers and traditional Blue Cross/Blue Shield providers for the employees of Massachusetts General Hospital, Boston. Of the 330 physicians surveyed, 202 (61%) responded. OUTCOMES MEASURES: Physician ratings of the effects of gatekeeping on 21 aspects of care, including administrative work, physician–patient interactions, decision making, appropriateness of resource use, cost, and quality of care. RESULTS: Physicians reported that

gatekeeping (compared with traditional care) had a positive effect on control of costs, frequency, and appropriateness of preventive services and knowledge of a patient's overall care (P less than .001). They also felt that gatekeeping increased paperwork and telephone calls and negatively affected the overall quality of care, access to specialists, ability to order expensive tests and procedures, freedom in clinical decisions, time spent with patients, physician–patient relationships, and appropriate use of hospitalizations and laboratory tests (P less than .001). Overall, 32% of physicians rated gatekeeping as better than traditional care, 40% the same, 21% gatekeeping as worse, and 7% were of mixed opinion. Positive ratings of gatekeeping were associated with fewer years in clinical practice, generalist training, and experience with gatekeeping and health maintenance organization plans. CONCLUSIONS: Physicians identified both positive and negative effects of gate-keeping. Overall, 72% of physicians thought gatekeeping was better than or comparable to traditional care arrangements.

Ham, Chris. Priority setting in health care: learning from international experience. *Health Policy.* 1997 Oct; 42(1): 49–66. 23 refs. BE57983.

advisory committees; biomedical technologies; common good; comparative studies; consensus; costs and benefits; *decision making; *economics; government financing; *health care; health care delivery; health personnel; indigents; *international aspects; justice; mass media; practice guidelines; public participation; *public policy; quality of life; *resource allocation; rights; selection for treatment; state government; technical expertise; technology assessment; *values; evidence-based medicine; *Great Britain; Medicaid; National Health Service; *Netherlands; *New Zealand; *Oregon; *Sweden; United States

Ham, Chris. Retracing the Oregon Trail: the experience of rationing and the Oregon health plan. *BMJ (British Medical Journal).* 1998 Jun 27; 316(7149): 1965–1969. 11 refs. BE58811.

advisory committees; aged; costs and benefits; decision making; disabled; employment; evaluation; *government financing; *health care delivery; health insurance; health maintenance organizations; *indigents; *managed care programs; physician's role; *practice guidelines; public participation; *public policy; *resource allocation; state government; technical expertise; values; evidence-based medicine; *Medicaid; *Oregon; Oregon Basic Health Services Act 1989; Oregon Health Services Commission

Hammes, Bernard J.; Webster, Stephen. Professional ethics and managed care in dermatology. *Archives of Dermatology.* 1996 Sep; 132(9): 1070–1073. 13 refs. BE55870.

alternatives; case studies; codes of ethics; conflict of interest; disclosure; *economics; *gatekeeping; health maintenance organizations; incentives; *managed care programs; *medical ethics; medical specialties; moral obligations; *patient advocacy; patient care; physician patient relationship; physician's role; *physicians; professional ethics; professional organizations; quality of health care; *referral and consultation; resource allocation; *withholding treatment; capitation fee; *dermatology; *undertreatment; United States

Heitman, Elizabeth; Bulger, Ruth Ellen. The healthcare ethics committee in the structural transformation of health care: administrative and organization ethics in changing times. *HEC (HealthCare Ethics Committee) Forum.* 1998 Jun; 10(2): 152–176. 40 refs. BE59064.

clinical ethics; *clinical ethics committees; committee membership; *economics; education; ethics consultation; federal government; government financing; health care delivery; health insurance; health maintenance organizations; hospitals; incentives; *institutional ethics; institutional policies; *managed care programs; *organization and administration; patients' rights; physicians; standards; business ethics; utilization review; Joint Commission on the Accreditation of Healthcare Organizations; Medicare; United States

Heller, Jan C.; Gerety, Jane. Catholic sponsorship and Medicare managed care: an uneasy alliance of faith and market. *HEC (HealthCare Ethics Committee) Forum.* 1998 Jun; 10(2): 186–200. 5 refs. 9 fn. BE59066.
 aged; common good; conflict of interest; disadvantaged; *economics; evaluation; *government financing; incentives; *institutional ethics; institutional policies; *managed care programs; organization and administration; *religious hospitals; resource allocation; *Roman Catholic ethics; value of life; values; Georgia; *Medicare; Saint Joseph's Health System (Atlanta, GA)

Hellinger, Fred J. The effect of managed care on quality: a review of recent evidence. *Archives of Internal Medicine.* 1998 Apr 27; 158(8): 833–841. 37 refs. BE58303.
 aged; attitudes; *empirical research; evaluation; health; health care delivery; *health maintenance organizations; health services research; indigents; *managed care programs; *patient satisfaction; patients; *quality of health care; referral and consultation; review; *social impact; *treatment outcome; *vulnerable populations; Medicare; United States
This article reviews recent evidence about the relationship between managed care and quality. With one exception, the studies reviewed represent observation periods that extend through 1990 or a more recent year. The review has led to the conclusion that managed care has not decreased the overall effectiveness of care. However, evidence suggests that managed care may adversely affect the health of some vulnerable subpopulations. Evidence also suggests that enrollees in managed care plans are less satisfied with their care and have more problems accessing specialized services. In addition, younger, wealthier, and healthier persons were more satisfied with their health plans than older, poorer, and sicker persons, even after adjusting for the type of health plans. The findings of the studies reviewed do not provide definitive results about the effect of managed care on quality. Indeed, relatively few studies include data from the 1990s, and little is known about the newer types of health maintenance organizations that invest heavily in information systems and rely on financial incentives to alter practice patterns. Furthermore, managed care is not a uniform method that is applied identically by all health plans, and research studying the different dimensions of managed care also is needed.

Himmelstein, David U.; Woolhandler, Steffie. Bound to gag. [Editorial]. *Archives of Internal Medicine.* 1997 Oct 13; 157(18): 2033. 15 refs. BE55866.
 *contracts; *disclosure; *economics; health maintenance organizations; insurance selection bias; *managed care programs; organizational policies; patient education; *physicians; proprietary information; United States

Hoffmann, Diane E. Managing the persistent patient with chronic pain. [Case study and commentary]. *HEC (HealthCare Ethics Committee) Forum.* 1997 Dec; 9(4): 365–372. 5 refs. Reprinted from *Ethics Rounds*, the ethics newsletter of Northern California Kaiser Permanente. BE58086.
 *behavior disorders; case studies; chronically ill; community services; *institutional ethics; legal aspects; *managed care programs; mentally ill; moral obligations; *pain; *patient compliance; patient discharge; physicians; referral and

consultation; refusal to treat; resource allocation; *health services misuse; patient abandonment; personal financing; *psychophysiologic disorders

Hoge, Steven K. APA resource document: I. The professional responsibilities of psychiatrists in evolving health care systems. *Bulletin of the American Academy of Psychiatry and the Law.* 1996; 24(3): 393–406. 11 refs. BE56208.
 autonomy; conflict of interest; contracts; *decision making; *disclosure; *economics; freedom; guidelines; *health care delivery; *health care reform; health insurance; health insurance reimbursement; incentives; legal aspects; *managed care programs; medical ethics; *mentally ill; *moral obligations; *patient advocacy; *patient care; *patient participation; physician patient relationship; *physicians; professional autonomy; professional competence; *psychiatry; psychotherapy; *quality of health care; referral and consultation; remuneration; *resource allocation; self regulation; trends; withholding treatment; continuity of patient care; personal financing; utilization review; American Psychiatric Association; *United States

Hoge, Steven K. APA resource document: II. Regulatory guidelines for protecting the interests of psychiatric patients in emerging health care systems. *Bulletin of the American Academy of Psychiatry and the Law.* 1996; 24(3): 407–418. 6 refs. BE56209.
 advertising; contracts; decision making; disclosure; due process; *economics; federal government; freedom; *government regulation; guidelines; *health care delivery; health care reform; health insurance reimbursement; incentives; *legal aspects; legal liability; legislation; malpractice; *managed care programs; medical ethics; mentally ill; model legislation; organization and administration; organizational policies; patient advocacy; patient participation; *physicians; professional autonomy; professional organizations; psychiatry; public policy; referral and consultation; *resource allocation; state government; torts; withholding treatment; utilization review; American Medical Association; American Psychiatric Association; Employee Retirement Income Security Act 1974 (ERISA); *United States

Holosko, Michael J.; Feit, Marvin D., eds. Health and Poverty. New York, NY: Haworth Press; 1997. 252 p. (Haworth health and social policy). Includes references. ISBN 0-7890-0228-0. BE58545.
 adults; AIDS; American Indians; blacks; children; economics; emergency care; federal government; females; health; *health care delivery; health care reform; HIV seropositivity; hospitals; *indigents; mass screening; morbidity; mothers; municipal government; newborns; patient transfer; pregnant women; primary health care; *public policy; resource allocation; state government; homeless persons; Canada; Early and Periodic Screening Diagnosis and Treatment Program (EPSDT); Medicaid; *United States

Iserson, Kenneth V.; Kastre, Tammy Y. Are emergency departments really a "safety net" for the medically indigent? *American Journal of Emergency Medicine.* 1996 Jan; 14(1): 1–5. 19 refs. BE55561.
 *emergency care; evaluation studies; family practice; *health care delivery; health insurance; *hospitals; *indigents; morbidity; *physicians; referral and consultation; *refusal to treat; selection for treatment; Arizona

Iserson, Kenneth V.; Jarrell, Bruce E. Financial relationships with patients. *In:* McCullough, Laurence B.; Jones, James W.; Brody, Baruch A., eds. Surgical Ethics. New York, NY: Oxford University Press; 1998: 322–341. 45 refs. ISBN 0-19-510347-5. BE58326.
 codes of ethics; conflict of interest; *economics; emergency care; ghost surgery; health facilities; health insurance

---

BE = bioethics accession number   fn. = footnotes   refs. = references

reimbursement; hospitals; indigents; institutional ethics; institutional policies; international aspects; legal obligations; managed care programs; medical ethics; medical specialties; moral obligations; organizational policies; patient advocacy; physician patient relationship; physician self-referral; *physicians; professional organizations; refusal to treat; *remuneration; review; *surgery; withholding treatment; health services misuse; undertreatment; American Medical Association; Hippocratic Oath; Medicaid; Medicare; United States

Iserson, Kenneth V. Staring at our future. *Cambridge Quarterly of Healthcare Ethics.* 1997 Spring; 6(2): 243-244. Reprinted in part from *World Press Review,* 1996; 43(7):34. BE56428.
　　*economics; *health care delivery; indigents; industry; malpractice; medical fees; misconduct; physicians; *private sector; *proprietary health facilities; public hospitals; public sector; quality of health care; strikes; health services misuse; *Sri Lanka; United States

If we only look elsewhere in the world, we may find what happens to entire medical systems when self-enrichment, cost-cutting, and unhampered privatization predominate. A recent letter by Dr. S. Bandara in the Colombo, Sri Lanka, *Daily News* (April 12, 1996) dramatically illustrates that.

Jecker, Nancy S.; Jonsen, Albert R. Managed care: a house of mirrors. *Journal of Clinical Ethics.* 1997 Fall; 8(3): 230-241. 35 fn. BE57564.
　　*attitudes; bioethics; communication; *conflict of interest; disclosure; economics; *empirical research; *gatekeeping; *incentives; literature; *managed care programs; medical ethics; medical specialties; patient advocacy; patient education; patients; physician patient relationship; *physicians; primary health care; professional autonomy; *quality of health care; referral and consultation; *social impact; survey; time factors; trust; withholding treatment; qualitative research; California; *Sacramento

Josefson, Deborah. Marketing of antipsychotic drugs attacked. [News]. *BMJ (British Medical Journal).* 1998 Feb 28; 316(7132): 648. BE57758.
　　*advertising; depressive disorder; *drug industry; economics; federal government; government regulation; incentives; *mass media; mentally ill; patient education; *psychoactive drugs; schizophrenia; *direct marketing; Eli Lilly; United States

Kaiser, Jocelyn. Furor over company deal roils AMA. [News]. *Science.* 1997 Oct 3; 278(5335): 26. BE56574.
　　administrators; *conflict of interest; contracts; guidelines; *industry; *medical devices; *organizational policies; *physicians; professional organizations; self regulation; *business ethics; *American Medical Association; Sunbeam Corporation

Kassirer, Jerome P. Managing care -- should we adopt a new ethic? [Editorial]. *New England Journal of Medicine.* 1998 Aug 6; 339(6): 397-398. 18 refs. BE59076.
　　*conflict of interest; disclosure; *economics; incentives; *managed care programs; *medical ethics; moral obligations; patient advocacy; *physician's role; quality of health care; resource allocation; utilitarianism; withholding treatment; capitation fee; utilization review

Kassirer, Jerome P.; Angell, Marcia. The high price of product endorsement. [Editorial]. *New England Journal of Medicine.* 1997 Sep 4; 337(10): 700. 2 refs. BE55911.
　　advertising; *conflict of interest; drugs; *economics; incentives; *industry; organizational policies; physicians; *professional organizations; remuneration; American Cancer Society; American Heart Association; *American Medical Association; *Sunbeam Corporation

Katz, Sheila Moriber. Medical education and managed care: keeping pace. *Journal of the American Geriatrics Society.* 1998 Mar; 46(3): 381-384. 30 refs. Paper presented at the 1996 Congress of Clinical Societies. BE56764.
　　accountability; conflict of interest; *curriculum; *economics; *financial support; government financing; health care delivery; hospitals; *managed care programs; *medical education; medical schools; physicians; Medicare; *United States

Khushf, George. A radical rupture in the paradigm of modern medicine: conflicts of interest, fiduciary obligations, and the scientific ideal. [Book review essay]. *Journal of Medicine and Philosophy.* 1998 Feb; 23(1): 98-122. 19 refs. 4 fn. BE57522.
　　accountability; bioethics; common good; *conflict of interest; costs and benefits; decision making; disclosure; *economics; entrepreneurship; government regulation; *health care delivery; health insurance; hospitals; iatrogenic disease; incentives; *institutional ethics; managed care programs; medical ethics; medicine; obligations to society; patient advocacy; patients; *physicians; professional organizations; remuneration; resource allocation; scarcity; self regulation; socioeconomic factors; surgery; health services misuse; *Balancing Act: The New Medical Ethics of New Economics (Morreim, H.); *Conflicts of Interest in Clinical Practice and Research (Spece, R. et al., eds.); *Medicine, Money and Morals: Physician's Conflicts of Interest (Rodwin, M.); United States

Conflicts of interest serve as a cipher for a radical rupture in the Flexnerian paradigm of medicine, and they can only be addressed if we recognize that health care is now practiced by institutions, not just individual physicians. By showing how "appropriate utilization of services" or "that which is medically indicated" is a function of socioeconomic factors related to institutional responsibilities, I point toward an administrative and organizational ethic as a needed component for addressing conflicts of interest. The argument is developed by reviewing three important books. First, I consider Mark Rodwin's attempt to configure the economic structures of medicine so that classical fiduciary and scientific ideals can be fostered. Second, I consider E. Haavi Morreim's attempt to modify the classical ideals in order to account for new economic realities. Finally, by considering essays in a recent volume on conflicts of interest edited by Spece, Shimm, and Buchanan, I argue for a constructive dialectic between the approaches of Rodwin and Morreim. In order to properly address conflicts of interest, there must be a radical reassessment of medicine that accounts for the interrelation between scientific, ethical, and economic concerns. Until institutions come into view and professional ethics is developed to account for their role, legitimate interests and obligations of diverse parties cannot be harmonized.

Khushf, George; Gifford, Robert. Understanding, assessing, and managing conflicts of interest. *In:* McCullough, Laurence B.; Jones, James W.; Brody, Baruch A., eds. Surgical Ethics. New York, NY: Oxford University Press; 1998: 342-366. 71 refs. ISBN 0-19-510347-5. BE58329.
　　biomedical research; *conflict of interest; *economics; entrepreneurship; faculty; ghost surgery; gifts; health facilities; health insurance reimbursement; historical aspects; hospitals; human experimentation; incentives; industry; investigators; *managed care programs; medical ethics; misconduct; *moral obligations; organizational policies; patents; *patient advocacy; patient care; physician patient relationship; physician self-referral; *physicians; professional organizations; referral and consultation; *remuneration;

---

review; selection of subjects; self regulation; social dominance; *surgery; trust; withholding treatment; capitation fee; health services misuse; undertreatment; American College of Surgeons; American Medical Association; Medicaid; Medicare; Nineteenth Century; Twentieth Century; United States

King, Leslie; Meyer, Madonna Harrington. The politics of reproductive benefits: U.S. insurance coverage of contraceptive and infertility treatments. *Gender and Society.* 1997 Feb; 11(1): 8–30. 83 refs. 3 fn. BE57686.
> age factors; *contraception; employment; eugenics; federal government; employment; *females; *government financing; health insurance; *health insurance reimbursement; indigents; infertility; political activity; politics; *public policy; *reproductive technologies; *socioeconomic factors; state government; survey; *women's health services; Illinois; Medicaid; *United States

Klein, Rudolph; Day, Patricia; Redmayne, Sharon. Managing Scarcity: Priority Setting and Rationing in the National Health Service. Philadelphia, PA: Open University Press; 1996. 161 p. (State of health series). Bibliography: p. 143–153. ISBN 0–335–19446–X. BE55699.
> accountability; administrators; age factors; biomedical technologies; *decision making; *economics; government financing; health care; *health care delivery; health care reform; international aspects; physician's role; physicians; politics; public participation; *public policy; quality adjusted life years; referral and consultation; refusal to treat; renal dialysis; reproductive technologies; *resource allocation; scarcity; *selection for treatment; self induced illness; standards; time factors; uncertainty; evidence–based medicine; geographic factors; *Great Britain; *National Health Service; Oregon; United States

Kuttner, Robert. Must good HMOs go bad? First of two parts: the commercialization of prepaid group health care. *New England Journal of Medicine.* 1998 May 21; 338(21): 1558–1563. 20 refs. BE57819.
> *economics; *entrepreneurship; gatekeeping; goals; *health maintenance organizations; *incentives; medical specialties; *organization and administration; organizational policies; *patient satisfaction; *physicians; preventive medicine; primary health care; quality of health care; referral and consultation; remuneration; withholding treatment; *nonprofit organizations; *proprietary organizations; United States

...In sum, although nonprofit status seems to be conducive to a less harsh form of managed care, it is no guarantee. The relentless pressure to cut costs will undoubtedly continue. The key question is whether counter–pressures will provide adequate checks and balances. In principle, counter–pressures can be generated by informed consumers with a meaningful choice of competing plans, professional ethics, the quality movement, industry self–regulation, and the growing bipartisan drive for government regulation. I will address these issues in Part 2 of this report.

Kuttner, Robert. Must good HMOs go bad? Second of two parts: the search for checks and balances. *New England Journal of Medicine.* 1998 May 28; 338(22): 1635–1639. 55 refs. BE58614.
> *conflict of interest; *economics; federal government; *government regulation; health care reform; *health maintenance organizations; incentives; *managed care programs; medical ethics; *organizational policies; *patient satisfaction; patients' rights; physicians; professional autonomy; professional organizations; *quality of health care; risk; *self regulation; standards; state government; treatment outcome; withholding treatment; *nonprofit organizations; *proprietary organizations; quality assurance; United States

La Puma, John. Managed Care Ethics: Essays on the Impact of Managed Care on Traditional Medical Ethics. New York, NY: Hatherleigh Press; 1998. 208 p. (A Hatherleigh CME book). Includes references. ISBN 57826–012–4. BE57205.
> accountability; advance directives; aged; alternative therapies; assisted suicide; autonomy; beneficence; clinical ethics committees; communication; confidentiality; disclosure; drugs; economics; ethics consultation; futility; goals; government financing; government regulation; home care; hospitals; incentives; informed consent; justice; legal liability; *managed care programs; medical ethics; medical records; minority groups; organ transplantation; patients; pharmacists; physician patient relationship; *physicians; preventive medicine; quality of health care; resource allocation; right to die; risk; selection for treatment; *social impact; state government; business ethics; integrity; outpatients; undertreatment; United States

Lahr, J. Gregory. What is the method to their "madness?" Experimental treatment exclusions in health insurance policies. [Comment]. *Journal of Contemporary Health Law and Policy.* 1997 Spring; 13(2): 613–636. 175 fn. BE56005.
> *contracts; decision making; ethical review; federal government; *health insurance; *health insurance reimbursement; human experimentation; industry; judicial action; *legal aspects; managed care programs; *organizational policies; patient care; peer review; research design; resource allocation; technology assessment; terminology; *therapeutic research; uncertainty; National Cancer Institute; *United States

Levinsky, Norman G. Truth or consequences. *New England Journal of Medicine.* 1998 Mar 26; 338(13): 913–915. 8 refs. BE57771.
> administrators; aged; alternatives; coercion; costs and benefits; deception; *decision making; *disclosure; *economics; health insurance reimbursement; hospitals; incentives; institutional policies; managed care programs; medical devices; moral obligations; organizational policies; patient advocacy; patient care; *physician's role; public policy; *resource allocation; withholding treatment; United States

Loewy, Erich H. What would a socialist health care system look like? A sketch. *Health Care Analysis.* 1997 Sep; 5(3): 195–204. 13 fn. BE55825.
> biomedical research; capitalism; communism; *decision making; *democracy; *economics; education; freedom; government financing; health care; *health care delivery; health personnel; historical aspects; international aspects; *justice; libertarianism; medical fees; *national health insurance; *obligations of society; *political systems; professional autonomy; public participation; resource allocation; rights; *socialism; *socioeconomic factors; standards; values; liberalism; personal financing; Europe; Nineteenth Century; Twentieth Century; *United States

In this paper I argue that, since institutions must reflect the societies in which they are placed, a socialist health–care system cannot be understood unless democratic socialism––which would assure all of basic necessities of existence, full education and health–care to all members of the community –– is not incompatible with a flourishing market for other products. In contrasting single with multiple tiered health care systems, I suggest that a single tiered system in which all have equal access to health care and none can buy more, is most consistent with the ideals of democratic socialism.

Love, Susan M.; Tuckfelt, Mark; Nicklin, David, et al. Rationing by any other name. [Letters and response]. *New England Journal of Medicine.* 1997 Nov 6; 337(19):

1395–1396. 3 refs. BE58267.
   costs and benefits; decision making; *economics;
   gatekeeping; *health care delivery; health insurance;
   indigents; managed care programs; patient care; *physicians;
   *resource allocation; rights; *withholding treatment; health
   services misuse; United States

Lynn, Joanne; Wilkinson, Anne; Cohn, Felicia, et al.
Capitated risk–bearing managed care systems could
improve end–of–life care. *Journal of the American
Geriatrics Society.* 1998 Mar; 46(3): 322–330. 46 refs.
Paper presented at the 1996 Congress of Clinical
Societies. BE56765.
   age factors; cancer; *chronically ill; critically ill; diagnosis;
   *economics; health care reform; health maintenance
   organizations; hospices; *managed care programs; morbidity;
   organization and administration; palliative care; patient
   advocacy; physicians; prognosis; *quality of health care; risk;
   selection for treatment; *terminal care; *terminally ill;
   trends; *capitation fee; *comprehensive health care;
   Medicare; Study to Understand Prognoses and Preferences
   for Outcomes and Risks of Treatments (SUPPORT); United
   States

McCarthy, Michael. Conflict of interest highlighted in
debate on calcium–channel blockers. [News]. *Lancet.*
1998 Jan 17; 351(9097): 191. BE57776.
   *biomedical research; *conflict of interest; disclosure; *drug
   industry; *drugs; economics; *financial support;
   *investigators

McCormick, Richard A. The end of Catholic hospitals?
America. 1998 Jul 4; 179(1): 5–6, 8–10, 12. BE58567.
   conflict of interest; dehumanization; economics; goals; health
   care delivery; indigents; *managed care programs; pastoral
   care; physician patient relationship; proprietary hospitals;
   public hospitals; *religious hospitals; *Roman Catholic
   ethics; social impact; trends; *United States

McCullough, Laurence B. Molecular medicine, managed
care, and the moral responsibilities of patients and
physicians. *Journal of Medicine and Philosophy.* 1998 Feb;
23(1): 3–9. 11 refs. BE57517.
   alcohol abuse; bioethics; biomedical technologies; *clinical
   ethics; disease; entrepreneurship; genetic information;
   genetic predisposition; genetic screening; goals; health;
   historical aspects; justice; *managed care programs;
   *medical ethics; *medicine; models, theoretical; *moral
   obligations; obligations to society; organ transplantation;
   patents; *patients; patients' rights; physician patient
   relationship; physician's role; *physicians; resource
   allocation; selection for treatment; self induced illness; social
   impact

McCullough, Laurence B. Preventive ethics, managed
practice, and the hospital ethics committee as a resource
for physician executives. *HEC (HealthCare Ethics
Committee) Forum.* 1998 Jun; 10(2): 136–151. 16 refs.
BE59063.
   accountability; *administrators; *clinical ethics committees;
   conflict of interest; costs and benefits; decision making;
   disclosure; *economics; health facilities; informed consent;
   *institutional ethics; institutional policies; *managed care
   programs; medicine; moral obligations; organization and
   administration; patient care; patients' rights; *physicians;
   private sector; public sector; quality of health care;
   remuneration; resource allocation; treatment outcome;
   *business ethics; *preventive ethics; United States

MacPherson, Peter. Is this where we want to go? *Hastings
Center Report.* 1997 Nov–Dec; 27(6): 17–22. 4 refs.
BE57855.
   *economics; *health care delivery; health insurance;
   *indigents; legislation; *managed care programs; morbidity;
   mortality; preventive medicine; *proprietary hospitals;

*public hospitals; quality of health care; *trends; *Las Vegas
(NV); Nevada; *United States

Macready, Norra. US doctors lie to help patients. [News].
BMJ (British Medical Journal). 1997 Jul 19; 315(7101):
148. BE58620.
   *attitudes; *deception; diagnosis; health care delivery;
   *health insurance; *misconduct; moral obligations; *patient
   advocacy; *physicians; remuneration; survey; United States

Mahlmeister, Laura. When cost–saving strategies are
unacceptable. *Pediatric Nursing.* 1996 Mar–Apr; 22(2):
130–132. 5 refs. BE55570.
   accountability; administrators; case studies; codes of ethics;
   *economics; *employment; government regulation; health
   care delivery; *hospitals; legal liability; *nurses; nursing
   ethics; organization and administration; *patient advocacy;
   patient care; pediatrics; professional organizations; *quality
   of health care; resource allocation; standards; American
   Nurses Association; United States

Mansheim, Bernard J. What care should be covered?
Kennedy Institute of Ethics Journal. 1997 Dec; 7(4):
331–336. BE59014.
   contracts; costs and benefits; *health insurance
   reimbursement; *managed care programs; patient care;
   practice guidelines; risks and benefits; evidence–based
   medicine; needs; United States
The answer to the question of what health care services
should be covered by a managed care plan is
straightforward; the plan should cover whatever the
consumer is willing to pay for. From the plan's
perspective, the consumer is the payer, that is, the
employer who negotiates the plan; not the individual
patient whose personal preferences and interests may be
quite different. Since managed care organizations
contract with payers to arrange for health care services
within a defined set of benefits, there is a broader
question as well: Within the benefits chosen by the payer,
what actually is covered? Criteria for determining
"medical necessity," which managed care plans
frequently use as the basis for coverage, are discussed.

Mariner, Wendy K. Mortal Peril: Our Inalienable Right
to Health Care? by Richard A. Epstein. [Book review
essay]. *JAMA.* 1998 Jan 28; 279(4): 330–331. BE57829.
   *autonomy; coercion; contracts; *economics; emergency
   care; freedom; government financing; *government
   regulation; *health care; *health care delivery; health
   insurance; justice; libertarianism; managed care programs;
   *public policy; *rights; Medicare; *Mortal Peril: Our
   Inalienable Right to Health Care? (Epstein, R.A.); *United
   States

Marwick, Charles. 'Bill of rights' for patients sent to
Clinton. [News]. *JAMA.* 1998 Jan 7; 279(1): 7–8. Includes
excerpts from text of "Patients' rights under the proposed
plan...and patients' responsibilities," p. 7. BE58060.
   advisory committees; decision making; dissent; *economics;
   health care delivery; health facilities; health insurance;
   *industry; legislation; *managed care programs; moral
   obligations; patient advocacy; patient participation;
   *patients' rights; politics; *public policy; *Advisory
   Commission on Consumer Protection and Quality in the
   Health Care Industry; U.S. Congress; *United States

Matthews, Merrill. Would physician–assisted suicide save
the healthcare system money? (Or, is Jack Kevorkian
doing all of us a favor?). *In:* Battin, Margaret P.; Rhodes,
Rosamond; Silvers, Anita, eds. Physician Assisted
Suicide: Expanding the Debate. New York, NY:
Routledge; 1998: 312–322. 24 fn. ISBN 0–415–92003–5.
BE58796.

---

age factors; *assisted suicide; *economics; government financing; guidelines; health care delivery; managed care programs; *physicians; public policy; resource allocation; *social impact; statistics; *terminal care; time factors; Medicaid; Medicare; Netherlands; *United States

Mehlman, Maxwell J.; Durchslag, Melvyn R.; Neuhauser, Duncan. When do health care decisions discriminate against persons with disabilities? *Journal of Health Politics, Policy and Law.* 1997 Dec; 22(6): 1385–1411. 25 refs. 26 fn. BE56747.
  anencephaly; carriers; *costs and benefits; *disabled; economics; employment; federal government; futility; genetic disorders; government financing; *government regulation; guidelines; health care; health insurance; *health insurance reimbursement; HIV seropositivity; hospitals; indigents; infertility; late–onset disorders; *legal aspects; minors; organ transplantation; physicians; prognosis; quality of life; *refusal to treat; reproduction; resource allocation; risks and benefits; scarcity; *selection for treatment; *social discrimination; state government; terminology; treatment outcome; withholding treatment; *Americans with Disabilities Act 1990; Civil Rights Act 1991; Equal Employment Opportunity Commission; Medicaid; Oregon; *Rehabilitation Act 1973; *United States
Recent interpretations of laws prohibiting discrimination against persons with disabilities indicate that these laws will play a greater role in health care decision making than previously anticipated. This article employs lessons from other areas of antidiscrimination law to examine these developments and to provide a framework for making health care decisions that are consistent with these new legal interpretations. This article addresses decisions in individual cases, treatment policies adopted by health care providers, and coverage programs of third–party payers, both public and private.

Miller, Tracy E. Managed care regulation: in the laboratory of the states. *JAMA.* 1997 Oct 1; 278(13): 1102–1109. 74 refs. BE55881.
  communication; conflict of interest; *disclosure; due process; *economics; employment; *government regulation; health care delivery; health insurance; health maintenance organizations; *incentives; legal rights; *managed care programs; patient care; physician patient relationship; *physicians; professional organizations; *public policy; social impact; *state government; withholding treatment; *continuity of patient care; American Medical Association; Employee Retirement Income Security Act 1974 (ERISA); Health Insurance Portability and Accountability Act 1996; *United States
In the wake of failed national health care system reform, the responsibility of crafting public policy to respond to changes in the health care system has fallen largely to state governments. Beginning in 1995, state policymakers focused intensively on managed care regulation, adopting policies on a broad array of issues with important implications for patients, physicians, and the physician–patient relationship. To a surprising degree, the regulatory activity in diverse health care markets across the nation has reflected a shared set of concerns about managed care practices and trends. An evaluation of the impact of these state policies will provide essential information about the most effective role for government in promoting the physician–patient relationship and the rights of patients and health care professionals in the era of managed care.

Mirvis, David M. Managed care, managing ethics. [Editorial]. *Journal of the American Geriatrics Society.* 1998 Mar; 46(3): 389–390. 17 refs. BE56767.
  conflict of interest; economics; health care delivery; *managed care programs; medical ethics; physician patient relationship; United States

Mirvis, David M.; Chang, Cyril F.; Morreim, E. Haavi. Protecting older people while managing their care. [Editorial]. *Journal of the American Geriatrics Society.* 1997 May; 45(5): 645–646. 12 refs. BE55826.
  advance care planning; *aged; attitudes; *coercion; conflict of interest; *costs and benefits; disclosure; *economics; futility; *health care delivery; incentives; insurance selection bias; *managed care programs; patient care; physicians; quality of life; resource allocation; stigmatization; uncertainty; *withholding treatment; Medicare; *United States

Moffic, H. Steven. The Ethical Way: Challenges and Solutions for Managed Behavioral Healthcare. San Francisco, CA: Jossey–Bass; 1997. 234 p. Bibliography: p. 219–220. ISBN 0–7879–0841–X. BE58547.
  administrators; confidentiality; decision making; economics; gatekeeping; health care delivery; health insurance reimbursement; health personnel; hospitals; incentives; informed consent; *managed care programs; mental health; *mentally ill; *patient care; patient discharge; psychoactive drugs; psychotherapy; treatment outcome; values; business ethics; utilization review; United States

Mohr, Wanda K. Ethics, nursing, and health care in the age of "re–form". *N and HC Perspectives on Community.* 1996 Jan–Feb; 17(1): 16–21. 30 refs. BE58305.
  administrators; capitalism; conflict of interest; *economics; employment; goals; *health care delivery; *health care reform; health insurance; incentives; managed care programs; *nurse's role; *nursing ethics; *private sector; *professional autonomy; *proprietary health facilities; quality of health care; *values; withholding treatment; *proprietary organizations; United States

Morain, William D. Patently unethical. [Editorial]. *Annals of Plastic Surgery.* 1996 Mar; 36(3): 334. BE56213.
  *biomedical technologies; cosmetic surgery; economics; entrepreneurship; federal government; government regulation; health care; medical ethics; *methods; *patents; physicians; *surgery; United States

Morgenlander, Keith H.; Greenwald, Devra E. Psychiatric DRGs: the legal and ethical impact. [Editorial]. *QRB/Quality Review Bulletin.* 1985 Jun; 11(6): 175–179. 25 refs. BE57068.
  *economics; health insurance reimbursement; involuntary commitment; legal aspects; *mental institutions; *mentally ill; patient admission; patient care; patient discharge; *psychiatric diagnosis; *remuneration; resource allocation; United States

Moros, Daniel A.; Rhodes, Rosamond. Putting universal healthcare on the religious agenda. [Editorial]. *Cambridge Quarterly of Healthcare Ethics.* 1998 Summer; 7(3): 233–234. BE58550.
  clergy; *health care delivery; *indigents; international aspects; national health insurance; obligations of society; political activity; *religious ethics; *socioeconomic factors; *United States

Morreim, E. Haavi. At the intersection of medicine, law, economics, and ethics: bioethics and the art of intellectual cross–dressing. *In:* Carson, Ronald A.; Burns, Chester R., eds. Philosophy of Medicine and Bioethics: A Twenty-Year Retrospective and Critical Appraisal. Boston, MA: Kluwer Academic; 1997: 299–325. 78 refs. 28 fn. ISBN 0–7923–3545–7. BE56544.
  bioethics; conflict of interest; contracts; *economics; ethics; *financial support; government financing; guidelines; *health care delivery; health insurance; health insurance reimbursement; indigents; industry; interdisciplinary communication; justice; law; legal aspects; legal liability; *legal obligations; *managed care programs; medical

specialties; medicine; *moral obligations; *patient advocacy; *patient care; *physician's role; *physicians; professional autonomy; professional organizations; quality of health care; referral and consultation; remuneration; *resource allocation; *standards; therapeutic research; torts; values; utilization review; United States

Morreim, E. Haavi. Medicine's monopoly: from trust busting to trust. *In:* Minogue, Brendan P.; Palmer-Fernández, Gabriel; Reagan, James E., eds. Reading Engelhardt: Essays on the Thought of H. Tristram Engelhardt, Jr. Boston, MA: Kluwer Academic; 1997: 45–75. 89 fn. ISBN 0-7923-4572-X. BE56547.
    allied health personnel; alternative therapies; autonomy; biomedical technologies; coercion; conflict of interest; decision making; disclosure; drugs; *economics; freedom; government regulation; health; *health care delivery; *health care reform; health insurance; health maintenance organizations; information dissemination; interprofessional relations; legal aspects; *medicine; paternalism; patient participation; physician patient relationship; *physician's role; *physicians; *professional autonomy; professional competence; professional patient relationship; resource allocation; rights; *social dominance; social impact; *sociology of medicine; standards; technical expertise; trends; trust; Engelhardt, H. Tristram; *United States

Morreim, E. Haavi. Revenue streams and clinical discretion. *Journal of the American Geriatrics Society.* 1998 Mar; 46(3): 331–337. 96 refs. Paper presented at the 1996 Congress of Clinical Societies. BE56768.
    communication; costs and benefits; *decision making; *economics; employment; health care delivery; health insurance; incentives; industry; interprofessional relations; *managed care programs; organization and administration; patient care; patient care team; patients; *physician patient relationship; *physicians; practice guidelines; *professional autonomy; risk; social impact; time factors; trust; capitation fee; continuity of patient care; *physician's practice patterns; utilization review; United States

Moskowitz, Ellen H. Clinical responsibility and legal liability in managed care. *Journal of the American Geriatrics Society.* 1998 Mar; 46(3): 373–377. 23 refs. Paper presented at the 1996 Congress of Clinical Societies. BE56769.
    accountability; administrators; *decision making; economics; federal government; government regulation; health insurance reimbursement; incentives; injuries; justice; *legal liability; legislation; malpractice; *managed care programs; *negligence; patient care; physicians; quality of health care; state government; withholding treatment; case managers; utilization review; Dukes v. U.S. Healthcare, Inc.; Employee Retirement Income Security Act 1974 (ERISA); Fox v. Health Net of California; Medi-Cal; *United States; Wickline v. State of California; Wilson v. Blue Cross of Southern California

Murphy, Donald J. The economics of futile interventions. *In:* Zucker, Marjorie B.; Zucker, Howard D., eds. Medical Futility and the Evaluation of Life-Sustaining Interventions. New York, NY: Cambridge University Press; 1997: 123–135. 37 refs. ISBN 0-521-56877-3. BE55985.
    advance directives; *age factors; aged; *biomedical technologies; *chronically ill; *common good; *costs and benefits; *critically ill; dementia; *economics; *futility; home care; hospices; *intensive care units; mortality; *palliative care; persistent vegetative state; prognosis; *prolongation of life; refusal to treat; *resource allocation; *selection for treatment; self induced illness; *social impact; *terminal care; *terminally ill; time factors; treatment outcome; treatment refusal; trends; uncertainty; *values; *health services misuse; Study to Understand Prognoses and Preferences for Outcomes and Risks of Treatments (SUPPORT); United

States

Murray-Garcia, Jann; Vietzke, Wesley M.; Wittkopp, George F., et al. Professionalism vs commercialism in managed care: the need for a National Council on Medical Care. [Letters and responses]. *JAMA.* 1997 Jul 2; 278(1): 20–22. 6 refs. BE56157.
    accountability; conflict of interest; *economics; *entrepreneurship; government regulation; *health care delivery; *managed care programs; minority groups; physicians; private sector; public sector; quality of health care; *regulation; selection for treatment; self regulation; standards; National Council on Medical Care; *United States

Mustard, Cameron A.; Kaufert, Patricia; Kozyrskyj, Anita, et al. Sex differences in the use of health care services. *New England Journal of Medicine.* 1998 Jun 4; 338(23): 1678–1683. 40 refs. BE58100.
    age factors; comparative studies; *economics; *females; *health care; hospitals; *males; mortality; national health insurance; patient care; physicians; reproduction; statistics; terminal care; Canada; *Manitoba
BACKGROUND: Sex differences in the use of health care services can be substantial at several stages of life. However, the extent to which differences in reproductive biology and mortality affect the use of health care services is unclear. METHODS: We studied age- and sex-specific per capita use of health care resources for a one-year period during 1994 and 1995 in the Canadian province of Manitoba, where there is universal insurance for a comprehensive range of health care services. Using information obtained from administrative records of physicians' services and acute hospital care, we tabulated the use of health care resources by male and female subjects in three categories: care for conditions specific to sex, care provided to persons who died during the study year, and care provided for all other conditions. RESULTS: The crude annual per capita use of health care resources (in Canadian dollars) was greater for female subjects ($1,164) than for male subjects ($918). Approximately 22 percent of health care expenditures for female subjects was associated with conditions specific to sex, including pregnancy and childbirth, as compared with 3 percent of expenditures for male subjects. An estimated 14 percent of health care expenditures for male subjects was consumed by persons who died during the study period, as compared with 10 percent of expenditures for female subjects. After adjustment for the use of health care associated with sex-specific conditions and differences in mortality, the female:male ratio in health care expenditures was reduced from 1.3 to 1.0. CONCLUSIONS: Expenditures for health care are similar for male and female subjects after differences in reproductive biology and higher age-specific mortality rates among men have been accounted for.

Neumann, Peter J. Should health insurance cover IVF? Issues and options. *Journal of Health Politics, Policy and Law.* 1997 Oct; 22(5): 1215–1239. 69 refs. 13 fn. BE56748.
    *adoption; alternatives; biomedical technologies; childbirth; comparative studies; *costs and benefits; embryo transfer; federal government; government regulation; guidelines; health facilities; *health insurance reimbursement; *in vitro fertilization; incentives; infertility; international aspects; legislation; multiple pregnancy; newborns; professional organizations; prognosis; public opinion; *public policy; *reproductive technologies; *resource allocation; risks and benefits; selection for treatment; standards; state government; personal financing; utilization review; American Society for Reproductive Medicine; Fertility Clinic Success Rate and Certification Act 1992; Society for Assisted Reproductive Technology; United States

---

BE = bioethics accession number   fn. = footnotes   refs. = references

An emotional debate has attended the question of whether health insurance should cover the cost of in vitro fertilization (IVF) for infertile couples. Some private health plans have opted to cover IVF, although most have not. Ten states have mandated that it be included or offered as a standard benefit for private health insurance plans. This article analyzes several key issues in the debate: the impact of insurance coverage; the cost–effectiveness of IVF; valuing the benefit of IVF; and adoption as an alternative. It recommends policy action in several areas: more efficiently allocating resources for IVF (by giving priority to couples with better chances of success, and by making more extensive use of facilities with higher success rates); ensuring that clear and reliable information about the effectiveness of IVF is available; and leveling the playing field between IVF and adoption.

Nightingale, Stuart L. New [FDA] rules require financial disclosure. [News]. *JAMA.* 1998 Apr 1; 279(13): 984. BE57775.
*conflict of interest; *disclosure; federal government; *financial support; *government regulation; human experimentation; industry; *investigators; *Food and Drug Administration; United States

Oppenheimer, Gerald M.; Padgug, Robert A. Health care financing. *In:* Chadwick, Ruth, ed. Encyclopedia of Applied Ethics, Volume 2. San Diego, CA: Academic Press; 1998: 539–549. 10 refs. ISBN 0–12–227067–3. BE56395.
accountability; disadvantaged; *economics; employment; federal government; *financial support; government financing; government regulation; guidelines; health care; *health care delivery; health care reform; *health insurance; industry; *managed care programs; *private sector; proprietary health facilities; *public policy; *public sector; risk; state government; trends; Blue Cross-Blue Shield; Medicaid; Medicare; *United States

Orentlicher, David. Practice guidelines: a limited role in resolving rationing decisions. *Journal of the American Geriatrics Society.* 1998 Mar; 46(3): 369–372. 27 refs. Paper presented at the 1996 Congress of Clinical Societies. BE56770.
alternatives; biomedical technologies; costs and benefits; decision making; evaluation; *guidelines; health insurance reimbursement; incentives; *managed care programs; physicians; *practice guidelines; *resource allocation; risks and benefits; treatment outcome; values; United States

Ozar, David T. The social obligations of health care practitioners. [Revised]. *In:* Monagle, John F.; Thomasma, David C., eds. Health Care Ethics: Issues Critical for the 21st Century. Gaithersburg, MD: Aspen Publishers; 1998: 378–391. 24 refs. ISBN 0–8342–0911–X. BE56292.
conflict of interest; contracts; disclosure; economics; freedom; *health care; human rights; libertarianism; *managed care programs; medical ethics; *moral obligations; *obligations to society; organ transplantation; *patient advocacy; *physician patient relationship; *physician's role; *physicians; public policy; resource allocation; selection for treatment; self regulation; social impact; standards; technical expertise; utilitarianism; values; withholding treatment; Golden Rule; Locke, John; Rawls, John; United States

Packer, Samuel. Medical ethics and the excimer laser. [Editorial]. *Archives of Ophthalmology.* 1997 May; 115(5): 666–667. 15 refs. BE57750.
advertising; biomedical technologies; *conflict of interest; disclosure; economics; *industry; informed consent; *ophthalmology; *physicians; *surgery; *keratotomy; *lasers

Pasztor, Andy; Lagnado, Lucette. Ethics czar aims to heal Columbia. [News]. *Wall Street Journal.* 1997 Nov 26: B1, B6. BE56343.
administrators; disclosure; federal government; *fraud; government regulation; *health care delivery; *industry; institutional policies; *private sector; *proprietary hospitals; *self regulation; voluntary programs; business ethics; *Columbia/HCA Healthcare Corporation; Medicare

Paton, Calum. Necessary conditions for a socialist health service. *Health Care Analysis.* 1997 Sep; 5(3): 205–216. 14 refs. BE55828.
capitalism; democracy; *economics; freedom; goals; government financing; health; health care; *health care delivery; health care reform; hospitals; international aspects; justice; national health insurance; organization and administration; political systems; politics; primary health care; private sector; public sector; resource allocation; *socialism; socioeconomic factors; standards; state medicine; personal financing; *Great Britain; *National Health Service
A socialist health service in a non–socialist society may be forced to stress care and rescue rather than prevention, health maintenance or the promotion of better health and more equal health status. A socialist health service ought to be 'integrated'. A socialist health service ought to provide universal and comprehensive care.

Patterson, W. Bradford; Emanuel, Ezekiel J.; Blumenthal, David. Physician–drug company conflict of interest. *Journal of Clinical Oncology.* 1996 Jan; 14(1): 316–320. 13 refs. BE55520.
biomedical research; *conflict of interest; *drug industry; *drugs; *financial support; *gifts; government financing; guidelines; hospitals; human experimentation; investigators; medical schools; *patient care; *physicians; professional organizations; referral and consultation; universities; teaching hospitals; American College of Physicians; American Medical Association; American Society of Clinical Oncology; United States

Pear, Robert. Presidential panel sees no need for a law on patient's rights. [News]. *New York Times.* 1998 Mar 13: A17. BE57730.
accountability; advisory committees; committee membership; federal government; government regulation; health care delivery; *health insurance; *patients' rights; *public policy; quality of health care; self regulation; *Advisory Commission on Consumer Protection and Quality in the Health Care Industry; *United States

Pearson, Steven D.; Sabin, James E.; Emanuel, Ezekiel J. Ethical guidelines for physician compensation based on capitation. *New England Journal of Medicine.* 1998 Sep 3; 339(10): 689–693. 30 refs. BE58660.
*conflict of interest; decision making; economics; *guidelines; *incentives; insurance; justice; *managed care programs; moral policy; physician patient relationship; *physicians; primary health care; quality of health care; *remuneration; resource allocation; risk; trust; withholding treatment; *capitation fee; United States

Pellegrino, Edmund D. Ethical issues in managed care: a Catholic Christian perspective. *Christian Bioethics.* 1997 Mar; 3(1): 55–73. 43 refs. Commented on by A.L. Smith, p. 74–84. BE56360.
administrators; autonomy; caring; Christian ethics; commodification; conflict of interest; *economics; ethics; gatekeeping; guidelines; *health care; *health care delivery; health insurance; indigents; institutional ethics; justice; love; *managed care programs; moral complicity; *moral obligations; morality; *obligations of society; patient advocacy; patient care; physician patient relationship; physicians; religious hospitals; resource allocation; *Roman

Catholic ethics; *values; vulnerable populations; withholding treatment; business ethics; institutional ethics; United States
A Christian analysis of the moral conflicts that exist among physicians and health care institutions requires a detailed treatment of the ethical issues in managed care. To be viable, managed care, as with any system of health care, must be economically sound and morally defensible. While managed care is *per se* a morally neutral concept, as it is currently practiced in the United States, it is morally dubious at best, and in many instances is antithetical to a Catholic Christian ethics of health care. The moral status of any system of managed care ought to be judged with respect to its congruence with Gospel teachings about the care of the sick, Papal Encyclicals, and the documents of the Second Vatican Council. In this essay, I look at the important conceptual or definitional issues of managed care, assess these concerns over against the source and content of a Catholic ethic of health care, and outline the necessary moral requirements of any licit system of health care.

Pellegrino, Edmund D. Managed care at the bedside: how do we look in the moral mirror? *Kennedy Institute of Ethics Journal.* 1997 Dec; 7(4): 321–330. 14 refs. BE59013.
    beneficence; biomedical technologies; *conflict of interest; contracts; disclosure; *economics; employment; gatekeeping; *managed care programs; *moral obligations; obligations to society; patient advocacy; patient care; *physician patient relationship; physician's role; *physicians; professional competence; quality of health care; *resource allocation; sociology of medicine; technical expertise; vulnerable populations; withholding treatment; continuity of patient care; gag clauses; *United States
Managed care per se is a morally neutral concept; however, as practiced today, it raises serious ethical issues at the clinical, managerial, and social levels. This essay focuses on the ethical issues that arise at the bedside, looking first at the ethical conflicts faced by the physician who is charged with responsibility for care of the patient and then turning to the way in which managed care exacts costs that are measured not in dollars but in compromises in the caring dimensions of the patient–physician relationship.

Philip, Donald J. Ethics of managed care: implications for group practice. *Medical Group Management Journal.* 1997 Nov–Dec; 44(6): 55–56, 58, 60–64, 66. 14 fn. BE58436.
    beneficence; conflict of interest; contracts; economics; health care; incentives; indigents; *managed care programs; medical ethics; physician patient relationship; physicians; religious ethics; rights; *withholding treatment; group practice; United States

Pike, Jon. Strikes. *In:* Chadwick, Ruth, ed. Encyclopedia of Applied Ethics, Volume 4. San Diego, CA: Academic Press; 1998: 239–247. 11 refs. ISBN 0-12-227069-X. BE56346.
    coercion; contracts; democracy; economics; employment; health personnel; moral obligations; public policy; rights; *strikes

Powers, Madison. Managed care: how economic incentive reforms went wrong. *Kennedy Institute of Ethics Journal.* 1997 Dec; 7(4): 353–360. 12 refs. BE59017.
    *accountability; biomedical technologies; comparative studies; *economics; employment; health; *health care delivery; *health care reform; health insurance; *incentives; *justice; *managed care programs; national health insurance; public policy; quality of health care; resource allocation; withholding treatment; managed competition; universal coverage; Canada; Clinton Health Security Plan; Europe;

*United States
In its response to pressures to rationalize health care resource allocation, the American health care system has embraced managed care without concurrent comprehensive health care reform, either in the form of the centralized tax-based systems found in Europe and Canada or that of the Clinton reform plan. What survives is managed care without managed competition, employer mandates, or universal access. Two problems inherent in the incentive structure of managed care plans developed in the absence of comprehensive health care reform work against the public interest. First, sacrifices in terms of medical innovation and quality of care may not be offset by greater equity in the distribution of health care. Second, such managed care plans fail to address the need for long-term accountability.

Pruchnicki, Alec. First, do no harm (pending prior approval). [Irony]. *New England Journal of Medicine.* 1997 Nov 27; 337(22): 1627–1628. BE56433.
    codes of ethics; confidentiality; disclosure; economics; *health maintenance organizations; institutional policies; medical ethics; physicians; withholding treatment; Hippocratic Oath; United States

Rasmussen, P. Elmegaard; Larsen, P. Munkholm; Nielsen, V.G., et al. Does physicians' knowledge of costing related to clinical decision making change the consumption of resources despite unchanged medical standards? *Scandinavian Journal of Gastroenterology.* 1985; 20(4): 401–406. 7 refs. BE57073.
    *biomedical technologies; comparative studies; decision making; drugs; *economics; evaluation studies; *hospitals; *knowledge, attitudes, practice; *patient care; *physicians; quality of health care; *resource allocation; *physician's practice patterns; *Denmark

Reinhardt, Uwe E. Wanted: a clearly articulated social ethic for American health care. *JAMA.* 1997 Nov 5; 278(17): 1446–1447. 18 refs. BE56051.
    attitudes; *economics; federal government; *health care; health care delivery; health insurance; *indigents; justice; minors; *public policy; quality of health care; *resource allocation; rights; *socioeconomic factors; *values; personal financing; Friedman, Milton; Mortal Peril: Our Inalienable Right to Health Care (Epstein, R.); *United States

Relman, Arnold S.; Lundberg, George D. Business and professionalism in medicine at the American Medical Association. *JAMA.* 1998 Jan 14; 279(2): 169–170. 1 fn. Statements by the editor-in-chief emeritus of the *New England Journal of Medicine* (Relman) and by the editor of *JAMA* (Lundberg) delivered during the AMA's interim meeting in Dallas, TX, on 7 Dec 1997. BE57972.
    advertising; *conflict of interest; economics; entrepreneurship; *industry; medical ethics; *organizational policies; physician patient relationship; *physicians; professional autonomy; professional organizations; *self regulation; trust; business ethics; *American Medical Association; Sunbeam Corporation

Relman, Arnold S. The economic future of health care: *False Hopes: Why America's Quest for Perfect Health Is a Recipe for Failure*, by Daniel Callahan, and *Life without Disease: The Pursuit of Medical Utopia*, by William B. Schwartz. [Book review essay]. *New England Journal of Medicine.* 1998 Jun 18; 338(25): 1855–1856. BE58630.
    attitudes; attitudes to death; biomedical technologies; costs and benefits; *economics; health; *health care delivery; *health care reform; industry; life extension; managed care programs; policy analysis; public policy; quality of life; *resource allocation; trends; values; *False Hopes: Why

---

BE = bioethics accession number   fn. = footnotes   refs. = references

America's Quest for Perfect Health Is a Recipe for Failure (Callahan, D.); *Life without Disease: The Pursuit of Medical Utopia (Schwartz, W.B.); Twenty-First Century; United States

Richmond, Caroline; Heasell, Stephen; Kahtan, Susannah, et al. Compensation for victims of medical accidents. [Letters]. *BMJ (British Medical Journal)*. 1998 Jan 3; 316(7124): 73–74. 2 refs. BE57973.
*compensation; economics; *health care; hospitals; iatrogenic disease; *injuries; legal aspects; *legal liability; *negligence; *patient care; *patients; physicians; *resource allocation; time factors; *Great Britain; National Health Service

Rodwin, Marc A. Conflicts of interest and accountability in managed care: the aging of medical ethics. *Journal of the American Geriatrics Society*. 1998 Mar; 46(3): 338–341. 43 refs. Paper presented at the 1996 Congress of Clinical Societies. BE56771.
*accountability; *conflict of interest; health care delivery; incentives; *managed care programs; medical ethics; medical fees; moral obligations; *physicians; professional autonomy; quality of health care; remuneration; resource allocation; risk; standards; trends; fee-for-service plans; United States

Rosner, Fred; Kark, Pieter; Packer, Samuel. Oregon's health care rationing plan. *Journal of General Internal Medicine*. 1996 Feb; 11(2): 104–108. 30 fn. BE57620.
biomedical technologies; costs and benefits; decision making; *government financing; government regulation; *health care delivery; health care reform; *indigents; justice; managed care programs; physician patient relationship; public participation; *public policy; quality of life; *resource allocation; social impact; standards; state government; values; *Medicaid; *Oregon; Oregon Basic Health Services Act 1989; Oregon Health Services Commission

Rosner, Fred; Widroff, Jacob. Physician's fees in Jewish law. *In:* Jewish Law Annual. Volume Twelve. Amsterdam, Netherlands: Harwood Academic Publishers; 1997: 115–126. 77 fn. ISBN 90-5702-551-5. BE58345.
historical aspects; indigents; *Jewish ethics; *medical fees; moral obligations; patient care; *physicians; *remuneration; technical expertise; value of life; Twentieth Century

Rothman, David J. Beginnings Count: The Technological Imperative in American Health Care. New York, NY: Oxford University Press; 1997. 189 p. 261 fn. A Twentieth Century Fund book. ISBN 0-19-511118-4. BE57280.
*biomedical technologies; costs and benefits; *economics; *government financing; *health care delivery; *health care reform; *health insurance; historical aspects; international aspects; *managed care programs; national health insurance; *patient satisfaction; political activity; politics; public opinion; *public policy; quality of life; renal dialysis; *resource allocation; rights; *socioeconomic factors; treatment outcome; ventilators; *Blue Cross; Health Security Act (1993 bill); Medicaid; *Medicare; Twentieth Century; *United States

Ruskin, Andrew. Capitation: the legal implications of using capitation to affect physician decision-making processes. *Journal of Contemporary Health Law and Policy*. 1997 Spring; 13(2): 391–421. 169 fn. BE56011.
alternatives; *decision making; *economics; federal government; government regulation; guidelines; *health care; health care delivery; *health maintenance organizations; *incentives; injuries; judicial action; *legal liability; *managed care programs; *negligence; *patient care; patient discharge; *physicians; practice guidelines; professional autonomy; referral and consultation; *remuneration; state government; suicide; *withholding

treatment; *capitation fee; *physician's practice patterns; relative value scales; utilization review; California; Employee Retirement Income Security Act 1974 (ERISA); Health Care Financing Administration; Medi-Cal; Medicare; National Association of Insurance Commissioners; *United States; Wickline v. State; Wilson v. Blue Cross of Southern California

Russell, Steven; Gilson, Lucy. User fee policies to promote health service access for the poor: a wolf in sheep's clothing? *International Journal of Health Services*. 1997; 27(2): 359–379. 29 refs. 1 fn. BE56012.
*developing countries; evaluation studies; goals; *health care delivery; *indigents; *international aspects; *medical fees; organization and administration; public health; *public policy; *public sector; quality of health care; resource allocation; social discrimination; survey; *health planning

Sabin, James E.; Daniels, Norman. Making insurance coverage for new technologies reasonable and accountable. [Editorial]. *JAMA*. 1998 Mar 4; 279(9): 703–704. 9 refs. BE57813.
*biomedical technologies; children; *decision making; *disclosure; growth disorders; health care reform; *health insurance reimbursement; hormones; *managed care programs; referral and consultation; *resource allocation; United States

Sandberg, Warren S.; Carlos, Ruth; Sandberg, Elisabeth H., et al. The effect of educational gifts from pharmaceutical firms on medical students' recall of company names or products. *Academic Medicine*. 1997 Oct; 72(10): 916–918. 10 refs. BE56632.
*advertising; *attitudes; *drug industry; drugs; evaluation studies; *gifts; hospitals; institutional policies; internship and residency; knowledge, attitudes, practice; *medical education; medical schools; motivation; physicians; recall; *social impact; *students; survey; Chicago; University of Chicago Pritzker School of Medicine

Schwartz, Jack. State regulation of managed care: fragments of reform. *Kennedy Institute of Ethics Journal*. 1997 Dec; 7(4): 345–351. 10 refs. 1 fn. BE59016.
*accountability; alternatives; *disclosure; federal government; gatekeeping; *government regulation; *health care reform; health insurance reimbursement; health personnel; hospitals; incentives; informed consent; legislation; *managed care programs; medical specialties; patient advocacy; patient care; patient discharge; physician patient relationship; *physicians; political activity; politics; primary health care; referral and consultation; risks and benefits; *state government; withholding treatment; gag clauses; Employee Retirement Income Security Act 1974 (ERISA); *United States
State legislatures consider numerous bills to regulate managed care organizations. After identifying the legal, political, and economic barriers to state reform efforts, the paper assesses recent types of state regulation, particularly mandated benefits and disclosure requirements. Two prerequisites to future reform, coalition building and the diffusion of information about managed care, are analyzed.

Sharpe, Virginia A. The politics, economics, and ethics of "appropriateness". *Kennedy Institute of Ethics Journal*. 1997 Dec; 7(4): 337–343. 8 refs. 1 fn. BE59015.
biomedical technologies; costs and benefits; *decision making; economics; empirical research; *health care; health insurance; *health insurance reimbursement; managed care programs; mass screening; *patient care; patients; physicians; public participation; public policy; *resource allocation; risks and benefits; *standards; treatment outcome; trends; evidence-based medicine; needs; *United States
The terms "appropriate" and "necessary" are crucial

determinants in decisions regarding the use and reimbursement of medical treatments. This paper encourages greater awareness of the political, economic, and normative assumptions that give meaning to these concepts.

Shickle, Darren. Resource allocation. *In:* Chadwick, Ruth, ed. Encyclopedia of Applied Ethics, Volume 3. San Diego, CA: Academic Press; 1998: 861–873. 13 refs. ISBN 0-12-227068-1. BE56273.
  *economics; *health care; health care reform; international aspects; justice; national health insurance; public opinion; public policy; random selection; *resource allocation; rights; selection for treatment; utilitarianism; value of life; Great Britain; Netherlands; New Zealand; United States

Shiell, Alan. Health outcomes are about choices and values: an economic perspective on the health outcomes movement. *Health Policy.* 1997 Jan; 39(1): 5–15. 51 refs. BE55607.
  costs and benefits; decision making; *economics; goals; health; *health care; health services research; incentives; patient participation; *public policy; quality adjusted life years; quality of life; resource allocation; standards; *treatment outcome; values; *outcome assessment (health care)

Shortell, Stephen M.; Waters, Teresa M.; Clarke, Kenneth W.B., et al. Physicians as double agents: maintaining trust in an era of multiple accountabilities. *JAMA.* 1998 Sep 23–30; 280(12): 1102–1108. 47 refs. BE58769.
  *accountability; administrators; *conflict of interest; costs and benefits; *economics; *incentives; information dissemination; *managed care programs; medical ethics; medical specialties; obligations to society; *organization and administration; patient advocacy; physician patient relationship; *physician's role; *physicians; practice guidelines; preventive medicine; primary health care; quality of health care; remuneration; resource allocation; social problems; *standards; survey; treatment outcome; trends; trust; withholding treatment; *physician's practice patterns; United States

Shuttleworth, John Sterling. Ethical issues of cost in long-term care. *Journal of the Medical Association of Georgia.* 1990 Nov; 79(11): 843–845. 5 refs. BE55642.
  administrators; *aged; *behavior control; communication; *economics; family members; government financing; *long-term care; *nursing homes; physicians; psychoactive drugs; *psychological stress; quality of life; personal financing; Medicare; United States

Siegel–Itzkovich, Judy. Doctors banned from drug company trip. [News]. *BMJ (British Medical Journal).* 1998 Aug 8; 317(7155): 370. BE58749.
  conflict of interest; *drug industry; *financial support; *gifts; *government regulation; international aspects; *physicians; public sector; *Israel; *Teva

Simon, Robert I. Psychiatrists' duties in discharging sicker and potentially violent inpatients in the managed care era. *Psychiatric Services.* 1998 Jan; 49(1): 62–67. 41 refs. BE58220.
  competence; *dangerousness; *disclosure; *duty to warn; health insurance reimbursement; informed consent; involuntary commitment; *legal liability; *legal obligations; *managed care programs; mandatory reporting; *mentally ill; *moral obligations; *patient advocacy; *patient care; *patient discharge; *physicians; *psychiatry; *quality of health care; *violence; utilization review; United States

Snyder, Jack W. Making Medical Spending Decisions: The Law, Ethics, and Economics of Rationing

Mechanisms, by Mark A. Hall. [Book review essay]. *Journal of Legal Medicine.* 1998 Mar; 19(1): 143–150. 16 fn. BE58930.
  costs and benefits; *decision making; disclosure; *economics; guidelines; *health care; health insurance; incentives; informed consent; managed care programs; patient participation; *physician's role; public participation; *resource allocation; standards; *Making Medical Spending Decisions (Hall, M.A.); United States

Snyder, Lois; Tooker, John. Obligations and opportunities: the role of clinical societies in the ethics of managed care. *Journal of the American Geriatrics Society.* 1998 Mar; 46(3): 378–380. 20 refs. Paper presented at the 1996 Congress of Clinical Societies. BE56773.
  conflict of interest; disclosure; health care delivery; incentives; *institutional ethics; *managed care programs; medical ethics; moral obligations; organizational policies; patient advocacy; patient care; physician patient relationship; physician's role; *physicians; *professional organizations; resource allocation; American College of Physicians; United States

Sorum, Paul C. Striking against managed care: the last gasp of *la medicine liberale*? *JAMA.* 1998 Aug 19; 280(7): 659–664. 36 refs. BE59001.
  *economics; government regulation; guidelines; *health care delivery; *health care reform; incentives; internship and residency; *managed care programs; medical education; medical fees; medical records; medical specialties; *national health insurance; patient access to records; *physicians; political systems; politics; practice guidelines; primary health care; *public policy; referral and consultation; sociology of medicine; *strikes; *France

The French health care system combines a strong tradition of autonomous private practice with nearly universal health care coverage through the social security system. The French state's responses to rising health care expenditures have included limitation of the number of medical students, control over physician fees, rules to prohibit certain clinical practices, experiments with generalist physicians coordinating care and access to specialists, and collective physician responsibility for expenditures beyond the health care budget. The failure of physicians' protests, including a strike of French residents and fellows in 1997, may signify the end of traditional private practice in the face of France's statist version of managed care.

Stelfox, Henry Thomas; Chua, Grace; O'Rourke, Keith, et al. Conflict of interest in the debate over calcium–channel antagonists. *New England Journal of Medicine.* 1998 Jan 8; 338(2): 101–105. 35 refs. BE56440.
  *attitudes; authorship; biomedical research; comparative studies; *conflict of interest; disclosure; *drug industry; *drugs; economics; editorial policies; evaluation studies; *financial support; guidelines; heart diseases; hypertension; *investigators; patient care; *physicians; *risks and benefits; survey; Canada; United States
  BACKGROUND: Physicians' financial relationships with the pharmaceutical industry are controversial because such relationships may pose a conflict of interest. It is unknown to what extent industry support of medical education and research influences the opinions and behavior of clinicians and researchers. The recent debate over the safety of calcium–channel antagonists provided an opportunity to examine the effect of financial conflicts of interest. METHODS: We searched the English–language medical literature published from March 1995 through September 1996 for articles examining the controversy about the safety of calcium–channel antagonists. Articles were reviewed

and classified as being supportive, neutral, or critical with respect to the use of calcium–channel antagonists. The authors of the articles were asked about their financial relationships with both manufacturers of calcium–channel antagonists and manufacturers of competing products (i.e., beta-blockers, angiotensin–converting–enzyme inhibitors, diuretics, and nitrates). We examined the authors' published positions on the safety of calcium–channel antagonists according to their financial relationships with pharmaceutical companies. RESULTS: Authors who supported the use of calcium–channel antagonists were significantly more likely than neutral or critical authors to have financial relationships with manufacturers of calcium–channel antagonists (96 percent, vs. 60 percent and 37 percent, respectively; P less than 0.001). Supportive authors were also more likely than neutral or critical authors to have financial relationships with any pharmaceutical manufacturer, irrespective of the product (100 percent, vs. 67 percent and 43 percent, respectively; P less than 0.001). CONCLUSIONS: Our results demonstrate a strong association between authors' published positions on the safety of calcium–channel antagonists and their financial relationships with pharmaceutical manufacturers. The medical profession needs to develop a more effective policy on conflict of interest. We support complete disclosure of relationships with pharmaceutical manufacturers for clinicians and researchers who write articles examining pharmaceutical products.

Stell, Lance K. Self–Interest and Universal Health Care: Why Well–Insured Americans Should Support Coverage for Everyone, by Larry J. Churchill. [Book review essay]. *Theoretical Medicine and Bioethics.* 1998 Apr; 19(2): 183–191. BE57596.
  age factors; *common good; communitarianism; *decision making; democracy; *economics; *goals; *health care delivery; *health care reform; justice; obligations of society; obligations to society; politics; public participation; public policy; *resource allocation; *Self–Interest and Universal Health Care (Churchill, L.J.); *United States

Stewart, F.E. *JAMA* 100 years ago: is it ethical for medical men to patent medical inventions? [Reprint]. *JAMA.* 1997 Sep 10; 278(10): 816. BE55942.
  *biomedical technologies; conflict of interest; drugs; *economics; *historical aspects; medical etiquette; *patents; patient care; *pharmacists; *physicians; *Nineteenth Century; United States

Stobo, John. Who should manage care? The case for providers. *Kennedy Institute of Ethics Journal.* 1997 Dec; 7(4): 387–389. 1 ref. BE59021.
  attitudes; costs and benefits; *decision making; economics; employment; *health care; health insurance; incentives; justice; *managed care programs; *patient participation; patients; *physicians; quality of health care; *resource allocation; treatment outcome; United States
Health care professionals should be the ones to make allocation decisions in the managed care setting because they are in the best position to assess outcomes, cost effectiveness, and quality of care.

Swee, David E. Health care system reform and the changing physician–patient relationship. *New Jersey Medicine.* 1995 May; 92(5): 313–317. 5 refs. BE55532.
  alternatives; autonomy; beneficence; confidentiality; conflict of interest; disclosure; health insurance; health maintenance organizations; justice; *managed care programs; models, theoretical; moral obligations; paternalism; patient advocacy; patients; *physician patient relationship; physicians; privacy;

professional autonomy; trends; withholding treatment; United States

Tanenbaum, Sandra J. Say the right thing: communication and physician accountability in the era of medical outcomes. *In:* Boyle, Philip J., ed. Getting Doctors to Listen: Ethics and Outcomes Data in Context. Washington, DC: Georgetown University Press; 1998: 204–223. 48 fn. ISBN 0–87840–654–9. BE57927.
  *accountability; *communication; decision making; disclosure; *economics; empirical research; guidelines; *health care; health care reform; health services research; methods; narrative ethics; *patient care; *patient satisfaction; *physician patient relationship; practice guidelines; referral and consultation; regulation; risks and benefits; standards; technical expertise; *treatment outcome; uncertainty; utilization review; United States

Teno, Joan; Lynn, Joanne; Connors, Alfred F., et al. The illusion of end–of–life resource savings with advance directives. [For the SUPPORT Investigators]. *Journal of the American Geriatrics Society.* 1997 Apr; 45(4): 513–518. 15 refs. BE57124.
  *advance directives; communication; comparative studies; control groups; *critically ill; *economics; *evaluation; evaluation studies; *hospitals; *medical records; patient admission; patients; research design; resource allocation; resuscitation; resuscitation orders; social impact; socioeconomic factors; *terminal care; treatment refusal; *seriously ill; Patient Self–Determination Act 1990; *Study to Understand Prognoses and Preferences for Outcomes and Risks of Treatments (SUPPORT); United States

Thomasma, David C. The ethics of managed care: challenges to the principles of relationship–centered care. *Journal of Allied Health.* 1996 Summer; 25(3): 233–246. 36 refs. BE57977.
  advance directives; autonomy; beneficence; conflict of interest; disclosure; economics; ethics committees; government financing; health care delivery; incentives; justice; *managed care programs; physician patient relationship; physicians; quality of health care; quality of life; resource allocation; withholding treatment; personal financing; Medicaid; Medicare; United States

Thompson, James N. Moral imperatives for academic medicine. *Academic Medicine.* 1997 Dec; 72(12): 1037–1042. 11 refs. BE56607.
  abortion, induced; bioethical issues; biomedical research; curriculum; *economics; euthanasia; financial support; goals; health care delivery; industry; *managed care programs; *medical education; *medical ethics; medical schools; medicine; patient advocacy; physician patient relationship; physician's role; quality of health care; religion; value of life; virtues; North Carolina; United States; Wake Forest University School of Medicine

U.S. Congress. Senate. A bill to prohibit the restriction of certain types of medical communications between a health care provider and a patient [Patient Right to Know Act]. S. 449, 105th Cong., 1st Sess. Introduced by Jon Kyl; 1997 Mar 17. 8 p. Referred to the Committee on Labor and Human Resources. BE57199.
  *communication; *contracts; *disclosure; government regulation; *health insurance; *health personnel; *legal aspects; legislation; managed care programs; patients; professional patient relationship; state government; *Patient Right to Know Act (1997 bill); *United States

U.S. General Accounting Office. Managed Care: Explicit Gag Clauses Not Found in HMO Contracts, but Physician Concerns Remain. Report to Congressional Requesters. Washington, DC: U.S. General Accounting Office; 1997 Aug. 23 p. 23 fn. GAO/HEHS–97–175.

BE = bioethics accession number   fn. = footnotes   refs. = references

BE58448.
    *alternatives; *communication; confidentiality; *contracts; *counseling; *disclosure; *health maintenance organizations; lawyers; *managed care programs; *patient care; physician patient relationship; *physicians; survey; *gag orders; *United States

Ubel, Peter A.; Arnold, Robert M.; Gramelspacher, Gregory P., et al. Acceptance of external funds by physician organizations: issues and policy options. *Journal of General Internal Medicine.* 1995 Nov; 10(11): 624–630. 22 refs. BE57513.
    *conflict of interest; *financial support; gifts; guidelines; industry; interprofessional relations; justice; *organizational policies; patient care; *physicians; *professional organizations; risks and benefits; integrity

van Schie, Tejo; Seedhouse, David. The importance of care. *Health Care Analysis.* 1997 Dec; 5(4): 283–291. 19 refs. BE58111.
    *caring; *economics; emotions; ethical theory; health; *health care; *health care delivery; health care reform; managed care programs; nurse patient relationship; nurses; public participation; resource allocation; *utilitarianism; *values; New Zealand
This paper is in three parts. In Part One we briefly explain that an unsophisticated form of utilitarianism -- economic rationalism (ER) -- has become dominant in many health systems. Its proponents argue that one of ER's most important effects is to increase consumer choice. However, evidence from New Zealand does not support this claim. Furthermore, the logic of ER requires the construction of systems which tend to restrict individual participation. In Part Two we argue that although some have advocated an 'ethic of care' in an attempt to counteract ER's utilitarianism, two decades of campaigning have had little influence on health policy. ER's pro-care adversaries have failed to make an impact because they have not developed a taxonomy of care -- they have not established a language compatible with, or as powerful as, ER's. In Part Three, in an attempt to raise the conceptual and practical status of caring in contemporary health systems, we distinguish four different forms of care. In opposition to those who believe the 'ethic of care' can adequately direct health care practice, we demonstrate that care is a secondary notion. We show that in order for a carer to decide which form of care to adopt in different situations she requires a more powerful idea. We contend further that health care ought to be governed by a theory of health, and suggest that 'the foundations theory of health' should be adopted by planners searching for a more humane alternative to ER. We conclude that ER's dominance can and must be challenged. However, only those arguments which offer detailed theoretical analyses of health care, as well as meticulously derived practical policies, have any chance of success.

van Weel, Chris; Michels, Joop. Dying, not old age, to blame for costs of health care. *Lancet.* 1997 Oct 18; 350(9085): 1159–1160. 6 refs. BE56217.
    *age factors; *aged; chronically ill; diagnosis; *economics; *health care; *morbidity; prevalence; stigmatization; *terminal care; terminally ill

Veatch, Robert M. Who should manage care? The case for patients. *Kennedy Institute of Ethics Journal.* 1997 Dec; 7(4): 391–401. 6 refs. BE59022.
    accountability; administrators; beneficence; conflict of interest; costs and benefits; *decision making; economics; gatekeeping; goals; *health care; health promotion; institutional policies; justice; *managed care programs; medicine; obligations to society; patient advocacy; *patient participation; *patients; physician's role; *physicians; prolongation of life; public policy; quality of health care; quality of life; *resource allocation; scarcity; treatment outcome; utilitarianism; value of life; withholding treatment; United States
After establishing that it is essential that health care be rationed in some fashion, the paper examines the arguments for and against clinicians as gatekeepers. It first argues that bedside clinicians do not have the information needed to make allocation decisions. Then it claims that physicians at the bedside can be expected to make the wrong choice for two reasons: their commitment to the Hippocratic ethic forces them to pursue the patient's best interest (even when resources will produce only very marginal benefit and could do much more good elsewhere) and their values will lead them to calculate the net value of treatments incorrectly. Alternative decision makers are considered. It is argued that both groups of physicians and administrators will also make allocations incorrectly and that leaving the allocation decisions to patients themselves is the best approach. Mechanisms for fair and efficient rationing by patients at the societal and individual level are examined.

Verhey, Allen. A Protestant perspective on access to healthcare. *Cambridge Quarterly of Healthcare Ethics.* 1998 Summer; 7(3): 247–253. 14 fn. BE58552.
    *compassion; consensus; *economics; *health care delivery; indigents; *justice; *Protestant ethics; *public policy; *resource allocation; scarcity; Good Samaritanism; United States

Wadman, Meredith. $100m payout after drug data withheld. [News]. *Nature.* 1997 Aug 21; 388(6644): 703. BE56353.
    *biomedical research; *compensation; contracts; costs and benefits; *drug industry; *drugs; economics; *financial support; human experimentation; *information dissemination; investigators; legal liability; *misconduct; patients; universities; Dong, Betty; *Knoll Pharmaceutical Co.; *Synthroid; United States; University of California, San Francisco

Warden, John. Crack down on drug inducements. [News]. *BMJ (British Medical Journal).* 1997 Aug 2; 315(7103): 273. BE56918.
    *conflict of interest; criminal law; *drug industry; *financial support; *gifts; *government regulation; legal liability; *pharmacists; *physicians; *Great Britain

Weber, Leonard. An HMO grievance committee: ethical challenges and opportunities for the organization. *HEC (HealthCare Ethics Committee) Forum.* 1998 Jun; 10(2): 201–212. 1 ref. BE59067.
    alternative therapies; autonomy; case studies; clinical ethics committees; contracts; *dissent; due process; ethical review; *health insurance reimbursement; *health maintenance organizations; institutional ethics; justice; patients' rights; resource allocation; *review committees; therapeutic research

Weil, Peter A. Opinions of health care executives on access to care. *Hospital and Health Services Administration.* 1987 Nov; 32(4): 421–437. 19 refs. BE56673.
    *administrators; *attitudes; biomedical technologies; *economics; emergency care; *financial support; *government financing; health care; *health care delivery; health insurance; *hospitals; *indigents; institutional ethics; justice; medical fees; obligations to society; patient care; physicians; primary health care; proprietary hospitals; survey; withholding treatment; American College of

Healthcare Executives; United States

Werner, Michael J.; American College of Physicians. Understanding the fraud and abuse laws: guidance for internists. *Annals of Internal Medicine.* 1998 Apr 15; 128(8): 678-684. Paper developed by the ACP Health and Public Policy Committee and approved by the ACP Board of Regents on 11 Jan 1998. BE58001.
 *conflict of interest; *economics; entrepreneurship; federal government; *fraud; government financing; *government regulation; guidelines; internal medicine; managed care programs; *physician self-referral; *physicians; professional organizations; proprietary health facilities; punishment; referral and consultation; remuneration; group practice; *American College of Physicians; Department of Health and Human Services; Ethics in Patient Referrals Act 1989; False Claims Act; Health Care Financing Administration; Medicare; *United States

Westfall, John M.; McCabe, Jennifer; Nicholas, Richard A. Personal use of drug samples by physicians and office staff. *JAMA.* 1997 Jul 9; 278(2): 141-143. 18 refs. BE58434.
 advertising; conflict of interest; *drug industry; *drugs; family practice; *gifts; health personnel; internship and residency; patient care; *physicians; statistics; survey; *self care; Colorado
 CONTEXT: Pharmaceutical samples are commonly used in ambulatory care settings. There is limited research on their use or impact on health care providers and patients. OBJECTIVE: To determine the extent of personal use of drug samples over a 1-year period by physicians and medical office staff. DESIGN, SUBJECTS, AND SETTING: An anonymous cross-sectional survey of all physicians, resident physicians, nursing staff, and office staff in a family practice residency. MAIN OUTCOME MEASURE: Quantity of drug samples taken for personal or family use. RESULTS: Of 55 surveys issued, 53 (96%) were returned. A total of 230 separate drug samples were reported taken in amounts ranging from 1 dose to greater than 1 month's supply. Two respondents reported no use of drug samples, while 4 respondents reported taking more than 10 different samples. CONCLUSION: Drug samples are commonly taken by physicians and office staff for personal and family use. The ethical implications of this practice warrant further discussion.

Whiteis, David G. Unhealthy cities: corporate medicine, community economic underdevelopment, and public health. *International Journal of Health Services.* 1997; 27(2): 227-242. 69 refs. BE56016.
 community services; *economics; financial support; government financing; *health care delivery; health care reform; *indigents; *industry; minority groups; politics; *private sector; proprietary health facilities; *public health; *public policy; public sector; *resource allocation; *social impact; *socioeconomic factors; *trends; *urban population; *United States

Whitman, Jeffrey P. Reclaiming the medical profession: the military profession as a model. *Professional Ethics.* 1995 Spring; 4(1): 3-22. 32 fn. BE55796.
 conflict of interest; conscience; *economics; entrepreneurship; *goals; *health care reform; killing; malpractice; *medical ethics; *medicine; *metaphor; *military personnel; misconduct; *moral obligations; morality; organizational policies; patient advocacy; *physician's role; *physicians; *professional autonomy; professional competence; *professional ethics; professional organizations; public opinion; remuneration; *resource allocation; *self regulation; trust; virtues; *war; *professional role; American Medical Association; United States

Wiener, Carolyn L.; Strauss, Anselm L., eds. Where Medicine Fails. Fifth Edition. New Brunswick, NJ: Transaction Publishers; 1997. 407 p. Includes references. With a new introduction by Carolyn L. Wiener. ISBN 1-56000-869-5. BE56191.
 advance directives; aged; AIDS; assisted suicide; attitudes to death; biomedical technologies; cancer; cesarean section; childbirth; chronically ill; drug abuse; *economics; fetal tissue donation; fetuses; government financing; *health care delivery; *health care reform; health hazards; health insurance; *hospitals; indigents; industry; managed care programs; medical ethics; patient care; patient discharge; physicians; pregnant women; proprietary hospitals; public hospitals; *public policy; resource allocation; values; homeless persons; Medicaid; Medicare; United States

Wildes, Keven Wm. Institutional identity, integrity, and conscience. *Kennedy Institute of Ethics Journal.* 1997 Dec; 7(4): 413-419. 9 refs. BE59024.
 accountability; *bioethics; *conscience; economics; *goals; guidelines; health care delivery; historical aspects; *institutional ethics; *institutional policies; justice; *managed care programs; medicine; models, theoretical; religious hospitals; Roman Catholic ethics; science; postmodernism; United States
 Bioethics has focused on the areas of individual ethical choices -- patient care -- or public policy and law. There are however, important arenas for ethical choices that have been overlooked. Health care is populated with intermediate arenas such as hospitals, nursing homes, hospices, and health care systems. This essay argues that bioethics needs to develop a language and concepts for institutional ethics. A first step in this direction is to think about institutional conscience.

Wildes, Kevin Wm.; Wallace, Robert B. Relationships with payers and institutions that manage and deliver patient services. *In:* McCullough, Laurence B.; Jones, James W.; Brody, Baruch A., eds. Surgical Ethics. New York, NY: Oxford University Press; 1998: 367-383. 18 refs. ISBN 0-19-510347-5. BE58339.
 administrators; advertising; autonomy; beneficence; clinical ethics committees; *conflict of interest; disclosure; *economics; goals; *health facilities; *health insurance; health insurance reimbursement; hospitals; incentives; informed consent; institutional ethics; institutional policies; *managed care programs; medical education; *moral obligations; *patient advocacy; *physician patient relationship; *physicians; practice guidelines; quality of health care; referral and consultation; remuneration; *resource allocation; *surgery; trust; withholding treatment; health services misuse; preventive ethics; undertreatment; United States

Wilson, Donna M. Administrative decision making in response to sudden health care agency funding reductions: is there a role for ethics? *Nursing Ethics.* 1998 Jul; 5(4): 319-329. 51 refs. BE58871.
 *administrators; *decision making; *economics; employment; *financial support; government financing; health care delivery; health facilities; institutional ethics; *organization and administration; *professional ethics; *public hospitals; resource allocation; survey; *Alberta

Wilson, Kumanan; Cook, Deborah J. Economics and the intensive care unit: a conflict of interests? *Journal of Critical Care.* 1997 Sep; 12(3): 147-151. 29 refs. BE58259.
 age factors; aged; cancer; *costs and benefits; *intensive care units; mortality; prognosis; quality adjusted life years; *resource allocation; selection for treatment; treatment outcome

Winslade, William J. Intellectual cross-dressing: an

BE = bioethics accession number   fn. = footnotes   refs. = references

eccentricity or a practical necessity? Commentary on Morreim. *In:* Carson, Ronald A.; Burns, Chester R., eds. Philosophy of Medicine and Bioethics: A Twenty-Year Retrospective and Critical Appraisal. Boston, MA: Kluwer Academic; 1997: 327–334. 3 refs. ISBN 0-7923-3545-7. BE56545.
> bioethics; conflict of interest; *economics; ethicist's role; financial support; *health care delivery; health education; legal liability; legal obligations; moral obligations; patient advocacy; patient care; patient education; physician patient relationship; *physician's role; *physicians; resource allocation; standards; United States

Wiseman, Virginia. Caring: the neglected health outcome? or input? *Health Policy.* 1997 Jan; 39(1): 43–53. 33 refs. BE55544.
> altruism; *caring; *economics; evaluation; family members; health; health care; models, theoretical; morality; *motivation; paternalism; patient care; social interaction; sociobiology; treatment outcome; utilitarianism

Wolf, Bruce L.; Westfall, John M.; McCabe, Jennifer, et al. Drug samples: benefit or bait? [Letter and response]. *JAMA.* 1998 Jun 3; 279(21): 1698–1699. 7 refs. BE58435.
> advertising; conflict of interest; *drug industry; *drugs; *economics; *gifts; indigents; patient care; *physicians

Wood, Joseph Patrick. Emergency physicians' obligations to managed care patients under COBRA. *Academic Emergency Medicine.* 1996 Aug; 3(8): 794–800. 34 refs. BE58110.
> *emergency care; federal government; *government regulation; hospitals; informed consent; institutional policies; *legal aspects; *legal liability; legal obligations; *managed care programs; *patient transfer; *physicians; *refusal to treat; selection for treatment; standards; *Consolidated Omnibus Budget Reconciliation Act (COBRA) 1985; Emergency Medical Treatment and Active Labor Act 1986; *United States

Yaes, Robert J.; Dveirin, Keith; Shelman, Keith, et al. Contempo 1997: economics. [Letters and response]. *JAMA.* 1997 Oct 8; 278(14): 1149–1150. 1 ref. BE55899.
> dehumanization; disclosure; *economics; employment; *entrepreneurship; health insurance; health maintenance organizations; incentives; industry; institutional ethics; medical ethics; moral obligations; motivation; patient advocacy; patients; physician patient relationship; *physicians; primary health care; professional autonomy; *property rights; *proprietary health facilities; practice management; United States

Young, Christopher J. Emergency! Says who?: analysis of the legal issues concerning managed care and emergency medical services. [Comment]. *Journal of Contemporary Health Law and Policy.* 1997 Spring; 13(2): 553–579. 207 fn. BE56017.
> diagnosis; *emergency care; federal government; gatekeeping; *government regulation; *health insurance reimbursement; *hospitals; *legal aspects; *managed care programs; patient discharge; patient transfer; physicians; referral and consultation; *standards; state government; Access to Emergency Medical Services Act 1997 (1995 bill); Emergency Medical Treatment and Active Labor Act 1986; Employee Retirement Income Security Act 1974 (ERISA); *United States

Yount, Lisa. How should health care be allocated? [Juvenile literature]. *In:* her Issues in Biomedical Ethics. San Diego, CA: Lucent Books; 1998: 17–35, 99–101. 33 fn. ISBN 1-56006-476-5. BE57679.
> administrators; biomedical technologies; common good; conflict of interest; *costs and benefits; *decision making;

economics; government financing; guidelines; *health care delivery; health insurance; incentives; indigents; managed care programs; morality; organ transplantation; patient advocacy; physicians; preventive medicine; prognosis; public opinion; public participation; *public policy; refusal to treat; *resource allocation; selection for treatment; self induced illness; social worth; standards; state government; life style; Medicaid; Oregon; United States

Zohar, Noam J. A Jewish perspective on access to healthcare. *Cambridge Quarterly of Healthcare Ethics.* 1998 Summer; 7(3): 260–265. 18 fn. BE58554.
> *economics; health care; *health care delivery; *Jewish ethics; managed care programs; *obligations of society; *resource allocation; United States

Zoloth-Dorfman, Laurie; Rubin, Susan B. "Medical futility": managed care and the powerful new vocabulary for clinical and public policy discourse. *Healthcare Forum Journal.* 1997 Mar–Apr; 40(2): 28, 30–33. BE57057.
> AIDS; allowing to die; biomedical technologies; case studies; clinical ethics committees; costs and benefits; cultural pluralism; *decision making; dissent; family members; *futility; *goals; health facilities; institutional policies; justice; *managed care programs; medicine; patient care team; persistent vegetative state; physicians; practice guidelines; *prolongation of life; public policy; *resource allocation; terminally ill; *values; *withholding treatment; evidence-based medicine; United States

HEALTH CARE/FOREIGN COUNTRIES

Brecher, Bob. What would a socialist health service look like? *Health Care Analysis.* 1997 Sep; 5(3): 217–225. 29 fn. BE55812.
> accountability; capitalism; democracy; economics; freedom; health; *health care delivery; health care reform; justice; obligations of society; paternalism; politics; private sector; public participation; public sector; resource allocation; *socialism; socioeconomic factors; standards; state medicine; values; liberalism; *Great Britain; Kant, Immanuel; *National Health Service; Rawls, John

A socialist health service cannot be a socialist island in a sea of capitalism, as the record of the British National Health Service shows. Nonetheless, since health is a basic need, it can be a key component of the advocacy of socialism. I propose two central socialist principles. On the basis of these I suggest that a socialist health system would emphasise care rather than service; insist on democratic structures and control of resources; and require the prohibition of private medicine.

Burgoyne, Carole B. Distributive justice and rationing in the NHS: framing effects in press coverage of a controversial decision. *Journal of Community and Applied Social Psychology.* 1997 Apr; 7(2): 119–136. 28 refs. BE57544.
> administrators; bone marrow; *children; costs and benefits; *decision making; *government financing; *health care delivery; justice; leukemia; *mass media; parents; physicians; prognosis; public opinion; *public sector; quality of life; *refusal to treat; *resource allocation; social worth; tissue transplantation; value of life; values; *withholding treatment; *Bowen, Jaymee; *Great Britain; *National Health Service; R v. Cambridge Health Authority

Coney, Sandra. Rationing in health care under scrutiny in New Zealand. [News]. *Lancet.* 1997 Oct 18; 350(9085): 1152. BE56182.
> dementia; guidelines; *health care delivery; health care reform; private sector; *public policy; public sector; refusal to treat; renal dialysis; *resource allocation; selection for treatment; withholding treatment; *New Zealand; Williams,

Rau

Coney, Sandra. To the uninformed: managed care means damaged ethics. [Letter]. *Health Care Analysis.* 1997 Sep; 5(3): 252–258. 6 refs. BE55816.
accountability; administrators; conflict of interest; decision making; disclosure; *economics; gatekeeping; government financing; guidelines; health care delivery; *health care reform; health promotion; hospitals; incentives; industry; insurance selection bias; international aspects; *managed care programs; physician patient relationship; physicians; primary health care; private sector; public participation; public policy; public sector; quality of health care; referral and consultation; resource allocation; *social impact; withholding treatment; capitation fee; personal financing; *New Zealand

Edgar, Andrew; Salek, Sam; Shickle, Darren, et al. The Ethical QALY: Ethical Issues in Healthcare Resource Allocations. Haslemere, Surrey, England: Euromed Communications; 1998. 168 p. Bibliography: p. 139–168. ISBN 1-899015-21-3. BE58582.
age factors; drug industry; economics; evaluation; health; *health care; *health care delivery; *international aspects; justice; legal aspects; methods; *moral policy; personhood; public health; *public policy; *quality adjusted life years; *quality of life; *resource allocation; scarcity; selection for treatment; social discrimination; social worth; time factors; trends; value of life; Czech Republic; Denmark; *Europe; France; Great Britain; Greece; Netherlands; New Zealand; Norway; Slovakia; Slovenia; Sweden

Fenigsen, Richard. Physician–assisted death in the Netherlands: impact on long–term care. *Issues in Law and Medicine.* 1995 Winter; 11(3): 283–297. 59 fn. BE58820.
*active euthanasia; adults; age factors; *aged; *allowing to die; assisted suicide; attitudes; children; congenital disorders; decision making; *disabled; Down syndrome; hospitals; infants; *involuntary euthanasia; *long–term care; mentally retarded; newborns; nurses; nursing homes; physicians; public opinion; *public policy; quality of health care; *social impact; *voluntary euthanasia; *withholding treatment; *Netherlands

Gillett, Grant. Justice and health care in a caring society. *BMJ (British Medical Journal).* 1998 Jul 4; 317(7150): 53–54. 2 refs. BE58813.
biomedical research; caring; commodification; common good; *government financing; health; *health care; *health care delivery; indigents; international aspects; *justice; private sector; *public policy; public sector; resource allocation; *rights; *socioeconomic factors; state medicine; values; *Great Britain; *National Health Service; *New Zealand

Gitanjali, B.; Shashindran, C.H.; Tripathi, K.D., et al. Are drug advertisements in Indian edition of BMJ unethical? [Article and commentary]. *BMJ (British Medical Journal).* 1997 Aug 23; 315(7106): 459–460. 12 refs. BE56649.
*advertising; alternative therapies; comparative studies; *deception; *drug industry; *drugs; *editorial policies; financial support; health personnel; *international aspects; *misconduct; *standards; survey; technical expertise; *BMJ (British Medical Journal); Great Britain; *India; World Health Organization

Ham, Chris. Priority setting in health care: learning from international experience. *Health Policy.* 1997 Oct; 42(1): 49–66. 23 refs. BE57983.
advisory committees; biomedical technologies; common good; comparative studies; consensus; costs and benefits; *decision making; *economics; government financing; *health care; health care delivery; health personnel;

indigents; *international aspects; justice; mass media; practice guidelines; public participation; *public policy; quality of life; *resource allocation; rights; selection for treatment; state government; technical expertise; technology assessment; *values; evidence–based medicine; *Great Britain; Medicaid; National Health Service; *Netherlands; *New Zealand; *Oregon; *Sweden; United States

Hunt, Geoffrey, ed. Whistleblowing in the Health Service: Accountability, Law and Professional Practice. London: Edward Arnold; 1995. 170 p. Includes references. ISBN 0-340-59234-6. BE55681.
*accountability; *administrators; confidentiality; democracy; employment; *government regulation; health care delivery; *health personnel; hospitals; information dissemination; international aspects; *legal aspects; malpractice; *misconduct; nurses; organization and administration; patient care; physicians; professional autonomy; *professional competence; *quality of health care; *self regulation; standards; values; *whistleblowing; *Great Britain; *National Health Service; United States

Kinmonth, Ann Louise; Reinhard, John; Bobrow, Martin, et al. The new genetics: implications for clinical services in Britain and the United States. *BMJ (British Medical Journal).* 1998 Mar 7; 316(7133): 767–770. 34 refs. BE57755.
comparative studies; computer communication networks; continuing education; data banks; genetic counseling; genetic disorders; genetic information; genetic predisposition; genetic research; genetic screening; *genetic services; genetics; guidelines; health care delivery; interdisciplinary communication; *international aspects; medical specialties; patient care team; patient education; physicians; *primary health care; private sector; referral and consultation; registries; risk; support groups; *Great Britain; Internet; National Health Service; *United States

Klein, Rudolph; Day, Patricia; Redmayne, Sharon. Managing Scarcity: Priority Setting and Rationing in the National Health Service. Philadelphia, PA: Open University Press; 1996. 161 p. (State of health series). Bibliography: p. 143–153. ISBN 0-335-19446-X. BE55699.
accountability; administrators; age factors; biomedical technologies; *decision making; *economics; government financing; health care; *health care delivery; health care reform; international aspects; physician's role; physicians; politics; public participation; *public policy; quality adjusted life years; referral and consultation; refusal to treat; renal dialysis; reproductive technologies; *resource allocation; scarcity; *selection for treatment; self induced illness; standards; time factors; uncertainty; evidence–based medicine; geographic factors; *Great Britain; *National Health Service; Oregon; United States

Light, Donald W. The real ethics of rationing. *BMJ (British Medical Journal).* 1997 Jul 12; 315(7100): 112–115. 19 refs. This article is a shortened version of the inaugural lecture given at the Institute of Medicine, Law, and Bioethics of the University of Manchester on 26 Mar 1997. BE55651.
accountability; administrators; costs and benefits; *government financing; *health care; *health care delivery; health insurance; insurance selection bias; justice; medical specialties; misconduct; *organization and administration; physician's role; private sector; public policy; *resource allocation; scarcity; selection for treatment; surgery; time factors; treatment outcome; evidence–based medicine; geographic factors; health services misuse; *Great Britain; *National Health Service

Marshall, Tom; St. Leger, Moya Frenz; Woodroffe, Caroline, et al. Rationing health care. [Letters]. *BMJ (British Medical Journal).* 1997 Jun 28; 314(7098):

1901–1902. 7 refs. BE56916.

    age factors; common good; costs and benefits; *goals; health; health care; *health care delivery; justice; moral policy; national health insurance; public health; *public policy; quality of life; *resource allocation; selection for treatment; social discrimination; utilitarianism; *Great Britain; *National Health Service

Morgan, Derek. Health rights, ethics and justice: the opportunity costs of rhetoric. *In:* McLean, Sheila A.M., ed. Contemporary Issues in Law, Medicine and Ethics. Brookfield, VT: Dartmouth; 1996: 15–27. 32 fn. ISBN 1-85521-586-1. BE57788.

    alternatives; confidentiality; cultural pluralism; disclosure; emergency care; government regulation; health; *health care; human rights; international aspects; *justice; legal rights; legislation; moral obligations; *moral policy; obligations of society; patient access to records; *patients' rights; physician patient relationship; public health; *public policy; referral and consultation; *resource allocation; *rights; risks and benefits; selection for treatment; socioeconomic factors; *standards; life style; European Union; *Great Britain; *National Health Service; Patient's Charter (Great Britain)

Mustard, Cameron A.; Kaufert, Patricia; Kozyrskyj, Anita, et al. Sex differences in the use of health care services. *New England Journal of Medicine.* 1998 Jun 4; 338(23): 1678–1683. 40 refs. BE58100.

    age factors; comparative studies; *economics; *females; *health care; hospitals; *males; mortality; national health insurance; patient care; physicians; reproduction; statistics; terminal care; Canada; *Manitoba

BACKGROUND: Sex differences in the use of health care services can be substantial at several stages of life. However, the extent to which differences in reproductive biology and mortality affect the use of health care services is unclear. METHODS: We studied age- and sex-specific per capita use of health care resources for a one-year period during 1994 and 1995 in the Canadian province of Manitoba, where there is universal insurance for a comprehensive range of health care services. Using information obtained from administrative records of physicians' services and acute hospital care, we tabulated the use of health care resources by male and female subjects in three categories: care for conditions specific to sex, care provided to persons who died during the study year, and care provided for all other conditions. RESULTS: The crude annual per capita use of health care resources (in Canadian dollars) was greater for female subjects ($1,164) than for male subjects ($918). Approximately 22 percent of health care expenditures for female subjects was associated with conditions specific to sex, including pregnancy and childbirth, as compared with 3 percent of expenditures for male subjects. An estimated 14 percent of health care expenditures for male subjects was consumed by persons who died during the study period, as compared with 10 percent of expenditures for female subjects. After adjustment for the use of health care associated with sex-specific conditions and differences in mortality, the female:male ratio in health care expenditures was reduced from 1.3 to 1.0. CONCLUSIONS: Expenditures for health care are similar for male and female subjects after differences in reproductive biology and higher age-specific mortality rates among men have been accounted for.

New, Bill; Le Grand, Julian. Rationing in the NHS: Principles and Pragmatism. London: King's Fund Publishing; 1996. 77 p. Bibliography: p. 73–77. ISBN 1-85717-113-6. BE59102.

    aged; costs and benefits; *decision making; drugs; economics;

goals; government financing; *health care delivery; health care reform; hospitals; justice; national health insurance; physician's role; public participation; *public policy; quality adjusted life years; *resource allocation; selection for treatment; self induced illness; standards; time factors; needs; *Great Britain; *National Health Service

Osborne, Judith A. Incarcerating Hippocrates. *Legal Medical Quarterly.* 1984–1985; 8–9: 1–8. 49 fn. BE55538.

    confidentiality; contracts; decision making; economics; *health care delivery; institutionalized persons; *legal aspects; legal rights; medical records; *organization and administration; physician patient relationship; physicians; *prisoners; *private sector; professional autonomy; professional competence; quality of health care; resource allocation; *British Columbia; Canada; United States

Paton, Calum. Necessary conditions for a socialist health service. *Health Care Analysis.* 1997 Sep; 5(3): 205–216. 14 refs. BE55828.

    capitalism; democracy; *economics; freedom; goals; government financing; health; health care; *health care delivery; health care reform; hospitals; international aspects; justice; national health insurance; organization and administration; political systems; politics; primary health care; private sector; public sector; resource allocation; *socialism; socioeconomic factors; standards; state medicine; personal financing; *Great Britain; *National Health Service

A socialist health service in a non-socialist society may be forced to stress care and rescue rather than prevention, health maintenance or the promotion of better health and more equal health status. A socialist health service ought to be 'integrated'. A socialist health service ought to provide universal and comprehensive care.

Rasmussen, P. Elmegaard; Larsen, P. Munkholm; Nielsen, V.G., et al. Does physicians' knowledge of costing related to clinical decision making change the consumption of resources despite unchanged medical standards? *Scandinavian Journal of Gastroenterology.* 1985; 20(4): 401–406. 7 refs. BE57073.

    *biomedical technologies; comparative studies; decision making; drugs; *economics; evaluation studies; *hospitals; *knowledge, attitudes, practice; *patient care; *physicians; quality of health care; *resource allocation; *physician's practice patterns; *Denmark

Richmond, Caroline; Heasell, Stephen; Kahtan, Susannah, et al. Compensation for victims of medical accidents. [Letters]. *BMJ (British Medical Journal).* 1998 Jan 3; 316(7124): 73–74. 2 refs. BE57973.

    *compensation; economics; *health care; hospitals; iatrogenic disease; *injuries; legal aspects; *legal liability; *negligence; *patient care; *patients; physicians; *resource allocation; time factors; *Great Britain; National Health Service

Robb, Merlin L.; Khambaroong, Chirasak; Nelson, Kenrad E., et al. Studies in Thailand of the vertical transmission of HIV. [Letters]. *New England Journal of Medicine.* 1998 Mar 19; 338(12): 843–844. 2 refs. BE57708.

    AIDS; *drugs; financial support; health care delivery; *HIV seropositivity; *human experimentation; informed consent; newborns; *nontherapeutic research; patient care; *pregnant women; *standards; *therapeutic research; time factors; *AZT; Chiang Mai University; Department of Defense; Johns Hopkins University; Ministry of Health (Thailand); National Institutes of Health; *Thailand; United States; Walter Reed Army Institute of Research

Sapru, R.P. Ethical concerns in modern medical practice. *Indian Heart Journal.* 1997 Jul–Aug; 49(4): 441–445. 23

BE = bioethics accession number   fn. = footnotes   refs. = references

refs. BE58562.

communication; confidentiality; continuing education; developing countries; disclosure; drug industry; drugs; economics; *health care; heart diseases; Hindu ethics; human experimentation; indigents; informed consent; medical education; *medical ethics; palliative care; *patient care; physician patient relationship; physician self-referral; physicians; *professional competence; quality of health care; regulation; surgery; *India

Sevenhuijsen, Selma. Feminist ethics and public health care policies: a case study on the Netherlands. *In:* DiQuinzio, Patrice; Young, Iris Marion, eds. Feminist Ethics and Social Policy. Bloomington, IN: Indiana University Press; 1997: 49–76. 43 refs. 17 fn. ISBN 0–253–21125–5. BE57285.

advisory committees; aged; autonomy; *caring; communitarianism; cosmetic surgery; cultural pluralism; democracy; ethical theory; *females; *feminist ethics; freedom; gatekeeping; health; *health care; *health care delivery; health care reform; health insurance reimbursement; home care; in vitro fertilization; industry; *justice; males; normality; obligations of society; obligations to society; policy analysis; private sector; *public participation; *public policy; public sector; resource allocation; rights; social control; social interaction; *standards; terminology; vulnerable populations; women's health services; empowerment; liberalism; *Choices in Health Care (Netherlands); Dunning Committee; *Netherlands

Sheaft, Rod. The Need for Healthcare. New York, NY: Routledge; 1996. 228 p. (Social ethics and policy series). Bibliography: p. 213–224. ISBN 0–415–10112–3. BE58649.

decision making; economics; ethical theory; health; *health care; *health care delivery; health personnel; incentives; international aspects; morality; motivation; normality; patients; physicians; professional autonomy; *public policy; resource allocation; scarcity; *needs; Europe; *Great Britain; *National Health Service; United States

Siegel–Itzkovich, Judy. Doctors banned from drug company trip. [News]. *BMJ (British Medical Journal).* 1998 Aug 8; 317(7155): 370. BE58749.

conflict of interest; *drug industry; *financial support; *gifts; *government regulation; international aspects; *physicians; public sector; *Israel; *Teva

Siegel–Itzkovich, Judy. Palestinian man shackled in Jerusalem hospital. [News]. *BMJ (British Medical Journal).* 1997 Sep 6; 315(7108): 568. BE56883.

dangerousness; dehumanization; hospitals; human rights; *patient care; *physical restraint; physicians; *prisoners; professional organizations; public policy; *Israel; Israel Medical Association; *Palestinians

Silver, Melanie H. Wilson. Patients' rights in England and the United States of America: *The Patient's Charter* and the New Jersey Patient Bill of Rights: a comparison. *Journal of Medical Ethics.* 1997 Aug; 23(4): 213–220. 16 fn. BE55925.

communication; comparative studies; due process; evaluation; *government regulation; health care; *health care delivery; health promotion; hospitals; human experimentation; informed consent; legal rights; minority groups; misconduct; patient care; *patients' rights; physically disabled; *public policy; quality of health care; resource allocation; *standards; state government; treatment refusal; hearing disorders; quality assurance; translating; *England; Great Britain; *National Health Service; *New Jersey; *New Jersey Patient Bill of Rights; *Patient's Charter (Great Britain); United States

The Patient's Charter has been in effect for nearly five years. This article considers the purpose and value of

the document through a comparison with the New Jersey Patient Bill of Rights. Patient rights statements have been posted in American hospitals for more than twenty years. However, the New Jersey document and the patient rights programme it established seven years ago, have proven to be economically effective, successful in their representation of patients and enforceable, due to the adoption of state legislation and regulation to oversee the process. Several examples of how the programme works are included in the comparison, with a similar review of The Patient's Charter. In the comparison the author argues that for the programme to succeed as it has done in New Jersey, the government will need to develop legislative backing to ensure enforcement, and an efficient system for monitoring compliance. The programme will need to become credible in the eyes of the health service user. The author suggests this may be best achieved by developing an efficient, accessible and user-friendly means of redress, should the patient consider his or her rights have been violated. A "mish-mash" of quality assurance standards and levels of care which patients can "expect" from the health service providers only serves to distract the health service user from the government's failure to commit the resources that would empower the patients rights portion of The Patient's Charter.

Sorum, Paul C. Striking against managed care: the last gasp of *la medicine liberale*? *JAMA.* 1998 Aug 19; 280(7): 659–664. 36 refs. BE59001.

*economics; government regulation; guidelines; *health care delivery; *health care reform; incentives; internship and residency; *managed care programs; medical education; medical fees; medical records; medical specialties; *national health insurance; patient access to records; *physicians; political systems; politics; practice guidelines; primary health care; *public policy; referral and consultation; sociology of medicine; *strikes; *France

The French health care system combines a strong tradition of autonomous private practice with nearly universal health care coverage through the social security system. The French state's responses to rising health care expenditures have included limitation of the number of medical students, control over physician fees, rules to prohibit certain clinical practices, experiments with generalist physicians coordinating care and access to specialists, and collective physician responsibility for expenditures beyond the health care budget. The failure of physicians' protests, including a strike of French residents and fellows in 1997, may signify the end of traditional private practice in the face of France's statist version of managed care.

Stronks, Karien; Strijbis, Anne-Margreet; Wendte, Johannes F., et al. Who should decide? Qualitative analysis of panel data from public, patients, healthcare professionals, and insurers on priorities in health care. *BMJ (British Medical Journal).* 1997 Jul 12; 315(7100): 92–96. 11 refs. BE55652.

aged; alternative therapies; breast cancer; circumcision; comparative studies; contraception; costs and benefits; *decision making; drugs; *government financing; *health care; health insurance; home care; hormones; in vitro fertilization; justice; mass screening; *national health insurance; organ transplantation; *patients; *physicians; *public participation; public policy; residential facilities; *resource allocation; selection for treatment; sports medicine; standards; survey; copayments; homeopathy; personal financing; qualitative research; *Netherlands

OBJECTIVE: To explore the arguments underlying the choices of patients, the public, general practitioners, specialists, and health insurers regarding priorities in

---

BE = bioethics accession number   fn. = footnotes   refs. = references

health care. DESIGN: A qualitative analysis of data gathered in a series of panels. Members were asked to economise on the publicly funded healthcare budget, exemplified by 10 services. RESULTS: From a medical point of view, both panels of healthcare professionals thought most services were necessary. The general practitioners tried to achieve the budget cuts by limiting access to services to those most in need of them or those who cannot afford to pay for them. The specialists emphasised the possibilities of reducing costs by increasing the efficiency within services and preventing inappropriate utilisation. The patients mainly economised by limiting universal access to preventive and acute services. The "public" panels excluded services that are relatively inexpensive for individual patients. Moreover, they emphasised the individual's own responsibility for health behaviour and the costs of health care, resulting in the choice for copayments. The health insurers emphasised the importance of including services that relate to a risk only, as well as feasibility aspects. CONCLUSIONS: There were substantial differences in the way the different groups approached the issue of what should be included in the basic package. Healthcare professionals seem to be most aware of the importance of maintaining equal access for everyone in need of health care.

Warden, John. Crack down on drug inducements. [News]. *BMJ (British Medical Journal).* 1997 Aug 2; 315(7103): 273. BE56918.
*conflict of interest; criminal law; *drug industry; *financial support; *gifts; *government regulation; legal liability; *pharmacists; *physicians; *Great Britain

Weale, Albert. Rationing health care: a logical solution to an inconsistent triad. [Editorial]. *BMJ (British Medical Journal).* 1998 Feb 7; 316(7129): 410. 5 refs. BE57851.
*health care delivery; *public policy; quality of health care; *resource allocation; values; *Great Britain; National Health Service; United States

Wells, John S.G. Health care rationing: nursing perspectives. *Journal of Advanced Nursing.* 1995 Oct; 22(4): 738–744. 59 refs. BE55780.
aged; beneficence; chronically ill; decision making; economics; guidelines; *health care delivery; hospitals; indigents; international aspects; justice; moral obligations; nurse's role; *nurses; nursing ethics; obligations to society; patient advocacy; *resource allocation; scarcity; selection for treatment; state medicine; values; *Great Britain; *National Health Service; United States

Wilson, Donna M. Administrative decision making in response to sudden health care agency funding reductions: is there a role for ethics? *Nursing Ethics.* 1998 Jul; 5(4): 319–329. 51 refs. BE58871.
*administrators; *decision making; *economics; employment; *financial support; government financing; health care delivery; health facilities; institutional ethics; *organization and administration; *professional ethics; *public hospitals; resource allocation; survey; *Alberta

Wise, Jacqui. British public wants free health care, whatever the cost. [News]. *BMJ (British Medical Journal).* 1998 May 16; 316(7143): 1478. BE58248.
aged; alternative therapies; *economics; government financing; *health care delivery; *public opinion; public participation; resource allocation; *Great Britain; National Health Service

HEALTH CARE RATIONING See RESOURCE ALLOCATION, SELECTION FOR

TREATMENT

HEALTH CARE/RIGHTS

Benatar, Solomon R. Just healthcare beyond individualism: challenges for North American bioethics. *Cambridge Quarterly of Healthcare Ethics.* 1997 Fall; 6(4): 397–415. 208 fn. Appendix: proposed World Medical Association statement on health and human rights, p. 414–415. Article based on a presentation at the World Medical Association Symposium, "Medical Ethics, Humanities' Needs: Formulating a Future Ethical Program for the WMA," held in Stockholm, Sep 1994, and on the Rosenstadt Lecture, University of Toronto, Mar 1995. BE56455.
autonomy; beneficence; *bioethics; *common good; communitarianism; cultural pluralism; democracy; developing countries; disadvantaged; *economics; ethicist's role; freedom; health; *health care; *health care delivery; health care reform; health promotion; *human rights; industry; institutional ethics; *international aspects; *justice; medical ethics; medicine; moral complicity; moral obligations; *obligations to society; organizational policies; physician patient relationship; *physician's role; political systems; professional organizations; public health; resource allocation; review; science; *socioeconomic factors; trends; values; non-Western World; Western World; United States; World Medical Organization

Consortium for Health and Human Rights. Writing Group. Health and human rights: a call to action on the 50th anniversary of the Universal Declaration of Human Rights. *JAMA.* 1998 Aug 5; 280(5): 462–464. 77 refs. BE58765.
ecology; freedom; guidelines; *health; *health care; health personnel; human experimentation; *human rights; *international aspects; public health; public policy; social discrimination; torture; war; women's rights; *Universal Declaration of Human Rights

Davis, Anne J.; Aroskar, Mila A.; Liaschenko, Joan, et al. Rights, responsibilities, and health care. *In: their* Ethical Dilemmas and Nursing Practice. Fourth Edition. Stamford, CT: Appleton and Lange; 1997: 83–103. 25 fn. ISBN 0-8385-2283-1. BE58594.
case studies; economics; *health care; health facilities; justice; legal aspects; *moral obligations; *nurses; *nursing ethics; *patient advocacy; *patients' rights; resource allocation; *rights; standards; United States

Dillon, Mary Ann. A dynamic force for change: the common good provides the rationale for a healthcare system for all. *Health Progress.* 1997 Mar–Apr; 78(2): 31–33, 42. 14 fn. BE56446.
*common good; disadvantaged; guidelines; *health care delivery; *health care reform; *human rights; justice; moral obligations; obligations of society; obligations to society; resource allocation; *Roman Catholic ethics; standards; theology; United States

Engelhardt, H. Tristram. Freedom and moral diversity: the moral failures of health care in the welfare state. *Social Philosophy and Policy.* 1997 Summer; 14(2): 180–196. 32 fn. BE55549.
age factors; coercion; costs and benefits; democracy; *economics; ethical relativism; females; *freedom; government financing; *health care delivery; health insurance; indigents; international aspects; *justice; males; moral obligations; *moral policy; morality; morbidity; mortality; obligations of society; *public policy; religion; resource allocation; *rights; risk; secularism; self induced illness; socioeconomic factors; standards; suffering; values; personal financing; postmodernism; rationality; Medicare;

United States

Gillett, Grant. Justice and health care in a caring society. *BMJ (British Medical Journal).* 1998 Jul 4; 317(7150): 53–54. 2 refs. BE58813.
   biomedical research; caring; commodification; common good; *government financing; health; *health care; *health care delivery; indigents; international aspects; *justice; private sector; *public policy; public sector; resource allocation; *rights; *socioeconomic factors; state medicine; values; *Great Britain; *National Health Service; *New Zealand

McCormick, Richard A. A Catholic perspective on access to healthcare. *Cambridge Quarterly of Healthcare Ethics.* 1998 Summer; 7(3): 254–259. 13 fn. BE58553.
   common good; *health care; health care delivery; health promotion; *human rights; indigents; justice; national health insurance; obligations of society; resource allocation; *Roman Catholic ethics; value of life; National Conference of Catholic Bishops; United States; Universal Declaration of Human Rights

Mariner, Wendy K. Mortal Peril: Our Inalienable Right to Health Care? by Richard A. Epstein. [Book review essay]. *JAMA.* 1998 Jan 28; 279(4): 330–331. BE57829.
   *autonomy; coercion; contracts; *economics; emergency care; freedom; government financing; *government regulation; *health care; *health care delivery; health insurance; justice; libertarianism; managed care programs; *public policy; *rights; Medicare; *Mortal Peril: Our Inalienable Right to Health Care? (Epstein, R.A.); *United States

Morgan, Derek. Health rights, ethics and justice: the opportunity costs of rhetoric. *In:* McLean, Sheila A.M., ed. Contemporary Issues in Law, Medicine and Ethics. Brookfield, VT: Dartmouth; 1996: 15–27. 32 fn. ISBN 1-85521-586-1. BE57788.
   alternatives; confidentiality; cultural pluralism; disclosure; emergency care; government regulation; health; *health care; human rights; international aspects; *justice; legal rights; legislation; moral obligations; *moral policy; obligations of society; patient access to records; *patients' rights; physician patient relationship; public health; *public policy; referral and consultation; *resource allocation; *rights; risks and benefits; selection for treatment; socioeconomic factors; *standards; life style; European Union; *Great Britain; *National Health Service; Patient's Charter (Great Britain)

Trappenburg, Margo J. Defining the medical sphere. *Cambridge Quarterly of Healthcare Ethics.* 1997 Fall; 6(4): 416–434. 39 fn. BE56481.
   aged; autonomy; *communitarianism; cultural pluralism; economics; health; *health care; health care delivery; human rights; *justice; medicine; morality; philosophy; physicians; professional autonomy; property rights; *resource allocation; *rights; selection for treatment; values; liberalism; Callahan, Daniel; Daniels, Norman; Dworkin, Ronald; Nozick, Robert; Rawls, John; *Spheres of Justice (Walzer, M.); United States; *Walzer, Michael

HEALTH ECONOMICS *See* HEALTH CARE/ECONOMICS, RESOURCE ALLOCATION

HEALTH PERSONNEL
See under
   AIDS/HEALTH PERSONNEL

HOSPICES
See under
   TERMINAL CARE/HOSPICES

HOSPITAL ETHICS COMMITTEES *See* ETHICISTS AND ETHICS COMMITTEES

HOST MOTHERS *See* SURROGATE MOTHERS

HUMAN EXPERIMENTATION

See also BEHAVIORAL RESEARCH, BIOMEDICAL RESEARCH, EMBRYO AND FETAL RESEARCH, GENETIC RESEARCH
See also under
   AIDS/HUMAN EXPERIMENTATION

Aarons, D. Research ethics. *West Indian Medical Journal.* 1995 Dec; 44(4): 115–118. 19 refs. BE55750.
   autonomy; beneficence; confidentiality; education; guidelines; *human experimentation; informed consent; international aspects; investigators; justice; nontherapeutic research; *research ethics committees; risks and benefits; scientific misconduct; selection of subjects; therapeutic research; West Indies

Ackerman, Terrence F. Choosing between Nuremberg and the National Commission: the balancing of moral principles in clinical research. *In:* Vanderpool, Harold Y., ed. The Ethics of Research Involving Human Subjects: Facing the 21st Century. Frederick, MD: University Publishing Group; 1996: 83–104. 27 fn. ISBN 1-55572-036-6. BE56983.
   advisory committees; codes of ethics; federal government; *government regulation; *guidelines; *human experimentation; informed consent; moral obligations; *moral policy; nontherapeutic research; obligations of society; research ethics committees; research subjects; risks and benefits; volunteers; vulnerable populations; Declaration of Helsinki; Department of Health and Human Services; *National Commission for the Protection of Human Subjects; *Nuremberg Code; United States

Ader, Mary. Investigational treatments: coverage, controversy, and consensus. *Annals of Health Law.* 1996; 5: 45–60. 20 fn. BE58363.
   biomedical technologies; contracts; financial support; *health insurance reimbursement; *legal aspects; public policy; risks and benefits; standards; technology assessment; terminally ill; *therapeutic research; evidence-based medicine; *investigational therapies; United States

Advisory Committee on Human Radiation Experiments. The Human Radiation Experiments: Final Report of the Advisory Committee. New York, NY: Oxford University Press; 1996. 620 p. 2,134 fn. "The Advisory Committee submitted its final report to the President in late 1995, and this book contains the entire text of the report issued by the U.S. Government Printing Office in October 1995. It also includes the full text of the President's remarks in acceptance of the report and a complete index." ISBN 0-19-510792-6. BE56500.
   *advisory committees; attitudes; blacks; children; codes of ethics; compensation; consent forms; deception; disclosure; ecology; ethical relativism; ethical review; *evaluation; evaluation studies; *federal government; government regulation; *guidelines; health hazards; *historical aspects; *human experimentation; information dissemination; informed consent; injuries; institutional policies; military personnel; nontherapeutic research; nuclear warfare;

BE = bioethics accession number   fn. = footnotes   refs. = references

occupational exposure; organization and administration; patients; policy analysis; prisoners; *public policy; *radiation; records; research institutes; research subjects; retrospective moral judgment; risks and benefits; *scientific misconduct; selection of subjects; *standards; survey; universities; volunteers; *Advisory Committee on Human Radiation Experiments; Atomic Energy Commission; Central Intelligence Agency; Cold War; Department of Defense; Department of Energy; Department of Health and Human Services; Department of Health, Education, and Welfare; National Aeronautics and Space Administration; Nuremberg Code; *Twentieth Century; *United States; Veterans Administration

Basketter, David; Reynolds, Fiona. The use of human volunteers for hazard and risk assessment of skin irritation. *In:* Close, Bryony; Combes, Robert; Hubbard, Anthony; Illingworth, John, eds. Volunteers in Research and Testing. Bristol, PA: Taylor and Francis; 1997: 117–127. 21 refs. ISBN 0–7484–0397–3. BE57036.
drugs; health hazards; *human experimentation; *nontherapeutic research; research design; risk; *toxicity; *volunteers

Behi, Ruhi; Nolan, Mike. Ethical issues in research. *British Journal of Nursing.* 1995 Jun 22–Jul 12; 4(12): 712–716. 15 refs. BE56854.
confidentiality; conflict of interest; cultural pluralism; deception; disclosure; ethical theory; guidelines; *human experimentation; informed consent; investigators; nurses; nursing research; research design; research ethics committees; risks and benefits; scientific misconduct; third party consent; vulnerable populations; Great Britain

Brody, Baruch A., comp. Appendixes: international research ethics policies; European transnational research ethics policies; U.S. research ethics policies; research ethics policies from other countries. *In: his* The Ethics of Biomedical Research: An International Perspective. New York, NY: Oxford University Press; 1998: 213–358. ISBN 0–19–509007–1. BE57677.
*animal experimentation; *biomedical research; codes of ethics; embryo research; federal government; fetal research; gene therapy; genetic research; genetic screening; genome mapping; government regulation; *guidelines; *human experimentation; *international aspects; patents; professional organizations; *research ethics; Australia; Canada; Council for International Organizations of Medical Sciences (CIOMS); Council of Europe; Declaration of Helsinki; Department of Health and Human Services; Europe; Food and Drug Administration; Great Britain; Japan; National Institutes of Health; Nuremberg Code; Public Health Service; United States; World Medical Association

Brody, Baruch A. Research on human subjects. *In: his* The Ethics of Biomedical Research: An International Perspective. New York, NY: Oxford University Press; 1998: 31–54, 363–364. 44 fn. ISBN 0–19–509007–1. BE57669.
coercion; committee membership; communication; compensation; confidentiality; consensus; consent forms; critically ill; disclosure; emergency care; epidemiology; ethical review; government regulation; guidelines; historical aspects; *human experimentation; informed consent; injuries; international aspects; moral policy; patients; privacy; public policy; remuneration; research design; research ethics committees; research subjects; review; risks and benefits; scientific misconduct; therapeutic research; vulnerable populations; Canada; Europe; United States

Brody, Baruch A. The Ethics of Biomedical Research: An International Perspective. New York, NY: Oxford University Press; 1998. 386 p. 393 fn. ISBN 0–19–509007–1. BE57667.
animal experimentation; *biomedical research; control

groups; drugs; embryo research; epidemiology; females; fetal research; genetic research; guidelines; *human experimentation; *international aspects; medical devices; mentally disabled; minority groups; minors; pregnant women; prisoners; public policy; random selection; regulation; research design; review; vulnerable populations; *research ethics; United States

Campbell, Duncan. Medicine needs its MI5. *BMJ (British Medical Journal).* 1997 Dec 20–27; 315(7123): 1677–1680. 2 refs. BE57651.
biomedical research; fraud; *human experimentation; *investigators; mass media; *misconduct; *patient care; *physicians; professional competence; *scientific misconduct; *self regulation; stigmatization; whistleblowing; medical audit; *General Medical Council (Great Britain); *Great Britain

Cassidy, Virginia R. Literary works as case studies for teaching human experimentation ethics. *Journal of Nursing Education.* 1996 Mar; 35(3): 142–144. 14 refs. BE55658.
behavioral research; case studies; *human experimentation; informed consent; investigator subject relationship; *literature; *nursing education; *nursing ethics; *teaching methods; Northern Illinois University

Chambers, Timothy. Questionable ethics –– whistle–blowing or tale–telling? *Journal of Medical Ethics.* 1997 Dec; 23(6): 382–383. 2 refs. BE57657.
case studies; disclosure; *editorial policies; informed consent; *kidney diseases; *nontherapeutic research; parental consent; patient care; peer review; physicians; prognosis; *scientific misconduct; *surgery; *whistleblowing; medical audit
Renal biopsy is a potentially hazardous procedure, generally performed for therapeutic reasons. An open renal biopsy was performed when there appeared to be no accepted clinical indication and its results published in a specialty journal, whose editors declined publication of subsequent correspondence, questioning the ethical propriety of such a procedure. The implications for clinical practice, authors, editors and readers are discussed.

Close, Bryony; Combes, Robert; Hubbard, Anthony, et al, eds. Volunteers in Research and Testing. Bristol, PA: Taylor and Francis; 1997. 198 p. 182 refs. 6 fn. Appendices: Declaration of Helsinki; list of examples of European national guidelines relating to clinical research; and main ethical guidelines relevant to the evaluation of clinical research in the UK. ISBN 0–7484–0397–3. BE57025.
animal experimentation; attitudes; codes of ethics; communication; compensation; consent forms; disadvantaged; drugs; guidelines; *human experimentation; injuries; international aspects; legal aspects; nontherapeutic research; regulation; remuneration; research design; research ethics committees; research subjects; risk; toxicity; volunteers; vulnerable populations; Declaration of Helsinki; Europe; Great Britain

Coughlin, Steven S. Ethics in Epidemiology and Public Health Practice: Collected Works. Columbus, GA: Quill Publications; 1997. 232 p. Includes references. ISBN 0–9661520–0–X. BE58542.
American Indians; autonomy; beneficence; biomedical research; cancer; case studies; confidentiality; control groups; curriculum; ecology; education; *epidemiology; ethical theory; ethics committees; federal government; females; government regulation; health hazards; health personnel; HIV seropositivity; human experimentation; informed consent; international aspects; investigators; justice; *preventive medicine; *professional ethics; professional organizations; *public health; random selection;

---

research design; research ethics committees; risks and benefits; scientific misconduct; selection of subjects; self regulation; socioeconomic factors; violence; vulnerable populations; professional role; Tuskegee Syphilis Study; United States

Daar, A.S.; Salomon, Daniel R.; Ferguson, Ronald M., et al. Xenotransplants: proceed with caution. [Letters]. *Nature.* 1998 Mar 5; 392(6671): 11–12. 6 refs. BE57765.
advisory committees; *animal organs; *attitudes; communicable diseases; consensus; government regulation; guidelines; *human experimentation; industry; information dissemination; *international aspects; mass media; *organ transplantation; organizational policies; physicians; professional organizations; public health; *public policy; *risk; risks and benefits; American Society of Transplant Physicians; American Society of Transplant Surgeons; European Union; Public Health Service; United States; World Health Organization

Dayan, Anthony. The volunteer subject, encouragement and protection. *In:* Close, Bryony; Combes, Robert; Hubbard, Anthony; Illingworth, John, eds. Volunteers in Research and Testing. Bristol, PA: Taylor and Francis; 1997: 5–21. 12 refs. ISBN 0–7484–0397–3. BE57026.
autoexperimentation; autonomy; beneficence; guidelines; historical aspects; *human experimentation; informed consent; international aspects; investigators; nontherapeutic research; organization and administration; research ethics committees; research subjects; rights; risks and benefits; scientific misconduct; social control; therapeutic research; volunteers; Great Britain

Dickens, Bernard M. Legal and ethical challenges in gene therapy. *Transfusion Science.* 1996 Mar; 17(1): 191–196. 10 refs. BE55671.
advisory committees; age factors; children; conflict of interest; cosmetic surgery; critically ill; disclosure; emergency care; ethical review; freedom; *gene therapy; genetic disorders; genetic enhancement; genetic research; germ cells; government regulation; health insurance reimbursement; human experimentation; industry; informed consent; investigators; *justice; paternalism; patient care; peer review; private sector; property rights; resource allocation; selection for treatment; *therapeutic research; withholding treatment; investigational therapies; seriously ill; Clothier Committee; Great Britain

Fayers, P.M.; Hand, D.J. Generalisation from phase III clinical trials: survival, quality of life, and health economics. *Lancet.* 1997 Oct 4; 350(9083): 1025–1027. 31 refs. BE56864.
cancer; costs and benefits; *economics; health care delivery; *human experimentation; investigational drugs; *mortality; patient care; patients; placebos; quality adjusted life years; *quality of life; random selection; research design; *therapeutic research; *treatment outcome

Frader, Joel E.; Caniano, Donna A. Research and innovation in surgery. *In:* McCullough, Laurence B.; Jones, James W.; Brody, Baruch A., eds. Surgical Ethics. New York, NY: Oxford University Press; 1998: 216–241. 65 refs. ISBN 0–19–510347–5. BE58324.
advisory committees; alternatives; children; comparative studies; conflict of interest; congenital disorders; control groups; disclosure; *evaluation; federal government; financial support; government regulation; heart diseases; historical aspects; *human experimentation; industry; infants; investigators; moral obligations; mortality; organ transplantation; palliative care; peer review; quality of life; random selection; research design; research ethics committees; research subjects; *risk; suffering; *surgery; *therapeutic research; vulnerable populations; *investigational therapies; sham surgery; unproven therapies;

United States

Freedman, Benjamin. The ethical analysis of clinical trials: new lessons for and from cancer research. *In:* Vanderpool, Harold Y., ed. The Ethics of Research Involving Human Subjects: Facing the 21st Century. Frederick, MD: University Publishing Group; 1996: 319–338. 17 fn. ISBN 1–55572–036–6. BE56992.
AIDS; autonomy; beneficence; *cancer; disclosure; ethical analysis; ethical review; guidelines; *human experimentation; informed consent; investigational drugs; justice; moral policy; nontherapeutic research; patients; political activity; research design; research ethics committees; research subjects; risks and benefits; selection of subjects; therapeutic research; toxicity; research ethics; Belmont Report; National Surgical Adjuvant Breast and Bowel Project

Freedman, Monroe H.; Hoenig, Leonard J.; Spiro, Howard M., et al. Nazi research: too evil to cite. [Letters]. *Hastings Center Report.* 1985 Aug; 15(4): 31–32. BE57827.
animal experimentation; *biomedical research; *editorial policies; historical aspects; *human experimentation; killing; moral complicity; *National Socialism; research subjects; *scientific misconduct; torture; utilitarianism; Germany; Twentieth Century

Giffels, J. Joseph. Clinical Trials: What You Should Know Before Volunteering to Be a Research Subject. [Pamphlet]. New York, NY: Demos Vermande; 1996. 43 p. ISBN 1–888799–02–1. BE57741.
alternatives; confidentiality; consent forms; disclosure; government regulation; *human experimentation; informed consent; injuries; investigators; *patient education; *patients; physician's role; placebos; research design; research ethics committees; *research subjects; risks and benefits; uncertainty; volunteers

Green, Ronald M.; Pascual–Leone, Alvaro; Wasserman, Eric M. Ethical guidelines for rTMS research. *IRB: A Review of Human Subjects Research.* 1997 Mar–Apr; 19(2): 1–7. 43 refs. BE58518.
data banks; depressive disorder; *electrical stimulation of the brain; evaluation; *guidelines; *human experimentation; informed consent; international aspects; investigators; *methods; nontherapeutic research; patients; registries; research subjects; *risks and benefits; selection of subjects; standards; therapeutic research; volunteers

Greenberg, Daniel S. Hidden data and abuse in research come to light in the USA. [News]. *Lancet.* 1997 Oct 11; 350(9084): 1083. BE56926.
cancer; compensation; *disclosure; federal government; government regulation; *health hazards; historical aspects; *human experimentation; industry; informed consent; mentally ill; *nuclear warfare; public health; *public policy; *radiation; research ethics committees; *scientific misconduct; Cold War; Twentieth Century; *United States

Hicks, Carolyn. Ethics in midwifery research. *In:* Frith, Lucy, ed. Ethics and Midwifery: Issues in Contemporary Practice. Boston, MA: Butterworth–Heinemann; 1996: 237–257. 14 refs. ISBN 0–7506–3056–6. BE58641.
behavioral research; confidentiality; deception; disclosure; ethical review; females; fetuses; *human experimentation; infants; informed consent; investigators; mothers; *nurse midwives; *nursing ethics; *nursing research; parental consent; placebos; pregnant women; prenatal diagnosis; privacy; research design; research subjects; risks and benefits; scientific misconduct; vulnerable populations; qualitative research

Holt, Bev. Recruitment, selection and compensation of volunteers for phase I studies. *In:* Close, Bryony;

BE = bioethics accession number   fn. = footnotes   refs. = references

Combes, Robert; Hubbard, Anthony; Illingworth, John, eds. Volunteers in Research and Testing. Bristol, PA: Taylor and Francis; 1997: 59–66. ISBN 0–7484–0397–3. BE57031.
    advertising; altruism; drugs; *human experimentation; incentives; informed consent; motivation; *nontherapeutic research; *remuneration; research ethics committees; *research subjects; *selection of subjects; students; *volunteers

Jonsen, Albert R., ed. The ethics of research with human subjects. *In:* Jonsen, Albert R.; Veatch, Robert M.; Walters, LeRoy, eds. Source Book in Bioethics: A Documentary History. Washington, DC: Georgetown University Press; 1998: 3–110. 3 refs. 31 fn. ISBN 0–87840–683–2. BE57890.
    aborted fetuses; advisory committees; children; *embryo research; ethical review; federal government; *fetal research; fetal tissue donation; government regulation; *guidelines; historical aspects; *human experimentation; in vitro fertilization; informed consent; international aspects; investigators; legal aspects; literature; nontherapeutic research; patients; physicians; professional organizations; research design; research ethics committees; research subjects; risks and benefits; scientific misconduct; self regulation; therapeutic research; volunteers; vulnerable populations; *Belmont Report; *Declaration of Helsinki; *DHEW Guidelines; *DHHS Guidelines; *Ethics Advisory Board; Germany; *Human Fetal Tissue Transplantation Research Panel; *National Commission for the Protection of Human Subjects; National Institutes of Health; Nineteenth Century; *Nuremberg Code; *Tuskegee Syphilis Study; *Twentieth Century; *United States

Jonsen, Albert R. The weight and weighing of ethical principles. *In:* Vanderpool, Harold Y., ed. The Ethics of Research Involving Human Subjects: Facing the 21st Century. Frederick, MD: University Publishing Group; 1996: 59–82. 23 fn. ISBN 1–55572–036–6. BE56982.
    advisory committees; autonomy; beneficence; bioethics; children; codes of ethics; ethical theory; fetal research; *guidelines; *human experimentation; informed consent; justice; *metaphor; *moral policy; nontherapeutic research; philosophy; public policy; research ethics committees; research subjects; risks and benefits; selection of subjects; therapeutic research; third party consent; Belmont Report; Declaration of Helsinki; National Commission for the Protection of Human Subjects; Nuremberg Code; United States

Kahn, Jeffrey P.; Mastroianni, Anna C.; Sugarman, Jeremy. Beyond Consent: Seeking Justice in Research. New York, NY: Oxford University Press; 1998. 190 p. 478 fn. ISBN 0–19–511353–5. BE58839.
    advisory committees; biomedical research; blacks; cancer; children; decision making; emergency care; federal government; females; government regulation; HIV seropositivity; *human experimentation; informed consent; institutionalized persons; international aspects; *justice; military personnel; nontherapeutic research; patients; prisoners; public policy; research subjects; resource allocation; review; risks and benefits; scientific misconduct; selection of subjects; social discrimination; standards; therapeutic research; vulnerable populations; *United States

Kahn, Jeffrey P.; Mastroianni, Anna C.; Sugarman, Jeremy. Implementing justice in a changing research environment. *In:* Kahn, Jeffrey P.; Mastroianni, Anna C.; Sugarman, Jeremy, eds. Beyond Consent: Seeking Justice in Research. New York, NY: Oxford University Press; 1998: 166–173. 5 fn. ISBN 0–19–511353–5. BE58849.
    *decision making; financial support; *human experimentation; incentives; information dissemination; informed consent; *justice; mass media; private sector; public

sector; research ethics committees; research subjects; selection of subjects; values; United States

Kerns, Thomas A. Jenner on Trial: An Ethical Examination of Vaccine Research in the Age of Smallpox and the Age of AIDS. Lanham, MD: University Press of America; 1997. 98 p. 71 fn. Appendix I: the Nuremberg Code; Appendix II: International Ethical Guidelines for Biomedical Research Involving Human Subjects (WHO/CIOMS). ISBN 0–7618–0719–5. BE57154.
    AIDS; codes of ethics; *communicable diseases; comparative studies; consent forms; disclosure; ethical review; family members; guidelines; *historical aspects; HIV seropositivity; *human experimentation; *immunization; informed consent; international aspects; investigator subject relationship; *investigators; minors; misconduct; National Socialism; parental consent; physicians; research design; research ethics committees; risks and benefits; selection of subjects; vulnerable populations; *smallpox; Germany; Great Britain; International Ethical Guidelines for Biomedical Research Involving Human Subjects; *Jenner, Edward; Nineteenth Century; Nuremberg Code

Lahr, J. Gregory. What is the method to their "madness?" Experimental treatment exclusions in health insurance policies. [Comment]. *Journal of Contemporary Health Law and Policy.* 1997 Spring; 13(2): 613–636. 175 fn. BE56005.
    *contracts; decision making; ethical review; federal government; *health insurance; *health insurance reimbursement; human experimentation; industry; judicial action; *legal aspects; managed care programs; *organizational policies; patient care; peer review; research design; resource allocation; technology assessment; terminology; *therapeutic research; uncertainty; National Cancer Institute; *United States

Lind, Stuart E. Financial issues and incentives related to clinical research and innovative therapies. *In:* Vanderpool, Harold Y., ed. The Ethics of Research Involving Human Subjects: Facing the 21st Century. Frederick, MD: University Publishing Group; 1996: 185–202. 27 fn. ISBN 1–55572–036–6. BE56987.
    conflict of interest; *financial support; health insurance; health insurance reimbursement; *human experimentation; *incentives; industry; informed consent; investigator subject relationship; *investigators; nontherapeutic research; *patients; *physicians; *remuneration; research ethics committees; *research subjects; *selection of subjects; therapeutic research; *volunteers; *investigational therapies; United States

London, Nancy L.; London, W. Thomas. A case of self-experimentation. [Editorial]. *Cancer Epidemiology, Biomarkers and Prevention.* 1997 Jul; 6(7): 475–476. 7 refs. BE58359.
    *autoexperimentation; historical aspects; *human experimentation; *investigators; physicians; research design; research ethics committees; research subjects; *risks and benefits; selection of subjects; toxicity; *volunteers

McCarthy, Charles R. The evolving story of justice in federal research policy. *In:* Kahn, Jeffrey P.; Mastroianni, Anna C.; Sugarman, Jeremy, eds. Beyond Consent: Seeking Justice in Research. New York, NY: Oxford University Press; 1998: 11–31. 67 fn. ISBN 0–19–511353–5. BE58841.
    advisory committees; AIDS; compensation; ethical review; *federal government; females; government financing; government regulation; historical aspects; *human experimentation; informed consent; *justice; legislation; nontherapeutic research; patients; peer review; *public policy; radiation; research subjects; risks and benefits; scientific misconduct; selection of subjects; therapeutic

research; volunteers; vulnerable populations; National Bioethics Advisory Commission; National Commission for the Protection of Human Subjects; National Institutes of Health; President's Commission for the Study of Ethical Problems; Public Health Service; Tuskegee Syphilis Study; Twentieth Century; U.S. Congress; *United States

McCarthy, Charles R. The rights of human research subjects and the necessity of conducting animal research as illuminated by the Nuremberg Code and the Declaration of Helsinki. *In:* Eder, G.; Kaiser, E.; King, F.A., eds. The Role of the Chimpanzee in Research. Symposium, Vienna, Austria, May 22–24, 1992. New York, NY: Karger; 1994: 1–6. 5 refs. ISBN 3–8055–5850–3. BE58156.
   *animal experimentation; autonomy; codes of ethics; deontological ethics; *guidelines; *human experimentation; human rights; informed consent; international aspects; nontherapeutic research; primates; research subjects; utilitarianism; *Declaration of Helsinki; *Nuremberg Code

McDevitt, Denis. Human volunteers in research: a physician's overview. *In:* Close, Bryony; Combes, Robert; Hubbard, Anthony; Illingworth, John, eds. Volunteers in Research and Testing. Bristol, PA: Taylor and Francis; 1997: 33–39. 1 ref. 1 fn. ISBN 0–7484–0397–3. BE57028.
   coercion; *human experimentation; medical schools; military personnel; *nontherapeutic research; patient advocacy; patients; physicians; remuneration; research ethics committees; *research subjects; risks and benefits; students; *volunteers

McNeill, Paul. Paying people to participate in research: why not? A response to Wilkinson and Moore. *Bioethics.* 1997 Oct; 11(5): 390–396. 6 fn. BE56334.
   autonomy; disadvantaged; *human experimentation; *incentives; informed consent; investigational drugs; justice; nontherapeutic research; paternalism; *remuneration; *research subjects; *risks and benefits; *volunteers
This paper argues against paying people to participate in research. Volunteering to participate as a subject in a research program is not like taking a job. The main difference is to do with the risks inherent in research. Experimentation on human beings is, by definition, trying out something with an unknown consequence and exposes people to risks of harm which cannot be known in advance. This is the main reason for independent review by committee of research programs. It is based on a recognition that researchers are not always capable of putting the interests of their subjects ahead of their research objectives. It is not simply a matter of individual autonomy. Society has an obligation, prior to the protection of individual freedom and autonomy, to establish basic safeguards that are equitable in their operation. Any inducement for participating in research would add to the difficulty subjects have in adequately assessing the risks of participating in research. An acceptance of inducement to participate in research would further increase the inequity of research conducted on the impecunious for the benefit of the well-off.

Marwick, Charles. Compensation for injured research subjects. [News]. *JAMA.* 1998 Jun 17; 279(23): 1854. BE58420.
   *compensation; federal government; *human experimentation; informed consent; *injuries; institutional ethics; institutional policies; insurance; medical schools; public policy; *research subjects; United States; University of Washington School of Medicine

Marwick, Charles. Volunteers in typhoid infection study

will aid future vaccine development. [News]. *JAMA.* 1998 May 13; 279(18): 1423–1424. BE57864.
   communicable diseases; compensation; consent forms; disclosure; federal government; government regulation; *human experimentation; *immunization; incentives; informed consent; injuries; international aspects; *nontherapeutic research; remuneration; research design; research subjects; risks and benefits; selection of subjects; *volunteers; *typhoid; Food and Drug Administration; United States; *University of Maryland School of Medicine

Mattson, Margaret E.; Curb, J. David; McArdle, Robert; Aspirin Myocardial Infarction Study (AMIS) Research Group; Beta–Blocker Heart Attack Trial (BHAT) Research Group. Participation in a clinical trial: the patients' point of view. *Controlled Clinical Trials.* 1985 Jun; 6(2): 156–167. 22 refs. BE56675.
   altruism; *attitudes; drugs; heart diseases; *human experimentation; *motivation; *patients; random selection; *research subjects; *risks and benefits; survey; multicenter studies; Aspirin Myocardial Infarction Study (AMIS); Beta–Blocker Heart Attack Trial (BHAT); United States

Moreno, Jonathan D. Reassessing the influence of the Nuremberg Code on American medical ethics. *Journal of Contemporary Health Law and Policy.* 1997 Spring; 13(2): 347–360. 74 fn. BE56008.
   cancer; *codes of ethics; comprehension; federal government; *guidelines; *historical aspects; *human experimentation; informed consent; international aspects; investigators; military personnel; nontherapeutic research; patients; physicians; professional organizations; *public policy; radiation; radiology; research subjects; scientific misconduct; *social impact; therapeutic research; trust; volunteers; American Medical Association; Armed Forces Medical Policy Council; Atomic Energy Commission; Beecher, Henry; Cold War; Declaration of Helsinki; Department of Defense; National Society for Medical Research; *Nuremberg Code; *Twentieth Century; *United States; World Medical Association

Orme, Michael. The risks of studies in healthy volunteers. *In:* Close, Bryony; Combes, Robert; Hubbard, Anthony; Illingworth, John, eds. Volunteers in Research and Testing. Bristol, PA: Taylor and Francis; 1997: 99–107. 4 refs. ISBN 0–7484–0397–3. BE57034.
   compensation; death; drugs; *human experimentation; informed consent; *injuries; medical education; *nontherapeutic research; physicians; remuneration; *research subjects; *risk; statistics; students; survey; *volunteers; Great Britain

Powers, Madison. Theories of justice in the context of research. *In:* Kahn, Jeffrey P.; Mastroianni, Anna C.; Sugarman, Jeremy, eds. Beyond Consent: Seeking Justice in Research. New York, NY: Oxford University Press; 1998: 147–165. 26 fn. ISBN 0–19–511353–5. BE58848.
   age factors; AIDS; autonomy; *biomedical research; critically ill; decision making; developing countries; disadvantaged; ecology; economics; emergency care; females; freedom; health care delivery; *human experimentation; informed consent; *justice; libertarianism; military personnel; *moral policy; nontherapeutic research; occupational medicine; political activity; prisoners; *public policy; research design; research ethics committees; research subjects; *resource allocation; *risks and benefits; selection of subjects; social discrimination; vulnerable populations; United States

Scandinavian Nursing Cooperative. Etiska riklinjer för omvårdnadsforskning i Norden [Ethical guidelines for nursing research]. *Vard i Norden.* 1987 Autumn; 7(3–4): 429–430. BE56633.
   *guidelines; *health services research; *human experimentation; informed consent; *nurses; *nursing ethics;

BE = bioethics accession number   fn. = footnotes   refs. = references

*nursing research; *organizational policies; professional organizations; research ethics committees; research subjects; Scandinavia; *Scandinavian Nursing Cooperative

Shuster, Evelyne. The Nuremberg Code: Hippocratic ethics and human rights. *Lancet.* 1998 Mar 28; 351(9107): 974–977. 29 refs. BE58563.
beneficence; codes of ethics; coercion; *developing countries; drugs; *guidelines; historical aspects; HIV seropositivity; *human experimentation; *human rights; informed consent; *international aspects; investigators; justice; medical ethics; *moral obligations; nontherapeutic research; *physicians; placebos; pregnant women; professional autonomy; professional organizations; *research subjects; scientific misconduct; therapeutic research; Alexander, Leo; Declaration of Helsinki; Hippocratic Oath; Ivy, Andrew; *Nuremberg Code; Twentieth Century; World Medical Association

Skolnick, Andrew A. Advisory committee report recommends that US make amends for human radiation experiments. [News]. *JAMA.* 1995 Sep 27; 274(12): 933. BE56668.
*advisory committees; compensation; *federal government; historical aspects; *human experimentation; *public policy; *radiation; research subjects; *scientific misconduct; *Advisory Committee on Human Radiation Experiments; Twentieth Century; *United States

Vanderpool, Harold Y., ed. The Ethics of Research Involving Human Subjects: Facing the 21st Century. Frederick, MD: University Publishing Group; 1996. 531 p. 806 fn. ISBN 1-55572-036-6. BE56980.
advisory committees; autonomy; bioethical issues; bioethics; children; conflict of interest; cultural pluralism; developing countries; embryo research; ethical relativism; federal government; fetal research; fetal tissue donation; financial support; genetic research; genome mapping; government regulation; guidelines; HIV seropositivity; *human experimentation; incentives; informed consent; international aspects; investigators; justice; moral policy; patients; physicians; public policy; remuneration; research ethics committees; research subjects; risks and benefits; selection of subjects; vulnerable populations; United States

Vanderpool, Harold Y. What's happening in research ethics? Commentary on Brody. *In:* Carson, Ronald A.; Burns, Chester R., eds. Philosophy of Medicine and Bioethics: A Twenty-Year Retrospective and Critical Appraisal. Boston, MA: Kluwer Academic; 1997: 287–297. 35 refs. 9 fn. ISBN 0-7923-3545-7. BE56543.
advisory committees; bioethical issues; bioethics; *biomedical research; drugs; education; *ethicist's role; ethicists; government regulation; *human experimentation; *literature; research design; research ethics committees; risks and benefits; scientific misconduct; *trends; *research ethics

Waters, W.E. Ethics and epidemiological research. *International Journal of Epidemiology.* 1985 Mar; 14(1): 48–51. 10 refs. BE56679.
*attitudes; *biomedical research; confidentiality; *epidemiology; *ethical review; health services research; *human experimentation; informed consent; *international aspects; *investigators; random selection; research design; research ethics committees; research subjects; survey

Weijer, Charles; Dickens, Bernard; Meslin, Eric M. Bioethics for clinicians: 10. Research ethics. *Canadian Medical Association Journal.* 1997 Apr 15; 156(8): 1153–1157. 44 refs. BE57358.
autonomy; beneficence; case studies; comprehension; confidentiality; conflict of interest; guidelines; *human experimentation; incentives; informed consent; *investigators; justice; legal aspects; physicians; placebos; professional ethics; remuneration; research design; research

subjects; risks and benefits; selection of subjects; research ethics; Canada; Medical Research Council of Canada

Weijer, Charles. Research methods and policies. *In:* Chadwick, Ruth, ed. Encyclopedia of Applied Ethics, Volume 3. San Diego, CA: Academic Press; 1998: 853–860. 11 refs. ISBN 0-12-227068-1. BE56272.
beneficence; codes of ethics; cultural pluralism; genetic research; government regulation; guidelines; *human experimentation; information dissemination; international aspects; justice; research design; risks and benefits; scientific misconduct; vulnerable populations

Wilkinson, Martin; Moore, Andrew. Inducement in research. *Bioethics.* 1997 Oct; 11(5): 373–389. 28 fn. Commented on by P. McNeill, p. 390–396. BE56339.
autonomy; coercion; freedom; guidelines; *human experimentation; *incentives; indigents; informed consent; *moral policy; nontherapeutic research; paternalism; *remuneration; research ethics committees; *research subjects; *risks and benefits; science; selection of subjects; *volunteers
Opposition to inducement payments for research subjects is an international orthodoxy amongst writers of ethics committee guidelines. We offer an argument in favour of these payments. We also critically evaluate the best arguments we can find or devise against such payments, and except in one very limited range of circumstances, we find these unconvincing.

Zucker, Arthur. Law and ethics: experimentation; assisted suicide. *Death Studies.* 1997 Mar–Apr; 21(2): 221–225. 6 refs. 1 fn. BE55545.
active euthanasia; *assisted suicide; children; drugs; government regulation; *human experimentation; informed consent; *legal aspects; mentally ill; physicians; placebos; research design; *right to die; scientific misconduct; Netherlands; United States

HUMAN EXPERIMENTATION/ETHICS COMMITTEES

Aarons, D. Research ethics. *West Indian Medical Journal.* 1995 Dec; 44(4): 115–118. 19 refs. BE55750.
autonomy; beneficence; confidentiality; education; guidelines; *human experimentation; informed consent; international aspects; investigators; justice; nontherapeutic research; *research ethics committees; risks and benefits; scientific misconduct; selection of subjects; therapeutic research; West Indies

Barker, E.M. Informed consent in medical research: the ethics committee's view. [Letter]. *BMJ (British Medical Journal).* 1998 Jan 31; 316(7128): 392–393. 3 refs. BE57800.
committee membership; deception; developing countries; ethical review; HIV seropositivity; *human experimentation; *informed consent; intensive care units; investigators; misconduct; motivation; *research ethics committees; selection for treatment; *South Africa

Benson, Paul R.; Roth, Loren H. Trends in the social control of medical and psychiatric research. *Law and Mental Health.* 1988; 4: 1–47. 227 refs. BE56609.
behavioral research; biomedical research; codes of ethics; competence; empirical research; *ethical review; evaluation; federal government; *government regulation; guidelines; historical aspects; *human experimentation; informed consent; international aspects; investigators; legal aspects; nontherapeutic research; organization and administration; physicians; professional autonomy; professional organizations; *research ethics committees; research subjects; review; scientific misconduct; self regulation;

*social control; state government; therapeutic research; trends; vulnerable populations; Canada; Central Intelligence Agency; Council for International Organizations of Medical Sciences; Declaration of Helsinki; Denmark; Department of Health, Education, and Welfare; Food and Drug Administration; Great Britain; National Institutes of Health; Nuremberg Code; Twentieth Century; *United States; World Health Organization

Berry, Jonathan. Local research ethics committees can audit ethical standards in research. *Journal of Medical Ethics.* 1997 Dec; 23(6): 379–381. 3 refs. BE57655.

comprehension; disclosure; *ethical review; *evaluation; evaluation studies; human experimentation; informed consent; recall; *research ethics committees; *research subjects; *standards; survey; *therapeutic research; questionnaires; *Great Britain

OBJECTIVES: To show that a Local Research Ethics Committee (LREC) can carry out an audit of ethical standards in research. To find out if a researcher met certain ethical standards in recruiting subjects for clinical trials and in obtaining their consent. DESIGN: Postal questionnaire. SETTING: Clinical research by one doctor during one year. SUBJECTS: Eleven patients entered in clinical trials. MAIN OUTCOME MEASURES: Success in ethics committee obtaining data. Achievement of ethical standards in recruitment of subjects and in obtaining consent. RESULTS: The audit was successfully carried out and standards were partly met. CONCLUSIONS: Local Research Ethics Committees can carry out audits of the conduct of research projects which they have approved. Provision for possible audits can be made at the time of application to the committee. Our committee thought the ethical standards in the research which we audited were acceptable.

Blunt, Jennifer; Savulescu, Julian; Watson, Alastair J.M. Meeting the challenges facing research ethics committees: some practical suggestions. *BMJ (British Medical Journal).* 1998 Jan 3; 316(7124): 58–61. 47 refs. BE57954.

committee membership; education; ethical review; fraud; human experimentation; information dissemination; investigators; *research ethics committees; standards; students; multicenter studies; *Great Britain

Campbell, Jean. Reforming the IRB process: towards new guidelines for quality and accountability in protecting human subjects. *In:* Shamoo, Adil E., ed. Ethics in Neurobiological Research with Human Subjects: The Baltimore Conference on Ethics. Amsterdam: Gordon and Breach; 1997: 299–303. ISBN 2–88449–161–9. BE57022.

accountability; communication; dehumanization; evaluation; family members; health services research; *human experimentation; *investigator subject relationship; investigators; *mentally ill; paternalism; *patient advocacy; *patient participation; patients; research design; *research ethics committees; research subjects; risks and benefits; stigmatization; United States

Collier, Joe. The future of ethics committees. *In:* Close, Bryony; Combes, Robert; Hubbard, Anthony; Illingworth, John, eds. Volunteers in Research and Testing. Bristol, PA: Taylor and Francis; 1997: 177–183. ISBN 0–7484–0397–3. BE57040.

clinical ethics committees; committee membership; ethicists; *ethics committees; hospitals; human experimentation; organization and administration; *research ethics committees; Europe; *Great Britain

European Forum for Good Clinical Practice. Ethics

Working Party. Guidelines and Recommendations for European Ethics Committees. Brussels, Belgium: European Forum for Good Clinical Practice; 1995. 17 p. 8 refs. BE58131.

committee membership; *guidelines; human experimentation; *international aspects; organization and administration; *research ethics committees; standards; *Europe

Foster, Claire. Research ethics committees. *In:* Chadwick, Ruth, ed. Encyclopedia of Applied Ethics, Volume 3. San Diego, CA: Academic Press; 1998: 845–852. 5 refs. ISBN 0–12–227068–1. BE56271.

committee membership; decision making; ethical review; evaluation; historical aspects; human experimentation; informed consent; moral obligations; nontherapeutic research; *research ethics committees; standards; therapeutic research; multicenter studies; Great Britain

Gordon, Bruce; Prentice, Ernest. Continuing review of research involving human subjects: approach to the problem and remaining areas of concern. *IRB: A Review of Human Subjects Research.* 1997 Mar–Apr; 19(2): 8–11. 7 refs. BE58516.

*ethical review; federal government; *government regulation; guidelines; *human experimentation; investigators; records; research design; *research ethics committees; risks and benefits; selection of subjects; *standards; time factors; universities; multicenter studies; Food and Drug Administration; Office for Protection from Research Risks; *United States; *University of Nebraska Medical Center (Omaha)

Gordon, Valery M.; Sugarman, Jeremy; Kass, Nancy. Toward a more comprehensive approach to protecting human subjects: the interface of data safety monitoring boards and institutional review boards in randomized clinical trials. *IRB: A Review of Human Subjects Research.* 1998 Jan–Feb; 20(1): 1–5. 28 refs. BE58517.

committee membership; drug industry; ethical review; federal government; government regulation; guidelines; *human experimentation; organization and administration; *random selection; *research design; *research ethics committees; *review committees; risks and benefits; *standards; *data monitoring committees; multicenter studies; National Institutes of Health; *United States

Häyry, Matti. Ethics committees, principles and consequences. *Journal of Medical Ethics.* 1998 Apr; 24(2): 81–85. 8 refs. BE58079.

*animal care committees; *animal experimentation; autonomy; beneficence; *human experimentation; infants; justice; *moral policy; pain; personhood; principle-based ethics; prisoners; *research ethics committees; research subjects; risks and benefits; speciesism; suffering; value of life

When ethics committees evaluate the research proposals submitted to them by biomedical scientists, they can seek guidance from laws and regulations, their own beliefs, values and experiences, and from the theories of philosophers. The starting point of this paper is that philosophers can only be helpful to the members of ethics committees if they take into account in their models both the basic moral intuitions that most of us share and the consequences of people's choices. A moral view which can be labelled as a consequentialist interpretation of mid-level principlism is developed, defended and applied to some real-life and hypothetical research proposals.

Jacobsen, Geir; Hals, Arild. Medical investigators' views about ethics and fraud in medical research. *Journal of the Royal College of Physicians of London.* 1995 Sep–Oct; 29(5): 405–409. 20 refs. BE55562.

advisory committees; age factors; *attitudes; *biomedical

BE = bioethics accession number   fn. = footnotes   refs. = references

research; *ethical review; evaluation; females; *fraud; freedom; historical aspects; human experimentation; information dissemination; *investigators; *knowledge, attitudes, practice; males; medical ethics; physicians; professional autonomy; professional ethics; regional ethics committees; *regulation; *research design; *research ethics committees; retrospective moral judgment; science; *scientific misconduct; *self regulation; statistics; survey; trends; *Norway; Twentieth Century

Klingmann, Ingrid. The European dimension. *In:* Close, Bryony; Combes, Robert; Hubbard, Anthony; Illingworth, John, eds. Volunteers in Research and Testing. Bristol, PA: Taylor and Francis; 1997: 169–175. 3 refs. ISBN 0-7484-0397-3. BE57039.
　　committee membership; compensation; guidelines; *human experimentation; injuries; *international aspects; regulation; remuneration; *research ethics committees; research subjects; volunteers; Austria; Belgium; *Europe; France; Germany; Great Britain; Spain; Sweden

McCarthy, Charles R. Challenges to IRBs in the coming decades. *In:* Vanderpool, Harold Y., ed. The Ethics of Research Involving Human Subjects: Facing the 21st Century. Frederick, MD: University Publishing Group; 1996: 127–144. 15 fn. ISBN 1-55572-036-6. BE56985.
　　advisory committees; AIDS; animal experimentation; autonomy; beneficence; compensation; cultural pluralism; ethical review; federal government; *government regulation; guidelines; *human experimentation; immunization; injuries; international aspects; investigational drugs; investigators; justice; professional ethics; *public policy; *research ethics committees; research subjects; review committees; risks and benefits; self regulation; trends; data monitoring committees; multicenter studies; research ethics; Belmont Report; Department of Health and Human Services; DHHS Guidelines; Office for Protection from Research Risks; *United States

McGough, Helen. OPRR and FDA propose revised expedited review categories. *IRB: A Review of Human Subjects Research.* 1998 Jan-Feb; 20(1): 9, 11. 2 refs. BE58520.
　　*ethical review; federal government; *government regulation; *human experimentation; informed consent; *research ethics committees; risk; *expedited review; *Food and Drug Administration; *Office for Protection from Research Risks; *United States

Marritt, Clive. Local research ethics committees: a view from the Department of Health. *In:* Close, Bryony; Combes, Robert; Hubbard, Anthony; Illingworth, John, eds. Volunteers in Research and Testing. Bristol, PA: Taylor and Francis; 1997: 53–58. 5 refs. 1 fn. ISBN 0-7484-0397-3. BE57030.
　　government regulation; guidelines; human experimentation; *organization and administration; *research ethics committees; standards; multicenter studies; *Department of Health (Great Britain); *Great Britain

Marshall, Eliot. NIH examines standards for consent. [News]. *Science.* 1998 Jun 12; 280(5370): 1688. BE58271.
　　bioethics; competence; conflict of interest; ethical review; evaluation; federal government; financial support; *government regulation; guidelines; *human experimentation; *informed consent; mentally ill; research design; *research ethics committees; research subjects; schizophrenia; *standards; withholding treatment; National Institute of Mental Health; *National Institutes of Health; *United States

Marshall, Eliot. Review boards: a system 'in jeopardy'? [News]. *Science.* 1998 Jun 19; 280(5371): 1830–1831. BE58270.
　　conflict of interest; economics; *ethical review; evaluation;

federal government; financial support; *government regulation; *human experimentation; private sector; *research ethics committees; standards; Department of Health and Human Services; *United States

Micetich, Kenneth. The IRB: current and future challenges. *In:* Monagle, John F.; Thomasma, David C., eds. Health Care Ethics: Critical Issues for the 21st Century. Gaithersburg, MD: Aspen Publishers; 1998: 265–276. 19 fn. ISBN 0-8342-0911-X. BE56286.
　　coercion; consent forms; drug industry; emergency care; employment; ethical review; federal government; financial support; government regulation; *human experimentation; incentives; informed consent; investigators; mentally disabled; nontherapeutic research; placebos; research design; *research ethics committees; risks and benefits; selection of subjects; technical expertise; therapeutic research; trends; volunteers; United States

Moutel, G.; Leroux, N.; Hervé, C. Analysis of a survey of 36 French research committees on intracytoplasmic sperm injection. *Lancet.* 1998 Apr 11; 351(9109): 1121–1123. 16 refs. BE58310.
　　embryo transfer; *ethical review; evaluation; health facilities; *human experimentation; in vitro fertilization; infertility; males; *methods; *reproductive technologies; research design; *research ethics committees; risks and benefits; *sperm; survey; technical expertise; therapeutic research; *intracytoplasmic sperm injection; *France
BACKGROUND: In France, when a new medical technology is to be applied experimentally to human beings, it must adhere to the principles stipulated by the Huriet–Sérusclat law on biomedical research. This law requires that the validation of a protocol applicable to human beings, with its corollary protection and information dimensions, is first submitted to a research committee, known as a Consultative Committee Protecting Persons in Biomedical Research (CCPPRB). We aimed to survey the competence of these committees in biotechnology, and whether or not intracytoplasmic sperm injection (ICSI) had been considered by the committees as being an innovative treatment. METHODS: We presented each of France's 48 CCPPRBs with a questionnaire to assess the choices and criteria for making decisions that arose at the time ICSI was implemented in the different centres in each region. FINDINGS: 36 committees took part. We found that ICSI had been largely introduced in settings outside the scope of the CCPPRBs and of the framework fixed by the law on biomedical research. Only three centres for medically assisted reproduction had submitted applications to a CCPPRB, although ICSI has been implemented in over 20 centres. 21 (58%) committees were of the opinion that the implementation of ICSI could have come under their supervision. 24 (67%) committees believed that, independently of their own involvement, evaluation procedures for ICSI should have been specified before centres decided to introduce it. INTERPRETATION: We observed important differences in the way CCPPRBs handled ICSI as being within or outside the medical research field. The status of the research committees is legally and identically defined. However, committees did not agree on the definition of the limits of their action, and, therefore, their handling of the same issue differed. An inquiry is needed to define how, now that ICSI is done in many centres, it should adhere to principles of evaluation and safety already in existence for other medical technologies.

Nicholson, Richard H. Seeking harmony in discord. [News]. *Hastings Center Report.* 1998 Jan-Feb; 28(1): 7.

BE = bioethics accession number   fn. = footnotes   refs. = references

BE57290.
ethical review; government regulation; *human experimentation; *international aspects; investigators; regional ethics committees; *research ethics committees; standards; multicenter studies; Europe; Great Britain; National Health Service; United States

Olson, Carin M.; Jobe, Kathleen A.; Rennie, Drummond, et al. Reporting institutional review board approval and patient consent. [Letter and response]. *JAMA.* 1997 Aug 13; 278(6): 477. 8 refs. BE55919.
*editorial policies; *ethical review; *human experimentation; *informed consent; records; *research ethics committees; BMJ (British Medical Journal)

Savulescu, Julian; Chalmers, Iain; Blunt, Jennifer. Does setting good practice standards for research ethics committees increase their legal liability? [Letter]. *BMJ (British Medical Journal).* 1997 Jun 21; 314(7097): 1833. 4 refs. BE56566.
accountability; injuries; *legal liability; *research ethics committees; research subjects; *standards; Great Britain

Scott, P.V.; Pinnock, C.A.; Stone, Peter G., et al. Local research ethics committees. [Letters]. *BMJ (British Medical Journal).* 1997 Jul 5; 315(7099): 60–61. 8 refs. BE55921.
ethical review; human experimentation; research design; *research ethics committees; *multicenter studies; *national ethics committees; *Great Britain

Silberner, Joanne. Remodelling IRBs. *Hastings Center Report.* 1998 Jul–Aug; 28(4): 5. BE58921.
committee membership; conflict of interest; *ethical review; *evaluation; federal government; government regulation; *human experimentation; *public policy; *research ethics committees; standards; state government; technical expertise; Department of Health and Human Services; *United States

Straw, Peggy. Consumer representation on IRBs -- how it should be done. *In:* Shamoo, Adil E., ed. Ethics in Neurobiological Research with Human Subjects: The Baltimore Conference on Ethics. Amsterdam: Gordon and Breach; 1997: 187–190. ISBN 2-88449-161-9. BE57016.
advisory committees; *committee membership; comprehension; consent forms; disclosure; *human experimentation; informed consent; *mentally ill; *patient advocacy; program descriptions; *public participation; *research ethics committees; research subjects; standards; Alliance for the Mentally Ill of New Hampshire; Dartmouth Medical School; *New Hampshire Division of Mental Health; United States

Talbot, D.; Reynolds, D.J.M.; Stone, Peter G., et al. Local research ethics committees. [Letters and response]. *BMJ (British Medical Journal).* 1997 Nov 29; 315(7120): 1464–1465. 10 refs. BE58222.
ethical review; guidelines; human experimentation; placebos; regional ethics committees; research design; *research ethics committees; medical audit; *multicenter studies; British Medical Association; *Great Britain

U.S. National Institutes of Health. Recombinant DNA research: proposed actions under the guidelines; notice. *Federal Register.* 1996 Nov 22; 61(227): 59726–59742. BE57536.
*advisory committees; committee membership; data banks; *ethical review; *federal government; *gene therapy; *government regulation; guidelines; *human experimentation; organization and administration; *public policy; recombinant DNA research; review committees; Food and Drug Administration; *Gene Therapy Policy Conferences; *National Institutes of Health; NIH Guidelines;

Office of Recombinant DNA Activities; Points to Consider: Transfer of Recombinant DNA into Human Subjects; *Recombinant DNA Advisory Committee; *United States

Verhoef, Marja J.; Lewkonia, Raymond M.; Kinsella, T. Douglas. Ethical issues concerning current human DNA banking practices in Canada: three perspectives. *In:* Knoppers, Bartha Maria, ed. Human DNA: Law and Policy: International and Comparative Perspectives. Proceedings of the First International Conference on DNA Sampling and Human Genetic Research: Ethical, Legal, and Policy Aspects, held in Montreal, Canada, 6–8 Sep 1996. Boston, MA: Kluwer Law International; 1997: 393–405. 17 fn. ISBN 90–411–0361–9. BE58196.
*administrators; comparative studies; confidentiality; consent forms; disclosure; *DNA data banks; donors; ethical review; evaluation; *genetic research; informed consent; *institutional policies; *investigators; *knowledge, attitudes, practice; organization and administration; organizational policies; professional organizations; property rights; *research ethics committees; research institutes; survey; tissue donation; *biological specimen banks; *Canada; Canadian College of Medical Genetics

LREC resigns unanimously [Basingstoke Local Research Ethics Committee]. [News]. *Bulletin of Medical Ethics.* 1997 May; No. 128: 3–6. BE55679.
administrators; dissent; ethical review; evaluation; interprofessional relations; *organization and administration; *professional competence; *regulation; *research ethics committees; standards; qualitative research; *Basingstoke Local Research Ethics Committee; England; *Great Britain; National Health Service; *North and Mid Hampshire Health Authority

HUMAN EXPERIMENTATION/FOREIGN COUNTRIES

Aaby, Peter; Babiker, Abdel; Darbyshire, Janet, et al. Ethics of HIV trials. [Letters]. *Lancet.* 1997 Nov 22; 350(9090): 1546–1547. 5 refs. BE58468.
*control groups; *developing countries; *drugs; economics; *HIV seropositivity; *human experimentation; international aspects; *placebos; *pregnant women; random selection; *research design; Africa; AZT

Addis, G.J.; London, D. The *BMJ*'s Nuremberg issue. [Letters]. *BMJ (British Medical Journal).* 1997 Apr 12; 314(7087): 1128. 2 refs. BE57240.
*conscience; *historical aspects; *human experimentation; *moral obligations; National Socialism; nontherapeutic research; *obligations to society; organizational policies; physicians; professional organizations; religion; *research subjects; *volunteers; *war; Germany; *Great Britain; Royal College of Physicians of London; Twentieth Century; *World War II

Association for Improvements in the Maternity Services (Great Britain); National Childbirth Trust (Great Britain); Maternity Alliance (Great Britain). A charter for ethical research in maternity care: Association for Improvements in the Maternity Services; the National Childbirth Trust. *Nursing Ethics.* 1998 May; 5(3): 256–262. 10 fn. Reprinted with permission from the Association for Improvements in the Maternity Services. BE58725.
behavioral research; childbirth; confidentiality; disclosure; *guidelines; *human experimentation; informed consent; *maternal health; mothers; newborns; organizational policies; *pregnant women; research design; research subjects; *Association for Improvements in the Maternity Services (Great Britain); *Great Britain; *National Childbirth Trust (Great Britain)

BE = bioethics accession number   fn. = footnotes   refs. = references

Ault, Alicia. USA accused of funding placebo–controlled AIDS trials. [News]. *Lancet.* 1997 May 3; 349(9061): 1305. BE56073.

> AIDS; *developing countries; drugs; federal government; government financing; *HIV seropositivity; *human experimentation; *newborns; *placebos; *pregnant women; public policy; withholding treatment; AZT; Centers for Disease Control and Prevention; National Institutes of Health; *United States

Barker, E.M. Informed consent in medical research: the ethics committee's view. [Letter]. *BMJ (British Medical Journal).* 1998 Jan 31; 316(7128): 392–393. 3 refs. BE57800.

> committee membership; deception; developing countries; ethical review; HIV seropositivity; *human experimentation; *informed consent; intensive care units; investigators; misconduct; motivation; *research ethics committees; selection for treatment; *South Africa

Bendall, Christine. Clinical research -- the relationship between law and guidelines. *In:* Close, Bryony; Combes, Robert; Hubbard, Anthony; Illingworth, John, eds. Volunteers in Research and Testing. Bristol, PA: Taylor and Francis; 1997: 41–52. 2 refs. 5 fn. ISBN 0-7484-0397-3. BE57029.

> compensation; confidentiality; ethical review; *guidelines; *human experimentation; informed consent; injuries; international aspects; law; *legal aspects; *regulation; research subjects; selection of subjects; *Europe; European Community; Great Britain

Bernard, Claire; Nassiry, Ladan; Knoppers, Bartha Maria, comps. Legal Aspects of Research and Clinical Practice with Human Beings: Selected Canadian Legal Bibliography, 1980–1992. Ottawa, ON: National Council on Bioethics in Human Research (NCBHR); 1992. 35 p. Text in English and in French. ISBN 0-9696111-2-9. BE56979.

> *human experimentation; *legal aspects; *Canada

Berry, Jonathan. Local research ethics committees can audit ethical standards in research. *Journal of Medical Ethics.* 1997 Dec; 23(6): 379–381. 3 refs. BE57655.

> comprehension; disclosure; *ethical review; *evaluation; evaluation studies; human experimentation; informed consent; recall; *research ethics committees; *research subjects; *standards; survey; *therapeutic research; questionnaires; *Great Britain

> OBJECTIVES: To show that a Local Research Ethics Committee (LREC) can carry out an audit of ethical standards in research. To find out if a researcher met certain ethical standards in recruiting subjects for clinical trials and in obtaining their consent. DESIGN: Postal questionnaire. SETTING: Clinical research by one doctor during one year. SUBJECTS: Eleven patients entered in clinical trials. MAIN OUTCOME MEASURES: Success in ethics committee obtaining data. Achievement of ethical standards in recruitment of subjects and in obtaining consent. RESULTS: The audit was successfully carried out and standards were partly met. CONCLUSIONS: Local Research Ethics Committees can carry out audits of the conduct of research projects which they have approved. Provision for possible audits can be made at the time of application to the committee. Our committee thought the ethical standards in the research which we audited were acceptable.

Bhagwanjee, Satish; Muckart, David J.J.; Jeena, Prakash M., et al. Does HIV status influence the outcome of patients admitted to a surgical intensive care

unit? A prospective double blind study. [Article, commentaries, and response]. *BMJ (British Medical Journal).* 1997 Apr 12; 314(7087): 1077–1084. 26 refs. BE55661.

> *AIDS serodiagnosis; anonymous testing; blacks; comparative studies; confidentiality; critically ill; developing countries; disadvantaged; disclosure; empirical research; *epidemiology; futility; *HIV seropositivity; hospitals; human experimentation; *informed consent; injuries; *intensive care units; justice; morbidity; mortality; patient admission; patient discharge; patients; research design; research ethics committees; *research subjects; resource allocation; scientific misconduct; *selection for treatment; surgery; *treatment outcome; prospective studies; *South Africa

> OBJECTIVES: (a) To assess the impact of HIV status (HIV negative, HIV positive, AIDS) on the outcome of patients admitted to intensive care units for diseases unrelated to HIV; (b) to decide whether a positive test result for HIV should be a criterion for excluding patients from intensive care for diseases unrelated to HIV. DESIGN: A prospective double blind study of all admissions over six months. HIV status was determined in all patients by enzyme linked immunosorbent assay (ELISA), immunofluorescence assay, western blotting, and flow cytometry. The ethics committee considered the clinical implications of the study important enough to waive patients' right to informed consent. Staff and patients were blinded to HIV results. On discharge patients could be advised of their HIV status if they wished. SETTING: A 16 bed surgical intensive care unit. SUBJECTS: All 267 men and 135 women admitted to the unit during the study period. INTERVENTIONS: None. MAIN OUTCOME MEASURES: APACHE II score (acute physiological, age, and chronic health evaluation), organ failure, septic shock, durations of intensive care unit and hospital stay, and intensive care unit and hospital mortality. RESULTS: No patient had AIDS. 52 patients were tested positive for HIV and 350 patients were tested negative. The two groups were similar in sex distribution but differed significantly in age, incidence of organ failure (37 (71%) v 171 (49%) patients), and incidence of septic shock (20 (38%) v 54 (15%)). After adjustment for age there were no differences in intensive care unit or hospital mortality or in the durations of stay in the intensive care unit or hospital. CONCLUSIONS: Morbidity was higher in HIV positive patients but there was no difference in mortality. In this patient population a positive HIV test result should not be a criterion for excluding a patient from intensive care.

Birchard, Karen. Irish research project abandoned after adverse publicity. [News]. *Lancet.* 1998 Feb 7; 351(9100): 426. BE58886.

> *human experimentation; *mentally ill; nutrition; *Ireland

Bloom, Barry R. The highest attainable standard: ethical issues in AIDS vaccines. *Science.* 1998 Jan 9; 279(5348): 186–188. 15 fn. BE58034.

> *AIDS; codes of ethics; *developing countries; drugs; economics; ethical review; goals; guidelines; *human experimentation; *immunization; informed consent; *international aspects; placebos; preventive medicine; research design; standards; *therapeutic research; Council for International Organizations of Medical Sciences; Declaration of Helsinki; International Ethical Guidelines for Biomedical Research Involving Human Subjects; UNAIDS; United Nations; World Health Organization

Blunt, Jennifer; Savulescu, Julian; Watson, Alastair J.M. Meeting the challenges facing research ethics

---

BE = bioethics accession number   fn. = footnotes   refs. = references

committees: some practical suggestions. *BMJ (British Medical Journal).* 1998 Jan 3; 316(7124): 58–61. 47 refs. BE57954.

committee membership; education; ethical review; fraud; human experimentation; information dissemination; investigators; *research ethics committees; standards; students; multicenter studies; *Great Britain

Brody, Baruch A. Research ethics: international perspectives. *Cambridge Quarterly of Healthcare Ethics.* 1997 Fall; 6(4): 376–384. 22 fn. BE56458.

adults; *animal experimentation; animal rights; bioethics; comparative studies; *consensus; *cultural pluralism; *dissent; *embryo research; embryos; ethical review; guidelines; *human experimentation; in vitro fertilization; informed consent; *international aspects; moral obligations; moral policy; regulation; research embryo creation; research subjects; speciesism; value of life; Asia; Australia; Europe; North America

Butler, Declan. Admission on Gulf War vaccines spurs debate on medical records. [News]. *Nature.* 1997 Nov 6; 390(6655): 3–4. BE56858.

biological warfare; epidemiology; *human experimentation; *immunization; injuries; medical records; *military personnel; *morbidity; *public policy; *war; whooping cough; *Great Britain; *Ministry of Defence (Great Britain); *Persian Gulf War

Butler, Declan. Spermatid injection fertilizes ethics debate. [News]. *Nature.* 1995 Sep 28; 377(6547): 277. BE56108.

animal experimentation; congenital disorders; *human experimentation; in vitro fertilization; infertility; investigators; males; *methods; ovum; *reproductive technologies; research design; risks and benefits; *sperm; *therapeutic research; *France; Testart, Jacques

Chen, Yuan–Fang. Japanese death factories and the American cover-up. *Cambridge Quarterly of Healthcare Ethics.* 1997 Spring; 6(2): 240–242. BE56425.

accountability; aliens; *biological warfare; communicable diseases; *historical aspects; *human experimentation; human rights; international aspects; investigators; killing; medical ethics; military personnel; moral complicity; National Socialism; physicians; *prisoners; *public policy; *research subjects; *scientific misconduct; torture; *war; China; Factories of Death (Harris, S.); Germany; Ishii, Shiro; *Japan; Twentieth Century; *United States; *World War II

Christakis, Nicolas A. The distinction between ethical pluralism and ethical relativism: implications for the conduct of transcultural clinical research. *In:* Vanderpool, Harold Y., ed. The Ethics of Research Involving Human Subjects: Facing the 21st Century. Frederick, MD: University Publishing Group; 1996: 261–280. 45 fn. ISBN 1-55572-036-6. BE56990.

AIDS; *cultural pluralism; developing countries; *ethical relativism; *guidelines; *human experimentation; humanism; informed consent; *international aspects; investigator subject relationship; investigators; medical ethics; *moral policy; morality; paternalism; personhood; research subjects; standards; values; non–Western World; research ethics; Western World

Clark, Peter A. The ethics of placebo–controlled trials for perinatal transmission of HIV in developing countries. *Journal of Clinical Ethics.* 1998 Summer; 9(2): 156–166. 44 fn. BE58961.

AIDS; alternatives; autonomy; beneficence; common good; comprehension; *control groups; costs and benefits; *developing countries; drugs; ethical analysis; ethical relativism; guidelines; *HIV seropositivity; *human experimentation; human rights; informed consent; international aspects; justice; *moral policy; morbidity;

*newborns; patient care; *placebos; *pregnant women; prevalence; public policy; *research design; research subjects; risks and benefits; socioeconomic factors; standards; vulnerable populations; AZT; United States

Cleaton–Jones, Peter E.; Busse, Peter; Emery, Sean, et al. Availability of antiretroviral therapy after clinical trials with HIV infected patients are ended: an ethical dilemma. [Article and commentaries]. *BMJ (British Medical Journal).* 1997 Mar 22; 314(7084): 887–891. 7 refs. BE58772.

*AIDS; communication; *developing countries; *drug industry; *drugs; economics; *financial support; government financing; guidelines; health care delivery; *HIV seropositivity; *human experimentation; *institutional ethics; investigators; patient advocacy; *patient care; private sector; research ethics committees; *research subjects; resource allocation; *therapeutic research; *continuity of patient care; Declaration of Helsinki; Medical Research Council (South Africa); *South Africa

Collier, Joe. The future of ethics committees. *In:* Close, Bryony; Combes, Robert; Hubbard, Anthony; Illingworth, John, eds. Volunteers in Research and Testing. Bristol, PA: Taylor and Francis; 1997: 177–183. ISBN 0-7484-0397-3. BE57040.

clinical ethics committees; committee membership; ethicists; *ethics committees; hospitals; human experimentation; organization and administration; *research ethics committees; Europe; *Great Britain

Darvall, Leanna. Gender and equity: emerging issues in Australian clinical drug trial regulatory policies. *In:* Petersen, Kerry, ed. Intersections: Women on Law, Medicine and Technology. Brookfield, VT: Ashgate; 1997: 185–200. 18 refs. 1 fn. ISBN 1-85521-882-8. BE57492.

age factors; AIDS; costs and benefits; *drugs; federal government; *females; *government regulation; *guidelines; *human experimentation; international aspects; justice; males; minority groups; *nontherapeutic research; pregnant women; prenatal injuries; *public policy; research design; *risks and benefits; *selection of subjects; toxicity; *Australia; Department of Health and Human Services; Food and Drug Administration; National Institutes of Health; *United States

Dyer, Clare. Consultant struck off over research fraud. [News]. *BMJ (British Medical Journal).* 1997 Jul 26; 315(7102): 205. BE58744.

consent forms; deception; drug industry; drugs; *fraud; *human experimentation; investigators; *physicians; punishment; records; regulation; *scientific misconduct; *Anderton, George; *General Medical Council (Great Britain); *Great Britain

European Forum for Good Clinical Practice. Ethics Working Party. Guidelines and Recommendations for European Ethics Committees. Brussels, Belgium: European Forum for Good Clinical Practice; 1995. 17 p. 8 refs. BE58131.

committee membership; *guidelines; human experimentation; *international aspects; organization and administration; *research ethics committees; standards; *Europe

Gambia. Medical Research Council Joint Ethical Committee. Ethical issues facing medical research in developing countries. *Lancet.* 1998 Jan 24; 351(9098): 286–287. 13 refs. BE57570.

AIDS; *developing countries; drugs; editorial policies; *ethical review; health care delivery; HIV seropositivity; *human experimentation; immunization; informed consent; peer review; placebos; public health; research design; research ethics committees; research subjects; resource

---

BE = bioethics accession number   fn. = footnotes   refs. = references

allocation; *socioeconomic factors; standards; national ethics committees; tuberculosis; Africa; *Gambia; Lancet; New England Journal of Medicine

Gold, Hal. Unit 731: Testimony -- Japan's Wartime Human Experimentation Program. Tokyo: Yenbooks; 1996. 256 p. Bibliography: p. 251-256. ISBN 4-900737-39-9. BE57996.
    *biological warfare; children; confidentiality; dehumanization; disclosure; federal government; females; historical aspects; *human experimentation; international aspects; investigators; killing; military personnel; *moral complicity; *prisoners; public policy; *scientific misconduct; torture; China; Cold War; Ishii, Shiro; *Japan; Manchuria; *Twentieth Century; *United States; USSR; *World War II

Goldbeck-Wood, Sandra. Denmark takes a lead on research ethics. [News]. *BMJ (British Medical Journal).* 1998 Apr 18; 316(7139): 1189. BE58619.
    disclosure; *ethical review; financial support; *government regulation; *human experimentation; research ethics committees; national ethics committees; *Denmark

Great Britain. Department of Health. Advisory Group on the Ethics of Xenotransplantation (Chair: Ian Kennedy). Animal Tissue into Humans: A Report by the Advisory Group on the Ethics of Xenotransplantation, 1996. London: Her Majesty's Stationery Office; 1997. 258 p. 92 fn. Appendixes include Glossary of terms; The consultation exercise; Report of the Workshop on Xenotransplantation and Infectious Disease; and Development of transgenic pigs. ISBN 0-11-321866-4. BE55999.
    advisory committees; alternatives; animal experimentation; *animal organs; animal rights; artificial organs; body parts and fluids; communicable diseases; ethical review; *evaluation; gene therapy; genetic intervention; *government regulation; *guidelines; health promotion; *human experimentation; informed consent; international aspects; legal aspects; organ donation; *organ transplantation; preventive medicine; primates; private sector; public health; *public policy; public sector; research ethics committees; resource allocation; *risks and benefits; scarcity; selection of subjects; suffering; therapeutic research; *tissue transplantation; *transgenic animals; swine; Advisory Group on the Ethics of Xenotransplantation (Great Britain); Animals (Scientific Procedures) Act 1986; Department of Health (Great Britain); *Great Britain

Guest, Stephen. Compensation for the subjects of medical research. [Letter]. *Journal of Medical Ethics.* 1997 Oct; 23(5): 328. 2 refs. BE58262.
    altruism; *compensation; government financing; *human experimentation; *injuries; insurance; legislation; negligence; public policy; *research subjects; torts; *Great Britain; National Health Service

Halsey, Neal A.; Sommer, Alfred; Henderson, Donald A., et al. Ethics and international research. [Editorial]. *BMJ (British Medical Journal).* 1997 Oct 18; 315(7114): 965-966. 8 refs. BE55908.
    *developing countries; *drugs; economics; *ethical relativism; guidelines; health care delivery; *HIV seropositivity; *human experimentation; *international aspects; *newborns; *placebos; *pregnant women; *research design; standards; *AZT; Centers for Disease Control and Prevention; Council for International Organizations of Medical Sciences; United States; World Health Organization

Horton, Richard. ICRF: from mayhem to meltdown. *Lancet.* 1997 Oct 11; 350(9084): 1043-1044. BE56927.
    *biomedical research; *breast cancer; *conflict of interest; editorial policies; epidemiology; females; *financial support;

*hormones; *human experimentation; *information dissemination; investigators; mass media; organizational policies; *risk; women's health; *estrogen replacement therapy; *Great Britain; *Imperial Cancer Research Fund; Lancet

IJesselmuiden, Carel B.; Faden, Ruth R. Medical research and the principle of respect for persons in non-Western cultures. *In:* Vanderpool, Harold Y., ed. The Ethics of Research Involving Human Subjects: Facing the 21st Century. Frederick, MD: University Publishing Group; 1996: 281-301. 48 fn. ISBN 1-55572-036-6. BE56991.
    AIDS; anthropology; *autonomy; beneficence; competence; *cultural pluralism; *developing countries; *ethical relativism; guidelines; *human experimentation; *informed consent; *international aspects; investigators; *moral policy; research subjects; third party consent; values; *non-Western World; Africa

Jacobsen, Geir; Hals, Arild. Medical investigators' views about ethics and fraud in medical research. *Journal of the Royal College of Physicians of London.* 1995 Sep-Oct; 29(5): 405-409. 20 refs. BE55562.
    advisory committees; age factors; *attitudes; *biomedical research; *ethical review; evaluation; females; *fraud; freedom; historical aspects; human experimentation; information dissemination; *investigators; *knowledge, attitudes, practice; males; medical ethics; physicians; professional autonomy; professional ethics; regional ethics committees; *regulation; *research design; *research ethics committees; retrospective moral judgment; science; *scientific misconduct; *self regulation; statistics; survey; trends; *Norway; Twentieth Century

Jayaraman, K.S. Inquiry looks into Indian cancer deaths. [News]. *Nature.* 1997 Dec 18-25; 390(6661): 653. BE57309.
    attitudes; *cancer; *disadvantaged; disclosure; *females; historical aspects; *human experimentation; *informed consent; investigators; retrospective moral judgment; *scientific misconduct; *withholding treatment; *India; Indian Council of Medical Research

Jayaraman, K.S. Policing ethical codes in India proves tough. [News]. *Nature.* 1997 Oct 16; 389(6652): 663. BE56308.
    advisory committees; bioethical issues; biomedical research; cancer; developing countries; females; genetics; *guidelines; *human experimentation; regulation; scientific misconduct; withholding treatment; *India

Josefson, Debbie. US journal attacks unethical HIV trials. [News]. *BMJ (British Medical Journal).* 1997 Sep 27; 315(7111): 765. BE56928.
    *developing countries; *drugs; economics; editorial policies; *HIV seropositivity; *human experimentation; *placebos; pregnant women; public policy; *research design; Africa; Asia; AZT; Latin America; New England Journal of Medicine; United States

Kaiser, Jocelyn. Flap on NEJM board over ethics articles. [News]. *Science.* 1997 Oct 10; 278(5336): 211. BE56066.
    *developing countries; dissent; *editorial policies; *HIV seropositivity; *human experimentation; interprofessional relations; investigators; *newborns; *placebos; *pregnant women; scientific misconduct; withholding treatment; *Ho, David; *New England Journal of Medicine; *Wilfert, Catherine

Kaiser, Jocelyn. UNAIDS to weigh vaccine ethics. [News]. *Science.* 1997 Sep 19; 277(5333): 1751. BE56067.
    *developing countries; drugs; *HIV seropositivity; *human experimentation; *immunization; *international aspects; newborns; patient care; placebos; pregnant women; AZT;

BE = bioethics accession number   fn. = footnotes   refs. = references

*UNAIDS; United Nations

Kigotho, Anderson Wachira. Another HIV-1 trial loses placebo control. [News]. *Lancet.* 1997 Dec 20–27; 350(9094): 1831. BE57861.
> control groups; *developing countries; *drugs; females; *HIV seropositivity; *human experimentation; *international aspects; mothers; newborns; *placebos; *pregnant women; *research design; *therapeutic research; AZT; *Ethiopia; Johns Hopkins University; United States

Klingmann, Ingrid. The European dimension. *In:* Close, Bryony; Combes, Robert; Hubbard, Anthony; Illingworth, John, eds. Volunteers in Research and Testing. Bristol, PA: Taylor and Francis; 1997: 169–175. 3 refs. ISBN 0-7484-0397-3. BE57039.
> committee membership; compensation; guidelines; *human experimentation; injuries; *international aspects; regulation; remuneration; *research ethics committees; research subjects; volunteers; Austria; Belgium; *Europe; France; Germany; Great Britain; Spain; Sweden

Kmietowicz, Zosia. MRC cleared of unethical research practices. [News]. *BMJ (British Medical Journal).* 1998 May 30; 316(7145): 1628. BE58278.
> financial support; *historical aspects; *human experimentation; informed consent; *radiation; research subjects; retrospective moral judgment; review committees; *scientific misconduct; standards; *Great Britain; *Medical Research Council (Great Britain); *Twentieth Century

Kondro, Wayne. Canada still seeking research code of ethics. [News]. *Lancet.* 1997 Sep 13; 350(9080): 794. BE56186.
> advisory committees; codes of ethics; dissent; *guidelines; *human experimentation; informed consent; investigators; *public policy; research ethics committees; self regulation; universities; *Canada; *Code of Conduct for Research Involving Humans; Medical Research Council of Canada; Natural Sciences and Engineering Research Council (Canada); Social Sciences and Humanities Research Council (Canada)

Kondro, Wayne. Leaked document indicates Canada's future stance on human research. [News]. *Lancet.* 1998 Jun 20; 351(9119): 1868. BE58416.
> cloning; drugs; *ethical review; gene therapy; germ cells; government regulation; guidelines; *human experimentation; hybrids; placebos; research embryo creation; research ethics committees; *Canada; *Medical Research Council of Canada; *Natural Sciences and Engineering Research Council (Canada); *Social Sciences and Humanities Research Council (Canada); *Tri-Council Policy Statement on Ethical Conduct for Research Involving Humans

Kondro, Wayne. New rules on human subjects could end debate in Canada. [News]. *Science.* 1998 Jun 5; 280(5369): 1521. BE58875.
> advisory committees; *behavioral research; biomedical research; committee membership; consensus; deception; dissent; ethical review; genetic research; *guidelines; *human experimentation; humanities; informed consent; interdisciplinary communication; lawyers; minority groups; *regulation; research ethics committees; research institutes; research subjects; science; social sciences; universities; community consent; *Canada; *Code of Conduct for Research Involving Humans; *Medical Research Council of Canada; *Natural Sciences and Engineering Research Council (Canada); *Social Sciences and Humanities Research Council (Canada)

Kumar, Sanjay. Hope, but little cheer, for India's revised code of ethics. [News]. *Lancet.* 1998 Jan 31; 351(9099): 347. BE57872.
> codes of ethics; *guidelines; *human experimentation;

informed consent; *India; *Indian Council of Medical Research

Kumar, Sanjay. India to ban use of quinacrine for sterilisation. [News]. *Lancet.* 1998 Mar 28; 351(9107): 968. BE58442.
> developing countries; *drugs; *females; *government regulation; *human experimentation; international aspects; *sterilization (sexual); women's health; *India; *quinacrine

Kumar, Sanjay. Sterilisation by quinacrine comes under fire in India. [News]. *Lancet.* 1997 May 17; 349(9063): 1460. BE55823.
> *drugs; *females; government regulation; *human experimentation; informed consent; involuntary sterilization; legal aspects; misconduct; physicians; *sterilization (sexual); *India; *quinacrine

Lantos, John D. Was the UK collaborative ECMO trial ethical? *Paediatric and Perinatal Epidemiology.* 1997 Jul; 11(3): 264–268. 7 refs. BE58033.
> alternatives; *biomedical technologies; coercion; congenital disorders; critically ill; *human experimentation; international aspects; mortality; *newborns; parental consent; *patient care; *random selection; *research design; risks and benefits; *technology assessment; *therapeutic research; time factors; *treatment outcome; uncertainty; *extracorporeal membrane oxygenation; *Great Britain

Lemaire, F.; Blanch, L.; Cohen, S.L.; European Society of Intensive Care Medicine. Working Group on Ethics. Informed consent for research purposes in intensive care patients in Europe -- part I: an official statement of the European Society of Intensive Care Medicine. *Intensive Care Medicine.* 1997 Mar; 23(3): 338–341. BE57653.
> competence; *critically ill; disclosure; *emergency care; family members; guidelines; *human experimentation; informed consent; *intensive care units; international aspects; legal guardians; *organizational policies; patients; physicians; *presumed consent; professional organizations; research subjects; *therapeutic research; *third party consent; *deferred consent; Council of Europe; *Europe; *European Society of Intensive Care Medicine; United States

Lemaire, F.; Blanch, L.; Cohen, S.L.; European Society of Intensive Care Medicine. Working Group on Ethics. Informed consent for research purposes in intensive care patients in Europe -- part II: an official statement of the European Society of Intensive Care Medicine. *Intensive Care Medicine.* 1997 Apr; 23(4): 435–439. 8 refs. BE57654.
> competence; *critically ill; *decision making; *emergency care; family members; government regulation; hospitals; *human experimentation; *informed consent; institutional policies; *intensive care units; *international aspects; investigators; *legal aspects; legal guardians; nontherapeutic research; patients; physicians; public policy; research ethics committees; research subjects; survey; therapeutic research; *third party consent; deferred consent; questionnaires; Austria; Belgium; Denmark; *Europe; *European Society of Intensive Care Medicine; Finland; France; Germany; Great Britain; Greece; Israel; Italy; Netherlands; Norway; Portugal; Spain; Sweden; Switzerland

Levine, Robert J. International codes and guidelines for research ethics: a critical appraisal. *In:* Vanderpool, Harold Y., ed. The Ethics of Research Involving Human Subjects: Facing the 21st Century. Frederick, MD: University Publishing Group; 1996: 235–259. 47 fn. ISBN 1-55572-036-6. BE56989.
> codes of ethics; *cultural pluralism; developing countries; disclosure; empirical research; *ethical relativism; *guidelines; *human experimentation; informed consent;

BE = bioethics accession number   fn. = footnotes   refs. = references

*international aspects; investigators; research subjects; risks and benefits; standards; *research ethics; Council for International Organizations of Medical Sciences; *Declaration of Helsinki; *International Ethical Guidelines for Biomedical Research Involving Human Subjects; *Nuremberg Code

Levine, Robert J. The "best proven therapeutic method" standard in clinical trials in technologically developing countries. [Editorial]. *IRB: A Review of Human Subjects Research.* 1998 Jan–Feb; 20(1): 5–9. 19 fn. BE58519.
    *control groups; *developing countries; *drugs; economics; guidelines; *HIV seropositivity; *human experimentation; international aspects; newborns; patient care; *placebos; *pregnant women; *research design; *standards; *AZT; Declaration of Helsinki

Lewith, George T. Ethical problems in evaluating complementary medicine. *Bulletin of Medical Ethics.* 1996 Aug; No. 120: 17–20. 15 refs. BE55879.
    *alternative therapies; chronically ill; control groups; *evaluation; guidelines; *human experimentation; placebos; *research design; research ethics committees; research subjects; selection of subjects; therapeutic research; treatment outcome; General Medical Council (Great Britain); *Great Britain

Macklin, Ruth. Justice in international research. *In:* Kahn, Jeffrey P.; Mastroianni, Anna C.; Sugarman, Jeremy, eds. Beyond Consent: Seeking Justice in Research. New York, NY: Oxford University Press; 1998: 131–146. 43 fn. ISBN 0-19-511353-5. BE58847.
    abortion, induced; contraception; cultural pluralism; *developing countries; drugs; ethical review; females; HIV seropositivity; *human experimentation; informed consent; *international aspects; investigational drugs; *justice; placebos; research design; research ethics committees; risks and benefits; standards; sterilization (sexual); trends; *vulnerable populations; Depo-provera; quinacrine; RU–486; United States

Marritt, Clive. Local research ethics committees: a view from the Department of Health. *In:* Close, Bryony; Combes, Robert; Hubbard, Anthony; Illingworth, John, eds. Volunteers in Research and Testing. Bristol, PA: Taylor and Francis; 1997: 53–58. 5 refs. 1 fn. ISBN 0-7484-0397-3. BE57030.
    government regulation; guidelines; human experimentation; *organization and administration; *research ethics committees; standards; multicenter studies; *Department of Health (Great Britain); *Great Britain

Marshall, Eliot. AIDS therapy: controversial trial offers hopeful result. [News]. *Science.* 1998 Feb 27; 279(5355): 1299. BE57260.
    costs and benefits; *developing countries; *drugs; *HIV seropositivity; *human experimentation; international aspects; newborns; *placebos; *pregnant women; *research design; therapeutic research; time factors; *Africa; *AZT; *Thailand

Marwick, Charles. Bioethics group considers transnational research. [News]. *JAMA.* 1998 May 13; 279(18): 1425. BE57862.
    advisory committees; *developing countries; *drugs; federal government; government financing; guidelines; *HIV seropositivity; *human experimentation; *international aspects; newborns; *placebos; *pregnant women; *public policy; *research design; scientific misconduct; *therapeutic research; *Africa; AZT; Declaration of Helsinki; National Bioethics Advisory Commission; *United States

Mbidde, Edward. Bioethics and local circumstances. [Editorial]. *Science.* 1998 Jan 9; 279(5348): 155. 5 fn.

BE58030.
    *developing countries; guidelines; health care; *HIV seropositivity; *human experimentation; international aspects; pregnant women; regulation; research design; socioeconomic factors; standards; Africa; Council for International Organizations of Medical Sciences; International Ethical Guidelines for Biomedical Research Involving Human Subjects

Miller, Judith. The Deschamps Report: controls for clinical research in Quebec. *International Journal of Bioethics.* 1997 Mar–Jun; 8(1–2): 79–85. 10 fn. BE59096.
    advisory committees; conflict of interest; drug industry; *evaluation; *government regulation; *human experimentation; misconduct; research ethics committees; Canada; *Deschamps Report; *Quebec

Montgomery, Jonathan. The position of the patient: consent to treatment; confidentiality and access to health care records; care for children; mental health; research. *In: his* Health Care Law. New York, NY: Oxford University Press; 1997: 225–356. 701 fn. ISBN 0-19-876260-7. BE56244.
    *adults; AIDS serodiagnosis; animal experimentation; coercion; compensation; competence; computers; *confidentiality; dangerousness; disclosure; dissent; duty to warn; genetic information; government regulation; *human experimentation; *informed consent; injuries; involuntary commitment; *legal aspects; legal guardians; legal liability; legislation; medical records; *mentally ill; *minors; parental consent; patient access to records; *patient care; patient discharge; patients' rights; research ethics committees; treatment refusal; *Great Britain; National Health Service

Moutel, G.; Leroux, N.; Hervé, C. Analysis of a survey of 36 French research committees on intracytoplasmic sperm injection. *Lancet.* 1998 Apr 11; 351(9109): 1121–1123. 16 refs. BE58310.
    embryo transfer; *ethical review; evaluation; health facilities; *human experimentation; in vitro fertilization; infertility; males; *methods; *reproductive technologies; research design; *research ethics committees; risks and benefits; *sperm; survey; technical expertise; therapeutic research; *intracytoplasmic sperm injection; *France
    BACKGROUND: In France, when a new medical technology is to be applied experimentally to human beings, it must adhere to the principles stipulated by the Huriet-Sérusclat law on biomedical research. This law requires that the validation of a protocol applicable to human beings, with its corollary protection and information dimensions, is first submitted to a research committee, known as a Consultative Committee Protecting Persons in Biomedical Research (CCPPRB). We aimed to survey the competence of these committees in biotechnology, and whether or not intracytoplasmic sperm injection (ICSI) had been considered by the committees as being an innovative treatment. METHODS: We presented each of France's 48 CCPPRBs with a questionnaire to assess the choices and criteria for making decisions that arose at the time ICSI was implemented in the different centres in each region. FINDINGS: 36 committees took part. We found that ICSI had been largely introduced in settings outside the scope of the CCPPRBs and of the framework fixed by the law on biomedical research. Only three centres for medically assisted reproduction had submitted applications to a CCPPRB, although ICSI has been implemented in over 20 centres. 21 (58%) committees were of the opinion that the implementation of ICSI could have come under their supervision. 24 (67%) committees believed that, independently of their own involvement, evaluation procedures for ICSI should have been specified before centres decided to introduce

---

BE = bioethics accession number   fn. = footnotes   refs. = references

it. INTERPRETATION: We observed important differences in the way CCPPRBs handled ICSI as being within or outside the medical research field. The status of the research committees is legally and identically defined. However, committees did not agree on the definition of the limits of their action, and, therefore, their handling of the same issue differed. An inquiry is needed to define how, now that ICSI is done in many centres, it should adhere to principles of evaluation and safety already in existence for other medical technologies.

Mudur, Ganapati. India to control foreign research involving Indian patients. [News]. *BMJ (British Medical Journal).* 1997 Jan 18; 314(7075): 165. BE58621.
     aborted fetuses; developing countries; eye diseases; fetal tissue donation; government financing; *government regulation; *human experimentation; *international aspects; investigators; *selection of subjects; tissue transplantation; *India; Indian Council of Medical Research; United States

Mudur, Ganapati. Indian study of women with cervical lesions called unethical. [News]. *BMJ (British Medical Journal).* 1997 Apr 12; 314(7087): 1065. BE56063.
     attitudes; *cancer; developing countries; *disadvantaged; disclosure; *females; historical aspects; *human experimentation; *informed consent; investigators; retrospective moral judgment; *scientific misconduct; withholding treatment; *India; Institute of Cytology and Preventive Oncology (New Delhi)

Nicholson, Richard H. Seeking harmony in discord. [News]. *Hastings Center Report.* 1998 Jan–Feb; 28(1): 7. BE57290.
     ethical review; government regulation; *human experimentation; *international aspects; investigators; regional ethics committees; *research ethics committees; standards; multicenter studies; Europe; Great Britain; National Health Service; United States

Ollila, Eeva; Hemminki, Elina. Does licensing of drugs in industrialized countries guarantee drug quality and safety for Third World countries? The case of Norplant licensing in Finland. *International Journal of Health Services.* 1997; 27(2): 309–328. 35 refs. BE56009.
     *contraception; *developing countries; drug industry; *drugs; *evaluation; *evaluation studies; females; government regulation; hormones; *human experimentation; information dissemination; *international aspects; patient care; patient education; *records; research design; research subjects; risks and benefits; *standards; *Finland; *Norplant; Sweden

Patel, Tara. Row over sterilisation divides India. [News]. *New Scientist.* 1997 Apr 5; 154(2076): 4. BE56188.
     developing countries; *drugs; *females; *human experimentation; international aspects; population control; public policy; risk; risks and benefits; *sterilization (sexual); *toxicity; *India; *quinacrine

Pfeffer, Naomi. Consumers' viewpoint. *In:* Close, Bryony; Combes, Robert; Hubbard, Anthony; Illingworth, John, eds. Volunteers in Research and Testing. Bristol, PA: Taylor and Francis; 1997: 23–31. 6 refs. 1 fn. ISBN 0-7484-0397-3. BE57027.
     *attitudes; coercion; communication; comprehension; disadvantaged; disclosure; *human experimentation; informed consent; motivation; nontherapeutic research; patient advocacy; patients; random selection; *research subjects; risks and benefits; scientific misconduct; uncertainty; *volunteers; *Consumers for Ethics in Research (CERES); *Great Britain

Phanuphak, Praphan; Vermund, Sten H. Ethical issues

for perinatal HIV trials in developing countries. [Editorial]. *Pediatric AIDS and HIV Infection.* 1996 Aug; 7(4): 236–238. 15 refs. BE57070.
     control groups; costs and benefits; *developing countries; drugs; ethical relativism; *HIV seropositivity; *human experimentation; *newborns; placebos; *pregnant women; preventive medicine; research design; therapeutic research; AZT

Phanuphak, Praphan. Ethical issues in studies in Thailand of the vertical transmission of HIV. *New England Journal of Medicine.* 1998 Mar 19; 338(12): 834–835. 5 refs. BE57707.
     AIDS; alternatives; control groups; *developing countries; *drugs; government financing; *HIV seropositivity; *human experimentation; international aspects; *newborns; *nontherapeutic research; *placebos; *pregnant women; *preventive medicine; private sector; *public policy; *research design; resource allocation; scientific misconduct; *therapeutic research; time factors; withholding treatment; *AZT; Centers for Disease Control and Prevention; National Institutes of Health; *Thailand; United States; Walter Reed Army Institute of Research

RAGE (Radiotherapy Action Group Exposure) National [Great Britain]. All treatment and trials must have informed consent. [Personal view]. *BMJ (British Medical Journal).* 1997 Apr 12; 314(7087): 1134–1135. BE55676.
     cancer; disclosure; *females; *human experimentation; *informed consent; *injuries; morbidity; patient participation; *patients; physicians; *political activity; *radiology; research ethics committees; risks and benefits; *scientific misconduct; trust; *Great Britain; *RAGE (Radiotherapy Action Group Exposure)

Robb, Merlin L.; Khambaroong, Chirasak; Nelson, Kenrad E., et al. Studies in Thailand of the vertical transmission of HIV. [Letters]. *New England Journal of Medicine.* 1998 Mar 19; 338(12): 843–844. 2 refs. BE57708.
     AIDS; *drugs; financial support; health care delivery; *HIV seropositivity; *human experimentation; informed consent; newborns; *nontherapeutic research; patient care; *pregnant women; *standards; *therapeutic research; time factors; *AZT; Chiang Mai University; Department of Defense; Johns Hopkins University; Ministry of Health (Thailand); National Institutes of Health; *Thailand; United States; Walter Reed Army Institute of Research

Rogers, Arthur. European drug industry concerned over proposed clinical-trial legislation. [News]. *Lancet.* 1997 Nov 29; 350(9091): 1609. BE57269.
     confidentiality; data banks; *drug industry; *drugs; ethical review; *government regulation; guidelines; *human experimentation; *international aspects; legislation; professional organizations; research ethics committees; *European Federation of Pharmaceutical Industries and Associations; *European Union; International Conference on Harmonisation; Japan; United States

Rolleston, Francis; Armour, Catherine; Stipich, Nina. Developing a Tri-Council code of conduct for research involving humans. *International Journal of Bioethics.* 1997 Mar–Jun; 8(1–2): 67–70. BE59097.
     accountability; biomedical research; consensus; ethical review; government regulation; *guidelines; *human experimentation; interdisciplinary communication; *regulation; research ethics committees; scientific misconduct; self regulation; *Canada; Medical Research Council of Canada; National Council on Bioethics in Human Research (Canada); Natural Sciences and Engineering Research Council (Canada); Social Sciences and Humanities Research Council (Canada); *Tri-Council Policy Statement on Ethical Conduct for Research Involving Humans

---

BE = bioethics accession number   fn. = footnotes   refs. = references

Sidley, Pat. AIDS drug scandal in South Africa continues. [News]. *BMJ (British Medical Journal)*. 1998 Mar 14; 316(7134): 800. BE57761.
administrators; *AIDS; conflict of interest; drug industry; *drugs; economics; ethical review; government financing; government regulation; *human experimentation; investigators; legal aspects; *politics; *scientific misconduct; *South Africa; *Virodene; Zuma, Nkosazana

Smith, Douglas. The limits of human studies. *In:* Close, Bryony; Combes, Robert; Hubbard, Anthony; Illingworth, John, eds. Volunteers in Research and Testing. Bristol, PA: Taylor and Francis; 1997: 135–143. ISBN 0-7484-0397-3. BE57038.
ethical review; government regulation; guidelines; health hazards; *human experimentation; *military personnel; nontherapeutic research; toxicity; volunteers; *Great Britain; *Institute of Naval Medicine (Great Britain)

Talbot, D.; Reynolds, D.J.M.; Stone, Peter G., et al. Local research ethics committees. [Letters and response]. *BMJ (British Medical Journal)*. 1997 Nov 29; 315(7120): 1464–1465. 10 refs. BE58222.
ethical review; guidelines; human experimentation; placebos; regional ethics committees; research design; *research ethics committees; medical audit; *multicenter studies; British Medical Association; *Great Britain

Tomossy, George F.; Weisstub, David N. The reform of adult guardianship laws: the case of non-therapeutic experimentation. *International Journal of Law and Psychiatry*. 1997 Winter; 20(1): 113–139. 123 fn. BE55533.
adults; advance directives; competence; dementia; disclosure; government regulation; guidelines; *human experimentation; *informed consent; investigators; *legal aspects; *legal guardians; *mentally disabled; *nontherapeutic research; research ethics committees; research subjects; risks and benefits; sterilization (sexual); *third party consent; vulnerable populations; *Canada; Re Eve

Varmus, Harold; Satcher, David. Ethical complexities of conducting research in developing countries. *New England Journal of Medicine*. 1997 Oct 2; 337(14): 1003–1005. 6 refs. BE55835.
AIDS; autonomy; beneficence; *control groups; *developing countries; *drugs; economics; ethical review; federal government; *HIV seropositivity; *human experimentation; international aspects; justice; *moral policy; *newborns; *placebos; *pregnant women; *preventive medicine; *public policy; *research design; risks and benefits; *therapeutic research; *AZT; Centers for Disease Control and Prevention; National Institutes of Health; *United States

Wadman, Meredith. Controversy flares over AIDS prevention trials in Third World. [News]. *Nature*. 1997 Oct 30; 389(6654): 894. BE56162.
*developing countries; *drugs; federal government; government financing; government regulation; *HIV seropositivity; *human experimentation; investigators; newborns; *placebos; *pregnant women; preventive medicine; *research design; therapeutic research; *AZT; Department of Health and Human Services; Johns Hopkins University; National Institutes of Health; Public Citizen; *United States

Watts, Jonathan. Japan taken to court over germ-warfare allegations. [News]. *Lancet*. 1998 Feb 28; 351(9103): 657. BE58264.
*biological warfare; *historical aspects; *human experimentation; international aspects; legal aspects; *scientific misconduct; war; China; *Japan; Twentieth Century; *World War II

Williams, Peter; Wallace, David. Unit 731: The Japanese Army's Secret of Secrets. London: Hodder and Stoughton; 1989. 366 p. 596 fn. ISBN 0-340-39463-3. BE57390.
*biological warfare; confidentiality; dehumanization; disclosure; federal government; *historical aspects; *human experimentation; international aspects; *investigators; killing; military personnel; *moral complicity; *prisoners; public policy; *scientific misconduct; technical expertise; torture; war; chemical warfare; Canada; China; France; Germany; Great Britain; Ishii, Shiro; *Japan; Korean War; Netherlands; Twentieth Century; *United States; USSR; *World War II

Wilmshurst, Peter. Scientific imperialism: if they won't benefit from the findings, poor people in the developing world shouldn't be used in research. [Editorial]. *BMJ (British Medical Journal)*. 1997 Mar 22; 314(7084): 840–841. 11 refs. BE58750.
advertising; AIDS; attitudes; *developing countries; drug industry; drugs; ethical review; financial support; HIV seropositivity; *human experimentation; institutional ethics; investigators; nontherapeutic research; patient care; research subjects; scientific misconduct; therapeutic research; toxicity; vulnerable populations

Wilson, Kerr. Volunteer studies using the Health and Safety Laboratory exposure chamber. *In:* Close, Bryony; Combes, Robert; Hubbard, Anthony; Illingworth, John, eds. Volunteers in Research and Testing. Bristol, PA: Taylor and Francis; 1997: 129–134. 5 refs. ISBN 0-7484-0397-3. BE57037.
animal experimentation; drugs; health hazards; *human experimentation; *nontherapeutic research; occupational exposure; research ethics committees; *toxicity; *volunteers; *Great Britain; *Health and Safety Executive (Great Britain)

Wise, Jacqui. New authority to monitor xenotransplantation experiments. [News]. *BMJ (British Medical Journal)*. 1997 Jan 25; 314(7076): 247. 1 ref. BE58703.
advisory committees; *animal organs; communicable diseases; *government regulation; *human experimentation; international aspects; *organ transplantation; *public policy; risk; self regulation; transgenic animals; transplant recipients; *swine; Advisory Group on the Ethics of Xenotransplantation (Great Britain); *Great Britain; United States; *Xenotransplantation Interim Regulatory Authority (Great Britain)

Zinn, Christopher. Australian orphans were used as guinea pigs. [News]. *BMJ (British Medical Journal)*. 1997 Jun 21; 314(7097): 1783. BE56129.
*children; historical aspects; *human experimentation; *immunization; *infants; institutionalized persons; research subjects; retrospective moral judgment; *scientific misconduct; vulnerable populations; *Australia; Commonwealth Serum Laboratories (Australia); Twentieth Century

Breast cancer: research without consent. [News]. *Journal of Medical Ethics*. 1997 Dec; 23(6): 372. BE57338.
*breast cancer; females; guidelines; *human experimentation; *informed consent; *patient advocacy; *Declaration of Helsinki; *Great Britain; Nuremberg Code; *UK Breast Cancer Coalition

LREC resigns unanimously [Basingstoke Local Research Ethics Committee]. [News]. *Bulletin of Medical Ethics*. 1997 May; No. 128: 3–6. BE55679.
administrators; dissent; ethical review; evaluation; interprofessional relations; *organization and administration; *professional competence; *regulation; *research ethics committees; standards; qualitative research; *Basingstoke Local Research Ethics Committee; England; *Great Britain;

BE = bioethics accession number   fn. = footnotes   refs. = references

National Health Service; *North and Mid Hampshire Health Authority

Pragmatism in codes of research ethics. [Editorial]. *Lancet.* 1998 Jan 24; 351(9098): 225. BE57817.
> codes of ethics; control groups; *developing countries; drugs; editorial policies; ethical relativism; guidelines; HIV seropositivity; *human experimentation; informed consent; *international aspects; *placebos; *research design; Lancet

Research without consent in South Africa. [News; title supplied]. *BMJ (British Medical Journal).* 1997 Jun 28; 314(7098): 1850. BE56128.
> *blacks; *human experimentation; *industry; informed consent; *occupational exposure; *occupational medicine; *scientific misconduct; *South Africa

HUMAN EXPERIMENTATION/INFORMED CONSENT

Agich, George J. Human experimentation and clinical consent. [Revised]. *In:* Monagle, John F.; Thomasma, David C., eds. Health Care Ethics: Critical Issues for the 21st Century. Gaithersburg, MD: Aspen Publishers; 1998: 228–238. 6 refs. 35 fn. ISBN 0-8342-0911-X. BE56284.
> competence; comprehension; disclosure; federal government; government regulation; *human experimentation; *informed consent; investigator subject relationship; legal aspects; nontherapeutic research; patients; physician patient relationship; research ethics committees; research subjects; risks and benefits; standards; therapeutic research; third party consent; investigational therapies; United States

Aller, Robert; Aller, Gregory. An institutional response to patient/family complaints. *In:* Shamoo, Adil E., ed. Ethics in Neurobiological Research with Human Subjects: The Baltimore Conference on Ethics. Amsterdam: Gordon and Breach; 1997: 155–172. 32 fn. This paper provides the viewpoints of a father and of his son, who was a research subject at the UCLA Clinical Research Center. ISBN 2-88449-161-9. BE57013.
> administrators; case studies; consent forms; *deception; *disclosure; family members; *human experimentation; iatrogenic disease; *informed consent; medical records; *mentally ill; patients; physician patient relationship; placebos; professional family relationship; *psychoactive drugs; *research design; research subjects; risks and benefits; *schizophrenia; *scientific misconduct; suicide; treatment outcome; universities; *withholding treatment; patient abandonment; *UCLA Neuropsychiatric Institute; United States; *University of California, Los Angeles

Alt–White, Anna C. Obtaining "informed" consent from the elderly. *Western Journal of Nursing Research.* 1995 Dec; 17(6): 700–705. 10 refs. 2 fn. BE55600.
> *aged; competence; comprehension; decision making; disabled; education; family members; *human experimentation; *informed consent; institutionalized persons; investigators; nursing research; recall; research subjects

American Association of Critical Care Nurses. Task Force on Ethics in Critical Care Research. Statement on ethics in critical care research. Part Two. *Focus on Critical Care.* 1985 Aug; 12(4): 58–63. 16 refs. BE56652.
> administrators; competence; *critically ill; disclosure; *guidelines; *human experimentation; *informed consent; investigators; *nurses; *organizational policies; patient care; professional organizations; research ethics committees; research subjects; *American Association of Critical Care Nurses; United States

Annas, George J.; Glantz, Leonard H. Informed consent to research on institutionalized mentally disabled persons: the dual problems of incapacity and voluntariness. *In:* Shamoo, Adil E., ed. Ethics in Neurobiological Research with Human Subjects: The Baltimore Conference on Ethics. Amsterdam: Gordon and Breach; 1997: 55–79. 46 fn. Appendices include the text of the Nuremberg Code and parts of the U.S. Department of Health, Education, and Welfare regulations proposed in 1978 on "protections pertaining to biomedical and behavioral research involving as subjects individuals institutionalized as mentally disabled." ISBN 2-88449-161-9. BE57009.
> behavior control; *coercion; *competence; comprehension; *decision making; federal government; government regulation; guidelines; hepatitis; *human experimentation; immunization; *informed consent; *institutionalized persons; involuntary commitment; judicial action; *legal aspects; *mentally disabled; *mentally ill; model legislation; nontherapeutic research; organ donation; patient advocacy; patient care; prisoners; psychoactive drugs; *regulation; research ethics committees; research subjects; scientific misconduct; state interest; sterilization (sexual); therapeutic research; *third party consent; treatment refusal; DHEW Guidelines; Nuremberg Code; *United States

Ault, Alicia. FDA may "pull the plug" on consent waiver. [News]. *Lancet.* 1997 Oct 11; 350(9084): 1084. BE57267.
> disclosure; *emergency care; federal government; *government regulation; hospitals; *human experimentation; *informed consent; public participation; research ethics committees; therapeutic research; *Food and Drug Administration; United States

Barker, E.M. Informed consent in medical research: the ethics committee's view. [Letter]. *BMJ (British Medical Journal).* 1998 Jan 31; 316(7128): 392–393. 3 refs. BE57800.
> committee membership; deception; developing countries; ethical review; HIV seropositivity; *human experimentation; *informed consent; intensive care units; investigators; misconduct; motivation; *research ethics committees; selection for treatment; *South Africa

Barnes, Patricia G. Beyond Nuremberg: fifty years later, the debate continues on informed consent. *ABA Journal: The Lawyer's Magazine.* 1997 Mar; 83: 24–27. BE58508.
> adults; competence; government regulation; *human experimentation; informed consent; institutionalized persons; *legal aspects; mental institutions; *mentally ill; minors; *nontherapeutic research; parental consent; psychoactive drugs; risk; state government; *third party consent; withholding treatment; New York; *T.D. v. New York State Office of Mental Health

Bartholome, William G. Ethical issues in pediatric research. *In:* Vanderpool, Harold Y., ed. The Ethics of Research Involving Human Subjects: Facing the 21st Century. Frederick, MD: University Publishing Group; 1996: 339–370. 61 fn. ISBN 1-55572-036-6. BE56993.
> advisory committees; age factors; *children; coercion; competence; comprehension; decision making; federal government; government regulation; growth disorders; guidelines; historical aspects; hormones; *human experimentation; *informed consent; moral policy; *nontherapeutic research; normality; parental consent; pediatrics; random selection; research ethics committees; research subjects; *risks and benefits; selection of subjects; *therapeutic research; McCormick, Richard; National Commission for the Protection of Human Subjects; Ramsey, Paul; United States

Baskin, Shari A.; Morris, Jane; Ahronheim, Judith C., et al. Barriers to obtaining consent in dementia research:

---

implications for surrogate decision–making. *Journal of the American Geriatrics Society.* 1998 Mar; 46(3): 287–290. 16 refs. BE56752.
    aged; comprehension; *decision making; *dementia; evaluation studies; *family members; health services research; hospitals; *human experimentation; institutionalized persons; legal guardians; minority groups; palliative care; single persons; terminally ill; *third party consent; vulnerable populations; absence of proxy; Mount Sinai Medical Center (New York City)

Benatar, David; Benatar, Solomon R. Informed consent and research. *BMJ (British Medical Journal).* 1998 Mar 28; 316(7136): 1008. 2 refs. BE57553.
    *AIDS serodiagnosis; *anonymous testing; biomedical research; confidentiality; epidemiology; *HIV seropositivity; *human experimentation; *informed consent; medical records; patients; research design; research subjects; South Africa

Berghmans, R.L.P. Advance directives for non–therapeutic dementia research: some ethical and policy considerations. *Journal of Medical Ethics.* 1998 Feb; 24(1): 32–37. 25 refs. BE57403.
    *advance directives; *competence; decision making; *dementia; *human experimentation; informed consent; moral policy; *nontherapeutic research; personhood; research subjects; selection of subjects; self concept; third party consent
This paper explores the use of advance directives in clinical dementia research. The focus is on advance consent to participation of demented patients in non–therapeutic research involving more than minimal risks and/or burdens. First, morally relevant differences between advance directives for treatment and care, and advance directives for dementia research are discussed. Then attention is paid to the philosophical issue of dementia and personal identity, and the implications for the moral authority of research advance directives. Thirdly, a number of practical shortcomings of advance directives for non–therapeutic dementia research are explored and attention is paid to the role of proxies. It is concluded that upon a closer look the initial attractiveness of advance directives for dementia research is lessened, and that it is doubtful whether these instruments can compensate for the lack of subject consent in case of non–therapeutic dementia research involving more than minimal risks and/or burdens for the incompetent demented subject.

Bhagwanjee, Satish; Muckart, David J.J.; Jeena, Prakash M., et al. Does HIV status influence the outcome of patients admitted to a surgical intensive care unit? A prospective double blind study. [Article, commentaries, and response]. *BMJ (British Medical Journal).* 1997 Apr 12; 314(7087): 1077–1084. 26 refs. BE55661.
    *AIDS serodiagnosis; anonymous testing; blacks; comparative studies; confidentiality; critically ill; developing countries; disadvantaged; disclosure; empirical research; *epidemiology; futility; *HIV seropositivity; hospitals; human experimentation; *informed consent; injuries; *intensive care units; justice; morbidity; mortality; patient admission; patient discharge; patients; research design; research ethics committees; *research subjects; resource allocation; scientific misconduct; *selection for treatment; surgery; *treatment outcome; prospective studies; *South Africa
OBJECTIVES: (a) To assess the impact of HIV status (HIV negative, HIV positive, AIDS) on the outcome of patients admitted to intensive care units for diseases unrelated to HIV; (b) to decide whether a positive test result for HIV should be a criterion for excluding

patients from intensive care for diseases unrelated to HIV. DESIGN: A prospective double blind study of all admissions over six months. HIV status was determined in all patients by enzyme linked immunosorbent assay (ELISA), immunofluorescence assay, western blotting, and flow cytometry. The ethics committee considered the clinical implications of the study important enough to waive patients' right to informed consent. Staff and patients were blinded to HIV results. On discharge patients could be advised of their HIV status if they wished. SETTING: A 16 bed surgical intensive care unit. SUBJECTS: All 267 men and 135 women admitted to the unit during the study period. INTERVENTIONS: None. MAIN OUTCOME MEASURES: APACHE II score (acute physiological, age, and chronic health evaluation), organ failure, septic shock, durations of intensive care unit and hospital stay, and intensive care unit and hospital mortality. RESULTS: No patient had AIDS. 52 patients were tested positive for HIV and 350 patients were tested negative. The two groups were similar in sex distribution but differed significantly in age, incidence of organ failure (37 (71%) v 171 (49%) patients), and incidence of septic shock (20 (38%) v 54 (15%)). After adjustment for age there were no differences in intensive care unit or hospital mortality or in the durations of stay in the intensive care unit or hospital. CONCLUSIONS: Morbidity was higher in HIV positive patients but there was no difference in mortality. In this patient population a positive HIV test result should not be a criterion for excluding a patient from intensive care.

Biros, Michelle H. Development of the multiorganizational document regarding emergency research consent. *Academic Emergency Medicine.* 1996 Feb; 3(2): 101–105. 15 refs. BE55707.
    consensus; critically ill; *decision making; *emergency care; federal government; government regulation; *human experimentation; *informed consent; interdisciplinary communication; investigators; models, theoretical; *organization and administration; *organizational policies; professional organizations; public policy; resuscitation; *consensus development conferences; American Heart Association; *Coalition Conference of Acute Resuscitation and Critical Care Researchers; Food and Drug Administration; National Institutes of Health; Office for Protection from Research Risks; Society for Academic Emergency Medicine; United States

Blenkinsop, Stanley. Whatever happened to plain English? The gobbledygook smokescreen that baffles research subjects. *In:* Close, Bryony; Combes, Robert; Hubbard, Anthony; Illingworth, John, eds. Volunteers in Research and Testing. Bristol, PA: Taylor and Francis; 1997: 89–98. 6 refs. 1 fn. ISBN 0–7484–0397–3. BE57033.
    *communication; comprehension; *consent forms; disclosure; drug industry; drugs; *human experimentation; informed consent; parental consent; *patient education; research subjects

Botkin, Jeffrey R.; McMahon, William M.; Smith, Ken R., et al. Privacy and confidentiality in the publication of pedigrees: a survey of investigators and biomedical journals. *JAMA.* 1998 Jun 10; 279(22): 1808–1812. 11 refs. BE58763.
    *attitudes; *confidentiality; *disclosure; *editorial policies; evaluation studies; *family members; *genetic information; *genetic research; genetic screening; guidelines; *informed consent; international aspects; *investigators; *knowledge, attitudes, practice; *privacy; *research subjects; survey; guideline adherence; medical illustration; *pedigree studies; publishing; International Committee of Medical Journal

---

BE = bioethics accession number   fn. = footnotes   refs. = references

Editors

CONTEXT: Pedigree diagrams efficiently communicate family information to genetics investigators; however, the publication of pedigrees poses a risk to the privacy and confidentiality of individuals depicted in the diagrams. Two sets of authoritative guidelines have been published to protect the privacy and confidentiality of subjects, but the influence of these guidelines on publication practices for pedigrees is unknown. OBJECTIVE: To determine the attitudes, practices, and experiences of investigators and journals with respect to privacy and confidentiality concerns in the publication of pedigrees. DESIGN: Investigators who have published pedigrees and editors of 26 biomedical journals were surveyed. Journals were reviewed for content in their "information for authors" sections and for documentation of informed consent in articles containing pedigrees. OUTCOME MEASURES: Practices regarding confidentiality and privacy reported by investigators and editors. RESULTS: Of 226 surveys sent to investigators, 177 were returned (78% response rate). Sixty-one investigators (36%) stated that family members were not informed that their pedigree would be published; 131 (78%) do not obtain informed consent specifically for pedigree publication and only 12 (28%) of the 43 who obtained consent obtained consent from all family members depicted. Thirty-two individuals (19%) reported having altered published pedigrees and 14 (45%) of 31 who had altered pedigrees stated that alterations were not disclosed to journals. Of the 14 journals that responded (54% response rate), only 3 reported written policies for managing potentially identifying information. Two journals reported having asked authors to alter pedigrees and 3 stated they had permitted alterations. A review of 5 genetics journals over a 2–year period revealed no documentation of consent for pedigree publication. CONCLUSIONS: Current practices in the publication of pedigrees do not conform with established recommendations and risk the privacy and confidentiality of subjects, often without informed consent. Attempts to address this problem through the alteration of data are being used, although this practice impairs the integrity of scientific communication.

Brody, Baruch A. Research on the vulnerable sick. *In:* Kahn, Jeffrey P.; Mastroianni, Anna C.; Sugarman, Jeremy, eds. Beyond Consent: Seeking Justice in Research. New York, NY: Oxford University Press; 1998: 32–46. 24 fn. ISBN 0–19–511353–5. BE58842.
   autonomy; *cancer; *critically ill; disclosure; *emergency care; federal government; government regulation; *HIV seropositivity; *human experimentation; *informed consent; investigational drugs; *justice; *nontherapeutic research; *patients; placebos; research design; research subjects; risks and benefits; terminally ill; *therapeutic research; third party consent; time factors; trends; values; vulnerable populations; deferred consent; Food and Drug Administration; United States

Clayton, Ellen Wright. Informed consent and genetic research. *In:* Rothstein, Mark A., ed. Genetic Secrets: Protecting Privacy and Confidentiality in the Genetic Era. New Haven, CT: Yale University Press; 1997: 126–136. 13 fn. ISBN 0–300–07251–1. BE58679.
   anonymous testing; confidentiality; disclosure; DNA data banks; family members; genetic information; *genetic research; genetic screening; *informed consent; insurance; mass screening; newborns; parental consent; records; *research subjects; risks and benefits; social discrimination; stigmatization; biological specimen banks; pedigree studies

Clayton, Ellen Wright. Prospective uses of DNA samples for research. *In:* Knoppers, Bartha Maria, ed. Human DNA: Law and Policy: International and Comparative Perspectives. Proceedings of the First International Conference on DNA Sampling and Human Genetic Research: Ethical, Legal, and Policy Aspects, held in Montreal, Canada, 6–8 Sep 1996. Boston, MA: Kluwer Law International; 1997: 291–301. 34 fn. ISBN 90–411–0361–9. BE58186.
   advisory committees; comparative studies; confidentiality; consent forms; decision making; disclosure; *DNA data banks; federal government; genetic information; *genetic materials; *genetic research; genetic screening; *government regulation; guidelines; *informed consent; *international aspects; model legislation; professional organizations; *public policy; research subjects; risk; tissue donation; *biological specimen banks; *Canada; Genetic Privacy Act; *Great Britain; Nuffield Council on Bioethics; *United States

Cox, Karen; Avis, Mark. Ethical and practical problems of early anti–cancer drug trials: a review of the literature. *European Journal of Cancer Care.* 1996 Jun; 5(2): 90–95. 55 refs. BE56301.
   attitudes; *cancer; comprehension; decision making; disclosure; drugs; empirical research; *human experimentation; *informed consent; motivation; *nontherapeutic research; nurses; patient participation; patients; research subjects; risk; risks and benefits; selection of subjects; terminally ill; qualitative research

Daugherty, C.K.; Ratain, M.J.; Siegler, M. Pushing the envelope: informed consent in phase I trials. [Editorial]. *Annals of Oncology.* 1995 Apr; 6(4): 321–323. 22 refs. BE55714.
   *cancer; *communication; *comprehension; consent forms; cultural pluralism; *disclosure; empirical research; *human experimentation; *informed consent; *investigational drugs; investigators; *nontherapeutic research; patients; physician patient relationship; physicians; research design; research subjects; *risks and benefits; terminally ill; *toxicity

Daugherty, Christopher; Ratain, Mark J.; Grochowski, Eugene, et al. Perceptions of cancer patients and their physicians involved in phase I trials. *Journal of Clinical Oncology.* 1995 May; 13(5): 1062–1072. 34 refs. Published erratum appears in *Journal of Clinical Oncology,* 1995 Sep; 13(9): 2476. BE56862.
   altruism; *attitudes; autonomy; *cancer; *comprehension; *decision making; disclosure; drugs; *human experimentation; *informed consent; *motivation; *nontherapeutic research; *patients; *physicians; research subjects; risks and benefits; survey; toxicity; trust; questionnaires; University of Chicago Medical Center

Davis, Anne J.; Aroskar, Mila A.; Liaschenko, Joan, et al. Ethical principles of informed consent. *In: their* Ethical Dilemmas and Nursing Practice. Fourth Edition. Stamford, CT: Appleton and Lange; 1997: 105–134. 144 fn. ISBN 0–8385–2283–1. BE58595.
   autonomy; behavioral research; beneficence; case studies; coercion; comprehension; disclosure; federal government; government regulation; guidelines; *human experimentation; *informed consent; investigator subject relationship; nurses; nursing research; patient care; research subjects; risks and benefits; scientific misconduct; trust; vulnerable populations; United States

Destro, Robert A. Government oversight. *In:* Shamoo, Adil E., ed. Ethics in Neurobiological Research with Human Subjects: The Baltimore Conference on Ethics. Amsterdam: Gordon and Breach; 1997: 81–99. 90 fn. ISBN 2–88449–161–9. BE57010.
   behavioral research; coercion; *competence; comprehension; conflict of interest; *disclosure; federal government;

BE = bioethics accession number   fn. = footnotes   refs. = references

*government regulation; *human experimentation; *informed consent; investigator subject relationship; investigators; *legal aspects; mentally disabled; minors; nontherapeutic research; professional ethics; research ethics committees; research subjects; state government; therapeutic research; *third party consent; *vulnerable populations; *United States

Doyal, Len. Informed consent -- a response to recent correspondence. *BMJ (British Medical Journal).* 1998 Mar 28; 316(7136): 1000–1001. 9 refs. BE57585.
   autonomy; biomedical research; epidemiology; *human experimentation; *informed consent; patients; research subjects; risks and benefits

Dresser, Rebecca; Whitehouse, Peter. Emergency research and research involving subjects with cognitive impairment: ethical connections and contrasts. [Editorial]. *Journal of the American Geriatrics Society.* 1997 Apr; 45(4): 521–523. 7 refs. BE57113.
   advance directives; *chronically ill; comparative studies; *competence; *critically ill; *decision making; *dementia; disclosure; *emergency care; family members; federal government; government regulation; *human experimentation; *informed consent; investigators; legal aspects; legal guardians; *mentally disabled; nontherapeutic research; patient participation; public participation; research ethics committees; *risks and benefits; therapeutic research; *third party consent; United States

Goodare, Heather. Studies that do not have informed consent from participants should not be published. *BMJ (British Medical Journal).* 1998 Mar 28; 316(7136): 1004–1005. 18 refs. BE57579.
   biomedical research; cancer; *editorial policies; epidemiology; guidelines; *human experimentation; *informed consent; minors; patients; research subjects; tissue donation; BMJ (British Medical Journal); Declaration of Helsinki

Haddad, Amy. Ethics in action: a cardiac patient has just signed a consent form agreeing to participate in a clinical trial testing a new drug for congestive heart failure -- what would you do? *RN.* 1996 Mar; 59(3): 17–19. 1 ref. BE56867.
   case studies; *comprehension; consent forms; heart diseases; *human experimentation; *informed consent; *investigational drugs; *nurse's role; patient advocacy; random selection

Haimowitz, Stephan; Delano, Susan J.; Oldham, John M. Uninformed decisionmaking: the case of surrogate research consent. *Hastings Center Report.* 1997 Nov–Dec; 27(6): 9–16. 26 fn. BE57854.
   adults; biomedical research; *competence; constitutional law; *decision making; dementia; family members; federal government; *government regulation; *human experimentation; *judicial action; *legal aspects; *mentally ill; minors; *nontherapeutic research; parental consent; patient advocacy; psychoactive drugs; research ethics committees; *risks and benefits; social impact; state government; suicide; therapeutic research; *third party consent; Department of Health and Human Services; Food and Drug Administration; *New York; Office of Mental Health (NY); *T.D. v. New York State Office of Mental Health; United States
A New York court recently struck down state Office of Mental Health regulations governing research involving subjects with impaired decisionmaking capacity. The court held that neither incapacitated adults nor minors could participate in any research protocol that contained a nontherapeutic element, irrespective of possible benefits to the subject or the importance of the knowledge to be gained. Although the decision rested

on a technical point of law and dealt only with psychiatric research, the court's holding has significantly broader implications.

Hansson, Mats O. Balancing the quality of consent. *Journal of Medical Ethics.* 1998 Jun; 24(3): 182–187. 7 fn. BE59114.
   autonomy; biomedical research; confidentiality; disclosure; *epidemiology; genetic materials; genetic research; human experimentation; *informed consent; *models, theoretical; patient care; presumed consent; research subjects; *standards; time factors; values
The rule that one must obtain informed consent is well established in medical ethics and an intrinsic part of clinical practice and of research in biomedicine. However, there is a tendency that the rule today is being applied too rigidly and with too little sensitivity to the values that are at stake in connection with different kinds of research protocols. It is here argued that the quality of consent needs to be balanced against variables such as degree of confidentiality and importance of values at stake, in order to be ethically acceptable. Appropriate information and consent procedures should be adjusted accordingly. Three levels are suggested, ranging from extensively informed consent with both written and oral information, through informed refusal with only a limited amount of information given to, at the other end of the scale, just making relevant information available.

Hirtle, Marie. Genetic screening and research revisited. *In:* Knoppers, Bartha Maria, ed. Human DNA: Law and Policy: International and Comparative Perspectives. Proceedings of the First International Conference on DNA Sampling and Human Genetic Research: Ethical, Legal, and Policy Aspects, held in Montreal, Canada, 6–8 Sep 1996. Boston, MA: Kluwer Law International; 1997: 333–340. 7 fn. ISBN 90–411–0361–9. BE58190.
   cancer; *carriers; cystic fibrosis; DNA data banks; federal government; genetic materials; *genetic research; *genetic screening; *informed consent; legal aspects; *newborns; *parental consent; prenatal diagnosis; presumed consent; thalassemia; biological specimen banks; Europe; National Center for Human Genome Research; United States

Hochhauser, Mark. Some overlooked aspects of consent form readability. *IRB: A Review of Human Subjects Research.* 1997 Sep–Oct; 19(5): 5–9. 23 refs. BE57138.
   *comprehension; *computers; *consent forms; education; *evaluation; human experimentation; informed consent; *research subjects

Hooker, Ellen Z. Can your research subjects read your study's informed consent form? *SCI Nursing.* 1995 Jun; 12(2): 57–58. 6 refs. BE55867.
   *comprehension; *consent forms; *human experimentation; *informed consent; nursing research; *research subjects; surgery; Europe; United States

IJesselmuiden, Carel B.; Faden, Ruth R. Medical research and the principle of respect for persons in non–Western cultures. *In:* Vanderpool, Harold Y., ed. The Ethics of Research Involving Human Subjects: Facing the 21st Century. Frederick, MD: University Publishing Group; 1996: 281–301. 48 fn. ISBN 1–55572–036–6. BE56991.
   AIDS; anthropology; *autonomy; beneficence; competence; *cultural pluralism; *developing countries; *ethical relativism; guidelines; *human experimentation; *informed consent; *international aspects; investigators; *moral policy; research subjects; third party consent; values; *non–Western World; Africa

---

BE = bioethics accession number   fn. = footnotes   refs. = references

Jayaraman, K.S. Inquiry looks into Indian cancer deaths. [News]. *Nature*. 1997 Dec 18–25; 390(6661): 653. BE57309.
> attitudes; *cancer; *disadvantaged; disclosure; *females; historical aspects; *human experimentation; *informed consent; investigators; retrospective moral judgment; *scientific misconduct; *withholding treatment; *India; Indian Council of Medical Research

Juengst, Eric T. Groups as gatekeepers to genomic research: conceptually confusing, morally hazardous, and practically useless. *Kennedy Institute of Ethics Journal*. 1998 June; 8(2): 183–200. 31 refs. BE58376.
> autonomy; *cultural pluralism; *decision making; epidemiology; eugenics; *genetic diversity; *genetic research; genetic screening; genome mapping; *informed consent; international aspects; minority groups; research design; research subjects; self concept; social discrimination; *vulnerable populations; *community consent; *population genetics; Human Genome Diversity Project

Some argue that human groups have a stake in the outcome of population–genomics research and that the decision to participate in such research should therefore be subject to group permission. It is not possible, however, to obtain prior group permission, because the actual human groups under study, human demes, are unidentifiable before research begins. Moreover, they lack moral standing. If identifiable social groups with moral standing are used as proxies for demes, group approval could be sought, but at the expense of unfairly exposing these surrogates to risks from which prior group approval is powerless to protect them. Unless population genomics can proceed without targeting socially defined groups, or can find other ways of protecting them, it may fall to individuals to protect the interests of the groups they care about, and to scientists to warn their subjects of the need to do so.

Kääriäinen, Helena. Genetic studies in populations. *In:* Knoppers, Bartha Maria, ed. Human DNA: Law and Policy: International and Comparative Perspectives. Proceedings of the First International Conference on DNA Sampling and Human Genetic Research: Ethical, Legal, and Policy Aspects, held in Montreal, Canada, 6–8 Sep 1996. Boston, MA: Kluwer Law International; 1997: 177–188. 9 fn. ISBN 90-411-0361-9. BE58177.
> cancer; DNA data banks; family members; *genetic predisposition; *genetic research; *genetic screening; human experimentation; *informed consent; mass screening; patients; asthma; biological specimen banks; *population genetics; *Finland

Keay, Timothy J. Approximating ethical research content. *In:* Shamoo, Adil E., ed. Ethics in Neurobiological Research with Human Subjects: The Baltimore Conference on Ethics. Amsterdam: Gordon and Breach; 1997: 149–153. 11 fn. ISBN 2-88449-161-9. BE57012.
> competence; conflict of interest; *human experimentation; *informed consent; injuries; investigator subject relationship; investigators; *mentally ill; physician patient relationship; psychoactive drugs; research design; research ethics committees; research subjects; risks and benefits; *schizophrenia; suicide; withholding treatment; United States

La Puma, John. Physicians' conflicts of interest in post–marketing research: what the public should know, and why industry should tell them. *In:* Vanderpool, Harold Y., ed. The Ethics of Research Involving Human Subjects: Facing the 21st Century. Frederick, MD: University Publishing Group; 1996: 203–219. 47 fn. ISBN 1-55572-036-6. BE56988.
> attitudes; *conflict of interest; disclosure; *drug industry; *drugs; ethical review; *financial support; *human experimentation; *informed consent; *investigators; *patients; physician patient relationship; *physicians; *remuneration; research ethics committees; research subjects; risks and benefits; *therapeutic research; *postmarketing research

Leikin, Sanford L. Beyond proforma consent for childhood cancer research. *Journal of Clinical Oncology*. 1985 Mar; 3(3): 420–428. 32 refs. BE57828.
> *cancer; comprehension; conflict of interest; disclosure; federal government; government regulation; *human experimentation; *informed consent; investigator subject relationship; *minors; *parental consent; *pediatrics; physician patient relationship; professional family relationship; psychological stress; random selection; standards; Department of Health and Human Services; United States

Lemaire, F.; Blanch, L.; Cohen, S.L.; European Society of Intensive Care Medicine. Working Group on Ethics. Informed consent for research purposes in intensive care patients in Europe -- part I: an official statement of the European Society of Intensive Care Medicine. *Intensive Care Medicine*. 1997 Mar; 23(3): 338–341. BE57653.
> competence; *critically ill; disclosure; *emergency care; family members; guidelines; *human experimentation; informed consent; *intensive care units; international aspects; legal guardians; *organizational policies; patients; physicians; *presumed consent; professional organizations; research subjects; *therapeutic research; *third party consent; *deferred consent; Council of Europe; *Europe; *European Society of Intensive Care Medicine; United States

Lemaire, F.; Blanch, L.; Cohen, S.L.; European Society of Intensive Care Medicine. Working Group on Ethics. Informed consent for research purposes in intensive care patients in Europe -- part II: an official statement of the European Society of Intensive Care Medicine. *Intensive Care Medicine*. 1997 Apr; 23(4): 435–439. 8 refs. BE57654.
> competence; *critically ill; *decision making; *emergency care; family members; government regulation; hospitals; *human experimentation; *informed consent; institutional policies; *intensive care units; *international aspects; investigators; *legal aspects; legal guardians; nontherapeutic research; patients; physicians; public policy; research ethics committees; research subjects; survey; therapeutic research; *third party consent; deferred consent; questionnaires; Austria; Belgium; Denmark; *Europe; *European Society of Intensive Care Medicine; Finland; France; Germany; Great Britain; Greece; Israel; Italy; Netherlands; Norway; Portugal; Spain; Sweden; Switzerland

Levine, Robert J. Adolescents as research subjects without permission of their parents or guardians: ethical considerations. *Journal of Adolescent Health*. 1995 Nov; 17(5): 287–297. 23 refs. BE55916.
> *adolescents; autonomy; behavioral research; beneficence; children; competence; epidemiology; federal government; government regulation; *guidelines; *human experimentation; *informed consent; investigational drugs; justice; nontherapeutic research; parental consent; paternalism; public participation; *public policy; random selection; regulation; research design; research subjects; risk; *risks and benefits; therapeutic research; Department of Health and Human Services; National Commission for the Protection of Human Subjects; United States

Lindley, Richard I. Thrombolytic treatment for acute ischaemic stroke: consent can be ethical. *BMJ (British Medical Journal)*. 1998 Mar 28; 316(7136): 1005–1007. 13 refs. BE57556.

BE = bioethics accession number   fn. = footnotes   refs. = references

attitudes; competence; consent forms; drugs; guidelines; *human experimentation; *informed consent; patients; *random selection; research design; research subjects; *risks and benefits; *therapeutic research; *cerebrovascular disorders; *thrombolytic therapy

Maloney, Dennis M. Federal agency's final rule says informed consent forms must be dated. [News]. *Human Research Report.* 1996 Dec; 11(12): 1-2. BE55627.
   *consent forms; federal government; *government regulation; *human experimentation; *informed consent; research ethics committees; research subjects; *time factors; *Food and Drug Administration; *United States

Marshall, Eliot. NIH examines standards for consent. [News]. *Science.* 1998 Jun 12; 280(5370): 1688. BE58271.
   bioethics; competence; conflict of interest; ethical review; evaluation; federal government; financial support; *government regulation; guidelines; *human experimentation; *informed consent; mentally ill; research design; *research ethics committees; research subjects; schizophrenia; *standards; withholding treatment; National Institute of Mental Health; *National Institutes of Health; *United States

Marwick, Charles. Assessment of exception to informed consent. [News]. *JAMA.* 1997 Nov 5; 278(17): 1392-1393. BE56166.
   community services; disclosure; *emergency care; evaluation; federal government; *government regulation; *human experimentation; information dissemination; *informed consent; mass media; minority groups; public participation; research ethics committees; third party consent; *Food and Drug Administration; United States

Marwick, Charles. Bioethics Commission examines informed consent from subjects who are 'decisionally incapable'. [News]. *JAMA.* 1997 Aug 27; 278(8): 618-619. BE56101.
   advisory committees; *competence; comprehension; disclosure; *human experimentation; *informed consent; *mentally disabled; psychoactive drugs; public policy; random selection; research design; research subjects; schizophrenia; standards; withholding treatment; National Bioethics Advisory Commission; United States

Mason, Su; Brown, Julia; Levene, Malcolm. What is this thing called "randomise"? [Editorial]. *Lancet.* 1997 Nov 15; 350(9089): 1416. 3 refs. BE57162.
   attitudes; *comprehension; control groups; critically ill; disclosure; empirical research; *human experimentation; informed consent; *newborns; *parental consent; parents; psychological stress; *random selection; research design; research subjects; selection of subjects; *therapeutic research; extracorporeal membrane oxygenation; qualitative research; Europe; European Union; Great Britain

Milner, Claire Alida. Gulf war guinea pigs: is informed consent optional during war? [Comment]. *Journal of Contemporary Health Law and Policy.* 1996 Fall; 13(1): 199-232. 249 fn. BE55791.
   *biological warfare; codes of ethics; federal government; *government regulation; health hazards; historical aspects; *human experimentation; iatrogenic disease; immunization; *informed consent; *investigational drugs; *legal aspects; legal liability; *military personnel; nontherapeutic research; occupational exposure; politics; *preventive medicine; psychoactive drugs; public policy; radiation; scientific misconduct; Supreme Court decisions; therapeutic research; toxicity; *war; *chemical warfare; Central Intelligence Agency; *Cold War; Declaration of Helsinki; Department of Defense; Federal Policy (Common Rule) for the Protection of Human Subjects 1991; *Food and Drug Administration; National Institutes of Health; Nuremberg Code; *Persian Gulf War; Twentieth Century; *United States

Moreno, Jonathan D.; Hurt, Valerie. How the Atomic Energy Commission discovered "informed consent." *In:* DeVries, Raymond; Subedi, Janardan, eds. Bioethics and Society: Constructing the Ethical Enterprise. Upper Saddle River, NJ: Prentice Hall; 1998: 78-93. 36 refs. 12 fn. ISBN 0-13-531252-3. BE58731.
   administrators; consent forms; *federal government; government regulation; *historical aspects; *human experimentation; *informed consent; interprofessional relations; investigators; nontherapeutic research; *public policy; *radiation; retrospective moral judgment; scientific misconduct; *standards; therapeutic research; volunteers; *Atomic Energy Commission; Cold War; *Twentieth Century; United States; Wilson, Carroll

Mudur, Ganapati. Indian study of women with cervical lesions called unethical. [News]. *BMJ (British Medical Journal).* 1997 Apr 12; 314(7087): 1065. BE56063.
   attitudes; *cancer; developing countries; *disadvantaged; disclosure; *females; historical aspects; *human experimentation; *informed consent; investigators; retrospective moral judgment; *scientific misconduct; withholding treatment; *India; Institute of Cytology and Preventive Oncology (New Delhi)

Nylenna, Magne. Details of patients' consent in studies should be reported. [Letter]. *BMJ (British Medical Journal).* 1997 Apr 12; 314(7087): 1127-1128. 4 refs. BE55918.
   aged; *editorial policies; ethical review; *human experimentation; *informed consent; records; research ethics committees

Olde Rikkert, Marcel G.M.; van den Bercken, John H.L.; ten Have, Henk A.M.J., et al. Experienced consent in geriatrics research: a new method to optimize the capacity to consent in frail elderly subjects. *Journal of Medical Ethics.* 1997 Oct; 23(5): 271-276. 24 refs. Appendix presents ten "multiple-choice questions asked of geriatric patients to assess their comprehension of relevant research information in a research project." BE57107.
   *aged; *competence; comprehension; dementia; depressive disorder; evaluation studies; *human experimentation; *informed consent; methods; nontherapeutic research; normality; research subjects; risks and benefits; time factors; Netherlands
   OBJECTIVES: Cognitive and sensory difficulties frequently jeopardize informed consent of frail elderly patients. This study is the first to test whether preliminary research experience could enhance geriatric patients' capacity to consent. DESIGN/SETTING: A step-wise consent procedure was introduced in a study on fluid balance in geriatric patients. Eligible patients providing verbal consent participated in a try-out of a week, during which bioelectrical impedance and weight measurements were performed daily. Afterwards, written informed consent was requested. Comprehension, risk and inconvenience scores (ranges: 0-10) were obtained before and after the try-out by asking ten questions about the study's essentials and by asking for a risk and inconvenience assessment on a ten-points rating scale. SUBJECTS AND RESULTS: Seventy of the 78 eligible subjects started the try-out and 53 (68%) provided written consent. The comprehension score increased from 5.0 (+/- 2.3) to 7.0 (+/- 1.9) following the try-out (P less than 0.001). The number of subjects capable of weighing risks and inconveniences increased from 32 to 48 (P less than 0.001). CONCLUSIONS: Research experience improved the capacity to consent, still enabling an acceptable participation rate. Therefore, experienced consent seems

---

BE = bioethics accession number   fn. = footnotes   refs. = references

a promising tool to optimize informed consent in frail elderly subjects.

Olson, Carin M.; Jobe, Kathleen A.; Rennie, Drummond, et al. Reporting institutional review board approval and patient consent. [Letter and response]. *JAMA.* 1997 Aug 13; 278(6): 477. 8 refs. BE55919.
*editorial policies; *ethical review; *human experimentation; *informed consent; records; *research ethics committees; BMJ (British Medical Journal)

Ondrusek, Nancy; Abramovitch, Rona; Pencharz, Paul, et al. Empirical examination of the ability of children to consent to clinical research. *Journal of Medical Ethics.* 1998 Jun; 24(3): 158–165. 6 refs. BE59112.
*adolescents; age factors; attitudes; blood specimen collection; *children; *competence; *comprehension; consent forms; evaluation studies; *informed consent; motivation; *nontherapeutic research; nutrition; research subjects; risks and benefits; questionnaires; Canada
This study examined the quality of children's assent to a clinical trial. In subjects younger than 9 years of age, understanding of most aspects of the study was found to be poor to non-existent. Understanding of procedures was poor in almost all subjects. In addition, voluntariness may have been compromised in many subjects by their belief that failure to complete the study would displease others. If the fact that a child's assent has been obtained is used to justify the exposure of that child to the potential harm of a non-therapeutic blood sample, the assent must be meaningful. In the nutrition study observed here, the quality of the assent of children younger than 9 years of age was very poor. The assent therefore did not provide a valid justification for requesting a blood sample from these children. This study indicates that most children younger than 9 years of age cannot be expected to consent or assent to clinical research in a meaningful way. The current age of 7 years for initiating assent (in addition to parental consent) is possibly not appropriate and should be reconsidered.

Ozar, David T. An alternative rationale for informed consent by human subjects. *American Psychologist.* 1983 Feb; 38(2): 230–232. BE57229.
decision making; *human experimentation; *informed consent; investigator subject relationship; trust; uncertainty

Philipson, Sandra J.; Doyle, Mary Anne; Gabram, Sheryl G.A., et al. Informed consent for research: a study to evaluate readability and processability to effect change. *Journal of Investigative Medicine.* 1995 Oct; 43(5): 459–467. 23 refs. BE55577.
*comprehension; *consent forms; disadvantaged; *evaluation; evaluation studies; hospitals; *human experimentation; informed consent; patients; research ethics committees; research subjects; socioeconomic factors; Connecticut; Hartford Hospital (CT)

Phillips, Jennifer M. Reducing postmortem examination refusal by families of research subjects. *IRB: A Review of Human Subjects Research.* 1997 Sep–Oct; 19(5): 10–11. BE57139.
*advance directives; *autopsies; *consent forms; death; family members; patients; *research subjects; *third party consent

Pierro, Agostino; Spitz, Lewis. Informed consent in clinical research: the crisis in paediatrics. [Letter]. *Lancet.* 1997 Jun 7; 349(9066): 1703. 5 refs. BE56880.
*children; critically ill; *dissent; *human experimentation; motivation; *nontherapeutic research; *parental consent; *parents; pediatrics; risks and benefits; trends; Ormond

Street Hospital for Children (London)

Power, Lisa. Trial subjects must be fully involved in design and approval of trials. *BMJ (British Medical Journal).* 1998 Mar 28; 316(7136): 1003–1004. BE57580.
*editorial policies; *human experimentation; *informed consent; patient participation; patients; research design; research subjects; *BMJ (British Medical Journal); Great Britain

Purtilo, Ruth; Sonnabend, Joseph; Purtilo, David T. Confidentiality, informed consent and untoward social consequences in research on a "new killer disease" (AIDS). *Clinical Research.* 1983 Oct; 31(4): 462–472. 31 refs. BE57233.
*AIDS; communication; *confidentiality; *epidemiology; *homosexuals; *informed consent; investigator subject relationship; investigators; public participation; research design; research subjects; *stigmatization; trust; *life style; United States

RAGE (Radiotherapy Action Group Exposure) National [Great Britain]. All treatment and trials must have informed consent. [Personal view]. *BMJ (British Medical Journal).* 1997 Apr 12; 314(7087): 1134–1135. BE55676.
cancer; disclosure; *females; *human experimentation; *informed consent; *injuries; morbidity; patient participation; *patients; physicians; *political activity; *radiology; research ethics committees; risks and benefits; *scientific misconduct; trust; *Great Britain; *RAGE (Radiotherapy Action Group Exposure)

Senn, Stephen; Ramsay, Lawrence E. Are placebo run ins justified? [Article and commentary]. *BMJ (British Medical Journal).* 1997 Apr 19; 314(7088): 1191–1193. 18 refs. BE56772.
*deception; disclosure; drugs; *human experimentation; *informed consent; patients; physicians; *placebos; random selection; *research design; research subjects

Speck, Peter. Consideration of consent in clinical research. *Palliative Medicine.* 1996 Apr; 10(2): 163–164. 2 refs. BE55892.
autonomy; cancer; competence; control groups; decision making; disclosure; *human experimentation; *informed consent; palliative care; physician patient relationship; placebos; random selection; research subjects; risks and benefits; selection of subjects; terminally ill; third party consent; uncertainty; Great Britain

Strauss, Evelyn. The tissue issue: losing oneself to science? *Science News.* 1997 Sep 20; 152(12): 190–191. BE56635.
*biomedical research; cadavers; confidentiality; consent forms; federal government; genetic research; government financing; government regulation; human experimentation; *informed consent; property rights; research ethics committees; time factors; *tissue banks; *tissue donation; United States

Tindall, Brett; Forde, Sally; Ross, Michael W., et al. Effects of two formats of informed consent on knowledge amongst persons with advanced HIV disease in a clinical trial of didanosine. *Patient Education and Counseling.* 1994 Dec; 24(3): 261–266. 14 refs. BE55776.
*AIDS; *communication; comparative studies; *comprehension; *consent forms; decision making; *drugs; evaluation; homosexuals; human experimentation; *informed consent; *knowledge, attitudes, practice; males; *methods; patient care; *patient education; *patients; physicians; recall; *research subjects; survey; *therapeutic research; Australia; DDI

Tobias, J.S. Changing the BMJ's position on informed

consent would be counterproductive. *BMJ (British Medical Journal)*. 1998 Mar 28; 316(7136): 1001–1002. 11 refs. BE57582.
   competence; *editorial policies; *human experimentation; *informed consent; paternalism; patient advocacy; patients; research subjects; *BMJ (British Medical Journal); Great Britain

Tomossy, George F.; Weisstub, David N. The reform of adult guardianship laws: the case of non–therapeutic experimentation. *International Journal of Law and Psychiatry*. 1997 Winter; 20(1): 113–139. 123 fn. BE55533.
   adults; advance directives; competence; dementia; disclosure; government regulation; guidelines; *human experimentation; *informed consent; investigators; *legal aspects; *legal guardians; *mentally disabled; *nontherapeutic research; research ethics committees; research subjects; risks and benefits; sterilization (sexual); *third party consent; vulnerable populations; *Canada; Re Eve

U.S. Congress. House. Committee on Government Reform and Oversight. Subcommittee on Human Resources. Oversight of NIH and FDA: Bioethics and the Adequacy of Informed Consent. Hearing, 8 May 1997. Washington, DC: U.S. Government Printing Office; 1997. Serial No. 105–49. ISBN 0–16–055827–1. BE58891.
   *advisory committees; bioethics; children; cloning; control groups; developing countries; disclosure; drugs; emergency care; *ethical review; evaluation; federal government; genetic research; government financing; *government regulation; hepatitis; HIV seropositivity; *human experimentation; immunization; *informed consent; international aspects; mentally ill; military personnel; parental consent; placebos; pregnant women; public policy; research design; research ethics committees; research subjects; scientific misconduct; *vulnerable populations; war; Africa; AZT; Centers for Disease Control and Prevention; Department of Defense; Food and Drug Administration; *National Bioethics Advisory Commission; National Institutes of Health; *United States

Veatch, Robert M. From Nuremberg through the 1990s: the priority of autonomy. *In:* Vanderpool, Harold Y., ed. The Ethics of Research Involving Human Subjects: Facing the 21st Century. Frederick, MD: University Publishing Group; 1996: 45–58. 14 fn. ISBN 1–55572–036–6. BE56981.
   advisory committees; *autonomy; beneficence; codes of ethics; disclosure; ethical review; freedom; guidelines; *human experimentation; *informed consent; investigational drugs; investigators; justice; moral obligations; public policy; research ethics committees; research subjects; rights; risks and benefits; therapeutic research; utilitarianism; investigational therapies; Belmont Report; Ethics Advisory Board; National Commission for the Protection of Human Subjects; Nuremberg Code; United States

Verheggen, Frank W.S.M.; Jonkers, Ruud; Kok, Gerjo. Patients' perceptions on informed consent and the quality of information disclosure in clinical trials. *Patient Education and Counseling*. 1996 Nov; 29(2): 137–153. 13 refs. BE57917.
   *attitudes; communication; comparative studies; comprehension; decision making; *disclosure; *evaluation; evaluation studies; *human experimentation; *informed consent; investigators; legal aspects; motivation; *patient satisfaction; *patients; physicians; risks and benefits; survey; time factors; Netherlands

Wadman, Meredith. 'Group debate' urged for gene studies. [News]. *Nature*. 1998 Jan 22; 391(6665): 314. BE57319.

advisory committees; attitudes; *genetic research; *human experimentation; *informed consent; investigators; Jews; minority groups; *public participation; *public policy; risks and benefits; *tissue banks; *tissue donation; *population genetics; *National Bioethics Advisory Commission; United States

Warnock, Mary. Informed consent — a publisher's duty. *BMJ (British Medical Journal)*. 1998 Mar 28; 316(7136): 1002–1003. BE57584.
   autonomy; biomedical research; *editorial policies; *human experimentation; *informed consent; patients; research subjects; wedge argument

Weir, Robert F. Differing perspectives on consent, choice and control. *In:* Knoppers, Bartha Maria, ed. Human DNA: Law and Policy: International and Comparative Perspectives. Proceedings of the First International Conference on DNA Sampling and Human Genetic Research: Ethical, Legal, and Policy Aspects, held in Montreal, Canada, 6–8 Sep 1996. Boston, MA: Kluwer Law International; 1997: 91–107. 31 fn. ISBN 90–411–0361–9. BE58170.
   attitudes; confidentiality; consent forms; *disclosure; *DNA data banks; donors; federal government; *genetic information; *genetic materials; *genetic research; genetic screening; government regulation; guidelines; *informed consent; model legislation; privacy; professional organizations; research ethics committees; *tissue banks; *tissue donation; *biological specimen banks; American College of Medical Genetics; American Society of Human Genetics; Centers for Disease Control and Prevention; Genetic Privacy Act; National Center for Human Genome Research; *United States

Wenger, Neil S.; Shapiro, Martin F. Consent and discontent. *Canadian Medical Association Journal*. 1997 Dec 15; 157(12): 1691–1692. 6 refs. BE59052.
   developing countries; emergency care; guidelines; *human experimentation; *informed consent; presumed consent; regulation; research ethics committees; scientific misconduct

Williams, Susan G. Research considerations: family opinions about elderly relatives in research. *Journal of Gerontological Nursing*. 1992 Dec; 18(12): 3–8. 11 refs. BE56636.
   *aged; *attitudes; dementia; disclosure; *family members; *human experimentation; informed consent; knowledge, attitudes, practice; nurses; nursing homes; nursing research; survey; *third party consent; questionnaires; United States

Williamson, Charlotte. Not gaining patients' consent in trials is deceitful. [Letter]. *BMJ (British Medical Journal)*. 1996 Jun 8; 312(7044): 1479. 3 refs. BE58155.
   deception; disclosure; *human experimentation; *informed consent; patients; therapeutic research

Wilson, John Robert. Clinical Trial Informed Consent: Outsiders and the Love–Justice Correlation. Ann Arbor, MI: University Microfilms International; 1992. 200 p. Bibliography: p. 194–200. Dissertation, Ph.D., Rice University, May 1992. Order No. 9234441. BE57448.
   Christian ethics; communication; consent forms; covenant; disclosure; drugs; ethicist's role; government regulation; *human experimentation; *informed consent; *investigator subject relationship; *justice; *love; models, theoretical; patient care; philosophy; physician patient relationship; research ethics committees; research subjects; rights; selection of subjects; *theology; uncertainty; *Ramsey, Paul; *Rawls, John

Breast cancer: research without consent. [News]. *Journal of Medical Ethics*. 1997 Dec; 23(6): 372. BE57338.
   *breast cancer; females; guidelines; *human experimentation;

---

*informed consent; *patient advocacy; *Declaration of Helsinki; *Great Britain; Nuremberg Code; *UK Breast Cancer Coalition

FDA seeks public comment on informed consent rules in combat situations. [News]. *Hastings Center Report.* 1997 Sep–Oct; 27(5): 43. BE56127.

*biological warfare; federal government; government regulation; *human experimentation; immunization; *informed consent; *investigational drugs; *military personnel; nontherapeutic research; public policy; toxicity; volunteers; *war; *chemical warfare; Department of Defense; *Food and Drug Administration; United States

HUMAN EXPERIMENTATION/MINORS

Bartholome, William G. Ethical issues in pediatric research. *In:* Vanderpool, Harold Y., ed. The Ethics of Research Involving Human Subjects: Facing the 21st Century. Frederick, MD: University Publishing Group; 1996: 339–370. 61 fn. ISBN 1-55572-036-6. BE56993.

advisory committees; age factors; *children; coercion; competence; comprehension; decision making; federal government; government regulation; growth disorders; guidelines; historical aspects; hormones; *human experimentation; *informed consent; moral policy; *nontherapeutic research; normality; parental consent; pediatrics; random selection; research ethics committees; research subjects; *risks and benefits; selection of subjects; *therapeutic research; McCormick, Richard; National Commission for the Protection of Human Subjects; Ramsey, Paul; United States

Bolster, Mary Catherine. Children as experimental subjects: a review of ethical and theological issues. *Linacre Quarterly.* 1998 May; 65(2): 6–32. 24 refs. BE58931.

advisory committees; age factors; Duchenne muscular dystrophy; federal government; gene therapy; government regulation; guidelines; *human experimentation; informed consent; *minors; nontherapeutic research; parental consent; research ethics committees; risk; *risks and benefits; *Roman Catholic ethics; theology; therapeutic research; Law, Peter; McCormick, Richard; *National Commission for the Protection of Human Subjects; Ramsey, Paul; Research Involving Children: Report and Recommendations; United States

Hilts, Philip J. Experiments on children are reviewed: research involved now–banned drug. [News]. *New York Times.* 1998 Apr 15: B3. BE57728.

advisory committees; aggression; *behavior disorders; behavioral genetics; behavioral research; blacks; *children; federal government; genetic predisposition; government regulation; Hispanic Americans; *human experimentation; males; *minority groups; *nontherapeutic research; patient advocacy; psychoactive drugs; scientific misconduct; social discrimination; vulnerable populations; Columbia University; *fenfluramine; Mount Sinai School of Medicine; National Bioethics Advisory Commission; *New York City; New York State Psychiatric Institute; Queens College

Langer, Dennis H. Children's legal rights as research subjects. *Journal of the American Academy of Child Psychiatry.* 1985 Sep; 24(5): 653–662. 28 refs. Paper presented at the Annual Meeting of the American Academy of Child Psychiatry, Toronto, Canada, October 1984. BE56971.

abortion, induced; *children; competence; contraception; due process; federal government; government regulation; guidelines; *human experimentation; *informed consent; involuntary commitment; *legal rights; parental consent; *patient care; patient participation; research ethics committees; *research subjects; *risks and benefits; Supreme Court decisions; treatment refusal; Department of Health,

Education, and Welfare; National Commission for the Protection of Human Subjects; United States

Lantos, John D. Was the UK collaborative ECMO trial ethical? *Paediatric and Perinatal Epidemiology.* 1997 Jul; 11(3): 264–268. 7 refs. BE58033.

alternatives; *biomedical technologies; coercion; congenital disorders; critically ill; *human experimentation; international aspects; mortality; *newborns; parental consent; *patient care; *random selection; *research design; risks and benefits; *technology assessment; *therapeutic research; time factors; *treatment outcome; uncertainty; *extracorporeal membrane oxygenation; *Great Britain

Leikin, Sanford L. Beyond proforma consent for childhood cancer research. *Journal of Clinical Oncology.* 1985 Mar; 3(3): 420–428. 32 refs. BE57828.

*cancer; comprehension; conflict of interest; disclosure; federal government; government regulation; *human experimentation; *informed consent; investigator subject relationship; *minors; *parental consent; *pediatrics; physician patient relationship; professional family relationship; psychological stress; random selection; standards; Department of Health and Human Services; United States

Levine, Robert J. Adolescents as research subjects without permission of their parents or guardians: ethical considerations. *Journal of Adolescent Health.* 1995 Nov; 17(5): 287–297. 23 refs. BE55916.

*adolescents; autonomy; behavioral research; beneficence; children; competence; epidemiology; federal government; government regulation; *guidelines; *human experimentation; *informed consent; investigational drugs; justice; nontherapeutic research; parental consent; paternalism; public participation; *public policy; *random selection; regulation; research design; research subjects; risk; *risks and benefits; therapeutic research; Department of Health and Human Services; National Commission for the Protection of Human Subjects; United States

Lowes, Lesley. Paediatric nursing and research ethics: is there a conflict? *Journal of Clinical Nursing.* 1996 Mar; 5(2): 91–97. 39 refs. BE55514.

age factors; caring; *children; competence; confidentiality; conflict of interest; disclosure; guidelines; *human experimentation; informed consent; investigators; moral development; moral obligations; nontherapeutic research; nurse patient relationship; nurse's role; *nurses; *nursing research; obligations to society; parental consent; parents; pediatrics; privacy; professional family relationship; professional organizations; research subjects; risks and benefits; therapeutic research; British Paediatric Association

Mason, Su; Brown, Julia; Levene, Malcolm. What is this thing called "randomise"? [Editorial]. *Lancet.* 1997 Nov 15; 350(9089): 1416. 3 refs. BE57162.

attitudes; *comprehension; control groups; critically ill; disclosure; empirical research; *human experimentation; informed consent; *newborns; *parental consent; parents; psychological stress; *random selection; research design; research subjects; selection of subjects; *therapeutic research; extracorporeal membrane oxygenation; qualitative research; Europe; European Union; Great Britain

Nelson, Robert M. Children as research subjects. *In:* Kahn, Jeffrey P.; Mastroianni, Anna C.; Sugarman, Jeremy, eds. Beyond Consent: Seeking Justice in Research. New York, NY: Oxford University Press; 1998: 47–66. 71 fn. ISBN 0-19-511353-5. BE58843.

advisory committees; *children; federal government; government regulation; growth disorders; hormones; *human experimentation; informed consent; institutionalized persons; *justice; mentally retarded; nontherapeutic research; parental consent; public policy; risk; *risks and benefits; scientific misconduct; *standards; trends; Belmont Report; National Commission for the Protection of Human Subjects; National Institutes of Health; United States

Ondrusek, Nancy; Abramovitch, Rona; Pencharz, Paul, et al. Empirical examination of the ability of children to consent to clinical research. *Journal of Medical Ethics.* 1998 Jun; 24(3): 158–165. 6 refs. BE59112.

*adolescents; age factors; attitudes; blood specimen collection; *children; *competence; *comprehension; consent forms; evaluation studies; *informed consent; motivation; *nontherapeutic research; nutrition; research subjects; risks and benefits; questionnaires; Canada

This study examined the quality of children's assent to a clinical trial. In subjects younger than 9 years of age, understanding of most aspects of the study was found to be poor to non-existent. Understanding of procedures was poor in almost all subjects. In addition, voluntariness may have been compromised in many subjects by their belief that failure to complete the study would displease others. If the fact that a child's assent has been obtained is used to justify the exposure of that child to the potential harm of a non-therapeutic blood sample, the assent must be meaningful. In the nutrition study observed here, the quality of the assent of children younger than 9 years of age was very poor. The assent therefore did not provide a valid justification for requesting a blood sample from these children. This study indicates that most children younger than 9 years of age cannot be expected to consent or assent to clinical research in a meaningful way. The current age of 7 years for initiating assent (in addition to parental consent) is possibly not appropriate and should be reconsidered.

Parkins, K.J.; Poets, C.F.; O'Brien, L.M., et al. Effect of exposure to 15% oxygen on breathing patterns and oxygen saturation in infants: interventional study. [Article, commentaries, and response]. *BMJ (British Medical Journal).* 1998 Mar 21; 316(7135): 887–894. 33 refs. BE57968.

disclosure; *human experimentation; *infants; *nontherapeutic research; parental consent; parents; research design; research ethics committees; *risk; *risks and benefits; intervention studies; Great Britain

OBJECTIVE: To assess the response of healthy infants to airway hypoxia (15% oxygen in nitrogen). DESIGN: Interventional study. SETTINGS: Infants' homes and paediatric ward. SUBJECTS: 34 healthy infants (20 boys) born at term; mean age at study 3.1 months. 13 of the infants had siblings whose deaths had been ascribed to the sudden infant death syndrome. INTERVENTION: Respiratory variables were measured in room air (pre-challenge), while infants were exposed to 15% oxygen (challenge), and after infants were returned to room air (post-challenge). MAIN OUTCOME MEASURES: Baseline oxygen saturation as measured by pulse oximetry, frequency of isolated and periodic apnoea, and frequency of desaturation (oxygen saturation less than or = 80% for greater than or = 4 s). Exposure to 15% oxygen was terminated if oxygen saturation fell to less than or = 80% for greater than or = 1 min. RESULTS: Mean duration of exposure to 15% oxygen was 6.3 (SD 2.9) hours. Baseline oxygen saturation fell from a median of 97.6% (range 94.0% to 100%) in room air to 92.8% (84.7% to 100%) in 15% oxygen. There was no correlation between baseline oxygen saturation in room air and the extent of the fall in baseline oxygen saturation on exposure to 15% oxygen. During exposure to 15% oxygen there was a reduction in the proportion of time spent in regular breathing pattern and a 3.5-fold increase in the proportion of time spent in periodic apnoea (P less than

0.001). There was an increase in the frequency of desaturation from 0 episodes per hour (range 0 to 0.2) to 0.4 episodes per hour (0 to 35) (P less than 0.001). In 4 infants exposure to hypoxic conditions was ended early because of prolonged and severe falls in oxygen saturation. CONCLUSIONS: A proportion of infants had episodes of prolonged (less than or = 80% for greater than or = 1 min) or recurrent shorter (less than or = 80% for greater than or = 4 s) desaturation, or both, when exposed to airway hypoxia. The quality and quantity of this response was unpredictable. These findings may explain why some infants with airway hypoxia caused by respiratory infection develop more severe hypoxaemia than others. Exposure to airway hypoxia similar to that experienced during air travel or on holiday at high altitude may be harmful to some infants.

Pear, Robert. Proposal to test drugs in children meets resistance. [News]. *New York Times.* 1997 Nov 30: 1, 28. BE55948.

age factors; *children; *drug industry; *drugs; economics; federal government; *government regulation; *human experimentation; therapeutic research; Food and Drug Administration; *United States

Pierro, Agostino; Spitz, Lewis. Informed consent in clinical research: the crisis in paediatrics. [Letter]. *Lancet.* 1997 Jun 7; 349(9066): 1703. 5 refs. BE56880.

*children; critically ill; *dissent; *human experimentation; motivation; *nontherapeutic research; *parental consent; *parents; pediatrics; risks and benefits; trends; Ormond Street Hospital for Children (London)

Rowell, Mary; Zlotkin, Stanley. The ethical boundaries of drug research in pediatrics. *Pediatric Clinics of North America.* 1997 Feb; 44(1): 27–40. 47 refs. BE57623.

brain death; cadavers; *children; competence; *drugs; economics; *human experimentation; information dissemination; informed consent; injuries; institutionalized persons; nontherapeutic research; parental consent; pediatrics; placebos; *risks and benefits; terminally ill; therapeutic research; toxicity; vulnerable populations

Snowdon, Claire; Garcia, Jo; Elbourne, Diana. Reactions of participants to the results of a randomised controlled trial: exploratory study. *BMJ (British Medical Journal).* 1998 Jul 4; 317(7150): 21–26. 12 refs. BE58814.

*attitudes; *communication; comparative studies; *control groups; *disclosure; *emotions; human experimentation; mortality; *newborns; *parents; psychological stress; *random selection; research subjects; survey; *therapeutic research; *treatment outcome; ventilators; *extracorporeal membrane oxygenation; *feedback; qualitative research; Great Britain

OBJECTIVES: To assess views of parents of babies who participated in a neonatal trial, about feedback of trial results. DESIGN: Qualitative analysis of interviews. SETTING: Parents' homes. SUBJECTS: Parents of 24 surviving babies enrolled in a UK randomised controlled trial comparing ventilatory support by extracorporeal membrane oxygenation with conventional management. MAIN OUTCOME MEASURES: Views about contents of results, reactions to results, effect of hindsight, and importance of feedback. RESULTS: Information about mortality was well understood by the parents but morbidity was less clearly reported. Even when the content was emotionally exacting, the information was still wanted as it removed uncertainty; provided an endpoint to difficult events; promoted further discussion within couples; and acknowledged their contribution to answering an important clinical

---

question. CONCLUSIONS: Feedback of trial results to participants should be a consideration of researchers, but a careful approach is required. This study was based on a highly selective group of parents within a particularly sensitive trial. More research is needed to assess the extent to which these results can be generalised to other trials or to groups such as bereaved parents.

Wadman, Meredith. Row erupts over child aggression study. [News]. *Nature.* 1998 Apr 23; 392(6678): 747. BE58075.
> *aggression; *behavioral research; blacks; *children; *drugs; ethical review; federal government; government regulation; Hispanic Americans; *human experimentation; indigents; males; *minority groups; *nontherapeutic research; research ethics committees; research subjects; scientific misconduct; selection of subjects; *fenfluramine; New York City; *New York State Psychiatric Institute (NYC); Office for Protection from Research Risks; United States

White, Robert J. Ethical issues in pediatric surgical research. *America.* 1997 Feb 8; 176(4): 17-20. BE58369.
> beginning of life; embryo research; embryos; fetal research; fetal therapy; fetuses; genetic research; *human experimentation; informed consent; *minors; *pediatrics; personhood; research design; research subjects; risks and benefits; Roman Catholic ethics; *surgery

Zinn, Christopher. Australian orphans were used as guinea pigs. [News]. *BMJ (British Medical Journal).* 1997 Jun 21; 314(7097): 1783. BE56129.
> *children; historical aspects; *human experimentation; *immunization; *infants; institutionalized persons; research subjects; retrospective moral judgment; *scientific misconduct; vulnerable populations; *Australia; Commonwealth Serum Laboratories (Australia); Twentieth Century

HUMAN EXPERIMENTATION/REGULATION

Ackerman, Terrence F. Choosing between Nuremberg and the National Commission: the balancing of moral principles in clinical research. *In:* Vanderpool, Harold Y., ed. The Ethics of Research Involving Human Subjects: Facing the 21st Century. Frederick, MD: University Publishing Group; 1996: 83-104. 27 fn. ISBN 1-55572-036-6. BE56983.
> advisory committees; codes of ethics; federal government; *government regulation; *guidelines; *human experimentation; informed consent; moral obligations; *moral policy; nontherapeutic research; obligations of society; research ethics committees; research subjects; risks and benefits; volunteers; vulnerable populations; Declaration of Helsinki; Department of Health and Human Services; *National Commission for the Protection of Human Subjects; *Nuremberg Code; United States

Annas, George J.; Glantz, Leonard H. Informed consent to research on institutionalized mentally disabled persons: the dual problems of incapacity and voluntariness. *In:* Shamoo, Adil E., ed. Ethics in Neurobiological Research with Human Subjects: The Baltimore Conference on Ethics. Amsterdam: Gordon and Breach; 1997: 55-79. 46 fn. Appendices include the text of the Nuremberg Code and parts of the U.S. Department of Health, Education, and Welfare regulations proposed in 1978 on "protections pertaining to biomedical and behavioral research involving as subjects individuals institutionalized as mentally disabled." ISBN 2-88449-161-9. BE57009.
> behavior control; *coercion; *competence; comprehension; *decision making; federal government; government regulation; guidelines; hepatitis; *human experimentation;

immunization; *informed consent; *institutionalized persons; involuntary commitment; judicial action; *legal aspects; *mentally disabled; *mentally ill; model legislation; nontherapeutic research; organ donation; patient advocacy; patient care; prisoners; psychoactive drugs; *regulation; research ethics committees; research subjects; scientific misconduct; state interest; sterilization (sexual); therapeutic research; *third party consent; treatment refusal; DHEW Guidelines; Nuremberg Code; *United States

Ault, Alicia. FDA may "pull the plug" on consent waiver. [News]. *Lancet.* 1997 Oct 11; 350(9084): 1084. BE57267.
> disclosure; *emergency care; federal government; *government regulation; hospitals; *human experimentation; *informed consent; public participation; research ethics committees; therapeutic research; *Food and Drug Administration; United States

Bendall, Christine. Clinical research -- the relationship between law and guidelines. *In:* Close, Bryony; Combes, Robert; Hubbard, Anthony; Illingworth, John, eds. Volunteers in Research and Testing. Bristol, PA: Taylor and Francis; 1997: 41-52. 2 refs. 5 fn. ISBN 0-7484-0397-3. BE57029.
> compensation; confidentiality; ethical review; *guidelines; *human experimentation; informed consent; injuries; international aspects; law; *legal aspects; *regulation; research subjects; selection of subjects; *Europe; European Community; Great Britain

Benson, Paul R.; Roth, Loren H. Trends in the social control of medical and psychiatric research. *Law and Mental Health.* 1988; 4: 1-47. 227 refs. BE56609.
> behavioral research; biomedical research; codes of ethics; competence; empirical research; *ethical review; evaluation; federal government; *government regulation; guidelines; historical aspects; *human experimentation; informed consent; international aspects; investigators; legal aspects; nontherapeutic research; organization and administration; physicians; professional autonomy; professional organizations; *research ethics committees; research subjects; review; scientific misconduct; self regulation; *social control; state government; therapeutic research; trends; vulnerable populations; Canada; Central Intelligence Agency; Council for International Organizations of Medical Sciences; Declaration of Helsinki; Denmark; Department of Health, Education, and Welfare; Food and Drug Administration; Great Britain; National Institutes of Health; Nuremberg Code; Twentieth Century; *United States; World Health Organization

Brody, Baruch. Whatever happened to research ethics? *In:* Carson, Ronald A.; Burns, Chester R., eds. Philosophy of Medicine and Bioethics: A Twenty-Year Retrospective and Critical Appraisal. Boston, MA: Kluwer Academic; 1997: 275-286. 25 refs. ISBN 0-7923-3545-7. BE56542.
> advisory committees; bioethical issues; bioethics; biomedical research; clinical ethics; control groups; drugs; education; *ethicist's role; ethicists; federal government; freedom; *government regulation; historical aspects; *human experimentation; international aspects; literature; moral policy; public policy; random selection; *research design; research ethics committees; risks and benefits; selection of subjects; time factors; *trends; values; *research ethics; Europe; Twentieth Century; United States

Brody, Baruch A. Research and the drug/device approval process. *In: his* The Ethics of Biomedical Research: An International Perspective. New York, NY: Oxford University Press; 1998: 161-183, 373-375. 41 fn. ISBN 0-19-509007-1. BE57675.
> adults; aged; alternatives; disclosure; *drugs; federal government; *government regulation; guidelines; historical aspects; *human experimentation; informed consent;

---

*international aspects; *medical devices; minors; motivation; nontherapeutic research; palliative care; patients; *public policy; research design; research subjects; risks and benefits; selection of subjects; standards; toxicity; Europe; Food and Drug Administration; United States

Darvall, Leanna. Gender and equity: emerging issues in Australian clinical drug trial regulatory policies. *In:* Petersen, Kerry, ed. Intersections: Women on Law, Medicine and Technology. Brookfield, VT: Ashgate; 1997: 185–200. 18 refs. 1 fn. ISBN 1–85521–882–8. BE57492.
> age factors; AIDS; costs and benefits; *drugs; federal government; *females; *government regulation; *guidelines; *human experimentation; international aspects; justice; males; minority groups; *nontherapeutic research; pregnant women; prenatal injuries; *public policy; research design; *risks and benefits; *selection of subjects; toxicity; *Australia; Department of Health and Human Services; Food and Drug Administration; National Institutes of Health; *United States

Destro, Robert A. Government oversight. *In:* Shamoo, Adil E., ed. Ethics in Neurobiological Research with Human Subjects: The Baltimore Conference on Ethics. Amsterdam: Gordon and Breach; 1997: 81–99. 90 fn. ISBN 2–88449–161–9. BE57010.
> behavioral research; coercion; *competence; comprehension; conflict of interest; *disclosure; federal government; *government regulation; *human experimentation; *informed consent; investigator subject relationship; investigators; *legal aspects; mentally disabled; minors; nontherapeutic research; professional ethics; research ethics committees; research subjects; state government; therapeutic research; *third party consent; *vulnerable populations; *United States

Fabick, Mary M. Ethical considerations for research on human subjects. *Plastic Surgical Nursing.* 1995 Winter; 15(4): 225–227, 231. 5 refs. BE55857.
> codes of ethics; competence; federal government; government regulation; *human experimentation; informed consent; international aspects; investigators; legal aspects; nurses; nursing research; *regulation; research ethics committees; scientific misconduct; state government; third party consent; American Hospital Association; American Nurses Association Code for Nurses; Declaration of Helsinki; Department of Health and Human Services; National Commission for the Protection of Human Subjects; Nuremberg Code; United States

Fletcher, John C.; Miller, Franklin G. The promise and perils of public bioethics. *In:* Vanderpool, Harold Y., ed. The Ethics of Research Involving Human Subjects: Facing the 21st Century. Frederick, MD: University Publishing Group; 1996: 155–184. 74 fn. ISBN 1–55572–036–6. BE56986.
> abortion, induced; accountability; *advisory committees; AIDS; *bioethical issues; *bioethics; biomedical research; embryo research; federal government; fetal research; fetal tissue donation; government financing; government regulation; health care delivery; historical aspects; *human experimentation; morality; politics; *public policy; *regulation; research institutes; scientific misconduct; Department of Health and Human Services; Ethics Advisory Board; National Bioethics Advisory Commission; National Commission for the Protection of Human Subjects; President's Commission for the Study of Ethical Problems; *United States

Fox, Jeffrey L. Green light for gene therapy in healthy volunteers. [News]. *Nature Biotechnology.* 1997 Apr; 15(4): 314. BE55858.
> advisory committees; federal government; *gene therapy; genetic research; *government regulation; *human

experimentation; investigators; *nontherapeutic research; *volunteers; Crystal, Ron; Food and Drug Administration; National Institutes of Health; *Recombinant DNA Advisory Committee; United States

Goldbeck–Wood, Sandra. Denmark takes a lead on research ethics. [News]. *BMJ (British Medical Journal).* 1998 Apr 18; 316(7139): 1189. BE58619.
> disclosure; *ethical review; financial support; *government regulation; *human experimentation; research ethics committees; national ethics committees; *Denmark

Gordon, Bruce; Prentice, Ernest. Continuing review of research involving human subjects: approach to the problem and remaining areas of concern. *IRB: A Review of Human Subjects Research.* 1997 Mar–Apr; 19(2): 8–11. 7 refs. BE58516.
> *ethical review; federal government; *government regulation; guidelines; *human experimentation; investigators; records; research design; *research ethics committees; risks and benefits; selection of subjects; *standards; time factors; universities; multicenter studies; Food and Drug Administration; Office for Protection from Research Risks; *United States; *University of Nebraska Medical Center (Omaha)

Great Britain. Department of Health. Advisory Group on the Ethics of Xenotransplantation (Chair: Ian Kennedy). Animal Tissue into Humans: A Report by the Advisory Group on the Ethics of Xenotransplantation, 1996. London: Her Majesty's Stationery Office; 1997. 258 p. 92 fn. Appendixes include Glossary of terms; The consultation exercise; Report of the Workshop on Xenotransplantation and Infectious Disease; and Development of transgenic pigs. ISBN 0–11–321866–4. BE55999.
> advisory committees; alternatives; animal experimentation; *animal organs; animal rights; artificial organs; body parts and fluids; communicable diseases; ethical review; *evaluation; gene therapy; genetic intervention; *government regulation; *guidelines; health promotion; *human experimentation; informed consent; international aspects; legal aspects; organ donation; *organ transplantation; preventive medicine; primates; private sector; public health; *public policy; public sector; research ethics committees; resource allocation; *risks and benefits; scarcity; selection of subjects; suffering; therapeutic research; *tissue transplantation; *transgenic animals; swine; Advisory Group on the Ethics of Xenotransplantation (Great Britain); Animals (Scientific Procedures) Act 1986; Department of Health (Great Britain); *Great Britain

Hamilton, Jean A. Women and health policy: on the inclusion of females in clinical trials. *In:* Sargent, Carolyn F.; Brettell, Caroline B., eds. Gender and Health: An International Perspective. Upper Saddle River, NJ: Prentice Hall; 1996: 292–325. 121 refs. 35 fn. ISBN 0–13–079427–9. BE58096.
> contraception; developing countries; *drugs; economics; federal government; *females; fetuses; *government regulation; guidelines; *human experimentation; informed consent; international aspects; investigators; males; minority groups; *public policy; research design; risks and benefits; *selection of subjects; *social discrimination; therapeutic research; *women's health; *Food and Drug Administration; *National Institutes of Health; U.S. Congress; *United States

Karlawish, Jason H.T.; Sachs, Greg A. Research on the cognitively impaired: lessons and warnings from the emergency research debate. *Journal of the American Geriatrics Society.* 1997 Apr; 45(4): 474–481. 65 refs. BE57116.
> advance directives; *dementia; *emergency care; family members; federal government; *government regulation;

BE = bioethics accession number   fn. = footnotes   refs. = references

*human experimentation; informed consent; judicial action; legal aspects; *mentally disabled; public participation; research ethics committees; research subjects; risk; risks and benefits; state government; *therapeutic research; *third party consent; Department of Health and Human Services; DHHS Guidelines; Food and Drug Administration; T.D. v. New York State Office of Mental Health; *United States

Kondro, Wayne. New rules on human subjects could end debate in Canada. [News]. *Science.* 1998 Jun 5; 280(5369): 1521. BE58875.
advisory committees; *behavioral research; biomedical research; committee membership; consensus; deception; dissent; ethical review; genetic research; *guidelines; *human experimentation; humanities; informed consent; interdisciplinary communication; lawyers; minority groups; *regulation; research ethics committees; research institutes; research subjects; science; social sciences; universities; community consent; *Canada; *Code of Conduct for Research Involving Humans; *Medical Research Council of Canada; *Natural Sciences and Engineering Research Council (Canada); *Social Sciences and Humanities Research Council (Canada)

Lehrman, Sally. Call for human subjects monitoring body. [News]. *Nature.* 1997 Jul 24; 388(6640): 313. BE56110.
advisory committees; confidentiality; *federal government; government financing; *government regulation; *human experimentation; informed consent; private sector; *public policy; public sector; research subjects; risks and benefits; National Bioethics Advisory Commission; *United States

McCarthy, Charles R. Challenges to IRBs in the coming decades. *In:* Vanderpool, Harold Y., ed. The Ethics of Research Involving Human Subjects: Facing the 21st Century. Frederick, MD: University Publishing Group; 1996: 127–144. 15 fn. ISBN 1-55572-036-6. BE56985.
advisory committees; AIDS; animal experimentation; autonomy; beneficence; compensation; cultural pluralism; ethical review; federal government; *government regulation; guidelines; *human experimentation; immunization; injuries; international aspects; investigational drugs; investigators; justice; professional ethics; *public policy; *research ethics committees; research subjects; review committees; risks and benefits; self regulation; trends; data monitoring committees; multicenter studies; research ethics; Belmont Report; Department of Health and Human Services; DHHS Guidelines; Office for Protection from Research Risks; *United States

McGough, Helen. OPRR and FDA propose revised expedited review categories. *IRB: A Review of Human Subjects Research.* 1998 Jan–Feb; 20(1): 9, 11. 2 refs. BE58520.
*ethical review; federal government; *government regulation; *human experimentation; informed consent; *research ethics committees; risk; *expedited review; *Food and Drug Administration; *Office for Protection from Research Risks; *United States

Maloney, Dennis M. Federal agency's final rule says informed consent forms must be dated. [News]. *Human Research Report.* 1996 Dec; 11(12): 1–2. BE55627.
*consent forms; federal government; *government regulation; *human experimentation; *informed consent; research ethics committees; research subjects; *time factors; *Food and Drug Administration; *United States

Marshall, Eliot. Review boards: a system 'in jeopardy'? [News]. *Science.* 1998 Jun 19; 280(5371): 1830–1831. BE58270.
conflict of interest; economics; *ethical review; evaluation; federal government; financial support; *government regulation; *human experimentation; private sector; *research ethics committees; standards; Department of

Health and Human Services; *United States

Marwick, Charles. Assessment of exception to informed consent. [News]. *JAMA.* 1997 Nov 5; 278(17): 1392–1393. BE56166.
community services; disclosure; *emergency care; evaluation; federal government; *government regulation; *human experimentation; information dissemination; *informed consent; mass media; minority groups; public participation; research ethics committees; third party consent; *Food and Drug Administration; United States

Marwick, Charles. Improved protection for human research subjects. [News]. *JAMA.* 1998 Feb 4; 279(5): 344–345. BE57863.
advisory committees; conflict of interest; ethical review; *federal government; *government regulation; *human experimentation; informed consent; Department of Health and Human Services; *National Bioethics Advisory Commission; National Institutes of Health; Office for Protection from Research Risks; *United States

Miller, Judith. The Deschamps Report: controls for clinical research in Quebec. *International Journal of Bioethics.* 1997 Mar–Jun; 8(1–2): 79–85. 10 fn. BE59096.
advisory committees; conflict of interest; drug industry; *evaluation; *government regulation; *human experimentation; misconduct; research ethics committees; Canada; *Deschamps Report; *Quebec

Mudur, Ganapati. India to control foreign research involving Indian patients. [News]. *BMJ (British Medical Journal).* 1997 Jan 18; 314(7075): 165. BE58621.
aborted fetuses; developing countries; eye diseases; fetal tissue donation; government financing; *government regulation; *human experimentation; *international aspects; investigators; *selection of subjects; tissue transplantation; *India; Indian Council of Medical Research; United States

Nightingale, Stuart L. New [FDA] rules require financial disclosure. [News]. *JAMA.* 1998 Apr 1; 279(13): 984. BE57775.
*conflict of interest; *disclosure; federal government; *financial support; *government regulation; human experimentation; industry; *investigators; *Food and Drug Administration; United States

Pear, Robert. Proposal to test drugs in children meets resistance. [News]. *New York Times.* 1997 Nov 30: 1, 28. BE55948.
age factors; *children; *drug industry; *drugs; economics; federal government; *government regulation; *human experimentation; therapeutic research; Food and Drug Administration; *United States

Pendergast, Mary K. Testimony of Mary K. Pendergast before the Subcommittee on Human Resources, Committee on Government Reform and Oversight, U.S. House of Representatives [re FDA regulation of human experimentation]. *In:* BioLaw: A Legal and Ethical Reporter on Medicine, Health Care, and Bioengineering. Special Sections, 2(11). Frederick, MD: University Publications of America; 1997 Nov: S355–S371. 5 fn. BE56648.
consent forms; critically ill; disclosure; education; *emergency care; federal government; *government regulation; guidelines; *human experimentation; informed consent; investigators; military personnel; research ethics committees; research subjects; war; Department of Defense; Department of Health and Human Services; *Food and Drug Administration; *United States

Rogers, Arthur. European drug industry concerned over proposed clinical–trial legislation. [News]. *Lancet.* 1997

BE = bioethics accession number   fn. = footnotes   refs. = references

Nov 29; 350(9091): 1609. BE57269.
confidentiality; data banks; *drug industry; *drugs; ethical review; *government regulation; guidelines; *human experimentation; *international aspects; legislation; professional organizations; research ethics committees; *European Federation of Pharmaceutical Industries and Associations; *European Union; International Conference on Harmonisation; Japan; United States

Rolleston, Francis; Armour, Catherine; Stipich, Nina. Developing a Tri-Council code of conduct for research involving humans. *International Journal of Bioethics.* 1997 Mar-Jun; 8(1-2): 67-70. BE59097.
accountability; biomedical research; consensus; ethical review; government regulation; *guidelines; *human experimentation; interdisciplinary communication; *regulation; research ethics committees; scientific misconduct; self regulation; *Canada; Medical Research Council of Canada; National Council on Bioethics in Human Research (Canada); Natural Sciences and Engineering Research Council (Canada); Social Sciences and Humanities Research Council (Canada); *Tri-Council Policy Statement on Ethical Conduct for Research Involving Humans

Ryan, Anne J. True protection for persons with severe mental disabilities, such as schizophrenia, involved as subjects in research? A look and consideration of the "Protection of Human Subjects." *Journal of Law and Health.* 1994-1995; 9(2): 349-376. 226 fn. BE57179.
disclosure; federal government; *government regulation; guidelines; historical aspects; *human experimentation; informed consent; *mentally ill; minors; patient advocacy; pregnant women; prisoners; psychoactive drugs; research ethics committees; research subjects; *schizophrenia; vulnerable populations; withholding treatment; *DHHS Guidelines; National Commission for the Protection of Human Subjects; Nuremberg Code; *United States; University of California, Los Angeles

Shuster, Evelyne. Fifty years later: the significance of the Nuremberg Code. *New England Journal of Medicine.* 1997 Nov 13; 337(20): 1436-1440. 25 refs. BE56438.
*codes of ethics; *guidelines; *historical aspects; *human experimentation; *human rights; informed consent; *international aspects; investigator subject relationship; investigators; medical ethics; misconduct; National Socialism; physician patient relationship; physician's role; *physicians; prisoners; professional organizations; *regulation; research design; research subjects; risks and benefits; scientific misconduct; social impact; Alexander, Leo; Declaration of Helsinki; Germany; Hippocratic Oath; Ivy, Andrew; Leibbrand, Werner; *Nuremberg Code; *Nuremberg Trials; *Twentieth Century; United States

Spurgeon, David. Trials sponsored by drug companies: review ordered. [News]. *BMJ (British Medical Journal).* 1998 Sep 5; 317(7159): 618. BE59078.
*biomedical research; confidentiality; contracts; *disclosure; *drug industry; *drugs; *financial support; *hospitals; *human experimentation; *institutional policies; *investigators; livers; minors; *regulation; *thalassemia; therapeutic research; *toxicity; *Apotex; Canada; *deferiprone; *Hospital for Sick Children (Toronto); *Olivieri, Nancy

Stecklow, Steve; Johannes, Laura. Drug makers relied on clinical researchers who now await trial. [News]. *Wall Street Journal.* 1997 Aug 15: A1, A6. BE55547.
competence; contracts; dementia; *drug industry; entrepreneurship; faculty; financial support; *fraud; government regulation; health personnel; human experimentation; *incentives; informed consent; *investigators; medical schools; physicians; psychoactive drugs; research subjects; schizophrenia; *scientific misconduct; *selection of subjects; *self regulation; technical expertise; guideline adherence; *Borison, Richard;

*Diamond, Bruce; Food and Drug Administration; Georgia; Medical College of Georgia

Sugarman, Jeremy; Mastroianni, Anna C.; Kahn, Jeffrey P., eds. Ethics of Research with Human Subjects: Selected Policies and Resources. Frederick, MD: University Publishing Group; 1998. 244 p. Bibliography: p. 229-244. ISBN 1-55572-057-9. BE59046.
adolescents; aged; children; codes of ethics; compensation; embryo research; emergency care; federal government; females; fetal research; genetic research; *government regulation; *guidelines; *human experimentation; incentives; informed consent; international aspects; mentally disabled; military personnel; minority groups; pregnant women; prisoners; *public policy; research ethics committees; students; volunteers; vulnerable populations; *United States

U.S. Congress. House. Committee on Government Reform and Oversight. Subcommittee on Human Resources. Oversight of NIH and FDA: Bioethics and the Adequacy of Informed Consent. Hearing, 8 May 1997. Washington, DC: U.S. Government Printing Office; 1997. Serial No. 105-49. ISBN 0-16-055827-1. BE58891.
*advisory committees; bioethics; children; cloning; control groups; developing countries; disclosure; drugs; emergency care; *ethical review; evaluation; federal government; genetic research; government financing; *government regulation; hepatitis; HIV seropositivity; *human experimentation; immunization; *informed consent; international aspects; mentally ill; military personnel; parental consent; placebos; pregnant women; public policy; research design; research ethics committees; research subjects; scientific misconduct; *vulnerable populations; war; Africa; AZT; Centers for Disease Control and Prevention; Department of Defense; Food and Drug Administration; *National Bioethics Advisory Commission; National Institutes of Health; *United States

U.S. National Institutes of Health. Recombinant DNA research: proposed actions under the guidelines; notice. *Federal Register.* 1996 Nov 22; 61(227): 59726-59742. BE57536.
*advisory committees; committee membership; data banks; *ethical review; *federal government; *gene therapy; *government regulation; guidelines; *human experimentation; organization and administration; *public policy; recombinant DNA research; review committees; Food and Drug Administration; *Gene Therapy Policy Conferences; *National Institutes of Health; NIH Guidelines; Office of Recombinant DNA Activities; Points to Consider: Transfer of Recombinant DNA into Human Subjects; *Recombinant DNA Advisory Committee; *United States

Vogel, Gretchen. Xenotransplants: no moratorium on clinical trials. [News]. *Science.* 1998 Jan 30; 279(5351): 648. BE57363.
advisory committees; *animal organs; communicable diseases; data banks; federal government; *government regulation; *human experimentation; *organ transplantation; primates; registries; risk; *therapeutic research; tissue banks; *tissue transplantation; transgenic animals; transplant recipients; swine; Centers for Disease Control and Prevention; *Food and Drug Administration; National Institutes of Health; *United States

Wadman, Meredith. FDA turns down moratorium demand on xenotransplants. [News]. *Nature.* 1998 Jan 29; 391(6666): 423. BE57362.
advisory committees; *animal organs; communicable diseases; data banks; federal government; *government regulation; guidelines; *human experimentation; investigators; *organ transplantation; primates; public participation; registries; risk; *therapeutic research; tissue

---

BE = bioethics accession number   fn. = footnotes   refs. = references

banks; tissue transplantation; swine; *Food and Drug Administration; National Institutes of Health; Public Health Service; *United States

Wadman, Meredith. Privacy bill under fire from researchers. [News]. *Nature.* 1998 Mar 5; 392(6671): 6. BE57258.
> biomedical research; *confidentiality; disclosure; *ethical review; federal government; *government regulation; *human experimentation; industry; informed consent; investigators; *legislation; *medical records; privacy; *private sector; research ethics committees; research subjects; expedited review; *Medical Information Protection Act 1998; *United States

Weiss, Rick. Bioethics group divided over research on mentally ill. [News]. *Washington Post.* 1998 Nov 16: A6. BE58997.
> advisory committees; family members; federal government; *government regulation; *human experimentation; informed consent; *mentally ill; nontherapeutic research; patient advocacy; *public policy; research subjects; risks and benefits; therapeutic research; third party consent; National Alliance for the Mentally Ill; *National Bioethics Advisory Commission; National Institutes of Health; Nuremberg Code; United States

Weiss, Rick. Research ethics panel urges new regulations to protect mentally ill. [News]. *Washington Post.* 1998 Nov 18: A11. BE58998.
> advisory committees; attitudes; family members; federal government; *government regulation; *human experimentation; informed consent; investigators; *mentally ill; nontherapeutic research; patient advocacy; *public policy; research subjects; risks and benefits; third party consent; American Psychiatric Association; Institute of Medicine; *National Bioethics Advisory Commission; National Institutes of Health; United States

Wise, Jacqui. New authority to monitor xenotransplantation experiments. [News]. *BMJ (British Medical Journal).* 1997 Jan 25; 314(7076): 247. 1 ref. BE58703.
> advisory committees; *animal organs; communicable diseases; *government regulation; *human experimentation; international aspects; *organ transplantation; *public policy; risk; self regulation; transgenic animals; transplant recipients; *swine; Advisory Group on the Ethics of Xenotransplantation (Great Britain); *Great Britain; United States; *Xenotransplantation Interim Regulatory Authority (Great Britain)

HUMAN EXPERIMENTATION/RESEARCH DESIGN

Aaby, Peter; Babiker, Abdel; Darbyshire, Janet, et al. Ethics of HIV trials. [Letters]. *Lancet.* 1997 Nov 22; 350(9090): 1546–1547. 5 refs. BE58468.
> *control groups; *developing countries; *drugs; economics; *HIV seropositivity; *human experimentation; international aspects; *placebos; *pregnant women; random selection; *research design; Africa; AZT

Alibhai, Shabbir M.H.; Weijer, Charles. The placebo effect. [Letter and response]. *Canadian Medical Association Journal.* 1997 Oct 15; 157(8): 1020, 1022. 5 refs. BE56582.
> competence; *human experimentation; investigational drugs; *nontherapeutic research; *placebos; *research design; standards; *therapeutic research; Canada

Aller, Robert; Aller, Gregory. An institutional response to patient/family complaints. *In:* Shamoo, Adil E., ed. Ethics in Neurobiological Research with Human

Subjects: The Baltimore Conference on Ethics. Amsterdam: Gordon and Breach; 1997: 155–172. 32 fn. This paper provides the viewpoints of a father and of his son, who was a research subject at the UCLA Clinical Research Center. ISBN 2-88449-161-9. BE57013.
> administrators; case studies; consent forms; *deception; *disclosure; family members; *human experimentation; iatrogenic disease; *informed consent; medical records; *mentally ill; patients; physician patient relationship; placebos; professional family relationship; *psychoactive drugs; *research design; research subjects; risks and benefits; *schizophrenia; *scientific misconduct; suicide; treatment outcome; universities; *withholding treatment; patient abandonment; *UCLA Neuropsychiatric Institute; United States; *University of California, Los Angeles

Ashcroft, Richard. Human research subjects, selection of. *In:* Chadwick, Ruth, ed. Encyclopedia of Applied Ethics, Volume 2. San Diego, CA: Academic Press; 1998: 627–639. 7 refs. ISBN 0-12-227067-3. BE56397.
> autonomy; competence; control groups; costs and benefits; females; guidelines; *human experimentation; incentives; informed consent; investigators; *justice; moral obligations; nontherapeutic research; obligations to society; paternalism; patient compliance; patients; random selection; remuneration; *research design; *research subjects; resource allocation; rights; risks and benefits; *selection of subjects; therapeutic research; vulnerable populations

Ault, Alicia. USA accused of funding placebo–controlled AIDS trials. [News]. *Lancet.* 1997 May 3; 349(9061): 1305. BE56073.
> AIDS; *developing countries; drugs; federal government; government financing; *HIV seropositivity; *human experimentation; *newborns; *placebos; *pregnant women; public policy; withholding treatment; AZT; Centers for Disease Control and Prevention; National Institutes of Health; *United States

Brody, Baruch. Whatever happened to research ethics? *In:* Carson, Ronald A.; Burns, Chester R., eds. Philosophy of Medicine and Bioethics: A Twenty–Year Retrospective and Critical Appraisal. Boston, MA: Kluwer Academic; 1997: 275–286. 25 refs. ISBN 0-7923-3545-7. BE56542.
> advisory committees; bioethical issues; bioethics; biomedical research; clinical ethics; control groups; drugs; education; *ethicist's role; ethicists; federal government; freedom; *government regulation; historical aspects; *human experimentation; international aspects; literature; moral policy; public policy; random selection; *research design; research ethics committees; risks and benefits; selection of subjects; time factors; *trends; values; *research ethics; Europe; Twentieth Century; United States

Brody, Baruch A. Clinical trials. *In: his* The Ethics of Biomedical Research: An International Perspective. New York, NY: Oxford University Press; 1998: 139–160, 372–373. 30 fn. ISBN 0-19-509007-1. BE57674.
> biomedical technologies; *control groups; guidelines; historical aspects; *human experimentation; international aspects; placebos; quality of life; *random selection; *research design; review; review committees; selection of subjects; therapeutic research; time factors; uncertainty; data monitoring committees

Burt, R.A.P.; Goldschmidt, Peter G.; Monaco, Grace Powers, et al. Investigational treatments: process, payment, and priorities. [Letters and response]. *JAMA.* 1997 Nov 5; 278(17): 1402–1404. 13 refs. BE57252.
> *biomedical technologies; decision making; *evaluation; *health insurance reimbursement; health maintenance organizations; human experimentation; patient care; random selection; *research design; review committees; risks and benefits; standards; *technology assessment; terminology;

*therapeutic research; *evidence-based medicine; *investigational therapies; United States

Carpenter, William T. Schizophrenia research: a challenge for constructive criticism. *In:* Shamoo, Adil E., ed. Ethics in Neurobiological Research with Human Subjects: The Baltimore Conference on Ethics. Amsterdam: Gordon and Breach; 1997: 215–228. 40 refs. ISBN 2-88449-161-9. BE57021.

attitudes; autonomy; *dissent; ethicists; evaluation; federal government; government regulation; *human experimentation; informed consent; injuries; investigators; *mentally ill; patient advocacy; patient care; patient compliance; patient transfer; patients; placebos; *psychoactive drugs; *research design; research subjects; *risks and benefits; *schizophrenia; scientific misconduct; toxicity; treatment outcome; *withholding treatment; patient abandonment; Maryland Psychiatric Research Center (Baltimore); National Alliance for the Mentally Ill; Office for Protection from Research Risks; United States

Carpenter, William T.; Schooler, Nina R.; Kane, John M. The rationale and ethics of medication-free research in schizophrenia. *Archives of General Psychiatry.* 1997 May; 54(5): 401–407. 58 refs. Commented on by F.A. Henn et al., p. 411–412, and by J.J. Fins and F.G. Miller, p. 415–416. BE57902.

*human experimentation; informed consent; *mentally ill; placebos; *psychoactive drugs; *research design; research subjects; *risks and benefits; *schizophrenia; selection of subjects; *withholding treatment

Clark, Peter A. The ethics of placebo-controlled trials for perinatal transmission of HIV in developing countries. *Journal of Clinical Ethics.* 1998 Summer; 9(2): 156–166. 44 fn. BE58961.

AIDS; alternatives; autonomy; beneficence; common good; comprehension; *control groups; costs and benefits; *developing countries; drugs; ethical analysis; ethical relativism; guidelines; *HIV seropositivity; *human experimentation; human rights; informed consent; international aspects; justice; *moral policy; morbidity; *newborns; patient care; *placebos; *pregnant women; prevalence; public policy; *research design; research subjects; risks and benefits; socioeconomic factors; standards; vulnerable populations; AZT; United States

Dixon, John. Catastrophic rights: vital public interests and civil liberties in conflict. *In:* Overall, Christine and Zion, William P., eds. Perspectives on AIDS: Ethical and Social Issues. New York, NY: Oxford University Press; 1991: 122–137. 9 refs. ISBN 0-19-540749-0. BE58291.

*AIDS; *autonomy; beneficence; coercion; *common good; control groups; government regulation; *HIV seropositivity; *human experimentation; *investigational drugs; investigators; *paternalism; patients; physicians; political activity; *public policy; random selection; *research design; resource allocation; *rights; *terminally ill; therapeutic research; treatment refusal; investigational therapies; AZT; Canada; United States

Edwards, S.J.L.; Lilford, R.J.; Braunholtz, David, et al. Why "underpowered" trials are not necessarily unethical. *Lancet.* 1997 Sep 13; 350(9080): 804–807. 26 refs. BE55852.

ethical analysis; financial support; government financing; *human experimentation; investigators; patients; random selection; *research design; research ethics committees; research subjects; *statistics; therapeutic research; evidence-based medicine; quality control; Great Britain; National Health Service

Emanuel, Ezekiel J.; Patterson, W. Bradford; Hellman, Samuel. Ethics of randomized clinical trials. *Journal of*

Clinical Oncology. 1998 Jan; 16(1): 365–371. 5 refs. BE58467.

alternatives; autonomy; breast cancer; coercion; communication; comprehension; conflict of interest; *decision making; disclosure; *human experimentation; informed consent; *investigational drugs; investigator subject relationship; investigators; patient advocacy; patient care; *patients; physician patient relationship; *physicians; prognosis; *random selection; rights; risks and benefits; *therapeutic research; toxicity; uncertainty; utilitarianism

Felten, David L. Cell transplantation and research design. [Letter]. *Science.* 1994 Mar 18; 263(5153): 1546. 2 refs. BE56222.

aged; *brain; central nervous system diseases; control groups; fetal research; fetal tissue donation; *human experimentation; informed consent; *placebos; random selection; *research design; *surgery; *tissue transplantation; Parkinson disease; *sham surgery

Fins, Joseph J.; Miller, Franklin G. The call of the sirens: navigating the ethics of medication-free research in schizophrenia. [Commentary]. *Archives of General Psychiatry.* 1997 May; 54(5): 415–416. 10 refs. Commentary by W.T. Carpenter et al., p. 401–407. BE57903.

*human experimentation; informed consent; *mentally ill; psychiatric wills; *psychoactive drugs; *research design; research subjects; *schizophrenia; *withholding treatment

Gordon, Valery M.; Sugarman, Jeremy; Kass, Nancy. Toward a more comprehensive approach to protecting human subjects: the interface of data safety monitoring boards and institutional review boards in randomized clinical trials. *IRB: A Review of Human Subjects Research.* 1998 Jan–Feb; 20(1): 1–5. 28 refs. BE58517.

committee membership; drug industry; ethical review; federal government; government regulation; guidelines; *human experimentation; organization and administration; *random selection; *research design; *research ethics committees; *review committees; risks and benefits; *standards; *data monitoring committees; multicenter studies; National Institutes of Health; *United States

Groudine, Scott; Lumb, Philip D. First, do no harm. *Journal of Medical Ethics.* 1997 Dec; 23(6): 377–378. BE57660.

cancer; case studies; *conflict of interest; *drugs; *human experimentation; injuries; *investigators; pain; paralysis; patient care; *physician's role; *placebos; *random selection; *research design; research subjects; risk; terminally ill; *therapeutic research; withholding treatment; paraplegia

When a physician acts as both doctor and researcher conflicts can develop. When a doctor does not know whether a patient is taking active drug or placebo, any new medical problems can result in a dilemma. Is the patient's suffering a side effect of the medication or is this a new medical problem? Mrs W's case demonstrates the problem that can occur when the physician is blinded in the name of research.

Halsey, Neal A.; Sommer, Alfred; Henderson, Donald A., et al. Ethics and international research. [Editorial]. *BMJ (British Medical Journal).* 1997 Oct 18; 315(7114): 965–966. 8 refs. BE55908.

*developing countries; *drugs; economics; *ethical relativism; guidelines; health care delivery; *HIV seropositivity; *human experimentation; *international aspects; *newborns; *placebos; *pregnant women; *research design; standards; *AZT; Centers for Disease Control and Prevention; Council for International Organizations of Medical Sciences; United States; World Health Organization

Henn, Fritz A.; Lader, Malcolm; Helmchen, Hanfried.

BE = bioethics accession number   fn. = footnotes   refs. = references

Medication-free research with schizophrenic patients: a European perspective. [Commentary]. *Archives of General Psychiatry.* 1997 May; 54(5): 412–413. 8 refs. Commentary on W.T. Carpenter et al., p. 401–407. BE57904.

*human experimentation; *mentally ill; placebos; *psychoactive drugs; *research design; risks and benefits; *schizophrenia; *withholding treatment; Europe

Irving, Dianne N.; Shamoo, Adil E. Washouts/relapses in patients participating in neurobiological research studies in schizophrenia. *In:* Shamoo, Adil E., ed. Ethics in Neurobiological Research with Human Subjects: The Baltimore Conference on Ethics. Amsterdam: Gordon and Breach; 1997: 119–127. 124 refs. ISBN 2-88449-161-9. BE57011.

decision making; *human experimentation; informed consent; injuries; international aspects; *mentally ill; *placebos; *psychoactive drugs; *research design; research subjects; risk; risks and benefits; *schizophrenia; suicide; third party consent; treatment outcome; *withholding treatment; Minneapolis; United States; University of California, Los Angeles

Jacobsen, Geir; Hals, Arild. Medical investigators' views about ethics and fraud in medical research. *Journal of the Royal College of Physicians of London.* 1995 Sep–Oct; 29(5): 405–409. 20 refs. BE55562.

advisory committees; age factors; *attitudes; *biomedical research; *ethical review; evaluation; females; *fraud; freedom; historical aspects; human experimentation; information dissemination; *investigators; *knowledge, attitudes, practice; males; medical ethics; physicians; professional autonomy; professional ethics; regional ethics committees; *regulation; *research design; *research ethics committees; retrospective moral judgment; science; *scientific misconduct; *self regulation; statistics; survey; trends; *Norway; Twentieth Century

Jaffe, Norman; van Eys, Jan; Gehan, Edmund, et al. Response to "Is it ethical not to conduct a prospectively controlled trial of adjuvant chemotherapy in osteosarcoma?" [Letter and response]. *Cancer Treatment Reports.* 1983 Jul–Aug; 67(7–8): 743–745. 7 refs. BE57232.

*cancer; children; *control groups; *drugs; *human experimentation; pediatrics; prognosis; random selection; research design; surgery; treatment outcome

Josefson, Debbie. US journal attacks unethical HIV trials. [News]. *BMJ (British Medical Journal).* 1997 Sep 27; 315(7111): 765. BE56928.

*developing countries; *drugs; economics; editorial policies; *HIV seropositivity; *human experimentation; *placebos; pregnant women; public policy; *research design; Africa; Asia; AZT; Latin America; New England Journal of Medicine; United States

Kadane, Joseph B., ed. Bayesian Methods and Ethics in a Clinical Trial Design. New York, NY: Wiley; 1996. 318 p. (Wiley series in probability and statistics). Includes references. ISBN 0-471-84680-5. BE56694.

alternatives; case studies; compensation; conflict of interest; decision analysis; disclosure; drugs; *human experimentation; hypertension; informed consent; injuries; investigators; legal aspects; legal liability; *methods; models, theoretical; *random selection; *research design; research subjects; standards; *statistics; technical expertise; uncertainty; Johns Hopkins Hospital; United States

Kairys, David. The law of clinical testing with human subjects: legal implications of the new and existing methodologies. *In:* Kadane, Joseph B., ed. Bayesian Methods and Ethics in a Clinical Trial Design. New

York, NY: Wiley; 1996: 223–249. 104 fn. ISBN 0-471-84680-5. BE56696.

compensation; disclosure; federal government; government regulation; *human experimentation; informed consent; injuries; investigators; *legal aspects; legal liability; legal obligations; legal rights; malpractice; *methods; physician patient relationship; physicians; *random selection; *research design; research ethics committees; research subjects; scientific misconduct; *standards; technical expertise; United States

Kaiser, Jocelyn. Bangkok study adds fuel to AIDS ethics debate. [News]. *Science.* 1997 Nov 28; 278(5343): 1553. BE56906.

AIDS; developing countries; *drugs; *HIV seropositivity; *human experimentation; *placebos; pregnant women; *research design; AZT; *Thailand

Kaiser, Jocelyn. Flap on NEJM board over ethics articles. [News]. *Science.* 1997 Oct 10; 278(5336): 211. BE56066.

*developing countries; dissent; *editorial policies; *HIV seropositivity; *human experimentation; interprofessional relations; investigators; *newborns; *placebos; *pregnant women; scientific misconduct; withholding treatment; *Ho, David; *New England Journal of Medicine; *Wilfert, Catherine

Kane, John M.; Borenstein, Michael. The use of placebo controls in psychiatric research. *In:* Shamoo, Adil E., ed. Ethics in Neurobiological Research with Human Subjects: The Baltimore Conference on Ethics. Amsterdam: Gordon and Breach; 1997: 207–213. 11 refs. ISBN 2-88449-161-9. BE57020.

control groups; *human experimentation; *mentally ill; *placebos; *psychoactive drugs; *research design; research subjects; risks and benefits; *schizophrenia; toxicity; *withholding treatment; United States

Kaptchuk, Ted J. Powerful placebo: the dark side of the randomised controlled trial. *Lancet.* 1998 Jun 6; 351(9117): 1722–1725. 42 refs. BE58860.

attitudes; biomedical research; control groups; deception; drugs; evaluation; *historical aspects; *human experimentation; informed consent; investigators; paternalism; patient care; physicians; *placebos; *random selection; *research design; research subjects; risks and benefits; Eighteenth Century; Nineteenth Century; *Twentieth Century

Karlawish, Jason H.T.; Lantos, John. Community equipoise and the architecture of clinical research. *Cambridge Quarterly of Healthcare Ethics.* 1997 Fall; 6(4): 385–396. 51 fn. BE56465.

AIDS; autonomy; biomedical research; breast cancer; consensus; *decision making; disclosure; drugs; emergency care; federal government; government regulation; *human experimentation; informed consent; investigator subject relationship; investigators; paternalism; *patient participation; physician patient relationship; physicians; placebos; public participation; random selection; *research design; research subjects; risks and benefits; standards; technical expertise; therapeutic research; *uncertainty; values; Food and Drug Administration; United States

We have argued for a revision of Freedman's concept of clinical equipoise to a broader sense of community that includes physicians and patients. Community equipoise is an essential condition for physicians and patients to answer these questions: Should there be a trial? If so, what kind? We have argued that community equipoise exists because of changes in the knowledge gap between physicians and patients and in the moral justification of medical decision-making. Finally, we have briefly examined the social aspect of medical knowledge to argue that it necessarily includes patients

---

BE = bioethics accession number   fn. = footnotes   refs. = references

and their values. In effect, community equipoise is not so much an effort to change things, as to explain the way they are. We suggest that patients can participate at a number of points in the process of drug study design and approval: (1) study design with attention to criteria for eligibility, endpoints, and choice of methodology, (2) research review and approval with attention to enhancing community participation in IRB activities, and (3) interim evaluation of ongoing studies with attention to including patient and clinician values in the decisionmaking. Clinical trials are a tool. Like a gun or a bomb or the very drugs they test, they are powerful tools to achieve their ends. The issue is how to properly use such tools as randomization, placebo controls, endpoints, and eligibility. To the extent that community equipoise exists prior to a trial, it means that clinical researchers and patients have collectively addressed the risk and benefit trade-offs that govern the decision to start and to end a clinical trial. In this way, trials can be both valid and valued.

Kigotho, Anderson Wachira. Another HIV-1 trial loses placebo control. [News]. *Lancet.* 1997 Dec 20-27; 350(9094): 1831. BE57861.
  control groups; *developing countries; *drugs; females; *HIV seropositivity; *human experimentation; *international aspects; mothers; newborns; *placebos; *pregnant women; *research design; *therapeutic research; AZT; *Ethiopia; Johns Hopkins University; United States

Klein, Donald F. Response to Rothman and Michels on placebo-controlled clinical trials. *Psychiatric Annals.* 1995 Jul; 25(7): 401-403. 6 refs. BE56232.
  control groups; depressive disorder; *drugs; *human experimentation; informed consent; *placebos; psychoactive drugs; *research design; *risks and benefits; *therapeutic research

Langer, Anatoly; Hopf, G. Early stopping of trials. [Letters]. *Lancet.* 1997 Sep 20; 350(9081): 890-891. 2 refs. BE56563.
  breast cancer; *drug industry; financial support; heart diseases; *human experimentation; patents; *research design; *time factors; Canada; Germany; Hoechst Marion Roussel; Liposome Co.; Pfizer Ltd.; Prospective Reinfarction Outcomes in the Thrombolytic Era Cardizem CD Trial (PROTECT); United States

Lantos, John D. Was the UK collaborative ECMO trial ethical? *Paediatric and Perinatal Epidemiology.* 1997 Jul; 11(3): 264-268. 7 refs. BE58033.
  alternatives; *biomedical technologies; coercion; congenital disorders; critically ill; *human experimentation; international aspects; mortality; *newborns; parental consent; *patient care; *random selection; *research design; risks and benefits; *technology assessment; *therapeutic research; time factors; *treatment outcome; uncertainty; *extracorporeal membrane oxygenation; *Great Britain

Levine, Robert J. The "best proven therapeutic method" standard in clinical trials in technologically developing countries. [Editorial]. *IRB: A Review of Human Subjects Research.* 1998 Jan-Feb; 20(1): 5-9. 19 fn. BE58519.
  *control groups; *developing countries; *drugs; economics; guidelines; *HIV seropositivity; *human experimentation; international aspects; newborns; patient care; *placebos; *pregnant women; *research design; *standards; *AZT; Declaration of Helsinki

Lewith, George T. Ethical problems in evaluating complementary medicine. *Bulletin of Medical Ethics.* 1996 Aug; No. 120: 17-20. 15 refs. BE55879.
  *alternative therapies; chronically ill; control groups;

*evaluation; guidelines; *human experimentation; placebos; *research design; research ethics committees; research subjects; selection of subjects; therapeutic research; treatment outcome; General Medical Council (Great Britain); *Great Britain

Lindley, Richard I. Thrombolytic treatment for acute ischaemic stroke: consent can be ethical. *BMJ (British Medical Journal).* 1998 Mar 28; 316(7136): 1005-1007. 13 refs. BE57556.
  attitudes; competence; consent forms; drugs; guidelines; *human experimentation; *informed consent; patients; *random selection; research design; research subjects; *risks and benefits; *therapeutic research; *cerebrovascular disorders; *thrombolytic therapy

Marshall, Eliot. AIDS therapy: controversial trial offers hopeful result. [News]. *Science.* 1998 Feb 27; 279(5355): 1299. BE57260.
  costs and benefits; *developing countries; *drugs; *HIV seropositivity; *human experimentation; international aspects; newborns; *placebos; *pregnant women; *research design; therapeutic research; time factors; *Africa; *AZT; *Thailand

Marwick, Charles. Bioethics group considers transnational research. [News]. *JAMA.* 1998 May 13; 279(18): 1425. BE57862.
  advisory committees; *developing countries; *drugs; federal government; government financing; guidelines; *HIV seropositivity; *human experimentation; *international aspects; newborns; *placebos; *pregnant women; *public policy; *research design; scientific misconduct; *therapeutic research; *Africa; AZT; Declaration of Helsinki; National Bioethics Advisory Commission; *United States

Mason, Su; Brown, Julia; Levene, Malcolm. What is this thing called "randomise"? [Editorial]. *Lancet.* 1997 Nov 15; 350(9089): 1416. 3 refs. BE57162.
  attitudes; *comprehension; control groups; critically ill; disclosure; empirical research; *human experimentation; informed consent; *newborns; *parental consent; parents; psychological stress; *random selection; research design; research subjects; selection of subjects; *therapeutic research; extracorporeal membrane oxygenation; qualitative research; Europe; European Union; Great Britain

Moore, Dale; Popp, A. John; Katz, Katheryn D., et al. Commentary I [and] Commentary II on "The law of clinical testing with human subjects," [and] Author's response. *In:* Kadane, Joseph B., ed. Bayesian Methods and Ethics in a Clinical Trial Design. New York, NY: Wiley; 1996: 251-266. 18 fn. ISBN 0-471-84680-5. BE56697.
  compensation; constitutional law; decision making; disclosure; drugs; evaluation; federal government; government regulation; *human experimentation; informed consent; injuries; investigators; *legal aspects; legal liability; malpractice; *methods; patients; *random selection; *research design; research subjects; risks and benefits; standards; vulnerable populations; United States

Narasimhan, Parthas; Kalra, Jagmohan; Warde, Padraig, et al. Ethical questions on the testicular seminoma study. [Letter and response]. *Journal of Clinical Oncology.* 1996 Feb; 14(2): 684. 5 refs. BE57512.
  *cancer; drugs; *human experimentation; *males; radiology; *research design; risk; risks and benefits; standards; withholding treatment

O'Fallon, Judith Rich. Policies for interim analysis and interim reporting of results. [Article and discussion]. *Cancer Treatment Reports.* 1985 Oct; 69(10): 1101-1106. 1 ref. BE57833.

BE = bioethics accession number   fn. = footnotes   refs. = references

cancer; *human experimentation; *information dissemination; *research design; time factors; treatment outcome; Mayo Comprehensive Cancer Center

Phanuphak, Praphan. Ethical issues in studies in Thailand of the vertical transmission of HIV. *New England Journal of Medicine.* 1998 Mar 19; 338(12): 834–835. 5 refs. BE57707.
AIDS; alternatives; control groups; *developing countries; *drugs; government financing; *HIV seropositivity; *human experimentation; international aspects; *newborns; *nontherapeutic research; *placebos; *pregnant women; *preventive medicine; private sector; *public policy; *research design; resource allocation; scientific misconduct; *therapeutic research; time factors; withholding treatment; *AZT; Centers for Disease Control and Prevention; National Institutes of Health; *Thailand; United States; Walter Reed Army Institute of Research

Schaffner, Kenneth F. Ethically optimizing clinical trials. *In:* Kadane, Joseph B., ed. Bayesian Methods and Ethics in a Clinical Trial Design. New York, NY: Wiley; 1996: 19–63. 95 refs. 49 fn. ISBN 0–471–84680–5. BE56695.
breast cancer; case studies; conflict of interest; critically ill; decision analysis; disclosure; drugs; ethical analysis; ethical theory; *human experimentation; hypertension; informed consent; investigators; methods; moral policy; patients; physician patient relationship; physicians; placebos; principle-based ethics; *random selection; *research design; research subjects; review; rights; surgery; uncertainty; values; National Surgical Adjuvant Breast and Bowel Project; United States

Schüklenk, Udo; Hogan, Carlton. AIDS clinical trials: ethical and design issues. *International Journal of Bioethics.* 1997 Sep; 8(3): 127–132. 29 refs. BE57432.
*AIDS; autonomy; coercion; *drugs; *human experimentation; patient compliance; patient participation; patients; political activity; random selection; *research design; research subjects; selection of subjects; terminally ill; *therapeutic research; uncertainty; volunteers

Senn, Stephen; Ramsay, Lawrence E. Are placebo run ins justified? [Article and commentary]. *BMJ (British Medical Journal).* 1997 Apr 19; 314(7088): 1191–1193. 18 refs. BE56772.
*deception; disclosure; drugs; *human experimentation; *informed consent; patients; physicians; *placebos; random selection; *research design; research subjects

Snowdon, Claire; Garcia, Jo; Elbourne, Diana. Reactions of participants to the results of a randomised controlled trial: exploratory study. *BMJ (British Medical Journal).* 1998 Jul 4; 317(7150): 21–26. 12 refs. BE58814.
*attitudes; *communication; comparative studies; *control groups; *disclosure; *emotions; human experimentation; mortality; *newborns; *parents; psychological stress; *random selection; research subjects; survey; *therapeutic research; *treatment outcome; ventilators; *extracorporeal membrane oxygenation; *feedback; qualitative research; Great Britain
OBJECTIVES: To assess views of parents of babies who participated in a neonatal trial, about feedback of trial results. DESIGN: Qualitative analysis of interviews. SETTING: Parents' homes. SUBJECTS: Parents of 24 surviving babies enrolled in a UK randomised controlled trial comparing ventilatory support by extracorporeal membrane oxygenation with conventional management. MAIN OUTCOME MEASURES: Views about contents of results, reactions to results, effect of hindsight, and importance of feedback. RESULTS: Information about mortality was well understood by the parents but morbidity was less clearly reported. Even when the content was emotionally exacting, the

information was still wanted as it removed uncertainty; provided an endpoint to difficult events; promoted further discussion within couples; and acknowledged their contribution to answering an important clinical question. CONCLUSIONS: Feedback of trial results to participants should be a consideration of researchers, but a careful approach is required. This study was based on a highly selective group of parents within a particularly sensitive trial. More research is needed to assess the extent to which these results can be generalised to other trials or to groups such as bereaved parents.

Taylor, Kathryn M.; Mehta, Cyrus; Patterson, Bradford, et al. The doctor's dilemma: physician participation in randomized clinical trials. [Article and discussion]. *Cancer Treatment Reports.* 1985 Oct; 69(10): 1095–1100. 6 refs. BE56963.
*attitudes; *human experimentation; informed consent; methods; physician patient relationship; *physicians; *random selection; research design; *selection of subjects; surgery; survey; uncertainty; Canada; *National Surgical Adjuvant Breast and Bowel Project; United States

UCLA Clinical Research Center. Statement of the UCLA Clinical Research Center. *In:* Shamoo, Adil E., ed. Ethics in Neurobiological Research with Human Subjects: The Baltimore Conference on Ethics. Amsterdam: Gordon and Breach; 1997: 173–174. ISBN 2–88449–161–9. BE57014.
advisory committees; *human experimentation; institutional policies; *mentally ill; professional family relationship; *program descriptions; *psychoactive drugs; *research design; research institutes; research subjects; *schizophrenia; scientific misconduct; withholding treatment; National Institutes of Health; Office for Protection from Research Risks; *UCLA Clinical Research Center; United States

Varmus, Harold; Satcher, David. Ethical complexities of conducting research in developing countries. *New England Journal of Medicine.* 1997 Oct 2; 337(14): 1003–1005. 6 refs. BE55835.
AIDS; autonomy; beneficence; *control groups; *developing countries; *drugs; economics; ethical review; federal government; *HIV seropositivity; *human experimentation; international aspects; justice; *moral policy; *newborns; *placebos; *pregnant women; *preventive medicine; *public policy; *research design; risks and benefits; *therapeutic research; *AZT; Centers for Disease Control and Prevention; National Institutes of Health; *United States

Wadman, Meredith. Controversy flares over AIDS prevention trials in Third World. [News]. *Nature.* 1997 Oct 30; 389(6654): 894. BE56162.
*developing countries; *drugs; federal government; government financing; government regulation; *HIV seropositivity; *human experimentation; investigators; newborns; *placebos; *pregnant women; preventive medicine; *research design; therapeutic research; *AZT; Department of Health and Human Services; Johns Hopkins University; National Institutes of Health; Public Citizen; *United States

Weymuller, Ernest A. A consideration of ethical issues in the design of clinical trials. *American Journal of Otolaryngology.* 1996 Jan–Feb; 17(1): 2–11. 26 refs. BE57350.
accountability; autonomy; ethical review; federal government; government regulation; historical aspects; *human experimentation; informed consent; international aspects; investigators; justice; *nontherapeutic research; physician's role; random selection; *research design; research ethics committees; research subjects; risk; risks and benefits; *therapeutic research; investigational therapies; Germany; United States

---

BE = bioethics accession number   fn. = footnotes   refs. = references

Young, Simon N.; Annable, Lawrence; Canadian College of Neuropsychopharmacology. The use of placebos in psychiatry: a response to the draft document prepared by the Tri–Council Working Group. [Position paper]. *Journal of Psychiatry and Neuroscience.* 1996 Jul; 21(4): 235–238. 15 refs. Approved at a meeting of the CCNP Council 2 Jun 1996 and at the CCNP Annual General Business Meeting 4 Jun 1996. BE57666.
    *depressive disorder; *human experimentation; *mentally ill; *organizational policies; physicians; *placebos; professional organizations; *psychiatry; *psychoactive drugs; *research design; Canada; *Canadian College of Neuropsychopharmacology; Code of Conduct for Research Involving Humans

Good manners for the pharmaceutical industry. [Editorial]. *Lancet.* 1997 Jun 7; 349(9066): 1635. BE56572.
    cancer; *coercion; *drug industry; drugs; *financial support; *human experimentation; international aspects; investigators; *research design; *therapeutic research; time factors; Bristol–Myers Squibb; Great Britain; International Collaboration on Ovarian Neoplasm (ICON3)

Pragmatism in codes of research ethics. [Editorial]. *Lancet.* 1998 Jan 24; 351(9098): 225. BE57817.
    codes of ethics; control groups; *developing countries; drugs; editorial policies; ethical relativism; guidelines; HIV seropositivity; *human experimentation; informed consent; *international aspects; *placebos; *research design; Lancet

HUMAN EXPERIMENTATION/SPECIAL POPULATIONS

Addis, G.J.; London, D. The *BMJ*'s Nuremberg issue. [Letters]. *BMJ (British Medical Journal).* 1997 Apr 12; 314(7087): 1128. 2 refs. BE57240.
    *conscience; *historical aspects; *human experimentation; *moral obligations; National Socialism; nontherapeutic research; *obligations to society; organizational policies; physicians; professional organizations; religion; *research subjects; *volunteers; *war; Germany; *Great Britain; Royal College of Physicians of London; Twentieth Century; *World War II

Adler, Martin W.; College on Problems of Drug Dependence. Human subject issues in drug abuse research. *Drug and Alcohol Dependence.* 1995 Feb; 37(2): 167–175. 29 refs. BE56200.
    competence; *drug abuse; federal government; government regulation; *human experimentation; informed consent; patient care; remuneration; research design; research ethics committees; risks and benefits; selection of subjects; volunteers; United States

Aller, Robert; Aller, Gregory. An institutional response to patient/family complaints. *In:* Shamoo, Adil E., ed. Ethics in Neurobiological Research with Human Subjects: The Baltimore Conference on Ethics. Amsterdam: Gordon and Breach; 1997: 155–172. 32 fn. This paper provides the viewpoints of a father and of his son, who was a research subject at the UCLA Clinical Research Center. ISBN 2–88449–161–9. BE57013.
    administrators; case studies; consent forms; *deception; *disclosure; family members; *human experimentation; iatrogenic disease; *informed consent; medical records; *mentally ill; patients; physician patient relationship; placebos; professional family relationship; *psychoactive drugs; *research design; research subjects; risks and benefits; *schizophrenia; *scientific misconduct; suicide; treatment outcome; universities; *withholding treatment; patient abandonment; *UCLA Neuropsychiatric Institute; United States; *University of California, Los Angeles

Alt–White, Anna C. Obtaining "informed" consent from the elderly. *Western Journal of Nursing Research.* 1995 Dec; 17(6): 700–705. 10 refs. 2 fn. BE55600.
    *aged; competence; comprehension; decision making; disabled; education; family members; *human experimentation; *informed consent; institutionalized persons; investigators; nursing research; recall; research subjects

American Association of Critical Care Nurses. Task Force on Ethics in Critical Care Research. Statement on ethics in critical care research. Part One. *Focus on Critical Care.* 1985 Jun; 12(3): 47–50. 16 refs. BE56651.
    administrators; *critically ill; *guidelines; *human experimentation; informed consent; *nurses; *organizational policies; patient care; peer review; professional organizations; research ethics committees; research subjects; vulnerable populations; *American Association of Critical Care Nurses; United States

American Association of Critical Care Nurses. Task Force on Ethics in Critical Care Research. Statement on ethics in critical care research. Part Two. *Focus on Critical Care.* 1985 Aug; 12(4): 58–63. 16 refs. BE56652.
    administrators; competence; *critically ill; disclosure; *guidelines; *human experimentation; *informed consent; investigators; *nurses; *organizational policies; patient care; professional organizations; research ethics committees; research subjects; *American Association of Critical Care Nurses; United States

Annas, George J.; Glantz, Leonard H. Informed consent to research on institutionalized mentally disabled persons: the dual problems of incapacity and voluntariness. *In:* Shamoo, Adil E., ed. Ethics in Neurobiological Research with Human Subjects: The Baltimore Conference on Ethics. Amsterdam: Gordon and Breach; 1997: 55–79. 46 fn. Appendices include the text of the Nuremberg Code and parts of the U.S. Department of Health, Education, and Welfare regulations proposed in 1978 on "protections pertaining to biomedical and behavioral research involving as subjects individuals institutionalized as mentally disabled." ISBN 2–88449–161–9. BE57009.
    behavior control; *coercion; *competence; comprehension; *decision making; federal government; government regulation; guidelines; hepatitis; *human experimentation; immunization; *informed consent; *institutionalized persons; involuntary commitment; judicial action; *legal aspects; *mentally disabled; *mentally ill; model legislation; nontherapeutic research; organ donation; patient advocacy; patient care; prisoners; psychoactive drugs; *regulation; research ethics committees; research subjects; scientific misconduct; state interest; sterilization (sexual); therapeutic research; *third party consent; treatment refusal; DHEW Guidelines; Nuremberg Code; *United States

Association for Improvements in the Maternity Services (Great Britain); National Childbirth Trust (Great Britain); Maternity Alliance (Great Britain). A charter for ethical research in maternity care: Association for Improvements in the Maternity Services; the National Childbirth Trust. *Nursing Ethics.* 1998 May; 5(3): 256–262. 10 fn. Reprinted with permission from the Association for Improvements in the Maternity Services. BE58725.
    behavioral research; childbirth; confidentiality; disclosure; *guidelines; *human experimentation; informed consent; *maternal health; mothers; newborns; organizational policies; *pregnant women; research design; research subjects; *Association for Improvements in the Maternity Services (Great Britain); *Great Britain; *National Childbirth Trust (Great Britain)

BE = bioethics accession number   fn. = footnotes   refs. = references

Ault, Alicia. USA accused of funding placebo–controlled AIDS trials. [News]. *Lancet.* 1997 May 3; 349(9061): 1305. BE56073.
> AIDS; *developing countries; drugs; federal government; government financing; *HIV seropositivity; *human experimentation; *newborns; *placebos; *pregnant women; public policy; withholding treatment; AZT; Centers for Disease Control and Prevention; National Institutes of Health; *United States

Avorn, Jerry. Including elderly people in clinical trials: better information could improve the effectiveness and safety of drug use. [Editorial]. *BMJ (British Medical Journal).* 1997 Oct 25; 315(7115): 1033–1034. 8 refs. BE56555.
> *aged; costs and benefits; drug industry; *drugs; *human experimentation; patient care; research design; *research subjects; risks and benefits; *selection of subjects; *postmarketing research

Babbs, Charles F. Falacious arguments against resuscitation research. *American Journal of Emergency Medicine.* 1985 Sep; 3(5): 461–466. 46 refs. BE56973.
> *critically ill; *emergency care; human experimentation; informed consent; morbidity; preventive medicine; *resuscitation; *risks and benefits; standards; terminally ill; *therapeutic research; treatment outcome

Barnes, Patricia G. Beyond Nuremberg: fifty years later, the debate continues on informed consent. *ABA Journal: The Lawyer's Magazine.* 1997 Mar; 83: 24–27. BE58508.
> adults; competence; government regulation; *human experimentation; informed consent; institutionalized persons; *legal aspects; mental institutions; *mentally ill; minors; *nontherapeutic research; parental consent; psychoactive drugs; risk; state government; *third party consent; withholding treatment; New York; *T.D. v. New York State Office of Mental Health

Baskin, Shari A.; Morris, Jane; Ahronheim, Judith C., et al. Barriers to obtaining consent in dementia research: implications for surrogate decision–making. *Journal of the American Geriatrics Society.* 1998 Mar; 46(3): 287–290. 16 refs. BE56752.
> aged; comprehension; *decision making; *dementia; evaluation studies; *family members; health services research; hospitals; *human experimentation; institutionalized persons; legal guardians; minority groups; palliative care; single persons; terminally ill; *third party consent; vulnerable populations; absence of proxy; Mount Sinai Medical Center (New York City)

Baylis, Françoise; Downie, Jocelyn; Sherwin, Susan. Reframing research involving humans. *In:* Sherwin, Susan, et al. The Politics of Women's Health: Exploring Agency and Autonomy. Philadelphia, PA: Temple University Press; 1998: 234–259. 20 fn. ISBN 1–56639–633–6. BE58400.
> advisory committees; attitudes; autonomy; behavioral research; federal government; *females; *feminist ethics; government regulation; *guidelines; *human experimentation; indigents; investigators; minority groups; occupational exposure; political activity; public policy; research design; research subjects; risks and benefits; scientific misconduct; *selection of subjects; social discrimination; Canada; Feminist Health Care Ethics Research Network (Canada); *Tri–Council Working Group (Canada); United States

Berghmans, R.L.P. Advance directives for non–therapeutic dementia research: some ethical and policy considerations. *Journal of Medical Ethics.* 1998 Feb; 24(1): 32–37. 25 refs. BE57403.
> *advance directives; *competence; decision making; *dementia; *human experimentation; informed consent; moral policy; *nontherapeutic research; personhood; research subjects; selection of subjects; self concept; third party consent
> This paper explores the use of advance directives in clinical dementia research. The focus is on advance consent to participation of demented patients in non–therapeutic research involving more than minimal risks and/or burdens. First, morally relevant differences between advance directives for treatment and care, and advance directives for dementia research are discussed. Then attention is paid to the philosophical issue of dementia and personal identity, and the implications for the moral authority of research advance directives. Thirdly, a number of practical shortcomings of advance directives for non–therapeutic dementia research are explored and attention is paid to the role of proxies. It is concluded that upon a closer look the initial attractiveness of advance directives for dementia research is lessened, and that it is doubtful whether these instruments can compensate for the lack of subject consent in case of non–therapeutic dementia research involving more than minimal risks and/or burdens for the incompetent demented subject.

Berghmans, Ron L.P.; ter Meulen, Rudd H.J. Ethical issues in research with dementia patients. *International Journal of Geriatric Psychiatry.* 1995 Aug; 10(8): 647–651. 15 refs. BE56610.
> aged; common good; competence; *dementia; future generations; goals; *human experimentation; moral policy; *nontherapeutic research; risks and benefits; science; *therapeutic research; third party consent

Bergsma, Jurrit. Response to "Ethical concerns about relapse studies" by Adil E. Shamoo and Timothy J. Keay: Research with vulnerable subjects. [Letter]. *Cambridge Quarterly of Healthcare Ethics.* 1997 Spring; 6(2): 233–234. 1 ref. Commentary on A.E. Shamoo and T.J. Keay, *CQ*, 1996 Summer; 5(3): 373–386. BE56423.
> beneficence; competence; conflict of interest; empirical research; *human experimentation; informed consent; interprofessional relations; *investigators; mentally ill; *patient advocacy; *physicians; placebos; psychoactive drugs; research design; research ethics committees; research subjects; schizophrenia; scientific misconduct; selection of subjects; *vulnerable populations; withholding treatment

Birchard, Karen. Irish research project abandoned after adverse publicity. [News]. *Lancet.* 1998 Feb 7; 351(9100): 426. BE58886.
> *human experimentation; *mentally ill; nutrition; *Ireland

Brakel, Samuel Jan. Considering behavioral and biomedical research on detainees in the mental health unit of an urban mega–jail. *New England Journal on Criminal and Civil Confinement.* 1996 Winter; 22(1): 1–27. 92 fn. BE57190.
> behavioral research; beneficence; coercion; competence; comprehension; confidentiality; federal government; government regulation; *human experimentation; incentives; informed consent; legal aspects; *mentally ill; nontherapeutic research; *prisoners; private sector; remuneration; research ethics committees; research subjects; right to treatment; selection of subjects; treatment refusal; Department of Health and Human Services; Isaac Ray Center (Cook County, IL); United States

Brody, Baruch A. Research involving vulnerable subjects. *In: his* The Ethics of Biomedical Research: An International Perspective. New York, NY: Oxford University Press; 1998: 119–138, 370–372. 45 fn. ISBN 0–19–509007–1. BE57673.

BE = bioethics accession number   fn. = footnotes   refs. = references

*adolescents; age factors; *children; coercion; comparative studies; competence; consensus; decision making; family members; government regulation; guidelines; historical aspects; *human experimentation; informed consent; institutionalized persons; *international aspects; legal guardians; *mentally disabled; *minors; nontherapeutic research; parental consent; *prisoners; research ethics committees; review; risks and benefits; scientific misconduct; therapeutic research; third party consent; *vulnerable populations; Canada; Europe; Great Britain; United States

Brody, Baruch A. Research involving women and members of minority groups. *In: his* The Ethics of Biomedical Research: An International Perspective. New York, NY: Oxford University Press; 1998: 185–196, 375–376. 23 fn. ISBN 0-19-509007-1. BE57676.

drugs; federal government; *females; fetuses; government regulation; guidelines; *human experimentation; international aspects; *minority groups; moral obligations; *pregnant women; *public policy; research design; therapeutic research; trust; women's health; community consent; *Canada; Food and Drug Administration; National Institutes of Health; *United States

Bugeja, G.; Kumar, A.; Banerjee, Arup K. Exclusion of elderly people from clinical research: a descriptive study of published reports. *BMJ (British Medical Journal).* 1997 Oct 25; 315(7115): 1059. 3 refs. BE56558.

*aged; disclosure; editorial policies; empirical research; *human experimentation; literature; patient care; *research subjects; *selection of subjects; social discrimination; survey; BMJ (British Medical Journal); Gut; Lancet; Thorax

Butler, Declan. Admission on Gulf War vaccines spurs debate on medical records. [News]. *Nature.* 1997 Nov 6; 390(6655): 3–4. BE56858.

biological warfare; epidemiology; *human experimentation; *immunization; injuries; medical records; *military personnel; *morbidity; *public policy; *war; whooping cough; *Great Britain; *Ministry of Defence (Great Britain); *Persian Gulf War

Campbell, Jean. Reforming the IRB process: towards new guidelines for quality and accountability in protecting human subjects. *In:* Shamoo, Adil E., ed. Ethics in Neurobiological Research with Human Subjects: The Baltimore Conference on Ethics. Amsterdam: Gordon and Breach; 1997: 299–303. ISBN 2-88449-161-9. BE57022.

accountability; communication; dehumanization; evaluation; family members; health services research; *human experimentation; *investigator subject relationship; investigators; *mentally ill; paternalism; *patient advocacy; *patient participation; patients; research design; *research ethics committees; research subjects; risks and benefits; stigmatization; United States

Carpenter, William T. Schizophrenia research: a challenge for constructive criticism. *In:* Shamoo, Adil E., ed. Ethics in Neurobiological Research with Human Subjects: The Baltimore Conference on Ethics. Amsterdam: Gordon and Breach; 1997: 215–228. 40 refs. ISBN 2-88449-161-9. BE57021.

attitudes; autonomy; *dissent; ethicists; evaluation; federal government; government regulation; *human experimentation; informed consent; injuries; investigators; *mentally ill; patient advocacy; patient care; patient compliance; patient transfer; patients; placebos; *psychoactive drugs; *research design; research subjects; *risks and benefits; *schizophrenia; scientific misconduct; toxicity; treatment outcome; *withholding treatment; patient abandonment; Maryland Psychiatric Research Center (Baltimore); National Alliance for the Mentally Ill; Office for Protection from Research Risks; United States

Carpenter, William T.; Schooler, Nina R.; Kane, John M. The rationale and ethics of medication-free research in schizophrenia. *Archives of General Psychiatry.* 1997 May; 54(5): 401–407. 58 refs. Commented on by F.A. Henn et al., p. 411–412, and by J.J. Fins and F.G. Miller, p. 415–416. BE57902.

*human experimentation; informed consent; *mentally ill; placebos; *psychoactive drugs; *research design; research subjects; *risks and benefits; *schizophrenia; selection of subjects; *withholding treatment

Cassel, Christine K. Research in nursing homes: ethical issues. *Journal of the American Geriatrics Society.* 1985 Nov; 33(11): 795–799. 11 refs. BE56961.

advisory committees; *aged; chronically ill; coercion; competence; confidentiality; conflict of interest; dementia; federal government; government regulation; *health services research; historical aspects; *human experimentation; informed consent; institutionalized persons; justice; long-term care; nontherapeutic research; *nursing homes; physicians; research design; research ethics committees; *research subjects; *risks and benefits; scientific misconduct; selection of subjects; therapeutic research; National Commission for the Protection of Human Subjects; Twentieth Century; United States

Chen, Yuan-Fang. Japanese death factories and the American cover-up. *Cambridge Quarterly of Healthcare Ethics.* 1997 Spring; 6(2): 240–242. BE56425.

accountability; aliens; *biological warfare; communicable diseases; *historical aspects; *human experimentation; human rights; international aspects; investigators; killing; medical ethics; military personnel; moral complicity; National Socialism; physicians; *prisoners; *public policy; *research subjects; *scientific misconduct; torture; *war; China; Factories of Death (Harris, S.); Germany; Ishii, Shiro; *Japan; Twentieth Century; *United States; *World War II

Clark, Peter A. The ethics of placebo-controlled trials for perinatal transmission of HIV in developing countries. *Journal of Clinical Ethics.* 1998 Summer; 9(2): 156–166. 44 fn. BE58961.

AIDS; alternatives; autonomy; beneficence; common good; comprehension; *control groups; costs and benefits; *developing countries; drugs; ethical analysis; ethical relativism; guidelines; *HIV seropositivity; *human experimentation; human rights; informed consent; international aspects; justice; *moral policy; morbidity; *newborns; patient care; *placebos; *pregnant women; prevalence; public policy; *research design; research subjects; risks and benefits; socioeconomic factors; standards; vulnerable populations; AZT; United States

Clinton, William J. Remarks by the president in apology for study done in Tuskegee. Washington, DC: The White House, Office of the Press Secretary, [Online]. Available: http://www1.whitehouse.gov/New/Remarks/Fri/199 70516-898.html; 1997 May 16. 3 p. Downloaded 22 Aug 1997. BE57692.

advisory committees; bioethics; *blacks; compensation; education; ethical review; federal government; *human experimentation; indigents; informed consent; *nontherapeutic research; *public policy; *research subjects; *scientific misconduct; selection of subjects; syphilis; trust; *withholding treatment; National Bioethics Advisory Commission; *Tuskegee Syphilis Study; *United States

Darvall, Leanna. Gender and equity: emerging issues in Australian clinical drug trial regulatory policies. *In:* Petersen, Kerry, ed. Intersections: Women on Law, Medicine and Technology. Brookfield, VT: Ashgate; 1997: 185–200. 18 refs. 1 fn. ISBN 1-85521-882-8. BE57492.

---

age factors; AIDS; costs and benefits; *drugs; federal government; *females; *government regulation; *guidelines; *human experimentation; international aspects; justice; males; minority groups; *nontherapeutic research; pregnant women; prenatal injuries; *public policy; research design; *risks and benefits; *selection of subjects; toxicity; *Australia; Department of Health and Human Services; Food and Drug Administration; National Institutes of Health; *United States

Destro, Robert A. Government oversight. *In:* Shamoo, Adil E., ed. Ethics in Neurobiological Research with Human Subjects: The Baltimore Conference on Ethics. Amsterdam: Gordon and Breach; 1997: 81–99. 90 fn. ISBN 2-88449-161-9. BE57010.
    behavioral research; coercion; *competence; comprehension; conflict of interest; *disclosure; federal government; *government regulation; *human experimentation; *informed consent; investigator subject relationship; investigators; *legal aspects; mentally disabled; minors; nontherapeutic research; professional ethics; research ethics committees; research subjects; state government; therapeutic research; *third party consent; *vulnerable populations; *United States

Dresser, Rebecca; Whitehouse, Peter. Emergency research and research involving subjects with cognitive impairment: ethical connections and contrasts. [Editorial]. *Journal of the American Geriatrics Society.* 1997 Apr; 45(4): 521–523. 7 refs. BE57113.
    advance directives; *chronically ill; comparative studies; *competence; *critically ill; *decision making; *dementia; disclosure; *emergency care; family members; federal government; government regulation; *human experimentation; *informed consent; investigators; legal aspects; legal guardians; *mentally disabled; nontherapeutic research; patient participation; public participation; research ethics committees; *risks and benefits; therapeutic research; *third party consent; United States

Farthing, Charles F. A necessary risk: why we doctors should volunteer to try an AIDS vaccine. *Washington Post.* 1997 Oct 19: C1, C6. BE57845.
    *AIDS; *autoexperimentation; historical aspects; *human experimentation; *immunization; *physicians; professional organizations; risks and benefits; *volunteers; International Association of Physicians in AIDS Care

Fins, Joseph J.; Miller, Franklin G. The call of the sirens: navigating the ethics of medication-free research in schizophrenia. [Commentary]. *Archives of General Psychiatry.* 1997 May; 54(5): 415–416. 10 refs. Commentary by W.T. Carpenter et al., p. 401–407. BE57903.
    *human experimentation; informed consent; *mentally ill; psychiatric wills; *psychoactive drugs; *research design; research subjects; *schizophrenia; *withholding treatment

Fisher, Celia B. A relational perspective on ethics–in–science decisionmaking for research with vulnerable populations. *IRB: A Review of Human Subjects Research.* 1997 Sep–Oct; 19(5): 1–4. 31 refs. BE57137.
    adolescents; attitudes; autonomy; behavioral research; beneficence; caring; confidentiality; *decision making; disadvantaged; disclosure; federal government; government regulation; guidelines; *human experimentation; informed consent; *investigator subject relationship; investigators; justice; mentally disabled; moral obligations; public policy; *research subjects; risks and benefits; third party consent; *vulnerable populations; United States

Fisher, Celia B. Presentation before the National Bioethics Advisory Commission Human Subjects Subcommittee: a relational perspective on ethics-in-science decision making. *In:* BioLaw: A Legal and Ethical Reporter on

Medicine, Health Care, and Bioengineering. Special Sections, 2(7–8). Frederick, MD: University Publications of America; 1997 Jul–Aug: S:153–S:159. 38 refs. BE55931.
    adolescents; advisory committees; behavioral research; caring; communication; confidentiality; *decision making; disadvantaged; federal government; government regulation; guidelines; *human experimentation; *investigator subject relationship; *investigators; justice; mentally disabled; minority groups; moral policy; public policy; *research subjects; risks and benefits; *vulnerable populations; National Bioethics Advisory Commission; United States

Frese, Frederick J. A consumer/professional's view of ethics in research. [Personal narrative]. *In:* Shamoo, Adil E., ed. Ethics in Neurobiological Research with Human Subjects: The Baltimore Conference on Ethics. Amsterdam: Gordon and Breach; 1997: 191–194. 3 refs. ISBN 2-88449-161-9. BE57017.
    advance directives; *attitudes; committee membership; competence; family members; health personnel; *human experimentation; informed consent; institutionalized persons; investigators; *mentally ill; patient participation; *patients; psychology; research ethics committees; research subjects; schizophrenia; third party consent; United States

Goodwin, Frederick K.; Hadley, Suzanne W. Enhancing the climate of trust in clinical psychiatric research. *In:* Shamoo, Adil E., ed. Ethics in Neurobiological Research with Human Subjects: The Baltimore Conference on Ethics. Amsterdam: Gordon and Breach; 1997: 309–314. 3 refs. ISBN 2-88449-161-9. BE57023.
    *communication; competence; family members; goals; government regulation; *human experimentation; informed consent; investigator subject relationship; *investigators; *mentally ill; moral obligations; nontherapeutic research; *patient advocacy; patient care; patients; psychiatric diagnosis; research ethics committees; *research subjects; risks and benefits; therapeutic research; *trust; National Alliance for the Mentally Ill; National Institute of Mental Health; United States

Haimowitz, Stephan; Delano, Susan J.; Oldham, John M. Uninformed decisionmaking: the case of surrogate research consent. *Hastings Center Report.* 1997 Nov–Dec; 27(6): 9–16. 26 fn. BE57854.
    adults; biomedical research; *competence; constitutional law; *decision making; dementia; family members; federal government; *government regulation; *human experimentation; *judicial action; *legal aspects; *mentally ill; minors; *nontherapeutic research; parental consent; patient advocacy; psychoactive drugs; research ethics committees; *risks and benefits; social impact; state government; suicide; therapeutic research; *third party consent; Department of Health and Human Services; Food and Drug Administration; *New York; Office of Mental Health (NY); *T.D. v. New York State Office of Mental Health; United States
A New York court recently struck down state Office of Mental Health regulations governing research involving subjects with impaired decisionmaking capacity. The court held that neither incapacitated adults nor minors could participate in any research protocol that contained a nontherapeutic element, irrespective of possible benefits to the subject or the importance of the knowledge to be gained. Although the decision rested on a technical point of law and dealt only with psychiatric research, the court's holding has significantly broader implications.

Halsey, Neal A.; Sommer, Alfred; Henderson, Donald A., et al. Ethics and international research. [Editorial]. *BMJ (British Medical Journal).* 1997 Oct 18; 315(7114): 965–966. 8 refs. BE55908.

BE = bioethics accession number   fn. = footnotes   refs. = references

*developing countries; *drugs; economics; *ethical relativism; guidelines; health care delivery; *HIV seropositivity; *human experimentation; *international aspects; *newborns; *placebos; *pregnant women; *research design; standards; *AZT; Centers for Disease Control and Prevention; Council for International Organizations of Medical Sciences; United States; World Health Organization

Hamilton, Jean A. Women and health policy: on the inclusion of females in clinical trials. *In:* Sargent, Carolyn F.; Brettell, Caroline B., eds. Gender and Health: An International Perspective. Upper Saddle River, NJ: Prentice Hall; 1996: 292–325. 121 refs. 35 fn. ISBN 0-13-079427-9. BE58096.
contraception; developing countries; *drugs; economics; federal government; *females; fetuses; *government regulation; guidelines; *human experimentation; informed consent; international aspects; investigators; males; minority groups; *public policy; research design; risks and benefits; *selection of subjects; *social discrimination; therapeutic research; *women's health; *Food and Drug Administration; *National Institutes of Health; U.S. Congress; *United States

Harris, Yvonne; Gorelick, Philip B.; Samuels, Patricia, et al. Why African Americans may not be participating in clinical trials. *Journal of the National Medical Association.* 1996 Oct; 88(10): 630–634. 19 refs. BE57569.
*attitudes; *blacks; communication; health; *human experimentation; morbidity; mortality; *research subjects; scientific misconduct; selection of subjects; socioeconomic factors; statistics; survey; trust; whites; cerebrovascular disorders; United States

Henn, Fritz A.; Lader, Malcolm; Helmchen, Hanfried. Medication-free research with schizophrenic patients: a European perspective. [Commentary]. *Archives of General Psychiatry.* 1997 May; 54(5): 412–413. 8 refs. Commentary on W.T. Carpenter et al., p. 401–407. BE57904.
*human experimentation; *mentally ill; placebos; *psychoactive drugs; *research design; risks and benefits; *schizophrenia; *withholding treatment; Europe

Hilts, Philip J. Experiments on children are reviewed: research involved now-banned drug. [News]. *New York Times.* 1998 Apr 15: B3. BE57728.
advisory committees; aggression; *behavior disorders; behavioral genetics; behavioral research; blacks; *children; federal government; genetic predisposition; government regulation; Hispanic Americans; *human experimentation; males; *minority groups; *nontherapeutic research; patient advocacy; psychoactive drugs; scientific misconduct; social discrimination; vulnerable populations; Columbia University; *fenfluramine; Mount Sinai School of Medicine; National Bioethics Advisory Commission; *New York City; New York State Psychiatric Institute; Queens College

Hope, Tony. Aging, research and families. [Editorial]. *Journal of Medical Ethics.* 1997 Oct; 23(5): 267–268. 3 refs. BE57105.
*aged; *competence; comprehension; *conflict of interest; *decision making; *dementia; *depressive disorder; *family members; *human experimentation; *informed consent; methods; patient advocacy; *patient care; physician patient relationship; *physicians; professional family relationship; time factors

Hornblum, Allen M. Acres of Skin: Human Experiments at Holmesburg Prison -- A True Story of Abuse and Exploitation in the Name of Medical Science. New York, NY: Routledge; 1998. 297 p. Bibliography: p. 271–284. ISBN 0-415-91990-8. BE58697.
administrators; blacks; disclosure; drug industry; federal government; government regulation; *historical aspects;

*human experimentation; *incentives; informed consent; institutionalized persons; *investigators; mass media; methods; National Socialism; *nontherapeutic research; *prisoners; psychoactive drugs; radiation; remuneration; research design; research subjects; risks and benefits; *scientific misconduct; state government; toxicity; volunteers; chemical warfare; dermatology; Atomic Energy Commission; Department of the Army; Environmental Protection Agency; Food and Drug Administration; *Holmesburg Prison (Philadelphia, PA); *Kligman, Albert; *Twentieth Century; *United States; University of Pennsylvania

Hornblum, Allen M. They were cheap and available: prisoners as research subjects in twentieth century America. *BMJ (British Medical Journal).* 1997 Nov 29; 315(7120): 1437–1441. 49 refs. BE57051.
attitudes; coercion; death; disclosure; drug industry; federal government; government regulation; guidelines; *historical aspects; *human experimentation; incentives; injuries; investigators; *nontherapeutic research; physicians; *prisoners; *public policy; research subjects; risk; *scientific misconduct; selection of subjects; trends; utilitarianism; volunteers; war; guideline adherence; Cold War; Nuremberg Code; *Twentieth Century; *United States; World War II

Irving, Dianne N.; Shamoo, Adil E. Washouts/relapses in patients participating in neurobiological research studies in schizophrenia. *In:* Shamoo, Adil E., ed. Ethics in Neurobiological Research with Human Subjects: The Baltimore Conference on Ethics. Amsterdam: Gordon and Breach; 1997: 119–127. 124 refs. ISBN 2-88449-161-9. BE57011.
decision making; *human experimentation; informed consent; injuries; international aspects; *mentally ill; *placebos; *psychoactive drugs; *research design; research subjects; risk; risks and benefits; *schizophrenia; suicide; third party consent; treatment outcome; *withholding treatment; Minneapolis; United States; University of California, Los Angeles

Jayaraman, K.S. Inquiry looks into Indian cancer deaths. [News]. *Nature.* 1997 Dec 18–25; 390(6661): 653. BE57309.
attitudes; *cancer; *disadvantaged; disclosure; *females; historical aspects; *human experimentation; *informed consent; investigators; retrospective moral judgment; *scientific misconduct; *withholding treatment; *India; Indian Council of Medical Research

Josefson, Deborah. Doctors volunteer to be guinea pigs for AIDS vaccine. [News]. *BMJ (British Medical Journal).* 1997 Oct 4; 315(7112): 833. BE56068.
AIDS; attitudes; *autoexperimentation; federal government; government regulation; *HIV seropositivity; *human experimentation; *immunization; international aspects; investigators; *physicians; risks and benefits; *volunteers; *International Association of Physicians in AIDS Care; National Institute of Allergy and Infectious Diseases; United Nations; United States

Josefson, Deborah. US admits radiation experiments on 20,000 veterans. [News]. *BMJ (British Medical Journal).* 1997 Sep 6; 315(7108): 566. BE56869.
compensation; *federal government; health hazards; historical aspects; *human experimentation; *military personnel; *public policy; *radiation; research subjects; scientific misconduct; *Department of Defense; Twentieth Century; *United States

Kahn, Jeffrey P.; Mastroianni, Anna C.; Sugarman, Jeremy. Changing claims about justice in research: an introduction and overview. *In:* Kahn, Jeffrey P.; Mastroianni, Anna C.; Sugarman, Jeremy, eds. Beyond Consent: Seeking Justice in Research. New York, NY:

Oxford University Press; 1998: 1–10. 12 fn. ISBN 0-19-511353-5. BE58840.

advisory committees; cancer; compensation; developing countries; federal government; females; government regulation; HIV seropositivity; *human experimentation; informed consent; institutionalized persons; international aspects; *justice; mentally retarded; minority groups; minors; prisoners; public policy; research subjects; risks and benefits; scientific misconduct; selection of subjects; therapeutic research; values; *vulnerable populations; National Commission for the Protection of Human Subjects; United States

Kaiser, Jocelyn. Flap on NEJM board over ethics articles. [News]. *Science.* 1997 Oct 10; 278(5336): 211. BE56066.

*developing countries; dissent; *editorial policies; *HIV seropositivity; *human experimentation; interprofessional relations; investigators; *newborns; *placebos; *pregnant women; scientific misconduct; withholding treatment; *Ho, David; *New England Journal of Medicine; *Wilfert, Catherine

Kane, John M.; Borenstein, Michael. The use of placebo controls in psychiatric research. *In:* Shamoo, Adil E., ed. Ethics in Neurobiological Research with Human Subjects: The Baltimore Conference on Ethics. Amsterdam: Gordon and Breach; 1997: 207–213. 11 refs. ISBN 2-88449-161-9. BE57020.

control groups; *human experimentation; *mentally ill; *placebos; *psychoactive drugs; *research design; research subjects; risks and benefits; *schizophrenia; toxicity; *withholding treatment; United States

Karlawish, Jason H.T.; Sachs, Greg A. Research on the cognitively impaired: lessons and warnings from the emergency research debate. *Journal of the American Geriatrics Society.* 1997 Apr; 45(4): 474–481. 65 refs. BE57116.

advance directives; *dementia; *emergency care; family members; federal government; *government regulation; *human experimentation; informed consent; judicial action; legal aspects; *mentally disabled; public participation; research ethics committees; research subjects; risk; risks and benefits; state government; *therapeutic research; *third party consent; Department of Health and Human Services; DHHS Guidelines; Food and Drug Administration; T.D. v. New York State Office of Mental Health; *United States

Kass, Nancy. Gender and research. *In:* Kahn, Jeffrey P.; Mastroianni, Anna C.; Sugarman, Jeremy, eds. Beyond Consent: Seeking Justice in Research. New York, NY: Oxford University Press; 1998: 67–87. 89 fn. ISBN 0-19-511353-5. BE58844.

aged; drugs; federal government; *females; feminist ethics; government regulation; heart diseases; HIV seropositivity; *human experimentation; *justice; legal liability; minority groups; pregnant women; prenatal injuries; *public policy; research subjects; risks and benefits; *selection of subjects; *social discrimination; trends; Food and Drug Administration; National Institutes of Health; *United States

Keay, Timothy J. Approximating ethical research content. *In:* Shamoo, Adil E., ed. Ethics in Neurobiological Research with Human Subjects: The Baltimore Conference on Ethics. Amsterdam: Gordon and Breach; 1997: 149–153. 11 fn. ISBN 2-88449-161-9. BE57012.

competence; conflict of interest; *human experimentation; *informed consent; injuries; investigator subject relationship; investigators; *mentally ill; physician patient relationship; psychoactive drugs; research design; research ethics committees; research subjects; risks and benefits; *schizophrenia; suicide; withholding treatment; United States

Keville, Terri D. The invisible woman: gender bias in medical research. *Women's Rights Law Reporter.* 1994; 15: 123–142. 209 fn. BE56661.

biomedical research; biomedical technologies; cancer; coercion; contraception; diagnosis; employment; federal government; *females; fetuses; government regulation; health hazards; health insurance; heart diseases; historical aspects; *human experimentation; *investigators; justice; *legal aspects; males; obstetrics and gynecology; occupational exposure; patient care; pregnant women; prenatal injuries; *public policy; research design; *research subjects; *selection of subjects; *social discrimination; treatment refusal; *women's health; International Union, UAW v. Johnson Controls, Inc.; National Institutes of Health; Office of Research on Women's Health; *United States; Women's Health Equity Act 1991

Kigotho, Anderson Wachira. Another HIV-1 trial loses placebo control. [News]. *Lancet.* 1997 Dec 20–27; 350(9094): 1831. BE57861.

control groups; *developing countries; *drugs; females; *HIV seropositivity; *human experimentation; *international aspects; mothers; newborns; *placebos; *pregnant women; *research design; *therapeutic research; AZT; *Ethiopia; Johns Hopkins University; United States

King, Patricia A. Race, justice, and research. *In:* Kahn, Jeffrey P.; Mastroianni, Anna C.; Sugarman, Jeremy, eds. Beyond Consent: Seeking Justice in Research. New York, NY: Oxford University Press; 1998: 88–110. 82 fn. ISBN 0-19-511353-5. BE58845.

*blacks; females; genetic screening; health care delivery; historical aspects; *human experimentation; informed consent; *justice; males; medical education; medicine; minority groups; public participation; public policy; research subjects; *scientific misconduct; selection of subjects; sickle cell anemia; *social discrimination; stigmatization; surgery; syphilis; trends; trust; vulnerable populations; whites; withholding treatment; slavery; Tuskegee Syphilis Study; United States

Kumar, Sanjay. India to ban use of quinacrine for sterilisation. [News]. *Lancet.* 1998 Mar 28; 351(9107): 968. BE58442.

developing countries; *drugs; *females; *government regulation; *human experimentation; international aspects; *sterilization (sexual); women's health; *India; *quinacrine

Kumar, Sanjay. Sterilisation by quinacrine comes under fire in India. [News]. *Lancet.* 1997 May 17; 349(9063): 1460. BE55823.

*drugs; *females; government regulation; *human experimentation; informed consent; involuntary sterilization; legal aspects; misconduct; physicians; *sterilization (sexual); *India; *quinacrine

Lemaire, F.; Blanch, L.; Cohen, S.L.; European Society of Intensive Care Medicine. Working Group on Ethics. Informed consent for research purposes in intensive care patients in Europe — part I: an official statement of the European Society of Intensive Care Medicine. *Intensive Care Medicine.* 1997 Mar; 23(3): 338–341. BE57653.

competence; *critically ill; disclosure; *emergency care; family members; guidelines; *human experimentation; informed consent; *intensive care units; international aspects; legal guardians; *organizational policies; patients; physicians; *presumed consent; professional organizations; research subjects; *therapeutic research; *third party consent; *deferred consent; Council of Europe; *Europe; *European Society of Intensive Care Medicine; United States

Lemaire, F.; Blanch, L.; Cohen, S.L.; European Society of Intensive Care Medicine. Working Group on

Ethics. Informed consent for research purposes in intensive care patients in Europe -- part II: an official statement of the European Society of Intensive Care Medicine. *Intensive Care Medicine.* 1997 Apr; 23(4): 435-439. 8 refs. BE57654.
> competence; *critically ill; *decision making; *emergency care; family members; government regulation; hospitals; *human experimentation; *informed consent; institutional policies; *intensive care units; *international aspects; investigators; *legal aspects; legal guardians; nontherapeutic research; patients; physicians; public policy; research ethics committees; research subjects; survey; therapeutic research; *third party consent; deferred consent; questionnaires; Austria; Belgium; Denmark; *Europe; *European Society of Intensive Care Medicine; Finland; France; Germany; Great Britain; Greece; Israel; Italy; Netherlands; Norway; Portugal; Spain; Sweden; Switzerland

Levine, Carol. Changing views of justice after Belmont: AIDS and the inclusion of "vulnerable" subjects. *In:* Vanderpool, Harold Y., ed. The Ethics of Research Involving Human Subjects: Facing the 21st Century. Frederick, MD: University Publishing Group; 1996: 105-126. 37 fn. ISBN 1-55572-036-6. BE56984.
> advisory committees; *AIDS; autonomy; beneficence; children; federal government; females; fetuses; government financing; government regulation; guidelines; *HIV seropositivity; *human experimentation; informed consent; investigational drugs; *justice; minority groups; patients; pregnant women; *public policy; research ethics committees; research subjects; risks and benefits; scientific misconduct; *selection of subjects; trends; *vulnerable populations; Belmont Report; Food and Drug Administration; National Commission for the Protection of Human Subjects; National Institutes of Health; Tuskegee Syphilis Study; United States

Levine, Robert J. The "best proven therapeutic method" standard in clinical trials in technologically developing countries. [Editorial]. *IRB: A Review of Human Subjects Research.* 1998 Jan-Feb; 20(1): 5-9. 19 fn. BE58519.
> *control groups; *developing countries; *drugs; economics; guidelines; *HIV seropositivity; *human experimentation; international aspects; newborns; patient care; *placebos; *pregnant women; *research design; *standards; *AZT; Declaration of Helsinki

Macklin, Ruth. Justice in international research. *In:* Kahn, Jeffrey P.; Mastroianni, Anna C.; Sugarman, Jeremy, eds. Beyond Consent: Seeking Justice in Research. New York, NY: Oxford University Press; 1998: 131-146. 43 fn. ISBN 0-19-511353-5. BE58847.
> abortion, induced; contraception; cultural pluralism; *developing countries; drugs; ethical review; females; HIV seropositivity; *human experimentation; informed consent; *international aspects; investigational drugs; *justice; placebos; research design; research ethics committees; risks and benefits; standards; sterilization (sexual); trends; *vulnerable populations; Depo-provera; quinacrine; RU-486; United States

Marshall, Eliot. AIDS therapy: controversial trial offers hopeful result. [News]. *Science.* 1998 Feb 27; 279(5355): 1299. BE57260.
> costs and benefits; *developing countries; *drugs; *HIV seropositivity; *human experimentation; international aspects; newborns; *placebos; *pregnant women; *research design; therapeutic research; time factors; *Africa; *AZT; *Thailand

Marwick, Charles. Bioethics Commission examines informed consent from subjects who are 'decisionally incapable'. [News]. *JAMA.* 1997 Aug 27; 278(8): 618-619. BE56101.
> advisory committees; *competence; comprehension; disclosure; *human experimentation; *informed consent; *mentally disabled; psychoactive drugs; public policy; random selection; research design; research subjects; schizophrenia; standards; withholding treatment; National Bioethics Advisory Commission; United States

Marwick, Charles. Bioethics group considers transnational research. [News]. *JAMA.* 1998 May 13; 279(18): 1425. BE57862.
> advisory committees; *developing countries; *drugs; federal government; government financing; guidelines; *HIV seropositivity; *human experimentation; *international aspects; newborns; *placebos; *pregnant women; *public policy; *research design; scientific misconduct; *therapeutic research; *Africa; AZT; Declaration of Helsinki; National Bioethics Advisory Commission; *United States

Melzer, David. New drug treatment for Alzheimer's disease: lessons for healthcare policy. *BMJ (British Medical Journal).* 1998 Mar 7; 316(7133): 762-764. 20 refs. BE57759.
> *advertising; aged; costs and benefits; *dementia; drug industry; editorial policies; government regulation; human experimentation; *information dissemination; *investigational drugs; nursing homes; *patient care; *public policy; research design; *risks and benefits; *technology assessment; *therapeutic research; *treatment outcome; *Aricept; Great Britain; National Health Service; United States

Milner, Claire Alida. Gulf war guinea pigs: is informed consent optional during war? [Comment]. *Journal of Contemporary Health Law and Policy.* 1996 Fall; 13(1): 199-232. 249 fn. BE55791.
> *biological warfare; codes of ethics; federal government; *government regulation; health hazards; historical aspects; *human experimentation; iatrogenic disease; immunization; *informed consent; *investigational drugs; *legal aspects; legal liability; *military personnel; nontherapeutic research; occupational exposure; politics; *preventive medicine; psychoactive drugs; public policy; radiation; scientific misconduct; Supreme Court decisions; therapeutic research; toxicity; *war; *chemical warfare; Central Intelligence Agency; *Cold War; Declaration of Helsinki; Department of Defense; Federal Policy (Common Rule) for the Protection of Human Subjects 1991; *Food and Drug Administration; National Institutes of Health; Nuremberg Code; *Persian Gulf War; Twentieth Century; *United States

Moreno, Jonathan D. Convenient and captive populations. *In:* Kahn, Jeffrey P.; Mastroianni, Anna C.; Sugarman, Jeremy, eds. Beyond Consent: Seeking Justice in Research. New York, NY: Oxford University Press; 1998: 111-130. 59 fn. ISBN 0-19-511353-5. BE58846.
> behavioral research; children; coercion; deception; federal government; government regulation; historical aspects; *human experimentation; informed consent; *institutionalized persons; *justice; mentally disabled; *military personnel; *prisoners; research subjects; scientific misconduct; social dominance; *students; trends; *vulnerable populations; United States

Mudur, Ganapati. Indian study of women with cervical lesions called unethical. [News]. *BMJ (British Medical Journal).* 1997 Apr 12; 314(7087): 1065. BE56063.
> attitudes; *cancer; developing countries; *disadvantaged; disclosure; *females; historical aspects; *human experimentation; *informed consent; investigators; retrospective moral judgment; *scientific misconduct; withholding treatment; *India; Institute of Cytology and Preventive Oncology (New Delhi)

Olde Rikkert, Marcel G.M.; van den Bercken, John H.L.; ten Have, Henk A.M.J., et al. Experienced consent in geriatrics research: a new method to optimize

the capacity to consent in frail elderly subjects. *Journal of Medical Ethics.* 1997 Oct; 23(5): 271–276. 24 refs. Appendix presents ten "multiple–choice questions asked of geriatric patients to assess their comprehension of relevant research information in a research project." BE57107.
  *aged; *competence; comprehension; dementia; depressive disorder; evaluation studies; *human experimentation; *informed consent; methods; nontherapeutic research; normality; research subjects; risks and benefits; time factors; Netherlands
OBJECTIVES: Cognitive and sensory difficulties frequently jeopardize informed consent of frail elderly patients. This study is the first to test whether preliminary research experience could enhance geriatric patients' capacity to consent. DESIGN/SETTING: A step–wise consent procedure was introduced in a study on fluid balance in geriatric patients. Eligible patients providing verbal consent participated in a try–out of a week, during which bioelectrical impedance and weight measurements were performed daily. Afterwards, written informed consent was requested. Comprehension, risk and inconvenience scores (ranges: 0–10) were obtained before and after the try–out by asking ten questions about the study's essentials and by asking for a risk and inconvenience assessment on a ten–points rating scale. SUBJECTS AND RESULTS: Seventy of the 78 eligible subjects started the try–out and 53 (68%) provided written consent. The comprehension score increased from 5.0 (+/- 2.3) to 7.0 (+/- 1.9) following the try–out (P less than 0.001). The number of subjects capable of weighing risks and inconveniences increased from 32 to 48 (P less than 0.001). CONCLUSIONS: Research experience improved the capacity to consent, still enabling an acceptable participation rate. Therefore, experienced consent seems a promising tool to optimize informed consent in frail elderly subjects.

Patel, Tara. Row over sterilisation divides India. [News]. *New Scientist.* 1997 Apr 5; 154(2076): 4. BE56188.
  developing countries; *drugs; *females; *human experimentation; international aspects; population control; public policy; risk; risks and benefits; *sterilization (sexual); *toxicity; *India; *quinacrine

Phanuphak, Praphan. Ethical issues in studies in Thailand of the vertical transmission of HIV. *New England Journal of Medicine.* 1998 Mar 19; 338(12): 834–835. 5 refs. BE57707.
  AIDS; alternatives; control groups; *developing countries; *drugs; government financing; *HIV seropositivity; *human experimentation; international aspects; *newborns; *nontherapeutic research; *placebos; *pregnant women; *preventive medicine; private sector; *public policy; *research design; resource allocation; scientific misconduct; *therapeutic research; time factors; withholding treatment; *AZT; Centers for Disease Control and Prevention; National Institutes of Health; *Thailand; United States; Walter Reed Army Institute of Research

Pinch, Winifred J. Research and nursing: ethical reflections. *N and HC Perspectives on Community.* 1996 Jan–Feb; 17(1): 26–31. 24 refs. BE58306.
  biomedical technologies; federal government; *females; feminist ethics; genetic intervention; government financing; *health services research; *human experimentation; informed consent; investigator subject relationship; *investigators; *nurse's role; nursing ethics; *nursing research; public policy; reproduction; research design; research subjects; resource allocation; selection of subjects; social discrimination; social impact; socioeconomic factors; women's health; qualitative research; National Institute for

Nursing Research; United States

RAGE (Radiotherapy Action Group Exposure) National [Great Britain]. All treatment and trials must have informed consent. [Personal view]. *BMJ (British Medical Journal).* 1997 Apr 12; 314(7087): 1134–1135. BE55676.
  cancer; disclosure; *females; *human experimentation; *informed consent; *injuries; morbidity; patient participation; *patients; physicians; *political activity; *radiology; research ethics committees; risks and benefits; *scientific misconduct; trust; *Great Britain; *RAGE (Radiotherapy Action Group Exposure)

Robb, Merlin L.; Khambaroong, Chirasak; Nelson, Kenrad E., et al. Studies in Thailand of the vertical transmission of HIV. [Letters]. *New England Journal of Medicine.* 1998 Mar 19; 338(12): 843–844. 2 refs. BE57708.
  AIDS; *drugs; financial support; health care delivery; *HIV seropositivity; *human experimentation; informed consent; newborns; *nontherapeutic research; patient care; *pregnant women; *standards; *therapeutic research; time factors; *AZT; Chiang Mai University; Department of Defense; Johns Hopkins University; Ministry of Health (Thailand); National Institutes of Health; *Thailand; United States; Walter Reed Army Institute of Research

Ryan, Anne J. True protection for persons with severe mental disabilities, such as schizophrenia, involved as subjects in research? A look and consideration of the "Protection of Human Subjects." *Journal of Law and Health.* 1994–1995; 9(2): 349–376. 226 fn. BE57179.
  disclosure; federal government; *government regulation; guidelines; *historical aspects; *human experimentation; informed consent; *mentally ill; minors; patient advocacy; pregnant women; prisoners; psychoactive drugs; research ethics committees; research subjects; *schizophrenia; vulnerable populations; withholding treatment; *DHHS Guidelines; National Commission for the Protection of Human Subjects; Nuremberg Code; *United States; University of California, Los Angeles

Satel, Sally L. Science by quota: P.C. medicine. *New Republic.* 1995 Feb 27; 212(9): 14, 16. BE57593.
  federal government; *females; *government financing; government regulation; guidelines; *human experimentation; legal aspects; *minority groups; *politics; public policy; research design; resource allocation; *selection of subjects; women's health; *National Institutes of Health; U.S. Congress; *United States

Shamoo, Adil E. Ethical considerations in medication–free research on the mentally ill. *In:* Shamoo, Adil E., ed. Ethics in Neurobiological Research with Human Subjects: The Baltimore Conference on Ethics. Amsterdam: Gordon and Breach; 1997: 195–199. 1 fn. ISBN 2–88449–161–9. BE57018.
  attitudes; federal government; government regulation; *human experimentation; investigators; *mentally ill; nontherapeutic research; placebos; *psychoactive drugs; public policy; research design; research subjects; risks and benefits; scientific misconduct; therapeutic research; treatment outcome; *withholding treatment; Belmont Report; National Institutes of Health; United States; University of California, Los Angeles

Shamoo, Adil E., ed. Ethics in Neurobiological Research with Human Subjects: The Baltimore Conference on Ethics. Amsterdam: Gordon and Breach; 1997. 335 p. 440 refs. 198 fn. Papers from the First National Conference on Ethics in Neurobiological Research with Human Subjects, Baltimore, MD, 7–9 Jan 1995. ISBN 2–88449–161–9. BE57008.

BE = bioethics accession number   fn. = footnotes   refs. = references

accountability; alternatives; coercion; committee membership; common good; competence; conflict of interest; disclosure; family members; goals; government regulation; *human experimentation; informed consent; institutionalized persons; investigator subject relationship; investigators; legal aspects; *mentally ill; moral obligations; nontherapeutic research; organizational policies; patient advocacy; patient participation; patients; physicians; placebos; psychoactive drugs; research design; research ethics committees; research subjects; review; risks and benefits; schizophrenia; scientific misconduct; standards; therapeutic research; third party consent; vulnerable populations; withholding treatment; Belmont Report; Maryland Psychiatric Research Center; National Alliance for the Mentally Ill; National Institute of Mental Health; Office for Protection from Research Risks; UCLA Clinical Research Center; *United States

Shamoo, Adil E.; Johnson, J. Rock; Honberg, Ron, et al. NAMI's standards for protection of individuals with severe mental illnesses who participate as human subjects in research. *In:* Shamoo, Adil E., ed. Ethics in Neurobiological Research with Human Subjects: The Baltimore Conference on Ethics. Amsterdam: Gordon and Breach; 1997: 325–328. ISBN 2–88449–161–9. BE57024.
alternatives; committee membership; communication; competence; comprehension; disclosure; education; family members; goals; *guidelines; *human experimentation; informed consent; investigators; *mentally ill; *organizational policies; *patient advocacy; patient participation; psychoactive drugs; research design; research ethics committees; research subjects; risks and benefits; third party consent; continuity of patient care; *National Alliance for the Mentally Ill; National Institute of Mental Health; United States

Shamoo, Adil E.; O'Sullivan, Joan L. The ethics of research on the mentally disabled. *In:* Monagle, John F.; Thomasma, David C., eds. Health Care Ethics: Critical Issues for the 21st Century. Gaithersburg, MD: Aspen Publishers; 1998: 239–250. 101 fn. ISBN 0–8342–0911–X. BE56285.
coercion; competence; comprehension; eugenics; federal government; government regulation; guidelines; historical aspects; *human experimentation; informed consent; international aspects; mentally disabled; *mentally ill; National Socialism; nontherapeutic research; psychoactive drugs; research design; research ethics committees; risks and benefits; schizophrenia; scientific misconduct; therapeutic research; third party consent; withholding treatment; Declaration of Helsinki; Germany; Nuremberg Code; Office for Protection from Research Risks; Twentieth Century; United States

Sharav, Vera Hassner. Independent family advocates challenge the fraternity of silence. *In:* Shamoo, Adil E., ed. Ethics in Neurobiological Research with Human Subjects: The Baltimore Conference on Ethics. Amsterdam: Gordon and Breach; 1997: 175–181. ISBN 2–88449–161–9. BE57015.
attitudes; *conflict of interest; deception; disclosure; drug industry; drugs; family members; federal government; financial support; government regulation; *human experimentation; iatrogenic disease; informed consent; institutionalized persons; *investigators; *mentally ill; *nontherapeutic research; *patient advocacy; physician's role; placebos; professional organizations; psychiatry; psychoactive drugs; research design; research ethics committees; research subjects; risks and benefits; schizophrenia; *scientific misconduct; state government; withholding treatment; *Alliance for the Mentally Ill of New York State; Bronx VA Medical Center (NY); National Institute of Mental Health; New York; Office for Protection from Research Risks; United States

Skirboll, Lana; Shore, David; Baruchin, Andrea, et al. National Institute of Mental Health human subject activities. *In:* Shamoo, Adil E., ed. Ethics in Neurobiological Research with Human Subjects: The Baltimore Conference on Ethics. Amsterdam: Gordon and Breach; 1997: 201–206. ISBN 2–88449–161–9. BE57019.
advisory committees; family members; federal government; government financing; government regulation; *human experimentation; informed consent; investigators; *mentally ill; patient education; patient participation; peer review; program descriptions; *public policy; research ethics committees; research subjects; American Psychiatric Association; National Alliance for the Mentally Ill; *National Institute of Mental Health; Office for Protection from Research Risks; United States

Smith, Douglas. The limits of human studies. *In:* Close, Bryony; Combes, Robert; Hubbard, Anthony; Illingworth, John, eds. Volunteers in Research and Testing. Bristol, PA: Taylor and Francis; 1997: 135–143. ISBN 0–7484–0397–3. BE57038.
ethical review; government regulation; guidelines; health hazards; *human experimentation; *military personnel; nontherapeutic research; toxicity; volunteers; *Great Britain; *Institute of Naval Medicine (Great Britain)

Straw, Peggy. Consumer representation on IRBs -- how it should be done. *In:* Shamoo, Adil E., ed. Ethics in Neurobiological Research with Human Subjects: The Baltimore Conference on Ethics. Amsterdam: Gordon and Breach; 1997: 187–190. ISBN 2–88449–161–9. BE57016.
advisory committees; *committee membership; comprehension; consent forms; disclosure; *human experimentation; informed consent; *mentally ill; *patient advocacy; program descriptions; *public participation; *research ethics committees; research subjects; standards; Alliance for the Mentally Ill of New Hampshire; Dartmouth Medical School; *New Hampshire Division of Mental Health; United States

U.S. Congress. Senate. Committee on Labor and Human Resources. Human Subjects Research: Radiation Experimentation. Hearing, 13 Jan 1994 (Waltham, MA). Washington, DC: U.S. Government Printing Office; 1994. 61 p. S. Hrg. 103–511. ISBN 0–16–044800–X. BE58699.
children; consent forms; deception; disclosure; *federal government; food; health hazards; *historical aspects; *human experimentation; informed consent; *institutionalized persons; *mentally retarded; nontherapeutic research; *radiation; records; research subjects; risks and benefits; *scientific misconduct; universities; vulnerable populations; Advisory Committee on Human Radiation Experiments; Fernald State School (MA); Massachusetts; Massachusetts Institute of Technology; *Twentieth Century; *United States

U.S. Congress. Senate. Committee on Labor and Human Resources. Women's Health: Ensuring Quality and Equity in Biomedical Research. Hearing, 29 Jun 1992. Washington, DC: U.S. Government Printing Office; 1992. 48 p. S. Hrg. 102–1180. BE58949.
*biomedical research; cancer; diagnosis; drugs; federal government; *females; government financing; heart diseases; *human experimentation; males; morbidity; mortality; patient care; *public policy; research subjects; selection of subjects; social discrimination; *women's health; ovaries; National Institutes of Health; Office of Research on Women's Health; *United States; Women's Health Initiative

UCLA Clinical Research Center. Statement of the UCLA Clinical Research Center. *In:* Shamoo, Adil E.,

ed. Ethics in Neurobiological Research with Human Subjects: The Baltimore Conference on Ethics. Amsterdam: Gordon and Breach; 1997: 173-174. ISBN 2-88449-161-9. BE57014.
advisory committees; *human experimentation; institutional policies; *mentally ill; professional family relationship; *program descriptions; *psychoactive drugs; *research design; research institutes; research subjects; *schizophrenia; scientific misconduct; withholding treatment; National Institutes of Health; Office for Protection from Research Risks; *UCLA Clinical Research Center; United States

Varmus, Harold; Satcher, David. Ethical complexities of conducting research in developing countries. *New England Journal of Medicine.* 1997 Oct 2; 337(14): 1003-1005. 6 refs. BE55835.
AIDS; autonomy; beneficence; *control groups; *developing countries; *drugs; economics; ethical review; federal government; *HIV seropositivity; *human experimentation; international aspects; justice; *moral policy; *newborns; *placebos; *pregnant women; *preventive medicine; *public policy; *research design; risks and benefits; *therapeutic research; *AZT; Centers for Disease Control and Prevention; National Institutes of Health; *United States

Vere, Duncan. Volunteers: the susceptible and the disadvantaged. *In:* Close, Bryony; Combes, Robert; Hubbard, Anthony; Illingworth, John, eds. Volunteers in Research and Testing. Bristol, PA: Taylor and Francis; 1997: 67-80. 44 refs. ISBN 0-7484-0397-3. BE57032.
cancer; children; coercion; compensation; competence; critically ill; *disadvantaged; disclosure; drugs; females; *human experimentation; informed consent; injuries; investigator subject relationship; mentally disabled; minority groups; paternalism; patients; research subjects; selection of subjects; *volunteers; *vulnerable populations; coma

Wadman, Meredith. Controversy flares over AIDS prevention trials in Third World. [News]. *Nature.* 1997 Oct 30; 389(6654): 894. BE56162.
*developing countries; *drugs; federal government; government financing; government regulation; *HIV seropositivity; *human experimentation; investigators; newborns; *placebos; *pregnant women; preventive medicine; *research design; therapeutic research; *AZT; Department of Health and Human Services; Johns Hopkins University; National Institutes of Health; Public Citizen; *United States

Wadman, Meredith. Mentally disabled research subjects 'need protection.' [News]. *Nature.* 1997 Oct 16; 389(6652): 652. BE56161.
advisory committees; federal government; government regulation; *human experimentation; informed consent; *mentally disabled; psychoactive drugs; *public policy; research subjects; *scientific misconduct; withholding treatment; National Bioethics Advisory Commission; National Institute of Mental Health; United States

Wadman, Meredith. Row erupts over child aggression study. [News]. *Nature.* 1998 Apr 23; 392(6678): 747. BE58075.
*aggression; *behavioral research; blacks; *children; *drugs; ethical review; federal government; government regulation; Hispanic Americans; *human experimentation; indigents; males; *minority groups; *nontherapeutic research; research ethics committees; research subjects; scientific misconduct; selection of subjects; *fenfluramine; New York City; *New York State Psychiatric Institute (NYC); Office for Protection from Research Risks; United States

Wadman, Meredith. US dispute over live AIDS vaccine trials. [News]. *Nature.* 1997 Oct 2; 389(6650): 426. BE56061.

*attitudes; *autoexperimentation; federal government; government regulation; *HIV seropositivity; *human experimentation; *immunization; *investigators; physicians; public policy; risks and benefits; *volunteers; *International Association of Physicians in AIDS Care; *National Institute of Allergy and Infectious Diseases; *United States

Weiss, Rick. Bioethics group divided over research on mentally ill. [News]. *Washington Post.* 1998 Nov 16: A6. BE58997.
advisory committees; family members; federal government; *government regulation; *human experimentation; informed consent; *mentally ill; nontherapeutic research; patient advocacy; *public policy; research subjects; risks and benefits; therapeutic research; third party consent; National Alliance for the Mentally Ill; *National Bioethics Advisory Commission; National Institutes of Health; Nuremberg Code; United States

Weiss, Rick. Research ethics panel urges new regulations to protect mentally ill. [News]. *Washington Post.* 1998 Nov 18: A11. BE58998.
advisory committees; attitudes; family members; federal government; *government regulation; *human experimentation; informed consent; investigators; *mentally ill; nontherapeutic research; patient advocacy; *public policy; research subjects; risks and benefits; third party consent; American Psychiatric Association; Institute of Medicine; *National Bioethics Advisory Commission; National Institutes of Health; United States

Williams, Peter; Wallace, David. Unit 731: The Japanese Army's Secret of Secrets. London: Hodder and Stoughton; 1989. 366 p. 596 fn. ISBN 0-340-39463-3. BE57390.
*biological warfare; confidentiality; dehumanization; disclosure; federal government; *historical aspects; *human experimentation; international aspects; *investigators; killing; military personnel; *moral complicity; *prisoners; public policy; *scientific misconduct; technical expertise; torture; war; chemical warfare; Canada; China; France; Germany; Great Britain; Ishii, Shiro; *Japan; Korean War; Netherlands; Twentieth Century; *United States; USSR; *World War II

Williams, Susan G. Research considerations: family opinions about elderly relatives in research. *Journal of Gerontological Nursing.* 1992 Dec; 18(12): 3-8. 11 refs. BE56636.
*aged; *attitudes; dementia; disclosure; *family members; *human experimentation; informed consent; knowledge, attitudes, practice; nurses; nursing homes; nursing research; survey; *third party consent; questionnaires; United States

Wolinsky, Howard. Steps still being taken to undo damage of "America's Nuremberg." [News]. *Annals of Internal Medicine.* 1997 Aug 15; 127(4): I43-I44. BE56100.
attitudes; *blacks; codes of ethics; compensation; drugs; federal government; historical aspects; *human experimentation; informed consent; males; National Socialism; organ donation; physicians; *research subjects; *scientific misconduct; social impact; *syphilis; trust; withholding treatment; Germany; *Nuremberg Code; Public Health Service; *Tuskegee Syphilis Study; Twentieth Century; *United States

Young, Simon N.; Annable, Lawrence; Canadian College of Neuropsychopharmacology. The use of placebos in psychiatry: a response to the draft document prepared by the Tri-Council Working Group. [Position paper]. *Journal of Psychiatry and Neuroscience.* 1996 Jul; 21(4): 235-238. 15 refs. Approved at a meeting of the CCNP Council 2 Jun 1996 and at the CCNP Annual General Business Meeting 4 Jun 1996. BE57666.
*depressive disorder; *human experimentation; *mentally ill;

BE = bioethics accession number   fn. = footnotes   refs. = references

*organizational policies; physicians; *placebos; professional organizations; *psychiatry; *psychoactive drugs; *research design; Canada; *Canadian College of Neuropsychopharmacology; Code of Conduct for Research Involving Humans

FDA seeks public comment on informed consent rules in combat situations. [News]. *Hastings Center Report.* 1997 Sep–Oct; 27(5): 43. BE56127.
*biological warfare; federal government; government regulation; *human experimentation; immunization; *informed consent; *investigational drugs; *military personnel; nontherapeutic research; public policy; toxicity; volunteers; *war; *chemical warfare; Department of Defense; *Food and Drug Administration; United States

Human rights begin at home. [Editorial]. *BMJ (British Medical Journal).* 1997 Nov 29; 315(7120): 1387. BE56915.
health personnel; *human experimentation; *human rights; investigators; mentally ill; *misconduct; patient care; *prisoners; *scientific misconduct; *torture; Great Britain; United Nations; United States; Universal Declaration of Human Rights

IMMUNIZATION

See also PUBLIC HEALTH

Allen, Arthur. Injection rejection: the dangerous backlash against vaccination. *New Republic.* 1998 Mar 23; 218(12): 20–23. BE57822.
attitudes; children; communicable diseases; compensation; disadvantaged; *dissent; federal government; health education; *immunization; injuries; mandatory programs; mortality; political activity; public health; *risks and benefits; treatment refusal; trust; whooping cough; United States

Bloom, Barry R. The highest attainable standard: ethical issues in AIDS vaccines. *Science.* 1998 Jan 9; 279(5348): 186–188. 15 fn. BE58034.
*AIDS; codes of ethics; *developing countries; drugs; economics; ethical review; goals; guidelines; *human experimentation; *immunization; informed consent; *international aspects; placebos; preventive medicine; research design; standards; *therapeutic research; Council for International Organizations of Medical Sciences; Declaration of Helsinki; International Ethical Guidelines for Biomedical Research Involving Human Subjects; UNAIDS; United Nations; World Health Organization

Butler, Declan. Admission on Gulf War vaccines spurs debate on medical records. [News]. *Nature.* 1997 Nov 6; 390(6655): 3–4. BE56858.
biological warfare; epidemiology; *human experimentation; *immunization; injuries; medical records; *military personnel; *morbidity; *public policy; *war; whooping cough; *Great Britain; *Ministry of Defence (Great Britain); *Persian Gulf War

Dare, Tim. Mass immunisation programmes: some philosophical issues. *Bioethics.* 1998 Apr; 12(2): 125–149. 33 fn. BE58624.
children; coercion; comparative studies; *decision making; health promotion; *immunization; *international aspects; *mandatory programs; moral policy; *parents; policy analysis; *public policy; risks and benefits; schools; time factors; uncertainty; utilitarianism; *voluntary programs; *New Zealand; *United States
Most countries promote mass immunisation programmes. The varying policy details raise a raft of philosophical issues. I have two broad aims in this paper. First, I hope to begin to remedy a rather curious philosophical neglect of immunisation. With this in mind, I take a broad

approach to the topic hoping to introduce rather than settle a range of philosophical issues. My second aim has two aspects: I argue that the states should have pro–immunisation policies, and I advance a view of the subsequent and more specific question as to which sorts of pro–immunisation policies they should prefer. I use the immunisation policies of the United States and New Zealand to frame my discussion of these substantive questions. Immunisation is effectively compulsory in the United States. New Zealand, by contrast, requires evidence not of immunisation but of immunisation status upon school enrolment: New Zealand's policy effectively makes immunisation choice compulsory. I argue that, as between the pro–immunisation policies of the United States and New Zealand, the latter should be preferred. Though the threshold question as to whether states should have pro–immunisation policies should be answered affirmatively, the move to compulsory immunisation cannot be justified.

Farthing, Charles F. A necessary risk: why we doctors should volunteer to try an AIDS vaccine. *Washington Post.* 1997 Oct 19: C1, C6. BE57845.
*AIDS; *autoexperimentation; historical aspects; *human experimentation; *immunization; *physicians; professional organizations; risks and benefits; *volunteers; International Association of Physicians in AIDS Care

Harding, Christine M. Whooping cough vaccination: the case presented by the British national press. *Child: Care, Health and Development.* 1985 Jan–Feb; 11(1): 21–30. 25 refs. BE56959.
*communicable diseases; comparative studies; *immunization; *mass media; *risks and benefits; survey; *whooping cough; *Great Britain

Josefson, Deborah. Doctors volunteer to be guinea pigs for AIDS vaccine. [News]. *BMJ (British Medical Journal).* 1997 Oct 4; 315(7112): 833. BE56068.
AIDS; attitudes; *autoexperimentation; federal government; government regulation; *HIV seropositivity; *human experimentation; *immunization; international aspects; investigators; *physicians; risks and benefits; *volunteers; *International Association of Physicians in AIDS Care; National Institute of Allergy and Infectious Diseases; United Nations; United States

Kaiser, Jocelyn. UNAIDS to weigh vaccine ethics. [News]. *Science.* 1997 Sep 19; 277(5333): 1751. BE56067.
*developing countries; drugs; *HIV seropositivity; *human experimentation; *immunization; *international aspects; newborns; patient care; placebos; pregnant women; AZT; *UNAIDS; United Nations

Kerns, Thomas A. Ethical Issues in HIV Vaccine Trials. New York, NY: St. Martin's Press; 1997. 249 p. Bibliography: p. 239–244. Appendices include texts of the Nuremberg Code, the International Ethical Guidelines for Biomedical Research Involving Human Subjects, a proposed Bill of Rights and Responsibilities for Participants in HIV Vaccine Trials, a test of understanding for informed consent, and proposed application forms for ethical review. ISBN 0–312–16397–5. BE57278.
*AIDS; autonomy; beneficence; coercion; common good; compensation; comprehension; confidentiality; control groups; counseling; developing countries; disclosure; economics; ethical review; forms; goals; guidelines; *HIV seropositivity; *human experimentation; *immunization; incentives; informed consent; injuries; investigators; justice; *moral policy; motivation; placebos; preventive medicine; research design; research ethics committees; research subjects; review; *risks and benefits; selection of subjects;

social discrimination; third party consent; *volunteers; vulnerable populations; Brazil; Council for International Organizations of Medical Sciences; International Ethical Guidelines for Biomedical Research Involving Human Subjects; Nuremberg Code; Thailand; Uganda; World Health Organization

Kerns, Thomas A. Jenner on Trial: An Ethical Examination of Vaccine Research in the Age of Smallpox and the Age of AIDS. Lanham, MD: University Press of America; 1997. 98 p. 71 fn. Appendix I: the Nuremberg Code; Appendix II: International Ethical Guidelines for Biomedical Research Involving Human Subjects (WHO/CIOMS). ISBN 0-7618-0719-5. BE57154.
AIDS; codes of ethics; *communicable diseases; comparative studies; consent forms; disclosure; ethical review; family members; guidelines; *historical aspects; HIV seropositivity; *human experimentation; *immunization; informed consent; international aspects; investigator subject relationship; *investigators; minors; misconduct; National Socialism; parental consent; physicians; research design; research ethics committees; risks and benefits; selection of subjects; vulnerable populations; *smallpox; Germany; Great Britain; International Ethical Guidelines for Biomedical Research Involving Human Subjects; *Jenner, Edward; Nineteenth Century; Nuremberg Code

McCarthy, Michael. AIDS doctors push for live-virus vaccine trials. Lancet. 1997 Oct 11; 350(9084): 1082. BE56930.
*AIDS; attitudes; autoexperimentation; dissent; HIV seropositivity; *human experimentation; *immunization; *physicians; preventive medicine; professional organizations; *risks and benefits; *volunteers; *International Association of Physicians in AIDS Care; United States

Marwick, Charles. Volunteers in typhoid infection study will aid future vaccine development. [News]. JAMA. 1998 May 13; 279(18): 1423-1424. BE57864.
communicable diseases; compensation; consent forms; disclosure; federal government; government regulation; *human experimentation; *immunization; incentives; informed consent; injuries; international aspects; *nontherapeutic research; remuneration; research design; research subjects; risks and benefits; selection of subjects; *volunteers; *typhoid; Food and Drug Administration; United States; *University of Maryland School of Medicine

Russell, Phillip K. Development of vaccines to meet public health needs: incentives and obstacles. Risk: Health, Safety and Environment. 1996 Summer; 7(3): 239-252. 2 fn. BE55939.
biomedical research; children; communicable diseases; compensation; decision making; *economics; federal government; *government regulation; iatrogenic disease; *immunization; *industry; *international aspects; *legal aspects; public health; public policy; Food and Drug Administration; National Institutes of Health; *United States

Severyn, Kristine M. Jacobson v. Massachusetts: impact on informed consent and vaccine policy. Journal of Pharmacy and Law. 1996; 5(2): 249-274. 160 fn. BE57592.
adults; child abuse; coercion; compensation; disclosure; drug industry; federal government; *government regulation; *immunization; information dissemination; *informed consent; injuries; *legal aspects; *mandatory programs; mandatory reporting; minors; parents; public health; public policy; state government; torts; treatment refusal; *Jacobson v. Massachusetts; National Childhood Vaccine Injury Act 1986; *United States

Wadman, Meredith. US dispute over live AIDS vaccine trials. [News]. Nature. 1997 Oct 2; 389(6650): 426. BE56061.

*attitudes; *autoexperimentation; federal government; government regulation; *HIV seropositivity; *human experimentation; *immunization; *investigators; physicians; public policy; risks and benefits; *volunteers; *International Association of Physicians in AIDS Care; *National Institute of Allergy and Infectious Diseases; *United States

Wehrwein, Peter; Morris, Kelly. HIV-1-vaccine-trial go-ahead reawakens ethics debate. [News]. Lancet. 1998 Jun 13; 351(9118): 1789. BE58863.
control groups; *developing countries; drug abuse; economics; federal government; government regulation; *HIV seropositivity; *human experimentation; *immunization; industry; *international aspects; placebos; preventive medicine; needle-exchange programs; Food and Drug Administration; Thailand; United States; VaxGen

Zinn, Christopher. Australian orphans were used as guinea pigs. [News]. BMJ (British Medical Journal). 1997 Jun 21; 314(7097): 1783. BE56129.
*children; historical aspects; *human experimentation; *immunization; *infants; institutionalized persons; research subjects; retrospective moral judgment; *scientific misconduct; vulnerable populations; *Australia; Commonwealth Serum Laboratories (Australia); Twentieth Century

Editorial [mass vaccination]. Bulletin of Medical Ethics. 1996 Jan; No. 114: 1. BE55853.
adolescents; children; coercion; communicable diseases; compensation; costs and benefits; hepatitis; iatrogenic disease; *immunization; infants; mandatory programs; parental consent; *public policy; rubella; treatment refusal; voluntary programs; measles; *Great Britain; Northern Ireland

IN VITRO FERTILIZATION

See also REPRODUCTIVE TECHNOLOGIES

Andersen, C. Yding; Westergaard, L.G.; Grinsted, J., et al. Frozen embryos: too cold to touch? Frozen pre-embryos in Denmark. Human Reproduction. 1996 Apr; 11(4): 703. 3 refs. BE56852.
*cryopreservation; *embryo disposition; embryo transfer; *embryos; *government regulation; *in vitro fertilization; legal aspects; statistics; time factors; *Denmark

Bleich, J. David. In vitro fertilization: questions of maternal identity and conversion. In: Feldman, Emanuel; Wolowelsky, Joel B., eds. Jewish Law and the New Reproductive Technologies. Hoboken, NJ: Ktav; 1997: 46-82. 46 fn. ISBN 0-88125-586-6. BE57456.
embryo transfer; *in vitro fertilization; *Jewish ethics; Jews; *mothers; *ovum donors; *parent child relationship; reproductive technologies; surrogate mothers; theology; Orthodox Judaism

Breitowitz, Yitzchok A. Halakhic approaches to the resolution of disputes concerning the disposition of preembryos. In: Feldman, Emanuel; Wolowelsky, Joel B., eds. Jewish Law and the New Reproductive Technologies. Hoboken, NJ: Ktav; 1997: 155-186. 95 fn. ISBN 0-88125-586-6. BE57461.
cryopreservation; death; *decision making; dissent; *embryo disposition; embryo research; embryo transfer; *embryos; fathers; *in vitro fertilization; *Jewish ethics; marital relationship; mothers; parent child relationship; property rights; reproductive technologies; surrogate mothers; theology; divorce; Orthodox Judaism

Franklin, Sarah. Embodied Progress: A Cultural Account of Assisted Conception. New York, NY: Routledge;

BE = bioethics accession number   fn. = footnotes   refs. = references

1997. 252 p. Bibliography: p. 230–245. ISBN 0–415–06767–7. BE58543.
    *anthropology; attitudes; *emotions; family relationship; females; feminist ethics; *in vitro fertilization; infertility; reproduction; *reproductive technologies; self concept; sexuality; social sciences; survey; ethnographic studies; hope; Great Britain

Greenfeld, Dorothy A.; Ort, Sharon I.; Greenfeld, David G., et al. Attitudes of IVF parents regarding the IVF experience and their children. *Journal of Assisted Reproduction and Genetics.* 1996 Mar; 13(3): 266–274. 18 refs. BE55860.
    age factors; *attitudes; children; *disclosure; *embryo transfer; fathers; health personnel; *in vitro fertilization; mothers; *parent child relationship; *parents; *patient satisfaction; psychology; survey; questionnaires; Connecticut; Yale University School of Medicine

Grubb, Andrew. The Human Fertilisation and Embryology (Statutory Storage Period for Embryos) Regulations 1996 (S.I. 1996 No. 375). [Comment]. *Medical Law Review.* 1996 Summer; 4(2): 211–215. BE56591.
    *cryopreservation; donors; *embryo disposition; embryo research; embryo transfer; *embryos; genetic disorders; *government regulation; guidelines; *in vitro fertilization; infertility; informed consent; legislation; patients; surrogate mothers; *time factors; *Great Britain; Human Fertilisation and Embryology Act 1990; *Human Fertilisation and Embryology Authority

Lehrman, Sally. University settles with patients over trade in 'stolen' embryos. [News]. *Nature.* 1997 Jul 31; 388(6641): 411. BE56064.
    *embryo transfer; human experimentation; *in vitro fertilization; informed consent; investigational drugs; investigators; *legal liability; *misconduct; physicians; *scientific misconduct; *universities; Asch, Ricardo; Balmaceda, Jose; California; Center for Reproductive Health (Irvine, CA); Stone, Sergio; *University of California, Irvine; *University of California, San Diego

May, William E. *Donum Vitae:* Catholic teaching concerning homologous *in vitro* fertilization. *In:* Wildes, Kevin Wm., ed. Infertility: A Crossroad of Faith, Medicine, and Technology. Boston, MA: Kluwer Academic; 1997: 73–92. 27 refs. 13 fn. ISBN 0–7923–4061–2. BE55992.
    children; embryo transfer; *in vitro fertilization; *marital relationship; married persons; *morality; personhood; reproduction; reproductive technologies; *Roman Catholic ethics; sexuality; *theology; value of life; dignity; Humanae Vitae; *Instruction on Respect for Human Life

Meldrum, David R.; Gardner, David K. Two–embryo transfer -- the future looks bright. [Editorial]. *New England Journal of Medicine.* 1998 Aug 27; 339(9): 624–625. 10 refs. BE58659.
    age factors; *embryo transfer; females; *in vitro fertilization; infertility; *multiple pregnancy; research design; risk; *treatment outcome; Great Britain

Neumann, Peter J. Should health insurance cover IVF? Issues and options. *Journal of Health Politics, Policy and Law.* 1997 Oct; 22(5): 1215–1239. 69 refs. 13 fn. BE56748.
    *adoption; alternatives; biomedical technologies; childbirth; comparative studies; *costs and benefits; embryo transfer; federal government; government regulation; guidelines; health facilities; *health insurance reimbursement; *in vitro fertilization; incentives; infertility; international aspects; legislation; multiple pregnancy; newborns; professional organizations; prognosis; public opinion; *public policy; *reproductive technologies; *resource allocation; risks and

benefits; selection for treatment; standards; state government; personal financing; utilization review; American Society for Reproductive Medicine; Fertility Clinic Success Rate and Certification Act 1992; Society for Assisted Reproductive Technology; United States
An emotional debate has attended the question of whether health insurance should cover the cost of in vitro fertilization (IVF) for infertile couples. Some private health plans have opted to cover IVF, although most have not. Ten states have mandated that it be included or offered as a standard benefit for private health insurance plans. This article analyzes several key issues in the debate: the impact of insurance coverage; the cost–effectiveness of IVF; valuing the benefit of IVF; and adoption as an alternative. It recommends policy action in several areas: more efficiently allocating resources for IVF (by giving priority to couples with better chances of success, and by making more extensive use of facilities with higher success rates); ensuring that clear and reliable information about the effectiveness of IVF is available; and leveling the playing field between IVF and adoption.

Pyers, Greg; Gott, Robert. Fertility Rights: The IVF Debate. Carlton, VIC, Australia: CIS Publishers; 1993. 49 p. (Australian issues series). ISBN 1–86391–102–2. BE57445.
    beginning of life; children; cryopreservation; economics; *embryo research; *embryo transfer; embryos; feminist ethics; *in vitro fertilization; infertility; legal aspects; *methods; *public policy; *reproductive technologies; *risks and benefits; social impact; terminology; treatment outcome; *Australia

Robertson, John A. Meaning what you sign. *Hastings Center Report.* 1998 Jul–Aug; 28(4): 22–23. 4 refs. BE58924.
    advance directives; autonomy; contracts; *cryopreservation; decision making; *embryo disposition; embryo research; *embryos; *in vitro fertilization; informed consent; *legal aspects; marital relationship; married persons; *property rights; *divorce; Davis v. Davis; *Kass v. Kass; *New York; Tennessee

Scritchfield, Shirley A. The infertility enterprise: IVF and the technological construction of reproductive impairments. *In:* Wertz, Dorothy C., ed. Research in the Sociology of Health Care: A Research Annual. Volume 8. Greenwich, CT: JAI Press; 1989: 61–97. 104 refs. 12 fn. ISBN 1–55938–043–8. BE57348.
    age factors; autonomy; disclosure; drugs; *economics; embryo research; embryos; employment; *females; goals; health hazards; *in vitro fertilization; *industry; *infertility; males; morality; motivation; parent child relationship; physician patient relationship; *physicians; prevalence; preventive medicine; professional autonomy; reproduction; *reproductive technologies; review; *risks and benefits; *social dominance; *social impact; socioeconomic factors; statistics; *treatment outcome; trends; values; women's health; United States

Tauer, Carol A. Donum Vitae: dissenting opinions on the "simple case" of in vitro fertilization. *In:* Wildes, Kevin Wm., ed. Infertility: A Crossroad of Faith, Medicine, and Technology. Boston, MA: Kluwer Academic; 1997: 125–146. 34 refs. ISBN 0–7923–4061–2. BE55995.
    biomedical technologies; consensus; contraception; dissent; females; *in vitro fertilization; justice; males; *marital relationship; *moral policy; newborns; reproduction; *Roman Catholic ethics; sexuality; social discrimination; *theology; *Instruction on Respect for Human Life

Tauer, Carol A. Embryo research and public policy: a philosopher's appraisal. *Journal of Medicine and*

BE = bioethics accession number   fn. = footnotes   refs. = references

Philosophy. 1997 Oct; 22(5): 423–439. 20 refs. 1 fn. BE56620.

advisory committees; beginning of life; committee membership; *embryo research; *embryos; federal government; fetal development; government financing; government regulation; *guidelines; human experimentation; *in vitro fertilization; *moral obligations; *moral policy; nontherapeutic research; ovum donors; parent child relationship; personhood; policy analysis; public opinion; *public policy; reproductive technologies; research embryo creation; risks and benefits; semen donors; twinning; value of life; values; Ethics Advisory Board; *Human Embryo Research Panel; National Institutes of Health; United States
The development of public policy on bioethical issues can be approached through substantive moral and philosophic reasoning, or through balancing perceived societal views as to what is ethically acceptable. The Human Embryo Research Panel had to apply the first approach to the question of the moral status of the preimplantation embryo. Only after concluding that the preimplantation embryo was not a full human subject could the panel consider the conditions under which embryo research was ethically acceptable, given a range of societal views, concerns, and interests.

Templeton, Allan; Morris, Joan K. Reducing the risk of multiple births by transfer of two embryos after in vitro fertilization. *New England Journal of Medicine.* 1998 Aug 27; 339(9): 573–577. 21 refs. BE58658.

age factors; *embryo transfer; evaluation studies; females; *in vitro fertilization; infertility; *multiple pregnancy; risk; time factors; *treatment outcome; Great Britain
BACKGROUND: In vitro fertilization is associated with a high risk of multiple births, which is a direct consequence of the number of embryos transferred. However, other factors that contribute to the risk are not well defined. METHODS: Using the data base established by the Human Fertilization and Embryology Authority in the United Kingdom, we studied the factors associated with an increased risk of multiple births in 44,236 cycles in 25,240 women. The factors included the woman's age, the cause and duration of infertility, previous attempts at in vitro fertilization, previous live births, number of eggs fertilized, and number of embryos transferred. RESULTS: Older age, tubal infertility, longer duration of infertility, and a higher number of previous attempts at in vitro fertilization were all associated with a significantly decreased chance of a birth and of multiple births. Previous live birth was associated with an increased chance of a birth but not of multiple births. The higher the number of eggs fertilized, the higher the likelihood of a live birth. When more than four eggs were fertilized, there was no increase in the birth rate for women receiving three transferred embryos as compared with those receiving two, but there was a considerable increase in the rate of multiple births when three were transferred (odds ratio, 1.6; 95 percent confidence interval, 1.5 to 1.8). CONCLUSIONS: Among women undergoing in vitro fertilization, the chances of a live birth are related to the number of eggs fertilized, presumably because of the greater selection of embryos for transfer. When more than four eggs are fertilized and available for transfer, the woman's chance of a birth is not diminished by transferring only two embryos. Transferring more embryos increases the risk of multiple births.

Trad, Fouad S.; Hornstein, Mark D.; Barbieri, Robert L. *In vitro* fertilization: a cost-effective alternative for infertile couples? *Journal of Assisted Reproduction and Genetics.* 1995 Aug; 12(7): 418–421. 22 refs. BE55582.

adoption; age factors; alternatives; childbirth; *costs and

benefits; *embryo transfer; *evaluation; evaluation studies; females; *in vitro fertilization; infertility; males; surgery; *treatment outcome; Brigham and Women's Hospital (Boston)

Aetna to charge extra for in vitro fertilization. [News]. *New York Times.* 1998 Jan 15: A15. BE57597.

*health insurance reimbursement; *in vitro fertilization; *reproductive technologies; *Aetna

INFANTICIDE

See also ALLOWING TO DIE/INFANTS, EUTHANASIA

Harris, John. Should we attempt to eradicate disability? *In:* Morscher, Edgar; Neumaier, Otto; Simons, Peter, eds. Applied Ethics in a Troubled World. Boston, MA: Kluwer Academic; 1998: 105–114. 24 fn. ISBN 0-7923-4965-2. BE58585.

active euthanasia; allowing to die; *congenital disorders; *disabled; embryo transfer; embryos; eugenics; fetuses; in vitro fertilization; *infanticide; intention; maternal health; newborns; personhood; political activity; quality of life; reproduction; *selective abortion; *social discrimination; therapeutic abortion; value of life; International Wittgenstein Symposium

Lester, David. Abortion laws and infanticide. *Psychological Reports.* 1995 Jun; 76(3, pt. 2): 1370. 3 refs. BE55513.

*abortion, induced; comparative studies; government regulation; *infanticide; infants; *international aspects; killing; *legal aspects; newborns; *social impact; statistics

INFANTS
See under
ALLOWING TO DIE/INFANTS

INFORMED CONSENT

See also TREATMENT REFUSAL
See also under
BEHAVIORAL RESEARCH/INFORMED CONSENT
HUMAN EXPERIMENTATION/INFORMED CONSENT

Ackerman, Terrence F. Chemically dependent physicians and informed consent disclosure. *Journal of Addictive Diseases.* 1996; 15(2): 25–42. 19 refs. BE55703.

*alcohol abuse; confidentiality; *disclosure; *drug abuse; employment; federal government; guidelines; HIV seropositivity; *informed consent; injuries; *legal aspects; legal liability; legal obligations; legal rights; organizational policies; patient care; *physicians; privacy; *professional competence; professional organizations; public opinion; *rehabilitation; *risk; *self regulation; *physician impairment; American Medical Association; Americans with Disabilities Act 1990; Centers for Disease Control and Prevention; United States

Agard, Ellen; Finkelstein, Daniel; Wallach, Edward. Cultural diversity and informed consent. [Case study]. *Journal of Clinical Ethics.* 1998 Summer; 9(2): 173–176. Commented on by M. d'Agostino, p. 177–178, and by E.G. Howe, p. 191–193. BE58962.

aliens; alternatives; *autonomy; case studies; clinical ethics committees; *coercion; *counseling; *cultural pluralism; *decision making; *females; human rights; infertility; *informed consent; males; *marital relationship; *married persons; motivation; *paternalism; *patient care team; physicians; reproduction; *risks and benefits; spousal

---

BE = bioethics accession number   fn. = footnotes   refs. = references

consent; *surgery; *values; women's rights

Agich, George J. Can the patient make treatment decisions? Evaluating decisional capacity. *Cleveland Clinic Journal of Medicine.* 1997 Oct; 64(9): 461–464. 6 refs. BE58350.
> advance directives; *competence; comprehension; decision making; disclosure; evaluation; *informed consent; physician's role; standards; third party consent; *treatment refusal; United States

Ardagh, Michael. May we practise endotracheal intubation on the newly dead? *Journal of Medical Ethics.* 1997 Oct; 23(5): 289–294. 40 refs. BE57100.
> advance directives; allied health personnel; alternatives; altruism; anesthesia; attitudes; attitudes to death; autopsies; *cadavers; cardiac death; communitarianism; emergency care; emotions; family members; human body; *informed consent; international aspects; legal aspects; *medical education; moral policy; organ donation; organizational policies; policy analysis; *presumed consent; professional organizations; property rights; *public policy; religion; *resuscitation; students; technical expertise; third party consent; utilitarianism; *intubation; *mandated choice

Endotracheal intubation (ETI) is a valuable procedure which must be learnt and practised, and performing ETI on cadavers is probably the best way to do this, although lesser alternatives do exist. Performing ETI on a cadaver is viewed with a real and reasonable repugnance and if it is done without proper authorisation it might be illegal. Some form of consent is required. Presumed consent would preferably be governed by statute and should only occur if the community is well informed and therefore in a position of being able to decline. Currently neither statute nor adequate informing exists. Endotracheal intubation on the newly dead may be justifiable according to a Guttman scale if the patient has already consented to organ donation and if further research supports the relevance of the Guttman scale to this question. A "mandated choice" with prior individual consent as a matter of public policy is the best of these solutions, however until such a solution is in place we may not practise endotracheal intubation on the newly dead.

Arnold, Robert M.; Shaw, Byers W.; Purtilo, Ruth. Acute, high risk patients: the case of transplantation. *In:* McCullough, Laurence B.; Jones, James W.; Brody, Baruch A., eds. Surgical Ethics. New York, NY: Oxford University Press; 1998: 97–115. 27 refs. ISBN 0–19–510347–5. BE58323.
> age factors; alcohol abuse; alternatives; body parts and fluids; *critically ill; disclosure; economics; hospitals; *informed consent; institutional policies; justice; livers; managed care programs; morbidity; mortality; organ donation; *organ transplantation; patients; *physicians; professional competence; prognosis; quality of health care; resource allocation; retreatment; risk; risks and benefits; scarcity; *selection for treatment; self induced illness; statistics; *surgery; time factors; treatment outcome; geographic factors; United Network for Organ Sharing; United States

Australia. Tasmania. An act (No. 44 of 1995) to enable persons with a disability to be represented by a guardian or administrator and to provide for medical and dental treatment for persons with a disability. Date of assent: 22 Sep 1995. [The Guardianship and Administration Act 1995]. *International Digest of Health Legislation.* 1996; 47(2): 174–178. BE57189.
> dentistry; *disabled; emergency care; *legal aspects; *legal guardians; *patient care; *third party consent; *Guardianship and Administration Act 1995 (Tasmania); *Tasmania

Aydin, Erdem. Informed consent in Turkey. [Letter]. *Journal of Medical Ethics.* 1997 Jun; 23(3): 192. 1 ref. BE55900.
> *communication; comprehension; *cultural pluralism; *informed consent; international aspects; *patients; physician patient relationship; terminology; non–Western World; Western World; *Turkey

Bailey, R. Norman. The doctor-patient relationship: communication, informed consent and the optometric patient. *Journal of the American Optometric Association.* 1994 Jun; 65(6): 418–422. 8 refs. BE55782.
> autonomy; *communication; decision making; *disclosure; eye diseases; *informed consent; legal aspects; paternalism; *patient care; *patient participation; *physician patient relationship; risks and benefits; trust; uncertainty; *optometry

Barnes, Donelle M.; Davis, Anne J.; Moran, Tracy, et al. Informed consent in a multicultural cancer patient population: implications for nursing practice. *Nursing Ethics.* 1998 Sep; 5(5): 412–423. 33 refs. BE58904.
> *Asian Americans; autonomy; *cancer; *communication; comprehension; *cultural pluralism; *decision making; diagnosis; disclosure; family relationship; females; goals; *Hispanic Americans; *informed consent; males; *minority groups; nurses; nursing research; paternalism; patient care; patient participation; physician patient relationship; physicians; prognosis; quality of life; survey; terminally ill; truth disclosure; *values; *whites; United States

Beauchamp, Tom L. Comparative studies: Japan and America. *In:* Hoshino, Kazumasa, ed. Japanese and Western Bioethics: Studies in Moral Diversity. Boston, MA: Kluwer Academic; 1997: 25–47. 62 refs. 17 fn. ISBN 0–7923–4112–0. BE57081.
> attitudes; *autonomy; bioethics; cancer; communication; comparative studies; competence; *cultural pluralism; decision making; *disclosure; *ethical relativism; historical aspects; human experimentation; human rights; *informed consent; *international aspects; investigator subject relationship; legal aspects; *morality; *paternalism; *patient care; patient compliance; physician patient relationship; physicians; research subjects; socioeconomic factors; time factors; truth disclosure; values; *Japan; Twentieth Century; *United States

Bernhardt, Barbara A.; Geller, Gail; Strauss, Misha, et al. Toward a model informed consent process for BRCA1 testing: a qualitative assessment of women's attitudes. *Journal of Genetic Counseling.* 1997 Jun; 6(2): 207–222. 16 refs. BE55666.
> adults; *breast cancer; children; comprehension; decision making; directive counseling; *disclosure; *females; *genetic counseling; *genetic predisposition; *genetic screening; guidelines; health education; *informed consent; insurance; *knowledge, attitudes, practice; models, theoretical; patient participation; physician patient relationship; physicians; public opinion; risk; *risks and benefits; social discrimination; socioeconomic factors; survey; trust; uncertainty; qualitative research; urban population; Baltimore

Billick, Stephen B.; Della Bella, Peter; Burgert, Woodward. Competency to consent to hospitalization in the medical patient. *Journal of the American Academy of Psychiatry and the Law.* 1997; 25(2): 191–196. 7 refs. BE55601.
> adolescents; adults; comparative studies; *competence; evaluation studies; hospitals; *informed consent; institutionalized persons; *mentally ill; *patient admission; *patients; psychiatric diagnosis; *voluntary admission; questionnaires; St. Vincent's Hospital and Medical Center (New York City)

Black, Douglas. Corporate tyranny. [Editorial]. *Journal of Medical Ethics.* 1997 Oct; 23(5): 269–270. 4 refs. BE56903.
>   *advisory committees; *artificial insemination; beneficence; *bioethical issues; *confidentiality; *consensus; death; *decision making; famous persons; *informed consent; married persons; *posthumous reproduction; regulation; *semen donors; suicide; *General Medical Council (Great Britain); Great Britain; *Human Fertilisation and Embryology Authority; Wingate, Orde

Bloche, M. Gregg. Managed care, medical privacy, and the paradigm of consent. *Kennedy Institute of Ethics Journal.* 1997 Dec; 7(4): 381–386. 2 refs. BE59020.
>   advertising; *computer communication networks; computers; *confidentiality; contracts; *disclosure; *informed consent; *managed care programs; *medical records; patient care; patients; *privacy; United States

The market success of managed health plans in the 1990s is bringing to medicine the easy availability of electronically stored information that is characteristic of the securities and consumer credit industries. Protection for medical confidentiality, however, has not kept pace with this information revolution. Employers, the managed care industry, and legal and ethics commentators frequently look to the concept of informed consent to justify particular uses of health information, but the elastic use of informed consent as a way of responding to managed care health plans' disclosure of information to third parties fails to address underlying questions involving substantive value choices.

Block, Marian R.; Schaffner, Kenneth F.; Coulehan, John L. Ethical problems of recording physician-patient interactions in family practice settings. *Journal of Family Practice.* 1985; 21(6): 467–472. 14 refs. BE57823.
>   *audiovisual aids; autonomy; coercion; competence; *confidentiality; *family practice; guidelines; *informed consent; *medical education; physician patient relationship; privacy; teaching methods; outpatients; *video recording

Blustein, Jeffrey; Robinson, Walter; Loeben, Gregory S., et al. Case vignette: placebos and informed consent. [Case study and commentaries]. *Ethics and Behavior.* 1998; 8(1): 89–98. 3 refs. BE58919.
>   autonomy; beneficence; chronically ill; deception; deontological ethics; disclosure; *informed consent; motivation; *pain; *patient care; patient participation; physician patient relationship; *placebos; psychology; teleological ethics; treatment outcome; trust

Bopp, James; Coleson, Richard E. A critique of family members as proxy decisionmakers without legal limits. *Issues in Law and Medicine.* 1996 Fall; 12(2): 133–165. 232 fn. BE58760.
>   adults; *allowing to die; artificial feeding; *autonomy; competence; *conflict of interest; congenital disorders; *decision making; *disabled; economics; emotions; *evaluation; *family members; family relationship; *legal aspects; legal rights; minors; motivation; newborns; parental consent; persistent vegetative state; physicians; prolongation of life; quality of life; *standards; state interest; *third party consent; value of life; withholding treatment; adult offspring; In re Lawrance; United States

Braaten, Ellen B.; Handelsman, Mitchell M. Client preferences for informed consent information. *Ethics and Behavior.* 1997; 7(4): 311–328. 57 refs. BE58663.
>   alternatives; *attitudes; autonomy; communication; comparative studies; confidentiality; consent forms; *counseling; *disclosure; health personnel; *informed consent; medical fees; *patients; professional competence;

professional patient relationship; psychology; *psychotherapy; risks and benefits; *students; survey; time factors; universities; United States

Thirty-five current therapy clients, 47 former clients, and 42 college students with no therapy experience rated 27 items in terms of importance for inclusion in informed consent discussions. The current and former client samples rated information about inappropriate therapeutic techniques, confidentiality, and the risks of alternative treatments as most important, and information about the personal characteristics of the therapist and the therapist's degree as least important. The results of this study provide evidence for differential informed consent disclosure practices.

Brahams, Diana. UK gynaecologist found guilty of serious professional misconduct. [News]. *Lancet.* 1997 Oct 4; 350(9083): 1014. BE56923.
>   females; *informed consent; *misconduct; *obstetrics and gynecology; *physicians; punishment; regulation; *surgery; *hysterectomy; *ovaries; General Medical Council (Great Britain); *Great Britain; *Studd, John

Brock, Dan W. An ethical framework for surrogate decision-making. *In:* Grubb, Andrew, ed. Decision-Making and Problems of Incompetence. New York, NY: Wiley; 1994: 41–52. 9 fn. ISBN 0-471-94236-7. BE57128.
>   adults; advance directives; *allowing to die; autonomy; *competence; *decision making; family members; informed consent; legal aspects; moral policy; patient care; physician's role; prolongation of life; quality of life; risks and benefits; *standards; *third party consent; treatment refusal; value of life; values; withholding treatment; *United States

Brock, Dan W. Informed consent. *In:* Borchert, Donald M., ed. The Encyclopedia of Philosophy. Supplement. New York, NY: Simon and Schuster Macmillan; 1996: 261–262. 2 refs. ISBN 0-02-864629-0. BE57223.
>   autonomy; competence; decision making; disclosure; *informed consent; patient care; patient participation; third party consent; treatment refusal

Buetow, Stephen; Cantrill, Judith; Sibbald, Bonnie. Risk communication in the patient-health professional relationship. *Health Care Analysis.* 1998 Sep; 6(3): 261–268. 42 refs. BE58929.
>   audiovisual aids; *communication; *disclosure; *informed consent; legal aspects; methods; patient care; quality of health care; *risk; risks and benefits; uncertainty

Cain, Paul. Using clients. *Nursing Ethics.* 1997 Nov; 4(6): 465–471. 1 ref. BE57415.
>   autonomy; confidentiality; disclosure; *informed consent; *moral obligations; nurse patient relationship; nurses; *nursing education; *nursing ethics; *nursing research; paternalism; *patients; privacy; *research subjects; *students; trust; utilitarianism; wedge argument

Cameron, Cheryl A. Mandatory consent to treatment by students in dental education: legal and policy considerations. *Journal of Dental Education.* 1995 Apr; 59(4): 495–501. 50 refs. BE56860.
>   contracts; *dentistry; dissent; *education; federal government; government regulation; *informed consent; *institutional policies; *legal rights; *mandatory programs; nontherapeutic research; *patient care; patients; privacy; property rights; *schools; *students; *dental schools; United States

Chambers, Tod. Letting the patient backstage: informed consent for HMO enrollees. *Journal of the American Geriatrics Society.* 1998 Mar; 46(3): 355–358. 10 refs.

BE = bioethics accession number   fn. = footnotes   refs. = references

Paper presented at the 1996 Congress of Clinical Societies. BE56755.
   administrators; alternatives; conflict of interest; contracts; decision making; *disclosure; economics; gatekeeping; *health maintenance organizations; incentives; *informed consent; *organizational policies; patient care; physician's role; physicians; referral and consultation; remuneration; risks and benefits; gag clauses; United States

d'Agostino, Monica. Respect for autonomy and a couple's decision. *Journal of Clinical Ethics.* 1998 Summer; 9(2): 177–178. Commentary on E. Agard et al., p. 173–176. BE58963.
   aliens; *autonomy; coercion; *counseling; *cultural pluralism; decision making; *informed consent; *marital relationship; *married persons; paternalism; physicians; reproduction; spousal consent; *surgery; values

Davis, Anne J.; Aroskar, Mila A.; Liaschenko, Joan, et al. Ethical principles of informed consent. *In: their* Ethical Dilemmas and Nursing Practice. Fourth Edition. Stamford, CT: Appleton and Lange; 1997: 105–134. 144 fn. ISBN 0-8385-2283-1. BE58595.
   autonomy; behavioral research; beneficence; case studies; coercion; comprehension; disclosure; federal government; government regulation; guidelines; *human experimentation; *informed consent; investigator subject relationship; nurses; nursing research; patient care; research subjects; risks and benefits; scientific misconduct; trust; vulnerable populations; United States

Dellasega, Cheryl; Frank, Lori; Smyer, Michael. Medical decision-making capacity in elderly hospitalized patients. *Journal of Ethics, Law, and Aging.* 1996 Fall–Winter; 2(2): 65–74. 28 refs. Commented on by D.J. Marson and K.K. Ingram, p. 59–63. BE57140.
   *aged; alternatives; *competence; comprehension; critically ill; *decision making; disclosure; *evaluation; evaluation studies; *hospitals; *informed consent; methods; patient admission; *patient care; patient discharge; *patients; physicians; risks and benefits; time factors; rationality; Patient Self-Determination Act 1990; Pennsylvania; United States

De Ville, Kenneth; Kaplan, Carl A. Treating the silent stranger: informed consent and defensive medicine in the critical care unit. *HEC (HealthCare Ethics Committee) Forum.* 1998 Mar; 10(1): 55–70. 20 refs. BE59058.
   biomedical technologies; case studies; communication; competence; *critically ill; decision making; diagnosis; *emergency care; iatrogenic disease; *informed consent; *intensive care units; legal liability; physicians; *presumed consent; quality of health care; third party consent; absence of proxy

Dickens, Bernard M. Choices, control, access -- the Canadian position. *In:* Knoppers, Bartha Maria, ed. Human DNA: Law and Policy: International and Comparative Perspectives. Proceedings of the First International Conference on DNA Sampling and Human Genetic Research: Ethical, Legal, and Policy Aspects, held in Montreal, Canada, 6–8 Sep 1996. Boston, MA: Kluwer Law International; 1997: 71–89. 59 fn. ISBN 90-411-0361-9. BE58169.
   *confidentiality; criminal law; *disclosure; *DNA data banks; DNA fingerprinting; employment; federal government; *genetic information; *genetic materials; *genetic research; *genetic screening; government regulation; health personnel; *informed consent; law enforcement; *legal aspects; legislation; mandatory testing; privacy; private sector; public sector; state government; tissue donation; *biological specimen banks; *Canada; *Privacy Act 1983 (Canada); Quebec

Draper, Heather. Consent in childbirth. *In:* Frith, Lucy, ed. Ethics and Midwifery: Issues in Contemporary Practice. Boston, MA: Butterworth–Heinemann; 1996: 17–35. 9 refs. ISBN 0-7506-3056-6. BE58632.
   *autonomy; beneficence; blood transfusions; cesarean section; *childbirth; coercion; competence; contracts; counseling; decision making; disclosure; fetuses; home care; *informed consent; Jehovah's Witnesses; moral obligations; *nurse midwives; nurse patient relationship; paternalism; *patient care; *pregnant women; risks and benefits; standards; treatment refusal; values; women's rights

Dresser, Rebecca; Astrow, Alan B. An alert and incompetent self: the irrelevance of advance directives. [Case study and commentaries]. *Hastings Center Report.* 1998 Jan–Feb; 28(1): 28–30. BE57295.
   *advance directives; *allowing to die; autonomy; case studies; clinical ethics committees; *competence; *critically ill; *decision making; *dissent; emotions; friends; *living wills; love; *patient care team; patient participation; patient transfer; physicians; professional patient relationship; prognosis; *prolongation of life; *third party consent; time factors; treatment refusal; *uncertainty; *ventilators

Dyer, Clare. Consultant suspended for not getting consent for cardiac procedure. [News]. *BMJ (British Medical Journal).* 1998 Mar 28; 316(7136): 955. BE58056.
   children; death; deception; hearts; *malpractice; *misconduct; *parental consent; *patient care; *physicians; punishment; surgery; General Medical Council (Great Britain); Jenkins, Debbie; London; *Taylor, James

Dyer, Clare. Gynaecologist admonished for removing ovaries without consent. [News]. *BMJ (British Medical Journal).* 1997 Oct 4; 315(7112): 832. BE56080.
   females; *informed consent; *misconduct; *obstetrics and gynecology; *physicians; punishment; self regulation; *surgery; *hysterectomy; *ovaries; Bartley, Jacqueline; General Medical Council (Great Britain); Great Britain; *Studd, John

Eller, Thomas R. Informed consent civil actions for post-abortion psychological trauma. *Notre Dame Law Review.* 1996; 71(4): 639–670. 214 fn. BE56659.
   *abortion, induced; alternatives; coercion; counseling; *disclosure; fetal development; government regulation; *informed consent; *legal aspects; *legal liability; legal rights; maternal health; mental health; paternalism; *physicians; *pregnant women; *psychological stress; *risk; state government; Supreme Court decisions; *Planned Parenthood of Southeastern Pennsylvania v. Casey; *United States

Espinoza, Leslie G. Dissecting women, dissecting law: the court-ordering of caesarean section operations and the failure of informed consent to protect women of color. *National Black Law Journal.* 1994; 13: 211–237. 211 fn. BE58974.
   Asian Americans; autonomy; blacks; *cesarean section; *coercion; communication; competence; cultural pluralism; decision making; *fetuses; Hispanic Americans; hospitals; indigents; *informed consent; judicial action; *legal aspects; legal rights; *minority groups; mother fetus relationship; physicians; *pregnant women; social discrimination; *state interest; terminally ill; *treatment refusal; *viability; District of Columbia; George Washington University Hospital; *In re A.C.; In re Madyun

Etchells, Edward; Sharpe, Gilbert; Dykeman, Mary Jane, et al. Bioethics for clinicians: 4. Voluntariness. *Canadian Medical Association Journal.* 1996 Oct 15; 155(8): 1083–1086. 29 refs. BE56152.
   aged; *autonomy; case studies; coercion; disclosure; *informed consent; institutionalized persons; legal aspects;

mentally ill; patient advocacy; patient care; physician patient relationship; treatment refusal; Canada

Faden, Ruth. Managed care and informed consent. *Kennedy Institute of Ethics Journal.* 1997 Dec; 7(4): 377–379. 7 refs. BE59019.

alternatives; contracts; *costs and benefits; *disclosure; economics; incentives; *informed consent; institutional policies; *managed care programs; medical specialties; patient care; physicians; withholding treatment; gag clauses; United States

Arguments for efficiency in health care delivery have been used to support some level of withholding of information about available treatment options from patients in managed care systems. To the extent that such arguments prevail, they may necessitate changes in the established understanding of and commitment to informed consent and the disclosure of information to patients.

Feenan, Dermot. Capable people: empowering the patient in the assessment of capacity. *Health Care Analysis.* 1997 Sep; 5(3): 227–236. 52 refs. BE55856.

*autonomy; *competence; *decision making; evaluation; health personnel; informed consent; mentally disabled; minors; paternalism; *patient advocacy; patient care; *patient participation; physician patient relationship; physician's role; social dominance; standards; treatment refusal; values; *empowerment; Great Britain

Fetters, Michael D. The family in medical decision making: Japanese perspectives. *Journal of Clinical Ethics.* 1998 Summer; 9(2): 132–146. 48 fn. BE58959.

age factors; attitudes to death; autonomy; beneficence; bioethics; Buddhist ethics; *cancer; clinical ethics; consensus; *cultural pluralism; *decision making; *diagnosis; economics; *family members; *family relationship; females; males; minority groups; models, theoretical; morality; paternalism; patient care; patient participation; physician patient relationship; physicians; public opinion; religion; social dominance; terminal care; *third party consent; trends; *truth disclosure; *values; Confucian ethics; non-Western World; preventive ethics; *Japan; United States

Flax, Robert A. Silicone breast implants: two stories of informed consent. *In:* BioLaw: A Legal and Ethical Reporter on Medicine, Health Care, and Bioengineering. Special Sections, 2(9). Frederick, MD: University Publications of America; 1997 Sep: S311–S330. 58 refs. BE56646.

autonomy; breast cancer; coercion; communication; comprehension; *cosmetic surgery; *disclosure; *federal government; *females; *government regulation; human experimentation; *industry; *information dissemination; *informed consent; legal liability; *medical devices; paternalism; patient care; *patient education; physicians; *risk; risks and benefits; standards; uncertainty; women's health; *breast implants; *Dow Corning; *Food and Drug Administration; United States

Foster, Peggy; Anderson, C. Mary. Reaching targets in the national cervical screening programme: are current practices unethical? *Journal of Medical Ethics.* 1998 Jun; 24(3): 151–157. 33 fn. BE59111.

age factors; autonomy; *cancer; coercion; disclosure; *females; goals; incentives; *informed consent; *mass screening; mortality; paternalism; physicians; *preventive medicine; primary health care; psychological stress; *public policy; remuneration; risk; *risks and benefits; socioeconomic factors; uncertainty; voluntary programs; *Great Britain; *National Health Service

The principle of informed consent is now well established within the National Health Service (NHS) in relation to any type of medical treatment. However,

this ethical principle appears to be far less well established in relation to medical screening programmes such as Britain's national cervical screening programme. This article will critically examine the case for health care providers vigorously pursuing women to accept an invitation to be screened. It will discuss the type of information which women would need in order to make an informed decision about whether or not to be screened. The lack of such information in current patient leaflets on the "smear test" will then be documented. Finally, the article will explore possible ways of maximising women's autonomy in relation to the cervical screening programme without sacrificing any of its main benefits.

Geller, Gail; Botkin, Jeffrey R.; Green, Michael J., et al. Genetic testing for susceptibility to adult–onset cancer: the process and content of informed consent. *JAMA.* 1997 May 14; 277(18): 1467–1474. 122 refs. BE55859.

adults; advisory committees; alternatives; audiovisual aids; *cancer; communication; comprehension; confidentiality; consent forms; decision making; *disclosure; DNA data banks; employment; *genetic counseling; genetic information; *genetic predisposition; *genetic screening; *guidelines; information dissemination; *informed consent; insurance; *late-onset disorders; minority groups; *patient education; privacy; professional patient relationship; psychology; *public policy; risks and benefits; social discrimination; teaching methods; time factors; NHGRI–funded publication; Cancer Genetics Studies Consortium; *Task Force on Informed Consent

OBJECTIVE: To provide guidance on informed consent to clinicians offering cancer susceptibility testing. PARTICIPANTS: The Task Force on Informed Consent is part of the Cancer Genetics Studies Consortium (CGSC), whose members were recipients of National Institutes of Health grants to assess the implications of cancer susceptibility testing. The 10 task force members represent a range of relevant backgrounds, including various medical specialties, social science, genetic counseling, and consumer advocacy. EVIDENCE: The CGSC held 3 public meetings from 1994 to 1996. At its first meeting, the task force jointly established a list of topics. The cochairs (G.G. and J.R.B) then developed an outline and assigned each topic to an appropriate writer and reviewer. Writers summarized the literature on their topics and drafted recommendations, which were then revised by the reviewers. The cochairs compiled and edited the entire manuscript. All members were involved in writing this report. CONSENSUS PROCESS: The first draft was distributed to task force members, after which a meeting was held to discuss its content and organization. Consensus was reached by voting. A subsequent draft was presented to the entire CGSC at its third meeting, and comments were incorporated. CONCLUSIONS: The task force recommends that informed consent for cancer susceptibility testing be an ongoing process of education and counseling in which (1) providers elicit participant, family, and community values and disclose their own, (2) decision making is shared, (3) the style of information disclosure is individualized, and (4) specific content areas are discussed.

Gevers, Sjef; Olsthoorn–Heim, Els. DNA sampling: Dutch and other European approaches to the issues of informed consent and confidentiality. *In:* Knoppers, Bartha Maria, ed. Human DNA: Law and Policy: International and Comparative Perspectives. Proceedings of the First International Conference on DNA Sampling and Human Genetic Research: Ethical,

---

BE = bioethics accession number   fn. = footnotes   refs. = references

Legal, and Policy Aspects, held in Montreal, Canada, 6–8 Sep 1996. Boston, MA: Kluwer Law International; 1997: 109–120. 18 fn. ISBN 90–411–0361–9. BE58171.
advisory committees; *confidentiality; *DNA data banks; *genetic information; *genetic materials; genetic research; *genetic screening; government regulation; guidelines; *informed consent; *international aspects; privacy; *public policy; *regulation; *tissue donation; *biological specimen banks; Council of Europe; *Europe; National Ethics Advisory Committee (France); *Netherlands; Nuffield Council on Bioethics

Giesen, Dieter. Comparative legal developments. *In:* Grubb, Andrew, ed. Decision–Making and Problems of Incompetence. New York, NY: Wiley; 1994: 7–26. 126 fn. ISBN 0–471–94236–7. BE57126.
adults; allowing to die; autonomy; *competence; *decision making; family members; *informed consent; international aspects; judicial action; *legal aspects; legal guardians; mentally disabled; minors; parental consent; *patient care; patients; physicians; quality of life; standards; *third party consent; *treatment refusal; value of life; withholding treatment; Australia; Canada; Germany; *Great Britain; United States

Goldblatt, A.D. You can't always get what you want. *Update Loma Linda University Center for Christian Bioethics.* 1997 Jul; 13(2): 5–7. 6 fn. Commentary on K.V. Iserson, "Life versus death: the ethical imperative to practice and teach using the newly dead," p. 2–4. BE57990.
alternatives; autonomy; *cadavers; consent forms; donor cards; emergency care; family members; freedom; *health personnel; hospitals; *informed consent; institutional policies; legal liability; legal rights; legislation; *medical education; organ donation; *presumed consent; *professional competence; property rights; *third party consent; required response; teaching hospitals

Gostin, Lawrence O. Personal privacy in the health care system: employer–sponsored insurance, managed care, and integrated delivery systems. *Kennedy Institute of Ethics Journal.* 1997 Dec; 7(4): 361–376. 27 refs. 3 fn. BE59018.
biomedical research; computer communication networks; computers; *confidentiality; data banks; *disclosure; *employment; *health care delivery; health facilities; *health insurance; health personnel; *informed consent; law; *managed care programs; *medical records; patient care; *privacy; public health; quality assurance; *United States
Widespread collection and use of identifiable information can promote social goods while, at the same time, infringing on personal privacy. Information systems are developing within the context of a fundamental transformation in the organization, delivery, and financing of health care. Changes in the health care system include rapid development of employer–sponsored health coverage, managed care organizations, and integrated delivery systems. These complex, multifaceted arrangements for delivering and paying for health care require ever–more–sophisticated information systems that facilitate extensive sharing of personal data. Systemic flows of sensitive health information occur both vertically and horizontally among employers, hospitals, insurers, laboratories, and suppliers. Beyond this complex web of vertical and horizontal sharing are the multiple demands for information management, quality assurance, research, governmental regulation, and public health. Theoretical problems exist with the law and ethics of informational privacy. The traditional method of exercising control over personal health information is through informed consent. Informed consent, however, within a modern health information infrastructure becomes highly complex. In this kind of environment, the doctrine of informed consent is flawed and does not provide sufficient control over personal information to assure adequate protection of privacy.

Grisso, Thomas; Appelbaum, Paul S. Assessing Competence to Consent to Treatment: A Guide for Physicians and Other Health Professionals. New York, NY: Oxford University Press; 1998. 211 p. 40 refs. ISBN 0–19–510372–6. BE57443.
adults; advance directives; autonomy; case studies; *competence; comprehension; *decision making; dementia; disclosure; *evaluation; family members; health personnel; *informed consent; judicial action; legal aspects; mentally disabled; *patient care; patient participation; patients; records; *standards; third party consent; treatment refusal; *MacArthur Competence Assessment Tool for Treatment (MacCat-T)

Grover, Bonnie Kae. From both sides now: informed consent, organ transplantation, and family–based disclosure. *Law and Policy.* 1995 Apr; 17(2): 188–209. 66 refs. 26 fn. Commented on by S. Wear and G. Logue, p. 210–216. BE58238.
autonomy; coercion; communicable diseases; decision making; disadvantaged; *disclosure; drugs; economics; *family members; *family relationship; hearts; *informed consent; *legal aspects; *organ transplantation; patient care; physician patient relationship; physicians; privacy; professional family relationship; risk; risks and benefits; social dominance; third party consent; toxicity; *transplant recipients

Grubb, Andrew, ed. Decision–Making and Problems of Incompetence. New York, NY: Wiley; 1994. 203 p. 508 fn. Papers presented at the first Annual Conference of the UK Forum on Health Care Ethics and the Law held under the auspices of the Centre of Medical Law and Ethics at King's College London in April 1991. ISBN 0–471–94236–7. BE57125.
adults; advance directives; AIDS; allowing to die; artificial feeding; autonomy; coercion; communication; *competence; comprehension; *decision making; family members; females; *informed consent; international aspects; involuntary sterilization; judicial action; *legal aspects; *mentally disabled; minors; outpatient commitment; paternalism; patient care; persistent vegetative state; physicians; reproduction; right to die; *standards; sterilization (sexual); *third party consent; treatment refusal; values; withholding treatment; Canada; *Great Britain; Law Commission (Great Britain); United States

Hawkins, Dana. A bloody mess at one federal lab. [News]. *U.S. News and World Report.* 1997 Jun 23; 122(24): 26–27. BE58044.
blacks; disclosure; *employment; federal government; females; Hispanic Americans; *informed consent; institutional policies; legal aspects; males; *mass screening; *minority groups; pregnant women; privacy; research institutes; sickle cell anemia; social discrimination; syphilis; Department of Energy; *Lawrence Berkeley National Laboratory; United States

Henley, L.; Benatar, S.R.; Robertson, B.A., et al. Informed consent -- a survey of doctors' practices in South Africa. *South African Medical Journal.* 1995 Dec; 85(12): 1273, 1275–1278. 25 refs. BE55557.
alternatives; comprehension; *disclosure; economics; guidelines; hospitals; *informed consent; *knowledge, attitudes, practice; legal aspects; medical education; medical ethics; parental consent; paternalism; patient care; patients; *physicians; professional organizations; risks and benefits; survey; values; *South Africa; University of Cape Town

---

BE = bioethics accession number   fn. = footnotes   refs. = references

Hern, H. Eugene; Koenig, Barbara A.; Moore, Lisa Jean, et al. The difference that culture can make in end–of–life decisionmaking. *Cambridge Quarterly of Healthcare Ethics.* 1998 Winter; 7(1): 27–40. 30 fn. BE58455.
　　alternative therapies; anthropology; *Asian Americans; *autonomy; *cancer; case studies; clinical ethics; *communication; *cultural pluralism; *decision making; *diagnosis; disclosure; *family members; *family relationship; females; *informed consent; *knowledge, attitudes, practice; *minority groups; models, theoretical; patient care; *patient care team; *patient participation; *patients; *physician patient relationship; physicians; *professional family relationship; *prognosis; risks and benefits; stigmatization; *terminal care; terminally ill; *third party consent; trust; *truth disclosure; *values; California; United States

Hirtle, Marie. Genetic screening and research revisited. *In:* Knoppers, Bartha Maria, ed. Human DNA: Law and Policy: International and Comparative Perspectives. Proceedings of the First International Conference on DNA Sampling and Human Genetic Research: Ethical, Legal, and Policy Aspects, held in Montreal, Canada, 6–8 Sep 1996. Boston, MA: Kluwer Law International; 1997: 333–340. 7 fn. ISBN 90–411–0361–9. BE58190.
　　cancer; *carriers; cystic fibrosis; DNA data banks; federal government; genetic materials; *genetic research; *genetic screening; *informed consent; legal aspects; *newborns; *parental consent; prenatal diagnosis; presumed consent; thalassemia; biological specimen banks; Europe; National Center for Human Genome Research; United States

Holland, Paul V. Consent for transfusion: is it informed? *Transfusion Medicine Reviews.* 1997 Oct; 11(4): 274–285. 64 refs. BE58978.
　　alternatives; *blood transfusions; consent forms; disclosure; drugs; human experimentation; *informed consent; legal aspects; patient care; risks and benefits; ambulatory care; United States

Hood, Catherine A.; Hope, Tony; Dove, Phillip. Videos, photographs, and patient consent. *BMJ (British Medical Journal).* 1998 Mar 28; 316(7136): 1009–1011. 13 refs. BE57555.
　　*audiovisual aids; *computer communication networks; *confidentiality; consent forms; editorial policies; *information dissemination; *informed consent; *patients; physicians; professional organizations; property rights; *medical illustration; *photography; Great Britain; Internet

Juengst, Eric T. Respecting human subjects in genome research: a preliminary policy agenda. *In:* Vanderpool, Harold Y., ed. The Ethics of Research Involving Human Subjects: Facing the 21st Century. Frederick, MD: University Publishing Group; 1996: 401–429. 74 fn. ISBN 1–55572–036–6. BE56995.
　　children; *confidentiality; *disclosure; employment; *family members; genetic information; genetic materials; genetic predisposition; *genetic research; *genome mapping; *informed consent; insurance; international aspects; mentally ill; minority groups; privacy; property rights; public policy; research subjects; *risks and benefits; *selection of subjects; stigmatization; truth disclosure; *pedigree studies; Human Genome Project; United States

Kaufert, Joseph M.; O'Neil, John D.; Koolage, William W. The cultural and political context of informed consent for Native Canadians. *Arctic Medical Research.* 1991; (Suppl.): 181–184. 5 refs. BE57060.
　　*American Indians; autonomy; case studies; coercion; *communication; competence; comprehension; *cultural pluralism; diagnosis; disclosure; health care delivery; *informed consent; *minority groups; *patient advocacy;

patient participation; physician patient relationship; risks and benefits; social dominance; social interaction; surgery; trust; values; *Eskimos; *Arctic Regions; *Canada

Kerns, Alice Fleury. Better to lay it out on the table rather than do it behind the curtain: hospitals need to obtain consent before using newly deceased patients to teach resuscitation procedures. [Comment]. *Journal of Contemporary Health Law and Policy.* 1997 Spring; 13(2): 581–612. 197 fn. BE56004.
　　advance directives; alternatives; attitudes; *cadavers; common good; criminal law; dehumanization; emergency care; *family members; hospitals; *institutional policies; internship and residency; *legal aspects; legal rights; *medical education; presumed consent; property rights; psychological stress; *public policy; *resuscitation; risks and benefits; students; *third party consent; intubation; United States

Keyserlingk, Edward W. Expanding the scope of clinical ethics: making informed consent healthier in the hospital context. *International Journal of Bioethics.* 1997 Mar–Jun; 8(1–2): 127–130. BE59100.
　　clinical ethics; *hospitals; *informed consent; institutional policies; *interdisciplinary communication; nurses; organization and administration; *patient care; *patient care team; physicians; teaching methods

Kotva, Joseph J.; Kotva, Carol S. Was this consent informed? *American Journal of Nursing.* 1997 May; 97(5): 23. 7 refs. BE56055.
　　aged; brain; case studies; communication; competence; decision making; *disclosure; family members; informed consent; *nurses; paternalism; physicians; professional family relationship; prognosis; risks and benefits; standards; surgery; *third party consent

Kravitz, Melva. Informed consent: must ethical responsibility conflict with professional conduct? *Nursing Management.* 1985 Nov; 16(11): 34A–34H. 26 fn. BE56972.
　　autonomy; decision making; *disclosure; human experimentation; *informed consent; interprofessional relations; legal aspects; *nurses; patient care; patient participation; patients; physicians; research subjects

Lane, Arline; Dubler, Nancy Neveloff. The health care agent: selected but neglected. *Bioethics Forum.* 1997 Summer; 13(2): 17–21. 3 refs. BE58282.
　　*advance directives; aged; allowing to die; artificial feeding; case studies; communication; *decision making; dementia; ethicists; *family members; legal aspects; patient care team; physicians; professional family relationship; prolongation of life; quality of life; risks and benefits; *third party consent; uncertainty; New York

Lescale, Keith B.; Inglis, Steven R.; Eddleman, Keith A., et al. Conflicts between physicians and patients in non–elective cesarean delivery: incidence and the adequacy of informed consent. *American Journal of Perinatology.* 1996 Apr; 13(3): 171–176. 9 refs. BE56470.
　　alternatives; *attitudes; autonomy; *cesarean section; childbirth; counseling; *decision making; *disclosure; *dissent; *informed consent; *mothers; *patient participation; *patient satisfaction; *patients; physician patient relationship; *physicians; *pregnant women; risks and benefits; statistics; survey; treatment refusal; preventive ethics; New York City; New York Hospital–Cornell Medical Center

Lundmark, Thomas. Surgery by an unauthorized surgeon as a battery. *Journal of Law and Health.* 1995–1996; 10(2): 287–296. 38 fn. BE57146.
　　autonomy; disclosure; *ghost surgery; *informed consent;

*legal aspects; *legal liability; paternalism; patients; physicians; *surgery; torts; *United States

Lustig, Andrew; Scardino, Peter. Elective patients. *In:* McCullough, Laurence B.; Jones, James W.; Brody, Baruch A., eds. Surgical Ethics. New York, NY: Oxford University Press; 1998: 133–151. 33 refs. ISBN 0–19–510347–5. BE58331.
  *alternatives; autonomy; beneficence; blood transfusions; chronically ill; competence; comprehension; conflict of interest; *decision making; directive counseling; economics; *informed consent; morbidity; mortality; paternalism; patient education; *patient participation; patients; *physicians; quality of life; referral and consultation; refusal to treat; resuscitation orders; review; risks and benefits; *surgery; time factors; treatment outcome; treatment refusal; *uncertainty; values; physician's practice patterns; prostate cancer

Lynn, Joanne; Teno, Joan. A care provider perspective on advance directives and surrogate decision making for incompetent adults in the United States. *In:* Sass, Hans–Martin; Veatch, Robert M.; Kimura, Rihito, eds. Advance Directives and Surrogate Decision Making in Health Care: United States, Germany, and Japan. Baltimore, MD: Johns Hopkins University Press; 1998: 3–33. 65 refs. ISBN 0–8018–5831–3. BE59035.
  advance care planning; *advance directives; aged; allowing to die; artificial feeding; case studies; chronically ill; communication; *competence; cultural pluralism; *decision making; empirical research; evaluation; *family members; legal aspects; *living wills; persistent vegetative state; physicians; prolongation of life; public policy; resuscitation orders; *risks and benefits; terminally ill; *third party consent; uncertainty; values; withholding treatment; cognition disorders; Patient Self-Determination Act 1990; United States

McCullough, Laurence B.; Jones, James W.; Brody, Baruch A. Informed consent: autonomous decision making of the surgical patient. *In:* McCullough, Laurence B.; Jones, James W.; Brody, Baruch A., eds. Surgical Ethics. New York, NY: Oxford University Press; 1998: 15–37. 23 refs. ISBN 0–19–510347–5. BE58334.
  adolescents; adults; alternatives; *autonomy; beneficence; children; *communication; competence; comprehension; *decision making; diagnosis; *disclosure; family members; goals; *informed consent; internship and residency; legal aspects; parental consent; patient care team; *patients; physician patient relationship; *physicians; psychiatric diagnosis; recall; religion; risks and benefits; standards; students; *surgery; third party consent; time factors; treatment refusal; trust; values; preventive ethics; United States

McFadzean, J.; Monson, J.P.; Watson, J.D., et al. The dilemma of the incapacitated patient who has previously refused consent for surgery. [Case study and commentaries]. *BMJ (British Medical Journal).* 1997 Dec 6; 315(7121): 1530–1532. 8 refs. BE57243.
  advance directives; autonomy; case studies; competence; *critically ill; decision making; emergency care; family members; *legal aspects; physicians; prognosis; *surgery; *third party consent; time factors; *treatment refusal; Great Britain
What should doctors do if a patient is critically ill and unable to give consent to a procedure that he or she has previously refused to consent to? Such a case is described below and discussed by a medicolegal specialist and by an ethicist.

McMillan, John. Competence to Consent, by Becky Cox White. [Book review essay]. *Theoretical Medicine and*

Bioethics. 1998 Apr; 19(2): 161–166. 1 ref. BE57595.
  *competence; comprehension; decision making; emotions; evaluation; *informed consent; mentally ill; patient care; patient participation; recall; standards; treatment refusal; *Competence to Consent (White, B.C.)

Magnusson, Roger S. Testing for HIV without specific consent: a short review. *Australian and New Zealand Journal of Public Health.* 1996 Feb; 20(1): 57–60. 33 refs. BE57964.
  *AIDS serodiagnosis; anonymous testing; autonomy; disclosure; epidemiology; *HIV seropositivity; *informed consent; legal aspects; patients; pregnant women; privacy; research subjects; Australia; New Zealand

Marson, Daniel; Ingram, Kellie K. Competency to consent to treatment: a growing field of research: commentary. *Journal of Ethics, Law, and Aging.* 1996 Fall–Winter; 2(2): 59–63. 41 refs. Commentary on Dellasega et al., p. 65–74. BE57141.
  advance directives; *aged; *competence; comprehension; decision making; disclosure; *empirical research; *evaluation; hospitals; *informed consent; methods; nursing homes; patient care; physicians; geographic factors; United States

Marta, Jan. Toward a bioethics for the twenty–first century: a Ricoeurian poststructuralist narrative hermeneutic approach to informed consent. *In:* Nelson, Hilde Lindemann, ed. Stories and Their Limits: Narrative Approaches to Bioethics. New York, NY: Routledge; 1997: 198–212. 20 fn. ISBN 0–415–91910–X. BE57471.
  bioethics; communication; *informed consent; models, theoretical; *narrative ethics; patient participation; personhood; physician patient relationship; physician's role; self concept; personal identity; *Ricoeur, Paul

Matheis–Kraft, Carol; Roberto, Karen A. Influence of a values discussion on congruence between elderly women and their families on critical health care decisions. *Journal of Women and Aging.* 1997; 9(4): 5–22. 33 refs. BE58970.
  *aged; allowing to die; artificial feeding; blood transfusions; *communication; comparative studies; competence; *decision making; dementia; drugs; evaluation studies; *family members; *females; *patient care; persistent vegetative state; renal dialysis; resuscitation; surgery; *third party consent; treatment refusal; *values; ventilators; *withholding treatment; women's health; United States

Meisel, Alan. Legal issues in decision making for incompetent patients: advance directives and surrogate decision making. *In:* Sass, Hans–Martin; Veatch, Robert M.; Kimura, Rihito, eds. Advance Directives and Surrogate Decision Making in Health Care: United States, Germany, and Japan. Baltimore, MD: Johns Hopkins University Press; 1998: 34–65. 62 refs. 11 fn. References include separate lists of court cases and legislation. ISBN 0–8018–5831–3. BE59036.
  *advance directives; *allowing to die; artificial feeding; case studies; *competence; conflict of interest; constitutional law; critically ill; *decision making; dementia; equal protection; *family members; futility; judicial action; *legal aspects; legal rights; legislation; *living wills; patients; persistent vegetative state; physically disabled; physicians; pregnant women; privacy; prolongation of life; right to die; risks and benefits; standards; state government; terminally ill; *third party consent; treatment refusal; uncertainty; values; withholding treatment; Patient Self-Determination Act 1990; *United States

Michielsen, Paul. Informed or presumed consent legislative models. *In:* Chapman, Jeremy R.; Deierhoi,

---

BE = bioethics accession number   fn. = footnotes   refs. = references

Mark; Wight, Celia, eds. Organ and Tissue Donation for Transplantation. New York, NY: Oxford University Press; 1997: 344–360. 52 refs. ISBN 0–340–61394–7. BE58232.

advance directives; attitudes; autonomy; autopsies; body parts and fluids; brain death; cadavers; cardiac death; computers; cultural pluralism; data banks; determination of death; donor cards; evaluation; family members; historical aspects; *informed consent; *international aspects; Islamic ethics; *legal aspects; *organ donation; physicians; *presumed consent; public opinion; registries; religion; social impact; third party consent; *tissue donation; values; mandated choice; Council of Europe; Europe; Japan; Singapore; United States; World Health Organization

Miller, Tracy E.; Coleman, Carl H.; Cugliari, Anna Maria. Treatment decisions for patients without surrogates: rethinking policies for a vulnerable population. *Journal of the American Geriatrics Society.* 1997 Mar; 45(3): 369–374. 35 refs. BE56473.

advisory committees; aged; *allowing to die; *alternatives; biomedical technologies; *clinical ethics committees; committee membership; *competence; *decision making; dementia; *ethics committees; guidelines; hospitals; indigents; *institutional policies; institutionalized persons; judicial action; legal aspects; legal guardians; managed care programs; mentally disabled; models, theoretical; *nursing homes; *patient advocacy; *patient care; patient care team; physician's role; physicians; referral and consultation; review committees; risks and benefits; single persons; standards; *third party consent; treatment refusal; *vulnerable populations; withholding treatment; *absence of proxy; New York State Task Force on Life and the Law; United States

Montgomery, Jonathan. The position of the patient: consent to treatment; confidentiality and access to health care records; care for children; mental health; research. *In: his* Health Care Law. New York, NY: Oxford University Press; 1997: 225–356. 701 fn. ISBN 0–19–876260–7. BE56244.

*adults; AIDS serodiagnosis; animal experimentation; coercion; compensation; competence; computers; *confidentiality; dangerousness; disclosure; dissent; duty to warn; genetic information; government regulation; *human experimentation; *informed consent; injuries; involuntary commitment; *legal aspects; legal guardians; legal liability; legislation; medical records; *mentally ill; *minors; parental consent; patient access to records; *patient care; patient discharge; patients' rights; research ethics committees; treatment refusal; *Great Britain; National Health Service

Moreno, Jonathan D.; Caplan, Arthur L.; Wolpe, Paul Root. Informed consent. *In:* Chadwick, Ruth, ed. Encyclopedia of Applied Ethics, Volume 2. San Diego, CA: Academic Press; 1998: 687–697. 11 refs. ISBN 0–12–227067–3. BE56399.

advance directives; autonomy; competence; cultural pluralism; disclosure; guidelines; historical aspects; human experimentation; *informed consent; investigator subject relationship; legal aspects; managed care programs; minority groups; paternalism; patient care; physician patient relationship; presumed consent; scientific misconduct; standards; terminology; third party consent; Declaration of Helsinki; Nuremberg Code; United States

Morrissey, James M. Informed consent: the New York approach. *New York State Journal of Medicine.* 1985 May; 85(5): 210–213. 26 fn. BE56958.

disclosure; *informed consent; *legal aspects; legal liability; physicians; risks and benefits; standards; state government; *New York

Multiple Organ Retrieval and Exchange (M.O.R.E.) Program of Ontario. Task Force on Presumed

Consent [and] Board of Directors. Organ Procurement Strategies: A Review of the Ethical Issues and Challenges. [Report]. Toronto, ON: Multiple Organ Retrieval and Exchange (M.O.R.E.) Program of Ontario; 1994 Nov. 31 p. 237 refs. 146 fn. BE57397.

alternatives; altruism; attitudes; autonomy; brain death; communitarianism; contracts; cultural pluralism; determination of death; donor cards; economics; education; family members; health personnel; human body; humanism; incentives; indigents; international aspects; legal aspects; legislation; libertarianism; mass media; *organ donation; physicians; policy analysis; *presumed consent; *public policy; religion; remuneration; required request; terminology; third party consent; trust; uncertainty; values; voluntary programs; mandated choice; unrelated donors; Belgium; Canada; France; *Ontario; Singapore; United States

Netherlands. Law of 17 November 1994 (Stb. 837) amending the Civil Code and certain other laws in connection with the adoption of provisions concerning the agreement to carry out procedures in the field of medicine. *International Digest of Health Legislation.* 1995; 46(2): 196–199. BE57182.

adults; confidentiality; disclosure; *informed consent; *legal aspects; medical records; minors; patient access to records; *patient care; *Netherlands

New York. Supreme Court, Appellate Division, Second Department. Hecht v. Kaplan. *New York Supplement, 2d Series.* 1996 Jun 17 (date of decision). 645: 51–54. BE56298.

*blood specimen collection; *communicable diseases; diagnosis; disclosure; duty to warn; human experimentation; *informed consent; *legal liability; leukemia; malpractice; married persons; *physicians; presumed consent; time factors; *Hecht v. Kaplan; New York

The New York Supreme Court, Appellate Division, reversed the lower trial court and dismissed a patient's complaint that the unauthorized testing of her blood for a contagious disease violated her bodily integrity, constituted unauthorized human research, and breached a duty to warn her husband. Trudy Hecht had consented to blood withdrawal for cytomegalovirus (CMV) testing. At the time, an additional tube of blood was drawn from the same needle and puncture site. The second vial, however, was not needed for the CMV test; instead, that blood was tested without the patient's consent for human T–cell leukemia virus (HTLV), a contagious disease. Hecht was not informed of the positive HTLV test until six months later. The court held that even if the testing is unauthorized, drawing extra blood did not violate the patient's bodily integrity where she had already and properly consented to the invasive part of the procedure. Furthermore, the court held that under state law human research did not mean testing performed only on tissues or fluids, like blood, which were already removed or drawn in the course of a standard medical procedure. Also, under state law the duty of a physician to warn household members of the risk of disease applied to a list of highly communicable diseases under the state sanitary code, and HTLV was not on that list. (KIE abstract)

Olver, Ian N.; Turrell, Susan J.; Olszewski, Nancy A., et al. Impact of an information and consent form on patients having chemotherapy. *Medical Journal of Australia.* 1995 Jan 16; 162(2): 82–83. 10 refs. BE55885.

*cancer; *comprehension; *consent forms; disclosure; *drugs; evaluation studies; *informed consent; *patient care; *patients; *recall; risks and benefits; survey; Australia

---

Page, David L.; Jensen, Roy A.; Geller, Gail, et al. Genetic testing and informed consent. [Letter and response]. *JAMA*. 1997 Sep 10; 278(10): 821–822. 2 refs. BE57315.
> biomedical research; *cancer; confidentiality; disclosure; DNA data banks; epidemiology; federal government; genetic information; *genetic predisposition; *genetic research; *genetic screening; government regulation; guidelines; health insurance; *informed consent; patients; research ethics committees; research subjects; risks and benefits; social discrimination; tissue banks; Office for Protection from Research Risks; United States

Pang, Mei–che Samantha. Information disclosure: the moral experience of nurses in China. *Nursing Ethics*. 1998 Jul; 5(4): 347–361. 64 refs. BE58873.
> active euthanasia; autonomy; beneficence; cancer; codes of ethics; compassion; conscience; *decision making; diagnosis; *disclosure; *family members; historical aspects; hospitals; *informed consent; *knowledge, attitudes, practice; literature; medical ethics; moral obligations; nurse patient relationship; *nurses; *nursing ethics; nursing research; paternalism; patient advocacy; patient care; patients' rights; physician nurse relationship; professional family relationship; *prognosis; survey; *terminal care; terminally ill; *third party consent; *truth disclosure; virtues; qualitative research; *China; Hong Kong

Parker, Lisa S. Beauty and breast implantation: how candidate selection affects autonomy and informed consent. *In:* DiQuinzio, Patrice; Young, Iris Marion, eds. Feminist Ethics and Social Policy. Bloomington, IN: Indiana University Press; 1997: 255–273. 47 refs. 9 fn. ISBN 0–253–21125–5. BE57287.
> *autonomy; breast cancer; competence; *cosmetic surgery; *decision making; *females; *feminist ethics; *informed consent; *medical devices; motivation; risks and benefits; *selection for treatment; self concept; *values; beauty; *breast implants; United States

Paterson, I.C.M. Consent to treatment: somebody's moved the goalposts. *Clinical Oncology (Royal College of Radiologists)*. 1994; 6(3): 179–182. 20 refs. BE56214.
> *cancer; consensus; consent forms; *disclosure; *informed consent; legal liability; patient care; physicians; referral and consultation; risks and benefits; *standards; treatment outcome; *oncology; Great Britain

Perkins, Henry S.; Supik, Josie D.; Hazuda, Helen P. Cultural differences among health professionals: a case illustration. *Journal of Clinical Ethics*. 1998 Summer; 9(2): 108–117. 35 fn. BE58956.
> *autonomy; case studies; cesarean section; comparative studies; counseling; critically ill; *cultural pluralism; *decision making; ethical relativism; family relationship; females; *health personnel; hospitals; *informed consent; *international aspects; mediation; paternalism; *patient care; pregnant women; spousal consent; survey; *treatment refusal; value of life; *values; voluntary sterilization; *non–Western World; qualitative research; *Western World; *Kenya

This study illustrates that cultural differences arise among similarly trained health professionals. Health professionals must learn to communicate sensitively with colleagues from other cultures, to respect their values, and to recognize and resolve cultural differences that affect patient care. In this shrinking, multicultural world, health professionals cannot afford the comfortable illusion that all similarly trained practitioners share the same values about the care of patients and professional conduct.

Power, Kevin J. The legal and ethical implications of consent to nursing procedures. *British Journal of Nursing.* 1997 Aug 14–Sep 10; 6(15): 885–888. 22 refs. BE58256.
> competence; disclosure; *informed consent; *legal aspects; *nurse's role; *patient care; standards; *Great Britain

Rankine, James J. Most patients don't read the BMJ. [Personal view]. *BMJ (British Medical Journal)*. 1998 Mar 28; 316(7136): 1026–1027. BE57581.
> biomedical research; *confidentiality; *editorial policies; *informed consent; *patients; physicians; *medical illustration; *publishing; *BMJ (British Medical Journal); Great Britain

Rowland, Heidi Fuhrman; Rowland, Adam B. Hospital Consents Manual. Volume 1. [Looseleaf format]. Gaithersburg, MD: Aspen Publishers; 1994. 1 v. ISBN 0–8342–0328–6. BE56514.
> aged; AIDS; biomedical technologies; competence; confidentiality; *consent forms; criminal law; *disclosure; emergency care; forms; guidelines; home care; *hospitals; human experimentation; *informed consent; institutional ethics; *institutional policies; internship and residency; judicial action; law enforcement; *legal aspects; legal liability; *legal obligations; medical specialties; minors; nurses; nursing homes; patient admission; physicians; *records; reproductive technologies; standards; third party consent; treatment refusal; *United States

Savulescu, Julian; Momeyer, Richard W. Should informed consent be based on rational beliefs? *Journal of Medical Ethics*. 1997 Oct; 23(5): 282–288. 17 fn. BE57109.
> *autonomy; *blood transfusions; communication; *competence; decision making; disclosure; *informed consent; *Jehovah's Witnesses; patient education; patients; physician patient relationship; *religion; *treatment refusal; *rationality

Our aim is to expand the regulative ideal governing consent. We argue that consent should not only be informed but also based on rational beliefs. We argue that holding true beliefs promotes autonomy. Information is important insofar as it helps a person to hold the relevant true beliefs. But in order to hold the relevant true beliefs, competent people must also think rationally. Insofar as information is important, rational deliberation is important. Just as physicians should aim to provide relevant information regarding the medical procedures prior to patients consenting to have those procedures, they should also assist patients to think more rationally. We distinguish between rational choice/action and rational belief. While autonomous choice need not necessarily be rational, it should be based on rational belief. The implication for the doctrine of informed consent and the practice of medicine is that, if physicians are to respect patient autonomy and help patients to choose and act more rationally, not only must they provide information, but they should care more about the theoretical rationality of their patients. They should not abandon their patients to irrationality. They should help their patients to deliberate more effectively and to care more about thinking rationally. We illustrate these arguments in the context of Jehovah's Witnesses refusing life–saving blood transfusions. Insofar as Jehovah's Witnesses should be informed of the consequences of their actions, they should also deliberate rationally about these consequences.

Schneiderman, Lawrence J.; Kaplan, Robert M.; Rosenberg, Esther, et al. Do physicians' own preferences for life–sustaining treatment influence their perceptions of patients' preferences? A second look. *Cambridge Quarterly of Healthcare Ethics*. 1997 Spring; 6(2): 131–137. 18 refs. BE56437.

---

advance directives; AIDS; *allowing to die; *attitudes; biomedical technologies; brain pathology; cancer; comparative studies; *consensus; *decision making; evaluation studies; pain; *patients; physician patient relationship; *physicians; prognosis; *prolongation of life; quality of life; survey; terminally ill; *third party consent; treatment refusal; values; withholding treatment; coma; California; University of California, San Diego Medical Center

Previous studies have documented the fallibility of attempts by surrogates and physicians to act in a substituted judgment capacity and predict end–of–life treatment decisions on behalf of patients. We previously reported that physicians misperceive their patients' preferences and substitute their own preferences for those of their patients with respect to four treatments: cardiopulmonary resuscitation (CPR) in the event of cardiac arrest, ventilator for an indefinite period of time, medical nutrition and hydration for an indefinite period of time, and hospitalization in the event of pneumonia. This paper extends our previous observations and reports on a different and larger population of subjects, employing a more detailed procedure–oriented advance directive instrument as well as a quality–of–life questionnaire. Our hypothesis remains the same, namely, that physicians' predictions of their patients' end–of–life treatment choices are closer to the choices they would make for themselves than to the choices expressed by their patients. Since physicians are the ones who ultimately exercise control over these important decisions, any unrecognized projection of personal preferences onto their patients would raise serious concerns about physicians acting in a substituted judgment capacity. It would also emphasize the importance of patients choosing surrogate decisionmakers carefully and, even more important, explicating clearly their directive instructions as part of advance care planning.

Sells, Robert A. Consent for organ donation: what are the ethical principles? *Transplantation Proceedings.* 1993 Feb; 25(1): 39–41. 10 refs. BE56634.
> altruism; body parts and fluids; cadavers; coercion; commodification; competence; developing countries; disclosure; family members; indigents; *informed consent; kidneys; legal aspects; *organ donation; *organ donors; presumed consent; *remuneration; risks and benefits; standards; third party consent; Great Britain

Shatz, David. Concepts of autonomy in Jewish medical ethics. *In:* Jewish Law Annual. Volume Twelve. Amsterdam, Netherlands: Harwood Academic Publishers; 1997: 3–43. 84 fn. ISBN 90–5702–551–5. BE58346.
> *allowing to die; altruism; *autonomy; *beneficence; bioethics; coercion; comparative studies; *decision making; disclosure; historical aspects; *informed consent; *Jewish ethics; medical ethics; moral obligations; *moral policy; pain; paternalism; patient compliance; prolongation of life; risks and benefits; secularism; *theology; treatment refusal; uncertainty; values; withholding treatment

Smith, Richard. Informed consent: edging forwards (and backwards). [Editorial]. *BMJ (British Medical Journal).* 1998 Mar 28; 316(7136): 949–951. 17 refs. Includes the text of the *BMJ*'s guidelines for "Publishing information that emerges from the doctor–patient relationship." BE58067.
> attitudes; *biomedical research; case studies; *confidentiality; death; *editorial policies; *guidelines; human experimentation; *informed consent; patient care; patients; physician patient relationship; privacy; research subjects; time factors; pedigree studies; photography; *BMJ (British

Medical Journal); General Medical Council (Great Britain); International Committee of Medical Journal Editors

Sprigler, Gail B. When the truth hurts. *Plastic Surgical Nursing.* 1996 Spring; 16(1): 51–53, 56. 15 refs. BE55890.
> alternatives; autonomy; beneficence; codes of ethics; deception; decision making; diagnosis; *disclosure; drugs; ethical theory; *informed consent; justice; moral obligations; *nurses; patient advocacy; patient care; physicians; placebos; prognosis; risks and benefits; terminal care; terminally ill; *truth disclosure; American Nurses Association; International Council of Nurses

Stadler, Holly A.; Morrissey, John; Rose, Teresa, et al. Patient capacity and judicial decisionmaking. *HEC (HealthCare Ethics Committee) Forum.* 1997 Sep; 9(3): 197–211. 23 refs. BE56177.
> advance directives; aged; *competence; *decision making; *evaluation; *informed consent; *judicial action; legal aspects; *legal guardians; mentally disabled; patient care; patient compliance; standards; survey; third party consent; treatment refusal; *judges; Missouri

Steinberg, Avraham. Informed consent: ethical and halakhic considerations. *In:* Jewish Law Annual. Volume Twelve. Amsterdam, Netherlands: Harwood Academic Publishers; 1997: 137–152. 41 fn. ISBN 90–5702–551–5. BE58349.
> alternatives; *autonomy; beneficence; coercion; competence; comprehension; decision making; *disclosure; family members; *informed consent; *Jewish ethics; moral obligations; paternalism; patient care; patient participation; physician patient relationship; psychological stress; risks and benefits; standards; therapeutic research; treatment refusal; uncertainty; *value of life; values

Sugarman, Jeremy; Harland, Robert. Acute yet non–emergent patients. *In:* McCullough, Laurence B.; Jones, James W.; Brody, Baruch A., eds. Surgical Ethics. New York, NY: Oxford University Press; 1998: 116–132. 18 refs. ISBN 0–19–510347–5. BE58337.
> advance directives; alternatives; beneficence; blood transfusions; *communication; comprehension; confidentiality; *critically ill; decision making; diagnosis; disclosure; family members; *informed consent; Jehovah's Witnesses; morbidity; patient care; patient education; patient participation; patients; *physicians; prognosis; referral and consultation; refusal to treat; review; risks and benefits; *surgery; treatment outcome; *treatment refusal; uncertainty; values; *seriously ill; Patient Self-Determination Act 1990; United States

Sulmasy, Daniel P.; Terry, Peter B.; Weisman, Carol S., et al. The accuracy of substituted judgments in patients with terminal diagnoses. *Annals of Internal Medicine.* 1998 Apr 15; 128(8): 621–629. 34 refs. BE57916.
> age factors; allowing to die; *attitudes; comparative studies; *consensus; *decision making; dementia; *evaluation; evaluation studies; *family members; *patients; prognosis; *prolongation of life; resuscitation; socioeconomic factors; *terminal care; *terminally ill; *third party consent; ventilators; coma; Baltimore; District of Columbia

BACKGROUND: Patients' loved ones often make end-of-life treatment decisions, but the accuracy of their substituted judgments and the factors associated with accuracy are poorly understood. OBJECTIVE: To assess the accuracy of judgments made by surrogate decision makers; ascertain the beliefs, practices, and clinical and sociodemographic factors associated with accuracy of surrogates' decisions; assess the preferences of patients for life-sustaining treatments; and compare differences in accuracy across diagnoses. DESIGN: Cross-sectional paired interviews. SETTING:

BE = bioethics accession number   fn. = footnotes   refs. = references

Outpatient practices of three university hospitals. PATIENTS: 250 patients with terminal diagnoses of congestive heart failure, AIDS, amyotrophic lateral sclerosis, lung cancer, and chronic obstructive pulmonary disease (50 patient–surrogate pairs in each group) and 50 general medical patients and their surrogates. MEASUREMENTS: The accuracy of surrogate predictions was measured by using scales based on 10 potential treatments in each of three hypothetical clinical scenarios. RESULTS: Preferences varied according to mode of treatment and scenario. On average, surrogates made correct predictions in 66% of instances. Accuracy was better for the permanent coma scenario than for the scenarios of severe dementia or coma with a small chance of recovery (P less than 0.001). In a binary logit model, the accuracy of substituted judgments was positively associated with the patient having spoken with the surrogate about end–of–life issues (odds ratio [OR], 1.9 [95% CI, 1.6 to 2.3]), the patient having private insurance (OR, 1.4 [CI, 1.1 to 1.7]), the surrogate's level of education (OR, 1.5 [CI, 1.2 to 1.9]), and the patient's level of education (OR, 1.7 [CI, 1.4 to 2.2]). Accuracy was negatively associated with the patient's belief that he or she would live longer than 10 years (OR, 0.6 [CI, 0.5 to 0.7]), surrogate experience with life–sustaining treatment (OR, 0.4 [CI, 0.3 to 0.5]), surrogate participation in religious services (OR, 0.67 [CI, 0.50 to 0.91]), and a diagnosis of heart failure (OR, 0.6 [CI, 0.5 to 0.8]). Age, ethnicity, marital status, religion, and advance directives were not associated with accuracy. CONCLUSIONS: The accuracy of substituted judgments is associated with multiple clinically apparent patient and surrogate factors. This information can help clinicians identify conditions under which substituted judgments are likely to be accurate or inaccurate and can help target populations for education designed to improve the accuracy of surrogate decision making.

Thompson, Carolyn R. HIV and the blood supply: assessing MANTRA [mandatory notification of transfusion alternatives] legislation. *Politics and the Life Sciences.* 1995 Aug; 14(2): 221–228. 33 refs. 12 fn. Includes list of cited legislation. BE55639.
    AIDS; *alternatives; blood donation; *blood transfusions; directed donation; *disclosure; economics; *government regulation; *HIV seropositivity; *informed consent; *legislation; mandatory programs; organizational policies; physicians; psychological stress; risk; *social impact; standards; *state government; voluntary programs; autologous blood transfusion; American Red Cross; United States

U.S. Court of Appeals, Sixth Circuit. Brotherton v. Cleveland. *Federal Reporter, 2d Series.* 1991 Jan 18 (date of decision). 923: 477–484. BE56742.
    body parts and fluids; *cadavers; constitutional law; *due process; *family members; federal government; hospitals; *legal aspects; legislation; *organ donation; *property rights; state government; *third party consent; corneas; *Brotherton v. Cleveland; Fourteenth Amendment; Ohio; Uniform Anatomical Gift Act
The U.S. Court of Appeals for the Sixth Circuit reversed the lower trial court and allowed a decedent's family to pursue a claim under the federal constitution for wrongful removal of the decedent's corneas. The hospital had documented Deborah Brotherton's refusal of any anatomical gift from her husband's body, but it failed to notify the coroner of her wishes. Furthermore, the coroner did not inquire about any objection to anatomical gifts before allowing an eyebank technician to remove Steven Brotherton's corneas. Deborah Brotherton alleged wrongful deprivation of property

under the due process clause. Based on state law allowing her a possessory right to the body, a right to control disposition of the body, and a claim for mishandling of the body, the court found the interest of the wife as next of kin in her dead husband's body to be substantial, and thus protected by the Fourteenth Amendment, even if it is not a property interest or quasi–property interest. (KIE abstract)

Veatch, Robert M. Ethical dimensions of advance directives and surrogate decision making in the United States. *In:* Sass, Hans–Martin; Veatch, Robert M.; Kimura, Rihito, eds. Advance Directives and Surrogate Decision Making in Health Care: United States, Germany, and Japan. Baltimore, MD: Johns Hopkins University Press; 1998: 66–91. 72 refs. 7 fn. ISBN 0–8018–5831–3. BE59037.
    adults; *advance directives; aged; *allowing to die; anencephaly; artificial feeding; *autonomy; beneficence; brain pathology; competence; consensus; *decision making; family members; freedom; futility; historical aspects; informed consent; judicial action; justice; *legal rights; living wills; mentally retarded; minors; moral policy; parents; paternalism; patients' rights; persistent vegetative state; physician patient relationship; physicians; professional autonomy; prolongation of life; refusal to treat; religion; *risks and benefits; Roman Catholic ethics; *third party consent; *treatment refusal; trends; ventilators; withholding treatment; liberalism; oral directives; values histories; Hippocratic Oath; In re Baby K; In re Conroy; In re Phillip B.; In re Quinlan; Twentieth Century; *United States

Veatch, Robert M., ed. Ethical issues in the changing health care system. *In:* Jonsen, Albert R.; Veatch, Robert M.; Walters, LeRoy, eds. Source Book in Bioethics: A Documentary History. Washington, DC: Georgetown University Press; 1998: 407–504. 8 fn. ISBN 0–87840–683–2. BE57894.
    advance directives; advisory committees; aliens; autonomy; body parts and fluids; cadavers; competence; *confidentiality; dangerousness; disclosure; *duty to warn; federal government; historical aspects; *informed consent; legal aspects; mentally ill; model legislation; *organ donation; organ donors; *organ transplantation; patient care; patients' rights; physician patient relationship; remuneration; selection for treatment; *third party consent; tissue donation; transplant recipients; *Canterbury v. Spence; National Organ Transplant Act 1984; President's Commission for the Study of Ethical Problems; *Tarasoff v. Regents of the University of California; *Task Force on Organ Transplantation; *Twentieth Century; *Uniform Anatomical Gift Act; *United States

Venn–Treloar, Josephine. Nuchal translucency -- screening without consent. [Personal view]. *BMJ (British Medical Journal).* 1998 Mar 28; 316(7136): 1027. BE57583.
    biomedical research; deception; Down syndrome; *informed consent; pregnant women; *prenatal diagnosis; *ultrasonography; Great Britain

Wainwright, Paul; Cain, Paul. Using clients: a response to Paul Cain. [Commentary and response]. *Nursing Ethics.* 1998 Jul; 5(4): 363–369. 3 refs. BE58881.
    autonomy; case studies; *confidentiality; *disclosure; hospitals; *informed consent; *moral obligations; nurse patient relationship; *nursing education; *nursing ethics; nursing research; paternalism; *patient care; *patients; privacy; research subjects; *students; teaching methods

Wear, Stephen; Logue, Gerald. Informed consent for organ transplantation: mandating the participation of the family. *Law and Policy.* 1995 Apr; 17(2): 210–216. Commentary on B.K. Grover, "From both sides now:

informed consent, organ transplantation, and family–based disclosure," p. 188–209. BE58246.
*disclosure; *family members; family relationship; *informed consent; *legal aspects; *mandatory programs; *organ transplantation; risks and benefits; third party consent; *transplant recipients

Wear, Stephen. Informed Consent: Patient Autonomy and Clinician Beneficence within Health Care. Second Edition. Washington, DC: Georgetown University Press; 1998. 200 p. (Clinical medical ethics). Bibliography: p. 181–196. ISBN 0-87840-706-5. BE59049.
alternatives; *autonomy; *beneficence; competence; comprehension; decision making; disclosure; emergency care; empirical research; freedom; *informed consent; legal aspects; models, theoretical; paternalism; patient care; *patient participation; physician patient relationship; review; rights; risks and benefits; standards; treatment refusal; values

Werner, D. Leonard. Informed consent in optometric institutions. *Journal of the American Optometric Association.* 1994 Jun; 65(6): 423–426. 19 refs. BE55795.
autonomy; *consent forms; disclosure; education; eye diseases; health facilities; health personnel; *informed consent; *institutional policies; patient care; *schools; survey; universities; *optometry; United States

Wilks, Ian. The debate over risk–related standards of competence. *Bioethics.* 1997 Oct; 11(5): 413–426. 26 fn. BE56340.
alternatives; autonomy; coercion; *competence; *decision making; *informed consent; *moral policy; patient care; *patients; *risks and benefits; *standards; treatment refusal
This discussion paper continues the debate over risk–related standards of mental competence which appears in Bioethics 5. Dan Brock there defends an approach to mental competence in patients which defines it as being relative to differing standards, more or less rigorous depending on the degree of risk involved in proposed treatment. But Mark Wicclair raises a problem for this approach: if significantly different levels of risk attach, respectively, to accepting and refusing the same treatment, then it is possible, on this account, for a patient to be considered competent to accept, but not refuse, the treatment, or vice versa. I argue that this puzzle does not constitute a genuine problem for a risk–related standard. To this end I focus on the situation where, of two mutually exclusive options, one is riskier, but offering more pronounced benefit, while the other is safer, but offering less benefit. I argue for this proposition: it can take far less insight to know that the safe option is good than to know that the risky option is better. Now say one is actually informed enough to know that the safe option is good, but not enough to know whether the risky option is better; in such a case one is competent to say yes to that first option (the safe one), but not to say yes to the other. (I argue in passing that Pascal's Wager can be interpreted as having precisely this deliberative structure.) I thus conclude that cases do indeed exist where one can be competent to say yes but not no, or vice versa; and that it is thus not an anomaly in the risk–related standard that it entails the existence of such cases.

Williams, F.G. Consent for transfusion. [Editorial]. *BMJ (British Medical Journal).* 1997 Aug 16; 315(7105): 380–381. 7 refs. BE57175.
*blood transfusions; disclosure; *informed consent; legal aspects; paternalism; patients; physicians; risk; standards; *Great Britain; United States

Williamson, Charlotte; Wilkie, Patricia. Teaching

medical students in general practice: respecting patients' rights. [Editorial]. *BMJ (British Medical Journal).* 1997 Nov 1; 315(7116): 1108–1109. 11 refs. BE56894.
attitudes; communication; *confidentiality; disclosure; family practice; *informed consent; *medical education; medical ethics; medical records; *patient care; patients; *students; Great Britain; National Health Service

Winslade, William J. Humanistic problem solving: the case of Mr. T. *Journal of Clinical Ethics.* 1997 Winter; 8(4): 389–397. 7 fn. BE57619.
aged; case studies; *communication; *competence; comprehension; *decision making; depressive disorder; emotions; *empathy; ethical theory; *ethicist's role; ethics consultation; expert testimony; family members; forensic psychiatry; *humanism; *interdisciplinary communication; interprofessional relations; *judicial action; lawyers; legal guardians; *mediation; patient advocacy; patient compliance; physicians; professional patient relationship; quality of life; surgery; *third party consent; *treatment refusal; *amputation; *judges; pragmatism; *professional role
...The following case provides an example of pragmatic humanism incorporated into a legal process. The case begins with Mr. T, an elderly gentleman, who resisted and refused numerous efforts to persuade him to have his gangrenous foot amputated. His family was intimidated by him; his physicians were exasperated; his attorney and the attorney for the government were bemused. I was appointed by a court to assess his situation, to be an independent legal and bioethics adviser to the court. My role went beyond what is currently called ethics consultation. I was also authorized to be a participant in the proceedings, to investigate, to examine witnesses at the hearing, and to report and make recommendations to the court. I accepted the invitation to explore the human problems, psychological, ethical, and legal, and to propose practical ways of solving them.

INFORMED CONSENT/MENTALLY DISABLED

Aller, Robert; Aller, Gregory. An institutional response to patient/family complaints. *In:* Shamoo, Adil E., ed. Ethics in Neurobiological Research with Human Subjects: The Baltimore Conference on Ethics. Amsterdam: Gordon and Breach; 1997: 155–172. 32 fn. This paper provides the viewpoints of a father and of his son, who was a research subject at the UCLA Clinical Research Center. ISBN 2-88449-161-9. BE57013.
administrators; case studies; consent forms; *deception; *disclosure; family members; *human experimentation; iatrogenic disease; *informed consent; medical records; *mentally ill; patients; physician patient relationship; placebos; professional family relationship; *psychoactive drugs; research design; research subjects; risks and benefits; *schizophrenia; *scientific misconduct; suicide; treatment outcome; universities; *withholding treatment; patient abandonment; *UCLA Neuropsychiatric Institute; United States; *University of California, Los Angeles

Annas, George J.; Glantz, Leonard H. Informed consent to research on institutionalized mentally disabled persons: the dual problems of incapacity and voluntariness. *In:* Shamoo, Adil E., ed. Ethics in Neurobiological Research with Human Subjects: The Baltimore Conference on Ethics. Amsterdam: Gordon and Breach; 1997: 55–79. 46 fn. Appendices include the text of the Nuremberg Code and parts of the U.S. Department of Health, Education, and Welfare regulations proposed in 1978 on "protections pertaining to biomedical and behavioral research involving as subjects individuals institutionalized as mentally disabled." ISBN 2-88449-161-9. BE57009.

BE = bioethics accession number   fn. = footnotes   refs. = references

behavior control; *coercion; *competence; comprehension; *decision making; federal government; government regulation; guidelines; hepatitis; *human experimentation; immunization; *informed consent; *institutionalized persons; involuntary commitment; judicial action; *legal aspects; *mentally disabled; *mentally ill; model legislation; nontherapeutic research; organ donation; patient advocacy; patient care; prisoners; psychoactive drugs; *regulation; research ethics committees; research subjects; scientific misconduct; state interest; sterilization (sexual); therapeutic research; *third party consent; treatment refusal; DHEW Guidelines; Nuremberg Code; *United States

Appelbaum, Paul S. Informed consent to psychotherapy: recent developments. *Psychiatric Services.* 1997 Apr; 48(4): 445–446. 7 refs. BE56201.
child abuse; confidentiality; *disclosure; government regulation; health personnel; *informed consent; *legal aspects; legal liability; mentally ill; *psychotherapy; recall; risks and benefits; sex offenses; state government; Osheroff v. Chestnut Lodge; *United States

Batten, Donald A.; Haliburn, Joan; Prager, Shirley. Informed consent by children and adolescents to psychiatric treatment. [Article and commentaries]. *Australian and New Zealand Journal of Psychiatry.* 1996 Oct; 30(5): 623–632. 26 refs. BE57953.
*adolescents; *children; coercion; *competence; comprehension; decision making; *informed consent; legal aspects; *mentally ill; parent child relationship; parental consent; *patient care; physician patient relationship; psychiatry; *psychotherapy; risks and benefits; treatment refusal; family therapy; Children Act 1989 (Great Britain); Great Britain

Billick, Stephen B.; Della Bella, Peter; Burgert, Woodward. Competency to consent to hospitalization in the medical patient. *Journal of the American Academy of Psychiatry and the Law.* 1997; 25(2): 191–196. 7 refs. BE55601.
adolescents; adults; comparative studies; *competence; evaluation studies; hospitals; *informed consent; institutionalized persons; *mentally ill; *patient admission; *patients; psychiatric diagnosis; *voluntary admission; questionnaires; St. Vincent's Hospital and Medical Center (New York City)

Dickenson, Donna. Ethical issues in long term psychiatric management. *Journal of Medical Ethics.* 1997 Oct; 23(5): 300–304. 18 fn. BE57104.
accountability; beneficence; case studies; chronically ill; coercion; *community services; *dangerousness; *deinstitutionalized persons; duration of commitment; *informed consent; involuntary commitment; legal aspects; *long-term care; *mentally ill; *outpatient commitment; paternalism; patient compliance; patient discharge; physicians; presumed consent; psychoactive drugs; resource allocation; *risk; *treatment refusal; *Great Britain; Mental Health Act 1983 (Great Britain)
Two general ethical problems in psychiatry are thrown into sharp relief by long term care. This article discusses each in turn, in the context of two anonymised case studies from actual clinical practice. First, previous mental health legislation soothed doubts about patients' refusal of consent by incorporating time limits on involuntary treatment. When these are absent, as in the provisions for long term care which have recently come into force, the justification for compulsory treatment and supervision becomes more obviously problematic. Second, Anglo-American law does not normally allow the preventive detention of someone who may be dangerous but has not actually committed any crime. The justification for detaining a possibly dangerous user of mental health services without his or her consent can

only be based on risk assessment, but this raises issues of moral luck. Is the psychiatrist who decides not to take out a supervision order for a possibly dangerous patient with an initial psychotic diagnosis morally at fault if that person harms someone in the community, or himself? Or is the psychiatrist merely unlucky?

Gadd, Elaine. Changing the law on decision making for mentally incapacitated adults: should advance directives have a statutory basis? [Editorial]. *BMJ (British Medical Journal).* 1998 Jan 10; 316(7125): 90. 8 refs. BE57306.
*advance directives; advisory committees; allowing to die; autonomy; *decision making; *informed consent; *legal aspects; *mentally disabled; nontherapeutic research; public policy; risks and benefits; *third party consent; treatment refusal; *Great Britain; Law Commission (Great Britain)

Glass, Kathleen Cranley. Refining definitions and devising instruments: two decades of assessing mental competence. *International Journal of Law and Psychiatry.* 1997 Winter; 20(1): 5–33. 107 fn. BE55550.
accountability; aged; autonomy; *competence; comprehension; decision making; dementia; emotions; *evaluation; *informed consent; intelligence; international aspects; *legal aspects; *mentally disabled; methods; patient advocacy; patients; psychiatric diagnosis; recall; risk; risks and benefits; *standards; treatment refusal; values; neuropsychology; psychological tests; Canada; Great Britain; United States

Grubb, Andrew, ed. Decision–Making and Problems of Incompetence. New York, NY: Wiley; 1994. 203 p. 508 fn. Papers presented at the first Annual Conference of the UK Forum on Health Care Ethics and the Law held under the auspices of the Centre of Medical Law and Ethics at King's College London in April 1991. ISBN 0–471–94236–7. BE57125.
adults; advance directives; AIDS; allowing to die; artificial feeding; autonomy; coercion; communication; *competence; comprehension; *decision making; family members; females; *informed consent; international aspects; involuntary sterilization; judicial action; *legal aspects; *mentally disabled; minors; outpatient commitment; paternalism; patient care; persistent vegetative state; physicians; reproduction; right to die; *standards; sterilization (sexual); *third party consent; treatment refusal; values; withholding treatment; Canada; *Great Britain; Law Commission (Great Britain); United States

Hale, Brenda. Mentally incapacitated adults and decision–making: the English perspective. *International Journal of Law and Psychiatry.* 1997 Winter; 20(1): 59–75. 122 fn. BE55554.
adults; advance directives; advisory committees; allowing to die; *competence; *decision making; guidelines; historical aspects; *informed consent; judicial action; *legal aspects; legal guardians; *mentally disabled; mentally retarded; nontherapeutic research; patient care; persistent vegetative state; public policy; sterilization (sexual); *third party consent; treatment refusal; vulnerable populations; Airedale NHS Trust v. Bland; *Great Britain; Law Commission (Great Britain); Mental Health Act 1959 (Great Britain); Re F (Mental Patient: Sterilisation)

Heginbotham, Christopher. Mental disorder and decision–making: respecting autonomy in substitute judgments. *In:* Grubb, Andrew, ed. Decision–Making and Problems of Incompetence. New York, NY: Wiley; 1994: 115–125. 9 refs. ISBN 0–471–94236–7. BE57133.
advance directives; autonomy; *competence; *decision making; *informed consent; *involuntary commitment; judicial action; legal guardians; *mentally ill; *outpatient commitment; paternalism; patient care; physicians; risks and benefits; *third party consent; Enduring Powers of Attorney

---

BE = bioethics accession number   fn. = footnotes   refs. = references

Act 1985 (Great Britain); *Great Britain; Mental Health Act 1983 (Great Britain)

Hoggett, Brenda. Mentally incapacitated adults and decision–making: the Law Commission's project. *In:* Grubb, Andrew, ed. Decision–Making and Problems of Incompetence. New York, NY: Wiley; 1994: 27–40. 34 fn. ISBN 0–471–94236–7. BE57127.
   adults; advisory committees; *competence; *decision making; family members; judicial action; *legal aspects; legislation; *mentally disabled; patient care; patients; physicians; *public policy; *standards; *third party consent; treatment refusal; England; *Great Britain; *Law Commission (Great Britain); Law Commission (Scotland); Wales

Hope, Tony. Aging, research and families. [Editorial]. *Journal of Medical Ethics.* 1997 Oct; 23(5): 267–268. 3 refs. BE57105.
   *aged; *competence; comprehension; *conflict of interest; *decision making; *dementia; *depressive disorder; *family members; *human experimentation; *informed consent; methods; patient advocacy; *patient care; physician patient relationship; *physicians; professional family relationship; time factors

Illinois. Appellate Court, Fourth District. In re Branning. *North Eastern Reporter, 2d Series.* 1996 Dec 18 (date of decision). 674: 463–472. BE58897.
   *decision making; *due process; *electroconvulsive therapy; institutionalized persons; judicial action; *legal aspects; *legal guardians; *mentally ill; psychosurgery; *third party consent; treatment refusal; *Illinois; *In re Branning
   The Appellate Court of Illinois, Fourth District, invalidated a law permitting a guardian, with court approval, to provide consent for a ward's participation in any medical procedure which the guardian deems to be in the best interests of the ward. Branning, age 70, had received electroconvulsive therapy (ECT) throughout her life, beginning at age 14 or 15, until two years ealier. Her guardian petitioned the court for approval of the guardian's consent to ECT. The court held that the law facially violated the due process rights of the patient. The court held that due process required, at a minimum, that the ward receive a hearing at which she be allowed to appear, present witnesses on her behalf, and cross–examine witnesses against her. She must also receive competent assistance at the hearing and she is entitled to an independent psychiatric examination. The ward must also be shown to be unable to make a reasoned decision about the treatment, and the treatment must be shown to be in her best interest and to be the least restrictive alternative. (KIE abstract)

Jones, Melinda; Marks, Lee Ann. Female and disabled: a human rights perspective on law and medicine. *In:* Petersen, Kerry, ed. Intersections: Women on Law, Medicine and Technology. Brookfield, VT: Ashgate; 1997: 49–71. 91 refs. 39 fn. ISBN 1–85521–882–8. BE57486.
   autonomy; competence; *decision making; *disabled; eugenics; *females; health care; heart diseases; *human rights; informed consent; international aspects; judicial action; *legal aspects; *mentally retarded; minors; parental consent; patient care; risks and benefits; state interest; *sterilization (sexual); surgery; *third party consent; transsexualism; treatment refusal; Australia; Great Britain

Keay, Timothy J. Approximating ethical research content. *In:* Shamoo, Adil E., ed. Ethics in Neurobiological Research with Human Subjects: The Baltimore Conference on Ethics. Amsterdam: Gordon and Breach; 1997: 149–153. 11 fn. ISBN 2–88449–161–9.

BE57012.
   competence; conflict of interest; *human experimentation; *informed consent; injuries; investigator subject relationship; investigators; *mentally ill; physician patient relationship; psychoactive drugs; research design; research ethics committees; research subjects; risks and benefits; *schizophrenia; suicide; withholding treatment; United States

Marson, Daniel C.; Hawkins, Lauren; McInturff, Bronwyn, et al. Cognitive models that predict physician judgments of capacity to consent in mild Alzheimer's disease. *Journal of the American Geriatrics Society.* 1997 Apr; 45(4): 458–464. 35 refs. BE57119.
   aged; *competence; consensus; *control groups; *decision making; *dementia; *evaluation; *informed consent; medical specialties; *models, theoretical; patients; *physicians; recall; standards; cognition disorders

Marson, Daniel C.; McInturff, Bronwyn; Hawkins, Lauren, et al. Consistency of physician judgments of capacity to consent in mild Alzheimer's disease. *Journal of the American Geriatrics Society.* 1997 Apr; 45(4): 453–457. 35 refs. BE57120.
   aged; *competence; consensus; *control groups; *decision making; *dementia; *evaluation; evaluation studies; *informed consent; medical education; medical specialties; patients; *physicians; standards; technical expertise

Marwick, Charles. Bioethics Commission examines informed consent from subjects who are 'decisionally incapable'. [News]. *JAMA.* 1997 Aug 27; 278(8): 618–619. BE56101.
   advisory committees; *competence; comprehension; disclosure; *human experimentation; *informed consent; *mentally disabled; psychoactive drugs; public policy; random selection; research design; research subjects; schizophrenia; standards; withholding treatment; National Bioethics Advisory Commission; United States

Meier, Diane E. Voiceless and vulnerable: dementia patients without surrogates in an era of capitation. [Editorial]. *Journal of the American Geriatrics Society.* 1997 Mar; 45(3): 375–377. 22 refs. BE56472.
   aged; allowing to die; *alternatives; biomedical technologies; clinical ethics committees; *competence; conflict of interest; *decision making; *dementia; economics; health care delivery; incentives; *institutional policies; *legal guardians; managed care programs; nursing homes; *patient advocacy; patient care; physicians; resource allocation; single persons; standards; *third party consent; treatment refusal; *vulnerable populations; *absence of proxy; undertreatment; United States

Montgomery, Jonathan. The position of the patient: consent to treatment; confidentiality and access to health care records; care for children; mental health; research. *In: his* Health Care Law. New York, NY: Oxford University Press; 1997: 225–356. 701 fn. ISBN 0–19–876260–7. BE56244.
   *adults; AIDS serodiagnosis; animal experimentation; coercion; compensation; competence; computers; *confidentiality; dangerousness; disclosure; dissent; duty to warn; genetic information; government regulation; *human experimentation; *informed consent; injuries; involuntary commitment; *legal aspects; legal guardians; legal liability; legislation; medical records; *mentally ill; *minors; parental consent; patient access to records; *patient care; patient discharge; patients' rights; research ethics committees; treatment refusal; *Great Britain; National Health Service

Muehleman, Thomas; Pickens, Bruce K.; Robinson, Franklin. Informing clients about the limits to confidentiality, risks, and their rights: is self–disclosure

---

BE = bioethics accession number   fn. = footnotes   refs. = references

inhibited? *Professional Psychology: Research and Practice.*
1985 Jun; 16(3): 385–397. 17 refs. BE56950.
  *confidentiality; consent forms; depressive disorder;
  *disclosure; evaluation studies; *informed consent;
  *psychotherapy; risks and benefits; students; universities

Munetz, Mark R.; Roth, Loren H. Informing patients
about tardive dyskinesia. *Archives of Internal Medicine.*
1985 Sep; 42(9): 866–871. 30 refs. BE56970.
  age factors; chronically ill; *communication; comparative
  studies; *comprehension; *consent forms; disclosure;
  iatrogenic disease; *informed consent; *mentally ill; patient
  care; patient compliance; physician patient relationship;
  *psychoactive drugs; *recall; risks and benefits;
  *schizophrenia; survey; *toxicity; follow-up studies;
  outpatients; *tardive dyskinesia; Pittsburgh

Noll, John O.; Haugan, Mark L. Informed consent to
psychotherapy: current practices at university-affiliated
psychology training clinics. *Law and Psychology Review.*
1985 Spring; 9: 57–66. 14 fn. BE56630.
  *administrators; alternatives; confidentiality; consent forms;
  *disclosure; education; employment; health facilities; health
  insurance; health personnel; *informed consent; *institutional
  policies; *knowledge, attitudes, practice; medical records;
  mentally ill; patient access to records; patient care; privacy;
  professional competence; professional ethics; *psychology;
  *psychotherapy; risks and benefits; *schools; stigmatization;
  survey; time factors; universities; questionnaires; United
  States

Roth, Loren; Lidz, Charles W.; Meisel, Alan, et al.
Competency to decide about treatment or research: an
overview of some empirical data. *International Journal
of Law and Psychiatry.* 1982; 5: 29–50. 31 refs. BE57433.
  *competence; *comprehension; consent forms; decision
  making; depressive disorder; disclosure; electroconvulsive
  therapy; *empirical research; human experimentation;
  *informed consent; institutionalized persons; *mentally ill;
  patient education; psychiatry; *treatment refusal; Western
  Psychiatric Institute and Clinic (Pittsburgh, PA)

Silberfeld, Michel; Grundstein–Amado, Rivka;
Stephens, Derek, et al. Family and physicians' views
of surrogate decision–making: the roles and how to
choose. *International Psychogeriatrics.* 1996 Winter; 8(4):
589–596. 11 refs. BE58463.
  adults; advance directives; aged; *attitudes; autonomy;
  comparative studies; competence; *decision making;
  *dementia; diagnosis; emotions; *family members; medical
  records; medical specialties; mentally disabled; *patient care;
  patient participation; *physicians; records; *schizophrenia;
  standards; survey; terminal care; *third party consent;
  Toronto

Silverman, Henry. The role of emotions in decisional
competence, standards of competency, and altruistic acts.
Journal of Clinical Ethics. 1997 Summer; 8(2): 171–175.
10 fn. Commentary on J. Spike, "What's love got to do
with it? The altruistic giving of organs," p. 165–170.
BE55954.
  *altruism; case studies; clinical ethics committees;
  *competence; comprehension; decision making; *directed
  donation; *emotions; *ethics consultation; family
  relationship; *informed consent; kidneys; love; *mentally
  retarded; motivation; *organ donation; *organ donors; risks
  and benefits; standards; *unrelated donors

Spike, Jeffrey. What's love got to do with it? The altruistic
giving of organs. *Journal of Clinical Ethics.* 1997 Summer;
8(2): 165–170. 4 fn. Commented on by H. Silverman,
p. 171–175. BE55955.
  *altruism; case studies; clinical ethics committees;
  *competence; comprehension; decision making; *directed

donation; disclosure; *ethics consultation; family members;
family relationship; *informed consent; kidneys; love;
*mentally retarded; *organ donation; *organ donors; risks
and benefits; self concept; *unrelated donors

Tomossy, George F.; Weisstub, David N. The reform
of adult guardianship laws: the case of non–therapeutic
experimentation. *International Journal of Law and
Psychiatry.* 1997 Winter; 20(1): 113–139. 123 fn. BE55533.
  adults; advance directives; competence; dementia;
  disclosure; government regulation; guidelines; *human
  experimentation; *informed consent; investigators; *legal
  aspects; *legal guardians; *mentally disabled;
  *nontherapeutic research; research ethics committees;
  research subjects; risks and benefits; sterilization (sexual);
  *third party consent; vulnerable populations; *Canada; Re
  Eve

Wisconsin. Court of Appeals. In re Guardianship of Ruth
E.J. *North Western Reporter, 2d Series.* 1995 Sep 6 (date
of decision). 540: 213–217. BE56744.
  *competence; constitutional law; critically ill; depressive
  disorder; *electroconvulsive therapy; equal protection;
  *informed consent; *legal aspects; legal guardians; legal
  rights; *legislation; *mentally ill; state government; *third
  party consent; *In re Guardianship of Ruth E.J.; *Wisconsin
The Wisconsin Court of Appeals allowed the guardian
of an incompetent ward to consent to electroconvulsive
therapy (ECT) because a state statute which required
the patient's consent prior to treatment in effect denied
the right to treatment to a patient who is incapable of
consent. Ruth E.J. suffered from severe depression and
was in danger of starvation and dehydration. Her doctor
had decided that she would likely die without ECT, yet
she was so ill that she could not make a decision
concerning treatment. The court concluded that the state
statute requiring "express and informed consent" for ECT
and other drastic treatment violated equal protection
under the federal and state constitutions because it
applied to all patients, including those unable to express
consent. (KIE abstract)

INFORMED CONSENT/MINORS

Bartholome, William G. Ethical issues in pediatric
research. *In:* Vanderpool, Harold Y., ed. The Ethics of
Research Involving Human Subjects: Facing the 21st
Century. Frederick, MD: University Publishing Group;
1996: 339–370. 61 fn. ISBN 1-55572-036-6. BE56993.
  advisory committees; age factors; *children; coercion;
  competence; comprehension; decision making; federal
  government; government regulation; growth disorders;
  guidelines; historical aspects; hormones; *human
  experimentation; *informed consent; moral policy;
  *nontherapeutic research; normality; parental consent;
  pediatrics; random selection; research ethics committees;
  research subjects; *risks and benefits; selection of subjects;
  *therapeutic research; McCormick, Richard; National
  Commission for the Protection of Human Subjects; Ramsey,
  Paul; United States

**Bartholome, William G.; Kohrman, Arthur F.; Frader,
Joel.** Informed consent, parental permission, and assent
in pediatric practice. [Letter and response]. *Pediatrics.*
1995 Nov; 96(5, Pt. 1): 981–982. 1 ref. BE55755.
  adolescents; *children; coercion; *decision making; dissent;
  *informed consent; *minors; organizational policies; parent
  child relationship; *parental consent; *parents; patient
  advocacy; *patient care; *patient participation; *pediatrics;
  physician patient relationship; physicians; professional
  organizations; treatment refusal; American Academy of
  Pediatrics

BE = bioethics accession number   fn. = footnotes   refs. = references

Batten, Donald A.; Haliburn, Joan; Prager, Shirley. Informed consent by children and adolescents to psychiatric treatment. [Article and commentaries]. *Australian and New Zealand Journal of Psychiatry.* 1996 Oct; 30(5): 623–632. 26 refs. BE57953.
*adolescents; *children; coercion; *competence; comprehension; decision making; *informed consent; legal aspects; *mentally ill; parent child relationship; parental consent; *patient care; physician patient relationship; psychiatry; *psychotherapy; risks and benefits; treatment refusal; family therapy; Children Act 1989 (Great Britain); Great Britain

Grubb, Andrew. Refusal of treatment: competent child and parents -- Houston, Applicant. [Comment]. *Medical Law Review.* 1997 Summer; 5(2): 237–239. BE57871.
*adolescents; coercion; *competence; dangerousness; *informed consent; involuntary commitment; *judicial action; *legal aspects; mental institutions; *mentally ill; *minors; *parental consent; *treatment refusal; *Great Britain; *Houston, Applicant; *Scotland

Hanna, Mark J. Consent for a minor. *Texas Dental Journal.* 1995 Apr; 112(4): 39, 41. BE55869.
*dentistry; family members; government regulation; *informed consent; *legal aspects; *minors; parental consent; state government; *third party consent; *Texas

Langer, Dennis H. Children's legal rights as research subjects. *Journal of the American Academy of Child Psychiatry.* 1985 Sep; 24(5): 653–662. 28 refs. Paper presented at the Annual Meeting of the American Academy of Child Psychiatry, Toronto, Canada, October 1984. BE56971.
abortion, induced; *children; competence; contraception; due process; federal government; government regulation; guidelines; *human experimentation; *informed consent; involuntary commitment; *legal rights; parental consent; *patient care; patient participation; research ethics committees; *research subjects; *risks and benefits; Supreme Court decisions; treatment refusal; Department of Health, Education, and Welfare; National Commission for the Protection of Human Subjects; United States

Levine, Robert J. Adolescents as research subjects without permission of their parents or guardians: ethical considerations. *Journal of Adolescent Health.* 1995 Nov; 17(5): 287–297. 23 refs. BE55916.
*adolescents; autonomy; behavioral research; beneficence; children; competence; epidemiology; federal government; government regulation; *guidelines; *human experimentation; *informed consent; investigational drugs; justice; nontherapeutic research; parental consent; paternalism; public participation; *public policy; random selection; regulation; research design; research subjects; risk; *risks and benefits; therapeutic research; Department of Health and Human Services; National Commission for the Protection of Human Subjects; United States

Montgomery, Jonathan. The position of the patient: consent to treatment; confidentiality and access to health care records; care for children; mental health; research. *In: his* Health Care Law. New York, NY: Oxford University Press; 1997: 225–356. 701 fn. ISBN 0–19–876260–7. BE56244.
*adults; AIDS serodiagnosis; animal experimentation; coercion; compensation; competence; computers; *confidentiality; dangerousness; disclosure; dissent; duty to warn; genetic information; government regulation; *human experimentation; informed consent; injuries; involuntary commitment; *legal aspects; legal guardians; legal liability; legislation; medical records; *mentally ill; *minors; parental consent; patient access to records; *patient care; patient discharge; patients' rights; research ethics committees; treatment refusal; *Great Britain; National Health Service

Morris, Kelly. UK GMC finds lack of consent merits serious–misconduct judgment. [News]. *Lancet.* 1998 Mar 28; 351(9107): 966. BE58748.
death; *minors; *misconduct; *parental consent; patient care; *physicians; punishment; *regulation; heart catheterization; *General Medical Council (Great Britain); *Great Britain; Jenkins, Deborah; *Taylor, James

Morris, Kelly. UK misconduct case raises informed–consent issues. [News]. *Lancet.* 1998 Mar 21; 351(9106): 885. BE58857.
children; death; heart diseases; informed consent; *misconduct; *parental consent; *physicians; surgery; *angioplasty; directive adherence; *Great Britain

Muscari, Mary E. When can an adolescent give consent? *American Journal of Nursing.* 1998 May; 98(5): 18–19. 4 refs. BE58800.
*adolescents; age factors; competence; confidentiality; decision making; *informed consent; legal aspects; *patient care; state government; United States

Nicholson, Richard. The greater the ignorance, the greater the dogmatism. *Hastings Center Report.* 1998 May–Jun; 28(3): 4. 3 refs. BE58605.
adolescents; age factors; children; *competence; *decision making; empirical research; *informed consent; international aspects; legal aspects; *minors; patient care; treatment refusal; Great Britain; United States

Ondrusek, Nancy; Abramovitch, Rona; Pencharz, Paul, et al. Empirical examination of the ability of children to consent to clinical research. *Journal of Medical Ethics.* 1998 Jun; 24(3): 158–165. 6 refs. BE59112.
*adolescents; age factors; attitudes; blood specimen collection; *children; *competence; *comprehension; consent forms; evaluation studies; *informed consent; motivation; *nontherapeutic research; nutrition; research subjects; risks and benefits; questionnaires; Canada
This study examined the quality of children's assent to a clinical trial. In subjects younger than 9 years of age, understanding of most aspects of the study was found to be poor to non–existent. Understanding of procedures was poor in almost all subjects. In addition, voluntariness may have been compromised in many subjects by their belief that failure to complete the study would displease others. If the fact that a child's assent has been obtained is used to justify the exposure of that child to the potential harm of a non–therapeutic blood sample, the assent must be meaningful. In the nutrition study observed here, the quality of the assent of children younger than 9 years of age was very poor. The assent therefore did not provide a valid justification for requesting a blood sample from these children. This study indicates that most children younger than 9 years of age cannot be expected to consent or assent to clinical research in a meaningful way. The current age of 7 years for initiating assent (in addition to parental consent) is possibly not appropriate and should be reconsidered.

Overbay, Jane Dring. Parental participation in treatment decisions for pediatric oncology ICU patients. *Dimensions of Critical Care Nursing.* 1996 Jan–Feb; 15(1): 16–24. 16 refs. BE56847.
*adolescents; allowing to die; alternatives; *cancer; case studies; *children; clinical ethics committees; *communication; consent forms; critically ill; *decision making; disclosure; ethical analysis; evaluation studies; infants; *intensive care units; interprofessional relations; medical records; *nurse's role; *nurses; nursing research; *parental consent; *parents; patient advocacy; *patient care; patient care team; pediatrics; physicians; *professional family relationship; prognosis; prolongation of life; psychological

---

BE = bioethics accession number   fn. = footnotes   refs. = references

stress; *records; referral and consultation; risks and benefits; terminally ill; treatment outcome; treatment refusal; truth disclosure; values; withholding treatment; retrospective studies; Midwestern United States

Robbennolt, Jennifer K.; Weisz, Victoria; Lawson, Craig M. Advancing the rights of children and adolescents to be altruistic: bone marrow donation by minors. *Journal of Law and Health.* 1994–1995; 9(2): 213–245. 156 fn. BE57148.
adolescents; altruism; attitudes; *bone marrow; competence; decision making; judicial action; *legal aspects; *minors; parental consent; psychology; risks and benefits; *siblings; *standards; students; survey; *third party consent; *tissue donation; United States

Ross, Lainie Friedman. Health care decisionmaking by children: is it in their best interest? *Hastings Center Report.* 1997 Nov–Dec; 27(6): 41–45. 19 refs. BE57859.
*adolescents; adults; *autonomy; *children; *competence; *decision making; dissent; *family relationship; freedom; *informed consent; organizational policies; parent child relationship; *parental consent; parents; paternalism; *patient care; patient participation; pediatrics; physicians; professional organizations; rights; *treatment refusal; American Academy of Pediatrics

The argument for children's rights in health care has been long in the making. The success of this position is reflected in the 1995 American Academy of Pediatrics recommendations for the role of children in health care decisionmaking, which suggest that children be given greater voice as they mature. But there are good moral and practical reasons for exercising caution in these health care situations, especially when the child and parents disagree. Parents need the moral and legal space within which to make decisions that will facilitate their child's long–term autonomy, not only her present–day autonomy. Moreover, third–party intrusion, by physicians or the state, should be resisted unless negligent and abusive decisions are in the making.

Weir, Robert F.; Peters, Charles. Affirming the decisions adolescents make about life and death. *Hastings Center Report.* 1997 Nov–Dec; 27(6): 29–40. 22 fn. BE57858.
*adolescents; *advance care planning; *advance directives; *age factors; allowing to die; autonomy; chronically ill; *communication; *competence; counseling; critically ill; *decision making; disclosure; dissent; empirical research; guidelines; *informed consent; legal aspects; legislation; organizational policies; parents; *patient advocacy; *patient care; *patient participation; pediatrics; physician patient relationship; physicians; practice guidelines; professional family relationship; professional organizations; prolongation of life; risks and benefits; state government; *terminal care; terminally ill; *treatment refusal; trust; American Academy of Pediatrics; Patient Self–Determination Act 1990; United States

Adolescents who are critically, chronically, and terminally ill traditionally have been given little voice in their health care treatment. But over the last three decades attitudes have begun to shift. The legal and medical professions as well as parents and children's advocates have started to recognize that cognitively normal adolescents have decisionmaking capacity and believe these patients ought to have the opportunity to participate in even the toughest of health treatment decisions. Advances directives, if used with sensitivity and care, could prove a valuable means of giving these older pediatric patients a say in their care.

INSTITUTIONAL REVIEW BOARDS See
BEHAVIORAL RESEARCH/ETHICS COMMITTEES, HUMAN

EXPERIMENTATION/ETHICS COMMITTEES

INVOLUNTARY COMMITMENT

Appelbaum, Paul S. Almost a revolution: an international perspective on the law of involuntary commitment. *Journal of the American Academy of Psychiatry and the Law.* 1997; 25(2): 135–147. 55 refs. BE55621.
comparative studies; dangerousness; decision making; evaluation; family members; historical aspects; *international aspects; *involuntary commitment; *legal aspects; legal rights; legislation; mental health; *mentally ill; physicians; social impact; *standards; Australia; France; Great Britain; Greece; India; Ireland; Israel; Italy; Japan; Mental Health Act 1983 (Great Britain); Mental Health Act 1983 (New South Wales); New Zealand; Scandinavia; Switzerland; *United States

Blank, Robert H. Mandating outpatient treatment for pregnant substance abusers: attractive but unfeasible. *Politics and the Life Sciences.* 1996 Mar; 15(1): 49–50. 3 refs. Commentary on D. Mathieu, "Mandating treatment for pregnant substance abusers: a compromise," *PLS* 1995 Aug; 14(2): 199–208. BE56021.
alcohol abuse; autonomy; children; *coercion; community services; criminal law; *drug abuse; government financing; health; indigents; mandatory programs; mother fetus relationship; obligations of society; *outpatient commitment; *pregnant women; *prenatal injuries; preventive medicine; public policy; rehabilitation; resource allocation; rights; smoking; social impact; state interest; treatment refusal; United States

Boling, Patricia. Mandating treatment for pregnant substance abusers is the wrong focus for public discussion. *Politics and the Life Sciences.* 1996 Mar; 15(1): 51–52. 5 refs. 1 fn. Commentary on D. Mathieu, "Mandating treatment for pregnant substance abusers: a compromise," *PLS* 1995 Aug; 14(2): 199–208. BE56022.
autonomy; blacks; *coercion; community services; disadvantaged; *drug abuse; freedom; health care delivery; health care reform; health education; indigents; legal aspects; obligations of society; *outpatient commitment; *pregnant women; *prenatal injuries; preventive medicine; public policy; social discrimination; stigmatization; United States

Chavkin, Wendy. Mandatory treatment for pregnant substance abusers: irrelevant and dangerous. *Politics and the Life Sciences.* 1996 Mar; 15(1): 53–54. 10 refs. 1 fn. Commentary on D. Mathieu, "Mandating treatment for pregnant substance abusers: a compromise," *PLS* 1995 Aug; 14(2): 199–208. BE56025.
*coercion; community services; disadvantaged; *drug abuse; government financing; health care delivery; indigents; obligations of society; *outpatient commitment; *pregnant women; *prenatal injuries; public policy; resource allocation; scarcity; United States

Daniels, Cynthia R. A million (missing) men: a commentary on Mathieu's compromise on pregnancy and substance abuse. *Politics and the Life Sciences.* 1996 Mar; 15(1): 54–56. 13 refs. Commentary on D. Mathieu, "Mandating treatment for pregnant substance abusers: a compromise," *PLS* 1995 Aug; 14(2): 199–208. BE56028.
accountability; blacks; *coercion; community services; *drug abuse; fathers; health care delivery; health hazards; indigents; legal aspects; obligations of society; obligations to society; *outpatient commitment; politics; *pregnant women; *prenatal injuries; rights; social discrimination; state interest; voluntary programs; United States

Geller, Jeffrey L. A biopsychosocial rationale for coerced community treatment in the management of

---

BE = bioethics accession number   fn. = footnotes   refs. = references

schizophrenia. *Psychiatric Quarterly.* 1995 Fall; 66(3): 219–235. 58 refs. BE56206.
  brain pathology; *coercion; community services; *deinstitutionalized persons; guidelines; incentives; *mentally ill; motivation; *outpatient commitment; *patient care; practice guidelines; rehabilitation; risks and benefits; *schizophrenia; selection for treatment; treatment outcome

Hendin, Herbert. Involuntary commitment. *In: his* Suicide in America. New and Expanded Edition. New York, NY: W.W. Norton; 1995: 214–235, 291–294. 45 fn. ISBN 0–393–31368–9. BE56134.
  dangerousness; deinstitutionalized persons; depressive disorder; due process; institutionalized persons; *involuntary commitment; legal aspects; legal rights; legislation; mental institutions; *mentally ill; model legislation; patient care; patient discharge; *psychiatric diagnosis; social impact; standards; state government; *suicide; treatment outcome; Lanterman–Petris–Short Act; Mental Health Law Project; United States

Hiday, Virginia Aldigé. Involuntary commitment as a psychiatric technology. *International Journal of Technology Assessment in Health Care.* 1996 Fall; 12(4): 585–603. 121 refs. 2 fn. BE55559.
  attitudes; *coercion; electroconvulsive therapy; *empirical research; international aspects; *involuntary commitment; legal aspects; mental institutions; *mentally ill; outpatient commitment; *patient care; patient compliance; patients; psychoactive drugs; psychosurgery; treatment outcome; treatment refusal; trends; voluntary admission; qualitative research; quantitative research

Madden, Robert G. Civil commitment for substance abuse by pregnant women? A view from the front lines. *Politics and the Life Sciences.* 1996 Mar; 15(1): 56–59. 13 refs. 4 fn. Commentary on D. Mathieu, "Mandating treatment for pregnant substance abusers: a compromise," *PLS* 1995 Aug; 14(2): 199–208. BE56033.
  behavior control; children; *coercion; community services; *drug abuse; fathers; goals; health; legal aspects; mandatory programs; *outpatient commitment; patient compliance; *pregnant women; *prenatal injuries; preventive medicine; public policy; rights; treatment refusal; voluntary programs; United States

Mathieu, Deborah. Mandating treatment for pregnant substance abusers: a compromise. *Politics and the Life Sciences.* 1995 Aug; 14(2): 199–208. 93 refs. 24 fn. Commented on in *PLS* 1996 Mar; 15(1): by R.H. Blank, p. 49–50; by P. Boling, p. 51–52; by W. Chavkin, p. 53–54; by C.R. Daniels, p. 54–56; by R.G. Madden, p. 56–59; by J.C. Merrick, p. 59–60; by E.H. Moskowitz, p. 61–63; by E.G. Patterson and A.B. Andrews, p. 64–66; by P. Peretz and J.R. Schroedel, p. 67–69; by R.A. Strickland, p. 70–72; by D.B. Wexler, 73–75; and by L.R. Woliver, p. 75–77; with a response by D. Mathieu, p. 77–81. BE56034.
  autonomy; children; *coercion; community services; *drug abuse; due process; fetuses; health; health education; indigents; low birth weight; mandatory programs; minority groups; newborns; obligations of society; *outpatient commitment; patient compliance; policy analysis; *pregnant women; *prenatal injuries; preventive medicine; *public policy; rehabilitation; residential facilities; *state interest; uncertainty; voluntary programs; United States

Mathieu, Deborah. Pregnant women in chains? [Response]. *Politics and the Life Sciences.* 1996 Mar; 15(1): 77–81. 8 refs. 9 fn. Response to twelve commentaries by R.H. Blank, p. 40–50; by P. Boling, p. 51–52; by W. Chavkin, p. 53–54; by C.R. Daniels, p. 54–56; by R.G. Madden, p. 56–59; by J.C. Merrick, p. 59–60; by E.H. Moskowitz, p. 61–63; by E.G. Patterson and A.B.

Andrews, p. 64–66; by P. Peretz and J.R. Schroedel, p. 67–69; by R.A. Strickland, p. 70–72; by D.B. Wexler, p. 73–75; and by L.R. Woliver, p. 75–77. BE56035.
  alcohol abuse; children; *coercion; community services; decision making; *drug abuse; due process; fetal development; fetuses; guidelines; health education; mandatory programs; moral obligations; *outpatient commitment; patient care; *pregnant women; *prenatal injuries; public policy; rights; state interest; stigmatization; voluntary programs; United States

Merrick, Janna C. Pregnancy and substance abuse: education or mandatory treatment? *Politics and the Life Sciences.* 1996 Mar; 15(1): 59–60. 7 refs. 1 fn. Commentary on D. Mathieu, "Mandating treatment for pregnant substance abusers: a compromise," *PLS* 1995 Aug; 14(2): 199–208. BE56036.
  alcohol abuse; blacks; children; *coercion; community services; criminal law; *drug abuse; fathers; fetal development; health care delivery; health education; legal aspects; *outpatient commitment; *pregnant women; *prenatal injuries; public policy; selection for treatment; smoking; social discrimination; United States

Moskowitz, Ellen H. Can government ever protect fetuses from substance abuse? *Politics and the Life Sciences.* 1996 Mar; 15(1): 61–63. 1 ref. Commentary on D. Mathieu, "Mandating treatment for pregnant substance abusers: a compromise," *PLS* 1995 Aug; 14(2): 199–208. BE56037.
  autonomy; community services; *drug abuse; fetuses; freedom; health care delivery; health education; incentives; legal aspects; moral obligations; *outpatient commitment; *pregnant women; *prenatal injuries; privacy; *public policy; rights; state interest; stigmatization; uncertainty; United States

Patterson, Elizabeth G.; Andrews, Arlene Bowers. Civil commitment for pregnant substance abusers: is it appropriate and is it enough? *Politics and the Life Sciences.* 1996 Mar; 15(1): 64–66. 12 refs. 2 fn. Commentary on D. Mathieu, "Mandating treatment for pregnant substance abusers: a compromise," *PLS* 1995 Aug; 14(2): 199–208. BE56039.
  alternatives; *coercion; community services; *drug abuse; fetuses; freedom; health care delivery; nutrition; obligations of society; *outpatient commitment; *pregnant women; *prenatal injuries; preventive medicine; punishment; rights; risk; United States

Peretz, Paul; Schroedel, Jean Reith. The road not to travel: a comment on Deborah Mathieu's proposal to mandate outpatient treatment for pregnant substance abusers. *Politics and the Life Sciences.* 1996 Mar; 15(1): 67–69. 24 refs. 3 fn. Commentary on D. Mathieu, "Mandating treatment for pregnant substance abusers: a compromise," *PLS* 1995 Aug; 14(2): 199–208. BE56040.
  children; *coercion; community services; criminal law; *drug abuse; fetuses; government regulation; health; mandatory programs; mass screening; obligations of society; *outpatient commitment; *pregnant women; *prenatal injuries; preventive medicine; privacy; public policy; resource allocation; rights; selection for treatment; social control; state interest; treatment outcome; uncertainty; utilitarianism; United States

Smith, Carol A. Use of involuntary outpatient commitment in community care of the seriously and persistently mentally ill patient. *Issues in Mental Health Nursing.* 1995 May–Jun; 16(3): 275–284. 20 refs. BE55891.
  chronically ill; coercion; community services; *evaluation; *government regulation; *legal aspects; *mentally ill; *nurses; *outpatient commitment; *patient advocacy; *patient care; patient compliance; patients' rights; social impact; state government; treatment outcome; *United

---

BE = bioethics accession number   fn. = footnotes   refs. = references

States

Strickland, Ruth Ann. The incivility of mandated drug treatment through civil commitments. *Politics and the Life Sciences.* 1996 Mar; 15(1): 70–72. 29 refs. Commentary on D. Mathieu, "Mandating treatment for pregnant substance abusers: a compromise," *PLS* 1995 Aug; 14(2): 199–208. BE56044.
    alcohol abuse; *coercion; community services; *drug abuse; equal protection; fathers; fetuses; health hazards; indigents; legal aspects; mandatory programs; moral obligations; occupational exposure; *outpatient commitment; paternalism; *pregnant women; *prenatal injuries; *public policy; smoking; *social control; social discrimination; uncertainty; United States

Swartz, Marvin S.; Burns, Barbara J.; George, Linda K., et al. The ethical challenges of a randomized controlled trial of involuntary outpatient commitment. *Journal of Mental Health Administration.* 1997 Winter; 24(1): 35–43. 27 refs. BE57762.
    *behavioral research; coercion; informed consent; legal aspects; *mentally ill; *outpatient commitment; patient compliance; *random selection; *research design; research subjects; selection of subjects; treatment outcome; North Carolina

Treffert, Darold A. The obviously ill patient in need of treatment: a fourth standard for civil commitment. *Hospital and Community Psychiatry.* 1985 Mar; 36(3): 259–264. 18 refs. BE56678.
    *competence; dangerousness; *decision making; due process; *involuntary commitment; *legal aspects; legal guardians; legal rights; legislation; *mentally ill; patient advocacy; *standards; Alliance for the Mentally Ill; *Wisconsin; Wisconsin Mental Health Act (1985 bill)

Wexler, David B. Some therapeutic jurisprudence implications of the outpatient civil commitment of pregnant substance abusers. *Politics and the Life Sciences.* 1996 Mar; 15(1): 73–75. 13 refs. 1 fn. Commentary on D. Mathieu, "Mandating treatment for pregnant substance abusers: a compromise," *PLS* 1995 Aug; 14(2): 199–208. BE56047.
    behavior control; *coercion; community services; contracts; decision making; *drug abuse; due process; legal aspects; mandatory programs; *outpatient commitment; patient compliance; patient participation; *pregnant women; *prenatal injuries; *public policy; treatment refusal; voluntary programs; United States

Woliver, Laura R. Policies to assist pregnant women and children should include a complete assessment of the realities of women's lives. *Politics and the Life Sciences.* 1996 Mar; 15(1): 75–77. 17 refs. Commentary on D. Mathieu, "Mandating treatment for pregnant substance abusers: a compromise," *PLS* 1995 Aug; 14(2): 199–208. BE56049.
    autonomy; blacks; *coercion; community services; disadvantaged; domestic violence; *drug abuse; fathers; federal government; females; government financing; health facilities; *outpatient commitment; *pregnant women; *prenatal injuries; *public policy; scarcity; *social control; *social discrimination; United States

INVOLUNTARY COMMITMENT/FOREIGN COUNTRIES

Appelbaum, Paul S. Almost a revolution: an international perspective on the law of involuntary commitment. *Journal of the American Academy of Psychiatry and the Law.* 1997; 25(2): 135–147. 55 refs. BE55621.
    comparative studies; dangerousness; decision making; evaluation; family members; historical aspects; *international aspects; *involuntary commitment; *legal aspects; legal rights; legislation; mental health; *mentally ill; physicians; social impact; *standards; Australia; France; Great Britain; Greece; India; Ireland; Israel; Italy; Japan; Mental Health Act 1983 (Great Britain); Mental Health Act 1983 (New South Wales); New Zealand; Scandinavia; Switzerland; *United States

Dickenson, Donna. Ethical issues in long term psychiatric management. *Journal of Medical Ethics.* 1997 Oct; 23(5): 300–304. 18 fn. BE57104.
    accountability; beneficence; case studies; chronically ill; coercion; *community services; *dangerousness; *deinstitutionalized persons; duration of commitment; *informed consent; involuntary commitment; legal aspects; *long-term care; *mentally ill; *outpatient commitment; paternalism; patient compliance; patient discharge; physicians; presumed consent; psychoactive drugs; resource allocation; *risk; *treatment refusal; *Great Britain; Mental Health Act 1983 (Great Britain)
Two general ethical problems in psychiatry are thrown into sharp relief by long term care. This article discusses each in turn, in the context of two anonymised case studies from actual clinical practice. First, previous mental health legislation soothed doubts about patients' refusal of consent by incorporating time limits on involuntary treatment. When these are absent, as in the provisions for long term care which have recently come into force, the justification for compulsory treatment and supervision becomes more obviously problematic. Second, Anglo–American law does not normally allow the preventive detention of someone who may be dangerous but has not actually committed any crime. The justification for detaining a possibly dangerous user of mental health services without his or her consent can only be based on risk assessment, but this raises issues of moral luck. Is the psychiatrist who decides not to take out a supervision order for a possibly dangerous patient with an initial psychotic diagnosis morally at fault if that person harms someone in the community, or himself? Or is the psychiatrist merely unlucky?

Dyer, Clare. High court detains girl with anorexia. [News]. *BMJ (British Medical Journal).* 1997 Mar 22; 314(7084): 850. BE58745.
    *adolescents; *behavior disorders; females; food; *involuntary commitment; *legal aspects; *minors; *anorexia nervosa; *Great Britain

Dyer, Clare. New safeguards planned for psychiatric patients. [News]. *BMJ (British Medical Journal).* 1998 Jul 4; 317(7150): 7. BE58617.
    competence; government regulation; *involuntary commitment; *legal aspects; *mentally disabled; patient admission; physicians; *Great Britain; Mental Health Act 1983 (Great Britain)

Dyer, Clare. Thousands of patients may be being detained illegally. [News]. *BMJ (British Medical Journal).* 1998 Feb 14; 316(7130): 497. BE57752.
    competence; government regulation; institutionalized persons; *involuntary commitment; *legal aspects; *mentally disabled; patient admission; guideline adherence; *Great Britain; National Health Service

Great Britain. England. High Court of Justice, Queen's Bench Division. R v. Canons Park Mental Health Review Tribunal, ex parte A. *All England Law Reports.* 1993 Jul 28 (date of decision). [1994] 1: 481–494. BE58999.
    decision making; duration of commitment; international

BE = bioethics accession number   fn. = footnotes   refs. = references

aspects; *involuntary commitment; *legal aspects; legal rights; *mentally ill; *patient discharge; psychiatric diagnosis; review committees; treatment refusal; European Human Rights Convention; *Great Britain; Mental Health Act 1983 (Great Britain); Mental Health Review Tribunals; *R v. Canons Park Mental Health Review Tribunal

England's High Court of Justice, Queen's Bench Division, quashed the decision of a mental health tribunal to detain for treatment an involuntary patient. Her refusal of appropriate treatment essentially made her untreatable, thus voiding any legal ground for commitment. The patient, a woman identified as A, had been involuntarily committed to a mental hospital for reactive depression in an impulsive personality. About seven months later, she sought release. Prior to the tribunal decision, her condition was reclassified to "psychopathic disorder." The law entitles those patients classified as psychopaths or mentally impaired, but not those patients classified as mentally ill or severely mentally impaired, to release from involuntary commitment unless a criminal offense is committed. The court determined that under the provisions of the 1983 Mental Health Act and the European Human Rights Convention, the tribunal's findings obliged its members to release A. (KIE abstract)

Heginbotham, Christopher. Mental disorder and decision–making: respecting autonomy in substitute judgments. *In:* Grubb, Andrew, ed. Decision–Making and Problems of Incompetence. New York, NY: Wiley; 1994: 115–125. 9 refs. ISBN 0–471–94236–7. BE57133.
    advance directives; autonomy; *competence; *decision making; *informed consent; *involuntary commitment; judicial action; legal guardians; *mentally ill; *outpatient commitment; paternalism; patient care; physicians; risks and benefits; *third party consent; Enduring Powers of Attorney Act 1985 (Great Britain); *Great Britain; Mental Health Act 1983 (Great Britain)

Hobson, Sarah. Legal aspects of dementia. [Letter]. *Lancet.* 1997 May 17; 349(9063): 1482. 5 refs. BE55896.
    *aged; *dementia; *involuntary commitment; *legal aspects; paternalism; *Great Britain; Law Commission (Great Britain); National Assistance Act 1948 (Great Britain)

Hobson, Sarah Jane. The ethics of compulsory removal under section 47 of the 1948 National Assistance Act. *Journal of Medical Ethics.* 1998 Feb; 24(1): 38–43. 26 refs. BE57407.
    aged; autonomy; beneficence; *coercion; competence; disadvantaged; hospitals; human rights; informed consent; *involuntary commitment; *legislation; morality; mortality; motivation; *paternalism; patient care; physically disabled; physician patient relationship; physicians; public opinion; risks and benefits; state interest; treatment refusal; trust; *Great Britain; National Assistance Act 1948 (Great Britain)
Orders for removal under Section 47 of the 1948 National Assistance Act are little discussed. However, they involve severe infringements of the civil liberties of those affected. It is argued that all previously presented justifications for the use of these orders fail. Repeal of the act is called for. The Law Commission has drafted alternative legislation, but this has not been enacted. Until this occurs local authorities, the Faculty of Public Health Medicine and individual public health physicians should refuse to be involved in its use.

Humphreys, Martin; Ryman, Ann. Knowledge of emergency compulsory detention procedures among general practitioners in Edinburgh: sample survey. *BMJ (British Medical Journal).* 1996 Jun 8; 312(7044): 1462–1463. 5 refs. BE57052.
    *emergency care; family practice; hospitals; *involuntary

commitment; *knowledge, attitudes, practice; *legal aspects; *legislation; *mentally ill; *physicians; survey; *Edinburgh; Scotland

Smith, Theresa C.; Oleszczuk, Thomas A. No Asylum: State Psychiatric Repression in the Former USSR. New York, NY: New York University Press; 1996. 289 p. Bibliography: p. 260–278. ISBN 0–8147–8061–X. BE56096.
    data banks; *dissent; empirical research; *involuntary commitment; legal aspects; mental institutions; misconduct; physicians; political activity; *politics; psychiatric diagnosis; psychiatry; public policy; social control; socioeconomic factors; statistics; trends; *USSR

INVOLUNTARY COMMITMENT/MINORS

Dyer, Clare. High court detains girl with anorexia. [News]. *BMJ (British Medical Journal).* 1997 Mar 22; 314(7084): 850. BE58745.
    *adolescents; *behavior disorders; females; food; *involuntary commitment; *legal aspects; *minors; *anorexia nervosa; *Great Britain

Hopcroft, Thomas. Civil commitment of minors to mental institutions in the Commonwealth of Massachusetts. [Note]. *New England Journal on Criminal and Civil Confinement.* 1995 Summer; 21(2): 543–574. 264 fn. BE55560.
    criminal law; decision making; *due process; health personnel; *involuntary commitment; *legal aspects; legal guardians; *legal rights; mental institutions; mentally ill; *minors; parental consent; paternalism; state government; third party consent; *voluntary admission; D.L. v. Commissioner of Social Services; *Massachusetts

INVOLUNTARY STERILIZATION *See* STERILIZATION

JUSTICE *See* HEALTH CARE/RIGHTS, RESOURCE ALLOCATION

LEGAL ASPECTS
See under
    ABORTION/LEGAL ASPECTS
    ALLOWING TO DIE/LEGAL ASPECTS
    CONFIDENTIALITY/LEGAL ASPECTS
    EUTHANASIA/LEGAL ASPECTS

LIVING WILLS *See* ADVANCE DIRECTIVES

MASS SCREENING

See also AIDS/TESTING AND SCREENING, GENETIC SCREENING, PUBLIC HEALTH

Chadwick, Ruth. Genetic screening. *In:* Chadwick, Ruth, ed. Encyclopedia of Applied Ethics, Volume 2. San Diego, CA: Academic Press; 1998: 445–449. 8 refs. ISBN 0–12–227067–3. BE56391.
    advisory committees; autonomy; communitarianism; confidentiality; decision making; disclosure; eugenics; family members; genetic counseling; genetic disorders; genetic information; genetic predisposition; *genetic screening; genetic services; guidelines; informed consent; international aspects; justice; mandatory programs; *mass screening; moral policy; normality; public health; risks and benefits; stigmatization; voluntary programs; incidental findings; Council of Europe; Danish Council of Ethics; Nuffield

---

BE = bioethics accession number   fn. = footnotes   refs. = references

Council on Bioethics

Clayton, Ellen Wright. Screening and treatment of newborns. *Houston Law Review.* 1992 Spring; 29(1): 85–148. 263 fn. BE56976.
　　carriers; congenital disorders; disclosure; empirical research; *family relationship; genetic counseling; genetic disorders; genetic information; *genetic screening; health insurance; insurance selection bias; late–onset disorders; *legal aspects; *mandatory testing; *mass screening; *newborns; *parents; privacy; psychological stress; public health; *public policy; reproduction; *risks and benefits; state government; *state interest; stigmatization; *voluntary programs; United States

Coughlin, Steven S. Implementing breast and cervical cancer prevention programs among the Houma Indians of southern Louisiana: cultural and ethical considerations. *Journal of Health Care for the Poor and Underserved.* 1998 Feb; 9(1): 30–41. 44 refs. BE58493.
　　*American Indians; attitudes; autonomy; beneficence; *breast cancer; *cancer; confidentiality; *cultural pluralism; epidemiology; *females; health; *health services research; informed consent; *mass screening; *preventive medicine; public participation; research design; research subjects; risks and benefits; socioeconomic factors; vulnerable populations; ethnographic studies; qualitative research; Louisiana

Dankert-Roelse, Jeannette E.; te Meerman, Gerard J. Screening for cystic fibrosis -- time to change our position? [Editorial]. *New England Journal of Medicine.* 1997 Oct 2; 337(14): 997–999. 10 refs. BE56407.
　　carriers; *costs and benefits; *cystic fibrosis; diagnosis; genetic counseling; *genetic screening; *mass screening; methods; *newborns; patient care; prognosis; public policy; reproduction; *risks and benefits; treatment outcome

Dhondt, Jean-Louis; Farriaux, Jean-Pierre. Impact of French legislation on neonatal screening. *In:* Knoppers, Bartha Maria, ed. Human DNA: Law and Policy: International and Comparative Perspectives.
Proceedings of the First International Conference on DNA Sampling and Human Genetic Research: Ethical, Legal, and Policy Aspects, held in Montreal, Canada, 6–8 Sep 1996. Boston, MA: Kluwer Law International; 1997: 285–289. 5 fn. ISBN 90–411–0361–9. BE58185.
　　costs and benefits; disclosure; DNA data banks; genetic disorders; genetic research; *genetic screening; guidelines; *legal aspects; legislation; *mass screening; *newborns; parental consent; professional organizations; biological specimen banks; Association for Neonatal Screening (France); *France

Doukas, David J.; Fetters, Michael; Ruffin, Mack T., et al. Ethical considerations in the provision of controversial screening tests. *Archives of Family Medicine.* 1997 Sep–Oct; 6(5): 486–490. 18 refs. BE57600.
　　beneficence; costs and benefits; disclosure; evaluation; guidelines; informed consent; *mass screening; patient advocacy; patient education; physicians; *preventive medicine; professional organizations; risk; *risks and benefits; standards; evidence-based medicine; United States

Durfy, Sharon J.; Page, Andrea; Eng, Barry, et al. Attitudes of high school students toward carrier screening and prenatal diagnosis of cystic fibrosis. *Journal of Genetic Counseling.* 1994 Jun; 3(2): 141–155. 23 refs. BE57379.
　　*adolescents; *attitudes; *carriers; *cystic fibrosis; disclosure; females; *genetic screening; males; *mass screening; *prenatal diagnosis; reproduction; self concept; social discrimination; *students; survey; uncertainty; voluntary programs; NCHGR–funded publication; *secondary schools; Ontario

Foster, Peggy; Anderson, C. Mary. Reaching targets in the national cervical screening programme: are current practices unethical? *Journal of Medical Ethics.* 1998 Jun; 24(3): 151–157. 33 fn. BE59111.
　　age factors; autonomy; *cancer; coercion; disclosure; *females; goals; incentives; *informed consent; *mass screening; mortality; paternalism; physicians; *preventive medicine; primary health care; psychological stress; *public policy; remuneration; risk; *risks and benefits; socioeconomic factors; uncertainty; voluntary programs; *Great Britain; *National Health Service
The principle of informed consent is now well established within the National Health Service (NHS) in relation to any type of medical treatment. However, this ethical principle appears to be far less well established in relation to medical screening programmes such as Britain's national cervical screening programme. This article will critically examine the case for health care providers vigorously pursuing women to accept an invitation to be screened. It will discuss the type of information which women would need in order to make an informed decision about whether or not to be screened. The lack of such information in current patient leaflets on the "smear test" will then be documented. Finally, the article will explore possible ways of maximising women's autonomy in relation to the cervical screening programme without sacrificing any of its main benefits.

Hawkins, Dana. A bloody mess at one federal lab. [News]. *U.S. News and World Report.* 1997 Jun 23; 122(24): 26–27. BE58044.
　　blacks; disclosure; *employment; federal government; females; Hispanic Americans; *informed consent; institutional policies; legal aspects; males; *mass screening; *minority groups; pregnant women; privacy; research institutes; sickle cell anemia; social discrimination; syphilis; Department of Energy; *Lawrence Berkeley National Laboratory; United States

Miller, Anthony B. The public health basis of cancer screening: principles and ethical aspects. *In:* Miller, A.B., ed. Advances in Cancer Screening. Boston, MA: Kluwer Academic; 1996: 1–7. 19 refs. (Cancer treatment and research: 86). ISBN 0–7923–4019–1. BE58112.
　　age factors; breast cancer; *cancer; costs and benefits; diagnosis; empirical research; females; health services research; informed consent; males; *mass screening; mortality; patient care; preventive medicine; psychological stress; public health; public policy; random selection; research design; resource allocation; risks and benefits; Canada; United States

Mosenkis, Ari. Genetic screening for breast cancer susceptibility: a Torah perspective. *Journal of Halacha and Contemporary Society.* 1997 Fall; No. 34: 5–26. 66 fn. BE57176.
　　adolescents; age factors; *breast cancer; carriers; confidentiality; disclosure; employment; females; genetic information; *genetic predisposition; *genetic screening; insurance; *Jewish ethics; *Jews; *mass screening; moral obligations; prevalence; preventive medicine; *psychological stress; reproduction; risk; *risks and benefits; self concept; single persons; social discrimination; stigmatization; Tay Sachs disease; uncertainty; Orthodox Judaism

Skupski, Daniel W.; Chervenak, Frank A.; McCullough, Laurence B. Routine obstetric ultrasound examination: a clinical and ethical evaluation. *In:* Chervenak, Frank A.; Kurjak, Asim, eds. Current Perspectives on the Fetus as a Patient. New York, NY: Parthenon Publishing Group; 1996: 203–212. 33 refs. ISBN 1–85070–742–1. BE57645.

BE = bioethics accession number　　　fn. = footnotes　　　refs. = references

alternatives; autonomy; beneficence; congenital disorders; costs and benefits; counseling; disclosure; ethical analysis; evaluation; fetuses; human experimentation; informed consent; justice; *mass screening; morbidity; mortality; physicians; *pregnant women; *prenatal diagnosis; random selection; *risks and benefits; technology assessment; *ultrasonography; Routine Antenatal Diagnostic Imaging with Ultrasound (RADIUS)

Spiegler, Gerard E.; Motulsky, Arno G. Genetic screening of adolescents. [Letter and response]. *New England Journal of Medicine.* 1997 Aug 28; 337(9): 639–640. 7 refs. BE59004.
    *adolescents; carriers; confidentiality; genetic counseling; genetic disorders; genetic information; *genetic screening; health insurance; *mass screening; national health insurance; patient compliance; risks and benefits; social discrimination; Montreal; United States

Sutton, Graham C. Will you still need me, will you still screen me, when I'm past 64? Breast screening policy is based on ageism. [Editorial]. *BMJ (British Medical Journal).* 1997 Oct 25; 315(7115): 1032–1033. 14 refs. BE56589.
    *age factors; *aged; *breast cancer; costs and benefits; empirical research; *females; *mass screening; *public policy; referral and consultation; risk; *selection for treatment; *social discrimination; *Great Britain; *National Health Service

Volk, Robert J.; Cantor, Scott B.; Spann, Stephen J., et al. Preferences of husbands and wives for prostate cancer screening. *Archives of Family Medicine.* 1997 Jan–Feb; 6(1): 72–76. 26 refs. BE56482.
    *attitudes; *cancer; comparative studies; decision analysis; *decision making; dissent; *females; guidelines; *males; *marital relationship; *married persons; *mass screening; *patient care; *patients; physicians; professional organizations; *quality of life; survey; *treatment outcome; uncertainty; *prostate cancer; American Cancer Society; American Urological Society; United States

Woolf, Steven H.; Lawrence, Robert S. Preserving scientific debate and patient choice: lessons from the Consensus Panel on Mammography Screening. *JAMA.* 1997 Dec 17; 278(23): 2105–2108. 41 refs. BE56320.
    advisory committees; *age factors; autonomy; *breast cancer; consensus; *decision making; *disclosure; *dissent; empirical research; federal government; *females; freedom; guidelines; information dissemination; interprofessional relations; investigators; *mass screening; paternalism; patient participation; physicians; political activity; *politics; practice guidelines; *public policy; research design; *risks and benefits; science; *uncertainty; values; women's health; *consensus development conferences; evidence-based medicine; *mammography; National Cancer Advisory Board; National Cancer Institute; National Institutes of Health; U.S. Congress; *United States

Woolf, Steven H. Should we screen for prostate cancer? Men over 50 have a right to decide for themselves. [Editorial]. *BMJ (British Medical Journal).* 1997 Apr 5; 314(7086): 989–990. 14 refs. BE56585.
    age factors; alternatives; autonomy; *cancer; costs and benefits; *decision making; *disclosure; *gatekeeping; government financing; *males; *mass screening; patient advocacy; patient care; patient education; *patient participation; *physicians; public policy; quality of life; resource allocation; *risks and benefits; technology assessment; treatment outcome; uncertainty; values; personal financing; *prostate cancer; *Great Britain; *National Health Service

Wright, D.S. Workplace urine screening for drug abuse. [Letter]. *Journal of Medical Ethics.* 1997 Jun; 23(3): 191.

5 refs. BE56897.
    administrators; body parts and fluids; *drug abuse; *employment; guidelines; industry; *legal aspects; *mandatory programs; *mass screening; *occupational medicine; organizational policies; patient access to records; *physician's role; physicians; professional organizations; technical expertise; Faculty of Occupational Medicine (Great Britain); *Great Britain

The screening muddle. [Editorial]. *Lancet.* 1998 Feb 14; 351(9101): 459. BE58225.
    *cancer; *diagnosis; disclosure; females; *mass screening; quality of health care; *risks and benefits; Great Britain

MEDICAL CARE *See* HEALTH CARE, PATIENT CARE, TERMINAL CARE

MEDICAL ETHICS

See also BIOETHICS, NURSING ETHICS, PROFESSIONAL ETHICS

Appelbaum, Paul S. A theory of ethics for forensic psychiatry. *Journal of the American Academy of Psychiatry and the Law.* 1997; 25(3): 233–247. 33 refs. 9 fn. BE57246.
    beneficence; capital punishment; coercion; confidentiality; conflict of interest; disclosure; duty to warn; ethical theory; expert testimony; *forensic psychiatry; informed consent; justice; law; *medical ethics; *moral obligations; physician patient relationship; *physician's role; physicians; prisoners; professional autonomy; professional ethics; standards; values; professional role

Ashley, Benedict M.; Veatch, Robert M. Basis for medical ethics: a triple contract theory. [Book review of R.M. Veatch's *A Theory of Medical Ethics*, with response]. *Hospital Progress.* 1983 Jan; 64(1): 58–61. BE57234.
    *contracts; covenant; deontological ethics; ethical theory; *medical ethics; principle-based ethics; public participation; religious ethics; *A Theory of Medical Ethics (Veatch, R.M.)

Berg, Robert N. The ethical practice of medicine. *Journal of the Medical Association of Georgia.* 1990 Nov; 79(11): 863–864. 8 fn. BE55648.
    codes of ethics; disclosure; guidelines; *legal aspects; *medical ethics; moral obligations; patient access to records; patient care; physician patient relationship; physician self-referral; physicians; professional organizations; proprietary health facilities; remuneration; *American Medical Association; Georgia

Bhagwati, Sanat N. Ethics, morality and practice of medicine in ancient India. *Child's Nervous System.* 1997 Aug–Sep; 13(8–9): 428–434. 17 refs. BE57560.
    allowing to die; *ancient history; brain death; Buddhist ethics; codes of ethics; determination of death; Hindu ethics; *historical aspects; medical education; *medical ethics; *medicine; organ donation; right to die; surgery; *India

Blakely, Robert L.; Harrington, Judith M., eds. Bones in the Basement: Postmortem Racism in Nineteenth-Century Medical Training. Washington, DC: Smithsonian Institution Press; 1997. 380 p. Includes references. ISBN 1-56098-750-2. BE57441.
    attitudes; autopsies; *blacks; *body parts and fluids; *cadavers; drugs; health; health care; *historical aspects; *human body; indigents; injuries; legal aspects; *medical education; medical ethics; medical schools; *misconduct; morbidity; nutrition; *physicians; social control; *social discrimination; sociology of medicine; students; *teaching methods; whites; ethnographic studies; slavery; Georgia;

BE = bioethics accession number   fn. = footnotes   refs. = references

Harris, Grandison; *Medical College of Georgia (Augusta); *Nineteenth Century; Twentieth Century; United States

Cassell, Jackie. Against medical ethics: opening the can of worms. *Journal of Medical Ethics.* 1998 Feb; 24(1): 8–12. 13 fn. BE57404.
*bioethics; deontological ethics; ethical theory; *ethics; medical education; *medical ethics; medical specialties; *medicine; morality; *philosophy; utilitarianism

In a controversial paper, David Seedhouse argues that medical ethics is not and cannot be a distinct discipline with it own field of study. He derives this claim from a characterization of ethics, which he states but does not defend. He claims further that the project of medical ethics as it exists and of moral philosophy do not overlap. I show that Seedhouse's views on ethics have wide implications which he does not declare, and in the light of this argue that Seedhouse owes us a defence of his characterization of ethics. Further, I show that his characterization of ethics, which he uses to attack medical ethics, is a committed position within moral philosophy. As a consequence of this, it does not allow the relation between moral philosophy and medical ethics to be discussed without prejudice to its outcome. Finally, I explore the relation between Seedhouse's position and naturalism, and its implications for medical epistemology. I argue that this shows us that Seedhouse's position, if it can be defended, is likely to lead to a fruitful and important line of inquiry which reconnects philosophy and medical ethics.

Chervenak, Frank A.; McCullough, Laurence B. What is obstetric ethics? *Journal of Perinatal Medicine.* 1995; 23(5): 331–341. 52 refs. BE57763.
autonomy; beneficence; clinical ethics; consensus; directive counseling; embryos; ethical analysis; ethical theory; fetal development; fetal therapy; *fetuses; informed consent; law; *medical ethics; moral obligations; *obstetrics and gynecology; *patient care; physicians; *pregnant women; prenatal diagnosis; religion; value of life; viability

Cook, E. David. The Medical Maze: A Christian Approach to Healthcare Ethics. London: Christian Medical Fellowship; 1991. 22 p. ISBN 0-906747-24-4. BE58130.
*active euthanasia; attitudes to death; *Christian ethics; compassion; conscience; cultural pluralism; decision making; *medical ethics; moral policy; *physicians; suffering; *theology; value of life

Downie, R.S. Professional ethics and business ethics. *In:* McLean, Sheila A.M., ed. Contemporary Issues in Law, Medicine and Ethics. Brookfield, VT: Dartmouth; 1996: 1–14. 14 fn. ISBN 1-85521-586-1. BE57787.
administrators; beneficence; confidentiality; decision making; disadvantaged; *economics; health care; *health care delivery; justice; *medical ethics; paternalism; patient advocacy; peer review; physician patient relationship; *professional ethics; *public policy; quality of health care; social dominance; trust; *business ethics; integrity; quality control; Great Britain; National Health Service

General Medical Council (Great Britain). Duties of a Doctor: Guidance from the General Medical Council. [Booklets]. London: The Council; 1995. portfolio of 4 booklets. BE57156.
advertising; AIDS serodiagnosis; biomedical research; *confidentiality; conflict of interest; disclosure; duty to warn; family practice; gifts; *guidelines; *HIV seropositivity; iatrogenic disease; informed consent; *interprofessional relations; *medical ethics; medical fees; medical specialties; occupational exposure; patient care; *physician patient relationship; *physicians; professional competence; referral

and consultation; refusal to treat; self regulation; traffic accidents; *General Medical Council (Great Britain); *Great Britain

Guinan, Patrick D. Has medicine lost the ethics battle? *Linacre Quarterly.* 1998 May; 65(2): 43–50. 2 refs. BE58933.
bioethics; decision making; ethical theory; ethicists; historical aspects; *medical ethics; natural law; physician patient relationship; *physicians; professional autonomy; technical expertise; trends; virtues

Gunderman, Richard. Medicine and the pursuit of wealth. *Hastings Center Report.* 1998 Jan–Feb; 28(1): 8–13. 3 refs. BE57291.
*altruism; *economics; *entrepreneurship; *goals; humanism; love; managed care programs; medical education; *medical ethics; *medicine; *motivation; physician patient relationship; *physicians; self concept; sociology of medicine; students; trends; trust; *values; virtues; *greed; Smith, Adam; United States

Hall, Mark A.; Berenson, Robert A. Ethical practice in managed care: a dose of realism. *Annals of Internal Medicine.* 1998 Mar 1; 128(5): 395–402. 72 refs. BE57850.
administrators; common good; conflict of interest; *decision making; disclosure; *economics; ethical analysis; *guidelines; health; health care delivery; health insurance reimbursement; *incentives; *managed care programs; *medical ethics; moral obligations; moral policy; patient advocacy; patient care; *physician patient relationship; physician's role; *physicians; practice guidelines; public policy; remuneration; *resource allocation; *trust; withholding treatment; capitation fee; United States

This article examines the ethics of medical practice under managed care from a pragmatic perspective that gives physicians more useful guidance than do existing ethical statements. The article begins with a framework for constructing a realistic set of ethical principles, namely, that medical ethics derives from physicians' role as healers; that ethical statements are primarily aspirational, not regulatory; and that preserving patient trust is the primary objective. The following concrete ethical guidelines are presented: Financial incentives should influence physicians to maximize the health of the group of patients under their care; physicians should not enter into incentive arrangements that they are embarrassed to describe accurately to their patients; physicians should treat each patient impartially without regard to source of payment, consistent with the physician's own treatment style; if physicians depart from this ideal, they should inform their patients honestly; and it is desirable, although not mandatory, to differentiate medical treatment recommendations from insurance coverage decisions by clearly assigning authority over these different roles and by physicians advocating for recommended treatment that is not covered.

Hammes, Bernard J.; Webster, Stephen. Professional ethics and managed care in dermatology. *Archives of Dermatology.* 1996 Sep; 132(9): 1070–1073. 13 refs. BE55870.
alternatives; case studies; codes of ethics; conflict of interest; disclosure; *economics; *gatekeeping; health maintenance organizations; incentives; *managed care programs; *medical ethics; medical specialties; moral obligations; *patient advocacy; patient care; physician patient relationship; physician's role; *physicians; professional ethics; professional organizations; quality of health care; *referral and consultation; resource allocation; *withholding treatment; capitation fee; *dermatology; *undertreatment; United States

Hattab, Jocelyn Y. Psychiatric ethics. *In:* Chadwick,

Ruth, ed. Encyclopedia of Applied Ethics, Volume 3. San Diego, CA: Academic Press; 1998: 703–726. 7 refs. ISBN 0–12–227068–1. BE56265.

aged; biomedical research; brain; brain pathology; confidentiality; disclosure; expert testimony; forensic psychiatry; freedom; human experimentation; iatrogenic disease; informed consent; involuntary commitment; legal aspects; medical education; *medical ethics; mental health; mentally ill; minors; misconduct; patient care; physician patient relationship; physicians; preventive medicine; psychiatric diagnosis; *psychiatry; psychoactive drugs; psychotherapy; research ethics committees; stigmatization; third party consent

Hawkins, Anne Hunsaker. Medical ethics and the epiphanic dimension of narrative. *In:* Nelson, Hilde Lindemann, ed. Stories and Their Limits: Narrative Approaches to Bioethics. New York, NY: Routledge; 1997: 153–170. 29 refs. 2 fn. ISBN 0–415–91910–X. BE57468.

bioethics; *comprehension; *decision making; empathy; *literature; medical education; *medical ethics; *medicine; *narrative ethics; physician patient relationship; *physicians; self concept; suffering; sick role; Joyce, James

Horner, J. Stuart. Medical ethics, history of. *In:* Chadwick, Ruth, ed. Encyclopedia of Applied Ethics, Volume 3. San Diego, CA: Academic Press; 1998: 165–175. 9 refs. ISBN 0–12–227068–1. BE56251.

advertising; alternative therapies; ancient history; bioethics; Christian ethics; codes of ethics; government regulation; *historical aspects; international aspects; interprofessional relations; *medical ethics; medical etiquette; medicine; professional competence; professional organizations; religion; self regulation; social control; Beddoes, Thomas; Eighteenth Century; *England; Europe; Gisborne, Thomas; Greece; Gregory, John; Hippocrates; Middle Ages; Nineteenth Century; Percival, Thomas; Twentieth Century

Houtepen, Rob. The social construction of euthanasia and medical ethics in the Netherlands. *In:* DeVries, Raymond; Subedi, Janardan, eds. Bioethics and Society: Constructing the Ethical Enterprise. Upper Saddle River, NJ: Prentice Hall; 1998: 117–144. 76 refs. 1 fn. ISBN 0–13–531252–3. BE58733.

accountability; active euthanasia; allowing to die; assisted suicide; attitudes; autonomy; bioethical issues; *bioethics; codes of ethics; *decision making; ethicists; *euthanasia; goals; guidelines; *historical aspects; *interdisciplinary communication; lawyers; *medical ethics; medicine; patients' rights; physician patient relationship; *physicians; professional autonomy; professional organizations; quality of life; *right to die; social control; *social sciences; *sociology of medicine; terminal care; terminology; treatment refusal; trends; value of life; *Netherlands; Royal Dutch Society of Physicians; *Twentieth Century

Hutchens, Michael P. Grave robbing and ethics in the 19th century. *JAMA.* 1997 Oct 1; 278(13): 1115. 7 refs. BE55868.

*cadavers; confidentiality; health insurance; *historical aspects; legal aspects; *medical education; medical ethics; *misconduct; *physicians; Great Britain; *Nineteenth Century

Junkerman, Charles; Schiedermayer, David. Practical Ethics for Students, Interns, and Residents: A Short Reference Manual. Second Edition. Frederick, MD: University Publishing Group; 1998. 73 p. Includes references. ISBN 1–55572–054–4. BE57923.

active euthanasia; advance directives; AIDS; allowing to die; assisted suicide; autopsies; *bioethical issues; brain death; clinical ethics committees; competence; confidentiality; determination of death; ethics consultation; futility; informed consent; legal aspects; managed care programs; *medical

ethics; organ donation; palliative care; patient care; patient compliance; pediatrics; persistent vegetative state; physician patient relationship; physician's role; refusal to treat; resource allocation; resuscitation orders; terminal care; third party consent; withholding treatment; United States

Kassirer, Jerome P. Managing care — should we adopt a new ethic? [Editorial]. *New England Journal of Medicine.* 1998 Aug 6; 339(6): 397–398. 18 refs. BE59076.

*conflict of interest; disclosure; *economics; incentives; *managed care programs; *medical ethics; moral obligations; patient advocacy; *physician's role; quality of health care; resource allocation; utilitarianism; withholding treatment; capitation fee; utilization review

Kelly, John H.; Emanuel, Linda. Doing what's best for patients: 1957 and 1997. [Letter and response]. *JAMA.* 1997 Oct 1; 278(13): 1061–1062. 2 refs. BE56871.

beneficence; codes of ethics; conflict of interest; historical aspects; *medical ethics; medical fees; medicine; patients' rights; physician patient relationship; physician's role; *physicians; *professional organizations; *American Medical Association

Lister, Graham D. Ethics in surgical practice. [Editorial]. *Plastic and Reconstructive Surgery.* 1996 Jan; 97(1): 185–193. 14 refs. BE55569.

advertising; autonomy; codes of ethics; disclosure; informed consent; internship and residency; *medical ethics; medical fees; morality; paternalism; patient advocacy; physician patient relationship; physicians; professional competence; quality of health care; resource allocation; *surgery; health services misuse

Lützén, Kim; Evertzon, Mats; Nordin, Conny. Moral sensitivity in psychiatric practice. *Nursing Ethics.* 1997 Nov; 4(6): 472–482. 13 refs. BE57418.

age factors; *attitudes; autonomy; beneficence; comparative studies; *decision making; *females; *males; *medical ethics; mentally ill; *moral development; paternalism; patient care; *physician patient relationship; *physicians; *psychiatry; survey; trust; values; *Sweden

McCullough, Laurence B. Molecular medicine, managed care, and the moral responsibilities of patients and physicians. *Journal of Medicine and Philosophy.* 1998 Feb; 23(1): 3–9. 11 refs. BE57517.

alcohol abuse; bioethics; biomedical technologies; *clinical ethics; disease; entrepreneurship; genetic information; genetic predisposition; genetic screening; goals; health; historical aspects; justice; *managed care programs; *medical ethics; *medicine; models, theoretical; *moral obligations; obligations to society; organ transplantation; patents; *patients; patients' rights; physician patient relationship; physician's role; *physicians; resource allocation; selection for treatment; self induced illness; social impact

McCullough, Laurence B.; Jones, James W.; Brody, Baruch A., eds. Surgical Ethics. New York, NY: Oxford University Press; 1998. 396 p. 642 refs. ISBN 0–19–510347–5. BE58322.

advance directives; autonomy; beneficence; competence; confidentiality; conflict of interest; determination of death; disclosure; emergency care; entrepreneurship; family members; health facilities; health insurance; indigents; informed consent; interprofessional relations; justice; managed care programs; *medical ethics; *moral obligations; organ transplantation; patient advocacy; *patient care; patients; physician patient relationship; *physicians; professional competence; professional organizations; remuneration; resource allocation; resuscitation orders; review; selection for treatment; self regulation; social discrimination; *surgery; terminal care; therapeutic research; third party consent; treatment refusal; health services misuse;

BE = bioethics accession number   fn. = footnotes   refs. = references

professional courtesy; undertreatment; American College of Surgeons; American Medical Association; United States

Mason, John Kenyon; McCall Smith, R.A. Law and Medical Ethics. Fourth Edition. London: Butterworths; 1994. 451 p. Includes references. Appendixes include the Hippocratic Oath, international codes and declarations, and a specimen living will. ISBN 0-406-02478-2. BE55694.
> abortion, induced; active euthanasia; aged; AIDS; allowing to die; *bioethical issues; brain death; codes of ethics; competence; confidentiality; contraception; determination of death; embryo research; fetal research; fetuses; forensic psychiatry; gene therapy; genetic counseling; homosexuals; human experimentation; informed consent; international aspects; involuntary commitment; *legal aspects; legal liability; *medical ethics; mentally ill; minors; negligence; newborns; nontherapeutic research; organ donation; organ transplantation; prenatal diagnosis; reproductive technologies; resource allocation; scientific misconduct; sex offenses; sexuality; sexually transmitted diseases; sterilization (sexual); transsexualism; wrongful life; *Great Britain

Mellsop, Graham. Issues in psychiatric ethics. *New Zealand Medical Journal.* 1983 Aug 10; 96(737): 616-619. 20 refs. Lecture delivered at the Ashburn Hall Centenary, 31 Oct 1983. BE57236.
> accountability; confidentiality; health personnel; human experimentation; informed consent; *medical ethics; misconduct; physician patient relationship; *psychiatry; psychotherapy

Montello, Martha. Narrative competence. *In:* Nelson, Hilde Lindemann, ed. Stories and Their Limits: Narrative Approaches to Bioethics. New York, NY: Routledge; 1997: 185-197. 51 refs. 2 fn. ISBN 0-415-91910-X. BE57470.
> clinical ethics; empathy; *literature; medical education; *medical ethics; medicine; *moral development; *narrative ethics; physician patient relationship; *physicians; *professional competence

Moreno, Jonathan D.; Lucente, Frank E. Patients who are family members, friends, colleagues, family members of colleagues. *In:* McCullough, Laurence B.; Jones, James W.; Brody, Baruch A., eds. Surgical Ethics. New York, NY: Oxford University Press; 1998: 198-215. 15 refs. ISBN 0-19-510347-5. BE58335.
> codes of ethics; communication; confidentiality; empirical research; *family members; friends; health insurance reimbursement; historical aspects; informed consent; *interprofessional relations; legal aspects; *medical ethics; *medical etiquette; medical fees; medical specialties; organizational policies; *patient care; *physician patient relationship; *physicians; *professional family relationship; professional organizations; review; *surgery; technical expertise; professional courtesy; American Medical Association; Hippocratic Oath; United States

Nathanson, Vivienne. Humanitarian action: the duty of all doctors. [Editorial]. *BMJ (British Medical Journal).* 1997 Nov 29; 315(7120): 1389-1390. 16 refs. BE56901.
> developing countries; disadvantaged; health care; human experimentation; *human rights; informed consent; *international aspects; medical ethics; *moral obligations; *obligations to society; *physicians; *political activity; politics; prisoners; war; Universal Declaration of Human Rights

Neeleman, J.; van Os, J. Ethical issues in European psychiatry. *European Psychiatry.* 1996; 11(1): 1-6. 55 refs. BE56415.
> assisted suicide; confidentiality; drug abuse; health care delivery; human experimentation; human rights; informed consent; *international aspects; involuntary commitment; law enforcement; legal aspects; medical education; *medical ethics; medical records; mentally ill; patient care; physicians; *psychiatry; research ethics committees; self regulation; standards; *Europe; *European Union

Pellegrino, Edmund D. Praxis as a keystone for the philosophy and professional ethics of medicine: the need for an arch-support: commentary on Toulmin and Wartofsky. *In:* Carson, Ronald A.; Burns, Chester R., eds. Philosophy of Medicine and Bioethics: A Twenty-Year Retrospective and Critical Appraisal. Boston, MA: Kluwer Academic; 1997: 69-84. 37 refs. ISBN 0-7923-3545-7. BE56527.
> bioethical issues; clinical ethics; *medical ethics; medical specialties; *medicine; metaethics; *philosophy; physician patient relationship

Pellegrino, Edmund D. The autopsy: some ethical reflections on the obligations of pathologists, hospitals, families, and society. *Archives of Pathology and Laboratory Medicine.* 1996 Aug; 120(8): 739-742. Presented at the College of American Pathologists/American Society of Clinical Pathologists/Association of Pathology Chairs Conference XXIX, Restructuring Autopsy Practice for Health Care Reform, 25 May 1995. BE55521.
> attitudes; *autopsies; cadavers; confidentiality; diagnosis; family members; hospitals; informed consent; medical ethics; *moral obligations; obligations of society; *physicians; technical expertise; *pathology

Peppin, John F. The Christian physician in the non-Christian institution: objections of conscience and physician value neutrality. *Christian Bioethics.* 1997 Mar; 3(1): 39-54. 33 refs. 16 fn. Commented on by A.L. Smith, p. 74-84. BE56359.
> abortion, induced; assisted suicide; autonomy; *Christian ethics; *conscience; government regulation; health facilities; institutional policies; legal rights; medical education; *medical ethics; moral complicity; morality; *patient care; physician patient relationship; *physicians; referral and consultation; refusal to treat; religious hospitals; *values; liberalism; United States

Christian physicians are in danger of losing the right of conscientious objection in situations they deem immoral. The erosion of this right is bolstered by the doctrine of "physician value neutrality" (PVN) which may be an impetus for the push to require physicians to refer for procedures they find immoral. It is only a small step from referral to compelling performance of these same procedures. If no one particular value is more morally correct than any other (a foundational PVN premise) and a physician ought to be value neutral, than conscientious objection to morally objectionable actions becomes a thing of the past. However, the argument for PVN fails. Therefore, Christian physicians should state their values openly, which would allow patients the ability to choose like-minded physicians. Some possible responses to this erosion of conscientious objection include, disengagement from non-Christian institutions, the formation of distinctly Christian medical institutions and political action. However, for the Christian the initial focus should be on a life of holiness which requires each of us to avoid evil.

Pierce, Susan Foley. A model for conceptualizing the moral dynamic in health care. *Nursing Ethics.* 1997 Nov; 4(6): 483-495. 13 refs. BE57419.
> autonomy; bioethical issues; caring; compassion; *decision making; emotions; empathy; ethical theory; females; justice; males; *medical ethics; *models, theoretical; *moral development; morality; nurse's role; *nurses; *nursing ethics; *patient care; patient care team; physician nurse relationship; physician's role; *physicians; professional patient

---

relationship; self concept; technical expertise; terminal care; *values; virtues

Pinkus, Rosa Lynn. Politics, paternalism, and the rise of the neurosurgeon: the evolution of moral reasoning. *Medical Humanities Review.* 1996 Fall; 10(2): 20–44. 81 fn. BE56598.
  accountability; brain pathology; case studies; coercion; decision making; dissent; *historical aspects; internship and residency; *interprofessional relations; medical education; *medical ethics; *medical specialties; newborns; paternalism; patient care; physician patient relationship; *physicians; politics; social dominance; standards; *surgery; technical expertise; truth disclosure; medical errors; *neurosurgery; *Cushing, Harvey; Dandy, Walter; Twentieth Century; United States

Poltawska, Wanda. The responsibility of the medical doctor and the life of the patient. *Dolentium Hominum: Church and Health in the World.* 1996; 31(11th Yr., No. 1): 137–140. 1 fn. BE57373.
  abortion, induced; attitudes to death; conscience; contraception; genetic intervention; killing; *medical ethics; *moral obligations; *physicians; professional competence; reproductive technologies; *Roman Catholic ethics; *Roman Catholics; sterilization (sexual); theology; value of life; dignity; Hippocratic Oath

Sapru, R.P. Ethical concerns in modern medical practice. *Indian Heart Journal.* 1997 Jul–Aug; 49(4): 441–445. 23 refs. BE58562.
  communication; confidentiality; continuing education; developing countries; disclosure; drug industry; drugs; economics; *health care; heart diseases; Hindu ethics; human experimentation; indigents; informed consent; medical education; *medical ethics; palliative care; *patient care; physician patient relationship; physician self-referral; physicians; *professional competence; quality of health care; regulation; surgery; *India

Seedhouse, David. What's the difference between health care ethics, medical ethics and nursing ethics? [Editorial]. *Health Care Analysis.* 1997 Dec; 5(4): 267–274. 16 refs. BE57543.
  *bioethics; caring; cultural pluralism; ethical theory; ethics; *goals; health; health care; health personnel; interdisciplinary communication; *medical ethics; medicine; nurses; *nursing ethics; philosophy; physicians; professional ethics; values

Thomasma, David C., ed. The Influence of Edmund D. Pellegrino's Philosophy of Medicine. Boston, MA: Kluwer Academic; 1997. 215 p. 561 fn. Reprinted from *Theoretical Medicine,* 18(1–2); 1997. ISBN 0–7923–4412–X. BE57642.
  allowing to die; assisted suicide; *bioethical issues; *bioethics; caring; clinical ethics; communitarianism; conflict of interest; covenant; cultural pluralism; decision making; disease; economics; *ethical theory; ethicists; health; international aspects; managed care programs; medical education; *medical ethics; *medicine; nursing ethics; patient advocacy; patient care; patient participation; *philosophy; *physician patient relationship; *physician's role; primary health care; principle-based ethics; psychiatry; public policy; quality of health care; religious ethics; resource allocation; secularism; sociology of medicine; trust; values; *virtues; voluntary euthanasia; *Pellegrino, Edmund; United States

Toaff, Elio. Judaism. *Dolentium Hominum: Church and Health in the World.* 1996; 31(11th Yr., No. 1): 78–81. BE57376.
  bioethics; biomedical technologies; compassion; *Jewish ethics; justice; love; *medical ethics; medicine; parent child relationship; physicians; religion; *reproductive technologies; self regulation; social impact; suffering;

theology; value of life; Italy

Toulmin, Stephen. The primacy of practice: medicine and postmodernism. *In:* Carson, Ronald A.; Burns, Chester R., eds. Philosophy of Medicine and Bioethics: A Twenty-Year Retrospective and Critical Appraisal. Boston, MA: Kluwer Academic; 1997: 41–53. 4 refs. ISBN 0–7923–3545–7. BE56525.
  ethics; historical aspects; interdisciplinary communication; international aspects; medical ethics; *medicine; *metaethics; *philosophy; *postmodernism; Twentieth Century

Tovey, Philip. Narrative and knowledge development in medical ethics. *Journal of Medical Ethics.* 1998 Jun; 24(3): 176–181. 29 refs. Commentary on R. Gillon, "Imagination, literature, medical ethics and medical practice," *JME,* 1997 Feb; 23(1) 3–4. BE59120.
  bioethics; *empirical research; ethical theory; health services research; *medical ethics; *methods; *narrative ethics; primary health care; science; social sciences; Great Britain; National Health Service

The role of individual life accounts has been promoted--largely through what has come to be described as narrative ethics--as important to the practice of medical ethics for a number of years. Beyond this the apparent incompatibility of personal stories with scientific procedure has limited their use. In this article I will argue that this represents a serious under-utilisation of a valuable method for researching ethical dilemmas and the settings in which these dilemmas are played out. Life stories need not simply provide a stimulus to scientific research but can in themselves yield intellectually robust evidence on the general as well as the particular. By drawing on the rigorous methods developed elsewhere, personal accounts not only allow us to "enter the world of the sick person" but allow us to do so in such a way as to contribute to empirical and theoretical knowledge.

Trotter, Griffin. The Loyal Physician: Roycean Ethics and the Practice of Medicine. Nashville, TN: Vanderbilt University Press; 1997. 299 p. Bibliography: p. 281–289. ISBN 0–8265–1291–7. BE58549.
  altruism; autonomy; beneficence; caring; decision making; economics; emergency care; entrepreneurship; gatekeeping; historical aspects; humanism; *medical ethics; *medicine; moral development; obligations to society; patient advocacy; patient care; *philosophy; physician patient relationship; *physicians; professional competence; professional ethics; resource allocation; self concept; standards; *virtues; pragmatism; MacIntyre, Alasdair; *Royce, Josiah; Twentieth Century

Udén, Giggi; Norberg, Astrid; Norberg, Siv. The stories of physicians, registered nurses and enrolled nurses about ethically difficult care episodes in surgical care. *Scandinavian Journal of Caring Sciences.* 1995; 9(4): 245–253. 36 refs. BE55834.
  allowing to die; *attitudes; attitudes to death; autonomy; bioethical issues; cancer; *clinical ethics; comparative studies; compassion; decision making; hospitals; interdisciplinary communication; *interprofessional relations; *medical ethics; moral development; narrative ethics; nurse patient relationship; *nurses; *nursing ethics; pain; palliative care; paternalism; patient advocacy; *patient care; *physician nurse relationship; physician patient relationship; *physicians; prognosis; psychological stress; quality of life; surgery; survey; terminal care; truth disclosure; withholding treatment; qualitative research; Sweden

Underwood, C.R. Of ethics -- of right and wrong. [Editorial]. *Journal of the Medical Association of Georgia.*

BE = bioethics accession number   fn. = footnotes   refs. = references

1990 Nov; 79(11): 800–803. BE55638.
    allowing to die; codes of ethics; conflict of interest; economics; historical aspects; *medical ethics; prolongation of life; proprietary health facilities; quality of life; value of life

Wartofsky, Marx W. What can the epistemologists learn from the endocrinologists? Or is the philosophy of medicine based on a mistake? *In:* Carson, Ronald A.; Burns, Chester R., eds. Philosophy of Medicine and Bioethics: A Twenty-Year Retrospective and Critical Appraisal. Boston, MA: Kluwer Academic; 1997: 55–68. 2 refs. 2 fn. ISBN 0–7923–3545–7. BE56526.
    biomedical technologies; medical specialties; *medicine; *metaethics; *philosophy

Whitman, Jeffrey P. Reclaiming the medical profession: the military profession as a model. *Professional Ethics.* 1995 Spring; 4(1): 3–22. 32 fn. BE55796.
    conflict of interest; conscience; *economics; entrepreneurship; *goals; *health care reform; killing; malpractice; *medical ethics; *medicine; *metaphor; *military personnel; misconduct; *moral obligations; morality; organizational policies; patient advocacy; *physician's role; *physicians; *professional autonomy; professional competence; *professional ethics; professional organizations; public opinion; remuneration; *resource allocation; *self regulation; trust; virtues; *war; *professional role; American Medical Association; United States

Wiesing, Urban. Medical ethics, use of historical evidence in. *In:* Chadwick, Ruth, ed. Encyclopedia of Applied Ethics, Volume 3. San Diego, CA: Academic Press; 1998: 177–184. 11 refs. ISBN 0–12–227068–1. BE56252.
    bioethics; ethics; *historical aspects; *medical ethics; medicine; *methods; moral development; morality; *philosophy; retrospective moral judgment; values

World Medical Association. Ethical issues concerning patients with mental illness. [Policy statement]. *Bulletin of Medical Ethics.* 1996 Aug; No. 120: 11. This statement was approved by the World Medical Association in Sep 1995. BE55943.
    alternatives; autonomy; competence; confidentiality; conflict of interest; disclosure; informed consent; *international aspects; involuntary commitment; *medical ethics; *mentally ill; military personnel; misconduct; obligations to society; *organizational policies; patient advocacy; *patient care; physician patient relationship; *physicians; prisoners; privacy; professional organizations; *psychiatry; risks and benefits; social discrimination; stigmatization; third party consent; trust; truth disclosure; *World Medical Association

Zribi, Ahmed. Medical ethics and Islam. *Dolentium Hominum: Church and Health in the World.* 1996; 31(11th Yr., No. 1): 82–85. 7 refs. BE57377.
    abortion, induced; active euthanasia; beneficence; *bioethical issues; cadavers; confidentiality; contraception; fetal development; freedom; gene therapy; genetic identity; genetic intervention; human experimentation; *Islamic ethics; justice; *medical ethics; organ donation; organ donors; organ transplantation; parent child relationship; reproductive technologies; *theology; Hippocrates

MEDICAL ETHICS/CODES OF ETHICS

American College of Physicians. Ethics and Human Rights Committee. Ethics manual. Fourth edition. [Position paper]. *Annals of Internal Medicine.* 1998 Apr 1; 128(7): 576–594. 66 refs. BE57323.
    active euthanasia; advance care planning; alternative therapies; artificial feeding; assisted suicide; biomedical research; clinical ethics committees; *codes of ethics;

communicable diseases; confidentiality; conflict of interest; determination of death; disclosure; economics; family members; genetic counseling; genetic screening; *guidelines; iatrogenic disease; information dissemination; informed consent; interprofessional relations; legal aspects; *medical ethics; medical records; misconduct; occupational exposure; organ donation; *organizational policies; patient access to records; patient care; persistent vegetative state; physician patient relationship; *physicians; professional organizations; referral and consultation; refusal to treat; reproduction; resource allocation; resuscitation orders; sexuality; terminal care; third party consent; withholding treatment; physician impairment; *American College of Physicians

Baker, Robert; Caplan, Arthur; Emanuel, Linda L., et al. Crisis, ethics, and the American Medical Association: 1847 and 1997. [Editorial]. *JAMA.* 1997 Jul 9; 278(2): 163–164. 4 refs. BE58402.
    *codes of ethics; economics; health care delivery; *historical aspects; *medical ethics; *physicians; *professional organizations; *trends; *American Medical Association; Council on Ethical and Judicial Affairs (AMA); *Nineteenth Century; *Twentieth Century; United States

Britton, Alison. Hippocrates: dead or alive? *In:* Petersen, Kerry, ed. Intersections: Women on Law, Medicine and Technology. Brookfield, VT: Ashgate; 1997: 1–23. 24 refs. 6 fn. ISBN 1–85521–882–8. BE57484.
    active euthanasia; ancient history; assisted suicide; beneficence; *codes of ethics; evaluation; health; health care; *historical aspects; *medical ethics; medicine; physician's role; physicians; sociology of medicine; trends; *Hippocratic Oath; Twentieth Century

Canadian Medical Association. Code of ethics of the Canadian Medical Association. *International Journal of Bioethics.* 1997 Mar–Jun; 8(1–2): 123–125. Approved by the CMA General Council, Aug 1996. BE59099.
    advance directives; *codes of ethics; confidentiality; human experimentation; informed consent; interprofessional relations; *medical ethics; medical etiquette; medical fees; obligations to society; peer review; physician patient relationship; physicians; professional competence; professional organizations; treatment refusal; physician impairment; *Canadian Medical Association

Canadian Medical Association. Code of Ethics of the Canadian Medical Association (approved by General Council, August 1996). *Canadian Medical Association Journal.* 1996 Oct 15; 155(8): 1176A–1176B. BE56150.
    *codes of ethics; communication; confidentiality; decision making; human experimentation; informed consent; *medical ethics; obligations to society; patient care; physician patient relationship; *physicians; professional organizations; Canada; *Canadian Medical Association

Fineschi, Vittorio; Turillazzi, Emanuela; Cateni, Cecilia. The new Italian code of medical ethics. *Journal of Medical Ethics.* 1997 Aug; 23(4): 239–244. 14 refs. BE55905.
    advance directives; advisory committees; autonomy; *bioethical issues; bioethics; *codes of ethics; competence; confidentiality; conscience; cultural pluralism; decision making; democracy; disclosure; government regulation; historical aspects; informed consent; legal aspects; *medical ethics; physician patient relationship; physicians; professional autonomy; professional organizations; reproductive technologies; selection for treatment; self regulation; *Italy; National Committee for Bioethics (Italy); Twentieth Century

In June 1995, the Italian code of medical ethics was revised in order that its principles should reflect the ever-changing relationship between the medical profession and society and between physicians and patients. The updated code is also a response to new

---

ethical problems created by scientific progress; the discussion of such problems often shows up a need for better understanding on the part of the medical profession itself. Medical deontology is defined as the discipline for the study of norms of conduct for the health care professions, including moral and legal norms as well as those pertaining more strictly to professional performance. The aim of deontology is therefore, the in-depth investigation and revision of the code of medical ethics. It is in the light of this conceptual definition that one should interpret a review of the different codes which have attempted, throughout the various periods of Italy's recent history, to adapt ethical norms to particular social and health care climates.

Hurwitz, Brian; Richardson, Ruth. Swearing to care: the resurgence in medical oaths. *BMJ (British Medical Journal).* 1997 Dec 20–27; 315(7123): 1671–1674. 27 refs. Includes the text of a draft revision of the Hippocratic Oath by the British Medical Association on behalf of the World Medical Association. BE57652.
    ancient history; *codes of ethics; conflict of interest; economics; *health personnel; historical aspects; international aspects; *medical ethics; medical schools; moral obligations; patient advocacy; patient care team; *physicians; *professional ethics; professional organizations; trends; virtues; British Medical Association; Declaration of Geneva; General Medical Council (Great Britain); Great Britain; *Hippocratic Oath; Twentieth Century; United States; World Medical Association

Kenny, Nuala P. The CMA Code of Ethics: more room for reflection. [Editorial]. *Canadian Medical Association Journal.* 1996 Oct 15; 155(8): 1063–1065. 6 refs. BE56156.
    *codes of ethics; *medical ethics; moral obligations; physician patient relationship; *physicians; professional organizations; Canada; *Canadian Medical Association

Keyserlingk, Edward W. Medical oaths and codes. *In:* Chadwick, Ruth, ed. Encyclopedia of Applied Ethics, Volume 3. San Diego, CA: Academic Press; 1998: 155–163. 10 refs. ISBN 0-12-227068-1. BE56250.
    autonomy; *codes of ethics; consensus; cultural pluralism; government regulation; guidelines; health personnel; historical aspects; human experimentation; international aspects; justice; *medical ethics; medical etiquette; morality; obligations to society; physician patient relationship; physicians; professional ethics; professional organizations; religion; rights; self regulation; standards; terminology; values; virtues; Declaration of Helsinki; Hippocratic Oath; Nuremberg Code; Twentieth Century

Kuhse, Helga. Confidentiality and the AMA's [Australian Medical Association] new code of ethics: an imprudent formulation? *Medical Journal of Australia.* 1996 Sep 16; 165(6): 327–329. 11 refs. BE58972.
    *codes of ethics; *confidentiality; dangerousness; disclosure; duty to warn; guidelines; *medical ethics; *physicians; *professional organizations; *Australia; *Australian Medical Association

Nutton, Vivian. What's in an oath? *Journal of the Royal College of Physicians of London.* 1995 Nov–Dec; 29(6): 518–524. 30 fn. Article based on a lecture given at the Royal College of Physicians, London, on 25 Jul 1995. BE57966.
    *codes of ethics; *historical aspects; medical education; *medical ethics; *physicians; public opinion; students; *Hippocratic Oath

Orr, Robert D.; Pang, Norman; Pellegrino, Edmund D., et al. Use of the Hippocratic oath: a review of twentieth century practice and a content analysis of oaths administered in medical schools in the U.S. and Canada in 1993. *Journal of Clinical Ethics.* 1997 Winter; 8(4): 377–388. 70 fn. BE57611.
    abortion, induced; accountability; ancient history; *codes of ethics; comparative studies; confidentiality; euthanasia; evaluation; historical aspects; *institutional policies; medical education; *medical ethics; *medical schools; medicine; physician patient relationship; physicians; professional organizations; religion; review; sexuality; statistics; survey; *trends; *values; virtues; *Canada; Declaration of Geneva; *Hippocratic Oath; Middle Ages; Oath of Lasagna; Osteopathic Oath; Prayer of Maimonides; *Twentieth Century; *United States; World Medical Association
The purposes of this empiric study, literature review, and analysis are to determine the current prevalence of oath taking in medical schools in North America, to compare the content of the oaths in use to that of the classical Hippocratic Oath, and to document changes in the practice and content during this century. From this review and analysis, we hope to make a case for the value of the Hippocratic tradition.

Pellegrino, Edmund D.; Caplan, Arthur L.; Goold, Susan Dorr. Doctors and ethics, morals and manuals. *Annals of Internal Medicine.* 1998 Apr 1; 128(7): 569–571. 6 refs. BE57328.
    *codes of ethics; conflict of interest; economics; *guidelines; historical aspects; *medical ethics; moral obligations; organizational policies; patient advocacy; physician patient relationship; *physicians; professional organizations; quality of health care; resource allocation; trust; *American College of Physicians

Rafuse, Jill. Revised Code of Ethics wins CMA approval. [News]. *Canadian Medical Association Journal.* 1996 Oct 15; 155(8): 1148–1149. BE56159.
    *codes of ethics; *medical ethics; *physicians; professional organizations; Canada; *Canadian Medical Association

Rothstein, Mark A. A proposed revision of the ACOEM [American College of Occupational and Environmental Medicine] code of ethics. *Journal of Occupational and Environmental Medicine.* 1997 Jul; 39(7): 616–622. 12 refs. BE57524.
    *codes of ethics; confidentiality; conflict of interest; disclosure; employment; evaluation; health personnel; international aspects; *medical ethics; *occupational medicine; physician patient relationship; *physicians; professional organizations; terminology; *American College of Occupational and Environmental Medicine; International Commission on Occupational Health

Royal Australasian College of Surgeons. Code of Ethics. *Archives of Surgery.* 1996 Aug; 131(8): 900–901. BE55524.
    *codes of ethics; confidentiality; conflict of interest; continuing education; human experimentation; industry; informed consent; medical education; *medical ethics; obligations to society; patient care; physician patient relationship; *physicians; professional organizations; *surgery; war; physician impairment; Australia; *Royal Australasian College of Surgeons

Williams, John R. The new code of ethics of the Canadian Medical Association. *International Journal of Bioethics.* 1997 Mar–Jun; 8(1–2): 119–122. 2 fn. BE59098.
    *codes of ethics; comparative studies; consensus; decision making; historical aspects; *medical ethics; moral obligations; obligations to society; physician patient relationship; *physicians; professional organizations; rights; *Canadian Medical Association

New code of medical ethics issued in Italy. [News]. *International Digest of Health Legislation.* 1993; 44(2): 353–354. BE57183.

BE = bioethics accession number   fn. = footnotes   refs. = references

*codes of ethics; dentistry; health personnel; *medical ethics; *professional ethics; professional organizations; Italy; *National Federation of the Associations of Physicians and Dentists (Italy)

MEDICAL ETHICS/EDUCATION

American College of Obstetricians and Gynecologists. Committee on Ethics. Ethical issues in obstetric-gynecologic education. ACOG Committee Opinion No. 181, April 1997. *International Journal of Gynaecology and Obstetrics.* 1997 Jun; 57(3): 327–330. 10 refs. BE57604.
communication; employment; faculty; institutional ethics; interprofessional relations; *medical education; medical ethics; obstetrics and gynecology; *organizational policies; patient care; physician patient relationship; professional organizations; social dominance; students; *American College of Obstetricians and Gynecologists

Ardagh, Michael. May we practise endotracheal intubation on the newly dead? *Journal of Medical Ethics.* 1997 Oct; 23(5): 289–294. 40 refs. BE57100.
advance directives; allied health personnel; alternatives; altruism; anesthesia; attitudes; attitudes to death; autopsies; *cadavers; cardiac death; communitarianism; emergency care; emotions; family members; human body; *informed consent; international aspects; legal aspects; *medical education; moral policy; organ donation; organizational policies; policy analysis; *presumed consent; professional organizations; property rights; *public policy; religion; *resuscitation; students; technical expertise; third party consent; utilitarianism; *intubation; *mandated choice
Endotracheal intubation (ETI) is a valuable procedure which must be learnt and practised, and performing ETI on cadavers is probably the best way to do this, although lesser alternatives do exist. Performing ETI on a cadaver is viewed with a real and reasonable repugnance and if it is done without proper authorisation it might be illegal. Some form of consent is required. Presumed consent would preferably be governed by statute and should only occur if the community is well informed and therefore in a position of being able to decline. Currently neither statute nor adequate informing exists. Endotracheal intubation on the newly dead may be justifiable according to a Guttman scale if the patient has already consented to organ donation and if further research supports the relevance of the Guttman scale to this question. A "mandated choice" with prior individual consent as a matter of public policy is the best of these solutions, however until such a solution is in place we may not practise endotracheal intubation on the newly dead.

Ashcroft, Richard; Baron, Dennis; Benatar, Solomon, et al. Teaching medical ethics and law within medical education: a model for the UK core curriculum. [Consensus statement by teachers of medical ethics and law in UK medical schools]. *Journal of Medical Ethics.* 1998 Jun; 24(3): 188–192. 1 ref. This consensus statement is also available at the *British Medical Journal* website: www.bmj.com. Additional authors: Jackson, Jennifer; Jessiman, Ian; Johnson, Alan; King, Jennifer; Lutrell, Steven; Matthews, Eric; Meakin, Richard; Parker, Michael; Portsmouth, O.; Schwartz, Lisa; Shenfield, Francoise; Snashall, David; Somerville, Ann; Steiner, Timothy; Vernon, Bryan; Ward, Christopher; Zander, Luke; de Zulueta, Paquita. BE59121.
*bioethical issues; bioethics; children; confidentiality; *consensus; *curriculum; *faculty; genetics; goals; human experimentation; informed consent; interprofessional relations; law; *medical education; *medical ethics; *medical

schools; mentally disabled; physician patient relationship; reproduction; resource allocation; *standards; teaching methods; terminal care; treatment refusal; General Medical Council (Great Britain); *Great Britain

Baldini, Massimo. The doctor-patient relationship in medical textbooks and manuals of the eighteenth and nineteenth centuries. *Dolentium Hominum: Church and Health in the World.* 1996; 31(11th Yr., No. 1): 88–92. 49 fn. BE57366.
alternative therapies; *communication; *historical aspects; *literature; *medical education; *medical ethics; *medical etiquette; medical schools; medicine; patient compliance; *physician patient relationship; *physicians; professional competence; public opinion; socioeconomic factors; students; trust; *virtues; *Eighteenth Century; Europe; *Nineteenth Century

Burack, Jeffrey H. Response to "Further exploration of the relationship between medical education and moral development" by Donnie J. Self, DeWitt C. Baldwin, Jr., and Frederic D. Wolinsky: Deriving "ought" from "*p*": methodological and theoretical pitfalls in quantitative ethics. *Cambridge Quarterly of Healthcare Ethics.* 1997 Spring; 6(2): 226–232. 12 refs. BE56424.
control groups; *empirical research; *evaluation; *evaluation studies; *medical education; medical ethics; *moral development; *research design; standards; *statistics; *students; time factors
In a recent issue of *CQ*, Self, Baldwin, and Wolinsky present data aimed at confirming their earlier observation that medical students fail to experience normal moral development during their four years of education. In the context of these authors' previous work, this represents an admirable effort to apply empiric techniques to a set of vexing measurement problems in the assessment and teaching of moral reasoning. However, as empiric studies begin to address such issues, readers of the ethics literature must be prepared to critically evaluate these studies, just as clinicians must evaluate the quality of published data intended to support the practice of evidence-based medicine. I will argue that Self and colleagues' conclusions about moral stagnation in medical school do not follow from the data presented. I will use a close examination of this study to illustrate some more general problems in the literature of empiric ethics, including attempting to prove negative hypotheses, interpreting small uncontrolled studies, and measuring such complex phenomena as moral development.

Clouser, K. Danner. Humanities in the service of medicine: three models. *In:* Carson, Ronald A.; Burns, Chester R., eds. Philosophy of Medicine and Bioethics: A Twenty-Year Retrospective and Critical Appraisal. Boston, MA: Kluwer Academic; 1997: 25–39. 2 refs. 2 fn. ISBN 0-7923-3545-7. BE56524.
goals; humanism; *humanities; *interdisciplinary communication; *medical education; *medicine; models, theoretical; values

Coles, Robert. The moral education of medical students. *Academic Medicine.* 1998 Jan; 73(1): 55–57. BE56613.
curriculum; humanism; *literature; *medical education; *medical ethics; United States

Conley, Frances K. Walking Out on the Boys. New York, NY: Farrar, Straus and Giroux; 1998. 245 p. 10 fn. ISBN 0-374-28621-3. BE58696.
administrators; attitudes; employment; faculty; *females; institutional policies; internship and residency; *interprofessional relations; legal aspects; *males; medical education; *medical schools; *physicians; self regulation; sex

offenses; *social discrimination; *social dominance; *sociology of medicine; students; *surgery; universities; women's rights; *neurosurgery; *Conley, Frances; *Stanford University School of Medicine; United States

Currie, Craig; Green, John; Davies, Steve, et al. Cost effectiveness of medical ethics training. [Letter]. *Journal of Medical Ethics.* 1997 Oct; 23(5): 328. 2 refs. BE58261.
*costs and benefits; empirical research; *medical education; *medical ethics; teaching methods; Great Britain

Doyal, Len; Gillon, Raanan. Medical ethics and law as a core subject in medical education: a core curriculum offers flexibility in how it is taught -- but not that it is taught. [Editorial]. *BMJ (British Medical Journal).* 1998 May 30; 316(7145): 1623-1624. 2 refs. BE58252.
*bioethical issues; consensus; *curriculum; law; *medical education; *medical ethics; *standards; *Great Britain

Gianakos, Dean. Accepting limits. *Archives of Internal Medicine.* 1998 May 25; 158(10): 1059-1061. 7 refs. BE58802.
communication; continuing education; *decision making; *disclosure; economics; faculty; incentives; interprofessional relations; *knowledge, attitudes, practice; managed care programs; *medical education; medical ethics; medical specialties; *patient care; physician patient relationship; *physicians; primary health care; *professional competence; referral and consultation; self concept; students; *technical expertise; trust; *uncertainty; evidence-based medicine

Goldblatt, A.D. You can't always get what you want. *Update Loma Linda University Center for Christian Bioethics.* 1997 Jul; 13(2): 5-7. 6 fn. Commentary on K.V. Iserson, "Life versus death: the ethical imperative to practice and teach using the newly dead," p. 2-4. BE57990.
alternatives; autonomy; *cadavers; consent forms; donor cards; emergency care; family members; freedom; *health personnel; hospitals; *informed consent; institutional policies; legal liability; legal rights; legislation; *medical education; organ donation; *presumed consent; *professional competence; property rights; *third party consent; required response; teaching hospitals

Gorton, Gregg E.; Samuel, Steven E. A national survey of training directors about education for prevention of psychiatrist-patient sexual exploitation. *Academic Psychiatry.* 1996 Summer; 20(2): 92-98. 15 refs. BE58119.
administrators; curriculum; faculty; *internship and residency; *medical education; medical ethics; *misconduct; *physician patient relationship; *psychiatry; *sexuality; survey; teaching methods; United States

Hope, Tony. Ethics and law for medical students: the core curriculum. [Editorial]. *Journal of Medical Ethics.* 1998 Jun; 24(3): 147-148. 2 refs. BE59115.
attitudes; *bioethical issues; bioethics; consensus; *curriculum; faculty; goals; law; *medical education; *medical ethics; physicians; teaching methods; General Medical Council (Great Britain); *Great Britain

Howe, K.R. Medical students' evaluations of different levels of medical ethics teaching: implications for curricula. *Medical Education.* 1987 Jul; 21(4): 340-349. 9 refs. BE56658.
*attitudes; clinical ethics; *curriculum; *evaluation; hospitals; *medical education; *medical ethics; medical schools; models, theoretical; *students; survey; *teaching methods; Michigan; *Michigan State University College of Human Medicine; *Michigan State University College of Osteopathic Medicine

Kane, Gregory C.; Leone, Frank T.; Rowane, Joseph,

et al. Nationwide perspective on the use of a formal ethics curriculum during critical care fellowship training. [Letter]. *Academic Medicine.* 1998 Jan; 73(1): 103. 1 ref. BE56627.
administrators; advance directives; allowing to die; attitudes; *bioethical issues; bioethics; biomedical technologies; critically ill; *curriculum; human experimentation; intensive care units; *medical education; *medical ethics; patient care; survey; withholding treatment; United States

Kerns, Alice Fleury. Better to lay it out on the table rather than do it behind the curtain: hospitals need to obtain consent before using newly deceased patients to teach resuscitation procedures. [Comment]. *Journal of Contemporary Health Law and Policy.* 1997 Spring; 13(2): 581-612. 197 fn. BE56004.
advance directives; alternatives; attitudes; *cadavers; common good; criminal law; dehumanization; emergency care; *family members; hospitals; *institutional policies; internship and residency; *legal aspects; legal rights; *medical education; presumed consent; property rights; psychological stress; *public policy; *resuscitation; risks and benefits; students; *third party consent; intubation; United States

Ladd, Rosalind Ekman; Forman, Edwin N. Pediatric ethics rounds: an evaluation -- the impact of ethics rounds on clinical decision-making is worthy of further exploration. *Rhode Island Medical Journal.* 1985 Oct; 68(10): 455-458. BE57438.
attitudes; *clinical ethics; decision making; *evaluation; goals; internship and residency; *medical education; *pediatrics; physicians; survey; Rhode Island Hospital (Providence)

Leaning, Jennifer. Human rights and medical education. [Editorial]. *BMJ (British Medical Journal).* 1997 Nov 29; 315(7120): 1390-1391. 13 refs. BE56900.
cultural pluralism; disadvantaged; guidelines; *human rights; *international aspects; *medical education; *medical ethics; *physician patient relationship; United Nations; *Universal Declaration of Human Rights

Lynch, Abbyann, ed. The Good Pediatrician: An Ethics Curriculum for Use in Canadian Pediatrics Residency Programs. Teacher's Handbook. [Looseleaf format]. Toronto, ON: Department of Bioethics, Hospital for Sick Children; 1996. 348 p. Includes references. ISBN 0-9690091-4-3. BE56510.
adolescents; allowing to die; bioethics; case studies; *children; confidentiality; cultural pluralism; *curriculum; decision making; ethical theory; evaluation; goals; historical aspects; human experimentation; interdisciplinary communication; *internship and residency; legal aspects; *medical education; *medical ethics; newborns; organ donation; organ transplantation; *patient care; *pediatrics; physician patient relationship; professional competence; professional family relationship; *teaching methods; terminal care; questionnaires; Canada

McCurdy, Layton; Goode, Leslie D.; Inui, Thomas S., et al. Fulfilling the social contract between medical schools and the public. *Academic Medicine.* 1997 Dec; 72(12): 1063-1070. 7 refs. BE56629.
*accountability; administrators; attitudes; biomedical research; consensus; contracts; faculty; *goals; government financing; health; hospitals; *institutional ethics; libertarianism; medical education; *medical schools; moral obligations; *obligations to society; patient care; public opinion; sociology of medicine; standards; students; survey; utilitarianism; teaching hospitals; Association of American Medical Colleges Working Group on Fulfilling the Social Contract; *United States

---

BE = bioethics accession number   fn. = footnotes   refs. = references

Nicholas, Barbara; Gillett, Grant. Doctors' stories, patients' stories: a narrative approach to teaching medical ethics. *Journal of Medical Ethics.* 1997 Oct; 23(5): 295–299. 13 fn. BE57106.

bioethics; caring; casuistry; *continuing education; ethical theory; goals; interprofessional relations; literature; *medical education; *medical ethics; *narrative ethics; physician patient relationship; physicians; principle–based ethics; *program descriptions; *teaching methods; New Zealand; *Otago University (Dunedin)

Many senior doctors have had little in the way of formal ethics training, but express considerable interest in extending their education in this area. This paper is the report of an initiative in continuing medical education in which doctors were introduced to narrative ethics. We review the theoretical basis of narrative ethics, and the structure of and response to the two–day workshop.

O'Flynn, Norma; Spencer, John; Jones, Roger. Consent and confidentiality in teaching in general practice: survey of patients' views on presence of students. *BMJ (British Medical Journal).* 1997 Nov 1; 315(7116): 1142. 5 refs. BE56225.

*attitudes; *confidentiality; *disclosure; *family practice; informed consent; *medical education; medical records; *patient care; *patient satisfaction; *patients; physicians; *privacy; referral and consultation; sexuality; *students; survey; group practice; outpatients; Great Britain

Orr, Robert D.; Pang, Norman; Pellegrino, Edmund D., et al. Use of the Hippocratic oath: a review of twentieth century practice and a content analysis of oaths administered in medical schools in the U.S. and Canada in 1993. *Journal of Clinical Ethics.* 1997 Winter; 8(4): 377–388. 70 fn. BE57611.

abortion, induced; accountability; ancient history; *codes of ethics; comparative studies; confidentiality; euthanasia; evaluation; historical aspects; *institutional policies; medical education; *medical ethics; *medical schools; medicine; physician patient relationship; physicians; professional organizations; religion; review; sexuality; statistics; survey; *trends; *values; virtues; *Canada; Declaration of Geneva; *Hippocratic Oath; Middle Ages; Oath of Lasagna; Osteopathic Oath; Prayer of Maimonides; *Twentieth Century; *United States; World Medical Association

The purposes of this empiric study, literature review, and analysis are to determine the current prevalence of oath taking in medical schools in North America, to compare the content of the oaths in use to that of the classical Hippocratic Oath, and to document changes in the practice and content during this century. From this review and analysis, we hope to make a case for the value of the Hippocratic tradition.

Pickering, Neil. Imaginary restrictions. *Journal of Medical Ethics.* 1998 Jun; 24(3): 171–175. 7 fn. Commentary on R. Gillon, "Imagination, literature, medical ethics and medical practice," *JME*, 1997 Feb; 23(1): 3–4. BE59119.

bioethics; case studies; empathy; ethical theory; *literature; *medical education; *medical ethics; *moral development; narrative ethics; philosophy; *physician patient relationship; *teaching methods

The role of literature and imagination in medicine and medical ethics is currently under discussion. This paper argues that the role of literature is not to furnish generalisable examples for guidance. Rather, engagement with literature parallels moral engagement with other people. The work of the imagination, in this context, is not to hypothesise, but to grant life to the characters and world of literature. In doing this, one may develop one's moral life.

Price, John; Price, David; Williams, Gail, et al. Changes in medical student attitudes as they progress through a medical course. *Journal of Medical Ethics.* 1998 Apr; 24(2): 110–117. 30 refs. BE58064.

aged; *attitudes; autonomy; beneficence; *bioethical issues; comparative studies; confidentiality; duty to warn; females; informed consent; justice; law enforcement; males; *medical education; *medical ethics; minority groups; misconduct; moral development; moral obligations; obligations to society; patient compliance; patients' rights; physicians; political activity; professional autonomy; resource allocation; self induced illness; social discrimination; *students; survey; *time factors; truth disclosure; value of life; *Australia; Queensland

OBJECTIVES: To explore the way ethical principles develop during a medical education course for three groups of medical students -- in their first year, at the beginning of their penultimate (fifth) year and towards the end of their final (sixth) year. DESIGN: Survey questionnaire administered to medical students in their first, fifth and final (sixth) year. SETTING: A large medical school in Queensland, Australia. SURVEY SAMPLE: Approximately half the students in each of three years (first, fifth and sixth) provided data on a voluntary basis, a total of 385 students. RESULTS: At the point of entry, minor differences were found between medical students and first year law and psychology students. More striking were differences between male and female medical students, suggesting early socialization had a substantial impact here. CONCLUSIONS: Results indicate that substantial changes in attitude have developed by the beginning of fifth year with little change thereafter. Gender difference persisted. Some difference in ethical attitudes were found when groups of different ethnic backgrounds were compared. The impact of a move to a graduate medical course, which gives high priority to ethics within a professional development domain, can now be evaluated.

Roberts, Alan; Fincher, Ruth–Marie E. Teaching third–year medical students how to handle ethical dilemmas. *Journal of the Medical Association of Georgia.* 1997 Nov; 86(4): 327–329. 13 refs. BE58851.

bioethical issues; case studies; clinical ethics; *curriculum; decision making; *medical education; *medical ethics; misconduct; physicians; *teaching methods; whistleblowing; *Medical College of Georgia School of Medicine

St. Onge, Joye. Medical education must make room for student-specific ethical dilemmas. *Canadian Medical Association Journal.* 1997 Apr 15; 156(8): 1175–1177. 12 refs. Third prize essay in the 1996 Dr. William Logie Medical Ethics Essay Contest for Canadian undergraduate medical students. BE57356.

*curriculum; interprofessional relations; *medical education; *medical ethics; misconduct; moral development; patient care; physician patient relationship; physicians; social dominance; *students; teaching methods; values; whistleblowing; Canada

Sandberg, Warren S.; Carlos, Ruth; Sandberg, Elisabeth H., et al. The effect of educational gifts from pharmaceutical firms on medical students' recall of company names or products. *Academic Medicine.* 1997 Oct; 72(10): 916–918. 10 refs. BE56632.

*advertising; *attitudes; *drug industry; drugs; evaluation studies; *gifts; hospitals; institutional policies; internship and residency; knowledge, attitudes, practice; *medical education; medical schools; motivation; physicians; recall; *social impact; *students; survey; Chicago; University of Chicago Pritzker School of Medicine

Seedhouse, David. Against medical ethics: a response to Cassell. *Journal of Medical Ethics.* 1998 Feb; 24(1): 13–17.

BE = bioethics accession number   fn. = footnotes   refs. = references

12 refs. BE57435.
*bioethics; curriculum; ethical theory; ethicists; *ethics; health personnel; *medical education; *medical ethics; medical specialties; medicine; morality; philosophy; physicians; Great Britain

Self, Donnie J.; Olivarez, Margie. Retention of moral reasoning skills over the four years of medical education. *Teaching and Learning in Medicine.* 1996; 8(4): 195–199. 38 refs. BE57691.
comparative studies; ethical analysis; evaluation studies; *medical education; *medical ethics; *moral development; morality; *recall; *students; time factors; Texas A&M University College of Medicine

Skolnick, Andrew A. End-of-life care movement growing. *JAMA.* 1997 Sep 24; 278(12): 967–969. BE55774.
advance care planning; attitudes; *continuing education; curriculum; *medical education; palliative care; patient advocacy; physicians; professional organizations; *program descriptions; quality of health care; teaching methods; *terminal care; American Institute of Life–Threatening Diseases; American Medical Association; Education for Physicians on End–of–Life Care (EPEC) Project; Health Decisions America; Last Acts: Care and Caring at the End of Life Initiative; United States

Stone, John. The medical ethics program at Emory. [Editorial]. *Journal of the Medical Association of Georgia.* 1990 Nov; 79(11): 811–812. BE55640.
*medical education; *medical ethics; medical schools; program descriptions; *Emory University

Thompson, James N. Moral imperatives for academic medicine. *Academic Medicine.* 1997 Dec; 72(12): 1037–1042. 11 refs. BE56607.
abortion, induced; bioethical issues; biomedical research; curriculum; *economics; euthanasia; financial support; goals; health care delivery; industry; *managed care programs; *medical education; *medical ethics; medical schools; medicine; patient advocacy; physician patient relationship; physician's role; quality of health care; religion; value of life; virtues; North Carolina; United States; Wake Forest University School of Medicine

Tiberius, Richard G.; Cleave–Hogg, Doreen. A data base for curriculum design in medical ethics. *Journal of Medical Education.* 1984 Jun; 59(6): 512–513. 3 refs. BE57493.
curriculum; *knowledge, attitudes, practice; *medical education; *medical ethics; *students; survey; University of Toronto

Tysinger, James W.; Klonis, Leah K.; Sadler, John Z., et al. Teaching ethics using small–group, problem–based learning. *Journal of Medical Ethics.* 1997 Oct; 23(5): 315–318. 11 fn. BE57110.
case studies; evaluation; faculty; goals; *medical education; *medical ethics; *program descriptions; students; *teaching methods; Texas; University of Texas Southwestern Medical School (Dallas)
Ethics is the emphasis of our first–year Introduction to Clinical Medicine–1 course. Introduction to Clinical Medicine–1 uses problem–based learning to involve groups of seven to nine students and two facilitators in realistic clinical cases. The cases emphasize ethics, but also include human behaviour, basic science, clinical medicine, and prevention learning issues. Three cases use written vignettes, while the other three cases feature standardized patients. Groups meet twice for each case. In session one, students read the case introduction, obtain data from the written case or standardized patient, identify the case's ethical problems, formulate learning

issues, discuss ways to resolve the moral conflicts, and assign research responsibilities. In session two, students discuss their assigned learning issues and specify and justify clinical actions to address the case's ethical dilemmas. Following three cases, groups write an essay discussing what they learned and describing how they would approach and resolve the case's learning issues.

Williamson, Charlotte; Wilkie, Patricia. Teaching medical students in general practice: respecting patients' rights. [Editorial]. *BMJ (British Medical Journal).* 1997 Nov 1; 315(7116): 1108–1109. 11 refs. BE56894.
attitudes; communication; *confidentiality; disclosure; family practice; *informed consent; *medical education; medical ethics; medical records; *patient care; patients; *students; Great Britain; National Health Service

MENTAL HEALTH
See also under
CONFIDENTIALITY/MENTAL HEALTH

Barker, Ann. Mental health and the law. *BMJ (British Medical Journal).* 1997 Sep 6; 315(7108): 590–592. 6 refs. BE57241.
adults; coercion; confidentiality; emergency care; informed consent; involuntary commitment; law enforcement; *legal aspects; legislation; *mental health; *mentally disabled; mentally ill; minors; parental consent; patient access to records; *patient care; physicians; psychiatry; treatment refusal; England; *Great Britain; Mental Health Act 1983 (Great Britain); Wales
The law relating to medical practice in general, and mental health in particular, is complex. This article provides a summary of the laws applying in England and Wales. Certain mental disorders are the only medical conditions for which the law permits treatment without the consent of the patient, but this can be undertaken only in a hospital or registered nursing home.

Coombes, Lindsey. Mental health. *In:* Chadwick, Ruth, ed. Encyclopedia of Applied Ethics, Volume 3. San Diego, CA: Academic Press; 1998: 197–212. 11 refs. ISBN 0–12–227068–1. BE56254.
autonomy; caring; community services; confidentiality; cultural pluralism; deinstitutionalized persons; disease; goals; health; health care delivery; health promotion; informed consent; *mental health; *mentally ill; *patient care; professional patient relationship; *psychotherapy; quality of life; social control; terminology; values

Fulford, K.W.M. Mental illness, concept of. *In:* Chadwick, Ruth, ed. Encyclopedia of Applied Ethics, Volume 3. San Diego, CA: Academic Press; 1998: 213–233. 12 refs. ISBN 0–12–227068–1. BE56255.
behavior disorders; health personnel; interprofessional relations; medical ethics; medicine; *mental health; *models, theoretical; patient care; philosophy; primary health care; professional patient relationship; *psychiatric diagnosis; psychiatry; psychotherapy; terminology; values

MENTALLY DISABLED

See also BEHAVIOR CONTROL,
ELECTROCONVULSIVE THERAPY,
INVOLUNTARY COMMITMENT,
PSYCHOSURGERY
See under
INFORMED CONSENT/MENTALLY
DISABLED
PATIENT CARE/MENTALLY DISABLED
PATIENTS' RIGHTS/MENTALLY DISABLED

BE = bioethics accession number   fn. = footnotes   refs. = references

STERILIZATION/MENTALLY DISABLED
TREATMENT REFUSAL/MENTALLY
    DISABLED

MERCY KILLING *See* EUTHANASIA

MINORS
    See under
        ABORTION/MINORS
        BEHAVIORAL RESEARCH/MINORS
        CONTRACEPTION/MINORS
        HUMAN EXPERIMENTATION/MINORS
        INFORMED CONSENT/MINORS
        INVOLUNTARY COMMITMENT/MINORS
        PATIENT CARE/MINORS
        TREATMENT REFUSAL/MINORS

MISCONDUCT *See* FRAUD AND MISCONDUCT

NURSE PATIENT RELATIONSHIP *See* NURSING
    ETHICS, PROFESSIONAL PATIENT
    RELATIONSHIP

NURSING CARE *See* PATIENT CARE, TERMINAL
    CARE

NURSING ETHICS

See also BIOETHICS, MEDICAL ETHICS,
    PROFESSIONAL ETHICS

American Nurses Association. American Nurses
Association position statements on ethics and human
rights. *In: its* Compendium of American Nurses
Association Position Statements. Washington, DC:
American Nurses Publishing; 1996: 79–118. Includes
references. ISBN 1–55810–123–3. BE57452.
    active euthanasia; advance directives; allowing to die;
    artificial feeding; assisted suicide; capital punishment; codes
    of ethics; cultural pluralism; health care; *human rights;
    legislation; nurse's role; *nurses; *nursing ethics;
    *organizational policies; pain; palliative care; patient
    advocacy; *patient care; professional organizations;
    resuscitation orders; *terminal care; treatment refusal;
    withholding treatment; *American Nurses Association;
    Patient Self–Determination Act 1990; United States

American Nurses Association. Compendium of American
Nurses Association Position Statements. Washington,
DC: American Nurses Publishing; 1996. 232 p. Includes
references. Pub. No. PR26–.75M–2/96. ISBN
1–55810–123–3. BE57450.
    active euthanasia; advance directives; aged; AIDS; AIDS
    serodiagnosis; alcohol abuse; allowing to die; artificial
    feeding; assisted suicide; *bioethical issues; capital
    punishment; codes of ethics; communicable diseases;
    computers; confidentiality; counseling; cultural pluralism;
    drug abuse; drugs; employment; financial support; health
    care delivery; health personnel; HIV seropositivity; human
    rights; iatrogenic disease; mass screening; medical records;
    *nurses; nursing education; *nursing ethics; nursing research;
    occupational exposure; *organizational policies; palliative
    care; patient care; pregnant women; prenatal injuries;
    primary health care; *professional organizations;
    resuscitation orders; *standards; terminal care; voluntary
    programs; women's health services; infection control;
    needle–exchange programs; tuberculosis; *American Nurses
    Association; United States

Artnak, Kathryn E.; Dimmitt, Jane H. Choosing a
framework for ethical analysis in advanced practice
settings: the case for casuistry. *Archives of Psychiatric
Nursing.* 1996 Feb; 10(1): 16–23. 12 refs. BE55660.
    adolescents; blacks; case studies; *casuistry; *clinical ethics;
    *confidentiality; *dangerousness; decision making;
    *disadvantaged; *domestic violence; *duty to warn; ethical
    analysis; family relationship; fathers; females; law
    enforcement; mentally ill; mothers; *nurses; *nursing ethics;
    patient care; patient participation; principle–based ethics;
    privacy; *psychotherapy; quality of life; sex offenses; *social
    problems; trust; values; *violence

Borawski, Deborah B. Ethical dilemmas for nurse
administrators. *Journal of Nursing Administration.* 1995
Jul–Aug; 25(7–8): 60–62. 6 refs. BE55757.
    *administrators; advertising; attitudes; conflict of interest;
    decision making; employment; hospitals; indigents;
    knowledge, attitudes, practice; *nurses; *nursing ethics;
    patient advocacy; patient care; physicians; professional
    competence; quality of health care; resource allocation;
    standards; statistics; survey; withholding treatment; North
    Carolina

Brown, J.M. Conscience: the professional and the
personal. *Journal of Nursing Management.* 1996 May;
4(3): 171–177. 24 refs. BE55759.
    *conscience; dissent; emotions; *morality; nurses; *nursing
    ethics; professional ethics; secularism; self concept; guilt;
    integrity

Chadwick, Ruth. Is nursing ethics distinct from medical
ethics? *In:* Morscher, Edgar; Neumaier, Otto; Simons,
Peter, eds. Applied Ethics in a Troubled World. Boston,
MA: Kluwer Academic; 1998: 115–125. 23 fn. ISBN
0–7923–4965–2. BE58586.
    accountability; caring; codes of ethics; females; medical
    ethics; *nurse's role; nurses; *nursing ethics; patient
    advocacy; physician nurse relationship; political activity

Chafey, Kathleen. "Caring" is not enough: ethical
paradigms for community–based care. *N and HC
Perspectives on Community.* 1996 Jan–Feb; 17(1): 10–15.
26 refs. BE58300.
    caring; children; community services; feminist ethics; *health
    care; health promotion; historical aspects; indigents; *justice;
    minority groups; *nurse's role; nurses; *nursing ethics;
    *obligations of society; political activity; public health;
    public policy; resource allocation; social impact; social
    problems; socioeconomic factors; values; women's health;
    Nineteenth Century; Twentieth Century; *United States;
    Wald, Lillian

**Davis, Anne J.; Aroskar, Mila A.; Liaschenko, Joan,
et al.** Ethical Dilemmas and Nursing Practice. Fourth
Edition. Stamford, CT: Appleton and Lange; 1997. 275
p. Includes references. ISBN 0–8385–2283–1. BE58588.
    abortion, induced; active euthanasia; allowing to die; assisted
    suicide; behavior control; bioethical issues; caring; case
    studies; codes of ethics; conflict of interest; employment;
    health care; historical aspects; human experimentation;
    informed consent; interprofessional relations; justice; legal
    aspects; mentally ill; mentally retarded; moral development;
    moral obligations; nurse patient relationship; nurse's role;
    nurses; *nursing ethics; obligations of society; patient
    advocacy; patient care; patients' rights; public policy;
    resource allocation; rights; social control; terminal care;
    values; vulnerable populations

**Davis, Anne J.; Aroskar, Mila A.; Liaschenko, Joan,
et al.** Professional ethics and institutional constraints in
nursing practice. *In: their* Ethical Dilemmas and Nursing
Practice. Fourth Edition. Stamford, CT: Appleton and
Lange; 1997: 63–81. 54 refs. ISBN 0–8385–2283–1.

BE58593.
administrators; codes of ethics; communication; conflict of interest; dissent; employment; historical aspects; *hospitals; institutional policies; interprofessional relations; moral obligations; nurse patient relationship; nurses; *nursing ethics; paternalism; patient advocacy; physician nurse relationship; *professional autonomy; rights; *social control; social dominance

Davis, Anne J.; Aroskar, Mila A.; Liaschenko, Joan, et al. Rights, responsibilities, and health care. *In: their* Ethical Dilemmas and Nursing Practice. Fourth Edition. Stamford, CT: Appleton and Lange; 1997: 83–103. 25 fn. ISBN 0–8385–2283–1. BE58594.
case studies; economics; *health care; health facilities; justice; legal aspects; *moral obligations; *nurses; *nursing ethics; *patient advocacy; *patients' rights; resource allocation; *rights; standards; United States

Davis, Anne J.; Aroskar, Mila A.; Liaschenko, Joan, et al. Selected ethical approaches: theories and concepts. *In: their* Ethical Dilemmas and Nursing Practice. Fourth Edition. Stamford, CT: Appleton and Lange; 1997: 45–61. 28 fn. ISBN 0–8385–2283–1. BE58592.
bioethics; caring; *decision making; deontological ethics; *ethical theory; nurses; *nursing ethics; principle-based ethics; utilitarianism; virtues

Davis, Anne J.; Aroskar, Mila A.; Liaschenko, Joan, et al. Values clarification, moral development, and other considerations in understanding health care ethics. *In: their* Ethical Dilemmas and Nursing Practice. Fourth Edition. Stamford, CT: Appleton and Lange; 1997: 35–44. 66 fn. ISBN 0–8385–2283–1. BE58591.
caring; females; *moral development; nurses; *nursing ethics; self concept; *values

Fowler, Marsha. Nursing's ethics. *In:* Davis, Anne J.; Aroskar, Mila A.; Liaschenko, Joan; Drought, Theresa S. Ethical Dilemmas and Nursing Practice. Fourth Edition. Stamford, CT: Appleton and Lange; 1997: 17–34. 64 refs. ISBN 0–8385–2283–1. BE58590.
codes of ethics; curriculum; *historical aspects; literature; moral development; moral obligations; nurse patient relationship; nurses; nursing education; *nursing ethics; professional organizations; students; values; virtues; American Nurses Association; Nineteenth Century; Twentieth Century; United States

Frith, Lucy, ed. Ethics and Midwifery: Issues in Contemporary Practice. Boston, MA: Butterworth–Heinemann; 1996. 282 p. Includes references. ISBN 0–7506–3056–6. BE58631.
aborted fetuses; allowing to die; autonomy; behavioral research; *bioethical issues; childbirth; conflict of interest; congenital disorders; decision making; drugs; fetal tissue donation; human experimentation; informed consent; intensive care units; moral policy; newborns; *nurse midwives; nurse patient relationship; *nursing ethics; nursing research; pain; patient advocacy; *patient care; physician nurse relationship; *pregnant women; prematurity; prenatal diagnosis; professional autonomy; public policy; regulation; reproductive technologies; risk; risks and benefits; selection for treatment; selective abortion; sexuality; standards; analgesia; ultrasonography; *Great Britain; United Kingdom Central Council for Nursing, Midwifery and Health Visiting

Gastmans, Chris. Challenges to nursing values in a changing nursing environment. *Nursing Ethics.* 1998 May; 5(3): 236–245. 22 refs. BE58723.
administrators; biomedical technologies; *caring; codes of ethics; employment; health care delivery; health facilities; institutional ethics; nurse patient relationship; *nurse's role; *nurses; *nursing ethics; *patient care; physician nurse relationship; physician's role; professional autonomy; professional organizations; trends; values

Godfrey, Nelda S.; Kuehne, Dale S.; Wildes, Kevin Wm. In the care of a nurse. [Case study and commentaries]. *Hastings Center Report.* 1997 Sep–Oct; 27(5): 23–24. BE56125.
active euthanasia; advance directives; *allowing to die; autonomy; case studies; *conscience; *deception; *decision making; *dissent; drugs; family members; hospitals; institutional ethics; institutional policies; intensive care units; *misconduct; moral obligations; *nurses; *nursing ethics; patient advocacy; *patient care team; *prolongation of life; terminally ill; treatment refusal; withholding treatment

Hicks, Carolyn. Ethics in midwifery research. *In:* Frith, Lucy, ed. Ethics and Midwifery: Issues in Contemporary Practice. Boston, MA: Butterworth–Heinemann; 1996: 237–257. 14 refs. ISBN 0–7506–3056–6. BE58641.
behavioral research; confidentiality; deception; disclosure; ethical review; females; fetuses; *human experimentation; infants; informed consent; investigators; mothers; *nurse midwives; *nursing ethics; *nursing research; parental consent; placebos; pregnant women; prenatal diagnosis; privacy; research design; research subjects; risks and benefits; scientific misconduct; vulnerable populations; qualitative research

Hughes, Katharine Kostbade; Dvorak, Eileen McQuaid. The use of decision analysis to examine ethical decision making by critical care nurses. *Heart and Lung.* 1997 May–Jun; 26(3): 238–248. 37 refs. BE57603.
alternatives; consensus; *decision analysis; *decision making; drug abuse; evaluation studies; intensive care units; interprofessional relations; models, theoretical; *nurses; nursing education; *nursing ethics; nursing research; *whistleblowing; *professional impairment

Hurry, Stephanie. Termination of pregnancy -- a nurse's right to choose. *British Journal of Theatre Nursing.* 1997 Oct; 7(7): 18–22. 15 refs. BE58357.
*abortion, induced; accountability; *conscience; emergency care; historical aspects; legal aspects; nurse patient relationship; *nurses; *nursing ethics; patient care; standards; Great Britain

Johnstone, Megan–Jane. Bioethics: A Nursing Perspective. Second Edition. Philadelphia, PA: W.B. Saunders; 1994. 574 p. Includes references and ten appendices of codes of ethics and patients' bills of rights. ISBN 0–7295–1421–8. BE56507.
abortion, induced; active euthanasia; allowing to die; *bioethical issues; *bioethics; clinical ethics committees; codes of ethics; confidentiality; conscience; cultural pluralism; decision making; ethical analysis; ethical relativism; ethical theory; feminist ethics; fetuses; informed consent; international aspects; legal aspects; misconduct; moral complicity; moral development; *moral policy; National Socialism; nurse patient relationship; *nurse's role; nursing education; *nursing ethics; organ donation; organ transplantation; patient advocacy; patients' rights; physician nurse relationship; political activity; pregnant women; professional organizations; quality of life; religious ethics; resuscitation orders; strikes; suicide; truth disclosure; Australia; New Zealand

Kendrick, Kevin. Should nurses always tell the truth? Honesty versus deception in healthcare. *Professional Nurse (London).* 1994 Jul; 9: 674–677. 10 refs. BE55787.
adults; beneficence; case studies; *deception; deontological ethics; domestic violence; minors; moral policy; motivation; nurse patient relationship; *nurses; *nursing ethics; prognosis; terminal care; terminally ill; trust; *truth disclosure; utilitarianism; virtues; personal integrity

---

BE = bioethics accession number   fn. = footnotes   refs. = references

Kuhse, Helga. A nursing ethics of care? Why caring is not enough. *In:* Morscher, Edgar; Neumaier, Otto; Simons, Peter, eds. Applied Ethics in a Troubled World. Boston, MA: Kluwer Academic; 1998: 127–142. 31 fn. ISBN 0-7923-4965-2. BE58587.
   *caring; case studies; communication; females; nurse patient relationship; nurses; *nursing ethics; patient advocacy; principle-based ethics; terminology

Kuhse, Helga. Caring: Nurses, Women and Ethics. Malden, MA: Blackwell; 1997. 296 p. Bibliography: p. 263–285. ISBN 0-631-20211-0. BE58546.
   allowing to die; autonomy; *caring; *decision making; ethical theory; *females; *feminist ethics; *justice; males; metaphor; moral development; nurse patient relationship; *nurse's role; nurses; *nursing ethics; palliative care; patient advocacy; patient care; *physician nurse relationship; physicians; professional autonomy; public policy; resuscitation orders; social dominance; *terminal care; terminally ill; truth disclosure; voluntary euthanasia; whistleblowing; withholding treatment; Cox, Nigel

Leners, Debra; Beardslee, Nancy Q. Suffering and ethical caring: incompatible entities. *Nursing Ethics.* 1997 Sep; 4(5): 361–369. 22 refs. BE56874.
   *attitudes; *caring; decision making; economics; employment; hospitals; institutional policies; nurse patient relationship; *nurses; *nursing ethics; pain; patient advocacy; *patient care; physician nurse relationship; risk; *suffering; terminally ill; values; ethnographic studies; qualitative research; Colorado

Lipp, Allyson. An enquiry into a combined approach for nursing ethics. *Nursing Ethics.* 1998 Mar; 5(2): 122–138. 44 refs. BE58474.
   autonomy; beneficence; caring; conscience; *decision making; ethical theory; evaluation studies; family relationship; institutional policies; interprofessional relations; justice; models, theoretical; nurse patient relationship; *nurses; nursing education; *nursing ethics; nursing research; paternalism; patient advocacy; patient care team; patients; physician nurse relationship; physician patient relationship; physicians; truth disclosure; qualitative research; Great Britain

Lützén, Kim; Nordin, Conny. Structuring moral meaning in psychiatric nursing practice. *Scandinavian Journal of Caring Sciences.* 1993; 7(3): 175–180. 20 refs. BE56413.
   alcohol abuse; autonomy; beneficence; *decision making; emotions; empathy; *mentally ill; moral development; nurse patient relationship; *nurses; *nursing ethics; *patient care; *psychiatry; suicide; Sweden

McAlpine, Heather. Critical reflections about professional ethical stances: have we lost sight of the major objectives? *Journal of Nursing Education.* 1996 Mar; 35(3): 119–126. 110 refs. BE55516.
   bioethics; *caring; dissent; ethical theory; feminist ethics; moral development; nurse patient relationship; nursing education; *nursing ethics; philosophy; psychology; Gilligan, Carol; Kohlberg, Lawrence; Noddings, Nel

McDaniel, Charlotte. Organizational culture and ethics work satisfaction. *Journal of Nursing Administration.* 1995 Nov; 25(11): 15–21. 22 refs. BE55571.
   *administrators; attitudes; clinical ethics committees; decision making; *employment; *hospitals; interprofessional relations; nurse's role; *nurses; *nursing ethics; *organization and administration; patient care; professional autonomy; retrospective studies; United States

Mahlmeister, Laura. When cost-saving strategies are unacceptable. *Pediatric Nursing.* 1996 Mar-Apr; 22(2): 130–132. 5 refs. BE55570.

accountability; administrators; case studies; codes of ethics; *economics; *employment; government regulation; health care delivery; *hospitals; legal liability; *nurses; nursing ethics; organization and administration; *patient advocacy; patient care; pediatrics; professional organizations; *quality of health care; resource allocation; standards; American Nurses Association; United States

Mohr, Wanda K. Ethics, nursing, and health care in the age of "re-form". *N and HC Perspectives on Community.* 1996 Jan-Feb; 17(1): 16–21. 30 refs. BE58305.
   administrators; capitalism; conflict of interest; *economics; employment; goals; *health care delivery; *health care reform; health insurance; incentives; managed care programs; *nurse's role; *nursing ethics; *private sector; *professional autonomy; *proprietary health facilities; quality of health care; *values; withholding treatment; *proprietary organizations; United States

Nortvedt, Per. Sensitive judgement: an inquiry into the foundations of nursing ethics. *Nursing Ethics.* 1998 Sep; 5(5): 385–392. 13 refs. BE58903.
   *emotions; *empathy; *nurse patient relationship; *nurses; *nursing ethics; patients; suffering; values

Pang, Mei-che Samantha. Information disclosure: the moral experience of nurses in China. *Nursing Ethics.* 1998 Jul; 5(4): 347–361. 64 refs. BE58873.
   active euthanasia; autonomy; beneficence; cancer; codes of ethics; compassion; conscience; *decision making; diagnosis; *disclosure; *family members; historical aspects; hospitals; *informed consent; *knowledge, attitudes, practice; literature; medical ethics; moral obligations; nurse patient relationship; *nurses; *nursing ethics; nursing research; paternalism; patient advocacy; patient care; patients' rights; physician nurse relationship; professional family relationship; *prognosis; survey; *terminal care; terminally ill; *third party consent; *truth disclosure; virtues; qualitative research; *China; Hong Kong

Penticuff, Joy Hinson. Nursing perspectives in bioethics. *In:* Hoshino, Kazumasa, ed. Japanese and Western Bioethics: Studies in Moral Diversity. Boston, MA: Kluwer Academic; 1997: 49–60. 30 refs. ISBN 0-7923-4112-0. BE57082.
   biomedical technologies; *caring; goals; institutional policies; international aspects; moral obligations; narrative ethics; *nurse patient relationship; nurses; *nursing ethics; principle-based ethics; professional autonomy; professional competence; psychological stress; values; United States

Pierce, Susan Foley. A model for conceptualizing the moral dynamic in health care. *Nursing Ethics.* 1997 Nov; 4(6): 483–495. 13 refs. BE57419.
   autonomy; bioethical issues; caring; compassion; *decision making; emotions; empathy; ethical theory; females; justice; males; *medical ethics; *models, theoretical; *moral development; morality; nurse's role; *nurses; *nursing ethics; *patient care; patient care team; physician nurse relationship; physician's role; *physicians; professional patient relationship; self concept; technical expertise; terminal care; *values; virtues

Pinch, Winifred J. Is caring a moral trap? *Nursing Outlook.* 1996 Mar-Apr; 44(2): 84–88. 56 refs. BE56010.
   *caring; females; moral development; morality; nurses; nursing ethics; values; virtues

Pritchard, Jane. Ethical decision-making and the positive use of codes. *In:* Frith, Lucy, ed. Ethics and Midwifery: Issues in Contemporary Practice. Boston, MA: Butterworth-Heinemann; 1996: 189–204. 13 refs. ISBN 0-7506-3056-6. BE58640.
   autonomy; beneficence; codes of ethics; decision making; ethical theory; guidelines; *nurse midwives; nursing

education; *nursing ethics; patients; professional autonomy; professional competence; professional organizations; *standards; values; *Great Britain; *United Kingdom Central Council for Nursing, Midwifery and Health Visiting

Scandinavian Nursing Cooperative. Etiska riklinjer för omvårdnadsforskning i Norden [Ethical guidelines for nursing research]. *Vard i Norden.* 1987 Autumn; 7(3-4): 429-430. BE56633.
  *guidelines; *health services research; *human experimentation; informed consent; *nurses; *nursing ethics; *nursing research; *organizational policies; professional organizations; research ethics committees; research subjects; Scandinavia; *Scandinavian Nursing Cooperative

Seedhouse, David. What's the difference between health care ethics, medical ethics and nursing ethics? [Editorial]. *Health Care Analysis.* 1997 Dec; 5(4): 267-274. 16 refs. BE57543.
  *bioethics; caring; cultural pluralism; ethical theory; ethics; *goals; health; health care; health personnel; interdisciplinary communication; *medical ethics; medicine; nurses; *nursing ethics; philosophy; physicians; professional ethics; values

Smurl, James F. Do ethical decisions leave you wondering: "Did I do the right thing?" Ethical decision making for everyday nursing problems. *Nursing Life.* 1983 May–Jun; 3(3): 48-53. 4 refs. BE57237.
  bioethical issues; case studies; conflict of interest; *decision making; ethical analysis; moral obligations; nurse patient relationship; *nurses; *nursing ethics; patients' rights; physician nurse relationship

Stanley, Teresa. Who is the moral agent? *AORN Journal (Association of Operating Room Nurses).* 1984 Sep; 40(3): 331, 334-335. 4 refs. BE57839.
  conscience; *decision making; dissent; interdisciplinary communication; nurses; *nursing ethics; patients; physicians; whistleblowing

Stillwell, Susan B. Ethical Issues in Critical Care Nursing. [Videorecording]. St. Louis, MO: Mosby; 1995. 1 videocassette; 36 min.; sd.; color; 1/2 in.; VHS. (Mosby's critical care nursing video series). Producer: David Smeltzer. Accompanied by a 7-page instructor's resource booklet, "Ethical Issues in Critical Care Nursing," by Mary E. Lough. BE57898.
  advance directives; autonomy; beneficence; critically ill; cultural pluralism; decision making; ethical theory; intensive care units; justice; nurse patient relationship; nurse's role; *nursing ethics; patient care; professional family relationship; religion; terminally ill; truth disclosure

Tadd, Win. Nurses' ethics. *In:* Chadwick, Ruth, ed. Encyclopedia of Applied Ethics, Volume 3. San Diego, CA: Academic Press; 1998: 367-380. 5 refs. ISBN 0-12-227068-1. BE56256.
  bioethics; caring; codes of ethics; compassion; ethical theory; females; historical aspects; justice; moral development; nurse patient relationship; nurses; *nursing ethics; patient advocacy; physician nurse relationship; professional autonomy; truth disclosure; values; *virtues; courage; honesty; integrity; Aristotle; Nightingale, Florence; Nineteenth Century; Twentieth Century

Tschudin, Verena. Myths, magic and reality in nursing ethics: a personal perspective. *Nursing Ethics.* 1998 Jan; 5(1): 52-58. 3 refs. BE58715.
  compassion; interprofessional relations; justice; nurse patient relationship; nurses; *nursing ethics; virtues

Udén, Giggi; Norberg, Astrid; Norberg, Siv. The stories of physicians, registered nurses and enrolled nurses about

ethically difficult care episodes in surgical care. *Scandinavian Journal of Caring Sciences.* 1995; 9(4): 245-253. 36 refs. BE55834.
  allowing to die; *attitudes; attitudes to death; autonomy; bioethical issues; cancer; *clinical ethics; comparative studies; compassion; decision making; hospitals; interdisciplinary communication; *interprofessional relations; *medical ethics; moral development; narrative ethics; nurse patient relationship; *nurses; *nursing ethics; pain; palliative care; paternalism; patient advocacy; *patient care; *physician nurse relationship; physician patient relationship; *physicians; prognosis; psychological stress; quality of life; surgery; survey; terminal care; truth disclosure; withholding treatment; qualitative research; Sweden

White, Gladys B. Philosophical ethics and nursing -- a word of caution. *In:* Chinn, Peggy L., ed. Advances in Nursing Theory Development. Rockville, MD: Aspen Systems Corp.; 1983: 35-46. 19 fn. Paper presented at the Hastings Center, Apr 1981. ISBN 0-89443-842-5. BE57473.
  bioethics; ethical analysis; *ethical theory; metaethics; nursing education; *nursing ethics; *philosophy; values

NURSING ETHICS/CODES OF ETHICS

Canadian Nurses Association. Code of ethics for registered nurses [1997]. *Nursing Ethics.* 1998 Jan; 5(1): 65-74. 8 refs. Updated 1997. Reprinted with permission from the Canadian Nurses Association (CNA). Includes a brief history of the CNA Code. BE58716.
  accountability; administrators; autonomy; *codes of ethics; confidentiality; health; historical aspects; interprofessional relations; justice; *nurses; nursing education; *nursing ethics; patient care; professional competence; professional organizations; standards; strikes; students; values; whistleblowing; Canada; *Canadian Nurses Association

Canadian Nurses Association. Everyday Ethics: Putting the Code into Practice. [Study Guide]. Ottawa, ON: The Association; 1998. 82 p. Bibliography: p. 76-80. ISBN 1-55119-027-3. BE58981.
  audiovisual aids; case studies; *codes of ethics; communication; *decision making; ethical analysis; ethical theory; models, theoretical; nurse patient relationship; *nursing education; *nursing ethics; values; Canada; *Canadian Nurses Association

Esterhuizen, Philip. Is the professional code still the cornerstone of clinical nursing practice? *Journal of Advanced Nursing.* 1996 Jan; 23(1): 25-31. 39 refs. BE58103.
  accountability; administrators; *codes of ethics; *decision making; employment; females; international aspects; males; moral development; *nurses; nursing education; *nursing ethics; patient advocacy; physician nurse relationship; professional autonomy; social dominance; whistleblowing; Great Britain; Netherlands; United States

International Council of Nurses. International Council of Nurses Code for Nurses: Ethical Concepts Applied to Nursing. [Pamphlet]. Available from the International Council of Nurses, Geneva, Switzerland; 1989. 7 p. Adopted by the ICN Council of National Representatives in Mexico City in May 1973 and reaffirmed in 1989. Available in English, French and Spanish. BE57277.
  *codes of ethics; international aspects; *nursing ethics; professional organizations; *International Council of Nurses

Rosenkoetter, Marlene Merifield. A code of ethics for nurse educators. *Nursing Outlook.* 1983 Sep-Oct; 31(5):

---

288. 2 refs. BE57238.
administrators; *codes of ethics; faculty; *nursing education; *nursing ethics

Scanlon, Colleen; Glover, Jacqueline. A professional code of ethics: providing a moral compass for turbulent times. *Oncology Nursing Forum.* 1995 Nov–Dec; 22(10): 1515–1521. 23 refs. BE57622.
cancer; *codes of ethics; decision making; economics; ethical analysis; health care delivery; interdisciplinary communication; nurses; nursing education; *nursing ethics; professional competence; professional organizations; quality of life; *values; *American Nurses Association Code for Nurses; *Oncology Nursing Society

NURSING ETHICS/EDUCATION

Andrews, Sam; Hutchinson, Sally A. Teaching nursing ethics: a practical approach. *Journal of Nursing Education.* 1981 Jan; 20(1): 6–11. 11 refs. BE57436.
attitudes; ethical analysis; informed consent; institutionalized persons; mentally ill; nurse patient relationship; *nursing education; *nursing ethics; risks and benefits; students; *teaching methods; values

Cain, Paul. Using clients. *Nursing Ethics.* 1997 Nov; 4(6): 465–471. 1 ref. BE57415.
autonomy; confidentiality; disclosure; *informed consent; *moral obligations; nurse patient relationship; nurses; *nursing education; *nursing ethics; *nursing research; paternalism; *patients; privacy; *research subjects; *students; trust; utilitarianism; wedge argument

Canadian Nurses Association. Everyday Ethics: Putting the Code into Practice. [Study Guide]. Ottawa, ON: The Association; 1998. 82 p. Bibliography: p. 76–80. ISBN 1–55119–027–3. BE58981.
audiovisual aids; case studies; *codes of ethics; communication; *decision making; ethical analysis; ethical theory; models, theoretical; nurse patient relationship; *nursing education; *nursing ethics; values; Canada; *Canadian Nurses Association

Cassidy, Virginia R. Literary works as case studies for teaching human experimentation ethics. *Journal of Nursing Education.* 1996 Mar; 35(3): 142–144. 14 refs. BE55658.
behavioral research; case studies; *human experimentation; informed consent; investigator subject relationship; *literature; *nursing education; *nursing ethics; *teaching methods; Northern Illinois University

Dierckx de Casterlé, Bernadette; Janssen, Piet J.; Grypdonck, Mieke. The relationship between education and ethical behavior of nursing students. *Western Journal of Nursing Research.* 1996 Jun; 18(3): 330–350. 29 refs. BE56863.
attitudes; curriculum; decision making; evaluation studies; *moral development; nurses; *nursing education; *nursing ethics; *students; time factors; Belgium

Mayo, Kelly. Social responsibility in nursing education. *Journal of Holistic Nursing.* 1996 Mar; 14(1): 24–43. 21 refs. BE56006.
attitudes; caring; *community services; curriculum; *disadvantaged; health care reform; *health promotion; minority groups; moral development; nurse patient relationship; *nursing education; nursing ethics; nursing research; *obligations to society; political activity; program descriptions; public health; schools; social problems; stigmatization; *students; *teaching methods; values; *homeless persons; qualitative research; Southeastern United States

Pang, Mei–che Samantha; Wong, Kwok–shing Thomas. Cultivating a moral sense of nursing through model emulation. *Nursing Ethics.* 1998 Sep; 5(5): 424–440. 73 refs. BE58905.
*caring; evaluation studies; faculty; *moral development; nurses; *nursing education; *nursing ethics; *students; *teaching methods; Confucian ethics; China; *Hong Kong

Plackowski, Linda C. Ethics in the Work Environment: Applied Bioethics in the Hospital for Delta's Nursing Students. Springfield, VA: ERIC Document Reproduction Service; 1993 Jul. 15 p. (ERIC reports; ED 362 249). Available from the ERIC Document Reproduction Service operated by DYNCORP I&ET, 7420 Fullerton Rd., Suite 110, Springfield, VA 22153–2852. Telephone: (800) 443–ERIC or (703) 440–1400; FAX: (703) 440–1408; Internet: edrs@inet.ed.gov. BE58134.
bioethics; case studies; communication; faculty; hospitals; *nursing education; *nursing ethics; nursing research; pediatrics; psychiatry; students; *teaching methods; *Delta College (University Center, MI)

Rich, Ann; Parker, David L. Reflection and critical incident analysis: ethical and moral implications of their use within nursing and midwifery education. *Journal of Advanced Nursing.* 1995 Dec; 22(6): 1050–1057. 52 refs. BE55772.
empirical research; interprofessional relations; malpractice; nurse midwives; nurses; *nursing education; *nursing ethics; patient advocacy; patient care; professional competence; psychological stress; students; *teaching methods; whistleblowing

Rosenkoetter, Marlene Merifield. A code of ethics for nurse educators. *Nursing Outlook.* 1983 Sep–Oct; 31(5): 288. 2 refs. BE57238.
administrators; *codes of ethics; faculty; *nursing education; *nursing ethics

Shotton, Leila. The ethics of teaching nursing ethics. *Health Care Analysis.* 1997 Sep; 5(3): 259–263. 16 fn. BE55830.
clinical ethics; curriculum; ethical theory; ethicists; ethics; faculty; interdisciplinary communication; literature; nurses; *nursing education; *nursing ethics; physician nurse relationship; *teaching methods

Simonson, Carol L.S. Teaching caring to nursing students. *Journal of Nursing Education.* 1996 Mar; 35(3): 100–104. 25 refs. BE55529.
*caring; cultural pluralism; faculty; interprofessional relations; minority groups; nurse patient relationship; *nursing education; *nursing ethics; nursing research; students; survey; teaching methods; values; qualitative research; University of New Mexico, Gallup

Sivberg, Bengt. Self-perception and value system as possible predictors of stress. *Nursing Ethics.* 1998 Mar; 5(2): 103–121. 33 refs. BE58477.
comparative studies; emotions; evaluation; interprofessional relations; *moral development; nurses; *nursing education; *nursing ethics; nursing research; self concept; social interaction; *students; universities; values; personality; *Sweden

Wainwright, Paul; Cain, Paul. Using clients: a response to Paul Cain. [Commentary and response]. *Nursing Ethics.* 1998 Jul; 5(4): 363–369. 3 refs. BE58881.
autonomy; case studies; *confidentiality; *disclosure; hospitals; *informed consent; *moral obligations; nurse patient relationship; *nursing education; *nursing ethics; nursing research; paternalism; *patient care; *patients;

BE = bioethics accession number   fn. = footnotes   refs. = references

privacy; research subjects; *students; teaching methods

OCCUPATIONAL HEALTH

See also PUBLIC HEALTH

Brandt-Rauf, Paul W.; Brandt-Rauf, Sherry I. Biomarkers -- scientific advances and societal implications. *In:* Rothstein, Mark A., ed. Genetic Secrets: Protecting Privacy and Confidentiality in the Genetic Era. New Haven, CT: Yale University Press; 1997: 184-196. 30 fn. ISBN 0-300-07251-1. BE58682.
> biomedical research; compensation; confidentiality; ecology; employment; *genetic predisposition; *genetic research; *genetic screening; *health hazards; *occupational exposure; toxicity; *genetic markers

Koh, D.; Jeyaratnam, J. Biomarkers, screening and ethics. *Occupational Medicine.* 1998 Jan; 48(1): 27-30. 10 refs. BE59077.
> *employment; *genetic predisposition; *genetic screening; guidelines; *health hazards; informed consent; medical ethics; *occupational exposure; *occupational medicine; preventive medicine; social discrimination

Murray, Thomas H. Genetic screening in the workplace: ethical issues. *Journal of Occupational Medicine.* 1983 Jun; 25(6): 451-454. BE57631.
> *employment; genetic predisposition; genetic research; *genetic screening; goals; health hazards; informed consent; *occupational exposure; social discrimination

Wright, D.S. Workplace urine screening for drug abuse. [Letter]. *Journal of Medical Ethics.* 1997 Jun; 23(3): 191. 5 refs. BE56897.
> administrators; body parts and fluids; *drug abuse; *employment; guidelines; industry; *legal aspects; *mandatory programs; *mass screening; *occupational medicine; organizational policies; patient access to records; *physician's role; physicians; professional organizations; technical expertise; Faculty of Occupational Medicine (Great Britain); *Great Britain

Research without consent in South Africa. [News; title supplied]. *BMJ (British Medical Journal).* 1997 Jun 28; 314(7098): 1850. BE56128.
> *blacks; *human experimentation; *industry; informed consent; *occupational exposure; *occupational medicine; *scientific misconduct; *South Africa

OPERANT CONDITIONING *See* BEHAVIOR CONTROL

ORGAN AND TISSUE DONATION

See also BLOOD DONATION, ORGAN AND TISSUE TRANSPLANTATION

Abbott, Alison. German law could boost prospects for organ transplants. [News]. *Nature.* 1997 Jul 3; 388(6637): 4. BE56072.
> body parts and fluids; *brain death; cadavers; *determination of death; *legal aspects; *organ donation; organ donors; remuneration; standards; Europe; Eurotransplant; *Germany

Akabayashi, Akira. Finally done -- Japan's decision on organ transplantation. [News]. *Hastings Center Report.* 1997 Sep-Oct; 27(5): 47. BE56123.
> brain death; cadavers; determination of death; donor cards; family members; informed consent; legal aspects; *legislation; *organ donation; organ transplantation; third

party consent; *Japan

Al, Joop. Comparative observations on some current medico-legal issues in Dutch law. *In:* Jewish Law Annual. Volume Twelve. Amsterdam, Netherlands: Harwood Academic Publishers; 1997: 167-215. 127 fn. ISBN 90-5702-551-5. BE58341.
> *active euthanasia; *allowing to die; assisted suicide; body parts and fluids; brain death; cadavers; cardiac death; competence; congenital disorders; criminal law; decision making; depressive disorder; *determination of death; donor cards; family members; futility; guidelines; involuntary euthanasia; *Jewish ethics; *legal aspects; newborns; *organ donation; *organ donors; organ transplantation; persistent vegetative state; physicians; professional organizations; *public policy; quality of life; referral and consultation; resource allocation; self regulation; suffering; voluntary euthanasia; withholding treatment; Austria; Belgium; Denmark; France; Germany; *Netherlands; Norway; Sweden

Alexander, J. Wesley. High-risk donors: diabetics, the elderly, and others. *Transplantation Proceedings.* 1992 Oct; 24(5): 2221-2222. 8 refs. BE56842.
> adults; *age factors; cadavers; cardiac death; diabetes; hypertension; *morbidity; *organ donation; *organ donors; organ transplantation; *risks and benefits; scarcity; treatment outcome; United States

Allmers, Henning; Kenwright, Simon. Ethics of cloning. [Letters]. *Lancet.* 1997 May 10; 349(9062): 1401. 1 ref. BE56851.
> bone marrow; cadavers; *cloning; cryopreservation; decision making; *directed donation; leukemia; motivation; *organ donation; parents; regulation; *reproduction; siblings; time factors; *tissue donation; transplant recipients; Ayala, Anissa; Ayala, Marissa; Great Britain; United States

Andrews, Lori B. The body as property: some philosophical reflections -- a response to J.F. Childress. *Transplantation Proceedings.* 1992 Oct; 24(5): 2149-2151. 8 refs. Commentary on J.F. Childress, p. 2143-2148. BE56823.
> advance directives; altruism; autonomy; *body parts and fluids; cadavers; coercion; commodification; gifts; informed consent; *organ donation; *organ donors; *property rights; *remuneration; risk; selection for treatment; social impact; transplant recipients; wedge argument

Aswad, Saleh; Souqiyyeh, M.Z.; Huraib, S., et al. Public attitudes toward organ donation in Saudi Arabia. *Transplantation Proceedings.* 1992 Oct; 24(5): 2056-2058. 7 refs. Presented at the First International Congress on Transplantation in Developing Countries, Singapore, 29 Apr-3 May 1992. BE56800.
> brain death; cadavers; directed donation; donor cards; family members; information dissemination; Islamic ethics; *kidneys; *knowledge, attitudes, practice; mass media; *organ donation; organ donors; *public opinion; public policy; remuneration; survey; *National Kidney Foundation (Saudi Arabia); *Saudi Arabia

Benjamin, Martin. Supply and demand for transplantable organs: the ethical perspective. *Transplantation Proceedings.* 1992 Oct; 24(5): 2139. BE56820.
> bioethical issues; interdisciplinary communication; moral policy; *organ donation; public policy

Bennett, Belinda. Gamete donation, reproductive technology and the law. *In:* Petersen, Kerry, ed. Intersections: Women on Law, Medicine and Technology. Brookfield, VT: Ashgate; 1997: 127-144. 54 refs. 9 fn. ISBN 1-85521-882-8. BE57489.
> artificial insemination; autonomy; confidentiality; disclosure;

BE = bioethics accession number   fn. = footnotes   refs. = references

family relationship; fathers; homosexuals; in vitro fertilization; international aspects; *legal aspects; married persons; mothers; *ovum donors; parent child relationship; reproduction; *reproductive technologies; rights; selection for treatment; *semen donors; single persons; surrogate mothers; *Australia; Great Britain

Bick, Ezra. Ovum donations: a rabbinic conceptual model of maternity. *In:* Feldman, Emanuel; Wolowelsky, Joel B., eds. Jewish Law and the New Reproductive Technologies. Hoboken, NJ: Ktav; 1997: 83–105. 19 fn. Commentary on J. David Bleich, p. 46–82; response by Bleich, p. 106–114. ISBN 0–88125–586–6. BE57457.
> *Jewish ethics; *mothers; *ovum donors; *parent child relationship; reproductive technologies; Orthodox Judaism

Bleich, J. David. In vitro fertilization: questions of maternal identity and conversion. *In:* Feldman, Emanuel; Wolowelsky, Joel B., eds. Jewish Law and the New Reproductive Technologies. Hoboken, NJ: Ktav; 1997: 46–82. 46 fn. ISBN 0–88125–586–6. BE57456.
> embryo transfer; *in vitro fertilization; *Jewish ethics; Jews; *mothers; *ovum donors; *parent child relationship; reproductive technologies; surrogate mothers; theology; Orthodox Judaism

Bleich, J. David. May tissue donations be compelled? *In: his* Contemporary Halakhic Problems. Volume IV. New York, NY: Ktav; 1995: 273–315. 111 fn. ISBN 0–88125–474–6. BE57748.
> *adults; blood donation; bone marrow; *coercion; compensation; competence; decision making; informed consent; injuries; *Jewish ethics; kidneys; legal aspects; legal guardians; *minors; moral obligations; organ donation; parental consent; risk; risks and benefits; siblings; standards; *theology; therapeutic abortion; third party consent; *tissue donation; value of life; Israel; Orthodox Judaism; United States

Blumstein, James F. The case for commerce in organ transplantation. *Transplantation Proceedings.* 1992 Oct; 24(5): 2190–2197. 27 refs. BE56834.
> advance directives; altruism; *autonomy; body parts and fluids; cadavers; commodification; common good; communitarianism; *contracts; decision making; directed donation; donor cards; *economics; family members; health care delivery; *incentives; *industry; *kidneys; libertarianism; *moral policy; *organ donation; *organ donors; policy analysis; property rights; *public policy; *remuneration; resource allocation; scarcity; third party consent; transplant recipients; utilitarianism; *values; Task Force on Organ Transplantation; Uniform Anatomical Gift Act; United Network for Organ Sharing; United States

Brahams, Diana. My kidney as property. [Commentary]. *Lancet.* 1998 Jul 18; 352(9123): 166. 7 refs. BE58862.
> biomedical research; *body parts and fluids; *cadavers; informed consent; international aspects; *kidneys; legal aspects; *organ donation; *property rights; remuneration; research subjects; Great Britain

Briggs, J.D.; Crombie, A.; Fabre, J., et al. Organ donation in the UK: a survey by a British Transplantation Society working party. *Nephrology, Dialysis, Transplantation.* 1997 Nov; 12(11): 2251–2257. 11 refs. BE58203.
> body parts and fluids; brain pathology; cadavers; cardiac death; determination of death; financial support; health personnel; hospitals; institutional policies; intensive care units; mortality; *organ donation; organ donors; prognosis; resuscitation; *scarcity; statistics; surgery; survey; ventilators; neurosurgery; *Great Britain

Burd, Larry; Gregory, Jennifer M.; Kerbeshian, Jacob.

The brain-mind quiddity: ethical issues in the use of human brain tissue for therapeutic and scientific purposes. *Journal of Medical Ethics.* 1998 Apr; 24(2): 118–122. 13 refs. BE58051.
> animal experimentation; *biomedical research; *brain; brain death; computers; electrical stimulation of the brain; *emotions; ethical review; human body; human experimentation; informed consent; laboratories; models, theoretical; *organ donation; *organ transplantation; *personhood; regulation; *tissue donation; *tissue transplantation; cell lines; personal identity

The use of human brain tissue in neuroscience research is increasing. Recent developments include transplanting neural tissue, growing or maintaining neural tissue in laboratories and using surgically removed tissue for experimentation. Also, it is likely that in the future there will be attempts at partial or complete brain transplants. A discussion of the ethical issues of using human brain tissue for research and brain transplantation has been organized around nine broadly defined topic areas. Criteria for human brain tissue transplantation and laboratory use of brain tissue are proposed.

Burdick, James F.; Turcotte, Jeremiah G.; Veatch, Robert M. Principles of organ and tissue allocation and donation by living donors. [Foreword]. *Transplantation Proceedings.* 1992 Oct; 24(5): 2226. Foreword to the Report on Organ Allocation (p. 2227–2235) and Living Donors (p. 2236–2237) by the 1991 Ethics Committee of the United Network for Organ Sharing, Richmond, VA. BE56844.
> committee membership; *ethics committees; *organ donation; *organ transplantation; organizational policies; *United Network for Organ Sharing; *United States

Burgio, Giuseppe Roberto; Nespoli, Luigi; Porta, Fulvio, et al. Programmed bone-marrow donor for a leukaemic sibling, 10 years on. [Letter]. *Lancet.* 1997 May 17; 349(9063): 1482. 5 refs. BE56857.
> blood donation; *bone marrow; *directed donation; family relationship; health; leukemia; motivation; parents; prenatal diagnosis; *reproduction; selective abortion; *siblings; stem cells; time factors; *tissue donation; transplant recipients; *treatment outcome; cord blood; Italy

Burrows, Beth. Second thoughts about U.S. Patent #4,438,032. *Bulletin of Medical Ethics.* 1997 Jan; No. 124: 11–14. 3 refs. BE55740.
> *biomedical research; *body parts and fluids; conflict of interest; deception; disclosure; drug industry; informed consent; *investigators; *legal aspects; *patents; *patients; *property rights; remuneration; *tissue donation; universities; *cell lines; California; Golde, David; *Moore v. Regents of the University of California; United States

Calne, Roy. Ethics in organ donation and transplantation: the position of the Transplantation Society (1996). *In:* Chapman, Jeremy R.; Deierhoi, Mark; Wight, Celia, eds. Organ and Tissue Donation for Transplantation. New York, NY: Oxford University Press; 1997: 62–66. 5 refs. ISBN 0–340–61394–7. BE58230.
> animal organs; brain death; cadavers; capital punishment; data banks; determination of death; family members; government regulation; *guidelines; human experimentation; informed consent; *international aspects; kidneys; livers; *organ donation; *organ donors; organ transplantation; *organizational policies; physician's role; prisoners; professional organizations; remuneration; tissue donation; transplant recipients; lungs; pancreases; unrelated donors; *Transplantation Society

Cantarovich, F. Legal aspects of transplantation in Argentina: a model to be considered for developing

countries. *Transplantation Proceedings.* 1992 Oct; 24(5): 2123–2124. 4 refs. Presented at the First International Congress on Transplantation in Developing Countries, Singapore, 29 Apr–3 May 1992. BE56819.
　　body parts and fluids; brain death; cadavers; developing countries; family members; government financing; informed consent; *legal aspects; *organ donation; organ donors; *organ transplantation; *public policy; remuneration; selection for treatment; third party consent; unrelated donors; *Argentina

Cantarovich, Felix. Current risks of organ commerce. *Transplantation Proceedings.* 1992 Oct; 24(5): 2091. 8 refs. Presented at the First International Congress on Transplantation in Developing Countries, Singapore, 29 Apr–3 May 1992. BE56804.
　　justice; motivation; *organ donation; *organ donors; organ transplantation; public policy; *remuneration; transplant recipients; *unrelated donors

Capron, Alexander M. More blessed to give than to receive? *Transplantation Proceedings.* 1992 Oct; 24(5): 2185–2187. 5 refs. Commentary on J. Muyskens, p. 2181–2184. BE56833.
　　*altruism; cadavers; coercion; commodification; *organ donation; *organ transplantation; *public policy; refusal to treat; resource allocation; *selection for treatment; social worth; *transplant recipients; refusal to donate; United States

Chadwick, Ruth; Schüklenk, Udo. Organ transplants and donors. *In:* Chadwick, Ruth, ed. Encyclopedia of Applied Ethics, Volume 3. San Diego, CA: Academic Press; 1998: 393–398. 12 refs. ISBN 0-12-227068-1. BE56257.
　　animal organs; cadavers; coercion; determination of death; *organ donation; organ donors; *organ transplantation; personhood; presumed consent; religion; remuneration; self concept; transplant recipients

Chelala, César. China's human–organ trade highlighted by US arrest of "salesman". [News]. *Lancet.* 1998 Mar 7; 351(9104): 735. BE58853.
　　*body parts and fluids; *cadavers; capital punishment; human rights; international aspects; kidneys; misconduct; *organ donation; *prisoners; *remuneration; *China; United States

Chelala, César. German dialysis firm quits Chinese interest. [News]. *Lancet.* 1998 Mar 14; 351(9105): 812. BE58443.
　　aliens; *cadavers; capital punishment; health facilities; industry; *international aspects; kidneys; *misconduct; moral complicity; *organ donation; organ transplantation; *prisoners; *renal dialysis; *China; *Fresenius Medical Care AG; Germany

Chelala, César. Prospect of discussions on prisoners' organs for sale in China. [News]. *Lancet.* 1997 Nov 1; 350(9087): 1307. BE57268.
　　body parts and fluids; cadavers; *capital punishment; disclosure; family members; human rights; informed consent; misconduct; *organ donation; *prisoners; public policy; *remuneration; Amnesty International; *China; Human Rights Watch/Asia; Singapore; Taiwan; United Nations

Childress, James F. The body as property: some philosophical reflections. *Transplantation Proceedings.* 1992 Oct; 24(5): 2143–2148. 23 refs. Commented on by L.B. Andrews, p. 2149–2151. BE56822.
　　*altruism; attitudes; autonomy; *body parts and fluids; *cadavers; coercion; commodification; compensation; economics; family members; *gifts; *human body; incentives; indigents; informed consent; libertarianism; moral

obligations; *moral policy; obligations to society; *organ donation; *organ donors; policy analysis; presumed consent; *property rights; *public policy; *remuneration; scarcity; selection for treatment; third party consent; transplant recipients; utilitarianism; National Organ Transplant Act 1984; Uniform Anatomical Gift Act; United States

Coghlan, Andy. Organs for research are on the cards. [News]. *New Scientist.* 1997 Apr 5; 154(2076): 5. BE56220.
　　*biomedical research; cadavers; *donor cards; drug industry; *organ donation; presumed consent; *public policy; *tissue donation; Department of Health (Great Britain); *Great Britain

Cohen, Carl. The case for presumed consent to transplant human organs after death. *Transplantation Proceedings.* 1992 Oct; 24(5): 2168–2172. 16 refs. BE56828.
　　attitudes; *autonomy; body parts and fluids; *cadavers; dissent; emotions; family members; informed consent; *organ donation; *presumed consent; *public policy; registries; religion; scarcity; third party consent; utilitarianism; refusal to donate; *United States

Cohen, Lloyd R. A futures market in cadaveric organs: would it work? *Transplantation Proceedings.* 1993 Feb; 25(1): 60–61. 1 ref. BE56612.
　　altruism; *body parts and fluids; *cadavers; contracts; donor cards; *economics; *incentives; motivation; *organ donation; *remuneration

Cooper, D.K.C. Xenotransplantation: benefits, risks and regulation. *Annals of the Royal College of Surgeons of England.* 1996 Mar; 78(2): 92–96. BE55760.
　　advisory committees; AIDS; anencephaly; animal experimentation; *animal organs; body parts and fluids; bone marrow; communicable diseases; diabetes; economics; government regulation; health hazards; human experimentation; informed consent; intelligence; newborns; *organ donation; *organ transplantation; patient advocacy; peer review; persistent vegetative state; primates; public health; public opinion; *public policy; quality of life; *regulation; research ethics committees; resource allocation; risk; *risks and benefits; scarcity; speciesism; technical expertise; therapeutic research; *tissue donation; *tissue transplantation; transgenic animals; swine; Institute of Medicine; United States

Craft, Ian. Should egg donors be paid? An "inconvenience allowance" would solve the egg shortage. *BMJ (British Medical Journal).* 1997 May 10; 314(7091): 1400–1401. 5 refs. BE55664.
　　government regulation; legal aspects; mass media; *ovum donors; *public policy; *remuneration; scarcity; semen donors; surrogate mothers; *Great Britain; Human Fertilisation and Embryology Act 1990; Human Fertilisation and Embryology Authority

Cranford, Ronald E. Anencephalic infants as organ donors. *Transplantation Proceedings.* 1992 Oct; 24(5): 2218–2220. 8 refs. BE56841.
　　*anencephaly; brain death; brain pathology; guidelines; hearts; institutional policies; international aspects; kidneys; killing; legal aspects; livers; moral policy; *newborns; *organ donation; organ transplantation; persistent vegetative state; professional organizations; public policy; therapeutic research; treatment outcome; Canada; Canadian Paediatric Society; Medical Task Force on Anencephaly; United States

Curriden, Mark. Inmate's last wish is to donate kidney. [News]. *ABA Journal: The Lawyer's Magazine.* 1996 Jun; 82: 26. BE57625.
　　autonomy; *capital punishment; kidneys; *legal aspects; *organ donation; *prisoners; *Georgia; *Lonchar, Larry

---

BE = bioethics accession number　　　　fn. = footnotes　　　　refs. = references

Daar, Abdallah S. Nonrelated donors and commercialism: a historical perspective. *Transplantation Proceedings.* 1992 Oct; 24(5): 2087-2090. 31 refs. Presented at the First International Congress on Transplantation in Developing Countries, Singapore, 29 Apr-3 May 1992. BE56803.
> altruism; attitudes; cadavers; compensation; gifts; historical aspects; incentives; international aspects; justice; *kidneys; medical fees; motivation; *organ donation; *organ donors; organ transplantation; organizational policies; physicians; professional organizations; *remuneration; standards; transplant recipients; treatment outcome; *unrelated donors; India; National Kidney Foundation; *Transplantation Society; United States; World Health Organization

Daar, Abdallah S. Paid organ donation: towards an understanding of the issues. *In:* Chapman, Jeremy R.; Deierhoi, Mark; Wight, Celia, eds. Organ and Tissue Donation for Transplantation. New York, NY: Oxford University Press; 1997: 46-61. 49 refs. ISBN 0-340-61394-7. BE58229.
> altruism; autonomy; body parts and fluids; cadavers; *developing countries; family members; gifts; historical aspects; human body; incentives; indigents; informed consent; *international aspects; *kidneys; legal aspects; married persons; morality; motivation; *organ donation; *organ donors; organizational policies; professional organizations; property rights; *public policy; *remuneration; *risks and benefits; scarcity; socioeconomic factors; transplant recipients; utilitarianism; *unrelated donors; Transplantation Society; Twentieth Century; World Health Organization

Daar, Abdallah S. Rewarded gifting. *Transplantation Proceedings.* 1992 Oct; 24(5): 2207-2211. 42 refs. BE56838.
> altruism; attitudes; body parts and fluids; cadavers; coercion; compensation; directed donation; family members; *gifts; *incentives; international aspects; *kidneys; *organ donation; *organ donors; organizational policies; physicians; professional organizations; regulation; *remuneration; scarcity; standards; wedge argument; unrelated donors; Council of Europe; India; Transplantation Society; United States; World Health Organization

de Burgh, Jane. Saving our bacon: the new animal farm [review of *Pig in the Middle*: A UK national touring play, written by Judy Upton, directed by Nigel Town]. *Lancet.* 1998 Mar 28; 351(9107): 993. BE58568.
> *animal organs; animal rights; education; *information dissemination; kidneys; mass media; *organ donation; *organ transplantation; schools; transgenic animals; universities; swine; *Great Britain; *Pig in the Middle (Upton, J.)

DePalma, Judith A.; Townsend, Ricard. Ethical issues in organ donation and transplantation: are we helping a few at the expense of many? *Critical Care Nursing Quarterly.* 1996 May; 19(1): 1-9. 15 refs. BE55715.
> altruism; attitudes; autonomy; beneficence; body parts and fluids; cadavers; case studies; coercion; decision making; donor cards; family members; government regulation; health care reform; health personnel; HIV seropositivity; incentives; informed consent; justice; *organ donation; *organ transplantation; patient participation; physicians; presumed consent; public opinion; *public policy; remuneration; required request; resource allocation; risk; risks and benefits; scarcity; selection for treatment; standards; state government; third party consent; transplant recipients; United Network for Organ Sharing; United States

de Witte, Joke I.; ten Have, Henk. Ownership of genetic material and information. *Social Science and Medicine.* 1997 Jul; 45(1): 51-60. 32 refs. BE58152.
> *autonomy; body parts and fluids; common good; DNA sequences; *donors; family members; genes; genetic counseling; *genetic information; *genetic materials; genetic screening; genome mapping; gifts; *human body; organ donation; patents; privacy; *property rights; remuneration; tissue donation; Bentham, Jeremy; Human Genome Project; Kant, Immanuel; Locke, John; Nozick, Robert

As a result of the International Human Genome Project genetic information is rapidly multiplying. To avoid some of the problems regarding the availability and use of genetic information, it is sometimes suggested to apply the concept of ownership. This article focuses on the clarification of the status of genetic material and genetic information, obtained as a result of screening and counseling of individual patients. First, some philosophical theories of ownership are examined for a justification of the use of the concept of ownership with regard to the human body. Next, arguments with regard to ownership of the human body are examined. The results of this analysis are applied to genetic material and genetic information.

Dickens, Bernard M. Legal aspects of transplantation -- judicial issues. *Transplantation Proceedings.* 1992 Oct; 24(5): 2118-2119. Presented at the First International Congress on Transplantation in Developing Countries, Singapore, 29 Apr-3 May 1992. BE56817.
> body parts and fluids; cadavers; contracts; decision making; directed donation; donor cards; family members; germ cells; gifts; international aspects; *judicial action; *legal aspects; legislation; minors; *organ donation; organ donors; property rights; remuneration; *tissue donation; Moore v. Regents of the University of California

Dickens, Bernard M.; Fluss, Sev S.; King, Ariel R. Legislation on organ and tissue donation. *In:* Chapman, Jeremy R.; Deierhoi, Mark; Wight, Celia, eds. Organ and Tissue Donation for Transplantation. New York, NY: Oxford University Press; 1997: 95-119. 11 refs. ISBN 0-340-61394-7. BE58231.
> aborted fetuses; adults; advance directives; anencephaly; autonomy; body parts and fluids; cadavers; competence; confidentiality; determination of death; family members; fetal tissue donation; *government regulation; *guidelines; informed consent; *international aspects; justice; *legal aspects; *legislation; minors; newborns; *organ donation; organ donors; organ transplantation; *organizational policies; presumed consent; professional organizations; remuneration; required request; selection for treatment; third party consent; *tissue donation; tissue transplantation; transplant recipients; refusal to donate; unrelated donors; Africa; Asia; Australia; Council of Europe; Europe; *France; Latin America; Middle East; *Portugal; *Russia; Transplantation Society; United States; *World Health Organization

Dorff, Elliot N. Jewish law and lore: the case of organ transplantation. *In:* Jewish Law Annual. Volume Twelve. Amsterdam, Netherlands: Harwood Academic Publishers; 1997: 65-114. 86 fn. ISBN 90-5702-551-5. BE58343.
> abortion, induced; advance directives; attitudes to death; beginning of life; brain death; cadavers; cardiac death; Christian ethics; communitarianism; compassion; *determination of death; donor cards; family members; fetal development; *human body; *Jewish ethics; justice; moral obligations; *organ donation; *organ donors; organ transplantation; philosophy; religion; risks and benefits; secularism; terminally ill; theology; third party consent; transplant recipients; *value of life; *values; United States

Dorozynski, Alexander. France creates opt out register for organ donation. [News]. *BMJ (British Medical Journal).* 1998 Jul 25; 317(7153): 234. BE58743.
> cadavers; computers; *data banks; family members; *organ donation; *presumed consent; *public policy; *registries; third party consent; *refusal to donate; *France

---

BE = bioethics accession number   fn. = footnotes   refs. = references

Dossetor, John B. Rewarded gifting: is it ever ethically acceptable? *Transplantation Proceedings.* 1992 Oct; 24(5): 2092–2094. 2 refs. Presented at the First International Congress on Transplantation in Developing Countries, Singapore, 29 Apr–3 May 1992. BE56805.
  *altruism; *developing countries; gifts; international aspects; *kidneys; *moral policy; *organ donation; *organ donors; paternalism; physicians; regulation; *remuneration; secularism; transplant recipients; unrelated donors; *Western World

Eaton, Stephanie. The subtle politics of organ donation: a proposal. *Journal of Medical Ethics.* 1998 Jun; 24(3): 166–170. 13 fn. BE59113.
  *cadavers; decision making; *family members; moral obligations; motivation; obligations to society; *organ donation; *organ donors; *organ transplantation; *presumed consent; *resource allocation; *selection for treatment; *third party consent; *transplant recipients; treatment outcome; withholding treatment; *refusal to donate; *Great Britain; Jarvis, Rupert
  Organs available for transplantation are scarce and valuable medical resources and decisions about who is to receive them should not be made more difficult by complicated calculations of desert. Consideration of likely clinical outcome must always take priority when allocating such a precious resource otherwise there is a danger of wasting that resource. However, desert may be a relevant concern in decision–making where the clinical risk is identical between two or more potential recipients of organs. Unlikely as this scenario is, such a decision procedure makes clear the interdependence of organ recipient and organ donor and hints at potential disadvantages for those who are willing to accept but unwilling to donate organs (free–riders). A combined opting–out and preference system weakens many of the objections to opting–out systems and may make the decision to donate organs on behalf of their deceased relatives easier for families.

Eisendrath, Charles R. Used body parts: buy, sell or swap? *Transplantation Proceedings.* 1992 Oct; 24(5): 2212–2214. 6 fn. BE56839.
  body parts and fluids; cadavers; data banks; donor cards; *economics; family members; *incentives; industry; *organ donation; organ donors; public participation; *public policy; registries; regulation; scarcity; transplant recipients; *values; United States

Elli, M.; Valeri, M.; Pisani, F., et al. Developing countries as the major future source of living donor renal transplants. *Transplantation Proceedings.* 1992 Oct; 24(5): 2110–2111. 4 refs. Presented at the First International Congress on Transplantation in Developing Countries, Singapore, 29 Apr–3 May 1992. BE56813.
  cadavers; comparative studies; *developing countries; economics; family members; international aspects; *kidneys; morbidity; organ donation; *organ donors; *organ transplantation; prognosis; *remuneration; statistics; *transplant recipients; *treatment outcome; *unrelated donors; Europe; *Italy; United States

Englert, Yvon, ed. Organ and Tissue Transplantation in the European Union: Management of Difficulties and Health Risks Linked to Donors. Boston, MA: Martinus Nijhoff; sold and distributed in the U.S. and Canada by Kluwer Academic Publishers; 1995. 202 p. 180 refs. ISBN 0-7923-3051-X. BE56196.
  aborted fetuses; accountability; altruism; autonomy; body parts and fluids; cadavers; cancer; children; communicable diseases; communication; computer communication networks; donor cards; donors; fetal tissue donation; government regulation; health personnel; information

dissemination; informed consent; *international aspects; misconduct; moral obligations; *organ donation; organ donors; *organ transplantation; organization and administration; presumed consent; *public policy; remuneration; risk; risks and benefits; scarcity; selection for treatment; standards; tissue banks; *tissue donation; *tissue transplantation; trends; mandated choice; Eastern Europe; *Europe; *European Union; Eurotransplant; Spain; Titmuss, Richard; Transplant European Computer Network

Fishman, Rachelle H.B. Israel proposes kidney swap to increase live donors for transplantation. [News]. *Lancet.* 1998 Mar 7; 351(9014): 735. BE58885.
  *directed donation; *family members; *incentives; *kidneys; *organ donation; *organ donors; *organ transplantation; public policy; *transplant recipients; *Israel

Fishman, Rachelle H.B. Israeli surgeon questioned over transplantation ethics. [News]. *Lancet.* 1998 Mar 14; 351(9105): 812. BE58440.
  international aspects; *kidneys; *misconduct; *organ donation; organ donors; organ transplantation; *physicians; *remuneration; *Israel; Romania; *Shapiro, Zaki

Fluss, Sev S. Legal aspects of transplantation: emerging trends in international action and national legislation. *Transplantation Proceedings.* 1992 Oct; 24(5): 2121–2122. 4 refs. Presented at the First International Congress on Transplantation in Developing Countries, Singapore, 29 Apr–3 May 1992. BE56818.
  body parts and fluids; guidelines; *international aspects; *legal aspects; legislation; *organ donation; *organ transplantation; organizational policies; professional organizations; public policy; regulation; remuneration; Council of Europe; World Health Assembly; World Health Organization

Fox, Renée C. Regulated commercialism of vital organ donation: a necessity? Con. *Transplantation Proceedings.* 1993 Feb; 25(1): 55–57. 17 refs. BE56614.
  *altruism; attitudes; *body parts and fluids; *cadavers; *commodification; common good; dehumanization; *economics; emotions; *gifts; health personnel; *human body; *incentives; *organ donation; organ transplantation; *remuneration; risks and benefits; scarcity; transplant recipients; treatment outcome

Gevers, Sjef; Olsthoorn–Heim, Els. DNA sampling: Dutch and other European approaches to the issues of informed consent and confidentiality. *In:* Knoppers, Bartha Maria, ed. Human DNA: Law and Policy: International and Comparative Perspectives. Proceedings of the First International Conference on DNA Sampling and Human Genetic Research: Ethical, Legal, and Policy Aspects, held in Montreal, Canada, 6–8 Sep 1996. Boston, MA: Kluwer Law International; 1997: 109–120. 18 fn. ISBN 90-411-0361-9. BE58171.
  advisory committees; *confidentiality; *DNA data banks; *genetic information; *genetic materials; genetic research; *genetic screening; government regulation; guidelines; *informed consent; *international aspects; privacy; *public policy; *regulation; *tissue donation; *biological specimen banks; Council of Europe; *Europe; National Ethics Advisory Committee (France); *Netherlands; Nuffield Council on Bioethics

Gillam, Lynn. Arguing by analogy in the fetal tissue debate. *Bioethics.* 1997 Oct; 11(5): 397–412. 18 fn. BE56328.
  *aborted fetuses; *abortion, induced; adults; attitudes; cadavers; *ethical analysis; ethical theory; *fetal tissue donation; government regulation; incentives; *killing; *moral complicity; *moral policy; organ donation; physicians; pregnant women; prisoners; public policy; social impact;

BE = bioethics accession number   fn. = footnotes   refs. = references

tissue transplantation
In the debate over fetal tissue use, an analogy is often drawn between removing organs from the body of a person who has been murdered to use for transplantation, and collecting tissue from an aborted fetus to use for the same purpose. The murder victim analogy is taken by its proponents to show that even if abortion is the moral equivalent of murder, there is still no good reason to refrain from using the fetal tissue, since as a society we do not see any problem about using organs from murder victims. However, I argue that the analogy between murder victims and aborted fetuses does not hold -- the two situations are not the same in all morally relevant respects. Thus the murder victim analogy does not provide an argument in favour of fetal tissue transplant. In conclusion, I point to some of the potential pitfalls of using analogies in ethical argument.

Goldstein, Amy. Woman alleges fiancé stole her heart, brother's kidney. [News]. *Washington Post.* 1997 Oct 21: A1, A10–A11. BE55947.
    *deception; *directed donation; family members; incentives; *kidneys; *organ donation; *organ donors; *organ transplantation; *transplant recipients; unrelated donors; Dahl, John; *McNutt, Richard; Minnesota; Zauhar, Dorothy

Gorman, Christine. Body parts for sale. [News]. *Time.* 1998 Mar 9; 151(9): 76. BE58043.
    *body parts and fluids; cadavers; *capital punishment; federal government; human rights; informed consent; *international aspects; legal aspects; *organ donation; *prisoners; *remuneration; *China; United States

Great Britain. Isle of Man. An act (Chapter No. 3) to prohibit commercial dealings in human organs intended for transplanting; to prohibit the transplanting of such organs between persons who are not genetically related; and for connected purposes. Dated 16 March 1993. (The Human Organ Transplants Act 1993). *International Digest of Health Legislation.* 1996; 47(2): 169–170. BE57187.
    advertising; body parts and fluids; cadavers; directed donation; *legal aspects; *organ donation; organ donors; *organ transplantation; remuneration; transplant recipients; *Great Britain; *Human Organ Transplants Act 1993 (Isle of Man); *Isle of Man

Grubb, Andrew. Adult incompetent: legality of non-therapeutic procedure -- Re Y. [Comment]. *Medical Law Review.* 1996 Summer; 4(2): 204–207. BE56483.
    adults; *bone marrow; competence; *decision making; family relationship; judicial action; *legal aspects; *mentally retarded; physically disabled; risks and benefits; *siblings; *tissue donation; *Great Britain; *Re Y

Guttmann, Astrid; Guttmann, Ronald D. Sale of kidneys for transplantation: attitudes of the health-care profession and the public. *Transplantation Proceedings.* 1992 Oct; 24(5): 2108–2109. 6 refs. Presented at the First International Congress on Transplantation in Developing Countries, Singapore, 29 Apr–3 May 1992. BE56812.
    *attitudes; case studies; economics; government regulation; informed consent; *kidneys; medical education; nurses; *organ donation; *organ donors; physicians; *public opinion; public policy; regulation; *remuneration; scarcity; students; survey; transplant recipients; *Canada; India

Guttmann, Ronald D. Future markets: claims and meanings. *Transplantation Proceedings.* 1992 Oct; 24(5): 2203. 6 refs. BE56836.
    altruism; cadavers; commodification; *contracts; *economics; *industry; *organ donation; *public policy; *remuneration; transplant recipients; values

Guttmann, Ronald D.; Guttmann, Astrid. Organ transplantation: duty reconsidered. *Transplantation Proceedings.* 1992 Oct; 24(5): 2179–2180. 7 refs. Commentary on P.T. Menzel, p. 2175–2178. BE56831.
    attitudes; cadavers; cultural pluralism; family members; health personnel; hospitals; informed consent; *moral obligations; motivation; obligations of society; obligations to society; *organ donation; *presumed consent; *public policy; resource allocation; scarcity; third party consent; refusal to donate; United States

Haberal, Mehmet; Altaca, G.; Tokyay, R., et al. Ethics in organ procurement in Turkey. *Transplantation Proceedings.* 1992 Oct; 24(5): 2100–2101. 7 refs. Presented at the First International Congress on Transplantation in Developing Countries, Singapore, 29 Apr–3 May 1992. BE56809.
    brain death; family members; informed consent; legal aspects; *organ donation; organ donors; *organ transplantation; public policy; remuneration; scarcity; third party consent; unrelated donors; *Turkey

Habgood, John; Spagnolo, Antonio G.; Sgreccia, Elio, et al. Religious views on organ and tissue donation. *In:* Chapman, Jeremy R.; Deierhoi, Mark; Wight, Celia, eds. Organ and Tissue Donation for Transplantation. New York, NY: Oxford University Press; 1997: 23–33. 25 refs. ISBN 0-340-61394-7. BE58227.
    aborted fetuses; altruism; anencephaly; animal organs; attitudes; body parts and fluids; brain death; Buddhist ethics; *cadavers; cardiac death; commodification; *cultural pluralism; determination of death; donor cards; family members; fetal tissue donation; germ cells; gifts; Hindu ethics; human body; informed consent; international aspects; *Islamic ethics; legal aspects; moral obligations; newborns; *organ donation; *organ donors; *Protestant ethics; public policy; *religious ethics; remuneration; *Roman Catholic ethics; third party consent; *tissue donation; transgenic animals; *values; voluntary programs; Anglican Church; Great Britain; India; Islamic Code of Medical Ethics; Japan; Middle East

Hersey, Jonathan. Enigma of the unborn mother: legal and ethical considerations of aborted fetal ovarian tissue and ova transplantations. *UCLA Law Review.* 1995 Oct; 43(1): 159–207. 228 fn. BE57196.
    *aborted fetuses; abortion, induced; advisory committees; conflict of interest; decision making; directed donation; federal government; females; fetal research; *fetal tissue donation; *government regulation; in vitro fertilization; infertility; informed consent; *legal aspects; legal rights; *organ donation; *ovum donors; property rights; *public policy; risks and benefits; scarcity; social impact; state government; *ovaries; Great Britain; National Organ Transplant Act 1984; Uniform Anatomical Gift Act; *United States

Hoffenberg, R.; Lock, M.; Tilney, N., et al. Should organs from patients in permanent vegetative state be used for transplantation? [For the International Forum for Transplant Ethics]. *Lancet.* 1997 Nov 1; 350(9087): 1320–1321. 7 refs. BE56463.
    allowing to die; anencephaly; body parts and fluids; brain; conscience; *determination of death; futility; health personnel; involuntary euthanasia; *killing; legal aspects; newborns; *organ donation; organizational policies; *persistent vegetative state; professional organizations; prolongation of life; withholding treatment; Airedale NHS Trust v. Bland; American Neurological Association; British Medical Association; Great Britain; United States

Holden, Constance. Tricky ethics of tissue samples. [News]. *Science.* 1998 Mar 13; 279(5357): 1621. BE57779.
    advisory committees; *biomedical research; blood donation; body parts and fluids; *donors; guidelines; informed consent;

---

legal rights; *public policy; stigmatization; *tissue donation; *community consent; *National Bioethics Advisory Commission; United States

Hoshino, Kazumasa. Bioethics in the light of Japanese sentiments. *In:* Hoshino, Kazumasa, ed. Japanese and Western Bioethics: Studies in Moral Diversity. Boston, MA: Kluwer Academic; 1997: 13-23. 5 refs. ISBN 0-7923-4112-0. BE57080.
autonomy; bioethical issues; cadavers; communication; *communitarianism; comparative studies; *decision making; diagnosis; family members; *family relationship; informed consent; legal aspects; *organ donation; *paternalism; patient care; patient compliance; *patients' rights; *physician patient relationship; *physicians; privacy; professional family relationship; prognosis; terminally ill; third party consent; *tissue donation; *truth disclosure; hope; non-Western World; Act of Donation of the Body for Medical and Dental Education 1983 (Japan); Cornea and Kidney Transplant Act 1979 (Japan); *Japan; United States

Ikels, Charlotte. Kidney failure and transplantation in China. *Social Science and Medicine.* 1997 May; 44(9): 1271-1283. 35 refs. BE58910.
aliens; artificial organs; attitudes; attitudes to death; brain death; Buddhist ethics; cadavers; capital punishment; determination of death; family members; incentives; kidney diseases; *kidneys; legal aspects; *organ donation; organ donors; organ transplantation; physicians; prisoners; public policy; renal dialysis; scarcity; terminally ill; third party consent; transplant recipients; withholding treatment; folk medicine; *China

The incidence of chronic renal failure in China is approximately 120,000 cases per year; the vast majority of these new cases will die within a very short time because of the shortage of funds, dialysis machines, and organs for transplantation. This paper focuses on the reasons behind the organ shortage and the strategies proposed by the Chinese medical profession to increase the supply of transplantable kidneys. The data were gathered on multiple trips to China, Hong Kong and Taiwan between August 1993 and January 1995. During these trips the author spoke formally with nephrologists, urologists, dialysis and transplant nurses, and other individuals active in the field of organ procurement, and informally with others familiar with general hospital practice. The author also draws heavily on articles published in leading Chinese journals. The kidney shortage in China is produced by the same sorts of problems as exist in other countries, but the shortage is aggravated by certain beliefs and practices specific to Chinese populations. Live donation is hampered by traditional beliefs about the function of the kidney, while cadaver donation is hampered by reluctance to cut a body and a host of beliefs about ghosts, labeled "feudal superstitions" by the authorities. Cadaver donation is further restrained by the lack of legal recognition of "brain death". In response to the organ shortage, the Chinese medical community has expanded the range of eligible sources to include those condemned to death as criminals, a practice itself usually condemned by the wider international community. At the same time it has advocated: (1) enhancing corpse donation through propaganda work, administrative work, legal work, and incentives; (2) encouraging live donation; (3) familiarizing the public with the benefits of organ transplantation, and (4) pursuing the development of artificial organs.

Indudhara, R.; Singh, S.K.; Minz, M. Opinion poll regarding knowledge, attitudes, and suggestions for developing a cadaver donor program. *Transplantation Proceedings.* 1992 Oct; 24(5): 2069. Presented at the First

International Congress on Transplantation in Developing Countries, Singapore, 29 Apr-3 May 1992. BE56801.
brain death; *cadavers; family members; health education; *health personnel; hospitals; institutional policies; kidneys; *knowledge, attitudes, practice; legislation; *organ donation; *organ transplantation; patients; public policy; renal dialysis; scarcity; survey; treatment outcome; *India

Ivanovski, Ninoslav; Stojkovski, Ljupco; Cakalaroski, Koco, et al. Renal transplantation from paid, unrelated donors in India -- it is not only unethical, it is also medically unsafe. [Letter]. *Nephrology, Dialysis, Transplantation.* 1997 Sep; 12(9): 2028-2029. 4 refs. BE58210.
developing countries; *kidneys; morbidity; *organ donation; *organ donors; organ transplantation; remuneration; risks and benefits; statistics; *transplant recipients; *treatment outcome; *unrelated donors; *India; *Macedonia

Johnson, Martin H. Should egg donors be paid? The culture of unpaid and voluntary egg donation should be strengthened. *BMJ (British Medical Journal).* 1997 May 10; 314(7091): 1401-1402. 10 refs. BE55650.
*altruism; blood donation; children; embryos; germ cells; *government regulation; incentives; informed consent; *legal aspects; motivation; *ovum donors; public opinion; *public policy; *remuneration; social impact; tissue donation; *Great Britain; Human Fertilisation and Embryology Act 1990; Human Fertilisation and Embryology Authority

Joralemon, Donald; Sharp, Lesley A. Authors' responses to commentaries. *Medical Anthropology Quarterly.* 1995 Sep; 9(3): 398-399. BE56590.
anthropology; cadavers; gifts; health personnel; *organ donation; *organ transplantation; self concept; socioeconomic factors; transplant recipients

Joralemon, Donald. Organ wars: the battle for body parts. *Medical Anthropology Quarterly.* 1995 Sep; 9(3): 335-356. 98 refs. 25 fn. Commented on by M. Lock, p. 390-393, and by B.A. Koenig and L.F. Hogle, p. 393-397. BE56581.
altruism; *anthropology; *attitudes; attitudes to death; autonomy; *body parts and fluids; brain death; *cadavers; *commodification; *cultural pluralism; determination of death; *economics; *emotions; family members; *gifts; *human body; *incentives; international aspects; legal aspects; mass media; metaphor; *organ donation; organ donors; *organ transplantation; *personhood; *property rights; *psychological stress; *psychology; public opinion; *remuneration; scarcity; *self concept; third party consent; *transplant recipients; *values; *United States

Josefson, Deborah. Two arrested in US for selling organs for transplantation. [News]. *BMJ (British Medical Journal).* 1998 Mar 7; 316(7133): 725. BE57705.
*body parts and fluids; *capital punishment; international aspects; *law enforcement; legal aspects; *organ donation; *prisoners; *remuneration; *tissue donation; China; United States

Kandela, Peter. Gulf countries to reconsider organ transplantation. [News]. *Lancet.* 1997 Aug 23; 350(9077): 574. BE56076.
*attitudes; cadavers; *Islamic ethics; *organ donation; organ donors; *public policy; *Gulf Co-operation Council; Kuwait; *Middle East; Saudi Arabia; United Arab Emirates

Kazem, R.; Thompson, L.A.; Hamilton, M.P., et al. Current attitudes towards egg donation among men and women. *Human Reproduction.* 1995 Jun; 10(6): 1543-1548. 19 refs. BE55565.
aborted fetuses; *attitudes; biomedical research; cadavers; comparative studies; *cryopreservation; embryos; fathers;

BE = bioethics accession number   fn. = footnotes   refs. = references

*females; fetal tissue donation; *infertility; knowledge, attitudes, practice; *males; mothers; *ovum; *ovum donors; patient care; patients; remuneration; reproduction; reproductive technologies; research embryo creation; semen donors; socioeconomic factors; sperm; survey; *tissue donation; ovum recipients; Great Britain

Kazim, E.; al-Rukaimi, M.; Fernandez, H., et al. Buying a kidney: the easy way out? *Transplantation Proceedings.* 1992 Oct; 24(5): 2112–2113. 4 refs. Presented at the First International Congress on Transplantation in Developing Countries, Singapore, 29 Apr–3 May 1992. BE56814.
*developing countries; *kidneys; morbidity; mortality; *organ donation; *organ donors; *organ transplantation; *remuneration; statistics; *transplant recipients; *treatment outcome; follow-up studies; *unrelated donors; India; Rashid Hospital (United Arab Emirates); United Arab Emirates

Kennedy, I.; Sells, R.A.; Daar, A.S., et al. The case for "presumed consent" in organ donation. [For the International Forum for Transplant Ethics]. *Lancet.* 1998 May 30; 351(9116): 1650–1652. 13 refs. BE58859.
*cadavers; family members; *international aspects; legal aspects; moral policy; *organ donation; *presumed consent; *public policy; social impact; statistics; third party consent; Europe

Kent, Bridie; Owens, R. Glynn. Conflicting attitudes to corneal and organ donation: a study of nurses' attitudes to organ donation. *International Journal of Nursing Studies.* 1995 Oct; 32(5): 484–492. 27 refs. BE55566.
*attitudes; body parts and fluids; donor cards; nurse's role; *nurses; *organ donation; survey; *tissue donation; *corneas; *Great Britain

Kinney, Joanna H. Restricting donative choice: fetal tissue transplantation and respect for human life. *Journal of Law and Health.* 1995–1996; 10(2): 259–285. 121 fn. BE57145.
*aborted fetuses; abortion, induced; casuistry; diabetes; *directed donation; fetal research; *fetal tissue donation; fetuses; government regulation; intention; *legal aspects; legal rights; moral obligations; motivation; pregnant women; state government; tissue transplantation; war; *United States

Koenig, Barbara A.; Hogle, Linda F. Organ transplantation (re)examined? Commentary. *Medical Anthropology Quarterly.* 1995 Sep; 9(3): 393–397. 17 refs. 2 fn. Commentary on D. Joralemon, p. 335–356, and on L.A. Sharp, p. 357–389. BE56468.
anthropology; attitudes; bioethics; biomedical technologies; body parts and fluids; cadavers; family members; gifts; health personnel; interdisciplinary communication; *organ donation; organ donors; *organ transplantation; personhood; self concept; social sciences; socioeconomic factors; transplant recipients

Kovac, Carl. Tissue trade in Hungary is investigated. [News]. *BMJ (British Medical Journal).* 1998 Feb 28; 316(7132): 647. BE57706.
body parts and fluids; cadavers; *hospitals; *industry; institutional policies; international aspects; *legal aspects; misconduct; *organ donation; presumed consent; *remuneration; *tissue donation; Europe; Germany; *Hungary; United States

Lamb, David. Ethics of fetal tissue transplants. *In:* Frith, Lucy, ed. Ethics and Midwifery: Issues in Contemporary Practice. Boston, MA: Butterworth–Heinemann; 1996: 156–169. 14 refs. ISBN 0-7506-3056-6. BE58638.
*aborted fetuses; abortion, induced; advisory committees; commodification; *fetal tissue donation; guidelines;

incentives; informed consent; *moral policy; pregnant women; public policy; risks and benefits; *Great Britain; Polkinghorne Report

Land, Walter; Cohen, B. Postmortem and living organ donation in Europe: transplant laws and activities. *Transplantation Proceedings.* 1992 Oct; 24(5): 2165–2167. 3 refs. BE56827.
*cadavers; comparative studies; disclosure; dissent; family members; informed consent; international aspects; kidneys; *legal aspects; *legislation; *organ donation; *organ donors; *presumed consent; social impact; statistics; Austria; Denmark; Eastern Europe; *Europe; Finland; France; Germany; Great Britain; Greece; Italy; Netherlands; Norway; Portugal; Spain; Sweden; Switzerland

Langston, J. William; Palfreman, Jon. The Case of the Frozen Addicts: Working at the Edge of the Mysteries of the Human Brain. New York, NY: Vintage Books; 1996. 309 p. ISBN 0-678-74708-7. BE56698.
*aborted fetuses; animal experimentation; biomedical research; *brain; *brain pathology; diagnosis; disadvantaged; *drug abuse; federal government; *fetal research; *fetal tissue donation; government financing; *heroin; human experimentation; international aspects; interprofessional relations; *investigators; moral complicity; *paralysis; patients; primates; research institutes; research subjects; risks and benefits; selection of subjects; therapeutic research; *tissue transplantation; *toxicity; *Parkinson disease; Human Fetal Tissue Transplantation Research Panel; *Langston, J. William; Lindvall, Olle; National Institutes of Health; Sweden; United States

Litman, Moe M. The legal status of genetic material. *In:* Knoppers, Bartha Maria, ed. Human DNA: Law and Policy: International and Comparative Perspectives. Proceedings of the First International Conference on DNA Sampling and Human Genetic Research: Ethical, Legal, and Policy Aspects, held in Montreal, Canada, 6–8 Sep 1996. Boston, MA: Kluwer Law International; 1997: 17–32. 76 fn. ISBN 90-411-0361-9. BE58165.
biomedical research; *body parts and fluids; commodification; *confidentiality; DNA data banks; economics; *genetic information; *genetic materials; *genetic research; international aspects; *legal aspects; patents; privacy; *property rights; public policy; *tissue donation; *Canada; Moore v. Regents of the University of California; *United States

Lockwood, G.M. Donating life: practical and ethical issues in gamete donation. *In:* Shenfield, F.; Sureau, C., eds. Ethical Dilemmas in Assisted Reproduction. New York, NY: Parthenon Pub. Group; 1997: 23–30. 9 refs. ISBN 1-85070-916-5. BE57943.
aborted fetuses; *altruism; brain death; cadavers; coercion; directed donation; family members; family relationship; females; *incentives; motivation; *ovum donors; public policy; *remuneration; reproductive technologies; risks and benefits; semen donors; socioeconomic factors; treatment outcome; Great Britain

Loewy, Erich H. Of sentiment, caring and anencephalics: a response to Sytsma. *Theoretical Medicine and Bioethics.* 1998 Jan; 19(1): 21–34. 19 refs. BE57312.
*anencephaly; autonomy; brain death; brain pathology; *caring; decision making; determination of death; emotions; *ethical analysis; ethical theory; justice; *moral obligations; *moral policy; *newborns; *organ donation; parental consent; parents; paternalism; persistent vegetative state; *personhood; prognosis; suffering; wedge argument; Kant, Immanuel

McEwen, Jean E. DNA sampling and banking: practices and procedures in the United States. *In:* Knoppers, Bartha Maria, ed. Human DNA: Law and Policy:

BE = bioethics accession number   fn. = footnotes   refs. = references

International and Comparative Perspectives. Proceedings of the First International Conference on DNA Sampling and Human Genetic Research: Ethical, Legal, and Policy Aspects, held in Montreal, Canada, 6–8 Sep 1996. Boston, MA: Kluwer Law International; 1997: 407–421. 76 fn. ISBN 90–411–0361–9. BE58197.
blood specimen collection; confidentiality; *DNA data banks; *DNA fingerprinting; family members; federal government; genetic research; genetic screening; government regulation; guidelines; informed consent; institutional policies; *law enforcement; legal aspects; mandatory programs; *military personnel; newborns; organization and administration; prisoners; privacy; professional organizations; public policy; regulation; state government; statistics; *tissue banks; *biological specimen banks; DNA Identification Act 1994; Human Genome Privacy Act; *United States

McLean, Sheila A.M. Transplantation and the 'nearly dead': the case of elective ventilation. *In:* McLean, Sheila A.M., ed. Contemporary Issues in Law, Medicine and Ethics. Brookfield, VT: Dartmouth; 1996: 143–162. 80 fn. ISBN 1–85521–586–1. BE57794.
*advance directives; altruism; beneficence; body parts and fluids; decision making; gifts; informed consent; intention; *legal aspects; moral policy; *organ donation; patients; physicians; *prolongation of life; public policy; resuscitation; risks and benefits; scarcity; *ventilators; *Great Britain; House of Lords Select Committee on Medical Ethics; Human Tissue Act 1961 (Great Britain); Law Commission (Great Britain)

Martin, Douglas K.; Singer, Peter A.; Siegler, Mark. Ethical considerations in liver transplantation. *In:* Boyer, J.L.; Ockner, R.K., eds. Progress in Liver Diseases, Vol. XII. Philadelphia, PA: Saunders; 1994: 215–229. 101 fn. BE55799.
age factors; alcohol abuse; animal organs; body parts and fluids; brain death; cadavers; cardiac death; determination of death; family members; informed consent; justice; *livers; *organ donation; organ donors; *organ transplantation; presumed consent; public policy; remuneration; required request; resource allocation; risks and benefits; scarcity; selection for treatment; therapeutic research; transplant recipients; United Network for Organ Sharing; United States

Mason, J.K. Contemporary issues in organ transplantation. *In:* McLean, Sheila A.M., ed. Contemporary Issues in Law, Medicine and Ethics. Brookfield, VT: Dartmouth; 1996: 117–141. 103 fn. ISBN 1–85521–586–1. BE57793.
aborted fetuses; anencephaly; animal organs; body parts and fluids; brain death; cadavers; cardiac death; criminal law; education; fetal tissue donation; health personnel; incentives; intensive care units; intention; kidneys; law enforcement; *legal aspects; *moral policy; newborns; *organ donation; organ donors; persistent vegetative state; presumed consent; primates; prolongation of life; public opinion; regulation; remuneration; scarcity; speciesism; terminally ill; third party consent; transgenic animals; ventilators; ovaries; unrelated donors; *Great Britain; Human Organ Transplants Act 1989 (Great Britain); Human Tissue Act 1961 (Great Britain)

Mazen, Noël–Jean. Human DNA on trial in French law. *In:* Knoppers, Bartha Maria, ed. Human DNA: Law and Policy: International and Comparative Perspectives. Proceedings of the First International Conference on DNA Sampling and Human Genetic Research: Ethical, Legal, and Policy Aspects, held in Montreal, Canada, 6–8 Sep 1996. Boston, MA: Kluwer Law International; 1997: 43–54. 45 fn. ISBN 90–411–0361–9. BE58168.
*biomedical technologies; body parts and fluids; DNA sequences; drugs; gene therapy; genetic intervention; *genetic materials; genetic research; gifts; *government regulation; informed consent; *legal aspects; legislation; *patents; *remuneration; *tissue donation; Europe; European

Community; *France

Menzel, Paul T. The moral duty to contribute and its implications for organ procurement policy. *Transplantation Proceedings.* 1992 Oct; 24(5): 2175–2178. 5 refs. Commented on by R.D. Guttmann and A. Guttmann, p. 2179–2180. BE56830.
altruism; autonomy; beneficence; cadavers; dissent; *moral obligations; obligations to society; *organ donation; *presumed consent; *public policy; transplant recipients; *refusal to donate; United States

Michielsen, Paul. Informed or presumed consent legislative models. *In:* Chapman, Jeremy R.; Deierhoi, Mark; Wight, Celia, eds. Organ and Tissue Donation for Transplantation. New York, NY: Oxford University Press; 1997: 344–360. 52 refs. ISBN 0–340–61394–7. BE58232.
advance directives; attitudes; autonomy; autopsies; body parts and fluids; brain death; cadavers; cardiac death; computers; cultural pluralism; data banks; determination of death; donor cards; evaluation; family members; historical aspects; *informed consent; *international aspects; Islamic ethics; *legal aspects; *organ donation; physicians; *presumed consent; public opinion; registries; religion; social impact; third party consent; *tissue donation; values; mandated choice; Council of Europe; Europe; Japan; Singapore; United States; World Health Organization

Miles, J.A.R. Organ transplants in China: use of organs from executed prisoners. *New Zealand Medical Journal.* 1995 May 10; 108(999): 178. 1 ref. BE58215.
body parts and fluids; *cadavers; capital punishment; deception; medical ethics; *organ donation; *physician's role; *prisoners; *public policy; *China

Miller, A.S.; Hagihara, A. Organ transplanting in Japan: the debate begins. *Public Health.* 1997 Nov; 111(6): 367–372. 29 refs. BE59011.
age factors; aliens; *attitudes; brain death; cadavers; determination of death; *organ donation; organ donors; *organ transplantation; prognosis; *public opinion; public participation; public policy; resource allocation; selection for treatment; self induced illness; survey; time factors; transplant recipients; *Japan

Mongoven, Ann. Federal hearings on liver transplant allocation and donation. *In:* BioLaw: A Legal and Ethical Reporter on Medicine, Health Care, and Bioengineering. Special Sections 2(12). Frederick, MD: University Publications of America; 1997 Dec: S:373–S:389. BE57643.
cadavers; chronically ill; computers; conflict of interest; consensus; critically ill; *decision making; determination of death; federal government; government regulation; health facilities; health insurance; justice; *livers; models, theoretical; *organ donation; *organ transplantation; patient advocacy; physicians; prognosis; public participation; *public policy; *resource allocation; scarcity; *selection for treatment; transplant recipients; treatment outcome; geographic factors; *Department of Health and Human Services; *United Network for Organ Sharing; *United States

Montgomery, Jonathan. Health care law and ethics: abortion; fertility; maternity care; selective treatment of the newborn; transplantation; terminal care and euthanasia. *In: his* Health Care Law. New York, NY: Oxford University Press; 1997: 357–456. 503 fn. ISBN 0–19–876260–7. BE56245.
*abortion, induced; active euthanasia; *adults; *allowing to die; assisted suicide; body parts and fluids; cadavers; childbirth; congenital disorders; conscience; contraception; family planning; fetuses; health personnel; *legal aspects;

BE = bioethics accession number   fn. = footnotes   refs. = references

legal liability; legislation; living wills; maternal health; minors; *newborns; *organ donation; organ donors; organ transplantation; *patient care; persistent vegetative state; *pregnant women; prenatal injuries; remuneration; *reproductive technologies; selective abortion; spousal consent; sterilization (sexual); surrogate mothers; terminal care; therapeutic abortion; treatment refusal; *Great Britain

Multiple Organ Retrieval and Exchange (M.O.R.E.) Program of Ontario. Task Force on Presumed Consent [and] Board of Directors. Organ Procurement Strategies: A Review of the Ethical Issues and Challenges. [Report]. Toronto, ON: Multiple Organ Retrieval and Exchange (M.O.R.E.) Program of Ontario; 1994 Nov. 31 p. 237 refs. 146 fn. BE57397.
   alternatives; altruism; attitudes; autonomy; brain death; communitarianism; contracts; cultural pluralism; determination of death; donor cards; economics; education; family members; health personnel; human body; humanism; incentives; indigents; international aspects; legal aspects; legislation; libertarianism; mass media; *organ donation; physicians; policy analysis; *presumed consent; *public policy; religion; remuneration; required request; terminology; third party consent; trust; uncertainty; values; voluntary programs; mandated choice; unrelated donors; Belgium; Canada; France; *Ontario; Singapore; United States

Muyskens, James. Should receiving depend upon willingness to give? *Transplantation Proceedings.* 1992 Oct; 24(5): 2181-2184. 5 refs. Commented on by A.M. Capron, p. 2185-2187. BE56832.
   altruism; cadavers; *organ donation; *organ donors; *organ transplantation; *public policy; *refusal to treat; resource allocation; scarcity; *selection for treatment; *transplant recipients; *refusal to donate; United States

Naqvi, Ali Anwar. Ethical issues in renal transplantation in developing countries. [Editorial]. *JPMA: Journal of the Pakistan Medical Association.* 1995 Sep; 45(9): 233-234. 13 refs. BE55517.
   body parts and fluids; cadavers; capital punishment; coercion; *developing countries; females; government regulation; indigents; informed consent; kidneys; *organ donation; *organ donors; organ transplantation; physicians; prisoners; remuneration; self regulation; China; India

Ohl, Dana A.; Park, John; Cohen, Carl, et al. Procreation after death or mental incompetence: medical advance or technology gone awry? *Fertility and Sterility.* 1996 Dec; 66(6): 889-895. 24 refs. BE56878.
   artificial insemination; brain death; *brain pathology; case studies; *competence; *cryopreservation; decision making; guidelines; informed consent; legal aspects; married persons; moral obligations; physicians; *posthumous reproduction; *reproductive technologies; *semen donors; single persons; *sperm; terminally ill; third party consent

Pechura, Constance M. Fetal and embryo research: a changing scientific, political, and ethical landscape. *In:* Vanderpool, Harold Y., ed. The Ethics of Research Involving Human Subjects: Facing the 21st Century. Frederick, MD: University Publishing Group; 1996: 371-400. 74 fn. ISBN 1-55572-036-6. BE56994.
   aborted fetuses; advisory committees; body parts and fluids; *embryo research; federal government; *fetal research; *fetal tissue donation; government financing; *government regulation; historical aspects; parental consent; pregnant women; prenatal diagnosis; professional organizations; *public policy; reproductive technologies; research embryo creation; risks and benefits; stem cells; tissue banks; trends; cord blood; American College of Obstetricians and Gynecologists; American Fertility Society; Biomedical Ethics Advisory Committee; Department of Health and Human Services; Ethics Advisory Board; Human Fetal

Tissue Transplantation Research Panel; National Advisory Board on Ethics in Reproduction (NABER); National Institutes of Health; Office of Technology Assessment; United States

Pennings, Guido. Should donors have the right to decide who receives their gametes? *Human Reproduction.* 1995 Oct; 10(10): 2736-2740. 24 refs. BE57507.
   age factors; attitudes; autonomy; confidentiality; cultural pluralism; *directed donation; females; homosexuals; informed consent; moral policy; *ovum donors; public opinion; public policy; remuneration; resource allocation; selection for treatment; *semen donors; single persons

Pike, Roseanne E.; Odell, J.A.; Kahn, D. Public attitudes to organ donation in South Africa. [Abstract]. *Transplantation Proceedings.* 1992 Oct; 24(5): 2102. Presented at the First International Congress on Transplantation in Developing Countries, Singapore, 29 Apr-3 May 1992. BE56810.
   *attitudes; *blacks; comparative studies; *organ donation; *public opinion; survey; *whites; rural population; urban population; *South Africa

Porter, John. Reason, law and medicine: anencephalics as organ donors. *In:* McLean, Sheila A.M., ed. Contemporary Issues in Law, Medicine and Ethics. Brookfield, VT: Dartmouth; 1996: 163-178. 28 fn. ISBN 1-85521-586-1. BE57795.
   allowing to die; *anencephaly; animal rights; body parts and fluids; brain death; *killing; *legal aspects; legal liability; moral obligations; morality; newborns; *organ donation; organ donors; persistent vegetative state; personhood; prolongation of life; ventilators; withholding treatment; Airedale NHS Trust v. Bland; *Great Britain

Potts, John T., et al.; Institute of Medicine. Non-Heart-Beating Organ Transplantation: Medical and Ethical Issues in Procurement. [Report]. Washington, DC: National Academy Press; 1997. 92 p. Bibliography: p. 65-72. Study funded by the U.S. Department of Health and Human Services. Study Director: Roger Herdman; Principal Investigator: John T. Potts. ISBN 0-309-06424-4. BE57745.
   body parts and fluids; *cadavers; *cardiac death; conflict of interest; costs and benefits; decision making; determination of death; drugs; family members; federal government; *guidelines; health facilities; *institutional policies; moral policy; *organ donation; organ transplantation; *organizational policies; physicians; policy analysis; public policy; review; scarcity; *standards; statistics; survey; third party consent; treatment outcome; withholding treatment; *Institute of Medicine; Organ Procurement and Transplantation Network; United States

Potts, Michael. Morals, metaphysics, and heart transplantation: reflections on Richard Selzer's "Whither Thou Goest". *Perspectives in Biology and Medicine.* 1998 Winter; 41(2): 212-223. 25 refs. 5 fn. BE59028.
   attitudes to death; bioethics; body parts and fluids; brain; *cadavers; *dehumanization; *emotions; *family members; *gifts; *hearts; *human body; literature; metaphor; *narrative ethics; *organ donation; *organ transplantation; personhood; *self concept; *transplant recipients; *personal identity; *Whither Thou Goest (Selzer, R.)

Provisional Commission for the Study on Brain Death and Organ Transplantation (Japan). Important Considerations with Respect to Brain Death and Organ Transplants, January 22, 1992. Tokyo: the Commission; translation issued by the Osaka Kidney Foundation; 1994 Jun. 39 p. English version of a report submitted to the Prime Minister. BE58449.
   advisory committees; *brain death; *cadavers; consensus;

---

*determination of death; dissent; informed consent; *organ donation; *organ transplantation; personhood; physicians; public policy; resource allocation; *standards; transplant recipients; trust; *Japan; *Provisional Commission for the Study on Brain Death and Organ Transplantation (Japan)

Quah, Stella R. Social and ethical aspects of organ donation. *Transplantation Proceedings.* 1992 Oct; 24(5): 2097–2098. 7 refs. Presented at the First International Congress on Transplantation in Developing Countries, Singapore, 29 Apr–3 May 1992. BE56807.
attitudes; body parts and fluids; cultural pluralism; *developing countries; health personnel; hospitals; intensive care units; international aspects; *organ donation; organ donors; *public policy; scarcity; socioeconomic factors; values

Quintana, Octavi. Human tissue banks in Europe. *In:* Knoppers, Bartha Maria, ed. Human DNA: Law and Policy: International and Comparative Perspectives. Proceedings of the First International Conference on DNA Sampling and Human Genetic Research: Ethical, Legal, and Policy Aspects, held in Montreal, Canada, 6–8 Sep 1996. Boston, MA: Kluwer Law International; 1997: 423–427. 11 fn. ISBN 90–411–0361–9. BE58198.
confidentiality; *DNA data banks; genetic research; informed consent; international aspects; medical devices; organization and administration; *regulation; *tissue banks; tissue donation; *biological specimen banks; *Europe; European Union; Group of Advisers on the Ethical Implications of Biotechnology (European Commission)

Radcliffe–Richards, J.; Daar, A.S.; Guttmann, R.D., et al. The case for allowing kidney sales. [For the International Forum for Transplant Ethics]. *Lancet.* 1998 Jun 27; 351(9120): 1950–1952. 15 refs. BE58471.
altruism; autonomy; coercion; developing countries; government regulation; *indigents; informed consent; *kidneys; *moral policy; *organ donation; *organ donors; *remuneration; risks and benefits; transplant recipients; wedge argument

Radin, Margaret Jane. Contested Commodities: The Trouble with Trade in Sex, Children, Body Parts, and Other Things. Cambridge, MA: Harvard University Press; 1996. 279 p. 437 fn. ISBN 0–674–16697–3. BE55801.
adoption; altruism; *body parts and fluids; children; coercion; *commodification; *dehumanization; *democracy; *economics; females; *feminist ethics; *freedom; *government regulation; indigents; *infants; justice; law; legal aspects; metaphor; minority groups; *organ donation; personhood; property rights; public policy; *remuneration; *sexuality; *surrogate mothers; torts; women's rights; liberalism; *prostitution

Rasheed, H.Z.A. Organ donation and transplantation -- a Muslim viewpoint. *Transplantation Proceedings.* 1992 Oct; 24(5): 2116–2117. Presented at the First International Congress on Transplantation in Developing Countries, Singapore, 29 Apr–3 May 1992. BE56816.
attitudes; donor cards; health education; informed consent; *Islamic ethics; *kidneys; *legal aspects; *organ donation; organ transplantation; presumed consent; *public policy; selection for treatment; uncertainty; *Muslims; Human Organ Transplant Act 1987 (Singapore); *Singapore

Robbennolt, Jennifer K.; Weisz, Victoria; Lawson, Craig M. Advancing the rights of children and adolescents to be altruistic: bone marrow donation by minors. *Journal of Law and Health.* 1994–1995; 9(2): 213–245. 156 fn. BE57148.
adolescents; altruism; attitudes; *bone marrow; competence; decision making; judicial action; *legal aspects; *minors;

parental consent; psychology; risks and benefits; *siblings; *standards; students; survey; *third party consent; *tissue donation; United States

Roleff, Tamara L., ed. Biomedical Ethics: Opposing Viewpoints. San Diego, CA: Greenhaven Press; 1998. 252 p. (Opposing viewpoints series). Includes references. ISBN 1–56510–792–6. BE59107.
age factors; animal organs; autonomy; beneficence; *bioethical issues; body parts and fluids; brain death; cadavers; capital punishment; childbirth; *cloning; eugenics; females; genes; *genetic intervention; *genetic research; genetic screening; genome mapping; government regulation; indigents; moral policy; *organ donation; organ transplantation; patents; personhood; posthumous reproduction; pregnant women; presumed consent; prisoners; public policy; remuneration; *reproductive technologies; risks and benefits; selection for treatment; surrogate mothers; transgenic animals

Sadler, Blair L. Presumed consent to organ transplantation: a different perspective. *Transplantation Proceedings.* 1992 Oct; 24(5): 2173–2174. 7 refs. BE56829.
body parts and fluids; cadavers; family members; health personnel; hospitals; informed consent; legal aspects; *organ donation; *presumed consent; *public policy; required request; scarcity; social impact; Uniform Anatomical Gift Act; *United States

Sauer, Mark V. Should egg donors be paid? Exploitation or a woman's right? *BMJ (British Medical Journal).* 1997 May 10; 314(7091): 1403. BE55665.
autonomy; drugs; health facilities; industry; infertility; informed consent; institutional policies; international aspects; *ovum donors; physicians; private sector; *remuneration; reproductive technologies; risk; self regulation; Great Britain; *United States

Schemo, Diana Jean. Death's new sting in Brazil: removal of organs. [News]. *New York Times.* 1998 Jan 15: A4. BE57736.
body parts and fluids; cadavers; *legal aspects; *organ donation; *presumed consent; *public opinion; scarcity; refusal to donate; *Brazil

Sehgal, Ashwini R.; LeBeau, Shane O.; Youngner, Stuart J. Dialysis patient attitudes toward financial incentives for kidney donation. *American Journal of Kidney Diseases.* 1997 Mar; 29(3): 410–418. 48 refs. BE57865.
age factors; *altruism; *attitudes; *blacks; *cadavers; chronically ill; *coercion; deontological ethics; *family members; females; *incentives; *indigents; *justice; *kidneys; males; morality; *organ donation; *patients; *remuneration; *renal dialysis; *risks and benefits; scarcity; social discrimination; *social impact; *socioeconomic factors; survey; third party consent; time factors; transplant recipients; utilitarianism; *whites; Ohio

Sells, Robert A. Consent for organ donation: what are the ethical principles? *Transplantation Proceedings.* 1993 Feb; 25(1): 39–41. 10 refs. BE56634.
altruism; body parts and fluids; cadavers; coercion; commodification; competence; developing countries; disclosure; family members; indigents; *informed consent; kidneys; legal aspects; *organ donation; *organ donors; presumed consent; *remuneration; risks and benefits; standards; third party consent; Great Britain

Sells, Robert A.; Ross, Lainie Friedman; Woodle, E. Steven, et al. Paired–kidney–exchange programs. [Letter and response]. *New England Journal of Medicine.* 1997 Nov 6; 337(19): 1392–1393. 6 refs. BE58426.
cadavers; directed donation; family members; incentives;

*kidneys; *legal aspects; *organ donation; *organ donors; *organ transplantation; public policy; *transplant recipients; *unrelated donors; *Great Britain

Sells, Robert A. The case against buying organs and a futures market in transplants. *Transplantation Proceedings.* 1992 Oct; 24(5): 2198–2202. 12 refs. BE56835.
*altruism; body parts and fluids; cadavers; coercion; commodification; *contracts; developing countries; *gifts; hospitals; *industry; international aspects; kidneys; legal aspects; minors; *organ donation; organ donors; parental consent; physicians; property rights; *public policy; *remuneration; scarcity; socioeconomic factors; terminally ill; third party consent; transplant recipients; ventilators; unrelated donors; Great Britain; India; Moore v. Regents of the University of California; United States; Western World

Sells, Robert A. Toward an affordable ethic. *Transplantation Proceedings.* 1992 Oct; 24(5): 2095–2096. 4 refs. Presented at the First International Congress on Transplantation in Developing Countries, Singapore, 29 Apr–3 May 1992. BE56806.
attitudes; developing countries; gifts; *kidneys; *organ donation; *organ donors; physicians; *regulation; *remuneration; social control; transplant recipients; *unrelated donors; *India

Sharp, Lesley A. Organ transplantation as a transformative experience: anthropological insights into the restructuring of the self. *Medical Anthropology Quarterly.* 1995 Sep; 9(3): 357–389. 113 refs. 18 fn. Commented on by M. Lock, p. 390–393, and by B.A. Koenig and L.F. Hogle, p. 393–397. BE56561.
*altruism; *anthropology; *attitudes; attitudes to death; *body parts and fluids; brain death; *cadavers; capitalism; *commodification; cultural pluralism; determination of death; disabled; economics; *emotions; *family members; *gifts; health personnel; *human body; metaphor; *organ donation; organ donors; *organ transplantation; *personhood; property rights; *psychological stress; *psychology; remuneration; scarcity; *self concept; social interaction; stigmatization; survey; third party consent; *transplant recipients; *values; ethnographic studies; Indiana; Mercy Memorial Hospital (Indianapolis); *United States

Siegler, Mark. Liver transplantation using living donors. *Transplantation Proceedings.* 1992 Oct; 24(5): 2223–2224. 2 refs. BE56843.
children; ethical review; infants; *livers; *organ donation; *organ donors; *organ transplantation; parents; program descriptions; *risk; *risks and benefits; surgery; therapeutic research; transplant recipients; *treatment outcome; University of Chicago

Silverman, Henry. The role of emotions in decisional competence, standards of competency, and altruistic acts. *Journal of Clinical Ethics.* 1997 Summer; 8(2): 171–175. 10 fn. Commentary on J. Spike, "What's love got to do with it? The altruistic giving of organs," p. 165–170. BE55954.
*altruism; case studies; clinical ethics committees; *competence; comprehension; decision making; *directed donation; *emotions; *ethics consultation; family relationship; *informed consent; kidneys; love; *mentally retarded; motivation; *organ donation; *organ donors; risks and benefits; standards; *unrelated donors

Simini, Bruno. Revolutionary swap of baby organs ends badly. [News]. *Lancet.* 1998 Feb 14; 351(9101): 503. BE58245.
*anencephaly; brain death; death; hearts; *newborns; *organ donation; *organ transplantation; transplant recipients; treatment outcome; Italy

Smith, Karen L.; Braslow, Judith B. Public attitudes toward organ and tissue donation. *In:* Chapman, Jeremy R.; Deierhoi, Mark; Wight, Celia, eds. Organ and Tissue Donation for Transplantation. New York, NY: Oxford University Press; 1997: 34–45. 18 refs. ISBN 0–340–61394–7. BE58228.
altruism; American Indians; Asian Americans; *attitudes; attitudes to death; blacks; body parts and fluids; communication; *cultural pluralism; determination of death; donor cards; empathy; family members; health education; health personnel; Hispanic Americans; hospitals; information dissemination; *knowledge, attitudes, practice; mass media; *minority groups; *organ donation; organ transplantation; presumed consent; professional family relationship; *public opinion; *public policy; religion; required request; scarcity; selection for treatment; *socioeconomic factors; third party consent; *tissue donation; transplant recipients; *trust; *values; withholding treatment; Uniform Anatomical Gift Act; United States

Spike, Jeffrey. What's love got to do with it? The altruistic giving of organs. *Journal of Clinical Ethics.* 1997 Summer; 8(2): 165–170. 4 fn. Commented on by H. Silverman, p. 171–175. BE55955.
*altruism; case studies; clinical ethics committees; *competence; comprehension; decision making; *directed donation; disclosure; *ethics consultation; family members; family relationship; *informed consent; kidneys; love; *mentally retarded; *organ donation; *organ donors; risks and benefits; self concept; *unrelated donors

Spital, Aaron. Do U.S. transplant centers encourage emotionally related kidney donation? *Transplantation.* 1996 Feb 15; 61(3): 374–377. 32 refs. BE56577.
*alternatives; altruism; cadavers; directed donation; emotions; family members; *friends; genetics; *hospitals; *institutional policies; *kidneys; *knowledge, attitudes, practice; *married persons; motivation; *organ donation; *organ donors; organ transplantation; risks and benefits; social interaction; survey; *transplant recipients; *unrelated donors; *United States

Spital, Aaron. Ethical and policy issues in altruistic living and cadaveric organ donation. *Clinical Transplantation.* 1997 Apr; 11(2): 77–87. 93 refs. BE57400.
advance directives; altruism; anencephaly; autonomy; beneficence; body parts and fluids; brain death; *cadavers; cardiac death; costs and benefits; decision making; family members; friends; informed consent; kidneys; mandatory programs; minors; mortality; motivation; newborns; *organ donation; *organ donors; paternalism; physicians; policy analysis; presumed consent; prolongation of life; risks and benefits; scarcity; terminally ill; transplant recipients; ventilators; withholding treatment; mandated choice; unrelated donors; Great Britain; Uniform Anatomical Gift Act; United States

Spital, Aaron L. Unrelated living donors: should they be used? *Transplantation Proceedings.* 1992 Oct; 24(5): 2215–2217. 22 refs. BE56840.
adults; *altruism; competence; friends; *hospitals; institutional policies; *kidneys; married persons; motivation; *organ donation; *organ donors; organ transplantation; *risks and benefits; self concept; transplant recipients; treatment outcome; volunteers; *unrelated donors; United States

Stempsey, William E. Paying people to give up their organs: the problem with commodification of body parts. *Medical Humanities Review.* 1996 Fall; 10(2): 45–55. 37 fn. BE56671.
altruism; *body parts and fluids; coercion; *commodification; dehumanization; disclosure; economics; human body; incentives; indigents; informed consent; international aspects; *justice; kidneys; motivation; *organ

donation; *organ donors; property rights; *remuneration; risk; social discrimination; transplant recipients

Stephenson, Joan. Ethics group drafts guidelines for control of genetic material and information. [News]. *JAMA.* 1998 Jan 21; 279(3): 184. BE58069.
  advisory committees; *confidentiality; disclosure; *DNA data banks; family members; *genetic information; *genetic materials; *genetic research; *guidelines; *international aspects; property rights; *tissue banks; *tissue donation; *biological specimen banks; *Ethical, Legal, and Social Issues Committee (HUGO-ELSI); *Human Genome Organization

Stevens, M.L. Tina. Redefining death in America, 1968. *Caduceus.* 1995 Winter; 11(3): 207-219. 41 fn. BE55530.
  allowing to die; *brain death; cadavers; *cardiac death; conflict of interest; *determination of death; hearts; historical aspects; human experimentation; killing; legal liability; motivation; *organ donation; organ transplantation; physicians; prolongation of life; public opinion; public policy; resuscitation; Roman Catholic ethics; standards; ventilators; withholding treatment; coma; Harvard Committee on Brain Death; Twentieth Century; United States

Strauss, Evelyn. The tissue issue: losing oneself to science? *Science News.* 1997 Sep 20; 152(12): 190-191. BE56635.
  *biomedical research; cadavers; confidentiality; consent forms; federal government; genetic research; government financing; government regulation; human experimentation; *informed consent; property rights; research ethics committees; time factors; *tissue banks; *tissue donation; United States

Sweden. Ministry of Health and Social Affairs. The Swedish Transplant Act. [Pamphlet]. Stockholm: Ministry of Health and Social Affairs; 1997. 52 p. Appendix: text of the Swedish Transplant Act 1995. BE57746.
  aborted fetuses; cadavers; economics; family members; *fetal tissue donation; informed consent; *legal aspects; legislation; mentally disabled; minors; *organ donation; organ donors; presumed consent; third party consent; tissue donation; *Sweden; *Transplant Act 1995 (Sweden)

Tedeschi, Christopher M. Foetal tissue transplantation research: scientific progress and the role of special interest groups. *Minerva.* 1995 Spring; 33(1): 45-66. 88 fn. BE57270.
  *aborted fetuses; abortion, induced; advisory committees; attitudes; federal government; *fetal research; *fetal tissue donation; *government financing; *government regulation; informed consent; investigators; legal aspects; mass media; moral policy; organizational policies; patient advocacy; *political activity; politics; pregnant women; professional organizations; *public policy; tissue transplantation; *Parkinson disease; American College of Obstetricians and Gynecologists; American Medical Association; *Department of Health and Human Services; Human Fetal Tissue Transplantation Research Panel; *National Institutes of Health; *United States

Teo, Bernard. Organ donation and transplantation: a Christian viewpoint. *Transplantation Proceedings.* 1992 Oct; 24(5): 2114-2115. 1 ref. Presented at the First International Congress on Transplantation in Developing Countries, Singapore, 29 Apr-3 May 1992. BE56815.
  accountability; altruism; cadavers; commodification; common good; developing countries; gifts; health personnel; human body; international aspects; justice; love; moral obligations; *organ donation; *organ transplantation; remuneration; resource allocation; *Roman Catholic ethics; selection for treatment

Thiel, G. Emotionally related living kidney donation: pro and contra. *Nephrology, Dialysis, Transplantation.* 1997 Sep; 12(9): 1820-1824. 35 refs. BE58223.
  beneficence; cadavers; coercion; gifts; health insurance reimbursement; international aspects; *kidneys; married persons; morbidity; mortality; *organ donation; *organ donors; patient advocacy; presumed consent; remuneration; *risks and benefits; scarcity; siblings; wedge argument; histocompatibility; *unrelated donors; *Europe

Toledo-Pereyra, Luis H. The problem of organ donation in minorities: some facts and incomplete answers. *Transplantation Proceedings.* 1992 Oct; 24(5): 2162-2164. 14 refs. BE56826.
  *attitudes; blacks; emotions; family members; Hispanic Americans; *minority groups; *organ donation; physicians; religion; selection for treatment; statistics; transplant recipients; trust; whites; Los Angeles; Miami; New York City

Toma, Tudor P. Romania adopts new transplant law. [News]. *BMJ (British Medical Journal).* 1997 Jun 21; 314(7097): 1784. BE55833.
  body parts and fluids; brain death; cadavers; criminal law; donor cards; informed consent; *legal aspects; minors; *organ donation; organ donors; parental consent; religion; remuneration; tissue banks; *Romania

Tomlinson, Tom. Inducements for donation: benign incentives or risky business? *Transplantation Proceedings.* 1992 Oct; 24(5): 2204-2206. 6 refs. BE56837.
  altruism; cadavers; contracts; dehumanization; economics; family members; *incentives; informed consent; morality; motivation; *organ donation; organ donors; *remuneration; risk; socioeconomic factors; third party consent; transplant recipients; United States

Torraco, Stephen F. Veritatis Splendor and the ethics of organ transplants. *Linacre Quarterly.* 1997 May; 64(2): 52-57. 4 refs. BE55619.
  altruism; *morality; motivation; *organ donation; *organ donors; *Roman Catholic ethics; self concept; theology

Turcotte, Jeremiah G. Supply, demand, and ethics of organ procurement: the medical perspective. *Transplantation Proceedings.* 1992 Oct; 24(5): 2140-2142. 7 refs. BE56821.
  body parts and fluids; indigents; *organ donation; *organ transplantation; patient advocacy; physician's role; scarcity; statistics; treatment outcome; withholding treatment; United States

U.S. Court of Appeals, Sixth Circuit. Brotherton v. Cleveland. *Federal Reporter, 2d Series.* 1991 Jan 18 (date of decision). 923: 477-484. BE56742.
  body parts and fluids; *cadavers; constitutional law; *due process; *family members; federal government; hospitals; *legal aspects; legislation; *organ donation; *property rights; state government; *third party consent; corneas; *Brotherton v. Cleveland; Fourteenth Amendment; Ohio; Uniform Anatomical Gift Act
The U.S. Court of Appeals for the Sixth Circuit reversed the lower trial court and allowed a decedent's family to pursue a claim under the federal constitution for wrongful removal of the decedent's corneas. The hospital had documented Deborah Brotherton's refusal of any anatomical gift from her husband's body, but it failed to notify the coroner of her wishes. Furthermore, the coroner did not inquire about any objection to anatomical gifts before allowing an eyebank technician to remove Steven Brotherton's corneas. Deborah Brotherton alleged wrongful deprivation of property under the due process clause. Based on state law

---

BE = bioethics accession number   fn. = footnotes   refs. = references

allowing her a possessory right to the body, a right to control disposition of the body, and a claim for mishandling of the body, the court found the interest of the wife as next of kin in her dead husband's body to be substantial, and thus protected by the Fourteenth Amendment, even if it is not a property interest or quasi-property interest. (KIE abstract)

U.S. General Accounting Office. NIH-Funded Research: Therapeutic Human Fetal Tissue Transplantation Projects Meet Federal Requirements. Report to the Chairmen and Ranking Minority Members, Committee on Labor and Human Resources, U.S. Senate, and Committee on Commerce, House of Representatives. Washington, DC: U.S. General Accounting Office; 1997 Mar. 8 p. 6 fn. GAO/HEHS-97-61. BE58135.
    *aborted fetuses; abortion, induced; donors; federal government; *fetal research; *fetal tissue donation; *government financing; *government regulation; guidelines; human experimentation; informed consent; investigators; research institutes; therapeutic research; tissue transplantation; transplant recipients; *guideline adherence; NIH Guidelines; NIH Revitalization Act 1993; *United States

United Methodist Church. Faithful Witness on Today's Issues: Genetic Science. [Pamphlet]. Washington, DC: General Board of Church and Society; 1992. 23 p. Includes General Conference resolutions on genetic science adopted 1992, and on organ and tissue donation adopted 1984. BE57388.
    Christian ethics; clergy; confidentiality; ecology; education; gene therapy; genes; genetic information; *genetic intervention; genetic research; genetic screening; genetic services; genome mapping; *organ donation; *organizational policies; patents; property rights; *Protestant ethics; public participation; public policy; resource allocation; risks and benefits; social impact; *tissue donation; agriculture; *Methodist Church; United States

United Network for Organ Sharing (UNOS). Ethics Committee. Ethics of organ transplantation from living donors. *Transplantation Proceedings.* 1992 Oct; 24(5): 2236-2237. 5 refs. BE56845.
    altruism; autonomy; beneficence; children; coercion; compensation; directed donation; *family members; *guidelines; hospitals; informed consent; moral policy; *organ donation; *organ donors; organ transplantation; organizational policies; parents; prisoners; risk; *risks and benefits; transplant recipients; treatment outcome; utilitarianism; *unrelated donors; *United Network for Organ Sharing; *United States

Valderrábano, Fernando. Cadaver transplantation as an ethical and cost-effective alternative to living donor transplantation: the Spanish experience. *Transplantation Proceedings.* 1992 Oct; 24(5): 2103-2105. 3 refs. Presented at the First International Congress on Transplantation in Developing Countries, Singapore, 29 Apr-3 May 1992. BE56811.
    brain death; *cadavers; costs and benefits; economics; education; family members; kidneys; legal aspects; *organ donation; organ donors; *organ transplantation; presumed consent; public opinion; public policy; quality of life; renal dialysis; statistics; technical expertise; third party consent; National Transplant Organization (Spain); *Spain

Veatch, Robert M., ed. Ethical issues in the changing health care system. *In:* Jonsen, Albert R.; Veatch, Robert M.; Walters, LeRoy, eds. Source Book in Bioethics: A Documentary History. Washington, DC: Georgetown University Press; 1998: 407-504. 8 fn. ISBN 0-87840-683-2. BE57894.

advance directives; advisory committees; aliens; autonomy; body parts and fluids; cadavers; competence; *confidentiality; dangerousness; disclosure; *duty to warn; federal government; historical aspects; *informed consent; legal aspects; mentally ill; model legislation; *organ donation; organ donors; *organ transplantation; patient care; patients' rights; physician patient relationship; remuneration; selection for treatment; *third party consent; tissue donation; transplant recipients; *Canterbury v. Spence; National Organ Transplant Act 1984; President's Commission for the Study of Ethical Problems; *Tarasoff v. Regents of the University of California; *Task Force on Organ Transplantation; *Twentieth Century; *Uniform Anatomical Gift Act; *United States

Virnig, Beth A.; Caplan, Arthur L. Required request: what difference has it made? *Transplantation Proceedings.* 1992 Oct; 24(5): 2155-2158. 10 refs. BE56824.
    *administrators; attitudes; cadavers; communication; education; evaluation studies; family members; federal government; health personnel; *hospitals; institutional policies; *legislation; medical records; *organ donation; physicians; public policy; *required request; *social impact; state government; survey; third party consent; *tissue donation; corneas; refusal to donate; Minneapolis; National Organ Transplant Act 1984; Pittsburgh; United States

Wade, Nicholas. Scientists cultivate cells at root of human life: hope for transplants and gene therapy -- ethics at issue. [News]. *New York Times.* 1998 Nov 6: A1, A24. BE59031.
    aborted fetuses; cloning; embryo disposition; *embryo research; federal government; *fetal tissue donation; gene therapy; government financing; government regulation; industry; investigators; private sector; risks and benefits; *stem cells; tissue transplantation; United States

Wadman, Meredith. 'Group debate' urged for gene studies. [News]. *Nature.* 1998 Jan 22; 391(6665): 314. BE57319.
    advisory committees; attitudes; *genetic research; *human experimentation; *informed consent; investigators; Jews; minority groups; *public participation; *public policy; risks and benefits; *tissue banks; *tissue donation; *population genetics; *National Bioethics Advisory Commission; United States

Walters, James W. What Is a Person? An Ethical Exploration. Urbana, IL: University of Illinois Press; 1997. 187 p. 344 fn. ISBN 0-252-02278-5. BE56192.
    allowing to die; *anencephaly; animal organs; animal rights; bioethics; brain death; *brain pathology; decision making; dementia; determination of death; Down syndrome; ethical theory; fetuses; human characteristics; legal aspects; moral obligations; *moral policy; *newborns; *organ donation; parents; patient care; persistent vegetative state; *personhood; philosophy; prolongation of life; public policy; religious ethics; risks and benefits; Roman Catholic ethics; secularism; *self concept; speciesism; *standards; theology; value of life; wedge argument; withholding treatment

Warwick, Ruth. Anonymity for unrelated bone marrow donors should remain. [Letter]. *BMJ (British Medical Journal).* 1997 Aug 30; 315(7107): 548-549. 3 refs. BE58224.
    *bone marrow; coercion; *confidentiality; directed donation; *donors; *privacy; retreatment; risks and benefits; siblings; *tissue donation; *unrelated donors; Great Britain

Weir, Robert F. Differing perspectives on consent, choice and control. *In:* Knoppers, Bartha Maria, ed. Human DNA: Law and Policy: International and Comparative Perspectives. Proceedings of the First International Conference on DNA Sampling and Human Genetic Research: Ethical, Legal, and Policy Aspects, held in

---

BE = bioethics accession number   fn. = footnotes   refs. = references

Montreal, Canada, 6–8 Sep 1996. Boston, MA: Kluwer Law International; 1997: 91–107. 31 fn. ISBN 90–411–0361–9. BE58170.
> attitudes; confidentiality; consent forms; *disclosure; *DNA data banks; donors; federal government; *genetic information; *genetic materials; *genetic research; genetic screening; government regulation; guidelines; *informed consent; model legislation; privacy; professional organizations; research ethics committees; *tissue banks; *tissue donation; *biological specimen banks; American College of Medical Genetics; American Society of Human Genetics; Centers for Disease Control and Prevention; Genetic Privacy Act; National Center for Human Genome Research; *United States

Weiss, Rick. Demand for organs fosters aggressive collection methods. [News]. *Washington Post.* 1997 Nov 24: A1, A16. BE55949.
> body parts and fluids; brain death; *cadavers; cardiac death; determination of death; drugs; family members; legal aspects; *organ donation; presumed consent; scarcity; statistics; terminally ill; third party consent; District of Columbia; United States

Werber, Stephen J. Ancient answers to modern questions: death, dying, and organ transplants -- a Jewish law perspective. *Journal of Law and Health.* 1996–1997; 11(1–2): 13–44. 139 fn. BE57589.
> *active euthanasia; *allowing to die; *assisted suicide; brain death; cadavers; chronically ill; *determination of death; hearts; *Jewish ethics; killing; *organ donation; organ donors; organ transplantation; physicians; *resuscitation orders; right to die; *suicide; terminally ill; tissue donation; treatment refusal; value of life; withholding treatment; Orthodox Judaism

Wise, Jacqui. Japan to allow organ transplants. [News]. *BMJ (British Medical Journal).* 1997 May 3; 314(7090): 1298. BE55928.
> attitudes; *brain death; *determination of death; *legal aspects; legislation; *organ donation; organ transplantation; *Japan

Youngner, Stuart J. Psychological impediments to procurement. *Transplantation Proceedings.* 1992 Oct; 24(5): 2159–2161. 3 refs. BE56825.
> allowing to die; *attitudes; body parts and fluids; brain death; cadavers; determination of death; *emotions; historical aspects; *human body; indigents; killing; medical education; motivation; *organ donation; physicians; prisoners; psychology; religion; scarcity; terminology; trust; uncertainty; *refusal to donate; Great Britain; Nineteenth Century

A ban on cells that could heal. [Editorial]. *New York Times.* 1998 Nov 7: 14. BE59094.
> aborted fetuses; embryo disposition; *embryo research; federal government; fetal tissue donation; government financing; *government regulation; industry; private sector; *stem cells; *tissue donation; tissue transplantation; *United States

Chinese deny organ trafficking. [News]. *Lancet.* 1998 Mar 28; 351(9107): 967. BE58742.
> cadavers; capital punishment; misconduct; *organ donation; *physicians; *prisoners; professional organizations; remuneration; *China; *Chinese Medical Association

Chinese doctors speak out against forced organ donation. [News]. *BMJ (British Medical Journal).* 1998 Mar 28; 316(7136): 956. BE58003.
> cadavers; capital punishment; international aspects; legal aspects; misconduct; *organ donation; *organizational policies; *physicians; *prisoners; professional organizations; remuneration; *China; *Chinese Medical Association; World

Medical Association

Guidelines are urged in using organs of heart–dead patients. [News]. *New York Times.* 1997 Dec 21: 38. BE56776.
> allowing to die; brain death; cadavers; *cardiac death; family members; federal government; *guidelines; *organ donation; public policy; third party consent; time factors; withholding treatment; Department of Health and Human Services; Institute of Medicine; United States

Jack Kevorkian. [News; title supplied]. *BMJ (British Medical Journal).* 1997 Nov 1; 315(7116): 1116. BE57342.
> *assisted suicide; cadavers; hearts; *organ donation; physicians; lungs; *Kevorkian, Jack

ORGAN AND TISSUE TRANSPLANTATION

See also ORGAN AND TISSUE DONATION

Abdulla, Sara. Xenotransplantation debate boils on. [News]. *Lancet.* 1997 Sep 20; 350(9081): 868. BE56081.
> *animal organs; communicable diseases; *organ transplantation; public health; *risk; risks and benefits; transgenic animals; transplant recipients; swine

Annas, George J. The dog and his shadow: a response to Overcast and Evans. *Law, Medicine and Health Care.* 1985 Jun; 13(3): 112–116, 129. 16 fn. BE56601.
> advisory committees; biomedical technologies; decision making; economics; federal government; government regulation; health care; hearts; hospitals; kidneys; legal aspects; livers; organ donation; *organ transplantation; *public policy; resource allocation; scarcity; state government; technology assessment; Massachusetts; *Massachusetts Task Force on Organ Transplantation; United States

Arnold, Robert M.; Shaw, Byers W.; Purtilo, Ruth. Acute, high risk patients: the case of transplantation. *In:* McCullough, Laurence B.; Jones, James W.; Brody, Baruch A., eds. Surgical Ethics. New York, NY: Oxford University Press; 1998: 97–115. 27 refs. ISBN 0–19–510347–5. BE58323.
> age factors; alcohol abuse; alternatives; body parts and fluids; *critically ill; disclosure; economics; hospitals; *informed consent; institutional policies; justice; livers; managed care programs; morbidity; mortality; organ donation; *organ transplantation; patients; *physicians; professional competence; prognosis; quality of health care; resource allocation; retreatment; risk; risks and benefits; scarcity; *selection for treatment; self induced illness; statistics; *surgery; time factors; treatment outcome; geographic factors; United Network for Organ Sharing; United States

Bach, F.H.; Fishman, J.A.; Daniels, N., et al. Uncertainty in xenotransplantation: individual benefit versus collective risk. *Nature Medicine.* 1998 Feb; 4(2): 141–144. 21 refs. BE57572.
> advisory committees; animal experimentation; *animal organs; communicable diseases; *decision making; guidelines; human experimentation; informed consent; *organ transplantation; public participation; public policy; regulation; risk; *risks and benefits; transgenic animals; transplant recipients; uncertainty; swine

Bach, Fritz H.; Fineberg, Harvey V. Call for moratorium on xenotransplants. [Letter]. *Nature.* 1998 Jan 22; 391(6665): 326. 4 refs. BE57769.
> *animal organs; biomedical research; communicable diseases; *government regulation; human experimentation; *organ transplantation; public health; public participation; public policy; *risk; tissue transplantation; *United States

Benjamin, Martin; Turcotte, Jeremiah G. Ethics,

alcoholism and liver transplantation. *In:* Lucey, Michael R.; Merion, Robert M.; Beresford, Thomas P., eds. Liver Transplantation and the Alcoholic Patient: Medical, Surgical and Psychosocial Issues. New York, NY: Cambridge University Press; 1994: 113–130. 12 refs. ISBN 0521–43332–0. BE56681.

accountability; *alcohol abuse; costs and benefits; disadvantaged; justice; *livers; moral obligations; *organ transplantation; patient compliance; preventive medicine; public policy; *resource allocation; scarcity; *selection for treatment; *self induced illness; social discrimination; stigmatization; *transplant recipients; treatment outcome; values; United States

Brown, Phyllida. Pig transplants 'should be banned.' [News]. *New Scientist.* 1997 Mar 1; 153(2071): 6. BE55649.

*animal organs; communicable diseases; federal government; guidelines; health hazards; *organ transplantation; *public policy; *risk; *swine; *Centers for Disease Control and Prevention; *Food and Drug Administration; *United States

Burd, Larry; Gregory, Jennifer M.; Kerbeshian, Jacob. The brain–mind quiddity: ethical issues in the use of human brain tissue for therapeutic and scientific purposes. *Journal of Medical Ethics.* 1998 Apr; 24(2): 118–122. 13 refs. BE58051.

animal experimentation; *biomedical research; *brain; brain death; computers; electrical stimulation of the brain; *emotions; ethical review; human body; human experimentation; informed consent; laboratories; models, theoretical; *organ donation; *organ transplantation; *personhood; regulation; *tissue donation; *tissue transplantation; cell lines; personal identity

The use of human brain tissue in neuroscience research is increasing. Recent developments include transplanting neural tissue, growing or maintaining neural tissue in laboratories and using surgically removed tissue for experimentation. Also, it is likely that in the future there will be attempts at partial or complete brain transplants. A discussion of the ethical issues of using human brain tissue for research and brain transplantation has been organized around nine broadly defined topic areas. Criteria for human brain tissue transplantation and laboratory use of brain tissue are proposed.

Burdick, James F.; Turcotte, Jeremiah G.; Veatch, Robert M. Principles of organ and tissue allocation and donation by living donors. [Foreword]. *Transplantation Proceedings.* 1992 Oct; 24(5): 2226. Foreword to the Report on Organ Allocation (p. 2227–2235) and Living Donors (p. 2236–2237) by the 1991 Ethics Committee of the United Network for Organ Sharing, Richmond, VA. BE56844.

committee membership; *ethics committees; *organ donation; *organ transplantation; organizational policies; *United Network for Organ Sharing; *United States

Butler, Declan. Last chance to stop and think on risks of xenotransplants. *Nature.* 1998 Jan 22; 391(6665): 320–324. Includes inset articles, "UK ahead in moves to regulate," p. 321; "Confronting the risks of 'xeno–havens'," p. 322; and "Primate risks 'still going unheeded'," p. 324. BE57768.

advisory committees; *animal organs; biomedical research; communicable diseases; decision making; federal government; financial support; *government regulation; guidelines; human experimentation; industry; international aspects; *organ transplantation; organizational policies; physicians; primates; public health; public participation; *public policy; *risk; risks and benefits; tissue transplantation; *transplant recipients; swine; American Society of Transplant Physicians; Centers for Disease

Control and Prevention; Europe; *Food and Drug Administration; Great Britain; National Institutes of Health; United States; World Health Organization; Xenotransplantation Interim Regulatory Authority (Great Britain)

Butler, Declan. Poll reveals backing for xenotransplants. [News]. *Nature.* 1998 Jan 22; 391(6665): 315. BE57767.

alternatives; *animal organs; attitudes; biomedical research; clergy; communicable diseases; drugs; human experimentation; information dissemination; investigators; knowledge, attitudes, practice; *organ transplantation; primates; public health; *public opinion; risk; statistics; transgenic animals; swine; European Union; *United States

Cantarovich, F. Legal aspects of transplantation in Argentina: a model to be considered for developing countries. *Transplantation Proceedings.* 1992 Oct; 24(5): 2123–2124. 4 refs. Presented at the First International Congress on Transplantation in Developing Countries, Singapore, 29 Apr–3 May 1992. BE56819.

body parts and fluids; brain death; cadavers; developing countries; family members; government financing; informed consent; *legal aspects; *organ donation; organ donors; *organ transplantation; *public policy; remuneration; selection for treatment; third party consent; unrelated donors; *Argentina

Capron, Alexander M. More blessed to give than to receive? *Transplantation Proceedings.* 1992 Oct; 24(5): 2185–2187. 5 refs. Commentary on J. Muyskens, p. 2181–2184. BE56833.

*altruism; cadavers; coercion; commodification; *organ donation; *organ donors; *organ transplantation; *public policy; refusal to treat; resource allocation; *selection for treatment; social worth; *transplant recipients; refusal to donate; United States

Chadwick, Ruth; Schüklenk, Udo. Organ transplants and donors. *In:* Chadwick, Ruth, ed. Encyclopedia of Applied Ethics, Volume 3. San Diego, CA: Academic Press; 1998: 393–398. 12 refs. ISBN 0–12–227068–1. BE56257.

animal organs; cadavers; coercion; determination of death; *organ donation; organ donors; *organ transplantation; personhood; presumed consent; religion; remuneration; self concept; transplant recipients

Cooper, D.K.C. Xenotransplantation: benefits, risks and regulation. *Annals of the Royal College of Surgeons of England.* 1996 Mar; 78(2): 92–96. BE55760.

advisory committees; AIDS; anencephaly; animal experimentation; *animal organs; body parts and fluids; bone marrow; communicable diseases; diabetes; economics; government regulation; health hazards; human experimentation; informed consent; intelligence; newborns; *organ donation; *organ transplantation; patient advocacy; peer review; persistent vegetative state; primates; public health; public opinion; *public policy; quality of life; *regulation; research ethics committees; resource allocation; risk; *risks and benefits; scarcity; speciesism; technical expertise; therapeutic research; *tissue donation; *tissue transplantation; transgenic animals; swine; Institute of Medicine; United States

Corley, Mary C.; Huff, Steven; Sayles, Linda, et al. Patient and nurse criteria for heart transplant candidacy. *Medsurg Nursing.* 1995 Jun; 4(3): 211–215. 20 refs. BE55712.

age factors; AIDS; alcohol abuse; aliens; *attitudes; behavior disorders; comparative studies; drug abuse; economics; family members; HIV seropositivity; mentally ill; mentally retarded; *nurses; *organ transplantation; patient compliance; *patients; prisoners; prognosis; resource allocation; *selection for treatment; *standards; survey;

*transplant recipients; United States

Daar, A.S. Ethics of xenotransplantation: animal issues, consent, and likely transformation of transplant ethics. *World Journal of Surgery.* 1997 Nov–Dec; 21(9): 975–982. 42 refs. BE58273.
    advisory committees; alternatives; animal experimentation; *animal organs; *animal rights; communicable diseases; conflict of interest; economics; federal government; gifts; *guidelines; human experimentation; industry; informed consent; *international aspects; medical devices; moral policy; organ donation; *organ transplantation; organizational policies; preventive medicine; primates; professional organizations; *public policy; religion; review; *risks and benefits; *social impact; transgenic animals; transplant recipients; swine; American Society of Transplant Physicians; Great Britain; Institute of Medicine; Public Health Service; Transplantation Society; United States; World Health Organization

Daar, A.S.; Salomon, Daniel R.; Ferguson, Ronald M., et al. Xenotransplants: proceed with caution. [Letters]. *Nature.* 1998 Mar 5; 392(6671): 11–12. 6 refs. BE57765.
    advisory committees; *animal organs; *attitudes; communicable diseases; consensus; government regulation; guidelines; *human experimentation; industry; information dissemination; *international aspects; mass media; *organ transplantation; organizational policies; physicians; professional organizations; public health; *public policy; *risk; risks and benefits; American Society of Transplant Physicians; American Society of Transplant Surgeons; European Union; Public Health Service; United States; World Health Organization

Daniels, Norman; Sabin, James E. Last chance therapies and managed care: pluralism, fair procedures, and legitimacy. *Hastings Center Report.* 1998 Mar–Apr; 28(2): 27–41. 19 fn. BE57541.
    accountability; autonomy; *biomedical technologies; *bone marrow; *breast cancer; cancer; case studies; communication; comparative studies; cultural pluralism; *decision making; democracy; *due process; females; government regulation; guidelines; health insurance; *health insurance reimbursement; historical aspects; industry; institutional policies; *justice; legal aspects; *managed care programs; *moral policy; paternalism; patient care; patients; physicians; policy analysis; political activity; *public participation; resource allocation; risks and benefits; state government; technology assessment; terminally ill; therapeutic research; *tissue transplantation; *investigational therapies; seriously ill; Aetna; Blue Cross-Blue Shield; Northern California Kaiser Permanente; Twentieth Century; United States

Dark, John H. Priorities for lung transplantation. *Lancet.* 1998 Jan 3; 351(9095): 4–5. 10 refs. BE57907.
    diagnosis; mortality; *organ transplantation; quality of life; *resource allocation; *selection for treatment; time factors; transplant recipients; *treatment outcome; *lungs; Great Britain

de Burgh, Jane. Saving our bacon: the new animal farm [review of *Pig in the Middle*: A UK national touring play, written by Judy Upton, directed by Nigel Town]. *Lancet.* 1998 Mar 28; 351(9107): 993. BE58568.
    *animal organs; animal rights; education; *information dissemination; kidneys; mass media; *organ donation; *organ transplantation; schools; transgenic animals; universities; swine; *Great Britain; *Pig in the Middle (Upton, J.)

DePalma, Judith A.; Townsend, Ricard. Ethical issues in organ donation and transplantation: are we helping a few at the expense of many? *Critical Care Nursing Quarterly.* 1996 May; 19(1): 1–9. 15 refs. BE55715.
    altruism; attitudes; autonomy; beneficence; body parts and fluids; cadavers; case studies; coercion; decision making; donor cards; family members; government regulation; health care reform; health personnel; HIV seropositivity; incentives; informed consent; justice; *organ donation; *organ transplantation; patient participation; physicians; presumed consent; public opinion; *public policy; remuneration; required request; resource allocation; risk; risks and benefits; scarcity; selection for treatment; standards; state government; third party consent; transplant recipients; United Network for Organ Sharing; United States

de Rave, Sjoerd. Allocation of donor organs. [Letter]. *Lancet.* 1997 Oct 11; 350(9084): 1107. 2 refs. BE58151.
    decision making; emergency care; *livers; *organ transplantation; *resource allocation; *selection for treatment; time factors; transplant recipients; Europe; Eurotransplant; France

Downie, Robin. Xenotransplantation. [Editorial]. *Journal of Medical Ethics.* 1997 Aug; 23(4): 205–206. 2 refs. BE55904.
    advisory committees; *animal organs; *animal rights; biomedical technologies; communicable diseases; costs and benefits; food; health hazards; *moral policy; *organ transplantation; public health; public policy; *risks and benefits; speciesism; suffering; transgenic animals; swine; Advisory Group on the Ethics of Xenotransplantation (Great Britain); Great Britain

Dyer, Clare. Doctors accused of refusing transplant on moral grounds. [News]. *BMJ (British Medical Journal).* 1997 May 10; 314(7091): 1370. BE55818.
    adolescents; behavior disorders; critically ill; decision making; *drug abuse; *livers; morality; *organ transplantation; patient compliance; *physicians; prognosis; *refusal to treat; *selection for treatment; social discrimination; transplant recipients; Edinburgh Royal Infirmary; *Great Britain; *Paul, Michelle; *Sanfey, Hilary

Eaton, Stephanie. The subtle politics of organ donation: a proposal. *Journal of Medical Ethics.* 1998 Jun; 24(3): 166–170. 13 fn. BE59113.
    *cadavers; decision making; *family members; moral obligations; motivation; obligations to society; *organ donation; *organ donors; *organ transplantation; *presumed consent; *resource allocation; *selection for treatment; *third party consent; *transplant recipients; treatment outcome; withholding treatment; *refusal to donate; *Great Britain; Jarvis, Rupert
Organs available for transplantation are scarce and valuable medical resources and decisions about who is to receive them should not be made more difficult by complicated calculations of desert. Consideration of likely clinical outcome must always take priority when allocating such a precious resource otherwise there is a danger of wasting that resource. However, desert may be a relevant concern in decision–making where the clinical risk is identical between two or more potential recipients of organs. Unlikely as this scenario is, such a decision procedure makes clear the interdependence of organ recipient and organ donor and hints at potential disadvantages for those who are willing to accept but unwilling to donate organs (free-riders). A combined opting–out and preference system weakens many of the objections to opting–out systems and may make the decision to donate organs on behalf of their deceased relatives easier for families.

Elli, M.; Valeri, M.; Pisani, F., et al. Developing countries as the major future source of living donor renal transplants. *Transplantation Proceedings.* 1992 Oct; 24(5): 2110–2111. 4 refs. Presented at the First International Congress on Transplantation in Developing Countries, Singapore, 29 Apr–3 May 1992. BE56813.

    BE = bioethics accession number   fn. = footnotes   refs. = references

cadavers; comparative studies; *developing countries; economics; family members; international aspects; *kidneys; morbidity; organ donation; *organ donors; *organ transplantation; prognosis; *remuneration; statistics; *transplant recipients; *treatment outcome; *unrelated donors; Europe; *Italy; United States

Englert, Yvon, ed. Organ and Tissue Transplantation in the European Union: Management of Difficulties and Health Risks Linked to Donors. Boston, MA: Martinus Nijhoff; sold and distributed in the U.S. and Canada by Kluwer Academic Publishers; 1995. 202 p. 180 refs. ISBN 0-7923-3051-X. BE56196.
   aborted fetuses; accountability; altruism; autonomy; body parts and fluids; cadavers; cancer; children; communicable diseases; communication; computer communication networks; donor cards; donors; fetal tissue donation; government regulation; health personnel; information dissemination; informed consent; *international aspects; misconduct; moral obligations; *organ donation; organ donors; *organ transplantation; organization and administration; presumed consent; *public policy; remuneration; risk; risks and benefits; scarcity; selection for treatment; standards; tissue banks; *tissue donation; *tissue transplantation; trends; mandated choice; Eastern Europe; *Europe; *European Union; Eurotransplant; Spain; Titmuss, Richard; Transplant European Computer Network

Felten, David L. Cell transplantation and research design. [Letter]. *Science.* 1994 Mar 18; 263(5153): 1546. 2 refs. BE56222.
   aged; *brain; central nervous system diseases; control groups; fetal research; fetal tissue donation; *human experimentation; informed consent; *placebos; random selection; *research design; *surgery; *tissue transplantation; Parkinson disease; *sham surgery

Field, Howard L. Organ allocation. [Letter; title supplied]. *Journal of Clinical Ethics.* 1997 Summer; 8(2): 208. BE57254.
   *alcohol abuse; critically ill; *decision making; depressive disorder; *drug abuse; *livers; *organ transplantation; *patient compliance; psychiatric diagnosis; referral and consultation; *refusal to treat; *resource allocation; *selection for treatment; *self induced illness; socioeconomic factors; *suicide; *transplant recipients

Fishman, Rachelle H.B. Israel proposes kidney swap to increase live donors for transplantation. [News]. *Lancet.* 1998 Mar 7; 351(9014): 735. BE58885.
   *directed donation; *family members; *incentives; *kidneys; *organ donation; *organ donors; *organ transplantation; public policy; *transplant recipients; *Israel

Fluss, Sev S. Legal aspects of transplantation: emerging trends in international action and national legislation. *Transplantation Proceedings.* 1992 Oct; 24(5): 2121-2122. 4 refs. Presented at the First International Congress on Transplantation in Developing Countries, Singapore, 29 Apr-3 May 1992. BE56818.
   body parts and fluids; guidelines; *international aspects; *legal aspects; legislation; *organ donation; *organ transplantation; organizational policies; professional organizations; public policy; regulation; remuneration; Council of Europe; World Health Assembly; World Health Organization

Glannon, Walter. Responsibility, alcoholism, and liver transplantation. *Journal of Medicine and Philosophy.* 1998 Feb; 23(1): 31-49. 40 refs. BE57519.
   accountability; *alcohol abuse; *autonomy; disease; drug abuse; *genetic determinism; *genetic predisposition; health care; *justice; *livers; moral obligations; *moral policy; *organ transplantation; patients; psychoactive drugs; *resource allocation; scarcity; *selection for treatment; *self

induced illness; transplant recipients; life style
Many believe that it is morally wrong to give lower priority for a liver transplant to alcoholics with end-stage liver disease than to patients whose disease is not alcohol-related. Presumably, alcoholism is a disease that results from factors beyond one's control and therefore one cannot be causally or morally responsible for alcoholism or the liver failure that results from it. Moreover, giving lower priority to alcoholics unfairly singles them out for the moral vice of heavy drinking. I argue that the etiology of alcoholism may involve enough control for the alcoholic to be responsible for his condition and accordingly have a weaker claim to receive a new liver than someone who acquires the disease through no fault of his own. In addition, I show why it is more plausible to reframe the question of priority in terms of control and responsibility rather than virtue and vice. Given that medical resources like livers are scarce, some people may justifiably be given lower priority than others in receiving these resources.

Golden, Frederic. Cock-a-doodle quail. [News]. *Time.* 1997 Mar 17; 149(11): 60. BE58042.
   *animal experimentation; *brain; embryo research; *embryos; *tissue transplantation; *animal behavior; Balaban, Evan; Neurosciences Institute (San Diego, CA)

Goldstein, Amy. Woman alleges fiancé stole her heart, brother's kidney. [News]. *Washington Post.* 1997 Oct 21: A1, A10-A11. BE55947.
   *deception; *directed donation; family members; incentives; *kidneys; *organ donation; *organ donors; *organ transplantation; *transplant recipients; unrelated donors; Dahl, John; *McNutt, Richard; Minnesota; Zauhar, Dorothy

Great Britain. Department of Health. Advisory Group on the Ethics of Xenotransplantation (Chair: Ian Kennedy). Animal Tissue into Humans: A Report by the Advisory Group on the Ethics of Xenotransplantation, 1996. London: Her Majesty's Stationery Office; 1997. 258 p. 92 fn. Appendixes include Glossary of terms; The consultation exercise; Report of the Workshop on Xenotransplantation and Infectious Disease; and Development of transgenic pigs. ISBN 0-11-321866-4. BE55999.
   advisory committees; alternatives; animal experimentation; *animal organs; animal rights; artificial organs; body parts and fluids; communicable diseases; ethical review; *evaluation; gene therapy; genetic intervention; *government regulation; *guidelines; health promotion; *human experimentation; informed consent; international aspects; legal aspects; organ donation; *organ transplantation; preventive medicine; primates; private sector; public health; *public policy; public sector; research ethics committees; resource allocation; *risks and benefits; scarcity; selection of subjects; suffering; therapeutic research; *tissue transplantation; *transgenic animals; swine; Advisory Group on the Ethics of Xenotransplantation (Great Britain); Animals (Scientific Procedures) Act 1986; Department of Health (Great Britain); *Great Britain

Great Britain. Isle of Man. An act (Chapter No. 3) to prohibit commercial dealings in human organs intended for transplanting; to prohibit the transplanting of such organs between persons who are not genetically related; and for connected purposes. Dated 16 March 1993. (The Human Organ Transplants Act 1993). *International Digest of Health Legislation.* 1996; 47(2): 169-170. BE57187.
   advertising; body parts and fluids; cadavers; directed donation; *legal aspects; *organ donation; organ donors; *organ transplantation; remuneration; transplant recipients;

BE = bioethics accession number   fn. = footnotes   refs. = references

*Great Britain; *Human Organ Transplants Act 1993 (Isle of Man); *Isle of Man

Grover, Bonnie Kae. From both sides now: informed consent, organ transplantation, and family-based disclosure. *Law and Policy.* 1995 Apr; 17(2): 188-209. 66 refs. 26 fn. Commented on by S. Wear and G. Logue, p. 210-216. BE58238.
autonomy; coercion; communicable diseases; decision making; disadvantaged; *disclosure; drugs; economics; *family members; *family relationship; hearts; *informed consent; *legal aspects; *organ transplantation; patient care; physician patient relationship; physicians; privacy; professional family relationship; risk; risks and benefits; social dominance; third party consent; toxicity; *transplant recipients

Gutmann, Thomas; Land, Walter. The ethics of organ allocation: the state of debate. *Transplantation Reviews.* 1997 Oct; 11(4): 191-207. 170 refs. BE58882.
age factors; *body parts and fluids; cadavers; decision making; deontological ethics; ethical theory; international aspects; *justice; *moral policy; organ donation; organ donors; *organ transplantation; public policy; quality of life; random selection; remuneration; *resource allocation; retreatment; review; scarcity; *selection for treatment; self induced illness; social discrimination; social worth; time factors; transplant recipients; utilitarianism; geographic factors; Europe; United States

Haberal, Mehmet; Altaca, G.; Tokyay, R., et al. Ethics in organ procurement in Turkey. *Transplantation Proceedings.* 1992 Oct; 24(5): 2100-2101. 7 refs. Presented at the First International Congress on Transplantation in Developing Countries, Singapore, 29 Apr-3 May 1992. BE56809.
brain death; family members; informed consent; legal aspects; *organ donation; organ donors; *organ transplantation; public policy; remuneration; scarcity; third party consent; unrelated donors; *Turkey

Hagihara, Akihito; Murakami, Masayoshi; Miller, Alan S., et al. Association between attitudes toward health promotion and opinions regarding organ transplants in Japan. *Health Policy.* 1997 Nov; 42(2): 157-170. 30 refs. BE57982.
*attitudes; *health promotion; *organ transplantation; preventive medicine; *public opinion; resource allocation; *self induced illness; survey; transplant recipients; *Japan

Hardy, K.J.; Milton, P.; Derham, P., et al. Attitudes towards liver transplantation in Victoria, Australia. *Australian and New Zealand Journal of Surgery.* 1993 Jul; 63(7): 520-524. 22 refs. BE55555.
*attitudes; family practice; *government financing; health care delivery; *knowledge, attitudes, practice; *livers; *organ transplantation; *physicians; *public opinion; *resource allocation; state government; survey; *Australia; *Victoria

Higgins, R.M.; West, N.; Edmunds, M.E., et al. Effect of a strict HLA matching policy on distribution of cadaveric kidney transplants to Indo-Asian and white European recipients: regional study. *BMJ (British Medical Journal).* 1997 Nov 22; 315(7119): 1354-1355. 3 refs. BE56553.
*cadavers; comparative studies; evaluation studies; *institutional policies; *kidneys; *minority groups; organ donation; *organ transplantation; renal dialysis; *resource allocation; *selection for treatment; *whites; *HLA matching; Great Britain

Hobbs, M. Nielsen. US Public Health Service sets out plan for xenotransplantation. [News]. *Lancet.* 1998 Jan 31; 351(9099): 343. BE58019.
advisory committees; *animal organs; data banks; federal government; *government regulation; guidelines; human experimentation; *organ transplantation; public policy; registries; tissue banks; transplant recipients; National Xenotransplantation Advisory Committee; *Public Health Service; *United States

Hughes, Jonathan. Xenografting: ethical issues. *Journal of Medical Ethics.* 1998 Feb; 24(1): 18-24. 25 fn. BE57408.
anencephaly; animal experimentation; *animal organs; animal rights; brain death; communicable diseases; genetic intervention; human experimentation; informed consent; mentally disabled; moral policy; newborns; organ donation; *organ transplantation; persistent vegetative state; presumed consent; public health; public policy; *risks and benefits; self concept; *social impact; therapeutic research; transplant recipients; nature; Great Britain
This paper considers the ethical issues raised by xenotransplantation under four headings: interfering with nature; effects on the recipient; effects on other humans; and effects on donor animals. The first two issues raise no insuperable problems: charges of unnaturalness are misguided, and the risks that xenotransplantation carries for the recipient are a matter for properly informed consent. The other two issues raise more serious problems, however, and it is argued that if we take seriously the risk of transferring new infectious agents from animal to human populations and the interests of donor animals, then a moratorium on xenotransplantation is called for. The paper finds that the recent Nuffield Council and Department of Health reports on xenotransplantation are insufficiently cautious in the conclusions that they draw from these considerations.

Indudhara, R.; Singh, S.K.; Minz, M. Opinion poll regarding knowledge, attitudes, and suggestions for developing a cadaver donor program. *Transplantation Proceedings.* 1992 Oct; 24(5): 2069. Presented at the First International Congress on Transplantation in Developing Countries, Singapore, 29 Apr-3 May 1992. BE56801.
brain death; *cadavers; family members; health education; *health personnel; hospitals; institutional policies; kidneys; *knowledge, attitudes, practice; legislation; *organ donation; *organ transplantation; patients; public policy; renal dialysis; scarcity; survey; treatment outcome; *India

Joralemon, Donald; Sharp, Lesley A. Authors' responses to commentaries. *Medical Anthropology Quarterly.* 1995 Sep; 9(3): 398-399. BE56590.
anthropology; cadavers; gifts; health personnel; *organ donation; *organ transplantation; self concept; socioeconomic factors; transplant recipients

Joralemon, Donald. Organ wars: the battle for body parts. *Medical Anthropology Quarterly.* 1995 Sep; 9(3): 335-356. 98 refs. 25 fn. Commented on by M. Lock, p. 390-393, and by B.A. Koenig and L.F. Hogle, p. 393-397. BE56581.
altruism; *anthropology; *attitudes; attitudes to death; autonomy; *body parts and fluids; brain death; *cadavers; *commodification; *cultural pluralism; determination of death; *economics; *emotions; family members; *gifts; *human body; *incentives; international aspects; legal aspects; mass media; metaphor; *organ donation; organ donors; *organ transplantation; *personhood; *property rights; *psychological stress; *psychology; public opinion; *remuneration; scarcity; *self concept; third party consent; *transplant recipients; *values; *United States

Kazim, E.; al-Rukaimi, M.; Fernandez, H., et al. Buying a kidney: the easy way out? *Transplantation Proceedings.* 1992 Oct; 24(5): 2112-2113. 4 refs. Presented at the First International Congress on Transplantation

---

BE = bioethics accession number   fn. = footnotes   refs. = references

in Developing Countries, Singapore, 29 Apr–3 May 1992. BE56814.

*developing countries; *kidneys; morbidity; mortality; *organ donation; *organ donors; *organ transplantation; *remuneration; statistics; *transplant recipients; *treatment outcome; follow–up studies; *unrelated donors; India; Rashid Hospital (United Arab Emirates); United Arab Emirates

Koenig, Barbara A.; Hogle, Linda F. Organ transplantation (re)examined? Commentary. *Medical Anthropology Quarterly.* 1995 Sep; 9(3): 393–397. 17 refs. 2 fn. Commentary on D. Joralemon, p. 335–356, and on L.A. Sharp, p. 357–389. BE56468.

anthropology; attitudes; bioethics; biomedical technologies; body parts and fluids; cadavers; family members; gifts; health personnel; interdisciplinary communication; *organ donation; organ donors; *organ transplantation; personhood; self concept; social sciences; socioeconomic factors; transplant recipients

Langston, J. William; Palfreman, Jon. The Case of the Frozen Addicts: Working at the Edge of the Mysteries of the Human Brain. New York, NY: Vintage Books; 1996. 309 p. ISBN 0–678–74708–7. BE56698.

*aborted fetuses; animal experimentation; biomedical research; *brain; *brain pathology; diagnosis; disadvantaged; *drug abuse; federal government; *fetal research; *fetal tissue donation; government financing; *heroin; human experimentation; international aspects; interprofessional relations; *investigators; moral complicity; *paralysis; patients; primates; research institutes; research subjects; risks and benefits; selection of subjects; therapeutic research; *tissue transplantation; *toxicity; *Parkinson disease; Human Fetal Tissue Transplantation Research Panel; *Langston, J. William; Lindvall, Olle; National Institutes of Health; Sweden; United States

Lock, Margaret. Transcending mortality: organ transplants and the practice of contradictions: commentary. *Medical Anthropology Quarterly.* 1995 Sep; 9(3): 390–393. Commentary on D. Joralemon, p. 335–356, and on L.A. Sharp, p. 357–389. BE56560.

anthropology; *attitudes; attitudes to death; body parts and fluids; cadavers; Down syndrome; emotions; mentally retarded; organ donation; *organ transplantation; resource allocation; selection for treatment; self concept; transplant recipients; Canada

Lucey, Michael R.; Beresford, Thomas P. Ethical considerations regarding orthotopic liver transplantation for alcoholic patients. *In:* Shelton, Wayne N.; Edwards, Rem B., eds. Advances in Bioethics. Volume 3: Values, Ethics, and Alcoholism. Greenwich, CT: JAI Press; 1997: 119–129. 33 refs. ISBN 0–7623–0219–4. BE57635.

accountability; *alcohol abuse; autonomy; beneficence; disclosure; disease; justice; *livers; moral obligations; *moral policy; obligations to society; *organ transplantation; patient compliance; patients; physicians; *prognosis; *public policy; referral and consultation; refusal to treat; *resource allocation; retreatment; risks and benefits; scarcity; *selection for treatment; *self induced illness; social discrimination; transplant recipients; treatment outcome; Great Britain

Maiorca, Rosario; Maggiore, Quirino; Mordacci, Roberto, et al. Ethical problems in dialysis and transplantation. *Nephrology, Dialysis, Transplantation.* 1996; 11(Suppl. 9): 100–112. BE57965.

age factors; aliens; allowing to die; cultural pluralism; decision making; developing countries; directed donation; economics; health care delivery; international aspects; *kidneys; organ donation; organ donors; *organ transplantation; physicians; professional autonomy; prolongation of life; quality of life; *renal dialysis; resource allocation; selection for treatment; treatment refusal;

withholding treatment; Europe; Great Britain; India; *Italy; United States

Marsh, J. Wallis; Dvorchik, Igor; Casavilla, Adrian, et al. Should reimbursement be denied for liver transplantation in patients with hepatocellular carcinoma? [Letter]. *JAMA.* 1997 Jul 16; 278(3): 203–205. 4 refs. BE55898.

*cancer; comparative studies; diagnosis; federal government; *government financing; *health insurance reimbursement; *livers; mortality; *organ transplantation; selection for treatment; treatment outcome; *Medicare; United States

Marshall, Patricia A. Boundary crossings: gender and power in clinical ethics consultations. *In:* Sargent, Carolyn F.; Brettell; Caroline B., eds. Gender and Health: An International Perspective. Upper Saddle River, NJ: Prentice Hall; 1996: 205–226. 88 refs. 5 fn. ISBN 0–13–079427–9. BE58097.

case studies; clinical ethics; *communication; *critically ill; *decision making; dissent; *ethicist's role; *ethics consultation; family members; family relationship; *females; *feminist ethics; futility; *narrative ethics; *organ transplantation; patient care team; patient transfer; *professional patient relationship; prognosis; psychological stress; *retreatment; self concept; social dominance; time factors; *uncertainty; values; sick role; Loyola University of Chicago Medical Center

Martin, Douglas K.; Singer, Peter A.; Siegler, Mark. Ethical considerations in liver transplantation. *In:* Boyer, J.L.; Ockner, R.K., eds. Progress in Liver Diseases, Vol. XII. Philadelphia, PA: Saunders; 1994: 215–229. 101 fn. BE55799.

age factors; alcohol abuse; animal organs; body parts and fluids; brain death; cadavers; cardiac death; determination of death; family members; informed consent; justice; *livers; *organ donation; organ donors; *organ transplantation; presumed consent; public policy; remuneration; required request; resource allocation; risks and benefits; scarcity; selection for treatment; therapeutic research; transplant recipients; United Network for Organ Sharing; United States

Mendez, R.; Aswad, S.; Dessouki, A., et al. Difficulties of foreigners seeking transplantation in the United States. *Transplantation Proceedings.* 1992 Oct; 24(5): 2075–2076. 4 refs. Presented at the First International Congress on Transplantation in Developing Countries, Singapore, 29 Apr–3 May 1992. BE56802.

*aliens; developing countries; *organ transplantation; psychological stress; public opinion; public policy; scarcity; selection for treatment; socioeconomic factors; transplant recipients; United Network for Organ Sharing; *United States

Merriken, Karen; Overcast, Thomas D. Governmental regulation of heart transplantation and the right to privacy. *Journal of Contemporary Law.* 1985; 11(2): 481–514. 123 fn. BE56662.

abortion, induced; alternative therapies; biomedical technologies; *constitutional law; contraception; federal government; freedom; *government financing; *government regulation; health care; *hearts; hospitals; *legal aspects; *legal rights; *organ transplantation; *privacy; public policy; resource allocation; standards; state interest; Supreme Court decisions; Laetrile; Medicaid; Medicare; *United States

Miller, A.S.; Hagihara, A. Organ transplanting in Japan: the debate begins. *Public Health.* 1997 Nov; 111(6): 367–372. 29 refs. BE59011.

age factors; aliens; *attitudes; brain death; cadavers; determination of death; *organ donation; organ donors; *organ transplantation; prognosis; *public opinion; public participation; public policy; resource allocation; selection for treatment; self induced illness; survey; time factors; transplant recipients; *Japan

Mintz, Benjamin. Analyzing the OPTN [Organ Procurement and Transplant Network] under the state action doctrine -- can UNOS's organ allocation criteria survive strict scrutiny? *Columbia Journal of Law and Social Problems.* 1995 Spring; 28(3): 339-396. 276 fn. BE57197.
    *blacks; body parts and fluids; equal protection; federal government; financial support; government regulation; *kidneys; *legal aspects; legal rights; *organ transplantation; organizational policies; public policy; *resource allocation; *selection for treatment; *social discrimination; standards; state government; Supreme Court decisions; *transplant recipients; treatment outcome; voluntary programs; *histocompatibility; Department of Health and Human Services; *Organ Procurement and Transplant Network; Organ Procurement Organizations; *United Network for Organ Sharing; *United States

Mongoven, Ann. Federal hearings on liver transplant allocation and donation. *In:* BioLaw: A Legal and Ethical Reporter on Medicine, Health Care, and Bioengineering. Special Sections 2(12). Frederick, MD: University Publications of America; 1997 Dec: S:373-S:389. BE57643.
    cadavers; chronically ill; computers; conflict of interest; consensus; critically ill; *decision making; determination of death; federal government; government regulation; health facilities; health insurance; justice; *livers; models, theoretical; *organ donation; *organ transplantation; patient advocacy; physicians; prognosis; public participation; *public policy; *resource allocation; scarcity; *selection for treatment; transplant recipients; treatment outcome; geographic factors; *Department of Health and Human Services; *United Network for Organ Sharing; *United States

Morris, Peter J. Pig transplants postponed: until we know more about graft rejection, physiology, and infectivity. [Editorial]. *BMJ (British Medical Journal).* 1997 Jan 25; 314(7076): 242. 15 refs. BE58701.
    advisory committees; *animal organs; biomedical research; communicable diseases; government regulation; human experimentation; *organ transplantation; public policy; risk; transgenic animals; *swine; Advisory Group on the Ethics of Xenotransplantation (Great Britain); *Great Britain

Muyskens, James. Should receiving depend upon willingness to give? *Transplantation Proceedings.* 1992 Oct; 24(5): 2181-2184. 5 refs. Commented on by A.M. Capron, p. 2185-2187. BE56832.
    altruism; cadavers; *organ donation; *organ donors; *organ transplantation; *public policy; *refusal to treat; resource allocation; scarcity; *selection for treatment; *transplant recipients; *refusal to donate; United States

Neuberger, James; Lake, John. Allocating donor livers. [Editorial]. *BMJ (British Medical Journal).* 1997 Apr 19; 314(7088): 1140-1141. 6 refs. BE57163.
    adults; age factors; children; consensus; critically ill; decision making; hospitals; institutional policies; *livers; models, theoretical; *organ transplantation; organizational policies; physicians; prognosis; *resource allocation; scarcity; *selection for treatment; self induced illness; *standards; time factors; treatment outcome; *Great Britain; United Network for Organ Sharing; *United States

Neuberger, James; Adams, David; MacMaster, Paul, et al. Assessing priorities for allocation of donor liver grafts: survey of public and clinicians. *BMJ (British Medical Journal).* 1998 Jul 18; 317(7152): 172-175. 26 refs. BE58816.

*age factors; *alcohol abuse; *attitudes; comparative studies; *drug abuse; employment; family practice; *livers; medical specialties; *organ transplantation; *physicians; *prisoners; prognosis; *public opinion; *resource allocation; scarcity; *selection for treatment; *self induced illness; *social worth; survey; *time factors; transplant recipients; *treatment outcome; gastroenterology; *Great Britain
OBJECTIVES: To compare the priorities of the general public, family doctors, and gastroenterologists in allocating donor livers to potential recipients of liver allograft. DESIGN: Representative quota sampling of 1000 members of the general public and 200 family doctors, and a postal questionnaire of 100 gastroenterologists. SUBJECTS: Respondents were given eight hypothetical case histories (based on real patients) and asked to select recipients for four donor livers. Cases were selected to identify controversial areas such as extremes of age, misuse of alcohol, and intravenous drugs. Respondents were also asked to select the least deserving case and which of seven possible factors (time on waiting list, outcome, age, value to society, return to work, previous use of illicit drugs, and involvement of alcohol in the liver damage) should be used to select patients already listed for transplantation. Focus groups were also held to explore further the reasons for the choices given. RESULTS: There were considerable differences between the three groups in the choice of the recipients, although alcohol use and antisocial behaviour always rated low. For selection of recipients the general public thought that, in decreasing order of importance, age, outcome, and time on the waiting list were the most important factors in selecting recipients; family doctors rated outcome, age, and likely work status after transplantation and the gastroenterologists outcome, work status, and non-involvement of alcohol in the cause of the liver disease as the most important factors. CONCLUSIONS: The views of the public are at variance with those of clinicians. Further debate is required to ensure an equitable and appropriate distribution of a scarce resource.

Newman, Joel D. Ethics committee offers criteria. *UNOS Update.* 1997 Jan-Feb: 8. BE56234.
    age factors; ethics committees; *guidelines; *organ transplantation; organizational policies; patient compliance; prognosis; resource allocation; retreatment; *selection for treatment; self induced illness; *transplant recipients; *United Network for Organ Sharing; United States

Post, Stephen G. Baboon livers and the human good. *Archives of Surgery.* 1993 Feb; 128(2): 131-133. 18 refs. BE57549.
    *animal organs; ecology; *human characteristics; livers; moral policy; *organ transplantation; primates; self concept; *speciesism

Potts, Michael. Morals, metaphysics, and heart transplantation: reflections on Richard Selzer's "Whither Thou Goest". *Perspectives in Biology and Medicine.* 1998 Winter; 41(2): 212-223. 25 refs. 5 fn. BE59028.
    attitudes to death; bioethics; body parts and fluids; brain; *cadavers; *dehumanization; *emotions; *family members; *gifts; *hearts; *human body; literature; metaphor; *narrative ethics; *organ donation; *organ transplantation; personhood; *self concept; *transplant recipients; *personal identity; *Whither Thou Goest (Selzer, R.)

Provisional Commission for the Study on Brain Death and Organ Transplantation (Japan). Important Considerations with Respect to Brain Death and Organ Transplants, January 22, 1992. Tokyo: the Commission;

BE = bioethics accession number   fn. = footnotes   refs. = references

translation issued by the Osaka Kidney Foundation; 1994 Jun. 39 p. English version of a report submitted to the Prime Minister. BE58449.

advisory committees; *brain death; *cadavers; consensus; *determination of death; dissent; informed consent; *organ donation; *organ transplantation; personhood; physicians; public policy; resource allocation; *standards; transplant recipients; trust; *Japan; *Provisional Commission for the Study on Brain Death and Organ Transplantation (Japan)

Qunibi, Wajeh; Abulrub, Daad; Shaheen, Faisal, et al. Attitudes of commercial renal transplant recipients toward renal transplantation in India. *Clinical Transplantation.* 1995 Aug; 9(4): 317–321. 14 refs. BE57971.

aliens; *attitudes; blood transfusions; hospitals; informed consent; *international aspects; *kidneys; motivation; organ donors; *organ transplantation; physicians; quality of health care; *remuneration; survey; *transplant recipients; unrelated donors; *India; *Saudi Arabia

Sampson, Mark T. Revised liver policy approved. *UNOS Update.* 1997 Jan–Feb: 5–7. BE56237.

*guidelines; *livers; minors; *organ transplantation; organizational policies; public participation; *resource allocation; *selection for treatment; transplant recipients; liver diseases; *United Network for Organ Sharing; United States

Schmidt, Volker H. Selection of recipients for donor organs in transplant medicine. *Journal of Medicine and Philosophy.* 1998 Feb; 23(1): 50–74. 45 refs. 20 fn. BE57520.

age factors; aged; alcohol abuse; deception; *decision making; due process; guidelines; health facilities; hearts; *institutional policies; justice; *kidneys; livers; moral policy; *organ transplantation; organization and administration; patient admission; patient advocacy; patient compliance; *physicians; prognosis; random selection; referral and consultation; *resource allocation; scarcity; *selection for treatment; social worth; statistics; time factors; *transplant recipients; uncertainty; utilitarianism; values; histocompatibility; Europe; *Eurotransplant; *Germany

This paper deals with a problem which has received a great deal of attention in the ethical literature, but about which very little is known empirically: the selection of recipients for organs in transplant medicine. Based on a larger study, it is shown how this problem is practically resolved in one European country, Germany. It is demonstrated that most of the criteria used to determine recipients are non-medical in nature, even though they generally tend to be rationalized in medical terms. Moreover, the choice of criteria depends as much on prognostic considerations as on personal indiosyncrasies and values held by individual physicians who are in charge at the various programs. Several examples of the extremely diverse policies in which this results are presented.

Sekela, Michael; Berk, Martin R.; Gallagher, Eugene B., et al. Cardiac transplantation: costs and ethics. *Hospital Practice (Office Edition).* 1996 Feb 15; 31(2): 127–130, 133–134, 136, 139. 3 refs. BE57401.

attitudes; case studies; *costs and benefits; faculty; government financing; heart diseases; *hearts; indigents; *organ transplantation; physicians; public policy; *resource allocation; risks and benefits; selection for treatment; social sciences; socioeconomic factors; transplant recipients; Kentucky; Medicaid

Sharp, Lesley A. Organ transplantation as a transformative experience: anthropological insights into the restructuring of the self. *Medical Anthropology Quarterly.*

1995 Sep; 9(3): 357–389. 113 refs. 18 fn. Commented on by M. Lock, p. 390–393, and by B.A. Koenig and L.F. Hogle, p. 393–397. BE56561.

*altruism; *anthropology; *attitudes; attitudes to death; *body parts and fluids; brain death; *cadavers; capitalism; *commodification; cultural pluralism; determination of death; disabled; economics; *emotions; *family members; *gifts; health personnel; *human body; metaphor; *organ donation; organ donors; *organ transplantation; *personhood; property rights; *psychological stress; *psychology; remuneration; scarcity; *self concept; social interaction; stigmatization; survey; third party consent; *transplant recipients; *values; ethnographic studies; Indiana; Mercy Memorial Hospital (Indianapolis); *United States

Shelton, Wayne N. Justice and alcoholism. *In:* Shelton, Wayne N.; Edwards, Rem B., eds. Advances in Bioethics. Volume 3: Values, Ethics, and Alcoholism. Greenwich, CT: JAI Press; 1997: 131–152. 26 refs. ISBN 0–7623–0219–4. BE57636.

*accountability; *alcohol abuse; autonomy; behavior control; *behavior disorders; biomedical technologies; coercion; *common good; *disease; freedom; health care delivery; *justice; *libertarianism; *livers; mental health; *models, theoretical; moral obligations; *moral policy; *organ transplantation; paternalism; patient care; *patient compliance; *public policy; *refusal to treat; *resource allocation; rights; scarcity; *selection for treatment; *self induced illness; stigmatization; treatment outcome; United States

Siegler, Mark. Liver transplantation using living donors. *Transplantation Proceedings.* 1992 Oct; 24(5): 2223–2224. 2 refs. BE56843.

children; ethical review; infants; *livers; *organ donation; *organ donors; *organ transplantation; parents; program descriptions; *risk; *risks and benefits; surgery; therapeutic research; transplant recipients; *treatment outcome; University of Chicago

Simini, Bruno. Revolutionary swap of baby organs ends badly. [News]. *Lancet.* 1998 Feb 14; 351(9101): 503. BE58245.

*anencephaly; brain death; death; hearts; *newborns; *organ donation; *organ transplantation; transplant recipients; treatment outcome; Italy

Spike, Jeffrey. Iatrogenic liver failure, transplantation, and prisoners. *Journal of Clinical Ethics.* 1997 Winter; 8(4): 398–404. 5 fn. BE57615.

blacks; case studies; decision making; drug abuse; drugs; ethics consultation; *iatrogenic disease; indigents; justice; *livers; males; moral obligations; moral policy; *organ transplantation; patient advocacy; patient care team; patient compliance; *prisoners; refusal to treat; resource allocation; risks and benefits; scarcity; *selection for treatment; social worth; socioeconomic factors; treatment outcome; tuberculosis; New York City

Stolberg, Sheryl Gay. U.S. orders sickest to be given priority on donated organs. [News]. *New York Times.* 1998 Mar 27: A16. BE57737.

attitudes; federal government; *government regulation; hospitals; *organ transplantation; patient advocacy; *resource allocation; *selection for treatment; *standards; time factors; transplant recipients; geographic factors; severity of illness index; *Department of Health and Human Services; United Network for Organ Sharing; *United States

Teo, Bernard. Organ donation and transplantation: a Christian viewpoint. *Transplantation Proceedings.* 1992 Oct; 24(5): 2114–2115. 1 ref. Presented at the First International Congress on Transplantation in Developing Countries, Singapore, 29 Apr–3 May 1992. BE56815.

accountability; altruism; cadavers; commodification; common good; developing countries; gifts; health personnel; human body; international aspects; justice; love; moral obligations; *organ donation; *organ transplantation; remuneration; resource allocation; *Roman Catholic ethics; selection for treatment

Thomas, G.; Ryall, M.; Taber, S.M. Ethical dilemmas in transplantation. *Transplantation Proceedings.* 1992 Oct; 24(5): 2099. Presented at the First International Congress on Transplantation in Developing Countries, Singapore, 29 Apr–3 May 1992. BE56808.

animal organs; economics; government regulation; HIV seropositivity; minors; organ donation; organ donors; *organ transplantation; parents; prolongation of life; remuneration; scarcity; selection for treatment; transplant recipients; treatment refusal; unrelated donors; Great Britain

Turcotte, Jeremiah G. Supply, demand, and ethics of organ procurement: the medical perspective. *Transplantation Proceedings.* 1992 Oct; 24(5): 2140–2142. 7 refs. BE56821.

body parts and fluids; indigents; *organ donation; *organ transplantation; patient advocacy; physician's role; scarcity; statistics; treatment outcome; withholding treatment; United States

Turcotte, Jeremiah G. Transplantation: a frontier for bioethics and bioscience. *In:* Phillips, Michael G., ed. Organ Procurement, Preservation and Distribution in Transplantation. Second Edition. Richmond, VA: UNOS; 1996: 13–22. 27 refs. ISBN 1-886651-12-4. BE57999.

autonomy; beneficence; bioethics; costs and benefits; economics; ethics committees; justice; organ donation; *organ transplantation; public policy; resource allocation; selection for treatment; United Network for Organ Sharing; United States

Ubel, Peter A.; Loewenstein, George. Distributing scarce livers: the moral reasoning of the general public. *Social Science and Medicine.* 1996 Apr; 42(7): 1049–1055. 29 refs. BE56889.

age factors; *attitudes; children; costs and benefits; justice; *livers; *organ transplantation; prognosis; *public opinion; public policy; *resource allocation; scarcity; *selection for treatment; survey; *transplant recipients; treatment outcome; *values; Pennsylvania

The transplant system has been criticized for not paying enough attention to efficiency in distributing scarce organs. But little research has been done to see how the general public views tradeoffs between efficiency and equity. We surveyed members of the general public to see how they would distribute organs among patients with varying chances of benefiting from them. In addition, we asked subjects to explain their decisions and to tell us about any other information they would have liked in order to make the decisions. We found that the public places a very high value on giving everyone a chance at receiving scarce resources, even if that means a significant decrease in the chance that available organs will save people's lives. Our results raise important questions about whether the aims of outcomes research and cost-effective studies agree with the values of the general public.

Ubel, Peter A.; Loewenstein, George. Public perceptions of the importance of prognosis in allocating transplantable livers to children. *Medical Decision Making.* 1996 Jul–Sep; 16(3): 234–241. 24 refs. BE57978.

adults; *children; *decision making; justice; *livers; *organ transplantation; *prognosis; *public opinion; public policy; *resource allocation; *selection for treatment; survey;

treatment outcome; values; *Pennsylvania; United States

Ubel, Peter A.; DeKay, M.; Baron, J., et al. Public preferences for efficiency and racial equity in kidney transplant allocation decisions. *Transplantation Proceedings.* 1996 Oct; 28(5): 2997–3002. 24 refs. BE57979.

*blacks; decision making; justice; *kidneys; *organ transplantation; *prognosis; *public opinion; *resource allocation; *selection for treatment; socioeconomic factors; survey; time factors; transplant recipients; treatment outcome; *whites; histocompatibility; *Philadelphia; United States

Ubel, Peter A.; Loewenstein, George. The efficacy and equity of retransplantation: an experimental survey of public attitudes. *Health Policy.* 1995 Nov; 34(2): 145–151. 12 refs. BE56602.

*attitudes; justice; *livers; morality; mortality; *organ transplantation; *prognosis; *public opinion; public policy; *resource allocation; *retreatment; *selection for treatment; survey; *transplant recipients; Pennsylvania; United States

United Network for Organ Sharing (UNOS). Ethics Committee. General principles for allocating human organs and tissues. *Transplantation Proceedings.* 1992 Oct; 24(5): 2227–2235. 6 fn. BE56846.

age factors; *autonomy; *beneficence; body parts and fluids; cultural pluralism; directed donation; *guidelines; *justice; *moral policy; organ donation; *organ transplantation; organizational policies; patient compliance; policy analysis; prognosis; *public policy; quality of life; remuneration; *resource allocation; retreatment; risks and benefits; *selection for treatment; self induced illness; social worth; time factors; *tissue transplantation; transplant recipients; treatment outcome; *utilitarianism; life style; National Organ Transplant Act 1984; *United Network for Organ Sharing; *United States

Valderrábano, Fernando. Cadaver transplantation as an ethical and cost-effective alternative to living donor transplantation: the Spanish experience. *Transplantation Proceedings.* 1992 Oct; 24(5): 2103–2105. 3 refs. Presented at the First International Congress on Transplantation in Developing Countries, Singapore, 29 Apr–3 May 1992. BE56811.

brain death; *cadavers; costs and benefits; economics; education; family members; kidneys; legal aspects; *organ donation; organ donors; *organ transplantation; presumed consent; public opinion; public policy; quality of life; renal dialysis; statistics; technical expertise; third party consent; National Transplant Organization (Spain); *Spain

Veatch, Robert M., ed. Ethical issues in the changing health care system. *In:* Jonsen, Albert R.; Veatch, Robert M.; Walters, LeRoy, eds. Source Book in Bioethics: A Documentary History. Washington, DC: Georgetown University Press; 1998: 407–504. 8 fn. ISBN 0-87840-683-2. BE57894.

advance directives; advisory committees; aliens; autonomy; body parts and fluids; cadavers; competence; *confidentiality; dangerousness; disclosure; *duty to warn; federal government; historical aspects; *informed consent; legal aspects; mentally ill; model legislation; *organ donation; organ donors; *organ transplantation; patient care; patients' rights; physician patient relationship; remuneration; selection for treatment; *third party consent; tissue donation; transplant recipients; *Canterbury v. Spence; National Organ Transplant Act 1984; President's Commission for the Study of Ethical Problems; *Tarasoff v. Regents of the University of California; *Task Force on Organ Transplantation; *Twentieth Century; *Uniform Anatomical Gift Act; *United States

---

BE = bioethics accession number   fn. = footnotes   refs. = references

Vogel, Gretchen. Xenotransplants: no moratorium on clinical trials. [News]. *Science.* 1998 Jan 30; 279(5351): 648. BE57363.
  advisory committees; *animal organs; communicable diseases; data banks; federal government; *government regulation; *human experimentation; *organ transplantation; primates; registries; risk; *therapeutic research; tissue banks; *tissue transplantation; transgenic animals; transplant recipients; swine; Centers for Disease Control and Prevention; *Food and Drug Administration; National Institutes of Health; *United States

Wadman, Meredith. FDA turns down moratorium demand on xenotransplants. [News]. *Nature.* 1998 Jan 29; 391(6666): 423. BE57362.
  advisory committees; *animal organs; communicable diseases; data banks; federal government; *government regulation; guidelines; *human experimentation; investigators; *organ transplantation; primates; public participation; registries; risk; *therapeutic research; tissue banks; tissue transplantation; swine; *Food and Drug Administration; National Institutes of Health; Public Health Service; *United States

Warden, John. Xenotransplantation moves ahead in UK. [News]. *BMJ (British Medical Journal).* 1998 Aug 8; 317(7155): 365. BE58836.
  *animal organs; *government regulation; human experimentation; *organ transplantation; *Great Britain; *Xenotransplantation Interim Regulatory Authority (Great Britain)

Wear, Stephen; Logue, Gerald. Informed consent for organ transplantation: mandating the participation of the family. *Law and Policy.* 1995 Apr; 17(2): 210–216. Commentary on B.K. Grover, "From both sides now: informed consent, organ transplantation, and family–based disclosure," p. 188–209. BE58246.
  *disclosure; *family members; family relationship; *informed consent; *legal aspects; *mandatory programs; *organ transplantation; risks and benefits; third party consent; *transplant recipients

Weiss, Robin A. Transgenic pigs and virus adaptation. *Nature.* 1998 Jan 22; 391(6665): 327–328. 20 refs. BE57770.
  *animal organs; *communicable diseases; methods; *organ transplantation; public health; regulation; *risk; risks and benefits; *transgenic animals; *transplant recipients; *swine
  Pigs offer the best hope of providing organs for transplantation to humans. But, in overcoming the problems of tissue rejection, we may be increasing our risk of injection from pig viruses.

Wilkes, Michael S.; Slavin, Stuart. Heart transplantation selection criteria: attitudes of ethnically diverse medical students. *Journal of Clinical Ethics.* 1998 Summer; 9(2): 147–155. 15 fn. BE58960.
  administrators; age factors; alcohol abuse; aliens; Asian Americans; *attitudes; blacks; comparative studies; curriculum; diagnosis; drug abuse; family relationship; females; health insurance; *hearts; Hispanic Americans; HIV seropositivity; homosexuals; indigents; males; medical education; medical schools; mentally disabled; *minority groups; morbidity; organ donation; *organ transplantation; patient compliance; patients; physicians; *resource allocation; retreatment; *selection for treatment; smoking; socioeconomic factors; *students; survey; *transplant recipients; whites; United States

Williams, Nigel. Paving the way for British xenotransplants. [News]. *Science.* 1998 Aug 7; 281(5378): 767. BE58827.
  *animal organs; *government regulation; guidelines; human experimentation; *organ transplantation; risks and benefits; *Great Britain; Xenotransplantation Interim Regulatory Authority (Great Britain)

Wise, Jacqui. New authority to monitor xenotransplantation experiments. [News]. *BMJ (British Medical Journal).* 1997 Jan 25; 314(7076): 247. 1 ref. BE58703.
  advisory committees; *animal organs; communicable diseases; *government regulation; *human experimentation; international aspects; *organ transplantation; *public policy; risk; self regulation; transgenic animals; transplant recipients; *swine; Advisory Group on the Ethics of Xenotransplantation (Great Britain); *Great Britain; United States; *Xenotransplantation Interim Regulatory Authority (Great Britain)

Changing the U.S. transplant system. [Editorial]. *Lancet.* 1998 Jul 11; 352(9122): 79. BE59070.
  body parts and fluids; *dissent; federal government; *government regulation; *organ transplantation; *organizational policies; *resource allocation; selection for treatment; standards; transplant recipients; *geographic factors; Department of Health and Human Services; *United Network for Organ Sharing; *United States

Halt the xeno–bandwagon. [Editorial]. *Nature.* 1998 Jan 22; 391(6665): 309. BE57766.
  *animal organs; communicable diseases; financial support; government regulation; human experimentation; industry; *organ transplantation; patient advocacy; public participation; public policy; *risk; risks and benefits

ORGAN PROCUREMENT *See* ORGAN AND TISSUE DONATION

OVUM DONORS *See* REPRODUCTIVE TECHNOLOGIES, SURROGATE MOTHERS

PALLIATIVE CARE *See* TERMINAL CARE

PARENTAL CONSENT *See* ABORTION/MINORS, ALLOWING TO DIE/INFANTS, HUMAN EXPERIMENTATION/MINORS, INFORMED CONSENT/MINORS, TREATMENT REFUSAL/MINORS

PASSIVE EUTHANASIA *See* ALLOWING TO DIE

PATENTING LIFE FORMS

See also GENETIC RESEARCH, RECOMBINANT DNA RESEARCH

Abbott, Alison. Euro–vote lifts block on biotech patents ... but Parliament wants closer scrutiny. [News]. *Nature.* 1997 Jul 24; 388(6640): 314–315. BE56422.
  biomedical technologies; ethical review; ethics committees; genes; *genetic intervention; *international aspects; legal aspects; *patents; political activity; *regulation; risks and benefits; transgenic animals; *transgenic organisms; agriculture; *Europe; *European Parliament; European Patent Office

Abbott, Alison. Europe's life patent moratorium may go. [News]. *Nature.* 1998 May 21; 393(6682): 200. Includes inset article by M. Wadman, "As US office claims right to rule on morality." BE58200.
  cloning; genes; genetic intervention; hybrids; *international

---

BE = bioethics accession number   fn. = footnotes   refs. = references

aspects; methods; morality; *patents; *regulation; *transgenic organisms; *Europe; *European Patent Office; Patent and Trademark Office; United States

Agius, Emmanuel. Patenting life: our responsibilities to present and future generations. *In:* Agius, Emmanuel; Busuttil, Salvino, eds. Germ–Line Intervention and Our Responsibilities to Future Generations. Boston, MA: Kluwer Academic; 1998: 67–83. 10 refs. 2 fn. ISBN 0-7923-4828-1. BE57880.

common good; *developing countries; ecology; evolution; freedom; *future generations; gene pool; gene therapy; genes; *genetic diversity; genetic enhancement; genetic intervention; *genetic research; germ cells; guidelines; human rights; industry; *international aspects; legal aspects; *moral obligations; *patents; *property rights; recombinant DNA research; *regulation; risks and benefits; *transgenic organisms; war; agriculture; *World Patent Convention on Biotechnological Inventions

Austin, Christopher P.; Tribble, Jack L. Gene patents and drug development: the perspective from Merck. *In:* Knoppers, Bartha Maria, ed. Human DNA: Law and Policy: International and Comparative Perspectives. Proceedings of the First International Conference on DNA Sampling and Human Genetic Research: Ethical, Legal, and Policy Aspects, held in Montreal, Canada, 6–8 Sep 1996. Boston, MA: Kluwer Law International; 1997: 379–383. 13 fn. ISBN 90–411–0361–9. BE58194.

*DNA sequences; *drug industry; drugs; federal government; financial support; *genes; genetic research; genome mapping; information dissemination; *patents; private sector; public sector; risks and benefits; Merck Gene Index; *Merck Inc.; *United States

Bruce, Donald M. Patenting human genes -- a Christian view. *Bulletin of Medical Ethics.* 1997 Jan; No. 124: 18–20. 10 fn. BE55738.

cloning; DNA sequences; drugs; *genes; *genetic materials; genetic research; industry; *moral policy; *patents; property rights; *Protestant ethics; regulation; theology; Europe; European Commission Biotechnology Directive; European Ecumenical Commission for Church and Society

Burrows, Beth. Second thoughts about U.S. Patent #4,438,032. *Bulletin of Medical Ethics.* 1997 Jan; No. 124: 11–14. 3 refs. BE55740.

*biomedical research; *body parts and fluids; conflict of interest; deception; disclosure; drug industry; informed consent; *investigators; *legal aspects; *patents; *patients; *property rights; remuneration; *tissue donation; universities; *cell lines; California; Golde, David; *Moore v. Regents of the University of California; United States

Cherniawsky, Kathy. Commercialization/patents. *In:* Knoppers, Bartha Maria, ed. Human DNA: Law and Policy: International and Comparative Perspectives. Proceedings of the First International Conference on DNA Sampling and Human Genetic Research: Ethical, Legal, and Policy Aspects, held in Montreal, Canada, 6–8 Sep 1996. Boston, MA: Kluwer Law International; 1997: 385–390. ISBN 90–411–0361–9. BE58195.

disclosure; DNA sequences; drug industry; *genetic materials; genetic research; *international aspects; *legal aspects; *patents; *Canada; *Europe; European Patent Office; *United States

Clinical Genetics Society (Great Britain); Clinical Molecular Genetics Society (Great Britain); Association of Clinical Cytogenetics (Great Britain); et al. Patenting and clinical genetics. [Joint statement]. *Bulletin of Medical Ethics.* 1997 Jan; No. 124: 8. BE55737.

cloning; common good; *DNA sequences; *genes; genetic

research; government financing; industry; *organizational policies; *patents; professional organizations; public sector; *Association of Clinical Cytogenetics (Great Britain); *Clinical Genetics Society (Great Britain); *Clinical Molecular Genetics Society (Great Britain); Genetic Nurses and Social Workers Association (Great Britain); Great Britain

Dickson, David. Legal fight looms over patent bid on human/animal chimaeras. [News]. *Nature.* 1998 Apr 2; 392(6675): 423–424. BE58055.

*hybrids; *legal aspects; methods; moral policy; motivation; *patents; *transgenic animals; Rifkin, Jeremy; United States

Eisenberg, Rebecca S. Genomic patents and product development incentives. *In:* Knoppers, Bartha Maria, ed. Human DNA: Law and Policy: International and Comparative Perspectives. Proceedings of the First International Conference on DNA Sampling and Human Genetic Research: Ethical, Legal, and Policy Aspects, held in Montreal, Canada, 6–8 Sep 1996. Boston, MA: Kluwer Law International; 1997: 373–378. 5 fn. ISBN 90–411–0361–9. BE58193.

*DNA sequences; federal government; *genome mapping; government financing; *incentives; *industry; *patents; private sector; *public policy; public sector; National Center for Human Genome Research; *United States

Eisenberg, Rebecca S. Proprietary rights and the norms of science in biotechnology research. *Yale Law Journal.* 1987 Dec; 97(2): 177–231. 261 fn. BE56488.

AIDS; *biomedical research; confidentiality; disclosure; editorial policies; federal government; financial support; government financing; incentives; industry; *information dissemination; investigators; *legal aspects; methods; microbiology; *patents; *property rights; *recombinant DNA research; *science; state government; Supreme Court decisions; transgenic organisms; universities; *values; Diamond v. Chakrabarty; Uniform Trade Secrets Act; *United States

Elles, R.G. Gene patenting. [Introduction to the joint statement of the four UK genetics societies]. *Bulletin of Medical Ethics.* 1997 Jan; No. 124: 9. BE55742.

common good; DNA sequences; *genes; genetic research; government financing; industry; international aspects; *organizational policies; *patents; professional organizations; property rights; public sector; Association of Clinical Cytogenetics (Great Britain); Clinical Genetics Society (Great Britain); Clinical Molecular Genetics Society (Great Britain); Genetic Nurses and Social Workers Association (Great Britain); *Great Britain

Fielder, John H. Patenting biotechnology: ethical and philosophical issues. *IEEE Engineering in Medicine and Biology Magazine.* 1997 Nov–Dec; 16(6): 118–120. 13 refs. BE58411.

animal rights; commodification; ecology; eugenics; food; *genetic intervention; industry; *patents; risk; social impact; *transgenic organisms; values

Galloux, Jean–Christophe. The patentability of the human genome: a European perspective. *In:* Knoppers, Bartha Maria, ed. Human DNA: Law and Policy: International and Comparative Perspectives. Proceedings of the First International Conference on DNA Sampling and Human Genetic Research: Ethical, Legal, and Policy Aspects, held in Montreal, Canada, 6–8 Sep 1996. Boston, MA: Kluwer Law International; 1997: 361–371. 20 fn. ISBN 90–411–0361–9. BE58192.

advisory committees; *DNA sequences; genes; *genome mapping; international aspects; *legal aspects; *patents; property rights; transgenic animals; *Europe; European Patent Convention; European Patent Office

---

BE = bioethics accession number   fn. = footnotes   refs. = references

Gannon, Philippa. Patenting human genetic material. *Bulletin of Medical Ethics.* 1997 Jan; No. 124: 33–36. 9 fn. BE55743.
  biomedical research; communitarianism; ethics committees; financial support; *genetic materials; incentives; industry; information dissemination; investigators; legal aspects; minority groups; *morality; *patents; private sector; property rights; public participation; public sector; science; tissue donation; Great Britain

Gavaghan, Helen. EU ends 10–year battle over biopatents. [News]. *Science.* 1998 May 22; 280(5367): 1188. BE58413.
  DNA sequences; genetic intervention; industry; international aspects; *legal aspects; *patents; recombinant DNA research; *transgenic organisms; Europe; *European Union

Hanson, Mark J. Religious voices in biotechnology: the case of gene patenting. *Hastings Center Report.* 1997 Nov–Dec; 27(6, Suppl.): S1–S21. 36 refs. 60 fn. BE57860.
  clergy; *commodification; common good; costs and benefits; DNA sequences; economics; *genes; genetic determinism; genetic identity; genetic intervention; *genetic materials; goals; incentives; *industry; interdisciplinary communication; *justice; law; legal aspects; moral obligations; *moral policy; *morality; *patents; personhood; *property rights; *public policy; recombinant DNA research; *religion; review; risks and benefits; science; secularism; suffering; *theology; transgenic organisms; utilitarianism; value of life; *values; dignity; Biotechnology Industry Organization; Patent and Trademark Office; Pharmaceutical Research and Manufacturers of America (PhRMA); United States

Hettinger, Ned. Patenting life: biotechnology, intellectual property, and environmental ethics. *Boston College Environmental Affairs Law Review.* 1995 Winter; 22(2): 267–305. 184 fn. BE57193.
  developing countries; *ecology; economics; financial support; genes; *genetic intervention; *genetic materials; genetic research; goals; government regulation; incentives; industry; investigators; legal aspects; *patents; private sector; property rights; public sector; rights; *risks and benefits; social impact; transgenic animals; *transgenic organisms; value of life; agriculture; transgenic plants; United States

Human Genome Organization. HUGO Statement on Patenting Issues Related to Early Release of Raw Sequence Data. London: HUGO; 1997 May. 2 p. Statement prepared by the Intellectual Property Rights Committee and approved by the Council of HUGO, 1997 May. BE58133.
  *DNA sequences; *genes; *genome mapping; information dissemination; *international aspects; legal aspects; *organizational policies; *patents; property rights; public policy; Europe; *Human Genome Organization (HUGO); United States

Kent, Alastair. Ethical aspects of the legal protection of biotechnological inventions and the principle of non-ownership of the human body. *Bulletin of Medical Ethics.* 1997 Jan; No. 124: 32–33. BE55744.
  body parts and fluids; DNA sequences; genes; *genetic materials; hormones; *human body; industry; legal aspects; *patents; *property rights

Kevles, Daniel J. Diamond v. Chakrabarty and beyond: the political economy of patenting life. *In:* Thackray, Arnold, ed. Private Science: Biotechnology and the Rise of the Molecular Sciences. Philadelphia, PA: University of Pennsylvania Press; 1998: 65–79. 38 fn. ISBN 0-8122-3428-6. BE57449.
  animal rights; biomedical research; economics; federal government; government regulation; *industry; *legal aspects; *microbiology; *patents; political activity;

recombinant DNA research; Supreme Court decisions; *transgenic animals; *universities; Diamond v. Chakrabarty; Ex parte Allen; Rifkin, Jeremy; *United States

King, David. Ethics and the oncomouse. *GenEthics News.* 1995 Sep–Oct; No. 8: 7. BE56231.
  animal rights; *patents; speciesism; *transgenic animals

Laurie, Graeme T. Biotechnology and intellectual property: a marriage of inconvenience? *In:* McLean, Sheila A.M., ed. Contemporary Issues in Law, Medicine and Ethics. Brookfield, VT: Dartmouth; 1996: 237–267. 151 fn. ISBN 1-85521-586-1. BE57798.
  *biomedical research; biomedical technologies; body parts and fluids; DNA sequences; donors; genome mapping; guidelines; human body; *industry; informed consent; international aspects; investigators; *legal aspects; *morality; *patents; property rights; *recombinant DNA research; standards; Supreme Court decisions; tissue donation; transgenic animals; cell lines; Diamond v. Chakrabarty; *Europe; European Patent Convention; European Patent Office; *Great Britain; Moore v. Regents of the University of California; National Institutes of Health; Patent and Trademark Office; *United States

Marusyk, Randall W.; Athanassiadis, Ariadni. Patenting of human genetic sequences in Canada. *In:* Knoppers, Bartha Maria, ed. Human DNA: Law and Policy: International and Comparative Perspectives. Proceedings of the First International Conference on DNA Sampling and Human Genetic Research: Ethical, Legal, and Policy Aspects, held in Montreal, Canada, 6–8 Sep 1996. Boston, MA: Kluwer Law International; 1997: 343–360. 78 fn. ISBN 90-411-0361-9. BE58191.
  disclosure; *DNA sequences; genetic materials; government regulation; informed consent; *legal aspects; legislation; *patents; *property rights; public policy; tissue donation; transgenic organisms; *Canada; Intellectual Property Improvement Act 1993 (Canada); Patent Act 1985 (Canada)

Mazen, Noël–Jean. Human DNA on trial in French law. *In:* Knoppers, Bartha Maria, ed. Human DNA: Law and Policy: International and Comparative Perspectives. Proceedings of the First International Conference on DNA Sampling and Human Genetic Research: Ethical, Legal, and Policy Aspects, held in Montreal, Canada, 6–8 Sep 1996. Boston, MA: Kluwer Law International; 1997: 43–54. 45 fn. ISBN 90-411-0361-9. BE58168.
  *biomedical technologies; body parts and fluids; DNA sequences; drugs; gene therapy; genetic intervention; *genetic materials; genetic research; gifts; *government regulation; informed consent; *legal aspects; legislation; *patents; *remuneration; *tissue donation; Europe; European Community; *France

Poste, George; Roberts, David; Gentry, Simon. Patents, ethics and improving healthcare. *Bulletin of Medical Ethics.* 1997 Jan; No. 124: 29–31. BE55745.
  *biomedical research; *drug industry; drugs; economics; genes; *genetic materials; health care; hormones; international aspects; legal aspects; *patents; risks and benefits

Reiss, Michael J. Is it right to patent DNA? *Bulletin of Medical Ethics.* 1997 Jan; No. 124: 21–24. 6 refs. BE55746.
  attitudes; autonomy; biomedical research; DNA sequences; genes; *genetic materials; industry; information dissemination; international aspects; legal aspects; *moral policy; *patents; property rights; religious ethics; utilitarianism; Europe; European Ecumenical Commission for Church and Society

Rogers, Arthur. European Parliament approves

intellectual property rights directive. [News]. *Lancet.* 1997 Jul 26; 350(9073): 272. BE56418.
> developing countries; *genetic intervention; *international aspects; *patents; property rights; *regulation; *transgenic organisms; *Europe; *European Parliament

Rogers, Arthur. European Union approves gene–patent directive. [News]. *Lancet.* 1998 May 16; 351(9114): 1500. BE58889.
> embryo research; *genetic materials; guidelines; international aspects; legal aspects; *patents; Europe; *European Union

Salgo, Reinhold C. Patenting the human genome. *Bulletin of Medical Ethics.* 1997 Jan; No. 124: 15–16. BE55747.
> DNA sequences; *genetic materials; *genome mapping; legal aspects; *patents; transgenic organisms; Europe; European Patent Convention; European Patent Office

Scott–Ram, Nicholas. Ethics and the directive for the legal protection of biotechnological inventions. *Bulletin of Medical Ethics.* 1997 Jan; No. 124: 25–28. 2 fn. BE55748.
> animal experimentation; biomedical research; ethical analysis; genetic intervention; *genetic materials; industry; information dissemination; legal aspects; *patents; property rights; *regulation; *transgenic organisms; Europe; *European Commission Biotechnology Directive; European Patent Convention

Sheppard, Julie. Patent and be damned! *Bulletin of Medical Ethics.* 1997 Jan; No. 124: 16–17. 2 refs. BE55749.
> attitudes; biomedical research; dissent; DNA sequences; financial support; genes; genetic disorders; genetic diversity; *genetic materials; genetic research; government financing; incentives; industry; information dissemination; international aspects; minority groups; *patents; patient advocacy; political activity; public opinion; tissue donation; orphan drugs

Sherry, Stephen F. The incentive of patents. *In:* Kilner, John F.; Pentz, Rebecca D.; Young, Frank E., eds. Genetic Ethics: Do the Ends Justify the Genes? Grand Rapids, MI: W.B. Eerdmans; 1997: 113–123. 36 fn. ISBN 0–8028–4428–6. BE56719.
> *Christian ethics; commodification; economics; hybrids; incentives; industry; legal aspects; microbiology; moral policy; *patents; public policy; *recombinant DNA research; regulation; Supreme Court decisions; *transgenic organisms; Diamond v. Chakrabarty; United States

Watson, Rory. EU approves rights to genetic material. [News]. *BMJ (British Medical Journal).* 1997 Dec 6; 315(7121): 1487. BE57346.
> biomedical technologies; cloning; embryo research; genetic intervention; *genetic materials; *genetic research; *international aspects; legislation; *patents; political activity; *regulation; *transgenic organisms; *Europe; *European Union

Watson, Rory. Patenting of genes moves one stage closer. [News]. *BMJ (British Medical Journal).* 1997 Jul 26; 315(7102): 207. BE58503.
> *genes; industry; *international aspects; *patents; politics; *regulation; *Europe; *European Union

Weiss, Rick. Patent sought on making of part–human creatures: scientist seeks to touch off ethics debate. [News]. *Washington Post.* 1998 Apr 2: A12. BE58048.
> *genetic intervention; government regulation; human experimentation; *hybrids; investigators; *legal aspects; *patents; primates; public policy; *Newman, Stuart; Patent and Trademark Office; United States

Williams, Nigel. European Parliament backs new

biopatent guidelines. [News]. *Science.* 1997 Jul 25; 277(5325): 472. BE56444.
> genes; *genetic intervention; industry; *international aspects; legal aspects; *patents; political activity; *regulation; risks and benefits; transgenic animals; *transgenic organisms; *Europe; *European Parliament

Wise, Jacqui. Doctors fight US company patent on umbilical cord blood. [News]. *BMJ (British Medical Journal).* 1997 Apr 19; 314(7088): 1146. BE56895.
> biomedical technologies; *blood banks; blood donation; blood transfusions; cryopreservation; *industry; *international aspects; *patents; *cord blood; *Biocyte; *Europe; *United States

Hard cases, bad laws: is patching human genes any more immoral than patenting nerve gases? [Editorial]. *New Scientist.* 1997 Jul 12; 155(2090): 3. BE55632.
> *genes; genetic intervention; genetic research; industry; international aspects; *patents; political activity; *regulation; risks and benefits; *Europe; *European Biotechnology Patent Directive; European Parliament; European Patent Office

Owning genes. [Editorial]. *Wall Street Journal.* 1998 May 14: A22. BE59109.
> animal experimentation; DNA sequences; economics; genome mapping; international aspects; *patents; property rights; regulation; *risks and benefits; *transgenic organisms; agriculture; Europe

Progress on patents, but more action is needed. [Editorial]. *Nature.* 1997 Jul 24; 388(6640): 309. BE56053.
> genes; genetic intervention; *genetic materials; genetic research; industry; *international aspects; *patents; political activity; regulation; *transgenic animals; transgenic organisms; *Europe; European Parliament; United States

PATERNALISM *See* PROFESSIONAL PATIENT RELATIONSHIP

PATIENT ACCESS TO RECORDS

See also CONFIDENTIALITY, TRUTH DISCLOSURE

American Medical Record Association. Confidentiality of Patient Health Information. *American Medical Record Association Journal.* 1985 Dec; 56(12): 4–14. BE57866.
> *confidentiality; *disclosure; forms; *health facilities; *institutional policies; *medical records; *organization and administration; *organizational policies; *patient access to records; professional organizations; *American Medical Record Association

Canada. Supreme Court. McInerney v. MacDonald. *Dominion Law Reports, 4th Series.* 1992 Jun 11 (date of decision). 93: 415–431. BE57393.
> confidentiality; interprofessional relations; *legal aspects; *medical records; *patient access to records; physician patient relationship; physicians; property rights; *Canada; *McInerney v. MacDonald

The Supreme Court of Canada dismissed an appeal by a physician who had challenged a patient's right of access to her complete medical record. Margaret MacDonald had gone to other doctors over the years before she became the patient of Dr. Elizabeth McInerney. After McInerney advised MacDonald to stop taking the thyroid pills prescribed by other doctors and she complied, MacDonald requested copies of her entire medical record. McInerney sent copies of all reports which she herself had prepared, but refused to send

---

BE = bioethics accession number   fn. = footnotes   refs. = references

copies of any reports on MacDonald from other physicians, believing that doing so would be unethical. She told MacDonald to contact each of the other physicians for release of their medical records. MacDonald's application for a court order directing McInerney to provide a copy of the entire medical file was granted. The Court determined that a fiduciary duty to provide access to medical records is based on the nature of the patient's interest in the records, and that the onus lies on the doctor to justify an exception to the general rule of access. (KIE abstract)

Cordner, Stephen; Ettershank, Kathy. Australian access to private medical records unchanged. [News]. *Lancet.* 1997 May 3; 349(9061): 1306. BE56587.
  government regulation; *legal aspects; *medical records; *patient access to records; *private sector; public sector; *Australia

Feenan, Dermot. Medical records: law, paternalism and harm. *Journal of the Royal College of Physicians of London.* 1995 Sep–Oct; 29(5): 401–404. 21 refs. BE56205.
  autonomy; counseling; *disclosure; *legal aspects; *medical records; mentally ill; *paternalism; *patient access to records; *psychological stress; psychotherapy; *risks and benefits; *Great Britain; *R v. Mid Glamorgan Family Health Services Authority, ex parte Martin

PATIENT CARE

See also HEALTH CARE, PROFESSIONAL PATIENT RELATIONSHIP, SELECTION FOR TREATMENT, TERMINAL CARE

Agich, George J.; May, Thomas. Alcoholism, moral agency, and paternalism: a theoretical framework. *In:* Shelton, Wayne N.; Edwards, Rem B., eds. Advances in Bioethics. Volume 3: Values, Ethics, and Alcoholism. Greenwich, CT: JAI Press; 1997: 103–118. 20 refs. ISBN 0-7623-0219-4. BE57634.
  *accountability; *alcohol abuse; *autonomy; *behavior control; *behavior disorders; beneficence; coercion; competence; dangerousness; disabled; *disease; freedom; goals; government regulation; *injuries; morality; *paternalism; *patient care; patient compliance; patients; *physicians; psychological stress; risk; *self induced illness; social interaction; traffic accidents; values; dependency; liberalism; rationality; Mills, John Stuart; Raz, Joseph

American College of Obstetricians and Gynecologists. Committee on Ethics. Ethical guidance for patient testing. ACOG Committee Opinion No. 159. *ACOG Committee Opinions.* 1995 Oct; No. 159: 3 p. BE56908.
  confidentiality; counseling; *diagnosis; disclosure; females; *guidelines; *obstetrics and gynecology; *organizational policies; *patient care; physicians; professional organizations; *American College of Obstetricians and Gynecologists

American Nurses Association. American Nurses Association position statements on ethics and human rights. *In: its* Compendium of American Nurses Association Position Statements. Washington, DC: American Nurses Publishing; 1996: 79–118. Includes references. ISBN 1-55810-123-3. BE57452.
  active euthanasia; advance directives; allowing to die; artificial feeding; assisted suicide; capital punishment; codes of ethics; cultural pluralism; health care; *human rights; legislation; nurse's role; *nurses; *nursing ethics; *organizational policies; pain; palliative care; patient advocacy; *patient care; professional organizations; resuscitation orders; *terminal care; treatment refusal; withholding treatment; *American Nurses Association;

Patient Self–Determination Act 1990; United States

Amu, Olubusola; Rajendran, Sasha; Bolaji, Ibrahim I., et al. Should doctors perform an elective caesarean section on request?: Yes, as long as the woman is fully informed; [and] Maternal choice alone should not determine method of delivery. *BMJ (British Medical Journal).* 1998 Aug 15; 317(7156): 462–465. 37 refs. BE58757.
  autonomy; *cesarean section; childbirth; competence; *decision making; disclosure; informed consent; morbidity; newborns; obstetrics and gynecology; *patient participation; *physicians; *pregnant women; risks and benefits; Great Britain

Angier, Natalie. Joined for life, and living life to the full. *New York Times.* 1997 Dec 23: F1, F5. BE56934.
  *attitudes; congenital disorders; decision making; parents; physically disabled; *quality of life; risks and benefits; selection for treatment; *surgery; *twins; *conjoined twins; Lakeberg twins; *Schappell twins

Asch, Adrienne. Distracted by disability. *Cambridge Quarterly of Healthcare Ethics.* 1998 Winter; 7(1): 77–87. 22 fn. BE58450.
  assisted suicide; *attitudes; autonomy; bioethics; chronically ill; communication; cultural pluralism; *decision making; depressive disorder; *disabled; goals; *health care; health facilities; *health personnel; medicine; minority groups; *moral obligations; motivation; *obligations of society; *patient care; *physically disabled; physician patient relationship; physicians; quality of life; rehabilitation; *resource allocation; social discrimination; *stigmatization; treatment refusal; withholding treatment; dependency

Astin, John A. Why patients use alternative medicine: results of a national study. *JAMA.* 1998 May 20; 279(19): 1548–1553. 34 refs. BE58401.
  *alternative therapies; attitudes; autonomy; health; health care; morbidity; *motivation; *patient satisfaction; *patients; socioeconomic factors; survey; values; holistic health; United States
  CONTEXT: Research both in the United States and abroad suggests that significant numbers of people are involved with various forms of alternative medicine. However, the reasons for such use are, at present, poorly understood. OBJECTIVE: To investigate possible predictors of alternative health care use. METHODS: Three primary hypotheses were tested. People seek out these alternatives because (1) they are dissatisfied in some way with conventional treatment; (2) they see alternative treatments as offering more personal autonomy and control over health care decisions; and (3) the alternatives are seen as more compatible with the patients' values, worldview, or beliefs regarding the nature and meaning of health and illness. Additional predictor variables explored included demographics and health status. DESIGN: A written survey examining use of alternative health care, health status, values, and attitudes toward conventional medicine. Multiple logistic regression analyses were used in an effort to identify predictors of alternative health care use. SETTING AND PARTICIPANTS: A total of 1035 individuals randomly selected from a panel who had agreed to participate in mail surveys and who live throughout the United States. MAIN OUTCOME MEASURE: Use of alternative medicine within the previous year. RESULTS: The response rate was 69%. The following variables emerged as predictors of alternative health care use: more education (odds ratio [OR], 1.2; 95% confidence interval [CI], 1.1–1.3); poorer health status (OR, 1.3; 95% CI, 1.1–1.5); a holistic orientation to health (OR, 1.4; 95% CI, 1.1–1.9); having had a

---

BE = bioethics accession number   fn. = footnotes   refs. = references

transformational experience that changed the person's worldview (OR, 1 .8; 95% CI, 1 .3–2.5); any of the following health problems: anxiety (OR, 3.1; 95% CI, 1.6–6.0); back problems (OR, 2.3; 95% CI, 1 .7–3.2); chronic pain (OR, 2.0; 95% CI, 1.1 –3.5); urinary tract problems (OR, 2.2; 95% CI, 1.3–3.5); and classification in a cultural group identifiable by their commitment to environmentalism, commitment to feminism, and interest in spirituality and personal growth psychology (OR, 2.0; 95% CI, 1.4–2.7). Dissatisfaction with conventional medicine did not predict use of alternative medicine. Only 4.4% of those surveyed reported relying primarily on alternative therapies. CONCLUSION: Along with being more educated and reporting poorer health status, the majority of alternative medicine users appear to be doing so not so much as a result of being dissatisfied with conventional medicine but largely because they find these health care alternatives to be more congruent with their own values, beliefs, and philosophical orientations toward health and life.

Balsamo, Anne. On the cutting edge: cosmetic surgery and new imaging technologies. *In: her:* Technologies of the Gendered Body: Reading Cyborg Women. Durham, NC: Duke University Press; 1996: 56–79, 177–184. 71 fn. ISBN 0–8223–1698–6. BE58521.
  *advertising; age factors; *audiovisual aids; *biomedical technologies; *commodification; *cosmetic surgery; counseling; *females; feminist ethics; human body; informed consent; males; motivation; normality; patient care; physician patient relationship; physicians; self concept; social control; standards; beauty; video recording

Barnard, David. Doctors and their suffering patients: commentary on Campbell. *In:* Carson, Ronald A.; Burns, Chester R., eds. Philosophy of Medicine and Bioethics: A Twenty–Year Retrospective and Critical Appraisal. Boston, MA: Kluwer Academic; 1997: 265–272. 17 refs. ISBN 0–7923–3545–7. BE56541.
  empathy; goals; *medicine; *pain; *palliative care; *patient care; *patients; physician's role; *suffering; values; undertreatment

Baylis, Françoise. Errors in medicine: nurturing truthfulness. *Journal of Clinical Ethics.* 1997 Winter; 8(4): 336–340. 10 fn. BE57605.
  attitudes; case studies; *disclosure; emotions; *iatrogenic disease; interprofessional relations; legal liability; medical ethics; moral obligations; motivation; *negligence; *patient care; physician patient relationship; *physicians; professional competence; risks and benefits; self regulation; *sociology of medicine; trust; *truth disclosure; uncertainty; whistleblowing; *medical errors
In "When a Physician Harms a Patient by a Medical Error," Finkelstein and colleagues maintain that patients have a right to the truth and that physicians have a corresponding obligation to be truthful. In their view, when an erroneous act or omission results in an adverse outcome for the patient, the physician should truthfully disclose the medical error, offer the patient a sincere apology, and explore the option of financial compensation. In the abstract, this seems reasonable –– and some might even argue uncontestable. Why then is it not common practice for physicians to routinely discuss their errors with their patients? In this article, I will critically examine some of the reasons given by physicians for non–disclosure or partial disclosure, and then consider what the medical profession should do to foster more respectful, open, and honest communication about errors with patients.

Beecham, Linda. GMC approves new ethical guidance.

[News]. *BMJ (British Medical Journal).* 1998 May 23; 316(7144): 1556. BE58275.
  death; *disclosure; *guidelines; *iatrogenic disease; negligence; *patient care; patients' rights; physician patient relationship; *physicians; *standards; *General Medical Council (Great Britain); *Good Medical Practice (General Medical Council); *Great Britain

Beisecker, Analee E.; Murden, Robert A.; Moore, William P., et al. Attitudes of medical students and primary care physicians regarding input of older and younger patients in medical decisions. *Medical Care.* 1996 Feb; 34(2): 126–137. 28 refs. BE55654.
  *adults; *age factors; *aged; alternatives; *attitudes; *autonomy; comparative studies; *decision making; diagnosis; drugs; faculty; family practice; females; hospitals; internal medicine; *internship and residency; males; medical education; medical schools; *paternalism; *patient care; *patient participation; *physician patient relationship; *physicians; primary health care; referral and consultation; *students; survey; Kansas; Ohio; Ohio State University Hospital; University of Kansas Medical Center

Bell, Marilynne; Mosher, Janet. (Re)fashioning medicine's response to wife abuse. *In:* Sherwin, Susan, et al. The Politics of Women's Health: Exploring Agency and Autonomy. Philadelphia, PA: Temple University Press; 1998: 205–233. 19 fn. ISBN 1–56639–633–6. BE58399.
  *attitudes; disclosure; *domestic violence; family relationship; *females; *feminist ethics; males; *medicine; *patient care; *physicians

Boyle, Philip J., ed. Getting Doctors to Listen: Ethics and Outcomes Data in Context. Washington, DC: Georgetown University Press; 1998. 234 p. (Hastings Center studies in ethics). 479 fn. ISBN 0–87840–654–9. BE57925.
  accountability; *biomedical technologies; bone marrow; cancer; communication; consensus; *decision making; drugs; economics; *evaluation; federal government; females; goals; *guidelines; health care; health insurance reimbursement; hormones; international aspects; knowledge, attitudes, practice; legal liability; medicine; moral obligations; *patient care; patient compliance; physician patient relationship; *physicians; political activity; *practice guidelines; professional autonomy; professional organizations; public participation; public policy; risks and benefits; science; *standards; surgery; technical expertise; *technology assessment; tissue transplantation; *treatment outcome; uncertainty; values; *guideline adherence; *investigational therapies; menopause; France; Great Britain; National Institutes of Health; Netherlands; *United States

Campbell, Courtney S. Must patients suffer? *In:* Carson, Ronald A.; Burns, Chester R., eds. Philosophy of Medicine and Bioethics: A Twenty–Year Retrospective and Critical Appraisal. Boston, MA: Kluwer Academic; 1997: 247–263. 22 refs. 1 fn. ISBN 0–7923–3545–7. BE56540.
  compassion; empathy; goals; human characteristics; *medicine; *pain; *palliative care; paternalism; *patient care; *patients; professional patient relationship; religion; self concept; *suffering; theology; *values

Campbell, Duncan. Medicine needs its MI5. *BMJ (British Medical Journal).* 1997 Dec 20–27; 315(7123): 1677–1680. 2 refs. BE57651.
  biomedical research; fraud; *human experimentation; *investigators; mass media; *misconduct; *patient care; *physicians; professional competence; *scientific misconduct; *self regulation; stigmatization; whistleblowing; medical audit; *General Medical Council (Great Britain); *Great Britain

Candib, Lucy M. Medicine and the Family: A Feminist Perspective. New York, NY: BasicBooks; 1995. 360 p. Bibliography: p. 307-350. ISBN 0-465-02374-6. BE56502.
  adults; autonomy; caring; children; communication; contracts; disclosure; domestic violence; empathy; family members; family practice; *family relationship; females; *feminist ethics; males; *medicine; parent child relationship; *patient care; patients; philosophy; *physician patient relationship; physicians; *professional family relationship; rape; self concept; sex offenses; social discrimination; *social dominance; incest; United States

Chan, Arlene; Woodruff, Roger K. Communicating with patients with advanced cancer. *Journal of Palliative Care.* 1997 Autumn; 13(3): 29-33. 21 refs. BE58052.
  adults; aged; *attitudes; *cancer; caring; *communication; comparative studies; *comprehension; *diagnosis; family practice; females; health maintenance organizations; hospitals; internship and residency; males; medical specialties; minority groups; *nurses; *pain; *palliative care; *patient care; *patient satisfaction; *patients; *physicians; professional patient relationship; *prognosis; quality of health care; quality of life; survey; terminal care; time factors; *truth disclosure; translating; Australia

Cher, Daniel J.; Lenert, Leslie A. Method of Medicare reimbursement and the rate of potentially ineffective care of critically ill patients. *JAMA.* 1997 Sep 24; 278(12): 1001-1007. 29 refs. Correction appears in *JAMA*, 1998 Jun 17; 279(23): 1876. BE55815.
  aged; allowing to die; biomedical technologies; comparative studies; *critically ill; *economics; *futility; *health maintenance organizations; hospitals; *intensive care units; *managed care programs; *mortality; *patient care; physicians; prolongation of life; quality of health care; remuneration; resource allocation; selection for treatment; *terminal care; time factors; *treatment outcome; withholding treatment; *fee-for-service plans; severity of illness index; *California; *Medicare
  CONTEXT: The worst outcome of critical care may not be death itself; rather, the worst may be an extended death process in which a patient's and his or her family's suffering has been prolonged by services that are ultimately impotent. We have previously used potentially ineffective care (PIC) as a proxy measure for this type of care. OBJECTIVE: To determine if PIC is delivered less often to Medicare patients enrolled in health maintenance organizations (HMOs) than those in traditional fee-for-service health plans. PATIENTS: All Medicare patients hospitalized in intensive care units in California during fiscal year 1994. OUTCOME: Potentially ineffective care was defined as the concurrence of in-hospital death or death within 100 days of hospital discharge and resource use (total hospital costs) above the 90th percentile. METHODS: Hospital costs were adjusted for institution-specific cost-to-charge ratios and local wage indices derived from Health Care Financing Administration cost reports. A multivariate regression model adjusted PIC rates for age, sex, race, elective admission to the hospital, Charlson index diseases, the 15 most common diagnosis related groups for death by 100 days, intensive care unit size, and number of residents at the hospital. RESULTS: A total of 3914 (4.8%) of 81,494 patients experienced PIC and used 21.6% of total intensive care unit resources. The occurrence of PIC was less common among HMO members (adjusted odds ratio, 0.75; 95% confidence interval, 0.65-0.87). However, HMO members were not more likely to experience in-hospital death (adjusted odds ratio, 0.99; 95% confidence interval, 0.91-1.07) and only slightly more likely to experience death by 100 days after hospital discharge (adjusted odds

ratio, 1.08; 95% confidence interval, 1.01-1.15). CONCLUSIONS: Patients who experience PIC outcomes are not uncommon in the Medicare population, and patients experiencing this outcome consume a disproportionate amount of medical resources. Medicare beneficiaries in HMO practice settings had a lower risk of experiencing PIC outcomes after adjusting for age, sex, diagnosis, comorbid conditions, and characteristics of the treating hospital. This suggests that HMO practices may be better at limiting or avoiding injudicious use of critical care near the end of life.

Chervenak, Frank A.; McCullough, Laurence B. What is obstetric ethics? *Journal of Perinatal Medicine.* 1995; 23(5): 331-341. 52 refs. BE57763.
  autonomy; beneficence; clinical ethics; consensus; directive counseling; embryos; ethical analysis; ethical theory; fetal development; fetal therapy; *fetuses; informed consent; law; *medical ethics; moral obligations; *obstetrics and gynecology; *patient care; physicians; *pregnant women; prenatal diagnosis; religion; value of life; viability

Cressey, David M.; Rigter, Henk; de Beaufort, Inez, et al. Ethical debate: too drunk to care? [Article and commentaries]. *BMJ (British Medical Journal).* 1998 May 16; 316(7143): 1515-1517. BE58301.
  *alcohol abuse; case studies; decision making; *emergency care; guidelines; moral obligations; *physicians; *professional competence; risks and benefits; *physician impairment; General Medical Council (Great Britain); Great Britain

Curran, William J.; Hall, Mark A.; Bobinski, Mary Anne, et al. Health Care Law and Ethics. Fifth Edition. New York, NY: Aspen Law and Business; 1998. 1,463 p. Includes references. ISBN 1-56706-809-X. BE57442.
  abortion, induced; adults; advance directives; AIDS serodiagnosis; allowing to die; alternative therapies; assisted suicide; *bioethical issues; brain death; communicable diseases; competence; confidentiality; conflict of interest; contact tracing; contraception; decision making; determination of death; drugs; economics; futility; government regulation; *health care delivery; health facilities; health personnel; HIV seropositivity; informed consent; *legal aspects; malpractice; managed care programs; mandatory programs; mentally ill; minors; organ donation; organ transplantation; *patient care; pregnant women; prenatal injuries; professional patient relationship; public health; reproduction; reproductive technologies; right to die; standards; third party consent; treatment refusal; *United States

Curran, William J. Legal history of emergency medicine from medieval common law to the AIDS epidemic. *American Journal of Emergency Medicine.* 1997 Nov; 15(7): 658-670. 88 refs. BE58355.
  *AIDS; *emergency care; federal government; government regulation; *historical aspects; *HIV seropositivity; *hospitals; judicial action; *legal aspects; *legal liability; *legal obligations; malpractice; organizational policies; patient admission; patient transfer; *physicians; professional organizations; *refusal to treat; review; social discrimination; standards; state government; torts; traffic accidents; Eighteenth Century; Emergency Medical Treatment and Active Labor Act 1986; England; Good Samaritanism; Nineteenth Century; *Twentieth Century; *United States

Curtis, J. Randall; Rubenfeld, Gordon D. Aggressive medical care at the end of life; does capitated reimbursement encourage the right care for the wrong reason? [Editorial]. *JAMA.* 1997 Sep 24; 278(12): 1025-1026. 12 refs. BE55814.
  biomedical technologies; *critically ill; decision making; *economics; *health maintenance organizations; hospitals; *intensive care units; *managed care programs; mortality;

---

*patient care; physicians; prolongation of life; quality of health care; remuneration; *terminal care; time factors; treatment outcome; withholding treatment; capitation fee; *fee-for-service plans; *Medicare; *United States

Davison, B. Joyce; Degner, Lesley F.; Morgan, Thomas R. Information and decision-making preferences of men with prostate cancer. *Oncology Nursing Forum.* 1995 Oct; 22(9): 1401-1408. 37 refs. BE55761.
*attitudes; *cancer; *decision making; *disclosure; informed consent; *males; married persons; *patient care; *patient participation; physician patient relationship; prognosis; quality of life; risks and benefits; single persons; survey; treatment outcome; *prostate cancer; Manitoba

Degner, Lesley F.; Kristjanson, Linda J.; Bowman, David, et al. Information needs and decisional preferences in women with breast cancer. *JAMA.* 1997 May 14; 277(18): 1485-1492. 36 refs. BE55849.
age factors; *attitudes; *breast cancer; communication; *decision making; disclosure; evaluation studies; *females; *patient care; *patient education; *patient participation; patients; *physician patient relationship; physicians; socioeconomic factors; survey; truth disclosure; Manitoba
OBJECTIVE: To determine the degree of involvement women with breast cancer wanted in medical decision making, extent to which they believed they had achieved their preferred level of involvement, and types of information they judged to be most important. DESIGN AND SETTING: Cross-sectional survey at 2 tertiary oncology referral clinics and 2 community hospital oncology clinics in Winnipeg, Manitoba. PATIENTS: Consecutive sample of 1012 women with a confirmed diagnosis of breast cancer who were scheduled for a visit at 1 of 4 hospital oncology clinics. MAIN OUTCOME MEASURES: The following measures were used: (1) Preferences about various levels of participation in treatment decision making; (2) the extent to which subjects believed they had achieved their preferred levels of involvement in decision making; and (3) priority needs for information and how these needs differed by selected sociodemographic, disease, and treatment variables. RESULTS: A total of 22% of women wanted to select their own cancer treatment, 44% wanted to select their treatment collaboratively with their physicians, and 34% wanted to delegate this responsibility to their physicians. Only 42% of women believed they had achieved their preferred level of control in decision making. The 2 most highly ranked types of information were related to knowing about chances of cure and spread of disease. Women younger than 50 years rated information about physical and sexual attractiveness as more important than did older women (P less than .001); women older than 70 years rated information about self-care as more important than did younger women (P=.002); and women who had a positive family history of breast cancer rated information about family risk as more important than did other women (P=.03). CONCLUSIONS: The substantial discrepancy between women's preferred and attained levels of involvement in treatment decision making suggests that systematic approaches to assess and respond to women's desired level of participation in treatment decision making need to be evaluated. Priorities for information identified in this study provide an empirical basis to guide communication with women seeking care for breast cancer.

Dreger, Alice Domurat. "Ambiguous sex" — or ambivalent medicine? Ethical issues in the treatment of intersexuality. *Hastings Center Report.* 1998 May-Jun; 28(3): 24-35. 45 fn. BE58610.

attitudes; circumcision; congenital disorders; *cosmetic surgery; deception; *decision making; diagnosis; *females; hormones; informed consent; *males; narrative ethics; newborns; *normality; parents; paternalism; *patient care; physicians; psychological stress; psychology; self concept; *sexuality; transsexualism; treatment outcome; truth disclosure; *uncertainty; personal identity; *sex differentiation disorders; United States

Elkins, Thomas E.; Brown, Douglas. Ethical issues in the utilization of cesarean section. *In:* Flamm, B.L.; Quilligan, E.J., eds. Cesarean Section: Guidelines for Appropriate Utilization. New York, NY: Springer-Verlag; 1995: 191-205. 69 refs. ISBN 0387-94238-6. BE56682.
autonomy; blood transfusions; *cesarean section; childbirth; *coercion; *decision making; developing countries; fetal therapy; *fetuses; informed consent; *judicial action; *legal aspects; maternal health; minority groups; *moral obligations; newborns; *obstetrics and gynecology; *organizational policies; *patient care; patient compliance; patient participation; physician patient relationship; *physicians; *pregnant women; privacy; professional organizations; prognosis; *risks and benefits; selection for treatment; socioeconomic factors; state interest; terminally ill; *treatment refusal; viability; *American Academy of Pediatrics; *American College of Obstetricians and Gynecologists; *American Medical Association; District of Columbia; *In re A.C.; *United States

Elliott, Carl. Why can't we go on as three? *Hastings Center Report.* 1998 May-Jun; 28(3): 36-39. 9 fn. BE58611.
attitudes; congenital disorders; *cosmetic surgery; cultural pluralism; deception; females; males; *normality; parents; patient care; physicians; self concept; *sexuality; transsexualism; *uncertainty; personal identity; *sex differentiation disorders

Elliston, Sarah. Life after death? Legal and ethical considerations of maintaining pregnancy in brain dead women. *In:* Petersen, Kerry, ed. Intersections: Women on Law, Medicine and Technology. Brookfield, VT: Ashgate; 1997: 145-164. 23 refs. 7 fn. ISBN 1-85521-882-8. BE57490.
advance directives; *autonomy; *brain death; cadavers; childbirth; *decision making; determination of death; *fetuses; informed consent; *legal aspects; models, theoretical; mother fetus relationship; *patient care; *pregnant women; *prolongation of life; treatment refusal; *withholding treatment; women's rights; *Great Britain

English, Dan C. Surgeon's role in ethical decisions. *American Surgeon.* 1985 Jul; 51(7): 423-425. 6 refs. BE57058.
autonomy; communication; competence; *decision making; disclosure; informed consent; *patient care; patient education; *patient participation; physician patient relationship; *physician's role; professional competence; professional family relationship; surgery; third party consent; treatment refusal; values; United States

Ferguson, Jeffrey A.; Weinberger, Morris; Westmoreland, Glenda R., et al. Racial disparity in cardiac decision making: results from patient focus groups. *Archives of Internal Medicine.* 1998 Jul 13; 158(13): 1450-1453. 25 refs. BE58807.
*attitudes; biomedical technologies; *blacks; caring; communication; comparative studies; comprehension; *decision making; family members; health care delivery; *heart diseases; hospitals; *patient care; *patients; physician patient relationship; physicians; religion; social discrimination; socioeconomic factors; survey; *trust; *whites; focus groups; qualitative research; teaching hospitals; Indiana; United States
BACKGROUND: While numerous studies suggest that

BE = bioethics accession number   fn. = footnotes   refs. = references

African Americans receive fewer invasive cardiac procedures than whites, the basis for these treatment differences is not understood. METHODS: We conducted focus group sessions with patients who had received treatment in the hospital or the emergency department within the preceding 3 months for ischemic heart disease at 2 urban, university–affiliated hospitals. RESULTS: Discussions with patients identified the following factors that influenced their decision making: clarity, simplicity, and consistency of treatment recommendations; advice from friends and family about whether to accept recommendations; availability to speak with others who accepted similar recommendations; and having honest and caring physicians. African American patients identified the following additional factors that influenced their decision making: perceptions of health care discrimination; perceptions of undesirable physician behavior; faith in God to control one's destiny; and patient–physician camaraderie. CONCLUSIONS: Participants identified common issues influencing health care decision making, regardless of race. However, additional factors were expressed only by African American participants. These factors conveyed racial differences in perceptions of the health care system that may, in part, contribute to differences in health care decision making and treatment.

Ferrell, Betty R. The role of ethics committees in responding to the moral outrage of unrelieved pain. *Bioethics Forum.* 1997 Fall; 13(3): 11–16. 20 refs. BE57528.
> accountability; *clinical ethics committees; drugs; government regulation; institutional ethics; interdisciplinary communication; *pain; *palliative care; patient care; patient education; placebos; *quality of health care; quality of life; standards; technical expertise; vulnerable populations

Ferris, Lorraine E.; Norton, Peter G.; Dunn, Earl V., et al. Guidelines for managing domestic abuse when male and female partners are patients of the same physician. [For the Delphi Panel and the Consulting Group]. *JAMA.* 1997 Sep 10; 278(10): 851–857. 59 refs. BE55854.
> communication; confidentiality; *conflict of interest; *domestic violence; females; *guidelines; males; *patient care; patient education; *patients; *physician patient relationship; physicians; *practice guidelines; primary health care; *professional family relationship; referral and consultation; risk

OBJECTIVE: To provide clinical guidelines for primary care physicians who are dealing with domestic abuse and who have both the abused woman and her partner as patients. PARTICIPANTS: A 15–member expert panel with members having experience in family practice, gynecology, emergency medicine, medical ethics, nursing, psychology, law, and social work; an 11–member consulting group with members representing medicine, consumers, police, psychology, social work, and nursing; and participants from focus groups including 48 previously abused women and 10 previously abusive men. Members of the expert panel and the consulting group were recruited by the research team. Focus group members were recruited through the agencies from which they were receiving services. EVIDENCE: Available research information, and opinions of the expert panel, the consulting group, and the focus group participants. CONSENSUS PROCESS: Scoring of 144 clinical scenarios was performed by the expert panel using a modified Delphi technique involving 4 iterations. Scenarios were rated in terms of best practice for primary care physicians dealing with

suspected and confirmed cases of physical abuse. Consulting group members and focus group participants then commented on the panel's results. Final guidelines were approved by the panel and the consulting group, with comments reserved in the guidelines for information from focus group participants. CONCLUSIONS: It is not a conflict of interest for the physician to deal with abuse of the female partner when both partners are patients. Both patients have a right to autonomy, confidentiality, honesty, and quality care. Patients should be dealt with independently, thereby facilitating assessment of the magnitude and severity of the victim's injuries. Physicians should not discuss the possibility of domestic abuse with the male partner without the prior consent of the abused female partner. Joint counseling is generally inadvisable and should be attempted only when the violence has ended, provided both partners give independent consent and the physician has adequate training and skills to deal with the situation without escalating the violence. If the physician feels unable to deal effectively with either patient because of the dual relationship, referral to another qualified physician is preferred.

Finkelstein, Daniel; Wu, Albert W.; Holtzman, Neil A., et al. When a physician harms a patient by a medical error: ethical, legal, and risk–management considerations. *Journal of Clinical Ethics.* 1997 Winter; 8(4): 330–335. 8 fn. BE57607.
> accountability; case studies; *communication; compensation; *disclosure; eye diseases; hospitals; *iatrogenic disease; interprofessional relations; legal aspects; *moral obligations; *negligence; patient care; peer review; physician patient relationship; *physicians; professional competence; referral and consultation; surgery; trust; whistleblowing; *medical errors; risk management

Errors that harm patients are infrequently brought to the attention of these patients. The full disclosure of such medical errors is in the best interest of patients because it allows them to understand what has occurred, and to gain appropriate compensation for the harm that they have suffered. Physicians have been given little guidance regarding how to conduct a relationship with the patient after such an injury. We argue that the physician must continue to respect the patient, and communicate honestly with him or her throughout their relationship, even after the patient has been injured. It is painful to admit our errors, especially to those who have been harmed by them. Nevertheless, offering an apology for harming a patient should be considered to be one of the ethical responsibilities of the profession of medicine. Monetary compensation alone is not to be offered as a charitable gesture; rather, it should be accompanied by an apology to demonstrate the responsibility of the physician to the trusting patient. Full and honest disclosure of errors is most consistent with the mutual respect and trust patients expect from their physicians. Clearly, physicians' ethical responsibilities sometimes differ from their legal and risk–management responsibilities.

Fins, Joseph J. Approximation and negotiation: clinical pragmatism and difference. *Cambridge Quarterly of Healthcare Ethics.* 1998 Winter; 7(1): 68–76. 17 fn. BE58453.
> attitudes to death; *blacks; *brain death; case studies; children; *clinical ethics; *communication; *consensus; *cultural pluralism; *decision making; *determination of death; diagnosis; *dissent; Jewish ethics; *Jews; *knowledge, attitudes, practice; legal aspects; *minority groups; parents; *patient care; *physicians; *professional family relationship; religion; secularism; terminal care; trust; *values;

---

*pragmatism; New York; Orthodox Judaism; United States

Franks, Peter; Clancy, Carolyn M.; Naumburg, Elizabeth H. Sex, access, and excess. [Editorial]. *Annals of Internal Medicine.* 1995 Oct 1; 123(7): 548–549. 20 refs. BE56106.
> biomedical technologies; diagnosis; *females; *health care; health services research; heart diseases; *males; *patient care; *patient satisfaction; preventive medicine; primary health care; quality of health care; referral and consultation; *selection for treatment; social discrimination; surgery; treatment outcome; women's health; continuity of patient care; United States

Frith, Lucy, ed. Ethics and Midwifery: Issues in Contemporary Practice. Boston, MA: Butterworth–Heinemann; 1996. 282 p. Includes references. ISBN 0–7506–3056–6. BE58631.
> aborted fetuses; allowing to die; autonomy; behavioral research; *bioethical issues; childbirth; conflict of interest; congenital disorders; decision making; drugs; fetal tissue donation; human experimentation; informed consent; intensive care units; moral policy; newborns; *nurse midwives; nurse patient relationship; *nursing ethics; nursing research; pain; patient advocacy; *patient care; physician nurse relationship; *pregnant women; prematurity; prenatal diagnosis; professional autonomy; public policy; regulation; reproductive technologies; risk; risks and benefits; selection for treatment; selective abortion; sexuality; standards; analgesia; ultrasonography; *Great Britain; United Kingdom Central Council for Nursing, Midwifery and Health Visiting

Gastmans, Chris. Challenges to nursing values in a changing nursing environment. *Nursing Ethics.* 1998 May; 5(3): 236–245. 22 refs. BE58723.
> administrators; biomedical technologies; *caring; codes of ethics; employment; health care delivery; health facilities; institutional ethics; nurse patient relationship; *nurse's role; *nurses; *nursing ethics; *patient care; physician nurse relationship; physician's role; professional autonomy; professional organizations; trends; values

Gianakos, Dean. Accepting limits. *Archives of Internal Medicine.* 1998 May 25; 158(10): 1059–1061. 7 refs. BE58802.
> communication; continuing education; *decision making; *disclosure; economics; faculty; incentives; interprofessional relations; *knowledge, attitudes, practice; managed care programs; *medical education; medical ethics; medical specialties; *patient care; physician patient relationship; *physicians; primary health care; *professional competence; referral and consultation; self concept; students; *technical expertise; trust; *uncertainty; evidence–based medicine

Giuffrida, Antonio; Torgerson, David J. Should we pay the patient? Review of financial incentives to enhance patient compliance. *BMJ (British Medical Journal).* 1997 Sep 20; 315(7110): 703–707. 64 refs. BE57308.
> *costs and benefits; *empirical research; health services research; *incentives; *patient care; *patient compliance; *remuneration; treatment outcome; United States
> OBJECTIVE: To determine whether financial incentives increase patients' compliance with healthcare treatments. DATA SOURCES: Systematic literature review of computer databases—Medline, Embase, PsychLit, EconLit, and the Cochrane Database of Clinical Trials. In addition, the reference list of each retrieved article was reviewed and relevant citations retrieved. STUDY SELECTION: Only randomised trials with quantitative data concerning the effect, of financial incentives (cash, vouchers, lottery tickets, or gifts) on compliance with medication, medical advice, or medical appointments were included in the review. Eleven papers were identified as meeting the selection

criteria. DATA EXTRACTION: Data on study populations, interventions, and outcomes were extracted and analysed using odds ratios and the number of patients needed to be treated to improve compliance by one patient. RESULTS: 10 of the 11 studies showed improvements in patient compliance with the use of financial incentives. CONCLUSIONS: Financial incentives can improve patient compliance.

Halevy, Amir; Baldwin, John C. Poor surgical risk patients. *In:* McCullough, Laurence B.; Jones, James W.; Brody, Baruch A., eds. Surgical Ethics. New York, NY: Oxford University Press; 1998: 152–170. 32 refs. ISBN 0–19–510347–5. BE58325.
> allowing to die; alternatives; autonomy; beneficence; competence; comprehension; *decision making; disclosure; dissent; futility; goals; HIV seropositivity; informed consent; interprofessional relations; justice; moral obligations; morbidity; mortality; occupational exposure; *patients; *physicians; professional autonomy; prolongation of life; quality of life; referral and consultation; refusal to treat; resource allocation; review; *risk; *risks and benefits; selection for treatment; *surgery; terminology; third party consent; treatment outcome; treatment refusal; values; withholding treatment; United States

Hanson, Mark J. The religious difference in clinical healthcare. *Cambridge Quarterly of Healthcare Ethics.* 1998 Winter; 7(1): 57–67. 24 fn. BE58454.
> attitudes to death; autonomy; beneficence; bioethical issues; bioethics; Christian Scientists; *clinical ethics; communication; *cultural pluralism; *decision making; goals; health; health care; health care delivery; *knowledge, attitudes, practice; medicine; morality; *patient care; *patients; physician patient relationship; *religion; religious ethics; secularism; self concept; suffering; terminal care; *values; faith healing

Harris, Cathleen M.; Mahowald, Mary B. Women and alcohol abuse. *In:* Shelton, Wayne N.; Edwards, Rem B., eds. Advances in Bioethics. Volume 3: Values, Ethics, and Alcoholism. Greenwich, CT: JAI Press; 1997: 153–170. 69 refs. ISBN 0–7623–0219–4. BE57637.
> accountability; *alcohol abuse; autonomy; *behavior control; *coercion; congenital disorders; criminal law; decision making; disease; *females; *fetuses; indigents; legal aspects; mandatory programs; minority groups; moral obligations; newborns; *patient care; *pregnant women; *prenatal injuries; privacy; psychological stress; public policy; reproduction; rights; self concept; sexuality; social discrimination; socioeconomic factors; state interest; *stigmatization; value of life; women's health services; women's rights; United States

Heilicser, Bernard; Stocking, Carol; Siegler, Mark. Ethical dilemmas in emergency medical services: the perspective of the emergency medical technician. *Annals of Emergency Medicine.* 1996 Feb; 27(2): 239–243. 11 refs. BE56550.
> advance directives; *allied health personnel; *attitudes; child abuse; *community services; competence; confidentiality; continuing education; decision making; *emergency care; evaluation studies; health maintenance organizations; information dissemination; informed consent; interprofessional relations; minors; organizational policies; patients; professional competence; resuscitation orders; selection for treatment; survey; terminally ill; treatment refusal; truth disclosure; health services misuse; outpatients; Illinois; South Cook County Emergency Medical Service System (IL)

Herwaldt, Loreen A. Ethical aspects of infection control. *Infection Control and Hospital Epidemiology.* 1996 Feb; 17(2): 108–113. 26 refs. BE56228.
> autonomy; *communicable diseases; confidentiality; decision

---

BE = bioethics accession number   fn. = footnotes   refs. = references

making; disclosure; economics; *epidemiology; guidelines; *health personnel; hepatitis; HIV seropositivity; *hospitals; *institutional policies; interprofessional relations; misconduct; patient care; patients; professional autonomy; *professional ethics; public health; quarantine; *infection control

Hoffmann, Diane E. Managing the persistent patient with chronic pain. [Case study and commentary]. *HEC (HealthCare Ethics Committee) Forum.* 1997 Dec; 9(4): 365–372. 5 refs. Reprinted from *Ethics Rounds*, the ethics newsletter of Northern California Kaiser Permanente. BE58086.
    *behavior disorders; case studies; chronically ill; community services; *institutional ethics; legal aspects; *managed care programs; mentally ill; moral obligations; *pain; *patient compliance; patient discharge; physicians; referral and consultation; refusal to treat; resource allocation; *health services misuse; patient abandonment; personal financing; *psychophysiologic disorders

Horton, Richard. Doctors, the General Medical Council, and Bristol. *Lancet.* 1998 May 23; 351(9115): 1525–1526. 5 refs. BE58239.
    administrators; biomedical research; disclosure; fraud; informed consent; mass media; *misconduct; mortality; *patient care; *physicians; *professional competence; quality of health care; risks and benefits; *self regulation; surgery; technical expertise; medical audit; *General Medical Council (Great Britain); Good Medical Practice (General Medical Council); *Great Britain

Howe, Edmund G. Commentary: "missing" patients by seeing only their cultures. *Journal of Clinical Ethics.* 1998 Summer; 9(2): 191–193. 5 fn. Commentary on E. Agard et al., p. 173–176, and on K.A. Culhane–Pera and D.E. Vawter, p. 179–190. BE58965.
    consensus; *cultural pluralism; *decision making; family members; *health personnel; *minority groups; *patient care; patient transfer; professional patient relationship; treatment refusal; trust

Howe, Edmund G. "Possible mistakes." *Journal of Clinical Ethics.* 1997 Winter; 8(4): 323–328. 35 fn. BE57608.
    *disclosure; empathy; *iatrogenic disease; interprofessional relations; legal liability; motivation; *negligence; *patient care; physician patient relationship; professional competence; psychological stress; risks and benefits; self concept; standards; *truth disclosure; uncertainty; whistleblowing; *medical errors; United States
What should a careprovider do if he or she has made a mistake that has harmed a patient? What if a careprovider learns that another's mistake has harmed a patient? Should a careprovider go so far as to tell a patient that he or she could sue? Several articles in this issue of *JCE* address these questions. In this introductory article, I shall ask a question that goes one step further: What should a careprovider do when he or she *may* have made a mistake? First I will discuss the arguments for and against disclosing such mistakes to patients. Then, because these arguments may not be conclusive in and of themselves, I shall also relate two somewhat surprising clinical findings that may help a careprovider facing this situation decide what to do.

Humber, James M.; Almeder, Robert F., eds. Alternative Medicine and Ethics. Totowa, NJ: Humana Press; 1998. 220 p. (Biomedical ethics reviews). Includes references. ISBN 0–89603–440–2. BE57206.
    *alternative therapies; biomedical research; children; drugs; evaluation; federal government; gatekeeping; government financing; health care delivery; health insurance; health insurance reimbursement; legal aspects; medicine; methods; parents; pharmacists; professional ethics; public policy; religion; resource allocation; risks and benefits; treatment refusal; faith healing; holistic health; National Institutes of Health; United States

Huston, Kathleen. Ethical decisions in treating battered women. *Professional Psychology: Research and Practice.* 1984 Dec; 15(6): 822–832. 31 refs. BE57239.
    autonomy; beneficence; competence; decision making; *directive counseling; *domestic violence; *females; health personnel; paternalism; patients; *professional patient relationship; psychology; *psychotherapy; professional role

International Federation of Gynecology and Obstetrics. Committee for the Study of Ethical Aspects of Human Reproduction. Recommendations on Ethical Issues in Obstetrics and Gynecology. London: FIGO; 1997 Jul. 117 p. Text in English, in French, and in Spanish. English text: p. 6–39. BE57742.
    allowing to die; anencephaly; cloning; congenital disorders; contraception; domestic violence; embryo research; embryos; *females; fetal tissue donation; gene therapy; genes; genetic enhancement; germ cells; HIV seropositivity; hormones; informed consent; multiple pregnancy; *newborns; *obstetrics and gynecology; organ donation; *organizational policies; ovum donors; parental consent; patents; *patient care; physician patient relationship; physicians; *pregnant women; prenatal diagnosis; professional organizations; remuneration; *reproduction; selective abortion; semen donors; sex determination; sexuality; surrogate mothers; viability; voluntary sterilization; withholding treatment; *International Federation of Gynecology and Obstetrics

Irving, Miles; Berwick, Donald M.; Rubin, Peter, et al. Five times: coincidence or something more serious? [Article and commentaries]. *BMJ (British Medical Journal).* 1998 Jun 6; 316(7146): 1736–1740. 8 refs. BE58368.
    interprofessional relations; *misconduct; mortality; *physicians; *professional competence; self regulation; *surgery; treatment outcome; *whistleblowing; medical audit; General Medical Council (Great Britain); Great Britain

Iserson, Kenneth V. Bioethical dilemmas in emergency medicine and prehospital care. [Revised]. *In:* Monagle, John F.; Thomasma, David C., eds. Health Care Ethics: Critical Issues for the 21st Century. Gaithersburg, MD: Aspen Publishers; 1998: 138–145. 24 fn. ISBN 0–8342–0911–X. BE56281.
    advance directives; allied health personnel; allowing to die; assisted suicide; autonomy; cadavers; competence; decision making; *emergency care; futility; gatekeeping; health care delivery; health insurance reimbursement; health personnel; indigents; informed consent; managed care programs; medical education; paternalism; patient advocacy; patient transfer; prolongation of life; refusal to treat; resource allocation; resuscitation orders; review; therapeutic research; third party consent; violence; United States

Jacobs, Joseph J. Alternative medicine and medical futility. *In:* Zucker, Marjorie B.; Zucker, Howard D., eds. Medical Futility and the Evaluation of Life–Sustaining Interventions. New York, NY: Cambridge University Press; 1997: 65–70. 7 refs. ISBN 0–521–56877–3. BE55980.
    AIDS; *alternative therapies; attitudes; cancer; caring; communication; evaluation; *futility; nutrition; *patient care; patients; physician patient relationship; physicians; prolongation of life; quality of life; risks and benefits; statistics; United States

Jakobovits, Yoel. Male infertility: halakhic issues in investigation and management. *In:* Feldman, Emanuel;

BE = bioethics accession number   fn. = footnotes   refs. = references

Wolowelsky, Joel B., eds. Jewish Law and the New Reproductive Technologies. Hoboken, NJ: Ktav; 1997: 115–138. 89 fn. ISBN 0-88125-586-6. BE57459.
*diagnosis; *infertility; *Jewish ethics; *males; methods; *patient care; reproduction; reproductive technologies; sperm; theology; Orthodox Judaism

Jecker, Nancy S.; Allen, Margaret D. Surgery and other medical specialties. In: McCullough, Laurence B.; Jones, James W.; Brody, Baruch A., eds. Surgical Ethics. New York, NY: Oxford University Press; 1998: 280–301. 41 refs. ISBN 0-19-510347-5. BE58327.
accountability; alternatives; conflict of interest; decision making; diagnosis; disclosure; dissent; economics; institutional policies; *interprofessional relations; managed care programs; medical ethics; *medical specialties; moral obligations; organ transplantation; organizational policies; *patient advocacy; patient care; patient participation; physician patient relationship; physician self-referral; *physicians; professional competence; professional organizations; quality of health care; *referral and consultation; sociology of medicine; *surgery; technical expertise; American College of Physicians; American College of Surgeons; United States

Johnson, Alan G. Surgery as a placebo. Lancet. 1994 Oct 22; 344(8930): 1140–1142. 14 refs. BE56578.
evaluation; physicians; *placebos; *risks and benefits; *surgery; time factors; treatment outcome; *sham surgery

Johnston, S.R.D.; Broadley, K.; Henson, G., et al. Management of metastatic melanoma during pregnancy. [Case study and commentaries]. BMJ (British Medical Journal). 1998 Mar 14; 316(7134): 848–851. 13 refs. BE57757.
altruism; *cancer; case studies; cesarean section; *childbirth; *decision making; drugs; fetal development; *fetuses; maternal health; morbidity; mortality; parents; *patient care; *pregnant women; *prognosis; radiology; *risks and benefits; terminally ill; *therapeutic abortion; viability

Jones, R. Scott; Fletcher, John C. Self-regulation of surgical practice and research. In: McCullough, Laurence B.; Jones, James W.; Brody, Baruch A., eds. Surgical Ethics. New York, NY: Oxford University Press; 1998: 255–279. 63 refs. ISBN 0-19-510347-5. BE58328.
*accountability; animal experimentation; authorship; beneficence; *biomedical research; conflict of interest; continuing education; economics; *goals; government regulation; guidelines; historical aspects; human experimentation; incentives; interprofessional relations; managed care programs; medical ethics; *medicine; *moral obligations; patient advocacy; peer review; physician patient relationship; *physicians; professional autonomy; professional competence; professional organizations; review; scientific misconduct; *self regulation; *surgery; whistleblowing; integrity; medical errors; physician impairment; United States

Kapp, Marshall B. Our Hands Are Tied: Legal Tensions and Medical Ethics. Westport, CT: Auburn House; 1998. 175 p. Includes references. ISBN 0-86569-276-9. BE57895.
administrators; allowing to die; autonomy; decision making; diagnosis; health care reform; health facilities; health insurance; informed consent; *knowledge, attitudes, practice; law; *legal aspects; legal guardians; *legal liability; *malpractice; medical ethics; medicine; palliative care; *patient care; physical restraint; physician patient relationship; *physicians; prolongation of life; public policy; quality of health care; resuscitation; social impact; terminal care; third party consent; health services misuse; risk management; *United States

Kirby, Dahlian. Transsexualism. In: Chadwick, Ruth, ed. Encyclopedia of Applied Ehtics, Volume 4. San Diego, CA: Academic Press; 1998: 409–412. 7 refs. ISBN 0-12-227069-X. BE56348.
cosmetic surgery; females; hormones; human body; males; morality; patient care; psychiatric diagnosis; self concept; surgery; *transsexualism

Klein, Rudolf. Competence, professional self regulation, and the public interest. BMJ (British Medical Journal). 1998 Jun 6; 316(7146): 1740–1742. 6 refs. BE58213.
children; heart diseases; hospitals; interprofessional relations; *misconduct; mortality; *pediatrics; *physicians; *professional competence; quality of health care; *self regulation; standards; *surgery; technical expertise; whistleblowing; medical audit; Bristol Royal Infirmary; *General Medical Council (Great Britain); *Great Britain; National Health Service

Koch, Tom. Principles and purpose: the patient surrogate's perspective and role. Cambridge Quarterly of Healthcare Ethics. 1997 Fall; 6(4): 461–469. 15 fn. BE56467.
adults; aged; alcohol abuse; bioethical issues; chronically ill; *computer communication networks; decision making; dementia; *family members; family relationship; *health education; *home care; human experimentation; *information dissemination; patient advocacy; *patient care; patients; *public participation; referral and consultation; third party consent; *self-help groups

Kokiko, Jeannine; Watts, Dorraine D. Ethical decision making in the emergency department: the R.O.L.E. acronym for four areas of consideration. Journal of Emergency Nursing. 1995 Jun; 21(3): 219–222. 8 refs. BE56605.
alcohol abuse; autonomy; beneficence; competence; dangerousness; *decision making; *emergency care; family members; hospitals; institutional policies; legal aspects; *nurses; nursing ethics; patient admission; patient discharge; physicians; quality of life; resuscitation; resuscitation orders; risks and benefits; treatment refusal

Konen, Joseph C. Whose life is it anyway? [Editorial]. Archives of Family Medicine. 1997 Jan–Feb; 6(1): 77–78. 6 refs. BE56469.
attitudes; cancer; coercion; consensus; counseling; *decision making; dissent; family members; *family practice; *females; informed consent; *males; *marital relationship; *married persons; mass screening; *patient care; *patients; physician patient relationship; *physician's role; *professional family relationship; quality of life; treatment outcome; uncertainty; values; prostate cancer

Kopelman, Loretta M.; Lannin, Donald R.; Kopelman, Arthur E. Preventing and managing unwarranted biases against patients. In: McCullough, Laurence B.; Jones, James W.; Brody, Baruch A., eds. Surgical Ethics. New York, NY: Oxford University Press; 1998: 242–254. 31 refs. ISBN 0-19-510347-5. BE58330.
aged; biomedical technologies; blacks; case studies; continuing education; cultural pluralism; curriculum; females; health facilities; Hispanic Americans; HIV seropositivity; human experimentation; humanities; indigents; institutional policies; medical ethics; *patient care; patients; *physician patient relationship; *physicians; prognosis; quality of health care; refusal to treat; risks and benefits; selection for treatment; selection of subjects; *social discrimination; *socioeconomic factors; *surgery; trust; United States

Leners, Debra; Beardslee, Nancy Q. Suffering and ethical caring: incompatible entities. Nursing Ethics. 1997 Sep; 4(5): 361–369. 22 refs. BE56874.
*attitudes; *caring; decision making; economics;

employment; hospitals; institutional policies; nurse patient relationship; *nurses; *nursing ethics; pain; patient advocacy; *patient care; physician nurse relationship; risk; *suffering; terminally ill; values; ethnographic studies; qualitative research; Colorado

Levin, Betty Wolder; Schiller, Nina Glick. Social class and medical decisionmaking: a neglected topic in bioethics. *Cambridge Quarterly of Healthcare Ethics.* 1998 Winter; 7(1): 41–56. 23 fn. BE58458.
    AIDS; allowing to die; attitudes; autonomy; *bioethics; case studies; *clinical ethics; *cultural pluralism; *decision making; ethicists; family relationship; females; health; health care delivery; health personnel; heart diseases; hearts; *indigents; justice; *knowledge, attitudes, practice; literature; minority groups; organ transplantation; *patient care; *patients; self concept; *social discrimination; social dominance; *socioeconomic factors; terminal care; treatment refusal; trust; values; *vulnerable populations; withholding treatment; United States

Lewis, Marcia A.; Tamparo, Carol D. Medical Law, Ethics, and Bioethics for Ambulatory Care. Fourth Edition. Philadelphia, PA: F.A. Davis; 1998. 295 p. Includes references and discussion questions. Appendix 1: Codes of ethics; Appendix 2: Sample documents for choices about health care, life, and death. ISBN 0–8036–0348–7. BE57279.
    abortion, induced; advance directives; AIDS; *allied health personnel; assisted suicide; *bioethical issues; case studies; codes of ethics; confidentiality; cultural pluralism; decision making; drugs; *employment; euthanasia; fetuses; genetic services; government regulation; health care delivery; health facilities; informed consent; interprofessional relations; law; *legal aspects; *legal liability; *legal obligations; malpractice; mandatory reporting; medical fees; medical records; negligence; *organization and administration; *patient care; *professional ethics; professional patient relationship; reproductive technologies; resource allocation; standards; terminal care; third party consent; *ambulatory care; United States

Lewison, Helen. Choices in childbirth: areas of conflict. *In:* Frith, Lucy, ed. Ethics and Midwifery: Issues in Contemporary Practice. Boston, MA: Butterworth–Heinemann; 1996: 36–50. 21 refs. ISBN 0–7506–3056–6. BE58633.
    alternatives; *autonomy; *childbirth; comprehension; conflict of interest; *decision making; disclosure; hospitals; informed consent; institutional policies; legal aspects; medical records; moral obligations; *nurse midwives; nurse patient relationship; organizational policies; patient access to records; patient advocacy; *patient care; patient education; practice guidelines; *pregnant women; professional autonomy; professional organizations; public participation; public policy; risks and benefits; standards; treatment refusal; *Great Britain; International Code of Ethics for Midwives; National Health Service; United Kingdom Central Council for Nursing, Midwifery and Health Visiting

Logmans, A.; Verhoeff, A.; Bol Raap, R., et al. Should doctors reconstruct the vaginal introitus of adolescent girls to mimic the virginal state? [Article and commentaries]. *BMJ (British Medical Journal).* 1998 Feb 7; 316(7129): 459–462. 22 refs. BE57963.
    adolescents; aliens; autonomy; *cultural pluralism; deception; *females; males; marital relationship; minority groups; moral complicity; moral obligations; physicians; psychological stress; refusal to treat; sex offenses; *sexuality; *surgery; women's rights; Netherlands

Loneck, Barry. How particular social environments affect alcoholics. *In:* Shelton, Wayne N.; Edwards, Rem B., eds. Advances in Bioethics. Volume 3: Values, Ethics,

and Alcoholism. Greenwich, CT: JAI Press; 1997: 171–205. 108 refs. ISBN 0–7623–0219–4. BE57638.
    accountability; adolescents; aged; *alcohol abuse; *autonomy; *beneficence; *coercion; dangerousness; disadvantaged; employment; family relationship; females; fetuses; genetic predisposition; injuries; involuntary commitment; *justice; mentally ill; models, theoretical; *moral policy; *paternalism; *patient care; physicians; pregnant women; prenatal injuries; psychological stress; *public policy; risk; social discrimination; social impact; social problems; traffic accidents; empowerment

Long, Ann; Long, Aishlinn; Smyth, Angus. Suicide: a statement of suffering. *Nursing Ethics.* 1998 Jan; 5(1): 3–15. 58 refs. BE58712.
    attitudes; autonomy; beneficence; caring; communication; competence; empathy; moral obligations; *nurse patient relationship; *nurse's role; *nurses; nursing ethics; paternalism; *patient care; professional family relationship; stigmatization; *suffering; *suicide; value of life

Lustig, Andrew; Scardino, Peter. Elective patients. *In:* McCullough, Laurence B.; Jones, James W.; Brody, Baruch A., eds. Surgical Ethics. New York, NY: Oxford University Press; 1998: 133–151. 33 refs. ISBN 0–19–510347–5. BE58331.
    *alternatives; autonomy; beneficence; blood transfusions; chronically ill; competence; comprehension; conflict of interest; *decision making; directive counseling; economics; *informed consent; morbidity; mortality; paternalism; patient education; *patient participation; patients; *physicians; quality of life; referral and consultation; refusal to treat; resuscitation orders; review; risks and benefits; *surgery; time factors; treatment outcome; treatment refusal; *uncertainty; values; physician's practice patterns; prostate cancer

McCullough, Laurence B.; Jones, James W.; Brody, Baruch A., eds. Surgical Ethics. New York, NY: Oxford University Press; 1998. 396 p. 642 refs. ISBN 0–19–510347–5. BE58322.
    advance directives; autonomy; beneficence; competence; confidentiality; conflict of interest; determination of death; disclosure; emergency care; entrepreneurship; family members; health facilities; health insurance; indigents; informed consent; interprofessional relations; justice; managed care programs; *medical ethics; *moral obligations; organ transplantation; patient advocacy; *patient care; patients; physician patient relationship; *physicians; professional competence; professional organizations; remuneration; resource allocation; resuscitation orders; review; selection for treatment; self regulation; social discrimination; *surgery; terminal care; therapeutic research; third party consent; treatment refusal; health services misuse; professional courtesy; undertreatment; American College of Surgeons; American Medical Association; United States

Mattox, Kenneth L.; Engelhardt, H. Tristram. Emerging patients: serious moral choices with limited time, information, and patient participation. *In:* McCullough, Laurence B.; Jones, James W.; Brody, Baruch A., eds. Surgical Ethics. New York, NY: Oxford University Press; 1998: 78–96. 14 refs. ISBN 0–19–510347–5. BE58333.
    advance directives; competence; conflict of interest; costs and benefits; critically ill; *decision making; economics; *emergency care; futility; goals; hospitals; informed consent; institutional policies; legal aspects; managed care programs; *moral obligations; patient advocacy; patients; *physicians; prognosis; quality of life; resuscitation orders; review; risks and benefits; *surgery; third party consent; time factors; treatment outcome; treatment refusal; withholding treatment

Mayer, Dan; Thibodeau, Lorraine. Ethical issues in alcohol-related emergencies and emergency care of

alcoholic and intoxicated patients. *In:* Shelton, Wayne N.; Edwards, Rem B., eds. Advances in Bioethics. Volume 3: Values, Ethics, and Alcoholism. Greenwich, CT: JAI Press; 1997: 287–308. 18 refs. ISBN 0-7623-0219-4. BE57639.
    adults; *alcohol abuse; autonomy; behavior control; beneficence; burns; competence; confidentiality; dangerousness; decision making; disadvantaged; drugs; *emergency care; hospitals; injuries; justice; law enforcement; legal aspects; minors; parental consent; paternalism; patient discharge; physical restraint; physicians; referral and consultation; suicide; time factors; traffic accidents; treatment refusal; homeless persons; Emergency Medical Treatment and Active Labor Act 1986; United States

Miller, Randolph A.; Goodman, Kenneth W. Ethical challenges in the use of decision–support software in clinical practice. *In:* Goodman, Kenneth W., ed. Ethics, Computing, and Medicine: Informatics and the Transformation of Health Care. New York, NY: Cambridge University Press; 1998: 102–115. 32 refs. ISBN 0-521-46905-8. BE57006.
    *computers; *decision making; guidelines; informed consent; medical education; *patient care; physician patient relationship; professional competence; referral and consultation; standards; technical expertise

Mollica, Richard F. Human rights reflections in daily medical practice. [Editorial]. *Medical Journal of Australia.* 1996 Dec 2–16; 165(11–12): 594–595. 9 refs. BE58973.
    *disadvantaged; *human rights; *misconduct; *obligations to society; *patient care; *physician's role; prisoners; public policy; *social problems; torture; violence; war

Montgomery, Jonathan. Health care law and ethics: abortion; fertility; maternity care; selective treatment of the newborn; transplantation; terminal care and euthanasia. *In: his* Health Care Law. New York, NY: Oxford University Press; 1997: 357–456. 503 fn. ISBN 0-19-876260-7. BE56245.
    *abortion, induced; active euthanasia; *adults; *allowing to die; assisted suicide; body parts and fluids; cadavers; childbirth; congenital disorders; conscience; contraception; family planning; fetuses; health personnel; *legal aspects; legal liability; legislation; living wills; maternal health; minors; *newborns; *organ donation; organ donors; organ transplantation; *patient care; persistent vegetative state; *pregnant women; prenatal injuries; remuneration; *reproductive technologies; selective abortion; spousal consent; sterilization (sexual); surrogate mothers; terminal care; therapeutic abortion; treatment refusal; *Great Britain

Morreim, E. Haavi. At the intersection of medicine, law, economics, and ethics: bioethics and the art of intellectual cross-dressing. *In:* Carson, Ronald A.; Burns, Chester R., eds. Philosophy of Medicine and Bioethics: A Twenty–Year Retrospective and Critical Appraisal. Boston, MA: Kluwer Academic; 1997: 299–325. 78 refs. 28 fn. ISBN 0-7923-3545-7. BE56544.
    bioethics; conflict of interest; contracts; *economics; ethics; *financial support; government financing; guidelines; *health care delivery; health insurance; health insurance reimbursement; indigents; industry; interdisciplinary communication; justice; law; legal aspects; legal liability; *legal obligations; *managed care programs; medical specialties; medicine; *moral obligations; *patient advocacy; *patient care; *physician's role; *physicians; professional autonomy; professional organizations; quality of health care; referral and consultation; remuneration; *resource allocation; *standards; therapeutic research; torts; values; utilization review; United States

Nyman, Deborah J.; Sprung, Charles L. International perspectives on ethics in critical care. *Critical Care Clinics.* 1997 Apr; 13(2): 409–415. 36 refs. BE58360.
    allowing to die; *critically ill; decision making; euthanasia; informed consent; *intensive care units; *international aspects; medical ethics; patient admission; *patient care; physicians; prognosis; quality of life; resource allocation; resuscitation orders; selection for treatment; values; withholding treatment

Peppin, John F. The Christian physician in the non–Christian institution: objections of conscience and physician value neutrality. *Christian Bioethics.* 1997 Mar; 3(1): 39–54. 33 refs. 16 fn. Commented on by A.L. Smith, p. 74–84. BE56359.
    abortion, induced; assisted suicide; autonomy; *Christian ethics; *conscience; government regulation; health facilities; institutional policies; legal rights; medical education; *medical ethics; moral complicity; morality; *patient care; physician patient relationship; *physicians; referral and consultation; refusal to treat; religious hospitals; *values; liberalism; United States
Christian physicians are in danger of losing the right of conscientious objection in situations they deem immoral. The erosion of this right is bolstered by the doctrine of "physician value neutrality" (PVN) which may be an impetus for the push to require physicians to refer for procedures they find immoral. It is only a small step from referral to compelling performance of these same procedures. If no one particular value is more morally correct than any other (a foundational PVN premise) and a physician ought to be value neutral, than conscientious objection to morally objectionable actions becomes a thing of the past. However, the argument for PVN fails. Therefore, Christian physicians should state their values openly, which would allow patients the ability to choose like-minded physicians. Some possible responses to this erosion of conscientious objection include, disengagement from non-Christian institutions, the formation of distinctly Christian medical institutions and political action. However, for the Christian the initial focus should be on a life of holiness which requires each of us to avoid evil.

Perkins, Henry S.; Supik, Josie D.; Hazuda, Helen P. Cultural differences among health professionals: a case illustration. *Journal of Clinical Ethics.* 1998 Summer; 9(2): 108–117. 35 fn. BE58956.
    *autonomy; case studies; cesarean section; comparative studies; counseling; critically ill; *cultural pluralism; *decision making; ethical relativism; family relationship; females; *health personnel; hospitals; *informed consent; *international aspects; mediation; paternalism; *patient care; pregnant women; spousal consent; survey; *treatment refusal; value of life; *values; voluntary sterilization; *non-Western World; qualitative research; *Western World; *Kenya
This study illustrates that cultural differences arise among similarly trained health professionals. Health professionals must learn to communicate sensitively with colleagues from other cultures, to respect their values, and to recognize and resolve cultural differences that affect patient care. In this shrinking, multicultural world, health professionals cannot afford the comfortable illusion that all similarly trained practitioners share the same values about the care of patients and professional conduct.

Pierce, Susan Foley. A model for conceptualizing the moral dynamic in health care. *Nursing Ethics.* 1997 Nov; 4(6): 483–495. 13 refs. BE57419.
    autonomy; bioethical issues; caring; compassion; *decision making; emotions; empathy; ethical theory; females; justice;

BE = bioethics accession number   fn. = footnotes   refs. = references

males; *medical ethics; *models, theoretical; *moral development; morality; nurse's role; *nurses; *nursing ethics; *patient care; patient care team; physician nurse relationship; physician's role; *physicians; professional patient relationship; self concept; technical expertise; terminal care; *values; virtues

Pinkus, Rosa Lynn. Politics, paternalism, and the rise of the neurosurgeon: the evolution of moral reasoning. *Medical Humanities Review.* 1996 Fall; 10(2): 20–44. 81 fn. BE56598.
　　accountability; brain pathology; case studies; coercion; decision making; dissent; *historical aspects; internship and residency; *interprofessional relations; medical education; *medical ethics; *medical specialties; newborns; paternalism; patient care; physician patient relationship; *physicians; politics; social dominance; standards; *surgery; technical expertise; truth disclosure; medical errors; *neurosurgery; *Cushing, Harvey; Dandy, Walter; Twentieth Century; United States

Plotnikoff, Gregory A. Spirituality, religion, and the physician: new ethical challenges in patient care. *Bioethics Forum.* 1997 Winter; 13(4): 25–30. 8 refs. BE58912.
　　case studies; communication; depressive disorder; moral obligations; pastoral care; paternalism; *patient care; physician patient relationship; *physicians; *religion; trust; values

Purtilo, Ruth; Shaw, Byers W.; Arnold, Robert. Obligations of surgeons to non-physician team members and trainees. *In:* McCullough, Laurence B.; Jones, James W.; Brody, Baruch A., eds. Surgical Ethics. New York, NY: Oxford University Press; 1998: 302–321. 41 refs. ISBN 0-19-510347-5. BE58336.
　　*accountability; communication; confidentiality; conflict of interest; disclosure; family members; goals; health personnel; informed consent; internship and residency; *interprofessional relations; legal obligations; medical education; *moral obligations; nurses; patient advocacy; *patient care team; patients; *physician's role; *physicians; professional autonomy; professional competence; quality of health care; review; self regulation; students; *surgery; technical expertise; truth disclosure; medical errors; professional impairment; United States

Reitemeier, Paul J. Musings on medical mistakes: a four-piece ensemble in search of an orchestra. *Journal of Clinical Ethics.* 1997 Winter; 8(4): 353–358. 5 fn. BE57612.
　　attitudes; bioethics; *clinical ethics; clinical ethics committees; communication; conscience; *disclosure; emotions; empirical research; *ethicist's role; ethics consultation; family members; *iatrogenic disease; legal liability; malpractice; moral obligations; moral policy; negligence; patient care; patients' rights; physician patient relationship; physicians; professional competence; quality of health care; standards; terminal care; *truth disclosure; virtues; whistleblowing; *medical errors

Rich, Ben A. A legacy of silence: bioethics and the culture of pain. *Journal of Medical Humanities.* 1997 Winter; 18(4): 233–259. 47 refs. BE57245.
　　assisted suicide; attitudes; bioethical issues; *bioethics; cancer; chronically ill; clinical ethics; drug abuse; drugs; ethical analysis; ethicists; goals; government regulation; historical aspects; hospices; legal aspects; medical education; medical ethics; medicine; moral obligations; morality; *pain; *palliative care; *patient care; physicians; quality of health care; review; self regulation; standards; state government; *suffering; technical expertise; *terminal care; terminally ill; Study to Understand Prognoses and Preferences for Outcomes and Risks of Treatments (SUPPORT); United States

For over 20 years the medical literature has carefully documented the undertreatment of all types of pain by physicians. During this same period, as the field of bioethics came of age, the phenomenon of undertreated pain received almost no attention from the bioethics literature. This article takes bioethicists to task for failing to recognize the undertreatment of pain as a major ethical, and not merely a clinical, failing of the medical profession. The nature and extent of the problem of undertreated pain is examined, as well as possible reasons for its disregard by bioethicists. The factors contributing to undertreated pain in the clinical setting are considered, as well as the hazards posed by recent failures to address ethically questionable clinical practices. Finally, suggestions are offered for refocusing the attention of bioethicists to this significant problem.

Richmond, Caroline; Heasell, Stephen; Kahtan, Susannah, et al. Compensation for victims of medical accidents. [Letters]. *BMJ (British Medical Journal).* 1998 Jan 3; 316(7124): 73–74. 2 refs. BE57973.
　　*compensation; economics; *health care; hospitals; iatrogenic disease; *injuries; legal aspects; *legal liability; *negligence; *patient care; *patients; physicians; *resource allocation; time factors; *Great Britain; National Health Service

Ruskin, Andrew. Capitation: the legal implications of using capitation to affect physician decision-making processes. *Journal of Contemporary Health Law and Policy.* 1997 Spring; 13(2): 391–421. 169 fn. BE56011.
　　alternatives; *decision making; *economics; federal government; government regulation; guidelines; *health care; health care delivery; *health maintenance organizations; *incentives; injuries; judicial action; *legal liability; *managed care programs; *negligence; *patient care; patient discharge; *physicians; practice guidelines; professional autonomy; referral and consultation; *remuneration; state government; suicide; *withholding treatment; *capitation fee; *physician's practice patterns; relative value scales; utilization review; California; Employee Retirement Income Security Act 1974 (ERISA); Health Care Financing Administration; Medi-Cal; Medicare; National Association of Insurance Commissioners; *United States; Wickline v. State; Wilson v. Blue Cross of Southern California

Salladay, Susan Anthony; Shelly, Judith Allen. Spirituality in nursing theory and practice: dilemmas for Christian bioethics. *Christian Bioethics.* 1997 Mar; 3(1): 20–38. 25 refs. 8 fn. Commented on by A.L. Smith, p. 74–84. BE56358.
　　alternative therapies; caring; *Christian ethics; *cultural pluralism; *goals; health; nurse patient relationship; *nurses; *pastoral care; *patient care; patient compliance; patients; philosophy; psychological stress; psychology; *religion; standards; stigmatization; terminology; treatment outcome; *values; holistic health

Moral strangerhood is due in part to competing worldviews. The profession of nursing is experiencing a paradigm shift which creates ethical dilemmas for both Christian nurses and Christian patients. Nursing's new focus on spirituality and spiritual care presents itself as broadly defining a desired state or patient outcome -- spiritual integrity -- supposed to be applicable to all patients of all faiths. Analysis of nursing's definition of spirituality reveals assumptions and values consistent with an Eastern/New Age worldview which may cause hostility towards Christian patients stereotyped as dogmatic or noncompliant.

Sapru, R.P. Ethical concerns in modern medical practice. *Indian Heart Journal.* 1997 Jul-Aug; 49(4): 441–445. 23

BE = bioethics accession number　　　fn. = footnotes　　　refs. = references

refs. BE58562.
 communication; confidentiality; continuing education; developing countries; disclosure; drug industry; drugs; economics; *health care; heart diseases; Hindu ethics; human experimentation; indigents; informed consent; medical education; *medical ethics; palliative care; *patient care; physician patient relationship; physician self-referral; physicians; *professional competence; quality of health care; regulation; surgery; *India

Schiedermayer, David. Holding Owen. *Journal of Clinical Ethics.* 1997 Winter; 8(4): 349–352. 1 fn. BE57613.
 aged; *patient care; patients; *physician patient relationship; physicians; professional competence; referral and consultation; technical expertise; truth disclosure; medical errors

Sharpe, Virginia A.; Faden, Alan I. Medical Harm: Historical, Conceptual, and Ethical Dimensions of Iatrogenic Illness. New York, NY: Cambridge University Press; 1998. 280 p. Bibliography: p. 248–270. ISBN 0–521–57133–2. BE57447.
 accountability; autonomy; beneficence; codes of ethics; drugs; economics; empirical research; ethical analysis; health; health care delivery; historical aspects; hospitals; human experimentation; *iatrogenic disease; informed consent; injuries; libertarianism; malpractice; medical ethics; medical etiquette; *medicine; negligence; paternalism; *patient care; patients' rights; physician patient relationship; physician's role; physicians; professional competence; professional organizations; quality of health care; regulation; risks and benefits; self regulation; standards; statistics; surgery; technical expertise; toxicity; trends; values; evidence-based medicine; health services misuse; infection control; medical errors; American Medical Association; Nineteenth Century; Twentieth Century; United States

Sharpe, Virginia A. The politics, economics, and ethics of "appropriateness". *Kennedy Institute of Ethics Journal.* 1997 Dec; 7(4): 337–343. 8 refs. 1 fn. BE59015.
 biomedical technologies; costs and benefits; *decision making; economics; empirical research; *health care; health insurance; *health insurance reimbursement; managed care programs; mass screening; *patient care; patients; physicians; public participation; public policy; *resource allocation; risks and benefits; *standards; treatment outcome; trends; evidence-based medicine; needs; *United States
The terms "appropriate" and "necessary" are crucial determinants in decisions regarding the use and reimbursement of medical treatments. This paper encourages greater awareness of the political, economic, and normative assumptions that give meaning to these concepts.

Sheldon, Sally; Wilkinson, Stephen. Conjoined twins: the legality and ethics of sacrifice. *Medical Law Review.* 1997 Summer; 5(2): 149–171. 57 fn. BE57874.
 criminal law; decision making; *double effect; drugs; *intention; *killing; legal aspects; *legal liability; *moral policy; newborns; organ donation; pain; palliative care; personhood; physicians; prognosis; prolongation of life; risks and benefits; *selection for treatment; *surgery; teleological ethics; terminally ill; *twins; *conjoined twins; *Great Britain

Shelton, Wayne N.; Edwards, Rem B., eds. Advances in Bioethics. Volume 3: Values, Ethics, and Alcoholism. Greenwich, CT: JAI Press; 1997. 314 p. (Advances in bioethics; v. 3) Includes references. ISBN 0–7623–0219–4. BE57632.
 *alcohol abuse; autonomy; behavior control; behavior disorders; beneficence; brain pathology; coercion; competence; diagnosis; disease; drugs; economics; emergency care; females; fetuses; genetic predisposition; justice; livers; models, theoretical; moral policy; morality;

organ transplantation; paternalism; *patient care; patient compliance; physician patient relationship; pregnant women; prenatal injuries; psychiatric diagnosis; psychotherapy; public policy; rehabilitation; resource allocation; retreatment; review; selection for treatment; self induced illness; social problems; socioeconomic factors; transplant recipients

Sherwin, Susan. A relational approach to autonomy in health care. *In:* Sherwin, Susan, et al. The Politics of Women's Health: Exploring Agency and Autonomy. Philadelphia, PA: Temple University Press; 1998: 19–47. 30 fn. ISBN 1–56639–633–6. BE58392.
 *autonomy; bioethics; coercion; competence; *decision making; disadvantaged; disclosure; females; *feminist ethics; *health care; health care delivery; informed consent; paternalism; *patient care; physician patient relationship; public policy; self concept; social discrimination; social dominance; social interaction; values; women's health; women's health services

Sherwin, Susan. Cancer and women: some feminist ethics concerns. *In:* Sargent, Carolyn F.; Brettell, Caroline B., eds. Gender and Health: An International Perspective. Upper Saddle River, NJ: Prentice Hall; 1996: 187–204. 28 refs. 1 fn. ISBN 0–13–079427–9. BE58099.
 bioethics; biomedical technologies; *breast cancer; *cancer; decision making; ethics; *females; *feminist ethics; genetic predisposition; health hazards; justice; palliative care; *patient care; physician patient relationship; political activity; preventive medicine; public policy; quality of life; self induced illness; social dominance; socioeconomic factors; violence; women's health; Canada; United States

Shotton, Leila; Seedhouse, David. Practical dignity in caring. *Nursing Ethics.* 1998 May; 5(3): 246–255. 6 refs. BE58724.
 aged; beneficence; *caring; dehumanization; disabled; health personnel; human rights; nursing ethics; *patient care; patients; prisoners; privacy; professional competence; professional patient relationship; *dignity

Siegel–Itzkovich, Judy. Palestinian man shackled in Jerusalem hospital. [News]. *BMJ (British Medical Journal).* 1997 Sep 6; 315(7108): 568. BE56883.
 dangerousness; dehumanization; hospitals; human rights; *patient care; *physical restraint; physicians; *prisoners; professional organizations; public policy; *Israel; Israel Medical Association; *Palestinians

Smith, Richard. Don't treat shackled patients: and keep trying to understand what the Nuremberg trials taught us. [Editorial]. *BMJ (British Medical Journal).* 1997 Jan 18; 314(7075): 164. 1 ref. BE58428.
 human rights; law enforcement; moral obligations; *physical restraint; *physicians; *political activity; *prisoners; *refusal to treat; Great Britain

Smith, Richard. Renegotiating medicine's contract with patients: the GMC is leading the way. [Editorial]. *BMJ (British Medical Journal).* 1998 May 30; 316(7145): 1622–1623. 9 refs. BE58251.
 contracts; *guidelines; iatrogenic disease; negligence; *patient care; patients' rights; physician patient relationship; *physicians; *professional competence; professional organizations; *self regulation; *standards; *General Medical Council (Great Britain); *Good Medical Practice (General Medical Council); *Great Britain

Sugarman, Jeremy; Harland, Robert. Acute yet non–emergent patients. *In:* McCullough, Laurence B.; Jones, James W.; Brody, Baruch A., eds. Surgical Ethics. New York, NY: Oxford University Press; 1998: 116–132. 18 refs. ISBN 0–19–510347–5. BE58337.

---

advance directives; alternatives; beneficence; blood transfusions; *communication; comprehension; confidentiality; *critically ill; decision making; diagnosis; disclosure; family members; *informed consent; Jehovah's Witnesses; morbidity; patient care; patient education; patient participation; patients; *physicians; prognosis; referral and consultation; refusal to treat; review; risks and benefits; *surgery; treatment outcome; *treatment refusal; uncertainty; values; *seriously ill; Patient Self-Determination Act 1990; United States

Sweet, Matthew P.; Bernat, James L. A study of the ethical duty of physicians to disclose errors. *Journal of Clinical Ethics.* 1997 Winter; 8(4): 341–348. 13 fn. BE57616.
   *attitudes; communication; conscience; death; deception; diagnosis; *disclosure; drugs; family members; hospitals; *iatrogenic disease; institutional policies; interprofessional relations; knowledge, attitudes, practice; legal liability; malpractice; medical ethics; *moral obligations; morbidity; *motivation; negligence; paralysis; patient care; patients' rights; physician patient relationship; *physicians; professional competence; psychological stress; referral and consultation; statistics; students; survey; *truth disclosure; *whistleblowing; *medical errors; Dartmouth-Hitchcock Medical Center (Lebanon, NH)

Tanenbaum, Sandra J. Say the right thing: communication and physician accountability in the era of medical outcomes. *In:* Boyle, Philip J., ed. Getting Doctors to Listen: Ethics and Outcomes Data in Context. Washington, DC: Georgetown University Press; 1998: 204–223. 48 fn. ISBN 0-87840-654-9. BE57927.
   *accountability; *communication; decision making; disclosure; *economics; empirical research; guidelines; *health care; health care reform; health services research; methods; narrative ethics; *patient care; *patient satisfaction; *physician patient relationship; practice guidelines; referral and consultation; regulation; risks and benefits; standards; technical expertise; *treatment outcome; uncertainty; utilization review; United States

Taylor, K.M.; Macdonald, K.G.; Bezjak, A., et al. Physicians' perspective on quality of life: an exploratory study of oncologists. *Quality of Life Research.* 1996 Feb; 5(1): 5–14. 47 refs. BE57248.
   *attitudes; *cancer; *decision making; human experimentation; *knowledge, attitudes, practice; medical specialties; palliative care; *patient care; patient participation; *physicians; prognosis; *quality of life; random selection; survey; treatment outcome; Canada; United States

Töyry, Eeva; Herve, Ritva; Mutka, Riitta, et al. Ethics in health care management: developing an instrument to assess humane caring. *Nursing Ethics.* 1998 May; 5(3): 228–235. 15 refs. BE58722.
   attitudes; *caring; emotions; *evaluation; *hospitals; humanism; institutional policies; nurses; *patient care; *patient satisfaction; *patients; physicians; privacy; professional patient relationship; *quality of health care; *standards; survey; *Finland

U.S. General Accounting Office. Managed Care: Explicit Gag Clauses Not Found in HMO Contracts, but Physician Concerns Remain. Report to Congressional Requesters. Washington, DC: U.S. General Accounting Office; 1997 Aug. 23 p. 23 fn. GAO/HEHS-97-175. BE58448.
   *alternatives; *communication; confidentiality; *contracts; *counseling; *disclosure; *health maintenance organizations; lawyers; *managed care programs; *patient care; physician patient relationship; *physicians; survey; *gag orders; *United States

Udén, Giggi; Norberg, Astrid; Norberg, Siv. The stories

of physicians, registered nurses and enrolled nurses about ethically difficult care episodes in surgical care. *Scandinavian Journal of Caring Sciences.* 1995; 9(4): 245–253. 36 refs. BE55834.
   allowing to die; *attitudes; attitudes to death; autonomy; bioethical issues; cancer; *clinical ethics; comparative studies; compassion; decision making; hospitals; interdisciplinary communication; *interprofessional relations; *medical ethics; moral development; narrative ethics; nurse patient relationship; *nurses; *nursing ethics; pain; palliative care; paternalism; patient advocacy; *patient care; *physician nurse relationship; physician patient relationship; *physicians; prognosis; psychological stress; quality of life; surgery; survey; terminal care; truth disclosure; withholding treatment; qualitative research; Sweden

Vazquez, Ma. Suarez. Technology and human dignity. *Dolentium Hominum: Church and Health in the World.* 1996; 33(11th Yr., No. 3): 29–34. 14 refs. BE57265.
   biomedical technologies; hospitals; humanism; *love; *nurse patient relationship; *nurses; *patient care; patient care team; physician patient relationship; *Roman Catholic ethics

Volk, Robert J.; Cantor, Scott B.; Spann, Stephen J., et al. Preferences of husbands and wives for prostate cancer screening. *Archives of Family Medicine.* 1997 Jan–Feb; 6(1): 72–76. 26 refs. BE56482.
   *attitudes; *cancer; comparative studies; decision analysis; *decision making; dissent; *females; guidelines; *males; *marital relationship; *married persons; *mass screening; *patient care; *patients; physicians; professional organizations; *quality of life; survey; *treatment outcome; uncertainty; *prostate cancer; American Cancer Society; American Urological Society; United States

Wallace, Ruth; Wiegand, Frances; Warren, Connie. Beneficence toward whom? Ethical decision-making in a maternal-fetal conflict. *AACN Clinical Issues in Critical Care Nursing.* 1997 Nov; 8(4): 586–594. 22 refs. BE58362.
   *beneficence; case studies; childbirth; critically ill; *decision making; drugs; ethical analysis; fetal development; *fetuses; informed consent; *leukemia; nurse's role; *patient care; patient participation; *pregnant women; prematurity; prenatal injuries; *prognosis; quality of life; *risks and benefits; time factors; toxicity; values; withholding treatment; *chemotherapy

Westall, Jessica. Shackling of prisoners denounced. [News]. *BMJ (British Medical Journal).* 1997 Feb 8; 314(7078): 393. BE58603.
   guidelines; *hospitals; institutional policies; patient care; *physical restraint; *prisoners; terminally ill; *Great Britain; Thomas, Geoffrey

Williamson, Charlotte; Wilkie, Patricia. Teaching medical students in general practice: respecting patients' rights. [Editorial]. *BMJ (British Medical Journal).* 1997 Nov 1; 315(7116): 1108–1109. 11 refs. BE56894.
   attitudes; communication; *confidentiality; disclosure; family practice; *informed consent; *medical education; medical ethics; medical records; *patient care; patients; *students; Great Britain; National Health Service

Wiseman, Virginia. Caring: the neglected health outcome? or input? *Health Policy.* 1997 Jan; 39(1): 43–53. 33 refs. BE55544.
   altruism; *caring; *economics; evaluation; family members; health; health care; models, theoretical; morality; *motivation; paternalism; patient care; social interaction; sociobiology; treatment outcome; utilitarianism

Younger-Lewis, Catherine. Genital mutilation may raise awkward issues for MDs after birth. [News]. *Canadian*

Medical Association Journal. 1997 Oct 15; 157(8): 1013. BE56583.

> *childbirth; *circumcision; *cultural pluralism; decision making; ethical relativism; *females; minority groups; *patient care; *physicians; *refusal to treat; sexuality; surgery; *women's health; emigration and immigration; *Canada

Zeman, Adam. Persistent vegetative state. *Lancet.* 1997 Sep 13; 350(9080): 795–799. 64 refs. BE56321.

> allowing to die; brain death; brain pathology; diagnosis; paralysis; patient care; *persistent vegetative state; *prognosis; terminology; time factors; treatment outcome; uncertainty; coma

PATIENT CARE/AGED

American Academy of Neurology. Ethics and Humanities Subcommittee. Ethical issues in the management of the demented patient. [Position statement]. *Neurology.* 1996 Apr; 46(4): 1180–1183. 20 refs. Statement approved by the Executive Board of the Academy 8 Jul 1995. BE55670.

> advance care planning; advance directives; *aged; decision making; *dementia; family members; home care; nursing homes; *organizational policies; palliative care; patient admission; *patient care; physical restraint; physician patient relationship; physicians; professional family relationship; professional organizations; stigmatization; third party consent; treatment refusal; *American Academy of Neurology; United States

American Geriatrics Society. Clinical Practice Committee. Management of cancer pain in older patients. *Journal of the American Geriatrics Society.* 1997 Oct; 45(10): 1273–1276. 7 refs. BE56450.

> *aged; *cancer; costs and benefits; diagnosis; double effect; *drugs; guidelines; informed consent; institutional policies; intention; *pain; *palliative care; pastoral care; *patient care; patient compliance; physicians; *practice guidelines; professional organizations; psychology; quality of health care; radiology; *risks and benefits; suffering; surgery; technical expertise; support groups; *American Geriatrics Society

American Psychiatric Association. Position statement on ensuring access and appropriate utilization of psychiatric services for the elderly. *American Journal of Psychiatry.* 1998 Mar; 155(3): 452. Statement developed by the APA's Committee on Access and Effectiveness of Psychiatric Services for the Elderly, approved by the APA Board of Trustees in Mar 1997, and by the APA Assembly in Nov 1997. BE57683.

> *aged; behavior control; *guidelines; health care delivery; *mentally ill; *organizational policies; *patient care; professional organizations; *psychiatry; *American Psychiatric Association

Bartoldus, Ellen Knapik. Medical futility: a nursing home perspective. *In:* Zucker, Marjorie B.; Zucker, Howard D., eds. Medical Futility and the Evaluation of Life-Sustaining Interventions. New York, NY: Cambridge University Press; 1997: 58–64. 8 refs. ISBN 0-521-56877-3. BE55979.

> *advance care planning; advance directives; *aged; allied health personnel; allowing to die; artificial feeding; caring; *communication; compassion; critically ill; *decision making; dementia; family members; *futility; institutionalized persons; *nursing homes; patient care; professional patient relationship; trust; *values; withholding treatment; Patient Self-Determination Act 1990; United States

Bernabei, Roberto; Gambassi, Giovanni; Lapane, Kate,

et al. Management of pain in elderly patients with cancer. [For the SAGE Study Group]. *JAMA.* 1998 Jun 17; 279(23): 1877–1882. 57 refs. BE58405.

> age factors; *aged; *cancer; comparative studies; dementia; depressive disorder; *drugs; females; males; minority groups; *nursing homes; *pain; *palliative care; *patient care; *quality of health care; statistics; survey; terminally ill; whites; *analgesia; *United States

CONTEXT: Cancer pain can be relieved with pharmacological agents as indicated by the World Health Organization (WHO). All too frequently pain management is reported to be poor. OBJECTIVE: To evaluate the adequacy of pain management in elderly and minority cancer patients admitted to nursing homes. DESIGN: Retrospective, cross-sectional study. SETTING: A total of 1492 Medicare-certified and/or Medicaid-certified nursing homes in 5 states participating in the Health Care Financing Administration's demonstration project, which evaluated the implementation of the Resident Assessment Instrument and its Minimum Data Set. STUDY POPULATION: A group of 13 625 cancer patients aged 65 years and older discharged from the hospital to any of the facilities from 1992 to 1995. Data were from the multilinked Systematic Assessment of Geriatric Drug Use via Epidemiology (SAGE) database. MAIN OUTCOME MEASURES: Prevalence and predictors of daily pain and of analgesic treatment. Pain assessment was based on patients' report and was completed by a multidisciplinary team of nursing home personnel that observed, over a 7-day period, whether each resident complained or showed evidence of pain daily. RESULTS: A total of 4003 patients (24%, 29%, and 38% of those aged greater than or = 85 years, 75 to 84 years, and 65 to 74 years, respectively) reported daily pain. Age, gender, race, marital status, physical function, depression, and cognitive status were all independently associated with the presence of pain. Of patients with daily pain, 16% received a WHO level 1 drug, 32% a WHO level 2 drug, and only 26% received morphine. Patients aged 85 years and older were less likely to receive either weak opiates or morphine than those aged 65 to 74 years (13% vs 38%, respectively). More than a quarter of patients (26%) in daily pain did not receive any analgesic agent. Patients older than 85 years in daily pain were also more likely to receive no analgesia (odds ratio [OR], 1.40; 95% confidence interval [CI], 1.13–1.73). Other independent predictors of failing to receive any analgesic agent were minority race (OR, 1.63; 95% CI, 1.18–2.26 for African Americans), low cognitive performance (OR, 1.23; 95% CI, 1.05–1.44), and the number of other medications received (OR, 0.65; 95% CI, 0.5–0.84 for 11 or more medications). CONCLUSIONS: Daily pain is prevalent among nursing home residents with cancer and is often untreated, particularly among older and minority patients.

Bradley, Elizabeth; Walker, Leslie; Blechner, Barbara, et al. Assessing capacity to participate in discussions of advance directives in nursing homes: findings from a study of the Patient Self-Determination Act. *Journal of the American Geriatrics Society.* 1997 Jan; 45(1): 79–83. 33 refs. BE55758.

> administrators; *advance care planning; *advance directives; *aged; attitudes; autonomy; communication; *competence; *decision making; *family members; health personnel; institutional policies; legislation; living wills; medical records; nurses; *nursing homes; patient admission; *patient education; *patient participation; *patients; psychological stress; social workers; survey; third party consent; time factors; qualitative research; retrospective studies; *Connecticut; *Patient Self-Determination Act 1990

BE = bioethics accession number   fn. = footnotes   refs. = references

Brocklehurst, J.; Dickinson, E. Cause for concern: autonomy for elderly people in long–term care. *Age and Ageing.* 1996 Jul; 25(4): 329–332. 9 refs. BE58101.
*aged; *autonomy; evaluation studies; *health facilities; hospitals; institutional policies; *long–term care; nursing homes; patient advocacy; patient participation; quality of health care; Great Britain

Cebik, L.B.; Graber, Glenn C.; Marsh, Frank H., eds. Advances in Bioethics. Volume 1: Violence, Neglect, and the Elderly. Greenwich, CT: JAI Press; 1996. 240 p. (Advances in bioethics; v. 1). 282 fn. ISBN 0–7623–0096–5. BE56680.
*aged; autonomy; children; competence; education; family members; health personnel; institutional policies; institutionalized persons; involuntary commitment; legal aspects; legal guardians; mandatory reporting; moral obligations; motivation; nursing homes; obligations of society; parent child relationship; paternalism; patient advocacy; *patient care; patients' rights; professional patient relationship; prolongation of life; property rights; public policy; quality of life; resuscitation orders; risk; social control; terminology; third party consent; treatment refusal; *violence; *elder abuse; United States

Daniels, Norman. Family responsibility initiatives and justice between age groups. *Law, Medicine and Health Care.* 1985 Sep; 13(4): 153–159. 25 fn. BE56702.
adults; *age factors; *aged; beneficence; biomedical technologies; children; *community services; disabled; economics; *family members; *family relationship; *financial support; *health care; health care delivery; home care; *justice; legal obligations; *long–term care; love; *moral obligations; *obligations of society; parents; patient care; private sector; *public policy; public sector; quality of life; *resource allocation; selection for treatment; socioeconomic factors; trends; prudence; United States

Dellasega, Cheryl; Frank, Lori; Smyer, Michael. Medical decision–making capacity in elderly hospitalized patients. *Journal of Ethics, Law, and Aging.* 1996 Fall–Winter; 2(2): 65–74. 28 refs. Commented on by D.J. Marson and K.K. Ingram, p. 59–63. BE57140.
*aged; alternatives; *competence; comprehension; critically ill; *decision making; disclosure; *evaluation; evaluation studies; *hospitals; *informed consent; methods; patient admission; *patient care; patient discharge; *patients; physicians; risks and benefits; time factors; rationality; Patient Self–Determination Act 1990; Pennsylvania; United States

Doolittle, Norma O.; Herrick, Charlotte A. Ethics in aging: a decision–making paradigm. *Educational Gerontology.* 1992 Jun; 18(4): 395–408. 52 refs. BE55933.
*advance care planning; *aged; autonomy; beneficence; confidentiality; *decision making; disclosure; family members; health personnel; informed consent; justice; *models, theoretical; *patient care; patients' rights; rights; risks and benefits; values

Dorner, Becky; Gallagher–Allred, Charlette; Deering, Carole P., et al. The "to feed or not to feed" dilemma. *Journal of the American Dietetic Association.* 1997 Oct; 97(10, Suppl. 2): S172–S176. 19 refs. BE58257.
advance directives; aged; allied health personnel; *allowing to die; *artificial feeding; *guidelines; *institutional policies; legal aspects; *nursing homes; *nutrition; *practice guidelines; risks and benefits; withholding treatment

Evans, Lois K.; Strumpf, Neville E.; Allen–Taylor, S. Lynne, et al. A clinical trial to reduce restraints in nursing homes. *Journal of the American Geriatrics Society.* 1997 Jun; 45(6): 675–681. 43 refs. BE55720.
*aged; *behavior control; comparative studies; *control groups; dementia; depressive disorder; *education; evaluation studies; *health personnel; injuries; nurses; *nursing homes; *patient care; *physical restraint; psychoactive drugs; *referral and consultation; time factors; continuing education; dependency; follow–up studies; Pennsylvania

Evans, Roger W. Limits of chronological age as a basis for rationing health care. *Dialysis and Transplantation.* 1994 Sep; 23(9): 506–507, 510–512+. 42 refs. BE57063.
*age factors; *aged; *economics; government financing; health; *health care; kidneys; morbidity; mortality; organ transplantation; patient care; *quality of life; rehabilitation; *renal dialysis; *resource allocation; *selection for treatment; statistics; *treatment outcome; Medicare; *United States

Felder, Stefan. Costs of dying: alternatives to rationing. *Health Policy.* 1997 Feb; 39(2): 167–176. 21 refs. 3 fn. Published erratum appears in *Health Policy* 1997 Jun; 40(3): 269. BE55605.
age factors; *aged; biomedical technologies; death; decision making; economic value of life; *economics; family members; *health care; *health insurance; health maintenance organizations; health personnel; incentives; justice; motivation; organ transplantation; prolongation of life; public policy; *resource allocation; risk; *terminal care; terminally ill; *personal financing

Fenigsen, Richard. Physician–assisted death in the Netherlands: impact on long–term care. *Issues in Law and Medicine.* 1995 Winter; 11(3): 283–297. 59 fn. BE58820.
*active euthanasia; adults; age factors; *aged; *allowing to die; assisted suicide; attitudes; children; congenital disorders; decision making; *disabled; Down syndrome; hospitals; infants; *involuntary euthanasia; *long–term care; mentally retarded; newborns; nurses; nursing homes; physicians; public opinion; *public policy; quality of health care; *social impact; *voluntary euthanasia; *withholding treatment; *Netherlands

Giugliano, Robert P.; Camargo, Carlos A.; Lloyd–Jones, Donald M., et al. Elderly patients receive less aggressive medical and invasive management of unstable angina: potential impact of practice guidelines. *Archives of Internal Medicine.* 1998 May 25; 158(10): 1113–1120. 69 refs. BE58804.
*age factors; *aged; diagnosis; drugs; evaluation studies; *guidelines; *heart diseases; hospitals; intensive care units; morbidity; *patient care; patients; *practice guidelines; quality of health care; referral and consultation; risk; *selection for treatment; surgery; withholding treatment; *guideline adherence; retrospective studies; Agency for Health Care Policy and Research; United States
BACKGROUND: The Agency for Health Care Policy and Research (AHCPR) released a practice guideline on the diagnosis and management of unstable angina in 1994. OBJECTIVE: To examine practice variation across the age spectrum in the management of patients hospitalized with unstable angina 2 years before release of the AHCPR guideline. DESIGN: Retrospective cohort. SETTING: Urban academic hospital. PATIENTS: All nonreferral patients diagnosed as having unstable angina who were hospitalized directly from the emergency department to the intensive care or telemetry unit between October 1, 1991, and September 30, 1992. MEASUREMENTS: Percentage of eligible patients receiving medical treatment concordant with 8 important AHCPR guideline recommendations. RESULTS: Half of the 280 patients were older than 66 years; women were older than men on average (70 vs 64 years; P less than .001). After excluding those with contraindications to therapy, patients in the oldest quartile (age, 75.20–93.37 years)

BE = bioethics accession number   fn. = footnotes   refs. = references

were less likely than younger patients to receive aspirin (P less than .009), beta–blockers (P less than .04), and referral for cardiac catheterization (P less than .001). Overall guideline concordance weighted for the number of eligible patients declined with increasing age (87.4%, 87.4%, 84.0%, and 74.9% for age quartiles 1 to 4, respectively; chi2, P less than .001). Increasing age, the presence of congestive heart failure at presentation, a history of congestive heart failure, previous myocardial infarction, increasing comorbidity, and elevated creatinine concentration were associated with care that was less concordant with AHCPR guideline recommendations; only age and congestive heart failure at presentation remained significant in the multivariate analysis (odds ratios, 1.28 per decade [95% confidence interval, 1.02–1.61] and 3.16 [95% confidence interval, 1.57–6.36], respectively). CONCLUSIONS: Older patients were less likely to receive standard therapies for unstable angina before release of the 1994 AHCPR guideline. Patients presenting with congestive heart failure also received care that was more discordant with guideline recommendations. The AHCPR guideline allows identification of patients who receive nonstandard care and, if applied to those patients with the greatest likelihood to benefit, could lead to improved health care delivery.

Gromb, Sophie; Manciet, Gerard; Descamps, Arnaud. Ethics and law in the field of medical care for the elderly in France. *Journal of Medical Ethics.* 1997 Aug; 23(4): 233–238. 9 refs. BE55907.
  *aged; allowing to die; artificial feeding; bioethical issues; clergy; clinical ethics committees; *competence; *decision making; dementia; depressive disorder; family members; freedom; hospitals; informed consent; interdisciplinary communication; lawyers; *legal aspects; *legal guardians; nurses; patient advocacy; *patient care; patient care team; patient participation; *physicians; prolongation of life; third party consent; withholding treatment; Bordeaux University Hospital; *France

The authors discuss law and ethics when medical decisions are to be taken by patients who are unable in any valid sense to express their own wishes. The main problem in legal terms is to protect an individual's free will as far as possible and ensure that his or her wishes, if known, are respected. If a patient's independent wishes cannot be known, then we must at least ensure that nothing is imposed which is not in his interest. Legal measures, however, are far from adequate in resolving all the concrete problems that emerge. The field of ethics does bring some better adapted solutions, but none is laid down in law. One such approach, involving a multidisciplinary advisory group in a department of geriatrics, is discussed.

Hantikainen, Virpi. Physical restraint: a descriptive study in Swiss nursing homes. *Nursing Ethics.* 1998 Jul; 5(4): 330–346. 30 refs. BE58872.
  *aged; allied health personnel; alternatives; *behavior control; competence; decision making; disclosure; *institutional policies; institutionalized persons; *knowledge; attitudes, practice; motivation; *nurses; *nursing homes; nursing research; *patient care; patient participation; *physical restraint; risks and benefits; statistics; survey; qualitative research; *Switzerland

Hesse, Katherine A. Ethical issues and terminal management of the old old. *Journal of Geriatric Psychiatry.* 1995; 28(1): 75–95. 64 refs. Paper presented at a meeting of the Boston Society for Gerontologic Psychiatry, Inc., "Older, Old People," 30 Oct 1993. BE55558.

advance directives; *age factors; *aged; *allowing to die; attitudes; autonomy; chronically ill; competence; decision making; dementia; family members; futility; patient participation; physicians; prognosis; prolongation of life; quality of life; refusal to treat; resuscitation; right to die; *terminal care; terminally ill; third party consent; treatment refusal; ventilators; withholding treatment; dignity

Hope, Tony. Aging, research and families. [Editorial]. *Journal of Medical Ethics.* 1997 Oct; 23(5): 267–268. 3 refs. BE57105.
  *aged; *competence; comprehension; *conflict of interest; *decision making; *dementia; *depressive disorder; *family members; *human experimentation; *informed consent; methods; patient advocacy; *patient care; physician patient relationship; *physicians; professional family relationship; time factors

Jones, D.G. Aging, dementia and care: setting limits on the allocation of health care resources to the aged. *New Zealand Medical Journal.* 1997 Dec 12; 110(1057): 466–468. 19 refs. BE58211.
  age factors; *aged; autonomy; beneficence; biomedical technologies; caring; *dementia; guidelines; health care; justice; *patient care; privacy; prolongation of life; quality of life; *resource allocation; dignity

Kane, Rosalie A. Ethical and legal issues in long–term care: food for futuristic thought. *Journal of Long–Term Care Administration.* 1993 Fall; 21(3): 66–74. 37 refs. BE56019.
  advance directives; *aged; allied health personnel; allowing to die; community services; competence; decision making; dementia; disabled; family members; government regulation; health personnel; home care; informed consent; institutionalized persons; legal aspects; legal guardians; *long–term care; *nursing homes; patient advocacy; *patient care; patient participation; patients' rights; physical restraint; privacy; resuscitation orders; state government; third party consent; withholding treatment; continuity of patient care; United States

Kane, Rosalie A.; Caplan, Arthur L.; Urv–Wong, Ene K., et al. Everyday matters in the lives of nursing home residents: wish for and perception of choice and control. *Journal of the American Geriatrics Society.* 1997 Sep; 45(9): 1086–1093. 31 refs. BE56309.
  *aged; *allied health personnel; *attitudes; *autonomy; freedom; *institutionalized persons; *nursing homes; *patient care; *patient satisfaction; *patients; quality of health care; survey; Arkansas; Los Angeles; Minnesota; New Mexico; New York City

Knight, James A. Ethics of care in caring for the elderly. *Southern Medical Journal.* 1994 Sep; 87(9): 909–917. 36 refs. BE58936.
  active euthanasia; age factors; *aged; allowing to die; assisted suicide; autonomy; beneficence; caring; coercion; competence; economics; nursing homes; patient admission; *patient care; physician patient relationship; resource allocation; social worth; stigmatization; suicide; rationality; United States

Lynn, Joanne; Cohn, Felicia; Pickering, John H., et al.; American Geriatrics Society. American Geriatrics Society on physician–assisted suicide: brief to the United States Supreme Court. *Journal of the American Geriatrics Society.* 1997 Apr; 45(4): 489–499. 70 fn. Background and brief of the American Geriatrics Society as amicus curiae urging reversal of the judgments below: Vacco v. Quill, No. 95–1858, and Washington v. Glucksberg, No. 96–110. BE57117.
  *aged; allowing to die; *assisted suicide; chronically ill; coercion; competence; constitutional law; economics;

BE = bioethics accession number   fn. = footnotes   refs. = references

government regulation; killing; *legal aspects; legal rights; moral complicity; obligations of society; *organizational policies; *palliative care; *physicians; *professional organizations; prognosis; *public policy; *quality of health care; resource allocation; social impact; suffering; Supreme Court decisions; *terminal care; terminally ill; treatment refusal; uncertainty; withholding treatment; *geriatrics; *American Geriatrics Society; *United States; *Vacco v. Quill; *Washington v. Glucksberg

Matheis-Kraft, Carol; Roberto, Karen A. Influence of a values discussion on congruence between elderly women and their families on critical health care decisions. *Journal of Women and Aging.* 1997; 9(4): 5–22. 33 refs. BE58970.
*aged; allowing to die; artificial feeding; blood transfusions; *communication; comparative studies; competence; *decision making; dementia; drugs; evaluation studies; *family members; *females; *patient care; persistent vegetative state; renal dialysis; resuscitation; surgery; *third party consent; treatment refusal; *values; ventilators; *withholding treatment; women's health; United States

Mazur, Dennis J. How older patient preferences are influenced by consideration of future health outcomes. *Journal of the American Geriatrics Society.* 1997 Jun; 45(6): 725–728. 11 refs. BE55727.
advance care planning; *aged; *allowing to die; *attitudes; brain pathology; decision making; family members; health; *males; married persons; mentally disabled; morbidity; *patient care; *patients; physically disabled; physicians; *prolongation of life; *quality of life; resuscitation; survey; *treatment outcome; *treatment refusal; *ventilators; withholding treatment; cerebrovascular disorders; *intubation; Oregon

Mead, Gillian E.; Pendleton, Neil; Pendleton, Deborah E., et al. High technology medical interventions: what do older people want? [Letter]. *Journal of the American Geriatrics Society.* 1997 Nov; 45(11): 1409–1411. 12 refs. BE56552.
*aged; allowing to die; *attitudes; *biomedical technologies; *cancer; critically ill; diagnosis; drugs; *heart diseases; *patient care; radiology; referral and consultation; surgery; survey; truth disclosure; *withholding treatment; Great Britain

Mirvis, David M.; Chang, Cyril F.; Morreim, E. Haavi. Protecting older people while managing their care. [Editorial]. *Journal of the American Geriatrics Society.* 1997 May; 45(5): 645–646. 12 refs. BE55826.
advance care planning; *aged; attitudes; *coercion; conflict of interest; *costs and benefits; disclosure; *economics; futility; *health care delivery; incentives; insurance selection bias; *managed care programs; patient care; physicians; quality of life; resource allocation; stigmatization; uncertainty; *withholding treatment; Medicare; *United States

O'Brien, Linda A.; Siegert, Elisabeth A.; Grisso, Jeane Ann, et al. Tube feeding preferences among nursing home residents. *Journal of General Internal Medicine.* 1997 Jun; 12(6): 364–371. 38 refs. BE58361.
advance directives; *aged; *allowing to die; *artificial feeding; *attitudes; blacks; brain pathology; communication; decision making; family members; females; health personnel; institutionalized persons; males; *nursing homes; *patient care; *patients; persistent vegetative state; physical restraint; *prolongation of life; survey; treatment refusal; whites; withholding treatment; Delaware; New Jersey; Pennsylvania

Phillips, Charles D.; Hawes, Catherine; Mor, Vince, et al. Facility and area variation affecting the use of physical restraints in nursing homes. *Medical Care.* 1996

Nov; 34(11): 1149–1162. 36 refs. BE59072.
*aged; *behavior control; evaluation studies; health personnel; institutional policies; *nursing homes; nursing research; *patient care; *physical restraint; resource allocation; selection for treatment; statistics; cognition disorders; *geographic factors; California; Connecticut; Iowa; Maryland; Minnesota; Ohio; Oregon; Tennessee; Texas; *United States; Virginia

Pinch, W.J. Ellenchild; Parsons, Mary E. Moral orientation of elderly persons: considering ethical dilemmas in health care. *Nursing Ethics.* 1997 Sep; 4(5): 380–393. 32 refs. BE56905.
*aged; *attitudes; bioethical issues; *caring; decision making; females; *justice; males; *moral development; nurses; nursing research; parent child relationship; patient care; physician patient relationship; survey; values; qualitative research; Midwestern United States

Piotrowski, Joseph J.; Akhrass, Rami; Alexander, J.J., et al. Rupture of known abdominal aortic aneurysms: an ethical dilemma. [Article and commentaries]. *American Surgeon.* 1995 Jul; 61(7): 556–559. 20 refs. BE56216.
*age factors; *aged; *critically ill; emergency care; morbidity; mortality; referral and consultation; *selection for treatment; *surgery; time factors; *treatment outcome; treatment refusal; withholding treatment; Cleveland (OH)

Rich, Ben A. The values history: restoring narrative identity to long-term care. *Journal of Ethics, Law, and Aging.* 1996 Fall-Winter; 2(2): 75–84. 29 refs. 7 fn. BE57143.
*advance directives; *aged; autonomy; *communication; competence; dehumanization; dementia; family members; health personnel; institutionalized persons; *long-term care; narrative ethics; *nursing homes; patient care; personhood; physician patient relationship; privacy; *quality of health care; *quality of life; self concept; time factors; value of life; *values; dignity; *personal identity; *values histories

Shaw, A.B. Ensuring equity and quality of care for elderly people: a critique of the College report. *Journal of the Royal College of Physicians of London.* 1995 Mar–Apr; 29(2): 89–91. 14 refs. BE56567.
*age factors; *aged; biomedical technologies; costs and benefits; health care; justice; public policy; *resource allocation; scarcity; *selection for treatment; Great Britain

Shuttleworth, John Sterling. Ethical issues of cost in long-term care. *Journal of the Medical Association of Georgia.* 1990 Nov; 79(11): 843–845. 5 refs. BE55642.
administrators; *aged; *behavior control; communication; *economics; family members; government financing; *long-term care; *nursing homes; physicians; psychoactive drugs; *psychological stress; quality of life; personal financing; Medicare; United States

Silverman, Myrna; McDowell, B. Joan; Musa, Donald, et al. To treat or not to treat: issues in decisions not to treat older persons with cognitive impairment, depression, and incontinence. *Journal of the American Geriatrics Society.* 1997 Sep; 45(9): 1094–1101. 35 refs. BE56316.
*aged; *decision making; *dementia; *depressive disorder; evaluation studies; *morbidity; *patient care; physicians; referral and consultation; *selection for treatment; treatment refusal; *withholding treatment; outpatients; Pennsylvania

Sutton, Graham C. Will you still need me, will you still screen me, when I'm past 64? Breast screening policy is based on ageism. [Editorial]. *BMJ (British Medical Journal).* 1997 Oct 25; 315(7115): 1032–1033. 14 refs.

BE56589.
*age factors; *aged; *breast cancer; costs and benefits; empirical research; *females; *mass screening; *public policy; referral and consultation; risk; *selection for treatment; *social discrimination; *Great Britain; *National Health Service

Thomas, A. Mathew; Cohen, Gene; Cook–Deegan, Robert M., et al. Alzheimer testing at Silver Years. *Cambridge Quarterly of Healthcare Ethics.* 1998 Summer; 7(3): 294–307. 38 fn. BE58557.
*aged; autonomy; beneficence; community services; contracts; *dementia; diagnosis; *economics; *genetic predisposition; *genetic screening; informed consent; *institutional policies; insurance selection bias; justice; late–onset disorders; legal aspects; *mandatory testing; *moral policy; nursing homes; *patient admission; *patient care; *residential facilities; *social discrimination; standards; Americans with Disabilities Act 1990; United States

Tsevat, Joel; Dawson, Neal V.; Wu, Albert W., et al. Health values of hospitalized patients 80 years or older. [For the HELP Investigators]. *JAMA.* 1998 Feb 4; 279(5): 371–375. 42 refs. BE57814.
*aged; *attitudes; comparative studies; depressive disorder; evaluation studies; family members; *health; hospitals; institutionalized persons; pain; palliative care; patient care; *patients; prognosis; prolongation of life; quality adjusted life years; *quality of life; resuscitation; survey; time factors; *value of life; *values; severity of illness index; Hospitalized Elderly Longitudinal Project (HELP)
CONTEXT: Health values (utilities or preferences for health states) are often incorporated into clinical decisions and health care policy when issues of quality vs length of life arise, but little is known about health values of the very old. OBJECTIVE: To assess health values of older hospitalized patients, compare their values with those of their surrogate decision makers, investigate possible determinants of health values, and determine whether health values change over time. DESIGN: A prospective, longitudinal, multicenter cohort study. SETTING: Four academic medical centers. PARTICIPANTS: Four hundred fourteen hospitalized patients aged 80 years or older and their surrogate decision makers who were interviewed and understood the task. MAIN OUTCOME MEASURES: Time–trade–off utilities, reflecting preferences for current health relative to a shorter but healthy life. RESULTS: On average, patients equated living 1 year in their current state of health with living 9.7 months in excellent health (mean [SD] utility, 0.81 [0.28]). Although only 126 patients (30.7%) rated their current quality of life as excellent or very good, 284 (68.6%) were willing to give up at most 1 month of 12 in exchange for excellent health (utility greater than or =0.92). At the other extreme, 25 (6.0%) were willing to live 2 weeks or less in excellent health rather than 1 year in their current state of health (utility less than or =0.04). Patients were willing to trade significantly less time for a healthy life than their surrogates assumed they would (mean difference, 0.05; P=.007); 61 surrogates (20.3%) underestimated the patient's time–trade–off score by 0.25 (3 months of 12) or more. Patients willing to trade less time for better health were more likely to want resuscitation and other measures to extend life. Time–trade–off score correlated only modestly with quality–of–life rating (r=0.28) and inversely with depression score (r=−0.27), but there were few other clinical or demographic predictors of health values. When patients who survived were asked the time–trade–off question again at 1 year, they were willing to trade less time for better health than at baseline

(mean difference, 0.04; P=.04). CONCLUSION: Very old hospitalized patients who could be interviewed were able, in most cases, to have their health values assessed using the time–trade–off technique. Most patients were unwilling to trade much time for excellent health, but preferences varied greatly. Because proxies and multivariable analyses cannot gauge health values of elderly hospitalized patients accurately, health values of the very old should be elicited directly from the patient.

van Weel, Chris; Michels, Joop. Dying, not old age, to blame for costs of health care. *Lancet.* 1997 Oct 18; 350(9085): 1159–1160. 6 refs. BE56217.
*age factors; *aged; chronically ill; diagnosis; *economics; *health care; *morbidity; prevalence; stigmatization; *terminal care; terminally ill

Veterans Affairs National Headquarters. Bioethics Committee. Ethical Issues in Long–Term Care: Committee Report. Issued by the VA National Center for Clinical Ethics, White River Junction, VT 05009; 1996 May. 30 p. 57 fn. Bibliography in appendix. BE56735.
advance care planning; advance directives; *aged; allowing to die; autonomy; beneficence; caring; chronically ill; competence; cultural pluralism; decision making; dementia; *disabled; education; evaluation; family members; health personnel; hospices; informed consent; institutional policies; legal guardians; *long–term care; mental institutions; *nursing homes; palliative care; pastoral care; *patient care; patient participation; patient transfer; public hospitals; resuscitation; suffering; terminal care; third party consent; treatment refusal; withholding treatment; *United States; *Veterans Health Administration

Williams, Carter Catlett; Finch, Caleb E. Physical restraint: not fit for woman, man, or beast. [Editorial]. *Journal of the American Geriatrics Society.* 1997 Jun; 45(6): 773–775. 27 refs. BE55735.
administrators; *aged; alternatives; *behavior control; brain pathology; dementia; education; empirical research; health personnel; injuries; *morbidity; *nursing homes; *patient care; *physical restraint; psychoactive drugs; psychological stress; referral and consultation; United States

PATIENT CARE/DRUGS

American College of Physicians. Health and Public Policy Committee. Drug therapy for severe, chronic pain in terminal illness. *Annals of Internal Medicine.* 1983 Dec; 99(6): 870–873. 29 refs. BE57230.
*drugs; goals; *organizational policies; *pain; *palliative care; physicians; professional organizations; technical expertise; *terminal care; *American College of Physicians

American Geriatrics Society. Clinical Practice Committee. Management of cancer pain in older patients. *Journal of the American Geriatrics Society.* 1997 Oct; 45(10): 1273–1276. 7 refs. BE56450.
*aged; *cancer; costs and benefits; diagnosis; double effect; *drugs; guidelines; informed consent; institutional policies; intention; *pain; *palliative care; pastoral care; *patient care; patient compliance; physicians; *practice guidelines; professional organizations; psychology; quality of health care; radiology; *risks and benefits; suffering; surgery; technical expertise; support groups; *American Geriatrics Society

Auguste, Valérie; Guérin, Corinne; Hervé, Christian, et al. Professional secret in hospitals: study conducted in a pharmacy department. *International Journal of Bioethics.* 1997 Dec; 8(4): 89–99. 12 refs. BE58366.

BE = bioethics accession number   fn. = footnotes   refs. = references

*attitudes; *confidentiality; disclosure; *drugs; *hospitals; *patient care; *patients; *pharmacists; *privacy; professional patient relationship; survey; *outpatients; *France

Bayer, Ronald; Stryker, Jeff. Ethical challenges posed by clinical progress in AIDS. *American Journal of Public Health.* 1997 Oct; 87(10): 1599–1602. 28 refs. BE56202.
*AIDS; autonomy; common good; developing countries; disadvantaged; *drugs; *economics; federal government; government financing; health care delivery; health insurance; *HIV seropositivity; *justice; paternalism; *patient care; *patient compliance; public health; public policy; *refusal to treat; socioeconomic factors; state government; withholding treatment; Medicaid; United States

Berger, John. Patient confidentiality in a high tech world. *Journal of Pharmacy and Law.* 1996; 5(1): 139–145. BE57591.
codes of ethics; computers; *confidentiality; disclosure; *drugs; federal government; government regulation; *legal aspects; legal liability; medical records; *patient care; *pharmacists; privacy; professional organizations; American Pharmaceutical Association; United States

Bernabei, Roberto; Gambassi, Giovanni; Lapane, Kate, et al. Management of pain in elderly patients with cancer. [For the SAGE Study Group]. *JAMA.* 1998 Jun 17; 279(23): 1877–1882. 57 refs. BE58405.
age factors; *aged; *cancer; comparative studies; dementia; depressive disorder; *drugs; females; males; minority groups; *nursing homes; *pain; *palliative care; *patient care; *quality of health care; statistics; survey; terminally ill; whites; *analgesia; *United States
CONTEXT: Cancer pain can be relieved with pharmacological agents as indicated by the World Health Organization (WHO). All too frequently pain management is reported to be poor. OBJECTIVE: To evaluate the adequacy of pain management in elderly and minority cancer patients admitted to nursing homes. DESIGN: Retrospective, cross-sectional study. SETTING: A total of 1492 Medicare-certified and/or Medicaid-certified nursing homes in 5 states participating in the Health Care Financing Administration's demonstration project, which evaluated the implementation of the Resident Assessment Instrument and its Minimum Data Set. STUDY POPULATION: A group of 13 625 cancer patients aged 65 years and older discharged from the hospital to any of the facilities from 1992 to 1995. Data were from the multilinked Systematic Assessment of Geriatric Drug Use via Epidemiology (SAGE) database. MAIN OUTCOME MEASURES: Prevalence and predictors of daily pain and of analgesic treatment. Pain assessment was based on patients' report and was completed by a multidisciplinary team of nursing home personnel that observed, over a 7-day period, whether each resident complained or showed evidence of pain daily. RESULTS: A total of 4003 patients (24%, 29%, and 38% of those aged greater than or = 85 years, 75 to 84 years, and 65 to 74 years, respectively) reported daily pain. Age, gender, race, marital status, physical function, depression, and cognitive status were all independently associated with the presence of pain. Of patients with daily pain, 16% received a WHO level 1 drug, 32% a WHO level 2 drug, and only 26% received morphine. Patients aged 85 years and older were less likely to receive either weak opiates or morphine than those aged 65 to 74 years (13% vs 38%, respectively). More than a quarter of patients (26%) in daily pain did not receive any analgesic agent. Patients older than 85 years in daily pain were also more likely to receive no analgesia (odds ratio [OR], 1.40; 95% confidence interval [CI],

1.13–1.73). Other independent predictors of failing to receive any analgesic agent were minority race (OR, 1.63; 95% CI, 1.18–2.26 for African Americans), low cognitive performance (OR, 1.23; 95% CI, 1.05–1.44), and the number of other medications received (OR, 0.65; 95% CI, 0.5–0.84 for 11 or more medications). CONCLUSIONS: Daily pain is prevalent among nursing home residents with cancer and is often untreated, particularly among older and minority patients.

Blustein, Jeffrey; Robinson, Walter; Loeben, Gregory S., et al. Case vignette: placebos and informed consent. [Case study and commentaries]. *Ethics and Behavior.* 1998; 8(1): 89–98. 3 refs. BE58919.
autonomy; beneficence; chronically ill; deception; deontological ethics; disclosure; *informed consent; motivation; *pain; *patient care; patient participation; physician patient relationship; *placebos; psychology; teleological ethics; treatment outcome; trust

Bremnes, R.M.; Andersen, K.; Wist, E.A. Cancer patients, doctors and nurses vary in their willingness to undertake cancer chemotherapy. *European Journal of Cancer.* 1995 Nov; 31A(12): 1955–1959. 27 refs. BE56199.
age factors; *attitudes; *cancer; comparative studies; *decision making; *drugs; family relationship; females; males; medical specialties; morbidity; *nurses; palliative care; *patient care; *patients; *physicians; prognosis; *risks and benefits; survey; toxicity; treatment outcome; *treatment refusal; Norway

Brodell, Robert T. Ethics and micromanaged care. *Archives of Dermatology.* 1996 Sep; 132(9): 1013–1015. 22 refs. BE55902.
*alternatives; case studies; *costs and benefits; decision making; disclosure; *drugs; *health insurance reimbursement; informed consent; *managed care programs; patient advocacy; *patient care; physicians; professional autonomy; quality of health care; *risks and benefits; dermatology; *formularies; *undertreatment; United States

Brook, C.G.D. Growth hormone: panacea or punishment for short stature? [Editorial]. *BMJ (British Medical Journal).* 1997 Sep 20; 315(7110): 692–693. 7 refs. BE57161.
*children; drugs; economics; *growth disorders; *hormones; *normality; *patient care; psychological stress; quality of life; selection for treatment; stigmatization; treatment outcome

Cleaton-Jones, Peter E.; Busse, Peter; Emery, Sean, et al. Availability of antiretroviral therapy after clinical trials with HIV infected patients are ended: an ethical dilemma. [Article and commentaries]. *BMJ (British Medical Journal).* 1997 Mar 22; 314(7084): 887–891. 7 refs. BE58772.
*AIDS; communication; *developing countries; *drug industry; *drugs; economics; *financial support; government financing; guidelines; health care delivery; *HIV seropositivity; *human experimentation; *institutional ethics; investigators; patient advocacy; *patient care; private sector; research ethics committees; *research subjects; resource allocation; *therapeutic research; *continuity of patient care; Declaration of Helsinki; Medical Research Council (South Africa); *South Africa

Cleeland, Charles S.; Gonin, René; Baez, Luis, et al. Pain and treatment of pain in minority patients with cancer: the Eastern Cooperative Oncology Group Minority Outpatient Pain Study. *Annals of Internal Medicine.* 1997 Nov 1; 127(9): 813–816. 17 refs. BE57050.
*blacks; *cancer; comparative studies; *drugs; evaluation studies; females; guidelines; health facilities; *Hispanic

---

BE = bioethics accession number   fn. = footnotes   refs. = references

Americans; males; *minority groups; *pain; *patient care; *quality of health care; whites; *analgesia; guideline adherence; outpatients; *undertreatment; United States

BACKGROUND: Clinics that primarily see members of ethnic minority groups have been found to provide inadequate treatment of cancer-related pain. The extent of undertreatment of pain in these patients and the factors that contribute to undertreatment are not known. OBJECTIVES: To evaluate the severity of cancer-related pain and the adequacy of prescribed analgesics in minority outpatients with cancer. DESIGN: Prospective clinical study. SETTING: Eastern Cooperative Oncology Group. PATIENTS: 281 minority outpatients with recurrent or metastatic cancer. MEASUREMENTS: Patients and physicians independently rated severity of pain, pain-related functional impairment, and pain relief obtained by taking analgesic drugs. Analgesic adequacy was determined on the basis of accepted guidelines. RESULTS: 77% of patients reported disease-related pain or took analgesics; 41% of patients reporting pain had severe pain. Sixty-five percent of minority patients did not receive guideline-recommended analgesic prescriptions compared with 50% of non-minority patients (P less than 0.001). Hispanic patients in particular reported less pain relief and had less adequate analgesia. CONCLUSIONS: The awareness that minority patients do not receive adequate pain control and that better assessment of pain is needed may improve control of cancer-related pain in this patient population.

Cleeland, Charles S. Undertreatment of cancer pain in elderly patients. [Editorial]. *JAMA.* 1998 Jun 17; 279(23): 1914–1915. 18 refs. BE58408.
age factors; aged; *cancer; *drugs; health personnel; minority groups; nursing homes; *pain; *palliative care; patient education; *quality of health care; *analgesia; United States

Crellin, John K. Alternative medicine: ethical challenges for the profession of pharmacy. *In:* Humber, James M.; Almeder, Robert F., eds. Alternative Medicine and Ethics. Totowa, NJ: Humana Press; 1998: 195–212. 26 fn. ISBN 0-89603-440-2. BE57208.
*alternative therapies; attitudes; autonomy; codes of ethics; conflict of interest; counseling; *drugs; paternalism; patient care; patients; *pharmacists; *professional ethics; professional organizations; risks and benefits; homeopathy; self care; American Pharmaceutical Association; Great Britain; North America; Royal Pharmaceutical Society of Great Britain

Crigger, Bette-Jane. Ask your doctor or pharmacist. *Hastings Center Report.* 1998 Mar–Apr; 28(2): 47. BE57542.
*advertising; developing countries; drug industry; *drugs; international aspects; mass media; United States

Davis, Kenneth M.; Clark, Doug; Koch, Karen E., et al. Physician marketing of nutritional supplements. [Letter and response]. *JAMA.* 1998 Sep 16; 280(11): 967–968. 9 refs. BE58768.
advertising; conflict of interest; counseling; *drug industry; *economics; *entrepreneurship; federal government; financial support; government regulation; medical ethics; *nutrition; patient care; *physicians; *vitamins; Food and Drug Administration; Rexall Showcase International; United States

Davis, Peter. Contested Ground: Public Purpose and Private Interest in the Regulation of Prescription Drugs. New York, NY: Oxford University Press; 1996. 262

p. Includes references. ISBN 0-19-509120-5. BE56787.
comparative studies; decision making; *drug industry; *drugs; economics; federal government; *government regulation; health care delivery; health insurance reimbursement; *international aspects; investigational drugs; managed care programs; mass media; mortality; national health insurance; patient care; physicians; political activity; public participation; *public policy; risks and benefits; self regulation; Australia; Europe; Food and Drug Administration; Great Britain; New Zealand; United States

Dawson, Angus. Psychopharmacology. *In:* Chadwick, Ruth, ed. Encyclopedia of Applied Ethics, Volume 3. San Diego, CA: Academic Press; 1998: 727–734. 14 refs. ISBN 0-12-227068-1. BE56266.
behavior control; competence; drug industry; empirical research; human experimentation; informed consent; *mentally ill; *patient care; *psychoactive drugs; risks and benefits; treatment refusal

Elliott, Thomas E.; Murray, David M.; Elliott, Barbara A., et al. Physician knowledge and attitudes about cancer pain management: a survey from the Minnesota Cancer Pain Project. *Journal of Pain and Symptom Management.* 1995 Oct; 10(7): 494–504. 30 refs. BE57621.
*cancer; *drugs; evaluation studies; *knowledge, attitudes, practice; medical specialties; *pain; *palliative care; *patient care; *physicians; primary health care; professional competence; quality of health care; survey; analgesia; opioids; *Minnesota

Fins, Joseph J. Drug benefits in managed care: seeking ethical guidance from the formulary? *Journal of the American Geriatrics Society.* 1998 Mar; 46(3): 346–350. 27 refs. Paper presented at the 1996 Congress of Clinical Societies. BE56759.
conflict of interest; costs and benefits; decision making; disclosure; drug industry; *drugs; *economics; guidelines; health insurance reimbursement; hospitals; informed consent; *managed care programs; organization and administration; *organizational policies; patient advocacy; patient care; physicians; professional autonomy; resource allocation; review committees; *standards; *formularies; *pharmacy and therapeutics committees; quality assurance; United States

Gitanjali, B.; Shashindran, C.H.; Tripathi, K.D., et al. Are drug advertisements in Indian edition of BMJ unethical? [Article and commentary]. *BMJ (British Medical Journal).* 1997 Aug 23; 315(7106): 459–460. 12 refs. BE56649.
*advertising; alternative therapies; comparative studies; *deception; *drug industry; *drugs; *editorial policies; financial support; health personnel; *international aspects; *misconduct; *standards; survey; technical expertise; *BMJ (British Medical Journal); Great Britain; *India; World Health Organization

Goldstein, Barry; Royal, Michael C.; Veatch, Robert M. Safety of an extemporaneously prepared injection. [Case study and commentaries]. *American Journal of Health-System Pharmacy.* 1996 Feb 15; 53(4): 414–417. 1 ref. BE56207.
*administrators; *alternatives; case studies; *costs and benefits; dissent; *drugs; economics; *hospitals; *interprofessional relations; moral policy; patient care; *pharmacists; *professional ethics; resource allocation; *risk; *risks and benefits; technical expertise; *morphine

Holm, Søren; Evans, Martyn. Product names, proper claims? More ethical issues in the marketing of drugs. *BMJ (British Medical Journal).* 1996 Dec 21–28; 313(7072): 1627–1629. 7 refs. Includes a list of drugs with allusive names. BE58809.

BE = bioethics accession number   fn. = footnotes   refs. = references

advertising; deception; *drug industry; *drugs; risks and benefits; survey; *terminology; *business ethics; Denmark; Great Britain
OBJECTIVES: To analyse the explicit or implicit claims embodied in the proprietary names of pharmaceutical products. DESIGN: Linguistic and ethical analysis of proprietary names of pharmaceutical products marketed in the UK and in Denmark. RESULTS AND CONCLUSIONS: A number of drugs have names that allude to their indication or actions. Such names may be problematic, however, because they often promise more than the drug can deliver. Taking into account, firstly, the type of allusion and its degree of sophistication, and, secondly, the seriousness of the indication may help in identifying the most problematic drug names.

Hsu, Irene; DuChane, Janeen; Veatch, Robert M. Recommendation of treatment that would allow parole -- Scenario; Position 1: pharmacist should recommend the hormonal treatment; Position 2: pharmacist should not recommend the hormonal treatment; Analysis and commentary. *American Journal of Health-System Pharmacy.* 1995 Apr 15; 52(8): 829-833. 5 refs. BE58105.
  *behavior control; case studies; codes of ethics; competence; freedom; government financing; health insurance reimbursement; HIV seropositivity; *hormones; legal aspects; mental institutions; mentally ill; obligations to society; patient compliance; patients' rights; *pharmacists; *prisoners; professional ethics; *selection for treatment; *sex offenses; sexuality; technical expertise; withholding treatment; professional role

Josefson, Deborah. Marketing of antipsychotic drugs attacked. [News]. *BMJ (British Medical Journal).* 1998 Feb 28; 316(7132): 648. BE57758.
  *advertising; depressive disorder; *drug industry; economics; federal government; government regulation; incentives; *mass media; mentally ill; patient education; *psychoactive drugs; schizophrenia; *direct marketing; Eli Lilly; United States

La Puma, John. Physicians' conflicts of interest in post-marketing research: what the public should know, and why industry should tell them. *In:* Vanderpool, Harold Y., ed. The Ethics of Research Involving Human Subjects: Facing the 21st Century. Frederick, MD: University Publishing Group; 1996: 203-219. 47 fn. ISBN 1-55572-036-6. BE56988.
  attitudes; *conflict of interest; disclosure; *drug industry; *drugs; ethical review; *financial support; *human experimentation; *informed consent; *investigators; *patients; physician patient relationship; *physicians; *remuneration; research ethics committees; research subjects; risks and benefits; *therapeutic research; *postmarketing research

McCarthy, Michael. Conflict of interest highlighted in debate on calcium-channel blockers. [News]. *Lancet.* 1998 Jan 17; 351(9097): 191. BE57776.
  *biomedical research; *conflict of interest; disclosure; *drug industry; *drugs; economics; *financial support; *investigators

Mander, Rosemary. Failure to deliver: ethical issues relating to epidural analgesia in uncomplicated labour. *In:* Frith, Lucy, ed. Ethics and Midwifery: Issues in Contemporary Practice. Boston, MA: Butterworth-Heinemann; 1996: 51-71. 59 refs. ISBN 0-7506-3056-6. BE58634.
  attitudes; autonomy; *childbirth; coercion; cultural pluralism; *decision making; disclosure; *drugs; empirical research; home care; hospitals; informed consent; *nurse

midwives; *pain; paternalism; *patient care; physicians; *pregnant women; professional patient relationship; *risks and benefits; social dominance; *analgesia; evidence-based medicine; Great Britain

Melzer, David. New drug treatment for Alzheimer's disease: lessons for healthcare policy. *BMJ (British Medical Journal).* 1998 Mar 7; 316(7133): 762-764. 20 refs. BE57759.
  *advertising; aged; costs and benefits; *dementia; drug industry; editorial policies; government regulation; human experimentation; *information dissemination; *investigational drugs; nursing homes; *patient care; *public policy; research design; *risks and benefits; *technology assessment; *therapeutic research; *treatment outcome; *Aricept; Great Britain; National Health Service; United States

Menkes, David B. Hazardous drugs in developing countries. [Editorial]. *BMJ (British Medical Journal).* 1997 Dec 13; 315(7122): 1557-1558. 14 refs. BE57557.
  advertising; *developing countries; *drug industry; *drugs; economics; entrepreneurship; fraud; *international aspects; public health

Moskop, John C.; Smith, Michael L.; De Ville, Kenneth. Ethical and legal aspects of teratogenic medications: the case of isotretinoin. *Journal of Clinical Ethics.* 1997 Fall; 8(3): 264-278. 57 fn. BE57565.
  adults; age factors; autonomy; beneficence; *congenital disorders; contraception; *decision making; disclosure; drug industry; *drugs; duty to warn; federal government; *females; fetuses; government regulation; *iatrogenic disease; informed consent; justice; *legal liability; negligence; paternalism; *patient care; patient compliance; *physicians; *pregnant women; *prenatal injuries; refusal to treat; risks and benefits; wrongful death; *wrongful life; dermatology; *Accutane; Food and Drug Administration; Roche Dermatologics; United States

Munetz, Mark R.; Roth, Loren H. Informing patients about tardive dyskinesia. *Archives of Internal Medicine.* 1985 Sep; 42(9): 866-871. 30 refs. BE56970.
  age factors; chronically ill; *communication; comparative studies; *comprehension; *consent forms; disclosure; iatrogenic disease; *informed consent; *mentally ill; patient care; patient compliance; physician patient relationship; *psychoactive drugs; *recall; risks and benefits; *schizophrenia; survey; *toxicity; follow-up studies; outpatients; *tardive dyskinesia; Pittsburgh

Naber, D.; Kircher, T.; Hessel, K. Schizophrenic patients' retrospective attitudes regarding involuntary psychopharmacological treatment and restraint. *European Psychiatry.* 1996; 11(1): 7-11. 20 refs. BE57064.
  *attitudes; *coercion; emotions; institutionalized persons; involuntary commitment; *mentally ill; *patient care; patient discharge; *patients; *physical restraint; *psychoactive drugs; recall; *schizophrenia; survey; *treatment refusal; retrospective studies; Germany

Ollila, Eeva; Hemminki, Elina. Does licensing of drugs in industrialized countries guarantee drug quality and safety for Third World countries? The case of Norplant licensing in Finland. *International Journal of Health Services.* 1997; 27(2): 309-328. 35 refs. BE56009.
  *contraception; *developing countries; drug industry; *drugs; *evaluation; *evaluation studies; females; government regulation; hormones; *human experimentation; information dissemination; *international aspects; patient care; patient education; *records; research design; research subjects; risks and benefits; *standards; *Finland; *Norplant; Sweden

Olver, Ian N.; Turrell, Susan J.; Olszewski, Nancy

A., et al. Impact of an information and consent form on patients having chemotherapy. *Medical Journal of Australia.* 1995 Jan 16; 162(2): 82–83. 10 refs. BE55885.
*cancer; *comprehension; *consent forms; disclosure; *drugs; evaluation studies; *informed consent; *patient care; *patients; *recall; risks and benefits; survey; Australia

Parens, Erik. Is better always good? The enhancement project. [Project on the Prospect of Technologies Aimed at the Enhancement of Human Capacities and Traits]. *Hastings Center Report.* 1998 Jan–Feb; 28(1): S1–S17. 35 fn. BE57294.
behavior control; *biomedical technologies; *cosmetic surgery; disabled; entrepreneurship; ethical analysis; females; *genetic enhancement; *goals; *health; *health care; health insurance reimbursement; *human characteristics; *justice; *medicine; moral complicity; *moral policy; motivation; *normality; preventive medicine; *psychoactive drugs; *public policy; resource allocation; *self concept; social control; social impact; social problems; socioeconomic factors; suffering; terminology; *values; authenticity; beauty; *enhancement technologies; life style; Hastings Center; *Project on the Prospect of Technologies Aimed at the Enhancement of Human Capabilities and Traits; Prozac
The following essay begins to say why and when it will sometimes make sense to worry about the prospect of aiming new biotechnologies at the enhancement of human capacities and traits. It grows out of a two–year, Hastings Center project, generously funded by the National Endowment for the Humanities.

Parnham, Michael J. Ethical Issues in Drug Research: Through a Glass Darkly. Washington, DC: IOS Press; 1996. 155 p. Includes references. ISBN 90–5199–279–3. BE55677.
advertising; animal experimentation; attitudes; *biomedical research; conscience; deception; developing countries; drug industry; *drugs; freedom; genetic research; government regulation; health; hormones; human experimentation; human rights; information dissemination; international aspects; investigators; pain; patents; patient care; psychoactive drugs; quality of life; research design; *risks and benefits; science; toxicity; universities; utilitarianism

Patterson, W. Bradford; Emanuel, Ezekiel J.; Blumenthal, David. Physician–drug company conflict of interest. *Journal of Clinical Oncology.* 1996 Jan; 14(1): 316–320. 13 refs. BE55520.
biomedical research; *conflict of interest; *drug industry; *drugs; *financial support; *gifts; government financing; guidelines; hospitals; human experimentation; investigators; medical schools; *patient care; *physicians; professional organizations; referral and consultation; universities; teaching hospitals; American College of Physicians; American Medical Association; American Society of Clinical Oncology; United States

Peppin, John F. An Engelhardtian analysis of interactions between pharmaceutical sales representatives and physicians. *Journal of Medicine and Philosophy.* 1997 Dec; 22(6): 623–641. 35 refs. 16 fn. BE57516.
advertising; autonomy; beneficence; coercion; *conflict of interest; democracy; disclosure; *drug industry; drugs; financial support; *freedom; gifts; informed consent; justice; *moral policy; organizational policies; patient care; philosophy; physician patient relationship; *physicians; principle–based ethics; professional organizations; secularism; standards; trust; *Engelhardt, H. Tristram
Physician conflict of interest has been of concern since Hippocrates and rarely is this concern more evident than in the relationship between pharmaceutical sales representatives (PSR) and physicians. Given the acrimonious public debates concerning this issue a careful exploration of the concerns at sake and the

conceptual arguments which support such concerns is called for. In this piece I will take as heuristic the conceptual philosophical framework argued for by H. Tristram Engelhardt. This framework would sanction interactions between PSRs and physicians given that such relationships are free and without coercion. Further, patients must be informed, uncoerced and free in choosing such relationships with physicians who engage in interactions with PSRs. I consider four major criticisms which claim that PSR–physician interactions are morally impermissible: 1) influence, 2) "patients do not choose, but they pay," 3) violation of ethical principles, and 4) erosion of the patient–physician relationship. Each is shown to be unpersuasive under Engelhardtian philosophy. As long as the principle of permission and informed consent obtain without coercion than the interaction between PSRs and physicians would be construed to be morally permissible.

Poikonen, John; Haupt, Bridget A.; Veatch, Robert M. Preferential service for a powerful physician –– Scenario; Position 1: pharmacist should serve physician immediately; Position 2: pharmacist should make physician wait; Analysis and commentary. *American Journal of Health–System Pharmacy.* 1996 Nov 1; 53(21): 2614–2618. 5 refs. BE58106.
case studies; codes of ethics; communication; drugs; employment; *interprofessional relations; justice; medical etiquette; moral obligations; patient advocacy; patient care; *pharmacists; *physicians; *professional ethics; *social dominance; time factors; utilitarianism

Prayle, David; Brazier, Margaret. Supply of medicines: paternalism, autonomy and reality. *Journal of Medical Ethics.* 1998 Apr; 24(2): 93–98. 30 fn. BE58081.
advertising; *autonomy; beneficence; counseling; drug industry; *drugs; economics; gatekeeping; *government regulation; information dissemination; injuries; legal liability; legal obligations; *paternalism; patients; *pharmacists; *professional ethics; *public policy; risks and benefits; *professional role; self care; European Community Directive; *Great Britain; Medicines Act 1968 (Great Britain); Medicines Control Agency (Great Britain); National Health Service
Radical changes are taking place in the United Kingdom in relation to the classification of, and access to, medicines. More and more medicines are being made available over the counter both in local pharmacies and in supermarkets. The provision of more open access to medicines may be hailed as a triumph for patient autonomy. This paper examines whether such a claim is real or illusory. It explores the ethical and legal implications of deregulating medicines. Do patients benefit? What is the impact on pharmacists? Are the true beneficiaries of change largely the pharmaceutical industries?

Robson, Philip. Cannabis as medicine: time for the phoenix to rise? [Editorial]. *BMJ (British Medical Journal).* 1998 Apr 4; 316(7137): 1034–1035. 9 refs. BE58219.
organizational policies; *palliative care; physicians; professional organizations; *psychoactive drugs; risks and benefits; *marijuana; British Medical Association; Great Britain; Royal Pharmaceutical Society (Great Britain); Therapeutic Uses of Cannabis (British Medical Association)

Royal Pharmaceutical Society of Great Britain. Medicines, Ethics and Practice: A Guide for Pharmacists. Number 17. London: The Society; 1996 Oct. 124 p. ISBN 0–85369–377–3. BE56092.
advertising; *codes of ethics; computers; confidentiality; continuing education; contraception; drug abuse; *drugs;

BE = bioethics accession number   fn. = footnotes   refs. = references

health facilities; health promotion; interprofessional relations; legal aspects; patient care team; patient education; *pharmacists; professional autonomy; professional competence; *professional ethics; professional organizations; records; *standards; computer security; *Great Britain; *Royal Pharmaceutical Society of Great Britain

Sandberg, Warren S.; Carlos, Ruth; Sandberg, Elisabeth H., et al. The effect of educational gifts from pharmaceutical firms on medical students' recall of company names or products. *Academic Medicine.* 1997 Oct; 72(10): 916–918. 10 refs. BE56632.
*advertising; *attitudes; *drug industry; drugs; evaluation studies; *gifts; hospitals; institutional policies; internship and residency; knowledge, attitudes, practice; *medical education; medical schools; motivation; physicians; recall; *social impact; *students; survey; Chicago; University of Chicago Pritzker School of Medicine

Stelfox, Henry Thomas; Chua, Grace; O'Rourke, Keith, et al. Conflict of interest in the debate over calcium–channel antagonists. *New England Journal of Medicine.* 1998 Jan 8; 338(2): 101–105. 35 refs. BE56440.
*attitudes; authorship; biomedical research; comparative studies; *conflict of interest; disclosure; *drug industry; *drugs; economics; editorial policies; evaluation studies; *financial support; guidelines; heart diseases; hypertension; *investigators; patient care; *physicians; *risks and benefits; survey; Canada; United States
BACKGROUND: Physicians' financial relationships with the pharmaceutical industry are controversial because such relationships may pose a conflict of interest. It is unknown to what extent industry support of medical education and research influences the opinions and behavior of clinicians and researchers. The recent debate over the safety of calcium–channel antagonists provided an opportunity to examine the effect of financial conflicts of interest. METHODS: We searched the English-language medical literature published from March 1995 through September 1996 for articles examining the controversy about the safety of calcium–channel antagonists. Articles were reviewed and classified as being supportive, neutral, or critical with respect to the use of calcium–channel antagonists. The authors of the articles were asked about their financial relationships with both manufacturers of calcium–channel antagonists and manufacturers of competing products (i.e., beta–blockers, angiotensin–converting–enzyme inhibitors, diuretics, and nitrates). We examined the authors' published positions on the safety of calcium–channel antagonists according to their financial relationships with pharmaceutical companies. RESULTS: Authors who supported the use of calcium–channel antagonists were significantly more likely than neutral or critical authors to have financial relationships with manufacturers of calcium–channel antagonists (96 percent, vs. 60 percent and 37 percent, respectively; P less than 0.001). Supportive authors were also more likely than neutral or critical authors to have financial relationships with any pharmaceutical manufacturer, irrespective of the product (100 percent, vs. 67 percent and 43 percent, respectively; P less than 0.001). CONCLUSIONS: Our results demonstrate a strong association between authors' published positions on the safety of calcium–channel antagonists and their financial relationships with pharmaceutical manufacturers. The medical profession needs to develop a more effective policy on conflict of interest. We support complete disclosure of relationships with pharmaceutical manufacturers for clinicians and researchers who write articles examining pharmaceutical products.

Stempsey, William E. The battle for medical marijuana in the war on drugs. *America.* 1998 Apr 11; 178(12): 14–16. BE58566.
*drug abuse; federal government; *palliative care; physicians; *psychoactive drugs; *public policy; terminally ill; *marijuana; *United States

Wadman, Meredith. $100m payout after drug data withheld. [News]. *Nature.* 1997 Aug 21; 388(6644): 703. BE56353.
*biomedical research; *compensation; contracts; costs and benefits; *drug industry; *drugs; economics; *financial support; human experimentation; *information dissemination; investigators; legal liability; *misconduct; patients; universities; Dong, Betty; *Knoll Pharmaceutical Co.; *Synthroid; United States; University of California, San Francisco

Washington. Supreme Court. Seeley v. State. *Pacific Reporter, 2d Series.* 1997 Jul 24 (date of decision). 940: 604–632. BE58671.
cancer; *constitutional law; due process; equal protection; federal government; *government regulation; *legal aspects; legal liability; legal rights; patient care; *psychoactive drugs; state government; state interest; *terminally ill; *marijuana; *Seeley v. State; *Washington
The Supreme Court of Washington refused to invalidate a Washington state law which classified marijuana as a controlled substance. Seeley was a terminally ill cancer patient who smoked marijuana to control the side effects of chemotherapy. The court rejected Seeley's argument that classifying marijuana as a controlled substance violated the privileges and immunities clause of the Washington constitution, which provides an express grant to the state to regulate the practice of medicine and the sale of drugs and medicines. The court found that the state's regulation of marijuana was rationally related to a legitimate state interest. The court also found that the recognition of a potential medical necessity defense for criminal liability of marijuana possession was not relevant in its equal protection analysis. The dissent, invoking U.S. Supreme Court precedent in abortion rights cases, argued that state classification of marijuana as a controlled substance violated Seeley's due process rights as it unduly burdened his medical treatment without an overriding state interest. (KIE abstract)

Weinstein, Bruce D. Teaching pharmacy ethics: the case study approach. *In:* Haddad, Amy Marie, ed. Teaching and Learning Strategies in Pharmacy Ethics. Second Edition. New York, NY: Pharmaceutical Products Press; 1997: 18–31. 21 refs. Co-published simultaneously in *Journal of Pharmacy Teaching,* 1997; 6(1/2): 18–31. ISBN 0–7890–0378–3. BE57930.
*case studies; *drugs; *education; ethical analysis; *patient care; *pharmacists; *professional ethics; *teaching methods

Welie, Jos V.M. Placebo treatment. *In:* Chadwick, Ruth, ed. Encyclopedia of Applied Ethics, Volume 3. San Diego, CA: Academic Press; 1998: 493–502. 9 refs. ISBN 0–12–227068–1. BE56260.
alternatives; autonomy; deception; drugs; human experimentation; informed consent; *patient care; physician patient relationship; *placebos; psychology; risks and benefits

Westfall, John M.; McCabe, Jennifer; Nicholas, Richard A. Personal use of drug samples by physicians and office staff. *JAMA.* 1997 Jul 9; 278(2): 141–143. 18 refs. BE58434.
advertising; conflict of interest; *drug industry; *drugs; family practice; *gifts; health personnel; internship and

---

BE = bioethics accession number   fn. = footnotes   refs. = references

residency; patient care; *physicians; statistics; survey; *self care; Colorado

CONTEXT: Pharmaceutical samples are commonly used in ambulatory care settings. There is limited research on their use or impact on health care providers and patients. OBJECTIVE: To determine the extent of personal use of drug samples over a 1-year period by physicians and medical office staff. DESIGN, SUBJECTS, AND SETTING: An anonymous cross-sectional survey of all physicians, resident physicians, nursing staff, and office staff in a family practice residency. MAIN OUTCOME MEASURE: Quantity of drug samples taken for personal or family use. RESULTS: Of 55 surveys issued, 53 (96%) were returned. A total of 230 separate drug samples were reported taken in amounts ranging from 1 dose to greater than 1 month's supply. Two respondents reported no use of drug samples, while 4 respondents reported taking more than 10 different samples. CONCLUSION: Drug samples are commonly taken by physicians and office staff for personal and family use. The ethical implications of this practice warrant further discussion.

Wolf, Bruce L.; Westfall, John M.; McCabe, Jennifer, et al. Drug samples: benefit or bait? [Letter and response]. *JAMA.* 1998 Jun 3; 279(21): 1698–1699. 7 refs. BE58435.

advertising; conflict of interest; *drug industry; *drugs; *economics; *gifts; indigents; patient care; *physicians

World Health Assembly. Ethical Criteria for Medicinal Drug Promotion. Geneva: World Health Organization; 1988. 16 p. ISBN 92-4-154239-X. BE56732.

*advertising; drug industry; *drugs; financial support; gifts; *guidelines; health personnel; information dissemination; *international aspects; mass media; organizational policies; patient education; physicians; public policy; postmarketing research; *World Health Organization

Pushing ethical pharmaceuticals direct to the public. [Editorial]. *Lancet.* 1998 Mar 28; 351(9107): 921. BE58506.

*advertising; *drug industry; *drugs; federal government; government regulation; information dissemination; mass media; patients; physicians; Food and Drug Administration; United States

PATIENT CARE/MENTALLY DISABLED

American Academy of Neurology. Ethics and Humanities Subcommittee. Ethical issues in the management of the demented patient. [Position statement]. *Neurology.* 1996 Apr; 46(4): 1180–1183. 20 refs. Statement approved by the Executive Board of the Academy 8 Jul 1995. BE55670.

advance care planning; advance directives; *aged; decision making; *dementia; family members; home care; nursing homes; *organizational policies; palliative care; patient admission; *patient care; physical restraint; physician patient relationship; physicians; professional family relationship; professional organizations; stigmatization; third party consent; treatment refusal; *American Academy of Neurology; United States

American Psychiatric Association. Position statement on ensuring access and appropriate utilization of psychiatric services for the elderly. *American Journal of Psychiatry.* 1998 Mar; 155(3): 452. Statement developed by the APA's Committee on Access and Effectiveness of Psychiatric Services for the Elderly, approved by the APA Board of Trustees in Mar 1997, and by the APA Assembly in Nov 1997. BE57683.

*aged; behavior control; *guidelines; health care delivery; *mentally ill; *organizational policies; *patient care; professional organizations; *psychiatry; *American Psychiatric Association

Anderson, Gail; Hill, Marcia, eds. Children's Rights, Therapists' Responsibilities: Feminist Commentaries. New York, NY: Harrington Park Press; 1997. 141 p. Includes references. Issued simultaneously, under the same title, as a special issue of the journal *Women and Therapy,* 1997; 20(2). ISBN 1-56023-100-9. BE58316.

*adolescents; American Indians; artificial insemination; autonomy; blacks; child abuse; *children; decision making; disabled; domestic violence; family relationship; females; *feminist ethics; health personnel; Hispanic Americans; homosexuals; *human rights; international aspects; males; models, theoretical; parent child relationship; patient care; professional patient relationship; *psychotherapy; semen donors; social dominance; socioeconomic factors; divorce; family therapy

Austad, Carol Shaw. Is Long-Term Psychotherapy Unethical? Toward a Social Ethic in an Era of Managed Care. San Francisco, CA: Jossey-Bass; 1996. 283 p. Includes references. ISBN 0-7879-0218-7. BE56093.

accountability; alternatives; behavior disorders; beneficence; case studies; confidentiality; conflict of interest; costs and benefits; economics; empirical research; evaluation; health care delivery; health care reform; health insurance; health personnel; justice; long-term care; *managed care programs; mental health; mentally ill; *patient care; practice guidelines; professional competence; professional ethics; professional patient relationship; psychoactive drugs; *psychotherapy; quality of health care; remuneration; *resource allocation; selection for treatment; standards; *time factors; treatment outcome; health services misuse; United States

Barker, Ann. Mental health and the law. *BMJ (British Medical Journal).* 1997 Sep 6; 315(7108): 590–592. 6 refs. BE57241.

adults; coercion; confidentiality; emergency care; informed consent; involuntary commitment; law enforcement; *legal aspects; legislation; *mental health; *mentally disabled; mentally ill; minors; parental consent; patient access to records; *patient care; physicians; psychiatry; treatment refusal; England; *Great Britain; Mental Health Act 1983 (Great Britain); Wales

The law relating to medical practice in general, and mental health in particular, is complex. This article provides a summary of the laws applying in England and Wales. Certain mental disorders are the only medical conditions for which the law permits treatment without the consent of the patient, but this can be undertaken only in a hospital or registered nursing home.

Coombes, Lindsey. Mental health. *In:* Chadwick, Ruth, ed. Encyclopedia of Applied Ethics, Volume 3. San Diego, CA: Academic Press; 1998: 197–212. 11 refs. ISBN 0-12-227068-1. BE56254.

autonomy; caring; community services; confidentiality; cultural pluralism; deinstitutionalized persons; disease; goals; health; health care delivery; health promotion; informed consent; *mental health; *mentally ill; *patient care; professional patient relationship; *psychotherapy; quality of life; social control; terminology; values

Crenshaw, Wesley B.; Cain, Kimberly A.; Francis, Paul S. An updated national survey on seclusion and restraint. *Psychiatric Services.* 1997 Mar; 48(3): 395–397. 2 refs. BE56861.

*behavior control; *institutionalized persons; *mental institutions; *mentally ill; *patient care; *physical restraint; statistics; survey; time factors; United States

---

BE = bioethics accession number   fn. = footnotes   refs. = references

Davis, Anne J.; Aroskar, Mila A.; Liaschenko, Joan, et al. Mental retardation. *In: their* Ethical Dilemmas and Nursing Practice. Fourth Edition. Stamford, CT: Appleton and Lange; 1997: 213–243. 133 fn. ISBN 0–8385–2283–1. BE58599.
case studies; diagnosis; females; genetic counseling; genetic disorders; genetic screening; historical aspects; involuntary commitment; justice; legal aspects; mass screening; *mentally retarded; nurses; obligations of society; patient care; personhood; phenylketonuria; public policy; refusal to treat; resource allocation; rights; social discrimination; sterilization (sexual); United States

Dawson, Angus. Psychopharmacology. *In:* Chadwick, Ruth, ed. Encyclopedia of Applied Ethics, Volume 3. San Diego, CA: Academic Press; 1998: 727–734. 14 refs. ISBN 0–12–227068–1. BE56266.
behavior control; competence; drug industry; empirical research; human experimentation; informed consent; *mentally ill; *patient care; *psychoactive drugs; risks and benefits; treatment refusal

d'Oronzio, Joseph C.; Reinders, Hans S.; Corsale, Massimo. Ethical obligations in the body politic: the case of normalization policy for marginal populations. [Introduction, article, and commentary]. *Cambridge Quarterly of Healthcare Ethics.* 1997 Fall; 6(4): 480–493. 27 fn. BE56460.
*community services; *deinstitutionalized persons; disadvantaged; family members; health care; international aspects; legal rights; mental health; *mentally disabled; normality; patient care; residential facilities; social discrimination; social interaction; *homeless persons

Dowbiggin, Ian Robert. Keeping America Sane: Psychiatry and Eugenics in the United States and Canada, 1880–1940. Ithaca, NY: Cornell University Press; 1997. 245 p. (Cornell studies in the history of psychiatry). 638 fn. ISBN 0–8014–3356–8. BE56505.
administrators; aliens; attitudes; behavior control; disadvantaged; *eugenics; females; government financing; health care reform; *historical aspects; institutionalized persons; international aspects; interprofessional relations; involuntary commitment; involuntary sterilization; legislation; males; mental institutions; *mentally ill; mentally retarded; National Socialism; patient care; *physician's role; *physicians; political activity; population control; professional organizations; *psychiatry; public health; public hospitals; public policy; reproduction; resource allocation; sexuality; social discrimination; socioeconomic factors; state government; emigration and immigration; American Medico-Psychological Association; Blumer, George; *Canada; Clarke, Charles; Nineteenth Century; Twentieth Century; *United States

Geller, Jeffrey L. A biopsychosocial rationale for coerced community treatment in the management of schizophrenia. *Psychiatric Quarterly.* 1995 Fall; 66(3): 219–235. 58 refs. BE56206.
brain pathology; *coercion; community services; *deinstitutionalized persons; guidelines; incentives; *mentally ill; motivation; *outpatient commitment; *patient care; practice guidelines; rehabilitation; risks and benefits; *schizophrenia; selection for treatment; treatment outcome

Great Britain. Lord Chancellor's Department. Who Decides? Making Decisions on Behalf of Mentally Incapacitated Adults. A Consultation Paper. London: The Stationery Office; 1997 Dec. 114 p. Cm 3803. A Green Paper presented to Parliament. ISBN 0–10–138032–1. BE58544.
adults; advance directives; allowing to die; artificial feeding; competence; *decision making; health facilities; human experimentation; *judicial action; *legal aspects; legal guardians; *mentally disabled; *patient advocacy; patient care; persistent vegetative state; sterilization (sexual); third party consent; tissue donation; treatment refusal; withholding treatment; *England; *Law Commission (Great Britain); *Wales

Grubb, Andrew. Treatment without consent (pregnancy): adult -- Tameside and Glossop Acute Services Trust v. C.H. [Comment]. *Medical Law Review.* 1996 Summer; 4(2): 193–198. 5 fn. BE56498.
*cesarean section; *coercion; competence; informed consent; *judicial action; *legal aspects; *mentally ill; *patient care; *pregnant women; psychoactive drugs; psychological stress; schizophrenia; *treatment refusal; *Great Britain; Mental Health Act 1983 (Great Britain); *Tameside and Glossop Acute Services Trust v. C.H.

Hattab, Jocelyn Y. Psychiatric ethics. *In:* Chadwick, Ruth, ed. Encyclopedia of Applied Ethics, Volume 3. San Diego, CA: Academic Press; 1998: 703–726. 7 refs. ISBN 0–12–227068–1. BE56265.
aged; biomedical research; brain; brain pathology; confidentiality; disclosure; expert testimony; forensic psychiatry; freedom; human experimentation; iatrogenic disease; informed consent; involuntary commitment; legal aspects; medical education; *medical ethics; mental health; mentally ill; minors; misconduct; patient care; physician patient relationship; physicians; preventive medicine; psychiatric diagnosis; *psychiatry; psychoactive drugs; psychotherapy; research ethics committees; stigmatization; third party consent

Hiday, Virginia Aldigé. Involuntary commitment as a psychiatric technology. *International Journal of Technology Assessment in Health Care.* 1996 Fall; 12(4): 585–603. 121 refs. 2 fn. BE55559.
attitudes; *coercion; electroconvulsive therapy; *empirical research; international aspects; *involuntary commitment; legal aspects; mental institutions; *mentally ill; outpatient commitment; *patient care; patient compliance; patients; psychoactive drugs; psychosurgery; treatment outcome; treatment refusal; trends; voluntary admission; qualitative research; quantitative research

Hoge, Steven K. APA resource document: I. The professional responsibilities of psychiatrists in evolving health care systems. *Bulletin of the American Academy of Psychiatry and the Law.* 1996; 24(3): 393–406. 11 refs. BE56208.
autonomy; conflict of interest; contracts; *decision making; *disclosure; *economics; freedom; guidelines; *health care delivery; *health care reform; health insurance; health insurance reimbursement; incentives; legal aspects; *managed care programs; medical ethics; *mentally ill; *moral obligations; *patient advocacy; *patient care; *patient participation; physician patient relationship; *physicians; professional autonomy; professional competence; *psychiatry; psychotherapy; *quality of health care; referral and consultation; remuneration; *resource allocation; self regulation; trends; withholding treatment; continuity of patient care; personal financing; utilization review; American Psychiatric Association; *United States

Holstein, Martha B. Ethics and Alzheimer's disease: widening the lens. *Journal of Clinical Ethics.* 1998 Spring; 9(1): 13–22. 27 fn. BE57710.
advance directives; aged; attitudes; autonomy; bioethics; competence; decision making; *dementia; diagnosis; disease; empathy; *family members; family relationship; females; genetic determinism; genetic identity; genetic predisposition; health personnel; interdisciplinary communication; long-term care; moral obligations; *patient care; personhood; professional patient relationship; public policy; quality of life; self concept; *social interaction; social sciences; socioeconomic factors; *stigmatization; United States

---

BE = bioethics accession number   fn. = footnotes   refs. = references

Hope, Tony. Aging, research and families. [Editorial]. *Journal of Medical Ethics.* 1997 Oct; 23(5): 267–268. 3 refs. BE57105.
   *aged; *competence; comprehension; *conflict of interest; *decision making; *dementia; *depressive disorder; *family members; *human experimentation; *informed consent; methods; patient advocacy; *patient care; physician patient relationship; *physicians; professional family relationship; time factors

Howe, Edmund G. Caring for patients with dementia: an indication for "emotional communism". *Journal of Clinical Ethics.* 1998 Spring; 9(1): 3–11. 30 fn. BE57709.
   aged; allowing to die; *dementia; *emotions; *health personnel; love; *patient care; *professional patient relationship; psychological stress; stigmatization; withholding treatment; grief

Howe, Edmund G. Deceiving patients for their own good. *Journal of Clinical Ethics.* 1997 Fall; 8(3): 211–216. 15 fn. BE57563.
   attitudes; *behavior disorders; behavioral research; compassion; *deception; *diagnosis; disclosure; emotions; medical ethics; mentally ill; nurses; patient care; *patients; physician patient relationship; *physicians; *placebos; *psychiatric diagnosis; *psychological stress; psychotherapy; research subjects; risks and benefits; self concept; *stigmatization; trust; debriefing; *psychophysiologic disorders; *sham procedures

Hurley, Ann C.; Volicer, Ladislav; Rempusheski, Veronica F., et al. Reaching consensus: the process of recommending treatment decisions for Alzheimer's patients. *Advances in Nursing Science.* 1995 Dec; 18(2): 33–43. 33 refs. BE57500.
   *advance care planning; aged; allowing to die; caring; competence; consensus; *decision making; *dementia; family members; hospices; models, theoretical; *nurse's role; *nurses; nursing education; *palliative care; *patient care; patient care team; professional family relationship; survey; *terminal care; third party consent; time factors; trust; withholding treatment; qualitative research

Jones, D.G. Aging, dementia and care: setting limits on the allocation of health care resources to the aged. *New Zealand Medical Journal.* 1997 Dec 12; 110(1057): 466–468. 19 refs. BE58211.
   age factors; *aged; autonomy; beneficence; biomedical technologies; caring; *dementia; guidelines; health care; justice; *patient care; privacy; prolongation of life; quality of life; *resource allocation; dignity

Kapp, Marshall B. Persons with dementia as "liability magnets": ethical implications. *Journal of Clinical Ethics.* 1998 Spring; 9(1): 66–70. 18 fn. BE57715.
   allowing to die; *attitudes; *autonomy; *behavior control; dangerousness; decision making; *dementia; *family members; *health facilities; *health personnel; hospices; human experimentation; injuries; legal guardians; *legal liability; motivation; *paternalism; *patient care; prolongation of life; quality of health care; refusal to treat; residential facilities; risk; selection of subjects; terminal care; *risk management

Kearney, Edmund M. Ethical dilemmas in the treatment of adolescent gang members. *Ethics and Behavior.* 1998; 8(1): 49–57. 27 refs. BE58917.
   *adolescents; aggression; *behavior disorders; confidentiality; dangerousness; disclosure; duty to warn; goals; health personnel; law enforcement; professional patient relationship; *psychotherapy; trust; values; *violence; United States
   Therapists treating adolescent gang members face unique ethical dilemmas. These dilemmas arise from clinical

issues that inevitably emerge in the treatment of this population. Clinical issues related to the adolescent gang member having great difficulty trusting, having experienced and observed much violence, and usually having participated in criminal activities are central to the treatment process. In this article I discuss the ethical problems that subsequently emerge: maintaining confidentiality, discharging one's duty to warn or protect, and imposing one's personal values. Suggestions for future research are offered.

Kelley, James L. Psychiatric Malpractice: Stories of Patients, Psychiatrists, and the Law. New Brunswick, NJ: Rutgers University Press; 1996. 229 p. Includes references. ISBN 0-8135-2323-0. BE56095.
   alternative therapies; confidentiality; duty to warn; expert testimony; health insurance; *health personnel; involuntary commitment; *legal liability; *malpractice; mental institutions; mentally ill; misconduct; negligence; patient discharge; *physicians; professional organizations; professional patient relationship; *psychiatry; *psychotherapy; quality of health care; sex offenses; sexuality; standards; suicide; violence; American Psychiatric Association; Bean-Bayog, Margaret; Lozano, Paul; Osheroff v. Chestnut Lodge; Tarasoff v. Regents; *United States

Kitwood, Tom. Toward a theory of dementia care: ethics and interaction. *Journal of Clinical Ethics.* 1998 Spring; 9(1): 23–34. 15 fn. BE57711.
   aged; behavior control; communication; decision making; *dementia; emotions; empathy; ethical theory; health personnel; historical aspects; misconduct; negligence; paternalism; *patient care; patient participation; patients; personhood; *professional patient relationship; *social interaction; stigmatization; empowerment

La Vigne, Gregory; Hassenfeld, Irwin N. The ethics of alcoholism treatment and rehabilitation. *In:* Shelton, Wayne N.; Edwards, Rem B., eds. Advances in Bioethics. Volume 3: Values, Ethics, and Alcoholism. Greenwich, CT: JAI Press; 1997: 81–101. 36 refs. ISBN 0-7623-0219-4. BE57633.
   *alcohol abuse; *autonomy; behavior control; *behavior disorders; brain pathology; *case studies; coercion; competence; dangerousness; decision making; *diagnosis; disabled; disease; family relationship; fetuses; genetic predisposition; health insurance reimbursement; involuntary commitment; justice; mental health; mentally ill; *models, theoretical; morality; normality; *paternalism; *patient care; *patient compliance; *physician's role; pregnant women; prenatal injuries; *psychiatric diagnosis; psychoactive drugs; psychotherapy; *rehabilitation; resource allocation; risk; *self induced illness; social problems; stigmatization; suicide; treatment outcome; treatment refusal; self-help groups; sick role

Lützén, Kim; Nordin, Conny. Structuring moral meaning in psychiatric nursing practice. *Scandinavian Journal of Caring Sciences.* 1993; 7(3): 175–180. 20 refs. BE56413.
   alcohol abuse; autonomy; beneficence; *decision making; emotions; empathy; *mentally ill; moral development; nurse patient relationship; *nurses; *nursing ethics; *patient care; *psychiatry; suicide; Sweden

Lyman, Karen A. Living with Alzheimer's disease: the creation of meaning among persons with dementia. *Journal of Clinical Ethics.* 1998 Spring; 9(1): 49–57. 30 fn. BE57713.
   aged; *attitudes; chronically ill; dehumanization; *dementia; disabled; disease; family members; health personnel; human experimentation; paternalism; patient care; patient participation; *patients; personhood; *quality of life; *self concept; social interaction; empowerment; *outpatients

---

BE = bioethics accession number   fn. = footnotes   refs. = references

McCurdy, David B. Personhood, spirituality, and hope in the care of human beings with dementia. *Journal of Clinical Ethics.* 1998 Spring; 9(1): 81–91. 60 fn. BE57717.
caring; communication; *dementia; *emotions; futility; *health personnel; humanism; long-term care; nursing homes; *patient care; *personhood; professional patient relationship; *religion; self concept; *social interaction; theology; value of life; dependency; dignity; *hope

Melzer, David. New drug treatment for Alzheimer's disease: lessons for healthcare policy. *BMJ (British Medical Journal).* 1998 Mar 7; 316(7133): 762–764. 20 refs. BE57759.
*advertising; aged; costs and benefits; *dementia; drug industry; editorial policies; government regulation; human experimentation; *information dissemination; *investigational drugs; nursing homes; *patient care; *public policy; research design; *risks and benefits; *technology assessment; *therapeutic research; *treatment outcome; *Aricept; Great Britain; National Health Service; United States

Moffic, H. Steven. The Ethical Way: Challenges and Solutions for Managed Behavioral Healthcare. San Francisco, CA: Jossey-Bass; 1997. 234 p. Bibliography: p. 219–220. ISBN 0-7879-0841-X. BE58547.
administrators; confidentiality; decision making; economics; gatekeeping; health care delivery; health insurance reimbursement; health personnel; hospitals; incentives; informed consent; *managed care programs; mental health; *mentally ill; *patient care; patient discharge; psychoactive drugs; psychotherapy; treatment outcome; values; business ethics; utilization review; United States

Morgenlander, Keith H.; Greenwald, Devra E. Psychiatric DRGs: the legal and ethical impact. [Editorial]. *QRB/Quality Review Bulletin.* 1985 Jun; 11(6): 175–179. 25 refs. BE57068.
*economics; health insurance reimbursement; involuntary commitment; legal aspects; *mental institutions; *mentally ill; patient admission; patient care; patient discharge; *psychiatric diagnosis; *remuneration; resource allocation; United States

Naber, D.; Kircher, T.; Hessel, K. Schizophrenic patients' retrospective attitudes regarding involuntary psychopharmacological treatment and restraint. *European Psychiatry.* 1996; 11(1): 7–11. 20 refs. BE57064.
*attitudes; *coercion; emotions; institutionalized persons; involuntary commitment; *mentally ill; *patient care; patient discharge; *patients; *physical restraint; *psychoactive drugs; recall; *schizophrenia; survey; *treatment refusal; retrospective studies; Germany

Nelson, James Lindemann. Reasons and feelings, duty and dementia. *Journal of Clinical Ethics.* 1998 Spring; 9(1): 58–65. 14 fn. BE57714.
case studies; *dementia; emotions; *family members; *family relationship; *females; *males; moral development; *moral obligations; motivation; narrative ethics; parents; *patient care; siblings; *adult offspring

Palermo, George B. The plight of the deinstitutionalized chronic schizophrenic: ethical considerations. [Revised]. *In:* Monagle, John F.; Thomasma, David C., eds. Health Care Ethics: Critical Issues for the 21st Century. Gaithersburg, MD: Aspen Publishers; 1998: 164–176. 63 fn. ISBN 0-8342-0911-X. BE56283.
*chronically ill; community services; dehumanization; *deinstitutionalized persons; freedom; goals; health care delivery; health care reform; historical aspects; involuntary commitment; law enforcement; mental institutions; *mentally ill; patient admission; *patient care; patient discharge; political activity; prisoners; psychiatric diagnosis;

quality of health care; quality of life; rights; *schizophrenia; *socioeconomic factors; stigmatization; homeless persons; patient abandonment; United States

Perlin, Terry M. Who will I be? Stephen G. Post's *The Moral Challenge of Alzheimer's kAlzheimerl Disease.* [Book review essay]. *Journal of Ethics, Law, and Aging.* 1996 Fall-Winter; 2(2): 85–86. 10 refs. 1 fn. BE57142.
advance directives; autonomy; behavior control; *dementia; diagnosis; empathy; family members; freedom; health personnel; home care; married persons; *patient care; *personhood; quality of life; *social interaction; time factors; treatment refusal; truth disclosure; value of life; dignity; *The Moral Challenge of Alzheimer Disease (Post, S.G.)

Post, Stephen G. Physician-assisted suicide in Alzheimer's disease. *Journal of the American Geriatrics Society.* 1997 May; 45(5): 647–651. 26 refs. BE55843.
active euthanasia; *advance directives; aged; *assisted suicide; attitudes; autonomy; beneficence; chronically ill; competence; *dementia; economics; health personnel; *hospices; international aspects; legal aspects; *long-term care; managed care programs; *palliative care; physicians; policy analysis; public opinion; *public policy; quality of life; resource allocation; self concept; social discrimination; social impact; suffering; *terminal care; terminally ill; wedge argument; withholding treatment; *United States

Post, Stephen G. The fear of forgetfulness: a grassroots approach to an ethics of Alzheimer's disease. *Journal of Clinical Ethics.* 1998 Spring; 9(1): 71–80. 47 fn. BE57716.
advance directives; allowing to die; artificial feeding; attitudes; autonomy; caring; *dementia; diagnosis; drugs; emotions; family members; genetic screening; guidelines; health personnel; palliative care; patient advocacy; *patient care; personhood; quality of life; risks and benefits; social interaction; social worth; *stigmatization; third party consent; *truth disclosure; value of life; withholding treatment; ELSI-funded publication; Alzheimer's Disease and Related Disorders Association; Aricept; United States

Russian Federation. Law of 2 July 1992 of the Russian Federation on psychiatric care and the safeguarding of citizens' rights in the dispensing of such care. *International Digest of Health Legislation.* 1993; 44(2): 267–281. BE57184.
adults; coercion; confidentiality; dangerousness; decision making; disclosure; health personnel; informed consent; institutionalized persons; involuntary commitment; judicial action; *legal aspects; legal rights; mental institutions; *mentally ill; minors; patient advocacy; *patient care; patient discharge; patient transfer; *patients' rights; professional competence; psychiatric diagnosis; psychiatry; right to treatment; third party consent; treatment refusal; voluntary admission; *Russia

Sabat, Steven R. Voices of Alzheimer's disease sufferers: a call for treatment based on personhood. *Journal of Clinical Ethics.* 1998 Spring; 9(1): 35–48. 36 fn. BE57712.
behavioral research; case studies; communication; dehumanization; *dementia; emotions; patient care; patient participation; *personhood; professional patient relationship; psychological stress; *self concept; *social interaction; stigmatization

Simon, Robert I. Psychiatrists' duties in discharging sicker and potentially violent inpatients in the managed care era. *Psychiatric Services.* 1998 Jan; 49(1): 62–67. 41 refs. BE58220.
competence; *dangerousness; *disclosure; *duty to warn; health insurance reimbursement; informed consent; involuntary commitment; *legal liability; *legal obligations; *managed care programs; mandatory reporting; *mentally ill; *moral obligations; *patient advocacy; *patient care;

BE = bioethics accession number   fn. = footnotes   refs. = references

*patient discharge; *physicians; *psychiatry; *quality of health care; *violence; utilization review; United States

Smith, Carol A. Use of involuntary outpatient commitment in community care of the seriously and persistently mentally ill patient. *Issues in Mental Health Nursing.* 1995 May–Jun; 16(3): 275–284. 20 refs. BE55891.
  chronically ill; coercion; community services; *evaluation; *government regulation; *legal aspects; *mentally ill; *nurses; *outpatient commitment; *patient advocacy; *patient care; patient compliance; patients' rights; social impact; state government; treatment outcome; *United States

Smith, Martin L.; Stagno, Susan J.; Dolske, Michelle, et al. Induction procedures for psychogenic seizures: ethical and clinical considerations. *Journal of Clinical Ethics.* 1997 Fall; 8(3): 217–229. 40 fn. BE57566.
  adults; alternatives; attitudes; *behavior disorders; children; *deception; *diagnosis; *disclosure; emotions; epilepsy; *health facilities; informed consent; *institutional policies; legal liability; medical ethics; *methods; pain; patient care; patients; physician patient relationship; physicians; *placebos; practice guidelines; *psychiatric diagnosis; psychological stress; *risks and benefits; standards; survey; trust; debriefing; *psychophysiologic disorders; *sham procedures; United States

Straker, Gillian. Ethical issues in working with children in war zones. *In:* Apfel, Roberta J.; Simon, Bennett, eds. Minefields in Their Hearts: The Mental Health of Children and Communal Violence. New Haven, CT: Yale University Press; 1996: 18–32. 17 refs. ISBN 0–300–06570–1. BE56147.
  *adolescents; autonomy; beneficence; case studies; *children; common good; confidentiality; cultural pluralism; developing countries; disclosure; *duty to warn; ethical relativism; *health personnel; human rights; international aspects; justice; mental health; moral complicity; *moral obligations; morality; *political activity; professional autonomy; professional ethics; professional patient relationship; *psychological stress; *psychotherapy; risks and benefits; social discrimination; torture; trust; *violence; *war; South Africa

Torrey, E. Fuller. Out of the Shadows: Confronting America's Mental Illness Crisis. New York, NY: Wiley; 1997. 244 p. Includes references. ISBN 0–471–24532–1. BE58948.
  accountability; biomedical research; brain pathology; dangerousness; *deinstitutionalized persons; economics; family members; federal government; government financing; *health care delivery; involuntary commitment; legal aspects; managed care programs; mental health; mental institutions; *mentally ill; patient care; politics; prisoners; proprietary health facilities; psychiatry; psychoactive drugs; public policy; schizophrenia; state government; stigmatization; treatment outcome; violence; homeless persons; nonprofit organizations; Medicaid; Medicare; Twentieth Century; *United States

Williams, Christopher J.; Pieri, Lorenzo; Sims, Andrew, et al. Does palliative care have a role in treatment of anorexia nervosa? We should strive to keep patients alive [and] Palliative care does not mean giving up. *BMJ (British Medical Journal).* 1998 Jul 18; 317(7152): 195–197. 10 refs. BE58817.
  *allowing to die; artificial feeding; *behavior disorders; chronically ill; competence; depressive disorder; drugs; force feeding; hospices; hospitals; *palliative care; *patient care; prognosis; *prolongation of life; terminally ill; treatment refusal; *anorexia nervosa; opiates

World Medical Association. Ethical issues concerning patients with mental illness. [Policy statement]. *Bulletin of Medical Ethics.* 1996 Aug; No. 120: 11. This statement was approved by the World Medical Association in Sep 1995. BE55943.
  alternatives; autonomy; competence; confidentiality; conflict of interest; disclosure; informed consent; *international aspects; involuntary commitment; *medical ethics; *mentally ill; military personnel; misconduct; obligations to society; *organizational policies; patient advocacy; *patient care; physician patient relationship; *physicians; prisoners; privacy; professional organizations; *psychiatry; risks and benefits; social discrimination; stigmatization; third party consent; trust; truth disclosure; *World Medical Association

PATIENT CARE/MINORS

Alderson, Priscilla; Goodey, Christopher. Doctors, ethics and special education. *Journal of Medical Ethics.* 1998 Feb; 24(1): 49–55. 11 fn. BE57402.
  *attitudes; beneficence; *children; comparative studies; decision making; diagnosis; *disabled; *education; faculty; historical aspects; justice; legal aspects; legislation; mentally retarded; parents; paternalism; pediatrics; *physician's role; *physicians; *referral and consultation; *schools; social discrimination; *technical expertise; *learning disorders; qualitative research; Education Act 1981 (Great Britain); *Great Britain
This discussion paper is drawn from a qualitative research project comparing the effect of special and ordinary schools on the lives of children, young people and their families. Special schools are recommended by health professionals who seldom know how ineffective these schools are. We question the beneficence and justice of health professionals' advice on education for children with disabilities and other difficulties. Cooperation with local education authorities (LEAs) plays a considerable part in the work of community paediatricians, clinical medical officers, therapists and other health professionals encountering children with "special needs". The "needs" range from physical disability and sensory impairment to learning difficulties and emotional or behavioural difficulties. This cooperation involves routine administrative problems, but it raises broad ethical issues too, particularly in respect of current tendencies in state schooling towards the integration or inclusion of these children in mainstream schools and classes.

American Academy of Pediatrics. Committee on Bioethics. Ethics and the care of critically ill infants and children. *Pediatrics.* 1996 Jul; 98(1): 149–152. 58 refs. BE55656.
  *allowing to die; children; congenital disorders; *critically ill; *decision making; federal government; futility; government regulation; *infants; *intensive care units; legal aspects; low birth weight; *newborns; *organizational policies; *parents; *patient care; *pediatrics; *physicians; prematurity; professional organizations; prognosis; *prolongation of life; public policy; resource allocation; selection for treatment; terminally ill; treatment outcome; uncertainty; withholding treatment; *American Academy of Pediatrics; United States

Anderson, Gail; Hill, Marcia, eds. Children's Rights, Therapists' Responsibilities: Feminist Commentaries. New York, NY: Harrington Park Press; 1997. 141 p. Includes references. Issued simultaneously, under the same title, as a special issue of the journal *Women and Therapy,* 1997; 20(2). ISBN 1–56023–100–9. BE58316.
  *adolescents; American Indians; artificial insemination; autonomy; blacks; child abuse; *children; decision making; disabled; domestic violence; family relationship; females; *feminist ethics; health personnel; Hispanic Americans;

homosexuals; *human rights; international aspects; males; models, theoretical; parent child relationship; patient care; professional patient relationship; *psychotherapy; semen donors; social dominance; socioeconomic factors; divorce; family therapy

Baxter, Rosario; Long, Ann; Sines, David. The legal and ethical status of children in health care in the UK. *Nursing Ethics.* 1998 May; 5(3): 189–199. 49 refs. BE58718.
age factors; autonomy; children; competence; decision making; health care delivery; human experimentation; human rights; informed consent; *legal aspects; *minors; nurses; parental consent; paternalism; patient advocacy; *patient care; Children Act 1989 (Great Britain); Declaration on the Rights of the Child; *Great Britain

Baylis, Françoise; Downie, Jocelyn. Child abuse and neglect: cross–cultural considerations. *In:* Nelson, Hilde Lindemann, ed. Feminism and Families. New York, NY: Routledge; 1997: 173–187. 22 fn. ISBN 0–415–91254–7. BE55840.
alternative therapies; *child abuse; children; circumcision; competence; critically ill; *cultural pluralism; decision making; emergency care; *ethical relativism; females; feminist ethics; injuries; intention; medical devices; *minority groups; normality; organ transplantation; *parents; patient advocacy; physically disabled; risks and benefits; social dominance; state interest; treatment refusal; values; cochlear implants; hearing disorders; non–Western World; Canada; United States

Brawn, W.J.; De Giovanni, J.V.; Hutchinson, S., et al. Hypoplastic left heart syndrome. [Letters]. *BMJ (British Medical Journal).* 1997 May 10; 314(7091): 1414. 4 refs. BE56855.
*allowing to die; *congenital disorders; *decision making; diagnosis; disabled; *heart diseases; mortality; *newborns; *palliative care; *parents; prenatal diagnosis; prognosis; program descriptions; *quality of life; selective abortion; *surgery; terminal care; *treatment outcome; uncertainty; *Great Britain; New York

Brook, C.G.D. Growth hormone: panacea or punishment for short stature? [Editorial]. *BMJ (British Medical Journal).* 1997 Sep 20; 315(7110): 692–693. 7 refs. BE57161.
*children; drugs; economics; *growth disorders; *hormones; *normality; *patient care; psychological stress; quality of life; selection for treatment; stigmatization; treatment outcome

Bulford, Rachel. Children have rights too. [Personal view]. *BMJ (British Medical Journal).* 1997 May 10; 314(7091): 1421–1422. BE55690.
competence; *decision making; health care; informed consent; *minors; nontherapeutic research; parents; *patient care; patients' rights; treatment refusal; truth disclosure; Great Britain

Calhoun, Byron C.; Reitman, James S.; Hoeldtke, Nathan J. Perinatal hospice: a response to partial birth abortion for infants with congenital defects. *Issues in Law and Medicine.* 1997 Fall; 13(2): 125–143. 86 fn. BE57805.
allowing to die; *alternatives; autonomy; *childbirth; *chromosome abnormalities; *congenital disorders; conscience; counseling; death; decision making; *fetal development; fetuses; health personnel; hospices; informed consent; methods; *newborns; *palliative care; parents; personhood; pregnant women; privacy; psychological stress; *selective abortion; suffering; theology; value of life; viability; *pregnancy trimesters

Dalton, John D.; Buick, R.G. Guidelines on

circumcision. [Letters]. *BMJ (British Medical Journal).* 1997 Sep 20; 315(7110): 750. 6 refs. BE58409.
*circumcision; guidelines; legal aspects; *males; *newborns; organizational policies; parental consent; physicians; professional organizations; risk; surgery; General Medical Council (Great Britain); Great Britain; North America

Fadiman, Anne. The Spirit Catches You and You Fall Down: A Hmong Child and Her American Doctors, and the Collision of Two Cultures. New York, NY: Farrar, Straus and Giroux; 1997. 339 p. Bibliography: p. 311–324. ISBN 0–374–26781–2. BE57048.
*alternative therapies; *Asian Americans; *attitudes; childbirth; *children; *communication; *cultural pluralism; *disease; *epilepsy; family relationship; *home care; hospitals; nurses; *parent child relationship; *patient care; *patient compliance; *persistent vegetative state; *physicians; *professional family relationship; *professional patient relationship; *religion; social workers; treatment refusal; ethnographic studies; *folk medicine; California; *Hmong; Laos; *Lee, Lia; *Merced Community Medical Center (CA); United States; Vietnam War

Finkelstein, Beth S.; Silvers, J.B.; Marrero, Ursula, et al. Insurance coverage, physician recommendations, and access to emerging treatments: growth hormone therapy for childhood short stature. *JAMA.* 1998 Mar 4; 279(9): 663–668. 37 refs. BE57809.
*children; costs and benefits; *decision making; *drugs; economics; family practice; *government financing; *growth disorders; health care delivery; *health insurance reimbursement; *health maintenance organizations; *hormones; medical specialties; *patient care; pediatrics; primary health care; *referral and consultation; selection for treatment; state government; survey; *physician's practice patterns; *Medicaid; United States

CONTEXT: There is concern in both the medical community and the general public about mechanisms of medical decision making and the interplay of physician and insurer decisions in determining access to care. OBJECTIVE: To examine the medical process influencing access to growth hormone (GH) therapy for childhood short stature by comparing coverage policies of US insurers with the treatment recommendations of US physicians. DESIGN AND PARTICIPANTS: Independent national representative surveys were mailed to insurers (private, Blue Cross/Blue Shield, health maintenance organizations, programs for Children with Special Health Care Needs, and Medicaid programs, n=113), primary care physicians (n=1504), and pediatric endocrinologists (n=534) with response rates of 75%, 60%, and 81%, respectively. Each survey included identical case scenarios. Primary care physicians were asked decisions about referrals to pediatric endocrinologists. Endocrinologists were asked GH treatment recommendations. Insurers were asked coverage decisions for GH therapy. MAIN OUTCOME MEASURES: Insurer coverage decisions for GH in specific case scenarios were compared with the recommendations of primary care physicians and pediatric endocrinologists. RESULTS: Physician recommendations and insurance coverage decisions differed strikingly. For example, while 96% of pediatric endocrinologists recommended GH therapy for children with Turner syndrome, insurer policies covered GH therapy for only 52% of these children. Overall, referral and treatment decisions by physicians resulted in recommendations for GH therapy in 78% of children with GH deficiency, Turner syndrome, or renal failure; of those recommended for treatment, 28% were denied coverage by insurers. Similarly, GH therapy would be recommended by physicians for only 9% of children with idiopathic short stature, but insurers would not

---

BE = bioethics accession number   fn. = footnotes   refs. = references

cover GH for the vast majority of these children. Furthermore, the data indicated considerable variation among insurers regarding coverage policies for GH (P less than .01). CONCLUSIONS: Access to GH therapy differs depending on the type of insurance coverage. The deep discord between physician recommendations and insurance coverage decisions, exemplified by these findings, represents a major challenge to mechanisms of health care decision making, access, and costs.

Ford, Carol A.; Millstein, Susan G.; Halpern-Felsher, Bonnie L., et al. Influence of physician confidentiality assurances on adolescents' willingness to disclose information and seek future health care: a randomized controlled trial. *JAMA.* 1997 Sep 24; 278(12): 1029-1034. 20 refs. BE56303.

*adolescents; alcohol abuse; *attitudes; communication; *confidentiality; contraception; depressive disorder; *disclosure; evaluation studies; females; males; mental health; *patient care; physician patient relationship; physicians; recall; sexuality; smoking; socioeconomic factors; suicide; survey; California

CONTEXT: Adolescents' concerns about privacy in clinical settings decrease their willingness to seek health care for sensitive problems and may inhibit their communication with physicians. OBJECTIVE: To investigate the influence of physicians' assurances of confidentiality on adolescents' willingness to disclose information and seek future health care. DESIGN: Randomized controlled trial. SETTING: Three suburban public high schools in California. PARTICIPANTS: The 562 participating adolescents represented 92% of students in mandatory classes. INTERVENTION: After random assignment to 1 of 3 groups, the adolescents listened to a standardized audiotape depiction of an office visit during which they heard a physician who assured unconditional confidentiality, a physician who assured conditional confidentiality, or a physician who did not mention confidentiality. MAIN OUTCOME MEASURES: Adolescents' willingness to disclose general information, willingness to disclose information about sensitive topics, intended honesty, and likelihood of return visits to the physician depicted in the scenario were assessed by anonymous written questionnaire. RESULTS: Assurances of confidentiality increased the number of adolescents willing to disclose sensitive information about sexuality, substance use, and mental health from 39% (68/175) to 46.5% (178/383) (beta = .10, P = .02) and increased the number willing to seek future health care from 53% (93/175) to 67% (259/386) (beta = .17, P less than .001). When comparing the unconditional with the conditional groups, assurances of unconditional confidentiality increased the number of adolescents willing to return for a future visit by 10 percentage points, from 62% (122/196) to 72% (137/190) (beta = .14, P = .001). CONCLUSIONS: Adolescents are more willing to communicate with and seek health care from physicians who assure confidentiality. Further investigation is needed to identify a confidentiality assurance statement that explains the legal and ethical limitations of confidentiality without decreasing adolescents' likelihood of seeking future health care for routine and nonreportable sensitive health concerns.

Goldberg, Allen I.; Faure, Eveline A.M.; O'Callaghan, John J. High-technology home care: critical issues and ethical choices. *In:* Monagle, John F.; Thomasma, David C., eds. Health Care Ethics: Critical Issues for the 21st Century. Gaithersburg, MD: Aspen Publishers; 1998: 146-163. 30 fn. ISBN 0-8342-0911-X. BE56282.

adults; autonomy; beneficence; *biomedical technologies; *children; *chronically ill; community services; *economics; family members; federal government; goals; government financing; *health care delivery; health care reform; health insurance reimbursement; health maintenance organizations; health personnel; historical aspects; *home care; justice; models, theoretical; moral policy; patient care team; private sector; public policy; resource allocation; state government; trends; values; ventilators; case managers; poliomyelitis; Medicaid; Twentieth Century; United States

Hemminki, Elina; Santalahti, Päivi; Louhiala, Pekka. Ethical conflicts in regulating the start of life. *Perspectives in Biology and Medicine.* 1997 Summer; 40(4): 586-591. 21 refs. BE56604.

abortion on demand; *abortion, induced; allowing to die; *beginning of life; biomedical technologies; congenital disorders; disabled; embryos; eugenics; fetuses; *intensive care units; multiple pregnancy; *newborns; patient care; personhood; prematurity; *prenatal diagnosis; *reproductive technologies; selective abortion; values

Kearney, Edmund M. Ethical dilemmas in the treatment of adolescent gang members. *Ethics and Behavior.* 1998; 8(1): 49-57. 27 refs. BE58917.

*adolescents; aggression; *behavior disorders; confidentiality; dangerousness; disclosure; duty to warn; goals; health personnel; law enforcement; professional patient relationship; *psychotherapy; trust; values; *violence; United States

Therapists treating adolescent gang members face unique ethical dilemmas. These dilemmas arise from clinical issues that inevitably emerge in the treatment of this population. Clinical issues related to the adolescent gang member having great difficulty trusting, having experienced and observed much violence, and usually having participated in criminal activities are central to the treatment process. In this article I discuss the ethical problems that subsequently emerge: maintaining confidentiality, discharging one's duty to warn or protect, and imposing one's personal values. Suggestions for future research are offered.

Lantos, John D. Was the UK collaborative ECMO trial ethical? *Paediatric and Perinatal Epidemiology.* 1997 Jul; 11(3): 264-268. 7 refs. BE58033.

alternatives; *biomedical technologies; coercion; congenital disorders; critically ill; *human experimentation; international aspects; mortality; *newborns; parental consent; *patient care; *random selection; *research design; risks and benefits; *technology assessment; *therapeutic research; time factors; *treatment outcome; uncertainty; *extracorporeal membrane oxygenation; *Great Britain

Lowenthal, Barbara; Getz, Marjorie; Kaye, Celia. The special educator and the hospital ethics committee. Available from the ERIC Document Reproduction Service, DYNCORP I&ET, 7420 Fullerton Rd., Suite 110, Springfield, VA 22153-2852; Document No. ED320338; EC231146; 1990 Feb. 40 p. 34 refs. Paper presented at the Conference of the Learning Disabilities Association, Anaheim, CA, 1990 February 21-24. BE57693.

*allowing to die; biomedical technologies; brain death; case studies; child abuse; children; *clinical ethics committees; committee membership; *congenital disorders; *decision making; determination of death; disabled; dissent; education; *ethics consultation; federal government; government regulation; hospitals; *infants; *institutional policies; legislation; low birth weight; mentally retarded; *newborns; organ donation; parents; *patient care; persistent vegetative state; *prolongation of life; psychological stress; *quality of life; suffering; surgery; treatment refusal; *value of life; ventilators; *withholding treatment; Department of Health and Human Services; Education of the Handicapped Act

---

BE = bioethics accession number   fn. = footnotes   refs. = references

Amendments 1986; *Lutheran General Hospital (Park Ridge, IL); United States

Lynch, Abbyann, ed. The Good Pediatrician: An Ethics Curriculum for Use in Canadian Pediatrics Residency Programs. Teacher's Handbook. [Looseleaf format]. Toronto, ON: Department of Bioethics, Hospital for Sick Children; 1996. 348 p. Includes references. ISBN 0-9690091-4-3. BE56510.
adolescents; allowing to die; bioethics; case studies; *children; confidentiality; cultural pluralism; *curriculum; decision making; ethical theory; evaluation; goals; historical aspects; human experimentation; interdisciplinary communication; *internship and residency; legal aspects; *medical education; *medical ethics; newborns; organ donation; organ transplantation; *patient care; *pediatrics; physician patient relationship; professional competence; professional family relationship; *teaching methods; terminal care; questionnaires; Canada

MacDougall, Jamie C. Adam and the implant. *Hastings Center Report.* 1998 Jul–Aug; 28(4): 47. BE58927.
attitudes; case studies; *children; communication; decision making; *medical devices; pain; parents; *physically disabled; *public policy; *surgery; uncertainty; *cochlear implants; *hearing disorders; Canada; *Saskatchewan

Meadow, William; Reimshisel, Tyler; Lantos, John. Birth weight–specific mortality for extremely low birth weight infants vanishes by four days of life: epidemiology and ethics in the neonatal intensive care unit. *Pediatrics.* 1996 May; 97(5): 636–643. 21 refs. BE58109.
allowing to die; decision making; epidemiology; institutional policies; *intensive care units; justice; *low birth weight; *mortality; *newborns; *prognosis; prolongation of life; resource allocation; resuscitation; selection for treatment; *time factors; treatment outcome; uncertainty; ventilators; retrospective studies; severity of illness index; University of Chicago Medical Center

Morley, Colin; Shabde, Neela; Craft, Alan W. Concerns about using and interpreting covert video surveillance. [Article and commentary]. *BMJ (British Medical Journal).* 1998 May 23; 316(7144): 1603–1605. 8 refs. BE58062.
*behavior disorders; *child abuse; children; *deception; *diagnosis; *forensic medicine; parent child relationship; *parents; risks and benefits; *covert monitoring; *Munchausen syndrome by proxy; *video recording; Children Act 1989 (Great Britain); *Great Britain

Price, Christopher. Male circumcision: an ethical and legal affront. *Bulletin of Medical Ethics.* 1997 May; No. 128: 13–19. 26 refs. BE55700.
child abuse; *circumcision; cultural pluralism; injuries; international aspects; *legal aspects; legal liability; legal rights; *males; *minors; newborns; pain; parental consent; parents; physicians; professional organizations; religion; risks and benefits; social discrimination; Australia; *Great Britain; Law Commission (Great Britain); Law Reform Commission of Queensland

Rosenbloom, Lewis; Sullivan, Peter B. The ethics and implications of treatment programmes for disabled children with feeding difficulties. *In:* Sullivan, Peter B.; Rosenbloom, Lewis, eds. Feeding the Disabled Child. New York, NY: Cambridge University Press; 1996: 151–156. 6 refs. (Clinics in developmental medicine; v. 140). ISBN 1898683085. BE57283.
adolescents; allowing to die; anesthesia; *artificial feeding; *children; communication; *disabled; infants; nutrition; parents; patient care; patient care team; quality of life; *risks and benefits; surgery; withholding treatment; Great Britain

Sachdeva, Ramesh C.; Jefferson, Larry S.; Coss–Bu, Jorge, et al. Resource consumption and the extent of futile care among patients in a pediatric intensive care unit setting. *Journal of Pediatrics.* 1996 Jun; 128(6): 742–747. 19 refs. BE57158.
adolescents; *children; diagnosis; evaluation studies; *futility; hospitals; *intensive care units; morbidity; mortality; *patient care; pediatrics; prognosis; prolongation of life; quality of life; *resource allocation; statistics; treatment outcome; prospective studies; Texas; *Texas Children's Hospital (Houston, TX)

Somerville, Margaret A.; Alwin, David M.; Scherger, Joseph E., et al. Lidocaine–prilocaine cream for pain during circumcision. [Letters]. *New England Journal of Medicine.* 1997 Aug 21; 337(8): 568–570. 11 refs. BE56163.
anesthesia; biomedical research; *circumcision; drugs; human experimentation; international aspects; *males; methods; *newborns; *pain; parental consent; placebos; risks and benefits; surgery

Spence, Kaye. Ethical issues for neonatal nurses. *Nursing Ethics.* 1998 May; 5(3): 206–217. 26 refs. BE58720.
allowing to die; *attitudes; chronically ill; congenital disorders; critically ill; *decision making; intensive care units; *newborns; *nurse's role; *nurses; nursing ethics; *patient advocacy; *patient care; patient transfer; prognosis; survey; withholding treatment; *Australia; Australian Capital Territory; New South Wales

Straker, Gillian. Ethical issues in working with children in war zones. *In:* Apfel, Roberta J.; Simon, Bennett, eds. Minefields in Their Hearts: The Mental Health of Children and Communal Violence. New Haven, CT: Yale University Press; 1996: 18–32. 17 refs. ISBN 0–300–06570–1. BE56147.
*adolescents; autonomy; beneficence; case studies; *children; common good; confidentiality; cultural pluralism; developing countries; disclosure; *duty to warn; ethical relativism; *health personnel; human rights; international aspects; justice; mental health; moral complicity; *moral obligations; morality; *political activity; professional autonomy; professional ethics; professional patient relationship; *psychological stress; *psychotherapy; risks and benefits; social discrimination; torture; trust; *violence; *war; South Africa

Tucker, Bonnie Poitras. Deaf culture, cochlear implants, and elective disability. *Hastings Center Report.* 1998 Jul–Aug; 28(4): 6–14. 35 fn. BE58922.
attitudes; *children; coercion; communication; *cultural pluralism; decision making; economics; international aspects; legal aspects; *medical devices; minority groups; moral obligations; *normality; obligations of society; *parents; *physically disabled; *political activity; risks and benefits; social discrimination; *surgery; *treatment refusal; *values; *cochlear implants; *hearing disorders; *language; Americans with Disabilities Act 1990; Great Britain; *National Association of the Deaf; United States

Verweij, Marcel; Kortmann, Frank. Moral assessment of growth hormone therapy for children with idiopathic short stature. *Journal of Medical Ethics.* 1997 Oct; 23(5): 305–309. 18 fn. BE57111.
*children; counseling; goals; *growth disorders; *hormones; informed consent; justice; medicine; *moral policy; *normality; parental consent; psychological stress; resource allocation; *risks and benefits; *selection for treatment; self concept; stigmatization; treatment outcome; uncertainty
The prescription of growth hormone therapy for children who are not growth hormone deficient is one of the controversies in contemporary paediatric endocrinology. Is it morally appropriate to enhance the

---

BE = bioethics accession number   fn. = footnotes   refs. = references

growth, by means of medical treatment, of a child wish idiopathic short stature? The medical, moral, and philosophical questions in this area are many. Data on the effects of human growth hormone (hGH) treatment will not on their own provide us with answers, as these effects have to be evaluated from a normative perspective. In this article we consider hGH treatment for children of idiopathic short stature from three normative perspectives: the goals of medicine, the good of the patient, and the public good. We argue that the prevention of psychological and social problems due to short stature (and not merely the enhancement of growth) should be the ultimate goal of medical treatment and research.

PATIENTS' RIGHTS

See also CONFIDENTIALITY, INFORMED CONSENT, TREATMENT REFUSAL, TRUTH DISCLOSURE

Annas, George J. A national bill of patients' rights. *New England Journal of Medicine.* 1998 Mar 5; 338(10): 695–699. 20 refs. BE57301.
　　accountability; advisory committees; autonomy; confidentiality; conflict of interest; decision making; disclosure; economics; emergency care; federal government; government regulation; health insurance; historical aspects; informed consent; *legal aspects; legal rights; managed care programs; patient access to records; patient advocacy; patient participation; *patients' rights; physician patient relationship; physician's role; privacy; *public policy; treatment refusal; Advisory Commission on Consumer Protection and Quality in the Health Care Industry; *United States

Davis, Anne J.; Aroskar, Mila A.; Liaschenko, Joan, et al. Rights, responsibilities, and health care. *In: their* Ethical Dilemmas and Nursing Practice. Fourth Edition. Stamford, CT: Appleton and Lange; 1997: 83–103. 25 fn. ISBN 0-8385-2283-1. BE58594.
　　case studies; economics; *health care; health facilities; justice; legal aspects; *moral obligations; *nurses; *nursing ethics; *patient advocacy; *patients' rights; resource allocation; *rights; standards; United States

Dickens, Bernard. Patients' rights. *In:* Chadwick, Ruth, ed. Encyclopedia of Applied Ethics, Volume 3. San Diego, CA: Academic Press; 1998: 459–471. 7 refs. ISBN 0-12-227068-1. BE56259.
　　autonomy; beneficence; bioethical issues; *ethical theory; ethics committees; feminist ethics; health care; human experimentation; human rights; justice; legal rights; natural law; paternalism; patient participation; *patients' rights; principle-based ethics; professional patient relationship; public health; utilitarianism

Hoshino, Kazumasa. Bioethics in the light of Japanese sentiments. *In:* Hoshino, Kazumasa, ed. Japanese and Western Bioethics: Studies in Moral Diversity. Boston, MA: Kluwer Academic; 1997: 13–23. 5 refs. ISBN 0-7923-4112-0. BE57080.
　　autonomy; bioethical issues; cadavers; communication; *communitarianism; comparative studies; *decision making; diagnosis; family members; *family relationship; informed consent; legal aspects; *organ donation; *paternalism; patient care; patient compliance; *patients' rights; *physician patient relationship; *physicians; professional family relationship; prognosis; terminally ill; third party consent; *tissue donation; *truth disclosure; hope; non-Western World; Act of Donation of the Body for Medical and Dental Education 1983 (Japan); Cornea and Kidney Transplant Act 1979 (Japan); *Japan; United States

Leino–Kilpi, Helena; Nyrhinen, Tarja; Katajisto, Jouko. Patients' rights in laboratory examinations: do they realize? *Nursing Ethics.* 1997 Nov; 4(6): 451–464. 36 refs. BE57417.
　　autonomy; confidentiality; decision making; *diagnosis; disclosure; evaluation studies; *hospitals; informed consent; institutional policies; *laboratories; misconduct; nurse's role; patient participation; *patients' rights; privacy; professional patient relationship; standards; survey; guideline adherence; *Finland

Marwick, Charles. 'Bill of rights' for patients sent to Clinton. [News]. *JAMA.* 1998 Jan 7; 279(1): 7–8. Includes excerpts from text of "Patients' rights under the proposed plan...and patients' responsibilities," p. 7. BE58060.
　　advisory committees; decision making; dissent; *economics; health care delivery; health facilities; health insurance; *industry; legislation; *managed care programs; moral obligations; patient advocacy; patient participation; *patients' rights; politics; *public policy; *Advisory Commission on Consumer Protection and Quality in the Health Care Industry; U.S. Congress; *United States

Morgan, Derek. Health rights, ethics and justice: the opportunity costs of rhetoric. *In:* McLean, Sheila A.M., ed. Contemporary Issues in Law, Medicine and Ethics. Brookfield, VT: Dartmouth; 1996: 15–27. 32 fn. ISBN 1-85521-586-1. BE57788.
　　alternatives; confidentiality; cultural pluralism; disclosure; emergency care; government regulation; health; *health care; human rights; international aspects; *justice; legal rights; legislation; moral obligations; *moral policy; obligations of society; patient access to records; *patients' rights; physician patient relationship; public health; *public policy; referral and consultation; *resource allocation; *rights; risks and benefits; selection for treatment; socioeconomic factors; *standards; life style; European Union; *Great Britain; *National Health Service; Patient's Charter (Great Britain)

Pear, Robert. Presidential panel sees no need for a law on patient's rights. [News]. *New York Times.* 1998 Mar 13: A17. BE57730.
　　accountability; advisory committees; committee membership; federal government; government regulation; health care delivery; *health insurance; *patients' rights; *public policy; quality of health care; self regulation; *Advisory Commission on Consumer Protection and Quality in the Health Care Industry; *United States

Savulescu, Julian; Marsden, Rachel; Hope, Tony, et al. Respect for privacy and the case of Mr. K. [Article and commentaries]. *BMJ (British Medical Journal).* 1998 Mar 21; 316(7135): 921–924. 4 refs. BE57974.
　　autonomy; case studies; *chronically ill; *drug abuse; *hospitals; *institutionalized persons; legal aspects; nurses; *patients; *patients' rights; *privacy; rehabilitation; *sexuality; social interaction; *marijuana; Great Britain

Silver, Melanie H. Wilson. Patients' rights in England and the United States of America: *The Patient's Charter* and the New Jersey Patient Bill of Rights: a comparison. *Journal of Medical Ethics.* 1997 Aug; 23(4): 213–220. 16 fn. BE55925.
　　communication; comparative studies; due process; evaluation; *government regulation; health care; *health care delivery; health promotion; hospitals; human experimentation; informed consent; legal rights; minority groups; misconduct; patient care; *patients' rights; physically disabled; *public policy; quality of health care; resource allocation; *standards; state government; treatment refusal; hearing disorders; quality assurance; translating; *England; Great Britain; *National Health Service; *New Jersey; *New Jersey Patient Bill of Rights; *Patient's Charter (Great Britain); United States

---

BE = bioethics accession number　　fn. = footnotes　　refs. = references

The Patient's Charter has been in effect for nearly five years. This article considers the purpose and value of the document through a comparison with the New Jersey Patient Bill of Rights. Patient rights statements have been posted in American hospitals for more than twenty years. However, the New Jersey document and the patient rights programme it established seven years ago, have proven to be economically effective, successful in their representation of patients and enforceable, due to the adoption of state legislation and regulation to oversee the process. Several examples of how the programme works are included in the comparison, with a similar review of The Patient's Charter. In the comparison the author argues that for the programme to succeed as it has done in New Jersey, the government will need to develop legislative backing to ensure enforcement, and an efficient system for monitoring compliance. The programme will need to become credible in the eyes of the health service user. The author suggests this may be best achieved by developing an efficient, accessible and user-friendly means of redress, should the patient consider his or her rights have been violated. A "mish-mash" of quality assurance standards and levels of care which patients can "expect" from the health service providers only serves to distract the health service user from the government's failure to commit the resources that would empower the patients rights portion of The Patient's Charter.

Worth-Staten, Patricia A.; Poniatowski, Larry. Advance directives and patient rights: a Joint Commission perspective. *Bioethics Forum.* 1997 Summer; 13(2): 47–50. 2 refs. BE58287.
    *advance directives; decision making; family members; *hospitals; informed consent; *institutional policies; patient participation; *patients' rights; *standards; terminal care; withholding treatment; *Joint Commission on Accreditation of Healthcare Organizations; United States

PATIENTS' RIGHTS/MENTALLY DISABLED

Levy, Robert M.; Rubenstein, Leonard S. The Rights of People with Mental Disabilites: The Authoritative ACLU Guide to the Rights of People with Mental Illness and Mental Retardation. Carbondale, IL: Southern Illinois University Press; 1996. 370 p. Includes references. ISBN 0-8093-1990-X. BE58645.
    advance directives; autonomy; behavior control; community services; competence; confidentiality; dangerousness; deinstitutionalized persons; disadvantaged; electroconvulsive therapy; employment; federal government; government financing; human experimentation; informed consent; institutionalized persons; involuntary commitment; judicial action; *legal aspects; legal guardians; *legal rights; *mentally disabled; *mentally ill; *mentally retarded; minors; nursing homes; outpatient commitment; patient admission; patient discharge; patient transfer; *patients' rights; physical restraint; prisoners; psychoactive drugs; psychosurgery; right to treatment; social discrimination; standards; state government; sterilization (sexual); third party consent; treatment refusal; withholding treatment; homeless persons; Americans with Disabilities Act 1990; *United States

Mowbray, Carol T.; Freddolino, Paul P.; Rhodes, Genice L., et al. Evaluation of a patient rights protection system: public policy implications. *Administration in Mental Health.* 1985 Summer; 12(4): 264–283. 16 refs. 7 fn. BE57830.
    *evaluation; *government regulation; health personnel; institutionalized persons; interprofessional relations; knowledge, attitudes, practice; *mental institutions; *mentally disabled; misconduct; *organization and administration; *patients' rights; public policy; state government; *Michigan

Russian Federation. Law of 2 July 1992 of the Russian Federation on psychiatric care and the safeguarding of citizens' rights in the dispensing of such care. *International Digest of Health Legislation.* 1993; 44(2): 267–281. BE57184.
    adults; coercion; confidentiality; dangerousness; decision making; disclosure; health personnel; informed consent; institutionalized persons; involuntary commitment; judicial action; *legal aspects; legal rights; mental institutions; *mentally ill; minors; patient advocacy; *patient care; patient discharge; patient transfer; *patients' rights; professional competence; psychiatric diagnosis; psychiatry; right to treatment; third party consent; treatment refusal; voluntary admission; *Russia

PERSONHOOD

Barlow, Bicka A. Severe penalties for the destruction of "potential life" -- cruel and unusual punishment? [Comment]. *University of San Francisco Law Review.* 1995 Winter; 29(2): 463–508. 401 fn. Appendix: [model] Fetal Homicide Statute. BE57274.
    abortion, induced; beginning of life; constitutional law; *criminal law; fetal development; *fetuses; intention; *killing; *legal liability; model legislation; *personhood; pregnant women; punishment; standards; state government; state interest; viability; violence; wrongful death; miscarriage; *Eighth Amendment; United States

Bermúdez, José Luis. The moral significance of birth. *Ethics.* 1996 Jan; 106(2): 378–403. 31 fn. BE55688.
    abortion, induced; beginning of life; *childbirth; *ethical analysis; fetal development; *fetuses; infanticide; killing; *moral policy; *newborns; *personhood; philosophy; prematurity; primates; psychology; *self concept; speciesism; *value of life

Burd, Larry; Gregory, Jennifer M.; Kerbeshian, Jacob. The brain-mind quiddity: ethical issues in the use of human brain tissue for therapeutic and scientific purposes. *Journal of Medical Ethics.* 1998 Apr; 24(2): 118–122. 13 refs. BE58051.
    animal experimentation; *biomedical research; *brain; brain death; computers; electrical stimulation of the brain; *emotions; ethical review; human body; human experimentation; informed consent; laboratories; models, theoretical; *organ donation; *organ transplantation; *personhood; regulation; *tissue donation; *tissue transplantation; cell lines; personal identity
The use of human brain tissue in neuroscience research is increasing. Recent developments include transplanting neural tissue, growing or maintaining neural tissue in laboratories and using surgically removed tissue for experimentation. Also, it is likely that in the future there will be attempts at partial or complete brain transplants. A discussion of the ethical issues of using human brain tissue for research and brain transplantation has been organized around nine broadly defined topic areas. Criteria for human brain tissue transplantation and laboratory use of brain tissue are proposed.

Csordas, Thomas J. A handmaid's tale: the rhetoric of personhood in American and Japanese healing of abortions. *In:* Sargent, Carolyn F.; Brettell, Caroline B., eds. Gender and Health: An International Perspective. Upper Saddle River, NJ: Prentice Hall; 1996: 227–241. 23 refs. 5 fn. ISBN 0-13-079427-9. BE58095.
    *aborted fetuses; *abortion, induced; *Buddhist ethics; comparative studies; emotions; *females; international aspects; mother fetus relationship; *personhood;

BE = bioethics accession number   fn. = footnotes   refs. = references

*psychological stress; psychology; *religion; *Roman Catholics; grief; guilt; *Japan; *Pentecostal Christians; *United States

Joralemon, Donald. Organ wars: the battle for body parts. *Medical Anthropology Quarterly.* 1995 Sep; 9(3): 335–356. 98 refs. 25 fn. Commented on by M. Lock, p. 390–393, and by B.A. Koenig and L.F. Hogle, p. 393–397. BE56581.

altruism; *anthropology; *attitudes; attitudes to death; autonomy; *body parts and fluids; brain death; *cadavers; *commodification; *cultural pluralism; determination of death; *economics; *emotions; family members; *gifts; *human body; *incentives; international aspects; legal aspects; mass media; metaphor; *organ donation; organ donors; *organ transplantation; *personhood; *property rights; *psychological stress; *psychology; public opinion; *remuneration; scarcity; *self concept; third party consent; *transplant recipients; *values; *United States

Khushf, George. Embryo research: the ethical geography of the debate. *Journal of Medicine and Philosophy.* 1997 Oct; 22(5): 495–519. 36 refs. 9 fn. BE56624.

abortion, induced; advisory committees; *beginning of life; consensus; *embryo research; *embryos; federal government; fetal development; *government financing; *government regulation; human experimentation; in vitro fertilization; informed consent; libertarianism; *moral obligations; *moral policy; nontherapeutic research; *personhood; *policy analysis; *politics; private sector; *public policy; reproductive technologies; research design; research embryo creation; risks and benefits; science; twinning; value of life; *Human Embryo Research Panel; United States

Three basic political positions on embryo research will be identified as libertarian, conservative, and social-democratic. The Human Embryo Research Panel will be regarded as an expression of the social-democratic position. A taxonomy of the ethical issues addressed by the Panel will then be developed at the juncture of political and ethical modes of reflection. Among the arguments considered will be those for the separability of the abortion and embryo research debates; arguments against the possibility of the preembryo being a person, especially arguments associated with totipotency and the significance of the primitive streak; and the various reasons for regulating embryo research, including those associated with respect for the preembryo, the protection of traditional views of human procreation, and the prevention of commercialization.

Klasing, Murphy S. Death of an unborn child: jurisprudential inconsistencies in wrongful death, criminal homicide, and abortion cases. *Pepperdine Law Review.* 1995; 22(3): 933–979. 385 fn. BE56670.

*abortion, induced; *beginning of life; criminal law; fetal development; *fetuses; judicial action; killing; *legal aspects; *legal liability; negligence; newborns; *personhood; prenatal injuries; *state government; Supreme Court decisions; torts; *viability; *wrongful death; *United States

Koch, Tom; Ridgley, Mark. Distanced perspectives: AIDS, anencephaly, and AHP [Analytic Hierarchy Process]. *Theoretical Medicine and Bioethics.* 1998 Jan; 19(1): 47–58. 26 fn. BE57311.

AIDS; *allowing to die; *anencephaly; *bioethical issues; brain pathology; *decision analysis; *decision making; equal protection; *futility; infants; *law; legal aspects; medicine; models, theoretical; *newborns; *personhood; prolongation of life; *quality of life; self concept; social interaction; speciesism; *standards; value of life; ventilators; withholding treatment; In re Baby K; In re T.A.C.P.; United States

Korein, Julius. Ontogenesis of the brain in the human organism: definitions of life and death of the human being and person. *In:* Edwards, Rem B., ed. Advances in Bioethics. Volume 2: New Essays on Abortion and Bioethics. Greenwich, CT: JAI Press; 1997: 1–74. 298 refs. ISBN 0-7623-0194-5. BE56789.

abortion, induced; adults; *anencephaly; *beginning of life; *brain; *brain death; children; *determination of death; diagnosis; embryos; *fetal development; *fetuses; infants; newborns; organ transplantation; persistent vegetative state; *personhood; prognosis; tissue transplantation

Loewy, Erich H. Of sentiment, caring and anencephalics: a response to Sytsma. *Theoretical Medicine and Bioethics.* 1998 Jan; 19(1): 21–34. 19 refs. BE57312.

*anencephaly; autonomy; brain death; brain pathology; *caring; decision making; determination of death; emotions; *ethical analysis; ethical theory; justice; *moral obligations; *moral policy; *newborns; *organ donation; parental consent; parents; paternalism; persistent vegetative state; *personhood; prognosis; suffering; wedge argument; Kant, Immanuel

Lusthaus, Evelyn W. Involuntary euthanasia and current attempts to define persons with mental retardation as less than human. *Mental Retardation.* 1985 Jun; 23(3): 148–154. 46 refs. BE56962.

*allowing to die; children; congenital disorders; *dehumanization; human characteristics; *involuntary euthanasia; legal aspects; *mentally retarded; *newborns; parents; *personhood; *quality of life; selection for treatment; treatment refusal; *value of life; withholding treatment; United States

McCurdy, David B. Personhood, spirituality, and hope in the care of human beings with dementia. *Journal of Clinical Ethics.* 1998 Spring; 9(1): 81–91. 60 fn. BE57717.

caring; communication; *dementia; *emotions; futility; *health personnel; humanism; long-term care; nursing homes; *patient care; *personhood; professional patient relationship; *religion; self concept; *social interaction; theology; value of life; dependency; dignity; *hope

Macready, Norra. US state rules that a viable fetus is a person. [News]. *BMJ (British Medical Journal).* 1997 Dec 6; 315(7121): 1488. BE57262.

child abuse; *drug abuse; *fetuses; *legal aspects; legal liability; *personhood; *pregnant women; *prenatal injuries; state government; *viability; *South Carolina; *Whitner, Cornelia

Miller, Hugh. DNA blueprints, personhood, and genetic privacy. *Health Matrix.* 1998 Summer; 8(2): 179–221. 105 fn. BE58953.

*autonomy; confidentiality; constitutional law; disclosure; *genetic determinism; *genetic identity; *genetic information; genetic research; genetic screening; legal aspects; *legal rights; *personhood; philosophy; *privacy; *personal identity; United States

Namihira, Emiko. The characteristics of Japanese concepts and attitudes with regard to human remains. *In:* Hoshino, Kazumasa, ed. Japanese and Western Bioethics: Studies in Moral Diversity. Boston, MA: Kluwer Academic; 1997: 61–69. 3 refs. ISBN 0-7923-4112-0. BE57083.

*attitudes; *attitudes to death; *cadavers; family members; family relationship; *human body; organ donation; *personhood; personal identity; *Japan

Patterson, Elizabeth G. Human rights and human life: an uneven fit. *Tulane Law Review.* 1994 Jun; 68(6): 1527–1561. 168 fn. BE55539.

abortion, induced; adults; allowing to die; *anencephaly;

BE = bioethics accession number   fn. = footnotes   refs. = references

autonomy; beginning of life; *brain death; cadavers; *competence; determination of death; equal protection; *fetuses; human rights; informed consent; *legal aspects; *legal rights; mentally disabled; *minors; newborns; *persistent vegetative state; *personhood; quality of life; Supreme Court decisions; third party consent; treatment refusal; *value of life; withholding treatment; *United States

Perlin, Terry M. Who will I be? Stephen G. Post's *The Moral Challenge of Alzheimer's kAlzheimerl Disease.* [Book review essay]. *Journal of Ethics, Law, and Aging.* 1996 Fall–Winter; 2(2): 85–86. 10 refs. 1 fn. BE57142.
   advance directives; autonomy; behavior control; *dementia; diagnosis; empathy; family members; freedom; health personnel; home care; married persons; *patient care; *personhood; quality of life; *social interaction; time factors; treatment refusal; truth disclosure; value of life; dignity; *The Moral Challenge of Alzheimer Disease (Post, S.G.)

Peters, Ted. Designer genes and selective abortion. *In: his* For the Love of Children: Genetic Technology and the Future of the Family. Louisville, KY: Westminster John Knox Press; 1996: 85–118, 193–199. 63 fn. ISBN 0–664–25468–3. BE55697.
   adoption; beginning of life; coercion; confidentiality; decision making; disabled; employment; eugenics; fetal development; *fetuses; genetic counseling; *genetic disorders; genetic information; *genetic predisposition; *genetic screening; government regulation; insurance; killing; legal rights; *personhood; pregnant women; prenatal diagnosis; privacy; Protestant ethics; public policy; risk; *Roman Catholic ethics; *selective abortion; *social discrimination; value of life; viability; dignity; Genetic Privacy Act 1994; United States

Prokes, Mary Timothy. Technology and the lived body. *In: her* Toward a Theology of the Body. Grand Rapids, MI: W.B. Eerdmans; 1996: 104–117. 10 fn. Includes references embedded in list at back of book. ISBN 0–8028–4339–5. BE56246.
   *biomedical technologies; conscience; contraception; embryos; eugenics; *human body; human characteristics; intention; marital relationship; mass media; moral obligations; morality; *personhood; reproduction; reproductive technologies; *Roman Catholic ethics; *theology; value of life; Humanae Vitae; Instruction on Respect for Human Life; Veritatis Splendor

Rich, Ben A. Prospective autonomy and critical interests: a narrative defense of the moral authority of advance directives. *Cambridge Quarterly of Healthcare Ethics.* 1997 Spring; 6(2): 138–147. 24 fn. BE56435.
   *advance directives; allowing to die; *autonomy; competence; *dementia; *moral policy; *narrative ethics; paternalism; *personhood; prolongation of life; public policy; quality of life; right to die; *self concept; treatment refusal; *personal identity; rationality; Dresser, Rebecca; Dworkin, Ronald; Parfit, Derek
In the mid to late 1980s a debate arose over the moral and legal authority of advance medical directives. At the center of this debate were two point–counterpoint law journal articles by Rebecca Dresser and Nancy Rhoden. What appeared to have the makings of an ongoing critical dialogue ended with the untimely death of Nancy Rhoden. Rebecca Dresser, however, has continued her challenge of advance directives in numerous publications, most recently in a critique of Ronald Dworkin's *Life's Dominion*. Like Rhoden, Dworkin has been a staunch advocate of advance directives as an exercise of what has come to be referred to as prospective or precedent autonomy. In this paper I will consider a number of the issues that Dresser has repeatedly raised about the infirmities of advance directives, and suggest that it is from an understanding

of and appreciation for the narrative dimension of the life of a person that advance directives draw one of their most powerful justifications.

Sabat, Steven R. Voices of Alzheimer's disease sufferers: a call for treatment based on personhood. *Journal of Clinical Ethics.* 1998 Spring; 9(1): 35–48. 36 fn. BE57712.
   behavioral research; case studies; communication; dehumanization; *dementia; emotions; patient care; patient participation; *personhood; professional patient relationship; psychological stress; *self concept; *social interaction; stigmatization

Schwartz, Lewis M. An essay on the moral status question. *In:* Edwards, Rem B., ed. Advances in Bioethics. Volume 2: New Essays on Abortion and Bioethics. Greenwich, CT: JAI Press; 1997: 267–301. 11 refs. ISBN 0–7623–0194–5. BE56797.
   *abortion, induced; adults; *fetal development; *fetuses; *killing; *moral obligations; *moral policy; pain; persistent vegetative state; *personhood; philosophy

Shannon, Thomas A. Fetal status: sources and implications. *Journal of Medicine and Philosophy.* 1997 Oct; 22(5): 415–422. 2 refs. BE56619.
   abortion, induced; *attitudes; beginning of life; biomedical technologies; cesarean section; coercion; drug abuse; embryo research; *embryos; fetal development; fetal therapy; fetal tissue donation; *fetuses; intensive care units; *moral obligations; newborns; *personhood; pregnant women; preimplantation diagnosis; prematurity; prenatal diagnosis; prenatal injuries; public policy; reproductive technologies; treatment refusal; utilitarianism; *value of life; viability; United States
This essay considers the ways in which the various contexts — abortion, prenatal diagnosis, fetal research, and the use of fetuses in transplantation — shape the American debate on the moral standing of the fetus. This discussion gives rise to several philosophical debates on the status of the preimplantation embryo, particularly the debate over when the preimplantation embryo becomes individuated. How that questions is resolved has critical ethical and policy implications.

Shannon, Thomas A. Response to Khushf. *Journal of Medicine and Philosophy.* 1997 Oct; 22(5): 525–527. 4 refs. BE56626.
   *beginning of life; embryo research; *embryos; fetal development; moral obligations; *personhood; twinning

Sharp, Lesley A. Organ transplantation as a transformative experience: anthropological insights into the restructuring of the self. *Medical Anthropology Quarterly.* 1995 Sep; 9(3): 357–389. 113 refs. 18 fn. Commented on by M. Lock, p. 390–393, and by B.A. Koenig and L.F. Hogle, p. 393–397. BE56561.
   *altruism; *anthropology; *attitudes; attitudes to death; *body parts and fluids; brain death; *cadavers; capitalism; *commodification; cultural pluralism; determination of death; disabled; economics; *emotions; *family members; *gifts; health personnel; *human body; metaphor; *organ donation; organ donors; *organ transplantation; *personhood; property rights; *psychological stress; *psychology; remuneration; scarcity; *self concept; social interaction; stigmatization; survey; third party consent; *transplant recipients; *values; ethnographic studies; Indiana; Mercy Memorial Hospital (Indianapolis); *United States

Singer, Peter. On comparing the value of human and nonhuman life. *In:* Morscher, Edgar; Neumaier, Otto; Simons, Peter, eds. Applied Ethics in a Troubled World. Boston, MA: Kluwer Academic; 1998: 93–104. 11 fn.

ISBN 0-7923-4965-2. BE58584.
> anencephaly; animal organs; *animal rights; brain death; comparative studies; ecology; fetuses; human characteristics; killing; mentally disabled; moral policy; National Socialism; newborns; organ donation; organ transplantation; *personhood; political activity; primates; religion; *speciesism; *value of life; wedge argument; Western World; International Wittgenstein Symposium

Strong, Carson. Response to Khushf. *Journal of Medicine and Philosophy.* 1997 Oct; 22(5): 521-523. 5 refs. BE56625.
> *beginning of life; embryo research; *embryos; *fetal development; moral obligations; *personhood; research embryo creation; value of life

Strong, Carson. The moral status of preembryos, embryos, fetuses, and infants. *Journal of Medicine and Philosophy.* 1997 Oct; 22(5): 457-478. 32 refs. 4 fn. BE56622.
> *beginning of life; embryo disposition; embryo research; *embryos; *fetal development; *fetuses; *human characteristics; legal aspects; *moral obligations; *moral policy; *newborns; *personhood; property rights; research embryo creation; risks and benefits; self concept; social interaction; teleological ethics; value of life; viability

Some have argued that embryos and fetuses have the moral status of personhood because of certain criteria that are satisfied during gestation. However, these attempts to base personhood during gestation on intrinsic characteristics have uniformly been unsuccessful. Within a secular framework, another approach to establishing a moral standing for embryos and fetuses is to argue that we ought to confer some moral status upon them. There appear to be two main approaches to defending conferred moral standing; namely, consequentialist and contractarian arguments. This article puts forward a consequentialist argument for the conferred moral standing of preembryos, embryos, fetuses, and infants. It states and defends an original version of the commonly-held view that moral standing increases during gestation. It also explores the implications of this viewpoint for several issues: what is involved in showing 'respect' for preembryos; and whether it is permissible to create preembryos solely for research.

Thomasma, David C.; Loewy, Erich H. A dialogue on species-specific rights: humans and animals in bioethics. *Cambridge Quarterly of Healthcare Ethics.* 1997 Fall; 6(4): 435-444. 12 fn. BE56479.
> animal experimentation; *animal rights; brain pathology; embryos; *human rights; mentally retarded; moral obligations; *moral policy; *personhood; religion; *rights; *speciesism; suffering; values; rationality

Verhey, Allen. Commodification, commercialization, and embodiment. *Women's Health Issues.* 1997 May-Jun; 7(3): 132-142. 12 refs. Paper presented at a workshop on "Assisted Reproductive Technologies, Ads, and Ethics: Philosophical, Ethical, and Clinical Perspectives on the Use of Advertising in Reproductive Medicine," held by the National Advisory Board on Ethics in Reproduction in Washington, DC on 19 Oct 1996. BE55952.
> children; coercion; *commodification; deception; dehumanization; *economics; embryo transfer; freedom; informed consent; misconduct; morality; ovum donors; *personhood; physicians; regulation; reproduction; *reproductive technologies; rights; treatment outcome; values; wedge argument; Asch, Ricardo

Walters, James W. What Is a Person? An Ethical Exploration. Urbana, IL: University of Illinois Press; 1997. 187 p. 344 fn. ISBN 0-252-02278-5. BE56192.
> allowing to die; *anencephaly; animal organs; animal rights;

bioethics; brain death; *brain pathology; decision making; dementia; determination of death; Down syndrome; ethical theory; fetuses; human characteristics; legal aspects; moral obligations; *moral policy; *newborns; *organ donation; parents; patient care; persistent vegetative state; *personhood; philosophy; prolongation of life; public policy; religious ethics; risks and benefits; Roman Catholic ethics; secularism; *self concept; speciesism; *standards; theology; value of life; wedge argument; withholding treatment

Warren, Mary Anne. Moral Status: Obligations to Persons and Other Living Things. New York, NY: Oxford University Press; 1997. 265 p. (Issues in biomedical ethics). Bibliography: p. 243-253. ISBN 0-19-823668-9. BE56996.
> abortion, induced; allowing to die; animal experimentation; *animal rights; assisted suicide; *bioethical issues; cultural pluralism; ecology; embryos; emotions; ethical relativism; ethical theory; euthanasia; fetal development; fetuses; food; freedom; genetic intervention; historical aspects; *human rights; infants; mentally disabled; *moral obligations; *moral policy; morality; pain; *personhood; religion; *rights; self concept; social interaction; speciesism; utilitarianism; *value of life; viability; women's rights; potentiality; rationality; Callicott, J. Baird; Kant, Immanuel; Regan, Tom

Werpehowski, William. Persons, practices, and the conception argument. *Journal of Medicine and Philosophy.* 1997 Oct; 22(5): 479-494. 18 refs. 6 fn. BE56623.
> *beginning of life; embryo research; *embryos; fetal development; genetic identity; justice; *moral obligations; moral policy; parent child relationship; *personhood; *Roman Catholic ethics; theology; twinning; value of life; Declaration on Procured Abortion; Instruction on Respect for Human Life

The argument that human life should be fully protected once conception is complete has been challenged by the claim that at that time such life is not genuinely individuated in the morally required sense. This essay analyzes the "conception versus individuation" exchange and directs attention to the communal contexts within which the relevant arguments and counter-arguments arise.

Whitehouse, Peter J. Readdressing our moral relationship to nonhuman creatures: commentary on "A dialogue on species-specific rights: humans and animals in bioethics." *Cambridge Quarterly of Healthcare Ethics.* 1997 Fall; 6(4): 445-448. 13 fn. BE56499.
> *animal rights; *bioethics; *ecology; *human rights; moral obligations; *moral policy; *personhood; religion; rights; *speciesism; rationality; Potter, Van Rensselear

Wisconsin. Supreme Court. State v. Kruzicki. *North Western Reporter, 2d Series.* 1997 Apr 22 (date of decision). 561: 729-749. BE56745.
> *behavior control; coercion; *criminal law; *drug abuse; *fetuses; government regulation; *legal aspects; *personhood; *pregnant women; *prenatal injuries; state government; treatment refusal; *viability; *Angela M.W.; *State v. Kruzicki; Wisconsin

The Wisconsin Supreme Court reversed the appellate court's denial of review of writs under which a pregnant woman sought release from the court's detention and protective custody of her viable fetus. Although she had given birth, the court considered the now moot issue of a child in need of protection or services. When Angela M.W. was thirty-six weeks pregnant, blood tests confirmed drug use in each of the preceding three months and it was decided that her continued use of drugs would cause the fetus serious harm. The county took protective custody of the fetus by a court order requiring that the woman be confined to an inpatient drug treatment facility. After considering the meanings

---

of "child" and "person", the court concluded that under state law a child is a human being born alive, not a fetus. The dissenting judge argued that the meanings of "child" and "person" include a viable fetus. (KIE abstract)

PHYSICIAN PATIENT RELATIONSHIP See MEDICAL ETHICS, PROFESSIONAL PATIENT RELATIONSHIP

POPULATION CONTROL

See also CONTRACEPTION

Callahan, Joan C. Birth control ethics. *In:* Chadwick, Ruth, ed. Encyclopedia of Applied Ethics, Volume 1. San Diego, CA: Academic Press; 1998: 335–351. 17 refs. ISBN 0–12–227066–5. BE56371.
   abortion on demand; *abortion, induced; attitudes; autonomy; beginning of life; coercion; congenital disorders; *contraception; drug abuse; eugenics; family planning; females; fetuses; government regulation; hormones; infanticide; international aspects; involuntary sterilization; males; medical devices; *methods; *moral policy; *morality; multiple pregnancy; personhood; physicians; politics; *population control; pregnant women; prenatal diagnosis; prenatal injuries; *public policy; religion; *reproduction; selective abortion; sex determination; sexuality; *social control; socioeconomic factors; voluntary sterilization; wedge argument; women's rights

Charo, R. Alta. The interaction between family planning policies and the introduction of new reproductive technologies. *In:* Petersen, Kerry, ed. Intersections: Women on Law, Medicine and Technology. Brookfield, VT: Ashgate; 1997: 73–97. 55 refs. 10 fn. ISBN 1–85521–882–8. BE57487.
   abortion, induced; autonomy; *contraception; decision making; drugs; eugenics; *family planning; *females; historical aspects; international aspects; legal aspects; physician's role; political activity; *population control; public health; public policy; *reproductive technologies; social dominance; women's health services; *women's rights; Nineteenth Century; RU–486; Twentieth Century; United States

David, Henry P.; Baban, Adriana. Women's health and reproductive rights: Romanian experience. *Patient Education and Counseling.* 1996 Aug; 28(3): 235–245. 25 refs. BE57259.
   *abortion, induced; adults; coercion; contraception; decision making; *family planning; *females; *government regulation; historical aspects; *illegal abortion; *knowledge, attitudes, practice; morbidity; mortality; mothers; motivation; *population control; pregnant women; psychological stress; *public policy; reproduction; sexuality; social control; *social impact; socioeconomic factors; survey; women's health; *women's rights; qualitative research; *Romania; Twentieth Century

Lee, Luke T. Population: the human rights approach. *Colorado Journal of International Environmental Law and Policy.* 1995 Summer; 6(2): 327–344. 85 fn. BE57194.
   abortion, induced; coercion; family planning; future generations; government regulation; *human rights; incentives; international aspects; *population control; *public policy; reproduction; United Nations International Conference on Population and Development

Neel, James V. Looking ahead: some genetic issues of the future. *Perspectives in Biology and Medicine.* 1997 Spring; 40(3): 328–347. 77 refs. Based on a presentation at the Ninth International Congress of Human Genetics

in Rio de Janeiro, 23 Aug 1996. BE59007.
   drug industry; ecology; eugenics; financial support; food; future generations; *gene pool; gene therapy; genetic disorders; genetic diversity; genetic predisposition; *genetic research; genetic screening; *genetics; health hazards; international aspects; investigators; *moral obligations; morbidity; nutrition; *population control; psychoactive drugs; public policy; radiation; social problems; trends; *population genetics; China

Rosenthal, Elisabeth. For one–child policy, China rethinks iron hand. [News]. *New York Times.* 1998 Nov 1: 1, 20. BE58996.
   contraception; *family planning; government regulation; law enforcement; minority groups; parents; *population control; *public policy; socioeconomic factors; sterilization (sexual); personal financing; rural population; urban population; *China

PRENATAL DIAGNOSIS

See also GENETIC COUNSELING, GENETIC SCREENING, SEX DETERMINATION

Allen, Jill S. Fonda; Mulhauser, Lynda C. Genetic counseling after abnormal prenatal diagnosis: facilitating coping in families who continue their pregnancies. *Journal of Genetic Counseling.* 1995 Dec; 4(4): 251–265. 43 refs. BE56020.
   allowing to die; *attitudes; case studies; *childbirth; decision making; disabled; fetuses; *genetic counseling; *genetic disorders; guidelines; marital relationship; motivation; newborns; parents; patient care; pregnant women; *prenatal diagnosis; prognosis; *psychological stress; risk; selective abortion; uncertainty; *values

Barnes, Frank L. Ethical considerations of preimplantation genetic diagnosis and embryo selection. *In:* Monagle, John F.; Thomasma, David C., eds. Health Care Ethics: Critical Issues for the 21st Century. Gaithersburg, MD: Aspen Publishers; 1998: 56–59. 10 fn. ISBN 0–8342–0911–X. BE56279.
   embryo transfer; embryos; gene therapy; *genetic disorders; genetic predisposition; *genetic screening; in vitro fertilization; methods; parents; *preimplantation diagnosis; selection for treatment

Beeson, Diane; Jennings, Patricia. Prenatal diagnosis of fetal disorders: ethical, legal, and social issues. *In:* Monagle, John F.; Thomasma, David C., eds. Health Care Ethics: Critical Issues for the 21st Century. Gaithersburg, MD: Aspen Publishers; 1998: 29–44. 86 fn. ISBN 0–8342–0911–X. BE56278.
   blacks; coercion; confidentiality; congenital disorders; disabled; eugenics; fetuses; genetic counseling; indigents; informed consent; legal liability; legal rights; minority groups; misconduct; mother fetus relationship; obligations to society; parents; pregnant women; *prenatal diagnosis; public opinion; quality of life; resource allocation; review; selective abortion; social control; social discrimination; socioeconomic factors; suffering; values; women's rights; wrongful life; United States

Cao, Antonio. Technical and social aspects of beta–thalassemia screening in Europe and developing countries. *In:* Knoppers, Bartha Maria, ed. Human DNA: Law and Policy: International and Comparative Perspectives. Proceedings of the First International Conference on DNA Sampling and Human Genetic Research: Ethical, Legal, and Policy Aspects, held in Montreal, Canada, 6–8 Sep 1996. Boston, MA: Kluwer Law International; 1997: 319–332. 36 refs. ISBN 90–411–0361–9. BE58189.

BE = bioethics accession number   fn. = footnotes   refs. = references

*carriers; communication; *developing countries; directive counseling; evaluation; genetic counseling; *genetic screening; health education; mass media; mass screening; *prenatal diagnosis; *preventive medicine; program descriptions; *thalassemia; *Europe; *Mediterranean Region; Middle East

Chervenak, F.A.; McCullough, L.B. Should sex identification be offered as part of the routine ultrasound examination? *Ultrasound in Obstetrics and Gynecology.* 1996 Nov; 8(5): 293–294. 5 refs. BE58879.
*autonomy; beneficence; disclosure; informed consent; justice; *pregnant women; *prenatal diagnosis; *sex determination; spousal consent; *ultrasonography

Donahue, James. Patenting of human DNA sequences -- implications for prenatal genetic testing. [Note]. *Journal of Family Law.* 1997–1998 Spring; 36(2): 267–283. 127 fn. BE58773.
*DNA sequences; eugenics; genetic counseling; genetic predisposition; genetic research; *genetic screening; genome mapping; indigents; industry; *legal aspects; negligence; *patents; physicians; *prenatal diagnosis; selective abortion; social impact; wrongful life; Patent and Trademark Office; *United States

Durfy, Sharon J.; Page, Andrea; Eng, Barry, et al. Attitudes of high school students toward carrier screening and prenatal diagnosis of cystic fibrosis. *Journal of Genetic Counseling.* 1994 Jun; 3(2): 141–155. 23 refs. BE57379.
*adolescents; *attitudes; *carriers; *cystic fibrosis; disclosure; females; *genetic screening; males; *mass screening; *prenatal diagnosis; reproduction; self concept; social discrimination; *students; survey; uncertainty; voluntary programs; NCHGR-funded publication; *secondary schools; Ontario

Glannon, Walter. Genes, embryos, and future people. *Bioethics.* 1998 Jul; 12(3): 187–211. 36 fn. BE58893.
beginning of life; *beneficence; children; *cryopreservation; *embryo disposition; *embryos; *eugenics; fetal therapy; fetuses; future generations; *gene therapy; *genetic disorders; genetic enhancement; *genetic intervention; *genetic screening; germ cells; *injuries; justice; late-onset disorders; mentally disabled; *moral obligations; *moral policy; pain; parents; personhood; physically disabled; posthumous reproduction; *preimplantation diagnosis; *quality of life; reproduction; reproductive technologies; risks and benefits; self concept; suffering; time factors; value of life; *wrongful life
Testing embryonic cells for genetic abnormalities gives us the capacity to predict whether and to what extent people will exist with disease and disability. Moreover, the freezing of embryos for long periods of time enables us to alter the length of a normal human lifespan. After highlighting the shortcomings of somatic-cell gene therapy and germ-line genetic alteration, I argue that the testing and selective termination of genetically defective embryos is the only medically and morally defensible way to prevent the existence of people with severe disability, pain and suffering that make their lives not worth living for them on the whole. In addition, I consider the possible harmful effects on children born from frozen embryos after the deaths of their biological parents, or when their parents are at an advanced age. I also explore whether embryos have moral status and whether the prospects for disease-preventing genetic alteration can justify long-term cryopreservation of embryos.

Hemminki, Elina; Santalahti, Päivi; Louhiala, Pekka. Ethical conflicts in regulating the start of life. *Perspectives in Biology and Medicine.* 1997 Summer; 40(4): 586–591.

21 refs. BE56604.
abortion on demand; *abortion, induced; allowing to die; *beginning of life; biomedical technologies; congenital disorders; disabled; embryos; eugenics; fetuses; *intensive care units; multiple pregnancy; *newborns; patient care; personhood; prematurity; *prenatal diagnosis; *reproductive technologies; selective abortion; values

Holt, Janet. Screening and the perfect baby. *In:* Frith, Lucy, ed. Ethics and Midwifery: Issues in Contemporary Practice. Boston, MA: Butterworth–Heinemann; 1996: 140–155. 14 refs. ISBN 0–7506–3056–6. BE58637.
attitudes; *congenital disorders; decision making; disabled; economics; eugenics; fetuses; genetic disorders; genetic predisposition; genetic screening; legal aspects; mass screening; nurse midwives; pregnant women; *prenatal diagnosis; public policy; risk; selection for treatment; *selective abortion; sex determination; social discrimination; social impact; teleological ethics; wedge argument; Great Britain

Jan, Sheau–Wen; Chen, Chih–Ping; Huang, Lian–Hua, et al. Attitudes toward maternal serum screening in Chinese women with positive results. *Journal of Genetic Counseling.* 1996 Dec; 5(4): 169–180. 33 refs. BE56329.
amniocentesis; *attitudes; decision making; *Down syndrome; females; *genetic counseling; *genetic screening; knowledge, attitudes, practice; *pregnant women; *prenatal diagnosis; survey; *alpha fetoproteins; *Taiwan

Juengst, Eric T. Prenatal diagnosis and the ethics of uncertainty. [Revised]. *In:* Monagle, John F.; Thomasma, David C., eds. Health Care Ethics: Critical Issues for the 21st Century. Gaithersburg, MD: Aspen Publishers; 1998: 15–28. 57 fn. ISBN 0–8342–0911–X. BE56277.
age factors; amniocentesis; autonomy; chorionic villi sampling; decision making; economics; fetal therapy; fetuses; genetic counseling; genetic predisposition; parents; physician patient relationship; pregnant women; *prenatal diagnosis; prognosis; public health; reproduction; risks and benefits; selection for treatment; selective abortion; sex determination; *uncertainty; United States

Lucassen, Emy. Prenatal genetic testing: the need for legislation. *In:* Doherty, Peter; Sutton, Agneta, eds. Man–Made Man: Ethical and Legal Issues in Genetics. Dublin, Ireland: Open Air; 1997: 98–112. 23 refs. ISBN 1–85182–278–X. BE58299.
amniocentesis; chorionic villi sampling; competence; disclosure; fetuses; genetic disorders; *genetic screening; government regulation; informed consent; *legal aspects; legal liability; physicians; pregnant women; *prenatal diagnosis; risks and benefits; selective abortion; torts; wrongful life; *Great Britain

Milliez, J.; Sureau, C. Pre-implantation diagnosis and the eugenics debate: our responsibility to future generations. *In:* Shenfield, F.; Sureau, C., eds. Ethical Dilemmas in Assisted Reproduction. New York, NY: Parthenon Pub. Group; 1997: 57–66. 26 refs. ISBN 1–85070–916–5. BE57947.
confidentiality; data banks; embryos; epidemiology; *eugenics; fetal therapy; future generations; gene therapy; genetic disorders; germ cells; informed consent; mandatory reporting; methods; *preimplantation diagnosis; risks and benefits; stem cells

Nelson, James Lindemann. The meaning of the act: reflections on the expressive force of reproductive decision making and policies. *Kennedy Institute of Ethics Journal.* 1998 June; 8(2): 165–182. 9 refs. 3 fn. BE58375.
abortion on demand; *congenital disorders; *decision making; *disabled; fetuses; genetic disorders; genetic screening; intention; *motivation; *pregnant women;

BE = bioethics accession number   fn. = footnotes   refs. = references

*prenatal diagnosis; quality of life; reproduction; rights; *selective abortion; social worth; *stigmatization; values; voluntary sterilization; ELSI-funded publication; Buchanan, Allen

Prenatal and preconceptual testing and screening programs provide information on the basis of which people can choose to avoid the birth of children likely to face disabilities. Some disabilities advocates have objected to such programs and to the decisions made within them, on the grounds that measures taken to avoid the birth of children with disabilities have an "expressive force" that conveys messages disrespectful to people with disabilities. Assessing such a claim requires careful attention to general considerations relating meaning, intention, and social practices; it has only begun to receive such attention. Building on work by Allen Buchanan, who has challenged this claim, I further consider the disabilities advocates' objection, ultimately concluding that it is misplaced; neither individual actions nor general practices of this type necessarily express disrespectful messages.

Proud, Jean. Ethical issues concerning ultrasound in pregnancy. *In:* Frith, Lucy, ed. Ethics and Midwifery: Issues in Contemporary Practice. Boston, MA: Butterworth-Heinemann; 1996: 72–85. 54 refs. ISBN 0-7506-3056-6. BE58635.
autonomy; beneficence; congenital disorders; *decision making; *disclosure; fetuses; informed consent; mass screening; moral policy; *nurse midwives; paternalism; patient care; *pregnant women; *prenatal diagnosis; professional autonomy; professional competence; psychological stress; *risks and benefits; selective abortion; truth disclosure; utilitarianism; women's rights; *ultrasonography; Great Britain

Rae, Scott B. Prenatal genetic testing, abortion, and beyond. *In:* Kilner, John F.; Pentz, Rebecca D.; Young, Frank E., eds. Genetic Ethics: Do the Ends Justify the Genes? Grand Rapids, MI: W.B. Eerdmans; 1997: 136–145. 12 fn. ISBN 0-8028-4428-6. BE56721.
*Christian ethics; disabled; embryos; fetal therapy; fetuses; genetic counseling; *genetic disorders; *genetic screening; genome mapping; late-onset disorders; personhood; *preimplantation diagnosis; *prenatal diagnosis; quality of life; *selective abortion; sex determination; uncertainty; value of life; United States

Rothenberg, Karen H. Genetic accountability and pregnant women. *Women's Health Issues.* 1997 Jul–Aug; 7(4): 215–219. 12 refs. BE55732.
*accountability; autonomy; coercion; conflict of interest; contraception; decision making; disabled; economics; eugenics; females; genetic counseling; genetic disorders; *genetic screening; genetic services; government financing; health education; health personnel; incentives; legal aspects; mandatory testing; medical education; obligations to society; *pregnant women; *prenatal diagnosis; public policy; *reproduction; selective abortion; state interest; *voluntary programs; wrongful life; ELSI-funded publication; United States

Saegusa, Asako. Japan okays test-tube baby gene tests. [News]. *Nature.* 1998 Jul 9; 394(6689): 110. BE58865.
*genetic screening; guidelines; in vitro fertilization; *organizational policies; physicians; *preimplantation diagnosis; professional organizations; *Japan; *Japan Society of Obstetrics and Gynecology

Salihu, Hamisu Mohammed. Genetic counselling among Muslims: questions remain unanswered. [Letter]. *Lancet.* 1997 Oct 4; 350(9083): 1035–1036. 2 refs. BE57359.
clergy; fetal development; *genetic counseling; genetic disorders; *genetic screening; *Islamic ethics;

*preimplantation diagnosis; *prenatal diagnosis; *selective abortion; socioeconomic factors; Cameroon; Great Britain

Sapin, Emmanuel. The horizons of fetal medicine and its ethical consequences. *Dolentium Hominum: Church and Health in the World.* 1996; 31(11th Yr., No. 1): 155–158. BE57374.
aborted fetuses; beginning of life; blood transfusions; congenital disorders; counseling; diabetes; drugs; eugenics; *fetal therapy; fetal tissue donation; fetuses; genetic disorders; neural tube defects; parents; pregnant women; prematurity; *prenatal diagnosis; preventive medicine; quality of life; selective abortion; value of life; vitamins

Saxton, Marsha; Anderson, Betsy; Blatt, Robin J.R., et al. Prenatal diagnosis and pregnancy options. *Genetic Resource.* 1991; 6(1): 31–42. 14 refs. Includes a list of resources for pregnant women who receive an abnormal prenatal test result. BE56042.
adoption; *alternatives; childbirth; community services; *congenital disorders; *counseling; *decision making; disabled; Down syndrome; *genetic counseling; genetic disorders; *guidelines; health personnel; parents; patient care; pregnant women; *prenatal diagnosis; psychological stress; referral and consultation; selective abortion; self-help groups; United States

Skupski, Daniel W.; Chervenak, Frank A.; McCullough, Laurence B. Routine obstetric ultrasound examination: a clinical and ethical evaluation. *In:* Chervenak, Frank A.; Kurjak, Asim, eds. Current Perspectives on the Fetus as a Patient. New York, NY: Parthenon Publishing Group; 1996: 203–212. 33 refs. ISBN 1-85070-742-1. BE57645.
alternatives; autonomy; beneficence; congenital disorders; costs and benefits; counseling; disclosure; ethical analysis; evaluation; fetuses; human experimentation; informed consent; justice; *mass screening; morbidity; mortality; physicians; *pregnant women; *prenatal diagnosis; random selection; *risks and benefits; technology assessment; *ultrasonography; Routine Antenatal Diagnostic Imaging with Ultrasound (RADIUS)

Venn–Treloar, Josephine. Nuchal translucency — screening without consent. [Personal view]. *BMJ (British Medical Journal).* 1998 Mar 28; 316(7136): 1027. BE57583.
biomedical research; deception; Down syndrome; *informed consent; pregnant women; *prenatal diagnosis; *ultrasonography; Great Britain

Viljoen, D.; Oosthuizen, C.; van der Westhuizen, S. Patient attitudes to prenatal screening and termination of pregnancy at Groote Schuur Hospital: a two year prospective study. *East African Medical Journal.* 1996 May; 73(5): 327–329. 6 refs. BE55535.
*attitudes; *congenital disorders; genetic counseling; genetic disorders; *pregnant women; *prenatal diagnosis; religion; *selective abortion; socioeconomic factors; survey; Muslims; prospective studies; Groote Schuur Hospital (Cape Town); *South Africa

PRENATAL INJURIES

See also FETUSES

Balsamo, Anne. Public pregnancies and cultural narratives of surveillance. *In: her:* Technologies of the Gendered Body: Reading the Cyborg Women. Durham, NC: Duke University Press; 1996: 80–115, 184–192. 72 fn. ISBN 0-8223-1698-6. BE58522.
biomedical technologies; coercion; cryopreservation; dehumanization; drug abuse; embryos; *females; *feminist

---

BE = bioethics accession number   fn. = footnotes   refs. = references

ethics; fetuses; human body; legal liability; legal rights; literature; minority groups; mothers; obstetrics and gynecology; patient care; *pregnant women; *prenatal injuries; privacy; property rights; *reproduction; *reproductive technologies; *social control; social discrimination; *social dominance; socioeconomic factors; stigmatization; The Handmaid's Tale (Atwood, M.); United States

Blank, Robert H. Mandating outpatient treatment for pregnant substance abusers: attractive but unfeasible. *Politics and the Life Sciences.* 1996 Mar; 15(1): 49–50. 3 refs. Commentary on D. Mathieu, "Mandating treatment for pregnant substance abusers: a compromise," *PLS* 1995 Aug; 14(2): 199–208. BE56021.
     alcohol abuse; autonomy; children; *coercion; community services; criminal law; *drug abuse; government financing; health; indigents; mandatory programs; mother fetus relationship; obligations of society; *outpatient commitment; *pregnant women; *prenatal injuries; preventive medicine; public policy; rehabilitation; resource allocation; rights; smoking; social impact; state interest; treatment refusal; United States

Boling, Patricia. Mandating treatment for pregnant substance abusers is the wrong focus for public discussion. *Politics and the Life Sciences.* 1996 Mar; 15(1): 51–52. 5 refs. 1 fn. Commentary on D. Mathieu, "Mandating treatment for pregnant substance abusers: a compromise," *PLS* 1995 Aug; 14(2): 199–208. BE56022.
     autonomy; blacks; *coercion; community services; disadvantaged; *drug abuse; freedom; health care delivery; health care reform; health education; indigents; legal aspects; obligations of society; *outpatient commitment; *pregnant women; *prenatal injuries; preventive medicine; public policy; social discrimination; stigmatization; United States

Capen, Karen. Mother's rights can't be infringed to protect fetus, Supreme Court's landmark ruling states. *Canadian Medical Association Journal.* 1997 Dec 1; 157(11): 1586–1587. 5 refs. BE57602.
     child abuse; coercion; *drug abuse; fetuses; freedom; *legal aspects; *legal rights; *mandatory programs; mandatory reporting; personhood; physicians; *pregnant women; *prenatal injuries; state interest; Supreme Court decisions; *Canada; *Manitoba; *Winnipeg Child and Family Services v. G.

Capron, Alexander Morgan. Punishing mothers. *Hastings Center Report.* 1998 Jan–Feb; 28(1): 31–33. 6 fn. BE57296.
     attitudes; *child abuse; *childbirth; congenital disorders; *drug abuse; embryo transfer; fetuses; government regulation; *legal liability; mass media; moral obligations; *multiple pregnancy; parents; personhood; physicians; *pregnant women; prematurity; *prenatal injuries; *reproductive technologies; risks and benefits; viability; wrongful death; McCaughey, Bobbi; South Carolina; Whitner v. State
What should society do when a woman, in producing children, exposes them to avoidable risks? That recurring question — which plunges one quickly and deeply into the murky waters of child protection, women's rights, and the far reaches of medical science — has been back on the front pages recently. Two very different stories illustrate how context affects our answer.

Chavkin, Wendy. Mandatory treatment for pregnant substance abusers: irrelevant and dangerous. *Politics and the Life Sciences.* 1996 Mar; 15(1): 53–54. 10 refs. 1 fn. Commentary on D. Mathieu, "Mandating treatment for pregnant substance abusers: a compromise," *PLS* 1995 Aug; 14(2): 199–208. BE56025.
     *coercion; community services; disadvantaged; *drug abuse;

government financing; health care delivery; indigents; obligations of society; *outpatient commitment; *pregnant women; *prenatal injuries; public policy; resource allocation; scarcity; United States

Daniels, Cynthia R. A million (missing) men: a commentary on Mathieu's compromise on pregnancy and substance abuse. *Politics and the Life Sciences.* 1996 Mar; 15(1): 54–56. 13 refs. Commentary on D. Mathieu, "Mandating treatment for pregnant substance abusers: a compromise," *PLS* 1995 Aug; 14(2): 199–208. BE56028.
     accountability; blacks; *coercion; community services; *drug abuse; fathers; health care delivery; health hazards; indigents; legal aspects; obligations of society; obligations to society; *outpatient commitment; politics; *pregnant women; *prenatal injuries; rights; social discrimination; state interest; voluntary programs; United States

Harris, Cathleen M.; Mahowald, Mary B. Women and alcohol abuse. *In:* Shelton, Wayne N.; Edwards, Rem B., eds. Advances in Bioethics. Volume 3: Values, Ethics, and Alcoholism. Greenwich, CT: JAI Press; 1997: 153–170. 69 refs. ISBN 0-7623-0219-4. BE57637.
     accountability; *alcohol abuse; autonomy; *behavior control; *coercion; congenital disorders; criminal law; decision making; disease; *females; *fetuses; indigents; legal aspects; mandatory programs; minority groups; moral obligations; newborns; *patient care; *pregnant women; *prenatal injuries; privacy; psychological stress; public policy; reproduction; rights; self concept; sexuality; social discrimination; socioeconomic factors; state interest; *stigmatization; value of life; women's health services; women's rights; United States

Inciardi, James A.; Surratt, Hilary L.; Saum, Christine A. Prenatal cocaine use and the prosecution of pregnant addicts. *In: their* Cocaine-Exposed Infants: Social, Legal, and Public Health Issues. Thousand Oaks, CA: Sage Publications; 1997: 62–85. References embedded in list at back of book. ISBN 0-8039-7087-0. BE57226.
     alcohol abuse; child abuse; constitutional law; criminal law; death; *drug abuse; due process; equal protection; *fetuses; health facilities; involuntary commitment; killing; *legal aspects; *legal liability; *legal rights; newborns; parents; personhood; *pregnant women; *prenatal injuries; privacy; punishment; state government; state interest; torts; viability; Alaska v. Grubbs; California; Eighth Amendment; Florida; Florida v. Johnson; Fourteenth Amendment; In re Ruiz; Ohio; People v. Stewart; Roe v. Wade; *United States; Webster v. Reproductive Health Services

Macready, Norra. US state rules that a viable fetus is a person. [News]. *BMJ (British Medical Journal).* 1997 Dec 6; 315(7121): 1488. BE57262.
     child abuse; *drug abuse; *fetuses; *legal aspects; legal liability; *personhood; *pregnant women; *prenatal injuries; state government; *viability; *South Carolina; *Whitner, Cornelia

Madden, Robert G. Civil commitment for substance abuse by pregnant women? A view from the front lines. *Politics and the Life Sciences.* 1996 Mar; 15(1): 56–59. 13 refs. 4 fn. Commentary on D. Mathieu, "Mandating treatment for pregnant substance abusers: a compromise," *PLS* 1995 Aug; 14(2): 199–208. BE56033.
     behavior control; children; *coercion; community services; *drug abuse; fathers; goals; health; legal aspects; mandatory programs; *outpatient commitment; patient compliance; *pregnant women; *prenatal injuries; preventive medicine; public policy; rights; treatment refusal; voluntary programs; United States

Mair, Jane. Maternal/foetal conflict: defined or defused? *In:* McLean, Sheila A.M., ed. Contemporary Issues in

---

Law, Medicine and Ethics. Brookfield, VT: Dartmouth; 1996: 79–97. 45 fn. ISBN 1-85521-586-1. BE57791.
autonomy; cesarean section; *coercion; communication; compensation; *drug abuse; *fetuses; freedom; guidelines; health; informed consent; international aspects; judicial action; *legal aspects; *legal liability; legal obligations; *legal rights; moral obligations; newborns; personhood; physicians; *pregnant women; *prenatal injuries; privacy; religion; state interest; torts; *treatment refusal; viability; women's rights; *Great Britain; United States

Mathieu, Deborah. Mandating treatment for pregnant substance abusers: a compromise. *Politics and the Life Sciences.* 1995 Aug; 14(2): 199–208. 93 refs. 24 fn. Commented on in *PLS* 1996 Mar; 15(1): by R.H. Blank, p. 49–50; by P. Boling, p. 51–52; by W. Chavkin, p. 53–54; by C.R. Daniels, p. 54–56; by R.G. Madden, p. 56–59; by J.C. Merrick, p. 59–60; by E.H. Moskowitz, p. 61–63; by E.G. Patterson and A.B. Andrews, p. 64–66; by P. Peretz and J.R. Schroedel, p. 67–69; by R.A. Strickland, p. 70–72; by D.B. Wexler, p. 73–75; and by L.R. Woliver, p. 75–77; with a response by D. Mathieu, p. 77–81. BE56034.
autonomy; children; *coercion; community services; *drug abuse; due process; fetuses; health; health education; indigents; low birth weight; mandatory programs; minority groups; newborns; obligations of society; *outpatient commitment; patient compliance; policy analysis; *pregnant women; *prenatal injuries; preventive medicine; *public policy; rehabilitation; residential facilities; *state interest; uncertainty; voluntary programs; United States

Mathieu, Deborah. Pregnant women in chains? [Response]. *Politics and the Life Sciences.* 1996 Mar; 15(1): 77–81. 8 refs. 9 fn. Response to twelve commentaries by R.H. Blank, p. 40–50; by P. Boling, p. 51–52; by W. Chavkin, p. 53–54; by C.R. Daniels, p. 54–56; by R.G. Madden, p. 56–59; by J.C. Merrick, p. 59–60; by E.H. Moskowitz, p. 61–63; by E.G. Patterson and A.B. Andrews, p. 64–66; by P. Peretz and J.R. Schroedel, p. 67–69; by R.A. Strickland, p. 70–72; by D.B. Wexler, p. 73–75; and by L.R. Woliver, p. 75–77. BE56035.
alcohol abuse; children; *coercion; community services; decision making; *drug abuse; due process; fetal development; fetuses; guidelines; health education; mandatory programs; moral obligations; *outpatient commitment; patient care; *pregnant women; *prenatal injuries; public policy; rights; state interest; stigmatization; voluntary programs; United States

Merchant, Jennifer. Biogenetics, artificial procreation, and public policy in the United States and France. *Technology in Society.* 1996; 18(1): 1–15. 26 fn. BE56595.
abortion, induced; advisory committees; biomedical research; cesarean section; coercion; comparative studies; criminal law; cryopreservation; drug abuse; embryo disposition; *embryo research; federal government; *fetal research; fetal therapy; *fetuses; *genetic research; genetic screening; genetic services; *government financing; in vitro fertilization; indigents; industry; international aspects; judicial action; *legal aspects; legal liability; legal rights; personhood; physicians; *pregnant women; preimplantation diagnosis; prenatal diagnosis; *prenatal injuries; private sector; *public policy; *reproductive technologies; state government; state interest; Supreme Court decisions; torts; treatment refusal; women's health services; women's rights; *wrongful life; Bonbrest v. Kotz; France; Roe v. Wade; *United States

Merrick, Janna C. Pregnancy and substance abuse: education or mandatory treatment? *Politics and the Life Sciences.* 1996 Mar; 15(1): 59–60. 7 refs. 1 fn. Commentary on D. Mathieu, "Mandating treatment for pregnant substance abusers: a compromise," *PLS* 1995

Aug; 14(2): 199–208. BE56036.
alcohol abuse; blacks; children; *coercion; community services; criminal law; *drug abuse; fathers; fetal development; health care delivery; health education; legal aspects; *outpatient commitment; *pregnant women; *prenatal injuries; public policy; selection for treatment; smoking; social discrimination; United States

Moskop, John C.; Smith, Michael L.; De Ville, Kenneth. Ethical and legal aspects of teratogenic medications: the case of isotretinoin. *Journal of Clinical Ethics.* 1997 Fall; 8(3): 264–278. 57 fn. BE57565.
adults; age factors; autonomy; beneficence; *congenital disorders; contraception; *decision making; disclosure; drug industry; *drugs; duty to warn; federal government; *females; fetuses; government regulation; *iatrogenic disease; informed consent; justice; *legal liability; negligence; paternalism; *patient care; patient compliance; *physicians; *pregnant women; *prenatal injuries; refusal to treat; risks and benefits; wrongful death; *wrongful life; dermatology; *Accutane; Food and Drug Administration; Roche Dermatologics; United States

Moskowitz, Ellen H. Can government ever protect fetuses from substance abuse? *Politics and the Life Sciences.* 1996 Mar; 15(1): 61–63. 1 ref. Commentary on D. Mathieu, "Mandating treatment for pregnant substance abusers: a compromise," *PLS* 1995 Aug; 14(2): 199–208. BE56037.
autonomy; community services; *drug abuse; fetuses; freedom; health care delivery; health education; incentives; legal aspects; moral obligations; *outpatient commitment; *pregnant women; *prenatal injuries; privacy; *public policy; rights; state interest; stigmatization; uncertainty; United States

Oberman, Michelle. Women, fetuses, physicians, and the state: pregnancy and medical ethics in the 21st century. *In:* Monagle, John F.; Thomasma, David C., eds. Health Care Ethics: Critical Issues for the 21st Century. Gaithersburg, MD: Aspen Publishers; 1998: 67–78. 33 fn. ISBN 0-8342-0911-X. BE56280.
advance directives; AIDS serodiagnosis; autonomy; biomedical technologies; cesarean section; coercion; confidentiality; drug abuse; fetuses; government regulation; historical aspects; *legal aspects; mandatory testing; obstetrics and gynecology; patient compliance; physician patient relationship; physician's role; *pregnant women; *prenatal injuries; socioeconomic factors; state interest; *treatment refusal; Twentieth Century; United States

Patterson, Elizabeth G.; Andrews, Arlene Bowers. Civil commitment for pregnant substance abusers: is it appropriate and is it enough? *Politics and the Life Sciences.* 1996 Mar; 15(1): 64–66. 12 refs. 2 fn. Commentary on D. Mathieu, "Mandating treatment for pregnant substance abusers: a compromise," *PLS* 1995 Aug; 14(2): 199–208. BE56039.
alternatives; *coercion; community services; *drug abuse; fetuses; freedom; health care delivery; nutrition; obligations of society; *outpatient commitment; *pregnant women; *prenatal injuries; preventive medicine; punishment; rights; risk; United States

Peretz, Paul; Schroedel, Jean Reith. The road not to travel: a comment on Deborah Mathieu's proposal to mandate outpatient treatment for pregnant substance abusers. *Politics and the Life Sciences.* 1996 Mar; 15(1): 67–69. 24 refs. 3 fn. Commentary on D. Mathieu, "Mandating treatment for pregnant substance abusers: a compromise," *PLS* 1995 Aug; 14(2): 199–208. BE56040.
children; *coercion; community services; criminal law; *drug abuse; fetuses; government regulation; health; mandatory programs; mass screening; obligations of society; *outpatient commitment; *pregnant women; *prenatal

---

BE = bioethics accession number   fn. = footnotes   refs. = references

injuries; preventive medicine; privacy; public policy; resource allocation; rights; selection for treatment; social control; state interest; treatment outcome; uncertainty; utilitarianism; United States

Roberts, Dorothy. Killing the Black Body: Race, Reproduction, and the Meaning of Liberty. New York, NY: Pantheon Books; 1997. 373 p. 1,073 fn. ISBN 0–679–44226–X. BE57998.
abortion, induced; adolescents; autonomy; *blacks; *coercion; *contraception; criminal law; deception; dehumanization; *drug abuse; eugenics; family relationship; *females; genetic identity; government financing; historical aspects; indigents; *involuntary sterilization; justice; legal aspects; misconduct; morality; parent child relationship; physicians; *pregnant women; *prenatal injuries; property rights; public policy; rape; *reproduction; *reproductive technologies; risks and benefits; sexuality; *social control; *social discrimination; socioeconomic factors; stigmatization; surrogate mothers; personal identity; slavery; Depo–provera; Medicaid; Nineteenth Century; Norplant; Twentieth Century; United States

Strickland, Ruth Ann. The incivility of mandated drug treatment through civil commitments. *Politics and the Life Sciences.* 1996 Mar; 15(1): 70–72. 29 refs. Commentary on D. Mathieu, "Mandating treatment for pregnant substance abusers: a compromise," *PLS* 1995 Aug; 14(2): 199–208. BE56044.
alcohol abuse; *coercion; community services; *drug abuse; equal protection; fathers; fetuses; health hazards; indigents; legal aspects; mandatory programs; moral obligations; occupational exposure; *outpatient commitment; paternalism; *pregnant women; *prenatal injuries; *public policy; smoking; *social control; social discrimination; uncertainty; United States

Wexler, David B. Some therapeutic jurisprudence implications of the outpatient civil commitment of pregnant substance abusers. *Politics and the Life Sciences.* 1996 Mar; 15(1): 73–75. 13 refs. 1 fn. Commentary on D. Mathieu, "Mandating treatment for pregnant substance abusers: a compromise," *PLS* 1995 Aug; 14(2): 199–208. BE56047.
behavior control; *coercion; community services; contracts; decision making; *drug abuse; due process; legal aspects; mandatory programs; *outpatient commitment; patient compliance; patient participation; *pregnant women; *prenatal injuries; *public policy; treatment refusal; voluntary programs; United States

Wisconsin. Supreme Court. State v. Kruzicki. *North Western Reporter, 2d Series.* 1997 Apr 22 (date of decision). 561: 729–749. BE56745.
*behavior control; coercion; *criminal law; *drug abuse; *fetuses; government regulation; *legal aspects; *personhood; *pregnant women; *prenatal injuries; state government; treatment refusal; *viability; *Angela M.W.; *State v. Kruzicki; Wisconsin

The Wisconsin Supreme Court reversed the appellate court's denial of review of writs under which a pregnant woman sought release from the court's detention and protective custody of her viable fetus. Although she had given birth, the court considered the now moot issue of a child in need of protection or services. When Angela M.W. was thirty-six weeks pregnant, blood tests confirmed drug use in each of the preceding three months and it was decided that her continued use of drugs would cause the fetus serious harm. The county took protective custody of the fetus by a court order requiring that the woman be confined to an inpatient drug treatment facility. After considering the meanings of "child" and "person", the court concluded that under state law a child is a human being born alive, not a fetus.

The dissenting judge argued that the meanings of "child" and "person" include a viable fetus. (KIE abstract)

Woliver, Laura R. Policies to assist pregnant women and children should include a complete assessment of the realities of women's lives. *Politics and the Life Sciences.* 1996 Mar; 15(1): 75–77. 17 refs. Commentary on D. Mathieu, "Mandating treatment for pregnant substance abusers: a compromise," *PLS* 1995 Aug; 14(2): 199–208. BE56049.
autonomy; blacks; *coercion; community services; disadvantaged; domestic violence; *drug abuse; fathers; federal government; females; government financing; health facilities; *outpatient commitment; *pregnant women; *prenatal injuries; *public policy; scarcity; *social control; *social discrimination; United States

Crack–using woman admits guilt in death of her fetus. [News]. *New York Times.* 1997 Dec 3: A33. BE58249.
child abuse; death; *drug abuse; fetuses; *legal liability; *pregnant women; *prenatal injuries; viability; *Garrick, Talitha; *South Carolina

PRIORITIES IN HEALTH CARE *See* RESOURCE ALLOCATION

PRIVILEGED COMMUNICATION *See* CONFIDENTIALITY

PROFESSIONAL ETHICS

See also BIOETHICS, FRAUD AND MISCONDUCT, MEDICAL ETHICS, NURSING ETHICS, PROFESSIONAL PATIENT RELATIONSHIP

Airaksinen, Timo. Professional ethics. *In:* Chadwick, Ruth, ed. Encyclopedia of Applied Ethics, Volume 3. San Diego, CA: Academic Press; 1998: 671–682. 9 refs. ISBN 0–12–227068–1. BE56264.
codes of ethics; ethical theory; goals; interprofessional relations; investigators; medicine; misconduct; moral obligations; paternalism; patients' rights; physician's role; professional autonomy; *professional ethics; rights; science; social control; social dominance; technical expertise; values; virtues; engineering; professional role

Andre, Judith. Speaking truth to employers. *Journal of Clinical Ethics.* 1997 Summer; 8(2): 199–203. 10 fn. BE56354.
clinical ethics committees; communication; *conflict of interest; *conscience; *dissent; *employment; *ethicist's role; *ethicists; ethics consultation; expert testimony; institutional policies; interprofessional relations; mass media; *moral obligations; patient advocacy; physicians; *professional ethics; truth disclosure; *virtues; whistleblowing; courage; *integrity

Badaway, Abdulla A.–B. Ethics in alcohol research and publishing. [Editorial]. *Alcohol and Alcoholism.* 1996 Jan; 31(1): 7–9. 10 refs. BE55753.
*alcohol abuse; *behavioral research; *biomedical research; codes of ethics; conflict of interest; disclosure; *editorial policies; financial support; *investigators; peer review; *professional ethics; scientific misconduct; *self regulation; universities; *journalism

Barnitt, Rosemary. Ethical dilemmas in occupational therapy and physical therapy: a survey of practitioners in the UK National Health Service. *Journal of Medical Ethics.* 1998 Jun; 24(3): 193–199. 32 fn. BE59116.
aged; *allied health personnel; *attitudes; behavior control;

BE = bioethics accession number   fn. = footnotes   refs. = references

comparative studies; dementia; mentally disabled; misconduct; patient care; patient discharge; professional competence; *professional ethics; professional patient relationship; *rehabilitation; resource allocation; survey; treatment outcome; truth disclosure; vulnerable populations; *occupational therapy; *physical therapy; *Great Britain; *National Health Service

OBJECTIVES: To identify ethical dilemmas experienced by occupational and physical therapists working in the UK National Health Service (NHS). To compare ethical contexts, themes and principles across the two groups. DESIGN: A structured questionnaire was circulated to the managers of occupational and physical therapy services in England and Wales. SUBJECTS: The questionnaires were given to 238 occupational and 249 physical therapists who conformed to set criteria. RESULTS: Ethical dilemmas experienced during the previous six months were reported by 118 occupational and 107 physical therapists. The two groups were similar in age, grade, and years of experience. Fifty of the occupational therapy dilemmas occurred in mental health settings but no equivalent setting emerged for physical therapy. Different ethical themes emerged between the two groups, with the most common in occupational therapy being difficult/dangerous behaviour in patients and unprofessional staff behaviour, and for physical therapists resource limitations and treatment effectiveness. No differences were found in the ethical principles used. CONCLUSION: The ethical dilemmas reported by the therapists were primarily concerned with health care ethics, rather than the more dramatic ethics reported in much of the biomedical ethics literature. Differences were found between the two professional groups when ethical contexts and themes were compared but not when ethical principles were compared. This suggests that educators and researchers need to be aware of work settings and the interdisciplinary nature of employment as well as ethical principles held by individual therapists.

Bass, Larry J.; DeMers, Stephen T.; Ogloff, James R.P., et al. Professional Conduct and Discipline in Psychology. Washington, DC; Montgomery, AL: American Psychological Association; Association of State and Provincial Psychology Boards; 1996. 330 p. Includes references. Appendixes include ASPPB and APA codes of conduct and Canadian Code of Ethics for Psychologists. ISBN 1-55798-372-0. BE57075.
*codes of ethics; confidentiality; economics; education; federal government; government regulation; health personnel; human experimentation; informed consent; legal aspects; legal liability; malpractice; *misconduct; professional competence; *professional ethics; professional organizations; professional patient relationship; *psychology; *regulation; self regulation; sexuality; *standards; state government; trends; American Psychological Association; Association of State and Provincial Psychology Boards; Canada; Canadian Psychological Association; United States

Bebeau, M.J.; Holt, S.C. Proceedings of a symposium, "Toward Responsible Research Conduct: The Role of Scientific Societies." [Introduction to a set of five papers and a consensus statement]. *Journal of Dental Research.* 1996 Feb; 75(2): 823-824. 2 refs. Paper presented at the symposium at the annual meeting of the American Association for Dental Research, held in San Antonio, TX, Mar 1995. BE56453.
biomedical research; codes of ethics; *dentistry; *investigators; organizational policies; *professional ethics; *professional organizations; *scientific misconduct; *self regulation; standards; *dental research; professional role; American Association for Dental Research

Bebeau, M.J.; Davis, E.L. Survey of ethical issues in dental research. *Journal of Dental Research.* 1996 Feb; 75(2): 845-855. 10 refs. Paper presented at the symposium, "Toward Responsible Research Conduct: The Role of Scientific Societies," during the annual meeting of the American Association for Dental Research, held in San Antonio, TX, Mar 1995. BE56452.
administrators; *attitudes; authorship; biomedical research; codes of ethics; *dentistry; education; ethics committees; *investigators; *professional ethics; professional organizations; *scientific misconduct; self regulation; standards; survey; *dental research; professional role; *American Association for Dental Research; International Association for Dental Research

Bebeau, Muriel J.; Holt, Stanley C.; American Association for Dental Research. Ethics Committee. The role of the AADR in promoting research integrity: perspectives and consensus statements. *Journal of Dental Research.* 1996 Feb; 75(2): 856-860. 9 refs. BE56454.
biomedical research; *codes of ethics; *dentistry; due process; education; ethics committees; goals; guidelines; *investigators; professional autonomy; *professional ethics; *professional organizations; *scientific misconduct; *self regulation; *standards; *dental research; professional role; *American Association for Dental Research; International Association for Dental Research

Benatar, Solomon R. Editorial ethics. [Personal view]. *BMJ (British Medical Journal).* 1998 Jan 10; 316(7125): 155-156. BE57772.
accountability; biomedical research; communication; *editorial policies; guidelines; investigators; peer review; *professional ethics; time factors; *journalism

Bersoff, D.N. Process and procedures for dealing with misconduct: a necessity or a nightmare? *Journal of Dental Research.* 1996 Feb; 75(2): 836-840. 14 refs. Paper presented at the symposium, "Toward Responsible Research Conduct: The Role of Scientific Societies," during the annual meeting of the American Association for Dental Research, held in San Antonio, TX, Mar 1995. BE56457.
biomedical research; codes of ethics; dentistry; *due process; economics; ethics committees; *investigators; *legal aspects; legal liability; *organizational policies; *professional ethics; *professional organizations; psychology; punishment; *science; *scientific misconduct; *self regulation; dental research; professional role; American Association for Dental Research; American Psychological Association

Berwick, Donald; Hiatt, Howard; Janeway, Penny, et al. An ethical code for everybody in health care. [Editorial]. *BMJ (British Medical Journal).* 1997 Dec 20-27; 315(7123): 1633-1634. 1 ref. BE57554.
administrators; *codes of ethics; confidentiality; economics; *health care; health care delivery; health facilities; health personnel; information dissemination; institutional ethics; interdisciplinary communication; international aspects; managed care programs; moral obligations; physicians; *professional ethics; rights; Great Britain; National Health Service

Betan, Ephi J. Toward a hermeneutic model of ethical decision making in clinical practice. *Ethics and Behavior.* 1997; 7(4): 347-365. 61 refs. BE58666.
autonomy; beneficence; codes of ethics; decision making; education; empirical research; ethical analysis; *health personnel; interprofessional relations; misconduct; *models, theoretical; *professional ethics; professional organizations; professional patient relationship; *psychology; *psychotherapy; self concept; sexuality; suicide; virtues; whistleblowing; American Psychological Association
Documented ethical violations and empirical research

have demonstrated that, despite professional standards and formal training in ethical principles, some psychotherapists engage in unethical behaviors that compromise the welfare of clients. It appears that competing values and interests that emerge in the therapeutic endeavor can interfere with therapists' considerations of ethical standards and their willingness to act ethically. Expanding current models of ethical decision making, this article offers a hermeneutic model that recognizes that in addition to moral reasoning, the context of the therapeutic relationship and the therapist's subjective responses are fundamental considerations in the interpretation and application of ethical interventions. Implications for understanding and training of ethics in psychotherapy in this broader context are explored.

Bird, Stephanie J.; Housman, David E. Conducting and reporting research. *Professional Ethics.* 1995 Spring–Summer; 4(3–4): 127–154. 4 fn. References embedded in back-of-issue bibliography. BE55692.
administrators; authorship; *biomedical research; contracts; financial support; information dissemination; interprofessional relations; *investigators; mass media; methods; obligations to society; peer review; *professional ethics; property rights; research design; *science; scientific misconduct; standards; students; United States

Bram, Anthony D. The physically ill or dying psychotherapist: a review of ethical and clinical considerations. *Psychotherapy.* 1995 Winter; 32(4): 568–580. 34 refs. BE56023.
attitudes to death; beneficence; codes of ethics; confidentiality; *disclosure; emotions; empirical research; guidelines; *health; *health personnel; patient care; patient transfer; patients; professional competence; *professional ethics; professional organizations; *professional patient relationship; psychology; *psychotherapy; referral and consultation; risks and benefits; *terminally ill; patient abandonment; patient care planning; professional impairment; *seriously ill; American Psychological Association

Brett, Allan S.; Raymond, James I.; Saunders, Donald E., et al. An ethics discussion series for hospital administrators. *HEC (HealthCare Ethics Committee) Forum.* 1998 Jun; 10(2): 177–185. 13 refs. BE59065.
*administrators; *communication; ethicists; evaluation; *hospitals; *institutional ethics; *institutional policies; *interprofessional relations; *professional ethics; *program descriptions; Richland Memorial Hospital (Columbia, SC); South Carolina; University of South Carolina

Brodeur, Dennis. Health care institutional ethics: broader than clinical ethics. [Revised]. *In:* Monagle, John F.; Thomasma, David C., eds. Health Care Ethics: Critical Issues for the 21st Century. Gaithersburg, MD: Aspen Publishers; 1998: 497–504. 16 fn. ISBN 0-8342-0911-X. BE56289.
*administrators; common good; economics; employment; goals; *health facilities; health personnel; indigents; *institutional ethics; institutional policies; organization and administration; *professional ethics; resource allocation; rights; social discrimination; standards; *values; business ethics; dignity; nonprofit health facilities; trustees; United States

Camenisch, P.F. The moral foundations of scientific ethics and responsibility. *Journal of Dental Research.* 1996 Feb; 75(2): 825–831. 16 refs. Paper presented at the symposium, "Toward Responsible Research Conduct: The Role of Scientific Societies," during the annual meeting of the American Association for Dental

Research, held in San Antonio, TX, Mar 1995. BE56459.
biomedical research; codes of ethics; common good; conflict of interest; *dentistry; disclosure; goals; information dissemination; *investigators; moral obligations; obligations to society; organizational policies; professional autonomy; professional competence; *professional ethics; *professional organizations; science; *scientific misconduct; *self regulation; trust; values; *dental research; professional role; *American Association for Dental Research; *International Association for Dental Research

Coughlin, Steven S.; Soskolne, Colin L.; Goodman, Kenneth W. Case Studies in Public Health Ethics. Washington, DC: American Public Health Association; 1997. 180 p. Includes references and instructor's guide. ISBN 0-87553-232-2. BE58580.
AIDS serodiagnosis; authorship; biomedical research; cancer; *case studies; confidentiality; conflict of interest; cultural pluralism; disclosure; drug abuse; epidemiology; ethical analysis; ethical theory; faculty; financial support; genetic screening; health hazards; HIV seropositivity; human experimentation; information dissemination; informed consent; international aspects; *investigators; law enforcement; privacy; *professional ethics; property rights; *public health; random selection; research design; research ethics committees; resource allocation; scientific misconduct; social discrimination; socioeconomic factors; vulnerable populations; United States

Coughlin, Steven S. Ethics in Epidemiology and Public Health Practice: Collected Works. Columbus, GA: Quill Publications; 1997. 232 p. Includes references. ISBN 0-9661520-0-X. BE58542.
American Indians; autonomy; beneficence; biomedical research; cancer; case studies; confidentiality; control groups; curriculum; ecology; education; *epidemiology; ethical theory; ethics committees; federal government; females; government regulation; health hazards; health personnel; HIV seropositivity; human experimentation; informed consent; international aspects; investigators; justice; *preventive medicine; *professional ethics; professional organizations; *public health; random selection; research design; research ethics committees; risks and benefits; scientific misconduct; selection of subjects; self regulation; socioeconomic factors; violence; vulnerable populations; professional role; Tuskegee Syphilis Study; United States

Crellin, John K. Alternative medicine: ethical challenges for the profession of pharmacy. *In:* Humber, James M.; Almeder, Robert F., eds. Alternative Medicine and Ethics. Totowa, NJ: Humana Press; 1998: 195–212. 26 fn. ISBN 0-89603-440-2. BE57208.
*alternative therapies; attitudes; autonomy; codes of ethics; conflict of interest; counseling; *drugs; paternalism; patient care; patients; *pharmacists; *professional ethics; professional organizations; risks and benefits; homeopathy; self care; American Pharmaceutical Association; Great Britain; North America; Royal Pharmaceutical Society of Great Britain

Crigger, Nancy J. What we owe the author: rethinking editorial peer review. *Nursing Ethics.* 1998 Sep; 5(5): 451–458. 20 refs. BE58907.
authorship; beneficence; biomedical research; codes of ethics; conflict of interest; editorial policies; interprofessional relations; moral obligations; nursing ethics; *nursing research; *peer review; *professional ethics; rights

Downie, R.S. Professional ethics and business ethics. *In:* McLean, Sheila A.M., ed. Contemporary Issues in Law, Medicine and Ethics. Brookfield, VT: Dartmouth; 1996: 1–14. 14 fn. ISBN 1-85521-586-1. BE57787.
administrators; beneficence; confidentiality; decision making; disadvantaged; *economics; health care; *health care

---

BE = bioethics accession number   fn. = footnotes   refs. = references

delivery; justice; *medical ethics; paternalism; patient advocacy; peer review; physician patient relationship; *professional ethics; *public policy; quality of health care; social dominance; trust; *business ethics; integrity; quality control; Great Britain; National Health Service

Dracy, David L.; Yutrzenka, Barbara A. Responses of direct–care paraprofessional mental health staff to hypothetical ethics violations. *Psychiatric Services.* 1997 Sep; 48(9): 1160–1163. 8 refs. BE55717.
  *allied health personnel; decision making; education; institutionalized persons; *interprofessional relations; *knowledge, attitudes, practice; *mental institutions; mentally ill; mentally retarded; *misconduct; patient care; *professional ethics; survey; *whistleblowing; Midwestern United States

Elliott, Deni. Researchers as professionals, professionals as researchers: a context for laboratory research ethics. *Professional Ethics.* 1995 Spring–Summer; 4(3–4): 5–16. 8 fn. References embedded in back-of-issue bibliography. BE55686.
  biomedical research; common good; conflict of interest; consensus; deception; goals; health hazards; injuries; *investigators; *laboratories; moral obligations; *morality; obligations to society; *professional ethics; research subjects; *science; self regulation; values; community consent; journalism; rationality

Fealy, Gerard M. Professional caring: the moral dimension. *Journal of Advanced Nursing.* 1995 Dec; 22(6): 1135–1140. 18 refs. BE56204.
  accountability; autonomy; *caring; codes of ethics; communitarianism; ethical theory; health personnel; justice; moral obligations; morality; *nurse patient relationship; nursing ethics; patient care; *professional ethics; *professional patient relationship; teleological ethics; virtues

Feldstein, Bruce D.; Ogle, Richard D. Satisfaction, managed ethics, and the duty to design. *HEC (HealthCare Ethics Committee) Forum.* 1997 Dec; 9(4): 333–354. 10 refs. BE58085.
  administrators; clinical ethics committees; decision making; economics; emergency care; goals; *health care delivery; *institutional ethics; institutional policies; interprofessional relations; *managed care programs; moral obligations; *organization and administration; *patient care team; *professional ethics; professional patient relationship; *quality of health care; time factors; *institutional ethics; myocardial infarction; thrombolytic therapy; Kaiser–Permanente Medical Center (Santa Clara, CA)
Healthcare ethics committee (HEC) members and healthcare professionals at all levels are facing a crisis in ethics as a result of the pervasive organizational, economic, scientific, and technological changes in medicine and healthcare. Our current approach to medical ethics does not effectively address the fundamental challenge this crisis poses: to provide ethically principled care to the satisfaction of all stakeholders. In this paper we present a new approach that extends the scope and understanding of ethics by building links between the disciplines of ethics, management, and design. We call such an approach "Managed Ethics and Design." After outlining the main tenets of this approach, we illustrate its application with a design-based quality improvement project at the Kaiser–Permanente Medical Center at Santa Clara, California, that successfully enhanced delivery of thrombolytic drugs to treat patients arriving with acute MI. We conclude that in order to provide and ensure ethically principled care to the satisfaction of all stakeholders, we have a "duty to design," a duty to improve, create and innovate new practices, processes, standards, and understandings of healthcare. Good

design can lead to new possibilities that will enable us to achieve higher, rather than lower, ethical standards. In the current era of organizational medicine and managed care, the duty to design is an inescapable moral imperative.

Foster, George E.; Bailey, R. Norman; Werner, D. Leonard, et al. Code of ethics: to keep the visual welfare of the patient uppermost at all times. *Journal of the American Optometric Association.* 1994 Jun; 65(6): 389, 391–395, 397–398+. 16 refs. Set of commentaries marking the 50th anniversary of the adoption of the American Optometric Association's Code of Ethics in 1944. BE56059.
  codes of ethics; confidentiality; education; eye diseases; *health personnel; indigents; interprofessional relations; medical records; patient care; professional competence; *professional ethics; professional organizations; referral and consultation; *standards; continuing education; *optometry; American Optometric Association; United States

Frankel, M.S. Developing ethical standards for responsible research: why? form? functions? process? outcomes? *Journal of Dental Research.* 1996 Feb; 75(2): 832–835. 6 refs. Paper presented at the symposium, "Toward Responsible Research Conduct: The Role of Scientific Societies," during the annual meeting of the American Association for Dental Research, held in San Antonio, TX, Mar 1995. BE56461.
  accountability; biomedical research; *codes of ethics; decision making; *dentistry; education; *investigators; professional autonomy; *professional ethics; *professional organizations; *science; *scientific misconduct; *self regulation; *standards; dental research; American Association for Dental Research

Garrett, Thomas M.; Baillie, Harold W.; Garrett, Rosellen M. Health Care Ethics: Principles and Problems. Third Edition. Upper Saddle River, NJ: Prentice Hall; 1998. 344 p. Bibliography: p. 323–338. ISBN 0-13-856634-8. BE56097.
  abortion, induced; active euthanasia; advance directives; allowing to die; assisted suicide; autonomy; beneficence; *bioethical issues; brain death; case studies; clinical ethics committees; cloning; confidentiality; determination of death; disclosure; fetal research; fetuses; gene therapy; genetic research; health care; *health personnel; hospitals; human experimentation; informed consent; institutional ethics; legal aspects; mass screening; moral obligations; organ donation; organ transplantation; paternalism; pregnant women; *professional ethics; professional organizations; quality of health care; reproductive technologies; resource allocation; resuscitation orders; selection for treatment; suicide; third party consent; treatment refusal; truth disclosure; withholding treatment

Goldstein, Barry; Royal, Michael C.; Veatch, Robert M. Safety of an extemporaneously prepared injection. [Case study and commentaries]. *American Journal of Health–System Pharmacy.* 1996 Feb 15; 53(4): 414–417. 1 ref. BE56207.
  *administrators; *alternatives; case studies; *costs and benefits; dissent; *drugs; economics; *hospitals; *interprofessional relations; moral policy; patient care; *pharmacists; *professional ethics; resource allocation; *risk; *risks and benefits; technical expertise; *morphine

Haffner, Alden N. The moral dignity of our profession. [Editorial]. *Journal of the American Optometric Association.* 1994 Jun; 65(6): 384. BE56226.
  codes of ethics; *health personnel; *professional ethics; professional organizations; *optometry; American Optometric Association

---

Herwaldt, Loreen A. Ethical aspects of infection control. *Infection Control and Hospital Epidemiology.* 1996 Feb; 17(2): 108–113. 26 refs. BE56228.

autonomy; *communicable diseases; confidentiality; decision making; disclosure; economics; *epidemiology; guidelines; *health personnel; hepatitis; HIV seropositivity; *hospitals; *institutional policies; interprofessional relations; misconduct; patient care; patients; professional autonomy; *professional ethics; public health; quarantine; *infection control

Holm, Søren. Ethical Problems in Clinical Practice -- A Study of the Ethical Reasoning of Health Care Professionals. Copenhagen: University of Copenhagen; 1996. 258 p. Includes references. Dissertation, Ph.D., University of Copenhagen, Dept. of Medical Philosophy and Clinical Theory. BE57888.

*bioethics; caring; case studies; *clinical ethics; *decision making; disclosure; education; empirical research; ethical analysis; ethical theory; health care delivery; *health personnel; hospitals; interprofessional relations; medical ethics; models, theoretical; *moral development; negligence; nurses; nursing ethics; philosophy; physicians; *professional ethics; science; sociology of medicine; survey; whistleblowing; medical errors; *qualitative research; *Denmark

Hunt, Geoffrey. The human condition of the professional: discretion and accountability. *Nursing Ethics.* 1997 Nov; 4(6): 519–526. 6 refs. BE57416.

*accountability; *conscience; *decision making; *misconduct; nursing ethics; *professional ethics; punishment; resuscitation

Kaiser, Jocelyn. Furor over company deal roils AMA. [News]. *Science.* 1997 Oct 3; 278(5335): 26. BE56574.

administrators; *conflict of interest; contracts; guidelines; *industry; *medical devices; *organizational policies; *physicians; professional organizations; self regulation; *business ethics; *American Medical Association; Sunbeam Corporation

Khushf, George. Administrative and organizational ethics. *HEC (HealthCare Ethics Committee) Forum.* 1997 Dec; 9(4): 299–309. 35 refs. BE58087.

accountability; *administrators; bioethics; *clinical ethics committees; decision making; goals; guidelines; *health facilities; *hospitals; *institutional ethics; institutional policies; managed care programs; *organization and administration; *professional ethics; regulation; religious hospitals; values; *institutional ethics; professional role; United States

Khushf, George. The scope of organizational ethics: editor's introduction. *HEC (HealthCare Ethics Committee) Forum.* 1998 Jun; 10(2): 127–135. 13 refs. 4 fn. BE59080.

clinical ethics; conflict of interest; economics; ethical theory; ethics consultation; health care delivery; *health facilities; incentives; *institutional ethics; organization and administration; professional ethics; professional organizations; standards; business ethics; evidence-based medicine; quality assurance; utilization review; American Society for Bioethics and Humanities; United States

Korenman, Stanley G.; Berk, Richard; Wenger, Neil S., et al. Evaluation of the research norms of scientists and administrators responsible for academic research integrity. *JAMA.* 1998 Jan 7; 279(1): 41–47. 28 refs. BE57816.

*administrators; *attitudes; authorship; biomedical research; comparative studies; *conflict of interest; financial support; fraud; industry; *information dissemination; interprofessional relations; *investigators; *professional ethics; punishment;

*scientific misconduct; survey; universities; *research ethics; United States

CONTEXT: The professional integrity of scientists is important to society as a whole and particularly to disciplines such as medicine that depend heavily on scientific advances for their progress. OBJECTIVE: To characterize the professional norms of active scientists and compare them with those of individuals with institutional responsibility for the conduct of research. DESIGN: A mailed survey consisting of 12 scenarios in 4 domains of research ethics. Respondents were asked whether an act was unethical and, if so, the degree to which they considered it unethical and to select responses and punishments for the act. PARTICIPANTS: A total of 924 National Science Foundation research grantees in 1993 or 1994 in molecular or cellular biology and 140 representatives from the researchers' institutions to the US Department of Health and Human Services Office of Research Integrity. MAIN OUTCOME MEASURES: Percentage of respondents considering an act unethical and the mean malfeasance rating on a scale of 1 to 10. RESULTS: A total of 606 research grantees and 91 institutional representatives responded to the survey (response rate of 69% of those who could be contacted). Respondents reported a hierarchy of unethical research behaviors. The mean malfeasance rating was unrelated to the characteristics of the investigator performing the hypothetical act or to its consequences. Fabrication, falsification, and plagiarism received malfeasance ratings higher than 8.6, and virtually all thought they were unethical. Deliberately misleading statements about a paper or failure to give proper attribution received ratings between 7 and 8. Sloppiness, oversights, conflicts of interest, and failure to share were less serious still, receiving malfeasance ratings between 5 and 6. Institutional representatives proposed more and different interventions and punishments than the scientists. CONCLUSIONS: Surveyed scientists and institutional representatives had strong and similar norms of professional behavior, but differed in their approaches to an unethical act.

Kuehnle, Kathryn. Ethics and the forensic expert: a case study of child custody involving allegations of child sexual abuse. *Ethics and Behavior.* 1998; 8(1): 1–18. 53 refs. BE58914.

age factors; case studies; *child abuse; children; *expert testimony; *forensic psychiatry; guidelines; *health personnel; marital relationship; parents; *professional competence; *professional ethics; professional family relationship; psychology; *sex offenses

Psychologists who participate as forensic evaluators in custody and visitation cases involving allegations of child sexual abuse must possess advanced assessment skills and a thorough knowledge of child development, child sexual abuse, and child interviewing techniques. This case study illustrates the types of problems that are inevitable when psychologists violate the boundaries of their role as an independent evaluator and fail to uphold their ethical obligation to be knowledgeable and competent in the area in which they profess expertise.

Kuhse, Helga; Singer, Peter; Rickard, Maurice, et al. Partial and impartial ethical reasoning in health care professionals. *Journal of Medical Ethics.* 1997 Aug; 23(4): 226–232. 28 fn. BE55914.

caring; *ethical analysis; family relationship; *females; justice; *males; *moral development; *nurses; *physicians; *professional ethics; selection for treatment; social worth; survey; qualitative research; Australia; Gilligan, Carol; Kohlberg, Lawrence; New South Wales; Victoria

---

BE = bioethics accession number   fn. = footnotes   refs. = references

OBJECTIVES: To determine the relationship between ethical reasoning and gender and occupation among a group of male and female nurses and doctors. DESIGN: Partialist and impartialist forms of ethical reasoning were defined and singled out as being central to the difference between what is known as the "care" moral orientation (Gilligan) and the "justice" orientation (Kohlberg). A structured questionnaire based on four hypothetical moral dilemmas involving combinations of (health care) professional, non-professional, life-threatening and non–life-threatening situations, was piloted and then mailed to a randomly selected sample of doctors and nurses. SETTING: 400 doctors from Victoria, and 200 doctors and 400 nurses from New South Wales. RESULTS: 178 doctors and 122 nurses returned completed questionnaires. 115 doctors were male, 61 female; 50 nurses were male and 72 were female. It was hypothesised that there would be an association between feminine subjects and partialist reasoning and masculine subjects and impartialist reasoning. It was also hypothesised that nurses would adopt a partialist approach to reasoning and doctors an impartialist approach. No relationship between any of these variables was observed.

Lewis, Marcia A.; Tamparo, Carol D. Medical Law, Ethics, and Bioethics for Ambulatory Care. Fourth Edition. Philadelphia, PA: F.A. Davis; 1998. 295 p. Includes references and discussion questions. Appendix 1: Codes of ethics; Appendix 2: Sample documents for choices about health care, life, and death. ISBN 0-8036-0348-7. BE57279.
   abortion, induced; advance directives; AIDS; *allied health personnel; assisted suicide; *bioethical issues; case studies; codes of ethics; confidentiality; cultural pluralism; decision making; drugs; *employment; euthanasia; fetuses; genetic services; government regulation; health care delivery; health facilities; informed consent; interprofessional relations; law; *legal aspects; *legal liability; *legal obligations; malpractice; mandatory reporting; medical fees; medical records; negligence; *organization and administration; *patient care; *professional ethics; professional patient relationship; reproductive technologies; resource allocation; standards; terminal care; third party consent; *ambulatory care; United States

McDaniel, Charlotte. Development and psychometric properties of the Ethics Environment Questionnaire. *Medical Care.* 1997 Sep; 35(9): 901–914. 32 refs. BE59071.
   accountability; *administrators; *attitudes; *evaluation; *health personnel; *health services research; *hospitals; *institutional ethics; institutional policies; misconduct; organization and administration; *professional ethics; *survey; whistleblowing; *questionnaires

Mandel, I.D. On being a scientist in a rapidly changing world. *Journal of Dental Research.* 1996 Feb; 75(2): 841–844. 18 refs. Paper presented at the symposium, "Toward Responsible Research Conduct: The Role of Scientific Societies," during the annual meeting of the American Association for Dental Research, held in San Antonio, TX, Mar 1995. BE56471.
   animal experimentation; biological warfare; *biomedical research; dentistry; economics; entrepreneurship; federal government; goals; government regulation; health hazards; *historical aspects; industry; *investigators; microbiology; political activity; *professional ethics; recombinant DNA research; research ethics committees; *science; scientific misconduct; self regulation; trends; universities; values; dental research; Twentieth Century; United States

Martin, Judith; Stent, Gunther S. Bioetiquette. *Perspectives in Biology and Medicine.* 1998 Winter; 41(2):

267–281. 11 refs. BE59029.
   *authorship; *biomedical research; ethics; guidelines; historical aspects; *information dissemination; *interprofessional relations; *investigators; law; *medical etiquette; morality; *peer review; *professional ethics; regulation; *science; scientific misconduct; smoking; *social interaction

Peterson, Andrew M.; Schwarz, Lewis R.; Veatch, Robert M. Asking a pharmacist to resign for making an error. [Case study and commentaries]. *American Journal of Health–System Pharmacy.* 1996 Apr 1; 53(7): 760–763. BE55768.
   *administrators; case studies; death; drugs; *hospitals; institutional policies; interprofessional relations; lawyers; negligence; obligations to society; organization and administration; *pharmacists; professional competence; *professional ethics; *punishment; terminally ill; virtues; culpability; *medical errors

Plant, Martin; Plant, Moira; Vernon, Bryan. Ethics, funding and alcohol research. *Alcohol and Alcoholism.* 1996 Jan; 31(1): 17–25. 36 refs. BE55770.
   *alcohol abuse; *behavioral research; *biomedical research; codes of ethics; *conflict of interest; disclosure; economics; editorial policies; *financial support; government financing; guidelines; industry; information dissemination; *investigators; peer review; *professional ethics; science; scientific misconduct; *self regulation; social sciences; universities; values; whistleblowing

Poikonen, John; Haupt, Bridget A.; Veatch, Robert M. Preferential service for a powerful physician –– Scenario; Position 1: pharmacist should serve physician immediately; Position 2: pharmacist should make physician wait; Analysis and commentary. *American Journal of Health–System Pharmacy.* 1996 Nov 1; 53(21): 2614–2618. 5 refs. BE58106.
   case studies; codes of ethics; communication; drugs; employment; *interprofessional relations; justice; medical etiquette; moral obligations; patient advocacy; patient care; *pharmacists; *physicians; *professional ethics; *social dominance; time factors; utilitarianism

Prayle, David; Brazier, Margaret. Supply of medicines: paternalism, autonomy and reality. *Journal of Medical Ethics.* 1998 Apr; 24(2): 93–98. 30 fn. BE58081.
   advertising; *autonomy; beneficence; counseling; drug industry; *drugs; economics; gatekeeping; *government regulation; information dissemination; injuries; legal liability; legal obligations; *paternalism; patients; *pharmacists; *professional ethics; *public policy; risks and benefits; *professional role; self care; European Community Directive; *Great Britain; Medicines Act 1968 (Great Britain); Medicines Control Agency (Great Britain); National Health Service
Radical changes are taking place in the United Kingdom in relation to the classification of, and access to, medicines. More and more medicines are being made available over the counter both in local pharmacies and in supermarkets. The provision of more open access to medicines may be hailed as a triumph for patient autonomy. This paper examines whether such a claim is real or illusory. It explores the ethical and legal implications of deregulating medicines. Do patients benefit? What is the impact on pharmacists? Are the true beneficiaries of change largely the pharmaceutical industries?

Ross, Lena B.; Roy, Manisha, eds. Cast the First Stone: Ethics in Analytic Practice. Wilmette, IL: Chiron Publications; 1995. 146 p. Includes references. ISBN 0-933029-89-6. BE58319.
   emotions; females; *health personnel; love; males;

BE = bioethics accession number   fn. = footnotes   refs. = references

*misconduct; morality; *professional ethics; *professional patient relationship; psychology; *psychotherapy; self concept; self regulation; *sexuality; values; Jung, Carl

Seiden, Dena J. Ethics for hospital administrators. *Hospital and Health Services Administration.* 1983 Mar–Apr; 28(2): 81–89. 1 fn. BE57499.
> *administrators; case studies; economics; *hospitals; indigents; institutional ethics; moral obligations; patient admission; *professional ethics; refusal to treat; resource allocation; professional role

Spencer, Edward M. A new role for institutional ethics committees: organizational ethics. *Journal of Clinical Ethics.* 1997 Winter; 8(4): 372–376. 12 fn. BE57614.
> administrators; *clinical ethics committees; codes of ethics; committee membership; economics; ethicist's role; *health facilities; *institutional ethics; managed care programs; moral obligations; *organization and administration; *professional ethics; proprietary health facilities; regulation; *standards; business ethics; *institutional ethics; *Joint Commission for Accreditation of Healthcare Organizations

New methods for financing and managing healthcare organizations have caused concerns regarding how these changes will affect the ethics of the care of patients. To address these concerns, the JCAHO has, for the first time, promulgated a standard requiring that each HCO develop and operate under a code of organizational ethics. This standard is now a part of the requirements that JCAHO will consider in its accreditation of HCOs. Development of the required code is mandatory for JCAHO subscribers and will, by necessity, need to be addressed by each institution. An IEC is the proper forum for undertaking this work.

Weil, Vivian; Arzbaecher, Robert. Ethics and relationships in laboratories and research communities. *Professional Ethics.* 1995 Spring–Summer; 4(3–4): 83–125. 17 fn. BE55673.
> accountability; administrators; authorship; *biomedical research; *case studies; communication; confidentiality; conflict of interest; deception; *faculty; females; financial support; goals; *interprofessional relations; *investigators; *laboratories; minority groups; organization and administration; peer review; professional autonomy; *professional ethics; property rights; *science; *scientific misconduct; self regulation; social control; social dominance; standards; *students; trust; values; Gallo, Robert; National Institutes of Health; Popovic, Mikulas; United States

Werhane, Patricia; Doering, Jeffrey. Conflicts of interest and conflicts of commitment. *Professional Ethics.* 1995 Spring–Summer; 4(3–4): 47–81. 4 fn. BE55672.
> accountability; administrators; *biomedical research; case studies; codes of ethics; *conflict of interest; disclosure; editorial policies; financial support; genome mapping; industry; information dissemination; institutional policies; interprofessional relations; *investigators; patents; *professional ethics; professional organizations; property rights; research subjects; *scientific misconduct; *self regulation; standards; trust; universities

Whitman, Jeffrey P. Reclaiming the medical profession: the military profession as a model. *Professional Ethics.* 1995 Spring; 4(1): 3–22. 32 fn. BE55796.
> conflict of interest; conscience; *economics; entrepreneurship; *goals; *health care reform; killing; malpractice; *medical ethics; *medicine; *metaphor; *military personnel; misconduct; *moral obligations; morality; organizational policies; patient advocacy; *physician's role; *physicians; *professional autonomy; professional competence; *professional ethics; professional organizations; public opinion; remuneration; *resource allocation; *self regulation; trust; virtues; *war; *professional role; American Medical Association; United States

Wilson, Donna M. Administrative decision making in response to sudden health care agency funding reductions: is there a role for ethics? *Nursing Ethics.* 1998 Jul; 5(4): 319–329. 51 refs. BE58871.
> *administrators; *decision making; *economics; employment; *financial support; government financing; health care delivery; health facilities; institutional ethics; *organization and administration; *professional ethics; *public hospitals; resource allocation; survey; *Alberta

Worthley, John Abbott. The Ethics of the Ordinary in Healthcare: Concepts and Cases. Chicago, IL: Health Administration Press; 1997. 332 p. Includes references. ISBN 1-56793-056-5. BE57077.
> *accountability; *administrators; bioethical issues; bioethics; case studies; codes of ethics; decision making; ethical analysis; *health care delivery; *health facilities; health insurance; *health personnel; hospitals; institutional ethics; interprofessional relations; misconduct; moral obligations; patient admission; *professional ethics; professional organizations; regulation; resource allocation; social dominance; standards; values; whistleblowing; microethics; American College of Healthcare Executives; American Hospital Association; United States

PROFESSIONAL ETHICS/CODES OF ETHICS

American Occupational Therapy Association (AOTA). Commission on Standards and Ethics. 1996 Occupational Therapy Code of Ethics Reference Guide. Bethesda, MD: American Occupational Therapy Association; 1996 Oct. Includes references. ISBN 1-56900-059-X. BE56140.
> *codes of ethics; confidentiality; contracts; employment; health personnel; interprofessional relations; managed care programs; misconduct; professional competence; *professional ethics; professional organizations; regulation; standards; whistleblowing; *occupational therapy; American Occupational Therapy Association

Bailey, R. Norman. The history of ethics in the American Optometric Association 1898–1994. *Journal of the American Optometric Association.* 1994 Jun; 65(6): 427–444. 54 refs. BE55783.
> advertising; *codes of ethics; economics; ethics committees; eye diseases; government regulation; *health personnel; *historical aspects; interprofessional relations; legal aspects; medical devices; medical fees; patents; patient care; *professional ethics; *professional organizations; professional patient relationship; referral and consultation; standards; state government; *optometry; American Association of Opticians; *American Optometric Association; Nineteenth Century; *Twentieth Century; United States

Commission on Rehabilitation Counselor Certification. Code of professional ethics for certified rehabilitation counselors and CRCC guidelines and procedures for processing complaints. *In:* Maki, Dennis R.; Riggar, T.F., eds. Rehabilitation Counseling: Profession and Practice. New York, NY: Springer Publishing; 1997: Appendix D, 300–321. Adopted also by the American Rehabilitation Counseling Association, the National Rehabilitation Counseling Association, and the National Council on Rehabilitation Education. ISBN 0-8261-9510-5. BE58437.
> *codes of ethics; confidentiality; *counseling; disabled; due process; *health personnel; interprofessional relations; misconduct; professional competence; *professional ethics; professional organizations; professional patient relationship; *rehabilitation; self regulation; standards; whistleblowing; *Commission on Rehabilitation Counselor Certification

Goodman, Kenneth W. Codes of ethics in occupational

and environmental health. [Editorial]. *Journal of Occupational and Environmental Medicine.* 1996 Sep; 38(9): 882–883. 6 refs. BE57523.
    *codes of ethics; evaluation; *occupational medicine; *professional ethics; professional organizations; values; professional role; International Commission on Occupational Health

Hurwitz, Brian; Richardson, Ruth. Swearing to care: the resurgence in medical oaths. *BMJ (British Medical Journal).* 1997 Dec 20–27; 315(7123): 1671–1674. 27 refs. Includes the text of a draft revision of the Hippocratic Oath by the British Medical Association on behalf of the World Medical Association. BE57652.
    ancient history; *codes of ethics; conflict of interest; economics; *health personnel; historical aspects; international aspects; *medical ethics; medical schools; moral obligations; patient advocacy; patient care team; *physicians; *professional ethics; professional organizations; trends; virtues; British Medical Association; Declaration of Geneva; General Medical Council (Great Britain); Great Britain; *Hippocratic Oath; Twentieth Century; United States; World Medical Association

Institute of Health Services Management (Great Britain). Code of professional practice of the Institute of Health Services Management. *Nursing Ethics.* 1998 Jan; 5(1): 75–77. Reprinted with permission of the Institute. BE58746.
    accountability; *administrators; *codes of ethics; confidentiality; gifts; health facilities; patients' rights; professional competence; *professional ethics; quality of health care; Great Britain; *Institute of Health Services Management (Great Britain); National Health Service

Pritchard, Jane. Codes of ethics. *In:* Chadwick, Ruth, ed. Encyclopedia of Applied Ethics, Volume 1. San Diego, CA: Academic Press; 1998: 527–533. 7 refs. ISBN 0–12–227066–5. BE56373.
    *codes of ethics; ethics; international aspects; medical ethics; nursing ethics; *professional ethics; review; risks and benefits

Royal Pharmaceutical Society of Great Britain. Medicines, Ethics and Practice: A Guide for Pharmacists. Number 17. London: The Society; 1996 Oct. 124 p. ISBN 0–85369–377–3. BE56092.
    advertising; *codes of ethics; computers; confidentiality; continuing education; contraception; drug abuse; *drugs; health facilities; health promotion; interprofessional relations; legal aspects; patient care team; patient education; *pharmacists; professional autonomy; professional competence; *professional ethics; professional organizations; records; *standards; computer security; *Great Britain; *Royal Pharmaceutical Society of Great Britain

Seitz, Joanne; O'Neill, Patrick. Ethical decision–making and the Code of Ethics of the Canadian Psychological Association. *Canadian Psychology.* 1996 Feb; 37(1): 23–30. 16 refs. BE55542.
    autonomy; caring; *codes of ethics; *decision making; education; evaluation studies; goals; obligations to society; principle–based ethics; *professional ethics; professional organizations; *psychology; *students; survey; universities; Canada; *Canadian Psychological Association

New code of medical ethics issued in Italy. [News]. *International Digest of Health Legislation.* 1993; 44(2): 353–354. BE57183.
    *codes of ethics; dentistry; health personnel; *medical ethics; *professional ethics; professional organizations; Italy; *National Federation of the Associations of Physicians and Dentists (Italy)

PROFESSIONAL ETHICS/EDUCATION

Becker, Evelyn S. Teaching ethics as a writing–intensive, ability–based course. *In:* Haddad, Amy Marie, ed. Teaching and Learning Strategies in Pharmacy Ethics. Second Edition. New York, NY: Pharmaceutical Products Press; 1997: 139–148. 4 refs. Co–published simultaneously in *Journal of Pharmacy Teaching*, 1997; 6(1/2): 139–148. ISBN 0–7890–0378–3. BE57939.
    attitudes; case studies; curriculum; *education; evaluation; *pharmacists; *professional ethics; program descriptions; students; *teaching methods; St. Louis College of Pharmacy

Buerki, Robert A. History and human values in ethics instruction. *In:* Haddad, Amy Marie, ed. Teaching and Learning Strategies in Pharmacy Ethics. Second Edition. New York, NY: Pharmaceutical Products Press; 1997: 65–75. 25 refs. Co–published simultaneously in *Journal of Pharmacy Teaching*, 1997; 6(1/2): 65–75. ISBN 0–7890–0378–3. BE57933.
    bioethics; biomedical technologies; codes of ethics; curriculum; *education; historical aspects; *pharmacists; *professional ethics; professional organizations; public opinion; *teaching methods; values; American Pharmaceutical Association

Coughlin, Steven S. Advancing professional ethics in epidemiology. *Journal of Epidemiology and Biostatistics.* 1996; 1(2): 71–77. 41 refs. BE58494.
    bioethics; biomedical research; conflict of interest; curriculum; *education; *epidemiology; ethical review; ethics committees; financial support; guidelines; historical aspects; international aspects; *investigators; *professional ethics; professional organizations; public health; schools; self regulation; American College of Epidemiology; International Epidemiological Association; Society for Epidemiologic Research; Twentieth Century; United States

Daly, Michael E. Alternative methods for the teaching of ethics. *In:* Haddad, Amy Marie, ed. Teaching and Learning Strategies in Pharmacy Ethics. Second Edition. New York, NY: Pharmaceutical Products Press; 1997: 77–86. 3 refs. Co–published simultaneously in *Journal of Pharmacy Teaching*, 1997; 6(1/2): 77–86. ISBN 0–7890–0378–3. BE57934.
    curriculum; *education; ethics; faculty; interdisciplinary communication; *professional ethics; program descriptions; *teaching methods; universities; University of New Mexico

Elliott, Deni. Case studies for teaching research ethics. *Professional Ethics.* 1995 Spring–Summer; 4(3–4): 179–198. 26 fn. References embedded in back–of–issue bibliography. BE55685.
    accountability; authorship; *biomedical research; *case studies; conflict of interest; *education; ethical analysis; financial support; fraud; industry; interprofessional relations; misconduct; *professional ethics; property rights; *science; *scientific misconduct; self regulation; students; *teaching methods; universities; whistleblowing

Giannetti, Vincent J. Experiential approach to teaching ethics. *In:* Haddad, Amy Marie, ed. Teaching and Learning Strategies in Pharmacy Ethics. Second Edition. New York, NY: Pharmaceutical Products Press; 1997: 87–99. 10 refs. Co–published simultaneously in *Journal of Pharmacy Teaching*, 1997; 6(1/2): 87–99. ISBN 0–7890–0378–3. BE57935.
    clinical ethics committees; decision making; *education; *pharmacists; *professional ethics; students; *teaching methods

Haddad, Amy Marie. Role playing and ethics instruction. *In:* Haddad, Amy Marie, ed. Teaching and Learning

---

BE = bioethics accession number   fn. = footnotes   refs. = references

Strategies in Pharmacy Ethics. Second Edition. New York, NY: Pharmaceutical Products Press; 1997: 49–63. 14 refs. Co-published simultaneously in *Journal of Pharmacy Teaching*, 1997; 6(1/2): 49–63. ISBN 0–7890–0378–3. BE57932.
  *education; interprofessional relations; *pharmacists; *professional ethics; social interaction; students; *teaching methods

Haddad, Amy Marie, ed. Teaching and Learning Strategies in Pharmacy Ethics. Second Edition. New York, NY: Pharmaceutical Products Press; 1997. 159 p. 121 refs. Co-published simultaneously as *Journal of Pharmacy Teaching*, 1997; 6(1/2). ISBN 0–7890–0378–3. BE57928.
  bioethical issues; case studies; codes of ethics; curriculum; decision making; drugs; *education; faculty; genetic intervention; legal aspects; patient care; *pharmacists; *professional ethics; professional organizations; social interaction; students; *teaching methods; American Pharmaceutical Association; United States

Homenko, Donna F. Overview of ethical issues perceived by allied health professionals in the workplace. *Journal of Allied Health.* 1997 Summer; 26(3): 97–103. 15 refs. BE58466.
  *allied health personnel; *bioethical issues; *bioethics; *education; hospitals; *knowledge, attitudes, practice; *professional ethics; survey; questionnaires; Midwestern United States

Plante, Thomas G. Training child clinical predoctoral interns and postdoctoral fellows in ethics and professional issues: an experimental model. *Professional Psychology: Research and Practice.* 1995 Dec; 26(6): 616–619. 4 refs. BE55644.
  children; *education; *professional ethics; program descriptions; *psychology; students; *Stanford University

Richardson, James D.; McCarthy, Robert L. The use of student-made vignettes in teaching pharmacy ethics. *In:* Haddad, Amy Marie, ed. Teaching and Learning Strategies in Pharmacy Ethics. Second Edition. New York, NY: Pharmaceutical Products Press; 1997: 127–138. 2 refs. Co-published simultaneously in *Journal of Pharmacy Teaching*, 1997; 6(1/2): 127–138. ISBN 0–7890–0378–3. BE57938.
  attitudes; *education; evaluation; faculty; *pharmacists; *professional ethics; program descriptions; social interaction; *students; *teaching methods; Massachusetts College of Pharmacy and Allied Health Sciences (Boston)

Rossignol, Annette MacKay; Goodmonson, Sharon. Are ethical topics in epidemiology included in the graduate epidemiology curricula? *American Journal of Epidemiology.* 1995 Dec 15; 142(12): 1265-1268. 38 refs. BE55523.
  *attitudes; *curriculum; *education; *epidemiology; *faculty; human experimentation; investigators; *professional ethics; public health; schools; survey; teaching methods; United States

Shannon, Michael C. Educating practitioners for ethical decision-making: current problems and future concerns. *In:* Haddad, Amy Marie, ed. Teaching and Learning Strategies in Pharmacy Ethics. Second Edition. New York, NY: Pharmaceutical Products Press; 1997: 101–109. 2 refs. Co-published simultaneously in *Journal of Pharmacy Teaching*, 1997; 6(1/2): 101–109. ISBN 0–7890–0378–3. BE57936.
  codes of ethics; decision making; *education; interprofessional relations; moral obligations; obligations to society; patient care; *pharmacists; *professional ethics;

professional organizations; professional patient relationship; professional role; American Pharmaceutical Association

Swazey, Judith P.; Bird, Stephanie J. Teaching and learning research ethics. *Professional Ethics.* 1995 Spring–Summer; 4(3–4): 155–178. 3 fn. References embedded in back-of-issue bibliography. BE55674.
  adults; *biomedical research; *case studies; communication; *education; ethical analysis; ethics; faculty; goals; interprofessional relations; moral development; *professional ethics; science; scientific misconduct; students; *teaching methods; universities; values

Veatch, Robert M. Case analysis in ethics instruction. *In:* Haddad, Amy Marie, ed. Teaching and Learning Strategies in Pharmacy Ethics. Second Edition. New York, NY: Pharmaceutical Products Press; 1997: 111–125. 11 refs. Co-published simultaneously in *Journal of Pharmacy Teaching*, 1997; 6(1/2): 111–125. ISBN 0–7890–0378–3. BE57937.
  bioethical issues; *case studies; casuistry; deception; drugs; *education; ethical analysis; misconduct; moral development; patient care; *pharmacists; philosophy; principle-based ethics; *professional ethics; students; *teaching methods

Vivian, Jesse C.; Brushwood, David B. Legal cases that raise ethical issues. *In:* Haddad, Amy Marie, ed. Teaching and Learning Strategies in Pharmacy Ethics. Second Edition. New York, NY: Pharmaceutical Products Press; 1997: 1–17. 4 refs. Co-published simultaneously in *Journal of Pharmacy Teaching*, 1997; 6(1/2): 1–17. ISBN 0–7890–0378–3. BE57929.
  *case studies; *education; *legal aspects; *pharmacists; *professional ethics; teaching methods; United States

Weinstein, Bruce D. Teaching pharmacy ethics: the case study approach. *In:* Haddad, Amy Marie, ed. Teaching and Learning Strategies in Pharmacy Ethics. Second Edition. New York, NY: Pharmaceutical Products Press; 1997: 18–31. 21 refs. Co-published simultaneously in *Journal of Pharmacy Teaching*, 1997; 6(1/2): 18–31. ISBN 0–7890–0378–3. BE57930.
  *case studies; *drugs; *education; ethical analysis; *patient care; *pharmacists; *professional ethics; *teaching methods

PROFESSIONAL PATIENT RELATIONSHIP

See also PATIENT CARE, PROFESSIONAL ETHICS

Allison, Althea; Ewens, Ann. Tensions in sharing client confidences while respecting autonomy: implications for interprofessional practice. *Nursing Ethics.* 1998 Sep; 5(5): 441–450. 19 refs. BE58906.
  autonomy; case studies; communication; *confidentiality; disclosure; health personnel; intention; *interprofessional relations; *patient care team; privacy; *professional patient relationship; referral and consultation; social workers

American College of Obstetricians and Gynecologists. Committee on Ethics. Sexual misconduct in the practice of obstetrics and gynecology: ethical considerations. ACOG Committee Opinion No. 144. *ACOG Committee Opinions.* 1994 Nov; No. 144: 3 p. 12 refs. BE56909.
  females; *guidelines; *misconduct; *obstetrics and gynecology; *organizational policies; patient care; *physician patient relationship; *physicians; professional organizations; *sexuality; *American College of Obstetricians and Gynecologists; American Medical Association; Society of Obstetricians and Gynecologists of Canada

Asai, Atsushi; Kishino, Minako; Tsuguya, Fukui, et al. A report from Japan: choices of Japanese patients in the face of disagreement. *Bioethics.* 1998 Apr; 12(2): 162–172. 11 refs. BE58626.

*attitudes; *autonomy; *cancer; communication; decision making; *diagnosis; *dissent; family members; family relationship; females; males; patient care; patient compliance; *patient participation; *patient satisfaction; *patients; *physician patient relationship; physicians; prognosis; survey; treatment refusal; *truth disclosure; *Japan

BACKGROUND: Patients in different countries have different attitudes toward self–determination and medical information. Little is known how much respect Japanese patients feel should be given for their wishes about medical care and for medical information, and what choices they would make in the face of disagreement. METHODS: Ambulatory patients in six clinics of internal medicine at a university hospital were surveyed using a self–administered questionnaire. RESULTS: A total of 307 patients participated in our survey. Of the respondents, 47% would accept recommendations made by physicians, even if such recommendations were against their wishes; 25% would try to persuade their physician to change their recommendations; and 14% would leave their physician to find a new one. Seventy–six percent of the respondents thought that physicians should routinely ask patients if they would want to know about a diagnosis of cancer, while 5% disagreed; 59% responded that physicians should inform them of the actual diagnosis, even against the request of their family not to do so, while 24% would want their physician to abide by their family's request and 14% could not decide. One–third of the respondents who initially said they would want to know the truth would yield to the desires of the family in a case of disagreement. INTERPRETATION: In the face of disagreement regarding medical care and disclosure, Japanese patients tend to respond in a diverse and unpredictable manner. Medical professionals should thus be prudent and ask their patients explicitly what they want regarding medical care and information.

Bailey, R. Norman. The doctor–patient relationship: communication, informed consent and the optometric patient. *Journal of the American Optometric Association.* 1994 Jun; 65(6): 418–422. 8 refs. BE55782.

autonomy; *communication; decision making; *disclosure; eye diseases; *informed consent; legal aspects; paternalism; *patient care; *patient participation; *physician patient relationship; risks and benefits; trust; uncertainty; *optometry

Baldini, Massimo. The doctor–patient relationship in medical textbooks and manuals of the eighteenth and nineteenth centuries. *Dolentium Hominum: Church and Health in the World.* 1996; 31(11th Yr., No. 1): 88–92. 49 fn. BE57366.

alternative therapies; *communication; *historical aspects; *literature; *medical education; *medical ethics; *medical etiquette; medical schools; medicine; patient compliance; *physician patient relationship; *physicians; professional competence; public opinion; socioeconomic factors; students; trust; *virtues; *Eighteenth Century; Europe; *Nineteenth Century

Bartlett, Peter. Doctors as fiduciaries: equitable regulation of the doctor–patient relationship. *Medical Law Review.* 1997 Summer; 5(2): 193–224. 104 fn. BE57867.

confidentiality; conflict of interest; disclosure; *economics; family practice; health care delivery; informed consent; international aspects; *legal aspects; legal obligations; malpractice; medical records; patient access to records; patient care; *physician patient relationship; remuneration;

torts; trust; *Great Britain; National Health Service

Baur, Susan. The Intimate Hour: Love and Sex in Psychotherapy. Boston, MA: Houghton Mifflin; 1997. 309 p. 50 refs. 275 fn. ISBN 0–395–82284–X. BE56239.

famous persons; females; health personnel; historical aspects; *love; males; misconduct; *professional patient relationship; *psychotherapy; *sexuality

Beisecker, Analee E.; Murden, Robert A.; Moore, William P., et al. Attitudes of medical students and primary care physicians regarding input of older and younger patients in medical decisions. *Medical Care.* 1996 Feb; 34(2): 126–137. 28 refs. BE55654.

*adults; *age factors; *aged; alternatives; *attitudes; *autonomy; comparative studies; *decision making; diagnosis; drugs; faculty; family practice; females; hospitals; internal medicine; *internship and residency; males; medical education; medical schools; *paternalism; *patient care; *patient participation; *physician patient relationship; *physicians; primary health care; referral and consultation; *students; survey; Kansas; Ohio; Ohio State University Hospital; University of Kansas Medical Center

Berg, Paula E. Lost in a doctrinal wasteland: the exceptionalism of doctor–patient speech within the Rehnquist Court's First Amendment jurisprudence. *Health Matrix.* 1998 Summer; 8(2): 153–177. 99 fn. BE58952.

abortion, induced; autonomy; *communication; constitutional law; counseling; federal government; *government regulation; informed consent; *legal aspects; *legal rights; paternalism; *physician patient relationship; *physicians; professional autonomy; psychoactive drugs; referral and consultation; religion; state government; *Supreme Court decisions; *gag clauses; marijuana; *First Amendment; Planned Parenthood of Southeastern Pennsylvania v. Casey; Rust v. Sullivan; *United States

Berkowitz, Sheldon T.; Boisaubin, Eugene V.; Perkins, Henry S., et al. Race and the delivery of care. [Letters and response]. *Hastings Center Report.* 1998 Jan–Feb; 28(1): 5–6. BE57289.

*allowing to die; *blacks; communication; *critically ill; *cultural pluralism; *decision making; *dissent; economics; emergency care; *family members; *futility; minority groups; *physicians; *professional family relationship; *prolongation of life; *social discrimination; *trust; whites; *United States

Blacksher, Erika. Desperately seeking difference. *Cambridge Quarterly of Healthcare Ethics.* 1998 Winter; 7(1): 11–16. 17 fn. BE58504.

bioethical issues; *clinical ethics; communication; consensus; *cultural pluralism; decision making; dissent; empirical research; ethical analysis; health care delivery; managed care programs; *minority groups; patient care; *professional patient relationship; self concept; stigmatization; terminal care; trust; truth disclosure; *values; United States

Bradby, Hannah; Gabe, Jonathan; Bury, Michael. 'Sexy docs' and 'busty blondes': press coverage of professional misconduct cases brought before the General Medical Council. *Sociology of Health and Illness.* 1995 Sep; 17(4): 458–476. 59 refs. 2 fn. BE55691.

*females; *males; marital relationship; *mass media; *misconduct; *patients; *physician patient relationship; *physicians; self regulation; *sex offenses; *sexuality; social discrimination; sociology of medicine; stigmatization; General Medical Council (Great Britain); *Great Britain

Bram, Anthony D. The physically ill or dying psychotherapist: a review of ethical and clinical considerations. *Psychotherapy.* 1995 Winter; 32(4):

568–580. 34 refs. BE56023.

> attitudes to death; beneficence; codes of ethics; confidentiality; *disclosure; emotions; empirical research; guidelines; *health; *health personnel; patient care; patient transfer; patients; professional competence; *professional ethics; professional organizations; *professional patient relationship; psychology; *psychotherapy; referral and consultation; risks and benefits; *terminally ill; patient abandonment; patient care planning; professional impairment; *seriously ill; American Psychological Association

Brody, Howard. Autonomy revisited: progress in medical ethics: discussion paper. *Journal of the Royal Society of Medicine.* 1985 May; 78(5): 380–387. 22 refs. BE57825.

> *autonomy; *beneficence; clinical ethics; ethical theory; informed consent; interdisciplinary communication; medical ethics; *medicine; *paternalism; *philosophy; *physician patient relationship; *physician's role; primary health care; trends

Candib, Lucy M. Medicine and the Family: A Feminist Perspective. New York, NY: BasicBooks; 1995. 360 p. Bibliography: p. 307–350. ISBN 0–465–02374–6. BE56502.

> adults; autonomy; caring; children; communication; contracts; disclosure; domestic violence; empathy; family members; family practice; *family relationship; females; *feminist ethics; males; *medicine; parent child relationship; *patient care; patients; philosophy; *physician patient relationship; physicians; *professional family relationship; rape; self concept; sex offenses; social discrimination; *social dominance; incest; United States

Cassell, Eric J. The future of the doctor–payer–patient relationship. *Journal of the American Geriatrics Society.* 1998 Mar; 46(3): 318–321. 5 refs. Paper presented at the 1996 Congress of Clinical Societies. BE56754.

> biomedical technologies; *chronically ill; commodification; diagnosis; disabled; disease; informed consent; *managed care programs; *medicine; patient care; *physician patient relationship; *physician's role; trends; self care; United States

Cohen, Jordan J. Remembering the real questions. *Annals of Internal Medicine.* 1998 Apr 1; 128(7): 563–566. 3 refs. BE57324.

> communication; cultural pluralism; *economics; genetic information; internal medicine; *managed care programs; medicine; organizational policies; *patient advocacy; patient care; patient education; *physician patient relationship; *physician's role; physicians; practice guidelines; prognosis; treatment outcome; evidence–based medicine; United States

College of Physicians and Surgeons of British Columbia. Committee on Physician Sexual Misconduct. Crossing the Boundaries. The Report of the Committee on Physician Sexual Misconduct. Issued by the College of Physicians and Surgeons of British Columbia, Vancouver, BC; 1992 Nov. 28 p. BE57276.

> attitudes; mandatory reporting; medical education; *misconduct; *organizational policies; patient advocacy; *patients; *physician patient relationship; *physicians; professional organizations; public opinion; public participation; *self regulation; *sexuality; social dominance; statistics; survey; *College of Physicians and Surgeons of British Columbia

Coverdale, John H.; Thomson, Alex N.; White, Gillian E. Social and sexual contact between general practitioners and patients in New Zealand: attitudes and prevalence. *British Journal of General Practice.* 1995 May; 45(394): 245–247. 16 refs. BE56554.

> *attitudes; family practice; *knowledge, attitudes, practice; *misconduct; *physician patient relationship; *physicians; risks and benefits; *sexuality; *social interaction; statistics; survey; *New Zealand

Cowart, Dax; Burt, Robert. Confronting death: who chooses, who controls? A dialogue between Dax Cowart and Robert Burt. *Hastings Center Report.* 1998 Jan–Feb; 28(1): 14–24. 1 ref. Commented on by D.G. Arnold and P.T. Menzel, p. 25–27. BE57292.

> *allowing to die; attitudes; *autonomy; *beneficence; *burns; *communication; competence; *decision making; *dissent; freedom; human rights; informed consent; nurses; *pain; palliative care; *paternalism; patient advocacy; *physically disabled; *physician patient relationship; physician's role; *prolongation of life; quality of life; *right to die; self concept; suffering; *time factors; *treatment refusal; values; *Cowart, Dax

On 21 November 1996, Dax Cowart and Robert Burt jointly delivered the Heather Koller Memorial Lecture at Pacific Lutheran University. This was the first time that they spoke together in a public forum. Dax Cowart now lives and practices law in Corpus Christi, Texas. In the summer of 1973, he was critically injured in a propane gas explosion that took his father's life and very deeply burned more than two–thirds of his own body. He was left blind and without the use of his hands. For more than a year Dax underwent extraordinarily painful treatments in the acute burn ward of two hospitals. Throughout his ordeal he demanded to die by refusing consent to his disinfectant treatments. Despite repeated declarations of competence by his psychiatrist, all his pleas were rejected. In 1974, while still hospitalized, he helped make the famous "Please Let Me Die" video, and in 1984 a second video, "Dax's Case." In 1986 Dax Cowart received a law degree from Texas Tech University. Burt and Cowart have corresponded over the course of several years on the subject of Dax's case and related issues. They met for the first time during their trip to Tacoma, Washington for the Koller Memorial Lecture. The following is an edited transcript of their public remarks.

Degner, Lesley F.; Kristjanson, Linda J.; Bowman, David, et al. Information needs and decisional preferences in women with breast cancer. *JAMA.* 1997 May 14; 277(18): 1485–1492. 36 refs. BE55849.

> age factors; *attitudes; *breast cancer; communication; *decision making; disclosure; evaluation studies; *females; *patient care; *patient education; *patient participation; patients; *physician patient relationship; physicians; socioeconomic factors; survey; truth disclosure; Manitoba

OBJECTIVE: To determine the degree of involvement women with breast cancer wanted in medical decision making, extent to which they believed they had achieved their preferred level of involvement, and types of information they judged to be most important. DESIGN AND SETTING: Cross–sectional survey at 2 tertiary oncology referral clinics and 2 community hospital oncology clinics in Winnipeg, Manitoba. PATIENTS: Consecutive sample of 1012 women with a confirmed diagnosis of breast cancer who were scheduled for a visit at 1 of 4 hospital oncology clinics. MAIN OUTCOME MEASURES: The following measures were used: (1) Preferences about various levels of participation in treatment decision making; (2) the extent to which subjects believed they had achieved their preferred levels of involvement in decision making; and (3) priority needs for information and how these needs differed by selected sociodemographic, disease, and treatment variables. RESULTS: A total of 22% of women wanted to select their own cancer treatment, 44% wanted to select their treatment collaboratively with their physicians, and 34% wanted to delegate this

---

BE = bioethics accession number   fn. = footnotes   refs. = references

responsibility to their physicians. Only 42% of women believed they had achieved their preferred level of control in decision making. The 2 most highly ranked types of information were related to knowing about chances of cure and spread of disease. Women younger than 50 years rated information about physical and sexual attractiveness as more important than did older women (P less than .001); women older than 70 years rated information about self-care as more important than did younger women (P=.002); and women who had a positive family history of breast cancer rated information about family risk as more important than did other women (P=.03). CONCLUSIONS: The substantial discrepancy between women's preferred and attained levels of involvement in treatment decision making suggests that systematic approaches to assess and respond to women's desired level of participation in treatment decision making need to be evaluated. Priorities for information identified in this study provide an empirical basis to guide communication with women seeking care for breast cancer.

Dehlendorf, Christine E.; Wolfe, Sidney M. Physicians disciplined for sex-related offenses. *JAMA.* 1998 Jun 17; 279(23): 1883–1888. 25 refs. BE58410.
   age factors; family practice; federal government; *government regulation; medical specialties; *misconduct; obstetrics and gynecology; *physician patient relationship; *physicians; psychiatry; *punishment; *self regulation; *sex offenses; *sexuality; state government; statistics; *United States

CONTEXT: Physicians who abuse their patients sexually cause immense harm, and, therefore, the discipline of physicians who commit any sex-related offenses is an important public health issue that should be examined. OBJECTIVES: To determine the frequency and severity of discipline against physicians who commit sex-related offenses and to describe the characteristics of these physicians. DESIGN AND SETTING: Analysis of sex-related orders from a national database of disciplinary orders taken by state medical boards and federal agencies. SUBJECTS: A total of 761 physicians disciplined for sex-related offenses from 1981 through 1996. MAIN OUTCOME MEASURES: Rate and severity of discipline over time for sex-related offenses and specialty, age, and board certification status of disciplined physicians. RESULTS: The number of physicians disciplined per year for sex-related offenses increased from 42 in 1989 to 147 in 1996, and the proportion of all disciplinary orders that were sex related increased from 2.1% in 1989 to 4.4% in 1996 (P less than .001 for trend). Discipline for sex-related offenses was significantly more severe (P less than .001) than for non-sex-related offenses, with 71.9% of sex-related orders involving revocation, surrender, or suspension of medical license. Of 761 physicians disciplined, the offenses committed by 567 (75%) involved patients, including sexual intercourse, rape, sexual molestation, and sexual favors for drugs. As of March 1997, 216 physicians (39.9%) disciplined for sex-related offenses between 1981 and 1994 were licensed to practice. Compared with all physicians, physicians disciplined for sex-related offenses were more likely to practice in the specialties of psychiatry, child psychiatry, obstetrics and gynecology, and family and general practice (all P less than .001) than in other specialties and were older than the national physician population, but were no different in terms of board certification status. CONCLUSIONS: Discipline against physicians for sex-related offenses is increasing over time and is relatively severe, although few physicians are

disciplined for sexual offenses each year. In addition, a substantial proportion of physicians disciplined for these offenses are allowed to either continue to practice or return to practice.

Epstein, Ronald M.; Morse, Diane S.; Frankel, Richard M., et al. Awkward moments in patient–physician communication about HIV risk. *Annals of Internal Medicine.* 1998 Mar 15; 128(6): 435–442. 50 refs. BE57305.
   *communication; *counseling; emotions; evaluation studies; family practice; *HIV seropositivity; internal medicine; knowledge, attitudes, practice; patients; *physician patient relationship; *physicians; *professional competence; *risk; New York

BACKGROUND: Physicians frequently encounter patients who are at risk for HIV infection, but they often evaluate risk behaviors ineffectively. OBJECTIVE: To describe the barriers to and facilitators of comprehensive HIV risk evaluation in primary care office visits. DESIGN: Qualitative thematic and sequential analysis of videotaped patient–physician discussions about HIV risk. Tapes were reviewed independently by physician and patient and were coded by the research team. SETTING: Physicians' offices. PARTICIPANTS: Convenience sample of 17 family physicians and general internists. Twenty-six consenting patients 18 to 45 years of age who indicated concern about or risks for HIV infection on a 10-item questionnaire administered before the physician visit were included. MEASUREMENTS: A thematic coding scheme and a five-level description of the depth of HIV-related discussion. RESULTS: In 73% of the encounters, physicians did not elicit enough information to characterize patients' HIV risk status. The outcome of HIV-related discussions was substantially influenced by the manner in which the physician introduced the topic, handled awkward moments, and dealt with problematic language and the extent to which the physician sought the patient's perspective. Feelings of ineffectiveness and strong emotions interfered with some physicians' ability to assess HIV risk. Physicians easily recognized problematic communication during reviews of their own videotapes. CONCLUSIONS: Comprehensive HIV risk discussions included providing a rationale for discussion, effectively negotiating awkward moments, repairing problematic language, persevering with the topic, eliciting the patient's perspective, responding to fears and expectations, and being empathic. Educational programs should use videotape review and should concentrate on physicians' personal reactions to discussing emotionally charged topics.

Fadiman, Anne. The Spirit Catches You and You Fall Down: A Hmong Child and Her American Doctors, and the Collision of Two Cultures. New York, NY: Farrar, Straus and Giroux; 1997. 339 p. Bibliography: p. 311–324. ISBN 0-374-26781-2. BE57048.
   *alternative therapies; *Asian Americans; *attitudes; childbirth; *children; *communication; *cultural pluralism; *disease; *epilepsy; family relationship; *home care; hospitals; nurses; *parent child relationship; *patient care; *patient compliance; *persistent vegetative state; *physicians; *professional family relationship; *professional patient relationship; *religion; social workers; treatment refusal; ethnographic studies; *folk medicine; California; *Hmong; Laos; *Lee, Lia; *Merced Community Medical Center (CA); United States; Vietnam War

Farber, Neil J.; Novack, Dennis H.; O'Brien, Mary K. Love, boundaries, and the patient–physician relationship. *Archives of Internal Medicine.* 1997 Nov 10;

BE = bioethics accession number   fn. = footnotes   refs. = references

157(20): 2291–2294. 37 refs. BE57159.
  communication; emotions; empathy; family relationship;
  females; gifts; love; males; medical education; motivation;
  patient care; patients; *physician patient relationship;
  physicians; psychological stress; *psychology; self concept;
  sexuality; social interaction; socioeconomic factors; trust
Physicians often use their relationships with patients to
promote specific therapeutic goals. Because of their
personal histories, values, and biases, patients may react
to physicians in ways that inhibit or enhance the
relationship. The feelings that are aroused may induce
physicians to become overly distant, engendering patient
and physician dissatisfaction, or to become overly
involved emotionally, which can have serious
psychological and clinical consequences. We explore
how a balance between clinical objectivity and bonding
with the patient is optimal and achievable. The nature
and origin of personal boundaries are described.
Boundary transgressions on the part of the patient are
discussed, and the means of preventing transgressions
by both patients and physicians through medical
education, the process of self-awareness, and an
exploration of family–of–origin issues are proposed.
Through attention to communication with patients, the
physician can maintain an empathetic yet objective
relationship with the patient.

Fealy, Gerard M. Professional caring: the moral
dimension. *Journal of Advanced Nursing.* 1995 Dec; 22(6):
1135–1140. 18 refs. BE56204.
  accountability; autonomy; *caring; codes of ethics;
  communitarianism; ethical theory; health personnel; justice;
  moral obligations; morality; *nurse patient relationship;
  nursing ethics; patient care; *professional ethics;
  *professional patient relationship; teleological ethics; virtues

Feinberg, Joel. Paternalism. *In:* Borchert, Donald M., ed.
The Encyclopedia of Philosophy. Supplement. New
York, NY: Simon and Schuster Macmillan; 1996:
390–392. 15 refs. ISBN 0-02-864629-0. BE57224.
  autonomy; beneficence; competence; *paternalism; physician
  patient relationship

**Ferris, Lorraine E.; Norton, Peter G.; Dunn, Earl V.,
et al.** Guidelines for managing domestic abuse when
male and female partners are patients of the same
physician. [For the Delphi Panel and the Consulting
Group]. *JAMA.* 1997 Sep 10; 278(10): 851–857. 59 refs.
BE55854.
  communication; confidentiality; *conflict of interest;
  *domestic violence; females; *guidelines; males; *patient
  care; patient education; *patients; *physician patient
  relationship; physicians; *practice guidelines; primary health
  care; *professional family relationship; referral and
  consultation; risk
OBJECTIVE: To provide clinical guidelines for primary
care physicians who are dealing with domestic abuse
and who have both the abused woman and her partner
as patients. PARTICIPANTS: A 15–member expert
panel with members having experience in family
practice, gynecology, emergency medicine, medical
ethics, nursing, psychology, law, and social work; an
11–member consulting group with members representing
medicine, consumers, police, psychology, social work,
and nursing; and participants from focus groups
including 48 previously abused women and 10 previously
abusive men. Members of the expert panel and the
consulting group were recruited by the research team.
Focus group members were recruited through the
agencies from which they were receiving services.
EVIDENCE: Available research information, and
opinions of the expert panel, the consulting group, and

the focus group participants. CONSENSUS PROCESS:
Scoring of 144 clinical scenarios was performed by the
expert panel using a modified Delphi technique involving
4 iterations. Scenarios were rated in terms of best
practice for primary care physicians dealing with
suspected and confirmed cases of physical abuse.
Consulting group members and focus group participants
then commented on the panel's results. Final guidelines
were approved by the panel and the consulting group,
with comments reserved in the guidelines for information
from focus group participants. CONCLUSIONS: It is
not a conflict of interest for the physician to deal with
abuse of the female partner when both partners are
patients. Both patients have a right to autonomy,
confidentiality, honesty, and quality care. Patients should
be dealt with independently, thereby facilitating
assessment of the magnitude and severity of the victim's
injuries. Physicians should not discuss the possibility of
domestic abuse with the male partner without the prior
consent of the abused female partner. Joint counseling
is generally inadvisable and should be attempted only
when the violence has ended, provided both partners
give independent consent and the physician has adequate
training and skills to deal with the situation without
escalating the violence. If the physician feels unable to
deal effectively with either patient because of the dual
relationship, referral to another qualified physician is
preferred.

Furst, Lilian R. Between Doctors and Patients: The
Changing Balance of Power. Charlottesville, VA:
University Press of Virginia; 1998. 287 p. Bibliography:
p. 267–277. ISBN 0-8139-1755-7. BE58943.
  biomedical research; biomedical technologies; codes of
  ethics; communication; females; *historical aspects; hospitals;
  interprofessional relations; laboratories; *literature; medical
  education; patient care; *physician patient relationship;
  *physicians; *social dominance; socioeconomic factors;
  *sociology of medicine; Europe; Nineteenth Century;
  Twentieth Century; United States

Gadow, Sally. Ethical narratives in practice. *Nursing
Science Quarterly.* 1996 Spring; 9(1): 8–9. 5 refs. BE55864.
  autonomy; *narrative ethics; *nurse patient relationship;
  nursing ethics; paternalism; patient care

General Medical Council (Great Britain). Duties of a
Doctor: Guidance from the General Medical Council.
[Booklets]. London: The Council; 1995. portfolio of 4
booklets. BE57156.
  advertising; AIDS serodiagnosis; biomedical research;
  *confidentiality; conflict of interest; disclosure; duty to warn;
  family practice; gifts; *guidelines; *HIV seropositivity;
  iatrogenic disease; informed consent; *interprofessional
  relations; *medical ethics; medical fees; medical specialties;
  occupational exposure; patient care; *physician patient
  relationship; *physicians; professional competence; referral
  and consultation; refusal to treat; self regulation; traffic
  accidents; *General Medical Council (Great Britain); *Great
  Britain

Gervais, Karen G. Changing society, changing medicine,
changing bioethics. *In:* DeVries, Raymond; Subedi,
Janardan, eds. Bioethics and Society: Constructing the
Ethical Enterprise. Upper Saddle River, NJ: Prentice
Hall; 1998: 216–232. 5 refs. 1 fn. ISBN 0-13-531252-3.
BE58737.
  autonomy; bioethics; *communication; conflict of interest;
  *cultural pluralism; *health care delivery; historical aspects;
  justice; *managed care programs; methods; *minority
  groups; patient care; *physician patient relationship;
  physicians; professional patient relationship; resource
  allocation; sociology of medicine; trends; trust; values;

BE = bioethics accession number   fn. = footnotes   refs. = references

non–Western World; Western World; *Hmong; Twentieth Century; United States

Gorton, Gregg E.; Samuel, Steven E. A national survey of training directors about education for prevention of psychiatrist–patient sexual exploitation. *Academic Psychiatry.* 1996 Summer; 20(2): 92–98. 15 refs. BE58119.
administrators; curriculum; faculty; *internship and residency; *medical education; medical ethics; *misconduct; *physician patient relationship; *psychiatry; *sexuality; survey; teaching methods; United States

Habermehl, Karl–Otto. The Hippocratic example of the neutrality and universality of medicine. *Dolentium Hominum: Church and Health in the World.* 1996; 31(11th Yr., No. 1): 124–126. BE57369.
biomedical technologies; costs and benefits; decision making; government regulation; humanism; *moral obligations; *patient advocacy; patient care; *physician patient relationship; *physicians; professional competence; psychological stress; resource allocation; sociology of medicine; *trust; truth disclosure; Hippocratic Oath

Hall, Mark A.; Berenson, Robert A. Ethical practice in managed care: a dose of realism. *Annals of Internal Medicine.* 1998 Mar 1; 128(5): 395–402. 72 refs. BE57850.
administrators; common good; conflict of interest; *decision making; disclosure; *economics; ethical analysis; *guidelines; health; health care delivery; health insurance reimbursement; *incentives; *managed care programs; *medical ethics; moral obligations; moral policy; patient advocacy; patient care; *physician patient relationship; physician's role; *physicians; practice guidelines; public policy; remuneration; *resource allocation; *trust; withholding treatment; capitation fee; United States
This article examines the ethics of medical practice under managed care from a pragmatic perspective that gives physicians more useful guidance than do existing ethical statements. The article begins with a framework for constructing a realistic set of ethical principles, namely, that medical ethics derives from physicians' role as healers; that ethical statements are primarily aspirational, not regulatory; and that preserving patient trust is the primary objective. The following concrete ethical guidelines are presented: Financial incentives should influence physicians to maximize the health of the group of patients under their care; physicians should not enter into incentive arrangements that they are embarrassed to describe accurately to their patients; physicians should treat each patient impartially without regard to source of payment, consistent with the physician's own treatment style; if physicians depart from this ideal, they should inform their patients honestly; and it is desirable, although not mandatory, to differentiate medical treatment recommendations from insurance coverage decisions by clearly assigning authority over these different roles and by physicians advocating for recommended treatment that is not covered.

Hern, H. Eugene; Koenig, Barbara A.; Moore, Lisa Jean, et al. The difference that culture can make in end–of–life decisionmaking. *Cambridge Quarterly of Healthcare Ethics.* 1998 Winter; 7(1): 27–40. 30 fn. BE58455.
alternative therapies; anthropology; *Asian Americans; *autonomy; *cancer; case studies; clinical ethics; *communication; *cultural pluralism; *decision making; *diagnosis; disclosure; *family members; *family relationship; females; *informed consent; *knowledge, attitudes, practice; *minority groups; models, theoretical; patient care; *patient care team; *patient participation; *patients; *physician patient relationship; physicians; *professional family relationship; *prognosis; risks and

benefits; stigmatization; *terminal care; terminally ill; *third party consent; trust; *truth disclosure; *values; California; United States

Higgs, Roger. Shaping our ends: the ethics of respect in a well–led NHS. *British Journal of General Practice.* 1997 Apr; 47(417): 245–249. 31 refs. Text based on the 1996 James Mackenzie lecture delivered at the annual general meeting of the Royal College of General Practitioners on 22 Nov 1996. BE57751.
autonomy; case studies; communication; *family practice; health care delivery; medical ethics; patient care; *physician patient relationship; suffering; terminally ill; Great Britain; National Health Service

Hoshino, Kazumasa. Bioethics in the light of Japanese sentiments. *In:* Hoshino, Kazumasa, ed. Japanese and Western Bioethics: Studies in Moral Diversity. Boston, MA: Kluwer Academic; 1997: 13–23. 5 refs. ISBN 0–7923–4112–0. BE57080.
autonomy; bioethical issues; cadavers; communication; *communitarianism; comparative studies; *decision making; diagnosis; family members; *family relationship; informed consent; legal aspects; *organ donation; *paternalism; patient care; patient compliance; *patients' rights; *physician patient relationship; *physicians; privacy; professional family relationship; prognosis; terminally ill; third party consent; *tissue donation; *truth disclosure; hope; non–Western World; Act of Donation of the Body for Medical and Dental Education 1983 (Japan); Cornea and Kidney Transplant Act 1979 (Japan); *Japan; United States

Howe, Edmund G. Caring for patients with dementia: an indication for "emotional communism". *Journal of Clinical Ethics.* 1998 Spring; 9(1): 3–11. 30 fn. BE57709.
aged; allowing to die; *dementia; *emotions; *health personnel; love; *patient care; *professional patient relationship; psychological stress; stigmatization; withholding treatment; grief

Howe, Edmund G. Deconstructing equity, autonomy, and ethical analysis. *Journal of Clinical Ethics.* 1998 Summer; 9(2): 99–107. 17 fn. BE58955.
advance directives; AIDS; assisted suicide; *autonomy; caring; clinical ethics; competence; control groups; cultural pluralism; decision making; developing countries; *emotions; empathy; *ethical analysis; family members; family relationship; genetic screening; health personnel; HIV seropositivity; human experimentation; *justice; mentally ill; minority groups; moral policy; paternalism; patient care; patient compliance; placebos; pregnant women; *professional patient relationship; psychological stress; public policy; research design; resource allocation; siblings; values; vulnerable populations

Huber, Ruth; Evans, Virginia Cox. Trust in physicians to honor death related instructions. *Omega: A Journal of Death and Dying.* 1997–1998; 36(1): 9–21. 39 refs. BE57720.
*advance directives; age factors; *aged; *allowing to die; assisted suicide; attitudes to death; comparative studies; *decision making; *institutionalized persons; *knowledge, attitudes, practice; *physician patient relationship; *physicians; *prolongation of life; *public opinion; residential facilities; *right to die; survey; *terminal care; treatment refusal; *trust; voluntary euthanasia; Kentucky

Huston, Kathleen. Ethical decisions in treating battered women. *Professional Psychology: Research and Practice.* 1984 Dec; 15(6): 822–832. 31 refs. BE57239.
autonomy; beneficence; competence; decision making; *directive counseling; *domestic violence; *females; health personnel; paternalism; patients; *professional patient relationship; psychology; *psychotherapy; professional role

---

Jehu, Derek. Patients as Victims: Sexual Abuse in Psychotherapy and Counselling. New York, NY: Wiley; 1994. 241 p. (Wiley series in psychotherapy and counselling). Bibliography: p. 225–238. ISBN 0–471–94398–3. BE55680.
> age factors; attitudes; *counseling; females; *health personnel; legal aspects; males; mentally ill; *misconduct; patient care; prevalence; professional ethics; *professional patient relationship; *psychotherapy; regulation; *sex offenses; *sexuality; statistics; Great Britain; United States

Jones, Hilary. Autonomy and paternalism: partners or rivals? *British Journal of Nursing.* 1996 Mar 28–Apr 10; 5(6): 378–381. 14 refs. BE55563.
> *autonomy; *nurse patient relationship; *paternalism; *professional patient relationship; social dominance; vulnerable populations; sick role

Kelly, Christine Kuehn. Patient–centered ethics reclaiming center stage. *Annals of Internal Medicine.* 1997 Aug 15; 127(4): I–45. 5 refs. Summary of an American Medical Association conference held in Philadelphia in March 1997. BE56171.
> industry; managed care programs; medical ethics; *patient advocacy; patient care; *physician patient relationship; *physicians; professional autonomy; professional organizations; public policy; resource allocation; American Medical Association; United States

Kitwood, Tom. Toward a theory of dementia care: ethics and interaction. *Journal of Clinical Ethics.* 1998 Spring; 9(1): 23–34. 15 fn. BE57711.
> aged; behavior control; communication; decision making; *dementia; emotions; empathy; ethical theory; health personnel; historical aspects; misconduct; negligence; paternalism; *patient care; patient participation; patients; personhood; *professional patient relationship; *social interaction; stigmatization; empowerment

Kopelman, Loretta M.; Lannin, Donald R.; Kopelman, Arthur E. Preventing and managing unwarranted biases against patients. *In:* McCullough, Laurence B.; Jones, James W.; Brody, Baruch A., eds. Surgical Ethics. New York, NY: Oxford University Press; 1998: 242–254. 31 refs. ISBN 0–19–510347–5. BE58330.
> aged; biomedical technologies; blacks; case studies; continuing education; cultural pluralism; curriculum; females; health facilities; Hispanic Americans; HIV seropositivity; human experimentation; humanities; indigents; institutional policies; medical ethics; *patient care; patients; *physician patient relationship; *physicians; prognosis; quality of health care; refusal to treat; risks and benefits; selection for treatment; selection of subjects; *social discrimination; *socioeconomic factors; *surgery; trust; United States

Koven, Suzanne J. The ungifted physician. [A piece of my mind]. *JAMA.* 1998 May 27; 279(20): 1607. BE58417.
> *gifts; health care delivery; *physician patient relationship; trends

Lazarus, Jeremy A. Ethical issues in doctor–patient sexual relationships. *Psychiatric Clinics of North America.* 1995 Mar; 18(1): 55–70. 37 refs. BE55512.
> codes of ethics; emotions; ethics committees; family members; females; health personnel; injuries; internship and residency; interprofessional relations; males; malpractice; medical ethics; mentally ill; *misconduct; patients; *physician patient relationship; *physicians; professional family relationship; professional organizations; *psychiatry; *psychotherapy; punishment; self regulation; sex offenses; *sexuality; time factors; American Medical Association; *American Psychiatric Association; United States

Leaning, Jennifer. Human rights and medical education. [Editorial]. *BMJ (British Medical Journal).* 1997 Nov 29; 315(7120): 1390–1391. 13 refs. BE56900.
> cultural pluralism; disadvantaged; guidelines; *human rights; *international aspects; *medical education; *medical ethics; *physician patient relationship; United Nations; *Universal Declaration of Human Rights

Long, Ann; Long, Aishlinn; Smyth, Angus. Suicide: a statement of suffering. *Nursing Ethics.* 1998 Jan; 5(1): 3–15. 58 refs. BE58712.
> attitudes; autonomy; beneficence; caring; communication; competence; empathy; moral obligations; *nurse patient relationship; *nurse's role; *nurses; nursing ethics; paternalism; *patient care; professional family relationship; stigmatization; *suffering; *suicide; value of life

Lupton, Deborah. Consumerism, reflexivity, and the medical encounter. *Social Science and Medicine.* 1997 Aug; 45(3): 373–381. 32 refs. BE58911.
> age factors; alternative therapies; *attitudes; autonomy; *patient participation; *patient satisfaction; patients; *physician patient relationship; physicians; professional competence; social dominance; socioeconomic factors; survey; trust; qualitative research; self care; Australia

Much emphasis has been placed recently in sociological, policy and popular discourses on changes in lay people's attitudes towards the medical profession that have been labelled by some as a move towards the embracing of "consumerism." Notions of consumerism tend to assume that lay people act as "rational" actors in the context of the medical encounter. They align with broader sociological concepts of the "reflexive self" as a product of late modernity; that is, the self who acts in a calculated manner to engage in self–improvement and who is sceptical about expert knowledges. To explore the ways that people think and feel about medicine and the medical profession, this article draws on findings from a study involving in–depth interviews with 60 lay people from a wide range of backgrounds living in Sydney. These data suggest that, in their interactions with doctors and other health care workers, lay people may pursue both the ideal–type "consumerist" and the "passive patient" subject position simultaneously or variously, depending on the context. The article concludes that late modernist notions of reflexivity as applied to issues of consumerism fail to recognize the complexity and changeable nature of the desires, emotions and needs that characterize the patient–doctor relationship.

Lützén, Kim; Evertzon, Mats; Nordin, Conny. Moral sensitivity in psychiatric practice. *Nursing Ethics.* 1997 Nov; 4(6): 472–482. 13 refs. BE57418.
> age factors; *attitudes; autonomy; beneficence; comparative studies; *decision making; *females; *males; *medical ethics; mentally ill; *moral development; paternalism; patient care; *physician patient relationship; *physicians; *psychiatry; survey; trust; values; *Sweden

McAliley, Lauren G.; Lambert, Sally A.; Ashenberg, Margaret D., et al. Therapeutic relations decision making: the Rainbow framework. *Pediatric Nursing.* 1996 May–Jun; 22(3): 199–203, 210. 5 refs. BE55515.
> children; communication; *decision making; emotions; gifts; goals; hospitals; institutional policies; interprofessional relations; *models, theoretical; *nurse patient relationship; *nurses; parents; patient care; pediatrics; professional family relationship; program descriptions; social interaction; utilitarianism; values; *Rainbow Babies and Children's Hospital (Cleveland, OH)

Madder, Hilary. Existential autonomy: why patients should make their own choices. *Journal of Medical*

BE = bioethics accession number   fn. = footnotes   refs. = references

Ethics. 1997 Aug; 23(4): 221–225. 5 refs. BE55917.
anesthesia; *autonomy; comprehension; *decision making; disclosure; informed consent; models, theoretical; *paternalism; patient care; *patient participation; *physician patient relationship; *physician's role; prognosis; surgery; technical expertise; treatment refusal; values; amputation; rationality; Savulescu, Julian

Savulescu has recently introduced the "rational non-interventional paternalist" model of the patient–doctor relationship. This paper addresses objections to such a model from the perspective of an anaesthetist. Patients need to make their own decisions if they are to be fully autonomous. Rational non-interventional paternalism undermines the importance of patient choice and so threatens autonomy. Doctors should provide an evaluative judgment of the best medical course of action, but ought to restrict themselves to helping patients to make their own choices rather than making such choices for them.

Marshall, Patricia A. Boundary crossings: gender and power in clinical ethics consultations. *In:* Sargent, Carolyn F.; Brettell; Caroline B., eds. Gender and Health: An International Perspective. Upper Saddle River, NJ: Prentice Hall; 1996: 205–226. 88 refs. 5 fn. ISBN 0–13–079427–9. BE58097.
case studies; clinical ethics; *communication; *critically ill; *decision making; dissent; *ethicist's role; *ethics consultation; family members; family relationship; *females; *feminist ethics; futility; *narrative ethics; *organ transplantation; patient care team; patient transfer; *professional patient relationship; prognosis; psychological stress; *retreatment; self concept; social dominance; time factors; *uncertainty; values; sick role; Loyola University of Chicago Medical Center

Martin, Geoffrey W. Communication breakdown or ideal speech situation: the problem of nurse advocacy. *Nursing Ethics.* 1998 Mar; 5(2): 147–157. 29 refs. BE58475.
*communication; empathy; employment; institutional policies; models, theoretical; *nurse patient relationship; *nurses; nursing ethics; nursing research; paternalism; *patient advocacy; patient care; patient participation; patients' rights; physician nurse relationship; professional family relationship; social dominance; survey; dependency; Great Britain

May, William E. The call to holiness and health care as service. *Linacre Quarterly.* 1997 May; 64(2): 66–73. 1 ref. Address to the 1996 annual meeting of the National Federation of Catholic Physicians. BE55614.
caring; confidentiality; decision making; emotions; moral development; *moral obligations; *patient care; patients; personhood; *physician patient relationship; physician's role; *physicians; professional competence; *Roman Catholic ethics; time factors; trust

Mitchell, Peter. Shared decision–making poses problems for UK. [News]. *Lancet.* 1997 May 3; 349(9061): 1306. BE56187.
accountability; *decision making; disclosure; economics; health care; patient care; *patient participation; *patient satisfaction; patients; *physician patient relationship; resource allocation; treatment outcome; Great Britain; National Health Service

Mitchinson, Wendy. Agency, diversity, and constraints: women and their physicians, Canada, 1850–1950. *In:* Sherwin, Susan, et al. The Politics of Women's Health: Exploring Agency and Autonomy. Philadelphia, PA: Temple University Press; 1998: 122–149. 43 fn. ISBN 1–56639–633–6. BE58396.
abortion, induced; attitudes; cesarean section; childbirth; contraception; decision making; *females; *historical aspects;

hospitals; human body; interprofessional relations; males; medicine; moral complicity; mortality; nurse midwives; obstetrics and gynecology; *physician patient relationship; physicians; pregnant women; *reproduction; social dominance; women's health services; women's rights; menopause; *Canada; *Nineteenth Century; *Twentieth Century

Moreno, Jonathan D.; Lucente, Frank E. Patients who are family members, friends, colleagues, family members of colleagues. *In:* McCullough, Laurence B.; Jones, James W.; Brody, Baruch A., eds. Surgical Ethics. New York, NY: Oxford University Press; 1998: 198–215. 15 refs. ISBN 0–19–510347–5. BE58335.
codes of ethics; communication; confidentiality; empirical research; *family members; friends; health insurance reimbursement; historical aspects; informed consent; *interprofessional relations; legal aspects; *medical ethics; *medical etiquette; medical fees; medical specialties; organizational policies; *patient care; *physician patient relationship; *physicians; *professional family relationship; professional organizations; review; *surgery; technical expertise; professional courtesy; American Medical Association; Hippocratic Oath; United States

Morreim, E. Haavi. Revenue streams and clinical discretion. *Journal of the American Geriatrics Society.* 1998 Mar; 46(3): 331–337. 96 refs. Paper presented at the 1996 Congress of Clinical Societies. BE56768.
communication; costs and benefits; *decision making; *economics; employment; health care delivery; health insurance; incentives; industry; interprofessional relations; *managed care programs; organization and administration; patient care; patient care team; patients; *physician patient relationship; *physicians; practice guidelines; *professional autonomy; risk; social impact; time factors; trust; capitation fee; continuity of patient care; *physician's practice patterns; utilization review; United States

Moseley, Kathryn L.; Truesdell, Sandra. A noncompliant patient? [Case study]. *Journal of Clinical Ethics.* 1997 Summer; 8(2): 176–177. Commented on by P.R. Muskin, p. 178–180. BE56351.
case studies; chronically ill; competence; diabetes; ethics consultation; females; food; insulin; patient care; *patient compliance; *patient discharge; *physician patient relationship; psychology; *treatment refusal; trust; self care

Muskin, Philip R. Care, support, and concern for noncompliant patients. *Journal of Clinical Ethics.* 1997 Summer; 8(2): 178–180. 3 fn. Commentary on K.L. Moseley and S. Truesdell, p. 176–177. BE56350.
age factors; autonomy; case studies; chronically ill; communication; competence; diabetes; family relationship; females; food; insulin; motivation; *patient compliance; *physician patient relationship; psychiatry; referral and consultation; *treatment refusal; self care

Nortvedt, Per. Sensitive judgement: an inquiry into the foundations of nursing ethics. *Nursing Ethics.* 1998 Sep; 5(5): 385–392. 13 refs. BE58903.
*emotions; *empathy; *nurse patient relationship; *nurses; *nursing ethics; patients; suffering; values

Overbay, Jane Dring. Parental participation in treatment decisions for pediatric oncology ICU patients. *Dimensions of Critical Care Nursing.* 1996 Jan-Feb; 15(1): 16–24. 16 refs. BE56847.
*adolescents; allowing to die; alternatives; *cancer; case studies; *children; clinical ethics committees; *communication; consent forms; critically ill; *decision making; disclosure; ethical analysis; evaluation studies; infants; *intensive care units; interprofessional relations; medical records; *nurse's role; *nurses; nursing research; *parental consent; *parents; patient advocacy; *patient care;

---

patient care team; pediatrics; physicians; *professional family relationship; prognosis; prolongation of life; psychological stress; *records; referral and consultation; risks and benefits; terminally ill; treatment outcome; treatment refusal; truth disclosure; values; withholding treatment; retrospective studies; Midwestern United States

Ozar, David T. The social obligations of health care practitioners. [Revised]. *In:* Monagle, John F.; Thomasma, David C., eds. Health Care Ethics: Issues Critical for the 21st Century. Gaithersburg, MD: Aspen Publishers; 1998: 378–391. 24 refs. ISBN 0–8342–0911–X. BE56292.
    conflict of interest; contracts; disclosure; economics; freedom; *health care; human rights; libertarianism; *managed care programs; medical ethics; *moral obligations; *obligations to society; organ transplantation; *patient advocacy; *physician patient relationship; *physician's role; *physicians; public policy; resource allocation; selection for treatment; self regulation; social impact; standards; technical expertise; utilitarianism; values; withholding treatment; Golden Rule; Locke, John; Rawls, John; United States

Ozar, David T. Three models of professionalism and professional obligation in dentistry. *Journal of the American Dental Association.* 1985 Feb; 110(2): 173–177. 4 refs. BE57834.
    autonomy; decision making; *dentistry; economics; education; entrepreneurship; *interprofessional relations; *models, theoretical; moral obligations; obligations to society; professional ethics; professional organizations; *professional patient relationship; technical expertise; *professional role

Parens, Erik. What differences make a difference? [Editorial]. *Cambridge Quarterly of Healthcare Ethics.* 1998 Winter; 7(1): 1–6. BE58486.
    advance directives; bioethical issues; *clinical ethics; consensus; *cultural pluralism; decision making; *disabled; dissent; empirical research; health care delivery; health personnel; justice; *minority groups; patient care; *professional patient relationship; religion; self concept; sexuality; *socioeconomic factors; stigmatization; terminal care; *values

Pellegrino, Edmund D. Managed care at the bedside: how do we look in the moral mirror? *Kennedy Institute of Ethics Journal.* 1997 Dec; 7(4): 321–330. 14 refs. BE59013.
    beneficence; biomedical technologies; *conflict of interest; contracts; disclosure; *economics; employment; gatekeeping; *managed care programs; *moral obligations; obligations to society; patient advocacy; patient care; *physician patient relationship; physician's role; *physicians; professional competence; quality of health care; *resource allocation; sociology of medicine; technical expertise; vulnerable populations; withholding treatment; continuity of patient care; gag clauses; *United States
Managed care per se is a morally neutral concept; however, as practiced today, it raises serious ethical issues at the clinical, managerial, and social levels. This essay focuses on the ethical issues that arise at the bedside, looking first at the ethical conflicts faced by the physician who is charged with responsibility for care of the patient and then turning to the way in which managed care exacts costs that are measured not in dollars but in compromises in the caring dimensions of the patient–physician relationship.

Penticuff, Joy Hinson. Nursing perspectives in bioethics. *In:* Hoshino, Kazumasa, ed. Japanese and Western Bioethics: Studies in Moral Diversity. Boston, MA: Kluwer Academic; 1997: 49–60. 30 refs. ISBN 0–7923–4112–0. BE57082.

biomedical technologies; *caring; goals; institutional policies; international aspects; moral obligations; narrative ethics; *nurse patient relationship; nurses; *nursing ethics; principle–based ethics; professional autonomy; professional competence; psychological stress; values; United States

Peppin, Patricia. Power and disadvantage in medical relationships. *Texas Journal of Women and the Law.* 1994 Spring; 3(2): 221–263. 233 fn. BE56664.
    aged; autonomy; biomedical research; coercion; decision making; disadvantaged; drugs; equal protection; *females; *feminist ethics; human experimentation; informed consent; *legal aspects; legal liability; legal rights; *males; medicine; metaphor; misconduct; paternalism; patient care; patient participation; *physician patient relationship; physicians; reproductive technologies; resource allocation; risks and benefits; sex offenses; social discrimination; *social dominance; social interaction; sociology of medicine; Supreme Court decisions; torts; vulnerable populations; women's health; *women's rights; *Canada; Canadian Charter of Rights and Freedoms; Norberg v. Wynrib

Pickering, Neil. Imaginary restrictions. *Journal of Medical Ethics.* 1998 Jun; 24(3): 171–175. 7 fn. Commentary on R. Gillon, "Imagination, literature, medical ethics and medical practice," *JME,* 1997 Feb; 23(1): 3–4. BE59119.
    bioethics; case studies; empathy; ethical theory; *literature; *medical education; *medical ethics; *moral development; narrative ethics; philosophy; *physician patient relationship; *teaching methods
The role of literature and imagination in medicine and medical ethics is currently under discussion. This paper argues that the role of literature is not to furnish generalisable examples for guidance. Rather, engagement with literature parallels moral engagement with other people. The work of the imagination, in this context, is not to hypothesise, but to grant life to the characters and world of literature. In doing this, one may develop one's moral life.

Poulson, Jane. Bitter pills to swallow. *New England Journal of Medicine.* 1998 Jun 18; 338(25): 1844–1846. BE58615.
    attitudes; cancer; *communication; drugs; emotions; empathy; human experimentation; medical education; *patients; *physician patient relationship; *physicians; *psychological stress; psychology; selection of subjects; suffering; time factors; toxicity; *truth disclosure; *seriously ill; *sick role

Putnam, Constance E. Who talks? Who listens? Who decides? Doctors and patients in discourse. *In:* van Eemeren, Frans H.; Grootendorst, Rob; Blair, J. Anthony; Willard, Charles A., eds. Special Fields and Cases: Proceedings of the Third ISSA [International Society for the Study of Argumentation] Conference on Argumentation, Volume IV. Amsterdam: International Centre for the Study of Argumentation; 1995: 412–423. 5 refs. Conference held 21–24 Jun 1994 at the University of Amsterdam. ISBN 90–74049–02–8. BE56683.
    attitudes; autonomy; caring; *communication; *decision making; diagnosis; goals; informed consent; models, theoretical; paternalism; patient care; *patient participation; *patient satisfaction; *physician patient relationship; *physician's role; professional competence; social dominance; survey; technical expertise; trust; values

Roman, Brenda; Kay, Jerald. Residency education on the prevention of physician–patient sexual misconduct. *Academic Psychiatry.* 1997 Spring; 21(1): 26–34. 34 refs. BE58123.
    curriculum; *internship and residency; *medical education; *misconduct; *physician patient relationship; *psychiatry; *psychotherapy; *sexuality; teaching methods

---

BE = bioethics accession number   fn. = footnotes   refs. = references

Ross, Lena B.; Roy, Manisha, eds. Cast the First Stone: Ethics in Analytic Practice. Wilmette, IL: Chiron Publications; 1995. 146 p. Includes references. ISBN 0-933029-89-6. BE58319.
   emotions; females; *health personnel; love; males; *misconduct; morality; *professional ethics; *professional patient relationship; psychology; *psychotherapy; self concept; self regulation; *sexuality; values; Jung, Carl

Rushton, Cindy Hylton; Armstrong, Linda; McEnhill, Marilyn. Establishing therapeutic boundaries as patient advocates. *Pediatric Nursing.* 1996 May–Jun; 22(3): 185–189. 16 refs. BE55525.
   case studies; *children; emotions; friends; misconduct; *nurse patient relationship; *nurses; parents; paternalism; *patient advocacy; pediatrics; professional family relationship; self regulation; social interaction; standards; empowerment

Schiedermayer, David. Holding Owen. *Journal of Clinical Ethics.* 1997 Winter; 8(4): 349–352. 1 fn. BE57613.
   aged; *patient care; patients; *physician patient relationship; physicians; professional competence; referral and consultation; technical expertise; truth disclosure; medical errors

Shaha, Maya. Racism and its implications in ethical–moral reasoning in nursing practice: a tentative approach to a largely unexplored topic. *Nursing Ethics.* 1998 Mar; 5(2): 139–146. 22 refs. BE58476.
   attitudes; cultural pluralism; empirical research; hospitals; *minority groups; *nurse patient relationship; *nurses; nursing research; patient advocacy; patient care; *patients; *social discrimination; stigmatization

Sledge, William H.; Feinstein, Alvan R. A clinimetric approach to the components of the patient–physician relationship. *JAMA.* 1997 Dec 17; 278(23): 2043–2048. 27 refs. BE56439.
   attitudes; chronically ill; *communication; *emotions; goals; mental health; models, theoretical; *patient care; patient compliance; patient participation; *patient satisfaction; *patients; *physician patient relationship; *physicians; psychological stress; *psychology; social interaction; socioeconomic factors; sick role; United States
Although patient–physician relationships have been expressed with diverse concepts and models, we have formulated a clinimetric classification derived from several years of observation and discussions at weekly house–staff conferences devoted to "difficult" patients. The observed phenomena are classified into the following components: (1) background factors intrinsic to patient and physician before they meet, (2) individual anticipations and hopes for what may happen, (3) extrinsic features of the setting, (4) individual reactions during the encounter, and (5) the consequences thereafter. These interacting components are usually too complex for characterizations based on single models for the relationship or single titles (such as "hateful" or "noncompliant") for the patient. The components can serve as a "review of systems" for identifying manifestations, sources, and solutions to such common problems as discordant hopes, the physician's unawareness of the patient's pertinent extramedical status, psychiatric and mental–status challenges, and cogent factors in chronic illness.

Smith, Sam. Postmodernity and a hypertensive patient: rescuing value from nihilism. *Journal of Medical Ethics.* 1998 Feb; 24(1): 25–31. 19 refs. BE57410.
   case studies; drugs; emotions; *hypertension; *medicine; *patient care; patient compliance; *philosophy; *physician patient relationship; practice guidelines; preventive medicine; values; *postmodernism

Much of postmodern philosophy questions the assumptions of Modernity, that period in the history of the Western world since the Enlightment. These assumptions are that truth is discoverable through human reason; that certain knowledge is possible; and furthermore, that such knowledge will provide a basis for the ineluctable progress of Mankind. The Enlightenment project is underwritten by the conviction that knowledge gained through the scientific method is secure. In so far as biomedicine inherits these assumptions it becomes fair game for postmodern deconstruction. Today, perhaps more than ever, plural values compete, and contradictory approaches to health, for instance, garner support and acquire supremacy through consumer choice and media manipulation rather than evidence-based science. Many doctors feel a tension between meeting the needs of the patient face to face, and working towards the broader health needs of the public at large. But if the very foundations of medical science are questioned, by patients, or by doctors themselves, wherein lies the value of their work? This paper examines the issues that the anti–foundationalist thrust of postmodernism raises, in the light of a case of mild hypertension. The strict application of medical protocol, derived from a nomothetic, statistical perspective, seems unlikely to furnish value in the treatment of an individual. The anything goes, consumerist approach, however, fares no better. The author argues that whilst value cannot depend on any rationally predetermined parameters, it can be rescued, and emerges from the process of the meeting with the patient.

Sommers–Flanagan, Rita; Elliott, Deni; Sommers–Flanagan, John. Exploring the edges: boundaries and breaks. *Ethics and Behavior.* 1998; 8(1): 37–48. 21 refs. BE58916.
   *counseling; health personnel; misconduct; motivation; *professional patient relationship; *psychotherapy; risks and benefits; social interaction
In this article, we examine conceptual and practical issues pertaining to relationship boundaries within the helping profession. Although our focus is primarily on relationships between mental health professionals and clients, there are considerable implications for a new approach to ethically structuring and understanding the construct of "required distance" in many human–interactive professions, such as teaching, religious leadership, public administration, and others. We define the concept of boundary as applied to human relationships, provide examples of boundary breaks, and raise questions regarding how to evaluate the significance and morality issues raised by specific boundary breaks. Questions and dilemmas are presented regarding boundary setting and accidental or deliberate boundary breaking. Representative dangers present in boundary breaks are identified, and examples are provided. Possible beneficial outcomes are also discussed. Finally, a suggested protocol for assessing a proposed boundary break is provided, much of which is drawn from the work and thinking of Laura Brown, applied more generally in this article, with additions from our perspectives.

Strain, James J.; Snyder, Stephen L.; Drooker, Martin. Conflict resolution: experience of consultation–liaison psychiatrists. *In:* Zucker, Marjorie B.; Zucker, Howard D., eds. Medical Futility and the Evaluation of Life-Sustaining Interventions. New York, NY: Cambridge University Press; 1997: 98–109. 8 refs. ISBN 0-521-56877-3. BE55983.

BE = bioethics accession number   fn. = footnotes   refs. = references

*allowing to die; caring; case studies; decision making; *dissent; emotions; *family members; *futility; goals; mediation; motivation; patient care team; patient transfer; *patients; *physician patient relationship; *physicians; professional family relationship; *prolongation of life; psychiatric diagnosis; *psychiatry; psychological stress; *psychology; *referral and consultation; refusal to treat; resource allocation; retreatment; terminal care; *treatment refusal; trust; guilt; health services misuse; patient abandonment; United States

Surbone, Antonella; Zwitter, Matjaž, eds.
Communication with the Cancer Patient: Information and Truth. New York, NY: New York Academy of Sciences; 1997. 540 p. (Annals of the New York Academy of Sciences; v. 809). 928 refs. 31 fn. ISBN 0-89766-986-X. BE56518.
adolescents; adults; attitudes; bone marrow; *cancer; children; *communication; continuing education; *cultural pluralism; decision making; developing countries; diagnosis; disclosure; disease; drugs; family members; historical aspects; HIV seropositivity; human experimentation; informed consent; *international aspects; metaphor; nurse's role; palliative care; parents; patient care; patient participation; patients; *physician patient relationship; physicians; prognosis; prolongation of life; quality of life; radiology; risks and benefits; socioeconomic factors; surgery; terminally ill; tissue transplantation; treatment outcome; *truth disclosure; values; hope; non-Western World; Western World; Africa; Asia; Australia; Europe; Latin America; Middle East; North America

Surbone, Antonella. The patient-doctor-family relationship: at the core of medical ethics. *In:* Baider, Lea; Cooper, Cary L.; Kaplan De-Nour, Atara, eds. Cancer and the Family. New York, NY: Wiley; 1996: 389-405. 42 refs. ISBN 0-471-95890-5. BE58898.
autonomy; beneficence; *cancer; caring; case studies; communication; cultural pluralism; emotions; family members; informed consent; justice; medical ethics; moral obligations; patient care; *physician patient relationship; physicians; *professional family relationship; self concept; suffering; truth disclosure

Swee, David E. Health care system reform and the changing physician-patient relationship. *New Jersey Medicine.* 1995 May; 92(5): 313-317. 5 refs. BE55532.
alternatives; autonomy; beneficence; confidentiality; conflict of interest; disclosure; health insurance; health maintenance organizations; justice; *managed care programs; models, theoretical; moral obligations; paternalism; patient advocacy; patients; *physician patient relationship; physicians; privacy; professional autonomy; trends; withholding treatment; United States

Tanenbaum, Sandra J. Say the right thing: communication and physician accountability in the era of medical outcomes. *In:* Boyle, Philip J., ed. Getting Doctors to Listen: Ethics and Outcomes Data in Context. Washington, DC: Georgetown University Press; 1998: 204-223. 48 fn. ISBN 0-87840-654-9. BE57927.
*accountability; *communication; decision making; disclosure; *economics; empirical research; guidelines; *health care; health care reform; health services research; methods; narrative ethics; *patient care; *patient satisfaction; *physician patient relationship; practice guidelines; referral and consultation; regulation; risks and benefits; standards; technical expertise; *treatment outcome; uncertainty; utilization review; United States

Taylor, Susan L. Quandary at the crossroads: paternalism versus advocacy surrounding end-of-treatment decisions. *American Journal of Hospice and Palliative Care.* 1995 Jul-Aug; 12(4): 43-46. 33 fn. BE57054.
allowing to die; *autonomy; caring; *decision making; *nurse

patient relationship; *nurse's role; paternalism; *patient advocacy; *patient participation; physician nurse relationship; physician patient relationship; right to die; *terminal care; values; withholding treatment; Twentieth Century; United States

Thomasma, David C., ed. The Influence of Edmund D. Pellegrino's Philosophy of Medicine. Boston, MA: Kluwer Academic; 1997. 215 p. 561 fn. Reprinted from *Theoretical Medicine*, 18(1-2); 1997. ISBN 0-7923-4412-X. BE57642.
allowing to die; assisted suicide; *bioethical issues; *bioethics; caring; clinical ethics; communitarianism; conflict of interest; covenant; cultural pluralism; decision making; disease; economics; *ethical theory; ethicists; health; international aspects; managed care programs; medical education; *medical ethics; *medicine; nursing ethics; patient advocacy; patient care; patient participation; *philosophy; *physician patient relationship; *physician's role; primary health care; principle-based ethics; psychiatry; public policy; quality of health care; religious ethics; resource allocation; secularism; sociology of medicine; trust; values; *virtues; voluntary euthanasia; *Pellegrino, Edmund; United States

Vazquez, Ma. Suarez. Technology and human dignity. *Dolentium Hominum: Church and Health in the World.* 1996; 33(11th Yr., No. 3): 29-34. 14 refs. BE57265.
biomedical technologies; hospitals; humanism; *love; *nurse patient relationship; *nurses; *patient care; patient care team; physician patient relationship; *Roman Catholic ethics

Ventres, William; Nichter, Mark; Reed, Richard, et al. Do-not-resuscitate discussions: a qualitative analysis. *Family Practice Research Journal.* 1992; 12(2): 157-169. 34 refs. BE56902.
*attitudes; clergy; *communication; *decision making; evaluation studies; family members; family practice; *health personnel; hospitals; internship and residency; nurses; *physician patient relationship; physicians; *professional family relationship; professional patient relationship; *resuscitation orders; social workers; survey; qualitative research; University of Arizona Medical School

Ward-Collins, Diana. "Noncompliant": isn't there a better way to say it? *American Journal of Nursing.* 1998 May; 98(5): 27-31. 7 refs. BE58801.
age factors; aged; autonomy; case studies; communication; cultural pluralism; interprofessional relations; *nurse patient relationship; patient advocacy; *patient compliance; social workers; terminology; values

Wilbers, Doaitse; Willibrord, C.M.; Schultz, Weijmar, et al. Sexual contact between doctors and patients. *In:* Lens, Peter; van der Wal, Gerrit, eds. Problem Doctors: A Conspiracy of Silence. Washington, DC: IOS Press; 1997: 75-85. 47 refs. ISBN 90-5199-287-4. BE56999.
continuing education; criminal law; emotions; international aspects; mass media; medical education; medical specialties; *misconduct; organizational policies; patients; *physician patient relationship; *physicians; prevalence; professional organizations; psychotherapy; risk; self regulation; *sexuality; social dominance; time factors; American Medical Association; Canada; Europe; Great Britain; United States

Wildes, Kevin Wm.; Wallace, Robert B. Relationships with payers and institutions that manage and deliver patient services. *In:* McCullough, Laurence B.; Jones, James W.; Brody, Baruch A., eds. Surgical Ethics. New York, NY: Oxford University Press; 1998: 367-383. 18 refs. ISBN 0-19-510347-5. BE58339.
administrators; advertising; autonomy; beneficence; clinical ethics committees; *conflict of interest; disclosure; *economics; goals; *health facilities; *health insurance;

BE = bioethics accession number   fn. = footnotes   refs. = references

health insurance reimbursement; hospitals; incentives; informed consent; institutional ethics; institutional policies; *managed care programs; medical education; *moral obligations; *patient advocacy; *physician patient relationship; *physicians; practice guidelines; quality of health care; referral and consultation; remuneration; *resource allocation; *surgery; trust; withholding treatment; health services misuse; preventive ethics; undertreatment; United States

Yarborough, Mark. The reluctant retained witness: alleged sexual misconduct in the doctor/patient relationship. *Journal of Medicine and Philosophy.* 1997 Aug; 22(4): 345–364. 10 refs. BE55930.
  bioethical issues; case studies; conflict of interest; *decision making; *ethicist's role; *ethicists; *expert testimony; faculty; interprofessional relations; judicial action; *legal aspects; *misconduct; *physician patient relationship; *physicians; professional ethics; remuneration; *sexuality; *technical expertise; uncertainty; universities; Colorado
Testifying as an expert ethics witness raises a number of important issues. These include: the prospect of generating adverse publicity for oneself and one's institution, avoiding bias, giving testimony that is at odds with testimony given by colleagues, potential conflicts of interest introduced by reimbursement, the need of those who hear the testimony of bioethicists to appreciate the nature of moral expertise, the difficulty of assessing the quality of legal evidence which emerges from adversarial legal proceedings, and the need to consider what weight should be assigned to expert ethics testimony. Along with these issues, what might constitute sexual misconduct is addressed in the essay so that readers can review the decision-making of the author in two cases.

Young, Marti; Klingle, Renee Storm. Silent partners in medical care: a cross-cultural study of patient participation. *Health Communication.* 1996; 8(1): 29–53. 84 refs. BE57726.
  *Asian Americans; *communication; comparative studies; *cultural pluralism; *decision making; females; obstetrics and gynecology; *patient care; *patient compliance; *patient participation; *patient satisfaction; patients; *physician patient relationship; survey; treatment outcome; trust; values; *whites

PROLONGATION OF LIFE *See* ALLOWING TO DIE

PROXY DECISION MAKING *See* ADVANCE DIRECTIVES, ALLOWING TO DIE, INFORMED CONSENT, RESUSCITATION ORDERS

PSYCHOSURGERY

See also BEHAVIOR CONTROL

Missa, Jean-Noël. Psychosurgery and physical brain manipulation. *In:* Chadwick, Ruth, ed. Encyclopedia of Applied Ethics, Volume 3. San Diego, CA: Academic Press; 1998: 735–744. 37 refs. ISBN 0–12–227068–1. BE56267.
  electroconvulsive therapy; historical aspects; human experimentation; informed consent; investigators; mentally ill; methods; misconduct; *psychosurgery; risks and benefits; selection for treatment; trends; Europe; Twentieth Century; United States

Pressman, Jack D. Last Resort: Psychosurgery and the

Limits of Medicine. New York, NY: Cambridge University Press; 1998. 555 p. 725 fn. ISBN 0–521–35371–8. BE58548.
  behavior control; evaluation; *historical aspects; human experimentation; investigators; *knowledge, attitudes, practice; mental institutions; mentally ill; patient care; *physicians; psychiatric diagnosis; *psychiatry; *psychosurgery; review; risks and benefits; selection for treatment; *sociology of medicine; statistics; technology assessment; treatment outcome; *Twentieth Century; *United States

PUBLIC HEALTH

See also AIDS, HEALTH, HEALTH CARE, IMMUNIZATION, MASS SCREENING, OCCUPATIONAL HEALTH

Brandt, Allan M.; Rozin, Paul. Morality and Health. New York, NY: Routledge; 1997. 416 p. Includes references. ISBN 0–415–91582–1. BE55841.
  adolescents; advertising; alcohol abuse; attitudes; behavior control; childbirth; communicable diseases; cultural pluralism; disadvantaged; disease; drug abuse; food; freedom; government regulation; *health; *health promotion; historical aspects; international aspects; mass media; metaphor; *morality; nutrition; *public health; public policy; religion; secularism; *self induced illness; sexuality; single persons; smoking; social problems; socioeconomic factors; stigmatization; suffering; life style; tuberculosis; China; Great Britain; India; Nineteenth Century; Twentieth Century; United States

Brazier, Margaret; Harris, John. Public health and private lives. *Medical Law Review.* 1996 Summer; 4(2): 171–192. 62 fn. BE56484.
  AIDS; autonomy; *coercion; *communicable diseases; confidentiality; *criminal law; dangerousness; freedom; HIV seropositivity; *legal aspects; *legal liability; legislation; mandatory reporting; moral obligations; obligations to society; *patients; privacy; *public health; quarantine; sexually transmitted diseases; *Great Britain; *Public Health (Control of Diseases) Act 1984 (Great Britain)

Burr, Chandler. The AIDS exception: privacy vs. public health. *Atlantic Monthly.* 1997 June; 279(6): 57–67. BE57989.
  *AIDS; AIDS serodiagnosis; anonymous testing; blood donation; *confidentiality; contact tracing; counseling; drugs; epidemiology; federal government; historical aspects; *HIV seropositivity; homosexuals; informed consent; *legal rights; mandatory reporting; mandatory testing; newborns; patient care; patients; *political activity; pregnant women; *privacy; *public health; *public policy; sexually transmitted diseases; social discrimination; state government; stigmatization; voluntary programs; Americans with Disabilities Act 1990; Centers for Disease Control and Prevention; United States

Burris, Scott; Gostin, Lawrence O. Genetic screening from a public health perspective: some lessons from the HIV experience. *In:* Rothstein, Mark A., ed. Genetic Secrets: Protecting Privacy and Confidentiality in the Genetic Era. New Haven, CT: Yale University Press; 1997: 137–158. 57 fn. ISBN 0–300–07251–1. BE58680.
  adults; AIDS serodiagnosis; costs and benefits; DNA data banks; epidemiology; *genetic information; genetic research; *genetic screening; *government regulation; guidelines; HIV seropositivity; informed consent; justice; legal aspects; mandatory reporting; mandatory testing; mass screening; moral policy; newborns; *privacy; *public health; *public policy; resource allocation; risks and benefits; social discrimination; socioeconomic factors; stigmatization; biological specimen banks; United States

---

BE = bioethics accession number   fn. = footnotes   refs. = references

Coughlin, Steven S.; Soskolne, Colin L.; Goodman, Kenneth W. Case Studies in Public Health Ethics. Washington, DC: American Public Health Association; 1997. 180 p. Includes references and instructor's guide. ISBN 0–87553–232–2. BE58580.

> AIDS serodiagnosis; authorship; biomedical research; cancer; *case studies; confidentiality; conflict of interest; cultural pluralism; disclosure; drug abuse; epidemiology; ethical analysis; ethical theory; faculty; financial support; genetic screening; health hazards; HIV seropositivity; human experimentation; information dissemination; informed consent; international aspects; *investigators; law enforcement; privacy; *professional ethics; property rights; *public health; random selection; research design; research ethics committees; resource allocation; scientific misconduct; social discrimination; socioeconomic factors; vulnerable populations; United States

Coughlin, Steven S. Ethics in Epidemiology and Public Health Practice: Collected Works. Columbus, GA: Quill Publications; 1997. 232 p. Includes references. ISBN 0–9661520–0–X. BE58542.

> American Indians; autonomy; beneficence; biomedical research; cancer; case studies; confidentiality; control groups; curriculum; ecology; education; *epidemiology; ethical theory; ethics committees; federal government; females; government regulation; health hazards; health personnel; HIV seropositivity; human experimentation; informed consent; international aspects; investigators; justice; *preventive medicine; *professional ethics; professional organizations; *public health; random selection; research design; research ethics committees; risks and benefits; scientific misconduct; selection of subjects; self regulation; socioeconomic factors; violence; vulnerable populations; professional role; Tuskegee Syphilis Study; United States

Davis, Michael. Arresting the white death: preventive detention, confinement for treatment, and medical ethics. *American Philosophical Association Newsletter on Philosophy and Medicine.* 1995 Spring; 94(2): 92–98. 35 fn. BE57261.

> coercion; *communicable diseases; dangerousness; government regulation; *mandatory programs; moral policy; municipal government; patient care; patient compliance; prisoners; *public health; *public policy; punishment; *quarantine; treatment refusal; *tuberculosis; New York City; United States

Gillon, Raanan. Doctors should not try to ban boxing -- but boxing's own ethics suggests reform. [Editorial]. *Journal of Medical Ethics.* 1998 Feb; 24(1): 3–4. 2 refs. BE57406.

> alternatives; autonomy; brain pathology; criminal law; government regulation; legal aspects; *organizational policies; paternalism; *physicians; preventive medicine; professional organizations; risk; *sports medicine; *British Medical Association; Great Britain

Illingworth, Patricia. Warning: AIDS health promotion programs may be hazardous to your autonomy. *In:* Overall, Christine and Zion, William P., eds. Perspectives on AIDS: Ethical and Social Issues. New York, NY: Oxford University Press; 1991: 138–154. 39 fn. ISBN 0–19–540749–0. BE58292.

> *AIDS; attitudes; *autonomy; *behavior control; *coercion; common good; drug abuse; *health education; *health promotion; HIV seropositivity; *information dissemination; methods; motivation; operant conditioning; preventive medicine; *public health; public policy; self concept; sexuality; social discrimination; social impact; Canada

Josefson, Deborah. US journal embroiled in another conflict of interest scandal. [News]. *BMJ (British Medical Journal).* 1998 Jan 24; 316(7127): 251. BE58120.

> authorship; cancer; *conflict of interest; *disclosure; *ecology; *editorial policies; employment; epidemiology; *health hazards; *industry; misconduct; *physicians; public health; *Berke, Jerry; Living Downstream: An Ecologist Looks at Cancer and the Environment (Steingraber, S.); *New England Journal of Medicine

Lupton, Deborah. The Imperative of Health: Public Health and the Regulated Body. Thousand Oaks, CA: Sage Publications; 1995. 181 p. Bibliography: p. 162–175. ISBN 0–8039–7936–3. BE56130.

> advertising; autonomy; *behavior control; diagnosis; freedom; health; health education; *health promotion; HIV seropositivity; mass media; mass screening; *public health; public policy; risk; self induced illness; *social control; social dominance; social sciences; uncertainty

Mindes, Paula. Tuberculosis quarantine: a review of legal issues in Ohio and other states. [Note]. *Journal of Law and Health.* 1995–1996; 10(2): 403–428. 160 fn. BE57147.

> *communicable diseases; due process; federal government; government regulation; historical aspects; involuntary commitment; *legal aspects; legal rights; *public health; *public policy; *quarantine; social discrimination; socioeconomic factors; state government; *tuberculosis; *Ohio; *United States

Morone, James A. Enemies of the people: the moral dimension to public health. *Journal of Health Politics, Policy and Law.* 1997 Aug; 22(4): 993–1020. 92 refs. 10 fn. BE57160.

> alcohol abuse; autonomy; blacks; communitarianism; criminal law; drug abuse; health care reform; historical aspects; indigents; law enforcement; mass media; minority groups; *morality; obligations of society; *politics; privacy; Protestant ethics; *public health; *public policy; review; rights; self concept; sexually transmitted diseases; *social control; *social discrimination; *social problems; *socioeconomic factors; *stigmatization; *values; liberalism; Eighteenth Century; Nineteenth Century; Twentieth Century; *United States

This essay explores the effects of morality on health policy. Moral images and stereotypes, I argue, have powerful political consequences. They are the differences between fighting poverty and fearing the poor, between expanding social welfare programs and cracking down on crime, between public health campaigns and drug wars. I begin by locating morality within traditional paradigms of American politics (which are designed to overlook the issue); I then suggest how moral stigmas are constructed; show how they are deployed in debates over public health issues, such as alcohol abuse and drug addiction; and briefly sketch an alternative approach to defining community and seeking public health.

Nikku, Nina; Eriksson, Bengt Erik. Preventive medicine. *In:* Chadwick, Ruth, ed. Encyclopedia of Applied Ethics, Volume 3. San Diego, CA: Academic Press; 1998: 643–648. 7 refs. ISBN 0–12–227068–1. BE56262.

> autonomy; behavior control; genetic information; health education; *health promotion; informed consent; mass screening; paternalism; *preventive medicine; *public health; risks and benefits; selection for treatment; self induced illness; social control; socioeconomic factors

Oscherwitz, Tom; Tulsky, Jacqueline Peterson; Roger, Steve, et al. Detention of persistently nonadherent patients with tuberculosis. *JAMA.* 1997 Sep 10; 278(10): 843–846. 13 refs. BE55887.

> *coercion; *communicable diseases; *criminal law; disadvantaged; drug abuse; government regulation; institutionalized persons; males; *mandatory programs;

mentally ill; minority groups; patient care; *patient compliance; prisoners; *public health; *public policy; quarantine; social control; socioeconomic factors; state government; time factors; treatment outcome; treatment refusal; *tuberculosis; California

CONTEXT: Patients with tuberculosis (TB) who are persistently nonadherent to treatment present a public health risk. In 1993, California created a new civil detention process and allowed detention of noninfectious but persistently nonadherent patients. OBJECTIVES: To determine (1) which patients TB controllers attempt to detain, (2) how often and where patients are detained, and (3) how many of these patients complete TB treatment. DESIGN: Case series with cross-sectional comparison to other adult TB patients in the study counties. SETTING: Twelve California counties with the largest number of new TB cases reported in 1994. SUBJECTS: All patients whom TB controllers sought to detain during 1994 and 1995 because of persistent nonadherence to treatment. DATA SOURCES: Public health records, interviews with county TB officials, and Reports of Verified Cases of Tuberculosis to the California Tuberculosis Control Branch. RESULTS: Tuberculosis controllers sought the civil detention or arrest of 67 patients during the study period (1.3% of adult TB patients with the same disease sites). Forty-six percent of these patients were homeless, 81% had drug or alcohol abuse, and 28% had mental illness. Tuberculosis controllers sought civil detention of 15 patients. Fourteen patients were detained (median length of detention, 14.5 days). Tuberculosis controllers sought to arrest 62 patients during the study period. Fifty-three patients were arrested (median time in jail, 83 days). In 10 cases, both civil and criminal detention were attempted. We analyzed completion of therapy after excluding patients who were not detained or who died or moved. Overall, 41 (84%) of the remaining 49 detained patients completed therapy. Of the patients who completed therapy, only 17 were detained until treatment was completed. Compared with other TB patients in these counties, detained patients had 4 times the proportion lost to follow-up and half the proportion completing therapy within 12 months. CONCLUSION: Further improvements in the care of persistently nonadherent patients may require more psychosocial services, appropriate facilities for civil detention, and detaining patients long enough to assure completion of treatment.

Reichman, Lee B. Defending the public's health against tuberculosis. [Editorial]. *JAMA.* 1997 Sep 10; 278(10): 865–867. 26 refs. BE55893.
coercion; *communicable diseases; criminal law; drugs; federal government; government financing; historical aspects; institutionalized persons; *mandatory programs; municipal government; patient care; *patient compliance; prevalence; prisoners; *public health; *public policy; quarantine; social control; treatment outcome; *tuberculosis; United States

Rom, Mark Carl. Fatal Extraction: The Story Behind the Florida Dentist Accused of Infecting His Patients with HIV and Poisoning Public Health. San Francisco, CA: Jossey-Bass Publishers; 1997. 226 p. 443 fn. ISBN 0-7879-0991-2. BE57924.
*AIDS; AIDS serodiagnosis; confidentiality; decision making; *dentistry; disclosure; family members; federal government; guidelines; *health personnel; *HIV seropositivity; *iatrogenic disease; *investigators; judicial action; legal aspects; mandatory testing; mass media; patient care; *patients; political activity; politics; professional competence; *public health; public policy; state government; trust; voluntary programs; infection control; retrospective

studies; *Acer, David; *Bergalis, Kimberly; *Centers for Disease Control and Prevention; Florida; United States

Rosner, Fred. Involuntary confinement for tuberculosis control: the Jewish view. *Mount Sinai Journal of Medicine.* 1996 Jan; 63(1): 44–48. 27 refs. BE56478.
coercion; common good; *communicable diseases; future generations; health; health facilities; incentives; *Jewish ethics; *moral obligations; obligations of society; obligations to society; *patient compliance; *public health; punishment; *quarantine; rights; socioeconomic factors; treatment refusal; value of life; *tuberculosis; United States

Schmidt, Terri A. When public health competes with individual needs. *Academic Emergency Medicine.* 1995 Mar; 2(3): 217–222. 31 refs. BE55528.
alcohol abuse; aliens; alternatives; case studies; *coercion; *communicable diseases; community services; drugs; guidelines; historical aspects; hospitals; immunization; patient care; *patient compliance; *public health; quality of life; quarantine; risk; homeless persons; *tuberculosis; Centers for Disease Control and Prevention; United States

Stryker, Jeff. Ethical issues in public health policy toward HIV disease. *In:* Cohen, P.T.; Sande, Merle A.; Volberding, Paul A., eds. The AIDS Knowledge Base: A Textbook on HIV Disease from the University of California, San Francisco, and the San Francisco General Hospital. Second Edition. Boston, MA: Little, Brown; 1994: 11.6-1 to 11.6-4. 17 refs. ISBN 0-316-77067-1. BE56644.
*AIDS; AIDS serodiagnosis; confidentiality; contact tracing; duty to warn; employment; *HIV seropositivity; mandatory reporting; moral obligations; physicians; *public health; *public policy; quarantine; risks and benefits; schools; social discrimination; United States

Warburton, Nigel. Freedom to box. *Journal of Medical Ethics.* 1998 Feb; 24(1): 56–60. 12 fn. BE57411.
adolescents; adults; *brain pathology; children; *criminal law; freedom; *government regulation; informed consent; injuries; intention; morality; *organizational policies; *paternalism; *physicians; preventive medicine; professional organizations; risk; *sports medicine; liberalism; *British Medical Association; *Great Britain

The British Medical Association wants to criminalise all boxing. This article examines the logic of the arguments it uses and finds them wanting. The move from medical evidence about the risk of brain damage to the conclusion that boxing should be banned is not warranted. The BMA's arguments are a combination of inconsistent paternalism and legal moralism. Consistent application of the principles implicit in the BMA's arguments would lead to absurd consequences and to severe limitations being put on individual freedom.

Whiteis, David G. Unhealthy cities: corporate medicine, community economic underdevelopment, and public health. *International Journal of Health Services.* 1997; 27(2): 227–242. 69 refs. BE56016.
community services; *economics; financial support; government financing; *health care delivery; health care reform; *indigents; *industry; minority groups; politics; *private sector; proprietary health facilities; *public health; *public policy; public sector; *resource allocation; *social impact; *socioeconomic factors; *trends; *urban population; *United States

RANDOM SELECTION *See* HUMAN EXPERIMENTATION/RESEARCH DESIGN

RATIONING OF HEALTH CARE *See* RESOURCE

BE = bioethics accession number   fn. = footnotes   refs. = references

ALLOCATION, SELECTION FOR
TREATMENT

RECOMBINANT DNA RESEARCH

See also GENE THERAPY, GENETIC
INTERVENTION, GENETIC RESEARCH,
PATENTING LIFE FORMS

Berg, Paul; Singer, Maxine. The recombinant DNA
controversy: twenty years later. *Bio/Technology.* 1995
Oct; 13(10): 1132–1134. 6 refs. BE57578.
 genetic intervention; genetic research; government
regulation; guidelines; investigators; public participation;
public policy; *recombinant DNA research; *risks and
benefits; self regulation; transgenic organisms; Asilomar
Conference

Dobson, Andrew. Genetic engineering and environmental
ethics. *Cambridge Quarterly of Healthcare Ethics.* 1997
Spring; 6(2): 205–221. 69 fn. BE56426.
 animal rights; communitarianism; *ecology; economics;
genetic identity; *genetic intervention; industry; justice;
microbiology; moral obligations; *moral policy; patents;
public participation; public policy; *recombinant DNA
research; regulation; review; rights; risks and benefits;
*speciesism; *transgenic animals; *transgenic organisms;
utilitarianism; *values; agriculture; *environmental ethics;
transgenic plants
 I shall be saying something about the ethical dilemmas
raised by genetic engineering in both these contexts —
that is to say, human and animal. But the bulk of what
I have to say refers to a field that covers both humans
and animals but extends beyond them — the field of
environmental ethics....

Eisenberg, Rebecca S. Proprietary rights and the norms
of science in biotechnology research. *Yale Law Journal.*
1987 Dec; 97(2): 177–231. 261 fn. BE56488.
 AIDS; *biomedical research; confidentiality; disclosure;
editorial policies; federal government; financial support;
government financing; incentives; industry; *information
dissemination; investigators; *legal aspects; methods;
microbiology; *patents; *property rights; *recombinant
DNA research; *science; state government; Supreme Court
decisions; transgenic organisms; universities; *values;
Diamond v. Chakrabarty; Uniform Trade Secrets Act;
*United States

Laurie, Graeme T. Biotechnology and intellectual
property: a marriage of inconvenience? *In:* McLean,
Sheila A.M., ed. Contemporary Issues in Law, Medicine
and Ethics. Brookfield, VT: Dartmouth; 1996: 237–267.
151 fn. ISBN 1-85521-586-1. BE57798.
 *biomedical research; biomedical technologies; body parts
and fluids; DNA sequences; donors; genome mapping;
guidelines; human body; *industry; informed consent;
international aspects; investigators; *legal aspects; *morality;
*patents; property rights; *recombinant DNA research;
standards; Supreme Court decisions; tissue donation;
transgenic animals; cell lines; Diamond v. Chakrabarty;
*Europe; European Patent Convention; European Patent
Office; *Great Britain; Moore v. Regents of the University
of California; National Institutes of Health; Patent and
Trademark Office; *United States

Reiss, Michael. Biotechnology. *In:* Chadwick, Ruth, ed.
Encyclopedia of Applied Ethics, Volume 1. San Diego,
CA: Academic Press; 1998: 319–333. 10 refs. ISBN
0-12-227066-5. BE56370.
 animal experimentation; animal rights; *biomedical
technologies; drugs; ecology; food; *gene therapy; genetic
enhancement; *genetic intervention; genetic materials; germ

cells; growth disorders; historical aspects; hormones;
international aspects; methods; moral policy; patents;
*recombinant DNA research; reproductive technologies;
risk; *risks and benefits; suffering; terminology; *transgenic
animals; *transgenic organisms; agriculture

Robb, J. Wesley. Reflections: ethics and the recombinant
DNA debate. *Journal of Craniofacial Genetics and
Developmental Biology.* 1982; 2(1): 51–63. 27 refs.
BE57497.
 conflict of interest; ethical analysis; freedom; genetic
intervention; government regulation; human
experimentation; *industry; information dissemination;
investigators; public policy; *recombinant DNA research;
*risks and benefits; social control; universities; United States

Sherry, Stephen F. The incentive of patents. *In:* Kilner,
John F.; Pentz, Rebecca D.; Young, Frank E., eds.
Genetic Ethics: Do the Ends Justify the Genes? Grand
Rapids, MI: W.B. Eerdmans; 1997: 113–123. 36 fn. ISBN
0-8028-4428-6. BE56719.
 *Christian ethics; commodification; economics; hybrids;
incentives; industry; legal aspects; microbiology; moral
policy; *patents; public policy; *recombinant DNA research;
regulation; Supreme Court decisions; *transgenic organisms;
Diamond v. Chakrabarty; United States

Singer, Maxine F. Genetics and the law: a scientist's view.
Yale Law and Policy Review. 1985 Spring; 3(2): 315–335.
44 fn. BE56497.
 biological warfare; clergy; education; evolution; federal
government; *genetic intervention; *genetic research;
*genetics; germ cells; government regulation;
*interdisciplinary communication; investigators; *law;
*lawyers; legal aspects; *political activity; political systems;
professional competence; public policy; *recombinant DNA
research; *risks and benefits; *science; self regulation;
technical expertise; transgenic organisms; agriculture;
Lysenko, T.D.; Rifkin, Jeremy; *United States; USSR

Wright, Susan; Sinsheimer, Robert L. Recombinant
DNA and biological warfare. *Bulletin of the Atomic
Scientists.* 1983 Nov; 39(9): 20–26. 35 fn. BE57498.
 *biological warfare; federal government; international
aspects; *recombinant DNA research; Biological Weapons
Convention; Department of Defense; *United States

RECOMBINANT DNA
RESEARCH/REGULATION

California. Berkeley. Hazardous biological research.
Berkeley Municipal Code. 1977 Oct 21 (date effective).
12.30.010 to 12.30.0100. BE57699.
 containment; *government regulation; guidelines; municipal
government; *recombinant DNA research; *Berkeley (CA);
California; NIH Guidelines

Gore, Albert; Owens, Steve. The challenge of
biotechnology. *Yale Law and Policy Review.* 1985 Spring;
3(2): 336–357. 88 fn. BE56491.
 advisory committees; ecology; federal government; gene
therapy; *genetic intervention; germ cells; *government
regulation; guidelines; historical aspects; industry;
investigators; *public policy; *recombinant DNA research;
*risks and benefits; self regulation; transgenic organisms;
Asilomar Conference; Department of Agriculture;
Environmental Protection Agency; National Institutes of
Health; NIH Guidelines; Recombinant DNA Advisory
Committee; Twentieth Century; U.S. Congress; *United
States

MacKenzie, Debora. Genes sans frontiéres. *New Scientist.*
1997 Mar 1; 153(2071): 50. BE55588.
 ecology; genes; government regulation; human

BE = bioethics accession number   fn. = footnotes   refs. = references

experimentation; immunization; *international aspects; microbiology; *recombinant DNA research; *regulation; *transgenic organisms; DNA; transgenic plants; Europe; *European Union; United States

Parrott, Robert H., et al.; American Academy of Pediatrics. Council on Research. Proposed guidelines on genetic engineering. *Pediatrics.* 1985 Jun; 75(6): 1159. BE56676.
federal government; genetic disorders; *genetic intervention; genetic research; germ cells; *government regulation; *guidelines; *organizational policies; pediatrics; physicians; professional organizations; public policy; *recombinant DNA research; risks and benefits; *American Academy of Pediatrics; National Institutes of Health; United States

U.S. National Institutes of Health. Guidelines for research involving recombinant DNA molecules. *Federal Register.* 1983 Jun 1; 48(106): 24556–24581. 20 fn. BE57587.
accountability; advisory committees; *containment; ecology; federal government; *government regulation; *guidelines; *recombinant DNA research; National Institutes of Health; *NIH Guidelines; Recombinant DNA Advisory Committee; *United States

Referendum's challenge to transgenic research [Switzerland]. [Editorial]. *Nature.* 1997 Sep 11; 389(6647): 103. BE56477.
*government regulation; industry; information dissemination; investigators; *legislation; mass media; morality; public opinion; *public participation; *recombinant DNA research; risks and benefits; social control; *transgenic animals; *Switzerland

REFUSAL OF TREATMENT *See* TREATMENT REFUSAL

REFUSAL TO TREAT *See* AIDS/HEALTH PERSONNEL, SELECTION FOR TREATMENT

REGULATION
See under
BEHAVIORAL RESEARCH/REGULATION
HUMAN EXPERIMENTATION/REGULATION
RECOMBINANT DNA
RESEARCH/REGULATION

RELIGIOUS ASPECTS
See under
ABORTION/RELIGIOUS ASPECTS
ALLOWING TO DIE/RELIGIOUS ASPECTS
EUTHANASIA/RELIGIOUS ASPECTS

RENAL DIALYSIS *See* BIOMEDICAL TECHNOLOGIES, RESOURCE ALLOCATION/BIOMEDICAL TECHNOLOGIES

REPRODUCTION

See also ABORTION, CONTRACEPTION, FETUSES, PRENATAL DIAGNOSIS, PRENATAL INJURIES, REPRODUCTIVE TECHNOLOGIES, STERILIZATION, WRONGFUL LIFE

Alcalá, Maria José; Family Care International.

Commitments to Sexual and Reproductive Health and Rights for All: Framework for Action. New York, NY: Family Care International; 1995. 64 p. 3 fn. Based on relevant international agreements and conventions, including the Beijing, Copenhagen, Cairo, and Vienna conferences. BE56148.
abortion, induced; adolescents; AIDS; autonomy; biomedical research; children; family planning; females; goals; *health; health care; health education; health services research; *human rights; indigents; *international aspects; justice; legal aspects; males; pregnant women; *public policy; quality of health care; regulation; *reproduction; resource allocation; *sexuality; sexually transmitted diseases; social discrimination; socioeconomic factors; standards; violence; voluntary programs; *women's health; *women's health services; *women's rights; *health planning; United Nations

Allmers, Henning; Kenwright, Simon. Ethics of cloning. [Letters]. *Lancet.* 1997 May 10; 349(9062): 1401. 1 ref. BE56851.
bone marrow; cadavers; *cloning; cryopreservation; decision making; *directed donation; leukemia; motivation; *organ donation; parents; regulation; *reproduction; siblings; time factors; *tissue donation; transplant recipients; Ayala, Anissa; Ayala, Marissa; Great Britain; United States

Andrews, Lori B. Mom, Dad, clone: implications for reproductive privacy. *Cambridge Quarterly of Healthcare Ethics.* 1998 Spring; 7(2): 176–186. 71 fn. BE58004.
children; *cloning; constitutional law; genetic determinism; genetic identity; genetic information; genetic screening; *government regulation; *legal rights; parent child relationship; privacy; *reproduction; risks and benefits; social discrimination; social impact; United States

Balsamo, Anne. Public pregnancies and cultural narratives of surveillance. *In: her:* Technologies of the Gendered Body: Reading the Cyborg Women. Durham, NC: Duke University Press; 1996: 80–115, 184–192. 72 fn. ISBN 0–8223–1698–6. BE58522.
biomedical technologies; coercion; cryopreservation; dehumanization; drug abuse; embryos; *females; *feminist ethics; fetuses; human body; legal liability; legal rights; literature; minority groups; mothers; obstetrics and gynecology; patient care; *pregnant women; *prenatal injuries; privacy; property rights; *reproduction; *reproductive technologies; *social control; social discrimination; *social dominance; socioeconomic factors; stigmatization; The Handmaid's Tale (Atwood, M.); United States

Beardsley, Tim. China syndrome: China's eugenics law makes trouble for science and business. *Scientific American.* 1997 Mar; 276(3): 33–34. BE56853.
*eugenics; *genetic disorders; genetic research; government regulation; human rights; industry; international aspects; investigators; legislation; *mandatory programs; political activity; *public policy; *reproduction; *China

Burgio, Giuseppe Roberto; Nespoli, Luigi; Porta, Fulvio, et al. Programmed bone–marrow donor for a leukaemic sibling, 10 years on. [Letter]. *Lancet.* 1997 May 17; 349(9063): 1482. 5 refs. BE56857.
blood donation; *bone marrow; *directed donation; family relationship; health; leukemia; motivation; parents; prenatal diagnosis; *reproduction; selective abortion; *siblings; stem cells; time factors; *tissue donation; transplant recipients; *treatment outcome; cord blood; Italy

Callahan, Joan C. Birth control ethics. *In:* Chadwick, Ruth, ed. Encyclopedia of Applied Ethics, Volume 1. San Diego, CA: Academic Press; 1998: 335–351. 17 refs. ISBN 0–12–227066–5. BE56371.
abortion on demand; *abortion, induced; attitudes;

BE = bioethics accession number   fn. = footnotes   refs. = references

autonomy; beginning of life; coercion; congenital disorders; *contraception; drug abuse; eugenics; family planning; females; fetuses; government regulation; hormones; infanticide; international aspects; involuntary sterilization; males; medical devices; *methods; *moral policy; *morality; multiple pregnancy; personhood; physicians; politics; *population control; pregnant women; prenatal diagnosis; prenatal injuries; *public policy; religion; *reproduction; selective abortion; sex determination; sexuality; *social control; socioeconomic factors; voluntary sterilization; wedge argument; women's rights

Cartwright, Will. The sterilisation of the mentally disabled: competence, the right to reproduce and discrimination. *In:* Grubb, Andrew, ed. Decision–Making and Problems of Incompetence. New York, NY: Wiley; 1994: 67–88. 32 fn. ISBN 0–471–94236–7. BE57130.
   autonomy; children; *competence; comprehension; *decision making; females; informed consent; *legal aspects; *legal rights; *mentally retarded; moral obligations; parent child relationship; quality of life; *reproduction; *social discrimination; standards; *sterilization (sexual)

De Koninck, Maria. Reflections on the transfer of "progress": the case of reproduction. *In:* Sherwin, Susan, et al. The Politics of Women's Health: Exploring Agency and Autonomy. Philadelphia, PA: Temple University Press; 1998: 150–177. 14 fn. ISBN 1–56639–633–6. BE58397.
   attitudes to death; cesarean section; childbirth; *developing countries; emergency care; family planning; *females; health personnel; indigents; international aspects; *mortality; nurse midwives; obstetrics and gynecology; patient care; physicians; *pregnant women; professional patient relationship; *reproduction; risk; *socioeconomic factors; *women's health; *women's health services; technology transfer; *Benin

Franklin, Sarah; Ragoné, Helena, eds. Reproducing Reproduction: Kinship, Power, and Technological Innovation. Philadelphia, PA: University of Pennsylvania Press; 1998. 245 p. Includes references. ISBN 0–8122–1584–2. BE58942.
   abortion, induced; anthropology; attitudes; children; computers; disabled; family relationship; genetic diversity; genome mapping; infertility; international aspects; legal aspects; legal rights; minority groups; normality; obstetrics and gynecology; ovum donors; parent child relationship; patents; political activity; pregnant women; prenatal diagnosis; privacy; *reproduction; *reproductive technologies; selective abortion; surrogate mothers; ethnographic studies; ultrasonography; Europe; Ireland; United States

Gibeaut, John. Class debates: reproductive, disability rights mix in KKK Act cases. *ABA Journal: The Lawyer's Magazine.* 1997 Aug; 83: 36–37. BE57626.
   due process; equal protection; historical aspects; hospitals; *involuntary sterilization; *legal aspects; legal liability; *legal rights; legislation; *mentally retarded; parents; physicians; *reproduction; social discrimination; Supreme Court decisions; Buck v. Bell; California; In re Valerie N.; *Ku Klux Klan Act 1871; *Lake v. Arnold; Pennsylvania; Twentieth Century; *United States

Hathout, Hassan. Islamic views on some reproductive issues. *In:* Teebi, Ahmad S.; Faraq, Talaat I., eds. Genetic Disorders Among Arab Populations. New York, NY: Oxford University Press; 1997: 469–473. 7 refs. ISBN 0–19–509305–4. BE58136.
   abortion, induced; adoption; contraception; fetuses; genetic intervention; *Islamic ethics; marital relationship; married persons; *reproduction; *reproductive technologies; rights

Horn, David G. Social Bodies: Science, Reproduction, and

Italian Modernity. Princeton, NJ: Princeton University Press; 1994. 189 p. (Princeton studies in culture/power/history). Bibliography: p. 159–181. ISBN 0–691–03720–5. BE56143.
   abortion, induced; anthropology; contraception; eugenics; family relationship; females; health; *historical aspects; human body; infertility; legal aspects; males; marital relationship; *political systems; population control; public policy; *reproduction; reproductive technologies; *social control; social problems; social sciences; socioeconomic factors; sociology of medicine; women's rights; *Italy; Twentieth Century

Ikemoto, Lisa C. Destabilizing thoughts on surrogacy legislation. [Commentary]. *University of San Francisco Law Review.* 1994 Spring; 28(3): 633–645. 57 fn. Commentary on A.D. Davis et al., p. 571–592. BE56938.
   abortion, induced; Asian Americans; blacks; contracts; fetal development; fetuses; *government regulation; homosexuals; *infertility; *legal aspects; legal rights; married persons; *model legislation; parent child relationship; *pregnant women; *reproduction; selection for treatment; *social discrimination; *socioeconomic factors; state interest; *surrogate mothers; women's rights; *California; Johnson v. Calvert

International Federation of Gynecology and Obstetrics. Recommendations on ethical issues in obstetrics and gynecology. [Official statement]. *Bulletin of Medical Ethics.* 1997 Nov; No. 133: 8–9. BE57629.
   circumcision; *contraception; disclosure; *females; government regulation; human rights; informed consent; international aspects; obstetrics and gynecology; *organizational policies; ovum donors; physicians; professional competence; professional organizations; remuneration; *reproduction; semen donors; sexuality; embryo donation; *International Federation of Gynecology and Obstetrics

International Federation of Gynecology and Obstetrics. Committee for the Study of Ethical Aspects of Human Reproduction. Recommendations on Ethical Issues in Obstetrics and Gynecology. London: FIGO; 1997 Jul. 117 p. Text in English, in French, and in Spanish. English text: p. 6–39. BE57742.
   allowing to die; anencephaly; cloning; congenital disorders; contraception; domestic violence; embryo research; embryos; *females; fetal tissue donation; gene therapy; genes; genetic enhancement; germ cells; HIV seropositivity; hormones; informed consent; multiple pregnancy; *newborns; *obstetrics and gynecology; organ donation; *organizational policies; ovum donors; parental consent; patents; *patient care; physician patient relationship; physicians; *pregnant women; prenatal diagnosis; professional organizations; remuneration; *reproduction; selective abortion; semen donors; sex determination; sexuality; surrogate mothers; viability; voluntary sterilization; withholding treatment; *International Federation of Gynecology and Obstetrics

Jamison, Tena. Should God be practicing medicine? *Human Rights.* 1995 Summer; 22(3): 10–13. BE55875.
   abortion, induced; clergy; contraception; females; government regulation; guidelines; *hospitals; legal aspects; prenatal diagnosis; public opinion; refusal to treat; *religious hospitals; *reproduction; *Roman Catholic ethics; state government; sterilization (sexual); *women's health services; *community hospitals; *health facility mergers; Amelia E. v. Public Health Council; California; Leonard Hospital (Troy, NY); Massachusetts; New York; Seton Health Systems (NY); St. Mary's Hospital (NY)

Kuhse, Helga; Singer, Peter. On the ethics of bringing people into existence. [Editorial]. *Bioethics.* 1998 Apr; 12(2): iii–v. 2 fn. BE58623.

BE = bioethics accession number   fn. = footnotes   refs. = references

bioethical issues; *cloning; *future generations; genetic intervention; genome mapping; moral obligations; population control; *quality of life; *reproduction; theology; *value of life

Lebacqz, Karen. Genes, justice, and clones. *In:* Cole-Turner, Ronald, ed. Human Cloning: Religious Responses. Louisville, KY: Westminster John Knox Press; 1997: 49–57. 21 fn. ISBN 0–664–25771–2. BE58143.
*cloning; disadvantaged; females; genetic identity; genetics; homosexuals; infertility; *justice; males; parent child relationship; *reproduction; reproductive technologies; resource allocation; *rights; social discrimination; socioeconomic factors

Lock, Margaret. Perfecting society: reproductive technologies, genetic testing, and the planned family in Japan. *In:* Lock, Margaret; Kaufert, Patricia A., eds. Pragmatic Women and Body Politics. New York, NY: Cambridge University Press; 1998: 206–239. 57 refs. ISBN 0–521–62929–2. BE58695.
abortion, induced; adoption; anthropology; *attitudes; autonomy; coercion; contraception; disabled; eugenics; family planning; family relationship; *females; feminist ethics; genetic disorders; *genetic screening; historical aspects; infanticide; married persons; paternalism; prenatal diagnosis; religion; *reproduction; *reproductive technologies; selective abortion; self concept; sex determination; single persons; social discrimination; *social dominance; social impact; stigmatization; women's rights; non-Western World; *Japan

Lombardo, Paul A. Medicine, eugenics, and the Supreme Court: from coercive sterilization to reproductive freedom. *Journal of Contemporary Health Law and Policy.* 1996 Fall; 13(1): 1–25. 180 fn. BE55766.
aliens; behavioral genetics; blacks; *constitutional law; criminal law; *eugenics; federal government; *genetic determinism; *genetic predisposition; historical aspects; *human rights; *involuntary sterilization; *legal aspects; legal rights; legislation; marital relationship; *mentally retarded; *prisoners; privacy; public health; *public policy; *reproduction; social discrimination; social problems; state government; *Supreme Court decisions; whites; *Buck v. Bell; Immigration Restriction Act 1924; Loving v. Commonwealth; *Skinner v. Oklahoma; *Twentieth Century; *United States; Virginia

Meyer, Cheryl L. The Wandering Uterus: Politics and the Reproductive Rights of Women. New York, NY: New York University Press; 1997. 226 p. 294 fn. ISBN 0–8147–5562–3. BE56511.
abortion, induced; age factors; artificial insemination; cesarean section; coercion; communicable diseases; contraception; contracts; cryopreservation; embryo transfer; embryos; employment; *females; fetuses; government regulation; guidelines; health hazards; in vitro fertilization; international aspects; *legal aspects; misconduct; multiple pregnancy; ovum donors; physicians; *politics; pregnant women; prematurity; prenatal injuries; professional organizations; property rights; remuneration; *reproduction; *reproductive technologies; risk; selection for treatment; self regulation; semen donors; *social control; *social discrimination; social dominance; surrogate mothers; treatment refusal; *women's health; *women's rights; hysterectomy; Davis v. Davis; In re A.C.; In re Baby M; International Union, UAW v. Johnson Controls, Inc.; Johnson v. Calvert; Roe v. Wade; RU–486; *United States

Mitchinson, Wendy. Agency, diversity, and constraints: women and their physicians, Canada, 1850–1950. *In:* Sherwin, Susan, et al. The Politics of Women's Health: Exploring Agency and Autonomy. Philadelphia, PA: Temple University Press; 1998: 122–149. 43 fn. ISBN

1–56639–633–6. BE58396.
abortion, induced; attitudes; cesarean section; childbirth; contraception; decision making; *females; *historical aspects; hospitals; human body; interprofessional relations; males; medicine; moral complicity; mortality; nurse midwives; obstetrics and gynecology; *physician patient relationship; physicians; pregnant women; *reproduction; social dominance; women's health services; women's rights; menopause; *Canada; *Nineteenth Century; *Twentieth Century

Peters, Ted. For the Love of Children: Genetic Technology and the Future of the Family. Louisville, KY: Westminster John Knox Press; 1996. 227 p. (The family, religion, and culture). 356 fn. ISBN 0–664–25468–3. BE55695.
children; *Christian ethics; *family relationship; fetal development; fetuses; genetic screening; humanism; libertarianism; *marital relationship; methods; natural law; ovum donors; parent child relationship; personhood; Protestant ethics; *reproduction; *reproductive technologies; Roman Catholic ethics; selective abortion; sexuality; surrogate mothers; theology; values

Rachels, Stuart. Is it good to make happy people? *Bioethics.* 1998 Apr; 12(2): 93–110. 35 fn. BE58628.
age factors; bioethical issues; congenital disorders; contraception; contracts; *ethical analysis; *future generations; *moral obligations; population control; prolongation of life; *quality of life; *reproduction; rights; suffering; teleological ethics; utilitarianism; *value of life
Would it be good, other things being equal, for additional people to exist whose lives would be worth living? I examine and reject several arguments for the answer that it would not be good; then I offer opposing arguments that I believe are more successful. Thus, I agree with utilitarians who say that it is better for there to be more happy people. Next I argue for the stronger claim that the happiness of potential people is as important as that of adults. Potential quality of life, then, matters in a host of bioethical issues: abortion, commercial surrogacy, the treatment of defective newborns, and so on. What is the practical upshot of all this? I reject the idea that we must do whatever is necessary to prolong life worth living. But I also reject the view that the side-effects of overpopulation always outweigh the value of realizing potential happiness. So I advocate a middle position, which I do not identify precisely. Even from this middle position, however, potential happiness is more important that is commonly assumed in bioethics.

Reichman, Edward. The rabbinic conception of conception: an exercise in fertility. *In:* Feldman, Emanuel; Wolowelsky, Joel B., eds. Jewish Law and the New Reproductive Technologies. Hoboken, NJ: Ktav; 1997: 1–35. 120 fn. ISBN 0–88125–586–6. BE57454.
*artificial insemination; embryos; females; germ cells; *historical aspects; *Jewish ethics; males; *reproduction; reproductive technologies; theology; Orthodox Judaism

Roberts, Dorothy. Killing the Black Body: Race, Reproduction, and the Meaning of Liberty. New York, NY: Pantheon Books; 1997. 373 p. 1,073 fn. ISBN 0–679–44226–X. BE57998.
abortion, induced; adolescents; autonomy; *blacks; *coercion; *contraception; criminal law; deception; dehumanization; *drug abuse; eugenics; family relationship; *females; genetic identity; government financing; historical aspects; indigents; *involuntary sterilization; justice; legal aspects; misconduct; morality; parent child relationship; physicians; *pregnant women; *prenatal injuries; property rights; public policy; rape; *reproduction; *reproductive technologies; risks and benefits; sexuality; *social control;

*social discrimination; socioeconomic factors; stigmatization; surrogate mothers; personal identity; slavery; Depo-provera; Medicaid; Nineteenth Century; Norplant; Twentieth Century; United States

Robertson, John A. Liberty, identity, and human cloning. *Texas Law Review.* 1998 May; 76(6): 1371–1456. 298 fn. BE57440.

adults; advisory committees; animal experimentation; autonomy; children; *cloning; disclosure; donors; embryo research; embryos; eugenics; family relationship; federal government; *freedom; genetic determinism; genetic enhancement; genetic identity; genetic intervention; genetic materials; *government regulation; guidelines; human experimentation; infertility; informed consent; intention; mandatory programs; methods; *moral policy; motivation; organ donation; parents; policy analysis; *public policy; remuneration; *reproduction; reproductive technologies; review; *rights; *risks and benefits; transgenic animals; twins; wrongful life; embryo donation; embryo splitting; nuclear transplantation; National Bioethics Advisory Commission; United States

Rothenberg, Karen H. Genetic accountability and pregnant women. *Women's Health Issues.* 1997 Jul–Aug; 7(4): 215–219. 12 refs. BE55732.

*accountability; autonomy; coercion; conflict of interest; contraception; decision making; disabled; economics; eugenics; females; genetic counseling; genetic disorders; *genetic screening; genetic services; government financing; health education; health personnel; incentives; legal aspects; mandatory testing; medical education; obligations to society; *pregnant women; *prenatal diagnosis; public policy; *reproduction; selective abortion; state interest; *voluntary programs; wrongful life; ELSI-funded publication; United States

Rush, Sharon Elizabeth. Breaking with tradition: surrogacy and gay fathers. *In:* Meyers, Diana Tietjens; Kipnis, Kenneth; Murphy, Cornelius F., eds. Kindred Matters: Rethinking the Philosophy of the Family. Ithaca, NY: Cornell University Press; 1993: 102–142. 62 refs. 79 fn. ISBN 0-8014-9909-7. BE55698.

adoption; behavioral genetics; children; contracts; *family relationship; *fathers; females; government regulation; *homosexuals; informed consent; *legal aspects; legal rights; *males; mass media; morality; *parent child relationship; paternalism; privacy; public opinion; public policy; remuneration; *reproduction; selection for treatment; sexuality; single persons; *stigmatization; Supreme Court decisions; *surrogate mothers; values; women's rights; United States

Schenker, Joseph G.; International Federation of Gynecology and Obstetrics. Committee for the Study of Ethical Aspects of Human Reproduction. Report of the FIGO Committee for the Study of Ethical Aspects of Human Reproduction. *International Journal of Gynaecology and Obstetrics.* 1997 Jun; 57(3): 333–337. 1 fn. BE57508.

*allowing to die; confidentiality; *congenital disorders; contraception; gene therapy; genetic enhancement; *genetic intervention; genetic materials; germ cells; guidelines; HIV seropositivity; informed consent; *newborns; organizational policies; quality of health care; remuneration; *reproduction; sexuality; withholding treatment; women's health services; women's rights; International Federation of Gynecology and Obstetrics

Shannon, Thomas A. Genetics, ethics, and theology: the Roman Catholic discussion. *In:* Peters, Ted, ed. Genetics: Issues of Social Justice. Cleveland, OH: Pilgrim Press; 1998: 144–179. 174 fn. ISBN 0-8298-1251-2. BE57478.

abortion, induced; autonomy; embryo research; embryos; eugenics; fetal research; gene therapy; genetic counseling;

*genetic intervention; genetic research; genetic screening; *genetics; genome mapping; human characteristics; marital relationship; moral obligations; morality; natural law; prenatal diagnosis; *reproduction; reproductive technologies; *Roman Catholic ethics; sexuality; sociobiology; *theology; value of life; Ashley, Benedict; Catholic Health Association; Curran, Charles; Haring, Bernard; Humanae Vitae; Instruction on Respect for Human Life; John Paul II, Pope; May, William; McCormick, Richard; O'Rourke, Kevin; Rahner, Karl; Vatican II

Tännsjö, Torbjörn. Compulsory sterilisation in Sweden. *Bioethics.* 1998 Jul; 12(3): 236–249. 1 fn. BE58892.

*autonomy; children; *coercion; *competence; congenital disorders; *disabled; *eugenics; genetic disorders; government regulation; historical aspects; informed consent; involuntary euthanasia; *involuntary sterilization; mandatory programs; mass media; mentally retarded; *moral policy; paternalism; politics; prenatal diagnosis; *public policy; quality of life; *reproduction; reproductive technologies; *rights; selective abortion; social discrimination; sterilization (sexual); suffering; third party consent; value of life; wedge argument; *Sweden; Twentieth Century

In the Fall of 1997 the leading Swedish newspaper, *Dagens Nyheter*, created a media hype over the Swedish policy of compulsory sterilisation that had been in operation between 1935 and 1975. In the discussion that followed, the moral condemnation of our medical past was unanimous. However, the reasons for rejecting what had gone on were varied and mutually inconsistent. Three strands of criticism were common: the argument from autonomy, the argument from caution, and the argument from biological scepticism. In the paper it is argued that what point of departure you choose in your criticism of the past should be of consequence also for your ideas about present and future medical practice. In particular, if you rely on the argument from autonomy, you should be prepared to accept a liberal (present and future) use of reproductive techniques.

Tooley, Michael. Value, obligation and the asymmetry question. *Bioethics.* 1998 Apr; 12(2): 111–124. 10 fn. BE58629.

bioethical issues; congenital disorders; deontological ethics; *ethical analysis; *future generations; killing; *moral obligations; *quality of life; *reproduction; suffering; teleological ethics; *value of life

Is there a prima facie obligation to produce additional individuals whose lives would be worth living? In his paper 'Is it good to make happy people?', Stuart Rachels argues not only that there is, but, also, that precisely as much weight should be assigned to the quality of life that would be enjoyed by such potential persons, if they were to be actualized, as to the quality of life enjoyed by actually existing persons. In response, I shall argue, first, that Rachels' view is exposed to very serious objections, and secondly, that his arguments in support of his position involve a crucial assumption, which cannot be sustained, concerning the relation between, on the one hand, propositions about good–making and bad–making properties, and, on the other, propositions about right–making and wrong–making ones. I shall then argue that there is a very plausible position concerning the conditions under which an action can be morally wrong which entails the following asymmetry: there is a prima facie obligation not to bring into existence individuals whose lives are not worth living, but there is no corresponding obligation to create additional individuals whose lives would be worth living.

Verhey, Allen. Theology after Dolly. *Christian Century.* 1997 Mar 19–26; 114(10): 285–286. BE56046.

autonomy; children; *cloning; *dehumanization; family

BE = bioethics accession number   fn. = footnotes   refs. = references

relationship; freedom; human body; motivation; parent child relationship; *reproduction; rights; risks and benefits; self concept; *theology; utilitarianism; personal identity; Lederberg, Joshua; *Ramsey, Paul

Water, Brent. One flesh? Cloning, procreation, and the family. *In:* Cole-Turner, Ronald, ed. Human Cloning: Religious Responses. Louisville, KY: Westminister John Knox Press; 1997: 78–90. 10 fn. ISBN 0–664–25771–2. BE58146.
    *cloning; *family relationship; freedom; love; motivation; parent child relationship; *reproduction; reproductive technologies; *rights; social impact

Woolfrey, Joan. What price reproductive potential? *Hastings Center Report.* 1998 Jan–Feb; 28(1): 47. BE57299.
    *compensation; hospitals; infertility; *legal liability; males; *negligence; property rights; records; *reproduction; semen donors; *sperm; *tissue banks; *Eubanks, Robert; *Legacy Emanuel Hospital (Portland, OR); United States

REPRODUCTIVE TECHNOLOGIES

See also ARTIFICIAL INSEMINATION, BIOMEDICAL TECHNOLOGIES, CLONING, GENETIC INTERVENTION, IN VITRO FERTILIZATION, REPRODUCTION, SEX PRESELECTION, SURROGATE MOTHERS

Aldhous, Peter. Surrogate fathers. [News]. *New Scientist.* 1998 Jan 31; 157(2119): 4. BE59092.
    animal experimentation; human experimentation; hybrids; infertility; *males; methods; *reproductive technologies; *sperm; tissue transplantation; *rodents; Short, Roger

Altman, Lawrence K. Health panel seeks sweeping changes in fertility therapy. [News]. *New York Times.* 1998 Apr 29: A1, A22. Includes inset article, "Toughen suggestions, dissenters say," by Charlie LeDuff, p. A22. BE57984.
    advisory committees; confidentiality; disclosure; donors; embryo disposition; *government regulation; health insurance reimbursement; human experimentation; informed consent; multiple pregnancy; parent child relationship; posthumous reproduction; public policy; *reproductive technologies; selection for treatment; selective abortion; self regulation; state government; surrogate mothers; New York; *New York State Task Force on Life and the Law

Andrews, Lori; Elster, Nanette; Gatter, Robert, et al.; Institute for Science, Law, and Technology Working Group. ART into science: regulation of fertility techniques. *Science.* 1998 Jul 31; 281(5377): 651–652. 27 fn. BE58909.
    children; disclosure; drugs; embryo transfer; federal government; government financing; *government regulation; guidelines; health facilities; health insurance reimbursement; health personnel; human experimentation; information dissemination; informed consent; legal liability; multiple pregnancy; records; *reproductive technologies; risk; standards; state government; treatment outcome; women's health; guideline adherence; Great Britain; *United States

Andrews, Lori B.; Elster, Nanette. Adoption, reproductive technologies, and genetic information. *Health Matrix.* 1998 Summer; 8(2): 125–151. 125 fn. BE58951.
    *adoption; artificial insemination; behavioral genetics; children; *confidentiality; *disclosure; *genetic information; *genetic screening; government regulation; informed consent; *legal aspects; ovum donors; parents; records;

registries; *reproductive technologies; semen donors; state government; *United States

Anleu, Sharyn L. Roach. Regulating new reproductive technologies: an examination of the emergence of legislation in two Australian states. *In:* Holstein, J.A.; Miller, G., eds. Perspectives on Social Problems: A Research Annual. Volume 8. Greenwich, CT: JAI Press; 1996: 175–197. 60 refs. 2 fn. ISBN 0–7623–0035–3. BE57747.
    advisory committees; artificial insemination; cryopreservation; embryo disposition; *embryo research; embryo transfer; embryos; *family relationship; feminist ethics; government financing; *government regulation; health insurance reimbursement; human experimentation; in vitro fertilization; infertility; *investigators; law; *legislation; married persons; mass media; medicine; national health insurance; personhood; political activity; professional autonomy; public policy; reproduction; *reproductive technologies; rights; selection for treatment; social dominance; social impact; surrogate mothers; *women's rights; Australia; Council on Reproductive Technology (South Australia); Medical Procedures (Infertility) Act 1984 (Victoria); Reproductive Technology Act 1988 (South Australia); *South Australia; *Victoria; Waller Committee

Anleu, Sharyn L. Roach. Reproductive autonomy and reproductive technology: gender, deviance and infertility. *In:* Petersen, Kerry, ed. Intersections: Women on Law, Medicine and Technology. Brookfield, VT: Ashgate; 1997: 99–125. 90 refs. 5 fn. ISBN 1–85521–882–8. BE57488.
    abortion, induced; attitudes; *autonomy; disabled; disclosure; *females; health; in vitro fertilization; *infertility; international aspects; legal aspects; males; normality; physicians; psychological stress; reproduction; *reproductive technologies; social control; social dominance; *stigmatization; women's rights; sick role

Annas, George J. The shadowlands — secrets, lies, and assisted reproduction. *New England Journal of Medicine.* 1998 Sep 24; 339(13): 935–939. 28 refs. BE59074.
    advisory committees; *children; confidentiality; contracts; cryopreservation; *embryo disposition; embryo research; embryo transfer; *embryos; federal government; government regulation; in vitro fertilization; informed consent; judicial action; *legal aspects; mothers; ovum donors; *parent child relationship; *public policy; records; *reproductive technologies; semen donors; standards; surrogate mothers; divorce; *Buzzanca v. Buzzanca; California; *Kass v. Kass; New York; *New York State Task Force on Life and the Law; *United States

Baird, P.A. Ethical issues of fertility and reproduction. *Annual Review of Medicine.* 1996; 47: 107–116. 12 refs. BE55754.
    age factors; artificial insemination; commodification; economics; embryo research; females; government regulation; homosexuals; in vitro fertilization; infertility; justice; ovum donors; public policy; remuneration; *reproductive technologies; resource allocation; selection for treatment; selective abortion; sex determination; sex preselection; single persons; surrogate mothers; North America

Baird, Patricia. Individual interests, societal interests, and reproductive technologies. *Perspectives in Biology and Medicine.* 1997 Spring; 40(3): 440–451. 22 refs. BE59008.
    age factors; *autonomy; children; coercion; commodification; *common good; costs and benefits; democracy; economics; embryo transfer; females; government financing; government regulation; in vitro fertilization; indigents; industry; *obligations to society; preimplantation diagnosis; prenatal diagnosis; private sector; *public policy; public sector; remuneration; reproduction;

*reproductive technologies; resource allocation; rights; risks and benefits; selection for treatment; selective abortion; sex determination; sex preselection; social impact; socioeconomic factors; surrogate mothers; North America

Balsamo, Anne. Public pregnancies and cultural narratives of surveillance. *In: her:* Technologies of the Gendered Body: Reading the Cyborg Women. Durham, NC: Duke University Press; 1996: 80–115, 184–192. 72 fn. ISBN 0-8223-1698-6. BE58522.
biomedical technologies; coercion; cryopreservation; dehumanization; drug abuse; embryos; *females; *feminist ethics; fetuses; human body; legal liability; legal rights; literature; minority groups; mothers; obstetrics and gynecology; patient care; *pregnant women; *prenatal injuries; privacy; property rights; *reproduction; *reproductive technologies; *social control; social discrimination; *social dominance; socioeconomic factors; stigmatization; The Handmaid's Tale (Atwood, M.); United States

Belkin, Lisa. Pregnant with complications. *New York Times Magazine.* 1997 Oct 26: 34–39, 48–49, 67–68. BE58039.
*age factors; children; embryo transfer; *females; health facilities; in vitro fertilization; institutional policies; maternal health; *ovum donors; parent child relationship; *reproductive technologies; risk; scarcity; *selection for treatment; menopause; United States

Ben–Meir, Yehoshua. Legal parenthood and genetic parenthood in Jewish law. *In:* Jewish Law Annual. Volume Twelve. Amsterdam, Netherlands: Harwood Academic Publishers; 1997: 153–166. 37 fn. ISBN 90-5702-551-5. BE58342.
aborted fetuses; aliens; artificial insemination; embryo transfer; *family relationship; fathers; fetal tissue donation; genetic identity; in vitro fertilization; *Jewish ethics; Jews; marital relationship; mothers; ovum donors; *parent child relationship; parents; religion; *reproductive technologies; semen donors; surrogate mothers

Benagiano, G.; Rowe, P.J. Assisted reproduction: a not so bright future? *Human Reproduction.* 1995 Jun; 10(6): 1324–1326. 9 refs. BE55756.
children; cryopreservation; disclosure; embryos; females; government regulation; health facilities; informed consent; multiple pregnancy; pregnant women; prematurity; records; *reproductive technologies; *risk; technology assessment; treatment outcome; World Health Organization

Bennett, Belinda. Gamete donation, reproductive technology and the law. *In:* Petersen, Kerry, ed. Intersections: Women on Law, Medicine and Technology. Brookfield, VT: Ashgate; 1997: 127–144. 54 refs. 9 fn. ISBN 1-85521-882-8. BE57489.
artificial insemination; autonomy; confidentiality; disclosure; family relationship; fathers; homosexuals; in vitro fertilization; international aspects; *legal aspects; married persons; mothers; *ovum donors; parent child relationship; reproduction; *reproductive technologies; rights; selection for treatment; *semen donors; single persons; surrogate mothers; *Australia; Great Britain

Bick, Ezra. Ovum donations: a rabbinic conceptual model of maternity. *In:* Feldman, Emanuel; Wolowelsky, Joel B., eds. Jewish Law and the New Reproductive Technologies. Hoboken, NJ: Ktav; 1997: 83–105. 19 fn. Commentary on J. David Bleich, p. 46–82; response by Bleich, p. 106–114. ISBN 0-88125-586-6. BE57457.
*Jewish ethics; *mothers; *ovum donors; *parent child relationship; reproductive technologies; Orthodox Judaism

Blake, Deborah D. Infertile couples: psychological needs,

social responsibilities. *In:* Wildes, Kevin Wm., ed. Infertility: A Crossroad of Faith, Medicine, and Technology. Boston, MA: Kluwer Academic; 1997: 149–166. 41 refs. ISBN 0-7923-4061-2. BE55996.
attitudes; *common good; economics; family relationship; females; freedom; government financing; *infertility; males; married persons; *moral obligations; obligations of society; obligations to society; *psychology; *public policy; *reproductive technologies; rights; *Roman Catholic ethics; social impact; socioeconomic factors; women's rights; United States

Bleich, J. David. Maternal identity revisited. *In:* Feldman, Emanuel; Wolowelsky, Joel B., eds. Jewish Law and the New Reproductive Technologies. Hoboken, NJ: Ktav; 1997: 106–114. 11 fn. Response to E. Bick, p. 83–105. ISBN 0-88125-586-6. BE57458.
*Jewish ethics; *mothers; ovum donors; *parent child relationship; *reproductive technologies; surrogate mothers; Orthodox Judaism

Bonduelle, M.; Joris, H.; Hofmans, K., et al. Mental development of 201 ICSI children at 2 years of age. *Lancet.* 1998 May 23; 351(9115): 1553. 4 refs. BE58312.
age factors; *children; comparative studies; embryo transfer; evaluation studies; in vitro fertilization; infertility; *intelligence; males; *methods; reproduction; *reproductive technologies; *sperm; *treatment outcome; follow-up studies; *intracytoplasmic sperm injection; Belgium

Bowen, Jennifer R.; Gibson, Frances L.; Leslie, Garth I., et al. Medical and developmental outcomes at 1 year for children conceived by intracytoplasmic sperm injection. *Lancet.* 1998 May 23; 315(9115): 1529–1534. 35 refs. BE58313.
age factors; *children; comparative studies; congenital disorders; embryo transfer; evaluation studies; health; in vitro fertilization; infertility; intelligence; males; *methods; reproduction; *reproductive technologies; *sperm; *treatment outcome; *intracytoplasmic sperm injection; Australia
BACKGROUND: Intracytoplasmic sperm injection (ICSI) was introduced as a new form of in–vitro fertilisation (IVF) in 1993 and is now accepted as the treatment of choice for severe male infertility in many centres around the world. However, there is little information about the long–term outcome of children conceived by ICSI. We aimed to find out the medical and developmental outcome of children conceived by ICSI at age 1 year. METHODS: In this prospective study, we compared the medical and developmental outcome at 1 year of 89 children conceived by ICSI with 84 children conceived by routine IVF, and with 80 children conceived naturally. Formal developmental assessment was done with Bayley Scales of Infant Development (2nd edition) from which a mental index (MDI) was derived. FINDINGS: There was no significant difference in the incidence of major congenital malformations or major health problems in the first year of life. However, the mean Bayley MDI was significantly lower for the children conceived by ICSI than for the children conceived by routine IVF or naturally (95.9 [SD 10.7], 101.8 [8.5] and 102.5 [7.6], respectively, p less than 0.0001). 15 (17%) of 89 children conceived by ICSI experienced mildly or significantly delayed development (MDI less than 85) at 1 year compared with two (2%) of the 84 children conceived by IVF and one (1%) of the 80 children conceived by natural conception (p less than 0.0001). INTERPRETATION: Although most children conceived by ICSI are healthy and develop normally, there is an increased risk of mild delays in development at 1 year when compared with children

---

conceived by routine IVF or conceived naturally. These findings support the need for ongoing developmental follow-up of children conceived by ICSI to see whether they are at increased risk of intellectual impairment or learning difficulties at school age.

Brown, Barry. Reconciling property law with advances in reproductive science. *Stanford Law and Policy Review.* 1995; 6(2): 73-88. 113 fn. BE56485.
   artificial insemination; body parts and fluids; confidentiality; *cryopreservation; death; decision making; dissent; *embryo disposition; *embryos; eugenics; females; future generations; gene therapy; genetic enhancement; genetic information; *genetic intervention; genetic screening; *germ cells; government regulation; in vitro fertilization; international aspects; *legal aspects; males; mandatory testing; parents; preimplantation diagnosis; privacy; *property rights; *public policy; reproduction; *reproductive technologies; state interest; divorce; Davis v. Davis; Hecht v. Superior Court (Kane); *United States

Butler, Declan. Spermatid injection fertilizes ethics debate. [News]. *Nature.* 1995 Sep 28; 377(6547): 277. BE56108.
   animal experimentation; congenital disorders; *human experimentation; in vitro fertilization; infertility; investigators; males; *methods; ovum; *reproductive technologies; research design; risks and benefits; *sperm; *therapeutic research; *France; Testart, Jacques

Callahan, Sidney. Gays, lesbians, and the use of alternate reproductive technologies. *In:* Nelson, Hilde Lindemann, ed. Feminism and Families. New York, NY: Routledge; 1997: 188-202. 16 fn. ISBN 0-415-91254-7. BE55839.
   adoption; children; commodification; confidentiality; disclosure; *family relationship; females; *feminist ethics; *homosexuals; males; parent child relationship; reproduction; *reproductive technologies; *selection for treatment; single persons; social discrimination; sociobiology

Canada. House of Commons. Human Reproductive and Genetic Technologies Act (an act respecting human reproductive technologies and commercial transactions relating to human reproduction): bill C-47. Bill C-47, 35th Parliament, 2d Sess. Introduced by the Minister of Health; 1996 Jun 14. 7 p. Text in English and in French. BE56738.
   cadavers; cloning; embryo research; embryo transfer; embryos; fetal tissue donation; fetuses; genetic intervention; *germ cells; *government regulation; hybrids; *legal aspects; remuneration; *reproductive technologies; sex determination; sex preselection; surrogate mothers; ectogenesis; *Canada; *Human Reproductive and Genetic Technologies Act (Canada)

Canada. Minister of Health. New Reproductive and Genetic Technologies: Setting Boundaries, Enhancing Health. Ottawa, ON: Minister of Supply and Services Canada; 1996 Jun. 48 p. Cat.H21-127/1996E. ISBN 0-662-24101-0. BE59032.
   accountability; advisory committees; children; cloning; disabled; embryo research; embryos; federal government; gene therapy; *genetic intervention; genetic screening; *government regulation; hybrids; industry; infertility; informed consent; moral policy; ovum donors; prenatal diagnosis; *public policy; registries; remuneration; *reproductive technologies; research embryo creation; selective abortion; semen donors; sex determination; standards; surrogate mothers; ectogenesis; Advisory Committee on the Interim Moratorium on Reproductive and Genetic Technologies (Canada); *Canada; *Human Reproductive and Genetic Technologies Act 1996 (Canada); *Royal Commission on New Reproductive Technologies (Canada)

Canada. Royal Commission on New Reproductive

Technologies. Update [on the work of the Royal Commission on New Reproductive Technologies -- includes letter from the chairperson and summary of the main topics in the final report, Proceed with Care]. Issued by the Commission, P.O. Box 1566, Station "B," Ottawa, ON, Canada K1P 5R5; 1993 Dec. 18 p. BE57781.
   adoption; advisory committees; artificial insemination; congenital disorders; drugs; economics; embryo research; embryo transfer; fetal tissue donation; gene therapy; genetic predisposition; germ cells; government regulation; guidelines; health care delivery; in vitro fertilization; *infertility; judicial action; late-onset disorders; ovum donors; prenatal diagnosis; prevalence; *public policy; *reproductive technologies; sex determination; sex preselection; surrogate mothers; *Canada; *Royal Commission on New Reproductive Technologies (Canada)

Capron, Alexander Morgan. Punishing mothers. *Hastings Center Report.* 1998 Jan-Feb; 28(1): 31-33. 6 fn. BE57296.
   attitudes; *child abuse; *childbirth; congenital disorders; *drug abuse; embryo transfer; fetuses; government regulation; *legal liability; mass media; moral obligations; *multiple pregnancy; parents; personhood; physicians; *pregnant women; prematurity; *prenatal injuries; *reproductive technologies; risks and benefits; viability; wrongful death; McCaughey, Bobbi; South Carolina; Whitner v. State
What should society do when a woman, in producing children, exposes them to avoidable risks? That recurring question -- which plunges one quickly and deeply into the murky waters of child protection, women's rights, and the far reaches of medical science -- has been back on the front pages recently. Two very different stories illustrate how context affects our answer.

Carlson, John W. Interventions upon gametes in assisting the conjugal act toward fertilization. *In:* Wildes, Kevin Wm., ed. Infertility: A Crossroad of Faith, Medicine, and Technology. Boston, MA: Kluwer Academic; 1997: 107-124. 23 refs. 21 fn. ISBN 0-7923-4061-2. BE55994.
   cryopreservation; gamete intrafallopian transfer; marital relationship; *methods; *ovum; reproduction; *reproductive technologies; *Roman Catholic ethics; sexuality; *sperm; *theology; *Instruction on Respect for Human Life

Charo, R. Alta. The interaction between family planning policies and the introduction of new reproductive technologies. *In:* Petersen, Kerry, ed. Intersections: Women on Law, Medicine and Technology. Brookfield, VT: Ashgate; 1997: 73-97. 55 refs. 10 fn. ISBN 1-85521-882-8. BE57487.
   abortion, induced; autonomy; *contraception; decision making; drugs; eugenics; *family planning; *females; historical aspects; international aspects; legal aspects; physician's role; political activity; *population control; public health; public policy; *reproductive technologies; social dominance; women's health services; *women's rights; Nineteenth Century; RU-486; Twentieth Century; United States

Cook, Rachel; Golombok, Susan; Bish, Alison, et al. Disclosure of donor insemination: parental attitudes. *American Journal of Orthopsychiatry.* 1995 Oct; 65(4): 549-559. 50 refs. BE55711.
   adoption; *artificial insemination; *attitudes; *children; comparative studies; *confidentiality; *disclosure; family members; fathers; genetic information; in vitro fertilization; infertility; mothers; motivation; parent child relationship; *parents; psychological stress; *reproductive technologies; semen donors; survey; Great Britain

Craft, Ian. Should egg donors be paid? An "inconvenience

---

allowance" would solve the egg shortage. *BMJ (British Medical Journal).* 1997 May 10; 314(7091): 1400–1401. 5 refs. BE55664.
> government regulation; legal aspects; mass media; *ovum donors; *public policy; *remuneration; scarcity; semen donors; surrogate mothers; *Great Britain; Human Fertilisation and Embryology Act 1990; Human Fertilisation and Embryology Authority

Curtis, Kimberley F. Hannah Arendt, feminist theorizing, and the debate over new reproductive technologies. *Polity.* 1995 Winter; 28(2): 159–187. 74 fn. BE57191.
> *autonomy; dissent; *ethical theory; females; *feminist ethics; *freedom; genetic intervention; *human characteristics; males; philosophy; political systems; reproduction; *reproductive technologies; social control; social dominance; women's rights; hope; *nature; *Arendt, Hannah

Dickens, B.M. Interfaces of assisted reproduction ethics and law. *In:* Shenfield, F.; Sureau, C., eds. Ethical Dilemmas in Assisted Reproduction. New York, NY: Parthenon Pub. Group; 1997: 77–81. 10 refs. ISBN 1–85070–916–5. BE57949.
> abortion, induced; embryo research; guidelines; infertility; international aspects; law; *legal aspects; *reproductive technologies; sex determination; social discrimination; Europe

Dolgin, Janet L. Defining the Family: Law, Technology, and Reproduction in an Uneasy Age. New York, NY: New York University Press; 1997. 287 p. Bibliography: p.273–281. ISBN 0–8147–1859–0. BE58581.
> anthropology; autonomy; children; contracts; cryopreservation; embryos; *family relationship; fathers; germ cells; judicial action; *law; *legal aspects; parent child relationship; posthumous reproduction; reproduction; *reproductive technologies; single persons; *social impact; Supreme Court decisions; *surrogate mothers; trends; *United States

Feldman, Emanuel; Wolowelsky, Joel B., eds. Jewish Law and the New Reproductive Technologies. Hoboken, NJ: Ktav; 1997. 186 p. 412 fn. ISBN 0–88125–586–6. BE57453.
> artificial insemination; cryopreservation; decision making; dissent; embryo disposition; embryo transfer; embryos; historical aspects; in vitro fertilization; infertility; *Jewish ethics; males; married persons; mothers; parent child relationship; reproduction; *reproductive technologies; sperm; surrogate mothers; theology; tissue banks; Orthodox Judaism

Franklin, Sarah. Embodied Progress: A Cultural Account of Assisted Conception. New York, NY: Routledge; 1997. 252 p. Bibliography: p. 230–245. ISBN 0–415–06767–7. BE58543.
> *anthropology; attitudes; *emotions; family relationship; females; feminist ethics; *in vitro fertilization; infertility; reproduction; *reproductive technologies; self concept; sexuality; social sciences; survey; ethnographic studies; hope; Great Britain

Franklin, Sarah; Ragoné, Helena, eds. Reproducing Reproduction: Kinship, Power, and Technological Innovation. Philadelphia, PA: University of Pennsylvania Press; 1998. 245 p. Includes references. ISBN 0–8122–1584–2. BE58942.
> abortion, induced; anthropology; attitudes; children; computers; disabled; family relationship; genetic diversity; genome mapping; infertility; international aspects; legal aspects; legal rights; minority groups; normality; obstetrics and gynecology; ovum donors; parent child relationship; patents; political activity; pregnant women; prenatal

diagnosis; privacy; *reproduction; *reproductive technologies; selective abortion; surrogate mothers; ethnographic studies; ultrasonography; Europe; Ireland; United States

Frith, Lucy. Reproductive technologies and midwifery. *In:* Frith, Lucy, ed. Ethics and Midwifery: Issues in Contemporary Practice. Boston, MA: Butterworth–Heinemann; 1996: 170–186. 28 refs. ISBN 0–7506–3056–6. BE58639.
> advisory committees; age factors; confidentiality; disclosure; embryo research; embryos; ethical review; government regulation; human experimentation; legal aspects; moral obligations; *nurse midwives; nurse's role; parent child relationship; patient care; practice guidelines; pregnant women; professional autonomy; public participation; *public policy; *reproductive technologies; risk; selection for treatment; single persons; treatment outcome; *Great Britain; Human Fertilisation and Embryology Act 1990; Human Fertilisation and Embryology Authority; Warnock Committee

Frith, Lucy. Reproductive technologies, overview. *In:* Chadwick, Ruth, ed. Encyclopedia of Applied Ethics, Volume 3. San Diego, CA: Academic Press; 1998: 817–827. 13 refs. ISBN 0–12–227068–1. BE56269.
> cryopreservation; embryo research; embryos; females; feminist ethics; genetic screening; infertility; informed consent; moral policy; ovum donors; parent child relationship; preimplantation diagnosis; remuneration; reproduction; *reproductive technologies; research embryo creation; rights; risks and benefits; selection for treatment; semen donors

Garcia, Jario E.; Katz, Michael. Panel two: reporting and advertising success rates — the Gordian Knot of assisted reproductive technology. [Articles followed by discussion]. *Women's Health Issues.* 1997 May–Jun; 7(3): 188–196. 5 refs. Papers presented and discussion at a workshop on "Assisted Reproductive Technologies, Ads, and Ethics: Philosophical, Ethical, and Clinical Perspectives on the Use of Advertising in Reproductive Medicine," held by the National Advisory Board on Ethics in Reproduction in Washington, DC on 19 Oct 1996. BE55861.
> accountability; *advertising; deception; *disclosure; economics; embryo transfer; federal government; *government regulation; guidelines; *health facilities; in vitro fertilization; infertility; *information dissemination; methods; *organizational policies; ovum donors; professional organizations; *reproductive technologies; risk; risks and benefits; self regulation; sperm; *treatment outcome; quality assurance; *Federal Trade Commission; *Society for Assisted Reproductive Technology; United States

Goldfarb, James; Kinzer, Donna J.; Boyle, Marian, et al. Attitudes of in vitro fertilization and intrauterine insemination couples toward multiple gestation pregnancy and multifetal pregnancy reduction. *Fertility and Sterility.* 1996 Apr; 65(4): 815–820. 18 refs. BE56462.
> artificial insemination; *attitudes; embryo transfer; females; hormones; in vitro fertilization; males; *married persons; *multiple pregnancy; *patients; *reproductive technologies; *selective abortion; survey; treatment outcome; Ohio; University Hospitals of Cleveland

Goldworth, Amnon; Verhey, Allen; Robertson, John A., et al. The commodification and advertising of infertility treatment. *Women's Health Issues.* 1997 May–Jun; 7(3): 149–152. 1 ref. Discussion following presentations by A. Verhey and A.R. Dyer at a workshop on "Assisted Reproductive Technologies, Ads, and Ethics: Philosophical, Ethical, and Clinical Perspectives on the Use of Advertising in Reproductive

---

BE = bioethics accession number   fn. = footnotes   refs. = references

Medicine," held by the National Advisory Board on Ethics in Reproduction in Washington, DC on 19 Oct 1996. BE55863.

*advertising; *commodification; *economics; freedom; managed care programs; morality; personhood; physician patient relationship; physicians; remuneration; *reproductive technologies; values; postmodernism

Great Britain. England. High Court of Justice, Queen's Bench Division. R v. Ethical Committee of St. Mary's Hospital (Manchester) ex parte H. *Family Law Reports.* 1987 Oct 26 (date of decision). [1988] 1: 512–520. BE58576.

adoption; *clinical ethics committees; *decision making; hospitals; in vitro fertilization; infertility; judicial action; *legal aspects; *physicians; referral and consultation; *refusal to treat; *reproductive technologies; *selection for treatment; sex offenses; standards; prostitution; *Great Britain; *National Health Service; *R v. Ethical Committee of St. Mary's Hospital (Manchester) ex parte H.

The Queen's Bench Division of England's High Court of Justice refused judicial review of a hospital ethics committee's decision that the medical team rather than the committee should determine denial of IVF services, in effect, refusal of treatment, to a patient and her husband. Because the patient, who was unable to conceive, had a past history of prostitution and poor understanding of the parental role, she and her husband were refused adoption and foster children by social services. They then sought IVF treatment and were put on a waiting list for services. After learning of the reasons for the adoption refusal, the consultant in obstetrics and gynecology decided that IVF should not be given and that the patient's name should be taken off the wait list. An ethics committee, which had been set up to provide advice and guidance on infertility services, as recommended by the Warnock Report, concluded that the decision on IVF services should be made by the medical consultant. Seeking judicial review, the patient claimed that once any matter is brought to the committee's attention, it was under a charge first to investigate and then to advise. The court found that the committtee with its "wide range of expertise" was intended to be advisory, not decision–making. In the court's opinion, the committee served as an informal forum for professionals. (KIE abstract)

Great Britain. Human Fertilisation and Embryology Authority. Code of Practice. London: The Authority; 1991. 1 v. 27 fn. BE58982.

accountability; advertising; confidentiality; conscience; counseling; cryopreservation; disclosure; embryo disposition; embryo research; embryos; family relationship; forms; germ cells; *government regulation; *guidelines; *health facilities; health personnel; informed consent; legal aspects; ovum donors; *practice guidelines; records; *reproductive technologies; selection for treatment; semen donors; *standards; *Great Britain; Human Fertilisation and Embryology Act 1990; *Human Fertilisation and Embryology Authority

Harris, John. Clones, Genes, and Immortality: Ethics and the Genetic Revolution. New York, NY: Oxford University Press; 1998. 328 p. Bibliography: p. 305–321. ISBN 0–19–288080–2. BE58945.

aborted fetuses; anencephaly; beginning of life; body parts and fluids; cadavers; cloning; confidentiality; DNA fingerprinting; embryo research; embryos; employment; eugenics; fetal tissue donation; future generations; gene therapy; genes; genetic diversity; genetic information; *genetic intervention; genetic screening; germ cells; hybrids; informed consent; injuries; insurance; justice; moral obligations; moral policy; morality; personhood; prenatal

diagnosis; property rights; remuneration; reproduction; *reproductive technologies; risks and benefits; selective abortion; social discrimination; tissue banks; tissue donation; transgenic organisms; wrongful life

Hathout, Hassan. Islamic views on some reproductive issues. *In:* Teebi, Ahmad S.; Faraq, Talaat I., eds. Genetic Disorders Among Arab Populations. New York, NY: Oxford University Press; 1997: 469–473. 7 refs. ISBN 0–19–509305–4. BE58136.

abortion, induced; adoption; contraception; fetuses; genetic intervention; *Islamic ethics; marital relationship; married persons; *reproduction; *reproductive technologies; rights

Hemminki, Elina; Santalahti, Päivi; Louhiala, Pekka. Ethical conflicts in regulating the start of life. *Perspectives in Biology and Medicine.* 1997 Summer; 40(4): 586–591. 21 refs. BE56604.

abortion on demand; *abortion, induced; allowing to die; *beginning of life; biomedical technologies; congenital disorders; disabled; embryos; eugenics; fetuses; *intensive care units; multiple pregnancy; *newborns; patient care; personhood; prematurity; *prenatal diagnosis; *reproductive technologies; selective abortion; values

Hollinger, Joan Heifetz. From coitus to commerce: legal and social consequences of noncoital reproduction. *University of Michigan Journal of Law Reform.* 1985 Summer; 18(4): 865–932. 246 fn. BE56951.

confidentiality; contracts; decision making; economics; government financing; government regulation; industry; informed consent; *legal aspects; parent child relationship; psychology; *regulation; *reproductive technologies; selection for treatment; semen donors; surrogate mothers; United States

Humphrey, Michael; Humphrey, Heather. New trends in human reproduction. *In: their* Families with a Difference: Varieties of Surrogate Parenthood. New York, NY: Routledge; 1988: 149–166, 182–183. 6 fn. ISBN 0–415–00690–2. BE56734.

artificial organs; cloning; fetuses; in vitro fertilization; legal aspects; ovum donors; parent child relationship; *reproductive technologies; sex preselection; *social impact; surrogate mothers; ectogenesis; uterus

Jakobovits, Yoel. Male infertility: halakhic issues in investigation and management. *In:* Feldman, Emanuel; Wolowelsky, Joel B., eds. Jewish Law and the New Reproductive Technologies. Hoboken, NJ: Ktav; 1997: 115–138. 89 fn. ISBN 0–88125–586–6. BE57459.

*diagnosis; *infertility; *Jewish ethics; *males; methods; *patient care; reproduction; reproductive technologies; sperm; theology; Orthodox Judaism

Johnson, Martin H. Should egg donors be paid? The culture of unpaid and voluntary egg donation should be strengthened. *BMJ (British Medical Journal).* 1997 May 10; 314(7091): 1401–1402. 10 refs. BE55650.

*altruism; blood donation; children; embryos; germ cells; *government regulation; incentives; informed consent; *legal aspects; motivation; *ovum donors; public opinion; *public policy; *remuneration; social impact; tissue donation; *Great Britain; Human Fertilisation and Embryology Act 1990; Human Fertilisation and Embryology Authority

Jones, Howard; Sher, Geoffrey; Robertson, John A., et al. Accountability in the advertising and marketing of assisted reproduction. *Women's Health Issues.* 1997 May–Jun; 7(3): 167–171. Discussion following presentations by G. Sher and M. Feinman and by J.A. Robertson at a workshop on "Assisted Reproductive Technologies, Ads, and Ethics: Philosophical, Ethical,

---

and Clinical Perspectives on the Use of Advertising in Reproductive Medicine," held by the National Advisory Board on Ethics in Reproduction in Washington, DC on 19 Oct 1996. BE55873.

*accountability; *advertising; age factors; conflict of interest; disclosure; *economics; embryo transfer; females; *health facilities; physicians; regulation; *reproductive technologies; risk; self regulation; *treatment outcome; *Pacific Fertility Medical Centers; Society for Assisted Reproductive Technology

Jung, Patricia Beattie. What price fertility? *In:* Wildes, Kevin Wm., ed. Infertility: A Crossroad of Faith, Medicine, and Technology. Boston, MA: Kluwer Academic; 1997: 167–180. 6 refs. 4 fn. ISBN 0-7923-4061-2. BE55997.

adoption; costs and benefits; disease; *economics; government financing; health care delivery; health insurance reimbursement; in vitro fertilization; *infertility; *justice; psychological stress; *public policy; *reproductive technologies; *resource allocation; rights; Roman Catholic ethics; socioeconomic factors; values; personal financing; Instruction on Respect for Human Life

Kalb, Claudia. How old is too old? *Newsweek.* 1997 May 5; 79(18): 64. BE58038.

*age factors; children; *females; mothers; ovum donors; *reproductive technologies; risks and benefits; *selection for treatment

Kazem, R.; Thompson, L.A.; Hamilton, M.P., et al. Current attitudes towards egg donation among men and women. *Human Reproduction.* 1995 Jun; 10(6): 1543–1548. 19 refs. BE55565.

aborted fetuses; *attitudes; biomedical research; cadavers; comparative studies; *cryopreservation; embryos; fathers; *females; fetal tissue donation; *infertility; knowledge, attitudes, practice; *males; mothers; *ovum; *ovum donors; patient care; patients; remuneration; reproduction; reproductive technologies; research embryo creation; semen donors; socioeconomic factors; sperm; survey; *tissue donation; ovum recipients; Great Britain

Keenan, James F. Moral horizons in health care: reproductive technologies and Catholic identity. *In:* Wildes, Kevin Wm., ed. Infertility: A Crossroad of Faith, Medicine, and Technology. Boston, MA: Kluwer Academic; 1997: 53–71. 69 refs. ISBN 0-7923-4061-2. BE55991.

attitudes; biomedical research; contraception; *health facilities; historical aspects; institutional policies; intention; marital relationship; moral policy; *religious hospitals; *reproductive technologies; *Roman Catholic ethics; sexuality; sterilization (sexual); *theology; Instruction on Respect for Human Life; Thomas Aquinas

King, Leslie; Meyer, Madonna Harrington. The politics of reproductive benefits: U.S. insurance coverage of contraceptive and infertility treatments. *Gender and Society.* 1997 Feb; 11(1): 8–30. 83 refs. 3 fn. BE57686.

age factors; *contraception; employment; eugenics; federal government; females; *government financing; health insurance; *health insurance reimbursement; indigents; infertility; political activity; politics; *public policy; *reproductive technologies; *socioeconomic factors; state government; survey; *women's health services; Illinois; Medicaid; *United States

Klotzko, Arlene Judith. Medical miracle or medical mischief? The saga of the McCaughey septuplets. *Hastings Center Report.* 1998 May–Jun; 28(3): 5–8. BE58606.

attitudes; bioethics; childbirth; drugs; fetuses; health insurance reimbursement; industry; infertility; informed

consent; international aspects; mass media; *multiple pregnancy; pregnant women; professional competence; regulation; religion; *reproductive technologies; *risks and benefits; selection for treatment; selective abortion; socioeconomic factors; treatment outcome; health services misuse; Allwood, Mandy; Christian Fundamentalists; Great Britain; *McCaughey, Bobbi; United States

Klotzko, Arlene Judith. Science fictions: cloning is bad and septuplets are good. *Washington Post.* 1997 Dec 14: C3. BE58498.

*cloning; mass media; *multiple pregnancy; *reproductive technologies; *risks and benefits

Kolata, Gina. Clinics selling embryos made for 'adoption'. [News]. *New York Times.* 1997 Nov 23: 1, 34. BE56185.

adoption; cryopreservation; economics; *embryo transfer; *embryos; eugenics; in vitro fertilization; industry; ovum donors; physician's role; remuneration; reproductive technologies; semen donors; *embryo creation; United States

Kolata, Gina. Scientists face new ethical quandaries in baby-making. [News]. *New York Times.* 1997 Aug 19: C1, C8. BE55537.

*embryo research; *methods; *ovum; physicians; *reproductive technologies; risks and benefits; trends; United States

Kondratowicz, Diane M. Approaches responsive to reproductive technologies: a need for critical assessment and directions for further study. *Cambridge Quarterly of Healthcare Ethics.* 1997 Spring; 6(2): 148–156. 49 fn. BE56429.

attitudes; autonomy; consensus; decision making; empirical research; *evaluation; feminist ethics; freedom; in vitro fertilization; infertility; justice; *morality; public participation; public policy; regulation; reproduction; *reproductive technologies; rights; risks and benefits; *social control; social impact; women's rights

Since its inception decades ago, technological intervention in human reproduction has been the subject of considerable attention and controversy. After identifying two focal points of debate, I focus in this paper upon an emerging body of literature responsive to a host of problematic issues that, scholars claim, reproductive technologies pose. Maintaining that critical assessment of this literature is necessary, I identify two areas of inquiry which deserve attention and, correspondingly, sketch directions which might guide further study.

Krebs, D. Rules and ethics concerning assisted procreation established by the government in Germany. *Journal of Assisted Reproduction and Genetics.* 1996 Mar; 13(3): 193–195. 3 refs. BE55876.

beginning of life; cloning; criminal law; *embryo research; embryo transfer; genetic disorders; genetic intervention; germ cells; *government regulation; hybrids; in vitro fertilization; informed consent; *legal aspects; multiple pregnancy; ovum donors; physicians; posthumous reproduction; preimplantation diagnosis; *reproductive technologies; semen donors; sex preselection; surrogate mothers; Embryo Protection Act 1990 (Germany); *Germany

Lemonick, Michael D. The new revolution in making babies. *Time.* 1997 Dec 1; 150(23): 40–46. BE58122.

adoption; age factors; cryopreservation; economics; embryos; females; infertility; males; methods; ovum; regulation; *reproductive technologies; treatment outcome; *trends; *United States

Levy, Michael J.; Kent-First, Marijo Greene; Zieselman, Kimberly. Panel one: marketing strategies and informing the patient/consumer. [Articles followed by discussion]. *Women's Health Issues.* 1997 May–Jun; 7(3): 172–187. 2 refs. Papers presented and discussion at a workshop on "Assisted Reproductive Technologies, Ads and Ethics: Philosophical, Ethical and Clinical Perspectives on the Use of Advertising in Reproductive Medicine," held by the National Advisory Board on Ethics in Reproduction in Washington, DC on 19 Oct 1996. BE55877.

> *advertising; *diagnosis; *disclosure; *economics; embryo transfer; genetic counseling; genetic disorders; genetic screening; genome mapping; *health facilities; health insurance reimbursement; *infertility; males; medical fees; methods; patient education; *patient satisfaction; prognosis; program descriptions; *reproductive technologies; *risk; *risks and benefits; *treatment outcome; personal financing; quality control; Shady Grove Fertility Center (Rockville, MD)

Lock, Margaret. Perfecting society: reproductive technologies, genetic testing, and the planned family in Japan. *In:* Lock, Margaret; Kaufert, Patricia A., eds. Pragmatic Women and Body Politics. New York, NY: Cambridge University Press; 1998: 206–239. 57 refs. ISBN 0–521–62929–2. BE58695.

> abortion, induced; adoption; anthropology; *attitudes; autonomy; coercion; contraception; disabled; eugenics; family planning; family relationship; *females; feminist ethics; genetic disorders; *genetic screening; historical aspects; infanticide; married persons; paternalism; prenatal diagnosis; religion; *reproduction; *reproductive technologies; selective abortion; self concept; sex determination; single persons; social discrimination; *social dominance; social impact; stigmatization; women's rights; non–Western World; *Japan

Lockwood, G.M. Donating life: practical and ethical issues in gamete donation. *In:* Shenfield, F.; Sureau, C., eds. Ethical Dilemmas in Assisted Reproduction. New York, NY: Parthenon Pub. Group; 1997: 23–30. 9 refs. ISBN 1–85070–916–5. BE57943.

> aborted fetuses; *altruism; brain death; cadavers; coercion; directed donation; family members; family relationship; females; *incentives; motivation; *ovum donors; public policy; *remuneration; reproductive technologies; risks and benefits; semen donors; socioeconomic factors; treatment outcome; Great Britain

Lublin, Nancy. Pandora's Box: Feminism Confronts Reproductive Technology. Lanham, MD: Rowman and Littlefield; 1998. 189 p. Bibliography: p. 171–182. ISBN 0–8476–8637–X. BE56785.

> abortion, induced; childbirth; contraception; dissent; ecology; equal protection; *females; *feminist ethics; infertility; justice; legal rights; political activity; prenatal diagnosis; privacy; religious ethics; reproduction; *reproductive technologies; sexuality; social discrimination; women's rights; Feminist International Network of Resistance to Reproductive and Genetic Engineering (FINRRAGE)

McClure, Mary Ann. Infertility. *In:* Chadwick, Ruth, ed. Encyclopedia of Applied Ethics, Volume 2. San Diego, CA: Academic Press; 1998: 673–678. 9 refs. ISBN 0–12–227067–3. BE56398.

> adoption; artificial insemination; autonomy; beginning of life; coercion; common good; contraception; costs and benefits; cryopreservation; embryos; in vitro fertilization; *infertility; involuntary sterilization; married persons; remuneration; reproduction; *reproductive technologies; risks and benefits; selection for treatment; single persons; surrogate mothers

Macklin, Ruth; White, Gladys B. Assisted reproductive technologies, ads, and ethics: philosophical, ethical, and

clinical perspectives on the use of advertising in reproductive medicine. [Conference report]. *Women's Health Issues.* 1997 May–Jun; 7(3): 127–131. Executive summary of a workshop held by the National Advisory Board on Ethics in Reproduction in Washington, DC on 19 Oct 1996. BE55882.

> accountability; *advertising; advisory committees; *economics; federal government; government regulation; industry; infertility; information dissemination; methods; professional organizations; regulation; *reproductive technologies; risk; *treatment outcome; quality assurance; Federal Trade Commission; National Advisory Board on Ethics in Reproduction (NABER); Society for Assisted Reproductive Technology; United States

Macklin, Ruth. Genetics and reproductive technologies. *In:* Borchert, Donald M., ed. The Encyclopedia of Philosophy. Supplement. New York, NY: Simon and Schuster and Macmillan; 1996: 217–220. 13 refs. ISBN 0–02–864629–0. BE57222.

> embryo disposition; eugenics; genetic counseling; genetic enhancement; genetic information; *genetic intervention; genetic predisposition; genetic screening; parent child relationship; *reproductive technologies

Maranto, Gina. Quest for Perfection: The Drive to Breed Better Human Beings. New York, NY: Scribner; 1996. 335 p. Bibliography: p. 303–315. ISBN 0–684–80029–2. BE56131.

> age factors; ancient history; anthropology; artificial insemination; attitudes; children; cloning; confidentiality; congenital disorders; cryopreservation; death; disabled; disclosure; embryo research; embryo transfer; embryos; *eugenics; females; gene therapy; genetic disorders; genetic enhancement; genetic intervention; genetic research; *historical aspects; in vitro fertilization; infanticide; infertility; international aspects; involuntary sterilization; legal aspects; males; medical specialties; minority groups; ovum donors; physicians; posthumous reproduction; preimplantation diagnosis; psychological stress; reproduction; *reproductive technologies; selection for treatment; semen donors; sex preselection; sociology of medicine; sperm; Eighteenth Century; Europe; Middle Ages; Nineteenth Century; Renaissance; Twentieth Century; United States

Mardesic, Tonko; Rezacova, Jitka; Ventruba, Pavel. The practice of assisted reproduction in the Czech Republic. *Journal of Assisted Reproduction and Genetics.* 1996 Mar; 13(3): 195–196. 4 refs. BE55883.

> data banks; government regulation; health facilities; registries; *reproductive technologies; self regulation; *Czech Republic

Merchant, Jennifer. Biogenetics, artificial procreation, and public policy in the United States and France. *Technology in Society.* 1996; 18(1): 1–15. 26 fn. BE56595.

> abortion, induced; advisory committees; biomedical research; cesarean section; coercion; comparative studies; criminal law; cryopreservation; drug abuse; embryo disposition; *embryo research; federal government; *fetal research; fetal therapy; *fetuses; *genetic research; genetic screening; genetic services; *government financing; in vitro fertilization; indigents; industry; international aspects; judicial action; *legal aspects; legal liability; legal rights; personhood; physicians; *pregnant women; preimplantation diagnosis; prenatal diagnosis; *prenatal injuries; private sector; *public policy; *reproductive technologies; state government; state interest; Supreme Court decisions; torts; treatment refusal; women's health services; women's rights; *wrongful life; Bonbrest v. Kotz; France; Roe v. Wade; *United States

Meyer, Cheryl L. The Wandering Uterus: Politics and the Reproductive Rights of Women. New York, NY:

New York University Press; 1997. 226 p. 294 fn. ISBN 0-8147-5562-3. BE56511.

abortion, induced; age factors; artificial insemination; cesarean section; coercion; communicable diseases; contraception; contracts; cryopreservation; embryo transfer; embryos; employment; *females; fetuses; government regulation; guidelines; health hazards; in vitro fertilization; international aspects; *legal aspects; misconduct; multiple pregnancy; ovum donors; physicians; *politics; pregnant women; prematurity; prenatal injuries; professional organizations; property rights; remuneration; *reproduction; *reproductive technologies; risk; selection for treatment; self regulation; semen donors; *social control; *social discrimination; social dominance; surrogate mothers; treatment refusal; *women's health; *women's rights; hysterectomy; Davis v. Davis; In re A.C.; In re Baby M; International Union, UAW v. Johnson Controls, Inc.; Johnson v. Calvert; Roe v. Wade; RU-486; *United States

Montgomery, Jonathan. Health care law and ethics: abortion; fertility; maternity care; selective treatment of the newborn; transplantation; terminal care and euthanasia. *In: his* Health Care Law. New York, NY: Oxford University Press; 1997: 357-456. 503 fn. ISBN 0-19-876260-7. BE56245.

*abortion, induced; active euthanasia; *adults; *allowing to die; assisted suicide; body parts and fluids; cadavers; childbirth; congenital disorders; conscience; contraception; family planning; fetuses; health personnel; *legal aspects; legal liability; legislation; living wills; maternal health; minors; *newborns; *organ donation; organ donors; organ transplantation; *patient care; persistent vegetative state; *pregnant women; prenatal injuries; remuneration; *reproductive technologies; selective abortion; spousal consent; sterilization (sexual); surrogate mothers; terminal care; therapeutic abortion; treatment refusal; *Great Britain

Mori, Takahide. Egg donation should be limited to women below 60 years of age. *Journal of Assisted Reproduction and Genetics.* 1995 Apr; 12(4): 229-230. 10 refs. BE55589.

*age factors; children; *embryo transfer; *females; *ovum; ovum donors; parent child relationship; *reproductive technologies; *selection for treatment; Japan

Moutel, G.; Leroux, N.; Hervé, C. Analysis of a survey of 36 French research committees on intracytoplasmic sperm injection. *Lancet.* 1998 Apr 11; 351(9109): 1121-1123. 16 refs. BE58310.

embryo transfer; *ethical review; evaluation; health facilities; *human experimentation; in vitro fertilization; infertility; males; *methods; *reproductive technologies; research design; *research ethics committees; risks and benefits; *sperm; survey; technical expertise; therapeutic research; *intracytoplasmic sperm injection; *France

BACKGROUND: In France, when a new medical technology is to be applied experimentally to human beings, it must adhere to the principles stipulated by the Huriet-Sérusclat law on biomedical research. This law requires that the validation of a protocol applicable to human beings, with its corollary protection and information dimensions, is first submitted to a research committee, known as a Consultative Committee Protecting Persons in Biomedical Research (CCPPRB). We aimed to survey the competence of these committees in biotechnology, and whether or not intracytoplasmic sperm injection (ICSI) had been considered by the committees as being an innovative treatment. METHODS: We presented each of France's 48 CCPPRBs with a questionnaire to assess the choices and criteria for making decisions that arose at the time ICSI was implemented in the different centres in each region. FINDINGS: 36 committees took part. We found that ICSI had been largely introduced in settings outside the scope of the CCPPRBs and of the framework fixed by

the law on biomedical research. Only three centres for medically assisted reproduction had submitted applications to a CCPPRB, although ICSI has been implemented in over 20 centres. 21 (58%) committees were of the opinion that the implementation of ICSI could have come under their supervision. 24 (67%) committees believed that, independently of their own involvement, evaluation procedures for ICSI should have been specified before centres decided to introduce it. INTERPRETATION: We observed important differences in the way CCPPRBs handled ICSI as being within or outside the medical research field. The status of the research committees is legally and identically defined. However, committees did not agree on the definition of the limits of their action, and, therefore, their handling of the same issue differed. An inquiry is needed to define how, now that ICSI is done in many centres, it should adhere to principles of evaluation and safety already in existence for other medical technologies.

New York State Task Force on Life and the Law. Assisted Reproductive Technologies: Analysis and Recommendations for Public Policy. New York, NY: The Task Force; 1998 Apr. 474 p. Includes references. ISBN 1-881268-03-9. BE57846.

advertising; advisory committees; age factors; Buddhist ethics; children; Christian ethics; cloning; counseling; cryopreservation; disclosure; embryo disposition; embryo research; embryos; federal government; genetic screening; government regulation; *guidelines; health insurance reimbursement; Hindu ethics; homosexuals; infertility; informed consent; Islamic ethics; Jewish ethics; legal aspects; multiple pregnancy; ovum donors; parent child relationship; posthumous reproduction; preimplantation diagnosis; psychology; *public policy; remuneration; reproduction; *reproductive technologies; review; risks and benefits; selection for treatment; semen donors; sex preselection; single persons; *standards; state government; surrogate mothers; treatment outcome; *New York; *New York State Task Force on Life and the Law; United States

Newman, Lucile F. Framing the ethical issues in new reproductive technologies. *Health Care for Women International.* 1987; 8(4): 287-292. 5 refs. BE56663.

autonomy; biomedical research; biomedical technologies; embryo research; females; human experimentation; human rights; justice; public policy; *reproductive technologies; resource allocation; risks and benefits; social control; values

Nisker, Jeffrey A. In quest of the perfect analogy for using in vitro fertilization patients as oocyte donors. *Women's Health Issues.* 1997 Jul-Aug; 7(4): 241-247. 31 refs. BE55730.

body parts and fluids; *coercion; *commodification; compassion; *dehumanization; *disadvantaged; *females; *in vitro fertilization; *indigents; international aspects; justice; literature; medical education; *narrative ethics; *ovum donors; patient compliance; *patients; *remuneration; reproductive technologies; risk; social dominance; teaching methods; women's rights

Ohl, Dana A.; Park, John; Cohen, Carl, et al. Procreation after death or mental incompetence: medical advance or technology gone awry? *Fertility and Sterility.* 1996 Dec; 66(6): 889-895. 24 refs. BE56878.

artificial insemination; brain death; *brain pathology; case studies; *competence; *cryopreservation; decision making; guidelines; informed consent; legal aspects; married persons; moral obligations; physicians; *posthumous reproduction; *reproductive technologies; *semen donors; single persons; *sperm; terminally ill; third party consent

Okonofua, Friday E. The case against new reproductive

technologies in developing countries. *British Journal of Obstetrics and Gynaecology.* 1996 Oct; 103(10): 957–962. 37 refs. BE56879.

> costs and benefits; *developing countries; evaluation; government financing; infertility; prevalence; *public policy; *reproductive technologies; resource allocation; risks and benefits; *Nigeria

Paulson, Richard J. Ethical considerations involving oocyte donation and gestational surrogacy. *Seminars in Reproductive Endocrinology.* 1995 Aug; 13(3): 225–230. 20 refs. BE55540.

> abortion, induced; age factors; coercion; conflict of interest; congenital disorders; ethics committees; females; fetuses; morbidity; mortality; newborns; organizational policies; *ovum donors; parent child relationship; political activity; pregnant women; religion; remuneration; reproduction; *reproductive technologies; rights; risk; selection for treatment; semen donors; *surrogate mothers; women's rights; American Fertility Society; Right to Life Movement

Pennings, Guido. Should donors have the right to decide who receives their gametes? *Human Reproduction.* 1995 Oct; 10(10): 2736–2740. 24 refs. BE57507.

> age factors; attitudes; autonomy; confidentiality; cultural pluralism; *directed donation; females; homosexuals; informed consent; moral policy; *ovum donors; public opinion; public policy; remuneration; resource allocation; selection for treatment; *semen donors; single persons

Peters, Ted. For the Love of Children: Genetic Technology and the Future of the Family. Louisville, KY: Westminster John Knox Press; 1996. 227 p. (The family, religion, and culture). 356 fn. ISBN 0–664–25468–3. BE55695.

> children; *Christian ethics; *family relationship; fetal development; fetuses; genetic screening; humanism; libertarianism; *marital relationship; methods; natural law; ovum donors; parent child relationship; personhood; Protestant ethics; *reproduction; *reproductive technologies; Roman Catholic ethics; selective abortion; sexuality; surrogate mothers; theology; values

Porter, Jean. Human need and natural law. *In:* Wildes, Kevin Wm., ed. Infertility: A Crossroad of Faith, Medicine, and Technology. Boston, MA: Kluwer Academic; 1997: 93–106. 5 refs. ISBN 0–7923–4061–2. BE55993.

> children; dissent; in vitro fertilization; *marital relationship; married persons; *natural law; reproduction; *reproductive technologies; *Roman Catholic ethics; sexuality; *theology; *Instruction on Respect for Human Life

Pyers, Greg; Gott, Robert. Fertility Rights: The IVF Debate. Carlton, VIC, Australia: CIS Publishers; 1993. 49 p. (Australian issues series). ISBN 1–86391–102–2. BE57445.

> beginning of life; children; cryopreservation; economics; *embryo research; *embryo transfer; embryos; feminist ethics; *in vitro fertilization; infertility; legal aspects; *methods; *public policy; *reproductive technologies; *risks and benefits; social impact; terminology; treatment outcome; *Australia

Ramogida, C. The views of the patients. *In:* Shenfield, F.; Sureau, C., eds. Ethical Dilemmas in Assisted Reproduction. New York, NY: Parthenon Pub. Group; 1997: 83–85. ISBN 1–85070–916–5. BE57950.

> attitudes; confidentiality; government regulation; *ovum donors; patients; *reproductive technologies; *semen donors; France

Roberts, Dorothy. Killing the Black Body: Race, Reproduction, and the Meaning of Liberty. New York, NY: Pantheon Books; 1997. 373 p. 1,073 fn. ISBN 0–679–44226–X. BE57998.

> abortion, induced; adolescents; autonomy; *blacks; *coercion; *contraception; criminal law; deception; dehumanization; *drug abuse; eugenics; family relationship; *females; genetic identity; government financing; historical aspects; indigents; *involuntary sterilization; justice; legal aspects; misconduct; morality; parent child relationship; physicians; *pregnant women; *prenatal injuries; property rights; public policy; rape; *reproduction; *reproductive technologies; risks and benefits; sexuality; *social control; *social discrimination; socioeconomic factors; stigmatization; surrogate mothers; personal identity; slavery; Depo-provera; Medicaid; Nineteenth Century; Norplant; Twentieth Century; United States

Robertson, John A. Ethical and legal issues in human embryo donation. *Fertility and Sterility.* 1995 Nov; 64(5): 885–894. 25 refs. BE57244.

> adoption; attitudes; children; commodification; compensation; confidentiality; counseling; disclosure; *donors; embryo research; *embryo transfer; *embryos; in vitro fertilization; informed consent; *legal aspects; legal liability; legal rights; motivation; organization and administration; *ovum donors; parent child relationship; remuneration; risks and benefits; *semen donors; United States

Robertson, John A. Innovations in infertility treatment and the rush to market. *Women's Health Issues.* 1997 May–Jun; 7(3): 162–166. Paper presented at a workshop on "Assisted Reproductive Technologies, Ads, and Ethics: Philosophical, Ethical, and Clinical Perspectives on the Use of Advertising in Reproductive Medicine," held by the National Advisory Board on Ethics in Reproduction in Washington, DC on 19 Oct 1996. BE55888.

> breast cancer; cryopreservation; ethical review; females; genetic screening; informed consent; males; *methods; *regulation; *reproductive technologies; risks and benefits; self regulation; sperm; standards; investigational therapies; ovaries; Great Britain; United States

Roleff, Tamara L., ed. Biomedical Ethics: Opposing Viewpoints. San Diego, CA: Greenhaven Press; 1998. 252 p. (Opposing viewpoints series). Includes references. ISBN 1–56510–792–6. BE59107.

> age factors; animal organs; autonomy; beneficence; *bioethical issues; body parts and fluids; brain death; cadavers; capital punishment; childbirth; *cloning; eugenics; females; genes; *genetic intervention; *genetic research; genetic screening; genome mapping; government regulation; indigents; moral policy; *organ donation; organ transplantation; patents; personhood; posthumous reproduction; pregnant women; presumed consent; prisoners; public policy; remuneration; *reproductive technologies; risks and benefits; selection for treatment; surrogate mothers; transgenic animals

Rowland, Robyn. A child at any price? An overview of issues in the use of the new reproductive technologies, and the threat to women. *Women's Studies International Forum.* 1985; 8(6): 539–546. 35 refs. 7 fn. BE57836.

> coercion; eugenics; *females; industry; investigators; males; regulation; reproduction; *reproductive technologies; resource allocation; risks and benefits; sex preselection; *social control; social discrimination; social impact; socioeconomic factors; *women's rights

Ryan, Maura Anne. Justice and Artificial Reproduction: A Catholic Feminist Analysis. Ann Arbor, MI: University Microfilms International; 1993. 214 p. Bibliography: p. 204–214. Order No. 9400369. Dissertation, Ph.D. in Philosophy, Yale University, May 1993. BE56516.

BE = bioethics accession number   fn. = footnotes   refs. = references

autonomy; common good; economics; ethical theory; family relationship; females; *feminist ethics; goals; health care; health insurance reimbursement; human rights; *indigents; *infertility; *justice; *moral policy; obligations of society; parent child relationship; population control; regulation; reproduction; *reproductive technologies; resource allocation; *Roman Catholic ethics; self concept; social impact; *socioeconomic factors; theology; women's rights; United States

Sauer, Mark V. Should egg donors be paid? Exploitation or a woman's right? *BMJ (British Medical Journal).* 1997 May 10; 314(7091): 1403. BE55665.
autonomy; drugs; health facilities; industry; infertility; informed consent; institutional policies; international aspects; *ovum donors; physicians; private sector; *remuneration; reproductive technologies; risk; self regulation; Great Britain; *United States

Scritchfield, Shirley A. The infertility enterprise: IVF and the technological construction of reproductive impairments. *In:* Wertz, Dorothy C., ed. Research in the Sociology of Health Care: A Research Annual. Volume 8. Greenwich, CT: JAI Press; 1989: 61–97. 104 refs. 12 fn. ISBN 1-55938-043-8. BE57348.
age factors; autonomy; disclosure; drugs; *economics; embryo research; embryos; employment; *females; goals; health hazards; *in vitro fertilization; *industry; *infertility; males; morality; motivation; parent child relationship; physician patient relationship; *physicians; prevalence; preventive medicine; professional autonomy; reproduction; *reproductive technologies; review; *risks and benefits; *social dominance; *social impact; socioeconomic factors; statistics; *treatment outcome; trends; values; women's health; United States

Selz, Michael. Birth business: industry races to aid infertile. [News]. *Wall Street Journal.* 1997 Nov 26: B1, B12. BE56189.
diagnosis; drug industry; *economics; entrepreneurship; in vitro fertilization; *industry; infertility; medical devices; physicians; *private sector; *reproductive technologies; personal financing; *United States

Serour, Gamal I.; Aboulghar, Mohamed A.; Mansour, Ragaa T. Reproductive health care policies around the world: bioethics in medically assisted conception in the Muslim world. *Journal of Assisted Reproduction and Genetics.* 1995 Oct; 12(9): 559–565. 68 refs. BE57687.
aborted fetuses; cryopreservation; developing countries; embryo research; embryos; fetal research; gene therapy; genetic enhancement; genetic research; infertility; *Islamic ethics; marital relationship; morality; multiple pregnancy; ovum donors; *reproductive technologies; research embryo creation; selective abortion; semen donors; surrogate mothers

Shenfield, F.; Sureau, C., eds. Ethical Dilemmas in Assisted Reproduction. New York, NY: Parthenon Pub. Group; 1997. 96 p. (Studies in profertility series; v.7). 161 refs. ISBN 1-85070-916-5. BE57940.
altruism; cultural pluralism; embryo research; eugenics; females; incentives; international aspects; legal aspects; males; methods; minority groups; multiple pregnancy; ovum donors; preimplantation diagnosis; remuneration; *reproductive technologies; resource allocation; selection for treatment; selective abortion; semen donors; sex determination; socioeconomic factors; sperm; surrogate mothers; Canada; Europe; Great Britain

Shenfield, F. Justice and access to fertility treatments. *In:* Shenfield, F.; Sureau, C., eds. Ethical Dilemmas in Assisted Reproduction. New York, NY: Parthenon Pub. Group; 1997: 7–14. 21 refs. ISBN 1-85070-916-5. BE57941.

age factors; deontological ethics; economics; *government financing; justice; *reproductive technologies; *resource allocation; rights; *selection for treatment; *socioeconomic factors; utilitarianism; *Great Britain; National Health Service

Sher, Geoffrey; Feinman, Michael. Accountability, representation, and advertising. *Women's Health Issues.* 1997 May–Jun; 7(3): 153–161. Paper presented at a workshop on "Assisted Reproductive Technologies, Ads, and Ethics: Philosophical, Ethical, and Clinical Perspectives on the Use of Advertising in Reproductive Medicine," held by the National Advisory Board on Ethics in Reproduction in Washington, DC on 19 Oct 1996. BE55924.
*accountability; *advertising; age factors; computers; *disclosure; *economics; females; *health facilities; health insurance reimbursement; in vitro fertilization; infertility; information dissemination; males; organizational policies; professional organizations; program descriptions; *reproductive technologies; *self regulation; *treatment outcome; personal financing; American Medical Association; *Pacific Fertility Medical Centers; Society for Assisted Reproductive Technology; United States

Shifman, Pinhas. New reproductive technologies and Jewish law. *In:* Jewish Law Annual. Volume Twelve. Amsterdam, Netherlands: Harwood Academic Publishers; 1997: 127–136. 19 fn. ISBN 90-5702-551-5. BE58347.
adoption; artificial insemination; disclosure; embryo transfer; genetic identity; government regulation; human rights; in vitro fertilization; *Jewish ethics; moral obligations; ovum donors; parent child relationship; patient care; privacy; records; reproduction; *reproductive technologies; semen donors; sexuality; single persons; surrogate mothers; *Israel; Sweden

Shildrick, Margrit. Leaky Bodies and Boundaries: Feminism, Postmodernism and (Bio)ethics. New York, NY: Routledge; 1997. 252 p. Bibliography: p. 231–244. ISBN 0-415-14617-8. BE56731.
autonomy; *bioethics; body parts and fluids; caring; cultural pluralism; *ethical theory; *females; *feminist ethics; health care; historical aspects; homosexuals; *human body; humanism; infertility; informed consent; males; medicine; moral development; mother fetus relationship; paternalism; *philosophy; physician patient relationship; pregnant women; reproduction; *reproductive technologies; risks and benefits; selection for treatment; *self concept; sexuality; social dominance; stigmatization; *postmodernism; rationality; Derrida, Jacques; Foucault, Michel; Irigaray, Luce

Silver, Lee M. Remaking Eden: Cloning and Beyond in a Brave New World. New York, NY: Avon Books; 1997. 317 p. Includes references. ISBN 0-380-97494-0. BE56517.
artificial insemination; beginning of life; *cloning; cryopreservation; embryos; eugenics; family relationship; fathers; females; fetal development; freedom; future generations; genetic enhancement; genetics; germ cells; government regulation; homosexuals; in vitro fertilization; infertility; males; mothers; motivation; ovum donors; parent child relationship; preimplantation diagnosis; religion; reproduction; *reproductive technologies; rights; semen donors; single persons; *social impact; socioeconomic factors; surrogate mothers; transgenic animals; *trends; United States

Simini, Bruno. Italy's assisted-reproduction clinics face restriction. [News]. *Lancet.* 1998 Jun 13; 351(9118): 1796. BE58883.
cloning; embryo research; germ cells; *government regulation; *health facilities; *legislation; *reproductive

---

BE = bioethics accession number   fn. = footnotes   refs. = references

technologies; selection for treatment; *Italy

Skovmand, Kaare. First–ever fertilisation bill passed in Denmark. [News]. *Lancet.* 1997 Jun 7; 349(9066): 1678. BE55831.
> age factors; cryopreservation; embryo transfer; embryos; females; government financing; *government regulation; homosexuals; in vitro fertilization; *legislation; private sector; proprietary health facilities; public sector; *reproductive technologies; selection for treatment; sex preselection; single persons; time factors; *Denmark

Stolberg, Sheryl Gay. U.S. publishes first guide to treatment of infertility. [News]. *New York Times.* 1997 Dec 19: A22. BE56943.
> federal government; *health facilities; *infertility; *information dissemination; multiple pregnancy; *reproductive technologies; statistics; *treatment outcome; Centers for Disease Control and Prevention; *United States

Talbot, Margaret. The egg women. *New Republic.* 1998 Mar 16; 218(11): 42. BE57841.
> advertising; attitudes; commodification; entrepreneurship; eugenics; *industry; motivation; *ovum donors; parents; remuneration; reproductive technologies; semen donors; socioeconomic factors; *donor selection

te Velde, E.R.; van Baar, A.L.; van Kooij, R.J. Concerns about assisted reproduction. *Lancet.* 1998 May 23; 351(9115): 1524–1525. 11 refs. BE58314.
> age factors; *children; chromosome abnormalities; comparative studies; congenital disorders; cryopreservation; embryo research; embryo transfer; embryos; *evaluation; evaluation studies; females; health; in vitro fertilization; infertility; intelligence; males; methods; regulation; reproduction; *reproductive technologies; *research design; *risk; *sperm; *treatment outcome; *intracytoplasmic sperm injection; Australia; Belgium; Sweden

Toaff, Elio. Judaism. *Dolentium Hominum: Church and Health in the World.* 1996; 31(11th Yr., No. 1): 78–81. BE57376.
> bioethics; biomedical technologies; compassion; *Jewish ethics; justice; love; *medical ethics; medicine; parent child relationship; physicians; religion; *reproductive technologies; self regulation; social impact; suffering; theology; value of life; Italy

Turiel, Judith Steinberg. Beyond Second Opinions: Making Choices About Fertility Treatment. Berkeley, CA: University of California Press; 1998. 393 p. Bibliography: 361–385. ISBN 0–520–20854–4. BE58321.
> advertising; age factors; cryopreservation; decision making; diagnosis; disclosure; drug industry; drugs; embryo research; embryos; entrepreneurship; federal government; gamete intrafallopian transfer; government financing; government regulation; iatrogenic disease; in vitro fertilization; industry; *infertility; information dissemination; informed consent; international aspects; managed care programs; mass media; misconduct; multiple pregnancy; ovum donors; patient care; *patient education; patient participation; physicians; professional competence; *reproductive technologies; retreatment; *risks and benefits; selective abortion; self regulation; surgery; technology assessment; time factors; uncertainty; *investigational therapies; United States

U.S. Court of Appeals, Eighth Circuit. Krauel v. Iowa Methodist Medical Center. *Federal Reporter, 3d Series.* 1996 Sep 11 (date of decision). 95: 674–681. BE58830.
> employment; federal government; females; government regulation; *health insurance reimbursement; infertility; *legal aspects; legal rights; legislation; *reproductive technologies; social discrimination; Americans with Disabilities Act 1990; Civil Rights Act 1964; Iowa; *Krauel v. Iowa Methodist Medical Center; Pregnancy

Discrimination Act; United States
> The U.S. Court of Appeals for the Eighth Circuit held that an employer–provided health insurance plan policy of denying coverage for infertility treatments does not violate the Americans with Disabilities Act (ADA), the Pregnancy Discrimination Act (PDA), or Title VII of the Civil Rights Act of 1964. Krauel underwent artificial insemination and GIFT (gamete intrafallopian tube transfer) prior to pregnancy and birth. She unsuccessfully sought reimbursement for those costs from her medical insurer. The court held that infertility does not substantially affect what are "major life activities" within the meaning of the ADA. The infertility exclusion applies equally to all insured employees, male of female, disabled or not, and thus does not thwart the purpose of the ADA, nor does it constitute a discriminatory sex–based classification under Title VII. Furthermore, infertility is not a medical condition related to pregnancy or childbirth, and so falls outside the scope of the PDA. (KIE abstract)

Van Steirteghem, A.; Tournaye, H.; Sureau, C., et al. Ethical considerations of intracytoplasmic sperm injection. *In:* Shenfield, F.; Sureau, C., eds. Ethical Dilemmas in Assisted Reproduction. New York, NY: Parthenon Pub. Group; 1997: 51–56. 23 refs. ISBN 1–85070–916–5. BE57946.
> children; disclosure; genetic counseling; genetic disorders; genetic screening; infertility; informed consent; males; *methods; parents; *reproductive technologies; risks and benefits; *sperm

Van Steirteghem, André. Outcome of assisted reproductive technology. [Editorial]. *New England Journal of Medicine.* 1998 Jan 15; 338(3): 194–195. 10 refs. BE56441.
> childbirth; chromosome abnormalities; congenital disorders; disclosure; embryo transfer; hybrids; in vitro fertilization; methods; multiple pregnancy; newborns; *reproductive technologies; risk; statistics; *treatment outcome; Great Britain; United States

Verhey, Allen. Commodification, commercialization, and embodiment. *Women's Health Issues.* 1997 May–Jun; 7(3): 132–142. 12 refs. Paper presented at a workshop on "Assisted Reproductive Technologies, Ads, and Ethics: Philosophical, Ethical, and Clinical Perspectives on the Use of Advertising in Reproductive Medicine," held by the National Advisory Board on Ethics in Reproduction in Washington, DC on 19 Oct 1996. BE55952.
> children; coercion; *commodification; deception; dehumanization; *economics; embryo transfer; freedom; informed consent; misconduct; morality; ovum donors; *personhood; physicians; regulation; reproduction; *reproductive technologies; rights; treatment outcome; values; wedge argument; Asch, Ricardo

Virginia. Status of children of assisted conception. *Code of Virginia Annotated.* 1997 Jul 1 (date effective). Sects. 20–156 to 20–165. 11 p. Sects. 20–156, 20–158, and 20–163 amended 1998. BE58895.
> children; *contracts; cryopreservation; embryos; *legal aspects; *parent child relationship; posthumous reproduction; remuneration; *reproductive technologies; *surrogate mothers; *Virginia

Wall, James M. A time to be born. *Christian Century.* 1997 May 14; 114(16): 467–468. BE57263.
> *age factors; autonomy; children; common good; *females; guidelines; public policy; *reproductive technologies; selection for treatment; time factors; United States

---

BE = bioethics accession number   fn. = footnotes   refs. = references

Walters, LeRoy, ed. Ethical issues arising from human reproductive technologies and arrangements. *In:* Jonsen, Albert R.; Veatch, Robert M.; Walters, LeRoy, eds. Source Book in Bioethics: A Documentary History. Washington, DC: Georgetown University Press; 1998: 335-406. 22 refs. ISBN 0-87840-683-2. BE57893.

   advisory committees; artificial insemination; contracts; embryo transfer; embryos; federal government; government regulation; guidelines; historical aspects; *in vitro fertilization; infertility; *international aspects; legal aspects; moral obligations; moral policy; organizational policies; ovum donors; professional organizations; public policy; remuneration; *reproductive technologies; Roman Catholic ethics; *surrogate mothers; value of life; *American College of Obstetricians and Gynecologists; *American Fertility Society; Canada; Ethics Advisory Board; Europe; *Glover Report; Great Britain; *In re Baby M; *Instruction on Respect for Human Life; *Office of Technology Assessment; *Royal Commission on New Reproductive Technologies (Canada); *Twentieth Century; United States; Victoria; *Waller Committee; *Warnock Committee

Wennerholm, Ulla-Britt; Albertsson-Wikland, Kerstin; Bergh, Christina, et al. Postnatal growth and health in children born after cryopreservation as embryos. *Lancet.* 1998 Apr 11; 351(9109): 1085-1090. 33 refs. BE58311.

   age factors; *children; chronically ill; communicable diseases; comparative studies; congenital disorders; *cryopreservation; *embryo transfer; *embryos; evaluation studies; health; *in vitro fertilization; infants; *morbidity; prevalence; reproduction; reproductive technologies; *treatment outcome; Sweden

   BACKGROUND: There is uncertainty about the health of children born from in-vitro fertilisation (IVF) with cryopreserved embryos. We investigated the postnatal growth and health (up to 18 months) of these children compared with those born after standard IVF with fresh embryos and those from spontaneous pregnancies. METHODS: 255 children from cryopreserved embryos were matched by maternal age, parity, single or twin pregnancy, and date of delivery with 255 children born after IVF with fresh embryos, and 252 children from spontaneous pregnancies. The main endpoint was growth; secondary endpoints were the prevalence of chronic illness, major malformations, cumulative incidence of common diseases, and development during the first 18 months. Growth was assessed by comparison with standard Swedish growth charts and by standard deviation scores. FINDINGS: Growth features were similar for both singletons and twins in the three groups. There were 6 (2.4%) of 255, 9 (3.5%) of 255, and 8 (3.2%) of 252 major malformations in the cryopreserved group, standard IVF, and spontaneous groups, respectively (p=0.6 between the cryopreserved and standard IVF group). The prevalence of chronic diseases did not differ between the three groups, with 18.0%, 15.3%, and 16.7% of children with a chronic illness in the cryopreserved group, standard IVF, and spontaneous groups, respectively. INTERPRETATION: The cryopreservation process does not adversely affect the growth and health of children during infancy and early childhood. Minor handicaps, behavioural disturbances, learning difficulties, and dysfunction of attention and perception cannot be ruled out at this age.

Wildes, Kevin Wm., ed. Infertility: A Crossroad of Faith, Medicine, and Technology. Boston, MA: Kluwer Academic; 1997. 243 p. (Philosophy and medicine; v. 53. Catholic studies in bioethics; v. 3). 293 refs. 99 fn. Includes appendix: Sacred Congregation for the Doctrine. *Instruction on Respect for Human Life in its*

Origin and on the Dignity of Procreation: Replies to Certain Questions of the Day. ISBN 0-7923-4061-2. BE55990.

   common good; dissent; economics; freedom; health facilities; in vitro fertilization; *infertility; marital relationship; methods; morality; natural law; psychology; public policy; reproduction; *reproductive technologies; resource allocation; *Roman Catholic ethics; secularism; sexuality; *theology; *Instruction on Respect for Human Life

Yovich, John L.; Matson, Phillip L. Legislation on the practice of assisted reproduction in Western Australia. *Journal of Assisted Reproduction and Genetics.* 1996 Mar; 13(3): 197-200. BE56074.

   advisory committees; committee membership; cryopreservation; embryos; ethical review; federal government; germ cells; *government regulation; *guidelines; health facilities; hybrids; laboratories; legislation; professional organizations; property rights; public policy; *regulation; *reproductive technologies; *self regulation; *standards; state government; time factors; *Australia; Fertility Society of Australia; *Human Reproductive Technology Act 1991 (Western Australia); National Health and Medical Research Council (Australia); *Reproductive Technology Accreditation Committee (Australia); *Western Australia; *Western Australian Reproductive Technology Council

Zohar, Noam J. Parenthood: natural fact and human society. *In: his* Alternatives in Jewish Bioethics. Albany, NY: State University of New York Press; 1997: 69-84. 26 fn. ISBN 0-7914-3274-2. BE57043.

   adoption; artificial insemination; Jewish ethics; parent child relationship; *reproductive technologies; semen donors; surrogate mothers; *theology

A woman who died may become a mother. [News]. *New York Times.* 1997 Dec 7: 33. BE58129.

   *cryopreservation; *embryos; *females; in vitro fertilization; *posthumous reproduction; *reproductive technologies; semen donors; surrogate mothers

Aetna to charge extra for in vitro fertilization. [News]. *New York Times.* 1998 Jan 15: A15. BE57597.

   *health insurance reimbursement; *in vitro fertilization; *reproductive technologies; *Aetna

Full exposure: eternal vigilance over reproductive technology is better than banning it. [Editorial]. *New Scientist.* 1998 Jan 31; 157(2119): 3. BE59091.

   animal experimentation; human experimentation; hybrids; infertility; males; *regulation; *reproductive technologies; risks and benefits; sperm; tissue transplantation; rodents

RESEARCH DESIGN
See under
   BEHAVIORAL RESEARCH/RESEARCH DESIGN
   HUMAN EXPERIMENTATION/RESEARCH DESIGN

RESEARCH ETHICS COMMITTEES *See* HUMAN EXPERIMENTATION/ETHICS COMMITTEES

RESOURCE ALLOCATION

See also SELECTION FOR TREATMENT

Asch, Adrienne. Distracted by disability. *Cambridge Quarterly of Healthcare Ethics.* 1998 Winter; 7(1): 77-87. 22 fn. BE58450.

   assisted suicide; *attitudes; autonomy; bioethics; chronically

---

BE = bioethics accession number   fn. = footnotes   refs. = references

ill; communication; cultural pluralism; *decision making; depressive disorder; *disabled; goals; *health care; health facilities; *health personnel; medicine; minority groups; *moral obligations; motivation; *obligations of society; *patient care; *physically disabled; physician patient relationship; physicians; quality of life; rehabilitation; *resource allocation; social discrimination; *stigmatization; treatment refusal; withholding treatment; dependency

Austad, Carol Shaw. Is Long–Term Psychotherapy Unethical? Toward a Social Ethic in an Era of Managed Care. San Francisco, CA: Jossey–Bass; 1996. 283 p. Includes references. ISBN 0–7879–0218–7. BE56093.
accountability; alternatives; behavior disorders; beneficence; case studies; confidentiality; conflict of interest; costs and benefits; economics; empirical research; evaluation; health care delivery; health care reform; health insurance; health personnel; justice; long–term care; *managed care programs; mental health; mentally ill; *patient care; practice guidelines; professional competence; professional ethics; professional patient relationship; psychoactive drugs; *psychotherapy; quality of health care; remuneration; *resource allocation; selection for treatment; standards; *time factors; treatment outcome; health services misuse; United States

Bodenheimer, Thomas. The Oregon Health Plan –– lessons for the nation. [First of two parts]. *New England Journal of Medicine.* 1997 Aug 28; 337(9): 651–655. 20 refs. BE59005.
decision making; disabled; *economics; employment; federal government; *government financing; government regulation; *health care delivery; health insurance; *indigents; *managed care programs; public participation; *public policy; quality of life; *resource allocation; social discrimination; state government; treatment outcome; capitation fee; *Medicaid; *Oregon; *Oregon Health Plan; Oregon Health Services Commission

Bodenheimer, Thomas S.; Grumbach, Kevin. Medical ethics and the rationing of health care. *In: their* Understanding Health Policy: A Clinical Approach. Stamford, CT: Appleton and Lange; 1995: 173–194. 45 refs. ISBN 0–8385–3678–6. BE56193.
allowing to die; autonomy; beneficence; case studies; costs and benefits; decision making; *economics; futility; gatekeeping; *health care; health insurance; indigents; intensive care units; *justice; medical ethics; organ transplantation; physician patient relationship; physicians; prolongation of life; public policy; *resource allocation; scarcity; selection for treatment; self induced illness; terminally ill; withholding treatment; Oregon; United States

Boyle, Philip J.; Moskowitz, Ellen. Making tough resource decisions. *Health Progress.* 1996 Nov–Dec; 77(6): 48–53. 3 refs. BE56322.
autonomy; common good; costs and benefits; *decision making; disclosure; due process; goals; guidelines; *hospitals; informed consent; *institutional policies; intensive care units; justice; patient care team; prognosis; *resource allocation; *selection for treatment; *values; severity of illness index

Burgoyne, Carole B. Distributive justice and rationing in the NHS: framing effects in press coverage of a controversial decision. *Journal of Community and Applied Social Psychology.* 1997 Apr; 7(2): 119–136. 28 refs. BE57544.
administrators; bone marrow; *children; costs and benefits; *decision making; *government financing; *health care delivery; justice; leukemia; *mass media; parents; physicians; prognosis; public opinion; *public sector; quality of life; *refusal to treat; *resource allocation; social worth; tissue transplantation; value of life; values; *withholding treatment; *Bowen, Jaymee; *Great Britain; *National Health Service; R v. Cambridge Health Authority

Calman, Kenneth C. Equity, poverty and health for all. *BMJ (British Medical Journal).* 1997 Apr 19; 314(7088): 1187–1191. 8 refs. BE56859.
*economics; *health; health care; *health care delivery; *indigents; international aspects; justice; public health; public policy; quality of life; *resource allocation; socioeconomic factors; Great Britain; National Health Service; World Health Organization

Casarett, David J.; Lantos, John D. Have we treated AIDS too well? Rationing and the future of AIDS exceptionalism. *Annals of Internal Medicine.* 1998 May 1; 128(9): 756–759. 29 refs. BE57906.
*AIDS; biomedical research; drugs; *economics; government financing; health care reform; health insurance; justice; patient care; political activity; *public policy; *resource allocation; stigmatization; AZT; Ryan White Comprehensive AIDS Resources Emergency Act 1990; *United States
During the past decade, medical therapy for AIDS has become more effective but also prohibitively expensive. A medical tragedy has been transformed into a financial crisis, and society has responded by establishing special programs and sources of funding for AIDS. These maneuvers parallel earlier approaches to HIV testing and reporting that have collectively come to be known as 'exceptionalism.' This paper suggests that exceptionalism in resource allocation is a fragile, short–term solution. In the long run, AIDS exceptionalism will create growing injustice and should be avoided. However, we should not eliminate the advances that this exceptionalism has already achieved. Instead, we need a working dialogue between these advances and public policy.

Cherry, Christopher. Health care, human worth and the limits of the particular. *Journal of Medical Ethics.* 1997 Oct; 23(5): 310–314. 10 fn. BE57103.
common good; costs and benefits; disabled; *health care; human characteristics; *managed care programs; physician patient relationship; quality adjusted life years; quality of life; *resource allocation; social worth; speciesism; *value of life
An ethics concerned with health care developments and systems must be historically continuous, especially as it concerns the application to managed structures of key moral–epistemic concepts such as care, love and empathy. These concepts are traditionally most at home in the personal, individual domain. Human beings have non–instrumental worth just because they are human beings and not by virtue of their capacities. Managed health care systems tend to abstract from this worth in respect of both individuals' distinctness and individual identity. The first, a common feature of quantitative approaches to health care assessment and delivery, is avoidable. The second, by contrast, is necessarily sacrificed in impersonally managed structures. Failure to distinguish the two encourages confusion and distress, and the demand for impossible medico–moral relationships.

Coney, Sandra. Rationing in health care under scrutiny in New Zealand. [News]. *Lancet.* 1997 Oct 18; 350(9085): 1152. BE56182.
dementia; guidelines; *health care delivery; health care reform; private sector; *public policy; public sector; refusal to treat; renal dialysis; *resource allocation; selection for treatment; withholding treatment; *New Zealand; Williams, Rau

Culyer, Anthony. Need: is a consensus possible? [Editorial]. *Journal of Medical Ethics.* 1998 Apr; 24(2):

77–80. 7 refs. BE58053.
biomedical research; biomedical technologies; consensus; costs and benefits; decision making; goals; health; *health care; health care delivery; health promotion; justice; *resource allocation; rights; terminology; *needs; Great Britain; National Health Service

Daniels, Norman. Family responsibility initiatives and justice between age groups. *Law, Medicine and Health Care.* 1985 Sep; 13(4): 153–159. 25 fn. BE56702.
adults; *age factors; *aged; beneficence; biomedical technologies; children; *community services; disabled; economics; *family members; *family relationship; *financial support; *health care; health care delivery; home care; *justice; legal obligations; *long-term care; love; *moral obligations; *obligations of society; parents; patient care; private sector; *public policy; public sector; quality of life; *resource allocation; selection for treatment; socioeconomic factors; trends; prudence; United States

Docker, Christopher. The way forward? *In:* McLean, Sheila A.M., ed. Death, Dying and the Law. Brookfield, VT: Dartmouth; 1996: 129–160. 99 fn. ISBN 1-85521-657-4. BE57217.
*active euthanasia; *advance directives; aged; *allowing to die; *assisted suicide; decision making; double effect; economics; hospices; legal aspects; living wills; pain; *palliative care; *persistent vegetative state; physicians; public policy; *resource allocation; selection for treatment; terminal care; withholding treatment; *Great Britain; National Health Service; Netherlands; United States

Dresser, Rebecca. Setting priorities for science support. *Hastings Center Report.* 1998 May–Jun; 28(3): 21–23. 7 fn. BE58609.
accountability; administrators; *biomedical research; *decision making; *federal government; *government financing; investigators; justice; politics; professional autonomy; public participation; public policy; *resource allocation; science; *National Institutes of Health; *U.S. Congress; *United States

Dworkin, Ronald. Justice in the distribution of health care. *McGill Law Journal.* 1993; 38(4): 883–898. 3 fn. The McGill Lecture in Jurisprudence and Public Policy, delivered at the Faculty of Law, McGill University, 17 Mar 1993. BE59026.
*economics; *health care; health care reform; health insurance; *justice; models, theoretical; obligations of society; public participation; public policy; *resource allocation; Canada; United States

Edgar, A. Health care allocation, public consultation and the concept of 'health'. *Health Care Analysis.* 1998 Sep; 6(3): 193–198. 10 refs. BE58980.
autonomy; commodification; democracy; economics; *health; *health care; *health care delivery; health insurance; health promotion; humanism; justice; libertarianism; managed care programs; *moral policy; obligations of society; public participation; *public policy; *resource allocation; self induced illness; state medicine; values; Great Britain; National Health Service; Oregon; United States

Edgar, Andrew. Quality of life indicators. *In:* Chadwick, Ruth, ed. Encyclopedia of Applied Ethics, Volume 3. San Diego, CA: Academic Press; 1998: 759–776. 16 refs. ISBN 0-12-227068-1. BE56268.
aged; contracts; costs and benefits; decision making; disabled; *evaluation; *health; health care; health services research; patient participation; physicians; prognosis; public participation; public policy; *quality adjusted life years; *quality of life; *resource allocation; social discrimination; *treatment outcome; utilitarianism; values; severity of illness index; Great Britain

Edgar, Andrew; Salek, Sam; Shickle, Darren, et al. The Ethical QALY: Ethical Issues in Healthcare Resource Allocations. Haslemere, Surrey, England: Euromed Communications; 1998. 168 p. Bibliography: p. 139–168. ISBN 1-899015-21-3. BE58582.
age factors; drug industry; economics; evaluation; health; *health care; *health care delivery; *international aspects; justice; legal aspects; methods; *moral policy; personhood; public health; *public policy; *quality adjusted life years; *quality of life; *resource allocation; scarcity; selection for treatment; social discrimination; social worth; time factors; trends; value of life; Czech Republic; Denmark; *Europe; France; Great Britain; Greece; Netherlands; New Zealand; Norway; Slovakia; Slovenia; Sweden

Farmer, Paul. Listening for prophetic voices in medicine. *America.* 1997 Jul 5; 177(1): 8–10, 12–13. BE55935.
AIDS; biomedical technologies; children; Christian ethics; communicable diseases; developing countries; drugs; *economics; females; *health care delivery; *indigents; industry; international aspects; *justice; obligations of society; patient compliance; prognosis; *resource allocation; selection of subjects; *social discrimination; *socioeconomic factors; suffering; therapeutic research; value of life; withholding treatment; tuberculosis; Haiti; Peru; United States

Fry, Sara T. Rationing health care: the ethics of cost containment. *Nursing Economics.* 1983 Nov–Dec; 1(3): 165–169. 11 refs. BE57495.
alternatives; decision making; *economics; federal government; government financing; *health care; health care delivery; health care reform; health insurance; justice; nurses; *public policy; *resource allocation; personal financing; Medicaid; Securing Access to Health Care (President's Commission for the Study of Ethical Problems); *United States

Gurewich, Victor; Johnson, James R.; Sobieraj, Jerry, et al. Truth or consequences. [Letters and response]. *New England Journal of Medicine.* 1998 Aug 6; 339(6): 410–412. 4 refs. BE58975.
alternatives; communication; costs and benefits; *disclosure; *economics; health insurance reimbursement; health maintenance organizations; incentives; patient care; *physician's role; *resource allocation; time factors; withholding treatment

Hackler, Chris. Is rationing of health care ethically defensible? *In:* Monagle, John F.; Thomasma, David C., eds. Health Care Ethics: Critical Issues for the 21st Century. Gaithersburg, MD: Aspen Publishers; 1998: 371–377. 12 fn. ISBN 0-8342-0911-X. BE56291.
*decision making; *economics; *health care; justice; public participation; public policy; *resource allocation; standards; terminology; values; United States

Hall, Mark A.; Berenson, Robert A. Ethical practice in managed care: a dose of realism. *Annals of Internal Medicine.* 1998 Mar 1; 128(5): 395–402. 72 refs. BE57850.
administrators; common good; conflict of interest; *decision making; disclosure; *economics; ethical analysis; *guidelines; health; health care delivery; health insurance reimbursement; *incentives; *managed care programs; *medical ethics; moral obligations; moral policy; patient advocacy; patient care; *physician patient relationship; physician's role; *physicians; practice guidelines; public policy; remuneration; *resource allocation; *trust; withholding treatment; capitation fee; United States
This article examines the ethics of medical practice under managed care from a pragmatic perspective that gives physicians more useful guidance than do existing ethical statements. The article begins with a framework for constructing a realistic set of ethical principles, namely,

---

BE = bioethics accession number   fn. = footnotes   refs. = references

that medical ethics derives from physicians' role as healers; that ethical statements are primarily aspirational, not regulatory; and that preserving patient trust is the primary objective. The following concrete ethical guidelines are presented: Financial incentives should influence physicians to maximize the health of the group of patients under their care; physicians should not enter into incentive arrangements that they are embarrassed to describe accurately to their patients; physicians should treat each patient impartially without regard to source of payment, consistent with the physician's own treatment style; if physicians depart from this ideal, they should inform their patients honestly; and it is desirable, although not mandatory, to differentiate medical treatment recommendations from insurance coverage decisions by clearly assigning authority over these different roles and by physicians advocating for recommended treatment that is not covered.

Halm, Ethan A.; Causino, Nancyanne; Blumenthal, David. Is gatekeeping better than traditional care? A survey of physicians' attitudes. *JAMA.* 1997 Nov 26; 278(20): 1677–1681. 23 refs. BE56305.

*attitudes; comparative studies; *economics; *evaluation; *gatekeeping; health insurance; knowledge, attitudes, practice; *managed care programs; organization and administration; patient care; physician patient relationship; *physicians; preventive medicine; primary health care; professional autonomy; *quality of health care; *referral and consultation; *resource allocation; *risks and benefits; *social impact; survey; time factors; continuity of patient care; outpatients; Boston; Massachusetts General Hospital

CONTEXT: Nearly all managed care plans rely on a physician "gatekeeper" to control use of specialty, hospital, and other expensive services. Gatekeeping is intended to reduce costs while maintaining or improving quality of care by increasing coordination and prevention and reducing duplicative or inappropriate care. Whether gatekeeping achieves these goals remains largely unproven. OBJECTIVE: To assess physicians' attitudes about the effects of gatekeeping compared with traditional care on administrative work, quality of patient care, appropriateness of resource use, and cost. DESIGN: Cross-sectional survey of primary care physicians. SETTING: Outpatient facilities in metropolitan Boston, Mass. PARTICIPANTS: All physicians who served as both primary care gatekeepers and traditional Blue Cross/Blue Shield providers for the employees of Massachusetts General Hospital, Boston. Of the 330 physicians surveyed, 202 (61%) responded. OUTCOMES MEASURES: Physician ratings of the effects of gatekeeping on 21 aspects of care, including administrative work, physician–patient interactions, decision making, appropriateness of resource use, cost, and quality of care. RESULTS: Physicians reported that gatekeeping (compared with traditional care) had a positive effect on control of costs, frequency, and appropriateness of preventive services and knowledge of a patient's overall care (P less than .001). They also felt that gatekeeping increased paperwork and telephone calls and negatively affected the overall quality of care, access to specialists, ability to order expensive tests and procedures, freedom in clinical decisions, time spent with patients, physician–patient relationships, and appropriate use of hospitalizations and laboratory tests (P less than .001). Overall, 32% of physicians rated gatekeeping as better than traditional care, 40% the same, 21% gatekeeping as worse, and 7% were of mixed opinion. Positive ratings of gatekeeping were associated with fewer years in clinical practice, generalist training, and experience with gatekeeping and health maintenance

organization plans. CONCLUSIONS: Physicians identified both positive and negative effects of gate-keeping. Overall, 72% of physicians thought gatekeeping was better than or comparable to traditional care arrangements.

Ham, Chris. Priority setting in health care: learning from international experience. *Health Policy.* 1997 Oct; 42(1): 49–66. 23 refs. BE57983.

advisory committees; biomedical technologies; common good; comparative studies; consensus; costs and benefits; *decision making; *economics; government financing; *health care; health care delivery; health personnel; indigents; *international aspects; justice; mass media; practice guidelines; public participation; *public policy; quality of life; *resource allocation; rights; selection for treatment; state government; technical expertise; technology assessment; *values; evidence-based medicine; *Great Britain; Medicaid; National Health Service; *Netherlands; *New Zealand; *Oregon; *Sweden; United States

Ham, Chris. Retracing the Oregon Trail: the experience of rationing and the Oregon health plan. *BMJ (British Medical Journal).* 1998 Jun 27; 316(7149): 1965–1969. 11 refs. BE58811.

advisory committees; aged; costs and benefits; decision making; disabled; employment; evaluation; *government financing; *health care delivery; health insurance; health maintenance organizations; *indigents; *managed care programs; physician's role; *practice guidelines; public participation; *public policy; *resource allocation; state government; technical expertise; values; evidence-based medicine; *Medicaid; *Oregon; Oregon Basic Health Services Act 1989; Oregon Health Services Commission

Hoge, Steven K. APA resource document: I. The professional responsibilities of psychiatrists in evolving health care systems. *Bulletin of the American Academy of Psychiatry and the Law.* 1996; 24(3): 393–406. 11 refs. BE56208.

autonomy; conflict of interest; contracts; *decision making; *disclosure; *economics; freedom; guidelines; *health care delivery; *health care reform; health insurance; health insurance reimbursement; incentives; legal aspects; *managed care programs; medical ethics; *mentally ill; *moral obligations; *patient advocacy; *patient care; *patient participation; physician patient relationship; *physicians; professional autonomy; professional competence; *psychiatry; psychotherapy; *quality of health care; referral and consultation; remuneration; *resource allocation; self regulation; trends; withholding treatment; continuity of patient care; personal financing; utilization review; American Psychiatric Association; *United States

Hoge, Steven K. APA resource document: II. Regulatory guidelines for protecting the interests of psychiatric patients in emerging health care systems. *Bulletin of the American Academy of Psychiatry and the Law.* 1996; 24(3): 407–418. 6 refs. BE56209.

advertising; contracts; decision making; disclosure; due process; *economics; federal government; freedom; *government regulation; guidelines; *health care delivery; health care reform; health insurance reimbursement; incentives; *legal aspects; legal liability; legislation; malpractice; *managed care programs; medical ethics; mentally ill; model legislation; organization and administration; organizational policies; patient advocacy; patient participation; *physicians; professional autonomy; professional organizations; psychiatry; public policy; referral and consultation; *resource allocation; state government; torts; withholding treatment; utilization review; American Medical Association; American Psychiatric Association; Employee Retirement Income Security Act 1974 (ERISA); *United States

---

BE = bioethics accession number   fn. = footnotes   refs. = references

Jones, D.G. Aging, dementia and care: setting limits on the allocation of health care resources to the aged. *New Zealand Medical Journal.* 1997 Dec 12; 110(1057): 466–468. 19 refs. BE58211.
> age factors; *aged; autonomy; beneficence; biomedical technologies; caring; *dementia; guidelines; health care; justice; *patient care; privacy; prolongation of life; quality of life; *resource allocation; dignity

Klein, Rudolph; Day, Patricia; Redmayne, Sharon. Managing Scarcity: Priority Setting and Rationing in the National Health Service. Philadelphia, PA: Open University Press; 1996. 161 p. (State of health series). Bibliography: p. 143–153. ISBN 0–335–19446–X. BE55699.
> accountability; administrators; age factors; biomedical technologies; *decision making; *economics; government financing; health care; *health care delivery; health care reform; international aspects; physician's role; physicians; politics; public participation; *public policy; quality adjusted life years; referral and consultation; refusal to treat; renal dialysis; reproductive technologies; *resource allocation; scarcity; *selection for treatment; self induced illness; standards; time factors; uncertainty; evidence-based medicine; geographic factors; *Great Britain; *National Health Service; Oregon; United States

Levinsky, Norman G. Truth or consequences. *New England Journal of Medicine.* 1998 Mar 26; 338(13): 913–915. 8 refs. BE57771.
> administrators; aged; alternatives; coercion; costs and benefits; deception; *decision making; *disclosure; *economics; health insurance reimbursement; hospitals; incentives; institutional policies; managed care programs; medical devices; moral obligations; organizational policies; patient advocacy; patient care; *physician's role; public policy; *resource allocation; withholding treatment; United States

Light, Donald W. The real ethics of rationing. *BMJ (British Medical Journal).* 1997 Jul 12; 315(7100): 112–115. 19 refs. This article is a shortened version of the inaugural lecture given at the Institute of Medicine, Law, and Bioethics of the University of Manchester on 26 Mar 1997. BE55651.
> accountability; administrators; costs and benefits; *government financing; *health care; *health care delivery; health insurance; insurance selection bias; justice; medical specialties; misconduct; *organization and administration; physician's role; private sector; public policy; *resource allocation; scarcity; selection for treatment; surgery; time factors; treatment outcome; evidence-based medicine; geographic factors; health services misuse; *Great Britain; *National Health Service

Love, Susan M.; Tuckfelt, Mark; Nicklin, David, et al. Rationing by any other name. [Letters and response]. *New England Journal of Medicine.* 1997 Nov 6; 337(19): 1395–1396. 3 refs. BE58267.
> costs and benefits; decision making; *economics; gatekeeping; *health care delivery; health insurance; indigents; managed care programs; patient care; *physicians; *resource allocation; rights; *withholding treatment; health services misuse; United States

Marshall, Tom; St. Leger, Moya Frenz; Woodroffe, Caroline, et al. Rationing health care. [Letters]. *BMJ (British Medical Journal).* 1997 Jun 28; 314(7098): 1901–1902. 7 refs. BE56916.
> age factors; common good; costs and benefits; *goals; health; health care; *health care delivery; justice; moral policy; national health insurance; public health; *public policy; quality of life; *resource allocation; selection for treatment; social discrimination; utilitarianism; *Great Britain;

*National Health Service

Mehlman, Maxwell J.; Botkin, Jeffrey R. Access to the Genome: The Challenge to Equality. Washington, DC: Georgetown University Press; 1998. 152 p. 231 fn. ISBN 0–87840–678–6. BE57386.
> carriers; communitarianism; disclosure; economics; employment; eugenics; gene pool; gene therapy; genetic counseling; genetic disorders; genetic enhancement; genetic information; *genetic intervention; genetic predisposition; genetic screening; *genetic services; *genome mapping; germ cells; health insurance reimbursement; insurance; *justice; late-onset disorders; libertarianism; managed care programs; mandatory testing; moral policy; newborns; policy analysis; prenatal diagnosis; *public policy; *resource allocation; rights; *risks and benefits; scarcity; selection for treatment; selective abortion; social discrimination; *social impact; social worth; stigmatization; utilitarianism; ELSI-funded publication; personal financing; *Human Genome Project; Medicaid; Medicare; National Center for Human Genome Research; United States

Meslin, Eric M.; Lemieux–Charles, Louise; Wortley, Jacinth Tracey. An ethics framework for assisting clinician–managers in resource allocation decision making. *Hospital and Health Services Administration.* 1997 Spring; 42(1): 33–48. 49 refs. 2 fn. BE58444.
> *administrators; *decision making; economics; ethical analysis; ethics consultation; *hospitals; *institutional policies; justice; nurses; obligations to society; patient admission; patient advocacy; patient care; *patient care team; physicians; referral and consultation; *resource allocation; selection for treatment; survey; terminal care; Canada; *Ontario

Morgan, Derek. Health rights, ethics and justice: the opportunity costs of rhetoric. *In:* McLean, Sheila A.M., ed. Contemporary Issues in Law, Medicine and Ethics. Brookfield, VT: Dartmouth; 1996: 15–27. 32 fn. ISBN 1–85521–586–1. BE57788.
> alternatives; confidentiality; cultural pluralism; disclosure; emergency care; government regulation; health; *health care; human rights; international aspects; *justice; legal rights; legislation; moral obligations; *moral policy; obligations of society; patient access to records; *patients' rights; physician patient relationship; public health; *public policy; referral and consultation; *resource allocation; *rights; risks and benefits; selection for treatment; socioeconomic factors; *standards; life style; European Union; *Great Britain; *National Health Service; Patient's Charter (Great Britain)

Morreim, E. Haavi. At the intersection of medicine, law, economics, and ethics: bioethics and the art of intellectual cross-dressing. *In:* Carson, Ronald A.; Burns, Chester R., eds. Philosophy of Medicine and Bioethics: A Twenty-Year Retrospective and Critical Appraisal. Boston, MA: Kluwer Academic; 1997: 299–325. 78 refs. 28 fn. ISBN 0–7923–3545–7. BE56544.
> bioethics; conflict of interest; contracts; *economics; ethics; *financial support; government financing; guidelines; *health care delivery; health insurance; health insurance reimbursement; indigents; industry; interdisciplinary communication; justice; law; legal aspects; legal liability; *legal obligations; *managed care programs; medical specialties; medicine; *moral obligations; *patient advocacy; *patient care; *physician's role; *physicians; professional autonomy; professional organizations; quality of health care; referral and consultation; remuneration; *resource allocation; *standards; therapeutic research; torts; values; utilization review; United States

New, Bill; Le Grand, Julian. Rationing in the NHS: Principles and Pragmatism. London: King's Fund Publishing; 1996. 77 p. Bibliography: p. 73–77. ISBN

1-85717-113-6. BE59102.

aged; costs and benefits; *decision making; drugs; economics; goals; government financing; *health care delivery; health care reform; hospitals; justice; national health insurance; physician's role; public participation; *public policy; quality adjusted life years; *resource allocation; selection for treatment; self induced illness; standards; time factors; needs; *Great Britain; *National Health Service

Nilstun, Tore; Ohlsson, Rolf. Should health care be rationed by age? *Scandinavian Journal of Social Medicine.* 1995 Jun; 23(2): 81–84. 18 refs. BE55518.

*age factors; autonomy; biomedical technologies; costs and benefits; *health care; justice; *moral policy; organ transplantation; *resource allocation; *scarcity; *selection for treatment; utilitarianism; Sweden

Orentlicher, David. Practice guidelines: a limited role in resolving rationing decisions. *Journal of the American Geriatrics Society.* 1998 Mar; 46(3): 369–372. 27 refs. Paper presented at the 1996 Congress of Clinical Societies. BE56770.

alternatives; biomedical technologies; costs and benefits; decision making; evaluation; *guidelines; health insurance reimbursement; incentives; *managed care programs; physicians; *practice guidelines; *resource allocation; risks and benefits; treatment outcome; values; United States

Pellegrino, Edmund D. Managed care at the bedside: how do we look in the moral mirror? *Kennedy Institute of Ethics Journal.* 1997 Dec; 7(4): 321–330. 14 refs. BE59013.

beneficence; biomedical technologies; *conflict of interest; contracts; disclosure; *economics; employment; gatekeeping; *managed care programs; *moral obligations; obligations to society; patient advocacy; patient care; *physician patient relationship; physician's role; *physicians; professional competence; quality of health care; *resource allocation; sociology of medicine; technical expertise; vulnerable populations; withholding treatment; continuity of patient care; gag clauses; *United States

Managed care per se is a morally neutral concept; however, as practiced today, it raises serious ethical issues at the clinical, managerial, and social levels. This essay focuses on the ethical issues that arise at the bedside, looking first at the ethical conflicts faced by the physician who is charged with responsibility for care of the patient and then turning to the way in which managed care exacts costs that are measured not in dollars but in compromises in the caring dimensions of the patient–physician relationship.

Pentz, Rebecca D. Expanding into organizational ethics: the experience of one clinical ethics committee. *HEC (HealthCare Ethics Committee) Forum.* 1998 Jun; 10(2): 213–219. 5 fn. BE59068.

bone marrow; cancer; case studies; *clinical ethics committees; costs and benefits; decision making; *economics; *ethics consultation; guidelines; hospitals; *institutional ethics; *institutional policies; justice; moral obligations; physicians; *resource allocation; tissue transplantation; treatment outcome; M.D. Anderson Cancer Center; Texas

Powers, Madison. Theories of justice in the context of research. *In:* Kahn, Jeffrey P.; Mastroianni, Anna C.; Sugarman, Jeremy, eds. Beyond Consent: Seeking Justice in Research. New York, NY: Oxford University Press; 1998: 147–165. 26 fn. ISBN 0-19-511353-5. BE58848.

age factors; AIDS; autonomy; *biomedical research; critically ill; decision making; developing countries; disadvantaged; ecology; economics; emergency care; females; freedom; health care delivery; *human experimentation; informed consent; *justice; libertarianism; military personnel; *moral policy; nontherapeutic research;

occupational medicine; political activity; prisoners; *public policy; research design; research ethics committees; research subjects; *resource allocation; *risks and benefits; selection of subjects; social discrimination; vulnerable populations; United States

Reiman, Jeffrey. On euthanasia and health care. *In:* his Critical Moral Liberalism: Theory and Practice. Lanham, MD: Rowman and Littlefield; 1997: 211–219. 8 fn. ISBN 0-8476-8314-1. BE57649.

*active euthanasia; age factors; aged; allowing to die; autonomy; *health care; *moral policy; personhood; public policy; quality of life; *resource allocation; *right to die; self concept; suffering; value of life; *voluntary euthanasia; wedge argument

Reinhardt, Uwe E. Wanted: a clearly articulated social ethic for American health care. *JAMA.* 1997 Nov 5; 278(17): 1446–1447. 18 refs. BE56051.

attitudes; *economics; federal government; *health care; health care delivery; health insurance; *indigents; justice; minors; *public policy; quality of health care; *resource allocation; rights; *socioeconomic factors; *values; personal financing; Friedman, Milton; Mortal Peril: Our Inalienable Right to Health Care (Epstein, R.); *United States

Relman, Arnold S. The economic future of health care: *False Hopes: Why America's Quest for Perfect Health Is a Recipe for Failure,* by Daniel Callahan, and *Life without Disease: The Pursuit of Medical Utopia,* by William B. Schwartz. [Book review essay]. *New England Journal of Medicine.* 1998 Jun 18; 338(25): 1855–1856. BE58630.

attitudes; attitudes to death; biomedical technologies; costs and benefits; *economics; health; *health care delivery; *health care reform; industry; life extension; managed care programs; policy analysis; public policy; quality of life; *resource allocation; trends; values; *False Hopes: Why America's Quest for Perfect Health Is a Recipe for Failure (Callahan, D.); *Life without Disease: The Pursuit of Medical Utopia (Schwartz, W.B.); Twenty-First Century; United States

Richmond, Caroline; Heasell, Stephen; Kahtan, Susannah, et al. Compensation for victims of medical accidents. [Letters]. *BMJ (British Medical Journal).* 1998 Jan 3; 316(7124): 73–74. 2 refs. BE57973.

*compensation; economics; *health care; hospitals; iatrogenic disease; *injuries; legal aspects; *legal liability; *negligence; *patient care; *patients; physicians; *resource allocation; time factors; *Great Britain; National Health Service

Rosner, Fred; Kark, Pieter; Packer, Samuel. Oregon's health care rationing plan. *Journal of General Internal Medicine.* 1996 Feb; 11(2): 104–108. 30 fn. BE57620.

biomedical technologies; costs and benefits; decision making; *government financing; government regulation; *health care delivery; health care reform; *indigents; justice; managed care programs; physician patient relationship; public participation; *public policy; quality of life; *resource allocation; social impact; standards; state government; values; *Medicaid; *Oregon; Oregon Basic Health Services Act 1989; Oregon Health Services Commission

Savulescu, Julian. Consequentialism, reasons, value and justice. *Bioethics.* 1998 Jul; 12(3): 212–235. 61 fn. BE58894.

age factors; autonomy; *health care; *justice; *moral policy; philosophy; *prognosis; *resource allocation; rights; *selection for treatment; *teleological ethics; *utilitarianism; values; rationality; *Harris, John

Over the past 10 years, John Harris has made important contributions to thinking about distributive justice in

---

health care. In his latest work, Harris controversially argues that clinicians should stop prioritising patients according to prognosis. He argues that the good or benefit of health care is providing each individual with an opportunity to live the best and longest life possible for him or her. I call this thesis, opportunism. For the purpose of distribution of resources in health care, Harris rejects welfarism (the thesis that the good of health care is well-being) and argues that utilitarianism in general may lead to de facto discrimination against groups of people needing health care. I argue that well-being is a superior theory of the good of health care to Harris' opportunism. Harris' concerns about utilitarianism can be better addressed by: (i) relating justice more closely to reasons for action; (ii) by conceptualising the relationship between reasons for action and the value of the consequences of those actions as a plateau rather than scalar relationship. Justice can be understood as satisfying as many equally rational claims on resources as possible. The rationality of a person's claim on health resources turns on the strength of that person's reasons to promote certain health-related states of affairs. I argue that the strength of that reason does not track the expected value of that state of affairs in a fully scalar fashion. Rather a person can have most reason to promote some state of affairs, even though he or she could promote other more valuable states of affairs. Thus there can be equal reason for a distributor of public resources to save either of two people, even though one will have a better and more valuable life. This approach, while addressing many of Harris' concerns about utilitarianism, does not imply that doctors should give up prioritising patients according to prognosis altogether, but it does allow that patients with lower but reasonable prognosis should have a share of public resources.

Sharpe, Virginia A. The politics, economics, and ethics of "appropriateness". *Kennedy Institute of Ethics Journal.* 1997 Dec; 7(4): 337–343. 8 refs. 1 fn. BE59015.
   biomedical technologies; costs and benefits; *decision making; economics; empirical research; *health care; health insurance; *health insurance reimbursement; managed care programs; mass screening; *patient care; patients; physicians; public participation; public policy; *resource allocation; risks and benefits; *standards; treatment outcome; trends; evidence-based medicine; needs; *United States
The terms "appropriate" and "necessary" are crucial determinants in decisions regarding the use and reimbursement of medical treatments. This paper encourages greater awareness of the political, economic, and normative assumptions that give meaning to these concepts.

Shaw, A.B. Ensuring equity and quality of care for elderly people: a critique of the College report. *Journal of the Royal College of Physicians of London.* 1995 Mar–Apr; 29(2): 89–91. 14 refs. BE56567.
   *age factors; *aged; biomedical technologies; costs and benefits; health care; justice; public policy; *resource allocation; scarcity; *selection for treatment; Great Britain

Sheehan, Myles N. Intergenerational justice: is it possible? *In:* Monagle, John F.; Thomasma, David C., eds. Health Care Ethics: Critical Issues for the 21st Century. Gaithersburg, MD: Aspen Publishers; 1998: 353–365. 14 fn. ISBN 0–8342–0911–X. BE56290.
   *age factors; *aged; caring; common good; compassion; disabled; extraordinary treatment; freedom; health care; human rights; indigents; *justice; love; *moral obligations; obligations of society; parent child relationship; public participation; public policy; *resource allocation; *Roman Catholic ethics; theology; value of life; United States

Shickle, Darren. Resource allocation. *In:* Chadwick, Ruth, ed. Encyclopedia of Applied Ethics, Volume 3. San Diego, CA: Academic Press; 1998: 861–873. 13 refs. ISBN 0–12–227068–1. BE56273.
   *economics; *health care; health care reform; international aspects; justice; national health insurance; public opinion; public policy; random selection; *resource allocation; rights; selection for treatment; utilitarianism; value of life; Great Britain; Netherlands; New Zealand; United States

Snyder, Jack W. Making Medical Spending Decisions: The Law, Ethics, and Economics of Rationing Mechanisms, by Mark A. Hall. [Book review essay]. *Journal of Legal Medicine.* 1998 Mar; 19(1): 143–150. 16 fn. BE58930.
   costs and benefits; *decision making; disclosure; *economics; guidelines; *health care; health insurance; incentives; informed consent; managed care programs; patient participation; *physician's role; public participation; *resource allocation; standards; *Making Medical Spending Decisions (Hall, M.A.); United States

Stell, Lance K. Self-Interest and Universal Health Care: Why Well-Insured Americans Should Support Coverage for Everyone, by Larry J. Churchill. [Book review essay]. *Theoretical Medicine and Bioethics.* 1998 Apr; 19(2): 183–191. BE57596.
   age factors; *common good; communitarianism; *decision making; democracy; *economics; *goals; *health care delivery; *health care reform; justice; obligations of society; obligations to society; politics; public participation; public policy; *resource allocation; *Self-Interest and Universal Health Care (Churchill, L.J.); *United States

Stobo, John. Who should manage care? The case for providers. *Kennedy Institute of Ethics Journal.* 1997 Dec; 7(4): 387–389. 1 ref. BE59021.
   attitudes; costs and benefits; *decision making; economics; employment; *health care; health insurance; incentives; justice; *managed care programs; *patient participation; patients; *physicians; quality of health care; *resource allocation; treatment outcome; United States
Health care professionals should be the ones to make allocation decisions in the managed care setting because they are in the best position to assess outcomes, cost effectiveness, and quality of care.

Stronks, Karien; Strijbis, Anne–Margreet; Wendte, Johannes F., et al. Who should decide? Qualitative analysis of panel data from public, patients, healthcare professionals, and insurers on priorities in health care. *BMJ (British Medical Journal).* 1997 Jul 12; 315(7100): 92–96. 11 refs. BE55652.
   aged; alternative therapies; breast cancer; circumcision; comparative studies; contraception; costs and benefits; *decision making; drugs; *government financing; *health care; health insurance; home care; hormones; in vitro fertilization; justice; mass screening; *national health insurance; organ transplantation; *patients; *physicians; *public participation; public policy; residential facilities; *resource allocation; selection for treatment; sports medicine; standards; survey; copayments; homeopathy; personal financing; qualitative research; *Netherlands
OBJECTIVE: To explore the arguments underlying the choices of patients, the public, general practitioners, specialists, and health insurers regarding priorities in health care. DESIGN: A qualitative analysis of data gathered in a series of panels. Members were asked to economise on the publicly funded healthcare budget, exemplified by 10 services. RESULTS: From a medical point of view, both panels of healthcare professionals thought most services were necessary. The general practitioners tried to achieve the budget cuts by limiting

---

BE = bioethics accession number   fn. = footnotes   refs. = references

access to services to those most in need of them or those who cannot afford to pay for them. The specialists emphasised the possibilities of reducing costs by increasing the efficiency within services and preventing inappropriate utilisation. The patients mainly economised by limiting universal access to preventive and acute services. The "public" panels excluded services that are relatively inexpensive for individual patients. Moreover, they emphasised the individual's own responsibility for health behaviour and the costs of health care, resulting in the choice for copayments. The health insurers emphasised the importance of including services that relate to a risk only, as well as feasibility aspects. CONCLUSIONS: There were substantial differences in the way the different groups approached the issue of what should be included in the basic package. Healthcare professionals seem to be most aware of the importance of maintaining equal access for everyone in need of health care.

Trappenburg, Margo J. Defining the medical sphere. *Cambridge Quarterly of Healthcare Ethics.* 1997 Fall; 6(4): 416–434. 39 fn. BE56481.
   aged; autonomy; *communitarianism; cultural pluralism; economics; health; *health care; health care delivery; human rights; *justice; medicine; morality; philosophy; physicians; professional autonomy; property rights; *resource allocation; *rights; selection for treatment; values; liberalism; Callahan, Daniel; Daniels, Norman; Dworkin, Ronald; Nozick, Robert; Rawls, John; *Spheres of Justice (Walzer, M.); United States; *Walzer, Michael

Ubel, Peter A.; Goold, Susan Dorr. 'Rationing' health care: not all definitions are created equal. *Archives of Internal Medicine.* 1998 Feb 9; 158(3): 209–214. 24 refs. BE57980.
   costs and benefits; decision making; *health care; health insurance; justice; physicians; *resource allocation; review; scarcity; *terminology; values; *withholding treatment; United States

University of Texas. M.D. Anderson Cancer Center. Ethical principles for allocating clinical resources. *HEC (HealthCare Ethics Committee) Forum.* 1998 Jun; 10(2): 220–221. BE59081.
   cancer; economics; *guidelines; *hospitals; *institutional ethics; *institutional policies; *resource allocation; selection for treatment; *treatment outcome; *M.D. Anderson Cancer Center; Texas

Veatch, Robert M. Who should manage care? The case for patients. *Kennedy Institute of Ethics Journal.* 1997 Dec; 7(4): 391–401. 6 refs. BE59022.
   accountability; administrators; beneficence; conflict of interest; costs and benefits; *decision making; economics; gatekeeping; goals; *health care; health promotion; institutional policies; justice; *managed care programs; medicine; obligations to society; patient advocacy; *patient participation; *patients; physician's role; *physicians; prolongation of life; public policy; quality of health care; quality of life; *resource allocation; scarcity; treatment outcome; utilitarianism; value of life; withholding treatment; United States
After establishing that it is essential that health care be rationed in some fashion, the paper examines the arguments for and against clinicians as gatekeepers. It first argues that bedside clinicians do not have the information needed to make allocation decisions. Then it claims that physicians at the bedside can be expected to make the wrong choice for two reasons: their commitment to the Hippocratic ethic forces them to pursue the patient's best interest (even when resources will produce only very marginal benefit and could do

much more good elsewhere) and their values will lead them to calculate the net value of treatments incorrectly. Alternative decision makers are considered. It is argued that both groups of physicians and administrators will also make allocations incorrectly and that leaving the allocation decisions to patients themselves is the best approach. Mechanisms for fair and efficient rationing by patients at the societal and individual level are examined.

Verhey, Allen. A Protestant perspective on access to healthcare. *Cambridge Quarterly of Healthcare Ethics.* 1998 Summer; 7(3): 247–253. 14 fn. BE58552.
   *compassion; consensus; *health care delivery; indigents; *justice; *Protestant ethics; *public policy; *resource allocation; scarcity; Good Samaritanism; United States

Weale, Albert. Rationing health care: a logical solution to an inconsistent triad. [Editorial]. *BMJ (British Medical Journal).* 1998 Feb 7; 316(7129): 410. 5 refs. BE57851.
   *health care delivery; *public policy; quality of health care; *resource allocation; values; *Great Britain; National Health Service; United States

Wells, John S.G. Health care rationing: nursing perspectives. *Journal of Advanced Nursing.* 1995 Oct; 22(4): 738–744. 59 refs. BE55780.
   aged; beneficence; chronically ill; decision making; economics; guidelines; *health care delivery; hospitals; indigents; international aspects; justice; moral obligations; nurse's role; *nurses; nursing ethics; obligations to society; patient advocacy; *resource allocation; scarcity; selection for treatment; state medicine; values; *Great Britain; *National Health Service; United States

Whiteis, David G. Unhealthy cities: corporate medicine, community economic underdevelopment, and public health. *International Journal of Health Services.* 1997; 27(2): 227–242. 69 refs. BE56016.
   community services; *economics; financial support; government financing; *health care delivery; health care reform; *indigents; *industry; minority groups; politics; *private sector; proprietary health facilities; *public health; *public policy; public sector; *resource allocation; *social impact; *socioeconomic factors; *trends; *urban population; *United States

Whitman, Jeffrey P. Reclaiming the medical profession: the military profession as a model. *Professional Ethics.* 1995 Spring; 4(1): 3–22. 32 fn. BE55796.
   conflict of interest; conscience; *economics; entrepreneurship; *goals; *health care reform; killing; malpractice; *medical ethics; *medicine; *metaphor; *military personnel; misconduct; *moral obligations; morality; organizational policies; patient advocacy; *physician's role; *physicians; *professional autonomy; professional competence; *professional ethics; professional organizations; public opinion; remuneration; *resource allocation; *self regulation; trust; virtues; *war; *professional role; American Medical Association; United States

Wildes, Kevin Wm.; Wallace, Robert B. Relationships with payers and institutions that manage and deliver patient services. *In:* McCullough, Laurence B.; Jones, James W.; Brody, Baruch A., eds. Surgical Ethics. New York, NY: Oxford University Press; 1998: 367–383. 18 refs. ISBN 0–19–510347–5. BE58339.
   administrators; advertising; autonomy; beneficence; clinical ethics committees; *conflict of interest; disclosure; *economics; goals; *health facilities; *health insurance; health insurance reimbursement; hospitals; incentives; informed consent; institutional ethics; institutional policies; *managed care programs; medical education; *moral

---

BE = bioethics accession number   fn. = footnotes   refs. = references

obligations; *patient advocacy; *physician patient relationship; *physicians; practice guidelines; quality of health care; referral and consultation; remuneration; *resource allocation; *surgery; trust; withholding treatment; health services misuse; preventive ethics; undertreatment; United States

Yount, Lisa. How should health care be allocated? [Juvenile literature]. *In:* her Issues in Biomedical Ethics. San Diego, CA: Lucent Books; 1998: 17–35, 99–101. 33 fn. ISBN 1-56006-476-5. BE57679.
administrators; biomedical technologies; common good; conflict of interest; *costs and benefits; *decision making; economics; government financing; guidelines; *health care delivery; health insurance; incentives; indigents; managed care programs; morality; organ transplantation; patient advocacy; physicians; preventive medicine; prognosis; public opinion; public participation; *public policy; refusal to treat; *resource allocation; selection for treatment; self induced illness; social worth; standards; state government; life style; Medicaid; Oregon; United States

Zohar, Noam J. A Jewish perspective on access to healthcare. *Cambridge Quarterly of Healthcare Ethics.* 1998 Summer; 7(3): 260–265. 18 fn. BE58554.
*economics; health care; *health care delivery; *Jewish ethics; managed care programs; *obligations of society; *resource allocation; United States

Zohar, Noam J. Allocating medical resources: global planning and immediate obligations. *In:* his Alternatives in Jewish Bioethics. Albany, NY: State University of New York Press; 1997: 143–152. 10 fn. ISBN 0-7914-3274-2. BE57044.
economics; health care; health personnel; humanism; *Jewish ethics; moral obligations; obligations of society; obligations to society; patient advocacy; *resource allocation; theology

Zoloth–Dorfman, Laurie; Rubin, Susan B. "Medical futility": managed care and the powerful new vocabulary for clinical and public policy discourse. *Healthcare Forum Journal.* 1997 Mar-Apr; 40(2): 28, 30–33. BE57057.
AIDS; allowing to die; biomedical technologies; case studies; clinical ethics committees; costs and benefits; cultural pluralism; *decision making; dissent; family members; *futility; *goals; health facilities; institutional policies; justice; *managed care programs; medicine; patient care team; persistent vegetative state; physicians; practice guidelines; *prolongation of life; public policy; *resource allocation; terminally ill; *values; *withholding treatment; evidence–based medicine; United States

RESOURCE ALLOCATION/BIOMEDICAL TECHNOLOGIES

Benjamin, Martin; Turcotte, Jeremiah G. Ethics, alcoholism and liver transplantation. *In:* Lucey, Michael R.; Merion, Robert M.; Beresford, Thomas P., eds. Liver Transplantation and the Alcoholic Patient: Medical, Surgical and Psychosocial Issues. New York, NY: Cambridge University Press; 1994: 113–130. 12 refs. ISBN 0521-43332-0. BE56681.
accountability; *alcohol abuse; costs and benefits; disadvantaged; justice; *livers; moral obligations; *organ transplantation; patient compliance; preventive medicine; public policy; *resource allocation; scarcity; *selection for treatment; *self induced illness; social discrimination; stigmatization; *transplant recipients; treatment outcome; values; United States

Daniels, Norman; Sabin, James. Closure, fair procedures, and setting limits within managed care organizations.

Journal of the American Geriatrics Society. 1998 Mar; 46(3): 351–354. 16 refs. Paper presented at the 1996 Congress of Clinical Societies. BE56756.
accountability; *biomedical technologies; costs and benefits; *decision making; democracy; disclosure; *economics; goals; health care delivery; health care reform; *health insurance reimbursement; industry; international aspects; justice; *managed care programs; medicine; organization and administration; *organizational policies; physicians; *resource allocation; risks and benefits; technology assessment; therapeutic research; withholding treatment; *United States

Daniels, Norman; Sabin, James. Limits to health care: fair procedures, democratic deliberation, and the legitimacy problem for insurers. *Philosophy and Public Affairs.* 1997 Fall; 26(4): 303–350. 32 fn. BE57340.
*accountability; alternatives; *biomedical technologies; bone marrow; breast cancer; common good; costs and benefits; *decision making; *democracy; disclosure; due process; economics; growth disorders; guidelines; health care; health care delivery; health insurance; *health insurance reimbursement; hormones; industry; *institutional ethics; *justice; law; *managed care programs; mediation; *moral policy; national health insurance; obligations of society; *private sector; *public participation; public policy; public sector; regulation; *resource allocation; risks and benefits; selection for treatment; technology assessment; therapeutic research; tissue transplantation; *investigational therapies; United States

Dark, John H. Priorities for lung transplantation. *Lancet.* 1998 Jan 3; 351(9095): 4–5. 10 refs. BE57907.
diagnosis; mortality; *organ transplantation; quality of life; *resource allocation; *selection for treatment; time factors; transplant recipients; *treatment outcome; *lungs; Great Britain

de Rave, Sjoerd. Allocation of donor organs. [Letter]. *Lancet.* 1997 Oct 11; 350(9084): 1107. 2 refs. BE58151.
decision making; emergency care; *livers; *organ transplantation; *resource allocation; *selection for treatment; time factors; transplant recipients; Europe; Eurotransplant; France

Eaton, Stephanie. The subtle politics of organ donation: a proposal. *Journal of Medical Ethics.* 1998 Jun; 24(3): 166–170. 13 fn. BE59113.
*cadavers; decision making; *family members; moral obligations; motivation; obligations to society; *organ donation; *organ donors; *organ transplantation; *presumed consent; *resource allocation; *selection for treatment; *third party consent; *transplant recipients; treatment outcome; withholding treatment; *refusal to donate; *Great Britain; Jarvis, Rupert
Organs available for transplantation are scarce and valuable medical resources and decisions about who is to receive them should not be made more difficult by complicated calculations of desert. Consideration of likely clinical outcome must always take priority when allocating such a precious resource otherwise there is a danger of wasting that resource. However, desert may be a relevant concern in decision–making where the clinical risk is identical between two or more potential recipients of organs. Unlikely as this scenario is, such a decision procedure makes clear the interdependence of organ recipient and organ donor and hints at potential disadvantages for those who are willing to accept but unwilling to donate organs (free–riders). A combined opting–out and preference system weakens many of the objections to opting–out systems and may make the decision to donate organs on behalf of their deceased relatives easier for families.

Evans, Roger W. Limits of chronological age as a basis for rationing health care. *Dialysis and Transplantation.* 1994 Sep; 23(9): 506–507, 510–512+. 42 refs. BE57063.
*age factors; *aged; *economics; government financing; health; *health care; kidneys; morbidity; mortality; organ transplantation; patient care; *quality of life; rehabilitation; *renal dialysis; *resource allocation; *selection for treatment; statistics; *treatment outcome; Medicare; *United States

Field, Howard L. Organ allocation. [Letter; title supplied]. *Journal of Clinical Ethics.* 1997 Summer; 8(2): 208. BE57254.
*alcohol abuse; critically ill; *decision making; depressive disorder; *drug abuse; *livers; *organ transplantation; *patient compliance; psychiatric diagnosis; referral and consultation; *refusal to treat; *resource allocation; *selection for treatment; *self induced illness; socioeconomic factors; *suicide; *transplant recipients

Frisho–Lima, P.; Gurman, G.; Schapira, A., et al. Rationing critical care -- what happens to patients who are not admitted? *Theoretical Surgery.* 1994 Dec; 9(4): 208–211. 17 refs. BE57548.
age factors; comparative studies; *critically ill; *hospitals; *intensive care units; *mortality; patient admission; prognosis; *quality of health care; *resource allocation; *selection for treatment; surgery; technology assessment; treatment outcome; withholding treatment; severity of illness index; teaching hospitals; *Israel

Furnham, Adrian; Ofstein, Abigail. Ethical ideology and the allocation of scarce medical resources. *British Journal of Medical Psychology.* 1997 Mar; 70 (Pt. 1): 51–63. 25 refs. BE57504.
age factors; allowing to die; *attitudes; decision making; deontological ethics; family relationship; females; guidelines; justice; kidney diseases; males; married persons; medical schools; *moral policy; parents; prognosis; public opinion; religion; *renal dialysis; *resource allocation; scarcity; *selection for treatment; single persons; social worth; socioeconomic factors; students; survey; teleological ethics; universities; utilitarianism; *values; virtues; England

Glannon, Walter. Responsibility, alcoholism, and liver transplantation. *Journal of Medicine and Philosophy.* 1998 Feb; 23(1): 31–49. 40 refs. BE57519.
accountability; *alcohol abuse; *autonomy; disease; drug abuse; *genetic determinism; *genetic predisposition; health care; *justice; *livers; moral obligations; *moral policy; *organ transplantation; patients; psychoactive drugs; *resource allocation; scarcity; *selection for treatment; *self induced illness; transplant recipients; life style
Many believe that it is morally wrong to give lower priority for a liver transplant to alcoholics with end-stage liver disease than to patients whose disease is not alcohol–related. Presumably, alcoholism is a disease that results from factors beyond one's control and therefore one cannot be causally or morally responsible for alcoholism or the liver failure that results from it. Moreover, giving lower priority to alcoholics unfairly singles them out for the moral vice of heavy drinking. I argue that the etiology of alcoholism may involve enough control for the alcoholic to be responsible for his condition and accordingly have a weaker claim to receive a new liver than someone who acquires the disease through no fault of his own. In addition, I show why it is more plausible to reframe the question of priority in terms of control and responsibility rather than virtue and vice. Given that medical resources like livers are scarce, some people may justifiably be given lower priority than others in receiving these resources.

Gutmann, Thomas; Land, Walter. The ethics of organ allocation: the state of debate. *Transplantation Reviews.* 1997 Oct; 11(4): 191–207. 170 refs. BE58882.
age factors; *body parts and fluids; cadavers; decision making; deontological ethics; ethical theory; international aspects; *justice; *moral policy; organ donation; organ donors; *organ transplantation; public policy; quality of life; random selection; remuneration; *resource allocation; retreatment; review; scarcity; *selection for treatment; self induced illness; social discrimination; social worth; time factors; transplant recipients; utilitarianism; geographic factors; Europe; United States

Hardy, K.J.; Milton, P.; Derham, P., et al. Attitudes towards liver transplantation in Victoria, Australia. *Australian and New Zealand Journal of Surgery.* 1993 Jul; 63(7): 520–524. 22 refs. BE55555.
*attitudes; family practice; *government financing; health care delivery; *knowledge, attitudes, practice; *livers; *organ transplantation; *physicians; *public opinion; *resource allocation; state government; survey; *Australia; *Victoria

Higgins, R.M.; West, N.; Edmunds, M.E., et al. Effect of a strict HLA matching policy on distribution of cadaveric kidney transplants to Indo–Asian and white European recipients: regional study. *BMJ (British Medical Journal).* 1997 Nov 22; 315(7119): 1354–1355. 3 refs. BE56553.
*cadavers; comparative studies; evaluation studies; *institutional policies; *kidneys; *minority groups; organ donation; *organ transplantation; renal dialysis; *resource allocation; *selection for treatment; *whites; *HLA matching; Great Britain

Hughes, David; Griffiths, Lesley. "But if you look at the coronary anatomy...": risk and rationing in cardiac surgery. *Sociology of Health and Illness.* 1996 Mar; 18(2): 172–197. 48 refs. 10 fn. BE56492.
*age factors; case studies; communication; *decision making; diagnosis; evaluation studies; *hearts; hospitals; *interprofessional relations; *minority groups; *physicians; prognosis; referral and consultation; *resource allocation; risk; *selection for treatment; *self induced illness; smoking; *social worth; *surgery; angioplasty; *coronary artery bypass; waiting lists; Great Britain

Jung, Patricia Beattie. What price fertility? *In:* Wildes, Kevin Wm., ed. Infertility: A Crossroad of Faith, Medicine, and Technology. Boston, MA: Kluwer Academic; 1997: 167–180. 6 refs. 4 fn. ISBN 0–7923–4061–2. BE55997.
adoption; costs and benefits; disease; *economics; government financing; health care delivery; health insurance reimbursement; in vitro fertilization; *infertility; *justice; psychological stress; *public policy; *reproductive technologies; *resource allocation; rights; Roman Catholic ethics; socioeconomic factors; values; personal financing; Instruction on Respect for Human Life

Lamke, Celia. Distributive justice and HIV disease in intensive care. *Critical Care Nursing Quarterly.* 1996 May; 19(1): 55–64. 23 refs. BE55724.
*AIDS; *decision making; *HIV seropositivity; *intensive care units; *justice; *nurses; patient admission; patient care team; patients; physicians; *resource allocation; *selection for treatment; standards

Levine, David Z. Would you deny this patient dialysis? [Editorial]. *American Journal of Kidney Diseases.* 1998 Jan; 31(1): 131–132. 11 refs. BE57551.
aged; allowing to die; attitudes; chronically ill; economics; international aspects; patient care; *physicians; quality of life; refusal to treat; *renal dialysis; *resource allocation;

*selection for treatment; withholding treatment; Canada; Great Britain; United States

Lucey, Michael R.; Beresford, Thomas P. Ethical considerations regarding orthotopic liver transplantation for alcoholic patients. *In:* Shelton, Wayne N.; Edwards, Rem B., eds. Advances in Bioethics. Volume 3: Values, Ethics, and Alcoholism. Greenwich, CT: JAI Press; 1997: 119–129. 33 refs. ISBN 0-7623-0219-4. BE57635.
accountability; *alcohol abuse; autonomy; beneficence; disclosure; disease; justice; *livers; moral obligations; *moral policy; obligations to society; *organ transplantation; patient compliance; patients; physicians; *prognosis; *public policy; referral and consultation; refusal to treat; *resource allocation; retreatment; risks and benefits; scarcity; *selection for treatment; *self induced illness; social discrimination; transplant recipients; treatment outcome; Great Britain

Mintz, Benjamin. Analyzing the OPTN [Organ Procurement and Transplant Network] under the state action doctrine -- can UNOS's organ allocation criteria survive strict scrutiny? *Columbia Journal of Law and Social Problems.* 1995 Spring; 28(3): 339–396. 276 fn. BE57197.
*blacks; body parts and fluids; equal protection; federal government; financial support; government regulation; *kidneys; *legal aspects; legal rights; *organ transplantation; organizational policies; public policy; *resource allocation; *selection for treatment; *social discrimination; standards; state government; Supreme Court decisions; *transplant recipients; treatment outcome; voluntary programs; *histocompatibility; Department of Health and Human Services; *Organ Procurement and Transplant Network; Organ Procurement Organizations; *United Network for Organ Sharing; *United States

Mongoven, Ann. Federal hearings on liver transplant allocation and donation. *In:* BioLaw: A Legal and Ethical Reporter on Medicine, Health Care, and Bioengineering. Special Sections 2(12). Frederick, MD: University Publications of America; 1997 Dec: S:373–S:389. BE57643.
cadavers; chronically ill; computers; conflict of interest; consensus; critically ill; *decision making; determination of death; federal government; government regulation; health facilities; health insurance; justice; *livers; models, theoretical; *organ donation; *organ transplantation; patient advocacy; physicians; prognosis; public participation; *public policy; *resource allocation; scarcity; *selection for treatment; transplant recipients; treatment outcome; geographic factors; *Department of Health and Human Services; *United Network for Organ Sharing; *United States

Murphy, Donald J. The economics of futile interventions. *In:* Zucker, Marjorie B.; Zucker, Howard D., eds. Medical Futility and the Evaluation of Life-Sustaining Interventions. New York, NY: Cambridge University Press; 1997: 123–135. 37 refs. ISBN 0-521-56877-3. BE55985.
advance directives; *age factors; aged; *biomedical technologies; *chronically ill; *common good; *costs and benefits; *critically ill; dementia; *economics; *futility; home care; hospices; *intensive care units; mortality; *palliative care; persistent vegetative state; prognosis; *prolongation of life; refusal to treat; *resource allocation; *selection for treatment; self induced illness; *social impact; *terminal care; *terminally ill; time factors; treatment outcome; treatment refusal; trends; uncertainty; *values; *health services misuse; Study to Understand Prognoses and Preferences for Outcomes and Risks of Treatments (SUPPORT); United States

Neuberger, James; Lake, John. Allocating donor livers. [Editorial]. *BMJ (British Medical Journal).* 1997 Apr 19;

314(7088): 1140–1141. 6 refs. BE57163.
adults; age factors; children; consensus; critically ill; decision making; hospitals; institutional policies; *livers; models, theoretical; *organ transplantation; organizational policies; physicians; prognosis; *resource allocation; scarcity; *selection for treatment; self induced illness; *standards; time factors; treatment outcome; *Great Britain; United Network for Organ Sharing; *United States

Neuberger, James; Adams, David; MacMaster, Paul, et al. Assessing priorities for allocation of donor liver grafts: survey of public and clinicians. *BMJ (British Medical Journal).* 1998 Jul 18; 317(7152): 172–175. 26 refs. BE58816.
*age factors; *alcohol abuse; *attitudes; comparative studies; *drug abuse; employment; family practice; *livers; medical specialties; *organ transplantation; *physicians; *prisoners; prognosis; *public opinion; *resource allocation; scarcity; *selection for treatment; *self induced illness; *social worth; survey; *time factors; transplant recipients; *treatment outcome; gastroenterology; *Great Britain
OBJECTIVES: To compare the priorities of the general public, family doctors, and gastroenterologists in allocating donor livers to potential recipients of liver allograft. DESIGN: Representative quota sampling of 1000 members of the general public and 200 family doctors, and a postal questionnaire of 100 gastroenterologists. SUBJECTS: Respondents were given eight hypothetical case histories (based on real patients) and asked to select recipients for four donor livers. Cases were selected to identify controversial areas such as extremes of age, misuse of alcohol, and intravenous drugs. Respondents were also asked to select the least deserving case and which of seven possible factors (time on waiting list, outcome, age, value to society, return to work, previous use of illicit drugs, and involvement of alcohol in the liver damage) should be used to select patients already listed for transplantation. Focus groups were also held to explore further the reasons for the choices given. RESULTS: There were considerable differences between the three groups in the choice of the recipients, although alcohol use and antisocial behaviour always rated low. For selection of recipients the general public thought that, in decreasing order of importance, age, outcome, and time on the waiting list were the most important factors in selecting recipients; family doctors rated outcome, age, and likely work status after transplantation and the gastroenterologists outcome, work status, and non-involvement of alcohol in the cause of the liver disease as the most important factors. CONCLUSIONS: The views of the public are at variance with those of clinicians. Further debate is required to ensure an equitable and appropriate distribution of a scarce resource.

Neumann, Peter J. Should health insurance cover IVF? Issues and options. *Journal of Health Politics, Policy and Law.* 1997 Oct; 22(5): 1215–1239. 69 refs. 13 fn. BE56748.
*adoption; alternatives; biomedical technologies; childbirth; comparative studies; *costs and benefits; embryo transfer; federal government; government regulation; guidelines; health facilities; *health insurance reimbursement; *in vitro fertilization; incentives; infertility; international aspects; legislation; multiple pregnancy; newborns; professional organizations; prognosis; public opinion; *public policy; *reproductive technologies; *resource allocation; risks and benefits; selection for treatment; standards; state government; personal financing; utilization review; American Society for Reproductive Medicine; Fertility Clinic Success Rate and Certification Act 1992; Society for Assisted Reproductive Technology; United States
An emotional debate has attended the question of

BE = bioethics accession number   fn. = footnotes   refs. = references

whether health insurance should cover the cost of in vitro fertilization (IVF) for infertile couples. Some private health plans have opted to cover IVF, although most have not. Ten states have mandated that it be included or offered as a standard benefit for private health insurance plans. This article analyzes several key issues in the debate: the impact of insurance coverage; the cost–effectiveness of IVF; valuing the benefit of IVF; and adoption as an alternative. It recommends policy action in several areas: more efficiently allocating resources for IVF (by giving priority to couples with better chances of success, and by making more extensive use of facilities with higher success rates); ensuring that clear and reliable information about the effectiveness of IVF is available; and leveling the playing field between IVF and adoption.

Pinch, Winifred J., et al. Allocation of scarce resources: critical care nursing dilemmas. [Case studies and commentaries]. *Dimensions of Critical Care Nursing.* 1985 May–Jun; 4(3): 164–173. 7 refs. Includes brief commentaries by Jeanne M. Yocke, Katherine W. Vestal, John M. Cloches, Joanne R. Duffy, Leah L. Curtin, Bernice Coleman, and Rebecca Hathaway. BE56953.
  case studies; critically ill; cultural pluralism; *decision making; deontological ethics; *ethical analysis; ethical theory; *intensive care units; *moral policy; patient admission; patient discharge; patient transfer; random selection; *resource allocation; rights; *selection for treatment; social worth; socioeconomic factors; utilitarianism; values

Rasmussen, P. Elmegaard; Larsen, P. Munkholm; Nielsen, V.G., et al. Does physicians' knowledge of costing related to clinical decision making change the consumption of resources despite unchanged medical standards? *Scandinavian Journal of Gastroenterology.* 1985; 20(4): 401–406. 7 refs. BE57073.
  *biomedical technologies; comparative studies; decision making; drugs; *economics; evaluation studies; *hospitals; *knowledge, attitudes, practice; *patient care; *physicians; quality of health care; *resource allocation; *physician's practice patterns; *Denmark

Rothman, David J. Beginnings Count: The Technological Imperative in American Health Care. New York, NY: Oxford University Press; 1997. 189 p. 261 fn. A Twentieth Century Fund book. ISBN 0-19-511118-4. BE57280.
  *biomedical technologies; costs and benefits; *economics; *government financing; *health care delivery; *health care reform; *health insurance; historical aspects; international aspects; *managed care programs; national health insurance; *patient satisfaction; political activity; politics; public opinion; *public policy; quality of life; renal dialysis; *resource allocation; rights; *socioeconomic factors; treatment outcome; ventilators; *Blue Cross; Health Security Act (1993 bill); Medicaid; *Medicare; Twentieth Century; *United States

Sabin, James E.; Daniels, Norman. Making insurance coverage for new technologies reasonable and accountable. [Editorial]. *JAMA.* 1998 Mar 4; 279(9): 703–704. 9 refs. BE57813.
  *biomedical technologies; children; *decision making; *disclosure; growth disorders; health care reform; *health insurance reimbursement; hormones; *managed care programs; referral and consultation; *resource allocation; United States

Sachdeva, Ramesh C.; Jefferson, Larry S.; Coss–Bu, Jorge, et al. Resource consumption and the extent of futile care among patients in a pediatric intensive care

unit setting. *Journal of Pediatrics.* 1996 Jun; 128(6): 742–747. 19 refs. BE57158.
  adolescents; *children; diagnosis; evaluation studies; *futility; hospitals; *intensive care units; morbidity; mortality; *patient care; pediatrics; prognosis; prolongation of life; quality of life; *resource allocation; statistics; treatment outcome; prospective studies; Texas; *Texas Children's Hospital (Houston, TX)

Sampson, Mark T. Revised liver policy approved. *UNOS Update.* 1997 Jan–Feb: 5–7. BE56237.
  *guidelines; *livers; minors; *organ transplantation; organizational policies; public participation; *resource allocation; *selection for treatment; transplant recipients; liver diseases; *United Network for Organ Sharing; United States

Schmidt, Volker H. Selection of recipients for donor organs in transplant medicine. *Journal of Medicine and Philosophy.* 1998 Feb; 23(1): 50–74. 45 refs. 20 fn. BE57520.
  age factors; aged; alcohol abuse; deception; *decision making; due process; guidelines; health facilities; hearts; *institutional policies; justice; *kidneys; livers; moral policy; *organ transplantation; organization and administration; patient admission; patient advocacy; patient compliance; *physicians; prognosis; random selection; referral and consultation; *resource allocation; scarcity; *selection for treatment; social worth; statistics; time factors; *transplant recipients; uncertainty; utilitarianism; values; histocompatibility; Europe; *Eurotransplant; *Germany
This paper deals with a problem which has received a great deal of attention in the ethical literature, but about which very little is known empirically: the selection of recipients for organs in transplant medicine. Based on a larger study, it is shown how this problem is practically resolved in one European country, Germany. It is demonstrated that most of the criteria used to determine recipients are non–medical in nature, even though they generally tend to be rationalized in medical terms. Moreover, the choice of criteria depends as much on prognostic considerations as on personal indiosyncrasies and values held by individual physicians who are in charge at the various programs. Several examples of the extremely diverse policies in which this results are presented.

Sekela, Michael; Berk, Martin R.; Gallagher, Eugene B., et al. Cardiac transplantation: costs and ethics. *Hospital Practice (Office Edition).* 1996 Feb 15; 31(2): 127–130, 133–134, 136, 139. 3 refs. BE57401.
  attitudes; case studies; *costs and benefits; faculty; government financing; heart diseases; *hearts; indigents; *organ transplantation; physicians; public policy; *resource allocation; risks and benefits; selection for treatment; social sciences; socioeconomic factors; transplant recipients; Kentucky; Medicaid

Shelton, Wayne N. Justice and alcoholism. *In:* Shelton, Wayne N.; Edwards, Rem B., eds. Advances in Bioethics. Volume 3: Values, Ethics, and Alcoholism. Greenwich, CT: JAI Press; 1997: 131–152. 26 refs. ISBN 0-7623-0219-4. BE57636.
  *accountability; *alcohol abuse; autonomy; behavior control; *behavior disorders; biomedical technologies; coercion; *common good; *disease; freedom; health care delivery; *justice; *libertarianism; *livers; mental health; *models, theoretical; moral obligations; *moral policy; *organ transplantation; paternalism; patient care; *patient compliance; *public policy; *refusal to treat; *resource allocation; rights; scarcity; *selection for treatment; *self induced illness; stigmatization; treatment outcome; United States

---

BE = bioethics accession number   fn. = footnotes   refs. = references

Shenfield, F. Justice and access to fertility treatments. *In:* Shenfield, F.; Sureau, C., eds. Ethical Dilemmas in Assisted Reproduction. New York, NY: Parthenon Pub. Group; 1997: 7–14. 21 refs. ISBN 1-85070-916-5. BE57941.

age factors; deontological ethics; economics; *government financing; justice; *reproductive technologies; *resource allocation; rights; *selection for treatment; *socioeconomic factors; utilitarianism; *Great Britain; National Health Service

Sidley, Pat. South African court rules against rationing decision. [News]. *BMJ (British Medical Journal)*. 1997 Feb 8; 314(7078): 396. BE58702.

hospitals; *legal aspects; *patient compliance; *refusal to treat; *renal dialysis; *resource allocation; Supreme Court decisions; Addington Hospital (Durban, SA); *Bock, Stephen; *South Africa

Sidley, Pat. South African row over denial of dialysis. [News]. *BMJ (British Medical Journal)*. 1997 Dec 13; 315(7122): 1562. BE57725.

*government financing; hospitals; indigents; institutional policies; kidneys; *legal aspects; organ transplantation; *public policy; *refusal to treat; *renal dialysis; *resource allocation; selection for treatment; Addington Hospital (Durban); Soobramoney, Thiagraj; *South Africa

Stolberg, Sheryl Gay. U.S. orders sickest to be given priority on donated organs. [News]. *New York Times.* 1998 Mar 27: A16. BE57737.

attitudes; federal government; *government regulation; hospitals; *organ transplantation; patient advocacy; *resource allocation; *selection for treatment; *standards; time factors; transplant recipients; geographic factors; severity of illness index; *Department of Health and Human Services; United Network for Organ Sharing; *United States

Ubel, Peter A.; Loewenstein, George. Distributing scarce livers: the moral reasoning of the general public. *Social Science and Medicine*. 1996 Apr; 42(7): 1049–1055. 29 refs. BE56889.

age factors; *attitudes; children; costs and benefits; justice; *livers; *organ transplantation; prognosis; *public opinion; public policy; *resource allocation; scarcity; *selection for treatment; survey; *transplant recipients; treatment outcome; *values; Pennsylvania

The transplant system has been criticized for not paying enough attention to efficiency in distributing scarce organs. But little research has been done to see how the general public views tradeoffs between efficiency and equity. We surveyed members of the general public to see how they would distribute organs among patients with varying chances of benefiting from them. In addition, we asked subjects to explain their decisions and to tell us about any other information they would have liked in order to make the decisions. We found that the public places a very high value on giving everyone a chance at receiving scarce resources, even if that means a significant decrease in the chance that available organs will save people's lives. Our results raise important questions about whether the aims of outcomes research and cost-effective studies agree with the values of the general public.

Ubel, Peter A.; Loewenstein, George. Public perceptions of the importance of prognosis in allocating transplantable livers to children. *Medical Decision Making*. 1996 Jul–Sep; 16(3): 234–241. 24 refs. BE57978.

adults; *children; *decision making; justice; *livers; *organ transplantation; *prognosis; *public opinion; public policy; *resource allocation; *selection for treatment; survey; treatment outcome; values; *Pennsylvania; United States

Ubel, Peter A.; DeKay, M.; Baron, J., et al. Public preferences for efficiency and racial equity in kidney transplant allocation decisions. *Transplantation Proceedings*. 1996 Oct; 28(5): 2997–3002. 24 refs. BE57979.

*blacks; decision making; justice; *kidneys; *organ transplantation; *prognosis; *public opinion; *resource allocation; *selection for treatment; socioeconomic factors; survey; time factors; transplant recipients; treatment outcome; *whites; histocompatibility; *Philadelphia; United States

Ubel, Peter A.; Loewenstein, George. The efficacy and equity of retransplantation: an experimental survey of public attitudes. *Health Policy*. 1995 Nov; 34(2): 145–151. 12 refs. BE56602.

*attitudes; justice; *livers; morality; mortality; *organ transplantation; *prognosis; *public opinion; public policy; *resource allocation; *retreatment; *selection for treatment; survey; *transplant recipients; Pennsylvania; United States

United Network for Organ Sharing (UNOS). Ethics Committee. General principles for allocating human organs and tissues. *Transplantation Proceedings*. 1992 Oct; 24(5): 2227–2235. 6 fn. BE56846.

age factors; *autonomy; *beneficence; body parts and fluids; cultural pluralism; directed donation; *guidelines; *justice; *moral policy; organ donation; *organ transplantation; organizational policies; patient compliance; policy analysis; prognosis; *public policy; quality of life; remuneration; *resource allocation; retreatment; risks and benefits; *selection for treatment; self induced illness; social worth; time factors; *tissue transplantation; transplant recipients; treatment outcome; *utilitarianism; life style; National Organ Transplant Act 1984; *United Network for Organ Sharing; *United States

Wilkes, Michael S.; Slavin, Stuart. Heart transplantation selection criteria: attitudes of ethnically diverse medical students. *Journal of Clinical Ethics*. 1998 Summer; 9(2): 147–155. 15 fn. BE58960.

administrators; age factors; alcohol abuse; aliens; Asian Americans; *attitudes; blacks; comparative studies; curriculum; diagnosis; drug abuse; family relationship; females; health insurance; *hearts; Hispanic Americans; HIV seropositivity; homosexuals; indigents; males; medical education; medical schools; mentally disabled; *minority groups; morbidity; organ donation; *organ transplantation; patient compliance; patients; physicians; *resource allocation; retreatment; *selection for treatment; smoking; socioeconomic factors; *students; survey; *transplant recipients; whites; United States

Wilson, Kumanan; Cook, Deborah J. Economics and the intensive care unit: a conflict of interests? *Journal of Critical Care*. 1997 Sep; 12(3): 147–151. 29 refs. BE58259.

age factors; aged; cancer; *costs and benefits; *intensive care units; mortality; prognosis; quality adjusted life years; *resource allocation; selection for treatment; treatment outcome

Changing the U.S. transplant system. [Editorial]. *Lancet.* 1998 Jul 11; 352(9122): 79. BE59070.

body parts and fluids; *dissent; federal government; *government regulation; *organ transplantation; *organizational policies; *resource allocation; selection for treatment; standards; transplant recipients; *geographic factors; Department of Health and Human Services; *United Network for Organ Sharing; *United States

RESUSCITATION ORDERS

See also ALLOWING TO DIE

BE = bioethics accession number   fn. = footnotes   refs. = references

Alexandrov, Andrei V.; Bladin, Christopher F.; Meslin, Eric M., et al. Do-not-resuscitate orders in acute stroke. *Neurology.* 1995 Apr; 45(4): 634–640. 39 refs. Appendix: "Provisional criteria for do-not-resuscitate orders in acute stroke," designed following recommendations of the U.S. Institute of Medicine and the Canadian Medical Association. BE56848.
advance directives; age factors; aged; artificial feeding; *brain pathology; competence; *critically ill; *decision making; evaluation studies; family members; futility; *guidelines; hospitals; informed consent; institutional policies; morbidity; mortality; patient care team; patients; physicians; *practice guidelines; prognosis; *resuscitation orders; statistics; third party consent; time factors; treatment outcome; *cerebrovascular disorders; *severity of illness index; Ontario; Sunnybrook Health Sciences Centre (ON)

Balentine, Jerry; Gaeta, Theodore; Rao, Narasinga, et al. Emergency department do-not-attempt-resuscitation orders: next-of-kin response to the emergency physician. *Academic Emergency Medicine.* 1996 Jan; 3(1): 54–57. 7 refs. BE55704.
*advance care planning; advance directives; *attitudes; chronically ill; *communication; critically ill; disadvantaged; *emergency care; *family members; *hospitals; internship and residency; nursing homes; *patient admission; patient transfer; *physicians; professional family relationship; *resuscitation orders; survey; terminally ill; *hospital emergency service; prospective studies; questionnaires; urban population

Bastron, R. Dennis. Ethical concerns in anesthetic care for patients with do-not-resuscitate orders. *Anesthesiology.* 1996 Nov; 85(5): 1190–1193. 17 refs. 3 fn. BE57502.
*anesthesia; attitudes; autonomy; decision making; forms; *guidelines; hospitals; informed consent; *institutional policies; patients; physicians; professional organizations; resuscitation; *resuscitation orders; *surgery; American Society of Anesthesiologists; *Scott and White Clinic and Memorial Hospital (Temple, TX)

Caniano, Donna A.; Hazebroek, Frans W.J.; DenBesten, Karen E., et al. End-of-life decisions for surgical neonates: experience in the Netherlands and United States. *Journal of Pediatric Surgery.* 1995 Oct; 30(10): 1420–1424. 13 refs. BE55659.
*allowing to die; artificial feeding; chromosome abnormalities; comparative studies; *congenital disorders; *decision making; drugs; evaluation studies; futility; *intensive care units; *international aspects; mortality; *newborns; nurses; parents; physicians; *prognosis; quality of life; *resuscitation orders; *surgery; time factors; treatment outcome; ventilators; *withholding treatment; antibiotics; *Netherlands; *United States

Cao, Lequn; Song, Wei. Do-not-resuscitate orders in critical care elderly: no age discrimination against elderly in a community hospital. [Letter]. *Archives of Internal Medicine.* 1998 May 25; 158(10): 1154. 2 refs. BE58805.
*adults; *age factors; *aged; decision making; hospitals; intensive care units; patient admission; patient participation; *resuscitation orders; statistics; survey; community hospitals

Curtin, Leah L. DNR in the OR: ethical concerns and hospital policies. *Nursing Management.* 1994 Feb; 25(2): 29–31. BE55713.
aged; AIDS; anesthesia; case studies; clinical ethics committees; coercion; disclosure; dissent; ethical analysis; hospitals; institutional policies; nurse's role; *nurses; patient care; physicians; *resuscitation orders; *surgery; terminally ill; withholding treatment

Gazelle, Gail. The slow code — should anyone rush to

its defense? *New England Journal of Medicine.* 1998 Feb 12; 338(7): 467–469. 25 refs. BE57307.
autonomy; *deception; decision making; dementia; family members; futility; *informed consent; *intention; methods; paternalism; persistent vegetative state; physicians; prognosis; *resuscitation; *resuscitation orders; terminally ill; United States

Ghusn, Husam F.; Teasdale, Thomas A.; Boyer, Kathryn. Characteristics of patients receiving or forgoing resuscitation at the time of cardiopulmonary arrest. *Journal of the American Geriatrics Society.* 1997 Sep; 45(9): 1118–1122. 17 refs. BE56304.
adults; *advance care planning; advance directives; age factors; aged; comparative studies; *critically ill; decision making; diagnosis; minority groups; *morbidity; physicians; public hospitals; quality of life; *resuscitation; *resuscitation orders; treatment outcome; treatment refusal; whites; Houston Veterans Affairs Medical Center; Texas

Ghusn, Husam F.; Teasdale, Thomas A.; Jordan, Darlene. Continuity of do-not resuscitate orders between hospital and nursing home settings. *Journal of the American Geriatrics Society.* 1997 Apr; 45(4): 465–469. 9 refs. BE57115.
*advance directives; aged; *communication; comparative studies; diagnosis; *hospitals; institutional policies; medical records; *nursing homes; *patient discharge; *patient transfer; *resuscitation orders; treatment refusal; continuity of patient care; Houston (TX); Texas

Gillon, Raanan. "Futility" -- too ambiguous and pejorative a term? [Editorial]. *Journal of Medical Ethics.* 1997 Dec; 23(6): 339–340. 5 fn. BE57659.
costs and benefits; *decision making; *dissent; family members; *futility; moral obligations; patients; physicians; psychological stress; refusal to treat; *resuscitation; *resuscitation orders; risks and benefits; selection for treatment; *terminology; uncertainty; values; withholding treatment

Goh, L.G. The do-not-resuscitate order. *Singapore Medical Journal.* 1995 Jun; 36(3): 258–259. 10 refs. BE55551.
communication; decision making; emergency care; family members; futility; *guidelines; international aspects; patient care team; patient participation; physicians; professional organizations; quality of life; referral and consultation; *resuscitation orders; treatment outcome; *Great Britain; *Royal College of Physicians of London; *Singapore

Hall, Spencer A.; Casarett, David; Ross, Lainie F. Overriding a patient's refusal of treatment after an iatrogenic complication. [Letter and response]. *New England Journal of Medicine.* 1997 Nov 13; 337(20): 1477. 4 refs. BE58414.
*iatrogenic disease; *resuscitation; *resuscitation orders; *treatment refusal

Heffner, John E.; Barbieri, Celia; Fracica, Phil, et al. Communicating do-not-resuscitate orders with a computer-based system. *Archives of Internal Medicine.* 1998 May 25; 158(10): 1090–1095. 19 refs. BE58803.
*communication; comparative studies; *computers; critically ill; *forms; hospitals; institutional policies; intensive care units; internship and residency; knowledge, attitudes, practice; medical records; *methods; *nurses; *patient care team; *physicians; *resuscitation orders; survey; *withholding treatment; questionnaires; St. Joseph's Hospital and Medical Center (Phoenix, AZ)
BACKGROUND: Do-not-resuscitate (DNR) orders for critically ill patients are frequently miscommunicated between attending physicians, house staff, and nurses. A computer-based system was developed to improve the communication of a procedure-specific DNR order

---

BE = bioethics accession number   fn. = footnotes   refs. = references

form. METHODS: Concordance of understanding of patients' DNR status was measured with the use of unstructured DNR orders (period 1), procedure-specific DNR order forms (period 2), and procedure-specific DNR order forms administered with a computer-based communication system (period 3). The 3 components of the DNR order assessed were (1) the clinical events to which the DNR order applied, (2) whether the DNR order withheld all elements of cardiopulmonary resuscitation, and (3) whether other treatments were to be withheld. RESULTS: For the 147 patients, the computer-based system in period 3 (n = 71) improved concordance for attending physicians and nurses or residents for all 3 of the DNR components compared with period 1 (n = 40) and some of the DNR components compared with period 2 (n = 36). Concordance was "substantial" or "almost perfect" as measured by the K statistic during period 3. The proportion of agreement for the composite of all 3 components of the DNR order increased during each period (P less than .001, period 3 vs period 1). Overall agreement between all caregivers for the composite DNR order also improved from period 1 (22.2%) to period 2 (47.8%) and period 3 (61.9%; P less than .001 vs period 1). Errors in order entry were detected by physicians because of the computer system and corrected in 9.9% of DNR orders in period 3. Progress note documentation of DNR status did not improve during period 3. The procedures of period 3 were considered acceptable by the physician and nursing staff. CONCLUSION: A computer-based system combined with a procedure-specific DNR order form improves communication of patients' DNR status in a critical care setting.

Hilberman, Mark; Kutner, Jean; Parsons, Debra, et al. Marginally effective medical care: ethical analysis of issues in cardiopulmonary resuscitation (CPR). *Journal of Medical Ethics.* 1997 Dec; 23(6): 361-367. 65 refs. BE57663.
    aged; autonomy; beneficence; *costs and benefits; *decision making; dementia; emergency care; evaluation; freedom; *futility; *guidelines; institutional policies; justice; legal aspects; moral policy; morbidity; mortality; nursing homes; patients; persistent vegetative state; physicians; *prognosis; quality of life; refusal to treat; *resuscitation; *resuscitation orders; *risks and benefits; *selection for treatment; statistics; terminally ill; *treatment outcome; treatment refusal; withholding treatment; United States
Outcomes from cardiopulmonary resuscitation (CPR) remain distressingly poor. Overuse of CPR is attributable to unrealistic expectations, unintended consequences of existing policies and failure to honour patient refusal of CPR. We analyzed the CPR outcomes literature using the bioethical principles of beneficence, non-maleficence, autonomy and justice and developed a proposal for selective use of CPR. Beneficence supports use of CPR when most effective. Non-maleficence argues against performing CPR when the outcomes are harmful or usage inappropriate. Additionally, policies which usurp good clinical judgment and moral responsibility, thereby contributing to inappropriate CPR usage, should be considered maleficent. Autonomy restricts CPR use when refused but cannot create a right to CPR. Justice requires that we define which medical interventions contribute sufficiently to health and happiness that they should be made universally available. This ordering is necessary whether one believes in the utilitarian standard or wishes medical care to be universally available on fairness grounds. Low-yield CPR fails justice criteria.

Cardiopulmonary resuscitation should be performed when justified by the extensive outcomes literature; not performed when not desired by the patient or not indicated; and performed infrequently when relatively contraindicated.

Hui, Elsie; Ho, Suzanne C.; Tsang, June, et al. Attitudes toward life-sustaining treatment of older persons in Hong Kong. *Journal of the American Geriatrics Society.* 1997 Oct; 45(10): 1232-1236. 27 refs. BE56464.
    age factors; *aged; *allowing to die; *attitudes; biomedical technologies; *decision making; disclosure; females; *hospitals; knowledge, attitudes, practice; *patients; *prolongation of life; *residential facilities; *resuscitation; resuscitation orders; single persons; survey; treatment outcome; treatment refusal; *Hong Kong

Konishi, Emiko. Nurses' attitudes towards developing a do not resuscitate policy in Japan. *Nursing Ethics.* 1998 May; 5(3): 218-227. 22 refs. BE58721.
    advance care planning; *attitudes; communication; decision making; family members; *hospitals; *institutional policies; nurse's role; *nurses; patient participation; physicians; *resuscitation orders; survey; time factors; *Japan

Lindon, James Lee. Consequences of End-of-Life Physician Orders: Economic and Hospital Policy Implications. Ann Arbor, MI: University Microfilms International; 1993. 108 p. Bibliography: p. 102-108. Dissertation, Ph.D. in Pharmacy, University of Arizona, 1993. Order No. 9328556. BE56699.
    advance directives; allowing to die; clinical ethics committees; communication; decision making; *economics; evaluation studies; family members; *forms; futility; *hospitals; *institutional policies; intensive care units; interdisciplinary communication; medical records; mortality; patient care team; patient participation; patients; physicians; records; *resuscitation orders; social impact; terminal care; third party consent; *withholding treatment; *University Medical Center (Tucson, AZ)

Loscalzo, John J.; Cooper, David J.; Arena, Francis P., et al. Do families understand "do not resuscitate" orders? *Oncology.* 1996 Apr; 10(4): 504, 507, 511. 6 refs. BE56876.
    artificial feeding; *comprehension; *decision making; drugs; *family members; motivation; palliative care; *resuscitation orders; survey; terminally ill; third party consent; ventilators; withholding treatment; antibiotics; New York

New York. Supreme Court, Queens County. Grand Jury. DNR Procedures: Purple Dots Revisited. Report of the Special January Third Additional 1983 Grand Jury Concerning "Do Not Resuscitate" Procedures at a Certain Hospital in Queens County. *Connecticut Medicine.* 1985 Jun; 49(6): 367-376. 4 fn. BE57831.
    accountability; *decision making; disclosure; *government regulation; *guidelines; *hospitals; *institutional policies; legal aspects; legal liability; medical records; nurses; patient participation; physicians; professional organizations; *records; *resuscitation orders; *standards; state government; ventilators; withholding treatment; Medical Society of the State of New York; *New York

Ohio. Court of Appeals, Hamilton County. Anderson v. St. Francis-St. George Hospital. *North Eastern Reporter, 2d Series.* 1992 Nov 18 (date of decision). 614: 841-847. BE56297.
    allowing to die; brain pathology; compensation; *hospitals; injuries; *legal liability; negligence; nurses; *prolongation of life; *resuscitation; *resuscitation orders; *right to die; torts; *treatment refusal; *wrongful life; *Anderson v. St. Francis-St. George Hospital; Ohio
The Ohio Court of Appeals for Hamilton County upheld

BE = bioethics accession number   fn. = footnotes   refs. = references

summary judgment on a claim for wrongful living, where the patient was resuscitated by a nurse contrary to his doctor's no code blue order and then later suffered a paralyzing stroke prior to his death. Wrongful living was the phrase coined by the appellant for the cause of action for the life that was forced on the decedent by resuscitation. The court noted that life was not a compensable harm in the state until the legislature or the highest court decides it is so. Because the patient had apparently expressly refused treatment in a medical emergency, the case could proceed under two other theories, battery or unauthorized touching, and negligence or breach of a duty of care. (KIE abstract)

Phillips, Russell S.; Wenger, Neil S.; Teno, Joan, et al. Choices of seriously ill patients about cardiopulmonary resuscitation: correlates and outcomes. [For the SUPPORT Investigators]. *American Journal of Medicine.* 1996 Feb; 100(2): 128–137. 38 refs. BE55578.
age factors; allowing to die; *attitudes; *communication; *critically ill; diagnosis; evaluation studies; females; hospitals; males; medical records; morbidity; *mortality; pain; palliative care; *patients; *physicians; prognosis; prolongation of life; quality of life; *resuscitation; *resuscitation orders; survey; *terminally ill; time factors; treatment outcome; treatment refusal; ventilators; coma; follow-up studies; severity of illness index; *Study to Understand Prognoses and Preferences for Outcomes and Risks of Treatments (SUPPORT); United States

Read, William Allan. Hospital's Role in Resuscitation Decisions. [Booklet]. Chicago, IL: Hospital Research and Educational Trust; 1983. 14 p. (Series on aging from the Office of Aging and Long-Term Care). 12 refs. 4 fn. Trust Catalog No. 630130. BE57446.
clinical ethics committees; competence; dissent; family members; guidelines; health personnel; *hospitals; informed consent; *institutional ethics; *institutional policies; legal aspects; living wills; medical records; minors; physician's role; *practice guidelines; *resuscitation orders; third party consent; treatment refusal; professional role

Rosin, Arnold J.; Sonnenblick, Moshe. Autonomy and paternalism in geriatric medicine: the Jewish ethical approach to issues of feeding terminally ill patients, and to cardiopulmonary resuscitation. *Journal of Medical Ethics.* 1998 Feb; 24(1): 44–48. 45 refs. BE57409.
*aged; *allowing to die; *artificial feeding; attitudes; *autonomy; decision making; *dementia; family members; futility; *Jewish ethics; palliative care; *paternalism; physicians; prognosis; *prolongation of life; religious hospitals; resuscitation; *resuscitation orders; risks and benefits; suffering; *terminal care; *terminally ill; treatment outcome; treatment refusal; *value of life; withholding treatment; *Israel; Orthodox Judaism; Shaare Zedek Medical Center (Jerusalem)
Respecting and encouraging autonomy in the elderly is basic to the practice of geriatrics. In this paper, we examine the practice of cardiopulmonary resuscitation (CPR) and "artificial" feeding in a geriatric unit in a general hospital subscribing to Jewish orthodox religious principles, in which the sanctity of life is a fundamental ethical guideline. The literature on the administration of food and water in terminal stages of illness, including dementia, still shows division of opinion on the morality of withdrawing nutrition. We uphold the principle that as long as feeding by naso-gastric (N–G) or percutaneous endoscopic gastrostomy (PEG) does not constitute undue danger or arouse serious opposition it should be given, without causing suffering to the patient. This is part of basic care, and the doctor has no mandate to withdraw this. The question of CPR still shows much discrepancy regarding elderly patients' wishes, and

doctors' opinions about its worthwhileness, although up to 10 percent survive. Our geriatric patients rarely discuss the subject, but it is openly ventilated with families who ask about it, who are then involved in the decision-making, and the decision about CPR or "do-not-resuscitate" (DNR) is based on clinical and prognostic considerations.

Sahadevan, S.; Pang, W.S. Do-not-resuscitate orders: towards a policy in Singapore. *Singapore Medical Journal.* 1995 Jun; 36(3): 267–270. 28 refs. BE55527.
clinical ethics committees; communication; competence; *decision making; dissent; emergency care; family members; futility; *guidelines; legal aspects; patient care team; patient participation; physicians; quality of life; *resuscitation orders; terminally ill; uncertainty; *Singapore

Sayers, Gwen M.; Schofield, Irene; Aziz, Michael. An analysis of CPR decision-making by elderly patients. *Journal of Medical Ethics.* 1997 Aug; 23(4): 207–212. 16 refs. BE55920.
*aged; attitudes; *autonomy; communication; *competence; comprehension; *decision making; disclosure; evaluation studies; hospitals; informed consent; *paternalism; *patient participation; *patients; physicians; psychological stress; quality of life; recall; *resuscitation; *resuscitation orders; risks and benefits; survey; treatment outcome; withholding treatment; Great Britain
Traditionally clinicians have determined their patients' resuscitation status without consultation. This has been condemned as morally indefensible in cases where not for resuscitation (NFR) orders are based on quality of life considerations and when the patient's true wishes are not known. Such instances would encompass most resuscitation decisions in elderly patients. Having previously involved patients in CPR decision-making, we chose formally to explore the reasons behind the choices made. Although the patients were not upset, and readily decided at the time of initial consultation, on later analysing the decision-making we found poor understanding of the procedure, poor recall of information given and in some cases evidence of harm. This may be attributed to impaired decision-making capacity of elderly hospitalised patients as previously shown, or to the discomfort precipitated by having to contemplate the apparent immediacy of cardiac arrest by these patients. We propose that subscribing to autonomy as a general principle needs to be balanced against particular cases where distress may be caused by, or result in, diminished competence and limited autonomy.

Sechriest, Kay; Payne, John; Jordan, Lynn, et al. Confronting the right to die: caught between a patient's will and a doctor's order. [Case study and commentaries]. *Journal of Christian Nursing.* 1985 Fall; 2(4): 5–10. BE56974.
attitudes; case studies; Christian ethics; *decision making; interprofessional relations; legal aspects; *living wills; *nurses; *patient advocacy; *physicians; *prolongation of life; *resuscitation orders; right to die

Shepardson, Laura B.; Youngner, Stuart J.; Speroff, Theodore, et al. Variation in the use of do-not-resuscitate orders in patients with stroke. *Archives of Internal Medicine.* 1997 Sep 8; 157(16): 1841–1847. 29 refs. BE55832.
age factors; blacks; *brain pathology; comparative studies; emergency care; evaluation studies; *hospitals; medical records; morbidity; nursing homes; patient admission; *resuscitation orders; statistics; survey; whites; *cerebrovascular disorders; coma; severity of illness index;

Cleveland (OH); Ohio
OBJECTIVES: To identify sociodemographic and clinical characteristics associated with the use of do–not–resuscitate (DNR) orders in hospitalized patients with stroke. To examine whether the use of DNR orders varies across hospitals. METHODS: This observational cohort study used data collected for 13337 consecutive eligible patients with a primary diagnosis of stroke. These patients were discharged in 1991 through 1994 from 30 hospitals in a large metropolitan area. Study data were abstracted from patients' hospital records using standard forms. Admission severity of illness was measured using a validated multivariable model. Sociodemographic and clinical factors independently associated with the use of DNR orders were identified using stepwise logistic regression. RESULTS: Do–not–resuscitate orders were written for 2898 patients (22%). Patient characteristics independently (P less than .01) associated with increased use of DNR orders included increasing age (odds ratio [OR], 1.06 per year); admission from a skilled nursing facility (OR, 2.44) or through the emergency department (OR, 1.49); cancer (OR, 2.73), intracerebral hemorrhage (OR, 2.12), coma (OR, 7.47), or lethargy or stupor on admission neurological assessment (OR, 3.38); and increasing admission severity (OR; 1.29 per decile). In contrast, African American race was associated with lower use of DNR orders (OR, 0.54). Although substantial variation in the use of DNR orders was observed across hospitals, with rates ranging from 12% to 32%, adjusting for the above patient characteristics eliminated much of this variation, including differences between major teaching and other hospitals and between hospitals with and without religious affiliations. CONCLUSIONS: In our community–based analysis of patients with stroke, the use of DNR orders was common and was strongly related to several patient characteristics. These factors explained much of the variation across hospitals. While our analysis did not account for differences in patient preferences for treatment, the differences we observed in the use of DNR orders across sociodemographic groups are suggestive of variations in care and may have important implications for the cost and quality of hospital care.

Smith, Thomas J.; Desch, Christopher E.; Hackney, Mary Helen, et al. How long does it take to get a "do not resuscitate" order? *Journal of Palliative Care.* 1997 Spring; 13(1): 5–8. 20 refs. BE55734.
attitudes; *cancer; *communication; decision making; evaluation studies; informed consent; patient education; patients; physicians; *resuscitation orders; terminally ill; *time factors; Virginia

Stewart, Kevin. Discussing cardiopulmonary resuscitation with patients and relatives. *Postgraduate Medical Journal.* 1995 Oct; 71(840): 585–589. 30 refs. BE55531.
advance directives; autonomy; beneficence; case studies; communication; competence; *decision making; dementia; disclosure; dissent; family members; futility; guidelines; informed consent; legal aspects; medical records; *patient participation; physicians; quality of life; resuscitation; *resuscitation orders; risks and benefits; treatment outcome; treatment refusal; withholding treatment; *Great Britain

Stewart, Kevin; Wagg, Adrian; Kinirons, Mark. When can elderly patients be excluded from discussing resuscitation? *Journal of the Royal College of Physicians of London.* 1996 Mar–Apr; 30(2): 133–135. 10 refs. BE56885.
advance care planning; *aged; *communication; *competence; comprehension; *decision making; *futility; *health personnel; hospitals; informed consent; institutional

policies; morbidity; *prognosis; resuscitation; *resuscitation orders; survey; Great Britain

Sulmasy, Daniel P.; Marx, Eric S. A computerized system for entering orders to limit treatment: implementation and evaluation. *Journal of Clinical Ethics.* 1997 Fall; 8(3): 258–263. 21 fn. BE57568.
advance directives; allowing to die; artificial feeding; attitudes; *computers; critically ill; *decision making; drugs; evaluation studies; health insurance; hospices; hospitals; *institutional policies; *intensive care units; internship and residency; morbidity; *organization and administration; palliative care; patient discharge; physicians; quality of health care; *records; *resuscitation orders; statistics; *terminal care; *withholding treatment; antibiotics; severity of illness index; *Georgetown University Medical Center

Taylor, E.M.; Parker, S.; Ramsay, M.P. Patients' receipt and understanding of written information about a resuscitation policy: report from New Zealand. *Bioethics.* 1998 Jan; 12(1): 65–76. 10 fn. BE58484.
*attitudes; *communication; *comprehension; disclosure; *hospitals; *information dissemination; informed consent; *institutional policies; patient admission; *patients; recall; *resuscitation orders; survey; *Dunedin Hospital (N.Z.); New Zealand

Teno, Joan; Lynn, Joanne; Wenger, Neil, et al. Advance directives for seriously ill hospitalized patients: effectiveness with the Patient Self–Determination Act and the SUPPORT intervention. [For the SUPPORT Investigators]. *Journal of the American Geriatrics Society.* 1997 Apr; 45(4): 500–507. 23 refs. BE57122.
advance care planning; *advance directives; *communication; comparative studies; *critically ill; *decision making; *evaluation; evaluation studies; family members; hospitals; living wills; medical records; patient education; patients; physician patient relationship; physician's role; physicians; prognosis; *resuscitation orders; terminal care; third party consent; retrospective studies; seriously ill; *Patient Self–Determination Act 1990; *Study to Understand Prognoses and Preferences for Outcomes and Risks of Treatments (SUPPORT); United States

Tulsky, James A.; Cassileth, Barrie R.; Bennett, Charles L. The effect of ethnicity on ICU use and DNR orders in hospitalized AIDS patients. *Journal of Clinical Ethics.* 1997 Summer; 8(2): 150–157. 18 fn. BE55777.
advance care planning; *AIDS; allowing to die; attitudes; *blacks; comparative studies; *Hispanic Americans; hospitals; *intensive care units; males; medical records; *minority groups; mortality; *patient admission; *patient care; patients; prolongation of life; *resuscitation orders; statistics; *terminal care; *time factors; treatment outcome; *whites; multicenter studies; retrospective studies; severity of illness index; Chicago; Los Angeles; Miami

van Delden, Johannes J.M. Do–not–resuscitate decisions. *In:* Chadwick, Ruth, ed. Encyclopedia of Applied Ethics, Volume 1. San Diego, CA: Academic Press; 1998: 839–847. 21 refs. ISBN 0–12–227066–5. BE56379.
advance directives; competence; *decision making; family members; futility; guidelines; hospitals; institutional policies; patient admission; patient participation; physicians; practice guidelines; prognosis; resuscitation; *resuscitation orders; risks and benefits; statistics; treatment outcome; withholding treatment; Netherlands; United States

Ventres, William; Nichter, Mark; Reed, Richard, et al. Do–not–resuscitate discussions: a qualitative analysis. *Family Practice Research Journal.* 1992; 12(2): 157–169. 34 refs. BE56902.
*attitudes; clergy; *communication; *decision making; evaluation studies; family members; family practice; *health

---

BE = bioethics accession number   fn. = footnotes   refs. = references

personnel; hospitals; internship and residency; nurses; *physician patient relationship; physicians; *professional family relationship; professional patient relationship; *resuscitation orders; social workers; survey; qualitative research; University of Arizona Medical School

Welch, Robyn Perlman. Characteristics related to DNR orders for pediatric ICU patients. *Dimensions of Critical Care Nursing.* 1996 May–Jun; 15(3): 142–149. 22 refs. BE56891.

adolescents; *children; communication; comparative studies; control groups; death; decision making; futility; guidelines; infants; *intensive care units; medical records; mortality; newborns; nurse's role; palliative care; parents; patient care; *pediatrics; practice guidelines; prognosis; quality of life; resuscitation; *resuscitation orders; risks and benefits; selection for treatment; statistics; time factors; treatment outcome; withholding treatment; retrospective studies; Florida

Wenger, Neil S.; Pearson, Marjorie L.; Desmond, Katherine A., et al. Changes over time in the use of do not resuscitate orders and the outcomes of patients receiving them. *Medical Care.* 1997 Apr; 35(4): 311–319. 27 refs. BE57571.

age factors; *aged; blacks; comparative studies; decision making; dementia; diagnosis; females; hospitals; indigents; males; morbidity; mortality; patient discharge; prognosis; *resuscitation orders; socioeconomic factors; statistics; terminal care; terminally ill; time factors; whites; Medicare; United States

Wenger, Neil S.; Greengold, Nancy L.; Oye, Robert K., et al. Patients with DNR orders in the operating room: surgery, resuscitation, and outcomes. [For the SUPPORT Investigators]. *Journal of Clinical Ethics.* 1997 Fall; 8(3): 250–257. 21 fn. BE57618.

aged; anesthesia; attitudes; autonomy; communication; *decision making; diagnosis; evaluation studies; guidelines; *hospitals; *institutional policies; medical records; mortality; palliative care; patient discharge; patients; physicians; *practice guidelines; prognosis; *resuscitation; *resuscitation orders; *selection for treatment; *standards; statistics; *surgery; *treatment outcome; severity of illness index; Study to Understand Prognoses and Preferences for Outcomes and Risks of Treatments (SUPPORT); United States

Werber, Stephen J. Ancient answers to modern questions: death, dying, and organ transplants -- a Jewish law perspective. *Journal of Law and Health.* 1996–1997; 11(1–2): 13–44. 139 fn. BE57589.

*active euthanasia; *allowing to die; *assisted suicide; brain death; cadavers; chronically ill; *determination of death; hearts; *Jewish ethics; killing; *organ donation; organ donors; organ transplantation; physicians; *resuscitation orders; right to die; *suicide; terminally ill; tissue donation; treatment refusal; value of life; withholding treatment; Orthodox Judaism

Yellin, Paul B.; Fleischman, Alan R. DNR in the DR? *Journal of Perinatology.* 1995 May–Jun; 15(3): 232–236. 16 refs. BE57700.

advance directives; *allowing to die; beneficence; *congenital disorders; *decision making; futility; moral policy; *newborns; parents; pediatrics; physicians; prematurity; prenatal diagnosis; prognosis; prolongation of life; *resuscitation; *resuscitation orders; uncertainty; *withholding treatment; neonatology

Youngner, Stuart J.; Shuck, Jerry M. Advance directives and the determination of death. *In:* McCullough, Laurence B.; Jones, James W.; Brody, Baruch A., eds. Surgical Ethics. New York, NY:

Oxford University Press; 1998: 57–77. 49 refs. ISBN 0–19–510347–5. BE58340.

advance care planning; *advance directives; brain death; cardiac death; *communication; decision making; *determination of death; family members; goals; guidelines; living wills; organ donation; palliative care; *physicians; professional autonomy; prolongation of life; quality of life; *resuscitation orders; *surgery; terminally ill; third party consent; treatment refusal; values; withholding treatment; Patient Self-Determination Act 1990; United States

RIGHT TO DIE *See* ALLOWING TO DIE, EUTHANASIA, SUICIDE

RIGHTS
See under
HEALTH CARE/RIGHTS

SCIENTIFIC MISCONDUCT *See* FRAUD AND MISCONDUCT

SELECTION FOR TREATMENT

See also ALLOWING TO DIE, PATIENT CARE, RESOURCE ALLOCATION

Arnold, Robert M.; Shaw, Byers W.; Purtilo, Ruth. Acute, high risk patients: the case of transplantation. *In:* McCullough, Laurence B.; Jones, James W.; Brody, Baruch A., eds. Surgical Ethics. New York, NY: Oxford University Press; 1998: 97–115. 27 refs. ISBN 0–19–510347–5. BE58323.

age factors; alcohol abuse; alternatives; body parts and fluids; *critically ill; disclosure; economics; hospitals; *informed consent; institutional policies; justice; livers; managed care programs; morbidity; mortality; organ donation; *organ transplantation; patients; *physicians; professional competence; prognosis; quality of health care; resource allocation; retreatment; risk; risks and benefits; scarcity; *selection for treatment; self induced illness; statistics; *surgery; time factors; treatment outcome; geographic factors; United Network for Organ Sharing; United States

Barnhart, J. Marie; Wassertheil–Smoller, Sylvia; Fowler, Cynthia, et al. Racial variation in the use of coronary–revascularization procedures. [Letters and response]. *New England Journal of Medicine.* 1997 Jul 10; 337(2): 131–132. 5 refs. BE55901.

blacks; comparative studies; *heart diseases; Hispanic Americans; *minority groups; morbidity; patient care; physicians; research design; *selection for treatment; social discrimination; socioeconomic factors; *surgery; whites; physician's practice patterns; United States

Belkin, Lisa. Pregnant with complications. *New York Times Magazine.* 1997 Oct 26: 34–39, 48–49, 67–68. BE58039.

*age factors; children; embryo transfer; *females; health facilities; in vitro fertilization; institutional policies; maternal health; *ovum donors; parent child relationship; *reproductive technologies; risk; scarcity; *selection for treatment; menopause; United States

Benjamin, Martin; Turcotte, Jeremiah G. Ethics, alcoholism and liver transplantation. *In:* Lucey, Michael R.; Merion, Robert M.; Beresford, Thomas P., eds. Liver Transplantation and the Alcoholic Patient: Medical, Surgical and Psychosocial Issues. New York, NY: Cambridge University Press; 1994: 113–130. 12 refs. ISBN 0521–43332–0. BE56681.

accountability; *alcohol abuse; costs and benefits;

BE = bioethics accession number   fn. = footnotes   refs. = references

disadvantaged; justice; *livers; moral obligations; *organ transplantation; patient compliance; preventive medicine; public policy; *resource allocation; scarcity; *selection for treatment; *self induced illness; social discrimination; stigmatization; *transplant recipients; treatment outcome; values; United States

Bhagwanjee, Satish; Muckart, David J.J.; Jeena, Prakash M., et al. Does HIV status influence the outcome of patients admitted to a surgical intensive care unit? A prospective double blind study. [Article, commentaries, and response]. *BMJ (British Medical Journal).* 1997 Apr 12; 314(7087): 1077–1084. 26 refs. BE55661.
　　*AIDS serodiagnosis; anonymous testing; blacks; comparative studies; confidentiality; critically ill; developing countries; disadvantaged; disclosure; empirical research; *epidemiology; futility; *HIV seropositivity; hospitals; human experimentation; *informed consent; injuries; *intensive care units; justice; morbidity; mortality; patient admission; patient discharge; patients; research design; research ethics committees; *research subjects; resource allocation; scientific misconduct; *selection for treatment; surgery; *treatment outcome; prospective studies; *South Africa
OBJECTIVES: (a) To assess the impact of HIV status (HIV negative, HIV positive, AIDS) on the outcome of patients admitted to intensive care units for diseases unrelated to HIV; (b) to decide whether a positive test result for HIV should be a criterion for excluding patients from intensive care for diseases unrelated to HIV. DESIGN: A prospective double blind study of all admissions over six months. HIV status was determined in all patients by enzyme linked immunosorbent assay (ELISA), immunofluorescence assay, western blotting, and flow cytometry. The ethics committee considered the clinical implications of the study important enough to waive patients' right to informed consent. Staff and patients were blinded to HIV results. On discharge patients could be advised of their HIV status if they wished. SETTING: A 16 bed surgical intensive care unit. SUBJECTS: All 267 men and 135 women admitted to the unit during the study period. INTERVENTIONS: None. MAIN OUTCOME MEASURES: APACHE II score (acute physiological, age, and chronic health evaluation), organ failure, septic shock, durations of intensive care unit and hospital stay, and intensive care unit and hospital mortality. RESULTS: No patient had AIDS. 52 patients were tested positive for HIV and 350 patients were tested negative. The two groups were similar in sex distribution but differed significantly in age, incidence of organ failure (37 (71%) v 171 (49%) patients), and incidence of septic shock (20 (38%) v 54 (15%)). After adjustment for age there were no differences in intensive care unit or hospital mortality or in the durations of stay in the intensive care unit or hospital. CONCLUSIONS: Morbidity was higher in HIV positive patients but there was no difference in mortality. In this patient population a positive HIV test result should not be a criterion for excluding a patient from intensive care.

Birchard, Karen. Irish doctors surveyed on treatment refusal. [News]. *Lancet.* 1997 Sep 20; 350(9081): 872. BE56083.
　　*attitudes; *physicians; *refusal to treat; resource allocation; *selection for treatment; *self induced illness; survey; *withholding treatment; life style; *Ireland

Boyle, Philip J.; Moskowitz, Ellen. Making tough resource decisions. *Health Progress.* 1996 Nov–Dec; 77(6): 48–53. 3 refs. BE56322.

autonomy; common good; costs and benefits; *decision making; disclosure; due process; goals; guidelines; *hospitals; informed consent; *institutional policies; intensive care units; justice; patient care team; prognosis; *resource allocation; *selection for treatment; *values; severity of illness index

Callahan, Sidney. Gays, lesbians, and the use of alternate reproductive technologies. *In:* Nelson, Hilde Lindemann, ed. Feminism and Families. New York, NY: Routledge; 1997: 188–202. 16 fn. ISBN 0–415–91254–7. BE55839.
　　adoption; children; commodification; confidentiality; disclosure; *family relationship; females; *feminist ethics; *homosexuals; males; parent child relationship; reproduction; *reproductive technologies; *selection for treatment; single persons; social discrimination; sociobiology

Capron, Alexander M. More blessed to give than to receive? *Transplantation Proceedings.* 1992 Oct; 24(5): 2185–2187. 5 refs. Commentary on J. Muyskens, p. 2181–2184. BE56833.
　　*altruism; cadavers; coercion; commodification; *organ donation; *organ donors; *organ transplantation; *public policy; refusal to treat; resource allocation; *selection for treatment; social worth; *transplant recipients; refusal to donate; United States

Corley, Mary C.; Huff, Steven; Sayles, Linda, et al. Patient and nurse criteria for heart transplant candidacy. *Medsurg Nursing.* 1995 Jun; 4(3): 211–215. 20 refs. BE55712.
　　age factors; AIDS; alcohol abuse; aliens; *attitudes; behavior disorders; comparative studies; drug abuse; economics; family members; *hearts; HIV seropositivity; mentally ill; mentally retarded; *nurses; *organ transplantation; patient compliance; *patients; prisoners; prognosis; resource allocation; *selection for treatment; *standards; survey; *transplant recipients; United States

Dark, John H. Priorities for lung transplantation. *Lancet.* 1998 Jan 3; 351(9095): 4–5. 10 refs. BE57907.
　　diagnosis; mortality; *organ transplantation; quality of life; *resource allocation; *selection for treatment; time factors; transplant recipients; *treatment outcome; *lungs; Great Britain

de Rave, Sjoerd. Allocation of donor organs. [Letter]. *Lancet.* 1997 Oct 11; 350(9084): 1107. 2 refs. BE58151.
　　decision making; emergency care; *livers; *organ transplantation; *resource allocation; *selection for treatment; time factors; transplant recipients; Europe; Eurotransplant; France

Dyer, Clare. Doctors accused of refusing transplant on moral grounds. [News]. *BMJ (British Medical Journal).* 1997 May 10; 314(7091): 1370. BE55818.
　　adolescents; behavior disorders; critically ill; decision making; *drug abuse; *livers; morality; *organ transplantation; patient compliance; *physicians; prognosis; *refusal to treat; *selection for treatment; social discrimination; transplant recipients; Edinburgh Royal Infirmary; *Great Britain; *Paul, Michelle; *Sanfey, Hilary

Eaton, Stephanie. The subtle politics of organ donation: a proposal. *Journal of Medical Ethics.* 1998 Jun; 24(3): 166–170. 13 fn. BE59113.
　　*cadavers; decision making; *family members; moral obligations; motivation; obligations to society; *organ donation; *organ donors; *organ transplantation; *presumed consent; *resource allocation; *selection for treatment; *third party consent; *transplant recipients; treatment outcome; withholding treatment; *refusal to donate; *Great Britain; Jarvis, Rupert
Organs available for transplantation are scarce and valuable medical resources and decisions about who is to receive them should not be made more difficult by

---

BE = bioethics accession number　　　　fn. = footnotes　　　　refs. = references

complicated calculations of desert. Consideration of likely clinical outcome must always take priority when allocating such a precious resource otherwise there is a danger of wasting that resource. However, desert may be a relevant concern in decision-making where the clinical risk is identical between two or more potential recipients of organs. Unlikely as this scenario is, such a decision procedure makes clear the interdependence of organ recipient and organ donor and hints at potential disadvantages for those who are willing to accept but unwilling to donate organs (free-riders). A combined opting-out and preference system weakens many of the objections to opting-out systems and may make the decision to donate organs on behalf of their deceased relatives easier for families.

Evans, Roger W. Limits of chronological age as a basis for rationing health care. *Dialysis and Transplantation.* 1994 Sep; 23(9): 506-507, 510-512+. 42 refs. BE57063.
*age factors; *aged; *economics; government financing; health; *health care; kidneys; morbidity; mortality; organ transplantation; patient care; *quality of life; rehabilitation; *renal dialysis; *resource allocation; *selection for treatment; statistics; *treatment outcome; Medicare; *United States

Field, Howard L. Organ allocation. [Letter; title supplied]. *Journal of Clinical Ethics.* 1997 Summer; 8(2): 208. BE57254.
*alcohol abuse; critically ill; *decision making; depressive disorder; *drug abuse; *livers; *organ transplantation; *patient compliance; psychiatric diagnosis; referral and consultation; *refusal to treat; *resource allocation; *selection for treatment; *self induced illness; socioeconomic factors; *suicide; *transplant recipients

Franks, Peter; Clancy, Carolyn M.; Naumburg, Elizabeth H. Sex, access, and excess. [Editorial]. *Annals of Internal Medicine.* 1995 Oct 1; 123(7): 548-549. 20 refs. BE56106.
biomedical technologies; diagnosis; *females; *health care; health services research; heart diseases; *males; *patient care; *patient satisfaction; preventive medicine; primary health care; quality of health care; referral and consultation; *selection for treatment; social discrimination; surgery; treatment outcome; women's health; continuity of patient care; United States

Frisho-Lima, P.; Gurman, G.; Schapira, A., et al. Rationing critical care -- what happens to patients who are not admitted? *Theoretical Surgery.* 1994 Dec; 9(4): 208-211. 17 refs. BE57548.
age factors; comparative studies; *critically ill; *hospitals; *intensive care units; *mortality; patient admission; prognosis; *quality of health care; *resource allocation; *selection for treatment; surgery; technology assessment; treatment outcome; withholding treatment; severity of illness index; teaching hospitals; *Israel

Furnham, Adrian; Ofstein, Abigail. Ethical ideology and the allocation of scarce medical resources. *British Journal of Medical Psychology.* 1997 Mar; 70 (Pt. 1): 51-63. 25 refs. BE57504.
age factors; allowing to die; *attitudes; decision making; deontological ethics; family relationship; females; guidelines; justice; kidney diseases; males; married persons; medical schools; *moral policy; parents; prognosis; public opinion; religion; *renal dialysis; *resource allocation; scarcity; *selection for treatment; single persons; social worth; socioeconomic factors; students; survey; teleological ethics; universities; utilitarianism; *values; virtues; England

Gaffney, B.; Kee, F. Are the economically active more deserving? *British Heart Journal.* 1995 Apr; 73(4):

385-389. 42 refs. BE55655.
*decision making; *diagnosis; employment; *heart diseases; *physicians; *referral and consultation; *selection for treatment; *socioeconomic factors; survey; *time factors; *heart catheterization; retrospective studies; *Northern Ireland

Gelder, Mark S. Life and death decisions in the intensive care unit. *Cancer.* 1995 Nov 15; 76(10, Suppl.): 2171-2175. 61 refs. BE56865.
age factors; aged; *allowing to die; *cancer; communication; costs and benefits; *decision making; family members; females; *intensive care units; mortality; patient admission; patient care; patient care team; physician patient relationship; prognosis; prolongation of life; resource allocation; resuscitation; *selection for treatment; treatment outcome; withholding treatment; severity of illness index; United States

Giugliano, Robert P.; Camargo, Carlos A.; Lloyd-Jones, Donald M., et al. Elderly patients receive less aggressive medical and invasive management of unstable angina: potential impact of practice guidelines. *Archives of Internal Medicine.* 1998 May 25; 158(10): 1113-1120. 69 refs. BE58804.
*age factors; *aged; diagnosis; drugs; evaluation studies; *guidelines; *heart diseases; hospitals; intensive care units; morbidity; *patient care; patients; *practice guidelines; quality of health care; referral and consultation; risk; *selection for treatment; surgery; withholding treatment; *guideline adherence; retrospective studies; Agency for Health Care Policy and Research; United States
BACKGROUND: The Agency for Health Care Policy and Research (AHCPR) released a practice guideline on the diagnosis and management of unstable angina in 1994. OBJECTIVE: To examine practice variation across the age spectrum in the management of patients hospitalized with unstable angina 2 years before release of the AHCPR guideline. DESIGN: Retrospective cohort. SETTING: Urban academic hospital. PATIENTS: All nonreferral patients diagnosed as having unstable angina who were hospitalized directly from the emergency department to the intensive care or telemetry unit between October 1, 1991, and September 30, 1992. MEASUREMENTS: Percentage of eligible patients receiving medical treatment concordant with 8 important AHCPR guideline recommendations. RESULTS: Half of the 280 patients were older than 66 years; women were older than men on average (70 vs 64 years; P less than .001). After excluding those with contraindications to therapy, patients in the oldest quartile (age, 75.20-93.37 years) were less likely than younger patients to receive aspirin (P less than .009), beta-blockers (P less than .04), and referral for cardiac catheterization (P less than .001). Overall guideline concordance weighted for the number of eligible patients declined with increasing age (87.4%, 87.4%, 84.0%, and 74.9% for age quartiles 1 to 4, respectively; chi2, P less than .001). Increasing age, the presence of congestive heart failure at presentation, a history of congestive heart failure, previous myocardial infarction, increasing comorbidity, and elevated creatinine concentration were associated with care that was less concordant with AHCPR guideline recommendations; only age and congestive heart failure at presentation remained significant in the multivariate analysis (odds ratios, 1.28 per decade [95% confidence interval, 1.02-1.61] and 3.16 [95% confidence interval, 1.57-6.36], respectively). CONCLUSIONS: Older patients were less likely to receive standard therapies for unstable angina before release of the 1994 AHCPR guideline. Patients presenting with congestive heart

---

failure also received care that was more discordant with guideline recommendations. The AHCPR guideline allows identification of patients who receive nonstandard care and, if applied to those patients with the greatest likelihood to benefit, could lead to improved health care delivery.

Glannon, Walter. Responsibility, alcoholism, and liver transplantation. *Journal of Medicine and Philosophy.* 1998 Feb; 23(1): 31-49. 40 refs. BE57519.
   accountability; *alcohol abuse; *autonomy; disease; drug abuse; *genetic determinism; *genetic predisposition; health care; *justice; *livers; moral obligations; *moral policy; *organ transplantation; patients; psychoactive drugs; *resource allocation; scarcity; *selection for treatment; *self induced illness; transplant recipients; life style
Many believe that it is morally wrong to give lower priority for a liver transplant to alcoholics with end-stage liver disease than to patients whose disease is not alcohol-related. Presumably, alcoholism is a disease that results from factors beyond one's control and therefore one cannot be causally or morally responsible for alcoholism or the liver failure that results from it. Moreover, giving lower priority to alcoholics unfairly singles them out for the moral vice of heavy drinking. I argue that the etiology of alcoholism may involve enough control for the alcoholic to be responsible for his condition and accordingly have a weaker claim to receive a new liver than someone who acquires the disease through no fault of his own. In addition, I show why it is more plausible to reframe the question of priority in terms of control and responsibility rather than virtue and vice. Given that medical resources like livers are scarce, some people may justifiably be given lower priority than others in receiving these resources.

Goodman, Kenneth W. Outcomes, futility, and health policy research. *In:* Goodman, Kenneth W., ed. Ethics, Computing, and Medicine: Informatics and the Transformation of Health Care. New York, NY: Cambridge University Press; 1998: 116-138. 61 refs. ISBN 0-521-46905-8. BE57007.
   allowing to die; *computers; *critically ill; *decision making; disclosure; economics; epidemiology; evaluation; family members; futility; human experimentation; informed consent; patient care; patients; practice guidelines; *prognosis; resource allocation; *selection for treatment; social discrimination; *treatment outcome; *uncertainty; withholding treatment; evidence-based medicine; severity of illness index

Great Britain. England. High Court of Justice, Queen's Bench Division. R v. Ethical Committee of St. Mary's Hospital (Manchester) ex parte H. *Family Law Reports.* 1987 Oct 26 (date of decision). [1988] 1: 512-520. BE58576.
   adoption; *clinical ethics committees; *decision making; hospitals; in vitro fertilization; infertility; judicial action; *legal aspects; *physicians; referral and consultation; *refusal to treat; *reproductive technologies; *selection for treatment; sex offenses; standards; prostitution; *Great Britain; *National Health Service; *R v. Ethical Committee of St. Mary's Hospital (Manchester) ex parte H.
The Queen's Bench Division of England's High Court of Justice refused judicial review of a hospital ethics committee's decision that the medical team rather than the committee should determine denial of IVF services, in effect, refusal of treatment, to a patient and her husband. Because the patient, who was unable to conceive, had a past history of prostitution and poor understanding of the parental role, she and her husband

were refused adoption and foster children by social services. They then sought IVF treatment and were put on a waiting list for services. After learning of the reasons for the adoption refusal, the consultant in obstetrics and gynecology decided that IVF should not be given and that the patient's name should be taken off the wait list. An ethics committee, which had been set up to provide advice and guidance on infertility services, as recommended by the Warnock Report, concluded that the decision on IVF services should be made by the medical consultant. Seeking judicial review, the patient claimed that once any matter is brought to the committee's attention, it was under a charge first to investigate and then to advise. The court found that the committtee with its "wide range of expertise" was intended to be advisory, not decision-making. In the court's opinion, the committee served as an informal forum for professionals. (KIE abstract)

Grubb, Andrew; Walsh, Pat; Lambe, Neil, et al. Doctors' Views on the Management of Patients in Persistent Vegetative State (PVS): A UK Study. London: Kings College London, Centre of Medical Law and Ethics; 1997. 68 p. (Occasional papers series; 1). 175 fn. ISBN 1-898484-20-1. BE59108.
   advance directives; age factors; *allowing to die; artificial feeding; *attitudes; brain pathology; comparative studies; *decision making; diagnosis; drugs; family members; home care; hospitals; knowledge, attitudes, practice; legal aspects; medical specialties; nursing homes; *patient care; patient care team; *persistent vegetative state; *physicians; prognosis; quality of life; rehabilitation; resource allocation; *selection for treatment; statistics; surgery; survey; terminology; time factors; treatment outcome; *withholding treatment; antibiotics; questionnaires; Airedale NHS Trust v. Bland; *Great Britain

Gutmann, Thomas; Land, Walter. The ethics of organ allocation: the state of debate. *Transplantation Reviews.* 1997 Oct; 11(4): 191-207. 170 refs. BE58882.
   age factors; *body parts and fluids; cadavers; decision making; deontological ethics; ethical theory; international aspects; *justice; *moral policy; organ donation; organ donors; *organ transplantation; public policy; quality of life; random selection; remuneration; *resource allocation; retreatment; review; scarcity; *selection for treatment; self induced illness; social discrimination; social worth; time factors; transplant recipients; utilitarianism; geographic factors; Europe; United States

Haas, Jennifer. The cost of being a woman. *New England Journal of Medicine.* 1998 Jun 4; 338(23): 1694-1695. 12 refs. BE58104.
   age factors; attitudes; biomedical technologies; chronically ill; *economics; *females; *health care; indigents; *males; morbidity; mortality; patient care; physicians; *selection for treatment; women's health; longevity; Canada; United States

Higgins, R.M.; West, N.; Edmunds, M.E., et al. Effect of a strict HLA matching policy on distribution of cadaveric kidney transplants to Indo-Asian and white European recipients: regional study. *BMJ (British Medical Journal).* 1997 Nov 22; 315(7119): 1354-1355. 3 refs. BE56553.
   *cadavers; comparative studies; evaluation studies; *institutional policies; *kidneys; *minority groups; organ donation; *organ transplantation; renal dialysis; *resource allocation; *selection for treatment; *whites; *HLA matching; Great Britain

Hilberman, Mark; Kutner, Jean; Parsons, Debra, et al. Marginally effective medical care: ethical analysis of issues in cardiopulmonary resuscitation (CPR).

Journal of Medical Ethics. 1997 Dec; 23(6): 361–367. 65 refs. BE57663.

aged; autonomy; beneficence; *costs and benefits; *decision making; dementia; emergency care; evaluation; freedom; *futility; *guidelines; institutional policies; justice; legal aspects; moral policy; morbidity; mortality; nursing homes; patients; persistent vegetative state; physicians; *prognosis; quality of life; refusal to treat; *resuscitation; *resuscitation orders; *risks and benefits; *selection for treatment; statistics; terminally ill; *treatment outcome; treatment refusal; withholding treatment; United States

Outcomes from cardiopulmonary resuscitation (CPR) remain distressingly poor. Overuse of CPR is attributable to unrealistic expectations, unintended consequences of existing policies and failure to honour patient refusal of CPR. We analyzed the CPR outcomes literature using the bioethical principles of beneficence, non–maleficence, autonomy and justice and developed a proposal for selective use of CPR. Beneficence supports use of CPR when most effective. Non–maleficence argues against performing CPR when the outcomes are harmful or usage inappropriate. Additionally, policies which usurp good clinical judgment and moral responsibility, thereby contributing to inappropriate CPR usage, should be considered maleficent. Autonomy restricts CPR use when refused but cannot create a right to CPR. Justice requires that we define which medical interventions contribute sufficiently to health and happiness that they should be made universally available. This ordering is necessary whether one believes in the utilitarian standard or wishes medical care to be universally available on fairness grounds. Low–yield CPR fails justice criteria. Cardiopulmonary resuscitation should be performed when justified by the extensive outcomes literature; not performed when not desired by the patient or not indicated; and performed infrequently when relatively contraindicated.

Hsu, Irene; DuChane, Janeen; Veatch, Robert M.
Recommendation of treatment that would allow parole -- Scenario; Position 1: pharmacist should recommend the hormonal treatment; Position 2: pharmacist should not recommend the hormonal treatment; Analysis and commentary. *American Journal of Health–System Pharmacy.* 1995 Apr 15; 52(8): 829–833. 5 refs. BE58105.

*behavior control; case studies; codes of ethics; competence; freedom; government financing; health insurance reimbursement; HIV seropositivity; *hormones; legal aspects; mental institutions; mentally ill; obligations to society; patient compliance; patients' rights; *pharmacists; *prisoners; professional ethics; *selection for treatment; *sex offenses; sexuality; technical expertise; withholding treatment; professional role

Hughes, David; Griffiths, Lesley. "But if you look at the coronary anatomy...": risk and rationing in cardiac surgery. *Sociology of Health and Illness.* 1996 Mar; 18(2): 172–197. 48 refs. 10 fn. BE56492.

*age factors; case studies; communication; *decision making; diagnosis; evaluation studies; *hearts; hospitals; *interprofessional relations; *minority groups; *physicians; prognosis; referral and consultation; *resource allocation; risk; *selection for treatment; *self induced illness; smoking; *social worth; *surgery; angioplasty; *coronary artery bypass; waiting lists; Great Britain

Kalb, Claudia. How old is too old? *Newsweek.* 1997 May 5; 79(18): 64. BE58038.

*age factors; children; *females; mothers; ovum donors; *reproductive technologies; risks and benefits; *selection for treatment

Klein, Rudolph; Day, Patricia; Redmayne, Sharon. Managing Scarcity: Priority Setting and Rationing in the National Health Service. Philadelphia, PA: Open University Press; 1996. 161 p. (State of health series). Bibliography: p. 143–153. ISBN 0–335–19446–X. BE55699.

accountability; administrators; age factors; biomedical technologies; *decision making; *economics; government financing; health care; *health care delivery; health care reform; international aspects; physician's role; physicians; politics; public participation; *public policy; quality adjusted life years; referral and consultation; refusal to treat; renal dialysis; reproductive technologies; *resource allocation; scarcity; *selection for treatment; self induced illness; standards; time factors; uncertainty; evidence–based medicine; geographic factors; *Great Britain; *National Health Service; Oregon; United States

Lamke, Celia. Distributive justice and HIV disease in intensive care. *Critical Care Nursing Quarterly.* 1996 May; 19(1): 55–64. 23 refs. BE55724.

*AIDS; *decision making; *HIV seropositivity; *intensive care units; *justice; nurses; patient admission; patient care team; patients; physicians; *resource allocation; *selection for treatment; standards

Levine, David Z. Would you deny this patient dialysis? [Editorial]. *American Journal of Kidney Diseases.* 1998 Jan; 31(1): 131–132. 11 refs. BE57551.

aged; allowing to die; attitudes; chronically ill; economics; international aspects; patient care; *physicians; quality of life; refusal to treat; *renal dialysis; *resource allocation; *selection for treatment; withholding treatment; Canada; Great Britain; United States

Lucey, Michael R.; Beresford, Thomas P. Ethical considerations regarding orthotopic liver transplantation for alcoholic patients. *In:* Shelton, Wayne N.; Edwards, Rem B., eds. Advances in Bioethics. Volume 3: Values, Ethics, and Alcoholism. Greenwich, CT: JAI Press; 1997: 119–129. 33 refs. ISBN 0–7623–0219–4. BE57635.

accountability; *alcohol abuse; autonomy; beneficence; disclosure; disease; justice; *livers; moral obligations; *moral policy; obligations to society; *organ transplantation; patient compliance; patients; physicians; *prognosis; *public policy; referral and consultation; refusal to treat; *resource allocation; retreatment; risks and benefits; scarcity; *selection for treatment; *self induced illness; social discrimination; transplant recipients; treatment outcome; Great Britain

Mehlman, Maxwell J.; Durchslag, Melvyn R.; Neuhauser, Duncan. When do health care decisions discriminate against persons with disabilities? *Journal of Health Politics, Policy and Law.* 1997 Dec; 22(6): 1385–1411. 25 refs. 26 fn. BE56747.

anencephaly; carriers; *costs and benefits; *disabled; economics; employment; federal government; futility; genetic disorders; government financing; *government regulation; guidelines; health care; health insurance; *health insurance reimbursement; HIV seropositivity; hospitals; indigents; infertility; late–onset disorders; *legal aspects; minors; organ transplantation; physicians; prognosis; quality of life; *refusal to treat; reproduction; resource allocation; risks and benefits; scarcity; *selection for treatment; *social discrimination; state government; terminology; treatment outcome; withholding treatment; *Americans with Disabilities Act 1990; Civil Rights Act 1991; Equal Employment Opportunity Commission; Medicaid; Oregon; *Rehabilitation Act 1973; *United States

Recent interpretations of laws prohibiting discrimination against persons with disabilities indicate that these laws will play a greater role in health care decision making than previously anticipated. This article employs lessons from other areas of antidiscrimination law to examine these developments and to provide a framework for

---

making health care decisions that are consistent with these new legal interpretations. This article addresses decisions in individual cases, treatment policies adopted by health care providers, and coverage programs of third-party payers, both public and private.

Miller, Pam. Ethical issues in neonatal intensive care. *In:* Frith, Lucy, ed. Ethics and Midwifery: Issues in Contemporary Practice. Boston, MA: Butterworth-Heinemann; 1996: 123-139. 24 refs. ISBN 0-7506-3056-6. BE58636.
> *allowing to die; artificial feeding; biomedical technologies; case studies; communication; *congenital disorders; *decision making; *intensive care units; moral policy; mothers; *newborns; *nurse midwives; *nurse's role; nurses; parents; patient advocacy; patient care; personhood; physicians; *prematurity; professional family relationship; prognosis; quality of life; resource allocation; risks and benefits; *selection for treatment; suffering; terminal care; treatment outcome; value of life; withholding treatment; Great Britain

Mintz, Benjamin. Analyzing the OPTN [Organ Procurement and Transplant Network] under the state action doctrine -- can UNOS's organ allocation criteria survive strict scrutiny? *Columbia Journal of Law and Social Problems.* 1995 Spring; 28(3): 339-396. 276 fn. BE57197.
> *blacks; body parts and fluids; equal protection; federal government; financial support; government regulation; *kidneys; *legal aspects; legal rights; *organ transplantation; organizational policies; public policy; *resource allocation; *selection for treatment; *social discrimination; standards; state government; Supreme Court decisions; *transplant recipients; treatment outcome; voluntary programs; *histocompatibility; Department of Health and Human Services; *Organ Procurement and Transplant Network; Organ Procurement Organizations; *United Network for Organ Sharing; *United States

Mongoven, Ann. Federal hearings on liver transplant allocation and donation. *In:* BioLaw: A Legal and Ethical Reporter on Medicine, Health Care, and Bioengineering. Special Sections 2(12). Frederick, MD: University Publications of America; 1997 Dec: S:373-S:389. BE57643.
> cadavers; chronically ill; computers; conflict of interest; consensus; critically ill; *decision making; determination of death; federal government; government regulation; health facilities; health insurance; justice; *livers; models, theoretical; *organ donation; *organ transplantation; patient advocacy; physicians; prognosis; public participation; *public policy; *resource allocation; scarcity; *selection for treatment; transplant recipients; treatment outcome; geographic factors; *Department of Health and Human Services; *United Network for Organ Sharing; *United States

Mori, Takahide. Egg donation should be limited to women below 60 years of age. *Journal of Assisted Reproduction and Genetics.* 1995 Apr; 12(4): 229-230. 10 refs. BE55589.
> *age factors; children; *embryo transfer; *females; *ovum; ovum donors; parent child relationship; *reproductive technologies; *selection for treatment; Japan

Murphy, Donald J. The economics of futile interventions. *In:* Zucker, Marjorie B.; Zucker, Howard D., eds. Medical Futility and the Evaluation of Life-Sustaining Interventions. New York, NY: Cambridge University Press; 1997: 123-135. 37 refs. ISBN 0-521-56877-3. BE55985.
> advance directives; *age factors; aged; *biomedical technologies; *chronically ill; *common good; *costs and benefits; *critically ill; dementia; *economics; *futility; home

care; hospices; *intensive care units; mortality; *palliative care; persistent vegetative state; prognosis; *prolongation of life; refusal to treat; *resource allocation; *selection for treatment; self induced illness; *social impact; *terminal care; *terminally ill; time factors; treatment outcome; treatment refusal; trends; uncertainty; *values; *health services misuse; Study to Understand Prognoses and Preferences for Outcomes and Risks of Treatments (SUPPORT); United States

Muyskens, James. Should receiving depend upon willingness to give? *Transplantation Proceedings.* 1992 Oct; 24(5): 2181-2184. 5 refs. Commented on by A.M. Capron, p. 2185-2187. BE56832.
> altruism; cadavers; *organ donation; *organ donors; *organ transplantation; *public policy; *refusal to treat; resource allocation; scarcity; *selection for treatment; *transplant recipients; *refusal to donate; United States

Neuberger, James; Lake, John. Allocating donor livers. [Editorial]. *BMJ (British Medical Journal).* 1997 Apr 19; 314(7088): 1140-1141. 6 refs. BE57163.
> adults; age factors; children; consensus; critically ill; decision making; hospitals; institutional policies; *livers; models, theoretical; *organ transplantation; organizational policies; physicians; prognosis; *resource allocation; scarcity; *selection for treatment; self induced illness; *standards; time factors; treatment outcome; *Great Britain; United Network for Organ Sharing; *United States

Neuberger, James; Adams, David; MacMaster, Paul, et al. Assessing priorities for allocation of donor liver grafts: survey of public and clinicians. *BMJ (British Medical Journal).* 1998 Jul 18; 317(7152): 172-175. 26 refs. BE58816.
> *age factors; *alcohol abuse; *attitudes; comparative studies; *drug abuse; employment; family practice; *livers; medical specialties; *organ transplantation; *physicians; *prisoners; prognosis; *public opinion; *resource allocation; scarcity; *selection for treatment; *self induced illness; *social worth; survey; *time factors; transplant recipients; *treatment outcome; gastroenterology; *Great Britain

OBJECTIVES: To compare the priorities of the general public, family doctors, and gastroenterologists in allocating donor livers to potential recipients of liver allograft. DESIGN: Representative quota sampling of 1000 members of the general public and 200 family doctors, and a postal questionnaire of 100 gastroenterologists. SUBJECTS: Respondents were given eight hypothetical case histories (based on real patients) and asked to select recipients for four donor livers. Cases were selected to identify controversial areas such as extremes of age, misuse of alcohol, and intravenous drugs. Respondents were also asked to select the least deserving case and which of seven possible factors (time on waiting list, outcome, age, value to society, return to work, previous use of illicit drugs, and involvement of alcohol in the liver damage) should be used to select patients already listed for transplantation. Focus groups were also held to explore further the reasons for the choices given. RESULTS: There were considerable differences between the three groups in the choice of the recipients, although alcohol use and antisocial behaviour always rated low. For selection of recipients the general public thought that, in decreasing order of importance, age, outcome, and time on the waiting list were the most important factors in selecting recipients; family doctors rated outcome, age, and likely work status after transplantation and the gastroenterologists outcome, work status, and non-involvement of alcohol in the cause of the liver disease as the most important factors. CONCLUSIONS: The views of the public are at variance with those of

---

BE = bioethics accession number   fn. = footnotes   refs. = references

clinicians. Further debate is required to ensure an equitable and appropriate distribution of a scarce resource.

Newman, Joel D. Ethics committee offers criteria. *UNOS Update.* 1997 Jan–Feb: 8. BE56234.
　　age factors; ethics committees; *guidelines; *organ transplantation; organizational policies; patient compliance; prognosis; resource allocation; retreatment; *selection for treatment; self induced illness; *transplant recipients; *United Network for Organ Sharing; United States

Nilstun, Tore; Ohlsson, Rolf. Should health care be rationed by age? *Scandinavian Journal of Social Medicine.* 1995 Jun; 23(2): 81–84. 18 refs. BE55518.
　　*age factors; autonomy; biomedical technologies; costs and benefits; *health care; justice; *moral policy; organ transplantation; *resource allocation; *scarcity; *selection for treatment; utilitarianism; Sweden

Parker, Lisa S. Beauty and breast implantation: how candidate selection affects autonomy and informed consent. *In:* DiQuinzio, Patrice; Young, Iris Marion, eds. Feminist Ethics and Social Policy. Bloomington, IN: Indiana University Press; 1997: 255–273. 47 refs. 9 fn. ISBN 0-253-21125-5. BE57287.
　　*autonomy; breast cancer; competence; *cosmetic surgery; *decision making; *females; *feminist ethics; *informed consent; *medical devices; motivation; risks and benefits; *selection for treatment; self concept; *values; beauty; *breast implants; United States

Pinch, Winifred J., et al. Allocation of scarce resources: critical care nursing dilemmas. [Case studies and commentaries]. *Dimensions of Critical Care Nursing.* 1985 May–Jun; 4(3): 164–173. 7 refs. Includes brief commentaries by Jeanne M. Yocke, Katherine W. Vestal, John M. Cloches, Joanne R. Duffy, Leah L. Curtin, Bernice Coleman, and Rebecca Hathaway. BE56953.
　　case studies; critically ill; cultural pluralism; *decision making; deontological ethics; *ethical analysis; ethical theory; *intensive care units; *moral policy; patient admission; patient discharge; patient transfer; random selection; *resource allocation; rights; *selection for treatment; social worth; socioeconomic factors; utilitarianism; values

Piotrowski, Joseph J.; Akhrass, Rami; Alexander, J.J., et al. Rupture of known abdominal aortic aneurysms: an ethical dilemma. [Article and commentaries]. *American Surgeon.* 1995 Jul; 61(7): 556–559. 20 refs. BE56216.
　　*age factors; *aged; *critically ill; emergency care; morbidity; mortality; referral and consultation; *selection for treatment; *surgery; time factors; *treatment outcome; treatment refusal; withholding treatment; Cleveland (OH)

Rapin, M. The ethics of intensive care. [Editorial]. *Intensive Care Medicine.* 1987; 13(5): 300–303. 7 refs. BE56631.
　　*allowing to die; *decision making; diagnosis; economics; family members; futility; *intensive care units; palliative care; *patient admission; patient care; patient care team; physicians; *prognosis; prolongation of life; resource allocation; *selection for treatment; *withholding treatment; *France

Sampson, Mark T. Revised liver policy approved. *UNOS Update.* 1997 Jan–Feb: 5–7. BE56237.
　　*guidelines; *livers; minors; *organ transplantation; organizational policies; public participation; *resource allocation; *selection for treatment; transplant recipients; liver diseases; *United Network for Organ Sharing; United States

Savulescu, Julian. Consequentialism, reasons, value and justice. *Bioethics.* 1998 Jul; 12(3): 212–235. 61 fn. BE58894.
　　age factors; autonomy; *health care; *justice; *moral policy; philosophy; *prognosis; *resource allocation; rights; *selection for treatment; *teleological ethics; *utilitarianism; values; rationality; *Harris, John

Over the past 10 years, John Harris has made important contributions to thinking about distributive justice in health care. In his latest work, Harris controversially argues that clinicians should stop prioritising patients according to prognosis. He argues that the good or benefit of health care is providing each individual with an opportunity to live the best and longest life possible for him or her. I call this thesis, opportunism. For the purpose of distribution of resources in health care, Harris rejects welfarism (the thesis that the good of health care is well-being) and argues that utilitarianism in general may lead to de facto discrimination against groups of people needing health care. I argue that well-being is a superior theory of the good of health care to Harris' opportunism. Harris' concerns about utilitarianism can be better addressed by: (i) relating justice more closely to reasons for action; (ii) by conceptualising the relationship between reasons for action and the value of the consequences of those actions as a plateau rather than scalar relationship. Justice can be understood as satisfying as many equally rational claims on resources as possible. The rationality of a person's claim on health resources turns on the strength of that person's reasons to promote certain health-related states of affairs. I argue that the strength of that reason does not track the expected value of that state of affairs in a fully scalar fashion. Rather a person can have most reason to promote some state of affairs, even though he or she could promote other more valuable states of affairs. Thus there can be equal reason for a distributor of public resources to save either of two people, even though one will have a better and more valuable life. This approach, while addressing many of Harris' concerns about utilitarianism, does not imply that doctors should give up prioritising patients according to prognosis altogether, but it does allow that patients with lower but reasonable prognosis should have a share of public resources.

Schmidt, Volker H. Selection of recipients for donor organs in transplant medicine. *Journal of Medicine and Philosophy.* 1998 Feb; 23(1): 50–74. 45 refs. 20 fn. BE57520.
　　age factors; aged; alcohol abuse; deception; *decision making; due process; guidelines; health facilities; hearts; *institutional policies; justice; *kidneys; livers; moral policy; *organ transplantation; organization and administration; patient admission; patient advocacy; patient compliance; *physicians; prognosis; random selection; referral and consultation; *resource allocation; scarcity; *selection for treatment; social worth; statistics; time factors; *transplant recipients; uncertainty; utilitarianism; values; histocompatibility; Europe; *Eurotransplant; *Germany

This paper deals with a problem which has received a great deal of attention in the ethical literature, but about which very little is known empirically: the selection of recipients for organs in transplant medicine. Based on a larger study, it is shown how this problem is practically resolved in one European country, Germany. It is demonstrated that most of the criteria used to determine recipients are non-medical in nature, even though they generally tend to be rationalized in medical terms. Moreover, the choice of criteria depends as much on prognostic considerations as on personal indiosyncrasies and values held by individual physicians who are in charge at the various programs. Several examples of the

---

BE = bioethics accession number   fn. = footnotes   refs. = references

extremely diverse policies in which this results are presented.

Schüppel, Reinhart; Büchele, Gisela; Batz, Lothar, et al. Sex differences in selection of pacemakers: retrospective observational study. [Article and commentary]. *BMJ (British Medical Journal).* 1998 May 16; 316(7143): 1492–1495. 24 refs. BE58307.

aged; data banks; *females; *heart diseases; *males; *medical devices; quality of health care; registries; *selection for treatment; *social discrimination; retrospective studies; undertreatment; *Germany

OBJECTIVE: To evaluate the effect of patients' sex on selection of pacemakers. DESIGN: Retrospective univariate and multivariate analysis of a large database. SETTING: German central pacemaker register. SUBJECTS: Records collected at the register for 1992 and 1993 (n=31 913), covering 64% of all implantations in Germany. MAIN OUTCOME MEASURE: Probability of receiving a single chamber, dual chamber, or rate responsive pacemaker in relation to sex. RESULTS: Univariate analysis showed that women were more likely to receive single chamber pacemakers and less likely to receive dual chamber or rate responsive systems than men. After demographic and clinical variables were controlled for, women were still more likely to receive a single chamber system (atrial pacing: odds ratio 0.89, 95% confidence interval 0.74 to 1.07; ventricular pacing: 0.85, 0.80 to 0.92) and less likely to receive a dual chamber (1.20, 1.12 to 1.30) or a rate responsive system (1.26, 1.17 to 1.37) than men. CONCLUSIONS: The data suggest sex differences in the selection of a pacemaker system which cannot be explained by the underlying cardiac disorder. Further research is needed to evaluate why guidelines for implanting pacemakers are not better adhered to.

Shaw, A.B. Ensuring equity and quality of care for elderly people: a critique of the College report. *Journal of the Royal College of Physicians of London.* 1995 Mar–Apr; 29(2): 89–91. 14 refs. BE56567.

*age factors; *aged; biomedical technologies; costs and benefits; health care; justice; public policy; *resource allocation; scarcity; *selection for treatment; Great Britain

Sheldon, Sally; Wilkinson, Stephen. Conjoined twins: the legality and ethics of sacrifice. *Medical Law Review.* 1997 Summer; 5(2): 149–171. 57 fn. BE57874.

criminal law; decision making; *double effect; drugs; *intention; *killing; legal aspects; *legal liability; *moral policy; newborns; organ donation; pain; palliative care; personhood; physicians; prognosis; prolongation of life; risks and benefits; *selection for treatment; *surgery; teleological ethics; terminally ill; *twins; *conjoined twins; *Great Britain

Sheldon, Tony. Dutch doctor refuses to treat smokers. [News]. *BMJ (British Medical Journal).* 1998 Jan 24; 316(7127): 250. BE57724.

legal aspects; *physicians; *refusal to treat; *self induced illness; *smoking; social discrimination; *Netherlands; *van Bunningen, Cees

Shelton, Wayne N. Justice and alcoholism. *In:* Shelton, Wayne N.; Edwards, Rem B., eds. Advances in Bioethics. Volume 3: Values, Ethics, and Alcoholism. Greenwich, CT: JAI Press; 1997: 131–152. 26 refs. ISBN 0–7623–0219–4. BE57636.

*accountability; *alcohol abuse; autonomy; behavior control; *behavior disorders; biomedical technologies; coercion; *common good; *disease; freedom; health care delivery; *justice; *libertarianism; *livers; mental health; *models,

theoretical; moral obligations; *moral policy; *organ transplantation; paternalism; patient care; *patient compliance; *public policy; *refusal to treat; *resource allocation; rights; scarcity; *selection for treatment; *self induced illness; stigmatization; treatment outcome; United States

Shenfield, F. Justice and access to fertility treatments. *In:* Shenfield, F.; Sureau, C., eds. Ethical Dilemmas in Assisted Reproduction. New York, NY: Parthenon Pub. Group; 1997: 7–14. 21 refs. ISBN 1–85070–916–5. BE57941.

age factors; deontological ethics; economics; *government financing; justice; *reproductive technologies; *resource allocation; rights; *selection for treatment; *socioeconomic factors; utilitarianism; *Great Britain; National Health Service

Silverman, Myrna; McDowell, B. Joan; Musa, Donald, et al. To treat or not to treat: issues in decisions not to treat older persons with cognitive impairment, depression, and incontinence. *Journal of the American Geriatrics Society.* 1997 Sep; 45(9): 1094–1101. 35 refs. BE56316.

*aged; *decision making; *dementia; *depressive disorder; evaluation studies; *morbidity; *patient care; physicians; referral and consultation; *selection for treatment; treatment refusal; *withholding treatment; outpatients; Pennsylvania

Sirmon, Maryella D. The combative patient: ethical issues in patient selection for chronic dialysis. *Seminars in Dialysis.* 1996 Jan–Feb; 9(1): 56–60. 38 refs. BE55798.

adolescents; adults; allowing to die; attitudes; case studies; chronically ill; costs and benefits; critically ill; *decision making; dementia; family members; guidelines; mentally retarded; palliative care; *patient compliance; persistent vegetative state; physicians; practice guidelines; professional organizations; *renal dialysis; resource allocation; risks and benefits; *selection for treatment; terminally ill; treatment refusal; *withholding treatment; United States

Slifkin, Robert F.; Charytan, Chaim. Ethical issues related to the provision or denial of renal services to non-citizens. [Case commentaries on ethical issues in dialysis]. *Seminars in Dialysis.* 1997 May–Jun; 10(3): 173–175. 5 refs. BE57921.

*aliens; emergency care; federal government; government financing; government regulation; *kidney diseases; obligations of society; *public policy; *refusal to treat; *renal dialysis; *selection for treatment; state government; Medicaid; *United States

Spike, Jeffrey. Iatrogenic liver failure, transplantation, and prisoners. *Journal of Clinical Ethics.* 1997 Winter; 8(4): 398–404. 5 fn. BE57615.

blacks; case studies; decision making; drug abuse; drugs; ethics consultation; *iatrogenic disease; indigents; justice; *livers; males; moral obligations; moral policy; *organ transplantation; patient advocacy; patient care team; patient compliance; *prisoners; refusal to treat; resource allocation; risks and benefits; scarcity; *selection for treatment; social worth; socioeconomic factors; treatment outcome; tuberculosis; New York City

Stolberg, Sheryl Gay. U.S. orders sickest to be given priority on donated organs. [News]. *New York Times.* 1998 Mar 27: A16. BE57737.

attitudes; federal government; *government regulation; hospitals; *organ transplantation; patient advocacy; *resource allocation; *selection for treatment; *standards; time factors; transplant recipients; geographic factors; severity of illness index; *Department of Health and Human Services; United Network for Organ Sharing; *United States

---

BE = bioethics accession number   fn. = footnotes   refs. = references

Sutton, Graham C. Will you still need me, will you still screen me, when I'm past 64? Breast screening policy is based on ageism. [Editorial]. *BMJ (British Medical Journal).* 1997 Oct 25; 315(7115): 1032–1033. 14 refs. BE56589.
> *age factors; *aged; *breast cancer; costs and benefits; empirical research; *females; *mass screening; *public policy; referral and consultation; risk; *selection for treatment; *social discrimination; *Great Britain; *National Health Service

Ubel, Peter A.; Loewenstein, George. Distributing scarce livers: the moral reasoning of the general public. *Social Science and Medicine.* 1996 Apr; 42(7): 1049–1055. 29 refs. BE56889.
> age factors; *attitudes; children; costs and benefits; justice; *livers; *organ transplantation; prognosis; *public opinion; public policy; *resource allocation; scarcity; *selection for treatment; survey; *transplant recipients; treatment outcome; *values; Pennsylvania

The transplant system has been criticized for not paying enough attention to efficiency in distributing scarce organs. But little research has been done to see how the general public views tradeoffs between efficiency and equity. We surveyed members of the general public to see how they would distribute organs among patients with varying chances of benefiting from them. In addition, we asked subjects to explain their decisions and to tell us about any other information they would have liked in order to make the decisions. We found that the public places a very high value on giving everyone a chance at receiving scarce resources, even if that means a significant decrease in the chance that available organs will save people's lives. Our results raise important questions about whether the aims of outcomes research and cost–effective studies agree with the values of the general public.

Ubel, Peter A.; Loewenstein, George. Public perceptions of the importance of prognosis in allocating transplantable livers to children. *Medical Decision Making.* 1996 Jul–Sep; 16(3): 234–241. 24 refs. BE57978.
> adults; *children; *decision making; justice; *livers; *organ transplantation; *prognosis; *public opinion; public policy; *resource allocation; *selection for treatment; survey; treatment outcome; values; *Pennsylvania; United States

Ubel, Peter A.; DeKay, M.; Baron, J., et al. Public preferences for efficiency and racial equity in kidney transplant allocation decisions. *Transplantation Proceedings.* 1996 Oct; 28(5): 2997–3002. 24 refs. BE57979.
> *blacks; decision making; justice; *kidneys; *organ transplantation; *prognosis; *public opinion; *resource allocation; *selection for treatment; socioeconomic factors; survey; time factors; transplant recipients; treatment outcome; *whites; histocompatibility; *Philadelphia; United States

Ubel, Peter A.; Loewenstein, George. The efficacy and equity of retransplantation: an experimental survey of public attitudes. *Health Policy.* 1995 Nov; 34(2): 145–151. 12 refs. BE56602.
> *attitudes; justice; *livers; morality; mortality; *organ transplantation; *prognosis; *public opinion; public policy; *resource allocation; *retreatment; *selection for treatment; survey; *transplant recipients; Pennsylvania; United States

United Network for Organ Sharing (UNOS). Ethics Committee. General principles for allocating human organs and tissues. *Transplantation Proceedings.* 1992 Oct; 24(5): 2227–2235. 6 fn. BE56846.
> age factors; *autonomy; *beneficence; body parts and fluids; cultural pluralism; directed donation; *guidelines; *justice; *moral policy; organ donation; *organ transplantation; organizational policies; patient compliance; policy analysis; prognosis; *public policy; quality of life; remuneration; *resource allocation; retreatment; risks and benefits; *selection for treatment; self induced illness; social worth; time factors; *tissue transplantation; transplant recipients; treatment outcome; *utilitarianism; life style; National Organ Transplant Act 1984; *United Network for Organ Sharing; *United States

Verweij, Marcel; Kortmann, Frank. Moral assessment of growth hormone therapy for children with idiopathic short stature. *Journal of Medical Ethics.* 1997 Oct; 23(5): 305–309. 18 fn. BE57111.
> *children; counseling; goals; *growth disorders; *hormones; informed consent; justice; medicine; *moral policy; *normality; parental consent; psychological stress; resource allocation; *risks and benefits; *selection for treatment; self concept; stigmatization; treatment outcome; uncertainty

The prescription of growth hormone therapy for children who are not growth hormone deficient is one of the controversies in contemporary paediatric endocrinology. Is it morally appropriate to enhance the growth, by means of medical treatment, of a child with idiopathic short stature? The medical, moral, and philosophical questions in this area are many. Data on the effects of human growth hormone (hGH) treatment will not on their own provide us with answers, as these effects have to be evaluated from a normative perspective. In this article we consider hGH treatment for children of idiopathic short stature from three normative perspectives: the goals of medicine, the good of the patient, and the public good. We argue that the prevention of psychological and social problems due to short stature (and not merely the enhancement of growth) should be the ultimate goal of medical treatment and research.

Wenger, Neil S.; Greengold, Nancy L.; Oye, Robert K., et al. Patients with DNR orders in the operating room: surgery, resuscitation, and outcomes. [For the SUPPORT Investigators]. *Journal of Clinical Ethics.* 1997 Fall; 8(3): 250–257. 21 fn. BE57618.
> aged; anesthesia; attitudes; autonomy; communication; *decision making; diagnosis; evaluation studies; guidelines; *hospitals; *institutional policies; medical records; mortality; palliative care; patient discharge; patients; physicians; *practice guidelines; prognosis; *resuscitation; *resuscitation orders; *selection for treatment; *standards; statistics; *surgery; *treatment outcome; severity of illness index; Study to Understand Prognoses and Preferences for Outcomes and Risks of Treatments (SUPPORT); United States

Wilkes, Michael S.; Slavin, Stuart. Heart transplantation selection criteria: attitudes of ethnically diverse medical students. *Journal of Clinical Ethics.* 1998 Summer; 9(2): 147–155. 15 fn. BE58960.
> administrators; age factors; alcohol abuse; aliens; Asian Americans; *attitudes; blacks; comparative studies; curriculum; diagnosis; drug abuse; family relationship; females; health insurance; *hearts; Hispanic Americans; HIV seropositivity; homosexuals; indigents; males; medical education; medical schools; mentally disabled; *minority groups; morbidity; organ donation; *organ transplantation; patient compliance; patients; physicians; *resource allocation; retreatment; *selection for treatment; smoking; socioeconomic factors; *students; survey; *transplant recipients; whites; United States

Wood, Joseph Patrick. Emergency physicians' obligations to managed care patients under COBRA. *Academic Emergency Medicine.* 1996 Aug; 3(8): 794–800. 34 refs.

BE58110.
*emergency care; federal government; *government regulation; hospitals; informed consent; institutional policies; *legal aspects; *legal liability; legal obligations; *managed care programs; *patient transfer; *physicians; *refusal to treat; selection for treatment; standards; *Consolidated Omnibus Budget Reconciliation Act (COBRA) 1985; Emergency Medical Treatment and Active Labor Act 1986; *United States

SEX DETERMINATION

See also PRENATAL DIAGNOSIS, SEX PRESELECTION

Chervenak, F.A.; McCullough, L.B. Should sex identification be offered as part of the routine ultrasound examination? *Ultrasound in Obstetrics and Gynecology.* 1996 Nov; 8(5): 293–294. 5 refs. BE58879.
*autonomy; beneficence; disclosure; informed consent; justice; *pregnant women; *prenatal diagnosis; *sex determination; spousal consent; *ultrasonography

Clark, Liana R. Sex preselection: the advent of the made-to-order child. *Pharos.* 1985 Fall; 48(4): 2–7. 17 refs. BE57071.
attitudes; females; males; methods; parents; physicians; prenatal diagnosis; reproduction; *risks and benefits; selective abortion; *sex determination; *sex preselection; social discrimination; *social impact; socioeconomic factors; women's rights

Kuhse, Helga; Singer, Peter. Choosing the sex, race and sexual orientation of our children. [Editorial]. *Bioethics.* 1998 Jan; 12(1): iii–v. BE58481.
blacks; children; females; genetic disorders; genetic intervention; homosexuals; males; minority groups; *motivation; *parents; reproductive technologies; *sex determination; *sex preselection; social discrimination; stigmatization; whites

Mao, Xin; Wertz, Dorothy C. China's genetic services providers' attitudes towards several ethical issues: a cross-cultural survey. *Clinical Genetics.* 1997 Aug; 52(2): 100–109. 38 refs. BE57506.
*attitudes; common good; confidentiality; congenital disorders; developing countries; *directive counseling; *disclosure; *DNA data banks; DNA fingerprinting; duty to warn; eugenics; *genetic counseling; *genetic disorders; *genetic information; genetic materials; genetic predisposition; genetic services; genome mapping; government regulation; *health personnel; informed consent; law enforcement; minority groups; population control; public policy; reproductive technologies; *selective abortion; *sex determination; socioeconomic factors; survey; *China

Netherlands. Health Council. Standing Committee on Medical Ethics and Health Law. Sex Selection for Non-Medical Reasons. Report of a Committee of the Health Council of the Netherlands. The Hague: Health Council of the Netherlands; 1995. 48 p. 78 refs. Pub. No. 1995/11E. ISBN 90–5549–102–0. BE56730.
children; embryo transfer; eugenics; females; males; methods; preimplantation diagnosis; prenatal diagnosis; selective abortion; *sex determination; *sex preselection; social discrimination; social impact; Netherlands

Nisker, J.A.; Jones, M. The ethics of sex selection. *In:* Shenfield, F.; Sureau, C., eds. Ethical Dilemmas in Assisted Reproduction. New York, NY: Parthenon Pub. Group; 1997: 41–50. 21 refs. ISBN 1–85070–916–5. BE57945.

aliens; attitudes; autonomy; *cultural pluralism; females; international aspects; *minority groups; obstetrics and gynecology; organizational policies; physicians; prenatal diagnosis; professional organizations; risk; selective abortion; *sex determination; sex preselection; socioeconomic factors; values; women's rights; ultrasonography; American Society for Reproductive Medicine; Asia; *Canada; Canadian Medical Association; International Federation of Gynecology and Obstetrics (FIGO); Society of Obstetricians and Gynaecologists of Canada; United States

Perry, Seymour. Reports from the Health Council of the Netherlands: sex selection for nonmedical reasons. *International Journal of Technology Assessment in Health Care.* 1996 Fall; 12(4): 756–759. BE55576.
advisory committees; artificial insemination; disclosure; embryo transfer; genetic disorders; government regulation; *motivation; parents; physicians; preimplantation diagnosis; prenatal diagnosis; public policy; reproductive technologies; selective abortion; *sex determination; *sex preselection; social impact; Committee on Medical Ethics and Health Law (Netherlands); *Netherlands

Stein, Edward. Choosing the sexual orientation of children. *Bioethics.* 1998 Jan; 12(1): 1–24. 57 fn. BE58483.
females; genetic determinism; genetic intervention; genetic research; *homosexuals; international aspects; justice; legal aspects; males; *moral policy; *parents; preimplantation diagnosis; prenatal diagnosis; *public policy; reproduction; reproductive technologies; rights; *selective abortion; *sex determination; *sex preselection; sexuality; social discrimination; social impact; *stigmatization; suffering; women's rights; India; United States

Ten, C.L. The use of reproductive technologies in selecting the sexual orientation, the race, and the sex of children. *Bioethics.* 1998 Jan; 12(1): 45–48. 1 fn. BE58485.
blacks; children; females; genetic intervention; *homosexuals; males; *minority groups; motivation; parents; reproductive technologies; *sex determination; *sex preselection; sexuality; social discrimination; *stigmatization; whites

SEX PRESELECTION

See also REPRODUCTIVE TECHNOLOGIES, SEX DETERMINATION

Berkowitz, Jonathan M.; Snyder, Jack W. Racism and sexism in medically assisted conception. *Bioethics.* 1998 Jan; 12(1): 25–44. 80 fn. BE58480.
blacks; disabled; females; genetic intervention; government regulation; males; minority groups; moral policy; motivation; *parents; physician's role; privacy; public policy; reproduction; reproductive technologies; rights; *sex preselection; sexuality; *social discrimination; *stigmatization; whites

Clark, Liana R. Sex preselection: the advent of the made-to-order child. *Pharos.* 1985 Fall; 48(4): 2–7. 17 refs. BE57071.
attitudes; females; males; methods; parents; physicians; prenatal diagnosis; reproduction; *risks and benefits; selective abortion; *sex determination; *sex preselection; social discrimination; *social impact; socioeconomic factors; women's rights

Kalaça, Cagri; Akin, Ayse. The issue of sex selection in Turkey. *Human Reproduction.* 1995 Jul; 10(7): 1631–1632. 10 refs. BE55510.
evaluation; family planning; females; *government regulation; males; *methods; *public policy; *sex preselection; sperm; *Turkey

---

BE = bioethics accession number   fn. = footnotes   refs. = references

Kuhse, Helga; Singer, Peter. Choosing the sex, race and sexual orientation of our children. [Editorial]. *Bioethics.* 1998 Jan; 12(1): iii–v. BE58481.
> blacks; children; females; genetic disorders; genetic intervention; homosexuals; males; minority groups; *motivation; *parents; reproductive technologies; *sex determination; *sex preselection; social discrimination; stigmatization; whites

Netherlands. Health Council. Standing Committee on Medical Ethics and Health Law. Sex Selection for Non-Medical Reasons. Report of a Committee of the Health Council of the Netherlands. The Hague: Health Council of the Netherlands; 1995. 48 p. 78 refs. Pub. No. 1995/11E. ISBN 90–5549–102–0. BE56730.
> children; embryo transfer; eugenics; females; males; methods; preimplantation diagnosis; prenatal diagnosis; selective abortion; *sex determination; *sex preselection; social discrimination; social impact; Netherlands

Perry, Seymour. Reports from the Health Council of the Netherlands: sex selection for nonmedical reasons. *International Journal of Technology Assessment in Health Care.* 1996 Fall; 12(4): 756–759. BE55576.
> advisory committees; artificial insemination; disclosure; embryo transfer; genetic disorders; government regulation; *motivation; parents; physicians; preimplantation diagnosis; prenatal diagnosis; public policy; reproductive technologies; selective abortion; *sex determination; *sex preselection; social impact; Committee on Medical Ethics and Health Law (Netherlands); *Netherlands

Stein, Edward. Choosing the sexual orientation of children. *Bioethics.* 1998 Jan; 12(1): 1–24. 57 fn. BE58483.
> females; genetic determinism; genetic intervention; genetic research; *homosexuals; international aspects; justice; legal aspects; males; *moral policy; *parents; preimplantation diagnosis; prenatal diagnosis; *public policy; reproduction; reproductive technologies; rights; *selective abortion; *sex determination; *sex preselection; sexuality; social discrimination; social impact; *stigmatization; suffering; women's rights; India; United States

Ten, C.L. The use of reproductive technologies in selecting the sexual orientation, the race, and the sex of children. *Bioethics.* 1998 Jan; 12(1): 45–48. 1 fn. BE58485.
> blacks; children; females; genetic intervention; *homosexuals; males; *minority groups; motivation; parents; reproductive technologies; *sex determination; *sex preselection; sexuality; social discrimination; *stigmatization; whites

SPECIAL POPULATIONS
See under
> BEHAVIORAL RESEARCH/SPECIAL POPULATIONS
> HUMAN EXPERIMENTATION/SPECIAL POPULATIONS

STERILIZATION

See also CONTRACEPTION

Armstrong, Claire. Thousands of women sterilised in Sweden without consent. [News]. *BMJ (British Medical Journal).* 1997 Sep 6; 315(7108): 563. BE57302.
> *eugenics; *females; historical aspects; institutionalized persons; *involuntary sterilization; legal aspects; mentally disabled; public policy; social problems; standards; sterilization (sexual); *Sweden; Twentieth Century

Broberg, Gunnar; Roll–Hansen, Nils, eds. Eugenics and

the Welfare State: Sterilization Policy in Denmark, Sweden, Norway, and Finland. East Lansing, MI: Michigan State University Press; 1996. 294 p. (Uppsala studies in history of science; v. 21). Bibliography: p. 273–280. ISBN 0–87013–413–2. BE57995.
> alcohol abuse; anthropology; coercion; consensus; democracy; *eugenics; family planning; females; *genetic disorders; genetic predisposition; *genetics; *historical aspects; informed consent; institutionalized persons; international aspects; investigators; *involuntary sterilization; *legal aspects; legislation; mentally ill; mentally retarded; minority groups; minors; National Socialism; physically disabled; physicians; *public policy; research institutes; secularism; sex offenses; sexuality; social control; social discrimination; social problems; social worth; socialism; *socioeconomic factors; *sterilization (sexual); third party consent; *voluntary sterilization; *Denmark; *Finland; Germany; Nineteenth Century; *Norway; *Scandinavia; *Sweden; *Twentieth Century; World War II

Butler, Declan. Eugenics scandal reveals silence of Swedish scientists. [News]. *Nature.* 1997 Sep 4; 389(6646): 9. BE55806.
> attitudes; disadvantaged; *eugenics; females; historical aspects; investigators; *involuntary sterilization; legal aspects; mentally disabled; misconduct; physicians; *public policy; *socioeconomic factors; statistics; *sterilization (sexual); *Sweden; *Twentieth Century

Kumar, Sanjay. India to ban use of quinacrine for sterilisation. [News]. *Lancet.* 1998 Mar 28; 351(9107): 968. BE58442.
> developing countries; *drugs; *females; *government regulation; *human experimentation; international aspects; *sterilization (sexual); women's health; *India; *quinacrine

Kumar, Sanjay. Sterilisation by quinacrine comes under fire in India. [News]. *Lancet.* 1997 May 17; 349(9063): 1460. BE55823.
> *drugs; *females; government regulation; *human experimentation; informed consent; involuntary sterilization; legal aspects; misconduct; physicians; *sterilization (sexual); *India; *quinacrine

McCartney, James J. Mergers and sterilization: ethics in the board room. *HEC (HealthCare Ethics Committee) Forum.* 1997 Sep; 9(3): 284–292. 2 refs. BE56174.
> conscience; contracts; cultural pluralism; *hospitals; managed care programs; moral complicity; organization and administration; *religious hospitals; *Roman Catholic ethics; *voluntary sterilization; women's health services; community hospitals; *health facility mergers; Ethical and Religious Directives for Catholic Health Care Services

Miller, Marvin D. Terminating the "Socially Inadequate": The American Eugenicists and the German Race Hygienists, California to Cold Spring Harbor, Long Island to Germany. Commack, NY: Malamud–Rose; 1996. 289 p. Bibliography: p. 245–280. ISBN 0–9610466–1–9. BE57153.
> active euthanasia; attitudes; blacks; contraception; *eugenics; financial support; genetic research; government regulation; *historical aspects; indigents; *international aspects; *interprofessional relations; investigators; *involuntary sterilization; Jews; legislation; mentally ill; mentally retarded; misconduct; National Socialism; physically disabled; political activity; professional organizations; reproduction; Roman Catholics; social discrimination; state government; *vulnerable populations; whites; pedigree studies; California; *Germany; Great Britain; *Twentieth Century; *United States

Mudur, Ganapati. India to ban female sterilisation with malaria drug. [News]. *BMJ (British Medical Journal).*

1998 Mar 28; 316(7136): 958. BE58093.
contraception; developing countries; *drugs; *females; *government regulation; human experimentation; international aspects; private sector; risks and benefits; *sterilization (sexual); toxicity; Chile; Costa Rica; *India; Indonesia; Iran; Pakistan; *quinacrine; Vietnam; World Health Organization

Patel, Tara. Row over sterilisation divides India. [News]. *New Scientist.* 1997 Apr 5; 154(2076): 4. BE56188.
developing countries; *drugs; *females; *human experimentation; international aspects; population control; public policy; risk; risks and benefits; *sterilization (sexual); *toxicity; *India; *quinacrine

Roberts, Dorothy. Killing the Black Body: Race, Reproduction, and the Meaning of Liberty. New York, NY: Pantheon Books; 1997. 373 p. 1,073 fn. ISBN 0–679–44226–X. BE57998.
abortion, induced; adolescents; autonomy; *blacks; *coercion; *contraception; criminal law; deception; dehumanization; *drug abuse; eugenics; family relationship; *females; genetic identity; government financing; historical aspects; indigents; *involuntary sterilization; justice; legal aspects; misconduct; morality; parent child relationship; physicians; *pregnant women; *prenatal injuries; property rights; public policy; rape; *reproduction; *reproductive technologies; risks and benefits; sexuality; *social control; *social discrimination; socioeconomic factors; stigmatization; surrogate mothers; personal identity; slavery; Depo-provera; Medicaid; Nineteenth Century; Norplant; Twentieth Century; United States

Savage, Wendy. Taking liberties with women: abortion, sterilization, and contraception. *International Journal of Health Services.* 1982; 12(2): 293–308. 27 refs. BE57235.
abortion, induced; coercion; *contraception; drug industry; informed consent; international aspects; involuntary sterilization; medical devices; methods; misconduct; morbidity; physicians; risks and benefits; socioeconomic factors; *sterilization (sexual); *women's health services; *women's rights; hysterectomy; intrauterine devices; Dalkon Shield; Depo-provera; Great Britain; National Health Service

Sills, E. Scott; Strider, William; Hyde, Henry J., et al. Gynaecology, forced sterilisation, and asylum in the USA. *Lancet.* 1998 Jun 6; 351(9117): 1729–1730. 9 refs. BE58861.
counseling; females; international aspects; *involuntary sterilization; physician's role; politics; population control; public policy; *emigration and immigration; *China; United States

Tännsjö, Torbjörn. Compulsory sterilisation in Sweden. *Bioethics.* 1998 Jul; 12(3): 236–249. 1 fn. BE58892.
*autonomy; children; *coercion; *competence; congenital disorders; *disabled; *eugenics; genetic disorders; government regulation; historical aspects; informed consent; involuntary euthanasia; *involuntary sterilization; mandatory programs; mass media; mentally retarded; *moral policy; paternalism; politics; prenatal diagnosis; *public policy; quality of life; *reproduction; reproductive technologies; *rights; selective abortion; social discrimination; sterilization (sexual); suffering; third party consent; value of life; wedge argument; *Sweden; Twentieth Century
In the Fall of 1997 the leading Swedish newspaper, *Dagens Nyheter,* created a media hype over the Swedish policy of compulsory sterilisation that had been in operation between 1935 and 1975. In the discussion that followed, the moral condemnation of our medical past was unanimous. However, the reasons for rejecting what had gone on were varied and mutually inconsistent. Three strands of criticism were common: the argument from autonomy, the argument from caution, and the

argument from biological scepticism. In the paper it is argued that what point of departure you choose in your criticism of the past should be of consequence also for your ideas about present and future medical practice. In particular, if you rely on the argument from autonomy, you should be prepared to accept a liberal (present and future) use of reproductive techniques.

Japan says forced sterilizations merit no payments, no apology. [News]. *New York Times.* 1997 Sep 18: A12. BE56219.
compensation; *disabled; females; historical aspects; *involuntary sterilization; legal aspects; political activity; *public policy; *Japan; Twentieth Century

STERILIZATION/MENTALLY DISABLED

Beaupré, Mylène. Decision-making and the sterilization of incompetent children. *In:* Grubb, Andrew, ed. Decision-Making and Problems of Incompetence. New York, NY: Wiley; 1994: 89–101. 34 fn. ISBN 0–471–94236–7. BE57131.
adults; alternatives; *decision making; females; human rights; *involuntary sterilization; judicial action; *legal aspects; legal rights; *mentally retarded; *minors; parental consent; physicians; *risks and benefits; *sterilization (sexual); *third party consent; *Canada; *England; *Re B (A Minor) (Wardship: Sterilisation); *Re Eve; Wales

Bosch, Xavier. "Voluntary" sterilisation in Spain clarified in new legislation. [News]. *Lancet.* 1998 Jul 11; 352(9122): 124. BE59083.
*decision making; family members; females; *legal aspects; legislation; *mentally retarded; physicians; *sterilization (sexual); third party consent; *Spain

Canada. British Columbia. Court of Appeal. Re K and Public Trustee. *Dominion Law Reports, 4th Series.* 1985 May 16 (date of decision). 19: 255–285. BE57392.
children; decision making; females; judicial action; *legal aspects; *mentally retarded; *minors; parents; psychological stress; risks and benefits; standards; *sterilization (sexual); *hysterectomy; *British Columbia; *Re K and Public Trustee
The British Columbia Court of Appeal allowed the mother who sought a court order to permit performance of a hysterectomy on her mentally disabled daughter to appeal the dismissal of her petition by the trial court. K was ten years old with a mental age of approximately twenty-six months. Because of her phobic or adverse reactions at the sight of her own blood, her parents sought a hysterectomy before the early onset of puberty characteristic of her disease. The trial court judge focused on the rights of the mentally disabled and interpreted the case as one involving substituted consent for nontherapeutic sterilization for contraceptive purposes. The appellate court viewed the operation as purely therapeutic, with the issue being what is in the best interests of the child. On appeal the question became whether or not a hysterectomy was in K's best interests based on a weighing of benefits and risks to her well-being. (KIE abstract)

Cartwright, Will. The sterilisation of the mentally disabled: competence, the right to reproduce and discrimination. *In:* Grubb, Andrew, ed. Decision-Making and Problems of Incompetence. New York, NY: Wiley; 1994: 67–88. 32 fn. ISBN 0–471–94236–7. BE57130.
autonomy; children; *competence; comprehension; *decision making; females; informed consent; *legal aspects; *legal rights; *mentally retarded; moral obligations; parent child relationship; quality of life; *reproduction; *social

---

BE = bioethics accession number   fn. = footnotes   refs. = references

discrimination; standards; *sterilization (sexual)

Dorozynski, Alexander. France to investigate illegal sterilisation of mentally ill patients. [News]. *BMJ (British Medical Journal).* 1997 Sep 20; 315(7110): 697. BE57170.
  *females; institutionalized persons; *involuntary sterilization; legal aspects; *mentally disabled; public policy; standards; sterilization (sexual); *France

Ettershank, Kathy. Report reveals Australia's illegal sterilisations. [News]. *Lancet.* 1998 Jan 3; 351(9095): 44. BE58018.
  criminal law; *females; government financing; hospitals; human rights; judicial action; *legal aspects; legal liability; *mentally retarded; misconduct; physicians; *sterilization (sexual); third party consent; guideline adherence; *Australia

Gibeaut, John. Class debates: reproductive, disability rights mix in KKK Act cases. *ABA Journal: The Lawyer's Magazine.* 1997 Aug; 83: 36–37. BE57626.
  due process; equal protection; historical aspects; hospitals; *involuntary sterilization; *legal aspects; legal liability; *legal rights; legislation; *mentally retarded; parents; physicians; *reproduction; social discrimination; Supreme Court decisions; Buck v. Bell; California; In re Valerie N.; *Ku Klux Klan Act 1871; *Lake v. Arnold; Pennsylvania; Twentieth Century; *United States

Jones, Melinda; Marks, Lee Ann. Female and disabled: a human rights perspective on law and medicine. *In:* Petersen, Kerry, ed. Intersections: Women on Law, Medicine and Technology. Brookfield, VT: Ashgate; 1997: 49–71. 91 refs. 39 fn. ISBN 1-85521-882-8. BE57486.
  autonomy; competence; *decision making; *disabled; eugenics; *females; health care; heart diseases; *human rights; informed consent; international aspects; judicial action; *legal aspects; *mentally retarded; minors; parental consent; patient care; risks and benefits; state interest; *sterilization (sexual); surgery; *third party consent; transsexualism; treatment refusal; Australia; Great Britain

Kondro, Wayne. Alberta retreats over sterilisation compensation. [News]. *Lancet.* 1998 Mar 21; 351(9106): 892. BE58887.
  *compensation; eugenics; *involuntary sterilization; *mentally retarded; *public policy; *Alberta

Lombardo, Paul A. Medicine, eugenics, and the Supreme Court: from coercive sterilization to reproductive freedom. *Journal of Contemporary Health Law and Policy.* 1996 Fall; 13(1): 1–25. 180 fn. BE55766.
  aliens; behavioral genetics; blacks; *constitutional law; criminal law; *eugenics; federal government; *genetic determinism; *genetic predisposition; historical aspects; *human rights; *involuntary sterilization; *legal aspects; legal rights; legislation; marital relationship; *mentally retarded; *prisoners; privacy; public health; *public policy; *reproduction; social discrimination; social problems; state government; *Supreme Court decisions; whites; *Buck v. Bell; Immigration Restriction Act 1924; Loving v. Commonwealth; *Skinner v. Oklahoma; *Twentieth Century; *United States; Virginia

Petersen, Kerry. Private decisions and public scrutiny: sterilisation and minors in Australia and England. *In:* McLean, Sheila A.M., ed. Contemporary Issues in Law, Medicine and Ethics. Brookfield, VT: Dartmouth; 1996: 57–77. 74 fn. ISBN 1-85521-586-1. BE57790.
  *alternatives; autonomy; beneficence; brain pathology; comparative studies; competence; contraception; *decision making; eugenics; expert testimony; *females; historical aspects; human rights; international aspects; involuntary sterilization; judicial action; *legal aspects; *mentally

retarded; *minors; *motivation; parental consent; paternalism; patients; physicians; professional autonomy; psychology; *risks and benefits; social workers; *sterilization (sexual); hysterectomy; menstruation; tubal ligation; *Australia; *Great Britain

Zumpano–Canto, Joe. Nonconsensual sterilization of the mentally disabled in North Carolina: an ethics critique of the statutory standard and its judicial interpretation. *Journal of Contemporary Health Law and Policy.* 1996 Fall; 13(1): 79–111. 138 fn. BE55797.
  autonomy; beneficence; common good; competence; conflict of interest; economics; ethics committees; eugenics; females; home care; indigents; informed consent; institutionalized persons; *involuntary sterilization; judicial action; *legal aspects; legal liability; legislation; *mentally retarded; motivation; parental consent; parents; public policy; rape; reproduction; risks and benefits; sexuality; social discrimination; standards; state government; state interest; technical expertise; unwanted children; *North Carolina; United States

SUICIDE

See also EUTHANASIA

Ackerman, Felicia. Assisted suicide, terminal illness, severe disability, and the double standard. *In:* Battin, Margaret P.; Rhodes, Rosamond; Silvers, Anita, eds. Physician Assisted Suicide: Expanding the Debate. New York, NY: Routledge; 1998: 149–161. 35 fn. ISBN 0-415-92003-5. BE58786.
  *adults; *assisted suicide; *autonomy; coercion; competence; disabled; equal protection; family members; government regulation; motivation; pain; physicians; prisoners; privacy; psychological stress; *public policy; quality of life; *right to die; socioeconomic factors; terminally ill; dependency; dignity; duty to die

Allen, William L.; Brushwood, David B. Pharmaceutically assisted death and the pharmacist's right of conscience. *Journal of Pharmacy and Law.* 1996; 5(1): 1–18. 76 fn. BE57590.
  accountability; *assisted suicide; attitudes; *conscience; *drugs; employment; *legal aspects; legal rights; moral obligations; patient care; *pharmacists; physicians; public policy; religion; state government; professional role; California Death with Dignity Act; Death with Dignity Act (OR); Initiative 119 (WA); United States

Angell, Marcia. Helping desperately ill people to die. *In:* Emanuel, Linda L., ed. Regulating How We Die: The Ethical, Medical, and Legal Issues Surrounding Physician–Assisted Suicide. Cambridge, MA: Harvard University Press; 1998: 3–20, 263–264. 19 fn. ISBN 0-674-66654-2. BE58531.
  *active euthanasia; *allowing to die; *assisted suicide; attitudes; autonomy; competence; critically ill; decision making; family members; government regulation; legal aspects; persistent vegetative state; physician's role; *physicians; public opinion; public policy; right to die; standards; state government; suffering; terminally ill; third party consent; treatment refusal; *voluntary euthanasia; wedge argument; withholding treatment; Brophy v. New England Sinai Hospital; In re Quinlan; Lane v. Candura; Netherlands; *United States

Annas, George J. The bell tolls for a constitutional right to physician–assisted suicide. *New England Journal of Medicine.* 1997 Oct 9; 337(15): 1098–1103. 21 refs. BE55805.
  abortion, induced; active euthanasia; advisory committees; allowing to die; *assisted suicide; autonomy; competence; *constitutional law; double effect; drugs; due process; equal

---

BE = bioethics accession number   fn. = footnotes   refs. = references

protection; freedom; government regulation; informed consent; intention; *legal aspects; *legal rights; legislation; palliative care; *physicians; privacy; right to die; state government; *state interest; suffering; suicide; *Supreme Court decisions; terminally ill; treatment refusal; wedge argument; withholding treatment; Cruzan v. Director, Missouri Department of Health; Fourteenth Amendment; New York; New York State Task Force on Life and the Law; Planned Parenthood of Southeastern Pennsylvania v. Casey; *United States; *Vacco v. Quill; Washington; *Washington v. Glucksberg

Annas, George J. The bell tolls for a right to suicide. *In:* Emanuel, Linda L., ed. Regulating How We Die: The Ethical, Medical, and Legal Issues Surrounding Physician–Assisted Suicide. Cambridge, MA: Harvard University Press; 1998: 203–233, 312–316. 22 fn. ISBN 0–674–66654–2. BE58539.
  abortion, induced; *assisted suicide; *constitutional law; double effect; drugs; *due process; *equal protection; *government regulation; *judicial action; killing; *legal aspects; *legal rights; pain; physician's role; physicians; prolongation of life; *right to die; state government; state interest; suffering; suicide; *Supreme Court decisions; terminal care; terminally ill; treatment refusal; value of life; wedge argument; sedatives; *Compassion in Dying v. State of Washington; Fourteenth Amendment; *Quill v. Vacco; *United States; *Vacco v. Quill; *Washington v. Glucksberg

Arras, John D. Physician–assisted suicide: a tragic view. *In:* Battin, Margaret P.; Rhodes, Rosamond; Silvers, Anita, eds. Physician Assisted Suicide: Expanding the Debate. New York, NY: Routledge; 1998: 279–300. 88 fn. ISBN 0–415–92003–5. BE58794.
  *active euthanasia; advance directives; allowing to die; *assisted suicide; autonomy; chronically ill; compassion; competence; constitutional law; cultural pluralism; depressive disorder; disabled; equal protection; government regulation; killing; legal aspects; legal rights; legislation; moral policy; pain; *palliative care; *physicians; policy analysis; professional family relationship; *public policy; quality of health care; risks and benefits; social impact; state government; suffering; Supreme Court decisions; terminally ill; theology; third party consent; treatment refusal; trust; *voluntary euthanasia; vulnerable populations; *wedge argument; withholding treatment; Compassion in Dying v. State of Washington; Quill v. Vacco; United States

Arras, John D. Physician–assisted suicide: a tragic view. *Journal of Contemporary Health Law and Policy.* 1997 Spring; 13(2): 361–389. 94 fn. BE56000.
  advance directives; *allowing to die; *assisted suicide; autonomy; chronically ill; coercion; competence; constitutional law; cultural pluralism; decision making; depressive disorder; due process; economics; equal protection; freedom; government regulation; intention; judicial action; killing; *legal aspects; legal rights; legislation; managed care programs; *moral policy; pain; *palliative care; physically disabled; physician patient relationship; *physicians; *public policy; religion; review; *right to die; secularism; *social impact; state government; suffering; terminally ill; third party consent; *voluntary euthanasia; vulnerable populations; *wedge argument; withholding treatment; Compassion in Dying v. State of Washington; Quill v. Vacco; *United States

Barondess, Jeremiah A.; New York Academy of Medicine. The position of the New York Academy of Medicine on physician–assisted suicide. *Bulletin of the New York Academy of Medicine.* 1997 Summer; 74(1): 109–113. Letter sent to the Justices of the U.S. Supreme Court in January 1997. BE57601.
  active euthanasia; *assisted suicide; disadvantaged; *legal aspects; legal rights; *organizational policies; palliative care; *physicians; professional organizations; *public policy; suffering; terminally ill; vulnerable populations; wedge

argument; *New York Academy of Medicine; United States

Barry, Robert. The biblical teachings on suicide. *Issues in Law and Medicine.* 1997 Winter; 13(3): 283–299. 58 fn. BE58705.
  *Christian ethics; compassion; historical aspects; Jewish ethics; killing; punishment; *suicide; *theology

Battin, Margaret P. Euthanasia: the way we do it, the way they do it. [Revised]. *In:* Monagle, John F.; Thomasma, David C., eds. Health Care Ethics: Critical Issues for the 21st Century. Gaithersburg, MD: Aspen Publishers; 1998: 311–322. 15 fn. ISBN 0–8342–0911–X. BE56288.
  active euthanasia; advance directives; *allowing to die; *assisted suicide; autonomy; *international aspects; involuntary euthanasia; legal aspects; national health insurance; physician patient relationship; physicians; policy analysis; *public policy; resource allocation; risks and benefits; *socioeconomic factors; standards; suffering; *terminally ill; third party consent; treatment refusal; *voluntary euthanasia; wedge argument; withholding treatment; German Society for Humane Dying; *Germany; *Netherlands; *United States

Battin, Margaret P. Is a physician ever obligated to help a patient die? *In:* Emanuel, Linda L., ed. Regulating How We Die: The Ethical, Medical, and Legal Issues Surrounding Physician–Assisted Suicide. Cambridge, MA: Harvard University Press; 1998: 21–47, 264–267. 15 fn. ISBN 0–674–66654–2. BE58532.
  *assisted suicide; autonomy; chronically ill; conscience; decision making; double effect; institutional policies; killing; legal obligations; moral complicity; *moral obligations; *moral policy; pain; palliative care; physician patient relationship; physician's role; *physicians; principle-based ethics; public policy; religion; religious ethics; *right to die; *rights; suffering; teleological ethics; terminal care; terminally ill; values; wedge argument; withholding treatment; Netherlands; United States

Battin, Margaret P.; Rhodes, Rosamond; Silvers, Anita, eds. Physician Assisted Suicide: Expanding the Debate. New York, NY: Routledge; 1998. 463 p. (Reflective bioethics). 736 fn. Appendixes include texts of two U.S. Supreme Court decisions, *Washington v. Glucksberg* and *Vacco v. Quill;* the "Philosophers' brief," in support of the respondents in the two Supreme Court decisions, by Ronald Dworkin, Thomas Nagel, Robert Nozick, John Rawls, Thomas Scanlon, and Judith Jarvis Thomson; and the Oregon Death with Dignity Act 1996. ISBN 0–415–92003–5. BE58777.
  *active euthanasia; aged; allowing to die; artificial feeding; *assisted suicide; attitudes to death; autonomy; blacks; compassion; contraception; disabled; drugs; economics; feminist ethics; hospitals; institutional policies; intention; Jewish ethics; killing; legal aspects; *moral policy; pain; palliative care; *physicians; Protestant ethics; psychological stress; *public policy; review; right to die; Roman Catholic ethics; social impact; suffering; suicide; Supreme Court decisions; terminal care; voluntary euthanasia; vulnerable populations; wedge argument; withholding treatment; women's rights; duty to die; sedatives; Death with Dignity Act (OR); United States; Vacco v. Quill; Washington v. Glucksberg

Battin, Margaret P. Physician-assisted suicide: safe, legal, rare? *In:* Battin, Margaret P.; Rhodes, Rosamond; Silvers, Anita, eds. Physician Assisted Suicide: Expanding the Debate. New York, NY: Routledge; 1998: 63–72. 8 fn. ISBN 0–415–92003–5. BE58780.
  advance care planning; allowing to die; *assisted suicide; attitudes to death; *autonomy; decision making; drugs; pain; palliative care; *physicians; prognosis; prolongation of life;

*right to die; suffering; terminal care; *terminally ill; time factors; treatment refusal; trends

Baumrin, Bernard. Physician, stay thy hand! *In:* Battin, Margaret P.; Rhodes, Rosamond; Silvers, Anita, eds. Physician Assisted Suicide: Expanding the Debate. New York, NY: Routledge; 1998: 177–181. ISBN 0-415-92003-5. BE58788.
> *assisted suicide; beneficence; codes of ethics; historical aspects; medical ethics; *physician's role; *physicians; trust; wedge argument; Hippocratic Oath

Beauchamp, Tom L. Physician-assisted suicide: a response to Edmund Pellegrino. *In:* Wildes, Kevin Wm.; Mitchell, Alan C., eds. Choosing Life: A Dialogue on *Evangelium Vitae.* Washington, DC: Georgetown University Press; 1997: 254–258. 3 fn. ISBN 0-87840-646-8. BE56692.
> *allowing to die; *assisted suicide; autonomy; intention; *killing; moral obligations; *moral policy; physician patient relationship; physicians; Protestant ethics; risks and benefits; Roman Catholic ethics; treatment refusal; *voluntary euthanasia; withholding treatment; Evangelium Vitae

Beecham, Linda. BMA opposes legalisation of euthanasia. [News]. *BMJ (British Medical Journal).* 1997 Jul 12; 315(7100): 80. BE55808.
> *active euthanasia; *assisted suicide; legal aspects; *organizational policies; physician's role; *physicians; professional organizations; public policy; terminal care; *British Medical Association; Great Britain

Berger, Douglas; Fukunishi, Isao; O'Dowd, Mary Alice, et al. A comparison of Japanese and American psychiatrists' attitudes towards patients wishing to die in the general hospital. *Psychotherapy and Psychosomatics.* 1997; 66(6): 319–328. 27 refs. BE59010.
> *active euthanasia; *allowing to die; *assisted suicide; *attitudes; comparative studies; competence; depressive disorder; hospitals; international aspects; mental health; motivation; *physicians; *psychiatry; quality of life; referral and consultation; right to die; suicide; survey; terminally ill; treatment refusal; truth disclosure; values; *voluntary euthanasia; rationality; *Japan; *United States

Berger, Douglas; Takahashi, Yoshitomo; Fukunishi, Isao, et al. Japanese psychiatrists' attitudes toward patients wishing to die in the general hospital: a cultural perspective. *Cambridge Quarterly of Healthcare Ethics.* 1997 Fall; 6(4): 470–479. 44 fn. BE56456.
> active euthanasia; *allowing to die; *assisted suicide; *attitudes; competence; *depressive disorder; *euthanasia; family members; family relationship; hospitals; patients; persistent vegetative state; *physicians; prolongation of life; *psychiatric diagnosis; *psychiatry; *quality of life; resuscitation orders; *right to die; suffering; *suicide; survey; terminally ill; third party consent; treatment refusal; voluntary euthanasia; withholding treatment; rationality; *Japan

Bernardin, Joseph. Euthanasia: ethical and legal challenge. *In:* Langan, John P., ed. Joseph Cardinal Bernardin: A Moral Vision for America. Washington, DC: Georgetown University Press; 1998: 59–69, 170. 1 fn. Reference embedded in list at back of book. Address at the Center for Clinical Medical Ethics, University of Chicago Hospital, 26 May 1988. ISBN 0-87840-675-1. BE58523.
> *active euthanasia; aged; allowing to die; artificial feeding; *assisted suicide; autonomy; biomedical technologies; common good; cultural pluralism; economics; hospices; indigents; legal aspects; *moral policy; obligations of society; privacy; prolongation of life; *public policy; resource allocation; Roman Catholic ethics; state interest; terminally ill; *value of life; *United States

Bernardin, Joseph. Euthanasia in the Catholic tradition. *In:* Langan, John P., ed. Joseph Cardinal Bernardin: A Moral Vision for America. Washington, DC: Georgetown University Press; 1998: 119–128. Visiting scholar lecture at Rockhurst College, Kansas City, MO, 1 Feb 1995. ISBN 0-87840-675-1. BE58525.
> *active euthanasia; *assisted suicide; attitudes; autonomy; biomedical technologies; international aspects; judicial action; legal aspects; legislation; *moral policy; physicians; *public policy; quality of life; *Roman Catholic ethics; state government; terminal care; *value of life; Europe; Kevorkian, Jack; Netherlands; *United States

Betzold, Michael. The selling of Doctor Death: how Jack Kevorkian became a national hero. *New Republic.* 1997 May 26; 216(21): 22–28. BE57545.
> accountability; active euthanasia; *assisted suicide; chronically ill; deception; depressive disorder; disabled; family relationship; informed consent; lawyers; legal aspects; *mass media; physician's role; *physicians; public opinion; quality of life; *right to die; suffering; terminally ill; *journalism; Fieger, Geoffrey; *Kevorkian, Jack; Michigan; United States

Bickenbach, Jerome E. Disability and life-ending decisions. *In:* Battin, Margaret P.; Rhodes, Rosamond; Silvers, Anita, eds. Physician Assisted Suicide: Expanding the Debate. New York, NY: Routledge; 1998: 123–132. 22 fn. ISBN 0-415-92003-5. BE58784.
> *assisted suicide; *autonomy; *coercion; *disabled; health care; legal aspects; paternalism; patient advocacy; *physically disabled; physicians; public policy; quality of life; resource allocation; right to die; *social discrimination; social worth; stigmatization; *suicide; third party consent; *value of life; Canada; United States

Biskupic, Joan. Oregon's assisted-suicide law lives on. [News]. *Washington Post.* 1997 Oct 15: A3. BE58233.
> *assisted suicide; depressive disorder; equal protection; *government regulation; *legal aspects; legal rights; legislation; right to die; state government; Supreme Court decisions; terminally ill; Lee v. Harcleroad; *Oregon

Blanck, Peter; Kirschner, Kristi; Bienen, Leigh. Socially-assisted dying and people with disabilities: some emerging legal, medical, and policy implications. *Mental and Physical Disability Law Reporter.* 1997 Jul–Aug; 21(4): 538–543. 26 refs. BE58354.
> active euthanasia; allowing to die; *assisted suicide; attitudes; autonomy; *disabled; government regulation; health care; *legal aspects; legal rights; palliative care; physicians; public policy; quality of life; right to die; social discrimination; state government; Supreme Court decisions; terminal care; terminology; Compassion in Dying v. State of Washington; Quill v. Vacco; *United States

Bopp, James; Coleson, Richard E. Roe v. Wade and the euthanasia debate. *Issues in Law and Medicine.* 1997 Spring; 12(4): 343–354. 38 fn. BE57802.
> abortion on demand; *abortion, induced; *assisted suicide; constitutional law; *due process; freedom; *government regulation; *legal aspects; legal rights; pregnant women; privacy; *right to die; state government; state interest; Supreme Court decisions; terminally ill; *wedge argument; Fourteenth Amendment; *Planned Parenthood of Southeastern Pennsylvania v. Casey; *Roe v. Wade; *United States

Bopp, James; Coleson, Richard E. The constitutional case against permitting physician-assisted suicide for competent adults with "terminal conditions". *Issues in Law and Medicine.* 1995 Winter; 11(3): 239–268. 130 fn. BE58819.
> aged; *assisted suicide; coercion; conscience; *constitutional

---

law; criminal law; depressive disorder; diagnosis; disabled; *due process; *equal protection; freedom; government regulation; indigents; *legal aspects; *legal rights; minority groups; motivation; pain; physician's role; physicians; privacy; psychiatric diagnosis; referral and consultation; state government; state interest; suffering; *terminally ill; treatment refusal; vulnerable populations; *Ballot Measure 16 (OR); Fourteenth Amendment; Oregon; *United States

Bostrom, Barry A. Lee v. Oregon. [Note]. *Issues in Law and Medicine.* 1997 Winter; 13(3): 333–338. BE58710.
*assisted suicide; constitutional law; equal protection; *legal aspects; legal rights; legislation; nursing homes; physicians; terminally ill; *Ballot Measure 16 (OR); *Death with Dignity Act (OR); First Amendment; Fourteenth Amendment; *Lee v. State of Oregon; *Oregon

Bostrom, Barry A. McIver v. Krischer. [Note]. *Issues in Law and Medicine.* 1997 Spring; 12(4): 385–389. BE57804.
*assisted suicide; constitutional law; equal protection; *legal aspects; legal liability; *legal rights; *physicians; privacy; *right to die; state government; *terminally ill; *Florida; *McIver v. Krischer

Bradley, Peter; Przygoda, Pablo; Saimovici, Javier, et al. Physician assisted suicide, euthanasia, and withdrawal of treatment. [Letters]. *BMJ (British Medical Journal).* 1998 Jan 3; 316(7124): 71–72. 9 refs. BE57955.
*active euthanasia; *allowing to die; *assisted suicide; attitudes; double effect; intention; moral policy; *physicians; survey; terminal care; terminology; wedge argument; withholding treatment; Argentina; Great Britain

Brody, Howard. Commentary on Billings and Block's "Slow euthanasia." *Journal of Palliative Care.* 1996 Winter; 12(4): 38–41. 11 refs. Commentary on J.A. Billings and S.D. Block, p. 21–30. BE55709.
*active euthanasia; allowing to die; *assisted suicide; decision making; double effect; drugs; *government regulation; intention; justice; killing; *legal aspects; *palliative care; physicians; resource allocation; suffering; *terminal care; *terminally ill; wedge argument; withholding treatment; morphine; Compassion in Dying v. State of Washington; Netherlands; United States

Brody, Howard; Vandekieft, Gregg K. Physician–assisted suicide: a very personal issue. [Editorial]. *American Family Physician.* 1997 May 15; 55(7): 2421–2427. 6 refs. BE57956.
*assisted suicide; *communication; disabled; hospices; palliative care; physician patient relationship; physicians; *terminal care; terminally ill

Bruder, Paul. Right to die -- duty to die: the growing debate over scarce resources. *Hospital Topics.* 1994 Winter; 72(1): 6–8. 6 refs. 1 fn. BE56402.
allowing to die; *assisted suicide; futility; moral obligations; pain; *right to die; rights; suffering; value of life; duty to die

Bursztajn, Harold; Gutheil, Thomas G.; Warren, Mark J., et al. Depression, self-love, time, and the "right" to suicide. *General Hospital Psychiatry.* 1986 Mar; 8(2): 91–95. 17 refs. BE57426.
allowing to die; autonomy; *competence; *depressive disorder; disabled; force feeding; hospitals; legal aspects; professional patient relationship; psychiatry; *right to die; *suicide; terminally ill; *time factors; treatment refusal; *Bouvia, Elizabeth

Burt, Robert A. The Supreme Court speaks -- not assisted suicide but a constitutional right to palliative care. *New England Journal of Medicine.* 1997 Oct 23; 337(17): 1234–1236. 23 fn. BE55803.

*assisted suicide; *constitutional law; double effect; *drugs; *government regulation; intention; *legal aspects; *legal rights; legislation; pain; *palliative care; *physicians; right to die; social impact; *state government; suffering; *Supreme Court decisions; *terminal care; *terminally ill; Institute of Medicine; New York; *United States; *Vacco v. Quill; Washington; *Washington v. Glucksberg

Bushong, Stephen K.; Balmer, Thomas A. Breathing life into the right to die: Oregon's Death with Dignity Act. *Issues in Law and Medicine.* 1995 Winter; 11(3): 269–282. 102 fn. BE58880.
*assisted suicide; *constitutional law; criminal law; due process; equal protection; freedom; *legal aspects; physicians; public policy; *right to die; state government; state interest; *terminally ill; vulnerable populations; *Death with Dignity Act (OR); Fourteenth Amendment; Oregon; United States

Callahan, Sydney. A feminist case against euthanasia. *Health Progress.* 1996 Nov-Dec; 77(6): 21–27, 29. 11 fn. BE56323.
aged; *assisted suicide; autonomy; coercion; communication; decision making; family relationship; females; *feminist ethics; informed consent; involuntary euthanasia; killing; palliative care; physicians; quality of life; *right to die; self concept; social discrimination; social impact; social interaction; suffering; suicide; third party consent; *value of life; *voluntary euthanasia; vulnerable populations; *wedge argument; women's rights; dependency; United States

Capron, Alexander Morgan. Death and the Court. *Hastings Center Report.* 1997 Sep-Oct; 27(5): 25–29. 12 fn. BE56118.
abortion, induced; allowing to die; *assisted suicide; autonomy; constitutional law; criminal law; *due process; *equal protection; freedom; government regulation; intention; killing; *legal aspects; *legal rights; pain; palliative care; physicians; privacy; quality of life; *right to die; state government; *state interest; *Supreme Court decisions; terminal care; terminally ill; treatment refusal; value of life; vulnerable populations; withholding treatment; Cruzan v. Director, Missouri Department of Health; Planned Parenthood of Southeastern Pennsylvania v. Casey; Roe v. Wade; *United States; *Vacco v. Quill; *Washington v. Glucksberg

Carlin, David R. Sing to me of the judge, muse, a man of twists and turns. *America.* 1997 May 3; 176(15): 9–13. BE55645.
ancient history; *assisted suicide; *attitudes; constitutional law; *historical aspects; *judicial action; legal rights; literature; motivation; philosophy; suicide; theology; stoicism; *Compassion in Dying v. State of Washington; Greece; Homer; Judas; *Reinhardt, Stephen; Socrates; Sophocles; St. Augustine; United States

Childress, James F. Religious viewpoints. *In:* Emanuel, Linda L., ed. Regulating How We Die: The Ethical, Medical, and Legal Issues Surrounding Physician–Assisted Suicide. Cambridge, MA: Harvard University Press; 1998: 120–147, 294–300. 54 fn. ISBN 0–674–66654–2. BE58536.
*active euthanasia; allowing to die; *assisted suicide; autonomy; covenant; dissent; double effect; extraordinary treatment; gifts; *Jewish ethics; killing; palliative care; *Protestant ethics; public policy; quality of life; *religious ethics; *Roman Catholic ethics; suffering; suicide; theology; value of life; voluntary euthanasia; wedge argument; withholding treatment; Evangelium Vitae; United States

Chochinov, Harvey Max; Wilson, Keith G.; Breitbart, William, et al. Assisted suicide for HIV patients. [Letter and response]. *American Journal of Psychiatry.*

BE = bioethics accession number   fn. = footnotes   refs. = references

1997 Feb; 154(2): 294–295. 2 refs. BE55813.
AIDS; *assisted suicide; *attitudes; depressive disorder; *HIV seropositivity; pain; palliative care; *patients; psychological stress; stigmatization; terminally ill; ambulatory care; undertreatment

Chochinov, Harvey Max; Wilson, Keith G. The euthanasia debate: attitudes, practices and psychiatric considerations. *Canadian Journal of Psychiatry.* 1995 Dec; 40(10): 593–602. 69 refs. BE56325.
*assisted suicide; *attitudes; cancer; competence; criminal law; depressive disorder; empirical research; family relationship; international aspects; *knowledge, attitudes, practice; legal aspects; mental health; mentally ill; palliative care; patients; *physician's role; *physicians; psychiatric diagnosis; *psychiatry; *public opinion; public policy; referral and consultation; suicide; terminal care; terminally ill; *voluntary euthanasia; wedge argument; Canada; Netherlands; United States

Churchill, Larry R.; King, Nancy M.P. Physician assisted suicide, euthanasia, or withdrawal of treatment. [Editorial]. *BMJ (British Medical Journal).* 1997 Jul 19; 315(7101): 137–138. 16 refs. BE58500.
*active euthanasia; *assisted suicide; government regulation; international aspects; *legal aspects; physicians; public policy; right to die; state government; Supreme Court decisions; treatment refusal; wedge argument; withholding treatment; Death with Dignity Act (OR); Great Britain; Netherlands; Northern Territory; Rights of the Terminally Ill Act (NT); *United States; Vacco v. Quill; Washington v. Glucksberg

Churchill, Larry R.; Callahan, Daniel; Linehan, Elizabeth A., et al. To die or not to die. [Letters and response]. *Hastings Center Report.* 1997 Nov–Dec; 27(6): 4–7. BE57852.
aged; allowing to die; *assisted suicide; decision making; economics; family members; *family relationship; *moral obligations; patient care; physicians; prolongation of life; public policy; religious ethics; *suicide; terminal care; terminally ill; treatment refusal; value of life; wedge argument; *duty to die

Claiborne, William. In Oregon, suicide option brings a kinder care. [News]. *Washington Post.* 1998 Apr 29: A1, A12. BE57844.
*assisted suicide; attitudes; decision making; drugs; hospices; hospitals; legal aspects; physicians; *social impact; state government; *terminal care; terminally ill; morphine; Death with Dignity Act (OR); *Oregon

Coatney, Caryn. Outback's assisted-suicide law: Australia delivers world's first dose of legal euthanasia. [News]. *Christian Science Monitor.* 1997 Jan 8: 1, 18. BE55736.
*active euthanasia; adults; *assisted suicide; attitudes; cultural pluralism; international aspects; *legislation; minority groups; physicians; public opinion; terminally ill; *voluntary euthanasia; *Australia; *Northern Territory

Coleson, Richard E. Krischer v. McIver. [Note]. *Issues in Law and Medicine.* 1997 Winter; 13(3): 329–332. BE58709.
allowing to die; *assisted suicide; constitutional law; equal protection; government regulation; *legal aspects; *legal rights; *physicians; *privacy; *right to die; state government; state interest; terminally ill; treatment refusal; *Florida; *Krischer v. McIver

Coleson, Richard E. The Glucksberg and Quill amicus curiae briefs: verbatim arguments opposing assisted suicide. *Issues in Law and Medicine.* 1997 Summer; 13(1): 3–102. 63 fn. BE56750.
active euthanasia; aged; allowing to die; *assisted suicide;

autonomy; Christian ethics; coercion; competence; conscience; *constitutional law; depressive disorder; disabled; due process; economics; equal protection; freedom; *government regulation; guidelines; hospices; informed consent; Jewish ethics; killing; *legal aspects; *legal rights; National Socialism; physicians; *right to die; state government; state interest; terminally ill; treatment refusal; value of life; wedge argument; withholding treatment; Fourteenth Amendment; Germany; Netherlands; New York; *United States; *Vacco v. Quill; Washington; *Washington v. Glucksberg

Coleson, Richard E. Vacco v. Quill. [Note]. *Issues in Law and Medicine.* 1997 Winter; 13(3): 323–328. 2 fn. BE58708.
allowing to die; *assisted suicide; *constitutional law; drugs; *equal protection; freedom; government regulation; *legal aspects; legal rights; physicians; *right to die; state government; state interest; Supreme Court decisions; terminally ill; treatment refusal; withholding treatment; Fourteenth Amendment; *New York; *United States; *Vacco v. Quill

Coleson, Richard E. Washington v. Glucksberg. [Note]. *Issues in Law and Medicine.* 1997 Winter; 13(3): 315–321. 4 fn. BE58707.
active euthanasia; *assisted suicide; *constitutional law; *due process; freedom; government regulation; *legal aspects; legal rights; physicians; quality of life; *right to die; state government; *state interest; suicide; Supreme Court decisions; terminally ill; treatment refusal; wedge argument; Fourteenth Amendment; *United States; *Washington; *Washington v. Glucksberg

Davis, Dena S. Why suicide is like contraception: a woman-centered view. *In:* Battin, Margaret P.; Rhodes, Rosamond; Silvers, Anita, eds. Physician Assisted Suicide: Expanding the Debate. New York, NY: Routledge; 1998: 113–122. 30 fn. ISBN 0-415-92003-5. BE58783.
aged; *assisted suicide; autonomy; common good; contraception; dementia; females; *feminist ethics; morality; physicians; public policy; reproduction; right to die; suffering; *suicide; terminally ill; voluntary sterilization; *women's rights; dependency; rationality

de Boer, Anthonius; Lau, Hong Sang; Porsius, Arijan. Physician-assisted death and pharmacy practice in the Netherlands. [Letter]. *New England Journal of Medicine.* 1997 Oct 9; 337(15): 1091–1092. 5 refs. BE57169.
*active euthanasia; *assisted suicide; *attitudes; *drugs; guidelines; hospitals; *knowledge, attitudes, practice; legal aspects; *pharmacists; physicians; practice guidelines; professional organizations; statistics; survey; *Netherlands; Royal Dutch Pharmaceutical Association

Devine, Philip E. Homicide, criminal versus justifiable. *In:* Chadwick, Ruth, ed. Encyclopedia of Applied Ethics, Volume 2. San Diego, CA: Academic Press; 1998: 587–595. 14 refs. ISBN 0-12-227067-3. BE56396.
*abortion, induced; *active euthanasia; assisted suicide; Christian ethics; criminal law; double effect; intention; involuntary euthanasia; *killing; moral policy; personhood; philosophy; public policy; secularism; speciesism; *suicide; theology; utilitarianism; voluntary euthanasia; wedge argument

Dixon, Kathleen Marie. The quality of mercy: reflections on provider-assisted suicide. *Journal of Clinical Ethics.* 1997 Fall; 8(3): 290–302. 47 fn. BE57561.
*assisted suicide; attitudes to death; communication; *compassion; counseling; disabled; empathy; *health personnel; love; moral obligations; *palliative care; patient care; physicians; professional patient relationship; quality of health care; referral and consultation; self concept;

BE = bioethics accession number   fn. = footnotes   refs. = references

*suffering; *terminal care; terminally ill; Levinas, Emmanuel

Docker, Christopher. The way forward? *In:* McLean, Sheila A.M., ed. Death, Dying and the Law. Brookfield, VT: Dartmouth; 1996: 129–160. 99 fn. ISBN 1-85521-657-4. BE57217.
*active euthanasia; *advance directives; aged; *allowing to die; *assisted suicide; decision making; double effect; economics; hospices; legal aspects; living wills; pain; *palliative care; *persistent vegetative state; physicians; public policy; *resource allocation; selection for treatment; terminal care; withholding treatment; *Great Britain; National Health Service; Netherlands; United States

Domino, George; Kempton, Susan; Cavender, Jim. Physician assisted suicide: a scale and some empirical findings. *Omega: A Journal of Death and Dying.* 1996–1997; 34(3): 247–257. 15 refs. BE56487.
aged; *assisted suicide; *attitudes; comparative studies; competence; *evaluation; family members; legal aspects; morality; *physicians; public policy; right to die; students; survey; terminally ill; universities; *voluntary euthanasia; *questionnaires; United States

Donovan, G. Kevin. Decisions at the end of life: Catholic tradition. *Christian Bioethics.* 1997 Dec; 3(3): 188–203. 22 refs. 4 fn. BE58488.
*active euthanasia; *allowing to die; artificial feeding; *assisted suicide; *attitudes to death; *brain death; cardiac death; costs and benefits; decision making; *determination of death; drugs; family members; informed consent; intention; organ donation; *pain; *palliative care; persistent vegetative state; prolongation of life; resuscitation; risks and benefits; *Roman Catholic ethics; *suffering; suicide; terminal care; *terminally ill; theology; third party consent; treatment outcome; treatment refusal; value of life; *withholding treatment; Congregation for the Doctrine of the Faith; National Conference of Catholic Bishops; United States

Medical decisions regarding end–of–life care have undergone significant changes in recent decades, driven by changes in both medicine and society. Catholic tradition in medical ethics offers clear guidance in many issues, and a moral framework accessible to those who do not share the same faith as well as to members of its faith community. In some areas, a Catholic perspective can be seen clearly and confidently, such as in teachings on the permissibility of suicide and euthanasia. In others, such as withdrawal of nutrition and hydration, the Church does not yet speak with one voice and has not closed out the discussion. Yet, it is not in the teaching on individual issues that a Catholic moral tradition offers the most help and comfort, but in its account of what it means to lead a life in Christ, and to prepare for a Christian death. As in the problem of pain and suffering, it is the spiritual support more than the ethical guidance that helps both patients and physicians bear the unbearable and fathom the unfathomable.

Dworkin, Ronald; Nagel, Thomas; Nozick, Robert, et al. Assisted suicide: the philosophers' brief. *New York Review of Books.* 1997 Mar 27: 41–47. 15 fn. BE57272.
allowing to die; *assisted suicide; autonomy; competence; *constitutional law; decision making; due process; equal protection; *freedom; *government regulation; *legal aspects; *legal rights; pain; palliative care; physicians; *right to die; state government; state interest; suffering; *terminally ill; treatment refusal; wedge argument; withholding treatment; New York; *United States; *Vacco v. Quill; Washington; *Washington v. Glucksberg

Egan, Timothy. Assisted suicide comes full circle, to Oregon. [News]. *New York Times.* 1997 Oct 26: 1, 25.

BE57842.
*assisted suicide; *legal aspects; physicians; political activity; Roman Catholics; state government; terminally ill; Death with Dignity Act (OR); *Oregon

Egan, Timothy. No one rushing in Oregon to use a new suicide law: doctors and pharmacists ponder their role. [News]. *New York Times.* 1998 Mar 15: 18. BE57729.
*assisted suicide; attitudes; drugs; government financing; indigents; legal aspects; nurses; pharmacists; physicians; public policy; state government; terminally ill; Death with Dignity Act (OR); Medicaid; *Oregon

Egan, Timothy. Right to die: in Oregon, opening a new front in the world of medicine. [News]. *New York Times.* 1997 Nov 6: A26. BE55944.
*assisted suicide; *attitudes; competence; drugs; *legal aspects; legal rights; organizational policies; palliative care; *physicians; political activity; professional organizations; public opinion; right to die; state government; terminally ill; American Medical Association; *Death with Dignity Act (OR); *Oregon; Right to Life Movement; United States

Egan, Timothy. Threat from Washington has chilling effect on Oregon law allowing assisted suicide. [News]. *New York Times.* 1997 Nov 19: A18. BE55945.
*assisted suicide; competence; *drugs; federal government; government regulation; *legal aspects; *legal liability; legislation; *physicians; state government; terminally ill; *Controlled Substances Act; *Death with Dignity Act (OR); Drug Enforcement Administration; Oregon; United States

Emanuel, Ezekiel. Whose right to die? *Atlantic Monthly.* 1997 Mar; 279(3): 73–79. BE57684.
accountability; allowing to die; *assisted suicide; attitudes; biomedical technologies; coercion; decision making; depressive disorder; economics; guidelines; historical aspects; international aspects; involuntary euthanasia; legal aspects; motivation; newborns; pain; physicians; psychological stress; public opinion; *public policy; *right to die; suffering; *voluntary euthanasia; vulnerable populations; wedge argument; dependency; dignity; duty to die; guideline adherence; Hippocratic Oath; *Netherlands; Nineteenth Century; Remmelink Commission; Twentieth Century; *United States

Emanuel, Ezekiel J.; Daniels, Elisabeth R.; Fairclough, Diane L., et al. The practice of euthanasia and physician–assisted suicide in the United States: adherence to proposed safeguards and effects on physicians. *JAMA.* 1998 Aug 12; 280(6): 507–513. 34 refs. BE58766.
*active euthanasia; *assisted suicide; *attitudes; *cancer; competence; decision making; drugs; empirical research; evaluation studies; family members; guidelines; hospices; involuntary euthanasia; *knowledge, attitudes, practice; medical specialties; motivation; pain; palliative care; physician patient relationship; *physicians; psychological stress; public policy; referral and consultation; religion; suffering; survey; terminal care; *terminally ill; *voluntary euthanasia; *guideline adherence; *oncology; *United States

CONTEXT: Despite intense debates about legalization, there are few data examining the details of actual euthanasia and physician–assisted suicide (PAS) cases in the United States. OBJECTIVE: To determine whether the practices of euthanasia and PAS are consistent with proposed safeguards and the effect on physicians of having performed euthanasia or PAS. DESIGN: Structured in–depth telephone interviews. SETTING AND PARTICIPANTS: Randomly selected oncologists in the United States. OUTCOME MEASURES: Adherence to primary and secondary safeguards for the practice of euthanasia and PAS; regret, comfort, and fear of prosecution from performing euthanasia or PAS. RESULTS: A total of 355 oncologists (72.6% response

---

BE = bioethics accession number   fn. = footnotes   refs. = references

rate) were interviewed on euthanasia and PAS. On 2 screening questions, 56 oncologists (15.8%) reported participating in euthanasia or PAS; 53 oncologists (94.6% response rate) participated in in-depth interviews. Thirty-eight of 53 oncologists described clearly defined cases of euthanasia or PAS. Twenty-three patients (60.5%) both initiated and repeated their request for euthanasia or PAS, but 6 patients (15.8%) did not participate in the decision for euthanasia or PAS. Thirty-seven patients (97.4%) were experiencing unremitting pain or such poor physical functioning they could not perform self-care. Physicians sought consultation in 15 cases (39.5%). Overall, oncologists adhered to all 3 main safeguards in 13 cases (34.2%): (1) having the patient initiate and repeat the request for euthanasia or PAS, (2) ensuring the patient was experiencing extreme physical pain or suffering, and (3) consulting with a colleague. Those who adhered to the safeguards had known their patients longer and tended to be more religious. In 28 cases (73.7%), the family supported the decision. In all cases of pain, patients were receiving narcotic analgesia. Fifteen patients (39.5%) were enrolled in a hospice. While 19 oncologists (52.6%) received comfort from having helped a patient with euthanasia or PAS, 9 (23.7%) regretted having performed euthanasia or PAS, and 15 (39.5%) feared prosecution. CONCLUSIONS: Intractable pain or poor physical functioning seem to be nearly absolute requirements for physicians to perform euthanasia or PAS. Only one third of cases are performed consistently with proposed safeguards. For some patients, end-of-life care that includes opioid analgesia and hospice care does not obviate their desire for euthanasia or PAS. While the majority of physicians seem comforted by their actions, some experience adverse consequences from having performed euthanasia or PAS.

Emanuel, Ezekiel J.; Battin, Margaret P. What are the potential cost savings from legalizing physician-assisted suicide? *New England Journal of Medicine.* 1998 Jul 16; 339(3): 167-172. 45 refs. BE58612.
    *assisted suicide; cancer; costs and benefits; *economics; *evaluation; government financing; health care; home care; hospices; hospitals; legal aspects; managed care programs; nursing homes; physicians; *public policy; *social impact; statistics; *terminal care; time factors; personal financing; Medicare; Netherlands; *United States

Emanuel, Ezekiel J. Why now? *In:* Emanuel, Linda L., ed. Regulating How We Die: The Ethical, Medical, and Legal Issues Surrounding Physician-Assisted Suicide. Cambridge, MA: Harvard University Press; 1998: 175-202, 307-312. 48 fn. ISBN 0-674-66654-2. BE58538.
    *active euthanasia; allowing to die; ancient history; *assisted suicide; attitudes; autonomy; economics; eugenics; *historical aspects; killing; legal aspects; moral obligations; pain; philosophy; physician patient relationship; *physicians; *public policy; social dominance; social worth; terminal care; terminally ill; values; voluntary euthanasia; wedge argument; Canada; Eighteenth Century; Europe; Nineteenth Century; Seventeenth Century; Sixteenth Century; Twentieth Century; United States

Emanuel, Linda. Physician-assisted suicide: a different approach. *Bioethics Forum.* 1997 Summer; 13(2): 13-16. BE58279.
    *advance care planning; alternatives; *assisted suicide; attitudes to death; communication; competence; depressive disorder; family members; legal aspects; *motivation; patients; physicians; right to die

Emanuel, Linda L. A question of balance. *In:* Emanuel, Linda L., ed. Regulating How We Die: The Ethical, Medical, and Legal Issues Surrounding Physician-Assisted Suicide. Cambridge, MA: Harvard University Press; 1998: 234-260. ISBN 0-674-66654-2. BE58540.
    *active euthanasia; *advance care planning; allowing to die; *assisted suicide; autonomy; compassion; cultural pluralism; decision making; health care delivery; intention; killing; legal rights; medical education; moral obligations; motivation; palliative care; physician's role; physicians; privacy; public policy; religious ethics; suffering; *terminal care; values; wedge argument; withholding treatment; dignity; Netherlands; United States

Emanuel, Linda L. Facing requests for physician-assisted suicide. *JAMA.* 1998 Aug 19; 280(7): 643-647. 50 refs. BE59000.
    advance care planning; artificial feeding; *assisted suicide; autonomy; communication; competence; depressive disorder; family members; food; freedom; goals; guidelines; hospices; legal rights; moral obligations; *palliative care; patients; *physicians; *practice guidelines; referral and consultation; suffering; *terminal care; treatment refusal; withholding treatment; sedatives
Requests for physician-assisted suicide are not a new phenomenon, and many physicians are likely to face this challenging situation. This article proposes for professionals an 8-step approach to respond to requests for physician-assisted suicide. The approach seeks to identify and treat the root causes of the request and aims to present a plan for consistent application of a set of clinical skills. Justification for the steps requires only 2 noncontentious principles: the patient should be free of unwanted intervention, and the physician is obligated to provide suffering patients with comfort care. Care based on these 2 principles alone does not include physician-assisted suicide. The approach does, however, justify patient refusal of oral intake in specific circumstances. The approach could resolve a majority of requests for physician-assisted suicide and should be tested further for clinical efficacy.

Emanuel, Linda L., ed. Regulating How We Die: The Ethical, Medical, and Legal Issues Surrounding Physician-Assisted Suicide. Cambridge, MA: Harvard University Press; 1998. 325 p. 401 fn. ISBN 0-674-66654-2. BE58530.
    *active euthanasia; adolescents; advance care planning; allowing to die; *assisted suicide; beneficence; capital punishment; children; critically ill; government regulation; historical aspects; Jewish ethics; *killing; legal aspects; legal rights; moral obligations; moral policy; physician's role; *physicians; Protestant ethics; public policy; religious ethics; right to die; Roman Catholic ethics; state government; *suffering; suicide; *terminally ill; Netherlands; United States

Faber-Langendoen, Kathy. Death by request: assisted suicide and the oncologist. [Editorial]. *Cancer.* 1998 Jan 1; 82(1): 35-41. 46 refs. BE58356.
    advance directives; *assisted suicide; attitudes; autonomy; *cancer; compassion; competence; economics; government regulation; international aspects; legal aspects; moral policy; organizational policies; pain; palliative care; physician patient relationship; *physicians; professional organizations; public opinion; public policy; state government; suffering; voluntary euthanasia; oncology; United States

Fairbairn, Gavin. Suicide. *In:* Chadwick, Ruth, ed. Encyclopedia of Applied Ethics, Volume 4. San Diego, CA: Academic Press; 1998: 259-273. 7 refs. ISBN 0-12-227069-X. BE56347.
    assisted suicide; autonomy; intention; killing; *moral policy;

BE = bioethics accession number   fn. = footnotes   refs. = references

morality; motivation; paternalism; philosophy; right to die; rights; social impact; *suicide; theology; voluntary euthanasia

Fenigsen, Richard. Dutch euthanasia revisited. *Issues in Law and Medicine.* 1997 Winter; 13(3): 301–311. 68 fn. BE58706.

*active euthanasia; adults; age factors; allowing to die; *assisted suicide; cancer; comparative studies; drugs; empirical research; guidelines; infants; *involuntary euthanasia; knowledge, attitudes, practice; legal liability; mandatory reporting; mentally ill; mortality; motivation; newborns; *physicians; referral and consultation; statistics; *trends; *voluntary euthanasia; wedge argument; withholding treatment; *guideline adherence; *Netherlands

FitzGibbon, Scott; Lai, Kwan Kew. The model physician–assisted suicide act and the jurisprudence of death. *Issues in Law and Medicine.* 1997 Fall; 13(2): 173–216. 194 fn. BE57807.

*assisted suicide; autonomy; coercion; conscience; decision making; economics; family members; government regulation; health facilities; hospices; insurance; involuntary euthanasia; *legal aspects; legal obligations; medical ethics; *model legislation; *moral policy; morality; motivation; nursing ethics; physician patient relationship; physicians; social impact; state government; suffering; terminally ill; utilitarianism; voluntary euthanasia; Netherlands; *United States

Fournier, Keith A.; Watkins, William D. In Defense of Life. Colorado Springs, CO: NavPress; 1996. 159 p. 352 fn. ISBN 08910–98801. BE56728.

aborted fetuses; *abortion, induced; *active euthanasia; aged; *allowing to die; *assisted suicide; beginning of life; body parts and fluids; brain death; *Christian ethics; commodification; congenital disorders; death; determination of death; disabled; economics; eugenics; fetal tissue donation; fetuses; government regulation; health personnel; historical aspects; human experimentation; infanticide; international aspects; judicial action; *killing; legal aspects; love; *morality; *newborns; organ donation; *political activity; population control; pregnant women; psychological stress; public policy; quality of life; rights; *value of life; *values; violence; hope; Humphry, Derek; Kevorkian, Jack; *Right to Life Movement; Roe v. Wade; Smith, Susan; United States

Francis, Leslie Pickering. Assisted suicide: are the elderly a special case? *In:* Battin, Margaret P.; Rhodes, Rosamond; Silvers, Anita, eds. Physician Assisted Suicide: Expanding the Debate. New York, NY: Routledge; 1998: 75–90. 36 fn. ISBN 0–415–92003–5. BE58781.

age factors; *aged; alternatives; *assisted suicide; autonomy; coercion; competence; decision making; depressive disorder; justice; palliative care; physically disabled; *physicians; public policy; resource allocation; suicide; terminally ill; values; vulnerable populations; cognition disorders; dependency; rationality

Fuller, Jon. Physician–assisted suicide: an unnecessary crisis. *America.* 1997 Jul 19; 177(2): 9–12. BE58564.

*assisted suicide; common good; conflict of interest; managed care programs; minority groups; physician patient relationship; *physicians; quality of health care; social impact; terminal care; trust; United States

Garrow, David J. The Oregon trail. *New York Times.* 1997 Nov 6: A31. BE55946.

*assisted suicide; competence; drugs; *legal aspects; *physicians; political activity; privacy; public opinion; *right to die; state government; terminally ill; *Death with Dignity Act (OR); Oregon; United States

Geis, Sally B.; Messer, Donald E., eds. How Shall We

Die?: Helping Christians Debate Assisted Suicide. Nashville, TN: Abingdon Press; 1997. 201 p. Annotated bibliography: p. 183–189. Appendices include generic forms for advance directives and for organ/tissue donation. ISBN 0–687–06140–7. BE57384.

*active euthanasia; advance directives; *allowing to die; *assisted suicide; attitudes to death; autonomy; beneficence; case studies; *Christian ethics; clergy; *decision making; diagnosis; drugs; ethics consultation; family members; forms; freedom; informed consent; killing; legal aspects; love; pain; palliative care; pastoral care; patients; physicians; prognosis; Protestant ethics; quality of life; resource allocation; right to die; Roman Catholic ethics; suffering; *suicide; terminally ill; *theology; treatment refusal; truth disclosure; value of life; voluntary euthanasia; wedge argument; withholding treatment; Compassion in Dying v. State of Washington; Death with Dignity Act (OR); New York; Quill v. Vacco; United States; Washington

Gert, Bernard; Culver, Charles M.; Clouser, K. Danner. An alternative to physician–assisted suicide: a conceptual and moral analysis. *In:* Battin, Margaret P.; Rhodes, Rosamond; Silvers, Anita, eds. Physician Assisted Suicide: Expanding the Debate. New York, NY: Routledge; 1998: 182–202. 25 fn. ISBN 0–415–92003–5. BE58789.

*active euthanasia; *allowing to die; alternatives; artificial feeding; *assisted suicide; competence; double effect; drugs; food; freedom; government regulation; informed consent; intention; *killing; legal aspects; model legislation; *moral obligations; *moral policy; pain; *palliative care; *physicians; policy analysis; prolongation of life; public policy; right to die; state government; suffering; suicide; Supreme Court decisions; terminal care; terminally ill; time factors; treatment refusal; *voluntary euthanasia; withholding treatment; analgesia; dehydration; rationality; United States; Vacco v. Quill; Washington v. Glucksberg

Gostin, Lawrence O. Deciding life and death in the courtroom: from Quinlan to Cruzan, Glucksberg, and Vacco -- a brief history and analysis of constitutional protection of the 'right to die'. *JAMA.* 1997 Nov 12; 278(18): 1523–1528. 60 refs. BE57164.

advance directives; *allowing to die; artificial feeding; *assisted suicide; autonomy; coercion; competence; *constitutional law; criminal law; decision making; double effect; drugs; due process; economics; equal protection; freedom; *historical aspects; intention; judicial action; killing; *legal aspects; legal liability; legal rights; legislation; *palliative care; patients; physician patient relationship; physician's role; *physicians; public opinion; review; *right to die; risks and benefits; social worth; state government; *state interest; *Supreme Court decisions; *terminally ill; third party consent; treatment refusal; value of life; values; vulnerable populations; wedge argument; withholding treatment; *Cruzan v. Director, Missouri Department of Health; Fourteenth Amendment; *In re Quinlan; New Jersey; New York; Patient Self–Determination Act 1990; *Twentieth Century; *United States; *Vacco v. Quill; Washington; *Washington v. Glucksberg

This article analyzes judicial determinations on the "right to die" from Quinlan to Cruzan, Glucksberg, and Vacco. The body of law known as right-to-die cases extends ordinary treatment refusal doctrine to end-of-life decisions. The courts, having affirmed a right to refuse life-sustaining treatment, held that certain categorical distinctions that had been drawn lacked a rational basis. No rational distinction could be made between competent vs incompetent patients, withholding vs withdrawing treatment, and ordinary vs extraordinary treatment. The courts, however, had persistently affirmed one categorical distinction: between withdrawing life-sustaining treatment on the one hand and active euthanasia or physician–assisted dying on the other. In Washington v Glucksberg and Vacco v Quill,

---

BE = bioethics accession number   fn. = footnotes   refs. = references

the Supreme Court unanimously held that physician–assisted suicide is not a fundamental liberty interest protected by the Constitution. Notably, five members of the Court wrote or joined in concurring opinions that took a more liberal view. The Court powerfully approved aggressive palliation of pain. The Supreme Court, hinting that it would find state legalization of physician–assisted suicide constitutional, invited the nation to pursue an earnest debate on physician assistance in the dying process.

Greenberg, Samuel I. Euthanasia and Assisted Suicide: Psychosocial Issues. Springfield, IL: Charles C. Thomas; 1997. 164 p. (American series in behavioral science and law). 113 refs. ISBN 0–398–06785–6. BE58317.
*active euthanasia; adults; advance directives; aged; allowing to die; *assisted suicide; attitudes; case studies; decision making; economics; ethicists; hospices; international aspects; judicial action; lawyers; legal rights; managed care programs; minors; newborns; nursing homes; organizational policies; pain; palliative care; physician patient relationship; physician's role; physicians; professional organizations; public policy; resuscitation orders; right to die; spina bifida; suffering; Supreme Court decisions; terminal care; treatment refusal; wedge argument; Germany; Great Britain; Kevorkian, Jack; Netherlands; *United States

Greenhouse, Linda. Assisted suicide clears a hurdle in highest court. [News]. *New York Times.* 1997 Oct 15: A1, A16. BE57843.
*assisted suicide; *legal aspects; legal rights; state government; Supreme Court decisions; terminally ill; *Death with Dignity Act (OR); *Lee v. Harcleroad; *Oregon

Gregory, Wilton. The Church and the public discussion of assisted suicide. *Health Progress.* 1997 Mar–Apr; 78(2): 48–50. BE56445.
active euthanasia; *assisted suicide; attitudes to death; double effect; drugs; extraordinary treatment; pain; physicians; public policy; *Roman Catholic ethics; suffering; *terminal care; theology; treatment refusal; United States

Hassan, Riaz. Euthanasia and the medical profession: an Australian study. *Australian Journal of Social Issues.* 1996 Aug; 31(3): 239–252. 12 refs. BE58274.
*active euthanasia; *allowing to die; *assisted suicide; *attitudes; family members; *knowledge, attitudes, practice; legal aspects; motivation; patients; *physicians; survey; *voluntary euthanasia; *Australia; Netherlands; *South Australia

Haverkate, Ilinka; van der Wal, Gerrit. Policies on assisted suicide in Dutch psychiatric facilities. *Psychiatric Services.* 1998 Jan; 49(1): 98–100. 10 refs. BE58209.
*assisted suicide; *hospitals; *institutional policies; *mental institutions; *mentally ill; survey; *hospital psychiatric units; *Netherlands

Heilig, Steve; Brody, Robert V. Physician–hastened death and end–of–life care: development of a community–wide consensus statement and guidelines. *Cambridge Quarterly of Healthcare Ethics.* 1998 Spring; 7(2): 223–225. 7 refs. BE57558.
*assisted suicide; *clinical ethics committees; committee membership; consensus; guidelines; physicians; *practice guidelines; program descriptions; public participation; regional ethics committees; *terminal care; *Bay Area Network of Ethics Committees; San Francisco

Hendin, Herbert. Assisted suicide and euthanasia. *In: his* Suicide in America. New and Expanded Edition. New York, NY: W.W. Norton; 1995: 236–277, 294–297. 43 fn. ISBN 0–393–31368–9. BE56135.
*active euthanasia; aged; *assisted suicide; attitudes to death; autonomy; behavior control; chronically ill; coercion; competence; depressive disorder; freedom; guidelines; involuntary euthanasia; legal aspects; motivation; paternalism; physicians; psychiatric diagnosis; psychotherapy; public policy; right to die; statistics; suffering; suicide; terminally ill; voluntary euthanasia; vulnerable populations; wedge argument; Chabot, Boudewijn; Netherlands; United States

Hendin, Herbert. Involuntary commitment. *In: his* Suicide in America. New and Expanded Edition. New York, NY: W.W. Norton; 1995: 214–235, 291–294. 45 fn. ISBN 0–393–31368–9. BE56134.
dangerousness; deinstitutionalized persons; depressive disorder; due process; institutionalized persons; *involuntary commitment; legal aspects; legal rights; legislation; mental institutions; *mentally ill; model legislation; patient care; patient discharge; *psychiatric diagnosis; social impact; standards; state government; *suicide; treatment outcome; Lanterman–Petris–Short Act; Mental Health Law Project; United States

Hendin, Herbert; Goold, Susan Dorr; Meier, Diane E., et al. Physician–assisted suicide and euthanasia in the United States. [Letters and response]. *New England Journal of Medicine.* 1998 Sep 10; 339(11): 775–776. 8 refs. BE59075.
*active euthanasia; *assisted suicide; drugs; females; government regulation; guidelines; *knowledge, attitudes, practice; legal aspects; males; *physicians; state government; voluntary euthanasia; guideline adherence; *Oregon; United States

Hendin, Herbert; Ganzini, Linda. Physician–assisted suicide: the Dutch case. [Letter and response]. *JAMA.* 1997 Nov 12; 278(18): 1492–1493. 6 refs. BE58822.
active euthanasia; *assisted suicide; competence; *decision making; double effect; drugs; guidelines; *physicians; psychiatry; *psychological stress; psychotherapy; referral and consultation; terminal care; guideline adherence; Netherlands; Oregon

Hentoff, Nat. Disabled, not dead. *Responsive Community.* 1996 Fall; 6(4): 4–6. BE55871.
*assisted suicide; *attitudes; chronically ill; *disabled; drugs; physicians; *political activity; quality of life; social discrimination; social worth; vulnerable populations; United States

Humphry, Derek. Final Exit: The Practicalities of Self–Deliverance and Assisted Suicide for the Dying. Second Edition. New York, NY: Dell Trade Paperback; 1996. 206 p. 25 refs. ISBN 0–440–50785–5. BE58643.
advance directives; allowing to die; *assisted suicide; autonomy; autopsies; dementia; depressive disorder; *drugs; family members; food; hospices; international aspects; legal liability; life insurance; *methods; model legislation; pain; physically disabled; physicians; privacy; quality of life; *right to die; suffering; *suicide; terminal care; terminally ill; terminology; toxicity; treatment refusal; *voluntary euthanasia; support groups; United States

Josefson, Deborah. U.S. sees first legal case of physician assisted suicide. [News]. *BMJ (British Medical Journal).* 1998 Apr 4; 316(7137): 1037. BE58107.
aged; *assisted suicide; breast cancer; *drugs; health personnel; *legal aspects; organizational policies; *physicians; professional organizations; terminally ill; *Death with Dignity Act (OR); *Oregon; United States

Kamisar, Yale. The reasons so many people support physician–assisted suicide –– and why these reasons are not convincing. *Issues in Law and Medicine.* 1996 Fall;

BE = bioethics accession number   fn. = footnotes   refs. = references

12(2): 113–131. 78 fn. BE58759.

allowing to die; artificial feeding; *assisted suicide; *attitudes; autonomy; coercion; due process; emotions; equal protection; government regulation; guidelines; *legal aspects; mass media; moral policy; physicians; policy analysis; *public policy; quality of life; religion; *right to die; risks and benefits; *social impact; suffering; terminally ill; treatment refusal; value of life; voluntary euthanasia; wedge argument; withholding treatment; guideline adherence; United States

Kamm, Frances M. Physician–assisted suicide, euthanasia, and intending death. *In:* Battin, Margaret P.; Rhodes, Rosamond; Silvers, Anita, eds. Physician Assisted Suicide: Expanding the Debate. New York, NY: Routledge; 1998: 28–62. 53 fn. ISBN 0–415–92003–5. BE58779.

accountability; *active euthanasia; *allowing to die; *assisted suicide; beneficence; *death; deontological ethics; *double effect; *drugs; *ethical analysis; *euthanasia; *intention; involuntary euthanasia; *killing; *moral obligations; *moral policy; morality; *pain; *palliative care; paralysis; personhood; *physicians; psychological stress; quality of life; right to die; suffering; suicide; terminal care; terminally ill; terminology; treatment refusal; value of life; *voluntary euthanasia; withholding treatment

Kass, Leon R.; Lund, Nelson. Courting death: assisted suicide, doctors, and the law. *Commentary.* 1996 Dec; 102(6): 17–29. 2 fn. BE57531.

abortion, induced; active euthanasia; allowing to die; *assisted suicide; attitudes; autonomy; codes of ethics; coercion; constitutional law; *dehumanization; double effect; drugs; economics; family members; government regulation; guidelines; intention; killing; *legal aspects; legal rights; medical ethics; medicine; *morality; palliative care; physician patient relationship; *physicians; policy analysis; privacy; professional organizations; *public policy; quality of health care; right to die; self regulation; social impact; state government; state interest; suffering; Supreme Court decisions; terminal care; treatment refusal; trust; value of life; vulnerable populations; *wedge argument; Hippocratic Oath; Netherlands; *United States

Kaveny, M. Cathleen. Assisted suicide, the Supreme Court, and the constitutive function of the law. *Hastings Center Report.* 1997 Sep–Oct; 27(5): 29–34. 19 fn. BE56119.

*assisted suicide; autonomy; common good; constitutional law; drugs; due process; empirical research; *equal protection; freedom; government regulation; involuntary euthanasia; judicial action; killing; law; *legal aspects; *legal rights; morality; pain; palliative care; philosophy; physicians; quality of life; *right to die; state government; state interest; suffering; *Supreme Court decisions; terminal care; terminally ill; value of life; voluntary euthanasia; vulnerable populations; wedge argument; dignity; guideline adherence; *United States; *Vacco v. Quill; *Washington v. Glucksberg

Kelly, Brian J.; Varghese, Francis T. Assisted suicide and euthanasia: what about the clinical issues? *Australian and New Zealand Journal of Psychiatry.* 1996 Feb; 30(1): 3–8. 34 refs. BE56870.

*active euthanasia; AIDS; *assisted suicide; autonomy; depressive disorder; medical education; mentally ill; palliative care; physician patient relationship; psychiatric diagnosis; psychiatry; quality of life; suffering; suicide; *terminal care; terminally ill; grief

Kelly, David F. Alternatives to physician–assisted suicide. *American Journal of Otolaryngology.* 1995 May–Jun; 16(3): 181–185. BE56211.

active euthanasia; *allowing to die; *assisted suicide; drugs; economics; killing; legal aspects; morality; pain; *palliative care; public policy; Roman Catholic ethics; *terminal care; terminally ill; treatment refusal; voluntary euthanasia; wedge

argument; withholding treatment; analgesia; United States

Kennedy, Randy. Doctor is arraigned in assisted suicide: veterinarian is said to admit role in terminally ill friend's death. [News]. *New York Times.* 1998 Oct 15: B3. BE58937.

*assisted suicide; criminal law; drugs; hospitals; law enforcement; *legal liability; terminally ill; Beigel, Cara; New York City; Zancope, Marco

King, Patricia A.; Wolf, Leslie E. Lessons for physician–assisted suicide from the African–American experience. *In:* Battin, Margaret P.; Rhodes, Rosamond; Silvers, Anita, eds. Physician Assisted Suicide: Expanding the Debate. New York, NY: Routledge; 1998: 91–112. 80 fn. A version of this paper, "Empowering and protecting patients: lessons for physician assisted suicide from the African–American experience," was published in the *Minnesota Law Review* 82(1998): 1015–1043. ISBN 0–415–92003–5. BE58782.

*assisted suicide; *attitudes; autonomy; autopsies; *blacks; coercion; *communication; cultural pluralism; eugenics; health; *health care delivery; historical aspects; human experimentation; medical education; medicine; morbidity; mortality; paternalism; physician patient relationship; *physicians; public policy; quality of health care; research subjects; scientific misconduct; selection for treatment; self concept; *social discrimination; social dominance; social worth; socioeconomic factors; *stigmatization; trust; voluntary euthanasia; vulnerable populations; whites; empowerment; Nineteenth Century; Tuskegee Syphilis Study; Twentieth Century; United States

Kinsella, T. Douglas; Verhoef, Marja J. Assisted suicide: opinions of Alberta physicians. *Clinical and Investigative Medicine.* 1995 Oct; 18(5): 406–412. 13 refs. BE55511.

age factors; *assisted suicide; *attitudes; criminal law; *legal aspects; *physicians; public policy; religion; statistics; survey; uncertainty; *voluntary euthanasia; *Alberta; Canada

Kleinman, Arthur. Intimations of solidarity? The popular culture responds to assisted suicide. *Hastings Center Report.* 1997 Sep–Oct; 27(5): 34–36. BE56120.

*assisted suicide; attitudes; depressive disorder; economics; health care delivery; international aspects; legal aspects; managed care programs; mass media; morality; palliative care; physicians; *public opinion; public policy; right to die; suffering; terminal care; trends; uncertainty; France; *United States

Kondro, Wayne. Canadian AIDS doctor convicted of physician–assisted suicide. [News]. *Lancet.* 1998 Jan 10; 351(9096): 121. BE57912.

*assisted suicide; drugs; HIV seropositivity; *legal liability; misconduct; *physicians; *Genereux, Maurice; Ontario

Kopala, Beverly; Kennedy, Susan Lorraine. Requests for assisted suicide: a nursing issue. *Nursing Ethics.* 1998 Jan; 5(1): 16–26. 31 refs. BE58713.

*assisted suicide; autonomy; beneficence; decision making; government regulation; legal aspects; mass media; motivation; nurse's role; *nurses; nursing ethics; organizational policies; professional organizations; risks and benefits; state government; terminally ill; American Nurses Association; Oregon Nurses Association; United States

Koval, Joseph C.; Rousseau, Paul; Coulehan, Jack. The man with stars inside. [Letter and response]. *Annals of Internal Medicine.* 1997 Dec 15; 127(12): 1137–1138. 6 refs. BE58214.

*assisted suicide; communication; empathy; medical education; pain; *palliative care; physician patient relationship; physicians; psychological stress; suffering; *terminal care; *terminally ill; patient abandonment

Kowalski, Edgar P.; Kowalski, Susan D.; Kirkland, Larry R., et al. Disability and physician–assisted suicide. [Letters and response]. *New England Journal of Medicine.* 1997 Dec 18; 337(25): 1852–1853. 9 refs. BE58304.
*assisted suicide; autonomy; economics; *legal rights; National Socialism; paternalism; patients' rights; *physically disabled; *physicians; *right to die; social discrimination; terminally ill; wedge argument; United States

Kowalski, Susan D. Assisted suicide: is there a future? Ethical and nursing considerations. *Critical Care Nursing Quarterly.* 1996 May; 19(1): 45–54. 10 refs. BE55723.
*active euthanasia; *allowing to die; artificial feeding; *assisted suicide; autonomy; case studies; chronically ill; common good; competence; double effect; economics; guidelines; *nurses; organizational policies; pain; palliative care; persistent vegetative state; physicians; professional organizations; professional patient relationship; quality of life; *right to die; suffering; terminal care; terminally ill; terminology; third party consent; treatment refusal; ventilators; *voluntary euthanasia; wedge argument; withholding treatment; American Nurses Association; Netherlands; United States

Kuhse, Helga. From intention to consent: learning from experience with euthanasia. *In:* Battin, Margaret P.; Rhodes, Rosamond; Silvers, Anita, eds. Physician Assisted Suicide: Expanding the Debate. New York, NY: Routledge; 1998: 252–266. 38 fn. ISBN 0–415–92003–5. BE58792.
*allowing to die; *assisted suicide; autonomy; comparative studies; *double effect; drugs; empirical research; informed consent; *intention; international aspects; involuntary euthanasia; killing; *knowledge, attitudes, practice; legal aspects; *moral policy; *palliative care; *physicians; policy analysis; *public policy; statistics; terminal care; *terminally ill; treatment refusal; *voluntary euthanasia; wedge argument; *withholding treatment; sedatives; *Australia; *Euthanasia Laws Act 1996 (Australia); *Netherlands; New York State Task Force on Life and the Law; United States

Lamberts, Robert J.; MacKie, Palmer; Loehrer, Patrick J. Physician–assisted suicide and euthanasia: a house staff debate. *Indiana Medicine.* 1995 May–Jun; 88(3): 192–195. BE56212.
*assisted suicide; attitudes; autonomy; futility; paternalism; physician's role; *physicians; public policy; social dominance; suffering; terminally ill; voluntary euthanasia; wedge argument; United States

Larson, Edward J.; Amundsen, Darrel W. A Different Death: Euthanasia and the Christian Tradition. Downers Grove, IL: InterVarsity Press; 1998. 288 p. 587 fn. ISBN 0–8308–1518–X. BE58946.
*active euthanasia; advance directives; allowing to die; ancient history; artificial feeding; *assisted suicide; attitudes to death; biomedical technologies; caring; *Christian ethics; due process; equal protection; freedom; *historical aspects; hospices; involuntary euthanasia; Jewish ethics; killing; legal aspects; palliative care; physicians; privacy; public opinion; public policy; *right to die; selection for treatment; state interest; suffering; *suicide; terminally ill; *theology; third party consent; treatment refusal; value of life; voluntary euthanasia; war; wedge argument; withholding treatment; Eighteenth Century; Europe; Middle Ages; Netherlands; Nineteenth Century; Seventeenth Century; Sixteenth Century; Twentieth Century; United States

Legemaate, Johan; Gevers, J.K.M. Physician–assisted suicide in psychiatry: developments in the Netherlands. *Cambridge Quarterly of Healthcare Ethics.* 1997 Spring;

6(2): 175–188. 45 fn. BE56430.
*active euthanasia; advisory committees; *assisted suicide; behavior disorders; competence; criminal law; depressive disorder; expert testimony; guidelines; judicial action; *legal aspects; legal liability; *mentally ill; *physicians; professional organizations; *psychiatry; *psychological stress; public policy; right to die; self regulation; *suffering; treatment refusal; *voluntary euthanasia; wedge argument; anorexia nervosa; Chabot, Boudewijn; *Netherlands
In this paper we give an overview of the legal developments in this area [physician–assisted suicide in psychiatry]. First, we will briefly outline the general legal situation in the Netherlands regarding euthanasia and assisted suicide. Second, we will analyze the case law on physician–assisted suicide in psychiatry. Third, we would like to give an impression of the debate outside the courtroom on physician–assisted suicide in psychiatry. That debate started even before publication of the first court ruling on this issue (by the Central Medical Disciplinary Board in 1990) and has not only continued but intensified as a result of subsequent decisions of criminal courts over the last four years. We sketch a general picture of the positions taken by different actors, mainly by referring to reports and statements of the most important organizations and advisory committees.

Lessenberry, Jack; Betzold, Michael. Grim reaper. [Letter and response]. *New Republic.* 1997 Jun 30; 216(26): 4. BE57546.
*assisted suicide; *mass media; *physicians; *journalism; *Kevorkian, Jack

Lester, David. Social characteristics of states which do not prohibit assisted–suicide. [Abstract]. *Perceptual and Motor Skills.* 1997 Oct; 85(2): 654. 2 refs. BE58419.
age factors; *assisted suicide; *government regulation; *socioeconomic factors; *state government; statistics; *United States

Lindsay, Ronald A. Assisted suicide: will the Supreme Court respect the autonomy rights of dying patients? *Free Inquiry.* 1996–1997 Winter; 17(1): 4–5. BE55788.
*assisted suicide; autonomy; constitutional law; equal protection; government regulation; *legal aspects; *legal rights; physicians; secularism; state government; state interest; Supreme Court decisions; terminally ill; withholding treatment; Fourteenth Amendment; *United States; Vacco v. Quill; Washington v. Glucksberg

Loewy, Erich H. Harming, healing, and euthanasia. *In:* Emanuel, Linda L., ed. Regulating How We Die: The Ethical, Medical, and Legal Issues Surrounding Physician–Assisted Suicide. Cambridge, MA: Harvard University Press; 1998: 48–67, 267–269. 18 fn. ISBN 0–674–66654–2. BE58533.
*active euthanasia; allowing to die; assisted suicide; autonomy; *capital punishment; health personnel; *killing; moral obligations; *moral policy; morality; National Socialism; physician patient relationship; *physician's role; physicians; prolongation of life; public policy; risks and benefits; *suffering; *suicide; terminal care; terminally ill; value of life; voluntary euthanasia; wedge argument; withholding treatment; Netherlands; United States

Long, Ann; Long, Aishlinn; Smyth, Angus. Suicide: a statement of suffering. *Nursing Ethics.* 1998 Jan; 5(1): 3–15. 58 refs. BE58712.
attitudes; autonomy; beneficence; caring; communication; competence; empathy; moral obligations; *nurse patient relationship; *nurse's role; *nurses; nursing ethics; paternalism; *patient care; professional family relationship; stigmatization; *suffering; *suicide; value of life

---

BE = bioethics accession number   fn. = footnotes   refs. = references

Lynn, Joanne; Cohn, Felicia; Pickering, John H., et al.; American Geriatrics Society. American Geriatrics Society on physician–assisted suicide: brief to the United States Supreme Court. *Journal of the American Geriatrics Society.* 1997 Apr; 45(4): 489–499. 70 fn. Background and brief of the American Geriatrics Society as amicus curiae urging reversal of the judgments below: Vacco v. Quill, No. 95–1858, and Washington v. Glucksberg, No. 96–110. BE57117.

> *aged; allowing to die; *assisted suicide; chronically ill; coercion; competence; constitutional law; economics; government regulation; killing; *legal aspects; legal rights; moral complicity; obligations of society; *organizational policies; *palliative care; *physicians; *professional organizations; prognosis; *public policy; *quality of health care; resource allocation; social impact; suffering; Supreme Court decisions; *terminal care; terminally ill; treatment refusal; uncertainty; withholding treatment; *geriatrics; *American Geriatrics Society; *United States; *Vacco v. Quill; *Washington v. Glucksberg

McGann, John R. To care for the dying. *Origins.* 1997 Mar 20; 26(39): 640–648. 99 fn. Text of a pastoral letter, "Comfort my people: finding peace as life ends," by Bishop John R. McGann of Rockville Centre, NY, 19 Feb 1997. BE56596.

> active euthanasia; *allowing to die; *assisted suicide; attitudes to death; biomedical technologies; clergy; coercion; compassion; depressive disorder; double effect; drugs; economics; emotions; family members; government regulation; health care; health personnel; hospices; intention; love; pain; *palliative care; pastoral care; patients; physician patient relationship; physician's role; physicians; prolongation of life; psychological stress; *Roman Catholic ethics; social interaction; suffering; *terminal care; terminally ill; trust; vulnerable populations; withholding treatment; dignity; United States

McGee, Ellen M. Can suicide intervention in hospice be ethical? *Journal of Palliative Care.* 1997 Spring; 13(1): 27–33. 50 refs. BE55728.

> assisted suicide; autonomy; beneficence; counseling; depressive disorder; goals; *hospices; *institutional policies; pain; palliative care; paternalism; physicians; psychological stress; suffering; *suicide; *terminal care; *terminally ill; *values; rationality

McLean, Sheila A.M., ed. Death, Dying and the Law. Brookfield, VT: Dartmouth; 1996. 185 p. (Medico–legal series). 531 fn. ISBN 1–85521–657–4. BE57209.

> *active euthanasia; *advance directives; *allowing to die; *assisted suicide; competence; decision making; disabled; futility; international aspects; legal aspects; palliative care; persistent vegetative state; *physicians; prognosis; public policy; resource allocation; suffering; *terminal care; treatment refusal; *voluntary euthanasia; withholding treatment; Airedale NHS Trust v. Bland; Death with Dignity Act (OR); *Great Britain; Netherlands; United States

Mann, Patricia S. Meanings of death. *In:* Battin, Margaret P.; Rhodes, Rosamond; Silvers, Anita, eds. Physician Assisted Suicide: Expanding the Debate. New York, NY: Routledge; 1998: 11–27. 26 fn. ISBN 0–415–92003–5. BE58778.

> aged; *assisted suicide; attitudes; *attitudes to death; autonomy; biomedical technologies; coercion; costs and benefits; cultural pluralism; *death; decision making; disadvantaged; family members; family relationship; freedom; legal aspects; managed care programs; medical ethics; metaphor; moral obligations; philosophy; physician patient relationship; physicians; prolongation of life; *public policy; *social impact; social interaction; socioeconomic factors; suicide; terminally ill; theology; uncertainty; values; dependency; duty to die; United States

Marquis, Don. The weakness of the case for legalising physician–assisted suicide. *In:* Battin, Margaret P.; Rhodes, Rosamond; Silvers, Anita, eds. Physician Assisted Suicide: Expanding the Debate. New York, NY: Routledge; 1998: 267–278. 22 fn. ISBN 0–415–92003–5. BE58793.

> advance directives; allowing to die; *assisted suicide; *autonomy; chronically ill; *compassion; disabled; drugs; moral obligations; *moral policy; motivation; pain; *physicians; psychological stress; *public policy; right to die; self concept; social worth; suffering; terminally ill; third party consent; treatment refusal; utilitarianism; wedge argument; *duty to die; United States

Matthews, Merrill. Would physician–assisted suicide save the healthcare system money? (Or, is Jack Kevorkian doing all of us a favor?). *In:* Battin, Margaret P.; Rhodes, Rosamond; Silvers, Anita, eds. Physician Assisted Suicide: Expanding the Debate. New York, NY: Routledge; 1998: 312–322. 24 fn. ISBN 0–415–92003–5. BE58796.

> age factors; *assisted suicide; *economics; government financing; guidelines; health care delivery; managed care programs; *physicians; public policy; resource allocation; *social impact; statistics; *terminal care; time factors; Medicaid; Medicare; Netherlands; *United States

Meier, Diane E.; Emmons, Carol–Ann; Wallenstein, Sylvan, et al. A national survey of physician–assisted suicide and euthanasia in the United States. *New England Journal of Medicine.* 1998 Apr 23; 338(17): 1193–1201. 23 refs. BE57820.

> *active euthanasia; *assisted suicide; *attitudes; family members; *knowledge, attitudes, practice; legal aspects; medical specialties; motivation; patients; *physicians; prognosis; survey; terminally ill; *voluntary euthanasia; *United States

BACKGROUND: Although there have been many studies of physician–assisted suicide and euthanasia in the United States, national data are lacking. METHODS: In 1996, we mailed questionnaires to a stratified probability sample of 3102 physicians in the 10 specialties in which doctors are most likely to receive requests from patients for assistance with suicide or euthanasia. We weighted the results to obtain nationally representative data. RESULTS: We received 1902 completed questionnaires (response rate, 61 percent). Eleven percent of the physicians said that under current legal constraints, there were circumstances in which they would be willing to hasten a patient's death by prescribing medication, and 7 percent said that they would provide a lethal injection; 36 percent and 24 percent, respectively, said that they would do so if it were legal. Since entering practice, 18.3 percent of the physicians (unweighted number, 320) reported having received a request from a patient for assistance with suicide and 11.1 percent (unweighted number, 196) had received a request for a lethal injection. Sixteen percent of the physicians receiving such requests (unweighted number, 42), or 3.3 percent of the entire sample, reported that they had written at least one prescription to be used to hasten death, and 4.7 percent (unweighted number, 59), said that they had administered at least one lethal injection. CONCLUSIONS: A substantial proportion of physicians in the United States report that they receive requests for physician–assisted suicide and euthanasia, and about 7 percent of those who responded to our survey have complied with such requests at least once.

Michigan. Commission on Death and Dying. Final Report of the Michigan Commission on Death and Dying. Lansing, MI: The Commission; 1994 Jun. 1 v.

BE = bioethics accession number   fn. = footnotes   refs. = references

37 refs. BE56729.

accountability; advance directives; advisory committees; *assisted suicide; autonomy; competence; consensus; criminal law; disabled; dissent; due process; government regulation; guidelines; hospices; insurance; involuntary euthanasia; killing; *legal aspects; legal liability; legal rights; mental health; model legislation; organizational policies; palliative care; physician's role; professional organizations; public participation; *public policy; quality of life; records; referral and consultation; right to die; social impact; state government; suffering; treatment refusal; wedge argument; Death with Dignity Act (MI); *Michigan; *Michigan Commission on Death and Dying; Netherlands

Miles, Steven H. The Oregon Death with Dignity Act: A Guidebook for Health Care Providers, edited by Kathleen Haley and Melinda Lee. [Book review essay]. *JAMA.* 1998 Jul 22–29; 280(4): 387–388. BE58445.

active euthanasia; advisory committees; *assisted suicide; government regulation; guidelines; *legal aspects; *physicians; state government; suffering; terminally ill; *Death with Dignity Act (OR); *Oregon; Task Force to Improve the Care of Terminally-Ill Oregonians

Miller, Franklin G.; Meier, Diane E. Voluntary death: a comparison of terminal dehydration and physician–assisted suicide. *Annals of Internal Medicine.* 1998 Apr 1; 128(7): 559–562. 29 refs. BE57327.

*alternatives; *artificial feeding; *assisted suicide; attitudes; autonomy; comparative studies; competence; decision making; family members; *food; legal aspects; palliative care; physicians; psychological stress; public policy; *terminal care; terminally ill; time factors; treatment refusal; *withholding treatment; *dehydration; integrity

Moreno, Jonathan D., ed. Arguing Euthanasia: The Controversy Over Mercy Killing, Assisted Suicide, and the "Right to Die." New York, NY: Simon and Schuster; 1995. 251 p. ISBN 0–684–80760–2. BE55810.

*active euthanasia; allowing to die; *assisted suicide; attitudes; autonomy; cultural pluralism; economics; family members; involuntary euthanasia; killing; legal aspects; moral policy; morality; pain; palliative care; physician's role; physicians; public opinion; public policy; religion; resource allocation; right to die; secularism; suffering; terminally ill; value of life; voluntary euthanasia; wedge argument; Death with Dignity Act (OR); Netherlands; United States

Morris, David C. Older adults' perceptions of Dr. Kevorkian in Middletown, U.S.A. *Omega: A Journal of Death and Dying.* 1997; 35(4): 405–412. 12 refs. BE57721.

*aged; *assisted suicide; *attitudes; criminal law; education; *legal liability; *physicians; politics; *public opinion; quality of life; religion; right to die; suffering; *suicide; survey; terminally ill; Indiana; *Kevorkian, Jack

Morrow, Elizabeth. Attitudes of women from vulnerable populations toward physician–assisted death: a qualitative approach. *Journal of Clinical Ethics.* 1997 Fall; 8(3): 279–289. 22 fn. BE57610.

aged; allowing to die; *assisted suicide; *attitudes; *autonomy; coercion; comparative studies; conflict of interest; *decision making; *disadvantaged; domestic violence; economics; family members; family relationship; *females; Hispanic Americans; indigents; physician patient relationship; physicians; public opinion; *public policy; referral and consultation; religion; social discrimination; social dominance; students; survey; terminally ill; third party consent; *trust; universities; *voluntary euthanasia; *vulnerable populations; empowerment; homeless persons; qualitative research; California; United States

Muller, M.T.; Onwuteaka–Philipsen, B.D.; Kriegsman, D.M.W., et al. Voluntary active euthanasia and doctor–assisted suicide: knowledge and attitudes of

Dutch medical students. *Medical Education.* 1996 Nov; 30(6): 428–433. 9 refs. BE57056.

*assisted suicide; *attitudes; females; guidelines; *knowledge, attitudes, practice; males; *medical education; *physicians; religion; *students; survey; *voluntary euthanasia; *Netherlands

Muller, Martien T.; van der Wal, Gerrit; van Eijk, Jacques Th.M., et al. Active euthanasia and physician–assisted suicide in Dutch nursing homes: patients' characteristics. *Age and Ageing.* 1995 Sep; 24(5): 429–433. 6 refs. BE56606.

age factors; *aged; *assisted suicide; cancer; central nervous system diseases; comparative studies; diagnosis; females; males; *nursing homes; *patients; *physicians; religion; socioeconomic factors; statistics; survey; time factors; *voluntary euthanasia; *Netherlands

Murphy, Patricia. Nursing's role in the assisted suicide debate. [Editorial]. *American Journal of Nursing.* 1997 Jun; 97(6): 80. BE55572.

*assisted suicide; *nurse's role; nurses; organizational policies; palliative care; professional organizations; public policy; American Nurses Association; United States

Muskin, Philip R. The request to die: role for a psychodynamic perspective on physician–assisted suicide. *JAMA.* 1998 Jan 28; 279(4): 323–328. 56 refs. BE57812.

*assisted suicide; autonomy; *communication; counseling; depressive disorder; *emotions; *motivation; pain; palliative care; *patients; physician patient relationship; *physician's role; physicians; psychiatric diagnosis; psychiatry; *psychological stress; referral and consultation; self concept; statistics; suffering; suicide; terminally ill; truth disclosure; voluntary euthanasia

Published reports indicate that 2.5% of deaths in the Netherlands are the result of euthanasia or physician–assisted suicide. It is not known how many patients make these requests in the United States, but the issue has gained considerable attention, including that of the Supreme Court. The focus of the writing and discussion regarding the request to die has been on a patient's capacity. There has not been an adequate focus on the possible meanings contained within the request to die. A patient's request to die is a situation that requires the physician to engage in a dialogue to understand what the request means, including whether the request arises from a clinically significant depression or inadequately treated pain. This article outlines some of the thoughts and emotions that could underlie the patient's request to die. Recommendations are made regarding the role of the primary care physician and the role of the psychiatric consultant in the exploration of the meaning of the request.

Norris, Patrick F. Palliative care and killing: understanding ethical distinctions. *Bioethics Forum.* 1997 Fall; 13(3): 25–30. 6 refs. 1 fn. BE57529.

*active euthanasia; *allowing to die; *assisted suicide; *double effect; drugs; *intention; *killing; moral policy; pain; *palliative care; suicide; *terminal care; terminally ill; withholding treatment; sedatives

Onwuteaka–Philipsen, B.D.; van der Wal, G. Cases of euthanasia and physician assisted suicide among AIDS patients reported to the Public Prosecutor in North Holland. *Public Health.* 1998 Jan; 112(1): 53–56. 17 refs. BE58216.

*AIDS; *assisted suicide; evaluation studies; females; males; mandatory reporting; medical specialties; mortality; *patients; physicians; referral and consultation; statistics; trends; *voluntary euthanasia; retrospective studies;

BE = bioethics accession number   fn. = footnotes   refs. = references

*Netherlands

Onwuteaka–Philipsen, Bregje D.; Muller, Martien T.; van der Wal, Gerrit, et al. Active voluntary euthanasia or physician–assisted suicide? *Journal of the American Geriatrics Society.* 1997 Oct; 45(10): 1208–1213. 18 refs. BE56474.
*assisted suicide; *attitudes; comparative studies; *family practice; *knowledge, attitudes, practice; morality; morbidity; *motivation; *nursing homes; *patients; *physicians; survey; *voluntary euthanasia; retrospective studies; *Netherlands

Onwuteaka–Philipsen, Bregje D.; Muller, Martien T.; van der Wal, Gerrit. Euthanasia and old age. *Age and Ageing.* 1997 Nov; 26(6): 487–492. 10 refs. BE57967.
*age factors; *aged; AIDS; *assisted suicide; cancer; *diagnosis; family practice; females; home care; hospitals; males; mandatory reporting; medical specialties; nursing homes; *physicians; *statistics; time factors; *voluntary euthanasia; cerebrovascular disorders; multiple sclerosis; retrospective studies; *Netherlands; North Holland

Orentlicher, David. The Supreme Court and physician–assisted suicide -- rejecting assisted suicide but embracing euthanasia. *New England Journal of Medicine.* 1997 Oct 23; 337(17): 1236–1239. 19 refs. BE55800.
*active euthanasia; artificial feeding; *assisted suicide; constitutional law; double effect; *drugs; intention; involuntary euthanasia; *legal aspects; *legal rights; pain; *palliative care; *physicians; right to die; suffering; *Supreme Court decisions; *terminal care; *terminally ill; wedge argument; withholding treatment; coma; *sedatives; *United States; *Vacco v. Quill; *Washington v. Glucksberg

Orentlicher, David. The Supreme Court and terminal sedation: an ethically inferior alternative to physician–assisted suicide. *In:* Battin, Margaret P.; Rhodes, Rosamond; Silvers, Anita, eds. Physician Assisted Suicide: Expanding the Debate. New York, NY: Routledge; 1998: 301–311. 29 fn. ISBN 0–415–92003–5. BE58795.
active euthanasia; *allowing to die; *artificial feeding; *assisted suicide; competence; double effect; drugs; food; *intention; involuntary euthanasia; *legal aspects; moral policy; *palliative care; *physicians; right to die; suffering; *Supreme Court decisions; terminally ill; vulnerable populations; wedge argument; *withholding treatment; *sedatives; United States; *Vacco v. Quill; *Washington v. Glucksberg

Otlowski, Margaret. Voluntary Euthanasia and the Common Law. New York, NY: Oxford University Press; 1997. 564 p. Bibliography: p. 520–552. ISBN 0–19–825996–4. BE57847.
active euthanasia; advisory committees; allowing to die; *assisted suicide; autonomy; constitutional law; *criminal law; double effect; drugs; *government regulation; informed consent; intention; *international aspects; knowledge, attitudes, practice; *legal aspects; legal liability; legislation; libertarianism; moral policy; morality; motivation; organizational policies; palliative care; physicians; policy analysis; professional organizations; public opinion; *public policy; terminally ill; treatment refusal; *voluntary euthanasia; withholding treatment; Appleton Consensus; *Australia; *Canada; Council of Europe; European Parliament; *Great Britain; *Netherlands; Netherlands State Commission on Euthanasia; Northern Territory; Remmelink Commission; Rights of the Terminally Ill Act (NT); Royal Dutch Medical Association; *United States

Paris, John J.; Moreland, Michael P. A Catholic perspective on physician–assisted suicide. *In:* Battin,

Margaret P.; Rhodes, Rosamond; Silvers, Anita, eds. Physician Assisted Suicide: Expanding the Debate. New York, NY: Routledge; 1998: 324–333. 32 fn. ISBN 0–415–92003–5. BE58797.
active euthanasia; allowing to die; *assisted suicide; attitudes to death; autonomy; intention; killing; legal aspects; physicians; prolongation of life; *Roman Catholic ethics; suffering; suicide; Supreme Court decisions; terminally ill; theology; treatment refusal; value of life; withholding treatment; Patient Self-Determination Act 1990; United States

Paris, John J. Autonomy and physician–assisted suicide. *America.* 1997 May 17; 176(17): 11–14. BE55792.
*active euthanasia; *allowing to die; *assisted suicide; attitudes to death; *autonomy; biomedical technologies; *killing; *morality; patients' rights; *physicians; prolongation of life; public opinion; quality of life; *right to die; *Roman Catholic ethics; sociology of medicine; suffering; treatment refusal; withholding treatment; United States

Pellegrino, Edmund D. Evangelium Vitae, euthanasia, and physician–assisted suicide: John Paul II's dialogue with the culture and ethics of contemporary medicine. *In:* Wildes, Kevin Wm.; Mitchell, Alan C., eds. Choosing Life: A Dialogue on *Evangelium Vitae.* Washington, DC: Georgetown University Press; 1997: 236–253. 35 fn. ISBN 0–87840–646–8. BE56691.
allowing to die; artificial feeding; *assisted suicide; autonomy; bioethics; compassion; determination of death; double effect; freedom; intention; killing; moral obligations; morality; natural law; organ donation; pain; palliative care; physician's role; *physicians; quality of life; *Roman Catholic ethics; suffering; *theology; value of life; *voluntary euthanasia; withholding treatment; dignity; *Evangelium Vitae; John Paul II, Pope

Pellegrino, Edmund D. The false promise of beneficent killing. *In:* Emanuel, Linda L., ed. Regulating How We Die: The Ethical, Medical, and Legal Issues Surrounding Physician–Assisted Suicide. Cambridge, MA: Harvard University Press; 1998: 71–91, 269–274. 48 fn. ISBN 0–674–66654–2. BE58534.
*active euthanasia; advance directives; aged; *assisted suicide; autonomy; *beneficence; coercion; compassion; decision making; depressive disorder; freedom; infants; informed consent; *killing; legal aspects; medical ethics; moral obligations; *moral policy; pain; palliative care; patients; physician's role; *physicians; privacy; prolongation of life; public policy; right to die; *suffering; terminal care; value of life; voluntary euthanasia; wedge argument; dignity; Netherlands; United States

Phillips, Pat. Views of assisted suicide from several nations. *JAMA.* 1997 Sep 24; 278(12): 969–970. Report of a conference entitled "Comparative Perspectives on Law and Medicine," held in the summer of 1997 in Dublin, Ireland under the sponsorship of Loyola University Chicago Institute for Health Law and the health law section of the American Bar Association in cooperation with the Irish Legal Education and Research Trust and the health law section of the Canadian Bar Association. BE55769.
active euthanasia; allowing to die; *assisted suicide; attitudes; autonomy; beneficence; criminal law; guidelines; *international aspects; *legal aspects; physician's role; *physicians; *public policy; suicide; withholding treatment; *Australia; British Columbia; *Canada; Criminal Code of Canada; Death with Dignity Act (OR); *Great Britain; *Ireland; *Oregon; Rights of the Terminally Ill Act (NT)

Podgers, James. Stepping carefully: [ABA] House of Delegates declines to endorse physician–assisted suicide. [Meeting report]. *ABA Journal: The Lawyer's Magazine.*

BE = bioethics accession number   fn. = footnotes   refs. = references

1997 Sep; 83: 94. BE57627.
  *assisted suicide; *lawyers; *organizational policies; physicians; professional organizations; *public policy; *state government; *American Bar Association; *United States

Portenoy, Russell K.; Coyle, Nessa; Kash, Kathryn M., et al. Determinants of the willingness to endorse assisted suicide: a survey of physicians, nurses, and social workers. *Psychosomatics.* 1997 May–Jun; 38(3): 277–287. 44 refs. BE58770.
  age factors; *assisted suicide; *attitudes; cancer; drugs; empathy; hospitals; knowledge, attitudes, practice; *nurses; pain; palliative care; *physicians; professional competence; psychological stress; religion; *social workers; survey; terminal care; terminally ill; toxicity; voluntary euthanasia; New York City

Post, Stephen G. Physician–assisted suicide in Alzheimer's disease. *Journal of the American Geriatrics Society.* 1997 May; 45(5): 647–651. 26 refs. BE55843.
  active euthanasia; *advance directives; aged; *assisted suicide; attitudes; autonomy; beneficence; chronically ill; competence; *dementia; economics; health personnel; *hospices; international aspects; legal aspects; *long–term care; managed care programs; *palliative care; physicians; policy analysis; public opinion; *public policy; quality of life; resource allocation; self concept; social discrimination; social impact; suffering; *terminal care; terminally ill; wedge argument; withholding treatment; *United States

President and Fellows of Harvard College. A model state act to authorize and regulate physician–assisted suicide. *Issues in Law and Medicine.* 1997 Fall; 13(2): 219–226. Reprinted from the Harvard Journal on Legislation, 1996 Jan: 33. BE57808.
  *assisted suicide; communication; conscience; counseling; law enforcement; *legal aspects; legal liability; medical records; *model legislation; physicians; records; referral and consultation; suffering; terminally ill; United States

Previn, Matthew P. Assisted suicide and religion: conflicting conceptions of the sanctity of human life. [Note]. *Georgetown Law Journal.* 1995 Feb; 84(3): 589–616. 163 fn. BE56701.
  active euthanasia; ancient history; *assisted suicide; autonomy; Christian ethics; compassion; competence; *constitutional law; freedom; government regulation; historical aspects; *humanism; *legal aspects; *legal rights; love; philosophy; physicians; *religion; *religious ethics; right to die; secularism; state government; state interest; suffering; suicide; terminally ill; theology; *value of life; *voluntary euthanasia; *United States

Quill, Timothy E. A physician's position on physician–assisted suicide. [Hearing testimony]. *Bulletin of the New York Academy of Medicine.* 1997 Summer; 74(1): 114–118. Testimony on "Assisted suicide in the United States" before the Subcommittee on the Constitution, Committee on the Judiciary, U.S. House of Representatives, 29 Apr 1996. BE57505.
  allowing to die; *assisted suicide; attitudes; guidelines; hospices; *legal aspects; palliative care; *physicians; public policy; suffering; terminal care; *terminally ill; treatment refusal; *United States

Quill, Timothy E.; Kimsma, Gerrit. End–of–life care in the Netherlands and the United States: a comparison of values, justifications, and practices. *Cambridge Quarterly of Healthcare Ethics.* 1997 Spring; 6(2): 189–204. 127 fn. BE56476.
  *allowing to die; *assisted suicide; autonomy; case studies; common good; comparative studies; competence; consensus; decision making; dissent; double effect; drugs; freedom; government regulation; guidelines; health care delivery; hospices; intention; *international aspects; *knowledge, attitudes, practice; legal aspects; mass media; obligations of society; *palliative care; physician patient relationship; *physicians; policy analysis; public opinion; *public policy; social control; socioeconomic factors; statistics; *suffering; *terminal care; *values; *voluntary euthanasia; *Netherlands; *United States

Voluntary active euthanasia (VAE) and physician–assisted suicide (PAS) remain technically illegal in the Netherlands, but the practices are openly tolerated provided that physicians adhere to carefully constructed guidelines. Harsh criticism of the Dutch practice by authors in the United States and Great Britain has made achieving a balanced understanding of its clinical, moral, and policy implications very difficult. Similar practice patterns probably exist in the United States, but they are conducted in secret because of a more uncertain legal and ethical climate. In this manuscript, we plan to compare end–of–life care in the United States and the Netherlands with regard to underlying values, justifications, and practices. We will explore the risks and benefits of each system for a real patient who was faced with a common end–of–life clinical dilemma, and close with challenges for public policies in both countries.

Quill, Timothy E.; Lo, Bernard; Brock, Dan W. Palliative options of last resort: a comparison of voluntarily stopping eating and drinking, terminal sedation, physician–assisted suicide, and voluntary active euthanasia. *JAMA.* 1997 Dec 17; 278(23): 2099–2104. 70 refs. BE56434.
  *active euthanasia; *allowing to die; artificial feeding; *assisted suicide; autonomy; beneficence; chronically ill; comparative studies; competence; conscience; diagnosis; double effect; *drugs; ethical analysis; family members; food; guidelines; informed consent; intention; legal aspects; *moral policy; pain; *palliative care; physician's role; physicians; prognosis; *public policy; suffering; *terminal care; terminally ill; treatment refusal; *voluntary euthanasia; *sedatives; United States

Palliative care is generally agreed to be the standard of care for the dying, but there remain some patients for whom intolerable suffering persists. In the face of ethical and legal controversy about the acceptability of physician–assisted suicide and voluntary active euthanasia, voluntarily stopping eating and drinking and terminal sedation have been proposed as ethically superior responses of last resort that do not require changes in professional standards or the law. The clinical and ethical differences and similarities between these 4 practices are critically compared in light of the doctrine of double effect, the active/passive distinction, patient voluntariness, proportionality between risks and benefits, and the physician's potential conflict of duties. Terminal sedation and voluntarily stopping eating and drinking would allow clinicians to remain responsive to a wide range of patient suffering, but they are ethically and clinically more complex and closer to physician–assisted suicide and voluntary active euthanasia than is ordinarily acknowledged. Safeguards are presented for any medical action that may hasten death, including determining that palliative care is ineffective, obtaining informed consent, ensuring diagnostic and prognostic clarity, obtaining an independent second opinion, and implementing reporting and monitoring processes. Explicit public policy about which of these practices are permissible would reassure the many patients who fear a bad death in their future and allow for a predictable response for the few whose suffering becomes intolerable in spite of optimal palliative care.

BE = bioethics accession number   fn. = footnotes   refs. = references

Quill, Timothy E.; Meier, Diane E.; Block, Susan D., et al. The debate over physician–assisted suicide: empirical data and convergent views. *Annals of Internal Medicine.* 1998 Apr 1; 128(7): 552–558. 100 refs. BE57329.
> allowing to die; *alternatives; *assisted suicide; conscience; consensus; depressive disorder; empirical research; food; health insurance; hospices; knowledge, attitudes, practice; legal aspects; motivation; pain; *palliative care; patients' rights; *physicians; public opinion; public policy; quality of health care; quality of life; standards; suffering; *terminal care; terminally ill; treatment refusal; withholding treatment; sedatives; United States

Quinn, Kevin P. Assisted suicide and equal protection: in defense of the distinction between killing and letting die. *Issues in Law and Medicine.* 1997 Fall; 13(2): 145–171. 129 fn. BE57806.
> *allowing to die; *assisted suicide; constitutional law; double effect; due process; *equal protection; government regulation; *intention; *killing; *legal aspects; legal rights; *moral policy; physicians; public policy; *right to die; state government; Supreme Court decisions; terminally ill; treatment refusal; withholding treatment; Compassion in Dying v. State of Washington; Cruzan v. Director, Missouri Department of Health; Fourteenth Amendment; *New York; *Quill v. Vacco; *United States; *Vacco v. Quill; *Washington; Washington v. Glucksberg

Reisner, Michelle; Damato, Anthony N. Attitudes of physicians regarding physician–assisted suicide. *New Jersey Medicine.* 1995 Oct; 92(10): 663–666. 20 refs. BE55522.
> *assisted suicide; *attitudes; competence; family members; knowledge, attitudes, practice; *legal aspects; patients; *physicians; survey; terminally ill; *New Jersey

Reitman, James S. The debate on assisted suicide -- redefining morally appropriate care for people with intractable suffering. *Issues in Law and Medicine.* 1995 Winter; 11(3): 299–329. 118 fn. BE58821.
> accountability; allowing to die; *assisted suicide; autonomy; caring; Christian ethics; compassion; competence; decision making; empathy; ethics consultation; hospices; moral policy; *palliative care; patient advocacy; *physically disabled; physician patient relationship; physician's role; *physicians; psychological stress; *religious ethics; *suffering; *terminal care; *terminally ill; value of life; dignity; hope; rationality

Rhodes, Rosamond. Physicians, assisted suicide, and the right to live or die. *In:* Battin, Margaret P.; Rhodes, Rosamond; Silvers, Anita, eds. Physician Assisted Suicide: Expanding the Debate. New York, NY: Routledge; 1998: 165–176. 20 fn. ISBN 0-415-92003-5. BE58787.
> advance directives; allowing to die; *assisted suicide; autonomy; *beneficence; caring; killing; medical ethics; *moral obligations; *moral policy; palliative care; physician patient relationship; *physician's role; *physicians; public policy; *right to die; *rights; suffering; suicide; third party consent; treatment refusal; trust; value of life; *voluntary euthanasia; withholding treatment; rationality

Roberts, John; Kjellstrand, Carl. Jack Kevorkian: a medical hero. [Editorial]. *BMJ (British Medical Journal).* 1996 Jun 8; 312(7044): 1434. 1 ref. BE56882.
> *assisted suicide; attitudes; morality; *physicians; suffering; *Kevorkian, Jack; United States

Roberts, John. Oregon reaffirms assisted suicide. [News]. *BMJ (British Medical Journal).* 1997 Nov 15; 315(7118): 1253. BE57168.
> *assisted suicide; competence; *legal aspects; legislation; physicians; politics; public opinion; state government; terminally ill; *Death with Dignity Act (OR); *Oregon; United States

Rosen, Jeffrey. What right to die? *New Republic.* 1996 Jun 24; 214(26): 28–31. BE57067.
> abortion, induced; allowing to die; *assisted suicide; attitudes; constitutional law; due process; equal protection; *government regulation; killing; *legal aspects; *legal rights; privacy; public opinion; public policy; *right to die; state government; terminally ill; treatment refusal; *Compassion in Dying v. State of Washington; New York; *Quill v. Vacco; *United States; Washington

Safranek, John P. Autonomy and assisted suicide: the execution of freedom. *Hastings Center Report.* 1998 Jul–Aug; 28(4): 32–36. 34 fn. BE58926.
> *assisted suicide; *autonomy; beneficence; *ethical analysis; ethical theory; *freedom; injuries; killing; legal aspects; value of life; wedge argument

Proponents of assisted suicide who base their arguments on autonomy err in ways that are little attended to. In the absence of a substantive theory of the good, in neither a descriptive nor an ascriptive sense can the concept of autonomy distinguish those acts that should be morally prohibited from those that may be permitted. And to impose a particular theory of the good, whether individual liberty or the sanctity of life, violates the autonomy of those who do not share a commitment to that theory.

Sandel, Michael J. The hard questions: last rights. *New Republic.* 1997 Apr 14; 216(16): 27. BE55541.
> *assisted suicide; *autonomy; ethicists; freedom; killing; legal rights; moral obligations; philosophy; public policy; *right to die; *social impact; *suicide; terminally ill; *value of life; vulnerable populations; Dworkin, Ronald; Kant, Immanuel; Locke, John; Nagel, Thomas; Nozick, Robert; Rawls, John; Scanlon, Thomas; Thomson, Judith; United States

Shanahan, Timothy; Wang, Robin. Suicide and euthanasia. *In: their* Reason and Insight: Western and Eastern Perspectives on the Pursuit of Moral Wisdom. Belmont, CA: Wadsworth; 1996: 396–425. Includes references, readings, and discussion questions. Designed as a textbook for college students. ISBN 0-534-23167-5. BE56142.
> *active euthanasia; *allowing to die; attitudes; attitudes to death; brain death; Buddhist ethics; determination of death; Hindu ethics; international aspects; *moral policy; *morality; physician's role; *suicide; non-Western World; rationality; Western World; India; Japan

Silvers, Anita. Protecting the innocents from physician–assisted suicide: disability discrimination and the duty to protect otherwise vulnerable groups. *In:* Battin, Margaret P.; Rhodes, Rosamond; Silvers, Anita, eds. Physician Assisted Suicide: Expanding the Debate. New York, NY: Routledge; 1998: 133–148. 25 fn. ISBN 0-415-92003-5. BE58785.
> aged; *assisted suicide; *autonomy; chronically ill; coercion; common good; competence; *disabled; government regulation; health care; legal rights; legislation; obligations of society; *paternalism; physicians; *public policy; quality of life; right to die; social discrimination; state interest; stigmatization; suffering; suicide; Supreme Court decisions; value of life; *vulnerable populations; Americans with Disabilities Act 1990; United States; Vacco v. Quill; Washington v. Glucksberg

Slome, Lee; Moulton, Jeffrey; Huffine, Carol, et al. Physicians' attitudes toward assisted suicide in AIDS. *Journal of Acquired Immune Deficiency Syndromes.* 1992; 5(7): 712–718. 30 refs. BE56238.

BE = bioethics accession number   fn. = footnotes   refs. = references

*AIDS; *assisted suicide; comparative studies; drugs; emotions; HIV seropositivity; homosexuals; intention; *knowledge, attitudes, practice; legal aspects; medical specialties; mental health; physician patient relationship; physician's role; *physicians; referral and consultation; suffering; survey; terminally ill; values; Hemlock Society; San Francisco; United States

Smith, Cheryl K. Safeguards for physician–assisted suicide: the Oregon Death with Dignity Act. *In:* McLean, Sheila A.M., ed. Death, Dying and the Law. Brookfield, VT: Dartmouth; 1996: 69–93. 56 fn. Appendix: Oregon Death with Dignity Act. ISBN 1–85521–657–4. BE57214.
alternatives; *assisted suicide; communication; competence; counseling; diagnosis; disclosure; drugs; *government regulation; informed consent; *legal aspects; legal liability; legal obligations; legislation; mandatory reporting; medical records; *physicians; prognosis; referral and consultation; standards; state government; terminally ill; time factors; Ballot Measure 16 (OR); *Death with Dignity Act (OR); *Oregon

Smith, Wesley J. "Inevitable" assisted suicide?: don't bet your life. *Human Life Review.* 1997 Spring; 23(2): 61–74. 37 fn. BE57431.
*active euthanasia; alternatives; *assisted suicide; autonomy; chronically ill; conflict of interest; congenital disorders; depressive disorder; disabled; economics; emotions; gatekeeping; guidelines; health maintenance organizations; hospices; involuntary euthanasia; legal aspects; managed care programs; mandatory reporting; mass media; newborns; palliative care; physicians; prolongation of life; proprietary health facilities; public opinion; *public policy; quality of life; referral and consultation; right to die; social impact; suffering; terminally ill; voluntary euthanasia; wedge argument; capitation fee; Compassion in Dying v. State of Washington; Death with Dignity Act (OR); *Netherlands; Oregon; Remmelink Commission; *United States

Sneiderman, Barney; Verhoef, Marja. Patient autonomy and the defence of medical necessity: five Dutch euthanasia cases. *Alberta Law Review.* 1996; 34(2): 374–415. 74 fn. BE59012.
*active euthanasia; *assisted suicide; autonomy; *beneficence; case studies; chronically ill; criminal law; depressive disorder; drugs; guidelines; killing; *legal aspects; *legal liability; mentally ill; motivation; physically disabled; physician patient relationship; *physicians; professional organizations; public policy; quality of life; *suffering; treatment refusal; *voluntary euthanasia; *Netherlands; Royal Dutch Medical Association

Stell, Lance K. Physician–assisted suicide: to decriminalize or legalize, that is the question. *In:* Battin, Margaret P.; Rhodes, Rosamond; Silvers, Anita, eds. Physician Assisted Suicide: Expanding the Debate. New York, NY: Routledge; 1998: 225–251. 49 fn. ISBN 0–415–92003–5. BE58791.
*allowing to die; *assisted suicide; autonomy; competence; criminal law; ethical analysis; government regulation; *intention; *killing; *legal aspects; *moral policy; physician patient relationship; physician's role; *physicians; policy analysis; *public policy; right to die; state interest; *suicide; Supreme Court decisions; terminally ill; treatment refusal; withholding treatment; Cruzan v. Director, Missouri Department of Health; United States; Vacco v. Quill; Washington v. Glucksberg

Stempsey, William E. End–of–life decisions: Christian perspectives. *Christian Bioethics.* 1997 Dec; 3(3): 249–261. 21 refs. 3 fn. BE58490.
*active euthanasia; *allowing to die; *assisted suicide; *attitudes to death; autonomy; *Christian ethics; conscience; constitutional law; costs and benefits; decision making;

*Eastern Orthodox ethics; human body; legal rights; libertarianism; moral obligations; morality; *natural law; personhood; physicians; prolongation of life; *Protestant ethics; risks and benefits; *Roman Catholic ethics; *secularism; suffering; Supreme Court decisions; *terminally ill; *theology; value of life; values; withholding treatment; *Methodist Church; United States; Vacco v. Quill; Washington v. Glucksberg
While legal rights to make medical treatment decisions at the end of one's life have been recognized by the courts, particular religious traditions put axiological and metaphysical meat on the bare bones of legal rights. Mere legal rights do not capture the full reality, meaning and importance of death. End–of–life decisions reflect not only the meaning we find in dying, but also the meaning we have found in living. The Christian religions bring particular understandings of the vision of life as a gift from God, human responsibility for stewardship of that life, the wholeness of the person, and the importance of the dying process in preparing spiritually for life beyond earthly life, to bear on end–of–life decisions.

Stryker, Jeff. Ethical issues in treating competent patients with HIV disease. *In:* Cohen, P.T.; Sande, Merle A.; Volberding, Paul A., eds. The AIDS Knowledge Base: A Textbook on HIV Disease from the University of California, San Francisco, and the San Francisco General Hospital. Second Edition. Boston, MA: Little, Brown; 1994: 11.2–1 to 11.2–5. 19 refs. ISBN 0–316–77067–1. BE56641.
advance directives; *AIDS; *allowing to die; *assisted suicide; communication; compassion; competence; *decision making; depressive disorder; drug abuse; futility; HIV seropositivity; homosexuals; intensive care units; *palliative care; *patient participation; patients; physicians; *prolongation of life; resuscitation orders; socioeconomic factors; *suicide; *terminally ill; treatment refusal; ventilators; withholding treatment; United States

Suarez–Almazor, Maria E.; Belzile, Michelle; Bruera, Eduardo. Euthanasia and physician–assisted suicide: a comparative study of physicians, terminally ill cancer patients, and the general population. *Journal of Clinical Oncology.* 1997 Feb; 15(2): 418–427. 37 refs. BE58258.
*active euthanasia; *assisted suicide; *attitudes; *cancer; comparative studies; family practice; medical specialties; *patients; *physicians; *public opinion; public policy; religion; socioeconomic factors; suffering; survey; *terminally ill; *Alberta

Sullivan, Mark; Rapp, Suzanne; Fitzgibbon, Dermot, et al. Pain and the choice to hasten death in patients with painful metastatic cancer. *Journal of Palliative Care.* 1997 Autumn; 13(3): 18–28. 34 refs. BE58070.
*active euthanasia; *allowing to die; artificial feeding; *assisted suicide; *attitudes; *cancer; depressive disorder; double effect; drugs; hospitals; living wills; *pain; *palliative care; *patients; physicians; *quality of life; resuscitation orders; right to die; suicide; survey; *terminal care; *terminally ill; treatment refusal; values; voluntary euthanasia; withholding treatment; analgesia; outpatients; United States; University of Washington Medical Center

Sullivan, Mark D.; Ganzini, Linda; Youngner, Stuart J. Should psychiatrists serve as gatekeepers for physician–assisted suicide? *Hastings Center Report.* 1998 Jul–Aug; 28(4): 24–31. 50 fn. BE58925.
abortion, induced; *assisted suicide; *competence; depressive disorder; *gatekeeping; historical aspects; *mandatory programs; mentally ill; morality; *physician's role; psychiatric diagnosis; *psychiatry; *referral and consultation; suicide; terminally ill; United States
Mandating psychiatric evaluation for patients who request physician–assisted suicide may not offer the

---

BE = bioethics accession number   fn. = footnotes   refs. = references

clearcut protection from possible coercion or other abuse that proponents assert. Competence itself is a complex concept and determinations of decisionmaking capacity are not straightforward, nor is the relationship between mental illness and decisionmaking capacity in dying patients clearly understood. And casting psychiatrists as gatekeepers in end–of–life decisions poses risks to the profession itself.

Sulmasy, Daniel P.; Linas, Benjamin P.; Gold, Karen F., et al. Physician resource use and willingness to participate in assisted suicide. *Archives of Internal Medicine.* 1998 May 11; 158(9): 974–978. 24 refs. BE57650.

> alternatives; *assisted suicide; *attitudes; comparative studies; competence; drugs; *economics; incentives; *internal medicine; pain; patient care; *physicians; resource allocation; survey; terminally ill; *physician's practice patterns; urban population; Atlanta; Chicago; District of Columbia; Los Angeles; New York City; Philadelphia; *United States

OBJECTIVE: To explore the relationship between general internists' tendency to conserve medical resources and their willingness to participate in physician–assisted suicide (PAS). DESIGN AND PARTICIPANTS: Survey of a random sample of general internists in 6 urban areas of the United States. MEASUREMENTS: We assessed the physicians' use of medical resources by constructing a scale based on 6 hypothetical clinical scenarios in which respondents were given a choice between resource-intensive and resource-conserving options. We then presented a scenario of a competent terminally ill patient with breast cancer making stable and persistent requests for PAS. RESULTS: Sixty–seven (33%) of the 206 respondents indicated that they would participate in the suicide of the depicted patient. In a multivariate model, physicians who were more conservative with resources were 6.4 times more likely than their resource-intensive counterparts to prescribe the requested drugs (P = .02); minority physicians were less willing than whites to participate in PAS (odds ratio, 0.34; P = .03). Physicians' number of years in practice, location, sex, reported percentage of fee-for-service patients, and self-reported strength and direction of financial incentives in the respondents' practices were not associated with willingness to prescribe drugs for PAS. CONCLUSIONS: Most general internists, especially minority physicians, are personally reluctant to participate in PAS. While the characteristics of their practices do not affect PAS, physicians who tend to practice resource-conserving medicine are significantly more likely than their resource-intensive counterparts to provide a lethal prescription at the request of a terminally ill patient.

Supanich, Barbara; Brody, Howard. Ethical issues concerning physician–assisted death. *In:* Monagle, John F.; Thomasma, David C., eds. Health Care Ethics: Critical Issues for the 21st Century. Gaithersburg, MD: Aspen Publishers; 1998: 302–310. 29 fn. ISBN 0–8342–0911–X. BE56287.

> *assisted suicide; autonomy; communication; compassion; competence; comprehension; decision making; disclosure; palliative care; patients; physician patient relationship; physician's role; public policy; quality of health care; referral and consultation; right to die; suffering; values; *voluntary euthanasia; wedge argument; United States

Teitelman, Michael. Not in the house: arguments for a policy of excluding physician–assisted suicide from the practice of hospital medicine. *In:* Battin, Margaret P.;

Rhodes, Rosamond; Silvers, Anita, eds. Physician Assisted Suicide: Expanding the Debate. New York, NY: Routledge; 1998: 203–222. 9 fn. ISBN 0–415–92003–5. BE58790.

> advance care planning; *assisted suicide; autonomy; coercion; communication; conscience; critically ill; depressive disorder; economics; home care; *hospitals; *institutional ethics; *institutional policies; institutionalized persons; involuntary euthanasia; managed care programs; minority groups; nursing homes; patient admission; patient care team; patient transfer; *physicians; privacy; professional patient relationship; psychiatric diagnosis; psychological stress; public policy; regulation; religious hospitals; *social impact; *sociology of medicine; suicide; terminal care; terminally ill; trust; voluntary euthanasia; wedge argument; seriously ill; United States

Thies, Winthrop Drake; Groth, Philip; Hyman, Lawrence, et al. Assisted suicide. [Letters and response]. *Commentary.* 1997 Apr; 103(4): 3–7. BE57532.

> active euthanasia; *assisted suicide; autonomy; coercion; freedom; government regulation; killing; legal aspects; medical ethics; morality; physicians; public policy; quality of life; religion; right to die; United States

Thobaben, James R. A United Methodist approach to end–of–life decisions: intentional ambiguity or ambiguous intentions. *Christian Bioethics.* 1997 Dec; 3(3): 222–248. 40 refs. 22 fn. BE58491.

> *active euthanasia; advance directives; *allowing to die; *assisted suicide; autonomy; *clergy; competence; *decision making; *dissent; family members; historical aspects; hospices; *organizational policies; pain; pastoral care; personhood; physicians; *Protestant ethics; quality of life; suffering; suicide; terminal care; *terminally ill; terminology; theology; third party consent; treatment refusal; uncertainty; vulnerable populations; withholding treatment; *Methodist Church; *Wesley, John

The position of the United Methodist Church on end–of–life decisions is best described as intentional ambiguity or ambiguous intentions or both. The paper analyzes the official position of the denomination and then considers the actions of a U.M.C. bishop who served as a foreman for a trial of Dr. Jack Kevorkian. In an effort to find some common ground within an increasingly divided denomination, the work concludes with a consideration of the work of John Wesley and his approach to human death.

Tilden, Virginia P.; Tolle, Susan W.; Lee, Melinda A., et al. Oregon's physician–assisted suicide vote: its effect on palliative care. *Nursing Outlook.* 1996 Mar–Apr; 44(2): 80–83. 17 refs. BE55775.

> *assisted suicide; attitudes; competence; continuing education; drugs; government regulation; health insurance reimbursement; health services research; hospices; legal aspects; legislation; *nurses; organizational policies; *palliative care; physicians; professional organizations; social impact; state government; *terminal care; terminally ill; Death with Dignity Act (OR); Oregon

U.S. Court of Appeals, Ninth Circuit. Lee v. State of Oregon. *Federal Reporter, 3d Series.* 1997 Feb 27 (date of decision). 107: 1382–1397. Decision amended March 21 and April 16. Appendix provides the text of the Oregon Death with Dignity Act. BE58831.

> *assisted suicide; depressive disorder; due process; equal protection; *legal aspects; legal rights; legislation; nursing homes; physicians; social discrimination; state government; *terminally ill; Americans with Disabilities Act 1990; *Death with Dignity Act (OR); First Amendment; Fourteenth Amendment; *Lee v. State of Oregon; *Oregon; Rehabilitation Act 1973; Religious Freedom Restoration Act 1993

BE = bioethics accession number		fn. = footnotes		refs. = references

The U.S. Court of Appeals for the Ninth Circuit ordered the dismissal of a challenge to Oregon's Death with Dignity Act because competent, terminally ill patients, physicians, and nursing homes all lacked standing. None were entitled to a judicial decision because all failed to assert an "injury in fact" resulting from violations against the Equal Protection or Due Process clauses, the Americans with Disabilities Act, or the Rehabilitation Act. The patient's claim of depression to the degree of being unable to make an informed decision about ending her life was too speculative. Nor would the conjectural nature of the claim have changed if it were asserted by either the doctors or the residential care facilities. (KIE abstract)

Ubel, Peter A.; Asch, David A. Semantic and moral debates about hastening death: a survey of bioethicists. *Journal of Clinical Ethics.* 1997 Fall; 8(3): 242–249. 24 fn. BE57617.
  *active euthanasia; *allowing to die; artificial feeding; *assisted suicide; *attitudes; case studies; competence; *consensus; *dissent; *double effect; *drugs; *ethicists; family members; intention; involuntary euthanasia; killing; *moral policy; *morality; pain; palliative care; physicians; survey; *terminology; third party consent; treatment refusal; ventilators; *voluntary euthanasia; *withholding treatment; American Association of Bioethics; United States

Uhlmann, Michael M., ed. Last Rights? Assisted Suicide and Euthanasia Debated. Washington, DC: Ethics and Public Policy Center; Grand Rapids, MI: W.B. Eerdmans; 1998. 667 p. 511 fn. ISBN 0-8028-4199-6. BE57202.
  *active euthanasia; *allowing to die; *assisted suicide; attitudes to death; autonomy; Christian ethics; coercion; compassion; competence; double effect; drugs; freedom; government regulation; historical aspects; intention; Jewish ethics; killing; legal aspects; medical ethics; model legislation; *moral policy; morality; natural law; pain; personhood; philosophy; physician's role; physicians; quality of life; review; *right to die; Roman Catholic ethics; state interest; suffering; *suicide; Supreme Court decisions; theology; treatment refusal; utilitarianism; value of life; vulnerable populations; wedge argument; withholding treatment; rationality; Western World; American Medical Association; Netherlands; United States; Vacco v. Quill; Washington v. Glucksberg

van der Arend, Arie J.G. An ethical perspective on euthanasia and assisted suicide in the Netherlands from a nursing point of view. *Nursing Ethics.* 1998 Jul; 5(4): 307–318. 16 refs. BE58870.
  active euthanasia; *assisted suicide; communication; *decision making; drugs; *empirical research; government regulation; guidelines; *knowledge, attitudes, practice; legal aspects; *nurse's role; nursing ethics; patient advocacy; physician nurse relationship; *physicians; professional organizations; referral and consultation; statistics; terminal care; *voluntary euthanasia; *Netherlands

van der Maas, Paul J.; Emanuel, Linda L. Factual findings. *In:* Emanuel, Linda L., ed. Regulating How We Die: The Ethical, Medical, and Legal Issues Surrounding Physician-Assisted Suicide. Cambridge, MA: Harvard University Press; 1998: 151–174, 300–307. 28 fn. ISBN 0-674-66654-2. BE58537.
  *active euthanasia; *assisted suicide; *attitudes; autonomy; cancer; coercion; cultural pluralism; decision making; depressive disorder; *empirical research; intention; international aspects; involuntary euthanasia; legal aspects; moral obligations; *motivation; organizational policies; pain; palliative care; physicians; professional organizations; *public opinion; public policy; suffering; terminally ill; value of life; voluntary euthanasia; wedge argument; withholding

treatment; dignity; Netherlands; United States

Verhey, Allen. A Protestant perspective on ending life: faithfulness in the face of death. *In:* Battin, Margaret P.; Rhodes, Rosamond; Silvers, Anita, eds. Physician Assisted Suicide: Expanding the Debate. New York, NY: Routledge; 1998: 347–361. 23 fn. ISBN 0-415-92003-5. BE58798.
  allowing to die; *assisted suicide; attitudes to death; autonomy; caring; coercion; compassion; cultural pluralism; freedom; goals; justice; killing; medicine; physician's role; *Protestant ethics; public policy; right to die; suffering; *suicide; terminally ill; theology; value of life; voluntary euthanasia; vulnerable populations; duty to die

Veterans Affairs National Headquarters. Bioethics Committee. Physician-Assisted Suicide: Committee Report. Issued by the VA National Center for Clinical Ethics, White River Junction, VT 05009; 1996 May. 5 p. 12 refs. BE56737.
  artificial feeding; *assisted suicide; coercion; counseling; federal government; institutional policies; medical education; *palliative care; *physicians; public hospitals; *public policy; *terminal care; treatment refusal; *United States; *Veterans Health Administration

Walker, Gail C. The right to die: healthcare workers' attitudes compared with a national public poll. *Omega: A Journal of Death and Dying.* 1997; 35(4): 339–345. 4 refs. BE57722.
  *active euthanasia; advance directives; *allowing to die; *attitudes; autonomy; clinical ethics committees; comparative studies; competence; congenital disorders; *decision making; drugs; family members; hospitals; newborns; *nurses; pain; palliative care; parents; patients; *public opinion; quality of life; *right to die; suffering; *suicide; survey; terminally ill; third party consent; treatment refusal; withholding treatment; dependency; New York; Times Mirror Center; United States

Walzer, Michael. The hard questions: feed the face. *New Republic.* 1997 Jun 9; 216(23): 29. BE57547.
  *assisted suicide; economics; freedom; *government regulation; health care delivery; *legal aspects; legal rights; palliative care; *quality of health care; right to die; state government; *terminal care; terminally ill; vulnerable populations; *United States; When Death Is Sought (New York State Task Force on Life and the Law)

Warren, Mary Anne. Euthanasia and the moral status of human beings. *In: her:* Moral Status: Obligations to Persons and Other Living Things. New York, NY: Oxford University Press; 1997: 185–200. 13 fn. ISBN 0-19-823668-9. BE56997.
  *active euthanasia; adults; advance directives; *allowing to die; anencephaly; *assisted suicide; brain death; children; coercion; competence; *euthanasia; *human rights; *involuntary euthanasia; killing; legal aspects; *moral obligations; *moral policy; newborns; persistent vegetative state; prolongation of life; public policy; quality of life; suffering; suicide; terminally ill; terminology; third party consent; treatment refusal; *value of life; *voluntary euthanasia; Netherlands; United States

Watler, Crosbie L.; Gervais, Laurent; Cameron, Stewart. Lessons from Amy. [Letters and response]. *Canadian Medical Association Journal.* 1997 Jul 1; 157(1): 13–14. 3 refs. BE55778.
  *competence; depressive disorder; psychiatric diagnosis; right to die; *suicide; *treatment refusal

Weakland, Rembert. Assisted suicide: bad public policy. *Origins.* 1997 May 29; 27(2): 22–24. Testimony before the Wisconsin Assembly's Health Committee during a

---

hearing on a proposed assisted-suicide bill, 29 Apr 1997. BE56597.
    *assisted suicide; freedom; legal aspects; legislation; pain; *public policy; right to die; *Roman Catholic ethics; state government; suffering; terminal care; terminally ill; value of life; wedge argument; withholding treatment; *Wisconsin; Wisconsin Catholic Conference

Werber, Stephen J. Ancient answers to modern questions: death, dying, and organ transplants -- a Jewish law perspective. *Journal of Law and Health*. 1996-1997; 11(1-2): 13-44. 139 fn. BE57589.
    *active euthanasia; *allowing to die; *assisted suicide; brain death; cadavers; chronically ill; *determination of death; hearts; *Jewish ethics; killing; *organ donation; organ donors; organ transplantation; physicians; *resuscitation orders; right to die; *suicide; terminally ill; tissue donation; treatment refusal; value of life; withholding treatment; Orthodox Judaism

Wolf, Susan. Facing assisted suicide and euthanasia in children and adolescents. *In:* Emanuel, Linda L., ed. Regulating How We Die: The Ethical, Medical, and Legal Issues Surrounding Physician-Assisted Suicide. Cambridge, MA: Harvard University Press; 1998: 92-119, 274-294. 154 fn. ISBN 0-674-66654-2. BE58535.
    abortion, induced; *active euthanasia; *adolescents; adults; age factors; allowing to die; *assisted suicide; autonomy; beneficence; *children; coercion; competence; congenital disorders; decision making; infanticide; infants; international aspects; involuntary euthanasia; killing; legal aspects; legal rights; National Socialism; newborns; palliative care; parental consent; physicians; public policy; quality of life; socioeconomic factors; state interest; treatment refusal; voluntary euthanasia; withholding treatment; Netherlands; United States

Woolfrey, Joan. What happens now? Oregon and physician-assisted suicide. *Hastings Center Report*. 1998 May-Jun; 28(3): 9-17. 6 fn. BE58607.
    active euthanasia; *assisted suicide; attitudes; coercion; communication; competence; confidentiality; conscience; consensus; decision making; disclosure; dissent; drugs; freedom; *guidelines; hospices; institutional policies; interprofessional relations; legislation; organizational policies; patient advocacy; pharmacists; physician patient relationship; *physician's role; *physicians; policy analysis; *practice guidelines; professional family relationship; professional organizations; *public policy; quality of health care; records; *social impact; terminal care; terminally ill; time factors; patient abandonment; *physician's practice patterns; *Death with Dignity Act (OR); *Oregon; Oregon Hospice Association; Oregon Medical Association; Physicians for Compassionate Care; Task Force to Improve Care of Terminally Ill Oregonians
With assisted suicide now legally sanctioned, health care professionals in Oregon face the challenge of implementing Oregon's Death with Dignity Act. Physicians, hospice professionals, pharmacists, and other caregivers may find their relationships with patients, families, and fellow professionals changing in unanticipated ways as all learn what it means to make aid in dying openly and compassionately available to patients at the end of life.

Yount, Lisa. Should doctors ever hasten patients' deaths? [Juvenile literature]. *In: her* Issues in Biomedical Ethics. San Diego, CA: Lucent Books; 1998: 36-55, 101-102. 29 fn. ISBN 1-56006-476-5. BE57680.
    *active euthanasia; *allowing to die; artificial feeding; *assisted suicide; attitudes; *autonomy; biomedical technologies; coercion; competence; constitutional law; *decision making; due process; economics; equal protection; food; freedom; judicial action; *legal aspects; legal rights; legislation; pain; persistent vegetative state; physically

disabled; physician patient relationship; physician's role; *physicians; prolongation of life; quality of life; *right to die; state government; state interest; suffering; Supreme Court decisions; terminal care; terminally ill; third party consent; treatment refusal; trust; value of life; ventilators; vulnerable populations; *wedge argument; withholding treatment; Bouvia, Elizabeth; Cruzan, Nancy; Death with Dignity Act (OR); Netherlands; New York; Oregon; Patient Self-Determination Act 1990; Quinlan, Karen; *United States; Washington

Zinn, Christopher. Australian doctor builds "coma machine." [News]. *BMJ (British Medical Journal)*. 1997 May 24; 314(7093): 1503. BE55837.
    *assisted suicide; death; *drugs; intention; legal aspects; medical devices; *methods; palliative care; *physicians; terminally ill; *coma; Australia; *Nitschke, Philip; Wild, Esther

Zinn, Christopher. Australian doctors renew battle over euthanasia. [News]. *BMJ (British Medical Journal)*. 1996 Jun 8; 312(7044): 1437. BE57347.
    *assisted suicide; attitudes; *decision making; *guidelines; *legal aspects; *organizational policies; *physicians; professional organizations; right to die; uncertainty; *voluntary euthanasia; *Australia; *Australian Medical Association; *Northern Territory; *Rights of the Terminally Ill Act (NT)

Zinn, Christopher. Australian voluntary euthanasia law is overturned. [News]. *BMJ (British Medical Journal)*. 1997 Apr 5; 314(7086): 994. BE55838.
    *assisted suicide; attitudes; federal government; government financing; *legislation; organizational policies; *palliative care; physicians; professional organizations; terminal care; *voluntary euthanasia; *Australia; Australian Medical Association; *Northern Territory; *Rights of the Terminally Ill Act (NT)

Zohar, Noam J. Death: natural process and human intervention. *In: his* Alternatives in Jewish Bioethics. Albany, NY: State University of New York Press; 1997: 37-68. 42 fn. ISBN 0-7914-3274-2. BE57042.
    *active euthanasia; allowing to die; *assisted suicide; death; deontological ethics; hospices; *Jewish ethics; killing; medicine; palliative care; prolongation of life; suffering; suicide; terminally ill; *theology; value of life; *voluntary euthanasia

Zohar, Noam J. Jewish deliberations on suicide: exceptions, toleration, and assistance. *In:* Battin, Margaret P.; Rhodes, Rosamond; Silvers, Anita, eds. Physician Assisted Suicide: Expanding the Debate. New York, NY: Routledge; 1998: 362-372. 18 fn. ISBN 0-415-92003-5. BE58799.
    *assisted suicide; compassion; conscience; consensus; cultural pluralism; dissent; *Jewish ethics; moral complicity; physician patient relationship; *physicians; suffering; *suicide; terminally ill; *theology; torture; value of life; values; voluntary euthanasia

Zucker, Arthur. Law and ethics: [assisted suicide]. *Death Studies*. 1997 Jan-Feb; 21(1): 107-110. 4 refs. BE55599.
    *assisted suicide; attitudes; disadvantaged; ethicists; legal aspects; motivation; patients; physicians; public policy; risks and benefits; wedge argument

Zucker, Arthur. Law and ethics: experimentation; assisted suicide. *Death Studies*. 1997 Mar-Apr; 21(2): 221-225. 6 refs. 1 fn. BE55545.
    active euthanasia; *assisted suicide; children; drugs; government regulation; *human experimentation; informed consent; *legal aspects; mentally ill; physicians; placebos; research design; *right to die; scientific misconduct; Netherlands; United States

---

BE = bioethics accession number   fn. = footnotes   refs. = references

Doctor assisted suicide needs to be discussed. [BMA Annual Meeting, July 1998]. *BMJ (British Medical Journal)*. 1998 Jul 18; 317(7152): 214. BE58510.
> *assisted suicide; organizational policies; palliative care; *physicians; professional organizations; *British Medical Association; Great Britain

Jack Kevorkian. [News; title supplied]. *BMJ (British Medical Journal)*. 1997 Nov 1; 315(7116): 1116. BE57342.
> *assisted suicide; cadavers; hearts; *organ donation; physicians; lungs; *Kevorkian, Jack

Philosophers reflect on suicide. [Editorial]. *America*. 1997 Apr 5; 176(11): 3. BE56235.
> *allowing to die; *assisted suicide; attitudes; competence; drugs; ethicists; legal aspects; moral policy; *physicians; public policy; terminally ill; withholding treatment; United States

Physicians divided on assisted suicide. *Iowa Medicine*. 1996 Jul–Aug; 86(6): 238–239. BE56215.
> allowing to die; *assisted suicide; *attitudes; guidelines; legal aspects; organizational policies; physician's role; *physicians; professional organizations; survey; American Medical Association; *Iowa

SURROGATE DECISION MAKING See
ALLOWING TO DIE, INFORMED CONSENT, RESUSCITATION ORDERS

SURROGATE MOTHERS

See also REPRODUCTIVE TECHNOLOGIES

Baker, Valerie L. Surrogacy: one physician's view of the role of law. [Commentary]. *University of San Francisco Law Review*. 1994 Spring; 28(3): 603–612. 28 fn. Commentary on A.D. Davis et al., p. 571–592. BE56936.
> adoption; children; contracts; counseling; *government regulation; infertility; *legal aspects; legislation; mandatory programs; model legislation; organizational policies; *parent child relationship; professional organizations; *surrogate mothers; American College of Obstetricians and Gynecologists; American Fertility Society

Brahams, Diana. Designating parents in surrogate pregnancies. *Lancet*. 1998 Jan 3; 351(9095): 8. 4 refs. BE57905.
> contracts; *legal aspects; ovum donors; *parent child relationship; posthumous reproduction; public policy; remuneration; *surrogate mothers; Great Britain

Brazier, Margaret. Hard cases make bad law? [Editorial]. *Journal of Medical Ethics*. 1997 Dec; 23(6): 341–343. 3 refs. BE57656.
> *artificial insemination; cesarean section; *coercion; compensation; *competence; cryopreservation; death; *decision making; *fetuses; government regulation; guidelines; informed consent; *judicial action; *legal aspects; legal rights; married persons; physicians; *posthumous reproduction; *pregnant women; professional organizations; remuneration; semen donors; sperm; *surrogate mothers; *treatment refusal; Blood, Diane; European Union; *Great Britain; Human Fertilisation and Embryology Act 1990; Human Fertilisation and Embryology Authority; In re MB (Caesarean Section); R v. Human Fertilisation and Embryology Authority (ex parte Blood); Re S (Adult: Medical Treatment); Royal College of Obstetricians and Gynaecologists

Davis, Adrienne D., et al. Surrogacy legislation in California: proposals and commentary. [Foreword and proposals]. *University of San Francisco Law Review*. 1994

Spring; 28(3): 571–592. 13 fn. Commented on by B. Kopytoff, p. 593–602; by V.L. Baker, p. 603–612; by M.M. Shultz, p. 613–625; by J.D. Miller, p. 627–632; by L.C. Ikemoto, p. 633–645; and by M.H. Shapiro, p. 647–680. BE56937.
> children; *contracts; *government regulation; *legal aspects; legal rights; *model legislation; *parent child relationship; parents; property rights; public policy; remuneration; state government; state interest; *surrogate mothers; *California

Dolgin, Janet L. Defining the Family: Law, Technology, and Reproduction in an Uneasy Age. New York, NY: New York University Press; 1997. 287 p. Bibliography: p.273–281. ISBN 0-8147-1859-0. BE58581.
> anthropology; autonomy; children; contracts; cryopreservation; embryos; *family relationship; fathers; germ cells; judicial action; *law; *legal aspects; parent child relationship; posthumous reproduction; reproduction; *reproductive technologies; single persons; *social impact; Supreme Court decisions; *surrogate mothers; trends; *United States

Dyer, Clare. Surrogate mother refuses to give up baby. [News]. *BMJ (British Medical Journal)*. 1997 Jan 25; 314(7076): 250. BE58618.
> criminal law; deception; *legal aspects; *surrogate mothers; Great Britain; *Richardson, Angela

English, V.; Sommerville, A.; Brinsden, P.R. Surrogacy. *In:* Shenfield, F.; Sureau, C., eds. Ethical Dilemmas in Assisted Reproduction. New York, NY: Parthenon Pub. Group; 1997: 31–40. 3 refs. ISBN 1-85070-916-5. BE57944.
> clinical ethics committees; counseling; embryo transfer; government regulation; legal aspects; legislation; parent child relationship; *surrogate mothers; *Great Britain; Human Fertilisation and Embryology Act 1990; Human Fertilisation and Embryology Authority; Surrogacy Arrangements Act 1985 (Great Britain)

Grubb, Andrew. Parental orders (Section 30) and parentage -- Re Q (Parental Order). [Comment]. *Medical Law Review*. 1996 Summer; 4(2): 207–211. BE56494.
> *fathers; *legal aspects; married persons; *parent child relationship; remuneration; semen donors; single persons; *surrogate mothers; *Great Britain; *Re Q (Parental Order)

Ikemoto, Lisa C. Destabilizing thoughts on surrogacy legislation. [Commentary]. *University of San Francisco Law Review*. 1994 Spring; 28(3): 633–645. 57 fn. Commentary on A.D. Davis et al., p. 571–592. BE56938.
> abortion, induced; Asian Americans; blacks; contracts; fetal development; fetuses; *government regulation; homosexuals; *infertility; *legal aspects; legal rights; married persons; *model legislation; parent child relationship; *pregnant women; *reproduction; selection for treatment; *social discrimination; *socioeconomic factors; state interest; *surrogate mothers; women's rights; *California; Johnson v. Calvert

Kandel, Randy Frances. Which came first: the mother or the egg? A kinship solution to gestational surrogacy. *Rutgers Law Review*. 1994 Fall; 47(1): 165–239. 325 fn. BE56660.
> adoption; anthropology; contracts; counseling; *cultural pluralism; *family relationship; genetics; homosexuals; international aspects; judicial action; legal aspects; mediation; mother fetus relationship; *mothers; natural law; *ovum donors; *parent child relationship; *surrogate mothers; Anna J. v. Mark C.; California; Uniform Parentage Act; United States

Kopytoff, Barbara. Explorations in the law of surrogacy. [Commentary]. *University of San Francisco Law Review*.

1994 Spring; 28(3): 593–602. 21 fn. Commentary on A.D. Davis et al., p. 571–592. BE56939.

>*contracts; *government regulation; *legal aspects; *model legislation; *parent child relationship; property rights; remuneration; state government; *surrogate mothers; California

Krim, Todd M. Beyond *Baby M*: international perspectives on gestational surrogacy and the demise of the unitary biological mother. *Annals of Health Law.* 1996; 5: 193–226. 120 fn. BE58365.

>advisory committees; contracts; embryo transfer; federal government; feminist ethics; *government regulation; in vitro fertilization; industry; intention; *international aspects; judicial action; *legal aspects; legal rights; mothers; ovum donors; *parent child relationship; remuneration; reproductive technologies; socioeconomic factors; state government; *surrogate mothers; women's rights; Australia; California; Canada; France; Germany; Great Britain; Israel; Johnson v. Calvert; Sweden; *United States

McLachlan, Hugh V. Defending commercial surrogate motherhood against Van Niekerk and Van Zyl. *Journal of Medical Ethics.* 1997 Dec; 23(6): 344–348. 6 fn. Commentary on A. van Niekerk and L. van Zyl, "The ethics of surrogacy: women's reproductive labour," *JME*, 1995 Dec; 21(6): 345–349. BE57664.

>autonomy; *commodification; *contracts; *dehumanization; emotions; females; human body; legal aspects; *moral policy; *morality; mother fetus relationship; parent child relationship; parents; pregnant women; *public policy; *remuneration; reproduction; *surrogate mothers

The arguments of Van Niekerk and Van Zyl that, on the grounds that it involves an inappropriate commodification and alienation of women's labour, commercial surrogate motherhood (CSM) is morally suspect are discussed and considered to be defective. In addition, doubt is cast on the notion that CSM should be illegal.

Miller, John D. A political review of alternative surrogacy proposals. [Commentary]. *University of San Francisco Law Review.* 1994 Spring; 28(3): 627–632. 12 fn. Commentary on A.D. Davis et al., p. 571–592. BE56940.

>*contracts; *government regulation; *legal aspects; *model legislation; *parent child relationship; politics; state government; *surrogate mothers; California

Mittwoch, Ursula. This womb for hire? *New Scientist.* 1997 Jun 28; 154(2088): 46. BE59085.

>attitudes; contracts; government regulation; remuneration; *surrogate mothers; Great Britain

New Hampshire. Surrogacy. *New Hampshire Revised Statutes Annotated.* 1995 Nov 1 (date effective). Sects. 168-13:1 to 168-13:31. 18 p. BE58574.

>artificial insemination; contracts; embryo transfer; fathers; in vitro fertilization; *legal aspects; mothers; parent child relationship; state government; *surrogate mothers; *New Hampshire

Paulson, Richard J. Ethical considerations involving oocyte donation and gestational surrogacy. *Seminars in Reproductive Endocrinology.* 1995 Aug; 13(3): 225–230. 20 refs. BE55540.

>abortion, induced; age factors; coercion; conflict of interest; congenital disorders; ethics committees; females; fetuses; morbidity; mortality; newborns; organizational policies; *ovum donors; parent child relationship; political activity; pregnant women; religion; remuneration; reproduction; *reproductive technologies; rights; risk; selection for treatment; semen donors; *surrogate mothers; women's rights; American Fertility Society; Right to Life Movement

Pennsylvania. Superior Court. Huddleston v. Infertility Center of America. *Atlantic Reporter, 2d Series.* 1997 Aug 20 (date of decision). 700: 453–462. BE58670.

>*child abuse; fathers; *health facilities; infertility; killing; *legal aspects; *legal liability; negligence; semen donors; *surrogate mothers; *wrongful death; *Huddleston v. Infertility Center of America; Pennsylvania

The Pennsylvania Superior Court held that a surrogate mother could sue a surrogacy clinic for the sperm-donor father's murder of the child she bore. One month after delivery, the child died from severe brain and head injuries caused by his biological father. The court held that a "special relationhsip" exists between a surrogacy business, its client-participants, and the child which is born. In this "special relationship" the surrogacy business has an affirmative duty to protect the surrogate mother and child from foreseeable harm. The court held that child abuse was a legally foreseeable harm in the surrogacy business, but whether child abuse leading to death is forseeable under a particular set of acts is a jury question. (KIE abstract)

Peters, Ted. Surrogate motherhood: an ethical puzzle. *In: his* For the Love of Children: Genetic Technology and the Future of the Family. Louisville, KY: Westminster John Knox Press; 1996: 58–84, 189–193. 62 fn. ISBN 0-664-25468-3. BE55696.

>children; commodification; contracts; disclosure; family relationship; feminist ethics; legal aspects; libertarianism; marital relationship; mother fetus relationship; ovum donors; parent child relationship; psychological stress; religion; remuneration; reproductive technologies; self concept; social discrimination; socioeconomic factors; standards; *surrogate mothers; women's rights; California; In re Baby M; Johnson v. Calvert; New Jersey; United States

Radin, Margaret Jane. Contested Commodities: The Trouble with Trade in Sex, Children, Body Parts, and Other Things. Cambridge, MA: Harvard University Press; 1996. 279 p. 437 fn. ISBN 0-674-16697-3. BE55801.

>adoption; altruism; *body parts and fluids; children; coercion; *commodification; *dehumanization; *democracy; *economics; females; *feminist ethics; *freedom; *government regulation; indigents; *infants; justice; law; legal aspects; metaphor; minority groups; *organ donation; personhood; property rights; public policy; *remuneration; *sexuality; *surrogate mothers; torts; women's rights; liberalism; *prostitution

Radin, Margaret Jane. What, if anything, is wrong with baby selling? *Pacific Law Journal.* 1995 Jan; 26(2): 135–145. 5 fn. Address to the student body of the McGeorge School of Law, 4 Mar 1994. BE55591.

>adoption; autonomy; *children; *commodification; constitutional law; due process; *economics; legal aspects; males; *parent child relationship; parents; personhood; *remuneration; rights; risks and benefits; self concept; semen donors; social discrimination; *surrogate mothers; unwanted children; *women's rights; prostitution; In re Baby M; United States

Rae, Scott B. Parental rights and the definition of motherhood in surrogate motherhood. *Southern California Review of Law and Women's Studies.* 1994 Spring; 3(2): 219–277. 239 fn. BE56665.

>adoption; artificial insemination; childbirth; *contracts; fathers; *genetic identity; in vitro fertilization; *legal aspects; *legal rights; *mother fetus relationship; *mothers; ovum donors; *parent child relationship; standards; *surrogate mothers; United States

Rosenfeld, Azriel. Generation, gestation, and Judaism. *In:*

Feldman, Emanuel; Wolowelsky, Joel B., eds. Jewish Law and the New Reproductive Technologies. Hoboken, NJ: Ktav; 1997: 36–45. 5 fn. ISBN 0-88125-586-6. BE57455.
*Jewish ethics; married persons; mothers; *parent child relationship; reproductive technologies; *surrogate mothers; Orthodox Judaism

Rush, Sharon Elizabeth. Breaking with tradition: surrogacy and gay fathers. *In:* Meyers, Diana Tietjens; Kipnis, Kenneth; Murphy, Cornelius F., eds. Kindred Matters: Rethinking the Philosophy of the Family. Ithaca, NY: Cornell University Press; 1993: 102–142. 62 refs. 79 fn. ISBN 0-8014-9909-7. BE55698.
adoption; behavioral genetics; children; contracts; *family relationship; *fathers; females; government regulation; *homosexuals; informed consent; *legal aspects; legal rights; *males; mass media; morality; *parent child relationship; paternalism; privacy; public opinion; public policy; remuneration; *reproduction; selection for treatment; sexuality; single persons; *stigmatization; Supreme Court decisions; *surrogate mothers; values; women's rights; United States

Shapiro, Michael H. How (not) to think about surrogacy and other reproductive innovations. [Commentary]. *University of San Francisco Law Review.* 1994 Spring; 28(3): 647–680. 108 fn. Commentary on A.D. Davis et al., p. 571–592. BE56941.
autonomy; biomedical technologies; children; coercion; commodification; contracts; fathers; genetic intervention; government regulation; informed consent; intention; *legal aspects; legal rights; model legislation; *moral policy; mothers; motivation; *parent child relationship; *risks and benefits; *surrogate mothers; terminology; value of life; California; In re Baby M; Johnson v. Calvert; Uniform Parentage Act; Uniform Status of Children of Assisted Conception Act

Shultz, Marjorie Maguire. Legislative regulation of surrogacy and reproductive technology. [Commentary]. *University of San Francisco Law Review.* 1994 Spring; 28(3): 613–625. 8 fn. Commentary on A.D. Davis et al., p. 571–592. BE56942.
autonomy; commodification; contracts; economics; family relationship; females; *government regulation; *legal aspects; legislation; males; *model legislation; *parent child relationship; *privacy; private sector; public policy; public sector; reproductive technologies; social control; social impact; *surrogate mothers; California; United States

Simini, Bruno. Italian surrogate "twins." *Lancet.* 1997 Nov 1; 350(9087): 1307. BE56931.
*multiple pregnancy; *surrogate mothers; twins; *Italy

Virginia. Status of children of assisted conception. *Code of Virginia Annotated.* 1997 Jul 1 (date effective). Sects. 20–156 to 20–165. 11 p. Sects. 20–156, 20–158, and 20–163 amended 1998. BE58895.
children; *contracts; cryopreservation; embryos; *legal aspects; *parent child relationship; posthumous reproduction; remuneration; *reproductive technologies; *surrogate mothers; *Virginia

Warden, John. Surrogacy to be reviewed in United Kingdom. [News]. *BMJ (British Medical Journal).* 1997 Jun 21; 314(7097): 1782. BE56588.
*advisory committees; contracts; criminal law; government regulation; industry; *legal aspects; remuneration; *surrogate mothers; *Great Britain

TECHNOLOGIES, BIOMEDICAL *See* BIOMEDICAL TECHNOLOGIES

TERMINAL CARE

See also ALLOWING TO DIE, PATIENT CARE, RESUSCITATION ORDERS

American College of Physicians. Health and Public Policy Committee. Drug therapy for severe, chronic pain in terminal illness. *Annals of Internal Medicine.* 1983 Dec; 99(6): 870–873. 29 refs. BE57230.
*drugs; goals; *organizational policies; *pain; *palliative care; physicians; professional organizations; technical expertise; *terminal care; *American College of Physicians

American Medical Association. Elements of Quality Care for Patients in the Last Phase of Life. Chicago, IL: American Medical Association; 1997 Jun 22. 1 p. BE57738.
advance directives; allowing to die; community services; family members; health facilities; organizational policies; palliative care; physicians; professional organizations; *standards; suffering; *terminal care; terminally ill; withholding treatment; patient abandonment; *American Medical Association

American Nurses Association. American Nurses Association position statements on ethics and human rights. *In: its* Compendium of American Nurses Association Position Statements. Washington, DC: American Nurses Publishing; 1996: 79–118. Includes references. ISBN 1-55810-123-3. BE57452.
active euthanasia; advance directives; allowing to die; artificial feeding; assisted suicide; capital punishment; codes of ethics; cultural pluralism; health care; *human rights; legislation; nurse's role; *nurses; *nursing ethics; *organizational policies; pain; palliative care; patient advocacy; *patient care; professional organizations; resuscitation orders; *terminal care; treatment refusal; withholding treatment; *American Nurses Association; Patient Self-Determination Act 1990; United States

Ayers, Elise; Harrold, Joan; Lynn, Joanne. A good death: improving care inch-by-inch. *Bioethics Forum.* 1997 Spring; 13(1): 38–40. 7 refs. BE55844.
advance care planning; aged; communication; death; dehumanization; family members; pain; palliative care; *patient satisfaction; physician patient relationship; professional competence; professional family relationship; psychological stress; quality of health care; quality of life; suffering; *terminal care; continuity of patient care; dignity; Study to Understand Prognoses and Preferences for Outcomes and Risks of Treatments (SUPPORT); United States

Billings, J. Andrew; Block, Susan D. Slow euthanasia. *Journal of Palliative Care.* 1996 Winter; 12(4): 21–30. 80 refs. Commented on by B. Mount, p. 31–37; by H. Brody, p. 38–41; by B.M. Dickens, p. 42–43; and by R.K. Portenoy, p. 44–46. BE55706.
*active euthanasia; allowing to die; *attitudes; beneficence; case studies; decision making; *double effect; *drugs; family members; hospices; informed consent; *intention; involuntary euthanasia; killing; pain; *palliative care; paternalism; patients; physicians; psychological stress; suffering; *terminal care; *terminally ill; time factors; voluntary euthanasia; withholding treatment; analgesia; *morphine; sedatives

Brahams, Diana. UK judge approves death free from mental pain. [News]. *Lancet.* 1997 Nov 8; 350(9088): 1376. BE57381.
*amyotrophic lateral sclerosis; criminal law; *double effect; *drugs; euthanasia; killing; *legal aspects; legal liability; pain; *palliative care; physicians; *psychological stress; right to die; *terminal care; *terminally ill; *Great Britain; *Lindsell,

---

BE = bioethics accession number   fn. = footnotes   refs. = references

Annie

Braun, Kathryn L.; Nichols, Rhea. Death and dying in four Asian American cultures: a descriptive study. *Death Studies.* 1997 Jul–Aug; 21(4): 327–359. 29 refs. BE56584.
active euthanasia; advance directives; allowing to die; *Asian Americans; assisted suicide; attitudes; *attitudes to death; Buddhist ethics; cadavers; comparative studies; cultural pluralism; drugs; family members; organ donation; pain; pastoral care; suicide; *terminal care; third party consent; treatment refusal; Hawaii; United States

Brody, Howard. Commentary on Billings and Block's "Slow euthanasia." *Journal of Palliative Care.* 1996 Winter; 12(4): 38–41. 11 refs. Commentary on J.A. Billings and S.D. Block, p. 21–30. BE55709.
*active euthanasia; allowing to die; *assisted suicide; decision making; double effect; drugs; *government regulation; intention; justice; killing; *legal aspects; *palliative care; physicians; resource allocation; suffering; *terminal care; *terminally ill; wedge argument; withholding treatment; morphine; Compassion in Dying v. State of Washington; Netherlands; United States

Brody, Howard; Vandekieft, Gregg K. Physician–assisted suicide: a very personal issue. [Editorial]. *American Family Physician.* 1997 May 15; 55(7): 2421–2427. 6 refs. BE57956.
*assisted suicide; *communication; disabled; hospices; palliative care; physician patient relationship; physicians; *terminal care; terminally ill

Burt, Robert A. The Supreme Court speaks -- not assisted suicide but a constitutional right to palliative care. *New England Journal of Medicine.* 1997 Oct 23; 337(17): 1234–1236. 23 fn. BE55803.
*assisted suicide; *constitutional law; double effect; *drugs; *government regulation; intention; *legal aspects; *legal rights; legislation; pain; *palliative care; *physicians; right to die; social impact; *state government; suffering; *Supreme Court decisions; *terminal care; *terminally ill; Institute of Medicine; New York; *United States; *Vacco v. Quill; Washington; *Washington v. Glucksberg

Calhoun, Byron C.; Reitman, James S.; Hoeldtke, Nathan J. Perinatal hospice: a response to partial birth abortion for infants with congenital defects. *Issues in Law and Medicine.* 1997 Fall; 13(2): 125–143. 86 fn. BE57805.
allowing to die; *alternatives; autonomy; *childbirth; *chromosome abnormalities; *congenital disorders; conscience; counseling; death; decision making; *fetal development; fetuses; health personnel; hospices; informed consent; methods; *newborns; *palliative care; parents; personhood; pregnant women; privacy; psychological stress; *selective abortion; suffering; theology; value of life; viability; *pregnancy trimesters

Cartwright, Colleen; Steinberg, Margaret; Williams, Ged, et al. Issues of death and dying: the perspective of critical care nurses. *Australian Critical Care.* 1997 Sep; 10(3): 81–84, 86–87. 14 refs. BE58250.
advance directives; allowing to die; assisted suicide; *attitudes; attitudes to death; communication; decision making; drugs; legal aspects; nurse's role; *nurses; palliative care; patient advocacy; survey; *terminal care; third party consent; voluntary euthanasia; *Australia; *Queensland

Catholic Health Association of the United States. Caring for Persons at the End of Life: A Facilitator's Guide to Educational Modules for Healthcare Leaders. [Looseleaf format manual]. St. Louis, MO: Catholic Health Association of the United States; 1993. 1 v. Bibliography: p. 203–211. Binder includes three earlier CHA publications: Care of the Dying: A Catholic

Perspective; Pain Management: Theological and Ethical Principles Governing the Use of Pain Relief for Dying Patients; and Principled and Virtuous Care of the Dying: A Catholic Response to Euthanasia. ISBN 0-87125-217-1. BE56504.
active euthanasia; administrators; advance directives; allowing to die; assisted suicide; attitudes to death; autonomy; caring; case studies; decision making; *education; health facilities; institutional policies; killing; legal aspects; nurses; pain; palliative care; pastoral care; physicians; resuscitation orders; right to die; *Roman Catholic ethics; suffering; teaching methods; *terminal care; truth disclosure; value of life; withholding treatment; United States

Cher, Daniel J.; Lenert, Leslie A. Method of Medicare reimbursement and the rate of potentially ineffective care of critically ill patients. *JAMA.* 1997 Sep 24; 278(12): 1001–1007. 29 refs. Correction appears in *JAMA*, 1998 Jun 17; 279(23): 1876. BE55815.
aged; allowing to die; biomedical technologies; comparative studies; *critically ill; *economics; *futility; *health maintenance organizations; hospitals; *intensive care units; *managed care programs; *mortality; *patient care; physicians; prolongation of life; quality of health care; remuneration; resource allocation; selection for treatment; *terminal care; time factors; *treatment outcome; withholding treatment; *fee-for-service plans; severity of illness index; *California; *Medicare

CONTEXT: The worst outcome of critical care may not be death itself; rather, the worst may be an extended death process in which a patient's and his or her family's suffering has been prolonged by services that are ultimately impotent. We have previously used potentially ineffective care (PIC) as a proxy measure for this type of care. OBJECTIVE: To determine if PIC is delivered less often to Medicare patients enrolled in health maintenance organizations (HMOs) than those in traditional fee-for-service health plans. PATIENTS: All Medicare patients hospitalized in intensive care units in California during fiscal year 1994. OUTCOME: Potentially ineffective care was defined as the concurrence of in-hospital death or death within 100 days of hospital discharge and resource use (total hospital costs) above the 90th percentile. METHODS: Hospital costs were adjusted for institution-specific cost-to-charge ratios and local wage indices derived from Health Care Financing Administration cost reports. A multivariate regression model adjusted PIC rates for age, sex, race, elective admission to the hospital, Charlson index diseases, the 15 most common diagnosis related groups for death by 100 days, intensive care unit size, and number of residents at the hospital. RESULTS: A total of 3914 (4.8%) of 81,494 patients experienced PIC and used 21.6% of total intensive care unit resources. The occurrence of PIC was less common among HMO members (adjusted odds ratio, 0.75; 95% confidence interval, 0.65–0.87). However, HMO members were not more likely to experience in-hospital death (adjusted odds ratio, 0.99; 95% confidence interval, 0.91–1.07) and only slightly more likely to experience death by 100 days after hospital discharge (adjusted odds ratio, 1.08; 95% confidence interval, 1.01–1.15). CONCLUSIONS: Patients who experience PIC outcomes are not uncommon in the Medicare population, and patients experiencing this outcome consume a disproportionate amount of medical resources. Medicare beneficiaries in HMO practice settings had a lower risk of experiencing PIC outcomes after adjusting for age, sex, diagnosis, comorbid conditions, and characteristics of the treating hospital. This suggests that HMO practices may be better at limiting or avoiding injudicious use of critical care near the end of life.

BE = bioethics accession number   fn. = footnotes   refs. = references

Claiborne, William. In Oregon, suicide option brings a kinder care. [News]. *Washington Post.* 1998 Apr 29: A1, A12. BE57844.
  *assisted suicide; attitudes; decision making; drugs; hospices; hospitals; legal aspects; physicians; *social impact; state government; *terminal care; terminally ill; morphine; Death with Dignity Act (OR); *Oregon

Cooke, Molly; Gourlay, Linda; Collette, Linda, et al. Informal caregivers and the intention to hasten AIDS-related death. *Archives of Internal Medicine.* 1998 Jan 12; 158(1): 69–75. 35 refs. BE56300.
  *active euthanasia; *AIDS; assisted suicide; *drugs; evaluation studies; family members; friends; HIV seropositivity; home care; homosexuals; hospices; hospitals; *intention; males; motivation; *palliative care; physician's role; psychological stress; survey; *terminal care; terminally ill; voluntary euthanasia; *caregivers; narcotics; prospective studies; sedatives; San Francisco
  OBJECTIVES: To determine the extent to which homosexual men dying of the acquired immunodeficiency syndrome (AIDS) receive medication intended to hasten death. To assess the impact on caregivers of administering medications intended to hasten death. METHODS: In a prospective study of caregiving partners of men with AIDS (n = 140), characteristics of the ill partner, the caregiver, and the relationship were assessed at baseline and 1 month before the ill partner's death. Three months after the death, caregivers were asked if they had increased their partner's narcotic and/or sedative-hypnotic medication dose and if so, what had been the objective of the increase, and their comfort with their medication decisions. RESULTS: Of 140 ill partners who died of AIDS, 17 (12.1%) received an increase in the use of medications immediately before death intended to hasten death. Diagnoses and care needs of ill partners who received increases in the use of medications to hasten death did not differ from those of ill partners receiving medication for symptoms. Fourteen increases (10%) in use of medications were administered by caregivers. These caregivers did not differ from those administering medication for symptom control in level of distress, caregiving burden, relationship characteristics, or comfort with the medication decision, but they reported more social support and positive meaning in caregiving. CONCLUSION: The decision to hasten death is not a rare event in this group of men. There is no evidence that it is the result of caregiver distress, poor relationship quality, or intolerable caregiving burden; and it does not cause excessive discomfort in the surviving partner. This study, although small, has implications for the policy debate on assisted suicide.

Coope, Christopher Miles. "Death with dignity." *Hastings Center Report.* 1997 Sep–Oct; 27(5): 37–38. BE56121.
  active euthanasia; allowing to die; assisted suicide; *attitudes to death; persistent vegetative state; *right to die; *terminal care; terminology; *dignity

Coppa, Seanda. Futile care: confronting the high costs of dying. *Journal of Nursing Administration.* 1996 Dec; 26(12): 18–23. 30 refs. BE58263.
  advance directives; allowing to die; assisted suicide; autonomy; beneficence; economics; *futility; government financing; health facilities; health personnel; hospices; institutional policies; justice; persistent vegetative state; prognosis; psychological stress; resource allocation; *terminal care; terminally ill; values; withholding treatment; Medicare; United States

Corner, Jessica. More openness needed in palliative care.

[Medicine and the media]. *BMJ (British Medical Journal).* 1997 Nov 8; 315(7117): 1242. BE56780.
  *double effect; drugs; *mass media; *palliative care; *paralysis; *physically disabled; physicians; right to die; suffering; *terminal care; *voluntary euthanasia; *Great Britain; *Lindsell, Annie

Curtis, J. Randall; Rubenfeld, Gordon D. Aggressive medical care at the end of life; does capitated reimbursement encourage the right care for the wrong reason? [Editorial]. *JAMA.* 1997 Sep 24; 278(12): 1025–1026. 12 refs. BE55814.
  biomedical technologies; *critically ill; decision making; *economics; *health maintenance organizations; hospitals; *intensive care units; *managed care programs; mortality; *patient care; physicians; prolongation of life; quality of health care; remuneration; *terminal care; time factors; treatment outcome; withholding treatment; capitation fee; *fee-for-service plans; *Medicare; *United States

Davis, Anne J.; Aroskar, Mila A.; Liaschenko, Joan, et al. Dying and death. *In: their* Ethical Dilemmas and Nursing Practice. Fourth Edition. Stamford, CT: Appleton and Lange; 1997: 159–183. 58 fn. ISBN 0-8385-2283-1. BE58597.
  *active euthanasia; adults; advance directives; *allowing to die; assisted suicide; caring; case studies; decision making; determination of death; hospices; legal aspects; newborns; *nurses; nursing ethics; resuscitation orders; right to die; suffering; suicide; *terminal care; third party consent; treatment refusal; withholding treatment; United States

Dickens, Bernard M. Commentary on "Slow euthanasia." *Journal of Palliative Care.* 1996 Winter; 12(4): 42–43. 4 refs. Commentary on J.A. Billings and S.D. Block, p. 21–30. BE55716.
  *active euthanasia; assisted suicide; criminal law; double effect; *drugs; intention; *legal aspects; motivation; *palliative care; physicians; suffering; *terminal care; terminally ill; withholding treatment; *morphine; Canada; Criminal Code of Canada

Dixon, Kathleen Marie. The quality of mercy: reflections on provider-assisted suicide. *Journal of Clinical Ethics.* 1997 Fall; 8(3): 290–302. 47 fn. BE57561.
  *assisted suicide; attitudes to death; communication; *compassion; counseling; disabled; empathy; *health personnel; love; moral obligations; *palliative care; patient care; physicians; professional patient relationship; quality of health care; referral and consultation; self concept; *suffering; *terminal care; terminally ill; Levinas, Emmanuel

Docker, Christopher. The way forward? *In:* McLean, Sheila A.M., ed. Death, Dying and the Law. Brookfield, VT: Dartmouth; 1996: 129–160. 99 fn. ISBN 1-85521-657-4. BE57217.
  *active euthanasia; *advance directives; aged; *allowing to die; *assisted suicide; decision making; double effect; economics; hospices; legal aspects; living wills; pain; *palliative care; *persistent vegetative state; physicians; public policy; *resource allocation; selection for treatment; terminal care; withholding treatment; *Great Britain; National Health Service; Netherlands; United States

Donaldson, Molla S.; Field, Marilyn J. Measuring quality of care at the end of life. *Archives of Internal Medicine.* 1998 Jan 26; 158(2): 121–128. 43 refs. BE56302.
  accountability; *evaluation; family members; health facilities; health services research; hospices; *palliative care; *patient satisfaction; prolongation of life; *quality of health care; quality of life; regulation; standards; *terminal care; treatment outcome; *quality assurance; United States
  Caring for patients at the end of life presents a series of quality-of-care problems to the health care system.

In the past, concern has focused on overaggressive treatment of dying patients. Given rapid changes in the financing and delivery of care, it is time to focus on a range of quality problems and address ways to improve care and achieve outcomes desired by patients and their families. We provide a framework for conceptualizing such a task. This article addresses the purposes of measurement, definition of the patient population, timing of measurement, use of surrogates in measurement, scope of services to be evaluated, and the choice of measures. It emphasizes the necessary links between quality measurement and quality improvement.

Dunphy, Kilian; Finlay, Ilora; Rathbone, Gillian, et al. Rehydration in palliative and terminal care: if not -- why not? *Palliative Medicine.* 1995 Jul; 9(3): 221-228. 32 refs. BE55718.
 advance directives; *artificial feeding; attitudes; decision making; family members; hospices; morbidity; *palliative care; physicians; prolongation of life; *risks and benefits; *terminal care; terminally ill; withholding treatment; *dehydration; *fluid therapy

Dyer, Clare. Court confirms right to palliative treatment for mental distress. [News]. *BMJ (British Medical Journal).* 1997 Nov 8; 315(7117): 1178. BE57351.
 *amyotrophic lateral sclerosis; criminal law; *double effect; *drugs; euthanasia; judicial action; killing; *legal aspects; legal liability; pain; *palliative care; physicians; *psychological stress; right to die; *terminal care; *terminally ill; *Great Britain; *Lindsell, Annie

Emanuel, Ezekiel J.; Battin, Margaret P. What are the potential cost savings from legalizing physician-assisted suicide? *New England Journal of Medicine.* 1998 Jul 16; 339(3): 167-172. 45 refs. BE58612.
 *assisted suicide; cancer; costs and benefits; *economics; *evaluation; government financing; health care; home care; hospices; hospitals; legal aspects; managed care programs; nursing homes; physicians; *public policy; *social impact; statistics; *terminal care; time factors; personal financing; Medicare; Netherlands; *United States

Emanuel, Linda L. A question of balance. *In:* Emanuel, Linda L., ed. Regulating How We Die: The Ethical, Medical, and Legal Issues Surrounding Physician-Assisted Suicide. Cambridge, MA: Harvard University Press; 1998: 234-260. ISBN 0-674-66654-2. BE58540.
 *active euthanasia; *advance care planning; allowing to die; *assisted suicide; autonomy; compassion; cultural pluralism; decision making; health care delivery; intention; killing; legal rights; medical education; moral obligations; motivation; palliative care; physician's role; physicians; privacy; public policy; religious ethics; suffering; *terminal care; values; wedge argument; withholding treatment; dignity; Netherlands; United States

Emanuel, Linda L. Facing requests for physician-assisted suicide. *JAMA.* 1998 Aug 19; 280(7): 643-647. 50 refs. BE59000.
 advance care planning; artificial feeding; *assisted suicide; autonomy; communication; competence; depressive disorder; family members; food; freedom; goals; guidelines; hospices; legal rights; moral obligations; *palliative care; patients; *physicians; *practice guidelines; referral and consultation; suffering; *terminal care; treatment refusal; withholding treatment; sedatives
Requests for physician-assisted suicide are not a new phenomenon, and many physicians are likely to face this challenging situation. This article proposes for professionals an 8-step approach to respond to requests for physician-assisted suicide. The approach seeks to

identify and treat the root causes of the request and aims to present a plan for consistent application of a set of clinical skills. Justification for the steps requires only 2 noncontentious principles: the patient should be free of unwanted intervention, and the physician is obligated to provide suffering patients with comfort care. Care based on these 2 principles alone does not include physician-assisted suicide. The approach does, however, justify patient refusal of oral intake in specific circumstances. The approach could resolve a majority of requests for physician-assisted suicide and should be tested further for clinical efficacy.

Emmott, David. Physicians, heroes, and palliative care. [Editorial]. *Bioethics Forum.* 1997 Fall; 13(3): 3-4. BE57527.
 attitudes to death; *palliative care; physician patient relationship; *physicians; *terminal care; *terminally ill; values

Fainsinger, Robin L.; Gramlich, Leah M. How often can we justify parenteral nutrition in terminally ill cancer patients? *Journal of Palliative Care.* 1997 Spring; 13(1): 48-51. 21 refs. BE55721.
 allowing to die; *artificial feeding; *cancer; case studies; costs and benefits; decision making; evaluation; home care; *palliative care; patient participation; prolongation of life; quality of life; *risks and benefits; selection for treatment; statistics; *terminal care; *terminally ill; withholding treatment; Canada

Farsides, Bobbie. Palliative care -- a euthanasia-free zone? [Editorial]. *Journal of Medical Ethics.* 1998 Jun; 24(3): 149-150. BE59110.
 *active euthanasia; communication; dissent; goals; health personnel; hospices; legal aspects; moral policy; *palliative care; patients; philosophy; quality of life; *terminal care

Faulkner, Ann. ABC of palliative care: communication with patients, families, and other professionals. *BMJ (British Medical Journal).* 1998 Jan 10; 316(7125): 130-132. 3 refs. BE57753.
 *communication; diagnosis; emotions; empathy; family members; interprofessional relations; palliative care; patient care team; patients; physician patient relationship; *physicians; professional family relationship; prognosis; psychological stress; *terminal care; *terminally ill; *truth disclosure

Felder, Stefan. Costs of dying: alternatives to rationing. *Health Policy.* 1997 Feb; 39(2): 167-176. 21 refs. 3 fn. Published erratum appears in *Health Policy* 1997 Jun; 40(3): 269. BE55605.
 age factors; *aged; biomedical technologies; death; decision making; economic value of life; *economics; family members; *health care; *health insurance; health maintenance organizations; health personnel; incentives; justice; motivation; organ transplantation; prolongation of life; public policy; *resource allocation; risk; *terminal care; terminally ill; *personal financing

Field, Marilyn J.; Cassel, Christine K., eds.; Institute of Medicine. Committee on Care at the End of Life. Approaching Death: Improving Care at the End of Life. [Report]. Washington, DC: National Academy Press; 1997. 437 p. Bibliography: p. 272-311. Appendices include an annotated list of "Examples of initiatives to improve care at the end of life," p. 327-357; outlines and summaries of workshops; and examples of medical education curricula. ISBN 0-309-06372-8. BE57046.
 accountability; advance care planning; advance directives; aged; assisted suicide; attitudes to death; communication; cultural pluralism; drugs; economics; education; evaluation;

BE = bioethics accession number   fn. = footnotes   refs. = references

family members; goals; government financing; guidelines; health care delivery; health services research; home care; hospices; hospitals; human experimentation; institutional policies; nursing homes; organization and administration; pain; *palliative care; patient care team; physician patient relationship; physicians; practice guidelines; prognosis; public participation; *public policy; *quality of health care; *quality of life; regulation; resource allocation; review; suffering; *terminal care; terminally ill; trends; truth disclosure; support groups; Institute of Medicine; Medicaid; Medicare; Patient Self-Determination Act 1990; *United States

Fins, Joseph J. Advance directives and SUPPORT. [Editorial]. *Journal of the American Geriatrics Society.* 1997 Apr; 45(4): 519–520. 23 refs. BE57114.
 *advance care planning; *advance directives; communication; control groups; decision making; economics; *evaluation studies; family members; hospitals; medical records; palliative care; physician patient relationship; physician's role; *research design; resuscitation orders; social impact; *terminal care; treatment refusal; continuity of patient care; *Study to Understand Prognoses and Preferences for Outcomes and Risks of Treatments (SUPPORT)

Gertner, Eric J.; Lukawski, Jolanta E.; Isaacson, Jeanne, et al. Care at the end of life. [Letters and response]. *Annals of Internal Medicine.* 1997 Oct 1; 127(7): 574–575. 5 refs. BE55895.
 advance directives; alternatives; *communication; *decision making; economics; goals; health services research; *palliative care; patient advocacy; patient education; patients; physician patient relationship; physicians; prolongation of life; *quality of health care; *terminal care; values; continuity of patient care; United States

Goldstein, Amy. Dying patients' care varies widely by place, study says. [News]. *Washington Post.* 1997 Oct 15: A1, A8. BE55663.
 aged; allowing to die; biomedical technologies; comparative studies; health care delivery; home care; hospitals; intensive care units; prolongation of life; statistics; *terminal care; *geographic factors; *United States

Goodlin, Sarah J.; Winzelberg, Gary S.; Teno, Joan M., et al. Death in the hospital. *Archives of Internal Medicine.* 1998 Jul 27; 158(14): 1570–1572. 12 refs. BE58808.
 advance directives; biomedical technologies; critically ill; death; diagnosis; drugs; evaluation studies; *hospitals; intensive care units; medical records; pain; palliative care; physical restraint; psychological stress; resuscitation; resuscitation orders; suffering; *terminal care; terminally ill; time factors; ventilators; analgesia; antibiotics; retrospective studies; Mary Hitchcock Memorial Hospital (NH); United States; White River Junction Veterans Affairs Medical Center (VT)
 OBJECTIVE: To examine symptoms and treatments among hospitalized adults in the last 2 days of life. METHODS: Review of 72 consecutive medical records of patients who died at an academic medical center and 32 consecutive medical records of patients who died at an affiliated Veterans Affairs hospital. Medical records were examined for documentation of symptoms, treatment, and orders to limit the use of life-sustaining interventions. RESULTS: The 104 patients who died had an average age of 68.9 years and 70 (68%) were men. The majority had neoplasms or acquired immunodeficiency syndrome, cardiovascular disease, and end-stage lung disease; the remainder died of other acute or chronic illnesses. In the last 2 days of life, pain was noted in 49 patients (46%). Dyspnea (n=53) and restlessness or agitation (n=50) were documented in

51% of the patients. In the last 48 hours of life 12 patients (12%) underwent an attempt at resuscitation, 26 patients (27%) were receiving ventilatory support, and 18% were restrained. Nearly half of the patients (48%) had an order or progress note specifying "comfort measures only" (CMO). Patients with CMO, compared with those without such orders, had similar levels of pain, agitation, and dyspnea. Patients with CMO were less likely to be in an intensive care unit (P=.001), receive ventilatory support (P=.001), receive antibiotics (P=.009), or be weighed (P=.001). CONCLUSIONS: Baseline information with which to begin improvement of care for dying individuals was obtained through a brief retrospective chart review. While patients with CMO receive less aggressive care, no specific process was used to provide comfort care. The evaluation and testing of processes of care for dying patients are necessary to begin the improvement of care. We provide baseline data about processes and outcomes of care in our hospitals.

Gregory, Wilton. The Church and the public discussion of assisted suicide. *Health Progress.* 1997 Mar–Apr; 78(2): 48–50. BE56445.
 active euthanasia; *assisted suicide; attitudes to death; double effect; drugs; extraordinary treatment; pain; physicians; public policy; *Roman Catholic ethics; suffering; *terminal care; theology; treatment refusal; United States

Guroian, Vigen. Life's Living toward Dying: A Theological and Medical–Ethical Study. Grand Rapids, MI: W.B. Eerdmans; 1996. 108 p. 130 fn. ISBN 0-8028-4190-2. BE55682.
 *active euthanasia; *allowing to die; *assisted suicide; *attitudes to death; autonomy; *Christian ethics; Eastern Orthodox ethics; human experimentation; infants; killing; *literature; medicine; morality; physician's role; prolongation of life; religion; right to die; secularism; social impact; suffering; *terminal care; terminally ill; *theology; trends; values; Baby Rena; Kevorkian, Jack

Hammes, Bernard J.; Rooney, Brenda L. Death and end-of-life planning in one midwestern community. *Archives of Internal Medicine.* 1998 Feb 23; 158(4): 383–390. 20 refs. BE57961.
 *advance care planning; *advance directives; aged; allowing to die; artificial feeding; death; *decision making; drugs; education; evaluation studies; family members; health facilities; medical records; palliative care; physicians; quality of life; resuscitation; statistics; survey; *terminal care; treatment refusal; ventilators; withholding treatment; retrospective studies; Wisconsin
 BACKGROUND: The major health care organizations in a geographically defined area implemented an extensive, collaborative advance directive education program approximately 2 years prior to this study. OBJECTIVES: To determine for a geographically defined population the prevalence and type of end-of-life planning and the relationship between end-of-life plans and decisions in all local health care organizations, including hospitals, medical clinics, long-term care facilities, home health agencies, hospices, and the county health department. METHODS: For more than 11 months, end-of-life planning and decisions were retrospectively studied for all adult decedents residing in areas within 5 ZIP codes. These decedents were mentally capable in the 10 years prior to death and died while under the care of the participating health care organizations. Data were collected from medical records and death certificates. Treating physicians and decedent proxies were also contacted for interviews. RESULTS: A total of 540 decedents were included in this study. The prevalence of written advance directives

was 85%. Almost all these documents (95%) were in the decedent's medical record. The median time between advance directive documentation and death was 1.2 years. Almost all advance directive documents requested that treatment be forgone as death neared. Treatment was forgone in 98% of the deaths. Treatment preferences expressed in advance directives seemed to be consistently followed while making end-of-life decisions.
CONCLUSIONS: This study provides a more complete picture of death, end-of-life planning, and decision making in a geographic area where an extensive advance directive education program exists. It indicates that advance planning can be prevalent and can effectively guide end-of-life decisions.

Hanson, Laura C.; Danis, Marion; Garrett, Joanne. What is wrong with end-of-life care? Opinions of bereaved family members. *Journal of the American Geriatrics Society.* 1997 Nov; 45(11): 1339-1344. 30 refs. BE56551.
    aged; *attitudes; communication; death; decision making; *family members; hospices; hospitals; intensive care units; morbidity; nurses; nursing homes; palliative care; physicians; professional family relationship; prolongation of life; *quality of health care; resuscitation; survey; *terminal care; treatment refusal; ventilators; North Carolina

Heilig, Steve; Brody, Robert V. Physician-hastened death and end-of-life care: development of a community-wide consensus statement and guidelines. *Cambridge Quarterly of Healthcare Ethics.* 1998 Spring; 7(2): 223-225. 7 refs. BE57558.
    *assisted suicide; *clinical ethics committees; committee membership; consensus; guidelines; physicians; *practice guidelines; program descriptions; public participation; regional ethics committees; *terminal care; *Bay Area Network of Ethics Committees; San Francisco

Hern, H. Eugene; Koenig, Barbara A.; Moore, Lisa Jean, et al. The difference that culture can make in end-of-life decisionmaking. *Cambridge Quarterly of Healthcare Ethics.* 1998 Winter; 7(1): 27-40. 30 fn. BE58455.
    alternative therapies; anthropology; *Asian Americans; *autonomy; *cancer; case studies; clinical ethics; *communication; *cultural pluralism; *decision making; *diagnosis; disclosure; *family members; family relationship; females; *informed consent; *knowledge, attitudes, practice; *minority groups; models, theoretical; patient care; *patient care team; *patient participation; *patients; *physician patient relationship; physicians; *professional family relationship; *prognosis; risks and benefits; stigmatization; *terminal care; terminally ill; *third party consent; trust; *truth disclosure; *values; California; United States

Hesse, Katherine A. Ethical issues and terminal management of the old old. *Journal of Geriatric Psychiatry.* 1995; 28(1): 75-95. 64 refs. Paper presented at a meeting of the Boston Society for Gerontologic Psychiatry, Inc., "Older, Old People," 30 Oct 1993. BE55558.
    advance directives; *age factors; *aged; *allowing to die; attitudes; autonomy; chronically ill; competence; decision making; dementia; family members; futility; patient participation; physicians; prognosis; prolongation of life; quality of life; refusal to treat; resuscitation; right to die; *terminal care; terminally ill; third party consent; treatment refusal; ventilators; withholding treatment; dignity

Hinohara, Shigeaki. Facing death the Japanese way -- customs and ethos. *In:* Hoshino, Kazumasa, ed. Japanese and Western Bioethics: Studies in Moral Diversity.

Boston, MA: Kluwer Academic; 1997: 145-154. 8 refs. ISBN 0-7923-4112-0. BE57090.
    *attitudes to death; cancer; family members; historical aspects; literature; physicians; religion; terminal care; terminally ill; truth disclosure; *Japan

Hoefler, James M. Managing Death: The First Guide for Patients, Family Members, and Care Providers on Forgoing Treatment at the End of Life. Boulder, CO: Westview Press; 1997. 206 p. Includes references. ISBN 0-8133-2816-0. BE57922.
    advance directives; advisory committees; aged; *allowing to die; artificial feeding; consensus; *decision making; dementia; drugs; economics; extraordinary treatment; family members; futility; guidelines; health personnel; hospices; legal aspects; legal rights; persistent vegetative state; physicians; professional organizations; prolongation of life; Protestant ethics; public opinion; quality of health care; resource allocation; right to die; Roman Catholic ethics; standards; *terminal care; treatment refusal; withholding treatment; antibiotics; dehydration; starvation; In re Fiori; United States

Holstein, Martha. Reflections on death and dying. *Academic Medicine.* 1997 Oct; 72(10): 848-855. 26 refs. BE56617.
    advance directives; *attitudes to death; caring; communication; compassion; dehumanization; empathy; family relationship; home care; hospices; hospitals; literature; medical education; narrative ethics; pain; palliative care; physician patient relationship; physician's role; professional family relationship; quality of health care; suffering; *terminal care; terminally ill; trends; dignity; United States

Huber, Ruth; Evans, Virginia Cox. Trust in physicians to honor death related instructions. *Omega: A Journal of Death and Dying.* 1997-1998; 36(1): 9-21. 39 refs. BE57720.
    *advance directives; age factors; *aged; *allowing to die; assisted suicide; attitudes to death; comparative studies; *decision making; *institutionalized persons; *knowledge, attitudes, practice; *physician patient relationship; *physicians; *prolongation of life; *public opinion; residential facilities; *right to die; survey; *terminal care; treatment refusal; *trust; voluntary euthanasia; Kentucky

Hurley, Ann C.; Volicer, Ladislav; Rempusheski, Veronica F., et al. Reaching consensus: the process of recommending treatment decisions for Alzheimer's patients. *Advances in Nursing Science.* 1995 Dec; 18(2): 33-43. 33 refs. BE57500.
    *advance care planning; aged; allowing to die; caring; competence; consensus; *decision making; *dementia; family members; hospices; models, theoretical; *nurse's role; *nurses; nursing education; *palliative care; *patient care; patient care team; professional family relationship; survey; *terminal care; third party consent; time factors; trust; withholding treatment; qualitative research

Jacobson, Jay A.; Francis, L.P.; Battin, Margaret P., et al. Dialogue to action: lessons learned from some family members of deceased patients at an interactive program in seven Utah hospitals. *Journal of Clinical Ethics.* 1997 Winter; 8(4): 359-371. 12 fn. BE57609.
    advance directives; allowing to die; *attitudes; autopsies; *clinical ethics committees; *communication; death; decision making; diagnosis; education; ethicist's role; *evaluation; *family members; health personnel; *hospitals; information dissemination; *institutional policies; pain; palliative care; *professional family relationship; prognosis; program descriptions; prolongation of life; *public participation; quality of health care; resuscitation; survey; *terminal care; truth disclosure; *Dialogue to Action (LDS Hospital, Salt Lake City, UT); Utah
Dialogue to Action is a program we developed to

establish a link between hospital ethics committees (HECs) and the public. We began Dialogue to Action in 1995 as a pilot program to consider how ethics committees should define their role. We described the format of this program and the results from the first Dialogue to Action in another publication. Now, the program has been completed at seven Utah hospitals, which has enabled us to validate the findings from the first program and learn substantially more information. In this article, we make our findings and methods available to others in the hope that they will benefit by using Dialogue to Action as a model for other programs.

Johnson, Linda; Potter, Robert Lyman. Professional and public community projects for developing medical futility guidelines. *In:* Zucker, Marjorie B.; Zucker, Howard D., eds. Medical Futility and the Evaluation of Life–Sustaining Interventions. New York, NY: Cambridge University Press; 1997: 155–167. 5 refs. ISBN 0–521–56877–3. BE55987.

advance directives; *allowing to die; clinical ethics committees; communication; consensus; cultural pluralism; *decision making; democracy; education; family members; *futility; goals; *guidelines; home care; hospices; *hospitals; *institutional policies; intensive care units; nursing homes; *organizational policies; *palliative care; patients; physicians; *program descriptions; *public participation; *public policy; refusal to treat; resource allocation; standards; *terminal care; terminally ill; terminology; withholding treatment; *community policies; Citywide Task Force on Medical Futility (Houston, TX); Collaborative Bioethics Working Group (Akron, OH); Colorado Collective for Medical Decisions; Extreme Care: Humane Options (ECHO) (Sacramento, CA); Guidelines for the Responsible Utilization of Intensive Care (Appleton, WI); Minnesota Center for Health Care Ethics; North Carolina Consortium to Set Limits in Medicine; Santa Monica UCLA Medical Center; Study to Understand Prognoses and Preferences for Outcomes and Risks of Treatments (SUPPORT); United States

Kelly, Brian J.; Varghese, Francis T. Assisted suicide and euthanasia: what about the clinical issues? *Australian and New Zealand Journal of Psychiatry.* 1996 Feb; 30(1): 3–8. 34 refs. BE56870.

*active euthanasia; AIDS; *assisted suicide; autonomy; depressive disorder; medical education; mentally ill; palliative care; physician patient relationship; psychiatric diagnosis; psychiatry; quality of life; suffering; suicide; *terminal care; terminally ill; grief

Kelly, David F. Alternatives to physician–assisted suicide. *American Journal of Otolaryngology.* 1995 May–Jun; 16(3): 181–185. BE56211.

active euthanasia; *allowing to die; *assisted suicide; drugs; economics; killing; legal aspects; morality; pain; *palliative care; public policy; Roman Catholic ethics; *terminal care; terminally ill; treatment refusal; voluntary euthanasia; wedge argument; withholding treatment; analgesia; United States

Kimura, Rihito. Death, dying, and advance directives in Japan: sociocultural and legal points of view. *In:* Sass, Hans–Martin; Veatch, Robert M.; Kimura, Rihito, eds. Advance Directives and Surrogate Decision Making in Health Care: United States, Germany, and Japan. Baltimore, MD: Johns Hopkins University Press; 1998: 187–208. 29 refs. ISBN 0–8018–5831–3. BE59042.

*active euthanasia; *advance directives; *allowing to die; assisted suicide; attitudes; *attitudes to death; cancer; common good; criminal law; decision making; diagnosis; drugs; family members; *family relationship; historical aspects; *legal aspects; living wills; model legislation; national health insurance; organ donation; organizational policies; pain; palliative care; paternalism; patient advocacy;

physician patient relationship; physicians; professional organizations; prognosis; prolongation of life; public opinion; *public policy; resuscitation orders; social dominance; *terminal care; terminally ill; third party consent; trends; trust; truth disclosure; *values; voluntary euthanasia; withholding treatment; oral directives; *Japan; Japan Medical Association; Japan Science Council; Japanese Society for Dying with Dignity

Koffman, Jonathan. There must be a better way. [Personal view]. *BMJ (British Medical Journal).* 1998 Jun 27; 316(7149): 1989–1990. BE58835.

*aged; attitudes to death; biomedical technologies; case studies; chronically ill; injuries; *palliative care; physicians; *prolongation of life; *suffering; *terminal care; *terminally ill

Koval, Joseph C.; Rousseau, Paul; Coulehan, Jack. The man with stars inside. [Letter and response]. *Annals of Internal Medicine.* 1997 Dec 15; 127(12): 1137–1138. 6 refs. BE58214.

*assisted suicide; communication; empathy; medical education; pain; *palliative care; physician patient relationship; physicians; psychological stress; suffering; *terminal care; *terminally ill; patient abandonment

Kuhse, Helga. Caring: Nurses, Women and Ethics. Malden, MA: Blackwell; 1997. 296 p. Bibliography: p. 263–285. ISBN 0–631–20211–0. BE58546.

allowing to die; autonomy; *caring; *decision making; ethical theory; *females; *feminist ethics; *justice; males; metaphor; moral development; nurse patient relationship; *nurse's role; nurses; *nursing ethics; palliative care; patient advocacy; patient care; *physician nurse relationship; physicians; professional autonomy; public policy; resuscitation orders; social dominance; *terminal care; terminally ill; truth disclosure; voluntary euthanasia; whistleblowing; withholding treatment; Cox, Nigel

Kuuppelomäki, Merja; Lauri, Sirkka. Ethical dilemmas in the care of patients with incurable cancer. *Nursing Ethics.* 1998 Jul; 5(4): 283–293. 24 refs. BE58868.

age factors; aged; artificial feeding; blood transfusions; *cancer; communication; decision making; *diagnosis; drugs; emotions; family members; hospitals; *knowledge, attitudes, practice; *nurses; pain; palliative care; patient care; *patient satisfaction; *patients; physician nurse relationship; physician patient relationship; *physicians; privacy; *prognosis; quality of health care; suffering; survey; *terminal care; *terminally ill; *truth disclosure; withholding treatment; antibiotics; chemotherapy; morphine; qualitative research; Finland

Lafrance, W. André; Singer, Peter A. Is it ethical to forgo treatment? [Letter and response]. *Canadian Medical Association Journal.* 1997 Dec 15; 157(12): 1740–1741. 1 ref. BE59053.

active euthanasia; *allowing to die; artificial feeding; assisted suicide; extraordinary treatment; *palliative care; quality of health care; *terminal care; *withholding treatment; Canada

Lynn, Joanne; Cohn, Felicia; Pickering, John H., et al.; American Geriatrics Society. American Geriatrics Society on physician–assisted suicide: brief to the United States Supreme Court. *Journal of the American Geriatrics Society.* 1997 Apr; 45(4): 489–499. 70 fn. Background and brief of the American Geriatrics Society as amicus curiae urging reversal of the judgments below: Vacco v. Quill, No. 95–1858, and Washington v. Glucksberg, No. 96–110. BE57117.

*aged; allowing to die; *assisted suicide; chronically ill; coercion; competence; constitutional law; economics; government regulation; killing; *legal aspects; legal rights; moral complicity; obligations of society; *organizational policies; *palliative care; *physicians; *professional organizations; prognosis; *public policy; *quality of health

---

care; resource allocation; social impact; suffering; Supreme Court decisions; *terminal care; terminally ill; treatment refusal; uncertainty; withholding treatment; *geriatrics; *American Geriatrics Society; *United States; *Vacco v. Quill; *Washington v. Glucksberg

Lynn, Joanne; Wilkinson, Anne; Cohn, Felicia, et al. Capitated risk-bearing managed care systems could improve end-of-life care. *Journal of the American Geriatrics Society.* 1998 Mar; 46(3): 322–330. 46 refs. Paper presented at the 1996 Congress of Clinical Societies. BE56765.
    age factors; cancer; *chronically ill; critically ill; diagnosis; *economics; health care reform; health maintenance organizations; hospices; *managed care programs; morbidity; organization and administration; palliative care; patient advocacy; physicians; prognosis; *quality of health care; risk; selection for treatment; *terminal care; *terminally ill; trends; *capitation fee; *comprehensive health care; Medicare; Study to Understand Prognoses and Preferences for Outcomes and Risks of Treatments (SUPPORT); United States

Lynn, Joanne. Legal and ethical issues in palliative health care. *Seminars in Oncology.* 1985 Dec; 12(4): 476–481. 24 refs. BE56952.
    advance directives; allowing to die; artificial feeding; autonomy; *cancer; communication; competence; *decision making; economics; family members; futility; goals; home care; hospices; hospitals; informed consent; legal aspects; legal guardians; *palliative care; physicians; professional competence; quality of health care; quality of life; resuscitation orders; *terminal care; *terminally ill; third party consent; values; withholding treatment; United States

Lynn, Joanne. Measuring Quality of Care at the End of Life: A Statement of Principles. *Journal of the American Geriatrics Society.* 1997 Apr; 45(4): 526–527. Signed by the Alzheimer's Association; American Academy of Hospice and Palliative Medicine; American Association of Critical-Care Nurses; American Association of Retired Persons; American Cancer Society; American College of Physicians; American Geriatrics Society; American Hospice Foundation; American Institute of Life-Threatening Illness and Loss; American Medical Association; American Nurses Association; American Pain Society; American Foundation for Suicide Prevention and others. BE57112.
    advance care planning; evaluation; family members; health services research; *organizational policies; *professional organizations; *quality of health care; quality of life; *standards; *terminal care; terminally ill; United States

McGann, John R. To care for the dying. *Origins.* 1997 Mar 20; 26(39): 640–648. 99 fn. Text of a pastoral letter, "Comfort my people: finding peace as life ends," by Bishop John R. McGann of Rockville Centre, NY, 19 Feb 1997. BE56596.
    active euthanasia; *allowing to die; *assisted suicide; attitudes to death; biomedical technologies; clergy; coercion; compassion; depressive disorder; double effect; drugs; economics; emotions; family members; government regulation; health care; health personnel; hospices; intention; love; pain; *palliative care; pastoral care; patients; physician patient relationship; physician's role; physicians; prolongation of life; psychological stress; *Roman Catholic ethics; social interaction; suffering; *terminal care; terminally ill; trust; vulnerable populations; withholding treatment; dignity; United States

McLean, Sheila A.M., ed. Death, Dying and the Law. Brookfield, VT: Dartmouth; 1996. 185 p. (Medico-legal series). 531 fn. ISBN 1-85521-657-4. BE57209.
    *active euthanasia; *advance directives; *allowing to die;

*assisted suicide; competence; decision making; disabled; futility; international aspects; legal aspects; palliative care; persistent vegetative state; *physicians; prognosis; public policy; resource allocation; suffering; *terminal care; treatment refusal; *voluntary euthanasia; withholding treatment; Airedale NHS Trust v. Bland; Death with Dignity Act (OR); *Great Britain; Netherlands; United States

Manni, Corrado. Palliative medicine and Christian eschatology. *Dolentium Hominum: Church and Health in the World.* 1996; 31(11th Yr., No. 1): 173–177. 13 refs. BE57371.
    active euthanasia; attitudes to death; caring; economics; family members; *moral obligations; *obligations of society; pain; *palliative care; physician patient relationship; *physicians; professional competence; prolongation of life; quality of life; *Roman Catholic ethics; self concept; suffering; *terminal care; *terminally ill; trust; vulnerable populations; *patient abandonment

Matthews, Merrill. Would physician-assisted suicide save the healthcare system money? (Or, is Jack Kevorkian doing all of us a favor?). *In:* Battin, Margaret P.; Rhodes, Rosamond; Silvers, Anita, eds. Physician Assisted Suicide: Expanding the Debate. New York, NY: Routledge; 1998: 312–322. 24 fn. ISBN 0-415-92003-5. BE58796.
    age factors; *assisted suicide; *economics; government financing; guidelines; health care delivery; managed care programs; *physicians; public policy; resource allocation; *social impact; statistics; *terminal care; time factors; Medicaid; Medicare; Netherlands; *United States

Miller, Franklin G.; Meier, Diane E. Voluntary death: a comparison of terminal dehydration and physician-assisted suicide. *Annals of Internal Medicine.* 1998 Apr 1; 128(7): 559–562. 29 refs. BE57327.
    *alternatives; *artificial feeding; *assisted suicide; attitudes; autonomy; comparative studies; competence; decision making; family members; *food; legal aspects; palliative care; physicians; psychological stress; public policy; *terminal care; terminally ill; time factors; treatment refusal; *withholding treatment; *dehydration; integrity

Miller, Patrick. Struggle. [Personal narrative]. *Bioethics Forum.* 1997 Spring; 13(1): 41–45. 7 refs. BE55884.
    advance care planning; aged; allowing to die; attitudes to death; caring; case studies; communication; compassion; competence; decision making; dementia; empathy; family members; nursing homes; palliative care; physician patient relationship; physicians; prognosis; prolongation of life; *terminal care; third party consent; truth disclosure; uncertainty

Mount, Balfour. Morphine drips, terminal sedation, and slow euthanasia: definitions and facts, not anecdotes. [Commentary]. *Journal of Palliative Care.* 1996 Winter; 12(4): 31–37. 27 refs. Commentary on J.A. Billings and S.D. Block, p. 21–30. BE55729.
    *active euthanasia; attitudes; case studies; *double effect; *drugs; empirical research; hospices; *intention; killing; pain; *palliative care; physicians; psychological stress; suffering; *terminal care; *terminally ill; time factors; *morphine; *sedatives

Murphy, Donald J. The economics of futile interventions. *In:* Zucker, Marjorie B.; Zucker, Howard D., eds. Medical Futility and the Evaluation of Life-Sustaining Interventions. New York, NY: Cambridge University Press; 1997: 123–135. 37 refs. ISBN 0-521-56877-3. BE55985.
    advance directives; *age factors; aged; *biomedical technologies; *chronically ill; *common good; *costs and

---

benefits; *critically ill; dementia; *economics; *futility; home care; hospices; *intensive care units; mortality; *palliative care; persistent vegetative state; prognosis; *prolongation of life; refusal to treat; *resource allocation; *selection for treatment; self induced illness; *social impact; *terminal care; *terminally ill; time factors; treatment outcome; treatment refusal; trends; uncertainty; *values; *health services misuse; Study to Understand Prognoses and Preferences for Outcomes and Risks of Treatments (SUPPORT); United States

National Council for Hospice and Specialist Palliative Care Services. Voluntary euthanasia: the Council's view. *Nursing Ethics.* 1998 Jul; 5(4): 371–374. 3 refs. 2 fn. Approved by the Council 17 Jul 1997. BE58874.
    advance directives; allowing to die; double effect; drugs; hospices; *organizational policies; *palliative care; public policy; *terminal care; treatment refusal; *voluntary euthanasia; Great Britain; House of Lords Select Committee on Medical Ethics; *National Council for Hospice and Specialist Palliative Care Services (Great Britain)

Neuberger, Julia. Death on camera. [Medicine and the media]. *BMJ (British Medical Journal).* 1998 Apr 4; 316(7137): 1100. BE58242.
    allowing to die; *attitudes to death; *death; famous persons; *mass media; privacy; terminal care; grief; Great Britain

Norris, Patrick F. Palliative care and killing: understanding ethical distinctions. *Bioethics Forum.* 1997 Fall; 13(3): 25–30. 6 refs. 1 fn. BE57529.
    *active euthanasia; *allowing to die; *assisted suicide; *double effect; drugs; *intention; *killing; moral policy; pain; *palliative care; suicide; *terminal care; terminally ill; withholding treatment; sedatives

Orentlicher, David. The Supreme Court and physician-assisted suicide -- rejecting assisted suicide but embracing euthanasia. *New England Journal of Medicine.* 1997 Oct 23; 337(17): 1236–1239. 19 refs. BE55800.
    *active euthanasia; artificial feeding; *assisted suicide; constitutional law; double effect; *drugs; intention; involuntary euthanasia; *legal aspects; *legal rights; pain; *palliative care; *physicians; right to die; suffering; *Supreme Court decisions; *terminal care; *terminally ill; wedge argument; withholding treatment; coma; *sedatives; *United States; *Vacco v. Quill; *Washington v. Glucksberg

Osuna, Eduardo; Pérez-Cárceles, Maria D.; Esteban, Miguel A., et al. The right to information for the terminally ill patient. *Journal of Medical Ethics.* 1998 Apr; 24(2): 106–109. 19 refs. BE58080.
    family members; home care; hospitals; *nurses; patient care team; *physicians; *prognosis; survey; *terminal care; *terminally ill; *truth disclosure; *Spain
    OBJECTIVES: To analyse the attitudes of medical personnel towards terminally ill patients and their right to be fully informed. DESIGN: Self-administered questionnaire composed of 56 closed questions. SETTING: Three general hospitals and eleven health centres in Granada (Spain). The sample comprised 168 doctors and 207 nurses. RESULTS: A high percentage of medical personnel (24.1%) do not think that informing the terminally ill would help them face their illness with greater serenity. Eighty-four per cent think the patient's own home is the best place to die: 8.9% of the subjects questioned state that the would not like to be informed of an incurable illness. CONCLUSION: In our opinion any information given should depend on the patient's personality, the stage of the illness and family circumstances. Our study confirms that a hospital is not the ideal environment for attending to the needs of the

terminally ill and their families.

Pace, Nicholas A. Law and ethics at the end of life: the practitioner's view. *In:* McLean, Sheila A.M., ed. Death, Dying and the Law. Brookfield, VT: Dartmouth; 1996: 3–18. 44 fn. ISBN 1-85521-657-4. BE57210.
    advance directives; aged; *allowing to die; autonomy; case studies; competence; *decision making; double effect; drugs; emergency care; extraordinary treatment; family members; futility; intensive care units; intention; international aspects; legal aspects; physicians; prognosis; quality of life; resource allocation; risks and benefits; Roman Catholic ethics; *terminal care; terminally ill; third party consent; withholding treatment; *Great Britain; United States

Pang, Mei-che Samantha. Information disclosure: the moral experience of nurses in China. *Nursing Ethics.* 1998 Jul; 5(4): 347–361. 64 refs. BE58873.
    active euthanasia; autonomy; beneficence; cancer; codes of ethics; compassion; conscience; *decision making; diagnosis; *disclosure; *family members; historical aspects; hospitals; *informed consent; *knowledge, attitudes, practice; literature; medical ethics; moral obligations; nurse patient relationship; *nurses; *nursing ethics; nursing research; paternalism; patient advocacy; patient care; patients' rights; physician nurse relationship; professional family relationship; *prognosis; survey; *terminal care; terminally ill; *third party consent; *truth disclosure; virtues; qualitative research; *China; Hong Kong

Paris, John J.; Muir, J. Cameron; Reardon, Frank E. Ethical and legal issues in intensive care. *Journal of Intensive Care Medicine.* 1997 Nov–Dec; 12(6): 298–309. 98 refs. BE58495.
    allowing to die; anencephaly; assisted suicide; autonomy; brain death; clinical ethics committees; *critically ill; *decision making; determination of death; dissent; family members; futility; guidelines; hospitals; infants; institutional policies; *intensive care units; judicial action; managed care programs; pain; patient care; physicians; prognosis; prolongation of life; quality of health care; quality of life; resuscitation orders; risks and benefits; surgery; *terminal care; terminally ill; treatment refusal; withholding treatment; seriously ill; Study to Understand Prognoses and Preferences for Outcomes and Risks of Treatments (SUPPORT); United States

Parkash, Ravi; Burge, Frederick. The family's perspective on issues of hydration in terminal care. *Journal of Palliative Care.* 1997 Winter; 13(4): 23–27. 16 refs. BE58823.
    *allowing to die; *artificial feeding; *attitudes; cancer; decision making; emotions; *family members; *palliative care; risks and benefits; suffering; survey; *terminal care; terminally ill; values; withholding treatment; *dehydration; qualitative research; Nova Scotia

Pellegrino, Edmund D. Emerging ethical issues in palliative care. [Contempo 1998]. *JAMA.* 1998 May 20; 279(19): 1521–1522. 25 refs. BE58424.
    accountability; *alternative therapies; autonomy; cancer; chronically ill; double effect; drugs; informed consent; intention; medical specialties; *pain; *palliative care; patient care team; prognosis; suffering; *terminal care; terminally ill; truth disclosure; analgesia; incurably ill; narcotics

Portenoy, Russell K. Morphine infusions at the end of life: the pitfalls in reasoning from anecdote. [Commentary]. *Journal of Palliative Care.* 1996 Winter; 12(4): 44–46. 12 refs. Commentary on J.A. Billings and S.D. Block, p. 21–30. BE55731.
    *active euthanasia; assisted suicide; attitudes; *double effect; *drugs; empirical research; intention; killing; *palliative care; physicians; suffering; *terminal care; terminally ill; *morphine; sedatives

---

BE = bioethics accession number   fn. = footnotes   refs. = references

Post, Linda Farber; Dubler, Nancy Neveloff. Palliative care: a bioethical definition, principles, and clinical guidelines. *Bioethics Forum.* 1997 Fall; 13(3): 17–24. 15 refs. BE57530.

artificial feeding; caring; communication; decision making; education; family members; *guidelines; health personnel; hospitals; institutional policies; moral obligations; pain; *palliative care; *practice guidelines; professional patient relationship; renal dialysis; technical expertise; *terminal care; terminally ill; terminology; truth disclosure; ventilators; withholding treatment; *Montefiore Medical Center (New York City)

Quill, Timothy E.; Kimsma, Gerrit. End–of–life care in the Netherlands and the United States: a comparison of values, justifications, and practices. *Cambridge Quarterly of Healthcare Ethics.* 1997 Spring; 6(2): 189–204. 127 fn. BE56476.

*allowing to die; *assisted suicide; autonomy; case studies; common good; comparative studies; competence; consensus; decision making; dissent; double effect; drugs; freedom; government regulation; guidelines; health care delivery; hospices; intention; *international aspects; *knowledge, attitudes, practice; legal aspects; mass media; obligations of society; *palliative care; physician patient relationship; *physicians; policy analysis; public opinion; *public policy; social control; socioeconomic factors; statistics; *suffering; *terminal care; *values; *voluntary euthanasia; *Netherlands; *United States

Voluntary active euthanasia (VAE) and physician–assisted suicide (PAS) remain technically illegal in the Netherlands, but the practices are openly tolerated provided that physicians adhere to carefully constructed guidelines. Harsh criticism of the Dutch practice by authors in the United States and Great Britain has made achieving a balanced understanding of its clinical, moral, and policy implications very difficult. Similar practice patterns probably exist in the United States, but they are conducted in secret because of a more uncertain legal and ethical climate. In this manuscript, we plan to compare end–of–life care in the United States and the Netherlands with regard to underlying values, justifications, and practices. We will explore the risks and benefits of each system for a real patient who was faced with a common end–of–life clinical dilemma, and close with challenges for public policies in both countries.

Quill, Timothy E.; Lo, Bernard; Brock, Dan W. Palliative options of last resort: a comparison of voluntarily stopping eating and drinking, terminal sedation, physician–assisted suicide, and voluntary active euthanasia. *JAMA.* 1997 Dec 17; 278(23): 2099–2104. 70 refs. BE56434.

*active euthanasia; *allowing to die; artificial feeding; *assisted suicide; autonomy; beneficence; chronically ill; comparative studies; competence; conscience; diagnosis; double effect; *drugs; ethical analysis; family members; food; guidelines; informed consent; intention; legal aspects; *moral policy; pain; *palliative care; physician's role; physicians; prognosis; *public policy; suffering; *terminal care; terminally ill; treatment refusal; *voluntary euthanasia; *sedatives; United States

Palliative care is generally agreed to be the standard of care for the dying, but there remain some patients for whom intolerable suffering persists. In the face of ethical and legal controversy about the acceptability of physician–assisted suicide and voluntary active euthanasia, voluntarily stopping eating and drinking and terminal sedation have been proposed as ethically superior responses of last resort that do not require changes in professional standards or the law. The clinical and ethical differences and similarities between these 4

practices are critically compared in light of the doctrine of double effect, the active/passive distinction, patient voluntariness, proportionality between risks and benefits, and the physician's potential conflict of duties. Terminal sedation and voluntarily stopping eating and drinking would allow clinicians to remain responsive to a wide range of patient suffering, but they are ethically and clinically more complex and closer to physician–assisted suicide and voluntary active euthanasia than is ordinarily acknowledged. Safeguards are presented for any medical action that may hasten death, including determining that palliative care is ineffective, obtaining informed consent, ensuring diagnostic and prognostic clarity, obtaining an independent second opinion, and implementing reporting and monitoring processes. Explicit public policy about which of these practices are permissible would reassure the many patients who fear a bad death in their future and allow for a predictable response for the few whose suffering becomes intolerable in spite of optimal palliative care.

Quill, Timothy E.; Meier, Diane E.; Block, Susan D., et al. The debate over physician–assisted suicide: empirical data and convergent views. *Annals of Internal Medicine.* 1998 Apr 1; 128(7): 552–558. 100 refs. BE57329.

allowing to die; *alternatives; *assisted suicide; conscience; consensus; depressive disorder; empirical research; food; health insurance; hospices; knowledge, attitudes, practice; legal aspects; motivation; pain; *palliative care; patients' rights; *physicians; public opinion; public policy; quality of health care; quality of life; standards; suffering; *terminal care; terminally ill; treatment refusal; withholding treatment; sedatives; United States

Quill, Timothy E.; Dresser, Rebecca; Brock, Dan W. The rule of double effect — a critique of its role in end–of–life decision making. *New England Journal of Medicine.* 1997 Dec 11; 337(24): 1768–1771. 42 refs. BE56475.

allowing to die; assisted suicide; autonomy; criminal law; cultural pluralism; *decision making; *double effect; drugs; informed consent; *intention; killing; legal liability; *moral policy; pain; *palliative care; physicians; suffering; *terminal care; terminally ill; treatment refusal; voluntary euthanasia; withholding treatment; narcotics; sedatives; United States

Reitman, James S. The debate on assisted suicide — redefining morally appropriate care for people with intractable suffering. *Issues in Law and Medicine.* 1995 Winter; 11(3): 299–329. 118 fn. BE58821.

accountability; allowing to die; *assisted suicide; autonomy; caring; Christian ethics; compassion; competence; decision making; empathy; ethics consultation; hospices; moral policy; *palliative care; patient advocacy; *physically disabled; physician patient relationship; physician's role; *physicians; psychological stress; *religious ethics; *suffering; *terminal care; *terminally ill; value of life; dignity; hope; rationality

Rich, Ben A. A legacy of silence: bioethics and the culture of pain. *Journal of Medical Humanities.* 1997 Winter; 18(4): 233–259. 47 refs. BE57245.

assisted suicide; attitudes; bioethical issues; *bioethics; cancer; chronically ill; clinical ethics; drug abuse; drugs; ethical analysis; ethicists; goals; government regulation; historical aspects; hospices; legal aspects; medical education; medical ethics; medicine; moral obligations; morality; *pain; *palliative care; *patient care; physicians; quality of health care; review; self regulation; standards; state government; *suffering; technical expertise; *terminal care; terminally ill; Study to Understand Prognoses and Preferences for Outcomes and Risks of Treatments (SUPPORT); United States

BE = bioethics accession number   fn. = footnotes   refs. = references

For over 20 years the medical literature has carefully documented the undertreatment of all types of pain by physicians. During this same period, as the field of bioethics came of age, the phenomenon of undertreated pain received almost no attention from the bioethics literature. This article takes bioethicists to task for failing to recognize the undertreatment of pain as a major ethical, and not merely a clinical, failing of the medical profession. The nature and extent of the problem of undertreated pain is examined, as well as possible reasons for its disregard by bioethicists. The factors contributing to undertreated pain in the clinical setting are considered, as well as the hazards posed by recent failures to address ethically questionable clinical practices. Finally, suggestions are offered for refocusing the attention of bioethicists to this significant problem.

Rich, Ben A. Advance directives: the next generation. *Journal of Legal Medicine.* 1998 Mar; 19(1): 63–97. 100 fn. BE58900.
    *advance care planning; *advance directives; allowing to die; artificial feeding; attitudes to death; autonomy; communication; *decision making; evaluation; forms; informed consent; judicial action; *legal aspects; legislation; living wills; palliative care; physician's role; *physicians; review; *terminal care; third party consent; treatment refusal; uncertainty; oral directives; values histories; Patient Self-Determination Act 1990; Study to Understand Prognoses and Preferences for Outcomes and Risks of Treatments (SUPPORT); United States

Rosin, Arnold J.; Sonnenblick, Moshe. Autonomy and paternalism in geriatric medicine: the Jewish ethical approach to issues of feeding terminally ill patients, and to cardiopulmonary resuscitation. *Journal of Medical Ethics.* 1998 Feb; 24(1): 44–48. 45 refs. BE57409.
    *aged; *allowing to die; *artificial feeding; attitudes; *autonomy; decision making; *dementia; family members; futility; *Jewish ethics; palliative care; *paternalism; physicians; prognosis; *prolongation of life; religious hospitals; resuscitation; *resuscitation orders; risks and benefits; suffering; *terminal care; *terminally ill; treatment outcome; treatment refusal; *value of life; withholding treatment; *Israel; Orthodox Judaism; Shaare Zedek Medical Center (Jerusalem)
Respecting and encouraging autonomy in the elderly is basic to the practice of geriatrics. In this paper, we examine the practice of cardiopulmonary resuscitation (CPR) and "artificial" feeding in a geriatric unit in a general hospital subscribing to Jewish orthodox religious principles, in which the sanctity of life is a fundamental ethical guideline. The literature on the administration of food and water in terminal stages of illness, including dementia, still shows division of opinion on the morality of withdrawing nutrition. We uphold the principle that as long as feeding by naso-gastric (N–G) or percutaneous endoscopic gastrostomy (PEG) does not constitute undue danger or arouse serious opposition it should be given, without causing suffering to the patient. This is part of basic care, and the doctor has no mandate to withdraw this. The question of CPR still shows much discrepancy regarding elderly patients' wishes, and doctors' opinions about its worthwhileness, although up to 10 percent survive. Our geriatric patients rarely discuss the subject, but it is openly ventilated with families who ask about it, who are then involved in the decision-making, and the decision about CPR or "do-not-resuscitate" (DNR) is based on clinical and prognostic considerations.

Rudberg, Mark A.; Teno, Joan M.; Lynn, Joanne; American Geriatrics Society. Ethics Committee.

Developing and implementing measures of quality of care at the end of life: a call for action. *Journal of the American Geriatrics Society.* 1997 Apr; 45(4): 528–530. 2 refs. BE57121.
    health services research; *quality of health care; standards; *terminal care; American Geriatrics Society; Measuring Quality of Care at the End of Life: A Statement of Principles; United States

Rye, Patricia D.; Wallston, Kenneth A.; Wallston, Barbara Strudler, et al. The desire to control terminal health care and attitudes toward living wills. *American Journal of Preventive Medicine.* 1985 May–Jun; 1(3): 56–60. 14 refs. BE56749.
    *adults; *attitudes; *autonomy; decision making; intention; *living wills; patients; survey; *terminal care; Tennessee

Skolnick, Andrew A. End-of-life care movement growing. *JAMA.* 1997 Sep 24; 278(12): 967–969. BE55774.
    advance care planning; attitudes; *continuing education; curriculum; *medical education; palliative care; patient advocacy; physicians; professional organizations; *program descriptions; quality of health care; teaching methods; *terminal care; American Institute of Life-Threatening Diseases; American Medical Association; Education for Physicians on End-of-Life Care (EPEC) Project; Health Decisions America; Last Acts: Care and Caring at the End of Life Initiative; United States

Skolnick, Andrew A. MediCaring Project to demonstrate, evaluate innovative end-of-life program for chronically ill. [News]. *JAMA.* 1998 May 20; 279(19): 1511–1512. BE58427.
    cancer; *chronically ill; dementia; economics; government financing; health care delivery; heart diseases; hospices; palliative care; prognosis; *terminal care; terminally ill; cerebrovascular disorders; continuity of patient care; lung diseases; severity of illness index; Medicare; *MediCaring; *United States

Smith, Anthony M.; Edmonds, Polly; Davies, Andrew, et al. More openness needed in palliative care. [Letters]. *BMJ (British Medical Journal).* 1998 Jan 31; 316(7128): 390–391. 6 refs. BE57801.
    *active euthanasia; *double effect; drugs; *intention; *palliative care; physicians; quality of life; *terminal care; Great Britain

Smith, Thomas J.; Swisher, Karen. Telling the truth about terminal cancer. [Editorial]. *JAMA.* 1998 Jun 3; 279(21): 1746–1748. 28 refs. BE58429.
    allowing to die; attitudes; autonomy; *cancer; communication; *decision making; drugs; informed consent; mortality; *palliative care; patient participation; patients; physicians; *prognosis; *prolongation of life; risks and benefits; *terminal care; *terminally ill; treatment outcome; *truth disclosure; Study to Understand Prognoses and Preferences for Outcomes and Risks of Treatments (SUPPORT)

Steinberg, M.A.; Parker, M.H.; Cartwright, C.M., et al. End-of-Life Decision-Making: Perspectives of General Practitioners and Patients. Report to the General Practice Evaluation Programme of the Department of Human Services and Health. Brisbane, QLD: University of Queensland Medical School, Department of Social and Preventive Medicine; 1996 Jul. 1 v. Bibliography: p. 128–130. BE58984.
    active euthanasia; advance directives; allowing to die; assisted suicide; *attitudes; autonomy; communication; comparative studies; decision making; family practice; home care; hospices; hospitals; legal aspects; pain; palliative care; patient participation; *patients; *physicians; religion; rights;

BE = bioethics accession number   fn. = footnotes   refs. = references

survey; *terminal care; terminally ill; third party consent; Australia; *Queensland

Steinberg, M.A.; Cartwright, C.M.; Najman, J., et al. Healthy Ageing, Healthy Dying: Community and Health Professional Perspectives on End-of-Life Decision-Making. Report to the Research and Development Grants Advisory Committee of the Department of Human Services and Health. Brisbane, QLD: University of Queensland Medical School, Department of Social and Preventive Medicine; 1996 Feb. 116 p. Bibliography: p.114–116. BE58985.
   active euthanasia; administrators; advance directives; allowing to die; assisted suicide; *attitudes; autonomy; comparative studies; decision making; *health personnel; home care; hospices; hospitals; legal aspects; nurses; nursing homes; pain; palliative care; persistent vegetative state; physicians; *public opinion; religion; resource allocation; resuscitation orders; rights; survey; *terminal care; terminally ill; third party consent; Australia; *Queensland

Steinberg, M.A.; Cartwright, C.M.; MacDonald, S.M., et al. Self-determination in terminal care: a comparison of GP and community members' responses. *Australian Family Physician.* 1997 Jun; 26(6): 703–705, 707. 11 refs. 8 fn. BE57552.
   *advance directives; age factors; *attitudes; autonomy; comparative studies; decision making; home care; hospices; hospitals; legal aspects; patient participation; *physicians; *public opinion; survey; *terminal care; Australia; *Queensland

Sullivan, Mark; Rapp, Suzanne; Fitzgibbon, Dermot, et al. Pain and the choice to hasten death in patients with painful metastatic cancer. *Journal of Palliative Care.* 1997 Autumn; 13(3): 18–28. 34 refs. BE58070.
   *active euthanasia; *allowing to die; artificial feeding; *assisted suicide; *attitudes; *cancer; depressive disorder; double effect; drugs; hospitals; living wills; *pain; *palliative care; *patients; physicians; *quality of life; resuscitation orders; right to die; suicide; survey; *terminal care; *terminally ill; treatment refusal; values; voluntary euthanasia; withholding treatment; analgesia; outpatients; United States; University of Washington Medical Center

Sulmasy, Daniel P.; Marx, Eric S. A computerized system for entering orders to limit treatment: implementation and evaluation. *Journal of Clinical Ethics.* 1997 Fall; 8(3): 258–263. 21 fn. BE57568.
   advance directives; allowing to die; artificial feeding; attitudes; *computers; critically ill; *decision making; drugs; evaluation studies; health insurance; hospices; hospitals; *institutional policies; *intensive care units; internship and residency; morbidity; *organization and administration; palliative care; patient discharge; physicians; quality of health care; *records; *resuscitation orders; statistics; *terminal care; *withholding treatment; antibiotics; severity of illness index; *Georgetown University Medical Center

Sulmasy, Daniel P.; Terry, Peter B.; Weisman, Carol S., et al. The accuracy of substituted judgments in patients with terminal diagnoses. *Annals of Internal Medicine.* 1998 Apr 15; 128(8): 621–629. 34 refs. BE57916.
   age factors; allowing to die; *attitudes; comparative studies; *consensus; *decision making; dementia; *evaluation; evaluation studies; *family members; *patients; prognosis; *prolongation of life; resuscitation; socioeconomic factors; *terminal care; *terminally ill; *third party consent; ventilators; coma; Baltimore; District of Columbia
   BACKGROUND: Patients' loved ones often make end-of-life treatment decisions, but the accuracy of their substituted judgments and the factors associated with accuracy are poorly understood. OBJECTIVE: To assess the accuracy of judgments made by surrogate decision makers; ascertain the beliefs, practices, and clinical and sociodemographic factors associated with accuracy of surrogates' decisions; assess the preferences of patients for life-sustaining treatments; and compare differences in accuracy across diagnoses. DESIGN: Cross-sectional paired interviews. SETTING: Outpatient practices of three university hospitals. PATIENTS: 250 patients with terminal diagnoses of congestive heart failure, AIDS, amyotrophic lateral sclerosis, lung cancer, and chronic obstructive pulmonary disease (50 patient-surrogate pairs in each group) and 50 general medical patients and their surrogates. MEASUREMENTS: The accuracy of surrogate predictions was measured by using scales based on 10 potential treatments in each of three hypothetical clinical scenarios. RESULTS: Preferences varied according to mode of treatment and scenario. On average, surrogates made correct predictions in 66% of instances. Accuracy was better for the permanent coma scenario than for the scenarios of severe dementia or coma with a small chance of recovery (P less than 0.001). In a binary logit model, the accuracy of substituted judgments was positively associated with the patient having spoken with the surrogate about end-of-life issues (odds ratio [OR], 1.9 [95% CI, 1.6 to 2.3]), the patient having private insurance (OR, 1.4 [CI, 1.1 to 1.7]), the surrogate's level of education (OR, 1.5 [CI, 1.2 to 1.9]), and the patient's level of education (OR, 1.7 [CI, 1.4 to 2.2]). Accuracy was negatively associated with the patient's belief that he or she would live longer than 10 years (OR, 0.6 [CI, 0.5 to 0.7]), surrogate experience with life-sustaining treatment (OR, 0.4 [CI, 0.3 to 0.5]), surrogate participation in religious services (OR, 0.67 [CI, 0.50 to 0.91]), and a diagnosis of heart failure (OR, 0.6 [CI, 0.5 to 0.8]). Age, ethnicity, marital status, religion, and advance directives were not associated with accuracy. CONCLUSIONS: The accuracy of substituted judgments is associated with multiple clinically apparent patient and surrogate factors. This information can help clinicians identify conditions under which substituted judgments are likely to be accurate or inaccurate and can help target populations for education designed to improve the accuracy of surrogate decision making.

Taylor, Robert M.; American Academy of Neurology. Ethics and Humanities Subcommittee. Palliative care in neurology. [Position statement]. *Neurology.* 1996 Mar; 46(3): 870–872. 6 refs. Approved by the AAN Executive Board 8 Jul 1995. BE56887.
   assisted suicide; *central nervous system diseases; chronically ill; goals; medicine; organizational policies; pain; *palliative care; professional organizations; quality of health care; quality of life; suffering; terminal care; treatment refusal; voluntary euthanasia; *neurology; *American Academy of Neurology

Taylor, Susan L. Quandary at the crossroads: paternalism versus advocacy surrounding end-of-treatment decisions. *American Journal of Hospice and Palliative Care.* 1995 Jul–Aug; 12(4): 43–46. 33 fn. BE57054.
   allowing to die; *autonomy; caring; *decision making; *nurse patient relationship; *nurse's role; paternalism; *patient advocacy; *patient participation; physician nurse relationship; physician patient relationship; right to die; *terminal care; values; withholding treatment; Twentieth Century; United States

ten Have, Henk A.M.J.; Janssens, Rien M.J.P.A. Regulating euthanasia in the Netherlands: ethics committees for review of euthanasia? *HEC (HealthCare*

Ethics Committee) Forum. 1997 Dec; 9(4): 393–399. 7 refs. BE58089.
    *active euthanasia; *clinical ethics committees; *decision making; disclosure; *ethics consultation; government regulation; legal aspects; *palliative care; physicians; *public policy; quality of health care; *regional ethics committees; technical expertise; *Netherlands
In this essay we critically review recent regulations with regard to euthanasia policy in The Netherlands. Euthanasia in Holland is formally structured under the penal code. However, because of court cases in which, from the beginning of the 1970s, conditions were formulated wherein euthanizing physicians would not be prosecuted, euthanasia could easily become part of the future standard of medical practice. Recently, new rules concerning the practice of euthanasia have been proposed by the Dutch government in order to adequately control euthanasia practice. These proposals mainly focus on retrospective review. Until now, relatively little attention was paid to preventability of euthanasia. In order to prevent euthanasia, prospective consultation with physicians considering to commit euthanasia would have to receive more attention. In the United States, ample experience has been acquired providing prospective consultative services in neonatalogy. In the aftermath of the "Baby Doe" case, infant care review committees (ICRCs) were established to enhance decisionmaking with regard to severely compromised newborns. These experiences provide interesting points of departure for the development of prospective consultative services in The Netherlands, particularly for physicians who are considering to euthanize patients.

Teno, Joan; Lynn, Joanne; Connors, Alfred F., et al.
The illusion of end–of–life resource savings with advance directives. [For the SUPPORT Investigators]. *Journal of the American Geriatrics Society.* 1997 Apr; 45(4): 513–518. 15 refs. BE57124.
    *advance directives; communication; comparative studies; control groups; *critically ill; *economics; *evaluation; evaluation studies; *hospitals; *medical records; patient admission; patients; research design; resource allocation; resuscitation; resuscitation orders; social impact; socioeconomic factors; *terminal care; treatment refusal; *seriously ill; Patient Self–Determination Act 1990; *Study to Understand Prognoses and Preferences for Outcomes and Risks of Treatments (SUPPORT); United States

Thomasma, David C. Ensuring a good death. *Bioethics Forum.* 1997 Winter; 13(4): 7–17. 50 refs. BE58913.
    active euthanasia; advance directives; *allowing to die; assisted suicide; attitudes to death; autonomy; biomedical technologies; double effect; economics; family members; *moral obligations; pain; palliative care; patients' rights; *physicians; *prolongation of life; *suffering; *terminal care; terminally ill; value of life; withholding treatment; United States

Tilden, Virginia P.; Tolle, Susan W.; Lee, Melinda A., et al. Oregon's physician–assisted suicide vote: its effect on palliative care. *Nursing Outlook.* 1996 Mar–Apr; 44(2): 80–83. 17 refs. BE55775.
    *assisted suicide; attitudes; competence; continuing education; drugs; government regulation; health insurance reimbursement; health services research; hospices; legal aspects; legislation; *nurses; organizational policies; *palliative care; physicians; professional organizations; social impact; state government; *terminal care; terminally ill; Death with Dignity Act (OR); Oregon

Tolle, Susan W. Care of the dying: clinical and financial lessons from the Oregon experience. [Editorial]. *Annals*

of Internal Medicine. 1998 Apr 1; 128(7): 567–568. 15 refs. BE57330.
    advance care planning; advance directives; assisted suicide; coercion; drugs; *economics; government financing; health insurance; hospices; hospitals; indigents; mortality; physicians; public policy; suffering; *terminal care; terminally ill; treatment refusal; Medicaid; *Oregon; United States

Tonelli, Mark. Beyond living wills. *Bioethics Forum.* 1997 Summer; 13(2): 6–12. 13 refs. 4 fn. BE58286.
    advance care planning; *advance directives; allowing to die; autonomy; decision making; evaluation; family members; futility; *living wills; physicians; prolongation of life; quality of health care; quality of life; resuscitation orders; standards; *terminal care; treatment refusal; withholding treatment

Tulsky, James A.; Cassileth, Barrie R.; Bennett, Charles L. The effect of ethnicity on ICU use and DNR orders in hospitalized AIDS patients. *Journal of Clinical Ethics.* 1997 Summer; 8(2): 150–157. 18 fn. BE55777.
    advance care planning; *AIDS; allowing to die; attitudes; *blacks; comparative studies; *Hispanic Americans; hospitals; *intensive care units; males; medical records; *minority groups; mortality; *patient admission; *patient care; patients; prolongation of life; *resuscitation orders; statistics; *terminal care; *time factors; treatment outcome; *whites; multicenter studies; retrospective studies; severity of illness index; Chicago; Los Angeles; Miami

van der Poel, Cornelius J. Ethical aspects in palliative care. *American Journal of Hospice and Palliative Care.* 1996 May–Jun; 13(3): 49–55. 9 fn. BE55534.
    double effect; drugs; futility; goals; pain; *palliative care; pastoral care; psychological stress; Roman Catholic ethics; suffering; *terminal care; terminology; value of life; sedatives

van Thiel, G.J.M.W.; van Delden, J.J.M.; de Haan, K., et al. Retrospective study of doctors' "end of life decisions" in caring for mentally handicapped people in institutions in the Netherlands. *BMJ (British Medical Journal).* 1997 Jul 12; 315(7100): 88–91. 8 refs. BE55583.
    *active euthanasia; *allowing to die; communication; competence; *decision making; drugs; family members; *institutionalized persons; *mentally retarded; mortality; motivation; nurses; *palliative care; *physicians; referral and consultation; statistics; suffering; survey; *terminal care; *terminally ill; withholding treatment; retrospective studies; *Netherlands
OBJECTIVES: To gain insight into the reasons behind and the prevalence of doctors' decisions at the end of life that might hasten a patient's death ("end of life decisions") in institutions caring for mentally handicapped people in the Netherlands, and to describe important aspects of the decisions making process. DESIGN: Survey of random sample of doctors caring for mentally handicapped people by means of self completed questionnaires and structured interviews. SUBJECTS: 89 of the 101 selected doctors completed the questionnaire. 67 doctors had taken an end of life decision and were interviewed about their most recent case. MAIN OUTCOME MEASURES: Prevalence of end of life decisions; types of decisions; characteristics of patients; reasons why the decision was taken; and the decision making process. RESULTS: The 89 doctors reported 222 deaths for 1995. An end of life decision was taken in 97 cases (44%); in 75 the decision was to withdraw or withhold treatment, and in 22 it was to relieve pain or symptoms with opiates in dosages that may have shortened life. In the 67 most recent cases with an end of life decision the patients were mostly incompetent (63) and under 65 years old (51). Only two patients explicitly asked to die, but in 23 cases there had

---

been some communication with the patient. In 60 cases the doctors discussed the decision with nursing staff and in 46 with a colleague. CONCLUSIONS: End of life decisions are an important aspect of the institutionalised care of mentally handicapped people. The proportion of such decisions in the total number of deaths is similar to that in other specialties. However, the discussion of such decisions is less open in the care of mental handicap than in other specialties. Because of distinctive features of care in this specialty an open debate about end of life decisions should not be postponed.

van Weel, Chris; Michels, Joop. Dying, not old age, to blame for costs of health care. *Lancet.* 1997 Oct 18; 350(9085): 1159–1160. 6 refs. BE56217.
*age factors; *aged; chronically ill; diagnosis; *economics; *health care; *morbidity; prevalence; stigmatization; *terminal care; terminally ill

Veterans Affairs National Headquarters. Bioethics Committee. Physician–Assisted Suicide: Committee Report. Issued by the VA National Center for Clinical Ethics, White River Junction, VT 05009; 1996 May. 5 p. 12 refs. BE56737.
artificial feeding; *assisted suicide; coercion; counseling; federal government; institutional policies; medical education; *palliative care; *physicians; public hospitals; *public policy; *terminal care; treatment refusal; *United States; *Veterans Health Administration

Viola, Raymond A.; Wells, George A.; Peterson, Joan. The effects of fluid status and fluid therapy on the dying: a systematic review. *Journal of Palliative Care.* 1997 Winter; 13(4): 41–52. 57 refs. BE58825.
*artificial feeding; *palliative care; *risks and benefits; *terminal care; *terminally ill; treatment outcome; withholding treatment; *fluid therapy

Wear, Stephen; Milch, Robert; Weaver, W. Lynn. Care of dying patients. *In:* McCullough, Laurence B.; Jones, James W.; Brody, Baruch A., eds. Surgical Ethics. New York, NY: Oxford University Press; 1998: 171–197. 15 refs. ISBN 0–19–510347–5. BE58338.
advance care planning; advance directives; artificial feeding; *communication; comprehension; *decision making; depressive disorder; diagnosis; family members; *goals; hospices; informed consent; intensive care units; mortality; pain; *palliative care; patient participation; patients; physician patient relationship; *physicians; professional family relationship; *prognosis; *prolongation of life; *quality of life; resuscitation orders; review; suffering; *surgery; *terminal care; *terminally ill; third party consent; treatment outcome; treatment refusal; *uncertainty; withholding treatment; health services misuse; preventive ethics; Study to Understand Prognoses and Preferences for Outcomes and Risks of Treatments (SUPPORT); United States

Weeks, Jane C.; Cook, E. Francis; O'Day, Steven J., et al. Relationship between cancer patients' predictions of prognosis and their treatment preferences. *JAMA.* 1998 Jun 3; 279(21): 1709–1714. 31 refs. BE58433.
adults; *allowing to die; *attitudes; *cancer; comparative studies; comprehension; *decision making; evaluation studies; hospitals; mortality; *palliative care; patient participation; *patients; physicians; *prognosis; *prolongation of life; risk; survey; *terminal care; *terminally ill; treatment outcome; truth disclosure; teaching hospitals; Study to Understand Prognoses and Preferences for Outcomes and Risks of Treatments (SUPPORT); United States
CONTEXT: Previous studies have documented that cancer patients tend to overestimate the probability of long-term survival. If patient preferences about the

trade-offs between the risks and benefits associated with alternative treatment strategies are based on inaccurate perceptions of prognosis, then treatment choices may not reflect each patient's true values. OBJECTIVE: To test the hypothesis that among terminally ill cancer patients an accurate understanding of prognosis is associated with a preference for therapy that focuses on comfort over attempts at life extension. DESIGN: Prospective cohort study. SETTING: Five teaching hospitals in the United States. PATIENTS: A total of 917 adults hospitalized with stage III or IV non–small cell lung cancer or colon cancer metastatic to liver in phases 1 and 2 of the Study to Understand Prognoses and Preferences for Outcomes and Risks of Treatments (SUPPORT). MAIN OUTCOME MEASURES: Proportion of patients favoring life-extending therapy over therapy focusing on relief of pain and discomfort, patient and physician estimates of the probability of 6-month survival, and actual 6-month survival. RESULTS: Patients who thought they were going to live for at least 6 months were more likely (odds ratio [OR], 2.6; 95% confidence interval [CI], 1.8–3.7) to favor life-extending therapy over comfort care compared with patients who thought there was at least a 10% chance that they would not live 6 months. This OR was highest (8.5; 95% CI, 3.0–24.0) among patients who estimated their 6-month survival probability at greater than 90% but whose physicians estimated it at 10% or less. Patients overestimated their chances of surviving 6 months, while physicians estimated prognosis quite accurately. Patients who preferred life-extending therapy were more likely to undergo aggressive treatment, but controlling for known prognostic factors, their 6-month survival was no better. CONCLUSIONS: Patients with metastatic colon and lung cancer overestimate their survival probabilities and these estimates may influence their preferences about medical therapies.

Weir, Robert F.; Peters, Charles. Affirming the decisions adolescents make about life and death. *Hastings Center Report.* 1997 Nov–Dec; 27(6): 29–40. 22 fn. BE57858.
*adolescents; *advance care planning; *advance directives; *age factors; allowing to die; autonomy; chronically ill; *communication; *competence; counseling; critically ill; *decision making; disclosure; dissent; empirical research; guidelines; *informed consent; legal aspects; legislation; organizational policies; parents; *patient advocacy; *patient care; *patient participation; pediatrics; physician patient relationship; physicians; practice guidelines; professional family relationship; professional organizations; prolongation of life; risks and benefits; state government; *terminal care; terminally ill; *treatment refusal; trust; American Academy of Pediatrics; Patient Self–Determination Act 1990; United States
Adolescents who are critically, chronically, and terminally ill traditionally have been given little voice in their health care treatment. But over the last three decades attitudes have begun to shift. The legal and medical professions as well as parents and children's advocates have started to recognize that cognitively normal adolescents have decisionmaking capacity and believe these patients ought to have the opportunity to participate in even the toughest of health treatment decisions. Advances directives, if used with sensitivity and care, could prove a valuable means of giving these older pediatric patients a say in their care.

White, W.D.; Prunier, Edward; Holmberg, Anders, et al. Clinical problem solving: when too much is too little. [Letters and response]. *New England Journal of Medicine.* 1997 May 15; 336(20): 1458–1459. 4 refs. BE56892.
allowing to die; assisted suicide; communication; home care;

hospices; hospitals; medical education; *palliative care; prolongation of life; quality of life; radiology; *terminal care; terminally ill; treatment refusal; withholding treatment; Medicaid; Medicare; United States

Wilson, Donna. A report of an investigation of end-of-life care practices in health care facilities and the influences on those practices. *Journal of Palliative Care.* 1997 Winter; 13(4): 34-40. 63 refs. BE58824.

age factors; artificial feeding; *biomedical technologies; death; decision making; family members; females; *health facilities; hospitals; intensive care units; males; palliative care; resuscitation; resuscitation orders; statistics; survey; *terminal care; terminally ill; ventilators; retrospective studies; *Alberta; Canada

Wrenn, Robert L.; Levinson, Dan; Papadatou, Danai. End of Life Decisions: Guidelines for the Health Care Provider. Tucson, AZ: University of Arizona College of Medicine, Arizona Health Services Center; 1996. 44 p. 65 refs. Includes bibliographies, world wide web resources and organizations of interest to health care providers, patients, and families. BE57391.

advance directives; alternative therapies; attitudes to death; cancer; case studies; *communication; competence; confidentiality; decision making; family members; guidelines; organ donation; patient care team; patients' rights; physician patient relationship; placebos; *practice guidelines; professional family relationship; professional patient relationship; psychological stress; psychology; suffering; suicide; *terminal care; terminally ill; terminology; treatment refusal; truth disclosure; uncertainty; grief; hope; United States

Yamazaki, Fumio. A thought on terminal care in Japan. *In:* Hoshino, Kazumasa, ed. Japanese and Western Bioethics: Studies in Moral Diversity. Boston, MA: Kluwer Academic; 1997: 131-134. ISBN 0-7923-4112-0. BE57088.

case studies; deception; decision making; drugs; family members; informed consent; interprofessional relations; killing; nurses; pain; palliative care; patient care team; physician nurse relationship; physicians; prognosis; prolongation of life; referral and consultation; social dominance; suffering; *terminal care; terminally ill; truth disclosure; coma; *Japan

Zerwekh, Joyce V. Do dying patients really need IV fluids? *American Journal of Nursing.* 1997 Mar; 97(3): 26-31. 9 refs. Includes an examination for continuing education credit, p. 31. BE56050.

allowing to die; *artificial feeding; attitudes; family members; health personnel; home care; hospices; patient advocacy; physicians; quality of life; *risks and benefits; suffering; *terminal care; *terminally ill; *dehydration; *fluid therapy

Zinn, Christopher. Australian voluntary euthanasia law is overturned. [News]. *BMJ (British Medical Journal).* 1997 Apr 5; 314(7086): 994. BE55838.

*assisted suicide; attitudes; federal government; government financing; *legislation; organizational policies; *palliative care; physicians; professional organizations; terminal care; *voluntary euthanasia; *Australia; Australian Medical Association; *Northern Territory; *Rights of the Terminally Ill Act (NT)

Zucker, Marjorie B.; Zucker, Howard D., eds. Medical Futility and the Evaluation of Life-Sustaining Interventions. New York, NY: Cambridge University Press; 1997. 201 p. 332 refs. 14 fn. ISBN 0-521-56877-3. BE55973.

advance directives; aged; *allowing to die; alternative therapies; attitudes to death; autonomy; children; clinical ethics committees; common good; communication;

consensus; cultural pluralism; *decision making; *dissent; economics; family members; *futility; goals; guidelines; intensive care units; judicial action; legal aspects; legislation; medicine; newborns; nursing homes; *palliative care; patients; physicians; professional autonomy; *prolongation of life; psychiatry; public participation; referral and consultation; refusal to treat; religion; resource allocation; resuscitation orders; *terminal care; terminology; treatment outcome; values; vulnerable populations; withholding treatment; community policies; United States

TERMINAL CARE/HOSPICES

Ackerman, Felicia. Response to "This porridge is too thin" by Gretchen M. Brown and "Demolishing a 'straw man'" by Elliott J. Rosen (*CQ* Vol. 7, No. 2). *Cambridge Quarterly of Healthcare Ethics.* 1998 Summer; 7(3): 323-325. 11 fn. BE58560.

alternatives; biomedical technologies; counseling; decision making; economics; *hospices; prolongation of life; *terminal care; terminally ill

Burke, James; Steel, R. Knight; Lynn, Joanne, et al. Contempo 1997: end-of-life care. [Letters and response]. *JAMA.* 1997 Oct 8; 278(14): 1150-1151. 5 refs. BE55894.

advance care planning; federal government; financial support; government financing; *hospices; *medical education; medical schools; *palliative care; *physicians; quality of health care; teaching methods; *terminal care; United States

Drane, James F. Caring to the End: Policy Suggestions and Ethics Education for Hospice and Home Health-Care Agencies. Erie, PA: Lake Area Health Education Center; 1997. 308 p. Includes references. Appendices include sample advance directives; a model for competency evaluation; what one hospice/home health-care agency did with the policy suggestions; and a glossary of terms. ISBN 0-9658342-0-4. BE58161.

advance directives; *allowing to die; artificial feeding; assisted suicide; blood transfusions; clinical ethics committees; competence; confidentiality; *decision making; double effect; economics; education; futility; health care delivery; health facilities; health personnel; *home care; *hospices; informed consent; *institutional policies; intention; killing; legal aspects; patient admission; patient transfer; physicians; prolongation of life; quality of life; religious ethics; renal dialysis; resuscitation orders; *terminal care; third party consent; values; ventilators; wedge argument; withholding treatment; United States

McGee, Ellen M. Can suicide intervention in hospice be ethical? *Journal of Palliative Care.* 1997 Spring; 13(1): 27-33. 50 refs. BE55728.

assisted suicide; autonomy; beneficence; counseling; depressive disorder; goals; *hospices; *institutional policies; pain; palliative care; paternalism; physicians; psychological stress; suffering; *suicide; *terminal care; *terminally ill; *values; rationality

McNeilly, Dennis P.; Hillary, Kristine. The hospice decision: psychosocial facilitators and barriers. *Omega: A Journal of Death and Dying.* 1997; 35(2): 193-217. 11 refs. BE56935.

*attitudes; cancer; communication; *decision making; *family members; family relationship; *health personnel; home care; *hospices; *knowledge, attitudes, practice; palliative care; *patient admission; *physicians; survey; *terminal care; terminally ill; truth disclosure

Meystre, Chantal J.N.; Burley, Neil M.J.; Ahmedzai, Sam. What investigations and procedures do patients in hospices want? Interview based survey of patients and

their nurses. *BMJ (British Medical Journal)*. 1997 Nov 8; 315(7117): 1202–1203. 5 refs. BE56766.
> *attitudes; biomedical technologies; *cancer; comparative studies; diagnosis; *hospices; *nurses; *patients; resuscitation; surgery; survey; *terminal care; *terminally ill; Great Britain

Post, Stephen G. Physician–assisted suicide in Alzheimer's disease. *Journal of the American Geriatrics Society*. 1997 May; 45(5): 647–651. 26 refs. BE55843.
> active euthanasia; *advance directives; aged; *assisted suicide; attitudes; autonomy; beneficence; chronically ill; competence; *dementia; economics; health personnel; *hospices; international aspects; legal aspects; *long-term care; managed care programs; *palliative care; physicians; policy analysis; public opinion; *public policy; quality of life; resource allocation; self concept; social discrimination; social impact; suffering; *terminal care; terminally ill; wedge argument; withholding treatment; *United States

Shapiro, Joseph P. Death be not swift enough: fraud fighters begin to probe the expense of hospice care. [News]. *U.S. News and World Report*. 1997 Mar 24; 122(11): 34–35. BE55794.
> diagnosis; *economics; federal government; *fraud; *government financing; *hospices; prognosis; proprietary health facilities; selection for treatment; *terminal care; terminally ill; time factors; Florida; *Medicare; *United States

Twycross, Robert. Palliative care. *In:* Chadwick, Ruth, ed. Encyclopedia of Applied Ethics, Volume 3. San Diego, CA: Academic Press; 1998: 419–433. 15 refs. ISBN 0-12-227068-1. BE56258.
> active euthanasia; allowing to die; artificial feeding; assisted suicide; drugs; goals; historical aspects; *hospices; international aspects; organization and administration; pain; *palliative care; pastoral care; patient care team; professional patient relationship; quality of life; rehabilitation; religion; *terminal care; dehydration; hope; *Great Britain; National Health Service; Poland; Saunders, Cicely; United States; World Health Organization

Volicer, Ladislav. Hospice care for dementia patients. [Editorial]. *Journal of the American Geriatrics Society*. 1997 Sep; 45(9): 1147–1149. 8 refs. BE56317.
> chronically ill; decision making; *dementia; guidelines; *hospices; nursing homes; pain; *palliative care; professional organizations; prognosis; referral and consultation; selection for treatment; standards; terminal care; terminally ill; National Hospice Organization

TEST TUBE FERTILIZATION See IN VITRO FERTILIZATION

TESTING AND SCREENING

See also GENETIC SCREENING, MASS SCREENING
See under
AIDS/TESTING AND SCREENING

THERAPEUTIC RESEARCH See HUMAN EXPERIMENTATION

THIRD PARTY CONSENT See ALLOWING TO DIE, INFORMED CONSENT, RESUSCITATION ORDERS

TISSUE DONATION See ORGAN AND TISSUE DONATION

TORTURE

Blachar, Yoram; Summerfield, Derek. The truth about Israeli medical ethics. [Letter and response]. *Lancet*. 1997 Oct 25; 350(9086): 1247. 3 refs. BE58406.
> *human rights; organizational policies; *physicians; prisoners; professional organizations; *torture; *Israel; *Israeli Medical Association; Palestinians

Bunce, Christina. Doctors involved in human rights' abuses in Kenya. [News]. *BMJ (British Medical Journal)*. 1997 Jan 18; 314(7075): 166. BE58741.
> death; deception; health care; human rights; medical records; *misconduct; physician's role; *physicians; *prisoners; *torture; Amnesty International; *Kenya

Geltman, Paul. Rwanda: physician complicity and rebuilding the medical community. *Lancet*. 1997 Jul 5; 350(9070): 64. 2 refs. BE56571.
> *human rights; *killing; *misconduct; moral complicity; *physician's role; physicians; *torture; *genocide; *Rwanda

Lee, Nick. Spotlight on South African medical profession. [News]. *Lancet*. 1997 Jul 5; 350(9070): 39. BE56593.
> blacks; historical aspects; *human rights; *misconduct; organizational policies; *physician's role; physicians; politics; prisoners; *professional organizations; social discrimination; *torture; Biko, Steve; *Medical Association of South Africa; *South Africa; Twentieth Century

Mansour, Paul. Turkish doctors collude in torture. [News]. *BMJ (British Medical Journal)*. 1997 Mar 8; 314(7082): 699. 1 ref. BE58747.
> dissent; fraud; human rights; medical records; *misconduct; organizational policies; physician's role; *physicians; *prisoners; professional organizations; *torture; Amnesty International; *Turkey; Turkish Medical Association

Prosor, Ron; Malnick, Stephen D.H.; Mahler, Ch., et al. Medical ethics: the Israeli Medical Association. [Letters and response]. *Lancet*. 1997 Aug 30; 350(9078): 669–670. 1 ref. BE56570.
> due process; *human rights; military personnel; misconduct; organizational policies; *physician's role; physicians; *political activity; prisoners; *professional organizations; public policy; *torture; violence; *Israel; *Israeli Medical Association; Palestinians

Sidley, Pat. South Africa Truth Commission calls doctors to account for their actions during the apartheid era. [News]. *BMJ (British Medical Journal)*. 1997 Jun 28; 314(7098): 1850. BE56594.
> blacks; *human rights; *misconduct; *physicians; political activity; prisoners; *social discrimination; *torture; *South Africa

Summerfield, Derek. Medical ethics: the Israeli Medical Association. *Lancet*. 1997 Jul 5; 350(9070): 63–64. 6 refs. BE56569.
> *human rights; military personnel; misconduct; organizational policies; *physician's role; physicians; *political activity; prisoners; *professional organizations; psychiatry; public policy; *torture; violence; Amnesty International; *Israel; *Israeli Medical Association; Palestinians; Physicians for Human Rights

Human rights begin at home. [Editorial]. *BMJ (British Medical Journal)*. 1997 Nov 29; 315(7120): 1387. BE56915.
> health personnel; *human experimentation; *human rights; investigators; mentally ill; *misconduct; patient care; *prisoners; *scientific misconduct; *torture; Great Britain; United Nations; United States; Universal Declaration of

---

BE = bioethics accession number   fn. = footnotes   refs. = references

Human Rights

TRANSGENIC ANIMALS *See* GENETIC
INTERVENTION, PATENTING LIFE FORMS,
RECOMBINANT DNA RESEARCH

TRANSPLANTATION *See* ORGAN AND TISSUE
TRANSPLANTATION

TREATMENT REFUSAL

See also ALLOWING TO DIE, ADVANCE
DIRECTIVES, INFORMED CONSENT,
PATIENTS' RIGHTS

Agich, George J. Can the patient make treatment
decisions? Evaluating decisional capacity. *Cleveland
Clinic Journal of Medicine.* 1997 Oct; 64(9): 461–464. 6
refs. BE58350.
 advance directives; *competence; comprehension; decision
making; disclosure; evaluation; *informed consent;
physician's role; standards; third party consent; *treatment
refusal; United States

Arnold, Denis G.; Menzel, Paul T. When comes "the
end of the day?" A comment on the dialogue between
Dax Cowart and Robert Burt. *Hastings Center Report.*
1998 Jan–Feb; 28(1): 25–27. 2 fn. Commentary on D.
Cowart and R. Burt, p. 14–24. BE57293.
 *allowing to die; *autonomy; burns; *communication;
competence; *decision making; *dissent; *pain; palliative
care; paternalism; patient advocacy; physician patient
relationship; prognosis; *prolongation of life; *right to die;
*time factors; *treatment refusal; Cowart, Dax

Bosek, Marcia Sue DeWolf. Doing good: an ethical
quandary. *Medsurg Nursing.* 1995 Apr; 4(2): 154–156. 5
refs. BE56401.
 aged; allowing to die; autonomy; beneficence; case studies;
coercion; communication; *competence; decision making;
diabetes; ethical theory; nurses; physicians; *surgery;
*treatment refusal; virtues; *amputation

Brazier, Margaret. Hard cases make bad law? [Editorial].
Journal of Medical Ethics. 1997 Dec; 23(6): 341–343. 3
refs. BE57656.
 *artificial insemination; cesarean section; *coercion;
compensation; *competence; cryopreservation; death;
*decision making; *fetuses; government regulation;
guidelines; informed consent; *judicial action; *legal aspects;
legal rights; married persons; physicians; *posthumous
reproduction; *pregnant women; professional organizations;
remuneration; semen donors; sperm; *surrogate mothers;
*treatment refusal; Blood, Diane; European Union; *Great
Britain; Human Fertilisation and Embryology Act 1990;
Human Fertilisation and Embryology Authority; In re MB
(Caesarean Section); R v. Human Fertilisation and
Embryology Authority (ex parte Blood); Re S (Adult:
Medical Treatment); Royal College of Obstetricians and
Gynaecologists

Bremnes, R.M.; Andersen, K.; Wist, E.A. Cancer
patients, doctors and nurses vary in their willingness to
undertake cancer chemotherapy. *European Journal of
Cancer.* 1995 Nov; 31A(12): 1955–1959. 27 refs. BE56199.
 age factors; *attitudes; *cancer; comparative studies;
*decision making; *drugs; family relationship; females;
males; medical specialties; morbidity; *nurses; palliative care;
*patient care; *patients; *physicians; prognosis; *risks and
benefits; survey; toxicity; treatment outcome; *treatment
refusal; Norway

Connecticut. Supreme Court. Stamford Hospital v. Vega.
Atlantic Reporter, 2d Series. 1996 Apr 16 (date of
decision). 674: 821–834. BE56198.
 autonomy; *blood transfusions; childbirth; coercion;
hospitals; *Jehovah's Witnesses; judicial action; *legal
aspects; legal rights; religion; state interest; *treatment
refusal; value of life; Connecticut; *Stamford Hospital v.
Vega
The Supreme Court of Connecticut held that a hospital's
interest in preserving a patient's life and in protecting
the medical profession's ethical integrity were not
sufficient to take priority over the common law right
of bodily self determination of a Jehovah's Witness to
refuse a blood transfusion. After giving birth to her first
child, Nelly Vega hemorrhaged and was in need of a
blood transfusion to save her life. In accord with her
beliefs as a Jehovah's Witness, she declined blood and
blood products. After an emergency hearing, the lower
court ordered the transfusion and Vega recovered. Her
case was not moot and went on to appeal because these
facts were capable of repetition, yet, due to their limited
duration in time, likely to evade judicial review. (KIE
abstract)

Cowart, Dax; Burt, Robert. Confronting death: who
chooses, who controls? A dialogue between Dax Cowart
and Robert Burt. *Hastings Center Report.* 1998 Jan–Feb;
28(1): 14–24. 1 ref. Commented on by D.G. Arnold and
P.T. Menzel, p. 25–27. BE57292.
 *allowing to die; attitudes; *autonomy; *beneficence; *burns;
*communication; competence; *decision making; *dissent;
freedom; human rights; informed consent; nurses; *pain;
palliative care; *paternalism; patient advocacy; *physically
disabled; *physician patient relationship; physician's role;
*prolongation of life; quality of life; *right to die; self
concept; suffering; *time factors; *treatment refusal; values;
*Cowart, Dax
On 21 November 1996, Dax Cowart and Robert Burt
jointly delivered the Heather Koller Memorial Lecture
at Pacific Lutheran University. This was the first time
that they spoke together in a public forum. Dax Cowart
now lives and practices law in Corpus Christi, Texas.
In the summer of 1973, he was critically injured in a
propane gas explosion that took his father's life and very
deeply burned more than two–thirds of his own body.
He was left blind and without the use of his hands. For
more than a year Dax underwent extraordinarily painful
treatments in the acute burn ward of two hospitals.
Throughout his ordeal he demanded to die by refusing
consent to his disinfectant treatments. Despite repeated
declarations of competence by his psychiatrist, all his
pleas were rejected. In 1974, while still hospitalized, he
helped make the famous "Please Let Me Die" video, and
in 1984 a second video, "Dax's Case." In 1986 Dax
Cowart received a law degree from Texas Tech
University. Burt and Cowart have corresponded over
the course of several years on the subject of Dax's case
and related issues. They met for the first time during
their trip to Tacoma, Washington for the Koller
Memorial Lecture. The following is an edited transcript
of their public remarks.

Culhane-Pera, Kathleen A.; Vawter, Dorothy E. A
study of healthcare professionals' perspectives about a
cross–cultural ethical conflict involving a Hmong patient
and her family. *Journal of Clinical Ethics.* 1998 Summer;
9(2): 179–190. 11 fn. Commented on by E.G. Howe, p.
191–193. BE58964.
 age factors; aged; allowing to die; *Asian Americans;
*attitudes; *autonomy; *beneficence; case studies; coercion;
competence; counseling; *critically ill; *cultural pluralism;
*decision making; dissent; *family members; *family

---

relationship; females; *health personnel; internship and residency; knowledge, attitudes, practice; males; *minority groups; nurses; *paternalism; patient transfer; *physicians; professional family relationship; professional patient relationship; students; *surgery; survey; third party consent; *treatment refusal; trust; values; ventilators; withholding treatment; adult offspring; questionnaires; *Hmong; Minnesota

Delany, Linda. Court-authorised caesareans: new guidance. *Health Care Analysis.* 1997 Sep; 5(3): 240-241, 243. 10 fn. BE55820.
autonomy; *cesarean section; coercion; *competence; *fetuses; guidelines; *judicial action; *legal aspects; legal rights; *pregnant women; *treatment refusal; *Great Britain; *Re MB (Caesarean Section)

Delany, Linda. Health care law: caesareans under duress. *Health Care Analysis.* 1997 Jun; 5(2): 160-163. 17 fn. BE55848.
*cesarean section; *coercion; competence; emergency care; fetuses; involuntary commitment; judicial action; *legal aspects; mentally ill; patient participation; *pregnant women; *treatment refusal; *Great Britain; Mental Health Act 1983 (Great Britain); Norfolk and Norwich Healthcare NHS Trust v. W; Re S (Adult: Refusal of Medical Treatment); Rochdale Healthcare NHS Trust v. C; Tameside and Glossop Acute Services Trust v. CH

Duffy, Barbara; Brent, Nancy J.; Pfaadt, Mary Joyce, et al. What to do about Harry? [Case study and commentaries]. *Home Healthcare Nurse.* 1996 Jun; 14(6): 420-426. 4 refs. BE55851.
administrators; *aged; autonomy; case studies; competence; disadvantaged; *home care; informed consent; legal aspects; legal liability; males; *nurses; *patient compliance; *treatment refusal; life style; patient abandonment

Dyer, Clare. Appeal court rules against compulsory caesarean sections. [News]. *BMJ (British Medical Journal).* 1997 Apr 5; 314(7086): 993. BE56556.
*cesarean section; *coercion; competence; death; fetuses; *judicial action; *legal aspects; *legal rights; organizational policies; physicians; *pregnant women; professional organizations; risk; *treatment refusal; *Great Britain; Royal College of Obstetricians and Gynaecologists

Dyer, Clare. Judge misled over call for caesarean operation. [News]. *BMJ (British Medical Journal).* 1998 Feb 21; 316(7131): 574. BE57773.
*cesarean section; *coercion; competence; judicial action; lawyers; *legal aspects; misconduct; *pregnant women; *treatment refusal; *Great Britain; *National Health Service

Dyer, Clare. Trusts face damages after forcing women to have ceasareans. [News]. *BMJ (British Medical Journal).* 1998 May 16; 316(7143): 1480. BE58236.
*cesarean section; *coercion; hospitals; involuntary commitment; judicial action; *legal aspects; *legal liability; *pregnant women; *treatment refusal; *Great Britain; Mental Health Act (Great Britain); National Health Service; Pathfinder Mental Health Services Trust; St. George's Hospital

Dyer, Clare. Woman can challenge hospital over forced caesarean. [News]. *BMJ (British Medical Journal).* 1997 Jul 12; 315(7100): 78. BE56586.
*cesarean section; *coercion; hospitals; *legal aspects; *legal liability; patient discharge; *pregnant women; social workers; *treatment refusal; *Great Britain; Mental Health Act 1983 (Great Britain); St. George's Healthcare Trust

Eiser, Arnold R. Withdrawal from dialysis: the role of autonomy and community-based values. *American Journal of Kidney Diseases.* 1996 Mar; 27(3): 451-457. 39 refs. BE56568.
*allowing to die; *autonomy; *beneficence; bioethical issues; *common good; *communitarianism; competence; consensus; cultural pluralism; *decision making; dissent; ethics consultation; family members; futility; guidelines; international aspects; judicial action; legal aspects; *libertarianism; minority groups; moral policy; paternalism; patients; persistent vegetative state; physician patient relationship; *physician's role; physicians; *prolongation of life; public participation; quality of life; *renal dialysis; *standards; third party consent; *treatment refusal; *values; *withholding treatment; undertreatment; Europe; *United States

Elkins, Thomas E.; Brown, Douglas. Ethical issues in the utilization of cesarean section. *In:* Flamm, B.L.; Quilligan, E.J., eds. Cesarean Section: Guidelines for Appropriate Utilization. New York, NY: Springer-Verlag; 1995: 191-205. 69 refs. ISBN 0-387-94238-6. BE56682.
autonomy; blood transfusions; *cesarean section; childbirth; *coercion; *decision making; developing countries; fetal therapy; *fetuses; informed consent; *judicial action; *legal aspects; maternal health; minority groups; *moral obligations; newborns; *obstetrics and gynecology; *organizational policies; *patient care; patient compliance; patient participation; physician patient relationship; *physicians; *pregnant women; privacy; professional organizations; prognosis; *risks and benefits; selection for treatment; socioeconomic factors; state interest; terminally ill; *treatment refusal; viability; *American Academy of Pediatrics; *American College of Obstetricians and Gynecologists; *American Medical Association; District of Columbia; *In re A.C.; *United States

Espinoza, Leslie G. Dissecting women, dissecting law: the court-ordering of caesarean section operations and the failure of informed consent to protect women of color. *National Black Law Journal.* 1994; 13: 211-237. 211 fn. BE58974.
Asian Americans; autonomy; blacks; *cesarean section; *coercion; communication; competence; cultural pluralism; decision making; *fetuses; Hispanic Americans; hospitals; indigents; *informed consent; judicial action; *legal aspects; legal rights; *minority groups; mother fetus relationship; physicians; *pregnant women; social discrimination; *state interest; terminally ill; *treatment refusal; *viability; District of Columbia; George Washington University Hospital; *In re A.C.; In re Madyun

Fishman, Rachelle H.B. Israeli courts intervene in medical issues. [News]. *Lancet.* 1997 Sep 20; 350(9081): 874. BE56489.
adults; allowing to die; children; compensation; *HIV seropositivity; hospitals; *judicial action; *legal aspects; mentally retarded; negligence; parents; renal dialysis; suffering; *treatment refusal; truth disclosure; *Israel

Flagler, Elizabeth; Baylis, Françoise; Rodgers, Sanda. Bioethics for clinicians: 12. Ethical dilemmas that arise in the care of pregnant women: rethinking "maternal-fetal conflicts." *Canadian Medical Association Journal.* 1997 Jun 15; 156(12): 1729-1732. 34 refs. BE57354.
AIDS serodiagnosis; autonomy; case studies; cesarean section; coercion; *fetuses; *legal aspects; legal rights; moral obligations; mother fetus relationship; obstetrics and gynecology; patient care; personhood; physicians; *pregnant women; *treatment refusal; *Canada

Garwin, Mark. The duty to care -- the right to refuse: changing roles of patients and physicians in end-of-life decision making. *Journal of Legal Medicine.* 1998 Mar; 19(1): 99-125. 95 fn. BE58901.

BE = bioethics accession number   fn. = footnotes   refs. = references

advance directives; *allowing to die; autonomy; beneficence; coercion; communication; competence; *decision making; disclosure; economics; emergency care; incentives; informed consent; judicial action; *legal aspects; *legal liability; legal rights; models, theoretical; physician patient relationship; *physicians; *prolongation of life; resuscitation orders; standards; state interest; terminal care; third party consent; torts; *treatment refusal; withholding treatment; directive adherence; Anderson v. St. Francis-St. George Hospital; *United States

Giesen, Dieter. Comparative legal developments. *In:* Grubb, Andrew, ed. Decision–Making and Problems of Incompetence. New York, NY: Wiley; 1994: 7–26. 126 fn. ISBN 0-471-94236-7. BE57126.
 adults; allowing to die; autonomy; *competence; *decision making; family members; *informed consent; international aspects; judicial action; *legal aspects; legal guardians; mentally disabled; minors; parental consent; *patient care; patients; physicians; quality of life; standards; *third party consent; *treatment refusal; value of life; withholding treatment; Australia; Canada; Germany; *Great Britain; United States

Guiles, Renée M.; Appelbaum, Paul S. Death in denial. [Case study and commentaries]. *Hastings Center Report.* 1997 Nov–Dec; 27(6): 23–25. BE57856.
 AIDS; case studies; *competence; death; drug abuse; *emergency care; emotions; females; health personnel; *hospitals; legal liability; motivation; *patient admission; patient advocacy; *patient compliance; smoking; *treatment refusal

Hall, Spencer A.; Casarett, David; Ross, Lainie F. Overriding a patient's refusal of treatment after an iatrogenic complication. [Letter and response]. *New England Journal of Medicine.* 1997 Nov 13; 337(20): 1477. 4 refs. BE58414.
 *iatrogenic disease; *resuscitation; *resuscitation orders; *treatment refusal

Hodgson, John. Rights of the terminally ill patient. *Annals of Health Law.* 1996; 5: 169–191. 93 fn. BE58364.
 *active euthanasia; adults; advance directives; *allowing to die; artificial feeding; assisted suicide; competence; *decision making; family members; informed consent; judicial action; *legal aspects; legal liability; *legal rights; minors; palliative care; *persistent vegetative state; physicians; quality of life; right to die; standards; *terminally ill; *third party consent; *treatment refusal; withholding treatment; Airedale NHS Trust v. Bland; *Great Britain; House of Lords Select Committee on Medical Ethics; Law Commission (Great Britain)

Howe, Edmund G. Biological drivenness: a relative indication for paternalism. *Journal of Clinical Ethics.* 1997 Fall; 8(3): 307–312. 23 fn. BE57562.
 advance directives; alcohol abuse; autonomy; *competence; *decision making; mentally ill; *paternalism; patient care; patient participation; *physicians; suicide; surgery; time factors; *treatment refusal; seriously ill; Ulysses contracts

Leavine, Barbara Ann. Court–ordered cesareans: can a pregnant woman refuse? *Houston Law Review.* 1992 Spring; 29(1): 185–218. 276 fn. BE56978.
 abortion, induced; autonomy; *cesarean section; coercion; decision making; *fetuses; *judicial action; *legal aspects; *legal rights; physicians; *pregnant women; privacy; *state interest; Supreme Court decisions; *treatment refusal; value of life; viability; *women's rights; District of Columbia; In re A.C.; Roe v. Wade; *United States

McFadzean, J.; Monson, J.P.; Watson, J.D., et al. The dilemma of the incapacitated patient who has previously refused consent for surgery. [Case study and

commentaries]. *BMJ (British Medical Journal).* 1997 Dec 6; 315(7121): 1530–1532. 8 refs. BE57243.
 advance directives; autonomy; case studies; competence; *critically ill; decision making; emergency care; family members; *legal aspects; physicians; prognosis; *surgery; *third party consent; time factors; *treatment refusal; Great Britain
What should doctors do if a patient is critically ill and unable to give consent to a procedure that he or she has previously refused to consent to? Such a case is described below and discussed by a medicolegal specialist and by an ethicist.

Mair, Jane. Maternal/foetal conflict: defined or defused? *In:* McLean, Sheila A.M., ed. Contemporary Issues in Law, Medicine and Ethics. Brookfield, VT: Dartmouth; 1996: 79–97. 45 fn. ISBN 1-85521-586-1. BE57791.
 autonomy; cesarean section; *coercion; communication; compensation; *drug abuse; *fetuses; freedom; guidelines; health; informed consent; international aspects; judicial action; *legal aspects; *legal liability; legal obligations; *legal rights; moral obligations; newborns; personhood; physicians; *pregnant women; *prenatal injuries; privacy; religion; state interest; torts; *treatment refusal; viability; women's rights; *Great Britain; United States

Malone, Ruth E.; Workman, Stephen. Caring for "difficult" patients. [Letters]. *Hastings Center Report.* 1998 Jul–Aug; 28(4): 4. BE58920.
 caring; case studies; emergency care; females; HIV seropositivity; *hospitals; *patient admission; *patient compliance; physician patient relationship; smoking; social worth; *treatment refusal

Mazur, Dennis J. How older patient preferences are influenced by consideration of future health outcomes. *Journal of the American Geriatrics Society.* 1997 Jun; 45(6): 725–728. 11 refs. BE55727.
 advance care planning; *aged; *allowing to die; *attitudes; brain pathology; decision making; family members; health; *males; married persons; mentally disabled; morbidity; *patient care; *patients; physically disabled; physicians; *prolongation of life; *quality of life; resuscitation; survey; *treatment outcome; *treatment refusal; *ventilators; withholding treatment; cerebrovascular disorders; *intubation; Oregon

Moseley, Kathryn L.; Truesdell, Sandra. A noncompliant patient? [Case study]. *Journal of Clinical Ethics.* 1997 Summer; 8(2): 176–177. Commented on by P.R. Muskin, p. 178–180. BE56351.
 case studies; chronically ill; competence; diabetes; ethics consultation; females; food; insulin; patient care; *patient compliance; *patient discharge; *physician patient relationship; psychology; *treatment refusal; trust; self care

Muramoto, Osamu. Medical ethics in the treatment of Jehovah's Witnesses. [Letter]. *Archives of Internal Medicine.* 1998 May 25; 158(10): 1155–1156. 4 refs. BE58806.
 *alternatives; *blood transfusions; clergy; conscience; *decision making; *Jehovah's Witnesses; organizational policies; patients; Protestant ethics; religion; *stem cells; tissue transplantation; *treatment refusal; Watch Tower Bible and Tract Society

Muskin, Philip R. Care, support, and concern for noncompliant patients. *Journal of Clinical Ethics.* 1997 Summer; 8(2): 178–180. 3 fn. Commentary on K.L. Moseley and S. Truesdell, p. 176–177. BE56350.
 age factors; autonomy; case studies; chronically ill; communication; competence; diabetes; family relationship; females; food; insulin; motivation; *patient compliance; *physician patient relationship; psychiatry; referral and

consultation; *treatment refusal; self care

Oberman, Michelle. Women, fetuses, physicians, and the state: pregnancy and medical ethics in the 21st century. *In:* Monagle, John F.; Thomasma, David C., eds. Health Care Ethics: Critical Issues for the 21st Century. Gaithersburg, MD: Aspen Publishers; 1998: 67–78. 33 fn. ISBN 0-8342-0911-X. BE56280.
 advance directives; AIDS serodiagnosis; autonomy; biomedical technologies; cesarean section; coercion; confidentiality; drug abuse; fetuses; government regulation; historical aspects; legal aspects; mandatory testing; obstetrics and gynecology; patient compliance; physician patient relationship; physician's role; *pregnant women; *prenatal injuries; socioeconomic factors; state interest; *treatment refusal; Twentieth Century; United States

Ohio. Court of Appeals, Hamilton County. Anderson v. St. Francis–St. George Hospital. *North Eastern Reporter, 2d Series.* 1992 Nov 18 (date of decision). 614: 841–847. BE56297.
 allowing to die; brain pathology; compensation; *hospitals; injuries; *legal liability; negligence; nurses; *prolongation of life; *resuscitation; *resuscitation orders; *right to die; torts; *treatment refusal; *wrongful life; *Anderson v. St. Francis–St. George Hospital; Ohio
The Ohio Court of Appeals for Hamilton County upheld summary judgment on a claim for wrongful living, where the patient was resuscitated by a nurse contrary to his doctor's no code blue order and then later suffered a paralyzing stroke prior to his death. Wrongful living was the phrase coined by the appellant for the cause of action for the life that was forced on the decedent by resuscitation. The court noted that life was not a compensable harm in the state until the legislature or the highest court decides it is so. Because the patient had apparently expressly refused treatment in a medical emergency, the case could proceed under two other theories, battery or unauthorized touching, and negligence or breach of a duty of care. (KIE abstract)

Perkins, Henry S.; Supik, Josie D.; Hazuda, Helen P. Cultural differences among health professionals: a case illustration. *Journal of Clinical Ethics.* 1998 Summer; 9(2): 108–117. 35 fn. BE58956.
 *autonomy; case studies; cesarean section; comparative studies; counseling; critically ill; *cultural pluralism; *decision making; ethical relativism; family relationship; females; *health personnel; hospitals; *informed consent; *international aspects; mediation; paternalism; *patient care; pregnant women; spousal consent; *treatment refusal; value of life; *values; voluntary sterilization; *non–Western World; qualitative research; *Western World; *Kenya
This study illustrates that cultural differences arise among similarly trained health professionals. Health professionals must learn to communicate sensitively with colleagues from other cultures, to respect their values, and to recognize and resolve cultural differences that affect patient care. In this shrinking, multicultural world, health professionals cannot afford the comfortable illusion that all similarly trained practitioners share the same values about the care of patients and professional conduct.

Pinkerton, JoAnn V.; Finnerty, James J.; Sosnowski, J. Richard. Resolving the clinical and ethical dilemma involved in fetal–maternal conflicts. [Article and discussion]. *American Journal of Obstetrics and Gynecology.* 1996 Aug; 175(2): 289–295. 28 refs. Presented at the Fifty-Eighth Annual Meeting of the South Atlantic Association of Obstetricians and Gynecologists,

27–30 Jan 1996. BE57969.
 allowing to die; *autonomy; *beneficence; *cesarean section; clinical ethics committees; *coercion; competence; counseling; *decision making; ethics consultation; fetal therapy; *fetuses; guidelines; *hospitals; informed consent; *institutional policies; *judicial action; moral obligations; moral policy; patient care team; patient transfer; *practice guidelines; *pregnant women; prolongation of life; religion; rights; risks and benefits; state interest; terminally ill; third party consent; *treatment refusal; viability; In re A.C.; In re Baby Boy Doe v. Mother Doe; In re Madgun; Jefferson v. Griffin Spalding Co. Hospital Authority; United States; *University of Virginia Health Services Center

Ramsay, Sarah. UK woman wins right to refuse caesarean section. [News]. *Lancet.* 1998 May 16; 351(9114): 1499. BE58888.
 *cesarean section; *fetuses; *legal aspects; *legal rights; *pregnant women; *treatment refusal; *Great Britain; *Re S; St. George's Hospital

Rossiter, Graham P. Contemporary transatlantic developments concerning compelled medical treatment of pregnant women. *Australian and New Zealand Journal of Obstetrics and Gynaecology.* 1995 May; 35(2): 132–138. 28 fn. BE55889.
 *autonomy; blood transfusions; cesarean section; *coercion; competence; decision making; emergency care; *fetuses; hospitals; informed consent; *international aspects; Jehovah's Witnesses; judicial action; *legal aspects; legal liability; legal rights; obstetrics and gynecology; physicians; *pregnant women; prognosis; religion; state interest; *treatment refusal; viability; women's rights; *Great Britain; In re A.C.; Jefferson v. Griffin Spalding Co. Hospital Authority; New Zealand; Re S (Adult: Refusal of Medical Treatment); Re T (Adult: Refusal of Medical Treatment); State of Illinois v. Bricci; *United States

Savulescu, Julian; Momeyer, Richard W. Should informed consent be based on rational beliefs? *Journal of Medical Ethics.* 1997 Oct; 23(5): 282–288. 17 fn. BE57109.
 *autonomy; *blood transfusions; communication; *competence; decision making; disclosure; *informed consent; *Jehovah's Witnesses; patient education; patients; physician patient relationship; *religion; *treatment refusal; *rationality
Our aim is to expand the regulative ideal governing consent. We argue that consent should not only be informed but also based on rational beliefs. We argue that holding true beliefs promotes autonomy. Information is important insofar as it helps a person to hold the relevant true beliefs. But in order to hold the relevant true beliefs, competent people must also think rationally. Insofar as information is important, rational deliberation is important. Just as physicians should aim to provide relevant information regarding the medical procedures prior to patients consenting to have those procedures, they should also assist patients to think more rationally. We distinguish between rational choice/action and rational belief. While autonomous choice need not necessarily be rational, it should be based on rational belief. The implication for the doctrine of informed consent and the practice of medicine is that, if physicians are to respect patient autonomy and help patients to choose and act more rationally, not only must they provide information, but they should care more about the theoretical rationality of their patients. They should not abandon their patients to irrationality. They should help their patients to deliberate more effectively and to care more about thinking rationally. We illustrate these arguments in the context of Jehovah's Witnesses refusing life-saving blood transfusions. Insofar as Jehovah's Witnesses should be informed of the consequences of

---

their actions, they should also deliberate rationally about these consequences.

Somerville, Margaret A. Refusal of medical treatment in "captive" circumstances. *Canadian Bar Review.* 1985; 63: 59–90. 105 fn. BE55594.
*aliens; coercion; *competence; force feeding; institutionalized persons; involuntary commitment; *judicial action; law enforcement; *legal aspects; legal rights; mental institutions; *mentally ill; motivation; patient care; *prisoners; psychoactive drugs; self induced illness; standards; suicide; *treatment refusal; rationality; Attorney–General of British Columbia v. Astaforoff; *Attorney–General of Canada v. Notre Dame Hospital; Niemiec; Bouvia v. County of Riverside; Canada; *Institut Philippe Pinel de Montreal v. Dion; *Quebec

Spike, Jeffrey. A paradox about capacity, alcoholism, and noncompliance. *Journal of Clinical Ethics.* 1997 Fall; 8(3): 303–306. 4 fn. BE57567.
*advance directives; *alcohol abuse; *autonomy; *competence; *decision making; family members; *paternalism; *patient care; *patient compliance; *patient participation; physician patient relationship; *physicians; *surgery; third party consent; time factors; *treatment refusal; values; rationality; Ulysses contracts

Strain, James J.; Snyder, Stephen L.; Drooker, Martin. Conflict resolution: experience of consultation–liaison psychiatrists. *In:* Zucker, Marjorie B.; Zucker, Howard D., eds. Medical Futility and the Evaluation of Life–Sustaining Interventions. New York, NY: Cambridge University Press; 1997: 98–109. 8 refs. ISBN 0–521–56877–3. BE55983.
*allowing to die; caring; case studies; decision making; *dissent; emotions; *family members; *futility; goals; mediation; motivation; patient care team; patient transfer; *patients; *physician patient relationship; *physicians; professional family relationship; *prolongation of life; psychiatric diagnosis; *psychiatry; psychological stress; *psychology; *referral and consultation; refusal to treat; resource allocation; retreatment; terminal care; *treatment refusal; trust; guilt; health services misuse; patient abandonment; United States

Sugarman, Jeremy; Harland, Robert. Acute yet non–emergent patients. *In:* McCullough, Laurence B.; Jones, James W.; Brody, Baruch A., eds. Surgical Ethics. New York, NY: Oxford University Press; 1998: 116–132. 18 refs. ISBN 0–19–510347–5. BE58337.
advance directives; alternatives; beneficence; blood transfusions; *communication; comprehension; confidentiality; *critically ill; decision making; diagnosis; disclosure; family members; *informed consent; Jehovah's Witnesses; morbidity; patient care; patient education; patient participation; patients; *physicians; prognosis; referral and consultation; refusal to treat; review; risks and benefits; *surgery; treatment outcome; *treatment refusal; uncertainty; values; *seriously ill; Patient Self–Determination Act 1990; United States

Tierney, William M.; Weinberger, Morris; Greene, James Y., et al. Jehovah's Witnesses and blood transfusion: physicians' attitudes and legal precedents. *Southern Medical Journal.* 1984 Apr; 77(4): 473–478. 31 refs. BE56672.
adults; age factors; *attitudes; autonomy; *blood transfusions; coercion; comparative studies; competence; *decision making; faculty; intention; internship and residency; *Jehovah's Witnesses; judicial action; knowledge, attitudes, practice; legal aspects; medical schools; medical specialties; minors; paternalism; *physicians; referral and consultation; students; suicide; surgery; *treatment refusal; Indiana; Indiana University Medical Center; Indiana University School of Medicine; United States

Veatch, Robert M. Ethical dimensions of advance directives and surrogate decision making in the United States. *In:* Sass, Hans–Martin; Veatch, Robert M.; Kimura, Rihito, eds. Advance Directives and Surrogate Decision Making in Health Care: United States, Germany, and Japan. Baltimore, MD: Johns Hopkins University Press; 1998: 66–91. 72 refs. 7 fn. ISBN 0–8018–5831–3. BE59037.
adults; *advance directives; aged; *allowing to die; anencephaly; artificial feeding; *autonomy; beneficence; brain pathology; competence; consensus; *decision making; family members; freedom; futility; historical aspects; informed consent; judicial action; justice; *legal rights; living wills; mentally retarded; minors; moral policy; parents; paternalism; patients' rights; persistent vegetative state; physician patient relationship; physicians; professional autonomy; prolongation of life; refusal to treat; religion; *risks and benefits; Roman Catholic ethics; *third party consent; *treatment refusal; trends; ventilators; withholding treatment; liberalism; oral directives; values histories; Hippocratic Oath; In re Baby K; In re Conroy; In re Phillip B.; In re Quinlan; Twentieth Century; *United States

Watler, Crosbie L.; Gervais, Laurent; Cameron, Stewart. Lessons from Amy. [Letters and response]. *Canadian Medical Association Journal.* 1997 Jul 1; 157(1): 13–14. 3 refs. BE55778.
*competence; depressive disorder; psychiatric diagnosis; right to die; *suicide; *treatment refusal

Wellman, Carl. The inalienable right to life and the durable power of attorney. *Law and Philosophy.* 1995; 14(2): 245–269. BE55598.
*advance directives; *allowing to die; communication; decision making; *freedom; informed consent; killing; legal rights; moral obligations; *moral policy; patient care; physicians; privacy; prolongation of life; right to die; *rights; third party consent; *treatment refusal; *value of life; withholding treatment

TREATMENT REFUSAL/MENTALLY DISABLED

Appelbaum, Paul S. Let my wife bleed to death. *Medical Ethics Newsletter.* 1997 Fall; 3(3): 3, 7. 2 refs. BE58114.
*allowing to die; case studies; competence; *critically ill; *depressive disorder; *emergency care; *family members; legal aspects; *mentally ill; physicians; spousal consent; suicide; *treatment refusal; withholding treatment

Berghmans, Ron L.P. Coercive treatment in psychiatry. *In:* Chadwick, Ruth, ed. Encyclopedia of Applied Ethics, Volume 1. San Diego, CA: Academic Press; 1998: 535–542. 12 refs. ISBN 0–12–227066–5. BE56374.
*autonomy; *behavior control; beneficence; *coercion; *competence; dangerousness; decision making; deinstitutionalized persons; incentives; institutionalized persons; international aspects; involuntary commitment; mental institutions; *mentally ill; *moral policy; outpatient commitment; *paternalism; *patient care; psychiatric diagnosis; psychiatric wills; *psychiatry; psychosurgery; review; risks and benefits; standards; suffering; *treatment refusal

Dickenson, Donna. Ethical issues in long term psychiatric management. *Journal of Medical Ethics.* 1997 Oct; 23(5): 300–304. 18 fn. BE57104.
accountability; beneficence; case studies; chronically ill; coercion; *community services; *dangerousness; *deinstitutionalized persons; duration of commitment; *informed consent; involuntary commitment; legal aspects; *long–term care; *mentally ill; *outpatient commitment; paternalism; patient compliance; patient discharge; physicians; presumed consent; psychoactive drugs; resource allocation; *risk; *treatment refusal; *Great Britain; Mental

---

BE = bioethics accession number   fn. = footnotes   refs. = references

Health Act 1983 (Great Britain)
Two general ethical problems in psychiatry are thrown into sharp relief by long term care. This article discusses each in turn, in the context of two anonymised case studies from actual clinical practice. First, previous mental health legislation soothed doubts about patients' refusal of consent by incorporating time limits on involuntary treatment. When these are absent, as in the provisions for long term care which have recently come into force, the justification for compulsory treatment and supervision becomes more obviously problematic. Second, Anglo-American law does not normally allow the preventive detention of someone who may be dangerous but has not actually committed any crime. The justification for detaining a possibly dangerous user of mental health services without his or her consent can only be based on risk assessment, but this raises issues of moral luck. Is the psychiatrist who decides not to take out a supervision order for a possibly dangerous patient with an initial psychotic diagnosis morally at fault if that person harms someone in the community, or himself? Or is the psychiatrist merely unlucky?

Dolan, Bridget; Parker, Camilla; Bewley, Susan, et al. Caesarean section: a treatment for mental disorder? Tameside and Glossop Acute Services Unit v CH (A Patient) [1996] 1 FLR 762. [Case report and commentaries]. *BMJ (British Medical Journal).* 1997 Apr 19; 314(7088): 1183–1187. 13 refs. BE56757.
case studies; *cesarean section; *coercion; competence; fetuses; informed consent; involuntary commitment; judicial action; *legal aspects; legal rights; *mentally ill; physical restraint; *pregnant women; schizophrenia; *treatment refusal; *Great Britain; Mental Health Act 1983 (Great Britain); *Tameside and Glossop Acute Services Trust v. CH

Draper, Heather. Treating anorexics without consent: some reservations. [Editorial]. *Journal of Medical Ethics.* 1998 Feb; 24(1): 5–7. 9 fn. BE57405.
*behavior disorders; competence; decision making; food; *force feeding; informed consent; legal aspects; prolongation of life; *treatment refusal; *anorexia nervosa; Great Britain

Goldbeck–Wood, Sandra. Women's autonomy in childbirth. [Editorial]. *BMJ (British Medical Journal).* 1997 Apr 19; 314(7088): 1143–1144. 4 refs. BE56763.
autonomy; *cesarean section; *coercion; fetuses; judicial action; *legal aspects; *mentally ill; *pregnant women; schizophrenia; *treatment refusal; *Great Britain; Mental Health Act 1983 (Great Britain); *Tameside and Glossop Acute Services Trust v. CH

Great Britain. England. Court of Appeal, Civil Division. B v. Croydon Health Authority. *All England Law Reports.* 1994 Nov 29 (date of decision). [1995] 1: 683–690. BE57784.
*artificial feeding; behavior disorders; coercion; emergency care; *food; *force feeding; informed consent; involuntary commitment; *legal aspects; *mentally ill; patient care; *treatment refusal; *B v. Croydon Health Authority; *Great Britain; *Mental Health Act 1983 (Great Britain)
England's Court of Appeal, Civil Division, dismissed the appeal of B, a mentally ill patient, and upheld the lower court's order allowing force feeding by a nasogastric tube. In an attempt to harm herself, B had refused to eat while she was involuntarily hospitalized. Under threat of tubal feeding, she accepted food. B argued that she could not be fed without her consent because, although the Mental Health Act did not require her consent for "any medical treatment" given for her mental illness, force feeding was not medical treatment in the

sense of psychotherapy. The court interpreted "medical treatment" to include ancillary acts such as "nursing and care concurrent with the core treatment or as a necessary prerequisite to such treatment or to prevent the patient from causing harm to himself or to alleviate the consequences of the disorder." A concurring judge agreed that "any medical treatment" included treatment to alleviate symptoms of the disorder as well as treatment to remedy the underlying cause of the disorder. (KIE abstract)

Grubb, Andrew. Treatment without consent (pregnancy): adult -- Tameside and Glossop Acute Services Trust v. C.H. [Comment]. *Medical Law Review.* 1996 Summer; 4(2): 193–198. 5 fn. BE56498.
*cesarean section; *coercion; competence; informed consent; *judicial action; *legal aspects; *mentally ill; *patient care; *pregnant women; psychoactive drugs; psychological stress; schizophrenia; *treatment refusal; *Great Britain; Mental Health Act 1983 (Great Britain); *Tameside and Glossop Acute Services Trust v. C.H.

Hoge, Steven K.; Gutheil, Thomas G.; Kaplan, Eric. The right to refuse treatment under Rogers v. Commissioner: preliminary empirical findings and comparisons. *Bulletin of the American Academy of Psychiatry and the Law.* 1987 Jun; 15(2): 163–169. 16 refs. BE56657.
*due process; economics; *institutionalized persons; *judicial action; legal aspects; mental institutions; *mentally ill; mentally retarded; psychoactive drugs; public hospitals; quality of health care; review committees; *social impact; state government; statistics; survey; *treatment refusal; *Massachusetts; *Rogers v. Commissioner of Department of Mental Health; United States

Jackson, Jennifer. Determining incompetence: problems with the function test. *In:* Grubb, Andrew, ed. Decision–Making and Problems of Incompetence. New York, NY: Wiley; 1994: 53–65. 20 fn. ISBN 0-471-94236-7. BE57129.
*autonomy; communication; *competence; comprehension; decision making; *evaluation; legal rights; paternalism; patient care; patients; physicians; presumed consent; *standards; *treatment refusal; values; vulnerable populations; rationality; Great Britain; Law Commission (Great Britain); President's Commission for the Study of Ethical Problems; United States

Knepper, Kathleen. The importance of establishing competence in cases involving the involuntary administration of psychotropic medications. *Law and Psychology Review.* 1996 Spring; 20: 97–137. 146 fn. BE55586.
adults; coercion; *competence; constitutional law; *decision making; *institutionalized persons; involuntary commitment; *judicial action; *legal aspects; legal guardians; *legal rights; mental institutions; *mentally ill; models, theoretical; *psychoactive drugs; risks and benefits; standards; state government; state interest; Supreme Court decisions; *treatment refusal; *Illinois; *In re C.E.; In re Guardianship of Roe; Massachusetts; *United States

Matthews, Eric. Paternalism, care and mental illness. *In:* Grubb, Andrew, ed. Decision–Making and the Problem of Incompetence. New York, NY: Wiley; 1994: 103–114. 5 fn. ISBN 0-471-94236-7. BE57132.
*autonomy; competence; decision making; *mentally ill; *paternalism; patients; *physicians; self concept; *treatment refusal; values; rationality; Great Britain; Mental Health Act 1983 (Great Britain)

Naber, D.; Kircher, T.; Hessel, K. Schizophrenic

patients' retrospective attitudes regarding involuntary psychopharmacological treatment and restraint.
European Psychiatry. 1996; 11(1): 7–11. 20 refs. BE57064.
  *attitudes; *coercion; emotions; institutionalized persons; involuntary commitment; *mentally ill; *patient care; patient discharge; *patients; *physical restraint; *psychoactive drugs; recall; *schizophrenia; survey; *treatment refusal; retrospective studies; Germany

Roth, Loren; Lidz, Charles W.; Meisel, Alan, et al. Competency to decide about treatment or research: an overview of some empirical data. *International Journal of Law and Psychiatry.* 1982; 5: 29–50. 31 refs. BE57433.
  *competence; *comprehension; consent forms; decision making; depressive disorder; disclosure; electroconvulsive therapy; *empirical research; human experimentation; *informed consent; institutionalized persons; *mentally ill; patient education; psychiatry; *treatment refusal; Western Psychiatric Institute and Clinic (Pittsburgh, PA)

Somerville, Margaret A. Refusal of medical treatment in "captive" circumstances. *Canadian Bar Review.* 1985; 63: 59–90. 105 fn. BE55594.
  *aliens; coercion; *competence; force feeding; institutionalized persons; involuntary commitment; *judicial action; law enforcement; *legal aspects; legal rights; mental institutions; *mentally ill; motivation; patient care; *prisoners; psychoactive drugs; self induced illness; standards; suicide; *treatment refusal; rationality; Attorney-General of British Columbia v. Astaforoff; *Attorney-General of Canada v. Notre Dame Hospital; Niemiec; Bouvia v. County of Riverside; Canada; *Institut Philippe Pinel de Montreal v. Dion; *Quebec

Winslade, William J. Humanistic problem solving: the case of Mr. T. *Journal of Clinical Ethics.* 1997 Winter; 8(4): 389–397. 7 fn. BE57619.
  aged; case studies; *communication; *competence; comprehension; *decision making; depressive disorder; emotions; *empathy; ethical theory; *ethicist's role; ethics consultation; expert testimony; family members; forensic psychiatry; *humanism; *interdisciplinary communication; interprofessional relations; *judicial action; lawyers; legal guardians; *mediation; patient advocacy; patient compliance; physicians; professional patient relationship; quality of life; surgery; *third party consent; *treatment refusal; *amputation; *judges; pragmatism; *professional role
...The following case provides an example of pragmatic humanism incorporated into a legal process. The case begins with Mr. T, an elderly gentleman, who resisted and refused numerous efforts to persuade him to have his gangrenous foot amputated. His family was intimidated by him; his physicians were exasperated; his attorney and the attorney for the government were bemused. I was appointed by a court to assess his situation, to be an independent legal and bioethics adviser to the court. My role went beyond what is currently called ethics consultation. I was also authorized to be a participant in the proceedings, to investigate, to examine witnesses at the hearing, and to report and make recommendations to the court. I accepted the invitation to explore the human problems, psychological, ethical, and legal, and to propose practical ways of solving them.

TREATMENT REFUSAL/MINORS

Canada. Ontario. Court of Appeal. Re B. and Children's Aid Society of Metropolitan Toronto. *Dominion Law Reports, 4th Series.* 1992 Sep 15 (date of decision). 96: 45–85. BE57783.
  autonomy; *blood transfusions; constitutional law; decision making; freedom; health; *infants; *Jehovah's Witnesses; legal aspects; *legal rights; parent child relationship;

*parents; quality of life; religion; *state interest; *treatment refusal; value of life; *Canada; *Canadian Charter of Rights and Freedoms; *Re B. v. Children's Aid Society of Metropolitan Toronto
Baby S. was born prematurely and required surgery to save her eyesight. Her parents had consented to all medical treatment, including life-support systems, but because of their religious beliefs as Jehovah's Witnesses, they objected to any blood transfusions. After a hearing, the infant was found to be a "child in need of protection" and made a temporary ward of a children's aid society in order to receive the blood transfusion. The court of appeal upheld the lower court's approach, "that the child has an individual right to have decisions made by the parents with respect to her health, but that there is no guaranteed right to 'family autonomy'" included in liberty under section 7 of the Canadian Charter of Rights and Freedoms. Because protection of a child's right to life and to health is a basic tenet of the Canadian legal system, the state has a strong interest in intervening when a parent's decision endangers the life or well-being of a child who lacks legal capacity to decide on his or her own. The court's parens patriae jurisdiction concerned not only life, but quality of life. The parents' right to choose medical treatment according to their religious beliefs is protected as long as it does not interfere with the state's interest in preservation of the life or health of the child. (KIE abstract)

Elliston, Sarah. If you know what's good for you: refusal of consent to medical treatment by children. *In:* McLean, Sheila A.M., ed. Contemporary Issues in Law, Medicine and Ethics. Brookfield, VT: Dartmouth; 1996: 29–55. 66 fn. ISBN 1-85521-586-1. BE57789.
  abortion, induced; *adolescents; adults; age factors; autonomy; behavior disorders; beneficence; blood transfusions; children; *competence; comprehension; *decision making; disclosure; human rights; informed consent; intelligence; Jehovah's Witnesses; judicial action; *legal aspects; mentally ill; *minors; parental consent; patient care; physicians; psychoactive drugs; quality of life; risks and benefits; *standards; *treatment refusal; value of life; anorexia nervosa; rationality; Age of Legal Capacity Act 1991 (Scotland); Children Act 1989 (Great Britain); *England; Family Law Reform Act 1969 (Great Britain); *Great Britain; Mental Health Act 1983 (Great Britain); *Scotland

Evans, Jennifer L. Are children competent to make decisions about their own deaths? *Behavioral Sciences and the Law.* 1995 Winter; 13(1): 27–41. 58 refs. BE55784.
  age factors; *allowing to die; autonomy; case studies; *competence; *decision making; *legal aspects; legislation; *minors; *parents; *patient participation; physicians; psychological stress; standards; state interest; terminally ill; *treatment refusal; truth disclosure; withholding treatment; United States

Garey, Christopher C.; Children's Legal Rights Journal. Editorial Staff. When parents refuse consent to medical care for their children: the role of the nurse. *Children's Legal Rights Journal.* 1996 Winter; 16(1): 11–16. 65 fn. BE56223.
  autonomy; beneficence; *blood transfusions; *Jehovah's Witnesses; *legal aspects; legal rights; *minors; *nurse's role; *parents; patient care; quality of life; *treatment refusal; United States

Grubb, Andrew. Re B (A Minor) (Treatment and Secure Accommodation). [Comment]. *Medical Law Review.* 1997 Summer; 5(2): 233–236. BE57870.
  *adolescents; coercion; *competence; drug abuse; hospitals; informed consent; *judicial action; *legal aspects; *minors;

patient care; pregnant women; prenatal injuries; *treatment refusal; Children Act 1989 (Great Britain); *Great Britain; *Re B (A Minor) (Treatment and Secure Accommodation)

Grubb, Andrew. Refusal of treatment: competent child and parents -- Houston, Applicant. [Comment]. *Medical Law Review.* 1997 Summer; 5(2): 237-239. BE57871.
    *adolescents; coercion; *competence; dangerousness; *informed consent; involuntary commitment; *judicial action; *legal aspects; mental institutions; *mentally ill; *minors; *parental consent; *treatment refusal; *Great Britain; *Houston, Applicant; *Scotland

Muram, David; Aiken, Margaret M.; Strong, Carson. Children's refusal of gynecologic examinations for suspected sexual abuse. *Journal of Clinical Ethics.* 1997 Summer; 8(2): 158-164. 12 fn. BE56352.
    age factors; case studies; *child abuse; coercion; competence; decision making; *diagnosis; law enforcement; legal aspects; *minors; obstetrics and gynecology; parental consent; patient compliance; patient participation; physicians; psychological stress; refusal to treat; risks and benefits; *sex offenses; *treatment refusal; United States

Neeley, G. Steven. Legal and ethical dilemmas surrounding prayer as a method of alternative healing for children. *In:* Humber, James M.; Almeder, Robert F., eds. Alternative Medicine and Ethics. Totowa, NJ: Humana Press; 1998: 163-194. 148 fn. ISBN 0-89603-440-2. BE57207.
    adults; *alternative therapies; child abuse; *children; *Christian Scientists; competence; due process; equal protection; federal government; government regulation; *legal aspects; legal rights; *parents; religion; state government; state interest; *treatment refusal; *faith healing; Child Abuse Prevention and Treatment Act 1984; Fifth Amendment; First Amendment; Fourteenth Amendment; *United States

Obernberger, Scott. When love and abuse are not mutually exclusive: the need for government intervention. *Issues in Law and Medicine.* 1997 Spring; 12(4): 355-381. 157 fn. BE57803.
    adults; advance directives; allowing to die; autonomy; child abuse; competence; *decision making; due process; federal government; futility; *government regulation; informed consent; judicial action; *legal aspects; legal rights; mandatory reporting; mentally retarded; *minors; parental consent; *parents; quality of life; standards; state government; state interest; third party consent; *treatment refusal; withholding treatment; Child Abuse Amendments 1984; *United States

Ross, Lainie Friedman. Health care decisionmaking by children: is it in their best interest? *Hastings Center Report.* 1997 Nov-Dec; 27(6): 41-45. 19 refs. BE57859.
    *adolescents; adults; *autonomy; *children; *competence; *decision making; dissent; *family relationship; freedom; *informed consent; organizational policies; parent child relationship; *parental consent; parents; paternalism; *patient care; patient participation; pediatrics; physicians; professional organizations; rights; *treatment refusal; American Academy of Pediatrics
The argument for children's rights in health care has been long in the making. The success of this position is reflected in the 1995 American Academy of Pediatrics recommendations for the role of children in health care decisionmaking, which suggest that children be given greater voice as they mature. But there are good moral and practical reasons for exercising caution in these health care situations, especially when the child and parents disagree. Parents need the moral and legal space within which to make decisions that will facilitate their child's long-term autonomy, not only her present-day

autonomy. Moreover, third-party intrusion, by physicians or the state, should be resisted unless negligent and abusive decisions are in the making.

Tucker, Bonnie Poitras. Deaf culture, cochlear implants, and elective disability. *Hastings Center Report.* 1998 Jul-Aug; 28(4): 6-14. 35 fn. BE58922.
    attitudes; *children; coercion; communication; *cultural pluralism; decision making; economics; international aspects; legal aspects; *medical devices; minority groups; moral obligations; *normality; obligations of society; *parents; *physically disabled; *political activity; risks and benefits; social discrimination; *surgery; *treatment refusal; *values; *cochlear implants; *hearing disorders; *language; Americans with Disabilities Act 1990; Great Britain; *National Association of the Deaf; United States

Webb, Sally L.; Marshall, Mary Faith; Boettcher, Flint, et al. Refusal of treatment by an adolescent: the deliverances of different consciences. *HEC (HealthCare Ethics Committee) Forum.* 1998 Mar; 10(1): 9-23. 15 refs. 3 fn. BE59054.
    *adolescents; advance directives; allowing to die; *blood transfusions; case studies; competence; *conscience; *decision making; dissent; *ethicists; ethics consultation; informed consent; *Jehovah's Witnesses; legal aspects; *parents; *physicians; religion; risks and benefits; surgery; third party consent; *treatment refusal; uncertainty; values

Weir, Robert F.; Peters, Charles. Affirming the decisions adolescents make about life and death. *Hastings Center Report.* 1997 Nov-Dec; 27(6): 29-40. 22 fn. BE57858.
    *adolescents; *advance care planning; *advance directives; *age factors; allowing to die; autonomy; chronically ill; *communication; *competence; counseling; critically ill; *decision making; disclosure; dissent; empirical research; guidelines; *informed consent; legal aspects; legislation; organizational policies; parents; *patient advocacy; *patient care; *patient participation; pediatrics; physician patient relationship; physicians; practice guidelines; professional family relationship; professional organizations; prolongation of life; risks and benefits; state government; *terminal care; terminally ill; *treatment refusal; trust; American Academy of Pediatrics; Patient Self-Determination Act 1990; United States
Adolescents who are critically, chronically, and terminally ill traditionally have been given little voice in their health care treatment. But over the last three decades attitudes have begun to shift. The legal and medical professions as well as parents and children's advocates have started to recognize that cognitively normal adolescents have decisionmaking capacity and believe these patients ought to have the opportunity to participate in even the toughest of health treatment decisions. Advances directives, if used with sensitivity and care, could prove a valuable means of giving these older pediatric patients a say in their care.

TRIAGE *See* SELECTION FOR TREATMENT

TRUTH DISCLOSURE

Adamolekun, Kemi. Openness of health professionals about death and terminal illness in a Nigerian teaching hospital. *Omega: A Journal of Death and Dying.* 1997-1998; 36(1): 23-32. 10 refs. BE57719.
    alternative therapies; attitudes to death; developing countries; *diagnosis; economics; *family members; hospices; hospitals; *knowledge, attitudes, practice; motivation; *nurses; patients; *physicians; *prognosis; psychological stress; risks and benefits; survey; terminal care; *terminally ill; *truth disclosure; *Nigeria

---

BE = bioethics accession number   fn. = footnotes   refs. = references

Asai, Atsushi; Kishino, Minako; Tsuguya, Fukui, et al. A report from Japan: choices of Japanese patients in the face of disagreement. *Bioethics.* 1998 Apr; 12(2): 162–172. 11 refs. BE58626.

*attitudes; *autonomy; *cancer; communication; decision making; *diagnosis; *dissent; family members; family relationship; females; males; patient care; patient compliance; *patient participation; *patient satisfaction; *patients; *physician patient relationship; physicians; prognosis; survey; treatment refusal; *truth disclosure; *Japan

BACKGROUND: Patients in different countries have different attitudes toward self–determination and medical information. Little is known how much respect Japanese patients feel should be given for their wishes about medical care and for medical information, and what choices they would make in the face of disagreement. METHODS: Ambulatory patients in six clinics of internal medicine at a university hospital were surveyed using a self–administered questionnaire. RESULTS: A total of 307 patients participated in our survey. Of the respondents, 47% would accept recommendations made by physicians, even if such recommendations were against their wishes; 25% would try to persuade their physician to change their recommendations; and 14% would leave their physician to find a new one. Seventy–six percent of the respondents thought that physicians should routinely ask patients if they would want to know about a diagnosis of cancer, while 5% disagreed; 59% responded that physicians should inform them of the actual diagnosis, even against the request of their family not to do so, while 24% would want their physician to abide by their family's request and 14% could not decide. One–third of the respondents who initially said they would want to know the truth would yield to the desires of the family in a case of disagreement. INTERPRETATION: In the face of disagreement regarding medical care and disclosure, Japanese patients tend to respond in a diverse and unpredictable manner. Medical professionals should thus be prudent and ask their patients explicitly what they want regarding medical care and information.

Asai, Atsushi; Fukuhara, Shunichi; Inoshita, Osamu, et al. Medical decisions concerning the end of life: a discussion with Japanese physicians. *Journal of Medical Ethics.* 1997 Oct; 23(5): 323–327. 5 refs. BE57101.

*advance directives; *allowing to die; *attitudes; cancer; *decision making; diagnosis; family members; knowledge, attitudes, practice; organizational policies; *physicians; professional organizations; prognosis; *prolongation of life; *resuscitation; resuscitation orders; survey; *terminally ill; *truth disclosure; *withholding treatment; patient abandonment; qualitative research; *Japan; Japan Medical Association

OBJECTIVES: Life–sustaining treatment at the end of life gives rise to many ethical problems in Japan. Recent surveys of Japanese physicians suggested that they tend to treat terminally ill patients aggressively. We studied why Japanese physicians were reluctant to withhold or withdraw life–support from terminally ill patients and what affected their decisions. DESIGN AND PARTICIPANTS: A qualitative study design was employed, using a focus group interview with seven physicians, to gain an in–depth understanding of attitudes and rationales in Japan regarding medical care at the end of life. RESULTS: Analysis revealed that physicians and patients' family members usually make decisions about life–sustaining treatment, while the patients' wishes are unavailable or not taken into account. Both physicians and family members tend to consider withholding or withdrawing life–sustaining treatment as abandonment or even killing. The strongest reason to start cardiopulmonary resuscitation –– and to continue it until patients' family members arrive –– seems to be the family members' desire to be at the bedside at the time of death. All physicians participating in our study regarded advance directives that provide information as to patients' wishes about life–sustaining treatment desirable. All expressed concern, however, that it would be difficult to forego or discontinue life–support based on a patient's advance directive, particularly when the patient's family opposed the directive. CONCLUSION: Our group interview suggested several possible barriers to death with dignity and the appropriate use of advance directives in Japan. Further qualitative and quantitative research in this regard is needed.

Baylis, Françoise. Errors in medicine: nurturing truthfulness. *Journal of Clinical Ethics.* 1997 Winter; 8(4): 336–340. 10 fn. BE57605.

attitudes; case studies; *disclosure; emotions; *iatrogenic disease; interprofessional relations; legal liability; medical ethics; moral obligations; motivation; *negligence; *patient care; physician patient relationship; *physicians; professional competence; risks and benefits; self regulation; *sociology of medicine; trust; *truth disclosure; uncertainty; whistleblowing; *medical errors

In "When a Physician Harms a Patient by a Medical Error," Finkelstein and colleagues maintain that patients have a right to the truth and that physicians have a corresponding obligation to be truthful. In their view, when an erroneous act or omission results in an adverse outcome for the patient, the physician should truthfully disclose the medical error, offer the patient a sincere apology, and explore the option of financial compensation. In the abstract, this seems reasonable –– and some might even argue uncontestable. Why then is it not common practice for physicians to routinely discuss their errors with their patients? In this article, I will critically examine some of the reasons given by physicians for non–disclosure or partial disclosure, and then consider what the medical profession should do to foster more respectful, open, and honest communication about errors with patients.

Blennerhassett, Mitzi; Tattersall, Martin; Ellis, Peter, et al. Truth, the first casualty. [Article and commentaries]. *BMJ (British Medical Journal).* 1998 Jun 20; 316(7148): 1890–1893. 14 refs. BE58050.

*cancer; case studies; *communication; decision making; diagnosis; disclosure; informed consent; pain; *patient care; patient care team; patient participation; physician patient relationship; prognosis; quality of health care; risks and benefits; *truth disclosure; Great Britain

Burgess, M.M.; Hayden, M.R. Patients' rights to laboratory data: trinucleotide repeat length in Huntington disease. [Editorial]. *American Journal of Medical Genetics.* 1996 Mar 1; 62(1): 6–9. 25 refs. BE55662.

autonomy; beneficence; decision making; *diagnosis; ethical analysis; *genetic counseling; *genetic information; genetic screening; *Huntington's disease; institutional policies; laboratories; late–onset disorders; paternalism; patient participation; professional patient relationship; risks and benefits; trust; *truth disclosure

Chan, Arlene; Woodruff, Roger K. Communicating with patients with advanced cancer. *Journal of Palliative Care.* 1997 Autumn; 13(3): 29–33. 21 refs. BE58052.

adults; aged; *attitudes; *cancer; caring; *communication; comparative studies; *comprehension; *diagnosis; family practice; females; health maintenance organizations; hospitals; internship and residency; males; medical specialties; minority groups; *nurses; *pain; *palliative care;

---

*patient care; *patient satisfaction; *patients; *physicians; professional patient relationship; *prognosis; quality of health care; quality of life; survey; terminal care; time factors; *truth disclosure; translating; Australia

Clafferty, R.A.; Brown, K.W.; McCabe, E. Under half of psychiatrists tell patients their diagnosis of Alzheimer's disease. [Letter]. *BMJ (British Medical Journal).* 1998 Aug 29; 317(7158): 603. 4 refs. BE59050.
*dementia; *knowledge, attitudes, practice; *physicians; *psychiatric diagnosis; *psychiatry; survey; *truth disclosure; National Health Service; *Scotland

Fallowfield, Lesley; Ford, Sarah; Lewis, Shon. No news is not good news: information preferences of patients with cancer. *Psycho-Oncology.* 1995 Oct; 4(3): 197-202. 29 refs. BE55622.
age factors; alternatives; *attitudes; *cancer; depressive disorder; diagnosis; females; patient care; *patients; prognosis; psychological stress; risks and benefits; survey; *truth disclosure; outpatients; *Great Britain

Faulkner, Ann. ABC of palliative care: communication with patients, families, and other professionals. *BMJ (British Medical Journal).* 1998 Jan 10; 316(7125): 130-132. 3 refs. BE57753.
*communication; diagnosis; emotions; empathy; family members; interprofessional relations; palliative care; patient care team; patients; physician patient relationship; *physicians; professional family relationship; prognosis; psychological stress; *terminal care; *terminally ill; *truth disclosure

Fetters, Michael D. The family in medical decision making: Japanese perspectives. *Journal of Clinical Ethics.* 1998 Summer; 9(2): 132-146. 48 fn. BE58959.
age factors; attitudes to death; autonomy; beneficence; bioethics; Buddhist ethics; *cancer; clinical ethics; consensus; *cultural pluralism; *decision making; *diagnosis; economics; *family members; *family relationship; females; males; minority groups; models, theoretical; morality; paternalism; patient care; patient participation; physician patient relationship; physicians; public opinion; religion; social dominance; terminal care; *third party consent; trends; *truth disclosure; *values; Confucian ethics; non-Western World; preventive ethics; *Japan; United States

Ford, Helen L.; Johnson, Michael H. Telling your patient he/she has multiple sclerosis. *Postgraduate Medical Journal.* 1995 Aug; 71(838): 449-452. 11 refs. BE55657.
case studies; *central nervous system diseases; *communication; *diagnosis; employment; guidelines; insurance; prognosis; psychological stress; risks and benefits; social discrimination; *truth disclosure; *uncertainty; *multiple sclerosis; British Society of Rehabilitation Medicine; Great Britain

Girgis, Afaf; Sanson-Fisher, Rob W. Breaking bad news: consensus guidelines for medical practitioners. *Journal of Clinical Oncology.* 1995 Sep; 13(9): 2449-2456. 69 refs. BE57909.
attitudes; cancer; communication; comprehension; diagnosis; emotions; guidelines; methods; patients; physicians; *practice guidelines; privacy; *prognosis; *truth disclosure

Helm, Ann. Truth telling, placebos, and deception: ethical and legal issues in practice. *Aviation, Space, and Environmental Medicine.* 1985 Jan; 56(1): 69-72. 22 refs. BE56956.
*deception; diagnosis; paternalism; *patient care; physicians; *placebos; prognosis; *risks and benefits; *truth disclosure

Hern, H. Eugene; Koenig, Barbara A.; Moore, Lisa

Jean, et al. The difference that culture can make in end-of-life decisionmaking. *Cambridge Quarterly of Healthcare Ethics.* 1998 Winter; 7(1): 27-40. 30 fn. BE58455.
alternative therapies; anthropology; *Asian Americans; *autonomy; *cancer; case studies; clinical ethics; *communication; *cultural pluralism; *decision making; *diagnosis; disclosure; *family members; *family relationship; females; *informed consent; *knowledge, attitudes, practice; *minority groups; models, theoretical; patient care; *patient care team; *patient participation; *patients; *physician patient relationship; physicians; *professional family relationship; *prognosis; risks and benefits; stigmatization; *terminal care; terminally ill; *third party consent; trust; *truth disclosure; *values; California; United States

Hoshino, Kazumasa. Bioethics in the light of Japanese sentiments. *In:* Hoshino, Kazumasa, ed. Japanese and Western Bioethics: Studies in Moral Diversity. Boston, MA: Kluwer Academic; 1997: 13-23. 5 refs. ISBN 0-7923-4112-0. BE57080.
autonomy; bioethical issues; cadavers; communication; *communitarianism; comparative studies; *decision making; diagnosis; family members; *family relationship; informed consent; legal aspects; *organ donation; *paternalism; patient care; patient compliance; *patients' rights; *physician patient relationship; *physicians; privacy; professional family relationship; prognosis; terminally ill; third party consent; *tissue donation; *truth disclosure; hope; non-Western World; Act of Donation of the Body for Medical and Dental Education 1983 (Japan); Cornea and Kidney Transplant Act 1979 (Japan); *Japan; United States

Howe, Edmund G. "Possible mistakes." *Journal of Clinical Ethics.* 1997 Winter; 8(4): 323-328. 35 fn. BE57608.
*disclosure; empathy; *iatrogenic disease; interprofessional relations; legal liability; motivation; *negligence; *patient care; physician patient relationship; professional competence; psychological stress; risks and benefits; self concept; standards; *truth disclosure; uncertainty; whistleblowing; *medical errors; United States
What should a careprovider do if he or she has made a mistake that has harmed a patient? What if a careprovider learns that another's mistake has harmed a patient? Should a careprovider go so far as to tell a patient that he or she could sue? Several articles in this issue of *JCE* address these questions. In this introductory article, I shall ask a question that goes one step further: What should a careprovider do when he or she *may* have made a mistake? First I will discuss the arguments for and against disclosing such mistakes to patients. Then, because these arguments may not be conclusive in and of themselves, I shall also relate two somewhat surprising clinical findings that may help a careprovider facing this situation decide what to do.

Kendrick, Kevin. Should nurses always tell the truth? Honesty versus deception in healthcare. *Professional Nurse (London).* 1994 Jul; 9: 674-677. 10 refs. BE55787.
adults; beneficence; case studies; *deception; deontological ethics; domestic violence; minors; moral policy; motivation; nurse patient relationship; *nurses; *nursing ethics; prognosis; terminal care; terminally ill; trust; *truth disclosure; utilitarianism; virtues; personal integrity

Keyserlingk, Edward W. Quality of life decisions and the hopelessly ill patient: the physician as moral agent and truth teller. *In:* Hoshino, Kazumasa, ed. Japanese and Western Bioethics: Studies in Moral Diversity. Boston, MA: Kluwer Academic; 1997: 103-116. 20 refs. ISBN 0-7923-4112-0. BE57086.
*allowing to die; *communication; *decision making; disclosure; extraordinary treatment; *family members;

BE = bioethics accession number   fn. = footnotes   refs. = references

*futility; goals; medicine; paternalism; patients; *persistent vegetative state; *physician's role; physicians; professional family relationship; prognosis; prolongation of life; *quality of life; refusal to treat; risks and benefits; suffering; *terminally ill; treatment outcome; treatment refusal; *truth disclosure; *values; withholding treatment; Canada; Japan; United States

Kuuppelomäki, Merja; Lauri, Sirkka. Ethical dilemmas in the care of patients with incurable cancer. *Nursing Ethics.* 1998 Jul; 5(4): 283–293. 24 refs. BE58868.

age factors; aged; artificial feeding; blood transfusions; *cancer; communication; decision making; *diagnosis; drugs; emotions; family members; hospitals; *knowledge, attitudes, practice; *nurses; pain; palliative care; patient care; *patient satisfaction; *patients; physician nurse relationship; physician patient relationship; *physicians; privacy; *prognosis; quality of health care; suffering; survey; *terminal care; *terminally ill; *truth disclosure; withholding treatment; antibiotics; chemotherapy; morphine; qualitative research; Finland

Ohi, Gen. Advance directives and the Japanese ethos. *In:* Sass, Hans-Martin; Veatch, Robert M.; Kimura, Rihito, eds. Advance Directives and Surrogate Decision Making in Health Care: United States, Germany, and Japan. Baltimore, MD: Johns Hopkins University Press; 1998: 175–186. 7 refs. ISBN 0-8018-5831-3. BE59041.

*advance directives; *attitudes; autonomy; cancer; case studies; common good; *communication; cultural pluralism; diagnosis; *family relationship; physician patient relationship; physicians; privacy; prognosis; psychological stress; *social interaction; socioeconomic factors; terminally ill; trust; *truth disclosure; *non-Western World; oral directives; Western World; Asia; *Japan

Ohi, Gen. Ethos and its changes: a commentary on 'facing death the Japanese way -- customs and ethos'. *In:* Hoshino, Kazumasa, ed. Japanese and Western Bioethics: Studies in Moral Diversity. Boston, MA: Kluwer Academic; 1997: 155–159. 1 ref. ISBN 0-7923-4112-0. BE57091.

aged; autonomy; beneficence; cancer; communitarianism; cultural pluralism; decision making; diagnosis; empathy; family members; hospices; intelligence; international aspects; paternalism; physician patient relationship; physicians; prognosis; social interaction; terminal care; terminally ill; trust; *truth disclosure; Africa; Asia; Europe; *Japan; United States

Osuna, Eduardo; Pérez–Cárceles, Maria D.; Esteban, Miguel A., et al. The right to information for the terminally ill patient. *Journal of Medical Ethics.* 1998 Apr; 24(2): 106–109. 19 refs. BE58080.

family members; home care; hospitals; *nurses; patient care team; *physicians; *prognosis; survey; *terminal care; *terminally ill; *truth disclosure; *Spain

OBJECTIVES: To analyse the attitudes of medical personnel towards terminally ill patients and their right to be fully informed. DESIGN: Self-administered questionnaire composed of 56 closed questions. SETTING: Three general hospitals and eleven health centres in Granada (Spain). The sample comprised 168 doctors and 207 nurses. RESULTS: A high percentage of medical personnel (24.1%) do not think that informing the terminally ill would help them face their illness with greater serenity. Eighty-four per cent think the patient's own home is the best place to die: 8.9% of the subjects questioned state that the would not like to be informed of an incurable illness. CONCLUSION: In our opinion any information given should depend on the patient's personality, the stage of the illness and family circumstances. Our study confirms that a hospital is not the ideal environment for attending to the needs of the terminally ill and their families.

Pang, Mei–che Samantha. Information disclosure: the moral experience of nurses in China. *Nursing Ethics.* 1998 Jul; 5(4): 347–361. 64 refs. BE58873.

active euthanasia; autonomy; beneficence; cancer; codes of ethics; compassion; conscience; *decision making; diagnosis; *disclosure; *family members; historical aspects; hospitals; *informed consent; *knowledge, attitudes, practice; literature; medical ethics; moral obligations; nurse patient relationship; *nurses; *nursing ethics; nursing research; paternalism; patient advocacy; patient care; patients' rights; physician nurse relationship; professional family relationship; *prognosis; survey; *terminal care; terminally ill; *third party consent; *truth disclosure; virtues; qualitative research; *China; Hong Kong

Parsons, Evelyn; Bradley, Don; Clarke, Angus. Disclosure of Duchenne muscular dystrophy after newborn screening. *Archives of Disease in Childhood.* 1996 Jun; 74(6): 550–553. 13 refs. BE56314.

attitudes; communication; *diagnosis; *Duchenne muscular dystrophy; evaluation; *genetic screening; informed consent; interdisciplinary communication; mass screening; *newborns; parents; patient care team; *patient satisfaction; professional patient relationship; program descriptions; time factors; *truth disclosure; voluntary programs; Wales

Post, Stephen G. The fear of forgetfulness: a grassroots approach to an ethics of Alzheimer's disease. *Journal of Clinical Ethics.* 1998 Spring; 9(1): 71–80. 47 fn. BE57716.

advance directives; allowing to die; artificial feeding; attitudes; autonomy; caring; *dementia; diagnosis; drugs; emotions; family members; genetic screening; guidelines; health personnel; palliative care; patient advocacy; *patient care; personhood; quality of life; risks and benefits; social interaction; social worth; *stigmatization; third party consent; *truth disclosure; value of life; withholding treatment; ELSI-funded publication; Alzheimer's Disease and Related Disorders Association; Aricept; United States

Poulson, Jane. Bitter pills to swallow. *New England Journal of Medicine.* 1998 Jun 18; 338(25): 1844–1846. BE58615.

attitudes; cancer; *communication; drugs; emotions; empathy; human experimentation; medical education; *patients; *physician patient relationship; *physicians; *psychological stress; psychology; selection of subjects; suffering; time factors; toxicity; *truth disclosure; *seriously ill; *sick role

Räikkä, Juha. Freedom and a right (not) to know. *Bioethics.* 1998 Jan; 12(1): 49–63. 21 fn. BE58482.

*autonomy; coercion; competence; *decision making; freedom; *genetic counseling; *genetic information; *moral obligations; *moral policy; *patient participation; *rights; *truth disclosure; *right not to know

Reitemeier, Paul J. Musings on medical mistakes: a four-piece ensemble in search of an orchestra. *Journal of Clinical Ethics.* 1997 Winter; 8(4): 353–358. 5 fn. BE57612.

attitudes; bioethics; *clinical ethics; clinical ethics committees; communication; conscience; *disclosure; emotions; empirical research; *ethicist's role; ethics consultation; family members; *iatrogenic disease; legal liability; malpractice; moral obligations; moral policy; negligence; patient care; patients' rights; physician patient relationship; physicians; professional competence; quality of health care; standards; terminal care; *truth disclosure; virtues; whistleblowing; *medical errors

Rhodes, Rosamond. Genetic links, family ties, and social bonds: rights and responsibilities in the face of genetic knowledge. *Journal of Medicine and Philosophy.* 1998 Feb; 23(1): 10–30. 42 refs. 19 fn. BE57518.

---

*autonomy; beneficence; case studies; confidentiality; decision making; directive counseling; disclosure; *family members; family relationship; friends; *genetic counseling; genetic disorders; *genetic information; genetic research; *genetic screening; Huntington's disease; *moral obligations; *moral policy; *obligations to society; patient participation; *patients; privacy; rights; social interaction; Tay Sachs disease; *truth disclosure; volunteers; pedigree studies; population genetics; *right not to know

Currently, some of the most significant moral issues involving genetic links relate to genetic knowledge. In this paper, instead of looking at the frequently addressed issues of responsibilities professionals or institutions have to individuals, I take up the question of what responsibilities individuals have to one another with respect to genetic knowledge. I address the questions of whether individuals have a moral right to pursue their own goals without contributing to society's knowledge of population genetics, without adding to their family's knowledge of its genetic history, and without discovering genetic information about themselves and their offspring. These questions lead to an examination of the presumed right to genetic ignorance and an exploration of a variety of social bonds. Analyzing cases in light of these considerations leads to a surprising conclusion about a widely accepted precept of genetic counseling, to some ethical insights into typical problems, and to some further unanswered questions about personal responsibility in the face of genetic knowledge.

Rosner, Fred. Informing the patient of a fatal illness. [Letter]. *Archives of Internal Medicine.* 1986 Feb; 146(2): 413. 4 refs. BE57059.
clergy; communication; compassion; diagnosis; *Jewish ethics; physicians; *prognosis; psychological stress; terminally ill; *truth disclosure; hope

Smith, Thomas J.; Swisher, Karen. Telling the truth about terminal cancer. [Editorial]. *JAMA.* 1998 Jun 3; 279(21): 1746–1748. 28 refs. BE58429.
allowing to die; attitudes; autonomy; *cancer; communication; *decision making; drugs; informed consent; mortality; *palliative care; patient participation; patients; physicians; *prognosis; *prolongation of life; risks and benefits; *terminal care; *terminally ill; treatment outcome; *truth disclosure; Study to Understand Prognoses and Preferences for Outcomes and Risks of Treatments (SUPPORT)

Spriggs, Merle. Autonomy in the face of a devastating diagnosis. *Journal of Medical Ethics.* 1998 Apr; 24(2): 123–126. 26 fn. BE58068.
*autonomy; cancer; decision making; dehumanization; diagnosis; freedom; goals; *literature; *patients; prisoners; *prognosis; *psychological stress; *self concept; *terminally ill; *truth disclosure; values; Cancer Ward (Solzhenitsyn, A.); Man's Search for Meaning (Frankl, V.); One Day in the Life of Ivan Denisovich (Solzhenitsyn, A.)

Literary accounts of traumatic events can be more informative and insightful than personal testimonials. In particular, reference to works of literature can give us a more vivid sense of what it is like to receive a devastating diagnosis. In turn this can lead us to question some common assumptions about the nature of autonomy, particularly for patients in these circumstances. The literature of concentration camp and labour camp experiences can help us understand what it is like to have one's life-plans altered utterly and unexpectedly. Contrary to common views of autonomy which have difficulty in characterising autonomous action when long-standing assumptions are suddenly lost, these examples show that autonomy is possible in

these circumstances. We need a theory of autonomy which can deal with traumatic events and is useful in the clinical context.

Sprigler, Gail B. When the truth hurts. *Plastic Surgical Nursing.* 1996 Spring; 16(1): 51–53, 56. 15 refs. BE55890.
alternatives; autonomy; beneficence; codes of ethics; deception; decision making; diagnosis; *disclosure; drugs; ethical theory; *informed consent; justice; moral obligations; *nurses; patient advocacy; patient care; physicians; placebos; prognosis; risks and benefits; terminal care; terminally ill; *truth disclosure; American Nurses Association; International Council of Nurses

Surbone, Antonella; Zwitter, Matjaž, eds. Communication with the Cancer Patient: Information and Truth. New York, NY: New York Academy of Sciences; 1997. 540 p. (Annals of the New York Academy of Sciences; v. 809). 928 refs. 31 fn. ISBN 0-89766-986-X. BE56518.
adolescents; adults; attitudes; bone marrow; *cancer; children; *communication; continuing education; *cultural pluralism; decision making; developing countries; diagnosis; disclosure; disease; drugs; family members; historical aspects; HIV seropositivity; human experimentation; informed consent; *international aspects; metaphor; nurse's role; palliative care; parents; patient care; patient participation; patients; *physician patient relationship; physicians; prognosis; prolongation of life; quality of life; radiology; risks and benefits; socioeconomic factors; surgery; terminally ill; tissue transplantation; treatment outcome; *truth disclosure; values; hope; non-Western World; Western World; Africa; Asia; Australia; Europe; Latin America; Middle East; North America

Sweet, Matthew P.; Bernat, James L. A study of the ethical duty of physicians to disclose errors. *Journal of Clinical Ethics.* 1997 Winter; 8(4): 341–348. 13 fn. BE57616.
*attitudes; communication; conscience; death; deception; diagnosis; *disclosure; drugs; family members; hospitals; *iatrogenic disease; institutional policies; interprofessional relations; knowledge, attitudes, practice; legal liability; malpractice; medical ethics; morbidity; *moral obligations; *motivation; negligence; paralysis; patient care; patients' rights; physician patient relationship; *physicians; professional competence; psychological stress; referral and consultation; statistics; students; survey; *truth disclosure; *whistleblowing; *medical errors; Dartmouth–Hitchcock Medical Center (Lebanon, NH)

Wachbroit, Robert. The question not asked: the challenge of pleiotropic genetic tests. *Kennedy Institute of Ethics Journal.* 1998 Jun; 8(2): 131–144. 10 refs. BE58372.
*dementia; *disclosure; double effect; genetic counseling; *genetic disorders; *genetic information; genetic predisposition; *genetic screening; *heart diseases; informed consent; moral obligations; moral policy; obligations to society; patients; physicians; policy analysis; psychological stress; risks and benefits; social discrimination; time factors; *truth disclosure; *incidental findings

Nearly all of the literature on the ethical, legal, or social issues surrounding genetic tests has proceeded on the assumption that any particular test for a gene mutation yields information about only one disease condition. Even though the phenomenon of pleiotropy, where a single gene has multiple, apparently unrelated phenotypic effects, is widely recognized in genetics, it has not had much significance for genetic testing until recently. In this article, I examine a moral dilemma created by one sort of pleiotropic testing, APOE genotyping, which can yield information about the risk of two different conditions -- coronary heart disease and Alzheimer's disease. A physician administering

---

BE = bioethics accession number   fn. = footnotes   refs. = references

APOE testing for the beneficial purpose of assessing the risk of heart disease may discover medically useless and socially harmful information about the patient's risk of Alzheimer's disease. I explore how much providers should disclose to patients about pleiotropic test results and whether patients are obligated to know as much about their genetic condition as possible.

Weaver, Kirke D. Genetic screening and the right not to know. *Issues in Law and Medicine.* 1997 Winter; 13(3): 243–281. 192 fn. BE58704.
coercion; dementia; disabled; *employment; federal government; genetic counseling; genetic disorders; genetic predisposition; *genetic screening; government regulation; health hazards; Huntington's disease; industry; *insurance; *legal aspects; *legal rights; legislation; *mandatory testing; occupational exposure; privacy; private sector; psychological stress; public sector; *risks and benefits; social discrimination; state interest; stigmatization; treatment refusal; *truth disclosure; voluntary programs; *right not to know; Americans with Disabilities Act 1990; Fourth Amendment; United States

WAR

Addis, G.J.; London, D. The *BMJ*'s Nuremberg issue. [Letters]. *BMJ (British Medical Journal).* 1997 Apr 12; 314(7087): 1128. 2 refs. BE57240.
*conscience; *historical aspects; *human experimentation; *moral obligations; National Socialism; nontherapeutic research; *obligations to society; organizational policies; physicians; professional organizations; religion; *research subjects; *volunteers; *war; Germany; *Great Britain; Royal College of Physicians of London; Twentieth Century; *World War II

Blinderman, Abraham. The physician and war: a layman's view. *New York State Journal of Medicine.* 1985 Feb; 85(2): 77–79. 27 refs. BE56967.
historical aspects; international aspects; moral obligations; *physician's role; political activity; *war; International Physicians for the Prevention of Nuclear War

Bond, Michael. Drugs firms fight biowar curbs. [News]. *New Scientist.* 1997 Mar 8; 153(2072): 8. BE55647.
*biological warfare; *drug industry; government regulation; *international aspects; microbiology; *regulation; Biological and Toxic Weapons Convention; Europe; European Union; United States

Butler, Declan. Admission on Gulf War vaccines spurs debate on medical records. [News]. *Nature.* 1997 Nov 6; 390(6655): 3–4. BE56858.
biological warfare; epidemiology; *human experimentation; *immunization; injuries; medical records; *military personnel; *morbidity; *public policy; *war; whooping cough; *Great Britain; *Ministry of Defence (Great Britain); *Persian Gulf War

Chen, Yuan-Fang. Japanese death factories and the American cover-up. *Cambridge Quarterly of Healthcare Ethics.* 1997 Spring; 6(2): 240–242. BE56425.
accountability; aliens; *biological warfare; communicable diseases; *historical aspects; *human experimentation; human rights; international aspects; investigators; killing; medical ethics; military personnel; moral complicity; National Socialism; physicians; *prisoners; *public policy; *research subjects; *scientific misconduct; torture; *war; China; Factories of Death (Harris, S.); Germany; Ishii, Shiro; *Japan; Twentieth Century; *United States; *World War II

Cohen, Maynard M. A Stand Against Tyranny: Norway's

Physicians and the Nazis. Detroit, MI: Wayne State University Press; 1997. 326 p. 355 fn. ISBN 0–8143–2603–X. BE57150.
*historical aspects; hospitals; human rights; Jews; killing; *National Socialism; patient care; *physician's role; *physicians; *political activity; prisoners; torture; *war; Germany; *Norway; Twentieth Century; *World War II

Coupland, Robin M. "Non-lethal" weapons: precipitating a new arms race. [Editorial]. *BMJ (British Medical Journal).* 1997 Jul 12; 315(7100): 72. 12 refs. BE56573.
biomedical technologies; physician's role; *war

Forrow, Lachlan; Blair, Bruce G.; Helfand, Ira, et al. Accidental nuclear war -- a post–Cold War assessment. *New England Journal of Medicine.* 1998 Apr 30; 338(18): 1326–1331. 67 refs. BE57818.
international aspects; *morbidity; *mortality; *nuclear warfare; *physician's role; political activity; professional organizations; public policy; radiation; risk; Abolition 2000; Russia; *United States
BACKGROUND: In the 1980s, many medical organizations identified the prevention of nuclear war as one of the medical profession's most important goals. An assessment of the current danger is warranted given the radically changed context of the post–Cold War era. METHODS: We reviewed the recent literature on the status of nuclear arsenals and the risk of nuclear war. We then estimated the likely medical effects of a scenario identified by leading experts as posing a serious danger: an accidental launch of nuclear weapons. We assessed possible measures to reduce the risk of such an event. RESULTS: U.S. and Russian nuclear–weapons systems remain on a high–level alert status. This fact, combined with the aging of Russian technical systems, has recently increased the risk of an accidental nuclear attack. As a conservative estimate, an accidental intermediate–sized launch of weapons from a single Russian submarine would result in the deaths of 6,838,000 persons from firestorms in eight U.S. cities. Millions of other people would probably be exposed to potentially lethal radiation from fallout. An agreement to remove all nuclear missiles from high–level alert status and eliminate the capability of a rapid launch would put an end to this threat. CONCLUSIONS: The risk of an accidental nuclear attack has increased in recent years, threatening a public health disaster of unprecedented scale. Physicians and medical organizations should work actively to help build support for the policy changes that would prevent such a disaster.

Forrow, Lachlan; Sidel, Victor W. Medicine and nuclear war: from Hiroshima to mutual assured destruction to Abolition 2000. *JAMA.* 1998 Aug 5; 280(5): 456–461. 97 refs. BE58764.
health hazards; historical aspects; *international aspects; morbidity; mortality; *nuclear warfare; *physician's role; *political activity; professional organizations; public policy; radiation; risk; *Abolition 2000; American Medical Association; Cold War; International Physicians for the Prevention of Nuclear War; Physicians for Social Responsibility; Twentieth Century; United States
To determine how physicians might participate in the prevention of nuclear war in the post–Cold War era, we review, from a medical perspective, the history of the nuclear weapons era since Hiroshima and the status of today's nuclear arsenals and dangers. In the 1950s, physicians were active partners in governmental civil defense planning. Since 1962, physicians have stressed prevention of nuclear war as the only effective medical intervention. Public advocacy by physicians helped end both atmospheric nuclear testing in the 1960s and

superpower plans for fighting a nuclear war in the 1980s. Today's dangers include nuclear arms proliferation, an increasing risk of nuclear terrorism, and the 35000 warheads that remain in superpower-nuclear arsenals, many still on hair-trigger alert. Physicians have recently joined with military and political leaders and over 1000 citizens' organizations in calling for the complete elimination of nuclear weapons. Global medical collaboration in support of a verifiable and enforceable Nuclear Weapons Convention would be a major contribution to safeguarding health in the 21st century.

Gold, Hal. Unit 731: Testimony -- Japan's Wartime Human Experimentation Program. Tokyo: Yenbooks; 1996. 256 p. Bibliography: p. 251–256. ISBN 4-900737-39-9. BE57996.
*biological warfare; children; confidentiality; dehumanization; disclosure; federal government; females; historical aspects; *human experimentation; international aspects; investigators; killing; military personnel; *moral complicity; *prisoners; public policy; *scientific misconduct; torture; China; Cold War; Ishii, Shiro; *Japan; Manchuria; *Twentieth Century; *United States; USSR; *World War II

Greenberg, Daniel S. Hidden data and abuse in research come to light in the USA. [News]. *Lancet.* 1997 Oct 11; 350(9084): 1083. BE56926.
cancer; compensation; *disclosure; federal government; government regulation; *health hazards; historical aspects; *human experimentation; industry; informed consent; mentally ill; *nuclear warfare; public health; *public policy; *radiation; research ethics committees; *scientific misconduct; Cold War; Twentieth Century; *United States

Ljubic, Bozo. War medicine. *Dolentium Hominum: Church and Health in the World.* 1996; 31(11th Yr., No. 1): 252–256. BE57370.
attitudes; bioethics; Christian ethics; dehumanization; epidemiology; ethics; international aspects; killing; *medicine; morality; philosophy; physicians; professional organizations; *war; *Bosnia-Herzegovina; *Croatia

Milner, Claire Alida. Gulf war guinea pigs: is informed consent optional during war? [Comment]. *Journal of Contemporary Health Law and Policy.* 1996 Fall; 13(1): 199–232. 249 fn. BE55791.
*biological warfare; codes of ethics; federal government; *government regulation; health hazards; historical aspects; *human experimentation; iatrogenic disease; immunization; *informed consent; *investigational drugs; *legal aspects; legal liability; *military personnel; nontherapeutic research; occupational exposure; politics; *preventive medicine; psychoactive drugs; public policy; radiation; scientific misconduct; Supreme Court decisions; therapeutic research; toxicity; *war; *chemical warfare; Central Intelligence Agency; *Cold War; Declaration of Helsinki; Department of Defense; Federal Policy (Common Rule) for the Protection of Human Subjects 1991; *Food and Drug Administration; National Institutes of Health; Nuremberg Code; *Persian Gulf War; Twentieth Century; *United States

Sidley, Pat. Doctors involved in South Africa's biological warfare programme. [News]. *BMJ (British Medical Journal).* 1998 Jun 20; 316(7148): 1852. BE58124.
*biological warfare; criminal law; historical aspects; investigators; *misconduct; *physicians; psychoactive drugs; public policy; *chemical warfare; Basson, Wouter; *South Africa; Twentieth Century

Straker, Gillian. Ethical issues in working with children in war zones. *In:* Apfel, Roberta J.; Simon, Bennett, eds.

Minefields in Their Hearts: The Mental Health of Children and Communal Violence. New Haven, CT: Yale University Press; 1996: 18–32. 17 refs. ISBN 0-300-06570-1. BE56147.
*adolescents; autonomy; beneficence; case studies; *children; common good; confidentiality; cultural pluralism; developing countries; disclosure; *duty to warn; ethical relativism; *health personnel; human rights; international aspects; justice; mental health; moral complicity; *moral obligations; morality; *political activity; professional autonomy; professional ethics; professional patient relationship; *psychological stress; *psychotherapy; risks and benefits; social discrimination; torture; trust; *violence; *war; South Africa

Watts, Jonathan. Japan taken to court over germ-warfare allegations. [News]. *Lancet.* 1998 Feb 28; 351(9103): 657. BE58264.
*biological warfare; *historical aspects; *human experimentation; international aspects; legal aspects; *scientific misconduct; war; China; *Japan; Twentieth Century; *World War II

Whitman, Jeffrey P. Reclaiming the medical profession: the military profession as a model. *Professional Ethics.* 1995 Spring; 4(1): 3–22. 32 fn. BE55796.
conflict of interest; conscience; *economics; entrepreneurship; *goals; *health care reform; killing; malpractice; *medical ethics; *medicine; *metaphor; *military personnel; misconduct; *moral obligations; morality; organizational policies; patient advocacy; *physician's role; *physicians; *professional autonomy; professional competence; *professional ethics; professional organizations; public opinion; remuneration; *resource allocation; *self regulation; trust; virtues; *war; *professional role; American Medical Association; United States

Williams, Peter; Wallace, David. Unit 731: The Japanese Army's Secret of Secrets. London: Hodder and Stoughton; 1989. 366 p. 596 fn. ISBN 0-340-39463-3. BE57390.
*biological warfare; confidentiality; dehumanization; disclosure; federal government; *historical aspects; *human experimentation; international aspects; *investigators; killing; military personnel; *moral complicity; *prisoners; public policy; *scientific misconduct; technical expertise; torture; war; chemical warfare; Canada; China; France; Germany; Great Britain; Ishii, Shiro; *Japan; Korean War; Netherlands; Twentieth Century; *United States; USSR; *World War II

Wright, Susan; Sinsheimer, Robert L. Recombinant DNA and biological warfare. *Bulletin of the Atomic Scientists.* 1983 Nov; 39(9): 20–26. 35 fn. BE57498.
*biological warfare; federal government; international aspects; *recombinant DNA research; Biological Weapons Convention; Department of Defense; *United States

Zilinskas, Raymond A. Bioethics and biological weapons. [Editorial]. *Science.* 1998 Jan 30; 279(5351): 635. BE57422.
*biological warfare; biomedical research; employment; financial support; *international aspects; *investigators; organizational policies; political activity; professional organizations; Iraq; Russia

FDA seeks public comment on informed consent rules in combat situations. [News]. *Hastings Center Report.* 1997 Sep–Oct; 27(5): 43. BE56127.
*biological warfare; federal government; government regulation; *human experimentation; immunization; *informed consent; *investigational drugs; *military personnel; nontherapeutic research; public policy; toxicity; volunteers; *war; *chemical warfare; Department of Defense; *Food and Drug Administration; United States

---

BE = bioethics accession number   fn. = footnotes   refs. = references

WITHHOLDING TREATMENT *See* ALLOWING TO DIE, RESUSCITATION ORDERS

WOMEN'S HEALTH *See* HEALTH

WRONGFUL BIRTH *See* WRONGFUL LIFE

WRONGFUL LIFE

Andrews, Lori B. Torts and the double helix: malpractice liability for failure to warn of genetic risks. *Houston Law Review.* 1992 Spring; 29(1): 149–184. 189 fn. BE56977.
  age factors; carriers; children; compensation; confidentiality; congenital disorders; disabled; *disclosure; *family members; *genetic counseling; *genetic disorders; *genetic information; *genetic predisposition; *genetic screening; *genetic services; health education; late–onset disorders; *legal aspects; *legal liability; legislation; mass media; minority groups; negligence; parents; *patients; *physicians; prenatal diagnosis; privacy; reproduction; risk; selective abortion; state government; torts; trends; *wrongful life; *recontact; *United States

Beaumont, Patricia M.A. Wrongful life and wrongful birth. *In:* McLean, Sheila A.M., ed. Contemporary Issues in Law, Medicine and Ethics. Brookfield, VT: Dartmouth; 1996: 99–115. 88 fn. ISBN 1–85521–586–1. BE57792.
  *children; compensation; congenital disorders; *disabled; disclosure; genetic counseling; genetic disorders; injuries; international aspects; judicial action; *legal aspects; *legal liability; *legal rights; legislation; *negligence; normality; *parents; *physicians; prenatal diagnosis; prenatal injuries; *public policy; quality of life; selective abortion; sterilization (sexual); torts; unwanted children; value of life; *wrongful life; Congenital Disabilities (Civil Liability) Act 1976 (Great Britain); Curlender v. Bio–Science Laboratories; England; *Great Britain; McKay v. Essex Area Health Authority and Dr. Gower–Davies; Scotland; *United States

Glannon, Walter. Genes, embryos, and future people. *Bioethics.* 1998 Jul; 12(3): 187–211. 36 fn. BE58893.
  beginning of life; *beneficence; children; *cryopreservation; *embryo disposition; *embryos; *eugenics; fetal therapy; fetuses; future generations; *gene therapy; *genetic disorders; genetic enhancement; *genetic intervention; *genetic screening; germ cells; *injuries; justice; late–onset disorders; mentally disabled; *moral obligations; *moral policy; pain; parents; personhood; physically disabled; posthumous reproduction; *preimplantation diagnosis; *quality of life; reproduction; reproductive technologies; risks and benefits; self concept; suffering; time factors; value of life; *wrongful life

Testing embryonic cells for genetic abnormalities gives us the capacity to predict whether and to what extent people will exist with disease and disability. Moreover, the freezing of embryos for long periods of time enables us to alter the length of a normal human lifespan. After highlighting the shortcomings of somatic–cell gene therapy and germ–line genetic alteration, I argue that the testing and selective termination of genetically defective embryos is the only medically and morally defensible way to prevent the existence of people with severe disability, pain and suffering that make their lives not worth living for them on the whole. In addition, I consider the possible harmful effects on children born from frozen embryos after the deaths of their biological parents, or when their parents are at an advanced age. I also explore whether embryos have moral status and whether the prospects for disease–preventing genetic alteration can justify long–term cryopreservation of embryos.

Jackson, Anthony. Wrongful life and wrongful birth: the English conception. *Journal of Legal Medicine.* 1996 Sep; 17(3): 349–381. 139 fn. BE58358.
  *children; compensation; congenital disorders; *disabled; genetic counseling; judicial action; *legal aspects; *legal liability; *negligence; *parents; *physicians; prenatal injuries; public policy; selective abortion; *wrongful life; Congenital Disabilities (Civil Liability) Act 1976 (Great Britain); *Great Britain; Human Fertilisation and Embryology Act 1990; *McKay v. Essex Area Health Authority and Dr. Gower–Davies

Lenke, Roger R.; Nemes, Joanne M. Wrongful birth, wrongful life: the doctor between a rock and a hard place. *Obstetrics and Gynecology.* 1985 Nov; 66(5): 719–722. 10 refs. BE56964.
  age factors; confidentiality; *congenital disorders; *disclosure; Down syndrome; informed consent; *legal liability; *negligence; newborns; *physicians; pregnant women; prenatal diagnosis; risk; *wrongful life; United States

Merchant, Jennifer. Biogenetics, artificial procreation, and public policy in the United States and France. *Technology in Society.* 1996; 18(1): 1–15. 26 fn. BE56595.
  abortion, induced; advisory committees; biomedical research; cesarean section; coercion; comparative studies; criminal law; cryopreservation; drug abuse; embryo disposition; *embryo research; federal government; *fetal research; fetal therapy; *fetuses; *genetic research; genetic screening; genetic services; *government financing; in vitro fertilization; indigents; industry; international aspects; judicial action; *legal aspects; legal liability; legal rights; personhood; physicians; *pregnant women; preimplantation diagnosis; prenatal diagnosis; *prenatal injuries; private sector; *public policy; *reproductive technologies; state government; state interest; Supreme Court decisions; torts; treatment refusal; women's health services; women's rights; *wrongful life; Bonbrest v. Kotz; France; Roe v. Wade; *United States

Moskop, John C.; Smith, Michael L.; De Ville, Kenneth. Ethical and legal aspects of teratogenic medications: the case of isotretinoin. *Journal of Clinical Ethics.* 1997 Fall; 8(3): 264–278. 57 fn. BE57565.
  adults; age factors; autonomy; beneficence; *congenital disorders; contraception; *decision making; disclosure; drug industry; *drugs; duty to warn; federal government; *females; fetuses; government regulation; *iatrogenic disease; informed consent; justice; *legal liability; negligence; paternalism; *patient care; patient compliance; *physicians; *pregnant women; *prenatal injuries; refusal to treat; risks and benefits; wrongful death; *wrongful life; dermatology; *Accutane; Food and Drug Administration; Roche Dermatologics; United States

Oddi, Samuel. The tort of interference with the right to die: the wrongful living cause of action. *Georgetown Law Journal.* 1986 Dec; 75(2): 625–665. 180 fn. BE56700.
  allowing to die; compensation; hospitals; *legal aspects; *legal liability; negligence; physicians; *prolongation of life; *right to die; state interest; *torts; treatment refusal; *wrongful life; *United States

Ohio. Court of Appeals, Hamilton County. Anderson v. St. Francis–St. George Hospital. *North Eastern Reporter, 2d Series.* 1992 Nov 18 (date of decision). 614: 841–847. BE56297.
  allowing to die; brain pathology; compensation; *hospitals; injuries; *legal liability; negligence; nurses; *prolongation of life; *resuscitation; *resuscitation orders; *right to die; torts; *treatment refusal; *wrongful life; *Anderson v. St. Francis–St. George Hospital; Ohio

The Ohio Court of Appeals for Hamilton County upheld summary judgment on a claim for wrongful living, where

---

BE = bioethics accession number   fn. = footnotes   refs. = references

the patient was resuscitated by a nurse contrary to his doctor's no code blue order and then later suffered a paralyzing stroke prior to his death. Wrongful living was the phrase coined by the appellant for the cause of action for the life that was forced on the decedent by resuscitation. The court noted that life was not a compensable harm in the state until the legislature or the highest court decides it is so. Because the patient had apparently expressly refused treatment in a medical emergency, the case could proceed under two other theories, battery or unauthorized touching, and negligence or breach of a duty of care. (KIE abstract)

Petersen, Kerry. Medical negligence and wrongful birth actions: Australian developments. *Journal of Medical Ethics.* 1997 Oct; 23(5): 319–322. 17 fn. BE57108.
  *abortion, induced; childbirth; diagnosis; health facilities; *legal aspects; *legal liability; *negligence; physicians; *pregnant women; quality of health care; social discrimination; state government; time factors; *wrongful life; diagnostic errors; *Australia; *CES v. Superclinics; New South Wales

Wrongful birth actions aim to compensate litigants who are negligently deprived by health professionals of their right to reproductive choice. Access to safe and legal abortion is integral to the action and wrongful birth claims in the United Kingdom have been facilitated by the Abortion Act 1967 (as amended). The recent Australian case CES v Superclinics (1995) 38 NSWLR 47 shows how judicial confusion about the legality of abortion can result in judges condoning medical negligence. The Superclinics case also suggests that doctors are not required to provide pregnant women with the same standard of care as other patients. These developments show that law can become incoherent and health professionals can act negligently with impunity when reproductive choice does not have a secure legal foundation.

AUTHOR INDEX

AUTHOR INDEX

A

Aaby, Peter; Babiker, Abdel; Darbyshire, Janet, et al. Ethics of HIV trials. [Letters]. *Lancet.* 1997 Nov 22; 350(9090): 1546–1547.
(AIDS/HUMAN EXPERIMENTATION; HUMAN EXPERIMENTATION/FOREIGN COUNTRIES; HUMAN EXPERIMENTATION/RESEARCH DESIGN)

Aarons, D. Research ethics. *West Indian Medical Journal.* 1995 Dec; 44(4): 115–118.
(HUMAN EXPERIMENTATION; HUMAN EXPERIMENTATION/ETHICS COMMITTEES)

Abbasi, Kamran. BMJ to act on media abuse. [News]. *BMJ (British Medical Journal).* 1998 Jan 17; 316(7126): 170.
(CONFIDENTIALITY/LEGAL ASPECTS)

Abbott, Alison. Euro-vote lifts block on biotech patents ... but Parliament wants closer scrutiny. [News]. *Nature.* 1997 Jul 24; 388(6640): 314–315.
(GENETIC INTERVENTION; PATENTING LIFE FORMS)

Abbott, Alison. Europe's life patent moratorium may go. [News]. *Nature.* 1998 May 21; 393(6682): 200.
(PATENTING LIFE FORMS)

Abbott, Alison. German law could boost prospects for organ transplants. [News]. *Nature.* 1997 Jul 3; 388(6637): 4.
(DETERMINATION OF DEATH/BRAIN DEATH; ORGAN AND TISSUE DONATION)

Abbott, Alison. Germany tightens grip on misconduct. [News]. *Nature.* 1997 Dec 4; 390(6659): 430.
(BIOMEDICAL RESEARCH; FRAUD AND MISCONDUCT)

Abbott, Alison. Germany's past still casts a long shadow. [News]. *Nature.* 1997 Oct 16; 389(6652): 660.
(BIOETHICS)

Abbott, Alison. Researcher sues over 'fraud' sanction. [News]. *Nature.* 1997 Dec 18–25; 390(6661): 652.
(BIOMEDICAL RESEARCH; FRAUD AND MISCONDUCT)

Abbott, David see **McGuire, John**

Abdulla, Sara. Xenotransplantation debate boils on. [News]. *Lancet.* 1997 Sep 20; 350(9081): 868.
(ORGAN AND TISSUE TRANSPLANTATION)

Aboulghar, Mohamed A. see **Serour, Gamal I.**

Abramovitch, Rona see **Ondrusek, Nancy**

Abrams, Donald see **Slome, Lee**

Abrams, Herbert see **Forrow, Lachlan**

Abulrub, Daad see **Qunibi, Wajeh**

Ackerman, Felicia. Assisted suicide, terminal illness, severe disability, and the double standard. *In:* Battin, Margaret P.; Rhodes, Rosamond; Silvers, Anita, eds. Physician Assisted Suicide: Expanding the Debate. New York, NY: Routledge; 1998: 149–161.
(SUICIDE)

Ackerman, Felicia. Response to "This porridge is too thin" by Gretchen M. Brown and "Demolishing a 'straw man'" by Elliott J. Rosen (*CQ* Vol. 7, No. 2). *Cambridge Quarterly of Healthcare Ethics.* 1998 Summer; 7(3): 323–325.
(TERMINAL CARE/HOSPICES)

Ackerman, Terrence F. Chemically dependent physicians and informed consent disclosure. *Journal of Addictive Diseases.* 1996; 15(2): 25–42.
(INFORMED CONSENT)

Ackerman, Terrence F. Choosing between Nuremberg and the National Commission: the balancing of moral principles in clinical research. *In:* Vanderpool, Harold Y., ed. The Ethics of Research Involving Human Subjects: Facing the 21st Century. Frederick, MD: University Publishing Group; 1996: 83–104.
(HUMAN EXPERIMENTATION; HUMAN EXPERIMENTATION/REGULATION)

Ackerman, Terrence F. Forsaking the spirit for the letter of the law: advance directives in nursing homes. *Journal of the American Geriatrics Society.* 1997 Jan; 45(1): 114–116.
(ADVANCE DIRECTIVES)

Ad Hoc Committee to Defend Health Care (Cambridge, MA). For our patients, not for profits: a Call to Action. *JAMA.* 1997 Dec 3; 278(21): 1733–1738.
(HEALTH CARE/ECONOMICS)

Adair, John G.; Dushenko, Terrance W.; Lindsay, R.C.L. Ethical regulations and their impact on research practice. *American Psychologist.* 1985 Jan; 40(1): 59–72.
(BEHAVIORAL RESEARCH/INFORMED CONSENT; BEHAVIORAL RESEARCH/REGULATION)

Adamolekun, Kemi. Openness of health professionals about death and terminal illness in a Nigerian teaching hospital. *Omega: A Journal of Death and Dying.* 1997–1998; 36(1): 23–32.
(TRUTH DISCLOSURE)

Adams, David see **Neuberger, James**

Adams, Wendy L. see **Gertner, Eric J.**

Addis, G.J.; London, D. The *BMJ*'s Nuremberg issue.

569

[Letters]. *BMJ (British Medical Journal).* 1997 Apr 12; 314(7087): 1128.
(HUMAN EXPERIMENTATION/FOREIGN COUNTRIES; HUMAN EXPERIMENTATION/SPECIAL POPULATIONS; WAR)

Ader, Mary. Investigational treatments: coverage, controversy, and consensus. *Annals of Health Law.* 1996; 5: 45–60.
(HEALTH CARE/ECONOMICS; HUMAN EXPERIMENTATION)

Adler, Martin W.; College on Problems of Drug Dependence. Human subject issues in drug abuse research. *Drug and Alcohol Dependence.* 1995 Feb; 37(2): 167–175.
(HUMAN EXPERIMENTATION/SPECIAL POPULATIONS)

Admiraal, Pieter. Voluntary euthanasia: the Dutch way. *In:* McLean, Sheila A.M., ed. Death, Dying and the Law. Brookfield, VT: Dartmouth; 1996: 113–127.
(EUTHANASIA)

Admiraal, Pieter V. Euthanasia in the Netherlands. *Free Inquiry.* 1996–1997 Winter; 17(1): 5–8.
(EUTHANASIA)

Adorno, D. see **Elli, M.**

Adshead, Gwen see **Dale, Ruth**

Advisory Committee on Human Radiation Experiments. The Human Radiation Experiments: Final Report of the Advisory Committee. New York, NY: Oxford University Press; 1996. 620 p.
(FRAUD AND MISCONDUCT; HUMAN EXPERIMENTATION)

Agard, Ellen; Finkelstein, Daniel; Wallach, Edward. Cultural diversity and informed consent. [Case study]. *Journal of Clinical Ethics.* 1998 Summer; 9(2): 173–176.
(INFORMED CONSENT)

Agich, George J. Can the patient make treatment decisions? Evaluating decisional capacity. *Cleveland Clinic Journal of Medicine.* 1997 Oct; 64(9): 461–464.
(INFORMED CONSENT; TREATMENT REFUSAL)

Agich, George J. Human experimentation and clinical consent. [Revised]. *In:* Monagle, John F.; Thomasma, David C., eds. Health Care Ethics: Critical Issues for the 21st Century. Gaithersburg, MD: Aspen Publishers; 1998: 228–238.
(HUMAN EXPERIMENTATION/INFORMED CONSENT)

Agich, George J.; May, Thomas. Alcoholism, moral agency, and paternalism: a theoretical framework. *In:* Shelton, Wayne N.; Edwards, Rem B., eds. Advances in Bioethics. Volume 3: Values, Ethics, and Alcoholism. Greenwich, CT: JAI Press; 1997: 103–118.
(BEHAVIOR CONTROL; PATIENT CARE)

Agich, George J.; Spielman, Bethany. Ethics expert testimony: against the skeptics. *Journal of Medicine and Philosophy.* 1997 Aug; 22(4): 381–403.
(BIOETHICS; ETHICISTS AND ETHICS COMMITTEES)

Agius, Emmanuel. Patenting life: our responsibilities to present and future generations. *In:* Agius, Emmanuel; Busuttil, Salvino, eds. Germ–Line Intervention and Our Responsibilities to Future Generations. Boston, MA: Kluwer Academic; 1998: 67–83.
(GENETIC RESEARCH; PATENTING LIFE FORMS)

Agius, Emmanuel; Busuttil, Salvino, eds. Germ–Line Intervention and Our Responsibilities to Future Generations. Boston, MA: Kluwer Academic; 1998. 174 p.
(GENETIC INTERVENTION)

Ahmedzai, Sam see **Meystre, Chantal J.N.**

Ahronheim, Judith C. see **Baskin, Shari A.**

Aiken, Margaret M. see **Muram, David**

Airaksinen, Timo. Professional ethics. *In:* Chadwick, Ruth, ed. Encyclopedia of Applied Ethics, Volume 3. San Diego, CA: Academic Press; 1998: 671–682.
(PROFESSIONAL ETHICS)

Aitkenhead, Marilyn; Dordoy, Jackie. What the subjects have to say. *British Journal of Social Psychology.* 1985 Nov; 24(Pt. 4): 293–305.
(BEHAVIORAL RESEARCH)

Akabayashi, Akira. Finally done -- Japan's decision on organ transplantation. [News]. *Hastings Center Report.* 1997 Sep–Oct; 27(5): 47.
(ORGAN AND TISSUE DONATION)

Akabayashi, Akira. The concept of happiness in Oriental thought and its significance in clinical medicine. *In:* Hoshino, Kazumasa, ed. Japanese and Western Bioethics: Studies in Moral Diversity. Boston, MA: Kluwer Academic; 1997: 161–164.
(BIOETHICS)

Akhrass, Rami see **Piotrowski, Joseph J.**

Akin, Ayse see **Kalaça, Cagri**

Akinsanya, J.A.; Rouse, Paul. Who Will Care? A Survey of the Knowledge and Attitudes of Hospital Nurses to People with HIV/AIDS: Report Submitted to the Department of Health. Chelmsford, Eng.: Anglia Polytechnic University, Faculty of Health and Social Work; 1991. 146 p.
(AIDS/HEALTH PERSONNEL)

Al, Joop. Comparative observations on some current medico–legal issues in Dutch law. *In:* Jewish Law Annual. Volume Twelve. Amsterdam, Netherlands: Harwood Academic Publishers; 1997: 167–215.
(DETERMINATION OF DEATH; EUTHANASIA/LEGAL ASPECTS; ORGAN AND TISSUE DONATION)

Alan Guttmacher Institute. Induced Abortion. [Fact sheet]. New York, NY: Alan Guttmacher Institute; 1996. 2 p.
(ABORTION)

Albertsson–Wikland, Kerstin see **Wennerholm, Ulla–Britt**

Alcalá, Maria José; Family Care International. Commitments to Sexual and Reproductive Health and Rights for All: Framework for Action. New York, NY: Family Care International; 1995. 64 p.
(HEALTH; HEALTH CARE; REPRODUCTION)

Alderson, Priscilla; Goodey, Christopher. Doctors, ethics and special education. *Journal of Medical Ethics.* 1998 Feb; 24(1): 49–55.
(PATIENT CARE/MINORS)

Alderson, Priscilla; Nicholson, Richard. Deciding when to withhold or withdraw life–sustaining treatment for children. *Bulletin of Medical Ethics.* 1997 Apr; No. 127: 13–20.
(ALLOWING TO DIE)

Aldhous, Peter. Surrogate fathers. [News]. *New Scientist.* 1998 Jan 31; 157(2119): 4.
(REPRODUCTIVE TECHNOLOGIES)

Alexander, J.J. see **Piotrowski, Joseph J.**

Alexander, J. Wesley. High–risk donors: diabetics, the elderly, and others. *Transplantation Proceedings.* 1992 Oct; 24(5): 2221–2222.
(ORGAN AND TISSUE DONATION)

Alexandrov, Andrei V.; Bladin, Christopher F.; Meslin, Eric M.; Norris, John W. Do–not–resuscitate orders in acute stroke. *Neurology.* 1995 Apr; 45(4): 634–640.
(RESUSCITATION ORDERS)

Alexis, Jeffrey D. see **Giugliano, Robert P.**

Alfurayh, Osman see **Qunibi, Wajeh**

Alibhai, Shabbir M.H.; Weijer, Charles. The placebo effect. [Letter and response]. *Canadian Medical Association Journal.* 1997 Oct 15; 157(8): 1020, 1022.
(HUMAN EXPERIMENTATION/RESEARCH DESIGN)

Alison, Dawn see **Williams, Christopher J.**

Allen, Anita L. Genetic privacy: emerging concepts and values. *In:* Rothstein, Mark A., ed. Genetic Secrets: Protecting Privacy and Confidentiality in the Genetic Era. New Haven, CT: Yale University Press; 1997: 31–59.
(CONFIDENTIALITY; GENETIC SCREENING)

Allen, Arthur. Injection rejection: the dangerous backlash against vaccination. *New Republic.* 1998 Mar 23; 218(12): 20–23.
(IMMUNIZATION)

Allen, Garland E. Genetics and behavior. *In:* Chadwick, Ruth, ed. Encyclopedia of Applied Ethics, Volume 2. San Diego, CA: Academic Press; 1998: 435–443.
(BEHAVIORAL GENETICS)

Allen, Jill S. Fonda; Mulhauser, Lynda C. Genetic counseling after abnormal prenatal diagnosis: facilitating coping in families who continue their pregnancies. *Journal of Genetic Counseling.* 1995 Dec; 4(4): 251–265.
(GENETIC COUNSELING; PRENATAL DIAGNOSIS)

Allen, Margaret D. see **Jecker, Nancy S.**

Allen–Taylor, S. Lynne see **Evans, Lois K.**

Allen, William L.; Brushwood, David B. Pharmaceutically assisted death and the pharmacist's right of conscience. *Journal of Pharmacy and Law.* 1996; 5(1): 1–18.
(SUICIDE)

Aller, Gregory see **Aller, Robert**

Aller, Robert; Aller, Gregory. An institutional response to patient/family complaints. *In:* Shamoo, Adil E., ed.

Ethics in Neurobiological Research with Human Subjects: The Baltimore Conference on Ethics. Amsterdam: Gordon and Breach; 1997: 155–172.
(FRAUD AND MISCONDUCT; HUMAN EXPERIMENTATION/INFORMED CONSENT; HUMAN EXPERIMENTATION/RESEARCH DESIGN; HUMAN EXPERIMENTATION/SPECIAL POPULATIONS; INFORMED CONSENT/MENTALLY DISABLED)

Allgeier, Elizabeth Rice see **Sensibaugh, Christine Cregan**

Allison, Althea; Ewens, Ann. Tensions in sharing client confidences while respecting autonomy: implications for interprofessional practice. *Nursing Ethics.* 1998 Sep; 5(5): 441–450.
(CONFIDENTIALITY; PROFESSIONAL PATIENT RELATIONSHIP)

Allmers, Henning; Kenwright, Simon. Ethics of cloning. [Letters]. *Lancet.* 1997 May 10; 349(9062): 1401.
(CLONING; ORGAN AND TISSUE DONATION; REPRODUCTION)

Almeder, Robert F. see **Humber, James M.**

Almeshari, Khalid see **Qunibi, Wajeh**

Alpers, Ann see **Oscherwitz, Tom**

Alpert, Hillel R.; Hoijtink, Herbert; Fischer, Gary S.; Emanuel, Linda. Psychometric analysis of an advance directive. *Medical Care.* 1996 Oct; 34(10): 1057–1065.
(ADVANCE DIRECTIVES)

Alpert, Sheri A. Health care information: access, confidentiality, and good practice. *In:* Goodman, Kenneth W., ed. Ethics, Computing, and Medicine: Informatics and the Transformation of Health Care. New York, NY: Cambridge University Press; 1998: 75–101.
(BIOMEDICAL TECHNOLOGIES; CONFIDENTIALITY; HEALTH CARE)

Alt–White, Anna C. Obtaining "informed" consent from the elderly. *Western Journal of Nursing Research.* 1995 Dec; 17(6): 700–705.
(HUMAN EXPERIMENTATION/INFORMED CONSENT; HUMAN EXPERIMENTATION/SPECIAL POPULATIONS)

Altaca, G. see **Haberal, Mehmet**

Altman, Lawrence K. AIDS experts leave journal after studies are criticized. [News]. *New York Times.* 1997 Oct 15: A10.
(AIDS/HUMAN EXPERIMENTATION)

Altman, Lawrence K. Health panel seeks sweeping changes in fertility therapy. [News]. *New York Times.* 1998 Apr 29: A1, A22.
(REPRODUCTIVE TECHNOLOGIES)

Altman, Lawrence K. Sex, privacy and tracking H.I.V. infections. [News]. *New York Times.* 1997 Nov 4: F1, F2.
(AIDS/CONFIDENTIALITY)

Altman, Stuart H.; Reinhardt, Uwe E.; Shields, Alexandra E., eds. The Future U.S. Healthcare System: Who Will Care for the Poor and Uninsured? Chicago, IL: Health Administration Press; Waltham, MA: Council on the Economic Impact of Health System Change; 1998.

426 p.
(HEALTH CARE/ECONOMICS)

Alvare, Helen M. A response to Leslie Griffin. *In:* Wildes, Kevin Wm.; Mitchell, Alan C., eds. Choosing Life: A Dialogue on *Evangelium Vitae.* Washington, DC: Georgetown University Press; 1997: 179–185.
(ABORTION/RELIGIOUS ASPECTS)

Alwin, David M. see **Somerville, Margaret A.**

Alzheimer's Disease International. Medical and Scientific Advisory Committee see **Brodaty, Henry**

Alzola, Carlos see **Teno, Joan**

American Academy of Neurology. Ethics and Humanities Subcommittee. Ethical issues in the management of the demented patient. [Position statement]. *Neurology.* 1996 Apr; 46(4): 1180–1183.
(PATIENT CARE/AGED; PATIENT CARE/MENTALLY DISABLED)

American Academy of Neurology. Ethics and Humanities Subcommittee see **Taylor, Robert M.**

American Academy of Pediatrics; American College of Obstetricians and Gynecologists. Joint Statement on Human Immunodeficiency Virus Screening. Issued by the American Academy of Pediatrics [and] by the American College of Obstetricians and Gynecologists, Washington, DC; 1995 Aug. 1 p.
(AIDS/TESTING AND SCREENING)

American Academy of Pediatrics. Committee on Bioethics. Ethics and the care of critically ill infants and children. *Pediatrics.* 1996 Jul; 98(1): 149–152.
(ALLOWING TO DIE/INFANTS; PATIENT CARE/MINORS)

American Academy of Pediatrics. Council on Research see **Parrott, Robert H.**

American Academy of Pediatrics. Task Force on Pediatric AIDS. Perinatal human immunodeficiency virus (HIV) testing. *Pediatrics.* 1992 Apr; 89(4, Pt.2): 791–794.
(AIDS/TESTING AND SCREENING)

American Association for Dental Research. Ethics Committee see **Bebeau, Muriel J.**

American Association of Critical Care Nurses. Task Force on Ethics in Critical Care Research. Statement on ethics in critical care research. Part One. *Focus on Critical Care.* 1985 Jun; 12(3): 47–50.
(HUMAN EXPERIMENTATION/SPECIAL POPULATIONS)

American Association of Critical Care Nurses. Task Force on Ethics in Critical Care Research. Statement on ethics in critical care research. Part Two. *Focus on Critical Care.* 1985 Aug; 12(4): 58–63.
(HUMAN EXPERIMENTATION/INFORMED CONSENT; HUMAN EXPERIMENTATION/SPECIAL POPULATIONS)

American Association of University Affiliated Programs for the Developmentally Disabled see **American Association on Mental Deficiency**

American Association on Mental Deficiency; Association for Persons with Severe Handicaps;

American Association of University Affiliated Programs for the Developmentally Disabled; et al. Brief of Amici Curiae in Support of Petitioner: Margaret M. Heckler v. American Hospital Association, No. 84–1529, on Writ of Certiorari to the U.S. Court of Appeals for the Second Circuit. Washington, DC: Filed in the Supreme Court of the United States, October term, 1985; 1985. 27 p.
(ALLOWING TO DIE/INFANTS; ALLOWING TO DIE/LEGAL ASPECTS)

American College of Obstetricians and Gynecologists see **American Academy of Pediatrics**

American College of Obstetricians and Gynecologists. Committee on Ethics. Endorsement of institutional ethics committees. ACOG Committee Opinion No. 46. *ACOG Committee Opinions.* 1985 Oct; No. 46: 3 p.
(ETHICISTS AND ETHICS COMMITTEES)

American College of Obstetricians and Gynecologists. Committee on Ethics. Ethical guidance for patient testing. ACOG Committee Opinion No. 159. *ACOG Committee Opinions.* 1995 Oct; No. 159: 3 p.
(PATIENT CARE)

American College of Obstetricians and Gynecologists. Committee on Ethics. Ethical issues in obstetric–gynecologic education. ACOG Committee Opinion No. 181, April 1997. *International Journal of Gynaecology and Obstetrics.* 1997 Jun; 57(3): 327–330.
(MEDICAL ETHICS/EDUCATION)

American College of Obstetricians and Gynecologists. Committee on Ethics. Guidelines for relationships with industry. ACOG Committee Opinion No. 182, April 1997 (replaces No. 45, October 1985). *International Journal of Gynaecology and Obstetrics.* 1997 Aug; 58(2): 255–256.
(HEALTH CARE/ECONOMICS)

American College of Obstetricians and Gynecologists. Committee on Ethics. Sexual misconduct in the practice of obstetrics and gynecology: ethical considerations. ACOG Committee Opinion No. 144. *ACOG Committee Opinions.* 1994 Nov; No. 144: 3 p.
(FRAUD AND MISCONDUCT; PROFESSIONAL PATIENT RELATIONSHIP)

American College of Obstetricians and Gynecologists. Committee on Obstetric Practice. Routine storage of umbilical cord blood for potential future transplantation. ACOG Committee Opinion No. 183, April 1997. *International Journal of Gynaecology and Obstetrics.* 1997 Aug; 58(2): 257–259.
(BLOOD DONATION)

American College of Physicians see **Werner, Michael J.**

American College of Physicians. Ethics and Human Rights Committee. Ethics manual. Fourth edition. [Position paper]. *Annals of Internal Medicine.* 1998 Apr 1; 128(7): 576–594.
(MEDICAL ETHICS/CODES OF ETHICS)

American College of Physicians. Health and Public Policy Committee. Drug therapy for severe, chronic pain in terminal illness. *Annals of Internal Medicine.* 1983 Dec; 99(6): 870–873.
(PATIENT CARE/DRUGS; TERMINAL CARE)

American Geriatrics Society see **Lynn, Joanne**

American Geriatrics Society. Clinical Practice Committee. Management of cancer pain in older patients. *Journal of the American Geriatrics Society.* 1997 Oct; 45(10): 1273–1276.
(PATIENT CARE/AGED; PATIENT CARE/DRUGS)

American Geriatrics Society. Ethics Committee see **Rudberg, Mark A.**

American Medical Association. Elements of Quality Care for Patients in the Last Phase of Life. Chicago, IL: American Medical Association; 1997 Jun 22. 1 p.
(TERMINAL CARE)

American Medical Association. Council on Ethical and Judicial Affairs. Multiplex genetic testing. [Policy statement]. *Hastings Center Report.* 1998 Jul–Aug; 28(4): 15–21.
(GENETIC SCREENING)

American Medical Association. Council on Ethical and Judicial Affairs. Sale of non–health–related goods from physicians' offices. *JAMA.* 1998 Aug 12; 280(6): 563.
(HEALTH CARE/ECONOMICS)

American Medical Record Association. Confidentiality of Patient Health Information. *American Medical Record Association Journal.* 1985 Dec; 56(12): 4–14.
(CONFIDENTIALITY; PATIENT ACCESS TO RECORDS)

American Nurses Association. American Nurses Association position statements on bloodborne and airborne diseases. *In: its* Compendium of American Nurses Association Position Statements. Washington, DC: American Nurses Publishing; 1996: 1–65.
(AIDS/HEALTH PERSONNEL)

American Nurses Association. American Nurses Association position statements on ethics and human rights. *In: its* Compendium of American Nurses Association Position Statements. Washington, DC: American Nurses Publishing; 1996: 79–118.
(NURSING ETHICS; PATIENT CARE; TERMINAL CARE)

American Nurses Association. Compendium of American Nurses Association Position Statements. Washington, DC: American Nurses Publishing; 1996. 232 p.
(BIOETHICS; NURSING ETHICS)

American Occupational Therapy Association (AOTA). Commission on Standards and Ethics. 1996 Occupational Therapy Code of Ethics Reference Guide. Bethesda, MD: American Occupational Therapy Association; 1996 Oct.
(PROFESSIONAL ETHICS/CODES OF ETHICS)

American Psychiatric Association. Position statement on ensuring access and appropriate utilization of psychiatric services for the elderly. *American Journal of Psychiatry.* 1998 Mar; 155(3): 452.
(PATIENT CARE/AGED; PATIENT CARE/MENTALLY DISABLED)

American Society of Human Genetics. Social Issues Subcommittee on Familial Disclosure. ASHG statement: professional disclosure of familial genetic information. *American Journal of Human Genetics.* 1998 Feb; 62(2): 474–483.
(CONFIDENTIALITY; GENETIC SCREENING)

Amos, Amanda see **Kerr, Anne**

Amu, Olubusola; Rajendran, Sasha; Bolaji, Ibrahim I.; Paterson–Brown, Sara. Should doctors perform an elective caesarean section on request?: Yes, as long as the woman is fully informed; [and] Maternal choice alone should not determine method of delivery. *BMJ (British Medical Journal).* 1998 Aug 15; 317(7156): 462–465.
(PATIENT CARE)

Amundsen, Darrel W. see **Larson, Edward J.**

Andereck, William S. see **Iserson, Kenneth V.**

Anderick, William see **Goldworth, Amnon**

Andersen, A. Nyboe see **Andersen, C. Yding**

Andersen, C. Yding; Westergaard, L.G.; Grinsted, J.; Petersen, K.; Andersen, A. Nyboe. Frozen embryos: too cold to touch? Frozen pre–embryos in Denmark. *Human Reproduction.* 1996 Apr; 11(4): 703.
(FETUSES; IN VITRO FERTILIZATION)

Andersen, K. see **Bremnes, R.M.**

Anderson, B. see **Bach, F.H.**

Anderson, Betsy see **Saxton, Marsha**

Anderson, C. Mary see **Foster, Peggy**

Anderson, David see **Brawn, W.J.**

Anderson, Gail; Hill, Marcia, eds. Children's Rights, Therapists' Responsibilities: Feminist Commentaries. New York, NY: Harrington Park Press; 1997. 141 p.
(PATIENT CARE/MENTALLY DISABLED; PATIENT CARE/MINORS)

Anderson, James G.; Aydin, Carolyn E. Evaluating medical information systems: social contexts and ethical challenges. *In:* Goodman, Kenneth W., ed. Ethics, Computing, and Medicine: Informatics and the Transformation of Health Care. New York, NY: Cambridge University Press; 1998: 57–74.
(BIOMEDICAL TECHNOLOGIES; HEALTH CARE)

Anderson, Jim see **Taylor, Kathryn M.**

Anderson, Kathryn see **Epstein, Ronald M.**

Andre, Judith. Goals of ethics consultation: toward clarity, utility, and fidelity. *Journal of Clinical Ethics.* 1997 Summer; 8(2): 193–198.
(ETHICISTS AND ETHICS COMMITTEES)

Andre, Judith. Speaking truth to employers. *Journal of Clinical Ethics.* 1997 Summer; 8(2): 199–203.
(ETHICISTS AND ETHICS COMMITTEES; PROFESSIONAL ETHICS)

Andre, Judith. The week of November seventh: bioethics as a practice. [Personal narrative]. *In:* Carson, Ronald A.; Burns, Chester R., eds. Philosophy of Medicine and Bioethics: A Twenty–Year Retrospective and Critical Appraisal. Boston, MA: Kluwer Academic; 1997: 153–172.
(BIOETHICS; ETHICISTS AND ETHICS COMMITTEES)

Andrews, Arlene Bowers see Patterson, Elizabeth G.

Andrews, Lori; Elster, Nanette; Gatter, Robert; Horwich, Terri Finesmith; Jaeger, Ami; Klock, Susan; Pergament, Eugene; Pizzulli, Francis; Shapiro, Robyn; Siegler, Mark; Smith, Peggie; Zager, Shirley; Institute for Science, Law, and Technology Working Group. ART into science: regulation of fertility techniques. *Science.* 1998 Jul 31; 281(5377): 651–652.
(REPRODUCTIVE TECHNOLOGIES)

Andrews, Lori; Nelkin, Dorothy. Whose body is it anyway? Disputes over body tissue in a biotechnology age. *Lancet.* 1998 Jan 3; 351(9095): 53–57.
(GENETIC RESEARCH)

Andrews, Lori B. Gen-etiquette: genetic information, family relationships, and adoption. *In:* Rothstein, Mark A., ed. Genetic Secrets: Protecting Privacy and Confidentiality in the Genetic Era. New Haven, CT: Yale University Press; 1997: 255–280.
(CONFIDENTIALITY; GENETIC SCREENING)

Andrews, Lori B. Genetic fallout: new technologies are changing the legal landscape. *Trial.* 1995 Dec; 31(12): 20–23, 25–27.
(CONFIDENTIALITY; GENETIC SCREENING)

Andrews, Lori B. Mom, Dad, clone: implications for reproductive privacy. *Cambridge Quarterly of Healthcare Ethics.* 1998 Spring; 7(2): 176–186.
(CLONING; REPRODUCTION)

Andrews, Lori B. The body as property: some philosophical reflections -- a response to J.F. Childress. *Transplantation Proceedings.* 1992 Oct; 24(5): 2149–2151.
(ORGAN AND TISSUE DONATION)

Andrews, Lori B. The genetic information superhighway: rules of the road for contacting relatives and recontacting former patients. *In:* Knoppers, Bartha Maria, ed. Human DNA: Law and Policy: International and Comparative Perspectives. Proceedings of the First International Conference on DNA Sampling and Human Genetic Research: Ethical, Legal, and Policy Aspects, held in Montreal, Canada, 6–8 Sep 1996. Boston, MA: Kluwer Law International; 1997: 133–143.
(CONFIDENTIALITY/LEGAL ASPECTS; GENETIC COUNSELING; GENETIC SCREENING)

Andrews, Lori B. Torts and the double helix: malpractice liability for failure to warn of genetic risks. *Houston Law Review.* 1992 Spring; 29(1): 149–184.
(GENETIC SERVICES; WRONGFUL LIFE)

Andrews, Lori B.; Elster, Nanette. Adoption, reproductive technologies, and genetic information. *Health Matrix.* 1998 Summer; 8(2): 125–151.
(CONFIDENTIALITY/LEGAL ASPECTS; GENETIC SCREENING; REPRODUCTIVE TECHNOLOGIES)

Andrews, Lori B.; Rothstein, Mark A.; Latham, Stephen R.; Garfinkel, Mark D.; Charo, R. Alta. The clone age. *ABA Journal: The Lawyer's Magazine.* 1997 Jul; 83: 68–73.
(CLONING)

Andrews, Sam; Hutchinson, Sally A. Teaching nursing ethics: a practical approach. *Journal of Nursing Education.* 1981 Jan; 20(1): 6–11.
(NURSING ETHICS/EDUCATION)

Angell, Marcia. Helping desperately ill people to die. *In:* Emanuel, Linda L., ed. Regulating How We Die: The Ethical, Medical, and Legal Issues Surrounding Physician–Assisted Suicide. Cambridge, MA: Harvard University Press; 1998: 3–20, 263–264.
(ALLOWING TO DIE; EUTHANASIA; SUICIDE)

Angell, Marcia; Kassirer, Jerome; Manson, JoAnn E.; Rothman, Kenneth J.; Cann, Christina. Conflict of interest. [Letter and responses]. *Epidemiology.* 1997 Nov; 8(6): 686–687.
(BIOMEDICAL RESEARCH; FRAUD AND MISCONDUCT)

Angell, Marcia see Kassirer, Jerome P.

Angier, Natalie. Joined for life, and living life to the full. *New York Times.* 1997 Dec 23: F1, F5.
(PATIENT CARE)

Anker, Deborah see Sills, E. Scott

Anleu, Sharyn L. Roach. Regulating new reproductive technologies: an examination of the emergence of legislation in two Australian states. *In:* Holstein, J.A.; Miller, G., eds. Perspectives on Social Problems: A Research Annual. Volume 8. Greenwich, CT: JAI Press; 1996: 175–197.
(EMBRYO AND FETAL RESEARCH; REPRODUCTIVE TECHNOLOGIES)

Anleu, Sharyn L. Roach. Reproductive autonomy and reproductive technology: gender, deviance and infertility. *In:* Petersen, Kerry, ed. Intersections: Women on Law, Medicine and Technology. Brookfield, VT: Ashgate; 1997: 99–125.
(REPRODUCTIVE TECHNOLOGIES)

Annable, Lawrence see Young, Simon N.

Annas, George J. A national bill of patients' rights. *New England Journal of Medicine.* 1998 Mar 5; 338(10): 695–699.
(PATIENTS' RIGHTS)

Annas, George J. Partial–birth abortion, Congress, and the Constitution. *New England Journal of Medicine.* 1998 Jul 23; 339(4): 279–283.
(ABORTION/LEGAL ASPECTS)

Annas, George J. The bell tolls for a constitutional right to physician–assisted suicide. *New England Journal of Medicine.* 1997 Oct 9; 337(15): 1098–1103.
(SUICIDE)

Annas, George J. The bell tolls for a right to suicide. *In:* Emanuel, Linda L., ed. Regulating How We Die: The Ethical, Medical, and Legal Issues Surrounding Physician–Assisted Suicide. Cambridge, MA: Harvard University Press; 1998: 203–233, 312–316.
(SUICIDE)

Annas, George J. The dog and his shadow: a response to Overcast and Evans. *Law, Medicine and Health Care.* 1985 Jun; 13(3): 112–116, 129.
(ORGAN AND TISSUE TRANSPLANTATION)

Annas, George J. The shadowlands -- secrets, lies, and assisted reproduction. *New England Journal of Medicine.* 1998 Sep 24; 339(13): 935–939.

(FETUSES; REPRODUCTIVE TECHNOLOGIES)

Annas, George J. Why we should ban human cloning. *New England Journal of Medicine.* 1998 Jul 9; 339(2): 122–125.
(CLONING)

Annas, George J.; Glantz, Leonard H. Informed consent to research on institutionalized mentally disabled persons: the dual problems of incapacity and voluntariness. *In:* Shamoo, Adil E., ed. Ethics in Neurobiological Research with Human Subjects: The Baltimore Conference on Ethics. Amsterdam: Gordon and Breach; 1997: 55–79.
(HUMAN EXPERIMENTATION/INFORMED CONSENT; HUMAN EXPERIMENTATION/REGULATION; HUMAN EXPERIMENTATION/SPECIAL POPULATIONS; INFORMED CONSENT/MENTALLY DISABLED)

Annas, George J.; Robertson, John A. Human cloning: should the United States legislate against it? Yes: individual dignity demands nothing less [Annas]; No: the potential for good is too compelling [Robertson]. *ABA Journal: The Lawyer's Magazine.* 1997 May; 83: 80–81.
(CLONING)

Annas, George J. see **Savulescu, Julian**

Appelbaum, Paul S. A "health information infrastructure" and the threat to confidentiality of health records. *Psychiatric Services.* 1998 Jan; 49(1): 27–28, 33.
(CONFIDENTIALITY/LEGAL ASPECTS; CONFIDENTIALITY/MENTAL HEALTH)

Appelbaum, Paul S. A theory of ethics for forensic psychiatry. *Journal of the American Academy of Psychiatry and the Law.* 1997; 25(3): 233–247.
(MEDICAL ETHICS)

Appelbaum, Paul S. Almost a revolution: an international perspective on the law of involuntary commitment. *Journal of the American Academy of Psychiatry and the Law.* 1997; 25(2): 135–147.
(INVOLUNTARY COMMITMENT; INVOLUNTARY COMMITMENT/FOREIGN COUNTRIES)

Appelbaum, Paul S. Informed consent to psychotherapy: recent developments. *Psychiatric Services.* 1997 Apr; 48(4): 445–446.
(INFORMED CONSENT/MENTALLY DISABLED)

Appelbaum, Paul S. Let my wife bleed to death. *Medical Ethics Newsletter.* 1997 Fall; 3(3): 3, 7.
(ALLOWING TO DIE; TREATMENT REFUSAL/MENTALLY DISABLED)

Appelbaum, Paul S.; Bourne, Richard; Candilis, Philip J.; Jorgenson, Linda Mabus. Case vignette: unanticipated propinquity. [Case study and commentaries]. *Ethics and Behavior.* 1997; 7(4): 377–388.
(CONFIDENTIALITY/MENTAL HEALTH)

Appelbaum, Paul S. see **Grisso, Thomas**

Appelbaum, Paul S. see **Guiles, Renée M.**

Appleby, Chuck. True values: while ethical decisionmaking and managed care aren't mutually exclusive, executives are struggling to find a common denominator. *Hospitals and Health Networks.* 1996 Jul 5; 70(13): 20–22, 26.
(HEALTH CARE/ECONOMICS)

Appleton, Susan Frelich. Doctors, patients and the Constitution: a theoretical analysis of the physician's role in "private" reproductive decisions. *Washington University Law Quarterly.* 1985 Summer; 63(2): 183–236.
(ABORTION/LEGAL ASPECTS)

Aragon, Alfredo S. see **Brody, Janet L.**

Archer, Luis. Genetic testing and gene therapy: the scientific and ethical background. *In:* Doherty, Peter; Sutton, Agneta, eds. Man–Made Man: Ethical and Legal Issues in Genetics. Dublin, Ireland: Open Air; 1997: 29–45.
(GENE THERAPY; GENETIC SCREENING)

Ard, Catherine see **Natowicz, Marvin R.**

Ardagh, Michael. May we practise endotracheal intubation on the newly dead? *Journal of Medical Ethics.* 1997 Oct; 23(5): 289–294.
(INFORMED CONSENT; MEDICAL ETHICS/EDUCATION)

Areen, Judith. Regulating human gene therapy. *West Virginia Law Review.* 1985 Fall; 88(2): 153–171.
(GENE THERAPY)

Arena, Francis P. see **Loscalzo, John J.**

Armour, Catherine see **Rolleston, Francis**

Armstrong, Claire. Thousands of women sterilised in Sweden without consent. [News]. *BMJ (British Medical Journal).* 1997 Sep 6; 315(7108): 563.
(EUGENICS; STERILIZATION)

Armstrong, Kerri; Weber, Kurt. Genetic engineering: a lesson on bioethics for the classroom. *American Biology Teacher.* 1991 May; 53(5): 294–297.
(BIOETHICS/EDUCATION; GENETIC INTERVENTION)

Armstrong, Linda see **Rushton, Cindy Hylton**

Armstrong, Mary Beth. Confidentiality, general issues of. *In:* Chadwick, Ruth, ed. Encyclopedia of Applied Ethics, Volume 1. San Diego, CA: Academic Press; 1998: 579–582.
(CONFIDENTIALITY)

Arno, Peter S.; Bonuck, Karen. The economics and financing of HIV disease. *In:* Cohen, P.T.; Sande, Merle A.; Volberding, Paul A., eds. The AIDS Knowledge Base: A Textbook on HIV Disease from the University of California, San Francisco, and the San Francisco General Hospital. Second Edition. Boston, MA: Little, Brown; 1994: 9.3–1 to 9.3–12.
(AIDS; HEALTH CARE/ECONOMICS)

Arnold, Denis G.; Menzel, Paul T. When comes "the end of the day?" A comment on the dialogue between Dax Cowart and Robert Burt. *Hastings Center Report.* 1998 Jan–Feb; 28(1): 25–27.
(ALLOWING TO DIE; TREATMENT REFUSAL)

Arnold, Robert see **Purtilo, Ruth**

Arnold, Robert M.; Shaw, Byers W.; Purtilo, Ruth. Acute, high risk patients: the case of transplantation. *In:* McCullough, Laurence B.; Jones, James W.; Brody, Baruch A., eds. Surgical Ethics. New York, NY: Oxford University Press; 1998: 97–115.
(INFORMED CONSENT; ORGAN AND TISSUE

TRANSPLANTATION; SELECTION FOR TREATMENT)

Arnold, Robert M. see **Aulisio, Mark P.**

Arnold, Robert M. see **Ubel, Peter A.**

Aroskar, Mila A. see **Davis, Anne J.**

Aroskar, Mila A. see **Kane, Rosalie A.**

Arras, John D. Physician–assisted suicide: a tragic view. *In:* Battin, Margaret P.; Rhodes, Rosamond; Silvers, Anita, eds. Physician Assisted Suicide: Expanding the Debate. New York, NY: Routledge; 1998: 279–300.
(EUTHANASIA; SUICIDE)

Arras, John D. Physician–assisted suicide: a tragic view. *Journal of Contemporary Health Law and Policy.* 1997 Spring; 13(2): 361–389.
(ALLOWING TO DIE/LEGAL ASPECTS; EUTHANASIA/LEGAL ASPECTS; SUICIDE)

Arruda, Monica see **McGee, Glenn**

Artnak, Kathryn E.; Dimmitt, Jane H. Choosing a framework for ethical analysis in advanced practice settings: the case for casuistry. *Archives of Psychiatric Nursing.* 1996 Feb; 10(1): 16–23.
(CONFIDENTIALITY/MENTAL HEALTH; NURSING ETHICS)

Arzbaecher, Robert see **Weil, Vivian**

Asai, Atsushi; Fukuhara, Shunichi; Inoshita, Osamu; Miura, Yasuhiko; Tanabe, Noboru; Kurokawa, Kiyoshi. Medical decisions concerning the end of life: a discussion with Japanese physicians. *Journal of Medical Ethics.* 1997 Oct; 23(5): 323–327.
(ADVANCE DIRECTIVES; ALLOWING TO DIE/ATTITUDES; TRUTH DISCLOSURE)

Asai, Atsushi; Kishino, Minako; Tsuguya, Fukui; Sakai, Masahiko; Yokota, Masako; Nakata, Kazumi; Sasakabe, Sumiko; Sawada, Kiyomi; Kaiji, Fumie. A report from Japan: choices of Japanese patients in the face of disagreement. *Bioethics.* 1998 Apr; 12(2): 162–172.
(PROFESSIONAL PATIENT RELATIONSHIP; TRUTH DISCLOSURE)

Asamen, Joy K. see **Childress, Craig A.**

Asch, Adrienne. Distracted by disability. *Cambridge Quarterly of Healthcare Ethics.* 1998 Winter; 7(1): 77–87.
(HEALTH CARE; PATIENT CARE; RESOURCE ALLOCATION)

Asch, D.A. see **Ubel, Peter A.**

Asch, David A.; Hansen–Flaschen, John; Lanken, Paul N. Decisions to limit or continue life-sustaining treatment by critical care physicians in the United States: conflicts between physicians' practices and patients' wishes. *American Journal of Respiratory and Critical Care Medicine.* 1995 Feb; 151(2, Pt. 1): 288–292.
(ALLOWING TO DIE/ATTITUDES)

Asch, David A. see **Love, Susan M.**

Asch, David A. see **Ubel, Peter A.**

Ashcroft, Richard. Human research subjects, selection of. *In:* Chadwick, Ruth, ed. Encyclopedia of Applied Ethics, Volume 2. San Diego, CA: Academic Press; 1998: 627–639.
(HUMAN EXPERIMENTATION/RESEARCH DESIGN)

Ashcroft, Richard; Baron, Dennis; Benatar, Solomon; Bewley, Susan; Boyd, Kenneth; Caddick, Jeremy; Campbell, Alastair; Cattan, A.; Clayden, Graham; Day, Albert; Dlugolecka, Maria; Dickenson, Donna; Doyal, Len; Draper, Heather; Farsides, Bobbie; von Fragstein, Martin; Fulford, Ken; Gillon, Raanan; Goodman, Danë; Harpwood, Vivienne; Harris, John; Haughton, Peter; Healy, Peter; Higgs, Roger; Hope, Anthony. Teaching medical ethics and law within medical education: a model for the UK core curriculum. [Consensus statement by teachers of medical ethics and law in UK medical schools]. *Journal of Medical Ethics.* 1998 Jun; 24(3): 188–192.
(BIOETHICS/EDUCATION; MEDICAL ETHICS/EDUCATION)

Ashenberg, Margaret D. see **McAliley, Lauren G.**

Ashley, Benedict M.; O'Rourke, Kevin D. Health Care Ethics: A Theological Analysis. Fourth Edition. Washington, DC: Georgetown University Press; 1997. 530 p.
(BIOETHICS)

Ashley, Benedict M.; Veatch, Robert M. Basis for medical ethics: a triple contract theory. [Book review of R.M. Veatch's *A Theory of Medical Ethics*, with response]. *Hospital Progress.* 1983 Jan; 64(1): 58–61.
(MEDICAL ETHICS)

Aspirin Myocardial Infarction Study (AMIS) Research Group see **Mattson, Margaret E.**

Association for Improvements in the Maternity Services (Great Britain); National Childbirth Trust (Great Britain); Maternity Alliance (Great Britain). A charter for ethical research in maternity care: Association for Improvements in the Maternity Services; the National Childbirth Trust. *Nursing Ethics.* 1998 May; 5(3): 256–262.
(HUMAN EXPERIMENTATION/FOREIGN COUNTRIES; HUMAN EXPERIMENTATION/SPECIAL POPULATIONS)

Association for Persons with Severe Handicaps see **American Association on Mental Deficiency**

Association of British Insurers. Genetic Testing: ABI Code of Practice. London: Association of British Insurers [online]. Internet Web Site: http://www.abi.org.uk/Industry/abikey/genetics/gentest97 [1998 April 29]; 1997 Dec. 23 p.
(GENETIC SCREENING)

Association of Clinical Cytogenetics (Great Britain) see **Clinical Genetics Society (Great Britain)**

Astarita, Joseph see **Thies, Winthrop Drake**

Astedt–Kurki, Päivi see **Paavilainen, Eija**

Astin, John A. Why patients use alternative medicine: results of a national study. *JAMA.* 1998 May 20; 279(19): 1548–1553.
(PATIENT CARE)

Astrow, Alan B. see **Dresser, Rebecca**

Aswad, S. see Mendez, R.

Aswad, Saleh; Souqiyyeh, M.Z.; Huraib, S.; El-Shihabi, R. Public attitudes toward organ donation in Saudi Arabia. *Transplantation Proceedings*. 1992 Oct; 24(5): 2056–2058.
(ORGAN AND TISSUE DONATION)

Athanassiadis, Ariadni see Marusyk, Randall W.

Atterstam, Inger. Karolinska Institute rocked by research misconduct. [News]. *Lancet*. 1997 Aug 30; 350(9078): 643.
(BIOMEDICAL RESEARCH; FRAUD AND MISCONDUCT)

Auguste, Valérie; Guérin, Corinne; Hervé, Christian; Hazebroucq, Georges. Professional secret in hospitals: study conducted in a pharmacy department. *International Journal of Bioethics*. 1997 Dec; 8(4): 89–99.
(CONFIDENTIALITY; PATIENT CARE/DRUGS)

Aulisio, Mark P.; Arnold, Robert M.; Youngner, Stuart J. Can there be educational and training standards for those conducting health care ethics consultation? *In:* Monagle, John F.; Thomasma, David C., eds. Health Care Ethics: Critical Issues for the 21st Century. Gaithersburg, MD: Aspen Publishers; 1998: 484–496.
(ETHICISTS AND ETHICS COMMITTEES)

Ault, Alicia. FDA may "pull the plug" on consent waiver. [News]. *Lancet*. 1997 Oct 11; 350(9084): 1084.
(HUMAN EXPERIMENTATION/INFORMED CONSENT; HUMAN EXPERIMENTATION/REGULATION)

Ault, Alicia. USA accused of funding placebo–controlled AIDS trials. [News]. *Lancet*. 1997 May 3; 349(9061): 1305.
(AIDS/HUMAN EXPERIMENTATION; HUMAN EXPERIMENTATION/FOREIGN COUNTRIES; HUMAN EXPERIMENTATION/RESEARCH DESIGN; HUMAN EXPERIMENTATION/SPECIAL POPULATIONS)

Austad, Carol Shaw. Is Long-Term Psychotherapy Unethical? Toward a Social Ethic in an Era of Managed Care. San Francisco, CA: Jossey-Bass; 1996. 283 p.
(HEALTH CARE/ECONOMICS; PATIENT CARE/MENTALLY DISABLED; RESOURCE ALLOCATION)

Austin, Christopher P.; Tribble, Jack L. Gene patents and drug development: the perspective from Merck. *In:* Knoppers, Bartha Maria, ed. Human DNA: Law and Policy: International and Comparative Perspectives. Proceedings of the First International Conference on DNA Sampling and Human Genetic Research: Ethical, Legal, and Policy Aspects, held in Montreal, Canada, 6–8 Sep 1996. Boston, MA: Kluwer Law International; 1997: 379–383.
(GENOME MAPPING; PATENTING LIFE FORMS)

Australia. New South Wales. Department of Health. Dying with Dignity: Interim Guidelines on Management. North Sydney, NSW: NSW Health; 1993 Mar 1. 6 p.
(ALLOWING TO DIE)

Australia. Tasmania. An act (No. 44 of 1995) to enable persons with a disability to be represented by a guardian or administrator and to provide for medical and dental treatment for persons with a disability. Date of assent: 22 Sep 1995. [The Guardianship and Administration Act 1995]. *International Digest of Health Legislation*. 1996; 47(2): 174–178.
(INFORMED CONSENT)

Avis, Mark see Cox, Karen

Avorn, Jerry. Including elderly people in clinical trials: better information could improve the effectiveness and safety of drug use. [Editorial]. *BMJ (British Medical Journal)*. 1997 Oct 25; 315(7115): 1033–1034.
(HUMAN EXPERIMENTATION/SPECIAL POPULATIONS)

Aydin, Carolyn E. see Anderson, James G.

Aydin, Erdem. Informed consent in Turkey. [Letter]. *Journal of Medical Ethics*. 1997 Jun; 23(3): 192.
(INFORMED CONSENT)

Ayers, Elise; Harrold, Joan; Lynn, Joanne. A good death: improving care inch–by–inch. *Bioethics Forum*. 1997 Spring; 13(1): 38–40.
(TERMINAL CARE)

Ayers, Karen see Saxton, Marsha

Aziz, Michael see Sayers, Gwen M.

B

Baban, Adriana see David, Henry P.

Babbs, Charles F. Falacious arguments against resuscitation research. *American Journal of Emergency Medicine*. 1985 Sep; 3(5): 461–466.
(HUMAN EXPERIMENTATION/SPECIAL POPULATIONS)

Babiker, Abdel see Aaby, Peter

Bacchetta, Matthew D.; Fins, Joseph J. The economics of clinical ethics programs: a quantitative justification. *Cambridge Quarterly of Healthcare Ethics*. 1997 Fall; 6(4): 451–460.
(ETHICISTS AND ETHICS COMMITTEES)

Bacchetta, Matthew D. see Miller, Franklin G.

Bach, F.H.; Fishman, J.A.; Daniels, N.; Proimos, J.; Anderson, B.; Carpenter, C.B.; Forrow, L.; Robson, S.C.; Fineberg, H.V. Uncertainty in xenotransplantation: individual benefit versus collective risk. *Nature Medicine*. 1998 Feb; 4(2): 141–144.
(ORGAN AND TISSUE TRANSPLANTATION)

Bach, Fritz H.; Fineberg, Harvey V. Call for moratorium on xenotransplants. [Letter]. *Nature*. 1998 Jan 22; 391(6665): 326.
(ORGAN AND TISSUE TRANSPLANTATION)

Badaway, Abdulla A.-B. Ethics in alcohol research and publishing. [Editorial]. *Alcohol and Alcoholism*. 1996 Jan; 31(1): 7–9.
(BEHAVIORAL RESEARCH; BIOMEDICAL RESEARCH; PROFESSIONAL ETHICS)

Badoux, John C.; Hunkeler, David; Waldner, Rosmarie; Greely, Henry T. Swiss democracy has its advantages. [Letters]. *Nature*. 1998 May 21; 393(6682): 205.
(GENETIC INTERVENTION)

Baez, Luis see Cleeland, Charles S.

Bailey, Keith; Ridgway, Anthony. A rational approach to regulation of gene therapy in Canada. *Transfusion*

Science. 1996 Mar; 17(1): 197–202.
(GENE THERAPY)

Bailey, Linda A. see **Samet, Jonathan M.**

Bailey, R. Norman. The doctor–patient relationship: communication, informed consent and the optometric patient. *Journal of the American Optometric Association.* 1994 Jun; 65(6): 418–422.
(INFORMED CONSENT; PROFESSIONAL PATIENT RELATIONSHIP)

Bailey, R. Norman. The history of ethics in the American Optometric Association 1898–1994. *Journal of the American Optometric Association.* 1994 Jun; 65(6): 427–444.
(PROFESSIONAL ETHICS/CODES OF ETHICS)

Bailey, R. Norman see **Foster, George E.**

Bailey, Ronald. What exactly is wrong with cloning people? *In:* McGee, Glenn, ed. The Human Cloning Debate. Berkeley, CA: Berkeley Hills Books; 1998: 181–188.
(CLONING)

Bailit, Howard. When the benefit is in doubt, who decides? *Journal of the American Geriatrics Society.* 1998 Mar; 46(3): 342–345.
(HEALTH CARE/ECONOMICS)

Baillie, Harold W. see **Garrett, Thomas M.**

Baird, P.A. Ethical issues of fertility and reproduction. *Annual Review of Medicine.* 1996; 47: 107–116.
(REPRODUCTIVE TECHNOLOGIES)

Baird, Patricia. Individual interests, societal interests, and reproductive technologies. *Perspectives in Biology and Medicine.* 1997 Spring; 40(3): 440–451.
(REPRODUCTIVE TECHNOLOGIES)

Baird, Patricia A. Registries, record linkage, and research in genetics: protecting privacy. *In:* Knoppers, Bartha Maria, ed. Human DNA: Law and Policy: International and Comparative Perspectives. Proceedings of the First International Conference on DNA Sampling and Human Genetic Research: Ethical, Legal, and Policy Aspects, held in Montreal, Canada, 6–8 Sep 1996. Boston, MA: Kluwer Law International; 1997: 165–175.
(CONFIDENTIALITY; GENETIC RESEARCH)

Baird, Rachel. Gene tests pose challenge for privacy guardian. [News]. *New Scientist.* 1997 Jun 28; 154(2088): 4.
(CONFIDENTIALITY/LEGAL ASPECTS; GENETIC SCREENING)

Baker, Robert; Caplan, Arthur; Emanuel, Linda L.; Latham, Stephen R. Crisis, ethics, and the American Medical Association: 1847 and 1997. [Editorial]. *JAMA.* 1997 Jul 9; 278(2): 163–164.
(MEDICAL ETHICS/CODES OF ETHICS)

Baker, Valerie L. Surrogacy: one physician's view of the role of law. [Commentary]. *University of San Francisco Law Review.* 1994 Spring; 28(3): 603–612.
(SURROGATE MOTHERS)

Balasubramaniam, R. see **Gitanjali, B.**

Baldini, Massimo. The doctor–patient relationship in medical textbooks and manuals of the eighteenth and nineteenth centuries. *Dolentium Hominum: Church and Health in the World.* 1996; 31(11th Yr., No. 1): 88–92.
(MEDICAL ETHICS/EDUCATION; PROFESSIONAL PATIENT RELATIONSHIP)

Baldwin, John C. see **Halevy, Amir**

Balentine, Jerry; Gaeta, Theodore; Rao, Narasinga; Brandon, Bernadette. Emergency department do–not–attempt–resuscitation orders: next–of–kin response to the emergency physician. *Academic Emergency Medicine.* 1996 Jan; 3(1): 54–57.
(RESUSCITATION ORDERS)

Ball, David see **Tyler, Audrey**

Balls, Michael; Goldberg, Alan M.; Fentem, Julia H.; Broadhead, Caren L.; Burch, Rex L.; Festing, Michael F.W.; Frazier, John M.; Hendriksen, Coenraad F.M.; Jennings, Margaret; van der Kamp, Margot D.O.; Morton, David B.; Rowan, Andrew N.; Russell, Claire; Russell, William M.S.; Spielmann, Horst; Stephens, Martin L.; Stokes, William S.; Straughan, Donald W.; Yager, James D.; Zurlo, Joanne; van Zutphen, Bert F.M. The three Rs: the way forward: the report and recommendations of ECVAM [European Centre for the Validation of Alternative Methods] Workshop 11. *ATLA: Alternatives to Laboratory Animals.* 1995 Nov–Dec; 23(6): 838–866.
(ANIMAL EXPERIMENTATION)

Balmer, Thomas A. see **Bushong, Stephen K.**

Balsamo, Anne. On the cutting edge: cosmetic surgery and new imaging technologies. *In: her:* Technologies of the Gendered Body: Reading Cyborg Women. Durham, NC: Duke University Press; 1996: 56–79, 177–184.
(BIOMEDICAL TECHNOLOGIES; PATIENT CARE)

Balsamo, Anne. Public pregnancies and cultural narratives of surveillance. *In: her:* Technologies of the Gendered Body: Reading the Cyborg Women. Durham, NC: Duke University Press; 1996: 80–115, 184–192.
(PRENATAL INJURIES; REPRODUCTION; REPRODUCTIVE TECHNOLOGIES)

Bancroft, Elizabeth A. see **Kowalski, Edgar P.**

Banerjee, Arup K. see **Bugeja, G.**

Bankowski, Zbigniew. International ethics guidelines and genetic epidemiology. *In:* Knoppers, Bartha Maria, ed. Human DNA: Law and Policy: International and Comparative Perspectives. Proceedings of the First International Conference on DNA Sampling and Human Genetic Research: Ethical, Legal, and Policy Aspects, held in Montreal, Cananda, 6–8 Sep 1996. Boston, MA: Kluwer Law International; 1997: 9–13.
(GENETIC RESEARCH; GENETIC SCREENING)

Barbieri, Celia see **Heffner, John E.**

Barbieri, Robert L. see **Trad, Fouad S.**

Barker, Ann. Mental health and the law. *BMJ (British Medical Journal).* 1997 Sep 6; 315(7108): 590–592.
(MENTAL HEALTH; PATIENT CARE/MENTALLY DISABLED)

Barker, E.M. Informed consent in medical research: the ethics committee's view. [Letter]. *BMJ (British Medical Journal)*. 1998 Jan 31; 316(7128): 392–393.
(HUMAN EXPERIMENTATION/ETHICS COMMITTEES; HUMAN EXPERIMENTATION/FOREIGN COUNTRIES; HUMAN EXPERIMENTATION/INFORMED CONSENT)

Barker, Steven see Tindall, Brett

Barlow, Bicka A. Severe penalties for the destruction of "potential life" -- cruel and unusual punishment? [Comment]. *University of San Francisco Law Review.* 1995 Winter; 29(2): 463–508.
(FETUSES; PERSONHOOD)

Barnard, David. Doctors and their suffering patients: commentary on Campbell. *In:* Carson, Ronald A.; Burns, Chester R., eds. Philosophy of Medicine and Bioethics: A Twenty-Year Retrospective and Critical Appraisal. Boston, MA: Kluwer Academic; 1997: 265–272.
(PATIENT CARE)

Barnes, Deborah E. see Green, Charles R.

Barnes, Donelle M.; Davis, Anne J.; Moran, Tracy; Portillo, Carmen J.; Koenig, Barbara A. Informed consent in a multicultural cancer patient population: implications for nursing practice. *Nursing Ethics.* 1998 Sep; 5(5): 412–423.
(INFORMED CONSENT)

Barnes, Donelle M. see Marshall, Patricia A.

Barnes, Frank L. Ethical considerations of preimplantation genetic diagnosis and embryo selection. *In:* Monagle, John F.; Thomasma, David C., eds. Health Care Ethics: Critical Issues for the 21st Century. Gaithersburg, MD: Aspen Publishers; 1998: 56–59.
(GENETIC SCREENING; PRENATAL DIAGNOSIS)

Barnes, Patricia G. Beyond Nuremberg: fifty years later, the debate continues on informed consent. *ABA Journal: The Lawyer's Magazine.* 1997 Mar; 83: 24–27.
(HUMAN EXPERIMENTATION/INFORMED CONSENT; HUMAN EXPERIMENTATION/SPECIAL POPULATIONS)

Barnhart, J. Marie; Wassertheil-Smoller, Sylvia; Fowler, Cynthia; Peterson, Eric D.; Shaw, Linda K.; DeLong, Elizabeth R. Racial variation in the use of coronary-revascularization procedures. [Letters and response]. *New England Journal of Medicine.* 1997 Jul 10; 337(2): 131–132.
(SELECTION FOR TREATMENT)

Barnitt, Rosemary. Ethical dilemmas in occupational therapy and physical therapy: a survey of practitioners in the UK National Health Service. *Journal of Medical Ethics.* 1998 Jun; 24(3): 193–199.
(PROFESSIONAL ETHICS)

Baron, Dennis see Ashcroft, Richard

Baron, J. see Ubel, Peter A.

Barondess, Jeremiah A.; New York Academy of Medicine. The position of the New York Academy of Medicine on physician-assisted suicide. *Bulletin of the New York Academy of Medicine.* 1997 Summer; 74(1): 109–113.
(SUICIDE)

Barr, Judith K. see Yedidia, Michael J.

Barr, Patricia A. see Holtzman, Neil A.

Barrett, Nicholas A. The medical student and the suicidal patient. *Journal of Medical Ethics.* 1997 Oct; 23(5): 277–281.
(CONFIDENTIALITY)

Barry, Robert. The biblical teachings on suicide. *Issues in Law and Medicine.* 1997 Winter; 13(3): 283–299.
(SUICIDE)

Barry, Robert. The Roman Catholic position on abortion. *In:* Edwards, Rem B., ed. Advances in Bioethics. Volume 2: New Essays on Abortion and Bioethics. Greenwich, CT: JAI Press; 1997: 151–182.
(ABORTION/RELIGIOUS ASPECTS)

Bartholome, William G. Ethical issues in pediatric research. *In:* Vanderpool, Harold Y., ed. The Ethics of Research Involving Human Subjects: Facing the 21st Century. Frederick, MD: University Publishing Group; 1996: 339–370.
(HUMAN EXPERIMENTATION/INFORMED CONSENT; HUMAN EXPERIMENTATION/MINORS; INFORMED CONSENT/MINORS)

Bartholome, William G.; Kohrman, Arthur F.; Frader, Joel. Informed consent, parental permission, and assent in pediatric practice. [Letter and response]. *Pediatrics.* 1995 Nov; 96(5, Pt. 1): 981–982.
(INFORMED CONSENT/MINORS)

Bartlett, Peter. Doctors as fiduciaries: equitable regulation of the doctor–patient relationship. *Medical Law Review.* 1997 Summer; 5(2): 193–224.
(PROFESSIONAL PATIENT RELATIONSHIP)

Bartoldus, Ellen Knapik. Medical futility: a nursing home perspective. *In:* Zucker, Marjorie B.; Zucker, Howard D., eds. Medical Futility and the Evaluation of Life-Sustaining Interventions. New York, NY: Cambridge University Press; 1997: 58–64.
(PATIENT CARE/AGED)

Bartolucci, Alfred see Marson, Daniel C.

Barton, Andrew see Talbot, D.

Barton, Roger see Dale, Ruth

Baruchin, Andrea see Skirboll, Lana

Basili, Laura see Patenaude, Andrea Farkas

Basketter, David; Reynolds, Fiona. The use of human volunteers for hazard and risk assessment of skin irritation. *In:* Close, Bryony; Combes, Robert; Hubbard, Anthony; Illingworth, John, eds. Volunteers in Research and Testing. Bristol, PA: Taylor and Francis; 1997: 117–127.
(HUMAN EXPERIMENTATION)

Baskin, Shari A.; Morris, Jane; Ahronheim, Judith C.; Meier, Diane E.; Morrison, R. Sean. Barriers to obtaining consent in dementia research: implications for surrogate decision-making. *Journal of the American Geriatrics Society.* 1998 Mar; 46(3): 287–290.
(HUMAN EXPERIMENTATION/INFORMED CONSENT; HUMAN EXPERIMENTATION/SPECIAL POPULATIONS)

Baskin, Shari A. see **Morrison, R. Sean**

Bass, Larry J.; DeMers, Stephen T.; Ogloff, James R.P.; Peterson, Christa; Pettifor, Jean L.; Reaves, Randolph P.; Rétfalvi, Teréz; Simon, Norma P.; Sinclair, Carole; Tipton, Robert M. Professional Conduct and Discipline in Psychology. Washington, DC; Montgomery, AL: American Psychological Association; Association of State and Provincial Psychology Boards; 1996. 330 p.
(FRAUD AND MISCONDUCT; PROFESSIONAL ETHICS)

Bassford, H.A. HIV testing and confidentiality. *In:* Overall, Christine and Zion, William P., eds. Perspectives on AIDS: Ethical and Social Issues. New York, NY: Oxford University Press; 1991: 106–121.
(AIDS/CONFIDENTIALITY; AIDS/TESTING AND SCREENING)

Bastian, Hilda see **Dolan, Bridget**

Bastron, R. Dennis. Ethical concerns in anesthetic care for patients with do-not-resuscitate orders. *Anesthesiology.* 1996 Nov; 85(5): 1190–1193.
(RESUSCITATION ORDERS)

Batavia, Andrew I. see **Kowalski, Edgar P.**

Bateman, Randall B. Attorneys on bioethics committees: unwelcome menace or valuable asset? *Journal of Law and Health.* 1994–1995; 9(2): 247–272.
(ETHICISTS AND ETHICS COMMITTEES)

Battcock, Timothy see **Zaman, Syed**

Batten, Donald A.; Haliburn, Joan; Prager, Shirley. Informed consent by children and adolescents to psychiatric treatment. [Article and commentaries]. *Australian and New Zealand Journal of Psychiatry.* 1996 Oct; 30(5): 623–632.
(INFORMED CONSENT/MENTALLY DISABLED; INFORMED CONSENT/MINORS)

Battin, Margaret P. Euthanasia: the way we do it, the way they do it. [Revised]. *In:* Monagle, John F.; Thomasma, David C., eds. Health Care Ethics: Critical Issues for the 21st Century. Gaithersburg, MD: Aspen Publishers; 1998: 311–322.
(ALLOWING TO DIE; EUTHANASIA; SUICIDE)

Battin, Margaret P. Is a physician ever obligated to help a patient die? *In:* Emanuel, Linda L., ed. Regulating How We Die: The Ethical, Medical, and Legal Issues Surrounding Physician–Assisted Suicide. Cambridge, MA: Harvard University Press; 1998: 21–47, 264–267.
(SUICIDE)

Battin, Margaret P. Physician–assisted suicide: safe, legal, rare? *In:* Battin, Margaret P.; Rhodes, Rosamond; Silvers, Anita, eds. Physician Assisted Suicide: Expanding the Debate. New York, NY: Routledge; 1998: 63–72.
(SUICIDE)

Battin, Margaret P.; Rhodes, Rosamond; Silvers, Anita, eds. Physician Assisted Suicide: Expanding the Debate. New York, NY: Routledge; 1998. 463 p.
(SUICIDE)

Battin, Margaret P. see **Emanuel, Ezekiel J.**

Battin, Margaret P. see **Jacobson, Jay A.**

Battin, Margaret P. see **Murphy, G. Don**

Baty, Bonnie J. see **McKinnon, Wendy C.**

Batz, Lothar see **Schüppel, Reinhart**

Baumrin, Bernard. Physician, stay thy hand! *In:* Battin, Margaret P.; Rhodes, Rosamond; Silvers, Anita, eds. Physician Assisted Suicide: Expanding the Debate. New York, NY: Routledge; 1998: 177–181.
(SUICIDE)

Baur, Susan. The Intimate Hour: Love and Sex in Psychotherapy. Boston, MA: Houghton Mifflin; 1997. 309 p.
(PROFESSIONAL PATIENT RELATIONSHIP)

Bausola, Adriano. The cultural anthropology of the right to life. *Dolentium Hominum: Church and Health in the World.* 1996; 31(11th Yr., No. 1): 146–149.
(ABORTION)

Baxter, Rosario; Long, Ann; Sines, David. The legal and ethical status of children in health care in the UK. *Nursing Ethics.* 1998 May; 5(3): 189–199.
(PATIENT CARE/MINORS)

Bayer, Ronald. Discrimination, informed consent, and the HIV infected clinician. [Editorial]. *BMJ (British Medical Journal).* 1997 Mar 29; 314(7085): 915–916.
(AIDS/HEALTH PERSONNEL)

Bayer, Ronald; Stryker, Jeff. Ethical challenges posed by clinical progress in AIDS. *American Journal of Public Health.* 1997 Oct; 87(10): 1599–1602.
(AIDS; PATIENT CARE/DRUGS)

Bayertz, Kurt. Ethical aspects of gene therapy and molecular genetic diagnostics. *Cytokines and Molecular Therapy.* 1996 Sep; 2(3): 207–211.
(GENE THERAPY; GENETIC SCREENING)

Bayertz, Kurt. The normative status of the human genome: a European perspective. *In:* Hoshino, Kazumasa, ed. Japanese and Western Bioethics: Studies in Moral Diversity. Boston, MA: Kluwer Academic; 1997: 167–180.
(GENETIC INTERVENTION)

Baylis, Françoise. Errors in medicine: nurturing truthfulness. *Journal of Clinical Ethics.* 1997 Winter; 8(4): 336–340.
(PATIENT CARE; TRUTH DISCLOSURE)

Baylis, Françoise; Downie, Jocelyn. Child abuse and neglect: cross–cultural considerations. *In:* Nelson, Hilde Lindemann, ed. Feminism and Families. New York, NY: Routledge; 1997: 173–187.
(PATIENT CARE/MINORS)

Baylis, Françoise; Downie, Jocelyn; Sherwin, Susan. Reframing research involving humans. *In:* Sherwin, Susan, et al. The Politics of Women's Health: Exploring Agency and Autonomy. Philadelphia, PA: Temple University Press; 1998: 234–259.
(HUMAN EXPERIMENTATION/SPECIAL POPULATIONS)

Baylis, Françoise see **Flagler, Elizabeth**

Beach, Doré. The Responsible Conduct of Research. Weinheim, Germany; New York, NY: VCH Publishers; 1996. 161 p.
(BIOMEDICAL RESEARCH)

Beardslee, Nancy Q. see **Leners, Debra**

Beardsley, Tim. China syndrome: China's eugenics law makes trouble for science and business. *Scientific American.* 1997 Mar; 276(3): 33–34.
(EUGENICS; REPRODUCTION)

Beauchamp, Tom L. Comparative studies: Japan and America. *In:* Hoshino, Kazumasa, ed. Japanese and Western Bioethics: Studies in Moral Diversity. Boston, MA: Kluwer Academic; 1997: 25–47.
(INFORMED CONSENT)

Beauchamp, Tom L. Opposing views on animal experimentation: do animals have rights? *Ethics and Behavior.* 1997; 7(2): 113–121.
(ANIMAL EXPERIMENTATION)

Beauchamp, Tom L. Physician–assisted suicide: a response to Edmund Pellegrino. *In:* Wildes, Kevin Wm.; Mitchell, Alan C., eds. Choosing Life: A Dialogue on *Evangelium Vitae.* Washington, DC: Georgetown University Press; 1997: 254–258.
(ALLOWING TO DIE; EUTHANASIA; SUICIDE)

Beauchamp, Tom L. see **Orlans, F. Barbara**

Beaumont, Patricia M.A. Wrongful life and wrongful birth. *In:* McLean, Sheila A.M., ed. Contemporary Issues in Law, Medicine and Ethics. Brookfield, VT: Dartmouth; 1996: 99–115.
(WRONGFUL LIFE)

Beaupré, Mylène. Decision–making and the sterilization of incompetent children. *In:* Grubb, Andrew, ed. Decision–Making and Problems of Incompetence. New York, NY: Wiley; 1994: 89–101.
(STERILIZATION/MENTALLY DISABLED)

Bebe, Judy see **Durna, Eva M.**

Bebeau, M.J.; Davis, E.L. Survey of ethical issues in dental research. *Journal of Dental Research.* 1996 Feb; 75(2): 845–855.
(BIOMEDICAL RESEARCH; FRAUD AND MISCONDUCT; PROFESSIONAL ETHICS)

Bebeau, M.J.; Holt, S.C. Proceedings of a symposium, "Toward Responsible Research Conduct: The Role of Scientific Societies." [Introduction to a set of five papers and a consensus statement] *Journal of Dental Research.* 1996 Feb; 75(2): 823–824.
(BIOMEDICAL RESEARCH; FRAUD AND MISCONDUCT; PROFESSIONAL ETHICS)

Bebeau, Muriel J.; Holt, Stanley C.; American Association for Dental Research. Ethics Committee. The role of the AADR in promoting research integrity: perspectives and consensus statements. *Journal of Dental Research.* 1996 Feb; 75(2): 856–860.
(BIOMEDICAL RESEARCH; FRAUD AND MISCONDUCT; PROFESSIONAL ETHICS)

Becker, Evelyn S. Ethical issues arising in biotechnology. *In:* Haddad, Amy Marie, ed. Teaching and Learning Strategies in Pharmacy Ethics. Second Edition. New York, NY: Pharmaceutical Products Press; 1997: 33–47.
(GENETIC INTERVENTION)

Becker, Evelyn S. Teaching ethics as a writing–intensive, ability–based course. *In:* Haddad, Amy Marie, ed. Teaching and Learning Strategies in Pharmacy Ethics. Second Edition. New York, NY: Pharmaceutical Products Press; 1997: 139–148.
(PROFESSIONAL ETHICS/EDUCATION)

Becker, Gerhold K., ed. Changing Nature's Course: The Ethical Challenge of Biotechnology. Hong Kong: Hong Kong University Press; 1996. 208 p.
(GENETIC INTERVENTION)

Beckman, Howard B. see **Epstein, Ronald M.**

Beckman, Linda J.; Harvey, S. Marie. Experience and acceptability of medical abortion with mifepristone and misoprostol among U.S. women. *Women's Health Issues.* 1997 Jul–Aug; 7(4): 253–262.
(ABORTION/ATTITUDES)

Beckwith, Francis J. Personal bodily rights, abortion, and unplugging the violinist. *International Philosophical Quarterly.* 1992 Mar; 32(1, Issue 125): 105–118.
(ABORTION)

Beecham, Linda. BMA opposes legalisation of euthanasia. [News]. *BMJ (British Medical Journal).* 1997 Jul 12; 315(7100): 80.
(EUTHANASIA; SUICIDE)

Beecham, Linda. BMA to consult on withdrawing treatment. [News]. *BMJ (British Medical Journal).* 1998 Jul 18; 317(7152): 165.
(ALLOWING TO DIE)

Beecham, Linda. GMC approves new ethical guidance. [News]. *BMJ (British Medical Journal).* 1998 May 23; 316(7144): 1556.
(PATIENT CARE)

Beeson, Diane. Nuance, complexity, and context: qualitative methods in genetic counseling research. *Journal of Genetic Counseling.* 1997 Mar; 6(1): 21–43.
(BEHAVIORAL RESEARCH/RESEARCH DESIGN; GENETIC COUNSELING)

Beeson, Diane; Jennings, Patricia. Prenatal diagnosis of fetal disorders: ethical, legal, and social issues. *In:* Monagle, John F.; Thomasma, David C., eds. Health Care Ethics: Critical Issues for the 21st Century. Gaithersburg, MD: Aspen Publishers; 1998: 29–44.
(PRENATAL DIAGNOSIS)

Begleiter, Michael L.; Rogers, Jill Cellars. Genetic counseling for a family with two distinct anomalies: a case report of a neural tube defect and 5p– syndrome in a fetus. *Journal of Genetic Counseling.* 1994 Jun; 3(2): 87–93.
(GENETIC COUNSELING)

Begley, Ann–Marie. Beneficent voluntary active euthanasia: a challenge to professionals caring for terminally ill patients. *Nursing Ethics.* 1998 Jul; 5(4): 294–306.
(EUTHANASIA)

Behi, Ruhi; Nolan, Mike. Ethical issues in research. *British Journal of Nursing.* 1995 Jun 22–Jul 12; 4(12):

712–716.
(HUMAN EXPERIMENTATION)

Beisecker, Analee E.; Murden, Robert A.; Moore, William P.; Graham, Deborah; Nelmig, Linda. Attitudes of medical students and primary care physicians regarding input of older and younger patients in medical decisions. *Medical Care.* 1996 Feb; 34(2): 126–137.
(PATIENT CARE; PROFESSIONAL PATIENT RELATIONSHIP)

Belkin, Lisa. Pregnant with complications. *New York Times Magazine.* 1997 Oct 26: 34–39, 48–49, 67–68.
(REPRODUCTIVE TECHNOLOGIES; SELECTION FOR TREATMENT)

Bell, Anthony J. see **Paris, John J.**

Bell, Bertrand M. see **DeGroot, Leslie J.**

Bell, Marilynne; Mosher, Janet. (Re)fashioning medicine's response to wife abuse. *In:* Sherwin, Susan, et al. The Politics of Women's Health: Exploring Agency and Autonomy. Philadelphia, PA: Temple University Press; 1998: 205–233.
(PATIENT CARE)

Bellamy, Paul see **Teno, Joan**

Belzile, Michelle see **Suarez–Almazor, Maria E.**

Bempong, Isaac see **Harris, Yvonne**

Ben–Meir, Yehoshua. Legal parenthood and genetic parenthood in Jewish law. *In:* Jewish Law Annual. Volume Twelve. Amsterdam, Netherlands: Harwood Academic Publishers; 1997: 153–166.
(REPRODUCTIVE TECHNOLOGIES)

Benagiano, G.; Rowe, P.J. Assisted reproduction: a not so bright future? *Human Reproduction.* 1995 Jun; 10(6): 1324–1326.
(REPRODUCTIVE TECHNOLOGIES)

Benatar, David; Benatar, Solomon R. Informed consent and research. *BMJ (British Medical Journal).* 1998 Mar 28; 316(7136): 1008.
(AIDS/HUMAN EXPERIMENTATION; AIDS/TESTING AND SCREENING; HUMAN EXPERIMENTATION/INFORMED CONSENT)

Benatar, S.R. see **Henley, L.**

Benatar, Solomon see **Ashcroft, Richard**

Benatar, Solomon R. Editorial ethics. [Personal view]. *BMJ (British Medical Journal).* 1998 Jan 10; 316(7125): 155–156.
(BIOMEDICAL RESEARCH; PROFESSIONAL ETHICS)

Benatar, Solomon R. Just healthcare beyond individualism: challenges for North American bioethics. *Cambridge Quarterly of Healthcare Ethics.* 1997 Fall; 6(4): 397–415.
(BIOETHICS; HEALTH CARE/RIGHTS)

Benatar, Solomon R. What makes a just healthcare system? Broader professional ethics, including consideration of the public interest and the common good. [Editorial]. *BMJ (British Medical Journal).* 1996 Dec 21–28; 313(7072): 1567–1568.

(HEALTH CARE)

Benatar, Solomon R. see **Benatar, David**

Bendall, Christine. Clinical research -- the relationship between law and guidelines. *In:* Close, Bryony; Combes, Robert; Hubbard, Anthony; Illingworth, John, eds. Volunteers in Research and Testing. Bristol, PA: Taylor and Francis; 1997: 41–52.
(HUMAN EXPERIMENTATION/FOREIGN COUNTRIES; HUMAN EXPERIMENTATION/REGULATION)

Benjamin, Martin. Supply and demand for transplantable organs: the ethical perspective. *Transplantation Proceedings.* 1992 Oct; 24(5): 2139.
(ORGAN AND TISSUE DONATION)

Benjamin, Martin; Turcotte, Jeremiah G. Ethics, alcoholism and liver transplantation. *In:* Lucey, Michael R.; Merion, Robert M.; Beresford, Thomas P., eds. Liver Transplantation and the Alcoholic Patient: Medical, Surgical and Psychosocial Issues. New York, NY: Cambridge University Press; 1994: 113–130.
(ORGAN AND TISSUE TRANSPLANTATION; RESOURCE ALLOCATION/BIOMEDICAL TECHNOLOGIES; SELECTION FOR TREATMENT)

Benjamin, Regina see **Scutchfield, F. Douglas**

Bennett, Allen J. see **Berger, Jeffrey T.**

Bennett, Belinda. Gamete donation, reproductive technology and the law. *In:* Petersen, Kerry, ed. Intersections: Women on Law, Medicine and Technology. Brookfield, VT: Ashgate; 1997: 127–144.
(ORGAN AND TISSUE DONATION; REPRODUCTIVE TECHNOLOGIES)

Bennett, Charles L. see **Tulsky, James A.**

Bennett, Robin L. see **McKinnon, Wendy C.**

Benson, Paul R.; Roth, Loren H. Trends in the social control of medical and psychiatric research. *Law and Mental Health.* 1988; 4: 1–47.
(HUMAN EXPERIMENTATION/ETHICS COMMITTEES; HUMAN EXPERIMENTATION/REGULATION)

Bent, Nuala see **Mead, Gillian E.**

Berenson, Robert A. see **Hall, Mark A.**

Beresford, Thomas P. see **Lucey, Michael R.**

Berg, Paul; Singer, Maxine. The recombinant DNA controversy: twenty years later. *Bio/Technology.* 1995 Oct; 13(10): 1132–1134.
(RECOMBINANT DNA RESEARCH)

Berg, Paula E. Lost in a doctrinal wasteland: the exceptionalism of doctor–patient speech within the Rehnquist Court's First Amendment jurisprudence. *Health Matrix.* 1998 Summer; 8(2): 153–177.
(PROFESSIONAL PATIENT RELATIONSHIP)

Berg, Robert N. The ethical practice of medicine. *Journal of the Medical Association of Georgia.* 1990 Nov; 79(11): 863–864.
(MEDICAL ETHICS)

Berger, Abi see **Schüppel, Reinhart**

Berger, Douglas; Fukunishi, Isao; O'Dowd, Mary Alice; Hosaka, Takashi; Kuboki, Tomifusa; Ishikawa, Yoshihiro. A comparison of Japanese and American psychiatrists' attitudes towards patients wishing to die in the general hospital. *Psychotherapy and Psychosomatics*. 1997; 66(6): 319–328.
(ALLOWING TO DIE/ATTITUDES; EUTHANASIA/ATTITUDES; SUICIDE)

Berger, Douglas; Takahashi, Yoshitomo; Fukunishi, Isao; Hosaka, Takashi; O'Dowd, Mary Alice; Ono, Yutaka; Kuboki, Tomifusa; Ishikawa, Yoshihiro. Japanese psychiatrists' attitudes toward patients wishing to die in the general hospital: a cultural perspective. *Cambridge Quarterly of Healthcare Ethics*. 1997 Fall; 6(4): 470–479.
(ALLOWING TO DIE/ATTITUDES; EUTHANASIA/ATTITUDES; SUICIDE)

Berger, Edward M.; Gert, Bernard. The institutional context for research. *Professional Ethics*. 1995 Spring–Summer; 4(3–4): 17–46.
(BIOMEDICAL RESEARCH; FRAUD AND MISCONDUCT)

Berger, Jeffrey T. Cultural discrimination in mechanisms for health decisions: a view from New York. *Journal of Clinical Ethics*. 1998 Summer; 9(2): 127–131.
(ADVANCE DIRECTIVES; ALLOWING TO DIE/LEGAL ASPECTS)

Berger, Jeffrey T.; Rosner, Fred; Potash, Joel; Kark, Pieter; Farnsworth, Peter; Bennett, Allen J. Medical futility: towards consensus on disagreement. *HEC (HealthCare Ethics Committee) Forum*. 1998 Mar; 10(1): 102–118.
(ALLOWING TO DIE)

Berger, John. Patient confidentiality in a high tech world. *Journal of Pharmacy and Law*. 1996; 5(1): 139–145.
(CONFIDENTIALITY/LEGAL ASPECTS; PATIENT CARE/DRUGS)

Bergh, Christina see Wennerholm, Ulla–Britt

Berghmans, R.L.P. Advance directives for non–therapeutic dementia research: some ethical and policy considerations. *Journal of Medical Ethics*. 1998 Feb; 24(1): 32–37.
(ADVANCE DIRECTIVES; HUMAN EXPERIMENTATION/INFORMED CONSENT; HUMAN EXPERIMENTATION/SPECIAL POPULATIONS)

Berghmans, Ron L.P. Coercive treatment in psychiatry. *In:* Chadwick, Ruth, ed. Encyclopedia of Applied Ethics, Volume 1. San Diego, CA: Academic Press; 1998: 535–542.
(BEHAVIOR CONTROL; TREATMENT REFUSAL/MENTALLY DISABLED)

Berghmans, Ron L.P.; ter Meulen, Rudd H.J. Ethical issues in research with dementia patients. *International Journal of Geriatric Psychiatry*. 1995 Aug; 10(8): 647–651.
(HUMAN EXPERIMENTATION/SPECIAL POPULATIONS)

Bergsma, Jurrit. Response to "Ethical concerns about relapse studies" by Adil E. Shamoo and Timothy J. Keay: Research with vulnerable subjects. [Letter] *Cambridge Quarterly of Healthcare Ethics*. 1997 Spring; 6(2): 233–234.
(HUMAN EXPERIMENTATION/SPECIAL POPULATIONS)

Berk, Martin R. see Sekela, Michael

Berk, Richard see Korenman, Stanley G.

Berkowitz, Jonathan M.; Snyder, Jack W. Racism and sexism in medically assisted conception. *Bioethics*. 1998 Jan; 12(1): 25–44.
(SEX PRESELECTION)

Berkowitz, Kenneth A. End-of-life decisionmaking in the Veterans Health Administration. *HEC (HealthCare Ethics Committee) Forum*. 1997 Jun; 9(2): 169–181.
(ALLOWING TO DIE)

Berkowitz, Sheldon T.; Boisaubin, Eugene V.; Perkins, Henry S.; Hazuda, Helen P.; Krakauer, Eric L. Race and the delivery of care. [Letters and response]. *Hastings Center Report*. 1998 Jan–Feb; 28(1): 5–6.
(ALLOWING TO DIE; PROFESSIONAL PATIENT RELATIONSHIP)

Bermúdez, José Luis. The moral significance of birth. *Ethics*. 1996 Jan; 106(2): 378–403.
(FETUSES; PERSONHOOD)

Bernabei, Roberto; Gambassi, Giovanni; Lapane, Kate; Landi, Francesco; Gatsonis, Constantine; Dunlop, Robert; Lipsitz, Lewis; Steel, Knight; Mor, Vincent. Management of pain in elderly patients with cancer. [For the SAGE Study Group]. *JAMA*. 1998 Jun 17; 279(23): 1877–1882.
(PATIENT CARE/AGED; PATIENT CARE/DRUGS)

Bernard, Claire; Nassiry, Ladan; Knoppers, Bartha Maria, comps. Legal Aspects of Research and Clinical Practice with Human Beings: Selected Canadian Legal Bibliography, 1980–1992. Ottawa, ON: National Council on Bioethics in Human Research (NCBHR); 1992. 35 p.
(HUMAN EXPERIMENTATION/FOREIGN COUNTRIES)

Bernardin, Joseph. Euthanasia: ethical and legal challenge. *In:* Langan, John P., ed. Joseph Cardinal Bernardin: A Moral Vision for America. Washington, DC: Georgetown University Press; 1998: 59–69, 170.
(EUTHANASIA; SUICIDE)

Bernardin, Joseph. Euthanasia in the Catholic tradition. *In:* Langan, John P., ed. Joseph Cardinal Bernardin: A Moral Vision for America. Washington, DC: Georgetown University Press; 1998: 119–128.
(EUTHANASIA/RELIGIOUS ASPECTS; SUICIDE)

Bernardin, Joseph. The consistent ethic of life after *Webster*. *In:* Langan, John P., ed. Joseph Cardinal Bernardin: A Moral Vision for America. Washington, DC: Georgetown University Press; 1998: 79–92.
(ABORTION/RELIGIOUS ASPECTS)

Bernat, James L. A defense of the whole–brain concept of death. *Hastings Center Report*. 1998 Mar–Apr; 28(2): 14–23.
(DETERMINATION OF DEATH/BRAIN DEATH)

Bernat, James L. Quality of neurological care: balancing cost control and ethics. *Archives of Neurology*. 1997 Nov; 54(11): 1341–1345.
(HEALTH CARE/ECONOMICS)

Bernat, James L.; Ringel, Steven P.; Vickrey, Barbara G.; Keran, Christopher. Attitudes of US neurologists concerning the ethical dimensions of managed care. *Neurology*. 1997 Jul; 49(1): 4–13.

(HEALTH CARE/ECONOMICS)

Bernat, James L. see **Sweet, Matthew P.**

Bernhardt, Barbara A.; Geller, Gail; Strauss, Misha; Helzlsouer, Kathy J.; Stefanek, Michael; Wilcox, Patti M.; Holtzman, Neil A. Toward a model informed consent process for BRCA1 testing: a qualitative assessment of women's attitudes. *Journal of Genetic Counseling.* 1997 Jun; 6(2): 207–222.
(GENETIC COUNSELING; GENETIC SCREENING; INFORMED CONSENT)

Bero, Lisa A. Disclosure policies for gifts from industry to academic faculty. [Editorial]. *JAMA.* 1998 Apr 1; 279(13): 1031–1032.
(BIOMEDICAL RESEARCH)

Bero, Lisa A. see **Green, Charles R.**

Berry, Carolyn A. see **Yedidia, Michael J.**

Berry, Jonathan. Local research ethics committees can audit ethical standards in research. *Journal of Medical Ethics.* 1997 Dec; 23(6): 379–381.
(HUMAN EXPERIMENTATION/ETHICS COMMITTEES; HUMAN EXPERIMENTATION/FOREIGN COUNTRIES)

Berry, Roberta M. The genetic revolution and the physician's duty of confidentiality: the role of the old Hippocratic virtues in the regulation of the new genetic intimacy. *Journal of Legal Medicine.* 1997 Dec; 18(4): 401–441.
(CONFIDENTIALITY/LEGAL ASPECTS; GENETIC SCREENING)

Bersoff, D.N. Process and procedures for dealing with misconduct: a necessity or a nightmare? *Journal of Dental Research.* 1996 Feb; 75(2): 836–840.
(BIOMEDICAL RESEARCH; FRAUD AND MISCONDUCT; PROFESSIONAL ETHICS)

Berwick, Donald; Hiatt, Howard; Janeway, Penny; Smith, Richard. An ethical code for everybody in health care. [Editorial]. *BMJ (British Medical Journal).* 1997 Dec 20–27; 315(7123): 1633–1634.
(HEALTH CARE; PROFESSIONAL ETHICS)

Berwick, Donald M. see **Irving, Miles**

Beta–Blocker Heart Attack Trial (BHAT) Research Group see **Aspirin Myocardial Infarction Study (AMIS) Research Group**

Betan, Ephi J. Toward a hermeneutic model of ethical decision making in clinical practice. *Ethics and Behavior.* 1997; 7(4): 347–365.
(PROFESSIONAL ETHICS)

Betzold, Michael. The selling of Doctor Death: how Jack Kevorkian became a national hero. *New Republic.* 1997 May 26; 216(21): 22–28.
(SUICIDE)

Betzold, Michael see **Lessenberry, Jack**

Bewley, Susan see **Ashcroft, Richard**

Bewley, Susan see **Dolan, Bridget**

Bezjak, A. see **Taylor, K.M.**

Bhagwanjee, Satish; Muckart, David J.J.; Jeena, Prakash M.; Moodley, Prushini; Kale, Rajendra; Seedat, Y.K. Does HIV status influence the outcome of patients admitted to a surgical intensive care unit? A prospective double blind study. [Article, commentaries, and response]. *BMJ (British Medical Journal).* 1997 Apr 12; 314(7087): 1077–1084.
(AIDS/HUMAN EXPERIMENTATION; AIDS/TESTING AND SCREENING; HUMAN EXPERIMENTATION/FOREIGN COUNTRIES; HUMAN EXPERIMENTATION/INFORMED CONSENT; SELECTION FOR TREATMENT)

Bhagwati, Sanat N. Ethics, morality and practice of medicine in ancient India. *Child's Nervous System.* 1997 Aug–Sep; 13(8–9): 428–434.
(MEDICAL ETHICS)

Bhopal, Raj. Spectre of racism in health and health care: lessons from history and the United States. *BMJ (British Medical Journal).* 1998 Jun 27; 316(7149): 1970–1973.
(HEALTH; HEALTH CARE)

Bhugra, Dinesh see **Logmans, A.**

Biagi, Enzo see **Maiorca, Rosario**

Bick, Ezra. Ovum donations: a rabbinic conceptual model of maternity. *In:* Feldman, Emanuel; Wolowelsky, Joel B., eds. Jewish Law and the New Reproductive Technologies. Hoboken, NJ: Ktav; 1997: 83–105.
(ORGAN AND TISSUE DONATION; REPRODUCTIVE TECHNOLOGIES)

Bickell, Nina A. Drug companies and continuing medical education. *Journal of General Internal Medicine.* 1995 Jul; 10(7): 392–394.
(HEALTH CARE/ECONOMICS)

Bickenbach, Jerome E. Disability and life–ending decisions. *In:* Battin, Margaret P.; Rhodes, Rosamond; Silvers, Anita, eds. Physician Assisted Suicide: Expanding the Debate. New York, NY: Routledge; 1998: 123–132.
(SUICIDE)

Bienen, Leigh see **Blanck, Peter**

Biermann, Carol A. What's a nice biology teacher like you doing teaching humanities? *American Biology Teacher.* 1990 Nov–Dec; 52(8): 487–490.
(BIOETHICS/EDUCATION)

Biesecker, Barbara B. see **Geller, Gail**

Biesecker, Barbara Bowles. Future directions in genetic counseling: practical and ethical considerations. *Kennedy Institute of Ethics Journal.* 1998 Jun; 8(2): 145–160.
(GENETIC COUNSELING)

Biesecker, Barbara Bowles. Privacy in genetic counseling. *In:* Rothstein, Mark A., ed. Genetic Secrets: Protecting Privacy and Confidentiality in the Genetic Era. New Haven, CT: Yale University Press; 1997: 108–125.
(CONFIDENTIALITY; GENETIC COUNSELING)

Bilgin, N. see **Haberal, Mehmet**

Billick, Stephen B.; Della Bella, Peter; Burgert, Woodward. Competency to consent to hospitalization in the medical patient. *Journal of the American Academy*

Bleich, J. David. Medical and life insurance: a halakhic mandate. *Tradition: A Journal of Orthodox Jewish Thought.* 1997 Spring; 31(3): 52–70.
(HEALTH CARE/ECONOMICS)

Bleich, J. David. Sperm banking in anticipation of infertility. *In:* Feldman, Emanuel; Wolowelsky, Joel B., eds. Jewish Law and the New Reproductive Technologies. Hoboken, NJ: Ktav; 1997: 139–154.
(ARTIFICIAL INSEMINATION)

Blenkinsop, Stanley. Whatever happened to plain English? The gobbledygook smokescreen that baffles research subjects. *In:* Close, Bryony; Combes, Robert; Hubbard, Anthony; Illingworth, John, eds. Volunteers in Research and Testing. Bristol, PA: Taylor and Francis; 1997: 89–98.
(HUMAN EXPERIMENTATION/INFORMED CONSENT)

Blennerhassett, Mitzi; Tattersall, Martin; Ellis, Peter; Metcalfe, D. Truth, the first casualty. [Article and commentaries]. *BMJ (British Medical Journal).* 1998 Jun 20; 316(7148): 1890–1893.
(TRUTH DISCLOSURE)

Blinderman, Abraham. The physician and war: a layman's view. *New York State Journal of Medicine.* 1985 Feb; 85(2): 77–79.
(WAR)

Bloche, M. Gregg. Cutting waste and keeping faith. [Editorial]. *Annals of Internal Medicine.* 1998 Apr 15; 128(8): 688–689.
(FRAUD AND MISCONDUCT; HEALTH CARE/ECONOMICS)

Bloche, M. Gregg. Managed care, medical privacy, and the paradigm of consent. *Kennedy Institute of Ethics Journal.* 1997 Dec; 7(4): 381–386.
(CONFIDENTIALITY; HEALTH CARE/ECONOMICS; INFORMED CONSENT)

Block, Marian R.; Schaffner, Kenneth F.; Coulehan, John L. Ethical problems of recording physician–patient interactions in family practice settings. *Journal of Family Practice.* 1985; 21(6): 467–472.
(CONFIDENTIALITY; INFORMED CONSENT)

Block, Susan D. see **Billings, J. Andrew**

Block, Susan D. see **Quill, Timothy E.**

Blogg, Colin E. see **Scott, P.V.**

Blogg, Colin E. see **Talbot, D.**

Blomquist, Glenn C. see **Sekela, Michael**

Bloom, Barry R. The highest attainable standard: ethical issues in AIDS vaccines. *Science.* 1998 Jan 9; 279(5348): 186–188.
(AIDS/HUMAN EXPERIMENTATION; HUMAN EXPERIMENTATION/FOREIGN COUNTRIES; IMMUNIZATION)

Blumenthal, David see **Campbell, Eric G.**

Blumenthal, David see **Halm, Ethan A.**

Blumenthal, David see **Patterson, W. Bradford**

Blumstein, James F. The case for commerce in organ transplantation. *Transplantation Proceedings.* 1992 Oct; 24(5): 2190–2197.
(ORGAN AND TISSUE DONATION)

Blunt, Jennifer; Savulescu, Julian; Watson, Alastair J.M. Meeting the challenges facing research ethics committees: some practical suggestions. *BMJ (British Medical Journal).* 1998 Jan 3; 316(7124): 58–61.
(HUMAN EXPERIMENTATION/ETHICS COMMITTEES; HUMAN EXPERIMENTATION/FOREIGN COUNTRIES)

Blunt, Jennifer see **Savulescu, Julian**

Blustein, Jeffrey. What bioethics needs to learn about families: The Worth of a Child, by Thomas Murray; The Patient in the Family: An Ethics of Medicine and Families, by Hilde Lindemann Nelson and James Lindemann Nelson. [Book review essay]. *Theoretical Medicine and Bioethics.* 1998 Apr; 19(2): 101–115.
(BIOETHICS)

Blustein, Jeffrey; Robinson, Walter; Loeben, Gregory S.; Wilfond, Benjamin S. Case vignette: placebos and informed consent. [Case study and commentaries]. *Ethics and Behavior.* 1998; 8(1): 89–98.
(INFORMED CONSENT; PATIENT CARE/DRUGS)

Bobinski, Mary Anne see **Curran, William J.**

Bobrow, Martin see **Kinmonth, Ann Louise**

Bobrow, Martin see **Marteau, Theresa**

Bobrow, Martin see **Michie, Susan**

Boccellari, Alicia see **Cooke, Molly**

Bodenheimer, Thomas. The Oregon Health Plan — lessons for the nation. [First of two parts]. *New England Journal of Medicine.* 1997 Aug 28; 337(9): 651–655.
(HEALTH CARE/ECONOMICS; RESOURCE ALLOCATION)

Bodenheimer, Thomas S.; Grumbach, Kevin. Medical ethics and the rationing of health care. *In: their* Understanding Health Policy: A Clinical Approach. Stamford, CT: Appleton and Lange; 1995: 173–194.
(HEALTH CARE/ECONOMICS; RESOURCE ALLOCATION)

Boettcher, Flint see **Webb, Sally L.**

Boisaubin, Eugene V. Nazi medicine: In the Shadow of the Reich: Nazi Medicine [videorecording], by John Michalczyk. [Audiovisual review essay]. *JAMA.* 1998 May 13; 279(18): 1496.
(EUGENICS; FRAUD AND MISCONDUCT)

Boisaubin, Eugene V. see **Berkowitz, Sheldon T.**

Bol Raap, R. see **Logmans, A.**

Bolaji, Ibrahim I. see **Amu, Olubusola**

Boling, Patricia. Mandating treatment for pregnant substance abusers is the wrong focus for public discussion. *Politics and the Life Sciences.* 1996 Mar; 15(1): 51–52.
(INVOLUNTARY COMMITMENT; PRENATAL INJURIES)

Bolster, Mary Catherine. Children as experimental subjects: a review of ethical and theological issues.

Linacre Quarterly. 1998 May; 65(2): 6–32.
(HUMAN EXPERIMENTATION/MINORS)

Bond, Michael. Drugs firms fight biowar curbs. [News]. *New Scientist.* 1997 Mar 8; 153(2072): 8.
(WAR)

Bonduelle, M.; Joris, H.; Hofmans, K.; Liebaers, I.; Van Steirteghem, A. Mental development of 201 ICSI children at 2 years of age. *Lancet.* 1998 May 23; 351(9115): 1553.
(REPRODUCTIVE TECHNOLOGIES)

Bonham, Vence L. see **Brody, Howard**

Bonn, Dorothy. Genome directory causes controversy. [News]. *Lancet.* 1995 Sep 30; 346(8979): 893.
(GENOME MAPPING)

Bonuck, Karen see **Arno, Peter S.**

Boonin–Vail, David. A defense of "A defense of abortion": on the responsibility objection to Thomson's argument. *Ethics.* 1997 Jan; 107(2): 286–313.
(ABORTION)

Boozang, Kathleen M. Deciding the fate of religious hospitals in the emerging health care market. *Houston Law Review.* 1995; 31: 1429–1516.
(HEALTH CARE)

Bopp, James; Coleson, Richard E. A critique of family members as proxy decisionmakers without legal limits. *Issues in Law and Medicine.* 1996 Fall; 12(2): 133–165.
(ALLOWING TO DIE/LEGAL ASPECTS; INFORMED CONSENT)

Bopp, James; Coleson, Richard E. Roe v. Wade and the euthanasia debate. *Issues in Law and Medicine.* 1997 Spring; 12(4): 343–354.
(ABORTION/LEGAL ASPECTS; SUICIDE)

Bopp, James; Coleson, Richard E. The constitutional case against permitting physician–assisted suicide for competent adults with "terminal conditions". *Issues in Law and Medicine.* 1995 Winter; 11(3): 239–268.
(SUICIDE)

Borawski, Deborah B. Ethical dilemmas for nurse administrators. *Journal of Nursing Administration.* 1995 Jul–Aug; 25(7–8): 60–62.
(NURSING ETHICS)

Borenstein, Michael see **Kane, John M.**

Borowsky, Steven J.; Davis, Margaret K.; Goertz, Christine; Lurie, Nicole. Are all health plans created equal? The physician's view. *JAMA.* 1997 Sep 17; 278(11): 917–921.
(HEALTH CARE)

Borres, Magnus P. see **Wennerholm, Ulla–Britt**

Borthwick, Christian J. The permanent vegetative state: ethical crux, medical fiction? *Issues in Law and Medicine.* 1996 Fall; 12(2): 167–185.
(ALLOWING TO DIE)

Borum, Randy see **Swartz, Marvin S.**

Bosch, Xavier. "Voluntary" sterilisation in Spain clarified in new legislation. [News]. *Lancet.* 1998 Jul 11; 352(9122): 124.
(STERILIZATION/MENTALLY DISABLED)

Bosek, Marcia Sue DeWolf. Doing good: an ethical quandary. *Medsurg Nursing.* 1995 Apr; 4(2): 154–156.
(TREATMENT REFUSAL)

Bosk, Charles L.; Frader, Joel. Institutional ethics committees: sociological oxymoron, empirical black box. *In:* DeVries, Raymond; Subedi, Janardan, eds. Bioethics and Society: Constructing the Ethical Enterprise. Upper Saddle River, NJ: Prentice Hall; 1998: 94–116.
(ETHICISTS AND ETHICS COMMITTEES)

Bostrom, Barry A. Lee v. Oregon. [Note]. *Issues in Law and Medicine.* 1997 Winter; 13(3): 333–338.
(SUICIDE)

Bostrom, Barry A. McIver v. Krischer. [Note]. *Issues in Law and Medicine.* 1997 Spring; 12(4): 385–389.
(SUICIDE)

Botkin, Jeffrey R.; McMahon, William M.; Smith, Ken R.; Nash, Jean E. Privacy and confidentiality in the publication of pedigrees: a survey of investigators and biomedical journals. *JAMA.* 1998 Jun 10; 279(22): 1808–1812.
(CONFIDENTIALITY; GENETIC RESEARCH; HUMAN EXPERIMENTATION/INFORMED CONSENT)

Botkin, Jeffrey R. see **Geller, Gail**

Botkin, Jeffrey R. see **Mehlman, Maxwell J.**

Botkin, Jeffrey R. see **Page, David L.**

Böttiger, Lars Erik. Scientific misconduct -- does it exist? [Editorial]. *Journal of Internal Medicine.* 1994 Feb; 235(2): 103–105.
(BIOMEDICAL RESEARCH; FRAUD AND MISCONDUCT)

Boulard, Nina see **Sigmon, Sandra T.**

Bourke, Leon H. Couture v. Couture. [Note]. *Issues in Law and Medicine.* 1990 Fall; 6(2): 201–204.
(ALLOWING TO DIE/LEGAL ASPECTS)

Bourne, Richard see **Appelbaum, Paul S.**

Bove, Catherine M.; Fry, Sara T.; MacDonald, Deborah J. Presymptomatic and predisposition genetic testing: ethical and social considerations. *Seminars in Oncology Nursing.* 1997 May; 13(2): 135–140.
(GENETIC SCREENING)

Bowden, M.F. see **Richmond, Caroline**

Bowen, Jennifer R.; Gibson, Frances L.; Leslie, Garth I.; Saunders, Douglas M. Medical and developmental outcomes at 1 year for children conceived by intracytoplasmic sperm injection. *Lancet.* 1998 May 23; 315(9115): 1529–1534.
(REPRODUCTIVE TECHNOLOGIES)

Bower, Hilary. Public consultation on human cloning launched. [News]. *BMJ (British Medical Journal).* 1998 Feb 7; 316(7129): 411.
(CLONING; EMBRYO AND FETAL RESEARCH)

Bowie, Cameron. Was the paper I wrote a fraud? [Personal view]. *BMJ (British Medical Journal)*. 1998 Jun 6; 316(7146): 1755–1756.
(BIOMEDICAL RESEARCH; FRAUD AND MISCONDUCT)

Bowling, Ann see Marshall, Tom

Bowman, David see Degner, Lesley F.

Boyce, Nell. In sickness and in health. [News]. *New Scientist*. 1997 Oct 25; 156(2105): 20–21.
(GENE THERAPY)

Boyd, Kenneth see Ashcroft, Richard

Boyd, Kenneth M. Little lamb, who made thee? A letter from Edinburgh. *Cambridge Quarterly of Healthcare Ethics*. 1998 Spring; 7(2): 199–202.
(CLONING)

Boyd, Kenneth M.; Higgs, Roger; Pinching, Anthony J., eds. The New Dictionary of Medical Ethics. London: BMJ Publishing Group; 1997. 285 p.
(BIOETHICS)

Boyd, Kenneth M. see Smith, Jane A.

Boyer, Kathryn see Ghusn, Husam F.

Boyle, Joseph. The Roman Catholic tradition and bioethics. *In:* Lustig, B. Andrew, ed.; Center for Medical Ethics and Health Policy (Houston, TX). Bioethics Yearbook, Volume 5: Theological Developments in Bioethics, 1992–1994. Boston, MA: Kluwer Academic; 1997: 11–32.
(BIOETHICS)

Boyle, Marian see Goldfarb, James

Boyle, Philip J., ed. Getting Doctors to Listen: Ethics and Outcomes Data in Context. Washington, DC: Georgetown University Press; 1998. 234 p.
(BIOMEDICAL TECHNOLOGIES; PATIENT CARE)

Boyle, Philip J.; Moskowitz, Ellen. Making tough resource decisions. *Health Progress*. 1996 Nov–Dec; 77(6): 48–53.
(RESOURCE ALLOCATION; SELECTION FOR TREATMENT)

Braaten, Ellen B.; Handelsman, Mitchell M. Client preferences for informed consent information. *Ethics and Behavior*. 1997; 7(4): 311–328.
(INFORMED CONSENT)

Bradby, Hannah; Gabe, Jonathan; Bury, Michael. 'Sexy docs' and 'busty blondes': press coverage of professional misconduct cases brought before the General Medical Council. *Sociology of Health and Illness*. 1995 Sep; 17(4): 458–476.
(FRAUD AND MISCONDUCT; PROFESSIONAL PATIENT RELATIONSHIP)

Bradley, Don see Parsons, Evelyn

Bradley, Elizabeth; Walker, Leslie; Blechner, Barbara; Wetle, Terrie. Assessing capacity to participate in discussions of advance directives in nursing homes: findings from a study of the Patient Self-Determination Act. *Journal of the American Geriatrics Society*. 1997 Jan; 45(1): 79–83.
(ADVANCE DIRECTIVES; PATIENT CARE/AGED)

Bradley, Peter; Przygoda, Pablo; Saimovici, Javier; Pollán, Javier; Figar, Silvana; Raithatha, Nick. Physician assisted suicide, euthanasia, and withdrawal of treatment. [Letters]. *BMJ (British Medical Journal)*. 1998 Jan 3; 316(7124): 71–72.
(ALLOWING TO DIE; EUTHANASIA; SUICIDE)

Bradley, Peter M.; Shenkin, Henry A.; Rivlin, Michael M.; Hobson, Sarah; Ryan, Christopher James; Burns-Cox, C.J. The ethics industry. [Letters]. *Lancet*. 1997 Nov 22; 350(9090): 1547–1549.
(BIOETHICS; ETHICISTS AND ETHICS COMMITTEES)

Brahams, Diana. Designating parents in surrogate pregnancies. *Lancet*. 1998 Jan 3; 351(9095): 8.
(SURROGATE MOTHERS)

Brahams, Diana. My kidney as property. [Commentary]. *Lancet*. 1998 Jul 18; 352(9123): 166.
(ORGAN AND TISSUE DONATION)

Brahams, Diana. UK gynaecologist found guilty of serious professional misconduct. [News]. *Lancet*. 1997 Oct 4; 350(9083): 1014.
(FRAUD AND MISCONDUCT; INFORMED CONSENT)

Brahams, Diana. UK judge approves death free from mental pain. [News]. *Lancet*. 1997 Nov 8; 350(9088): 1376.
(TERMINAL CARE)

Brakel, Samuel Jan. Considering behavioral and biomedical research on detainees in the mental health unit of an urban mega-jail. *New England Journal on Criminal and Civil Confinement*. 1996 Winter; 22(1): 1–27.
(HUMAN EXPERIMENTATION/SPECIAL POPULATIONS)

Bram, Anthony D. The physically ill or dying psychotherapist: a review of ethical and clinical considerations. *Psychotherapy*. 1995 Winter; 32(4): 568–580.
(HEALTH; PROFESSIONAL ETHICS; PROFESSIONAL PATIENT RELATIONSHIP)

Bramblett, Michael T. see DeGroot, Leslie J.

Brandon, Bernadette see Balentine, Jerry

Brandt, Allan M.; Rozin, Paul. Morality and Health. New York, NY: Routledge; 1997. 416 p.
(HEALTH; PUBLIC HEALTH)

Brandt, C.P. see Piotrowski, Joseph J.

Brandt-Rauf, Paul W.; Brandt-Rauf, Sherry I. Biomarkers -- scientific advances and societal implications. *In:* Rothstein, Mark A., ed. Genetic Secrets: Protecting Privacy and Confidentiality in the Genetic Era. New Haven, CT: Yale University Press; 1997: 184–196.
(GENETIC RESEARCH; GENETIC SCREENING; OCCUPATIONAL HEALTH)

Brandt-Rauf, Sherry I. see Brandt-Rauf, Paul W.

Brannigan, Michael. On asking the right questions: personal death vs. brain death in Japan. *Death Studies*. 1998 Mar–Apr; 22(2): 157–169.
(DETERMINATION OF DEATH/BRAIN DEATH)

Brantigan, Charles O. see DeGroot, Leslie J.

Braslow, Judith B. see **Smith, Karen L.**

Braun, Barbara see **Elliott, Thomas E.**

Braun, Kathryn L.; Nichols, Rhea. Death and dying in four Asian American cultures: a descriptive study. *Death Studies*. 1997 Jul–Aug; 21(4): 327–359.
(TERMINAL CARE)

Braunholtz, David see **Edwards, S.J.L.**

Brawn, W.J.; De Giovanni, J.V.; Hutchinson, S.; Sethia, B.; Silove, E.D.; Stumper, O.; Wright, J.G.C.; Simpson, John; Sharland, Gurleen; Anderson, David; Murdoch, Ian; Tynan, Michael; Thwaites, Richard. Hypoplastic left heart syndrome. [Letters]. *BMJ (British Medical Journal)*. 1997 May 10; 314(7091): 1414.
(ALLOWING TO DIE/INFANTS; PATIENT CARE/MINORS)

Brazier, Margaret. Hard cases make bad law? [Editorial]. *Journal of Medical Ethics*. 1997 Dec; 23(6): 341–343.
(ARTIFICIAL INSEMINATION; FETUSES; SURROGATE MOTHERS; TREATMENT REFUSAL)

Brazier, Margaret; Harris, John. Public health and private lives. *Medical Law Review*. 1996 Summer; 4(2): 171–192.
(PUBLIC HEALTH)

Brazier, Margaret see **David, T.J.**

Brazier, Margaret see **Prayle, David**

Brecher, Bob. What would a socialist health service look like? *Health Care Analysis*. 1997 Sep; 5(3): 217–225.
(HEALTH CARE/ECONOMICS; HEALTH CARE/FOREIGN COUNTRIES)

Breitbart, William see **Chochinov, Harvey Max**

Breitowitz, Yitzchok A. Halakhic approaches to the resolution of disputes concerning the disposition of preembryos. *In:* Feldman, Emanuel; Wolowelsky, Joel B., eds. Jewish Law and the New Reproductive Technologies. Hoboken, NJ: Ktav; 1997: 155–186.
(FETUSES; IN VITRO FERTILIZATION)

Bremnes, R.M.; Andersen, K.; Wist, E.A. Cancer patients, doctors and nurses vary in their willingness to undertake cancer chemotherapy. *European Journal of Cancer*. 1995 Nov; 31A(12): 1955–1959.
(PATIENT CARE/DRUGS; TREATMENT REFUSAL)

Brent, Nancy J. see **Duffy, Barbara**

Brescia, Frank see **Portenoy, Russell K.**

Brestrup, Craig. Experimenting on animals. *In: his* Disposable Animals: Ending the Tragedy of Throwaway Pets. Leander, TX: Camino Bay Books; 1997: 115–128.
(ANIMAL EXPERIMENTATION)

Brett, Allan S.; Raymond, James I.; Saunders, Donald E.; Khushf, George. An ethics discussion series for hospital administrators. *HEC (HealthCare Ethics Committee) Forum*. 1998 Jun; 10(2): 177–185.
(HEALTH CARE; PROFESSIONAL ETHICS)

Brettell, Caroline B. see **Sargent, Carolyn F.**

Breyer, Stephen. The interdependence of science and law. *Science*. 1998 Apr 24; 280(5363): 537–538.
(BIOMEDICAL RESEARCH)

Briggs, J.D.; Crombie, A.; Fabre, J.; Major, E.; Thorogood, J.; Veitch, P.S. Organ donation in the UK: a survey by a British Transplantation Society working party. *Nephrology, Dialysis, Transplantation*. 1997 Nov; 12(11): 2251–2257.
(ORGAN AND TISSUE DONATION)

Brinsden, P.R. see **English, V.**

British Medical Association see **Sommerville, Ann**

Britton, Alison. Hippocrates: dead or alive? *In:* Petersen, Kerry, ed. Intersections: Women on Law, Medicine and Technology. Brookfield, VT: Ashgate; 1997: 1–23.
(MEDICAL ETHICS/CODES OF ETHICS)

Broaddus, Barbara see **Thies, Winthrop Drake**

Broadhead, Caren L. see **Balls, Michael**

Broadley, K. see **Johnston, S.R.D.**

Broberg, Gunnar; Roll-Hansen, Nils, eds. Eugenics and the Welfare State: Sterilization Policy in Denmark, Sweden, Norway, and Finland. East Lansing, MI: Michigan State University Press; 1996. 294 p.
(EUGENICS; STERILIZATION)

Brock, Dan W. An ethical framework for surrogate decision–making. *In:* Grubb, Andrew, ed. Decision–Making and Problems of Incompetence. New York, NY: Wiley; 1994: 41–52.
(ALLOWING TO DIE; INFORMED CONSENT)

Brock, Dan W. Informed consent. *In:* Borchert, Donald M., ed. The Encyclopedia of Philosophy. Supplement. New York, NY: Simon and Schuster Macmillan; 1996: 261–262.
(INFORMED CONSENT)

Brock, Dan W. see **Quill, Timothy E.**

Brockett, Patrick L.; Tankersley, E. Susan. The genetics revolution, economics, ethics, and insurance. *Journal of Business Ethics*. 1997 Nov; 16(15): 1661–1676.
(GENETIC SCREENING; GENOME MAPPING)

Brocklehurst, J.; Dickinson, E. Cause for concern: autonomy for elderly people in long–term care. *Age and Ageing*. 1996 Jul; 25(4): 329–332.
(PATIENT CARE/AGED)

Brockman, Bea see **Humphreys, Martin**

Brodaty, Henry; Alzheimer's Disease International. Medical and Scientific Advisory Committee. Consensus statement on predictive testing for Alzheimer disease. *Alzheimer Disease and Associated Disorders*. 1995 Winter; 9(4): 182–187.
(GENETIC SCREENING)

Brodell, Robert T. Ethics and micromanaged care. *Archives of Dermatology*. 1996 Sep; 132(9): 1013–1015.
(HEALTH CARE/ECONOMICS; PATIENT CARE/DRUGS)

Brodeur, Dennis. Health care institutional ethics: broader

than clinical ethics. [Revised]. *In:* Monagle, John F.; Thomasma, David C., eds. Health Care Ethics: Critical Issues for the 21st Century. Gaithersburg, MD: Aspen Publishers; 1998: 497–504.
(PROFESSIONAL ETHICS)

Brodeur, Dennis. Redefining long–term care, personal choices and "futile care." *Journal of Long–Term Care Administration.* 1993 Fall; 21(3): 78–80.
(HEALTH CARE)

Brodsky, Archie see **Bursztajn, Harold**

Brody, Baruch. Medical futility: philosophical reflections on death. *In:* Hoshino, Kazumasa, ed. Japanese and Western Bioethics: Studies in Moral Diversity. Boston, MA: Kluwer Academic; 1997: 135–144.
(ALLOWING TO DIE/ATTITUDES)

Brody, Baruch. Whatever happened to research ethics? *In:* Carson, Ronald A.; Burns, Chester R., eds. Philosophy of Medicine and Bioethics: A Twenty–Year Retrospective and Critical Appraisal. Boston, MA: Kluwer Academic; 1997: 275–286.
(ETHICISTS AND ETHICS COMMITTEES; HUMAN EXPERIMENTATION/REGULATION; HUMAN EXPERIMENTATION/RESEARCH DESIGN)

Brody, Baruch A., comp. Appendixes: international research ethics policies; European transnational research ethics policies; U.S. research ethics policies; research ethics policies from other countries. *In: his* The Ethics of Biomedical Research: An International Perspective. New York, NY: Oxford University Press; 1998: 213–358.
(ANIMAL EXPERIMENTATION; BIOMEDICAL RESEARCH; HUMAN EXPERIMENTATION)

Brody, Baruch A. Clinical trials. *In: his* The Ethics of Biomedical Research: An International Perspective. New York, NY: Oxford University Press; 1998: 139–160, 372–373.
(HUMAN EXPERIMENTATION/RESEARCH DESIGN)

Brody, Baruch A. Epidemiological research. *In: his* The Ethics of Biomedical Research: An International Perspective. New York, NY: Oxford University Press; 1998: 55–75, 364–366.
(BIOMEDICAL RESEARCH)

Brody, Baruch A. Genetic research. *In: his* The Ethics of Biomedical Research: An International Perspective. New York, NY: Oxford University Press; 1998: 77–97, 366–368.
(GENETIC RESEARCH)

Brody, Baruch A. Reproductive and fetal research. *In: his* The Ethics of Biomedical Research: An International Perspective. New York, NY: Oxford University Press; 1998: 99–118, 368–370.
(EMBRYO AND FETAL RESEARCH)

Brody, Baruch A. Research and the drug/device approval process. *In: his* The Ethics of Biomedical Research: An International Perspective. New York, NY: Oxford University Press; 1998: 161–183, 373–375.
(HUMAN EXPERIMENTATION/REGULATION)

Brody, Baruch A. Research ethics: international perspectives. *Cambridge Quarterly of Healthcare Ethics.* 1997 Fall; 6(4): 376–384.
(ANIMAL EXPERIMENTATION; EMBRYO AND FETAL RESEARCH; HUMAN EXPERIMENTATION/FOREIGN

COUNTRIES)

Brody, Baruch A. Research involving vulnerable subjects. *In: his* The Ethics of Biomedical Research: An International Perspective. New York, NY: Oxford University Press; 1998: 119–138, 370–372.
(HUMAN EXPERIMENTATION/SPECIAL POPULATIONS)

Brody, Baruch A. Research involving women and members of minority groups. *In: his* The Ethics of Biomedical Research: An International Perspective. New York, NY: Oxford University Press; 1998: 185–196, 375–376.
(HUMAN EXPERIMENTATION/SPECIAL POPULATIONS)

Brody, Baruch A. Research on human subjects. *In: his* The Ethics of Biomedical Research: An International Perspective. New York, NY: Oxford University Press; 1998: 31–54, 363–364.
(HUMAN EXPERIMENTATION)

Brody, Baruch A. Research on the vulnerable sick. *In:* Kahn, Jeffrey P.; Mastroianni, Anna C.; Sugarman, Jeremy, eds. Beyond Consent: Seeking Justice in Research. New York, NY: Oxford University Press; 1998: 32–46.
(AIDS/HUMAN EXPERIMENTATION; HUMAN EXPERIMENTATION/INFORMED CONSENT)

Brody, Baruch A. The Ethics of Biomedical Research: An International Perspective. New York, NY: Oxford University Press; 1998. 386 p.
(BIOMEDICAL RESEARCH; HUMAN EXPERIMENTATION)

Brody, Baruch A. The use of animals in research. *In: his* The Ethics of Biomedical Research: An International Perspective. New York, NY: Oxford University Press; 1998: 11–30, 361–362.
(ANIMAL EXPERIMENTATION)

Brody, Baruch A. see **McCullough, Laurence B.**

Brody, Baruch A. see **Sachdeva, Ramesh C.**

Brody, Howard. Autonomy revisited: progress in medical ethics: discussion paper. *Journal of the Royal Society of Medicine.* 1985 May; 78(5): 380–387.
(PROFESSIONAL PATIENT RELATIONSHIP)

Brody, Howard. Bringing clarity to the futility debate: don't use the wrong cases. *Cambridge Quarterly of Healthcare Ethics.* 1998 Summer; 7(3): 269–273.
(ALLOWING TO DIE)

Brody, Howard. Commentary on Billings and Block's "Slow euthanasia." *Journal of Palliative Care.* 1996 Winter; 12(4): 38–41.
(EUTHANASIA/LEGAL ASPECTS; SUICIDE; TERMINAL CARE)

Brody, Howard. Is there a treatment for cynicism? Expanding moral conversation from health care to the public sphere. *Medical Humanities Review.* 1996 Fall; 10(2): 9–19.
(HEALTH CARE)

Brody, Howard. Medical futility: a useful concept? *In:* Zucker, Marjorie B.; Zucker, Howard D., eds. Medical Futility and the Evaluation of Life–Sustaining Interventions. New York, NY: Cambridge University Press; 1997: 1–14.
(ALLOWING TO DIE)

Brody, Howard. Who gets to tell the story? Narrative in postmodern bioethics. *In:* Nelson, Hilde Lindemann, ed. Stories and Their Limits: Narrative Approaches to Bioethics. New York, NY: Routledge; 1997: 18–30.
(BIOETHICS)

Brody, Howard; Bonham, Vence L. Gag rules and trade secrets in managed care contracts: ethical and legal concerns. *Archives of Internal Medicine.* 1997 Oct 13; 157(18): 2037–2043.
(HEALTH CARE/ECONOMICS)

Brody, Howard; Vandekieft, Gregg K. Physician–assisted suicide: a very personal issue. [Editorial]. *American Family Physician.* 1997 May 15; 55(7): 2421–2427.
(SUICIDE; TERMINAL CARE)

Brody, Howard see **Supanich, Barbara**

Brody, Janet L.; Gluck, John P.; Aragon, Alfredo S. Participants' understanding of the process of psychological research: informed consent. *Ethics and Behavior.* 1997; 7(4): 285–298.
(BEHAVIORAL RESEARCH/INFORMED CONSENT)

Brody, Robert V. see **Heilig, Steve**

Brook, C.G.D. Growth hormone: panacea or punishment for short stature? [Editorial]. *BMJ (British Medical Journal).* 1997 Sep 20; 315(7110): 692–693.
(PATIENT CARE/DRUGS; PATIENT CARE/MINORS)

Brooke, Deborah see **Dale, Ruth**

Brooks, Chandler McC. A consideration of the ethics of brain death. *Sangyo Ika Daigaku Zasshi/Journal of University of Occupational and Environmental Health.* 1985 Jun 1; 7(2): 139–150.
(DETERMINATION OF DEATH/BRAIN DEATH)

Brooks, Timothy Paul. State v. Forrest: mercy killing and malice in North Carolina. [Note]. *North Carolina Law Review.* 1988 Sep; 66(6): 1160–1176.
(EUTHANASIA/LEGAL ASPECTS)

Brophy, Patricia. Death with dignity. [Personal narrative]. *In:* Zucker, Marjorie B.; Zucker, Howard D., eds. Medical Futility and the Evaluation of Life–Sustaining Interventions. New York, NY: Cambridge University Press; 1997: 15–23.
(ALLOWING TO DIE)

Brown, Barry. Reconciling property law with advances in reproductive science. *Stanford Law and Policy Review.* 1995; 6(2): 73–88.
(FETUSES; GENETIC INTERVENTION; REPRODUCTIVE TECHNOLOGIES)

Brown, Douglas see **Elkins, Thomas E.**

Brown, Iona Jane; Gannon, Philippa. Confidentiality and the Human Genome Project: a prophecy for conflict. *In:* McLean, Sheila A.M., ed. Contemporary Issues in Law, Medicine and Ethics. Brookfield, VT: Dartmouth; 1996: 215–236.
(CONFIDENTIALITY/LEGAL ASPECTS; GENETIC SCREENING)

Brown, J.M. Conscience: the professional and the personal. *Journal of Nursing Management.* 1996 May;

4(3): 171–177.
(NURSING ETHICS)

Brown, Julia see **Mason, Su**

Brown, Julie B. see **Gallagher, Eugene B.**

Brown, K.W. see **Clafferty, R.A.**

Brown, Lawrence D. Health reform in America: the mystery of the missing moral momentum. *Cambridge Quarterly of Healthcare Ethics.* 1998 Summer; 7(3): 239–246.
(HEALTH CARE/ECONOMICS)

Brown, Lee K. see **Heffner, John E.**

Brown, Phyllida. Pig transplants 'should be banned.' [News]. *New Scientist.* 1997 Mar 1; 153(2071): 6.
(ORGAN AND TISSUE TRANSPLANTATION)

Broyde, Michael J. Cloning people and Jewish law: a preliminary analysis. *Journal of Halacha and Contemporary Society.* 1997 Fall; No. 34: 27–65.
(CLONING)

Bruce, Donald M. A view from Edinburgh. *In:* Cole–Turner, Ronald, ed. Human Cloning: Religious Responses. Louisville, KY: Westminister John Knox Press; 1997: 1–11.
(CLONING)

Bruce, Donald M. Patenting human genes –– a Christian view. *Bulletin of Medical Ethics.* 1997 Jan; No. 124: 18–20.
(PATENTING LIFE FORMS)

Bruder, Paul. Right to die –– duty to die: the growing debate over scarce resources. *Hospital Topics.* 1994 Winter; 72(1): 6–8.
(SUICIDE)

Bruera, Eduardo see **Suarez–Almazor, Maria E.**

Brunner, E.J.; Sheppard, J.; Ravetz, J. Public is concerned about gene testing. [Letter]. *BMJ (British Medical Journal).* 1997 May 24; 314(7093): 1552–1553.
(GENETIC RESEARCH; GENETIC SCREENING)

Brushwood, David B. see **Allen, William L.**

Brushwood, David B. see **Vivian, Jesse C.**

Buchanan, Allen E. The limits of proxy decisionmaking for incompetents. *UCLA Law Review.* 1981; 29(2): 386–408.
(ALLOWING TO DIE/LEGAL ASPECTS)

Buchanan, James P. Future–perfect? Biotechnology and the ethics of the unknown: an afterword. *In:* Becker, Gerhold K., ed. Changing Nature's Course: The Ethical Challenge of Biotechnology. Hong Kong: Hong Kong University Press; 1996: 185–201.
(GENETIC INTERVENTION)

Büchele, Gisela see **Schüppel, Reinhart**

Buck, Gene. An open letter to Dr. Seed. [Satire]. *JAMA.* 1998 Apr 1; 279(10): 977.
(CLONING)

Bucur, Maria. Disciplining the Future: Eugenics and Modernization in Interwar Romania. Ann Arbor, MI: University Microfilms International; 1996. 315 p.
(EUGENICS)

Budetti, Peter P. see **Shortell, Stephen M.**

Budowle, Bruce see **Murch, Randall S.**

Budziszewski, J. Why we kill the weak. *Human Life Review.* 1997 Fall; 23(4): 67–74.
(ABORTION; ALLOWING TO DIE; EUTHANASIA)

Buerki, Robert A. History and human values in ethics instruction. *In:* Haddad, Amy Marie, ed. Teaching and Learning Strategies in Pharmacy Ethics. Second Edition. New York, NY: Pharmaceutical Products Press; 1997: 65–75.
(PROFESSIONAL ETHICS/EDUCATION)

Buetow, Stephen; Cantrill, Judith; Sibbald, Bonnie. Risk communication in the patient–health professional relationship. *Health Care Analysis.* 1998 Sep; 6(3): 261–268.
(INFORMED CONSENT)

Bugeja, G.; Kumar, A.; Banerjee, Arup K. Exclusion of elderly people from clinical research: a descriptive study of published reports. *BMJ (British Medical Journal).* 1997 Oct 25; 315(7115): 1059.
(HUMAN EXPERIMENTATION/SPECIAL POPULATIONS)

Buick, R.G. see **Dalton, John D.**

Bulfield, Grahame see **Klotzko, Arlene Judith**

Bulford, Rachel. Children have rights too. [Personal view]. *BMJ (British Medical Journal).* 1997 May 10; 314(7091): 1421–1422.
(PATIENT CARE/MINORS)

Bulger, Ruth Ellen see **Heitman, Elizabeth**

Bunce, Christina. Doctors involved in human rights' abuses in Kenya. [News]. *BMJ (British Medical Journal).* 1997 Jan 18; 314(7075): 166.
(FRAUD AND MISCONDUCT; TORTURE)

Burack, Jeffrey H. Response to "Further exploration of the relationship between medical education and moral development" by Donnie J. Self, DeWitt C. Baldwin, Jr., and Frederic D. Wolinsky: Deriving "ought" from "*p*": methodological and theoretical pitfalls in quantitative ethics. *Cambridge Quarterly of Healthcare Ethics.* 1997 Spring; 6(2): 226–232.
(MEDICAL ETHICS/EDUCATION)

Burch, Rex L. The progress of humane experimental technique since 1959: a personal view. *ATLA: Alternatives to Laboratory Animals.* 1995 Nov–Dec; 23(6): 776–783.
(ANIMAL EXPERIMENTATION)

Burch, Rex L. see **Balls, Michael**

Burd, Larry; Gregory, Jennifer M.; Kerbeshian, Jacob. The brain–mind quiddity: ethical issues in the use of human brain tissue for therapeutic and scientific purposes. *Journal of Medical Ethics.* 1998 Apr; 24(2): 118–122.
(BIOMEDICAL RESEARCH; ORGAN AND TISSUE DONATION; ORGAN AND TISSUE TRANSPLANTATION; PERSONHOOD)

Burdick, James F.; Turcotte, Jeremiah G.; Veatch, Robert M. Principles of organ and tissue allocation and donation by living donors. [Foreword]. *Transplantation Proceedings.* 1992 Oct; 24(5): 2226.
(ETHICISTS AND ETHICS COMMITTEES; ORGAN AND TISSUE DONATION; ORGAN AND TISSUE TRANSPLANTATION)

Burge, Frederick see **Parkash, Ravi**

Burgert, Tania see **Eng, Christine M.**

Burgert, Woodward see **Billick, Stephen B.**

Burgess, M.M.; Hayden, M.R. Patients' rights to laboratory data: trinucleotide repeat length in Huntington disease. [Editorial]. *American Journal of Medical Genetics.* 1996 Mar 1; 62(1): 6–9.
(GENETIC COUNSELING; TRUTH DISCLOSURE)

Burgio, Giuseppe Roberto; Nespoli, Luigi; Porta, Fulvio; Locatelli, Franco. Programmed bone–marrow donor for a leukaemic sibling, 10 years on. [Letter]. *Lancet.* 1997 May 17; 349(9063): 1482.
(ORGAN AND TISSUE DONATION; REPRODUCTION)

Burgoyne, Carole B. Distributive justice and rationing in the NHS: framing effects in press coverage of a controversial decision. *Journal of Community and Applied Social Psychology.* 1997 Apr; 7(2): 119–136.
(HEALTH CARE/ECONOMICS; HEALTH CARE/FOREIGN COUNTRIES; RESOURCE ALLOCATION)

Burke, James; Steel, R. Knight; Lynn, Joanne; Sulmasy, Daniel P. Contempo 1997: end–of–life care. [Letters and response]. *JAMA.* 1997 Oct 8; 278(14): 1150–1151.
(TERMINAL CARE/HOSPICES)

Burleigh, Michael. Ethics and Extermination: Reflections on Nazi Genocide. New York, NY: Cambridge University Press; 1997. 261 p.
(EUGENICS; EUTHANASIA; FRAUD AND MISCONDUCT)

Burleigh, Michael. Psychiatry, German society, and the Nazi "euthanasia" programme. *Social History of Medicine.* 1994 Aug; 7(2): 213–228.
(EUGENICS; EUTHANASIA)

Burleigh, Michael. Saving money, spending lives: psychiatry, society and the 'euthanasia' programme. *In:* Burleigh, Michael, ed. Confronting the Nazi Past: New Debates on Modern German History. New York, NY: St. Martin's Press; 1996: 98–111.
(EUGENICS; EUTHANASIA; FRAUD AND MISCONDUCT)

Burley, Neil M.J. see **Meystre, Chantal J.N.**

Burns, Barbara J. see **Swartz, Marvin S.**

Burns, Chester R. see **Carson, Ronald A.**

Burns–Cox, C.J. see **Bradley, Peter M.**

Burr, Chandler. The AIDS exception: privacy vs. public health. *Atlantic Monthly.* 1997 June; 279(6): 57–67.
(AIDS/CONFIDENTIALITY; PUBLIC HEALTH)

Burris, Scott. Driving the epidemic underground? A new look at law and the social risk of HIV testing. *AIDS and Public Policy Journal.* 1997 Summer; 12(2): 66–78.

Perone, Anne M.; Evers, Joseph C.; Traynor, Richard J. Quinlan re-examined. *Linacre Quarterly*. 1997 May; 64(2): 58–65.
(ALLOWING TO DIE)

Byrnes, Timothy A. see Segers, Mary C.

C

Caddick, Jeremy see Ashcroft, Richard

Cadieux, Mary Martin see Jones, Howard

Cahill, Lisa Sowle. The status of the embryo and policy discourse. *Journal of Medicine and Philosophy*. 1997 Oct; 22(5): 407–414.
(EMBRYO AND FETAL RESEARCH)

Cain, Kevin C. see Pearlman, Robert A.

Cain, Kimberly A. see Crenshaw, Wesley B.

Cain, Paul. The limits of confidentiality. *Nursing Ethics*. 1998 Mar; 5(2): 158–165.
(CONFIDENTIALITY)

Cain, Paul. Using clients. *Nursing Ethics*. 1997 Nov; 4(6): 465–471.
(INFORMED CONSENT; NURSING ETHICS/EDUCATION)

Cain, Paul see Wainwright, Paul

Cakalaroski, Koco see Ivanovski, Ninoslav

Calhoun, Byron C.; Reitman, James S.; Hoeldtke, Nathan J. Perinatal hospice: a response to partial birth abortion for infants with congenital defects. *Issues in Law and Medicine*. 1997 Fall; 13(2): 125–143.
(ABORTION; PATIENT CARE/MINORS; TERMINAL CARE)

Califf, Robert see Phillips, Russell S.

California. Human cloning. *California Health and Safety Code (West)*. 1997 Oct 4 (date enacted). Sects. 24185, 24187, 24189. 2 p.
(CLONING)

California. Berkeley. Hazardous biological research. *Berkeley Municipal Code*. 1977 Oct 21 (date effective). 12.30.010 to 12.30.0100.
(RECOMBINANT DNA RESEARCH/REGULATION)

California. Court of Appeal, Second District, Division 7. Hecht v. Superior Court (Kane). *California Reporter, 2d Series*. 1996 Nov 13 (date of decision; modified Nov 19). 59: 222–229.
(ARTIFICIAL INSEMINATION)

Callahan, Daniel. Cloning: the work not done. *Hastings Center Report*. 1997 Sep–Oct; 27(5): 18–20.
(BIOMEDICAL RESEARCH; CLONING)

Callahan, Daniel. Cloning: then and now. *Cambridge Quarterly of Healthcare Ethics*. 1998 Spring; 7(2): 141–144.
(BIOETHICS; CLONING)

Callahan, Daniel. Communitarian bioethics: a pious hope? *Responsive Community*. 1996 Fall; 6(4): 26–33.
(BIOETHICS)

Callahan, Daniel. False Hopes: Why America's Quest for Perfect Health Is a Recipe for Failure. New York, NY: Simon and Schuster; 1998. 330 p.
(HEALTH CARE)

Callahan, Daniel. International perspectives. *Hastings Center Report*. 1998 Jan–Feb; 28(1): 45–46.
(BIOETHICS)

Callahan, Daniel. Managed care and the goals of medicine. *Journal of the American Geriatrics Society*. 1998 Mar; 46(3): 385–388.
(HEALTH CARE/ECONOMICS)

Callahan, Daniel see Churchill, Larry R.

Callahan, Joan C. Birth control ethics. *In:* Chadwick, Ruth, ed. Encyclopedia of Applied Ethics, Volume 1. San Diego, CA: Academic Press; 1998: 335–351.
(ABORTION; CONTRACEPTION; POPULATION CONTROL; REPRODUCTION)

Callahan, Sidney. Gays, lesbians, and the use of alternate reproductive technologies. *In:* Nelson, Hilde Lindemann, ed. Feminism and Families. New York, NY: Routledge; 1997: 188–202.
(REPRODUCTIVE TECHNOLOGIES; SELECTION FOR TREATMENT)

Callahan, Sydney. A feminist case against euthanasia. *Health Progress*. 1996 Nov–Dec; 77(6): 21–27, 29.
(EUTHANASIA; SUICIDE)

Calman, Kenneth C. Equity, poverty and health for all. *BMJ (British Medical Journal)*. 1997 Apr 19; 314(7088): 1187–1191.
(HEALTH; HEALTH CARE/ECONOMICS; RESOURCE ALLOCATION)

Calne, Roy. Ethics in organ donation and transplantation: the position of the Transplantation Society (1996). *In:* Chapman, Jeremy R.; Deierhoi, Mark; Wight, Celia, eds. Organ and Tissue Donation for Transplantation. New York, NY: Oxford University Press; 1997: 62–66.
(ORGAN AND TISSUE DONATION)

Camargo, Carlos A. see Giugliano, Robert P.

Camenisch, P.F. The moral foundations of scientific ethics and responsibility. *Journal of Dental Research*. 1996 Feb; 75(2): 825–831.
(BIOMEDICAL RESEARCH; FRAUD AND MISCONDUCT; PROFESSIONAL ETHICS)

Cameron, Cheryl A. Mandatory consent to treatment by students in dental education: legal and policy considerations. *Journal of Dental Education*. 1995 Apr; 59(4): 495–501.
(INFORMED CONSENT)

Cameron, Stewart see Watler, Crosbie L.

Campbell, Alastair see Ashcroft, Richard

Campbell, Courtney S. Ecclesiology and ethics: an LDS response. *In:* Lustig, B. Andrew, ed.; Center for Medical Ethics and Health Policy (Houston, TX). Bioethics Yearbook, Volume 5: Theological Developments in Bioethics, 1992–1994. Boston, MA: Kluwer Academic; 1997: 33–53.
(BIOETHICS)

Campbell, Courtney S. Must patients suffer? *In:* Carson, Ronald A.; Burns, Chester R., eds. Philosophy of Medicine and Bioethics: A Twenty–Year Retrospective and Critical Appraisal. Boston, MA: Kluwer Academic; 1997: 247–263.
(PATIENT CARE)

Campbell, Courtney S. Prophecy and policy. *Hastings Center Report.* 1997 Sep–Oct; 27(5): 15–17.
(CLONING)

Campbell, Courtney S. The crumbling foundations of medical ethics: Rethinking Life and Death: The Collapse of Our Traditional Ethics, by Peter Singer; The Foundations of Bioethics, by H. Tristram Engelhardt; Deciding Together: Bioethics and Moral Consensus, by Jonathan D. Moreno. [Book review essay]. *Theoretical Medicine and Bioethics.* 1998 Apr; 19(2): 143–152.
(BIOETHICS)

Campbell, Donald D. see **Byrne, Paul A.**

Campbell, Duncan. Medicine needs its MI5. *BMJ (British Medical Journal).* 1997 Dec 20–27; 315(7123): 1677–1680.
(FRAUD AND MISCONDUCT; HUMAN EXPERIMENTATION; PATIENT CARE)

Campbell, Eric G.; Louis, Karen Seashore; Blumenthal, David. Looking a gift horse in the mouth: corporate gifts supporting life sciences research. *JAMA.* 1998 Apr 1; 279(13): 995–999.
(BIOMEDICAL RESEARCH)

Campbell, Jean. Reforming the IRB process: towards new guidelines for quality and accountability in protecting human subjects. *In:* Shamoo, Adil E., ed. Ethics in Neurobiological Research with Human Subjects: The Baltimore Conference on Ethics. Amsterdam: Gordon and Breach; 1997: 299–303.
(HUMAN EXPERIMENTATION/ETHICS COMMITTEES; HUMAN EXPERIMENTATION/SPECIAL POPULATIONS)

Campbell, Keith see **Klotzko, Arlene Judith**

Campbell, Stuart see **Simms, Madeleine**

Campion, Peter see **Chapple, Alison**

Canada. Alberta. Advance Directives Act. Bill 58, 23rd Legislature, 2d Sess. Introduced by Ms. Haley.; 1994. 16 p.
(ADVANCE DIRECTIVES)

Canada. British Columbia. Court of Appeal. Re K and Public Trustee. *Dominion Law Reports, 4th Series.* 1985 May 16 (date of decision). 19: 255–285.
(STERILIZATION/MENTALLY DISABLED)

Canada. House of Commons. Human Reproductive and Genetic Technologies Act (an act respecting human reproductive technologies and commercial transactions relating to human reproduction): bill C–47. Bill C–47, 35th Parliament, 2d Sess. Introduced by the Minister of Health; 1996 Jun 14. 7 p.
(REPRODUCTIVE TECHNOLOGIES)

Canada. Manitoba. Health Care Directives Act. 1993 Jul 26 (date of proclamation). *International Digest of Health Legislation.* 1995; 46(2): 195–196.
(ADVANCE DIRECTIVES)

Canada. Medical Research Council of Canada; Canada. Natural Sciences and Engineering Research Council of Canada; Canada. Social Sciences and Humanities Research Council of Canada. Integrity in Research and Scholarship: A Tri–Council Policy Statement. Ottawa, ON: Medical Research Council of Canada; 1994 Jan. 4 p.
(BIOMEDICAL RESEARCH; FRAUD AND MISCONDUCT)

Canada. Minister of Health. New Reproductive and Genetic Technologies: Setting Boundaries, Enhancing Health. Ottawa, ON: Minister of Supply and Services Canada; 1996 Jun. 48 p.
(GENETIC INTERVENTION; REPRODUCTIVE TECHNOLOGIES)

Canada. Natural Sciences and Engineering Research Council of Canada see **Canada. Medical Research Council of Canada**

Canada. Ontario. Court of Appeal. Re B. and Children's Aid Society of Metropolitan Toronto. *Dominion Law Reports, 4th Series.* 1992 Sep 15 (date of decision). 96: 45–85.
(TREATMENT REFUSAL/MINORS)

Canada. Royal Commission on New Reproductive Technologies. Update [on the work of the Royal Commission on New Reproductive Technologies –– includes letter from the chairperson and summary of the main topics in the final report, Proceed with Care]. Issued by the Commission, P.O. Box 1566, Station "B," Ottawa, ON, Canada K1P 5R5; 1993 Dec. 18 p.
(REPRODUCTIVE TECHNOLOGIES)

Canada. Social Sciences and Humanities Research Council of Canada see **Canada. Medical Research Council of Canada**

Canada. Supreme Court. McInerney v. MacDonald. *Dominion Law Reports, 4th Series.* 1992 Jun 11 (date of decision). 93: 415–431.
(PATIENT ACCESS TO RECORDS)

Canadian College of Medical Geneticists. China's eugenics law: position statement of the Canadian College of Medical Geneticists. *Journal of Medical Genetics.* 1997 Nov; 34(11): 960.
(EUGENICS)

Canadian College of Neuropsychopharmacology see **Young, Simon N.**

Canadian HIV/AIDS Legal Network and Canadian AIDS Society. Joint Project on Legal and Ethical Issues see **Elliott, Richard**

Canadian Medical Association. Code of ethics of the Canadian Medical Association. *International Journal of Bioethics.* 1997 Mar–Jun; 8(1–2): 123–125.
(MEDICAL ETHICS/CODES OF ETHICS)

Canadian Medical Association. Code of Ethics of the Canadian Medical Association (approved by General Council, August 1996). *Canadian Medical Association Journal.* 1996 Oct 15; 155(8): 1176A–1176B.
(MEDICAL ETHICS/CODES OF ETHICS)

Canadian Nurses Association. Code of ethics for registered nurses [1997]. *Nursing Ethics.* 1998 Jan; 5(1):

Carlson, John W. Interventions upon gametes in assisting the conjugal act toward fertilization. *In:* Wildes, Kevin Wm., ed. Infertility: A Crossroad of Faith, Medicine, and Technology. Boston, MA: Kluwer Academic; 1997: 107–124.
(REPRODUCTIVE TECHNOLOGIES)

Carlson, John W. On the justification and limits of medical research: a response to Kevin Wildes. *In:* Wildes, Kevin Wm.; Mitchell, Alan C., eds. Choosing Life: A Dialogue on *Evangelium Vitae.* Washington, DC: Georgetown University Press; 1997: 199–205.
(BIOMEDICAL RESEARCH; EMBRYO AND FETAL RESEARCH; GENETIC RESEARCH)

Carlyle, Ruth see **Savulescu, Julian**

Carnall, Douglas. Report urges widespread reform of handling of NHS data. [News]. *BMJ (British Medical Journal).* 1997 Dec 13; 315(7122): 1562.
(CONFIDENTIALITY)

Carpenter, C.B. see **Bach, F.H.**

Carpenter, William T. Schizophrenia research: a challenge for constructive criticism. *In:* Shamoo, Adil E., ed. Ethics in Neurobiological Research with Human Subjects: The Baltimore Conference on Ethics. Amsterdam: Gordon and Breach; 1997: 215–228.
(HUMAN EXPERIMENTATION/RESEARCH DESIGN; HUMAN EXPERIMENTATION/SPECIAL POPULATIONS)

Carpenter, William T.; Schooler, Nina R.; Kane, John M. The rationale and ethics of medication–free research in schizophrenia. *Archives of General Psychiatry.* 1997 May; 54(5): 401–407.
(HUMAN EXPERIMENTATION/RESEARCH DESIGN; HUMAN EXPERIMENTATION/SPECIAL POPULATIONS)

Carriere, K.C. see **Degner, Lesley F.**

Carse, Alisa L. Impartial principle and moral context: securing a place for the particular in ethical theory. *Journal of Medicine and Philosophy.* 1998 Apr; 23(2): 153–169.
(BIOETHICS)

Carson, Ronald A. Medical ethics as reflective practice. *In:* Carson, Ronald A.; Burns, Chester R., eds. Philosophy of Medicine and Bioethics: A Twenty–Year Retrospective and Critical Appraisal. Boston, MA: Kluwer Academic; 1997: 181–191.
(BIOETHICS)

Carson, Ronald A.; Burns, Chester R., eds. Philosophy of Medicine and Bioethics: A Twenty–Year Retrospective and Critical Appraisal. Boston, MA: Kluwer Academic; 1997. 341 p.
(BIOETHICS)

Carson, Sandra A. see **Simpson, Joe Leigh**

Cartwright, C.M. see **Steinberg, M.A.**

Cartwright, Colleen; Steinberg, Margaret; Williams, Ged; Najman, Jake; Williams, Gail. Issues of death and dying: the perspective of critical care nurses. *Australian Critical Care.* 1997 Sep; 10(3): 81–84, 86–87.
(TERMINAL CARE)

Cartwright, Will. The sterilisation of the mentally disabled:

competence, the right to reproduce and discrimination. *In:* Grubb, Andrew, ed. Decision–Making and Problems of Incompetence. New York, NY: Wiley; 1994: 67–88.
(REPRODUCTION; STERILIZATION/MENTALLY DISABLED)

Casabona, C. see **Hoffenberg, R.**

Casarett, David see **Hall, Spencer A.**

Casarett, David J.; Lantos, John D. Have we treated AIDS too well? Rationing and the future of AIDS exceptionalism. *Annals of Internal Medicine.* 1998 May 1; 128(9): 756–759.
(AIDS; RESOURCE ALLOCATION)

Casavilla, Adrian see **Marsh, J. Wallis**

Casciani, C.U. see **Elli, M.**

Cass, Alvah R. see **Volk, Robert J.**

Cassel, Christine see **Forrow, Lachlan**

Cassel, Christine K. Policy implications of the Human Genome Project for women. *Women's Health Issues.* 1997 Jul–Aug; 7(4): 225–229.
(GENETIC SERVICES; HEALTH; HEALTH CARE)

Cassel, Christine K. Research in nursing homes: ethical issues. *Journal of the American Geriatrics Society.* 1985 Nov; 33(11): 795–799.
(HUMAN EXPERIMENTATION/SPECIAL POPULATIONS)

Cassel, Christine K. see **Field, Marilyn J.**

Cassel, Christine K. see **Meier, Diane E.**

Cassel, Christine K. see **White, W.D.**

Cassell, Eric J. The future of the doctor–payer–patient relationship. *Journal of the American Geriatrics Society.* 1998 Mar; 46(3): 318–321.
(HEALTH CARE/ECONOMICS; PROFESSIONAL PATIENT RELATIONSHIP)

Cassell, Jackie. Against medical ethics: opening the can of worms. *Journal of Medical Ethics.* 1998 Feb; 24(1): 8–12.
(BIOETHICS; MEDICAL ETHICS)

Cassidy, Virginia R. Literary works as case studies for teaching human experimentation ethics. *Journal of Nursing Education.* 1996 Mar; 35(3): 142–144.
(HUMAN EXPERIMENTATION; NURSING ETHICS/EDUCATION)

Cassileth, Barrie R. see **Tulsky, James A.**

Castellani, Betty C. Medical ethics: prolonging life or protracting death? *Journal of the Medical Association of Georgia.* 1990 Nov; 79(11): 835–837.
(ALLOWING TO DIE)

Castledine, George. Whistleblowing guidelines for nursing colleagues. *British Journal of Nursing.* 1997 Jun 12–25; 6(11): 654.
(FRAUD AND MISCONDUCT)

Cateni, Cecilia see **Fineschi, Vittorio**

Catholic Health Association of the United States.

Caring for Persons at the End of Life: A Facilitator's Guide to Educational Modules for Healthcare Leaders. [Looseleaf format manual]. St. Louis, MO: Catholic Health Association of the United States; 1993. 1 v.
(TERMINAL CARE)

Cattan, A. see **Ashcroft, Richard**

Causino, Nancyanne see **Halm, Ethan A.**

Cavalli-Sforza, L. Luca. Human genome diversity: where is the project now? *In:* Knoppers, Bartha Maria, ed. Human DNA: Law and Policy: International and Comparative Perspectives. Proceedings of the First International Conference on DNA Sampling and Human Genetic Research: Ethical, Legal, and Policy Aspects, held in Montreal, Canada, 6-8 Sep 1996. Boston, MA: Kluwer Law International; 1997: 219-227.
(GENOME MAPPING)

Cavanagh, Denis. Legal abortion in America: factors in the dynamics of change. *Liberty, Life and Family.* 1996; 2(2): 309-317.
(ABORTION)

Cavender, Jim see **Domino, George**

Cebik, L.B.; Graber, Glenn C.; Marsh, Frank H., eds. Advances in Bioethics. Volume 1: Violence, Neglect, and the Elderly. Greenwich, CT: JAI Press; 1996. 240 p.
(PATIENT CARE/AGED)

Center for Medical Ethics and Health Policy (Houston, TX) see **Lustig, B. Andrew**

Chadwick, Ruth. Genetic screening. *In:* Chadwick, Ruth, ed. Encyclopedia of Applied Ethics, Volume 2. San Diego, CA: Academic Press; 1998: 445-449.
(GENETIC SCREENING; MASS SCREENING)

Chadwick, Ruth. Is nursing ethics distinct from medical ethics? *In:* Morscher, Edgar; Neumaier, Otto; Simons, Peter, eds. Applied Ethics in a Troubled World. Boston, MA: Kluwer Academic; 1998: 115-125.
(NURSING ETHICS)

Chadwick, Ruth. The status of human genetic material -- European approaches. *In:* Knoppers, Bartha Maria, ed. Human DNA: Law and Policy: International and Comparative Perspectives. Proceedings of the First International Conference on DNA Sampling and Human Genetic Research: Ethical, Legal, and Policy Aspects, held in Montreal, Canada, 6-8 Sep 1996. Boston, MA: Kluwer Law International; 1997: 55-62.
(GENETIC RESEARCH; GENETIC SCREENING)

Chadwick, Ruth; Schüklenk, Udo. Organ transplants and donors. *In:* Chadwick, Ruth, ed. Encyclopedia of Applied Ethics, Volume 3. San Diego, CA: Academic Press; 1998: 393-398.
(ORGAN AND TISSUE DONATION; ORGAN AND TISSUE TRANSPLANTATION)

Chafey, Kathleen. "Caring" is not enough: ethical paradigms for community-based care. *N and HC Perspectives on Community.* 1996 Jan-Feb; 17(1): 10-15.
(HEALTH CARE; NURSING ETHICS)

Chalmers, Iain see **Savulescu, Julian**

Chambers, Timothy. Questionable ethics -- whistle-blowing or tale-telling? *Journal of Medical Ethics.* 1997 Dec; 23(6): 382-383.
(FRAUD AND MISCONDUCT; HUMAN EXPERIMENTATION)

Chambers, Tod. Letting the patient backstage: informed consent for HMO enrollees. *Journal of the American Geriatrics Society.* 1998 Mar; 46(3): 355-358.
(HEALTH CARE/ECONOMICS; INFORMED CONSENT)

Chambers, Tod. What to expect from an ethics case (and what it expects from you). *In:* Nelson, Hilde Lindemann, ed. Stories and Their Limits: Narrative Approaches to Bioethics. New York, NY: Routledge; 1997: 171-184.
(BIOETHICS)

Chan, Arlene; Woodruff, Roger K. Communicating with patients with advanced cancer. *Journal of Palliative Care.* 1997 Autumn; 13(3): 29-33.
(PATIENT CARE; TRUTH DISCLOSURE)

Chan, Kevin W. Jaffee v. Redmond: making the courts a tool of injustice? *Journal of the American Academy of Psychiatry and the Law.* 1997; 25(3): 383-389.
(CONFIDENTIALITY/LEGAL ASPECTS; CONFIDENTIALITY/MENTAL HEALTH)

Chang, Cyril F. see **Mirvis, David M.**

Chang, Patricia L. see **Durfy, Sharon J.**

Chantler, Cyril; Chantler, Shireen. Dealing with research misconduct in the United Kingdom: deception: difficulties and initiatives. *BMJ (British Medical Journal).* 1998 Jun 6; 316(7146): 1731-1732.
(BIOMEDICAL RESEARCH; FRAUD AND MISCONDUCT)

Chantler, Shireen see **Chantler, Cyril**

Chapman, C. Richard see **Sullivan, Mark**

Chapple, Alison; May, Carl; Campion, Peter. Lay understanding of genetic disease: a British study of families attending a genetic counseling service. *Journal of Genetic Counseling.* 1995 Dec; 4(4): 281-300.
(GENETIC COUNSELING)

Charo, R. Alta. The interaction between family planning policies and the introduction of new reproductive technologies. *In:* Petersen, Kerry, ed. Intersections: Women on Law, Medicine and Technology. Brookfield, VT: Ashgate; 1997: 73-97.
(CONTRACEPTION; POPULATION CONTROL; REPRODUCTIVE TECHNOLOGIES)

Charo, R. Alta see **Andrews, Lori B.**

Charytan, Chaim see **Slifkin, Robert F.**

Chavkin, Wendy. Mandatory treatment for pregnant substance abusers: irrelevant and dangerous. *Politics and the Life Sciences.* 1996 Mar; 15(1): 53-54.
(INVOLUNTARY COMMITMENT; PRENATAL INJURIES)

Chelala, César. China's human-organ trade highlighted by US arrest of "salesman". [News]. *Lancet.* 1998 Mar 7; 351(9104): 735.
(ORGAN AND TISSUE DONATION)

Chelala, César. German dialysis firm quits Chinese interest. [News]. *Lancet.* 1998 Mar 14; 351(9105): 812.

(BIOMEDICAL TECHNOLOGIES; FRAUD AND MISCONDUCT; ORGAN AND TISSUE DONATION)

Chelala, César. Prospect of discussions on prisoners' organs for sale in China. [News]. *Lancet.* 1997 Nov 1; 350(9087): 1307.
(CAPITAL PUNISHMENT; ORGAN AND TISSUE DONATION)

Chen, Chih-Ping see **Jan, Sheau-Wen**

Chen, Yuan-Fang. Japanese death factories and the American cover-up. *Cambridge Quarterly of Healthcare Ethics.* 1997 Spring; 6(2): 240–242.
(FRAUD AND MISCONDUCT; HUMAN EXPERIMENTATION/FOREIGN COUNTRIES; HUMAN EXPERIMENTATION/SPECIAL POPULATIONS; WAR)

Cheng, Tsung O. see **O'Connor, Nancy K.**

Cher, Daniel J.; Lenert, Leslie A. Method of Medicare reimbursement and the rate of potentially ineffective care of critically ill patients. *JAMA.* 1997 Sep 24; 278(12): 1001–1007.
(BIOMEDICAL TECHNOLOGIES; HEALTH CARE/ECONOMICS; PATIENT CARE; TERMINAL CARE)

Cherniawsky, Kathy. Commercialization/patents. *In:* Knoppers, Bartha Maria, ed. Human DNA: Law and Policy: International and Comparative Perspectives. Proceedings of the First International Conference on DNA Sampling and Human Genetic Research: Ethical, Legal, and Policy Aspects, held in Montreal, Canada, 6–8 Sep 1996. Boston, MA: Kluwer Law International; 1997: 385–390.
(PATENTING LIFE FORMS)

Cherry, Christopher. Health care, human worth and the limits of the particular. *Journal of Medical Ethics.* 1997 Oct; 23(5): 310–314.
(HEALTH CARE; RESOURCE ALLOCATION)

Cherry, Mark J. Moral strangers: a humanity that does not bind. *In:* Hoshino, Kazumasa, ed. Japanese and Western Bioethics: Studies in Moral Diversity. Boston, MA: Kluwer Academic; 1997: 201–223.
(BIOETHICS)

Chervenak, F.A.; McCullough, L.B. Should sex identification be offered as part of the routine ultrasound examination? *Ultrasound in Obstetrics and Gynecology.* 1996 Nov; 8(5): 293–294.
(PRENATAL DIAGNOSIS; SEX DETERMINATION)

Chervenak, Frank A.; McCullough, Laurence B. Common ethical dilemmas encountered in the management of HIV-infected women and newborns. *Clinical Obstetrics and Gynecology.* 1996 Jun; 39(2): 411–419.
(AIDS)

Chervenak, Frank A.; McCullough, Laurence B. What is obstetric ethics? *Journal of Perinatal Medicine.* 1995; 23(5): 331–341.
(FETUSES; MEDICAL ETHICS; PATIENT CARE)

Chervenak, Frank A.; McCullough, Laurence B.; Kurjak, Asim. An essential clinical ethical concept. *In:* Chervenak, Frank A.; Kurjak, Asim, eds. Current Perspectives on the Fetus as a Patient. New York, NY: Parthenon Publishing Group; 1996: 1–9.
(FETUSES)

Chervenak, Frank A. see **Lescale, Keith B.**

Chervenak, Frank A. see **Simms, Madeleine**

Chervenak, Frank A. see **Skupski, Daniel W.**

Chesney, Margaret A. see **Cooke, Molly**

Children's Legal Rights Journal. Editorial Staff see **Garey, Christopher C.**

Childress, Craig A.; Asamen, Joy K. The emerging relationship of psychology and the Internet: proposed guidelines for conducting Internet intervention research. *Ethics and Behavior.* 1998; 8(1): 19–35.
(BEHAVIORAL RESEARCH)

Childress, James F. Conscience and conscientious actions in the context of MCOs. *Kennedy Institute of Ethics Journal.* 1997 Dec; 7(4): 403–411.
(HEALTH CARE/ECONOMICS)

Childress, James F. Narrative(s) versus norm(s): a misplaced debate in bioethics. *In:* Nelson, Hilde Lindemann, ed. Stories and Their Limits: Narrative Approaches to Bioethics. New York, NY: Routledge; 1997: 252–271.
(BIOETHICS)

Childress, James F. Religious viewpoints. *In:* Emanuel, Linda L., ed. Regulating How We Die: The Ethical, Medical, and Legal Issues Surrounding Physician-Assisted Suicide. Cambridge, MA: Harvard University Press; 1998: 120–147, 294–300.
(EUTHANASIA/RELIGIOUS ASPECTS; SUICIDE)

Childress, James F. The body as property: some philosophical reflections. *Transplantation Proceedings.* 1992 Oct; 24(5): 2143–2148.
(ORGAN AND TISSUE DONATION)

Childress, James F. The challenges of public ethics: reflections on NBAC's report. *Hastings Center Report.* 1997 Sep–Oct; 27(5): 9–11.
(CLONING; ETHICISTS AND ETHICS COMMITTEES)

Childs, Brian H. see **Ehleben, Carole M.**

Cho, Mildred. Disclosing conflicts of interest. [Letter]. *Lancet.* 1997 Jul 5; 350(9070): 72–73.
(BIOMEDICAL RESEARCH)

Cho, Mildred K.; Merz, Jon F. Patients and patents. [Letter]. *Nature.* 1997 Nov 20; 390(6657): 221.
(GENOME MAPPING)

Chochinov, Harvey Max; Wilson, Keith G. The euthanasia debate: attitudes, practices and psychiatric considerations. *Canadian Journal of Psychiatry.* 1995 Dec; 40(10): 593–602.
(EUTHANASIA/ATTITUDES; SUICIDE)

Chochinov, Harvey Max; Wilson, Keith G.; Breitbart, William; Rosenfeld, Barry D.; Passik, Steven D. Assisted suicide for HIV patients. [Letter and response]. *American Journal of Psychiatry.* 1997 Feb; 154(2): 294–295.
(AIDS; SUICIDE)

Chokevivat, Vichai see **Schüklenk, Udo**

Cholewinska, Anna see **Gallagher, Eugene B.**

Christakis, Nicolas A. The distinction between ethical pluralism and ethical relativism: implications for the conduct of transcultural clinical research. *In:* Vanderpool, Harold Y., ed. The Ethics of Research Involving Human Subjects: Facing the 21st Century. Frederick, MD: University Publishing Group; 1996: 261–280.
(HUMAN EXPERIMENTATION/FOREIGN COUNTRIES)

Christensen, Kate; Miles, Steven H. The ethical importance of differences between managed care systems. *HEC (HealthCare Ethics Committee) Forum.* 1997 Dec; 9(4): 313–322.
(HEALTH CARE/ECONOMICS)

Christo, G.G. see **Gitanjali, B.**

Chua, Grace see **Stelfox, Henry Thomas**

Church of England. Board for Social Responsibility. Abortion and the Church: What are the Issues? London: Church House Publishing; 1993 Jan. 31 p.
(ABORTION/FOREIGN COUNTRIES; ABORTION/LEGAL ASPECTS; ABORTION/RELIGIOUS ASPECTS)

Churchill, Larry R. Bioethics in social context. *In:* Carson, Ronald A.; Burns, Chester R., eds. Philosophy of Medicine and Bioethics: A Twenty-Year Retrospective and Critical Appraisal. Boston, MA: Kluwer Academic; 1997: 137–151.
(BIOETHICS)

Churchill, Larry R.; Callahan, Daniel; Linehan, Elizabeth A.; Thal, Anne E.; Graves, Frances A.; Prendergast, Alice V.; Flory, Donald G.; Hardwig, John. To die or not to die. [Letters and response]. *Hastings Center Report.* 1997 Nov–Dec; 27(6): 4–7.
(SUICIDE)

Churchill, Larry R.; King, Nancy M.P. Physician assisted suicide, euthanasia, or withdrawal of treatment. [Editorial]. *BMJ (British Medical Journal).* 1997 Jul 19; 315(7101): 137–138.
(EUTHANASIA/LEGAL ASPECTS; SUICIDE)

Ciarleglio, Leslie see **Saxton, Marsha**

Cicciarelli, J. see **Mendez, R.**

Clafferty, R.A.; Brown, K.W.; McCabe, E. Under half of psychiatrists tell patients their diagnosis of Alzheimer's disease. [Letter]. *BMJ (British Medical Journal).* 1998 Aug 29; 317(7158): 603.
(TRUTH DISCLOSURE)

Claiborne, William. In Oregon, suicide option brings a kinder care. [News]. *Washington Post.* 1998 Apr 29: A1, A12.
(SUICIDE; TERMINAL CARE)

Clancy, Carolyn M. see **Franks, Peter**

Clarity, James F. Irish girl, 13, to abort baby in England. [News]. *New York Times.* 1997 Dec 2: A7.
(ABORTION/FOREIGN COUNTRIES)

Clark, Doug see **Davis, Kenneth M.**

Clark, Jack see **Markson, Lawrence**

Clark, Liana R. Sex preselection: the advent of the made-to-order child. *Pharos.* 1985 Fall; 48(4): 2–7.
(SEX DETERMINATION; SEX PRESELECTION)

Clark, Peter A. The ethics of placebo-controlled trials for perinatal transmission of HIV in developing countries. *Journal of Clinical Ethics.* 1998 Summer; 9(2): 156–166.
(AIDS/HUMAN EXPERIMENTATION; HUMAN EXPERIMENTATION/FOREIGN COUNTRIES; HUMAN EXPERIMENTATION/RESEARCH DESIGN; HUMAN EXPERIMENTATION/SPECIAL POPULATIONS)

Clarke, Angus. Genetic counseling. *In:* Chadwick, Ruth, ed. Encyclopedia of Applied Ethics, Volume 2. San Diego, CA: Academic Press; 1998: 391–405.
(GENETIC COUNSELING)

Clarke, Angus see **Parsons, Evelyn**

Clarke, Angus see **Tyler, Audrey**

Clarke, Angus J. see **Harper, Peter S.**

Clarke, Joe T.R.; Ray, Peter N. Look-back: the duty to update genetic counselling. *In:* Knoppers, Bartha Maria, ed. Human DNA: Law and Policy: International and Comparative Perspectives. Proceedings of the First International Conference on DNA Sampling and Human Genetic Research: Ethical, Legal, and Policy Aspects, held in Montreal, Canada, 6–8 Sep 1996. Boston, MA: Kluwer Law International; 1997: 121–132.
(GENETIC COUNSELING; GENETIC SCREENING)

Clarke, Kenneth W.B. see **Shortell, Stephen M.**

Clarridge, Brian R. see **Emanuel, Ezekiel J.**

Classé, John G. see **Foster, George E.**

Clayden, Graham see **Ashcroft, Richard**

Clayton, Ellen Wright. Informed consent and genetic research. *In:* Rothstein, Mark A., ed. Genetic Secrets: Protecting Privacy and Confidentiality in the Genetic Era. New Haven, CT: Yale University Press; 1997: 126–136.
(GENETIC RESEARCH; HUMAN EXPERIMENTATION/INFORMED CONSENT)

Clayton, Ellen Wright. Prospective uses of DNA samples for research. *In:* Knoppers, Bartha Maria, ed. Human DNA: Law and Policy: International and Comparative Perspectives. Proceedings of the First International Conference on DNA Sampling and Human Genetic Research: Ethical, Legal, and Policy Aspects, held in Montreal, Canada, 6–8 Sep 1996. Boston, MA: Kluwer Law International; 1997: 291–301.
(GENETIC RESEARCH; HUMAN EXPERIMENTATION/INFORMED CONSENT)

Clayton, Ellen Wright. Screening and treatment of newborns. *Houston Law Review.* 1992 Spring; 29(1): 85–148.
(GENETIC SCREENING; MASS SCREENING)

Cleaton-Jones, Peter E.; Busse, Peter; Emery, Sean; Cooper, David A.; McLean, G.R.; King, Peter. Availability of antiretroviral therapy after clinical trials with HIV infected patients are ended: an ethical

dilemma. [Article and commentaries]. *BMJ (British Medical Journal)*. 1997 Mar 22; 314(7084): 887–891.
(AIDS/HUMAN EXPERIMENTATION; HUMAN EXPERIMENTATION/FOREIGN COUNTRIES; PATIENT CARE/DRUGS)

Cleave–Hogg, Doreen see **Tiberius, Richard G.**

Cleeland, Charles S. Undertreatment of cancer pain in elderly patients. [Editorial]. *JAMA*. 1998 Jun 17; 279(23): 1914–1915.
(PATIENT CARE/DRUGS)

Cleeland, Charles S.; Gonin, René; Baez, Luis; Loehrer, Patrick; Pandya, Kishan J. Pain and treatment of pain in minority patients with cancer: the Eastern Cooperative Oncology Group Minority Outpatient Pain Study. *Annals of Internal Medicine*. 1997 Nov 1; 127(9): 813–816.
(PATIENT CARE/DRUGS)

Clinical Genetics Society (Great Britain); Clinical Molecular Genetics Society (Great Britain); Association of Clinical Cytogenetics (Great Britain); et al. Patenting and clinical genetics. [Joint statement]. *Bulletin of Medical Ethics*. 1997 Jan; No. 124: 8.
(PATENTING LIFE FORMS)

Clinical Molecular Genetics Society (Great Britain) see **Clinical Genetics Society (Great Britain)**

Clinton, William J. Remarks by the president in apology for study done in Tuskegee. Washington, DC: The White House, Office of the Press Secretary, [Online]. Available: http://www1.whitehouse.gov/New/Remarks/Fri/199 70516-898.html; 1997 May 16. 3 p.
(FRAUD AND MISCONDUCT; HUMAN EXPERIMENTATION/SPECIAL POPULATIONS)

Close, Bryony; Combes, Robert; Hubbard, Anthony; Illingworth, John, eds. Volunteers in Research and Testing. Bristol, PA: Taylor and Francis; 1997. 198 p.
(HUMAN EXPERIMENTATION)

Clouser, K. Danner. Biomedical ethics. *In:* Borchert, Donald M., ed. The Encyclopedia of Philosophy. Supplement. New York, NY: Simon and Schuster Macmillan; 1996: 61–67.
(BIOETHICS)

Clouser, K. Danner. Humanities in the service of medicine: three models. *In:* Carson, Ronald A.; Burns, Chester R., eds. Philosophy of Medicine and Bioethics: A Twenty-Year Retrospective and Critical Appraisal. Boston, MA: Kluwer Academic; 1997: 25–39.
(MEDICAL ETHICS/EDUCATION)

Clouser, K. Danner see **Gert, Bernard**

Coakley, J.H. see **McFadzean, J.**

Coatney, Caryn. Outback's assisted-suicide law: Australia delivers world's first dose of legal euthanasia. [News]. *Christian Science Monitor*. 1997 Jan 8: 1, 18.
(EUTHANASIA; SUICIDE)

Coghlan, Andy. Organs for research are on the cards. [News]. *New Scientist*. 1997 Apr 5; 154(2076): 5.
(BIOMEDICAL RESEARCH; ORGAN AND TISSUE DONATION)

Coghlan, Andy. Silent slaughter. [News]. *New Scientist*. 1997 Oct 25; 156(2105): 25.
(ANIMAL EXPERIMENTATION)

Cohen–Almagor, Raphael. Autonomy, life as an intrinsic value, and the right to die in dignity. *Science and Engineering Ethics*. 1995; 1(3): 261–272.
(ALLOWING TO DIE)

Cohen, B. see **Land, Walter**

Cohen, Carl. Do animals have rights? *Ethics and Behavior*. 1997; 7(2): 91–102.
(ANIMAL EXPERIMENTATION)

Cohen, Carl. Ethical aspects of animal research. *In:* Eder, G.; Kaiser, E.; King, F.A., eds. The Role of the Chimpanzee in Research. Symposium, Vienna, Austria, May 22–24, 1992. New York, NY: Karger; 1994: 18–25.
(ANIMAL EXPERIMENTATION)

Cohen, Carl. The case for presumed consent to transplant human organs after death. *Transplantation Proceedings*. 1992 Oct; 24(5): 2168–2172.
(ORGAN AND TISSUE DONATION)

Cohen, Carl see **Ohl, Dana A.**

Cohen, Cynthia see **Jones, Howard**

Cohen, Cynthia B. Wrestling with the future: should we test children for adult-onset genetic conditions? *Kennedy Institute of Ethics Journal*. 1998 Jun; 8(2): 111–130.
(GENETIC SCREENING)

Cohen, Cynthia B.; McCloskey, Elizabeth Leibold. Introduction [to a set of five articles and one commentary on genetic information]. *Kennedy Institute of Ethics Journal*. 1998 Jun; 8(2): vii–x.
(GENETIC COUNSELING; GENETIC SCREENING)

Cohen, David see **Edgar, Andrew**

Cohen, Gene see **Thomas, A. Mathew**

Cohen, Jordan J. Remembering the real questions. *Annals of Internal Medicine*. 1998 Apr 1; 128(7): 563–566.
(HEALTH CARE/ECONOMICS; PROFESSIONAL PATIENT RELATIONSHIP)

Cohen, Lloyd R. A futures market in cadaveric organs: would it work? *Transplantation Proceedings*. 1993 Feb; 25(1): 60–61.
(ORGAN AND TISSUE DONATION)

Cohen, Maynard M. A Stand Against Tyranny: Norway's Physicians and the Nazis. Detroit, MI: Wayne State University Press; 1997. 326 p.
(WAR)

Cohen, Pamela E.; Wertz, Dorothy C.; Nippert, Irmgard; Wolff, Gerhard. Genetic counseling practices in Germany: a comparison between East German and West German geneticists. *Journal of Genetic Counseling*. 1997 Mar; 6(1): 61–80.
(GENETIC COUNSELING)

Cohen, Philip. Cult's bizarre vision rekindles cloning debate. [News]. *New Scientist*. 1997 May 31; 154(2084): 12.
(CLONING)

Cohen, S.L. see **Lemaire, F.**

Cohn, Felicia see Lynn, Joanne

Cole, A.P. see Howard, Philip J.

Cole, Thomas R. Toward a humanist bioethics: commentary on Churchill and Andre. *In:* Carson, Ronald A.; Burns, Chester R., eds. Philosophy of Medicine and Bioethics: A Twenty–Year Retrospective and Critical Appraisal. Boston, MA: Kluwer Academic; 1997: 173–179.
(BIOETHICS)

Cole–Turner, Ronald. At the beginning. *In:* Cole–Turner, Ronald, ed. Human Cloning: Religious Responses. Louisville, KY: Westminister John Knox Press; 1997: 119–130.
(CLONING)

Cole–Turner, Ronald, ed. Human Cloning: Religious Responses. Louisville, KY: Westminister John Knox Press; 1997. 151 p.
(CLONING)

Cole, William G. see Pearlman, Robert A.

Coleman, Carl H. see Miller, Tracy E.

Coles, Matthew. Discrimination, insurance, health care decisions, and wills. *In:* Cohen, P.T.; Sande, Merle A.; Volberding, Paul A., eds. The AIDS Knowledge Base: A Textbook on HIV Disease from the University of California, San Francisco, and the San Francisco General Hospital. Second Edition. Boston, MA: Little, Brown; 1994: 9.2–1 to 9.2–13.
(AIDS)

Coles, Matthew. The law and health care workers: confidentiality, testing, and treatment. *In:* Cohen, P.T.; Sande, Merle A.; Volberding, Paul A., eds. The AIDS Knowledge Base: A Textbook on HIV Disease from the University of California, San Francisco, and the San Francisco General Hospital. Second Edition. Boston, MA: Little, Brown; 1994: 9.1–1 to 9.1–11.
(AIDS/CONFIDENTIALITY; AIDS/HEALTH PERSONNEL; AIDS/TESTING AND SCREENING)

Coles, Robert. The moral education of medical students. *Academic Medicine.* 1998 Jan; 73(1): 55–57.
(MEDICAL ETHICS/EDUCATION)

Coles, William H. see Wear, Stephen E.

Coleson, Richard E. Krischer v. McIver. [Note]. *Issues in Law and Medicine.* 1997 Winter; 13(3): 329–332.
(SUICIDE)

Coleson, Richard E. The Glucksberg and Quill amicus curiae briefs: verbatim arguments opposing assisted suicide. *Issues in Law and Medicine.* 1997 Summer; 13(1): 3–102.
(SUICIDE)

Coleson, Richard E. Vacco v. Quill. [Note]. *Issues in Law and Medicine.* 1997 Winter; 13(3): 323–328.
(SUICIDE)

Coleson, Richard E. Washington v. Glucksberg. [Note]. *Issues in Law and Medicine.* 1997 Winter; 13(3): 315–321.
(SUICIDE)

Coleson, Richard E. see Bopp, James

College of Physicians and Surgeons of British Columbia. Committee on Physician Sexual Misconduct. Crossing the Boundaries. The Report of the Committee on Physician Sexual Misconduct. Issued by the College of Physicians and Surgeons of British Columbia, Vancouver, BC; 1992 Nov. 28 p.
(FRAUD AND MISCONDUCT; PROFESSIONAL PATIENT RELATIONSHIP)

College on Problems of Drug Dependence see Adler, Martin W.

Collette, Linda see Cooke, Molly

Collier, Joe. The future of ethics committees. *In:* Close, Bryony; Combes, Robert; Hubbard, Anthony; Illingworth, John, eds. Volunteers in Research and Testing. Bristol, PA: Taylor and Francis; 1997: 177–183.
(ETHICISTS AND ETHICS COMMITTEES; HUMAN EXPERIMENTATION/ETHICS COMMITTEES; HUMAN EXPERIMENTATION/FOREIGN COUNTRIES)

Collins, Francis S. The Human Genome Project. *In:* Kilner, John F.; Pentz, Rebecca D.; Young, Frank E., eds. Genetic Ethics: Do the Ends Justify the Genes? Grand Rapids, MI: W.B. Eerdmans; 1997: 95–103.
(GENOME MAPPING)

Collins, Francis S. see Kahn, Mary Jo Ellis

Combes, Robert see Close, Bryony

Combs, Elmer W. Home health, AIDS, and refusal to care. *Home Healthcare Nurse.* 1996 Mar; 14(3): 188–194.
(AIDS/HEALTH PERSONNEL)

Commission on Rehabilitation Counselor Certification. Code of professional ethics for certified rehabilitation counselors and CRCC guidelines and procedures for processing complaints. *In:* Maki, Dennis R.; Riggar, T.F., eds. Rehabilitation Counseling: Profession and Practice. New York, NY: Springer Publishing; 1997: Appendix D, 300–321.
(PROFESSIONAL ETHICS/CODES OF ETHICS)

Coney, Sandra. Rationing in health care under scrutiny in New Zealand. [News]. *Lancet.* 1997 Oct 18; 350(9085): 1152.
(HEALTH CARE/FOREIGN COUNTRIES; RESOURCE ALLOCATION)

Coney, Sandra. To the uninformed: managed care means damaged ethics. [Letter]. *Health Care Analysis.* 1997 Sep; 5(3): 252–258.
(HEALTH CARE/ECONOMICS; HEALTH CARE/FOREIGN COUNTRIES)

Conley, Frances K. Walking Out on the Boys. New York, NY: Farrar, Straus and Giroux; 1998. 245 p.
(MEDICAL ETHICS/EDUCATION)

Connecticut. Supreme Court. Stamford Hospital v. Vega. *Atlantic Reporter, 2d Series.* 1996 Apr 16 (date of decision). 674: 821–834.
(TREATMENT REFUSAL)

Connors, Alfred F. see Phillips, Russell S.

Connors, Alfred F. see Teno, Joan

Connors, Alfred F. see Teno, Joan M.

Connors, Alfred F. see Weeks, Jane C.

Connors, Alfred F. see Wenger, Neil S.

Conrad, Peter see DeVries, Raymond

Conroy, Cathy see Dolan, Bridget

Consortium for Health and Human Rights. Writing Group. Health and human rights: a call to action on the 50th anniversary of the Universal Declaration of Human Rights. *JAMA*. 1998 Aug 5; 280(5): 462–464.
(HEALTH CARE/RIGHTS)

Cook, Deborah J. see Wilson, Kumanan

Cook–Deegan, Robert M. see Thomas, A. Mathew

Cook–Deegan, Robert Mullan. Confidentiality, collective resources, and commercial genomics. *In:* Rothstein, Mark A., ed. Genetic Secrets: Protecting Privacy and Confidentiality in the Genetic Era. New Haven, CT: Yale University Press; 1997: 161–183.
(CONFIDENTIALITY; GENETIC RESEARCH; GENOME MAPPING)

Cook, E. David. The Medical Maze: A Christian Approach to Healthcare Ethics. London: Christian Medical Fellowship; 1991. 22 p.
(EUTHANASIA/RELIGIOUS ASPECTS; MEDICAL ETHICS)

Cook, E. Francis see Tsevat, Joel

Cook, E. Francis see Weeks, Jane C.

Cook, Elizabeth Adell; Jelen, Ted G.; Wilcox, Clyde. Measuring public attitudes on abortion: methodological and substantive considerations. *Family Planning Perspectives*. 1993 May–Jun; 25(3): 118–121, 145.
(ABORTION/ATTITUDES)

Cook, Rachel; Golombok, Susan; Bish, Alison; Murray, Clare. Disclosure of donor insemination: parental attitudes. *American Journal of Orthopsychiatry*. 1995 Oct; 65(4): 549–559.
(ARTIFICIAL INSEMINATION; CONFIDENTIALITY; REPRODUCTIVE TECHNOLOGIES)

Cooke, Molly; Gourlay, Linda; Collette, Linda; Boccellari, Alicia; Chesney, Margaret A.; Folkman, Susan. Informal caregivers and the intention to hasten AIDS–related death. *Archives of Internal Medicine*. 1998 Jan 12; 158(1): 69–75.
(AIDS; EUTHANASIA; TERMINAL CARE)

Coombes, Lindsey. Mental health. *In:* Chadwick, Ruth, ed. Encyclopedia of Applied Ethics, Volume 3. San Diego, CA: Academic Press; 1998: 197–212.
(MENTAL HEALTH; PATIENT CARE/MENTALLY DISABLED)

Coon, Stephanie M.; Keyes, Denis W. Attitudes and Opinions of Preservice Professionals: Withholding Life–Sustaining Treatment from Infants with Severe Disabilities. Available from ERIC Document Reproduction Service, DYNCORP I&ET, 7420 Fullerton Rd., Suite 110, Springfield, VA 22153–2852; Document No. ED374635; EC303360; 1994 Jun 2. 55 p.
(ALLOWING TO DIE/INFANTS)

Coope, Christopher Miles. "Death with dignity." *Hastings*

Center Report. 1997 Sep–Oct; 27(5): 37–38.
(TERMINAL CARE)

Cooper, D.K.C. Xenotransplantation: benefits, risks and regulation. *Annals of the Royal College of Surgeons of England*. 1996 Mar; 78(2): 92–96.
(ORGAN AND TISSUE DONATION; ORGAN AND TISSUE TRANSPLANTATION)

Cooper, David A. see Cleaton–Jones, Peter E.

Cooper, David A. see Tindall, Brett

Cooper, David J. see Loscalzo, John J.

Cooper, J.E. Ethics and laboratory animals. *Veterinary Record*. 1985 Jun 1; 116(22): 594–595.
(ANIMAL EXPERIMENTATION)

Cooper–Mahkorn, Déirdre. Many journals have not retracted "fraudulent" research. [News]. *BMJ (British Medical Journal)*. 1998 Jun 20; 316(7148): 1850.
(BIOMEDICAL RESEARCH; FRAUD AND MISCONDUCT)

Copeland, Edward M. see McCurdy, Layton

Copeland, Peter see Hamer, Dean

Coppa, Seanda. Futile care: confronting the high costs of dying. *Journal of Nursing Administration*. 1996 Dec; 26(12): 18–23.
(TERMINAL CARE)

Cordner, Stephen; Ettershank, Kathy. Australian access to private medical records unchanged. [News]. *Lancet*. 1997 May 3; 349(9061): 1306.
(PATIENT ACCESS TO RECORDS)

Cordner, Stephen; Ettershank, Kathy. Australian doctors charged over abortion. [News]. *Lancet*. 1998 Feb 21; 351(9102): 578.
(ABORTION/FOREIGN COUNTRIES; ABORTION/LEGAL ASPECTS)

Cordner, Stephen see Loff, Bebe

Corley, Mary C.; Huff, Steven; Sayles, Linda; Short, Lynette. Patient and nurse criteria for heart transplant candidacy. *Medsurg Nursing*. 1995 Jun; 4(3): 211–215.
(ORGAN AND TISSUE TRANSPLANTATION; SELECTION FOR TREATMENT)

Corner, Jessica. More openness needed in palliative care. [Medicine and the media]. *BMJ (British Medical Journal)*. 1997 Nov 8; 315(7117): 1242.
(EUTHANASIA; TERMINAL CARE)

Corsale, Massimo see d'Oronzio, Joseph C.

Coss–Bu, Jorge see Sachdeva, Ramesh C.

Cotler, Miriam P. Dimensions of time in managed care: metaphor or measure? *HEC (HealthCare Ethics Committee) Forum*. 1997 Dec; 9(4): 323–332.
(HEALTH CARE/ECONOMICS)

Coughlin, Steven S. Advancing professional ethics in epidemiology. *Journal of Epidemiology and Biostatistics*. 1996; 1(2): 71–77.
(BIOMEDICAL RESEARCH; PROFESSIONAL ETHICS/EDUCATION)

Coughlin, Steven S. Ethics in Epidemiology and Public Health Practice: Collected Works. Columbus, GA: Quill Publications; 1997. 232 p.
(BIOMEDICAL RESEARCH; HUMAN EXPERIMENTATION; PROFESSIONAL ETHICS; PUBLIC HEALTH)

Coughlin, Steven S. Implementing breast and cervical cancer prevention programs among the Houma Indians of southern Louisiana: cultural and ethical considerations. *Journal of Health Care for the Poor and Underserved.* 1998 Feb; 9(1): 30–41.
(BIOMEDICAL RESEARCH; MASS SCREENING)

Coughlin, Steven S. Invited commentary: on the role of ethics committees in epidemiology professional societies. *American Journal of Epidemiology.* 1997 Aug 1; 146(3): 209–213.
(ETHICISTS AND ETHICS COMMITTEES)

Coughlin, Steven S.; Soskolne, Colin L.; Goodman, Kenneth W. Case Studies in Public Health Ethics. Washington, DC: American Public Health Association; 1997. 180 p.
(PROFESSIONAL ETHICS; PUBLIC HEALTH)

Coulehan, Jack see **Koval, Joseph C.**

Coulehan, John L. see **Block, Marian R.**

Council for Responsible Genetics. Position statement on cloning. *Bulletin of Medical Ethics.* 1997 Sep; No. 131: 10–11.
(CLONING)

Coupland, Robin M. "Non-lethal" weapons: precipitating a new arms race. [Editorial]. *BMJ (British Medical Journal).* 1997 Jul 12; 315(7100): 72.
(WAR)

Coverdale, John H.; Thomson, Alex N.; White, Gillian E. Social and sexual contact between general practitioners and patients in New Zealand: attitudes and prevalence. *British Journal of General Practice.* 1995 May; 45(394): 245–247.
(FRAUD AND MISCONDUCT; PROFESSIONAL PATIENT RELATIONSHIP)

Cowart, Dax; Burt, Robert. Confronting death: who chooses, who controls? A dialogue between Dax Cowart and Robert Burt. *Hastings Center Report.* 1998 Jan–Feb; 28(1): 14–24.
(ALLOWING TO DIE; PROFESSIONAL PATIENT RELATIONSHIP; TREATMENT REFUSAL)

Cox, Karen; Avis, Mark. Ethical and practical problems of early anti-cancer drug trials: a review of the literature. *European Journal of Cancer Care.* 1996 Jun; 5(2): 90–95.
(HUMAN EXPERIMENTATION/INFORMED CONSENT)

Coyle, Nessa see **Portenoy, Russell K.**

Cozby, Dimitri. Prolonging life: an Orthodox Christian perspective. *Christian Bioethics.* 1997 Dec; 3(3): 204–221.
(ALLOWING TO DIE/RELIGIOUS ASPECTS)

Craft, Alan W. see **Morley, Colin**

Craft, Ian. Should egg donors be paid? An "inconvenience allowance" would solve the egg shortage. *BMJ (British Medical Journal).* 1997 May 10; 314(7091): 1400–1401.
(ORGAN AND TISSUE DONATION; REPRODUCTIVE TECHNOLOGIES)

Crain, Madeleine. A cross–cultural study of beliefs, attitudes and values in Chinese–born American and non–Chinese frail homebound elderly. *Journal Of Long Term Home Health Care.* 1996 Winter; 15(1): 9–18.
(ALLOWING TO DIE/ATTITUDES)

Cranford, Ronald E. Anencephalic infants as organ donors. *Transplantation Proceedings.* 1992 Oct; 24(5): 2218–2220.
(ORGAN AND TISSUE DONATION)

Craufurd, D. see **Hartley, N.E.**

Crawford, Cromwell. Hindu developments in bioethics. *In:* Lustig, B. Andrew, ed.; Center for Medical Ethics and Health Policy (Houston, TX). Bioethics Yearbook, Volume 5: Theological Developments in Bioethics, 1992–1994. Boston, MA: Kluwer Academic; 1997: 55–74.
(BIOETHICS)

Creasey, Larry see **Foster, George E.**

Creighton, F. see **Logmans, A.**

Creighton, Susan see **Gallagher, Bernard**

Crellin, John K. Alternative medicine: ethical challenges for the profession of pharmacy. *In:* Humber, James M.; Almeder, Robert F., eds. Alternative Medicine and Ethics. Totowa, NJ: Humana Press; 1998: 195–212.
(PATIENT CARE/DRUGS; PROFESSIONAL ETHICS)

Crenshaw, Wesley B.; Cain, Kimberly A.; Francis, Paul S. An updated national survey on seclusion and restraint. *Psychiatric Services.* 1997 Mar; 48(3): 395–397.
(BEHAVIOR CONTROL; PATIENT CARE/MENTALLY DISABLED)

Cressey, David M.; Rigter, Henk; de Beaufort, Inez; Rees, Gareth; Walsh, Pat. Ethical debate: too drunk to care? [Article and commentaries]. *BMJ (British Medical Journal).* 1998 May 16; 316(7143): 1515–1517.
(PATIENT CARE)

Crigger, Bette–Jane. As time goes by: an intellectual ethnography of bioethics. *In:* DeVries, Raymond; Subedi, Janardan, eds. Bioethics and Society: Constructing the Ethical Enterprise. Upper Saddle River, NJ: Prentice Hall; 1998: 192–215.
(BIOETHICS)

Crigger, Bette–Jane. Ask your doctor or pharmacist. *Hastings Center Report.* 1998 Mar–Apr; 28(2): 47.
(PATIENT CARE/DRUGS)

Crigger, Bette–Jane. Bioethnography: fieldwork in the lands of medical ethics. [Book review essay]. *Medical Anthropology Quarterly.* 1995 Sep; 9(3): 400–417.
(BIOETHICS)

Crigger, Nancy J. What we owe the author: rethinking editorial peer review. *Nursing Ethics.* 1998 Sep; 5(5): 451–458.
(PROFESSIONAL ETHICS)

Crombie, A. see **Briggs, J.D.**

Crosland, Ann see **Jones, Roger**

Crowther, C.A. see **Gunning, K.F.**

Croyle, Robert T. see **Marteau, Theresa M.**

Csikai, Ellen L. The status of hospital ethics committees in Pennsylvania. *Cambridge Quarterly of Healthcare Ethics.* 1998 Winter; 7(1): 104–107.
(ETHICISTS AND ETHICS COMMITTEES)

Csordas, Thomas J. A handmaid's tale: the rhetoric of personhood in American and Japanese healing of abortions. *In:* Sargent, Carolyn F.; Brettell, Caroline B., eds. Gender and Health: An International Perspective. Upper Saddle River, NJ: Prentice Hall; 1996: 227–241.
(ABORTION/FOREIGN COUNTRIES; ABORTION/RELIGIOUS ASPECTS; FETUSES; PERSONHOOD)

Cugliari, Anna Maria see **Miller, Tracy E.**

Culhane-Pera, Kathleen A.; Vawter, Dorothy E. A study of healthcare professionals' perspectives about a cross-cultural ethical conflict involving a Hmong patient and her family. *Journal of Clinical Ethics.* 1998 Summer; 9(2): 179–190.
(TREATMENT REFUSAL)

Culver, Charles M. see **Gert, Bernard**

Culyer, Anthony. Need: is a consensus possible? [Editorial]. *Journal of Medical Ethics.* 1998 Apr; 24(2): 77–80.
(HEALTH CARE/ECONOMICS; RESOURCE ALLOCATION)

Cunningham, Brian C. Impact of the Human Genome Project at the interface between patent and FDA laws. *Risk: Health, Safety and Environment.* 1996 Summer; 7(3): 253–266.
(GENETIC RESEARCH)

Cunningham-Burley, Sarah see **Kerr, Anne**

Curb, J. David see **Mattson, Margaret E.**

Curran, William J. Legal history of emergency medicine from medieval common law to the AIDS epidemic. *American Journal of Emergency Medicine.* 1997 Nov; 15(7): 658–670.
(AIDS/HEALTH PERSONNEL; PATIENT CARE)

Curran, William J.; Hall, Mark A.; Bobinski, Mary Anne; Orentlicher, David. Health Care Law and Ethics. Fifth Edition. New York, NY: Aspen Law and Business; 1998. 1,463 p.
(BIOETHICS; HEALTH CARE; PATIENT CARE)

Curriden, Mark. Inmate's last wish is to donate kidney. [News]. *ABA Journal: The Lawyer's Magazine.* 1996 Jun; 82: 26.
(CAPITAL PUNISHMENT; ORGAN AND TISSUE DONATION)

Currie, Craig; Green, John; Davies, Steve; Morgan, Christopher. Cost effectiveness of medical ethics training. [Letter]. *Journal of Medical Ethics.* 1997 Oct; 23(5): 328.
(MEDICAL ETHICS/EDUCATION)

Curtin, Leah L. DNR in the OR: ethical concerns and hospital policies. *Nursing Management.* 1994 Feb; 25(2): 29–31.
(RESUSCITATION ORDERS)

Curtis, David see **Kellett, John M.**

Curtis, J. Randall; Rubenfeld, Gordon D. Aggressive medical care at the end of life; does capitated reimbursement encourage the right care for the wrong reason? [Editorial]. *JAMA.* 1997 Sep 24; 278(12): 1025–1026.
(BIOMEDICAL TECHNOLOGIES; HEALTH CARE/ECONOMICS; PATIENT CARE; TERMINAL CARE)

Curtis, Kimberley F. Hannah Arendt, feminist theorizing, and the debate over new reproductive technologies. *Polity.* 1995 Winter; 28(2): 159–187.
(REPRODUCTIVE TECHNOLOGIES)

Cuschieri, Alfred. Screening for genetic diseases: what are the moral constraints? *In:* Agius, Emmanuel; Busuttil, Salvino, eds. Germ-Line Intervention and Our Responsibilities to Future Generations. Boston, MA: Kluwer Academic; 1998: 3–11.
(GENETIC INTERVENTION; GENETIC SCREENING)

Cuttler, Leona see **Finkelstein, Beth S.**

D

Daar, A.S. Ethics of xenotransplantation: animal issues, consent, and likely transformation of transplant ethics. *World Journal of Surgery.* 1997 Nov–Dec; 21(9): 975–982.
(ORGAN AND TISSUE TRANSPLANTATION)

Daar, A.S.; Salomon, Daniel R.; Ferguson, Ronald M.; Helderman, J. Harold; Macchiarini, Paolo. Xenotransplants: proceed with caution. [Letters]. *Nature.* 1998 Mar 5; 392(6671): 11–12.
(HUMAN EXPERIMENTATION; ORGAN AND TISSUE TRANSPLANTATION)

Daar, A.S. see **Hoffenberg, R.**

Daar, A.S. see **Kennedy, I.**

Daar, A.S. see **Radcliffe-Richards, J.**

Daar, Abdallah S. Nonrelated donors and commercialism: a historical perspective. *Transplantation Proceedings.* 1992 Oct; 24(5): 2087–2090.
(ORGAN AND TISSUE DONATION)

Daar, Abdallah S. Paid organ donation: towards an understanding of the issues. *In:* Chapman, Jeremy R.; Deierhoi, Mark; Wight, Celia, eds. Organ and Tissue Donation for Transplantation. New York, NY: Oxford University Press; 1997: 46–61.
(ORGAN AND TISSUE DONATION)

Daar, Abdallah S. Rewarded gifting. *Transplantation Proceedings.* 1992 Oct; 24(5): 2207–2211.
(ORGAN AND TISSUE DONATION)

Daar, Abdallah S. see **Habgood, John**

Dabul, Amy J. see **Russo, Nancy Felipe**

d'Agostino, Monica. Respect for autonomy and a couple's decision. *Journal of Clinical Ethics.* 1998 Summer; 9(2): 177–178.
(INFORMED CONSENT)

Dale, Ruth; Barton, Roger; Shepherd, Jonathan; Burrows, Andrew; Brooke, Deborah; Adshead,

Gwen. Why are doctors ambivalent about patients who misuse alcohol? [Case study and commentaries]. *BMJ (British Medical Journal).* 1997 Nov 15; 315(7118): 1297–1300.
(CONFIDENTIALITY/LEGAL ASPECTS)

Dalton, John D.; Buick, R.G. Guidelines on circumcision. [Letters]. *BMJ (British Medical Journal).* 1997 Sep 20; 315(7110): 750.
(PATIENT CARE/MINORS)

Dalton, Rex. Collins' student sanctioned over 'most severe' case of fraud. [News]. *Nature.* 1997 Jul 24; 388(6640): 313.
(BIOMEDICAL RESEARCH; FRAUD AND MISCONDUCT)

Dalton, Rex. Neuroscientist accused of misconduct turns on his accusers. [News]. *Nature.* 1998 Apr 2; 392(6675): 424.
(BIOMEDICAL RESEARCH; FRAUD AND MISCONDUCT)

Daly, Mary B. see **Geller, Gail**

Daly, Michael E. Alternative methods for the teaching of ethics. *In:* Haddad, Amy Marie, ed. Teaching and Learning Strategies in Pharmacy Ethics. Second Edition. New York, NY: Pharmaceutical Products Press; 1997: 77–86.
(PROFESSIONAL ETHICS/EDUCATION)

Damato, Anthony N. see **Reisner, Michelle**

Daniels, Cynthia R. A million (missing) men: a commentary on Mathieu's compromise on pregnancy and substance abuse. *Politics and the Life Sciences.* 1996 Mar; 15(1): 54–56.
(INVOLUNTARY COMMITMENT; PRENATAL INJURIES)

Daniels, Elisabeth R. see **Emanuel, Ezekiel J.**

Daniels, Jo; McGuffin, Peter; Owen, Mike. Molecular genetic research on IQ: can it be done? Should it be done? *Journal of Biosocial Science.* 1996 Oct; 28(4): 491–507.
(BEHAVIORAL GENETICS; GENETIC RESEARCH)

Daniels, Ken; Lalos, Othon. The Swedish insemination act and the availability of donors. *Human Reproduction.* 1995 Jul; 10(7): 1871–1874.
(ARTIFICIAL INSEMINATION; CONFIDENTIALITY)

Daniels, N. see **Bach, F.H.**

Daniels, Norman. Family responsibility initiatives and justice between age groups. *Law, Medicine and Health Care.* 1985 Sep; 13(4): 153–159.
(HEALTH CARE/ECONOMICS; PATIENT CARE/AGED; RESOURCE ALLOCATION)

Daniels, Norman; Sabin, James. Closure, fair procedures, and setting limits within managed care organizations. *Journal of the American Geriatrics Society.* 1998 Mar; 46(3): 351–354.
(HEALTH CARE/ECONOMICS; RESOURCE ALLOCATION/BIOMEDICAL TECHNOLOGIES)

Daniels, Norman; Sabin, James. Limits to health care: fair procedures, democratic deliberation, and the legitimacy problem for insurers. *Philosophy and Public Affairs.* 1997 Fall; 26(4): 303–350.
(HEALTH CARE/ECONOMICS; RESOURCE

ALLOCATION/BIOMEDICAL TECHNOLOGIES)

Daniels, Norman; Sabin, James E. Last chance therapies and managed care: pluralism, fair procedures, and legitimacy. *Hastings Center Report.* 1998 Mar–Apr; 28(2): 27–41.
(BIOMEDICAL TECHNOLOGIES; HEALTH CARE/ECONOMICS; ORGAN AND TISSUE TRANSPLANTATION)

Daniels, Norman see **Sabin, James E.**

Danis, Marion see **Gertner, Eric J.**

Danis, Marion see **Hanson, Laura C.**

Dankert-Roelse, Jeannette E.; te Meerman, Gerard J. Screening for cystic fibrosis — time to change our position? [Editorial]. *New England Journal of Medicine.* 1997 Oct 2; 337(14): 997–999.
(GENETIC SCREENING; MASS SCREENING)

Danziger, Renée; Gill, Nöel. HIV testing and HIV prevention in Sweden. [Article and commentary]. *BMJ (British Medical Journal).* 1998 Jan 24; 316(7127): 293–296.
(AIDS/TESTING AND SCREENING)

Darbyshire, Janet, et al. see **Aaby, Peter**

Dare, Tim. Mass immunisation programmes: some philosophical issues. *Bioethics.* 1998 Apr; 12(2): 125–149.
(IMMUNIZATION)

Dark, John H. Priorities for lung transplantation. *Lancet.* 1998 Jan 3; 351(9095): 4–5.
(ORGAN AND TISSUE TRANSPLANTATION; RESOURCE ALLOCATION/BIOMEDICAL TECHNOLOGIES; SELECTION FOR TREATMENT)

Darragh, Martina, comp. Ethical issues in managed care: selected bibliography. *Kennedy Institute of Ethics Journal.* 1997 Dec; 7(4): 421–426.
(HEALTH CARE/ECONOMICS)

Darvall, Leanna. Gender and equity: emerging issues in Australian clinical drug trial regulatory policies. *In:* Petersen, Kerry, ed. Intersections: Women on Law, Medicine and Technology. Brookfield, VT: Ashgate; 1997: 185–200.
(HUMAN EXPERIMENTATION/FOREIGN COUNTRIES; HUMAN EXPERIMENTATION/REGULATION; HUMAN EXPERIMENTATION/SPECIAL POPULATIONS)

Daugherty, C.K.; Ratain, M.J.; Siegler, M. Pushing the envelope: informed consent in phase I trials. [Editorial]. *Annals of Oncology.* 1995 Apr; 6(4): 321–323.
(HUMAN EXPERIMENTATION/INFORMED CONSENT)

Daugherty, Christopher; Ratain, Mark J.; Grochowski, Eugene; Stocking, Carol; Kodish, Eric; Mick, Rosemarie; Siegler, Mark. Perceptions of cancer patients and their physicians involved in phase I trials. *Journal of Clinical Oncology.* 1995 May; 13(5): 1062–1072.
(HUMAN EXPERIMENTATION/INFORMED CONSENT)

Daugherty, Robert M. see **McCurdy, Layton**

David, Henry P.; Baban, Adriana. Women's health and reproductive rights: Romanian experience. *Patient Education and Counseling.* 1996 Aug; 28(3): 235–245.
(ABORTION/FOREIGN COUNTRIES; POPULATION

Davis, Dena S. Why suicide is like contraception: a woman-centered view. *In:* Battin, Margaret P.; Rhodes, Rosamond; Silvers, Anita, eds. Physician Assisted Suicide: Expanding the Debate. New York, NY: Routledge; 1998: 113–122.
(SUICIDE)

Davis, E.L. see **Bebeau, M.J.**

Davis, Fran; Post, Edward R.; Rogers, Connie S.; Depp, Michael; Ferrell, Peter; Worthy, Jane. What could have saved John Worthy? *Hastings Center Report.* 1998 Jul–Aug; 28(4): S1–S17.
(HEALTH CARE/ECONOMICS)

Davis, Helen R.; Mitrius, Janice V. Recent legislation on genetics and insurance. [Note]. *Jurimetrics Journal.* 1996 Fall; 37(1): 69–82.
(CONFIDENTIALITY/LEGAL ASPECTS; GENETIC SCREENING)

Davis, Kenneth M.; Clark, Doug; Koch, Karen E.; Schofield, David J. Physician marketing of nutritional supplements. [Letter and response]. *JAMA.* 1998 Sep 16; 280(11): 967–968.
(HEALTH CARE/ECONOMICS; PATIENT CARE/DRUGS)

Davis, Margaret K. see **Borowsky, Steven J.**

Davis, Michael. Arresting the white death: preventive detention, confinement for treatment, and medical ethics. *American Philosophical Association Newsletter on Philosophy and Medicine.* 1995 Spring; 94(2): 92–98.
(PUBLIC HEALTH)

Davis, N. Ann. Not drowning but waving: reflections on swimming through the shark-infested waters of the abortion debate. *In:* Edwards, Rem B., ed. Advances in Bioethics. Volume 2: New Essays on Abortion and Bioethics. Greenwich, CT: JAI Press; 1997: 227–265.
(ABORTION/ATTITUDES)

Davis, Owen K. see **Sills, E. Scott**

Davis, Peter. Contested Ground: Public Purpose and Private Interest in the Regulation of Prescription Drugs. New York, NY: Oxford University Press; 1996. 262 p.
(PATIENT CARE/DRUGS)

Davison, B. Joyce; Degner, Lesley F.; Morgan, Thomas R. Information and decision-making preferences of men with prostate cancer. *Oncology Nursing Forum.* 1995 Oct; 22(9): 1401–1408.
(PATIENT CARE)

Davison, Sandy see **Maiorca, Rosario**

Dawson, Angus. Psychopharmacology. *In:* Chadwick, Ruth, ed. Encyclopedia of Applied Ethics, Volume 3. San Diego, CA: Academic Press; 1998: 727–734.
(PATIENT CARE/DRUGS; PATIENT CARE/MENTALLY DISABLED)

Dawson, Neal V. see **Tsevat, Joel**

Dawson, Neal V. see **Weeks, Jane C.**

Day, Albert see **Ashcroft, Richard**

Day, Patricia see **Klein, Rudolph**

Dayan, Anthony. The volunteer subject, encouragement and protection. *In:* Close, Bryony; Combes, Robert; Hubbard, Anthony; Illingworth, John, eds. Volunteers in Research and Testing. Bristol, PA: Taylor and Francis; 1997: 5–21.
(HUMAN EXPERIMENTATION)

Dean, Peter see **Payne–James, Jason**

de Beaufort, Inez see **Cressey, David M.**

Deber, Raisa see **Silberfeld, Michel**

de Boer, Anthonius; Lau, Hong Sang; Porsius, Arijan. Physician-assisted death and pharmacy practice in the Netherlands. [Letter]. *New England Journal of Medicine.* 1997 Oct 9; 337(15): 1091–1092.
(EUTHANASIA/ATTITUDES; SUICIDE)

de Bousingen, Denis Durand. Exhumation angers French ethicists. [News]. *Lancet.* 1997 Nov 15; 350(9089): 1458.
(DNA FINGERPRINTING)

de Bousingen, Denis Durand. French Medical Association apologises to Jews. [News]. *Lancet.* 1997 Oct 18; 350(9085): 1153.
(FRAUD AND MISCONDUCT)

de Burgh, Jane. Saving our bacon: the new animal farm [review of *Pig in the Middle*: A UK national touring play, written by Judy Upton, directed by Nigel Town]. *Lancet.* 1998 Mar 28; 351(9107): 993.
(ORGAN AND TISSUE DONATION; ORGAN AND TISSUE TRANSPLANTATION)

de Carvalho, Carlos Alberto see **Byrne, Paul A.**

De Cock, Kevin M.; Johnson, Anne M. From exceptionalism to normalisation: a reappraisal of attitudes and practice around HIV testing. *BMJ (British Medical Journal).* 1998 Jan 24; 316(7127): 290–293.
(AIDS/TESTING AND SCREENING)

Deepandung, Attajinda; Noonpakdee, Wilai T. The moral status of the human genome. *In:* Agius, Emmanuel; Busuttil, Salvino, eds. Germ-Line Intervention and Our Responsibilities to Future Generations. Boston, MA: Kluwer Academic; 1998: 13–18.
(GENE THERAPY; GENETIC SCREENING; GENOME MAPPING)

Deering, Carole P. see **Dorner, Becky**

Defanti, C.A. Brain death. *In:* Chadwick, Ruth, ed. Encyclopedia of Applied Ethics, Volume 1. San Diego, CA: Academic Press; 1998: 369–376.
(DETERMINATION OF DEATH/BRAIN DEATH)

DeFries, John C. see **Sherman, Stephanie L.**

DeGandt, Olivier see **Butler, Declan**

Degani, Naushaba see **Ferris, Lorraine E.**

De Giovanni, J.V. see **Brawn, W.J.**

Degner, Lesley F.; Kristjanson, Linda J.; Bowman, David; Sloan, Jeffrey A.; Carriere, K.C.; O'Neil, John; Bilodeau, Barbara; Watson, Peter; Mueller, Bryan. Information needs and decisional preferences in women with breast cancer. *JAMA.* 1997 May 14; 277(18):

1485–1492.
(PATIENT CARE; PROFESSIONAL PATIENT RELATIONSHIP)

Degner, Lesley F. see **Davison, B. Joyce**

Degnin, Francis Dominic. Max Weber on ethics case consultation: a methodological critique of the Conference on Evaluation of Ethics Consultation. *Journal of Clinical Ethics.* 1997 Summer; 8(2): 181–192.
(ETHICISTS AND ETHICS COMMITTEES)

DeGroot, Leslie J.; St. Germain, Donald L.; Ridgway, E. Chester; Gordon, Benjamin D.; Bell, Bertrand M.; Donohoe, Martin; Brantigan, Charles O.; Dreyer, Nancy A.; Lankin, Kenneth M.; Birnbaum, Ron; Dong, Betty J.; Gambertoglio, John G.; Greenspan, Francis S.; Hauck, Walter W.; Rennie, Drummond; Bramblett, Michael T.; Fontanarosa, Phil B.; Glass, Richard M.; Murphy, Peter J. Bioequivalence of levothyroxine preparations: issues of science, publication, and advertising. [Letters and responses]. *JAMA.* 1997 Sep 17; 278(11): 895–900.
(BIOMEDICAL RESEARCH; HEALTH CARE/ECONOMICS)

de Haan, K. see **van Thiel, G.J.M.W.**

Dehlendorf, Christine E.; Wolfe, Sidney M. Physicians disciplined for sex–related offenses. *JAMA.* 1998 Jun 17; 279(23): 1883–1888.
(FRAUD AND MISCONDUCT; PROFESSIONAL PATIENT RELATIONSHIP)

Deichmann, Ute; Müller–Hill, Benno. The fraud of Abderhalden's enzymes. *Nature.* 1998 May 14; 393(6681): 109–111.
(BIOMEDICAL RESEARCH; FRAUD AND MISCONDUCT)

DeKay, M. see **Ubel, Peter A.**

De Koninck, Maria. Reflections on the transfer of "progress": the case of reproduction. *In:* Sherwin, Susan, et al. The Politics of Women's Health: Exploring Agency and Autonomy. Philadelphia, PA: Temple University Press; 1998: 150–177.
(HEALTH; REPRODUCTION)

de Langavant, Ghislaine Cleret see **Roy, David J.**

Delano, Susan J. see **Haimowitz, Stephan**

Delany, Linda. Bending the statutory rules: the case of Mrs. Blood. *Health Care Analysis.* 1997 Sep; 5(3): 238–240, 243.
(ARTIFICIAL INSEMINATION)

Delany, Linda. Court–authorised caesareans: new guidance. *Health Care Analysis.* 1997 Sep; 5(3): 240–241, 243.
(FETUSES; TREATMENT REFUSAL)

Delany, Linda. Health care law: caesareans under duress. *Health Care Analysis.* 1997 Jun; 5(2): 160–163.
(TREATMENT REFUSAL)

Delany, Linda. Withholding life–sustaining treatment: the case of Miss D. *Health Care Analysis.* 1997 Sep; 5(3): 237–238, 242.
(ALLOWING TO DIE/LEGAL ASPECTS)

Delaware. Supreme Court. In re Tavel. *Atlantic Reporter,*

2d Series. 1995 Aug 2 (date of decision). 661: 1061–1072.
(ALLOWING TO DIE/LEGAL ASPECTS)

deLeon, Dennis M. see **Orr, Robert D.**

Della Bella, Peter see **Billick, Stephen B.**

Dellasega, Cheryl; Frank, Lori; Smyer, Michael. Medical decision–making capacity in elderly hospitalized patients. *Journal of Ethics, Law, and Aging.* 1996 Fall–Winter; 2(2): 65–74.
(INFORMED CONSENT; PATIENT CARE/AGED)

Dell'Oro, Roberto; Viafora, Corrado, eds. History of Bioethics: International Perspectives. San Francisco, CA: International Scholars Publications; 1996. 313 p.
(BIOETHICS)

Del Mar, C.B. see **Steinberg, M.A.**

DeLong, Elizabeth R. see **Barnhart, J. Marie**

del Rio, Carlos see **Schüklenk, Udo**

Deluzio, Charles see **Rinchuse, Daniel J.**

Demartis, Francesco. Mass pre–embryo adoption. *Cambridge Quarterly of Healthcare Ethics.* 1998 Winter; 7(1): 101–103.
(FETUSES)

DeMers, Stephen T. see **Bass, Larry J.**

DeMichele, Sarah Gelbach see **Morrison, Mary F.**

DenBesten, Karen E. see **Caniano, Donna A.**

DePalma, Anthony. Canadian gets light term in child's death. [News]. *New York Times.* 1997 Dec 2: A8.
(EUTHANASIA/LEGAL ASPECTS)

DePalma, Anthony. Father's killing of Canadian girl: mercy or murder? [News]. *New York Times.* 1997 Dec 1: A3.
(EUTHANASIA/LEGAL ASPECTS)

DePalma, Judith A.; Townsend, Ricard. Ethical issues in organ donation and transplantation: are we helping a few at the expense of many? *Critical Care Nursing Quarterly.* 1996 May; 19(1): 1–9.
(ORGAN AND TISSUE DONATION; ORGAN AND TISSUE TRANSPLANTATION)

De Paolis, P. see **Elli, M.**

DePetrillo, A.D. see **Taylor, K.M.**

Depp, Michael see **Davis, Fran**

de Rave, Sjoerd. Allocation of donor organs. [Letter]. *Lancet.* 1997 Oct 11; 350(9084): 1107.
(ORGAN AND TISSUE TRANSPLANTATION; RESOURCE ALLOCATION/BIOMEDICAL TECHNOLOGIES; SELECTION FOR TREATMENT)

DeRenzo, Evan G.; Strauss, Michelle. A feminist model for clinical ethics consultation: increasing attention to context and narrative. *HEC (HealthCare Ethics Committee) Forum.* 1997 Sep; 9(3): 212–227.
(BIOETHICS; ETHICISTS AND ETHICS COMMITTEES)

Derham, P. see Hardy, K.J.

Desbiens, Norman see Phillips, Russell S.

Desbiens, Norman see Teno, Joan

Desbiens, Norman see Teno, Joan M.

Desbiens, Norman A. see Wenger, Neil S.

Descamps, Arnaud see Gromb, Sophie

Desch, Christopher E. see Smith, Thomas J.

Desmond, Katherine A. see Wenger, Neil S.

Desnick, Robert J. see Eng, Christine M.

Dessouki, A. see Mendez, R.

Destro, Robert A. Government oversight. *In:* Shamoo, Adil E., ed. Ethics in Neurobiological Research with Human Subjects: The Baltimore Conference on Ethics. Amsterdam: Gordon and Breach; 1997: 81–99.
(HUMAN EXPERIMENTATION/INFORMED CONSENT; HUMAN EXPERIMENTATION/REGULATION; HUMAN EXPERIMENTATION/SPECIAL POPULATIONS)

Detsky, Allan S. see Stelfox, Henry Thomas

De Ville, Kenneth; Kaplan, Carl A. Treating the silent stranger: informed consent and defensive medicine in the critical care unit. *HEC (HealthCare Ethics Committee) Forum.* 1998 Mar; 10(1): 55–70.
(INFORMED CONSENT)

De Ville, Kenneth see Moskop, John C.

Devine, Philip E. 'Conservative' views of abortion. *In:* Edwards, Rem B., ed. Advances in Bioethics. Volume 2: New Essays on Abortion and Bioethics. Greenwich, CT: JAI Press; 1997: 183–202.
(ABORTION)

Devine, Philip E. Homicide, criminal versus justifiable. *In:* Chadwick, Ruth, ed. Encyclopedia of Applied Ethics, Volume 2. San Diego, CA: Academic Press; 1998: 587–595.
(ABORTION; EUTHANASIA; SUICIDE)

Devins, Neal. Shaping Constitutional Values: Elected Government, the Supreme Court, and the Abortion Debate. Baltimore, MD: Johns Hopkins University Press; 1996. 193 p.
(ABORTION/LEGAL ASPECTS)

Devlin, Maureen M. In re Fiori. [Note]. *Issues in Law and Medicine.* 1996 Fall; 12(2): 189–190.
(ALLOWING TO DIE/LEGAL ASPECTS)

DeVries, Raymond; Conrad, Peter. Why bioethics needs sociology. *In:* DeVries, Raymond; Subedi, Janardan, eds. Bioethics and Society: Constructing the Ethical Enterprise. Upper Saddle River, NJ: Prentice Hall; 1998: 233–257.
(BIOETHICS; ETHICISTS AND ETHICS COMMITTEES)

DeVries, Raymond; Subedi, Janardan, eds. Bioethics and Society: Constructing the Ethical Enterprise. Upper Saddle River, NJ: Prentice Hall; 1998. 276 p.
(BIOETHICS)

DeVries, Raymond see Fox, Renée C.

de Wachter, Maurice A.M. DNA sampling and duties to relatives -- looking back: European approaches. *In:* Knoppers, Bartha Maria, ed. Human DNA: Law and Policy: International and Comparative Perspectives. Proceedings of the First International Conference on DNA Sampling and Human Genetic Research: Ethical, Legal, and Policy Aspects, held in Montreal, Canada, 6–8 Sep 1996. Boston, MA: Kluwer Law International; 1997: 145–156.
(GENETIC SCREENING)

de Wachter, Maurice A.M.; Knoppers, Bartha M.; Monti, Chantal LeGris. Ethical decision-making by hospital committees. [Letter]. *Canadian Medical Association Journal.* 1984 Oct 1; 131(7): 713–714.
(ETHICISTS AND ETHICS COMMITTEES)

de Wert, G.M.W.R. see Tibben, A.

de Witte, Joke I.; ten Have, Henk. Ownership of genetic material and information. *Social Science and Medicine.* 1997 Jul; 45(1): 51–60.
(GENOME MAPPING; ORGAN AND TISSUE DONATION)

Dexter, Paul R.; Wolinsky, Fredric D.; Gramelspacher, Gregory P.; Zhou, Xiao-Hua; Eckert, George J.; Waisburd, Marina; Tierney, William M. Effectiveness of computer-generated reminders for increasing discussions about advance directives and completion of advance directive forms: a randomized, controlled trial. *Annals of Internal Medicine.* 1998 Jan 15; 128(2): 102–110.
(ADVANCE DIRECTIVES)

Dhondt, Jean-Louis; Farriaux, Jean-Pierre. Impact of French legislation on neonatal screening. *In:* Knoppers, Bartha Maria, ed. Human DNA: Law and Policy: International and Comparative Perspectives. Proceedings of the First International Conference on DNA Sampling and Human Genetic Research: Ethical, Legal, and Policy Aspects, held in Montreal, Canada, 6–8 Sep 1996. Boston, MA: Kluwer Law International; 1997: 285–289.
(GENETIC SCREENING; MASS SCREENING)

Diamond, Eugene F. Reflections on the 50th anniversary of the Nuremberg doctors' trials. *Linacre Quarterly.* 1997 May; 64(2): 17–20.
(EMBRYO AND FETAL RESEARCH)

Dickens, B. Canadian developments [bioethics and the law]. [News]. *International Journal of Bioethics.* 1997 Mar–Jun; 8(1–2): 131–134.
(BIOETHICS)

Dickens, B.M. Interfaces of assisted reproduction ethics and law. *In:* Shenfield, F.; Sureau, C., eds. Ethical Dilemmas in Assisted Reproduction. New York, NY: Parthenon Pub. Group; 1997: 77–81.
(REPRODUCTIVE TECHNOLOGIES)

Dickens, Bernard. Patients' rights. *In:* Chadwick, Ruth, ed. Encyclopedia of Applied Ethics, Volume 3. San Diego, CA: Academic Press; 1998: 459–471.
(PATIENTS' RIGHTS)

Dickens, Bernard see Weijer, Charles

Dickens, Bernard M. Choices, control, access -- the

Canadian position. *In:* Knoppers, Bartha Maria, ed. Human DNA: Law and Policy: International and Comparative Perspectives. Proceedings of the First International Conference on DNA Sampling and Human Genetic Research: Ethical, Legal, and Policy Aspects, held in Montreal, Canada, 6–8 Sep 1996. Boston, MA: Kluwer Law International; 1997: 71–89.
(CONFIDENTIALITY/LEGAL ASPECTS; GENETIC RESEARCH; GENETIC SCREENING; INFORMED CONSENT)

Dickens, Bernard M. Commentary on "Slow euthanasia." *Journal of Palliative Care.* 1996 Winter; 12(4): 42–43.
(EUTHANASIA/LEGAL ASPECTS; TERMINAL CARE)

Dickens, Bernard M. Legal and ethical challenges in gene therapy. *Transfusion Science.* 1996 Mar; 17(1): 191–196.
(GENE THERAPY; HUMAN EXPERIMENTATION)

Dickens, Bernard M. Legal aspects of transplantation — judicial issues. *Transplantation Proceedings.* 1992 Oct; 24(5): 2118–2119.
(ORGAN AND TISSUE DONATION)

Dickens, Bernard M.; Fluss, Sev S.; King, Ariel R. Legislation on organ and tissue donation. *In:* Chapman, Jeremy R.; Deierhoi, Mark; Wight, Celia, eds. Organ and Tissue Donation for Transplantation. New York, NY: Oxford University Press; 1997: 95–119.
(ORGAN AND TISSUE DONATION)

Dickenson, Donna. Ethical issues in long term psychiatric management. *Journal of Medical Ethics.* 1997 Oct; 23(5): 300–304.
(INFORMED CONSENT/MENTALLY DISABLED; INVOLUNTARY COMMITMENT/FOREIGN COUNTRIES; TREATMENT REFUSAL/MENTALLY DISABLED)

Dickenson, Donna see **Ashcroft, Richard**

Dickinson, E. see **Brocklehurst, J.**

Dickson, David. Biosafety code gathers pace through bilateral agreements. [News]. *Nature.* 1995 Sep 14; 377(6545): 94.
(GENETIC INTERVENTION)

Dickson, David. Legal fight looms over patent bid on human/animal chimaeras. [News]. *Nature.* 1998 Apr 2; 392(6675): 423–424.
(PATENTING LIFE FORMS)

Dickson, David. Physicians prepare guidelines on use of human genome data. [News]. *Nature.* 1995 Sep 28; 377(6547): 279.
(GENETIC SCREENING)

Dickson, David. UK consults public on clones for research. [News]. *Nature.* 1998 Feb 5; 391(6667): 523.
(CLONING; EMBRYO AND FETAL RESEARCH)

Dickson, David. UK takes pride in 'principled pragmatism'. [News]. *Nature.* 1997 Oct 16; 389(6652): 663.
(BIOETHICS)

Dickson, David; Wadman, Meredith. Genome effort 'still in need of support.' [News]. *Nature.* 1998 May 21; 393(6682): 201.
(GENOME MAPPING)

Dierckx de Casterlé, Bernadette; Janssen, Piet J.;

Grypdonck, Mieke. The relationship between education and ethical behavior of nursing students. *Western Journal of Nursing Research.* 1996 Jun; 18(3): 330–350.
(NURSING ETHICS/EDUCATION)

Dillon, Mary Ann. A dynamic force for change: the common good provides the rationale for a healthcare system for all. *Health Progress.* 1997 Mar–Apr; 78(2): 31–33, 42.
(HEALTH CARE/RIGHTS)

Dillon, Michele. Cultural differences in the abortion discourse of the Catholic Church: evidence from four countries. *Sociology of Religion.* 1996 Spring; 57(1): 25–36.
(ABORTION/FOREIGN COUNTRIES; ABORTION/RELIGIOUS ASPECTS)

Dimmitt, Jane H. see **Artnak, Kathryn E.**

El–Din, A.B. Shehab see **Qunibi, Wajeh**

Di Noia, J. Augustine. The virtues of the Good Samaritan: health care ethics in the perspective of a renewed moral theology. *Dolentium Hominum: Church and Health in the World.* 1996; 31(11th Yr., No. 1): 211–214.
(BIOETHICS)

Dixon, John. Catastrophic rights: vital public interests and civil liberties in conflict. *In:* Overall, Christine and Zion, William P., eds. Perspectives on AIDS: Ethical and Social Issues. New York, NY: Oxford University Press; 1991: 122–137.
(AIDS/HUMAN EXPERIMENTATION; HUMAN EXPERIMENTATION/RESEARCH DESIGN)

Dixon, Kathleen Marie. The quality of mercy: reflections on provider–assisted suicide. *Journal of Clinical Ethics.* 1997 Fall; 8(3): 290–302.
(SUICIDE; TERMINAL CARE)

Djikova, Sonja see **Ivanovski, Ninoslav**

Dlugolecka, Maria see **Ashcroft, Richard**

Dobson, Andrew. Genetic engineering and environmental ethics. *Cambridge Quarterly of Healthcare Ethics.* 1997 Spring; 6(2): 205–221.
(GENETIC INTERVENTION; RECOMBINANT DNA RESEARCH)

Docker, Chris. Advance directives/living wills. *In:* McLean, Sheila A.M., ed. Contemporary Issues in Law, Medicine and Ethics. Brookfield, VT: Dartmouth; 1996: 179–214.
(ADVANCE DIRECTIVES)

Docker, Christopher. The way forward? *In:* McLean, Sheila A.M., ed. Death, Dying and the Law. Brookfield, VT: Dartmouth; 1996: 129–160.
(ADVANCE DIRECTIVES; ALLOWING TO DIE; EUTHANASIA; RESOURCE ALLOCATION; SUICIDE; TERMINAL CARE)

Doering, Jeffrey see **Werhane, Patricia**

Doherty, Peter; Sutton, Agneta, eds. Man–Made Man: Ethical and Legal Issues in Genetics. Dublin, Ireland: Open Air; 1997. 116 p.
(GENE THERAPY; GENETIC INTERVENTION; GENETIC SCREENING)

Dolan, Bridget; Parker, Camilla; Bewley, Susan; Whitfield, Adrian; Bastian, Hilda; Conroy, Cathy. Caesarean section: a treatment for mental disorder? Tameside and Glossop Acute Services Unit v CH (A Patient) [1996] 1 FLR 762. [Case report and commentaries]. *BMJ (British Medical Journal).* 1997 Apr 19; 314(7088): 1183–1187.
(TREATMENT REFUSAL/MENTALLY DISABLED)

Dolgin, Janet L. Defining the Family: Law, Technology, and Reproduction in an Uneasy Age. New York, NY: New York University Press; 1997. 287 p.
(REPRODUCTIVE TECHNOLOGIES; SURROGATE MOTHERS)

Doll, John J. The patenting of DNA. *Science.* 1998 May 1; 280(5364): 689–690.
(GENOME MAPPING)

Dolske, Michelle see **Smith, Martin L.**

Dombrowski, Daniel A. Babies and Beasts: The Argument from Marginal Cases. Urbana, IL: University of Illinois Press; 1997. 221 p.
(ANIMAL EXPERIMENTATION)

Domino, George; Kempton, Susan; Cavender, Jim. Physician assisted suicide: a scale and some empirical findings. *Omega: A Journal of Death and Dying.* 1996–1997; 34(3): 247–257.
(EUTHANASIA/ATTITUDES; SUICIDE)

Donahue, James. Patenting of human DNA sequences -- implications for prenatal genetic testing. [Note]. *Journal of Family Law.* 1997–1998 Spring; 36(2): 267–283.
(GENETIC SCREENING; PRENATAL DIAGNOSIS)

Donaldson, Molla S.; Field, Marilyn J. Measuring quality of care at the end of life. *Archives of Internal Medicine.* 1998 Jan 26; 158(2): 121–128.
(TERMINAL CARE)

Dong, Betty J. see **DeGroot, Leslie J.**

Donohoe, Martin see **DeGroot, Leslie J.**

Donovan, G. Kevin. Decisions at the end of life: Catholic tradition. *Christian Bioethics.* 1997 Dec; 3(3): 188–203.
(ALLOWING TO DIE/RELIGIOUS ASPECTS; DETERMINATION OF DEATH/BRAIN DEATH; EUTHANASIA/RELIGIOUS ASPECTS; SUICIDE)

Doolittle, Norma O.; Herrick, Charlotte A. Ethics in aging: a decision-making paradigm. *Educational Gerontology.* 1992 Jun; 18(4): 395–408.
(PATIENT CARE/AGED)

Dordoy, Jackie see **Aitkenhead, Marilyn**

Dorff, Elliot N. A methodology for Jewish medical ethics. *In:* Dorff, Elliot N.; Newman, Louis E., eds. Contemporary Jewish Ethics and Morality: A Reader. New York, NY: Oxford University Press; 1995: 161–176.
(BIOETHICS)

Dorff, Elliot N. Jewish law and lore: the case of organ transplantation. *In:* Jewish Law Annual. Volume Twelve. Amsterdam, Netherlands: Harwood Academic Publishers; 1997: 65–114.
(DETERMINATION OF DEATH; ORGAN AND TISSUE DONATION)

Dorff, Elliot N. Review of recent work in Jewish bioethics. *In:* Lustig, B. Andrew, ed.; Center for Medical Ethics and Health Policy (Houston, TX). Bioethics Yearbook, Volume 5: Theological Developments in Bioethics, 1992–1994. Boston, MA: Kluwer Academic; 1997: 75–91.
(BIOETHICS)

Dorhofer, Diana see **Sigmon, Sandra T.**

Dorner, Becky; Gallagher-Allred, Charlette; Deering, Carole P.; Posthauer, Mary Ellen. The "to feed or not to feed" dilemma. *Journal of the American Dietetic Association.* 1997 Oct; 97(10, Suppl. 2): S172–S176.
(ALLOWING TO DIE; PATIENT CARE/AGED)

d'Oronzio, Joseph C.; Reinders, Hans S.; Corsale, Massimo. Ethical obligations in the body politic: the case of normalization policy for marginal populations. [Introduction, article, and commentary]. *Cambridge Quarterly of Healthcare Ethics.* 1997 Fall; 6(4): 480–493.
(PATIENT CARE/MENTALLY DISABLED)

Dorozynski, Alexander. France creates opt out register for organ donation. [News]. *BMJ (British Medical Journal).* 1998 Jul 25; 317(7153): 234.
(ORGAN AND TISSUE DONATION)

Dorozynski, Alexander. France to investigate illegal sterilisation of mentally ill patients. [News]. *BMJ (British Medical Journal).* 1997 Sep 20; 315(7110): 697.
(STERILIZATION/MENTALLY DISABLED)

Dorozynski, Alexander. French doctors apologise for wartime antisemitism. [News]. *BMJ (British Medical Journal).* 1997 Nov 1; 315(7116): 1116.
(FRAUD AND MISCONDUCT)

Dorozynski, Alexander. Scandal unfolds over blood donation in French prisons. [News]. *BMJ (British Medical Journal).* 1998 Jan 17; 316(7126): 171.
(AIDS; FRAUD AND MISCONDUCT)

Dorozynski, Alexander. Yves Montand to be exhumed to test paternity. [News]. *BMJ (British Medical Journal).* 1997 Nov 29; 315(7120): 1398.
(DNA FINGERPRINTING)

Dossetor, John B. Human values in health care: trying to get it right. *Canadian Medical Association Journal.* 1997 Dec 15; 157(12): 1689–1690.
(BIOETHICS)

Dossetor, John B. Rewarded gifting: is it ever ethically acceptable? *Transplantation Proceedings.* 1992 Oct; 24(5): 2092–2094.
(ORGAN AND TISSUE DONATION)

Dougherty, Charles J. How to avoid flying blind: to truly improve U.S. healthcare, leaders must consider seven moral values. *Health Progress.* 1997 Mar–Apr; 78(2): 20–22.
(HEALTH CARE)

Dougherty, Charles J. Tradition, mission, and the market: faith in ultimate purposefulness makes Catholic healthcare different. *Health Progress.* 1997 Jul–Aug; 78(4): 44–51.
(HEALTH CARE)

Doukas, David J.; Fetters, Michael; Ruffin, Mack T.;

McCullough, Laurence B. Ethical considerations in the provision of controversial screening tests. *Archives of Family Medicine.* 1997 Sep–Oct; 6(5): 486–490.
(MASS SCREENING)

Dove, Phillip see **Hood, Catherine A.**

Dowbiggin, Ian Robert. Keeping America Sane: Psychiatry and Eugenics in the United States and Canada, 1880-1940. Ithaca, NY: Cornell University Press; 1997. 245 p.
(EUGENICS; PATIENT CARE/MENTALLY DISABLED)

Dowey, J.A. Child B: A Personal View. *BMJ (British Medical Journal).* 1997 Jan 18; 314(7075): 200.
(ALLOWING TO DIE)

Downie, Jocelyn see **Baylis, Françoise**

Downie, R.S. Professional ethics and business ethics. *In:* McLean, Sheila A.M., ed. Contemporary Issues in Law, Medicine and Ethics. Brookfield, VT: Dartmouth; 1996: 1–14.
(HEALTH CARE/ECONOMICS; MEDICAL ETHICS; PROFESSIONAL ETHICS)

Downie, Robin. Xenotransplantation. [Editorial]. *Journal of Medical Ethics.* 1997 Aug; 23(4): 205–206.
(ORGAN AND TISSUE TRANSPLANTATION)

Doyal, Len. Informed consent -- a response to recent correspondence. *BMJ (British Medical Journal).* 1998 Mar 28; 316(7136): 1000–1001.
(HUMAN EXPERIMENTATION/INFORMED CONSENT)

Doyal, Len. Need for moral audit in evaluating quality in health care. *Quality in Health Care.* 1992 Sep; 1(3): 178–183.
(HEALTH CARE)

Doyal, Len; Gillon, Raanan. Medical ethics and law as a core subject in medical education: a core curriculum offers flexibility in how it is taught -- but not that it is taught. [Editorial]. *BMJ (British Medical Journal).* 1998 May 30; 316(7145): 1623–1624.
(BIOETHICS/EDUCATION; MEDICAL ETHICS/EDUCATION)

Doyal, Len see **Ashcroft, Richard**

Doyle, Mary Anne see **Philipson, Sandra J.**

Dracy, David L.; Yutrzenka, Barbara A. Responses of direct–care paraprofessional mental health staff to hypothetical ethics violations. *Psychiatric Services.* 1997 Sep; 48(9): 1160–1163.
(FRAUD AND MISCONDUCT; PROFESSIONAL ETHICS)

Drake, Harriet; Reid, Margaret; Marteau, Theresa. Attitudes towards termination for fetal abnormality: comparisons in three European countries. *Clinical Genetics.* 1996 Mar; 49(3): 134–140.
(ABORTION/ATTITUDES; ABORTION/FOREIGN COUNTRIES)

Drake, Harriet see **Marteau, Theresa**

Drane, James F. Caring to the End: Policy Suggestions and Ethics Education for Hospice and Home Health–Care Agencies. Erie, PA: Lake Area Health Education Center; 1997. 308 p.
(ALLOWING TO DIE; TERMINAL CARE/HOSPICES)

Draper, Elaine Alma. Social issues of genome innovation and intellectual property. *Risk: Health, Safety and Environment.* 1996 Summer; 7(3): 201–229.
(GENETIC SCREENING)

Draper, Heather. Consent in childbirth. *In:* Frith, Lucy, ed. Ethics and Midwifery: Issues in Contemporary Practice. Boston, MA: Butterworth–Heinemann; 1996: 17–35.
(INFORMED CONSENT)

Draper, Heather. Euthanasia. *In:* Chadwick, Ruth, ed. Encyclopedia of Applied Ethics, Volume 2. San Diego, CA: Academic Press; 1998: 175–187.
(ALLOWING TO DIE; EUTHANASIA)

Draper, Heather. Treating anorexics without consent: some reservations. [Editorial]. *Journal of Medical Ethics.* 1998 Feb; 24(1): 5–7.
(FORCE FEEDING; TREATMENT REFUSAL/MENTALLY DISABLED)

Draper, Heather see **Ashcroft, Richard**

Dreger, Alice Domurat. "Ambiguous sex" -- or ambivalent medicine? Ethical issues in the treatment of intersexuality. *Hastings Center Report.* 1998 May–Jun; 28(3): 24–35.
(PATIENT CARE)

Dresser, Rebecca. Missing persons: legal perceptions of incompetent patients. *Rutgers Law Review.* 1994 Winter; 46(2): 609–719.
(ALLOWING TO DIE/LEGAL ASPECTS)

Dresser, Rebecca. Scientists in the sunshine. *Hastings Center Report.* 1997 Nov–Dec; 27(6): 26–28.
(ANIMAL EXPERIMENTATION; BIOMEDICAL RESEARCH; ETHICISTS AND ETHICS COMMITTEES)

Dresser, Rebecca. Setting priorities for science support. *Hastings Center Report.* 1998 May–Jun; 28(3): 21–23.
(BIOMEDICAL RESEARCH; RESOURCE ALLOCATION)

Dresser, Rebecca; Astrow, Alan B. An alert and incompetent self: the irrelevance of advance directives. [Case study and commentaries]. *Hastings Center Report.* 1998 Jan–Feb; 28(1): 28–30.
(ADVANCE DIRECTIVES; ALLOWING TO DIE; INFORMED CONSENT)

Dresser, Rebecca; Whitehouse, Peter. Emergency research and research involving subjects with cognitive impairment: ethical connections and contrasts. [Editorial]. *Journal of the American Geriatrics Society.* 1997 Apr; 45(4): 521–523.
(HUMAN EXPERIMENTATION/INFORMED CONSENT; HUMAN EXPERIMENTATION/SPECIAL POPULATIONS)

Dresser, Rebecca see **Orlans, F. Barbara**

Dresser, Rebecca see **Quill, Timothy E.**

Dreyer, Nancy A. see **DeGroot, Leslie J.**

Drooker, Martin see **Strain, James J.**

Drought, Theresa S. see **Davis, Anne J.**

Dubler, Nancy Neveloff. Mediation and managed care. *Journal of the American Geriatrics Society.* 1998 Mar;

46(3): 359–364.
(HEALTH CARE/ECONOMICS)

Dubler, Nancy Neveloff see Lane, Arline

Dubler, Nancy Neveloff see Post, Linda Farber

DuChane, Janeen see Hsu, Irene

DudokdeWit, A.C.; Tibben, A.; Duivenvoorden, H.J.; Frets, P.G.; Zoeteweij, M.W.; Losekoot, M.; van Haeringen, A.; Niermeijer, M.F.; Passchier, J. Psychological distress in applicants for predictive DNA testing for autosomal dominant, heritable, late onset disorders. [For the Rotterdam/Leiden Genetics Workgroup]. *Journal of Medical Genetics.* 1997 May; 34(5): 382–390.
(GENETIC SCREENING)

Duffy, Barbara; Brent, Nancy J.; Pfaadt, Mary Joyce; Rooney, Anne L. What to do about Harry? [Case study and commentaries]. *Home Healthcare Nurse.* 1996 Jun; 14(6): 420–426.
(TREATMENT REFUSAL)

Duivenvoorden, H.J. see DudokdeWit, A.C.

Dukes, D.C. see Higgins, R.M.

Dull, Susan M. see McAliley, Lauren G.

Dunea, George. Death by Injection. *BMJ (British Medical Journal).* 1998 May 2; 316(7141): 1394.
(CAPITAL PUNISHMENT)

Dunlop, Robert see Bernabei, Roberto

Dunn, Earl V. see Ferris, Lorraine E.

Dunn, Patrick M. see White, Jocelyn C.

Dunphy, Kilian; Finlay, Ilora; Rathbone, Gillian; Gilbert, James; Hicks, Fiona. Rehydration in palliative and terminal care: if not -- why not? *Palliative Medicine.* 1995 Jul; 9(3): 221–228.
(TERMINAL CARE)

Durand, Andre Mark see Love, Susan M.

Durant, John, ed. Biotechnology in Public: A Review of Recent Research. London: Science Museum for the European Federation of Biotechnology; 1992. 201 p.
(GENETIC INTERVENTION)

Durchslag, Melvyn R. see Mehlman, Maxwell J.

Durfy, Sharon J.; Page, Andrea; Eng, Barry; Chang, Patricia L.; Waye, John S. Attitudes of high school students toward carrier screening and prenatal diagnosis of cystic fibrosis. *Journal of Genetic Counseling.* 1994 Jun; 3(2): 141–155.
(GENETIC SCREENING; MASS SCREENING; PRENATAL DIAGNOSIS)

Durna, Eva M.; Bebe, Judy; Steigrad, Stephen J.; Leader, Leo R.; Garrett, Don G. Donor insemination: attitudes of parents towards disclosure. *Medical Journal of Australia.* 1997 Sep 1; 167(5): 256–259.
(ARTIFICIAL INSEMINATION)

Dushenko, Terrance W. see Adair, John G.

Duster, Troy. Persistence and continuity in human genetics and social stratification. *In:* Peters, Ted, ed. Genetics: Issues of Social Justice. Cleveland, OH: Pilgrim Press; 1998: 218–238.
(BEHAVIORAL GENETICS; EUGENICS)

Dveirin, Keith see Yaes, Robert J.

Dvorak, Eileen McQuaid see Hughes, Katharine Kostbade

Dvorchik, Igor see Marsh, J. Wallis

Dworkin, Ronald. Justice in the distribution of health care. *McGill Law Journal.* 1993; 38(4): 883–898.
(HEALTH CARE/ECONOMICS; RESOURCE ALLOCATION)

Dworkin, Ronald; Nagel, Thomas; Nozick, Robert; Rawls, John; Scanlon, Thomas; Thomson, Judith Jarvis. Assisted suicide: the philosophers' brief. *New York Review of Books.* 1997 Mar 27: 41–47.
(SUICIDE)

Dwyer, Susan; Feinberg, Joel. The Problem of Abortion. Third Edition. Belmont, CA: Wadsworth; 1997. 243 p.
(ABORTION)

Dyck, Arthur J. Eugenics in historical and ethical perspective. *In:* Kilner, John F.; Pentz, Rebecca D.; Young, Frank E., eds. Genetic Ethics: Do the Ends Justify the Genes? Grand Rapids, MI: W.B. Eerdmans; 1997: 25–39.
(EUGENICS)

Dyer, Allen R. Ethics, advertising, and assisted reproduction: the goals and methods of advertising. *Women's Health Issues.* 1997 May–Jun; 7(3): 143–148.
(HEALTH CARE/ECONOMICS)

Dyer, Allen R. see Goldworth, Amnon

Dyer, Clare. Appeal court rules against compulsory caesarean sections. [News]. *BMJ (British Medical Journal).* 1997 Apr 5; 314(7086): 993.
(TREATMENT REFUSAL)

Dyer, Clare. British court allows terminally ill baby to die. [News]. *BMJ (British Medical Journal).* 1997 Nov 29; 315(7120): 1398.
(ALLOWING TO DIE/INFANTS)

Dyer, Clare. Cardiologist admits research misconduct. [News]. *BMJ (British Medical Journal).* 1997 May 24; 314(7093): 1501.
(FRAUD AND MISCONDUCT)

Dyer, Clare. Consultant struck off over research fraud. [News]. *BMJ (British Medical Journal).* 1997 Jul 26; 315(7102): 205.
(FRAUD AND MISCONDUCT; HUMAN EXPERIMENTATION/FOREIGN COUNTRIES)

Dyer, Clare. Consultant suspended for not getting consent for cardiac procedure. [News]. *BMJ (British Medical Journal).* 1998 Mar 28; 316(7136): 955.
(FRAUD AND MISCONDUCT; INFORMED CONSENT)

Dyer, Clare. Court confirms right to palliative treatment

for mental distress. [News]. *BMJ (British Medical Journal).* 1997 Nov 8; 315(7117): 1178.
(TERMINAL CARE)

Dyer, Clare. Doctors accused of refusing transplant on moral grounds. [News]. *BMJ (British Medical Journal).* 1997 May 10; 314(7091): 1370.
(ORGAN AND TISSUE TRANSPLANTATION; SELECTION FOR TREATMENT)

Dyer, Clare. Government reviews law on "posthumous conceptions." [News]. *BMJ (British Medical Journal).* 1997 Oct 4; 315(7112): 834.
(ARTIFICIAL INSEMINATION)

Dyer, Clare. Gynaecologist admonished for removing ovaries without consent. [News]. *BMJ (British Medical Journal).* 1997 Oct 4; 315(7112): 832.
(FRAUD AND MISCONDUCT; INFORMED CONSENT)

Dyer, Clare. High court detains girl with anorexia. [News]. *BMJ (British Medical Journal).* 1997 Mar 22; 314(7084): 850.
(INVOLUNTARY COMMITMENT/FOREIGN COUNTRIES; INVOLUNTARY COMMITMENT/MINORS)

Dyer, Clare. Hillsborough survivor emerges from permanent vegetative state. [News]. *BMJ (British Medical Journal).* 1997 Apr 5; 314(7086): 996.
(ALLOWING TO DIE)

Dyer, Clare. Judge misled over call for caesarean operation. [News]. *BMJ (British Medical Journal).* 1998 Feb 21; 316(7131): 574.
(TREATMENT REFUSAL)

Dyer, Clare. Living wills put on statutory footing. [News]. *BMJ (British Medical Journal).* 1998 Jan 3; 316(7124): 9.
(ADVANCE DIRECTIVES)

Dyer, Clare. New safeguards planned for psychiatric patients. [News]. *BMJ (British Medical Journal).* 1998 Jul 4; 317(7150): 7.
(INVOLUNTARY COMMITMENT/FOREIGN COUNTRIES)

Dyer, Clare. Newcastle GP charged with murder. [News]. *BMJ (British Medical Journal).* 1998 Jun 20; 316(7148): 1849.
(EUTHANASIA/LEGAL ASPECTS)

Dyer, Clare. PVS criteria put under spotlight. [News]. *BMJ (British Medical Journal).* 1997 Mar 29; 314(7085): 919.
(ALLOWING TO DIE/LEGAL ASPECTS)

Dyer, Clare. Scottish inquiry vindicates decision not to resuscitate baby. [News]. *BMJ (British Medical Journal).* 1997 Jul 5; 315(7099): 9.
(ALLOWING TO DIE/INFANTS)

Dyer, Clare. Surrogate mother refuses to give up baby. [News]. *BMJ (British Medical Journal).* 1997 Jan 25; 314(7076): 250.
(SURROGATE MOTHERS)

Dyer, Clare. Thousands of patients may be being detained illegally. [News]. *BMJ (British Medical Journal).* 1998 Feb 14; 316(7130): 497.
(INVOLUNTARY COMMITMENT/FOREIGN COUNTRIES)

Dyer, Clare. Tobacco company set up network of sympathetic scientists. [News]. *BMJ (British Medical Journal).* 1998 May 23; 316(7144): 1555.
(BIOMEDICAL RESEARCH)

Dyer, Clare. Trusts face damages after forcing women to have ceasareans. [News]. *BMJ (British Medical Journal).* 1998 May 16; 316(7143): 1480.
(TREATMENT REFUSAL)

Dyer, Clare. Two doctors confess to helping patients to die. [News]. *BMJ (British Medical Journal).* 1997 Jul 26; 315(7102): 206.
(EUTHANASIA)

Dyer, Clare. UK public calls for legislation over living wills. [News]. *BMJ (British Medical Journal).* 1998 Mar 28; 316(7136): 959.
(ADVANCE DIRECTIVES)

Dyer, Clare. Woman can challenge hospital over forced caesarean. [News]. *BMJ (British Medical Journal).* 1997 Jul 12; 315(7100): 78.
(TREATMENT REFUSAL)

Dykeman, Mary Jane see **Etchells, Edward**

Dyson, Anthony O. Reflections on method in theology and genetics: from suspicion to critical cooperation. *In:* Becker, Gerhold K., ed. Changing Nature's Course: The Ethical Challenge of Biotechnology. Hong Kong: Hong Kong University Press; 1996: 159–169.
(BIOETHICS; GENETIC INTERVENTION)

E

Eagle, Kim A. see **Giugliano, Robert P.**

Eaton, Stephanie. The subtle politics of organ donation: a proposal. *Journal of Medical Ethics.* 1998 Jun; 24(3): 166–170.
(ORGAN AND TISSUE DONATION; ORGAN AND TISSUE TRANSPLANTATION; RESOURCE ALLOCATION/BIOMEDICAL TECHNOLOGIES; SELECTION FOR TREATMENT)

Eber, George. End-of-life decision making: an authentic Christian death. *Christian Bioethics.* 1997 Dec; 3(3): 183–187.
(ALLOWING TO DIE/RELIGIOUS ASPECTS)

Eberle, Catherine see **Gertner, Eric J.**

Eckert, George J. see **Dexter, Paul R.**

Eddleman, Keith A. see **Lescale, Keith B.**

Eddy, David M. see **Burt, R.A.P.**

Edgar, A. Health care allocation, public consultation and the concept of 'health'. *Health Care Analysis.* 1998 Sep; 6(3): 193–198.
(HEALTH; HEALTH CARE; RESOURCE ALLOCATION)

Edgar, Andrew. Quality of life indicators. *In:* Chadwick, Ruth, ed. Encyclopedia of Applied Ethics, Volume 3. San Diego, CA: Academic Press; 1998: 759–776.
(HEALTH; RESOURCE ALLOCATION)

Edgar, Andrew; Salek, Sam; Shickle, Darren; Cohen, David. The Ethical QALY: Ethical Issues in Healthcare

Resource Allocations. Haslemere, Surrey, England: Euromed Communications; 1998. 168 p.
(HEALTH CARE/FOREIGN COUNTRIES; RESOURCE ALLOCATION)

Edmonds, Polly see **Smith, Anthony M.**

Edmunds, M.E. see **Higgins, R.M.**

Edwards, Griffith. Should industry sponsor research? If the drinks industry does not clean up its act, pariah status is inevitable. *BMJ (British Medical Journal).* 1998 Aug 1; 317(7154): 336.
(BIOMEDICAL RESEARCH)

Edwards, Rem B., ed. Advances in Bioethics. Volume 2: New Essays on Abortion and Bioethics. Greenwich, CT: JAI Press; 1997. 346 p.
(ABORTION)

Edwards, Rem B. Public funding of abortions and abortion counseling for poor women. *In:* Edwards, Rem B., ed. Advances in Bioethics. Volume 2: New Essays on Abortion and Bioethics. Greenwich, CT: JAI Press; 1997: 303–334.
(ABORTION/FINANCIAL SUPPORT)

Edwards, Rem B. see **Shelton, Wayne N.**

Edwards, S.J.L.; Lilford, R.J.; Braunholtz, David; Jackson, Jennifer. Why "underpowered" trials are not necessarily unethical. *Lancet.* 1997 Sep 13; 350(9080): 804–807.
(HUMAN EXPERIMENTATION/RESEARCH DESIGN)

Egan, Timothy. Assisted suicide comes full circle, to Oregon. [News]. *New York Times.* 1997 Oct 26: 1, 25.
(SUICIDE)

Egan, Timothy. No one rushing in Oregon to use a new suicide law: doctors and pharmacists ponder their role. [News]. *New York Times.* 1998 Mar 15: 18.
(SUICIDE)

Egan, Timothy. Right to die: in Oregon, opening a new front in the world of medicine. [News]. *New York Times.* 1997 Nov 6: A26.
(SUICIDE)

Egan, Timothy. Threat from Washington has chilling effect on Oregon law allowing assisted suicide. [News]. *New York Times.* 1997 Nov 19: A18.
(SUICIDE)

Egbert, Lawrence D. Physicians and the death penalty. *America.* 1998 Mar 7; 178(7): 15–16.
(CAPITAL PUNISHMENT)

Ehleben, Carole M.; Childs, Brian H.; Saltzman, Steven L. HEC self assessment: what is it exactly that you do? A "snapshot" of an ethicist at work. *HEC (HealthCare Ethics Committee) Forum.* 1998 Mar; 10(1): 71–74.
(ETHICISTS AND ETHICS COMMITTEES)

Eidelman, Leonid A. see **Sprung, Charles L.**

Eisenberg, Rebecca S. Genomic patents and product development incentives. *In:* Knoppers, Bartha Maria, ed. Human DNA: Law and Policy: International and Comparative Perspectives. Proceedings of the First International Conference on DNA Sampling and Human Genetic Research: Ethical, Legal, and Policy Aspects, held in Montreal, Canada, 6–8 Sep 1996. Boston, MA: Kluwer Law International; 1997: 373–378.
(GENOME MAPPING; PATENTING LIFE FORMS)

Eisenberg, Rebecca S. Proprietary rights and the norms of science in biotechnology research. *Yale Law Journal.* 1987 Dec; 97(2): 177–231.
(BIOMEDICAL RESEARCH; PATENTING LIFE FORMS; RECOMBINANT DNA RESEARCH)

Eisenberg, Rebecca S. see **Heller, Michael A.**

Eisenberg, Ruth see **Rubenstein, William B.**

Eisendrath, Charles R. Used body parts: buy, sell or swap? *Transplantation Proceedings.* 1992 Oct; 24(5): 2212–2214.
(ORGAN AND TISSUE DONATION)

Eiser, Arnold R. Withdrawal from dialysis: the role of autonomy and community-based values. *American Journal of Kidney Diseases.* 1996 Mar; 27(3): 451–457.
(ALLOWING TO DIE; TREATMENT REFUSAL)

Elbourne, Diana see **Snowdon, Claire**

Elder, Janet see **Goldberg, Carey**

Elkins, Thomas E.; Brown, Douglas. Ethical issues in the utilization of cesarean section. *In:* Flamm, B.L.; Quilligan, E.J., eds. Cesarean Section: Guidelines for Appropriate Utilization. New York, NY: Springer-Verlag; 1995: 191–205.
(FETUSES; PATIENT CARE; TREATMENT REFUSAL)

Eller, Thomas R. Informed consent civil actions for post-abortion psychological trauma. *Notre Dame Law Review.* 1996; 71(4): 639–670.
(ABORTION/LEGAL ASPECTS; INFORMED CONSENT)

Elles, R.G. Gene patenting. [Introduction to the joint statement of the four UK genetics societies]. *Bulletin of Medical Ethics.* 1997 Jan; No. 124: 9.
(PATENTING LIFE FORMS)

Elli, M.; Valeri, M.; Pisani, F.; Tisone, G.; Utzeri, G.; De Paolis, P.; Manca di Villahermosa, S.; Adorno, D.; Famulari, A.; Casciani, C.U. Developing countries as the major future source of living donor renal transplants. *Transplantation Proceedings.* 1992 Oct; 24(5): 2110–2111.
(ORGAN AND TISSUE DONATION; ORGAN AND TISSUE TRANSPLANTATION)

Elliott, Barbara A. see **Elliott, Thomas E.**

Elliott, Carl. Hedgehogs and hermaphrodites: toward a more anthropological bioethics. *In:* Carson, Ronald A.; Burns, Chester R., eds. Philosophy of Medicine and Bioethics: A Twenty-Year Retrospective and Critical Appraisal. Boston, MA: Kluwer Academic; 1997: 197–211.
(BIOETHICS)

Elliott, Carl. On being unprincipled: Principles of Health Care Ethics, edited by Raanan Gillon and Ann Lloyd; A Matter of Principles? Ferment in U.S. Bioethics, by Edwin R. DuBose, Ron Hamel, and Laurence J. O'Connell. [Book review essay]. *Theoretical Medicine and Bioethics.* 1998 Apr; 19(2): 153–159.

Emmons, Carol-Ann see **Meier, Diane E.**

Emmott, David. Physicians, heroes, and palliative care. [Editorial]. *Bioethics Forum.* 1997 Fall; 13(3): 3-4.
(TERMINAL CARE)

Emson, Harry E. The right to die: withdrawal of tube feeding in the persistent vegetative state in Canada. *In:* Grubb, Andrew, ed. Decision-Making and Problems of Incompetence. New York, NY: Wiley; 1994: 181-186.
(ADVANCE DIRECTIVES; ALLOWING TO DIE/LEGAL ASPECTS)

Endocrine Society. Ethical guidelines for publications of research. *Journal of Clinical Endocrinology and Metabolism.* 1996 Jan; 81(1): R1-R2.
(BIOMEDICAL RESEARCH; FRAUD AND MISCONDUCT)

Eng, Barry see **Durfy, Sharon J.**

Eng, Christine M.; Schechter, Clyde; Robinowitz, Jane; Fulop, George; Burgert, Tania; Levy, Brynn; Zinberg, Randi; Desnick, Robert J. Prenatal genetic carrier testing using triple disease screening. *JAMA.* 1997 Oct 15; 278(15): 1268-1272.
(GENETIC COUNSELING; GENETIC SCREENING)

Engelberg, Joseph see **Sekela, Michael**

Engelhardt, H. Tristram. Bioethics and the philosophy of medicine reconsidered. *In:* Carson, Ronald A.; Burns, Chester R., eds. Philosophy of Medicine and Bioethics: A Twenty-Year Retrospective and Critical Appraisal. Boston, MA: Kluwer Academic; 1997: 85-103.
(BIOETHICS)

Engelhardt, H. Tristram. Freedom and moral diversity: the moral failures of health care in the welfare state. *Social Philosophy and Policy.* 1997 Summer; 14(2): 180-196.
(HEALTH CARE/ECONOMICS; HEALTH CARE/RIGHTS)

Engelhardt, H. Tristram. Holiness, virtue, and social justice: contrasting understandings of the moral life. *Christian Bioethics.* 1997 Mar; 3(1): 3-19.
(HEALTH CARE)

Engelhardt, H. Tristram. Human nature genetically re-engineered: moral responsibilities to future generations. *In:* Agius, Emmanuel; Busuttil, Salvino, eds. Germ-Line Intervention and Our Responsibilities to Future Generations. Boston, MA: Kluwer Academic; 1998: 51-63.
(GENE THERAPY; GENETIC INTERVENTION)

Engelhardt, H. Tristram. Japanese and Western bioethics: studies in moral diversity. *In:* Hoshino, Kazumasa, ed. Japanese and Western Bioethics: Studies in Moral Diversity. Boston, MA: Kluwer Academic; 1997: 1-10.
(BIOETHICS)

Engelhardt, H. Tristram. Medical decisions in a context of conflicts. *Chest.* 1985 Sep; 88(3, Suppl.): 172S-174S.
(ALLOWING TO DIE)

Engelhardt, H. Tristram. Moral puzzles concerning the human genome: Western taboos, intuitions, and beliefs at the end of the Christian era. *In:* Hoshino, Kazumasa, ed. Japanese and Western Bioethics: Studies in Moral Diversity. Boston, MA: Kluwer Academic; 1997: 181-186.

(BIOETHICS; GENETIC INTERVENTION)

Engelhardt, H. Tristram see **Mattox, Kenneth L.**

Englert, Yvon, ed. Organ and Tissue Transplantation in the European Union: Management of Difficulties and Health Risks Linked to Donors. Boston, MA: Martinus Nijhoff; sold and distributed in the U.S. and Canada by Kluwer Academic Publishers; 1995. 202 p.
(ORGAN AND TISSUE DONATION; ORGAN AND TISSUE TRANSPLANTATION)

English, Dan C. Surgeon's role in ethical decisions. *American Surgeon.* 1985 Jul; 51(7): 423-425.
(PATIENT CARE)

English, V.; Sommerville, A.; Brinsden, P.R. Surrogacy. *In:* Shenfield, F.; Sureau, C., eds. Ethical Dilemmas in Assisted Reproduction. New York, NY: Parthenon Pub. Group; 1997: 31-40.
(SURROGATE MOTHERS)

Enríquez, Juan. Genomics and the world's economy. [News]. *Science.* 1998 Aug 14; 281(5379): 925-926.
(GENETIC RESEARCH)

Enserink, Martin. Dutch pull the plug on cow cloning. [News]. *Science.* 1998 Mar 6; 279(5356): 1444.
(CLONING; GENETIC INTERVENTION)

Enserink, Martin. Physicians wary of scheme to pool Icelanders' genetic data. [News]. *Science.* 1998 Aug 14; 281(5379): 890-891.
(GENETIC RESEARCH)

Ensink, K. see **Henley, L.**

Entwistle, Vikki A.; Renfrew, Mary J.; Yearley, Steven; Forrester, John; Lamont, Tara. Lay perspectives: advantages for health research. *BMJ (British Medical Journal).* 1998 Feb 7; 316(7129): 463-466.
(HEALTH CARE)

Epstein, Ronald M.; Morse, Diane S.; Frankel, Richard M.; Frarey, Lisabeth; Anderson, Kathryn; Beckman, Howard B. Awkward moments in patient-physician communication about HIV risk. *Annals of Internal Medicine.* 1998 Mar 15; 128(6): 435-442.
(AIDS/HEALTH PERSONNEL; PROFESSIONAL PATIENT RELATIONSHIP)

Erickson-Nesmith, Sharon see **Lewthwaite, Barbara**

Eriksson, Bengt Erik see **Nikku, Nina**

Ernst, Edzard. Killing in the name of healing: the active role of the German medical profession during the Third Reich. *American Journal of Medicine.* 1996 May; 100(5): 579-581.
(EUGENICS; FRAUD AND MISCONDUCT)

Espinoza, Leslie G. Dissecting women, dissecting law: the court-ordering of caesarean section operations and the failure of informed consent to protect women of color. *National Black Law Journal.* 1994; 13: 211-237.
(FETUSES; INFORMED CONSENT; TREATMENT REFUSAL)

Esteban, Miguel A. see **Osuna, Eduardo**

Esterhuizen, Philip. Is the professional code still the cornerstone of clinical nursing practice? *Journal of*

Advanced Nursing. 1996 Jan; 23(1): 25–31.
(NURSING ETHICS/CODES OF ETHICS)

Etchells, Edward; Sharpe, Gilbert; Dykeman, Mary Jane; Meslin, Eric M.; Singer, Peter A. Bioethics for clinicians: 4. Voluntariness. *Canadian Medical Association Journal.* 1996 Oct 15; 155(8): 1083–1086.
(INFORMED CONSENT)

Ettershank, Kathy. Report reveals Australia's illegal sterilisations. [News]. *Lancet.* 1998 Jan 3; 351(9095): 44.
(STERILIZATION/MENTALLY DISABLED)

Ettershank, Kathy see Cordner, Stephen

European Commission. Group of Advisers on the Ethical Implications of Biotechnology. Ethical aspects of cloning techniques. *Journal of Medical Ethics.* 1997 Dec; 23(6): 349–352.
(CLONING)

European Commission. Group of Advisers on the Ethical Implications of Biotechnology see Lenoir, Noëlle

European Commission. Group of Advisers on the Ethical Implications of Biotechnology see McLaren, Anne

European Commission. Group of Advisers on the Ethical Implications of Biotechnology see Schroten, Egbert

European Forum for Good Clinical Practice. Ethics Working Party. Guidelines and Recommendations for European Ethics Committees. Brussels, Belgium: European Forum for Good Clinical Practice; 1995. 17 p.
(HUMAN EXPERIMENTATION/ETHICS COMMITTEES; HUMAN EXPERIMENTATION/FOREIGN COUNTRIES)

European Parliament. Cloning animals and human beings. [Resolution of 12 March 1997]. *Bulletin of Medical Ethics.* 1997 May; No. 128: 10–11.
(CLONING)

European Society of Intensive Care Medicine. Working Group on Ethics see Lemaire, F.

Evans, Abigail Rian. Saying no to human cloning. *In:* Cole-Turner, Ronald, ed. Human Cloning: Religious Responses. Louisville, KY: Westminister John Knox Press; 1997: 25–34.
(CLONING)

Evans, Imogen. Dealing with research misconduct in the United Kingdom: conduct unbecoming -- the MRC's approach. *BMJ (British Medical Journal).* 1998 Jun 6; 316(7146): 1728–1729.
(BIOMEDICAL RESEARCH; FRAUD AND MISCONDUCT)

Evans, Jennifer L. Are children competent to make decisions about their own deaths? *Behavioral Sciences and the Law.* 1995 Winter; 13(1): 27–41.
(ALLOWING TO DIE/LEGAL ASPECTS; TREATMENT REFUSAL/MINORS)

Evans, Lois K.; Strumpf, Neville E.; Allen-Taylor, S. Lynne; Capezuti, Elizabeth; Maislin, Greg; Jacobsen, Barbara. A clinical trial to reduce restraints in nursing homes. *Journal of the American Geriatrics Society.* 1997 Jun; 45(6): 675–681.
(BEHAVIOR CONTROL; PATIENT CARE/AGED)

Evans, Lois K. see O'Brien, Linda A.

Evans, Martyn see Holm, Søren

Evans, Roger W. Limits of chronological age as a basis for rationing health care. *Dialysis and Transplantation.* 1994 Sep; 23(9): 506–507, 510–512+.
(HEALTH CARE/ECONOMICS; PATIENT CARE/AGED; RESOURCE ALLOCATION/BIOMEDICAL TECHNOLOGIES; SELECTION FOR TREATMENT)

Evans, Virginia Cox see Huber, Ruth

Evers, Joseph C. see Byrne, Paul A.

Evertzon, Mats see Lützén, Kim

Ewart, Wendy R.; Winikoff, Beverly. Toward safe and effective medical abortion. *Science.* 1998 Jul 24; 281(5376): 520–521.
(ABORTION)

Ewens, Ann see Allison, Althea

F

Faber-Langendoen, Kathy. Death by request: assisted suicide and the oncologist. [Editorial]. *Cancer.* 1998 Jan 1; 82(1): 35–41.
(SUICIDE)

Fabick, Mary M. Ethical considerations for research on human subjects. *Plastic Surgical Nursing.* 1995 Winter; 15(4): 225–227, 231.
(HUMAN EXPERIMENTATION/REGULATION)

Fabre, J. see Briggs, J.D.

Faden, Alan I. see Sharpe, Virginia A.

Faden, Ruth. Managed care and informed consent. *Kennedy Institute of Ethics Journal.* 1997 Dec; 7(4): 377–379.
(HEALTH CARE/ECONOMICS; INFORMED CONSENT)

Faden, Ruth R. see IJesselmuiden, Carel B.

Fadiman, Anne. The Spirit Catches You and You Fall Down: A Hmong Child and Her American Doctors, and the Collision of Two Cultures. New York, NY: Farrar, Straus and Giroux; 1997. 339 p.
(PATIENT CARE/MINORS; PROFESSIONAL PATIENT RELATIONSHIP)

Fainsinger, Robin L.; Gramlich, Leah M. How often can we justify parenteral nutrition in terminally ill cancer patients? *Journal of Palliative Care.* 1997 Spring; 13(1): 48–51.
(TERMINAL CARE)

Fairbairn, Gavin. Suicide. *In:* Chadwick, Ruth, ed. Encyclopedia of Applied Ethics, Volume 4. San Diego, CA: Academic Press; 1998: 259–273.
(SUICIDE)

Fairclough, Diane L. see Emanuel, Ezekiel J.

Fairclough, Diane L. see Patenaude, Andrea Farkas

Falasca, Gerald F. see Kowalski, Edgar P.

Fallowfield, Lesley; Ford, Sarah; Lewis, Shon. No news is not good news: information preferences of patients with cancer. *Psycho–Oncology.* 1995 Oct; 4(3): 197–202.
(TRUTH DISCLOSURE)

Fals, Juan C. see Orr, Robert D.

Family Care International see Alcalá, Maria José

Famulari, A. see Elli, M.

Fan, Ruiping. Three levels of problems in cross–cultural explorations of bioethics: a methodological approach. *In:* Hoshino, Kazumasa, ed. Japanese and Western Bioethics: Studies in Moral Diversity. Boston, MA: Kluwer Academic; 1997: 189–199.
(BIOETHICS)

Fanos, Joanna H.; Johnson, John P. Barriers to carrier testing for adult cystic fibrosis sibs: the importance of not knowing. *American Journal of Medical Genetics.* 1995 Oct 23; 59(1): 85–91.
(GENETIC SCREENING)

Farber, Neil J.; Novack, Dennis H.; O'Brien, Mary K. Love, boundaries, and the patient–physician relationship. *Archives of Internal Medicine.* 1997 Nov 10; 157(20): 2291–2294.
(PROFESSIONAL PATIENT RELATIONSHIP)

Farmer, Paul. Listening for prophetic voices in medicine. *America.* 1997 Jul 5; 177(1): 8–10, 12–13.
(HEALTH CARE/ECONOMICS; RESOURCE ALLOCATION)

Farnsworth, Peter see Berger, Jeffrey T.

Farriaux, Jean–Pierre see Dhondt, Jean–Louis

Farsides, Bobbie. Palliative care -- a euthanasia–free zone? [Editorial]. *Journal of Medical Ethics.* 1998 Jun; 24(3): 149–150.
(EUTHANASIA; TERMINAL CARE)

Farsides, Bobbie see Ashcroft, Richard

Farthing, Charles F. A necessary risk: why we doctors should volunteer to try an AIDS vaccine. *Washington Post.* 1997 Oct 19: C1, C6.
(AIDS/HEALTH PERSONNEL; AIDS/HUMAN EXPERIMENTATION; HUMAN EXPERIMENTATION/SPECIAL POPULATIONS; IMMUNIZATION)

Farthing, Michael J.G. Dealing with research misconduct in the United Kingdom: an editor's response to fraudsters. *BMJ (British Medical Journal).* 1998 Jun 6; 316(7146): 1729–1731.
(BIOMEDICAL RESEARCH; FRAUD AND MISCONDUCT)

Faulkner, Ann. ABC of palliative care: communication with patients, families, and other professionals. *BMJ (British Medical Journal).* 1998 Jan 10; 316(7125): 130–132.
(TERMINAL CARE; TRUTH DISCLOSURE)

Faure, Eveline A.M. see Goldberg, Allen I.

Fayers, P.M.; Hand, D.J. Generalisation from phase III clinical trials: survival, quality of life, and health economics. *Lancet.* 1997 Oct 4; 350(9083): 1025–1027.
(HUMAN EXPERIMENTATION)

Fealy, Gerard M. Professional caring: the moral dimension. *Journal of Advanced Nursing.* 1995 Dec; 22(6): 1135–1140.
(PROFESSIONAL ETHICS; PROFESSIONAL PATIENT RELATIONSHIP)

Feenan, Dermot. Capable people: empowering the patient in the assessment of capacity. *Health Care Analysis.* 1997 Sep; 5(3): 227–236.
(INFORMED CONSENT)

Feenan, Dermot. Medical records: law, paternalism and harm. *Journal of the Royal College of Physicians of London.* 1995 Sep–Oct; 29(5): 401–404.
(PATIENT ACCESS TO RECORDS)

Fein, Esther B. Hospital deals raise concern on abortion. [News]. *New York Times.* 1997 Oct 14: B1, B10.
(ABORTION/RELIGIOUS ASPECTS)

Fein, Esther B. Medical professionals with H.I.V. keep silent, fearing reprisals. [News]. *New York Times.* 1997 Dec 21: 41, 45.
(AIDS/CONFIDENTIALITY; AIDS/HEALTH PERSONNEL)

Feinberg, Joel. Paternalism. *In:* Borchert, Donald M., ed. The Encyclopedia of Philosophy. Supplement. New York, NY: Simon and Schuster Macmillan; 1996: 390–392.
(PROFESSIONAL PATIENT RELATIONSHIP)

Feinberg, Joel see Dwyer, Susan

Feinberg, John S. A theological basis for genetic intervention. *In:* Kilner, John F.; Pentz, Rebecca D.; Young, Frank E., eds. Genetic Ethics: Do the Ends Justify the Genes? Grand Rapids, MI: W.B. Eerdmans; 1997: 183–192.
(GENE THERAPY; GENETIC INTERVENTION)

Feinman, Michael see Sher, Geoffrey

Feinstein, Alvan R. see Sledge, William H.

Feit, Marvin D. see Holosko, Michael J.

Felder, Michael. Bioethics and the HMO. *HEC (HealthCare Ethics Committee) Forum.* 1997 Dec; 9(4): 355–364.
(ETHICISTS AND ETHICS COMMITTEES)

Felder, Stefan. Costs of dying: alternatives to rationing. *Health Policy.* 1997 Feb; 39(2): 167–176.
(HEALTH CARE/ECONOMICS; PATIENT CARE/AGED; TERMINAL CARE)

Feldman, Emanuel; Wolowelsky, Joel B., eds. Jewish Law and the New Reproductive Technologies. Hoboken, NJ: Ktav; 1997. 186 p.
(REPRODUCTIVE TECHNOLOGIES)

Feldmann, Bruce Max. The immorality of nonhuman animal research. *Journal of the American Veterinary Medical Association.* 1996 Jun 1; 208(11): 1798–1801.
(ANIMAL EXPERIMENTATION)

Feldstein, Bruce D.; Ogle, Richard D. Satisfaction,

managed ethics, and the duty to design. *HEC (HealthCare Ethics Committee) Forum.* 1997 Dec; 9(4): 333–354.
(HEALTH CARE/ECONOMICS; PROFESSIONAL ETHICS)

Felice, Alex E. Guardianship by peer review in genetic engineering and biotechnology. *In:* Agius, Emmanuel; Busuttil, Salvino, eds. Germ–Line Intervention and Our Responsibilities to Future Generations. Boston, MA: Kluwer Academic; 1998: 117–129.
(GENETIC INTERVENTION; GENETIC RESEARCH)

Felten, David L. Cell transplantation and research design. [Letter]. *Science.* 1994 Mar 18; 263(5153): 1546.
(HUMAN EXPERIMENTATION/RESEARCH DESIGN; ORGAN AND TISSUE TRANSPLANTATION)

Fenigsen, Richard. Dutch euthanasia revisited. *Issues in Law and Medicine.* 1997 Winter; 13(3): 301–311.
(EUTHANASIA; SUICIDE)

Fenigsen, Richard. Physician–assisted death in the Netherlands: impact on long–term care. *Issues in Law and Medicine.* 1995 Winter; 11(3): 283–297.
(ALLOWING TO DIE; EUTHANASIA; HEALTH CARE/FOREIGN COUNTRIES; PATIENT CARE/AGED)

Fentem, Julia H. see **Balls, Michael**

Fenwick, Andrea J. Applying best interests to persistent vegetative state –– a principled distortion? *Journal of Medical Ethics.* 1998 Apr; 24(2): 86–92.
(ALLOWING TO DIE/LEGAL ASPECTS)

Ferguson, James R. Biomedical research and insider trading. *New England Journal of Medicine.* 1997 Aug 28; 337(9): 631–634.
(BIOMEDICAL RESEARCH; CONFIDENTIALITY/LEGAL ASPECTS)

Ferguson, Jeffrey A.; Weinberger, Morris; Westmoreland, Glenda R.; Mamlin, Lorrie A.; Segar, Douglas S.; Greene, James Y.; Martin, Douglas K.; Tierney, William M. Racial disparity in cardiac decision making: results from patient focus groups. *Archives of Internal Medicine.* 1998 Jul 13; 158(13): 1450–1453.
(PATIENT CARE)

Ferguson, Pamela R. Causing death or allowing to die? Developments in the law. *Journal of Medical Ethics.* 1997 Dec; 23(6): 368–372.
(ALLOWING TO DIE/LEGAL ASPECTS; EUTHANASIA/LEGAL ASPECTS)

Ferguson, Ronald M. see **Daar, A.S.**

Fernandez, H. see **Kazim, E.**

Ferrell, Betty R. The role of ethics committees in responding to the moral outrage of unrelieved pain. *Bioethics Forum.* 1997 Fall; 13(3): 11–16.
(ETHICISTS AND ETHICS COMMITTEES; PATIENT CARE)

Ferrell, Peter see **Davis, Fran**

Ferris, Lorraine E. Protecting the public from risk of harm: Ontario's forthcoming regulatory law protects doctors, public, and the patient. [Editorial]. *BMJ (British Medical Journal).* 1998 Apr 4; 316(7137): 1033–1034.
(CONFIDENTIALITY/LEGAL ASPECTS)

Ferris, Lorraine E.; Norton, Peter G.; Dunn, Earl V.; Gort, Elaine H.; Degani, Naushaba. Guidelines for managing domestic abuse when male and female partners are patients of the same physician. [For the Delphi Panel and the Consulting Group]. *JAMA.* 1997 Sep 10; 278(10): 851–857.
(PATIENT CARE; PROFESSIONAL PATIENT RELATIONSHIP)

Festing, Michael F.W. see **Balls, Michael**

Fetters, Michael see **Doukas, David J.**

Fetters, Michael D. The family in medical decision making: Japanese perspectives. *Journal of Clinical Ethics.* 1998 Summer; 9(2): 132–146.
(INFORMED CONSENT; TRUTH DISCLOSURE)

Field, Howard L. Organ allocation. [Letter; title supplied]. *Journal of Clinical Ethics.* 1997 Summer; 8(2): 208.
(ORGAN AND TISSUE TRANSPLANTATION; RESOURCE ALLOCATION/BIOMEDICAL TECHNOLOGIES; SELECTION FOR TREATMENT)

Field, Marilyn J.; Cassel, Christine K., eds.; Institute of Medicine. Committee on Care at the End of Life. Approaching Death: Improving Care at the End of Life. [Report]. Washington, DC: National Academy Press; 1997. 437 p.
(TERMINAL CARE)

Field, Marilyn J. see **Donaldson, Molla S.**

Fielder, John. Ethical experts and *Dr. Ethics. IEEE Engineering in Medicine and Biology Magazine.* 1993 Dec; 12(4): 116–119.
(BIOETHICS/EDUCATION)

Fielder, John H. Patenting biotechnology: ethical and philosophical issues. *IEEE Engineering in Medicine and Biology Magazine.* 1997 Nov–Dec; 16(6): 118–120.
(GENETIC INTERVENTION; PATENTING LIFE FORMS)

Fielding, Ellen Wilson. Fear of cloning. *Human Life Review.* 1997 Spring; 23(2): 15–22.
(CLONING)

Figar, Silvana see **Bradley, Peter**

Finch, Caleb E. see **Williams, Carter Catlett**

Finch, Michael see **Kane, Rosalie A.**

Fincher, Ruth–Marie E. see **Roberts, Alan**

Fine, Beth A. Genetic counseling and women. *Women's Health Issues.* 1997 Jul–Aug; 7(4): 220–224.
(GENETIC COUNSELING)

Fineberg, H.V. see **Bach, F.H.**

Fineberg, Harvey V. see **Bach, Fritz H.**

Fineschi, Vittorio; Turillazzi, Emanuela; Cateni, Cecilia. The new Italian code of medical ethics. *Journal of Medical Ethics.* 1997 Aug; 23(4): 239–244.
(BIOETHICS; MEDICAL ETHICS/CODES OF ETHICS)

Finetti, Marco. Second careers of the Nazis' doctors. [Book review essay]. *Nature.* 1997 Dec 4; 390(6659): 457–458.

Foster, Claire. Research ethics committees. *In:* Chadwick, Ruth, ed. Encyclopedia of Applied Ethics, Volume 3. San Diego, CA: Academic Press; 1998: 845–852.
(HUMAN EXPERIMENTATION/ETHICS COMMITTEES)

Foster, F. Gordon see **Roth, Loren**

Foster, George E.; Bailey, R. Norman; Werner, D. Leonard; Roth, Michael S.; Sterling, John; Classé, John G.; Haffner, Alden N.; Creasey, Larry; Walls, Lesley L.; Marenco, Marc. Code of ethics: to keep the visual welfare of the patient uppermost at all times. *Journal of the American Optometric Association.* 1994 Jun; 65(6): 389, 391–395, 397–398+.
(PROFESSIONAL ETHICS)

Foster, Peggy; Anderson, C. Mary. Reaching targets in the national cervical screening programme: are current practices unethical? *Journal of Medical Ethics.* 1998 Jun; 24(3): 151–157.
(INFORMED CONSENT; MASS SCREENING)

Fournier, Keith A.; Watkins, William D. In Defense of Life. Colorado Springs, CO: NavPress; 1996. 159 p.
(ABORTION/RELIGIOUS ASPECTS; ALLOWING TO DIE/INFANTS; ALLOWING TO DIE/RELIGIOUS ASPECTS; EUTHANASIA/RELIGIOUS ASPECTS; SUICIDE)

Fowler, Cynthia see **Barnhart, J. Marie**

Fowler, Marsha. Nursing's ethics. *In:* Davis, Anne J.; Aroskar, Mila A.; Liaschenko, Joan; Drought, Theresa S. Ethical Dilemmas and Nursing Practice. Fourth Edition. Stamford, CT: Appleton and Lange; 1997: 17–34.
(NURSING ETHICS)

Fox, Daniel M. Managed care: the third reorganization of health care. *Journal of the American Geriatrics Society.* 1998 Mar; 46(3): 314–317.
(HEALTH CARE/ECONOMICS)

Fox, Jeffrey L. Green light for gene therapy in healthy volunteers. [News]. *Nature Biotechnology.* 1997 Apr; 15(4): 314.
(GENE THERAPY; HUMAN EXPERIMENTATION/REGULATION)

Fox, Mark D.; McGee, Glenn; Caplan, Arthur. Paradigms for clinical ethics consultation practice. *Cambridge Quarterly of Healthcare Ethics.* 1998 Summer; 7(3): 308–314.
(BIOETHICS; ETHICISTS AND ETHICS COMMITTEES)

Fox, Michael W. Genetic engineering and biomedical research. *In: his* Eating with Conscience: The Bioethics of Food. Troutdale, OR: NewSage Press; 1997: 85–103, 185.
(GENETIC INTERVENTION)

Fox, Renée C. Regulated commercialism of vital organ donation: a necessity? Con. *Transplantation Proceedings.* 1993 Feb; 25(1): 55–57.
(ORGAN AND TISSUE DONATION)

Fox, Renée C.; DeVries, Raymond. Afterword: the sociology of bioethics. *In:* DeVries, Raymond; Subedi, Janardan, eds. Bioethics and Society: Constructing the Ethical Enterprise. Upper Saddle River, NJ: Prentice Hall; 1998: 270–276.

(BIOETHICS)

Fracica, Phil see **Heffner, John E.**

Frader, Joel see **Bartholome, William G.**

Frader, Joel see **Bosk, Charles L.**

Frader, Joel E.; Caniano, Donna A. Research and innovation in surgery. *In:* McCullough, Laurence B.; Jones, James W.; Brody, Baruch A., eds. Surgical Ethics. New York, NY: Oxford University Press; 1998: 216–241.
(HUMAN EXPERIMENTATION)

Frader, Joel E.; Watchko, Jon. Futility issues in pediatrics. *In:* Zucker, Marjorie B.; Zucker, Howard D., eds. Medical Futility and the Evaluation of Life–Sustaining Interventions. New York, NY: Cambridge University Press; 1997: 48–57.
(ALLOWING TO DIE; ALLOWING TO DIE/INFANTS)

France. National Ethics Advisory Committee for the Biological and Health Sciences (Comité Consultatif National d'Éthique pour les Sciences de la Vie et de la Santé). Reply to the President of the French Republic on the Subject of Reproductive Cloning [Report No. 54]. [English translation]. Internet Web Site: http://www.ccne-ethique.org/ccne—uk/avis/a—054.htm; 1997 Apr 22 [online]. 25 p.
(CLONING)

Francis, L.P. see **Jacobson, Jay A.**

Francis, Leslie Pickering. Assisted suicide: are the elderly a special case? *In:* Battin, Margaret P.; Rhodes, Rosamond; Silvers, Anita, eds. Physician Assisted Suicide: Expanding the Debate. New York, NY: Routledge; 1998: 75–90.
(SUICIDE)

Francis, Paul S. see **Crenshaw, Wesley B.**

Frank, Arthur W. Enacting illness stories: when, what, and why. *In:* Nelson, Hilde Lindemann, ed. Stories and Their Limits: Narrative Approaches to Bioethics. New York, NY: Routledge; 1997: 31–49.
(BIOETHICS)

Frank, Lori see **Dellasega, Cheryl**

Frankel, M.S. Developing ethical standards for responsible research: why? form? functions? process? outcomes? *Journal of Dental Research.* 1996 Feb; 75(2): 832–835.
(BIOMEDICAL RESEARCH; FRAUD AND MISCONDUCT; PROFESSIONAL ETHICS)

Frankel, Richard see **Ventres, William**

Frankel, Richard M. see **Epstein, Ronald M.**

Franklin, Sarah. Dolly: a new form of transgenic breedwealth. *Environmental Values.* 1997 Nov; 6(4): 427–437.
(CLONING; GENETIC INTERVENTION)

Franklin, Sarah. Embodied Progress: A Cultural Account of Assisted Conception. New York, NY: Routledge; 1997. 252 p.
(IN VITRO FERTILIZATION; REPRODUCTIVE

of Medical Psychology. 1997 Mar; 70 (Pt. 1): 51–63.
(RESOURCE ALLOCATION/BIOMEDICAL TECHNOLOGIES; SELECTION FOR TREATMENT)

Furst, Lilian R. Between Doctors and Patients: The Changing Balance of Power. Charlottesville, VA: University Press of Virginia; 1998. 287 p.
(PROFESSIONAL PATIENT RELATIONSHIP)

Fuster, Valentin see **Giugliano, Robert P.**

G

Gabe, Jonathan see **Bradby, Hannah**

Gabram, Sheryl G.A. see **Philipson, Sandra J.**

Gadd, Elaine. Changing the law on decision making for mentally incapacitated adults: should advance directives have a statutory basis? [Editorial]. *BMJ (British Medical Journal).* 1998 Jan 10; 316(7125): 90.
(ADVANCE DIRECTIVES; INFORMED CONSENT/MENTALLY DISABLED)

Gadow, Sally. Ethical narratives in practice. *Nursing Science Quarterly.* 1996 Spring; 9(1): 8–9.
(PROFESSIONAL PATIENT RELATIONSHIP)

Gaeta, Theodore see **Balentine, Jerry**

Gaffney, B.; Kee, F. Are the economically active more deserving? *British Heart Journal.* 1995 Apr; 73(4): 385–389.
(SELECTION FOR TREATMENT)

Gallagher–Allred, Charlette see **Dorner, Becky**

Gallagher, Bernard; Creighton, Susan; Gibbons, Jane. Ethical dilemmas in social research: no easy solutions. *British Journal of Social Work.* 1995 Jun; 25(3): 295–311.
(BEHAVIORAL RESEARCH)

Gallagher, Eugene B.; Schlomann, Pamela; Sloan, Rebecca S.; Mesman, Jessica; Brown, Julie B.; Cholewinska, Anna. To enrich bioethics, add one part social to one part clinical. *In:* DeVries, Raymond; Subedi, Janardan, eds. Bioethics and Society: Constructing the Ethical Enterprise. Upper Saddle River, NJ: Prentice Hall; 1998: 166–191.
(BIOETHICS)

Gallagher, Eugene B. see **Sekela, Michael**

Gallagher, Hugh Gregory. FDR's Splendid Deception: The Moving Story of Roosevelt's Massive Disability –– and the Intense Efforts to Conceal It from the Public. Revised Edition. Arlington, VA: Vandamere Press; 1994. 242 p.
(CONFIDENTIALITY; HEALTH)

Galloux, Jean–Christophe. The patentability of the human genome: a European perspective. *In:* Knoppers, Bartha Maria, ed. Human DNA: Law and Policy: International and Comparative Perspectives. Proceedings of the First International Conference on DNA Sampling and Human Genetic Research: Ethical, Legal, and Policy Aspects, held in Montreal, Canada, 6–8 Sep 1996. Boston, MA: Kluwer Law International; 1997: 361–371.
(GENOME MAPPING; PATENTING LIFE FORMS)

Galton, Clare J. see **Galton, David J.**

Galton, David J.; Galton, Clare J. Francis Galton and eugenics today. *Journal of Medical Ethics.* 1998 Apr; 24(2): 99–105.
(EUGENICS; GENETIC SCREENING)

Gambassi, Giovanni see **Bernabei, Roberto**

Gambertoglio, John G. see **DeGroot, Leslie J.**

Gambia. Medical Research Council Joint Ethical Committee. Ethical issues facing medical research in developing countries. *Lancet.* 1998 Jan 24; 351(9098): 286–287.
(HUMAN EXPERIMENTATION/FOREIGN COUNTRIES)

Gannon, Philippa. Patenting human genetic material. *Bulletin of Medical Ethics.* 1997 Jan; No. 124: 33–36.
(PATENTING LIFE FORMS)

Gannon, Philippa see **Brown, Iona Jane**

Ganzini, Linda see **Hendin, Herbert**

Ganzini, Linda see **Sullivan, Mark D.**

Garcia, Jario E.; Katz, Michael. Panel two: reporting and advertising success rates –– the Gordian Knot of assisted reproductive technology. [Articles followed by discussion]. *Women's Health Issues.* 1997 May–Jun; 7(3): 188–196.
(REPRODUCTIVE TECHNOLOGIES)

Garcia, Jo see **Snowdon, Claire**

Gardner, David K. see **Meldrum, David R.**

Garey, Christopher C.; Children's Legal Rights Journal. Editorial Staff. When parents refuse consent to medical care for their children: the role of the nurse. *Children's Legal Rights Journal.* 1996 Winter; 16(1): 11–16.
(TREATMENT REFUSAL/MINORS)

Garfinkel, Mark D. see **Andrews, Lori B.**

Garrett, Don G. see **Durna, Eva M.**

Garrett, Joanne see **Hanson, Laura C.**

Garrett, Rosellen M. see **Garrett, Thomas M.**

Garrett, Thomas M.; Baillie, Harold W.; Garrett, Rosellen M. Health Care Ethics: Principles and Problems. Third Edition. Upper Saddle River, NJ: Prentice Hall; 1998. 344 p.
(BIOETHICS; PROFESSIONAL ETHICS)

Garrow, David J. The Oregon trail. *New York Times.* 1997 Nov 6: A31.
(SUICIDE)

Garthwaite, Thomas L. see **Lomax, Karen J.**

Garwin, Mark. The duty to care –– the right to refuse: changing roles of patients and physicians in end–of–life decision making. *Journal of Legal Medicine.* 1998 Mar; 19(1): 99–125.
(ALLOWING TO DIE/LEGAL ASPECTS; TREATMENT

REFUSAL)

Gastmans, Chris. Challenges to nursing values in a changing nursing environment. *Nursing Ethics.* 1998 May; 5(3): 236–245.
(NURSING ETHICS; PATIENT CARE)

Gastmans, Chris. Contemporary challenges in health care ethics. *Nursing Ethics.* 1998 Jan; 5(1): 81–83.
(BIOETHICS/EDUCATION)

Gatsonis, Constantine see **Bernabei, Roberto**

Gatter, Robert see **Andrews, Lori**

Gauthier, Candace see **Foglio, John**

Gavaghan, Helen. EU ends 10–year battle over biopatents. [News]. *Science.* 1998 May 22; 280(5367): 1188.
(PATENTING LIFE FORMS)

Gávai, M. see **Simms, Madeleine**

Gavazov, M. see **Mendez, R.**

Gazelle, Gail. The slow code -- should anyone rush to its defense? *New England Journal of Medicine.* 1998 Feb 12; 338(7): 467–469.
(RESUSCITATION ORDERS)

Gehan, Edmund see **Jaffe, Norman**

Geis, Sally B.; Messer, Donald E., eds. How Shall We Die?: Helping Christians Debate Assisted Suicide. Nashville, TN: Abingdon Press; 1997. 201 p.
(ALLOWING TO DIE/RELIGIOUS ASPECTS; EUTHANASIA/RELIGIOUS ASPECTS; SUICIDE)

Gelder, Mark S. Life and death decisions in the intensive care unit. *Cancer.* 1995 Nov 15; 76(10, Suppl.): 2171–2175.
(ALLOWING TO DIE; SELECTION FOR TREATMENT)

Geller, Gail; Botkin, Jeffrey R.; Green, Michael J.; Press, Nancy; Biesecker, Barbara B.; Wilfond, Benjamin; Grana, Generosa; Daly, Mary B.; Schneider, Katherine; Kahn, Mary Jo Ellis. Genetic testing for susceptibility to adult–onset cancer: the process and content of informed consent. *JAMA.* 1997 May 14; 277(18): 1467–1474.
(GENETIC COUNSELING; GENETIC SCREENING; INFORMED CONSENT)

Geller, Gail see **Bernhardt, Barbara A.**

Geller, Gail see **Page, David L.**

Geller, Jeffrey L. A biopsychosocial rationale for coerced community treatment in the management of schizophrenia. *Psychiatric Quarterly.* 1995 Fall; 66(3): 219–235.
(INVOLUNTARY COMMITMENT; PATIENT CARE/MENTALLY DISABLED)

Gelo, Florence; O'Connor, Bonnie; Vaught, Wayne. Should we protect families from patients? [Case study and commentaries]. *Hastings Center Report.* 1998 May–Jun; 28(3): 18–21.
(AIDS/CONFIDENTIALITY)

Geltman, Paul. Rwanda: physician complicity and rebuilding the medical community. *Lancet.* 1997 Jul 5; 350(9070): 64.
(FRAUD AND MISCONDUCT; TORTURE)

General Medical Council (Great Britain). Duties of a Doctor: Guidance from the General Medical Council. [Booklets]. London: The Council; 1995. portfolio of 4 booklets.
(AIDS/HEALTH PERSONNEL; CONFIDENTIALITY; MEDICAL ETHICS; PROFESSIONAL PATIENT RELATIONSHIP)

Genetic Nurses and Social Workers Association (Great Britain) see **Clinical Genetics Society (Great Britain)**

Gentry, Simon see **Poste, George**

George, James E.; Quattrone, Madelyn S.; Goldstone, Marc. A pediatric right to die? *Journal of Emergency Nursing.* 1995 Aug; 21(4): 341–342.
(ALLOWING TO DIE/LEGAL ASPECTS)

George, Linda K. see **Swartz, Marvin S.**

Georgia. Court of Appeals. Velez v. Bethune. *South Eastern Reporter, 2d Series.* 1995 Dec 5 (date of decision). 466: 627–635.
(ALLOWING TO DIE/INFANTS; ALLOWING TO DIE/LEGAL ASPECTS)

Gerety, Jane see **Heller, Jan C.**

German, L.G. The beginning of individual human life. *Linacre Quarterly.* 1997 May; 64(2): 94–95.
(FETUSES)

Gert, Bernard. Euthanasia. *In:* Borchert, Donald M., ed. The Encyclopedia of Philosophy. Supplement. New York, NY: Simon and Schuster Macmillan; 1996: 155–158.
(ALLOWING TO DIE; EUTHANASIA)

Gert, Bernard; Culver, Charles M.; Clouser, K. Danner. An alternative to physician–assisted suicide: a conceptual and moral analysis. *In:* Battin, Margaret P.; Rhodes, Rosamond; Silvers, Anita, eds. Physician Assisted Suicide: Expanding the Debate. New York, NY: Routledge; 1998: 182–202.
(ALLOWING TO DIE; EUTHANASIA; SUICIDE)

Gert, Bernard see **Berger, Edward M.**

Gert, Heather J. Viability. *In:* Dwyer, Susan; Feinberg, Joel, eds. The Problem of Abortion. Third Edition. Belmont, CA: Wadsworth; 1997: 118–126.
(ABORTION)

Gertner, Eric J.; Lukawski, Jolanta E.; Isaacson, Jeanne; Adams, Wendy L.; Eberle, Catherine; Hanson, Laura C.; Danis, Marion; Tulsky, James A. Care at the end of life. [Letters and response]. *Annals of Internal Medicine.* 1997 Oct 1; 127(7): 574–575.
(TERMINAL CARE)

Gervais, Karen G. Changing society, changing medicine, changing bioethics. *In:* DeVries, Raymond; Subedi, Janardan, eds. Bioethics and Society: Constructing the Ethical Enterprise. Upper Saddle River, NJ: Prentice Hall; 1998: 216–232.
(HEALTH CARE/ECONOMICS; PROFESSIONAL PATIENT RELATIONSHIP)

Gervais, Karen G. see **Burt, R.A.P.**

Gervais, Laurent see **Watler, Crosbie L.**

Getz, Marjorie see **Lowenthal, Barbara**

Gevers, J.K.M. see **Legemaate, Johan**

Gevers, Sjef; Olsthoorn-Heim, Els. DNA sampling: Dutch and other European approaches to the issues of informed consent and confidentiality. *In:* Knoppers, Bartha Maria, ed. Human DNA: Law and Policy: International and Comparative Perspectives. Proceedings of the First International Conference on DNA Sampling and Human Genetic Research: Ethical, Legal, and Policy Aspects, held in Montreal, Canada, 6–8 Sep 1996. Boston, MA: Kluwer Law International; 1997: 109–120.
(CONFIDENTIALITY; GENETIC SCREENING; INFORMED CONSENT; ORGAN AND TISSUE DONATION)

Ghusn, Husam F.; Teasdale, Thomas A.; Boyer, Kathryn. Characteristics of patients receiving or forgoing resuscitation at the time of cardiopulmonary arrest. *Journal of the American Geriatrics Society.* 1997 Sep; 45(9): 1118–1122.
(RESUSCITATION ORDERS)

Ghusn, Husam F.; Teasdale, Thomas A.; Jordan, Darlene. Continuity of do-not resuscitate orders between hospital and nursing home settings. *Journal of the American Geriatrics Society.* 1997 Apr; 45(4): 465–469.
(ADVANCE DIRECTIVES; RESUSCITATION ORDERS)

Gianakos, Dean. Accepting limits. *Archives of Internal Medicine.* 1998 May 25; 158(10): 1059–1061.
(MEDICAL ETHICS/EDUCATION; PATIENT CARE)

Giannetti, Vincent J. Experiential approach to teaching ethics. *In:* Haddad, Amy Marie, ed. Teaching and Learning Strategies in Pharmacy Ethics. Second Edition. New York, NY: Pharmaceutical Products Press; 1997: 87–99.
(PROFESSIONAL ETHICS/EDUCATION)

Gibbons, Ann. Which of our genes makes us human? [News]. *Science.* 1998 Sep 4; 281(5382): 1432–1434.
(GENOME MAPPING)

Gibbons, Jane see **Gallagher, Bernard**

Gibeaut, John. Class debates: reproductive, disability rights mix in KKK Act cases. *ABA Journal: The Lawyer's Magazine.* 1997 Aug; 83: 36–37.
(REPRODUCTION; STERILIZATION/MENTALLY DISABLED)

Gibson, Frances L. see **Bowen, Jennifer R.**

Gibson, Susanne. Abortion. *In:* Chadwick, Ruth, ed. Encyclopedia of Applied Ethics, Volume 1. San Diego, CA: Academic Press; 1998: 1–8.
(ABORTION)

Gibson, Susanne. Acts and omissions. *In:* Chadwick, Ruth, ed. Encyclopedia of Applied Ethics, Volume 1. San Diego, CA: Academic Press; 1998: 23–28.
(ALLOWING TO DIE; EUTHANASIA)

Giesen, Dieter. Comparative legal developments. *In:* Grubb, Andrew, ed. Decision-Making and Problems of Incompetence. New York, NY: Wiley; 1994: 7–26.
(INFORMED CONSENT; TREATMENT REFUSAL)

Giffels, J. Joseph. Clinical Trials: What You Should Know Before Volunteering to Be a Research Subject. [Pamphlet]. New York, NY: Demos Vermande; 1996. 43 p.
(HUMAN EXPERIMENTATION)

Gifford, Robert see **Khushf, George**

Gilbert, James see **Dunphy, Kilian**

Giles, Scott see **Neff-Smith, Martha**

Gill, Nöel see **Danziger, Renée**

Gillam, Lynn. Arguing by analogy in the fetal tissue debate. *Bioethics.* 1997 Oct; 11(5): 397–412.
(FETUSES; ORGAN AND TISSUE DONATION)

Gillett, Grant. Justice and health care in a caring society. *BMJ (British Medical Journal).* 1998 Jul 4; 317(7150): 53–54.
(HEALTH CARE/FOREIGN COUNTRIES; HEALTH CARE/RIGHTS)

Gillett, Grant. "We be of one blood, you and I": commentary on Kopelman. *In:* Carson, Ronald A.; Burns, Chester R., eds. Philosophy of Medicine and Bioethics: A Twenty-Year Retrospective and Critical Appraisal. Boston, MA: Kluwer Academic; 1997: 239–245.
(BIOETHICS)

Gillett, Grant see **Nicholas, Barbara**

Gillis, Jonathan. When lifesaving treatment in children is not the answer. [Editorial]. *BMJ (British Medical Journal).* 1997 Nov 15; 315(7118): 1246–1247.
(ALLOWING TO DIE)

Gillon, Raanan. Bioethics, overview. *In:* Chadwick, Ruth, ed. Encyclopedia of Applied Ethics, Volume 1. San Diego, CA: Academic Press; 1998: 305–317.
(BIOETHICS)

Gillon, Raanan. Clinical ethics committees -- pros and cons. [Editorial]. *Journal of Medical Ethics.* 1997 Aug; 23(4): 203–204.
(ETHICISTS AND ETHICS COMMITTEES)

Gillon, Raanan. Doctors should not try to ban boxing -- but boxing's own ethics suggests reform. [Editorial]. *Journal of Medical Ethics.* 1998 Feb; 24(1): 3–4.
(PUBLIC HEALTH)

Gillon, Raanan. "Futility" -- too ambiguous and pejorative a term? [Editorial]. *Journal of Medical Ethics.* 1997 Dec; 23(6): 339–340.
(RESUSCITATION ORDERS)

Gillon, Raanan. Persistent vegetative state, withdrawal of artificial nutrition and hydration, and the patient's "best interests". [Editorial]. *Journal of Medical Ethics.* 1998 Apr; 24(2): 75–76.
(ALLOWING TO DIE/LEGAL ASPECTS)

Gillon, Raanan see **Ashcroft, Richard**

Gillon, Raanan see **Doyal, Len**

Gillott, John. Germ line gene therapy — why not? *GenEthics News.* 1995 Nov–Dec; No. 9: 6.
(GENE THERAPY)

Gilson, Lucy see **Russell, Steven**

Ginsburg, Ruth Bader. Some thoughts on autonomy and equality in relation to Roe v. Wade. *North Carolina Law Review.* 1985 Jan; 63(2): 375–386.
(ABORTION/LEGAL ASPECTS)

Ginzburg, Harold M. The legal perspective: the duty to notify. *Pediatric AIDS and HIV Infection.* 1996 Aug; 7(4): 269–272.
(AIDS)

Girgis, Afaf; Sanson–Fisher, Rob W. Breaking bad news: consensus guidelines for medical practitioners. *Journal of Clinical Oncology.* 1995 Sep; 13(9): 2449–2456.
(TRUTH DISCLOSURE)

Gitanjali, B.; Shashindran, C.H.; Tripathi, K.D.; Sethuraman, K.R.; Christo, G.G.; Balasubramaniam, R. Are drug advertisements in Indian edition of BMJ unethical? [Article and commentary]. *BMJ (British Medical Journal).* 1997 Aug 23; 315(7106): 459–460.
(FRAUD AND MISCONDUCT; HEALTH CARE/ECONOMICS; HEALTH CARE/FOREIGN COUNTRIES; PATIENT CARE/DRUGS)

Giuffrida, Antonio; Torgerson, David J. Should we pay the patient? Review of financial incentives to enhance patient compliance. *BMJ (British Medical Journal).* 1997 Sep 20; 315(7110): 703–707.
(HEALTH CARE/ECONOMICS; PATIENT CARE)

Giugliano, Robert P.; Camargo, Carlos A.; Lloyd–Jones, Donald M.; Zagrodsky, Jason D.; Alexis, Jeffrey D.; Eagle, Kim A.; Fuster, Valentin; O'Donnell, Christopher J. Elderly patients receive less aggressive medical and invasive management of unstable angina: potential impact of practice guidelines. *Archives of Internal Medicine.* 1998 May 25; 158(10): 1113–1120.
(PATIENT CARE/AGED; SELECTION FOR TREATMENT)

Glannon, Walter. Genes, embryos, and future people. *Bioethics.* 1998 Jul; 12(3): 187–211.
(GENE THERAPY; GENETIC INTERVENTION; GENETIC SCREENING; PRENATAL DIAGNOSIS; WRONGFUL LIFE)

Glannon, Walter. Responsibility, alcoholism, and liver transplantation. *Journal of Medicine and Philosophy.* 1998 Feb; 23(1): 31–49.
(ORGAN AND TISSUE TRANSPLANTATION; RESOURCE ALLOCATION/BIOMEDICAL TECHNOLOGIES; SELECTION FOR TREATMENT)

Glantz, Leonard see **Markson, Lawrence**

Glantz, Leonard H. Legal issues in withholding or withdrawing medical treatment. [Article and discussion]. *Chest.* 1985 Sep; 88(3, Suppl.): 175S–182S.
(ALLOWING TO DIE/LEGAL ASPECTS)

Glantz, Leonard H. see **Annas, George J.**

Glass, James M. "Life Unworthy of Life": Racial Phobia and Mass Murder in Hitler's Germany. New York, NY: Basic Books; 1997. 252 p.
(EUGENICS)

Glass, Kathleen Cranley. Challenging the paradigm: stored tissue samples and access to genetic information. *In:* Knoppers, Bartha Maria, ed. Human DNA: Law and Policy: International and Comparative Perspectives. Proceedings of the First International Conference on DNA Sampling and Human Genetic Research: Ethical, Legal, and Policy Aspects, held in Montreal, Canada, 6–8 Sep 1996. Boston, MA: Kluwer Law International; 1997: 157–162.
(GENETIC SCREENING)

Glass, Kathleen Cranley. Refining definitions and devising instruments: two decades of assessing mental competence. *International Journal of Law and Psychiatry.* 1997 Winter; 20(1): 5–33.
(INFORMED CONSENT/MENTALLY DISABLED)

Glass, Nigel. Austrian medicine encouraged to confront its Nazi past. [News]. *Lancet.* 1998 Feb 7; 351(9100): 427.
(FRAUD AND MISCONDUCT)

Glass, Richard M. see **DeGroot, Leslie J.**

Glass, Richard M. see **Olson, Carin M.**

Glen, Sally. Confidentiality: a critique of the traditional view. *Nursing Ethics.* 1997 Sep; 4(5): 403–406.
(CONFIDENTIALITY)

Glover, Jacqueline see **Scanlon, Colleen**

Glover, John L. see **Piotrowski, Joseph J.**

Gluck, John P. Harry F. Harlow and animal research: reflection on the ethical paradox. *Ethics and Behavior.* 1997; 7(2): 149–161.
(ANIMAL EXPERIMENTATION; FRAUD AND MISCONDUCT)

Gluck, John P.; Orlans, F. Barbara. Institutional animal care and use committees: a flawed paradigm or work in progress? *Ethics and Behavior.* 1997; 7(4): 329–336.
(ANIMAL EXPERIMENTATION)

Gluck, John P.; Shapiro, Kenneth J. Behavioral research and animal welfare. [Case study and commentaries]. *Ethics and Behavior.* 1997; 7(2): 185–192.
(ANIMAL EXPERIMENTATION)

Gluck, John P. see **Brody, Janet L.**

Gluck, John P. see **Orlans, F. Barbara**

Godard, Béatrice; Kinsella, T. Douglas. DNA sampling and banking: practices and procedures. *In:* Knoppers, Bartha Maria, ed. Human DNA: Law and Policy: International and Comparative Perspectives.
Proceedings of the First International Conference on DNA Sampling and Human Genetic Research: Ethical, Legal, and Policy Aspects, held in Montreal, Canada, 6–8 Sep 1996. Boston, MA: Kluwer Law International; 1997: 429–434.
(GENETIC RESEARCH; GENETIC SCREENING)

Godfrey, Nelda S.; Kuehne, Dale S.; Wildes, Kevin Wm. In the care of a nurse. [Case study and commentaries]. *Hastings Center Report.* 1997 Sep–Oct; 27(5): 23–24.
(ALLOWING TO DIE; FRAUD AND MISCONDUCT; NURSING ETHICS)

Goertz, Christine see **Borowsky, Steven J.**

Goh, L.G. The do–not–resuscitate order. *Singapore Medical Journal.* 1995 Jun; 36(3): 258–259.
(RESUSCITATION ORDERS)

Gold, Hal. Unit 731: Testimony –– Japan's Wartime Human Experimentation Program. Tokyo: Yenbooks; 1996. 256 p.
(FRAUD AND MISCONDUCT; HUMAN EXPERIMENTATION/FOREIGN COUNTRIES; WAR)

Gold, Karen F. see **Sulmasy, Daniel P.**

Goldbeck–Wood, Sandra. Denmark takes a lead on research ethics. [News]. *BMJ (British Medical Journal).* 1998 Apr 18; 316(7139): 1189.
(HUMAN EXPERIMENTATION/FOREIGN COUNTRIES; HUMAN EXPERIMENTATION/REGULATION)

Goldbeck–Wood, Sandra. Scientists call for whistleblowers' charter. [News]. *BMJ (British Medical Journal).* 1997 Nov 15; 315(7118): 1252.
(BIOMEDICAL RESEARCH; FRAUD AND MISCONDUCT)

Goldbeck–Wood, Sandra. Women's autonomy in childbirth. [Editorial]. *BMJ (British Medical Journal).* 1997 Apr 19; 314(7088): 1143–1144.
(TREATMENT REFUSAL/MENTALLY DISABLED)

Goldberg, Alan M. see **Balls, Michael**

Goldberg, Allen I.; Faure, Eveline A.M.; O'Callaghan, John J. High–technology home care: critical issues and ethical choices. *In:* Monagle, John F.; Thomasma, David C., eds. Health Care Ethics: Critical Issues for the 21st Century. Gaithersburg, MD: Aspen Publishers; 1998: 146–163.
(BIOMEDICAL TECHNOLOGIES; HEALTH CARE/ECONOMICS; PATIENT CARE/MINORS)

Goldberg, Carey; Elder, Janet. Public still backs abortion, but wants limits, poll says. [News]. *New York Times.* 1998 Jan 16: A1, A16.
(ABORTION/ATTITUDES)

Goldblatt, A.D. You can't always get what you want. *Update Loma Linda University Center for Christian Bioethics.* 1997 Jul; 13(2): 5–7.
(INFORMED CONSENT; MEDICAL ETHICS/EDUCATION)

Golden, Frederic. Cock-a-doodle quail. [News]. *Time.* 1997 Mar 17; 149(11): 60.
(ANIMAL EXPERIMENTATION; ORGAN AND TISSUE TRANSPLANTATION)

Goldfarb, James; Kinzer, Donna J.; Boyle, Marian; Kurit, Doris. Attitudes of in vitro fertilization and intrauterine insemination couples toward multiple gestation pregnancy and multifetal pregnancy reduction. *Fertility and Sterility.* 1996 Apr; 65(4): 815–820.
(ABORTION/ATTITUDES; REPRODUCTIVE TECHNOLOGIES)

Goldfinger, Dennis. Controversies in transfusion medicine: directed blood donations –– pro. *Transfusion.* 1989 Jan–Feb; 29(1): 70–74.
(BLOOD DONATION)

Goldman, David. Interdisciplinary perceptions of genetics and behavior. *Politics and the Life Sciences.* 1996 Mar; 15(1): 97–98.
(BEHAVIORAL GENETICS; GENETIC RESEARCH)

Goldschmidt, Peter G. see **Burt, R.A.P.**

Goldstein, Amy. Dying patients' care varies widely by place, study says. [News]. *Washington Post.* 1997 Oct 15: A1, A8.
(TERMINAL CARE)

Goldstein, Amy. Woman alleges fiancé stole her heart, brother's kidney. [News]. *Washington Post.* 1997 Oct 21: A1, A10–A11.
(ORGAN AND TISSUE DONATION; ORGAN AND TISSUE TRANSPLANTATION)

Goldstein, Barry; Royal, Michael C.; Veatch, Robert M. Safety of an extemporaneously prepared injection. [Case study and commentaries]. *American Journal of Health–System Pharmacy.* 1996 Feb 15; 53(4): 414–417.
(PATIENT CARE/DRUGS; PROFESSIONAL ETHICS)

Goldstein, David see **Tindall, Brett**

Goldstone, Marc see **George, James E.**

Goldworth, Amnon; Verhey, Allen; Robertson, John A.; Turiel, Judy; Dyer, Allen R.; Macklin, Ruth; Scheckle, Darren; Anderick, William. The commodification and advertising of infertility treatment. *Women's Health Issues.* 1997 May–Jun; 7(3): 149–152.
(REPRODUCTIVE TECHNOLOGIES)

Goldworth, Amnon; White, Robert J.; Truog, Robert. On brain death. [Letters and response]. *Hastings Center Report.* 1997 Sep–Oct; 27(5): 4–5.
(DETERMINATION OF DEATH/BRAIN DEATH)

Golombok, Susan see **Cook, Rachel**

Golub, Edward S. Ethical considerations arising from economic aspects of human genetics. *In:* Becker, Gerhold K., ed. Changing Nature's Course: The Ethical Challenge of Biotechnology. Hong Kong: Hong Kong University Press; 1996: 71–83.
(GENETIC SCREENING)

Gonin, René see **Cleeland, Charles S.**

Gonsoulin, Thomas P. Ethical issues raised by managed care. *Laryngoscope.* 1997 Nov; 107(11, Part 1): 1425–1428.
(HEALTH CARE/ECONOMICS)

Goodare, Heather. Studies that do not have informed consent from participants should not be published. *BMJ (British Medical Journal).* 1998 Mar 28; 316(7136): 1004–1005.
(HUMAN EXPERIMENTATION/INFORMED CONSENT)

Goode, Leslie D. see **McCurdy, Layton**

Goodey, Chris. Genes that are all in the mind. *New Scientist.* 1997 Jun 7; 154(2085): 49.
(BEHAVIORAL GENETICS)

Goodey, Chris. Genetic markers for intelligence. *Bulletin of Medical Ethics.* 1996 Aug; No. 120: 13–16.
(BEHAVIORAL GENETICS; GENETIC RESEARCH)

Goodey, Christopher see **Alderson, Priscilla**

Goodhall, Lesley. Tube feeding dilemmas: can artificial nutrition and hydration be legally or ethically withheld

or withdrawn? *Journal of Advanced Nursing.* 1997 Feb; 25(2): 217–222.
(ALLOWING TO DIE)

Goodlin, Sarah J.; Winzelberg, Gary S.; Teno, Joan M.; Whedon, Marie; Lynn, Joanne. Death in the hospital. *Archives of Internal Medicine.* 1998 Jul 27; 158(14): 1570–1572.
(TERMINAL CARE)

Goodman, Danë see **Ashcroft, Richard**

Goodman, Karen see **Ohl, Dana A.**

Goodman, Kenneth W. Bioethics and health informatics: an introduction. *In:* Goodman, Kenneth W., ed. Ethics, Computing, and Medicine: Informatics and the Transformation of Health Care. New York, NY: Cambridge University Press; 1998: 1–31.
(BIOETHICS; BIOMEDICAL TECHNOLOGIES; HEALTH CARE)

Goodman, Kenneth W. Codes of ethics in occupational and environmental health. [Editorial]. *Journal of Occupational and Environmental Medicine.* 1996 Sep; 38(9): 882–883.
(PROFESSIONAL ETHICS/CODES OF ETHICS)

Goodman, Kenneth W., ed. Ethics, Computing, and Medicine: Informatics and the Transformation of Health Care. New York, NY: Cambridge University Press; 1998. 180 p.
(BIOMEDICAL TECHNOLOGIES; HEALTH CARE)

Goodman, Kenneth W. Outcomes, futility, and health policy research. *In:* Goodman, Kenneth W., ed. Ethics, Computing, and Medicine: Informatics and the Transformation of Health Care. New York, NY: Cambridge University Press; 1998: 116–138.
(BIOMEDICAL TECHNOLOGIES; SELECTION FOR TREATMENT)

Goodman, Kenneth W. see **Coughlin, Steven S.**

Goodman, Kenneth W. see **Miller, Randolph A.**

Goodmonson, Sharon see **Rossignol, Annette MacKay**

Goodwin, Frederick K.; Hadley, Suzanne W. Enhancing the climate of trust in clinical psychiatric research. *In:* Shamoo, Adil E., ed. Ethics in Neurobiological Research with Human Subjects: The Baltimore Conference on Ethics. Amsterdam: Gordon and Breach; 1997: 309–314.
(HUMAN EXPERIMENTATION/SPECIAL POPULATIONS)

Goold, Susan Dorr. Is distance critical for clinical ethicists? A reply to Glenn McGee. *HEC (HealthCare Ethics Committee) Forum.* 1997 Sep; 9(3): 280–283.
(BIOETHICS; ETHICISTS AND ETHICS COMMITTEES)

Goold, Susan Dorr see **Hendin, Herbert**

Goold, Susan Dorr see **Pellegrino, Edmund D.**

Goold, Susan Dorr see **Ubel, Peter A.**

Görbe, É. see **Simms, Madeleine**

Gordon, Benjamin D. see **DeGroot, Leslie J.**

Gordon, Bruce; Prentice, Ernest. Continuing review of research involving human subjects: approach to the

problem and remaining areas of concern. *IRB: A Review of Human Subjects Research.* 1997 Mar–Apr; 19(2): 8–11.
(HUMAN EXPERIMENTATION/ETHICS COMMITTEES; HUMAN EXPERIMENTATION/REGULATION)

Gordon, Valery M.; Sugarman, Jeremy; Kass, Nancy. Toward a more comprehensive approach to protecting human subjects: the interface of data safety monitoring boards and institutional review boards in randomized clinical trials. *IRB: A Review of Human Subjects Research.* 1998 Jan–Feb; 20(1): 1–5.
(HUMAN EXPERIMENTATION/ETHICS COMMITTEES; HUMAN EXPERIMENTATION/RESEARCH DESIGN)

Gore, Albert; Owens, Steve. The challenge of biotechnology. *Yale Law and Policy Review.* 1985 Spring; 3(2): 336–357.
(GENETIC INTERVENTION; RECOMBINANT DNA RESEARCH/REGULATION)

Gore, M.E. see **Johnston, S.R.D.**

Gorelick, Philip B. see **Harris, Yvonne**

Gorman, Christine. Body parts for sale. [News]. *Time.* 1998 Mar 9; 151(9): 76.
(CAPITAL PUNISHMENT; ORGAN AND TISSUE DONATION)

Gorman, Christine. To ban or not to ban? [News]. *Time.* 1997 Jun 16; 149(24): 66.
(CLONING)

Gort, Elaine H. see **Ferris, Lorraine E.**

Gorter, Robert see **Slome, Lee**

Gorton, Gregg E.; Samuel, Steven E. A national survey of training directors about education for prevention of psychiatrist–patient sexual exploitation. *Academic Psychiatry.* 1996 Summer; 20(2): 92–98.
(FRAUD AND MISCONDUCT; MEDICAL ETHICS/EDUCATION; PROFESSIONAL PATIENT RELATIONSHIP)

Gospodarowicz, Mary see **Narasimhan, Parthas**

Gostin, Lawrence. Health care information and the protection of personal privacy: ethical and legal considerations. *Annals of Internal Medicine.* 1997 Oct 15; 127(8, Pt. 2): 683–690.
(CONFIDENTIALITY/LEGAL ASPECTS)

Gostin, Lawrence O. Deciding life and death in the courtroom: from Quinlan to Cruzan, Glucksberg, and Vacco -- a brief history and analysis of constitutional protection of the 'right to die'. *JAMA.* 1997 Nov 12; 278(18): 1523–1528.
(ALLOWING TO DIE/LEGAL ASPECTS; SUICIDE)

Gostin, Lawrence O. Personal privacy in the health care system: employer–sponsored insurance, managed care, and integrated delivery systems. *Kennedy Institute of Ethics Journal.* 1997 Dec; 7(4): 361–376.
(CONFIDENTIALITY; HEALTH CARE/ECONOMICS; INFORMED CONSENT)

Gostin, Lawrence O.; Webber, David W. HIV infection and AIDS in the public health and health care systems: the role of law and litigation. *JAMA.* 1998 Apr 8; 279(14): 1108–1113.
(AIDS)

Gostin, Lawrence O. see **Burris, Scott**

Gostin, Lawrence O. see **Rubenstein, William B.**

Gott, Robert see **Pyers, Greg**

Gottesman, Irving I. see **Carey, Gregory**

Gottesman, Irving I. see **Sherman, Stephanie L.**

Gough, Pippa see **Savulescu, Julian**

Gourlay, Linda see **Cooke, Molly**

Graber, Glenn C. Basic theories in medical ethics. [Revised]. *In:* Monagle, John F.; Thomasma, David C., eds. Health Care Ethics: Critical Issues for the 21st Century. Gaithersburg, MD: Aspen Publishers; 1998: 515–526.
(BIOETHICS)

Graber, Glenn C. The moral status of gametes and embryos: storage and surrogacy. *In:* Monagle, John F.; Thomasma, David C., eds. Health Care Ethics: Critical Issues for the 21st Century. Gaithersburg, MD: Aspen Publishers; 1998: 8–14.
(FETUSES)

Graber, Glenn C. see **Cebik, L.B.**

Grace, Eric S. Ethical issues. *In: his* Biotechnology Unzipped: Promises and Realities. Washington, DC: Joseph Henry Press; 1997: 191–224, 237.
(GENETIC INTERVENTION)

Graham, Deborah see **Beisecker, Analee E.**

Graham, Elizabeth see **Wilkie, Tom**

Gramelspacher, Gregory P. see **Dexter, Paul R.**

Gramelspacher, Gregory P. see **Ubel, Peter A.**

Gramlich, Leah M. see **Fainsinger, Robin L.**

Grammes, C. see **Jacobson, Jay A.**

Grana, Generosa see **Geller, Gail**

Granbois, Judith A.; Smith, David H. The Anglican Communion and bioethics. *In:* Lustig, B. Andrew, ed.; Center for Medical Ethics and Health Policy (Houston, TX). Bioethics Yearbook, Volume 5: Theological Developments in Bioethics, 1992–1994. Boston, MA: Kluwer Academic; 1997: 93–122.
(BIOETHICS)

Grandjean, P. Ethical aspects of genetic predisposition to disease. *In:* Grandjean, Phillippe, ed. Ecogenetics: Genetic Predisposition to the Toxic Effects of Chemicals. New York, NY: Chapman and Hall on behalf of the World Health Organization, Regional Office for Europe; 1991: 237–251.
(GENETIC SCREENING)

Granger, Ellen see **Runkle, Deborah**

Grassin, Marc see **Howard, Philip J.**

Grassin, Marc see **Pochard, Frédéric**

Graves, Frances A. see **Churchill, Larry R.**

Grayson, Lesley. Scientific Deception: An Overview and Guide to the Literature of Misconduct and Fraud in Scientific Research. London: British Library, Science Reference and Information Service; 1995. 107 p.
(FRAUD AND MISCONDUCT)

Great Britain. Department of Health. Protection and Use of Patient Information: Guidance from the Department of Health. London: The Department; 1996 Mar. 24 p.
(CONFIDENTIALITY/LEGAL ASPECTS)

Great Britain. Department of Health. Advisory Group on the Ethics of Xenotransplantation (Chair: Ian Kennedy). Animal Tissue into Humans: A Report by the Advisory Group on the Ethics of Xenotransplantation, 1996. London: Her Majesty's Stationery Office; 1997. 258 p.
(GENETIC INTERVENTION; HUMAN EXPERIMENTATION/FOREIGN COUNTRIES; HUMAN EXPERIMENTATION/REGULATION; ORGAN AND TISSUE TRANSPLANTATION)

Great Britain. England. Court of Appeal, Civil Division. B v. Croydon Health Authority. *All England Law Reports.* 1994 Nov 29 (date of decision). [1995] 1: 683–690.
(FORCE FEEDING; TREATMENT REFUSAL/MENTALLY DISABLED)

Great Britain. England. Court of Appeal, Civil Division. R v. Human Fertilisation and Embryology Authority, ex parte Blood. *All England Law Reports.* 1997 Feb 6 (date of decision). [1997] 2: 687–704.
(ARTIFICIAL INSEMINATION)

Great Britain. England. Court of Appeal, Civil Division. Re B (A Minor) (Wardship: Medical Treatment). *All England Law Reports.* 1981 Aug 7 (date of decision). [1990] 3: 927–930.
(ALLOWING TO DIE/INFANTS; ALLOWING TO DIE/LEGAL ASPECTS)

Great Britain. England. Court of Appeal, Civil Division. Re J (A Minor) (Wardship: Medical Treatment). *All England Law Reports.* 1992 Jun 10 (date of decision). [1992] 4: 614–626.
(ALLOWING TO DIE/INFANTS; ALLOWING TO DIE/LEGAL ASPECTS)

Great Britain. England. Court of Appeal, Civil Division. W v. Egdell. *All England Law Reports.* 1989 Nov 9 (date of decision). [1990] 1: 835–853.
(CONFIDENTIALITY/MENTAL HEALTH)

Great Britain. England. High Court of Justice, Queen's Bench Division. R v. Canons Park Mental Health Review Tribunal, ex parte A. *All England Law Reports.* 1993 Jul 28 (date of decision). [1994] 1: 481–494.
(INVOLUNTARY COMMITMENT/FOREIGN COUNTRIES)

Great Britain. England. High Court of Justice, Queen's Bench Division. R v. Ethical Committee of St. Mary's Hospital (Manchester) ex parte H. *Family Law Reports.* 1987 Oct 26 (date of decision). [1988] 1: 512–520.
(ETHICISTS AND ETHICS COMMITTEES; REPRODUCTIVE TECHNOLOGIES; SELECTION FOR TREATMENT)

Great Britain. Human Fertilisation and Embryology Authority. Code of Practice. London: The Authority;

1991. 1 v.
(REPRODUCTIVE TECHNOLOGIES)

Great Britain. Isle of Man. An act (Chapter No. 3) to prohibit commercial dealings in human organs intended for transplanting; to prohibit the transplanting of such organs between persons who are not genetically related; and for connected purposes. Dated 16 March 1993. (The Human Organ Transplants Act 1993). *International Digest of Health Legislation.* 1996; 47(2): 169–170.
(ORGAN AND TISSUE DONATION; ORGAN AND TISSUE TRANSPLANTATION)

Great Britain. Lord Chancellor's Department. Who Decides? Making Decisions on Behalf of Mentally Incapacitated Adults. A Consultation Paper. London: The Stationery Office; 1997 Dec. 114 p.
(PATIENT CARE/MENTALLY DISABLED)

Great Britain. Parliamentary Office of Science and Technology. The Use of Animals in Research, Development and Testing. London: Parliamentary Office of Science and Technology; 1992 Sep. 92 p.
(ANIMAL EXPERIMENTATION)

Greely, Henry T. The ethics of the Human Genome Diversity Project: the North American Regional Committee's proposed model ethical protocol. *In:* Knoppers, Bartha Maria, ed. Human DNA: Law and Policy: International and Comparative Perspectives. Proceedings of the First International Conference on DNA Sampling and Human Genetic Research: Ethical, Legal, and Policy Aspects, held in Montreal, Canada, 6–8 Sep 1996. Boston, MA: Kluwer Law International; 1997: 239–256.
(GENETIC RESEARCH; GENOME MAPPING)

Greely, Henry T. The Human Genome Diversity Project: ethical, legal, and social issues. *In:* Peters, Ted, ed. Genetics: Issues of Social Justice. Cleveland, OH: Pilgrim Press; 1998: 71–81.
(GENETIC RESEARCH; GENOME MAPPING)

Greely, Henry T. see **Badoux, John C.**

Green, Charles R.; Barnes, Deborah E.; Bero, Lisa A. Industry-funded research and conflict of interest: funding by the Center for Indoor Air Research [title supplied]. [Letter and response]. *Journal of Health Politics, Policy and Law.* 1997 Oct; 22(5): 1279–1293.
(BIOMEDICAL RESEARCH)

Green, David J. see **Jacobson, Jay A.**

Green, J.M. see **Hallowell, N.**

Green, John see **Currie, Craig**

Green, Michael J. see **Geller, Gail**

Green, Ronald M.; Pascual-Leone, Alvaro; Wasserman, Eric M. Ethical guidelines for rTMS research. *IRB: A Review of Human Subjects Research.* 1997 Mar–Apr; 19(2): 1–7.
(HUMAN EXPERIMENTATION)

Green, Ronald M.; Thomas, A. Mathew. Whose gene is it? A case discussion about familial conflict over genetic testing for breast cancer. *Journal of Genetic Counseling.* 1997 Jun; 6(2): 245–254.
(GENETIC SCREENING)

Green, Ronald M. see **Thomas, A. Mathew**

Greenberg, Daniel S. Hidden data and abuse in research come to light in the USA. [News]. *Lancet.* 1997 Oct 11; 350(9084): 1083.
(FRAUD AND MISCONDUCT; HUMAN EXPERIMENTATION; WAR)

Greenberg, Henry M. American medicine is on the right track. *JAMA.* 1998 Feb 11; 279(6): 426–428.
(HEALTH CARE/ECONOMICS)

Greenberg, Samuel I. Euthanasia and Assisted Suicide: Psychosocial Issues. Springfield, IL: Charles C. Thomas; 1997. 164 p.
(EUTHANASIA; SUICIDE)

Greene, James Y. see **Ferguson, Jeffrey A.**

Greene, James Y. see **Tierney, William M.**

Greenfeld, David G. see **Greenfeld, Dorothy A.**

Greenfeld, Dorothy A.; Ort, Sharon I.; Greenfeld, David G.; Jones, Ervin E.; Olive, David L. Attitudes of IVF parents regarding the IVF experience and their children. *Journal of Assisted Reproduction and Genetics.* 1996 Mar; 13(3): 266–274.
(IN VITRO FERTILIZATION)

Greenfield, Arnold L. see **Mowbray, Carol T.**

Greengold, Nancy L. see **Wenger, Neil S.**

Greenhouse, Linda. Assisted suicide clears a hurdle in highest court. [News]. *New York Times.* 1997 Oct 15: A1, A16.
(SUICIDE)

Greenhouse, Linda. Overturning of late-term abortion ban is let stand. [News]. *New York Times.* 1998 Mar 24: A15.
(ABORTION/LEGAL ASPECTS)

Greenhouse, Linda. U.S. appellate panel rules Ohio ban on late-term abortion is unconstitutional. [News]. *New York Times.* 1997 Nov 19: A24.
(ABORTION/LEGAL ASPECTS)

Greenspan, Francis S. see **DeGroot, Leslie J.**

Greenwald, Devra E. see **Morgenlander, Keith H.**

Gregory, Jennifer M. see **Burd, Larry**

Gregory, Wilton. The Church and the public discussion of assisted suicide. *Health Progress.* 1997 Mar–Apr; 78(2): 48–50.
(SUICIDE; TERMINAL CARE)

Greisdorf, Eliezer see **Thies, Winthrop Drake**

Grey, William. Playing God. *In:* Chadwick, Ruth, ed. Encyclopedia of Applied Ethics, Volume 3. San Diego, CA: Academic Press; 1998: 525–530.
(BIOETHICS; GENETIC INTERVENTION)

Griffin, Gilly. Alternatives in Canada. *ATLA: Alternatives to Laboratory Animals.* 1995 Nov–Dec; 23(6): 824–826.
(ANIMAL EXPERIMENTATION)

Griffin, Leslie C. Evangelium Vitae: abortion. *In:* Wildes, Kevin Wm.; Mitchell, Alan C., eds. Choosing Life: A Dialogue on *Evangelium Vitae.* Washington, DC: Georgetown University Press; 1997: 159–173.
(ABORTION/RELIGIOUS ASPECTS)

Griffiths, Lesley see Hughes, David

Grim, Pamela. The price of life. *Discover.* 1997 Sep; 18(9): 39, 41–43.
(HEALTH CARE/ECONOMICS)

Grinnell, Frederick. Truth, fairness, and the definition of scientific misconduct. *Journal of Laboratory and Clinical Medicine.* 1997 Feb; 129(2): 189–192.
(BIOMEDICAL RESEARCH; FRAUD AND MISCONDUCT)

Grinsted, J. see Andersen, C. Yding

Grisez, Germain. Difficult moral questions: may a physician remain in a group that provides immoral services? *Linacre Quarterly.* 1997 May; 64(2): 21–25.
(ABORTION/RELIGIOUS ASPECTS; CONTRACEPTION)

Grisso, Jeane Ann see O'Brien, Linda A.

Grisso, Thomas; Appelbaum, Paul S. Assessing Competence to Consent to Treatment: A Guide for Physicians and Other Health Professionals. New York, NY: Oxford University Press; 1998. 211 p.
(INFORMED CONSENT)

Grochowski, Eugene see Daugherty, Christopher

Groenhout, Ruth. Care theory and the ideal of neutrality in public moral discourse. *Journal of Medicine and Philosophy.* 1998 Apr; 23(2): 170–189.
(BIOETHICS)

Gromb, Sophie; Manciet, Gerard; Descamps, Arnaud. Ethics and law in the field of medical care for the elderly in France. *Journal of Medical Ethics.* 1997 Aug; 23(4): 233–238.
(PATIENT CARE/AGED)

Gross, Mortimer D. What do patients express as their preferences in advance directives? *Archives of Internal Medicine.* 1998 Feb 23; 158(4): 363–365.
(ADVANCE DIRECTIVES; ALLOWING TO DIE/ATTITUDES)

Gross, Rita M. see Ravindra, Ravi

Groth, Philip see Thies, Winthrop Drake

Groudine, Scott; Lumb, Philip D. First, do no harm. *Journal of Medical Ethics.* 1997 Dec; 23(6): 377–378.
(HUMAN EXPERIMENTATION/RESEARCH DESIGN)

Grover, Bonnie Kae. From both sides now: informed consent, organ transplantation, and family-based disclosure. *Law and Policy.* 1995 Apr; 17(2): 188–209.
(INFORMED CONSENT; ORGAN AND TISSUE TRANSPLANTATION)

Groves, Julian McAllister. Hearts and Minds: The Controversy over Laboratory Animals. Philadelphia, PA: Temple University Press; 1997. 230 p.
(ANIMAL EXPERIMENTATION)

Grubb, Andrew. Adult incompetent: legality of non–therapeutic procedure -- Re Y. [Comment]. *Medical*

Law Review. 1996 Summer; 4(2): 204–207.
(ORGAN AND TISSUE DONATION)

Grubb, Andrew, ed. Decision–Making and Problems of Incompetence. New York, NY: Wiley; 1994. 203 p.
(INFORMED CONSENT; INFORMED CONSENT/MENTALLY DISABLED)

Grubb, Andrew. Incompetent patient (PVS): decision–making, courts and the family -- In re Tavel. [Comment]. *Medical Law Review.* 1997 Summer; 5(2): 245–250.
(ALLOWING TO DIE/LEGAL ASPECTS)

Grubb, Andrew. Incompetent patient (PVS): withdrawal of feeding and compliance with RCP guidelines -- Re D. [Comment]. *Medical Law Review.* 1997 Summer; 5(2): 225–227.
(ALLOWING TO DIE/LEGAL ASPECTS)

Grubb, Andrew. Parental orders (Section 30) and parentage -- Re Q (Parental Order). [Comment]. *Medical Law Review.* 1996 Summer; 4(2): 207–211.
(SURROGATE MOTHERS)

Grubb, Andrew. Re B (A Minor) (Treatment and Secure Accommodation). [Comment]. *Medical Law Review.* 1997 Summer; 5(2): 233–236.
(TREATMENT REFUSAL/MINORS)

Grubb, Andrew. Refusal of treatment: competent child and parents -- Houston, Applicant. [Comment]. *Medical Law Review.* 1997 Summer; 5(2): 237–239.
(INFORMED CONSENT/MINORS; TREATMENT REFUSAL/MINORS)

Grubb, Andrew. The Human Fertilisation and Embryology (Statutory Storage Period for Embryos) Regulations 1996 (S.I. 1996 No. 375). [Comment]. *Medical Law Review.* 1996 Summer; 4(2): 211–215.
(FETUSES; IN VITRO FERTILIZATION)

Grubb, Andrew. Treatment without consent (pregnancy): adult -- Tameside and Glossop Acute Services Trust v. C.H. [Comment]. *Medical Law Review.* 1996 Summer; 4(2): 193–198.
(PATIENT CARE/MENTALLY DISABLED; TREATMENT REFUSAL/MENTALLY DISABLED)

Grubb, Andrew; Walsh, Pat; Lambe, Neil; Murrell, Trevor; Robinson, Sarah. Doctors' Views on the Management of Patients in Persistent Vegetative State (PVS): A UK Study. London: Kings College London, Centre of Medical Law and Ethics; 1997. 68 p.
(ALLOWING TO DIE/ATTITUDES; SELECTION FOR TREATMENT)

Grumbach, Kevin see Bodenheimer, Thomas S.

Grundstein–Amado, Rivka see Silberfeld, Michel

Grypdonck, Mieke see Dierckx de Casterlé, Bernadette

Guérin, Corinne see Auguste, Valérie

Guest, Stephen. Compensation for the subjects of medical research. [Letter]. *Journal of Medical Ethics.* 1997 Oct; 23(5): 328.
(HUMAN EXPERIMENTATION/FOREIGN COUNTRIES)

Guiles, Renée M.; Appelbaum, Paul S. Death in denial. [Case study and commentaries]. *Hastings Center Report.*

1997 Nov–Dec; 27(6): 23–25.
(TREATMENT REFUSAL)

Guillemin, Jeanne. Bioethics and the coming of the corporation to medicine. *In:* DeVries, Raymond; Subedi, Janardan, eds. Bioethics and Society: Constructing the Ethical Enterprise. Upper Saddle River, NJ: Prentice Hall; 1998: 60–77.
(BIOETHICS; HEALTH CARE/ECONOMICS)

Guinan, Patrick D. Has medicine lost the ethics battle? *Linacre Quarterly.* 1998 May; 65(2): 43–50.
(MEDICAL ETHICS)

Gulgolgarn, Vilaivan see **Robb, Merlin L.**

Gully, J. see **Jacobson, Jay A.**

Gunderman, Richard. Medicine and the pursuit of wealth. *Hastings Center Report.* 1998 Jan–Feb; 28(1): 8–13.
(HEALTH CARE/ECONOMICS; MEDICAL ETHICS)

Gunning, K.F.; Crowther, C.A. End of life decisions. [Letters]. *BMJ (British Medical Journal).* 1997 Nov 1; 315(7116): 1164–1165.
(EUTHANASIA)

Gunning-Schepers, Louise J. see **Stronks, Karien**

Guo, Sun-Wei; Zheng, Chang-Jiang; Li, C.C. "Gene war of the century?" [Letter]. *Science.* 1997 Dec 5; 278(5344): 1693–1694.
(GENETIC RESEARCH)

Gurewich, Victor; Johnson, James R.; Sobieraj, Jerry; McCall, Timothy B.; Levinsky, Norman G. Truth or consequences. [Letters and response]. *New England Journal of Medicine.* 1998 Aug 6; 339(6): 410–412.
(HEALTH CARE/ECONOMICS; RESOURCE ALLOCATION)

Gurman, G. see **Frisho-Lima, P.**

Guroian, Vigen. Life's Living toward Dying: A Theological and Medical-Ethical Study. Grand Rapids, MI: W.B. Eerdmans; 1996. 108 p.
(ALLOWING TO DIE/RELIGIOUS ASPECTS; EUTHANASIA/RELIGIOUS ASPECTS; TERMINAL CARE)

Gustafson, James M. Ethics: an American growth industry. *Perspectives in Biology and Medicine.* 1998 Winter; 41(2): 191–199.
(BIOETHICS)

Gustafson, James M. Where theologians and geneticists meet. *Dialog: A Journal of Theology.* 1994 Winter; 33(1): 7–16.
(GENETIC INTERVENTION)

Gutheil, Thomas G. see **Bursztajn, Harold**

Gutheil, Thomas G. see **Hoge, Steven K.**

Gutierrez, Ed. Japan's House of Representatives passes brain-death bill. [News]. *Lancet.* 1997 May 3; 349(9061): 1304.
(DETERMINATION OF DEATH/BRAIN DEATH)

Gutmann, Thomas; Land, Walter. The ethics of organ allocation: the state of debate. *Transplantation Reviews.* 1997 Oct; 11(4): 191–207.
(ORGAN AND TISSUE TRANSPLANTATION; RESOURCE

ALLOCATION/BIOMEDICAL TECHNOLOGIES; SELECTION FOR TREATMENT)

Gutscher, Heinz. Informed consent in the social sciences: agreeing to being deceived. *In:* Berthoud, Gérald; Sitter-Liver, Beat, eds. The Responsible Scholar: Ethical Considerations in the Humanities and Social Sciences. Canton, MA: Watson Publishing International; 1996: 255–269.
(BEHAVIORAL RESEARCH/INFORMED CONSENT)

Guttmann, Astrid; Guttmann, Ronald D. Sale of kidneys for transplantation: attitudes of the health-care profession and the public. *Transplantation Proceedings.* 1992 Oct; 24(5): 2108–2109.
(ORGAN AND TISSUE DONATION)

Guttmann, Astrid see **Guttmann, Ronald D.**

Guttmann, R.D. see **Hoffenberg, R.**

Guttmann, R.D. see **Kennedy, I.**

Guttmann, R.D. see **Radcliffe-Richards, J.**

Guttmann, Ronald D. Future markets: claims and meanings. *Transplantation Proceedings.* 1992 Oct; 24(5): 2203.
(ORGAN AND TISSUE DONATION)

Guttmann, Ronald D.; Guttmann, Astrid. Organ transplantation: duty reconsidered. *Transplantation Proceedings.* 1992 Oct; 24(5): 2179–2180.
(ORGAN AND TISSUE DONATION)

Guttmann, Ronald D. see **Guttmann, Astrid**

Guyer, Ruth Levy. When decisions are life-and-death: patients and their families are increasingly turning to hospital ethicists to help them make tough calls on treatments. *USA Weekend.* 1998 Feb 6–8: 26.
(ETHICISTS AND ETHICS COMMITTEES)

H

Haas, Jennifer. The cost of being a woman. *New England Journal of Medicine.* 1998 Jun 4; 338(23): 1694–1695.
(HEALTH CARE/ECONOMICS; SELECTION FOR TREATMENT)

Haas-Wilson, Deborah. The impact of state abortion restrictions on minors' demand for abortions. *Journal of Human Resources.* 1996 Winter; 31(1): 140–158.
(ABORTION/LEGAL ASPECTS; ABORTION/MINORS)

Haas-Wilson, Deborah. Women's reproductive choices: the impact of Medicaid funding restrictions. *Family Planning Perspectives.* 1997 Sep–Oct; 29(5): 228–233.
(ABORTION/FINANCIAL SUPPORT; ABORTION/LEGAL ASPECTS)

Haberal, Mehmet; Altaca, G.; Tokyay, R.; Bilgin, N. Ethics in organ procurement in Turkey. *Transplantation Proceedings.* 1992 Oct; 24(5): 2100–2101.
(ORGAN AND TISSUE DONATION; ORGAN AND TISSUE TRANSPLANTATION)

Habermehl, Karl-Otto. The Hippocratic example of the neutrality and universality of medicine. *Dolentium Hominum: Church and Health in the World.* 1996; 31(11th Yr., No. 1): 124–126.
(PROFESSIONAL PATIENT RELATIONSHIP)

Habgood, John; Spagnolo, Antonio G.; Sgreccia, Elio; Daar, Abdallah S. Religious views on organ and tissue donation. *In:* Chapman, Jeremy R.; Deierhoi, Mark; Wight, Celia, eds. Organ and Tissue Donation for Transplantation. New York, NY: Oxford University Press; 1997: 23–33.
(ORGAN AND TISSUE DONATION)

Hackler, Chris. Is rationing of health care ethically defensible? *In:* Monagle, John F.; Thomasma, David C., eds. Health Care Ethics: Critical Issues for the 21st Century. Gaithersburg, MD: Aspen Publishers; 1998: 371–377.
(HEALTH CARE/ECONOMICS; RESOURCE ALLOCATION)

Hackney, Mary Helen see **Smith, Thomas J.**

Haddad, Amy. Ethics in action: a cardiac patient has just signed a consent form agreeing to participate in a clinical trial testing a new drug for congestive heart failure -- what would you do? *RN.* 1996 Mar; 59(3): 17–19.
(HUMAN EXPERIMENTATION/INFORMED CONSENT)

Haddad, Amy. Ethics in action: you've recently been assigned to care for a post-trauma patient who has been in a persistent vegetative state for a month -- what would you do? *RN.* 1996 May; 59(5): 21–22, 24.
(ALLOWING TO DIE)

Haddad, Amy Marie. Role playing and ethics instruction. *In:* Haddad, Amy Marie, ed. Teaching and Learning Strategies in Pharmacy Ethics. Second Edition. New York, NY: Pharmaceutical Products Press; 1997: 49–63.
(PROFESSIONAL ETHICS/EDUCATION)

Haddad, Amy Marie, ed. Teaching and Learning Strategies in Pharmacy Ethics. Second Edition. New York, NY: Pharmaceutical Products Press; 1997. 159 p.
(PROFESSIONAL ETHICS/EDUCATION)

Hadley, Suzanne W. see **Goodwin, Frederick K.**

Haffner, Alden N. The moral dignity of our profession. [Editorial]. *Journal of the American Optometric Association.* 1994 Jun; 65(6): 384.
(PROFESSIONAL ETHICS)

Haffner, Alden N. see **Foster, George E.**

Hagihara, A. see **Miller, A.S.**

Hagihara, Akihito; Murakami, Masayoshi; Miller, Alan S.; Nobutomo, Koichi. Association between attitudes toward health promotion and opinions regarding organ transplants in Japan. *Health Policy.* 1997 Nov; 42(2): 157–170.
(HEALTH; ORGAN AND TISSUE TRANSPLANTATION)

Haglund, Keith. Ninety-day wonder. [Editorial]. *Journal of NIH Research.* 1997 Jul; 9(7): 10.
(CLONING)

Haimowitz, Stephan; Delano, Susan J.; Oldham, John M. Uninformed decisionmaking: the case of surrogate research consent. *Hastings Center Report.* 1997 Nov–Dec; 27(6): 9–16.
(HUMAN EXPERIMENTATION/INFORMED CONSENT; HUMAN EXPERIMENTATION/SPECIAL POPULATIONS)

Hale, Brenda. Mentally incapacitated adults and decision–making: the English perspective. *International Journal of Law and Psychiatry.* 1997 Winter; 20(1): 59–75.
(INFORMED CONSENT/MENTALLY DISABLED)

Hale, Paul N. see **Napper, Stan A.**

Halevy, Amir; Baldwin, John C. Poor surgical risk patients. *In:* McCullough, Laurence B.; Jones, James W.; Brody, Baruch A., eds. Surgical Ethics. New York, NY: Oxford University Press; 1998: 152–170.
(PATIENT CARE)

Haley, Sarah see **Stadler, Holly A.**

Haliburn, Joan see **Batten, Donald A.**

Hall, Mark A.; Berenson, Robert A. Ethical practice in managed care: a dose of realism. *Annals of Internal Medicine.* 1998 Mar 1; 128(5): 395–402.
(HEALTH CARE/ECONOMICS; MEDICAL ETHICS; PROFESSIONAL PATIENT RELATIONSHIP; RESOURCE ALLOCATION)

Hall, Mark A. see **Curran, William J.**

Hall, Spencer A.; Casarett, David; Ross, Lainie F. Overriding a patient's refusal of treatment after an iatrogenic complication. [Letter and response]. *New England Journal of Medicine.* 1997 Nov 13; 337(20): 1477.
(RESUSCITATION ORDERS; TREATMENT REFUSAL)

Haller, Karen B. see **Sulmasy, Daniel P.**

Hallowell, N.; Murton, F.; Statham, H.; Green, J.M.; Richards, M.P.M. Women's need for information before attending genetic counselling for familial breast or ovarian cancer: a questionnaire, interview, and observational study. *BMJ (British Medical Journal).* 1997 Jan 25; 314(7076): 281–283.
(GENETIC COUNSELING)

Halm, Ethan A.; Causino, Nancyanne; Blumenthal, David. Is gatekeeping better than traditional care? A survey of physicians' attitudes. *JAMA.* 1997 Nov 26; 278(20): 1677–1681.
(HEALTH CARE/ECONOMICS; RESOURCE ALLOCATION)

Halpern–Felsher, Bonnie L. see **Ford, Carol A.**

Hals, Arild see **Jacobsen, Geir**

Halsey, Neal A.; Sommer, Alfred; Henderson, Donald A.; Black, Robert E. Ethics and international research. [Editorial]. *BMJ (British Medical Journal).* 1997 Oct 18; 315(7114): 965–966.
(AIDS/HUMAN EXPERIMENTATION; HUMAN EXPERIMENTATION/FOREIGN COUNTRIES; HUMAN EXPERIMENTATION/RESEARCH DESIGN; HUMAN EXPERIMENTATION/SPECIAL POPULATIONS)

Ham, Chris. Priority setting in health care: learning from international experience. *Health Policy.* 1997 Oct; 42(1): 49–66.
(HEALTH CARE/ECONOMICS; HEALTH CARE/FOREIGN COUNTRIES; RESOURCE ALLOCATION)

Ham, Chris. Retracing the Oregon Trail: the experience of rationing and the Oregon health plan. *BMJ (British Medical Journal).* 1998 Jun 27; 316(7149): 1965–1969.
(HEALTH CARE/ECONOMICS; RESOURCE ALLOCATION)

Hamberger, Lars see **Wennerholm, Ulla–Britt**

Hamer, Dean; Copeland, Peter. Engineering temperament: cloning and the future politics of personality. *In: their* Living with Our Genes: Why They Matter More Than You Think. New York, NY: Doubleday; 1998: 295–316, 344.
(BEHAVIORAL GENETICS; CLONING; GENETIC INTERVENTION)

Hamilton, Jean A. Women and health policy: on the inclusion of females in clinical trials. *In:* Sargent, Carolyn F.; Brettell, Caroline B., eds. Gender and Health: An International Perspective. Upper Saddle River, NJ: Prentice Hall; 1996: 292–325.
(HUMAN EXPERIMENTATION/REGULATION; HUMAN EXPERIMENTATION/SPECIAL POPULATIONS)

Hamilton, M.P. see **Kazem, R.**

Hammes, Bernard J.; Rooney, Brenda L. Death and end–of–life planning in one midwestern community. *Archives of Internal Medicine.* 1998 Feb 23; 158(4): 383–390.
(ADVANCE DIRECTIVES; TERMINAL CARE)

Hammes, Bernard J.; Webster, Stephen. Professional ethics and managed care in dermatology. *Archives of Dermatology.* 1996 Sep; 132(9): 1070–1073.
(HEALTH CARE/ECONOMICS; MEDICAL ETHICS)

Hammond, Robert see **Johnston, S.R.D.**

Hampton, Stephanie see **Stadler, Holly A.**

Hanafin, Patrick. Last Rights: Death, Dying and the Law in Ireland. Cork, Ireland: Cork University Press; 1997. 114 p.
(ALLOWING TO DIE/LEGAL ASPECTS; EUTHANASIA/LEGAL ASPECTS)

Hand, D.J. see **Fayers, P.M.**

Handelsman, Mitchell M. see **Braaten, Ellen B.**

Hanley, Ruth Ann. Hoffmeister v. Satz. [Note]. *Issues in Law and Medicine.* 1990 Fall; 6(2): 205–206.
(ALLOWING TO DIE/LEGAL ASPECTS)

Hanna, Mark J. Consent for a minor. *Texas Dental Journal.* 1995 Apr; 112(4): 39, 41.
(INFORMED CONSENT/MINORS)

Hannum, Hurst. Should industry sponsor research? Condemning the drinks industry rules out potentially useful research. *BMJ (British Medical Journal).* 1998 Aug 1; 317(7154): 335–336.
(BIOMEDICAL RESEARCH)

Hansen–Flaschen, John see **Asch, David A.**

Hansen–Flaschen, John see **McFadzean, J.**

Hanson, Laura C.; Danis, Marion; Garrett, Joanne. What is wrong with end–of–life care? Opinions of bereaved family members. *Journal of the American Geriatrics Society.* 1997 Nov; 45(11): 1339–1344.
(TERMINAL CARE)

Hanson, Laura C. see **Gertner, Eric J.**

Hanson, Mark J. Religious voices in biotechnology: the case of gene patenting. *Hastings Center Report.* 1997 Nov–Dec; 27(6, Suppl.): S1–S21.
(PATENTING LIFE FORMS)

Hanson, Mark J. The religious difference in clinical healthcare. *Cambridge Quarterly of Healthcare Ethics.* 1998 Winter; 7(1): 57–67.
(BIOETHICS; PATIENT CARE)

Hansson, Mats O. Balancing the quality of consent. *Journal of Medical Ethics.* 1998 Jun; 24(3): 182–187.
(HUMAN EXPERIMENTATION/INFORMED CONSENT)

Hantikainen, Virpi. Physical restraint: a descriptive study in Swiss nursing homes. *Nursing Ethics.* 1998 Jul; 5(4): 330–346.
(BEHAVIOR CONTROL; PATIENT CARE/AGED)

Hardacre, Helen. Marketing the Menacing Fetus in Japan. Berkeley, CA: University of California Press; 1997. 310 p.
(ABORTION/ATTITUDES; ABORTION/FOREIGN COUNTRIES; ABORTION/RELIGIOUS ASPECTS)

Harding, Christine M. Whooping cough vaccination: the case presented by the British national press. *Child: Care, Health and Development.* 1985 Jan–Feb; 11(1): 21–30.
(IMMUNIZATION)

Hardwig, John see **Churchill, Larry R.**

Hardy, K.J.; Milton, P.; Derham, P.; Fletcher, D.R.; MacLellan, D.G.; Jones, R.McL.; Shulkes, A. Attitudes towards liver transplantation in Victoria, Australia. *Australian and New Zealand Journal of Surgery.* 1993 Jul; 63(7): 520–524.
(ORGAN AND TISSUE TRANSPLANTATION; RESOURCE ALLOCATION/BIOMEDICAL TECHNOLOGIES)

Harland, Robert see **Sugarman, Jeremy**

Harper, Peter S.; Clarke, Angus J. Genetics, Society, and Clinical Practice. Herndon, VA: BIOS Scientific Publishers; 1997. 253 p.
(GENETIC COUNSELING; GENETIC SCREENING; GENETIC SERVICES)

Harpwood, Vivienne see **Ashcroft, Richard**

Harrell, Frank E. see **Weeks, Jane C.**

Harrell, Lindy E. see **Marson, Daniel C.**

Harrington, Judith M. see **Blakely, Robert L.**

Harris, Cathleen M.; Mahowald, Mary B. Women and alcohol abuse. *In:* Shelton, Wayne N.; Edwards, Rem B., eds. Advances in Bioethics. Volume 3: Values, Ethics, and Alcoholism. Greenwich, CT: JAI Press; 1997: 153–170.
(BEHAVIOR CONTROL; FETUSES; PATIENT CARE; PRENATAL INJURIES)

Harris, H. see **Hartley, N.E.**

Harris, John. Clones, Genes, and Immortality: Ethics and the Genetic Revolution. New York, NY: Oxford University Press; 1998. 328 p.
(GENETIC INTERVENTION; REPRODUCTIVE TECHNOLOGIES)

Harris, John. Cloning and bioethical thinking. [Letter]. *Nature.* 1997 Oct 2; 389(6650): 433.

(CLONING)

Harris, John. Cloning and human dignity. *Cambridge Quarterly of Healthcare Ethics.* 1998 Spring; 7(2): 163–167.
(CLONING)

Harris, John. "Goodbye Dolly?" The ethics of human cloning. *Journal of Medical Ethics.* 1997 Dec; 23(6): 353–360.
(CLONING)

Harris, John. Should we attempt to eradicate disability? *In:* Morscher, Edgar; Neumaier, Otto; Simons, Peter, eds. Applied Ethics in a Troubled World. Boston, MA: Kluwer Academic; 1998: 105–114.
(ABORTION; INFANTICIDE)

Harris, John see **Ashcroft, Richard**

Harris, John see **Brazier, Margaret**

Harris, R. see **Hartley, N.E.**

Harris, Yvonne; Gorelick, Philip B.; Samuels, Patricia; Bempong, Isaac. Why African Americans may not be participating in clinical trials. *Journal of the National Medical Association.* 1996 Oct; 88(10): 630–634.
(HUMAN EXPERIMENTATION/SPECIAL POPULATIONS)

Harrison, Helen. Need exists for advance directives from parents. [Letter; title supplied]. *Journal of Perinatology.* 1995 Nov–Dec; 15(6): 522.
(ADVANCE DIRECTIVES; ALLOWING TO DIE/INFANTS)

Harrold, Joan see **Ayers, Elise**

Hart, C.B. Legal control of use of animals for scientific purposes. *In:* Tuffery, A.A., ed. Laboratory Animals: An Introduction for Experimenters. Second Edition. New York, NY: Wiley; 1995: 37–65.
(ANIMAL EXPERIMENTATION)

Hartley, N.E.; Scotcher, D.; Harris, H.; Williamson, P.; Wallace, A.; Craufurd, D.; Harris, R. The uptake and acceptability to patients of cystic fibrosis carrier testing offered in pregnancy by the GP. *Journal of Medical Genetics.* 1997 Jun; 34(6): 459–464.
(GENETIC SCREENING)

Harvey, S. Marie see **Beckman, Linda J.**

Hassan, Riaz. Euthanasia and the medical profession: an Australian study. *Australian Journal of Social Issues.* 1996 Aug; 31(3): 239–252.
(ALLOWING TO DIE/ATTITUDES; EUTHANASIA/ATTITUDES; SUICIDE)

Hassenfeld, Irwin N. see **La Vigne, Gregory**

Hathout, Hassan. Islamic views on some reproductive issues. *In:* Teebi, Ahmad S.; Faraq, Talaat I., eds. Genetic Disorders Among Arab Populations. New York, NY: Oxford University Press; 1997: 469–473.
(REPRODUCTION; REPRODUCTIVE TECHNOLOGIES)

Hattab, Jocelyn Y. Psychiatric ethics. *In:* Chadwick, Ruth, ed. Encyclopedia of Applied Ethics, Volume 3. San Diego, CA: Academic Press; 1998: 703–726.
(MEDICAL ETHICS; PATIENT CARE/MENTALLY DISABLED)

Hauck, Walter W. see **DeGroot, Leslie J.**

Hauerwas, Stanley; Shuman, Joel. Cloning the human body. *In:* Cole–Turner, Ronald, ed. Human Cloning: Religious Responses. Louisville, KY: Westminister John Knox Press; 1997: 58–65.
(CLONING)

Hauerwas, Stanley M. How Christian ethics became medical ethics: the case of Paul Ramsey. *In: his:* Wilderness Wanderings: Probing Twentieth–Century Theology and Philosophy. Boulder, CO: Westview Press; 1997: 124–140.
(ETHICISTS AND ETHICS COMMITTEES)

Haugan, Mark L. see **Noll, John O.**

Haughton, Peter see **Ashcroft, Richard**

Haupt, Bridget A. see **Poikonen, John**

Haverkate, Ilinka; van der Wal, Gerrit. Policies on assisted suicide in Dutch psychiatric facilities. *Psychiatric Services.* 1998 Jan; 49(1): 98–100.
(SUICIDE)

Hawes, Catherine see **Phillips, Charles D.**

Hawkins, Anne Hunsaker. Medical ethics and the epiphanic dimension of narrative. *In:* Nelson, Hilde Lindemann, ed. Stories and Their Limits: Narrative Approaches to Bioethics. New York, NY: Routledge; 1997: 153–170.
(BIOETHICS; MEDICAL ETHICS)

Hawkins, Dana. A bloody mess at one federal lab. [News]. *U.S. News and World Report.* 1997 Jun 23; 122(24): 26–27.
(INFORMED CONSENT; MASS SCREENING)

Hawkins, Lauren see **Marson, Daniel C.**

Hayden, M.R. see **Burgess, M.M.**

Häyry, Heta see **Häyry, Matti**

Häyry, Matti. Ethics committees, principles and consequences. *Journal of Medical Ethics.* 1998 Apr; 24(2): 81–85.
(ANIMAL EXPERIMENTATION; HUMAN EXPERIMENTATION/ETHICS COMMITTEES)

Häyry, Matti; Häyry, Heta. Genetic engineering. *In:* Chadwick, Ruth, ed. Encyclopedia of Applied Ethics, Volume 2. San Diego, CA: Academic Press; 1998: 407–417.
(GENETIC INTERVENTION)

Hazebroek, Frans W.J. see **Caniano, Donna A.**

Hazebroucq, Georges see **Auguste, Valérie**

Hazuda, Helen P. see **Berkowitz, Sheldon T.**

Hazuda, Helen P. see **Perkins, Henry S.**

Healton, Cheryl see **Nakchbandi, Inaam A.**

Healy, Bernadine. BRCA genes — bookmaking, fortunetelling, and medical care. [Editorial]. *New England Journal of Medicine.* 1997 May 15; 336(20):

1448–1449.
(GENETIC SCREENING)

Healy, Peter see **Ashcroft, Richard**

Heasell, Stephen see **Richmond, Caroline**

Hecht, Barbara K.; Hecht, Frederick. Murder of son with a genital malformation. [Letter]. *American Journal of Medical Genetics.* 1995 Sep 25; 58(4): 381.
(EUTHANASIA)

Hecht, Frederick see **Hecht, Barbara K.**

Hecker, Lorna see **Schlossberger, Eugene**

Hedgecoe, Adam. Genetic Catch–22: testing, risk and private health insurance. *Business and Professional Ethics Journal.* 1996 Summer; 15(2): 69–86.
(GENETIC SCREENING)

Hedgecoe, Adam M. Gene therapy. *In:* Chadwick, Ruth, ed. Encyclopedia of Applied Ethics, Volume 2. San Diego, CA: Academic Press; 1998: 383–390.
(GENE THERAPY)

Hedgecoe, Adam M. Genome analysis. *In:* Chadwick, Ruth, ed. Encyclopedia of Applied Ethics, Volume 2. San Diego, CA: Academic Press; 1998: 463–470.
(GENOME MAPPING)

Hedley, A.J.; Whidden, Phillip. The tobacco industry and scientific publications. [Letters]. *BMJ (British Medical Journal).* 1997 May 3; 314(7090): 1350–1351.
(BIOMEDICAL RESEARCH)

Heffner, John E.; Barbieri, Celia; Fracica, Phil; Brown, Lee K. Communicating do–not–resuscitate orders with a computer–based system. *Archives of Internal Medicine.* 1998 May 25; 158(10): 1090–1095.
(RESUSCITATION ORDERS)

Hefner, Philip. Determinism, freedom, and moral failure. *Dialog: A Journal of Theology.* 1994 Winter; 33(1): 23–29.
(BEHAVIORAL GENETICS; GENETIC INTERVENTION; GENOME MAPPING)

Heginbotham, Christopher. Mental disorder and decision–making: respecting autonomy in substitute judgments. *In:* Grubb, Andrew, ed. Decision–Making and Problems of Incompetence. New York, NY: Wiley; 1994: 115–125.
(INFORMED CONSENT/MENTALLY DISABLED; INVOLUNTARY COMMITMENT/FOREIGN COUNTRIES)

Heilicser, Bernard; Stocking, Carol; Siegler, Mark. Ethical dilemmas in emergency medical services: the perspective of the emergency medical technician. *Annals of Emergency Medicine.* 1996 Feb; 27(2): 239–243.
(PATIENT CARE)

Heilig, Steve; Brody, Robert V. Physician–hastened death and end–of–life care: development of a community-wide consensus statement and guidelines. *Cambridge Quarterly of Healthcare Ethics.* 1998 Spring; 7(2): 223–225.
(ETHICISTS AND ETHICS COMMITTEES; SUICIDE; TERMINAL CARE)

Heimler, Audrey; Zanko, Andrea. Huntington disease: a case study describing the complexities and nuances of predictive testing of monozygotic twins. *Journal of Genetic Counseling.* 1995 Jun; 4(2): 125–137.
(GENETIC COUNSELING; GENETIC SCREENING)

Heimler, Audrey see **Reich, Elsa**

Hein, Karen. Aligning science with politics and policy in HIV prevention. *Science.* 1998 Jun 19; 280(5371): 1905–1906.
(AIDS)

Heitman, Elizabeth. The public's role in the evaluation of health care technology: the conflict over ECT. *International Journal of Technology Assessment in Health Care.* 1996 Fall; 12(4): 657–672.
(ELECTROCONVULSIVE THERAPY)

Heitman, Elizabeth; Bulger, Ruth Ellen. The healthcare ethics committee in the structural transformation of health care: administrative and organization ethics in changing times. *HEC (HealthCare Ethics Committee) Forum.* 1998 Jun; 10(2): 152–176.
(ETHICISTS AND ETHICS COMMITTEES; HEALTH CARE/ECONOMICS)

Helderman, J. Harold see **Daar, A.S.**

Helfand, Ira see **Forrow, Lachlan**

Heller, Jan C.; Gerety, Jane. Catholic sponsorship and Medicare managed care: an uneasy alliance of faith and market. *HEC (HealthCare Ethics Committee) Forum.* 1998 Jun; 10(2): 186–200.
(HEALTH CARE/ECONOMICS)

Heller, Michael A.; Eisenberg, Rebecca S. Can patents deter innovation? The anticommons in biomedical research. *Science.* 1998 May 1; 280(5364): 698–701.
(BIOMEDICAL RESEARCH; GENOME MAPPING)

Hellinger, Fred J. The effect of managed care on quality: a review of recent evidence. *Archives of Internal Medicine.* 1998 Apr 27; 158(8): 833–841.
(HEALTH CARE/ECONOMICS)

Hellman, Samuel see **Emanuel, Ezekiel J.**

Helm, Ann. Truth telling, placebos, and deception: ethical and legal issues in practice. *Aviation, Space, and Environmental Medicine.* 1985 Jan; 56(1): 69–72.
(TRUTH DISCLOSURE)

Helmchen, Hanfried see **Henn, Fritz A.**

Helzlsouer, Kathy J. see **Bernhardt, Barbara A.**

Hemlock Society. Mercy killing: a position statement regarding David Rodriguez. *Issues in Law and Medicine.* 1997 Winter; 13(3): 341–342.
(EUTHANASIA/LEGAL ASPECTS)

Hemminki, Elina; Santalahti, Päivi; Louhiala, Pekka. Ethical conflicts in regulating the start of life. *Perspectives in Biology and Medicine.* 1997 Summer; 40(4): 586–591.
(ABORTION; PATIENT CARE/MINORS; PRENATAL DIAGNOSIS; REPRODUCTIVE TECHNOLOGIES)

Hemminki, Elina see **Ollila, Eeva**

Henderson, Donald A. see **Halsey, Neal A.**

Hendin, Herbert. Assisted suicide and euthanasia. *In:* his Suicide in America. New and Expanded Edition. New York, NY: W.W. Norton; 1995: 236–277, 294–297.
(EUTHANASIA; SUICIDE)

Hendin, Herbert. Involuntary commitment. *In:* his Suicide in America. New and Expanded Edition. New York, NY: W.W. Norton; 1995: 214–235, 291–294.
(INVOLUNTARY COMMITMENT; SUICIDE)

Hendin, Herbert; Ganzini, Linda. Physician–assisted suicide: the Dutch case. [Letter and response]. *JAMA.* 1997 Nov 12; 278(18): 1492–1493.
(SUICIDE)

Hendin, Herbert; Goold, Susan Dorr; Meier, Diane E.; Morrison, R. Sean; Wallenstein, Sylvan. Physician–assisted suicide and euthanasia in the United States. [Letters and response]. *New England Journal of Medicine.* 1998 Sep 10; 339(11): 775–776.
(EUTHANASIA; SUICIDE)

Hendin, Herbert see **O'Connor, Nancy K.**

Hendriksen, Coenraad F.M. see **Balls, Michael**

Henk, M. see **Johnston, S.R.D.**

Henley, L.; Benatar, S.R.; Robertson, B.A.; Ensink, K. Informed consent -- a survey of doctors' practices in South Africa. *South African Medical Journal.* 1995 Dec; 85(12): 1273, 1275–1278.
(INFORMED CONSENT)

Henn, Fritz A.; Lader, Malcolm; Helmchen, Hanfried. Medication–free research with schizophrenic patients: a European perspective. [Commentary]. *Archives of General Psychiatry.* 1997 May; 54(5): 412–413.
(HUMAN EXPERIMENTATION/RESEARCH DESIGN; HUMAN EXPERIMENTATION/SPECIAL POPULATIONS)

Henn, Wolfram. Predictive diagnosis and genetic screening: manipulation of fate? *Perspectives in Biology and Medicine.* 1998 Winter; 41(2): 282–289.
(GENETIC COUNSELING; GENETIC SCREENING)

Henry, David see **Kerridge, Ian**

Henson, G. see **Johnston, S.R.D.**

Hentoff, Nat. Disabled, not dead. *Responsive Community.* 1996 Fall; 6(4): 4–6.
(SUICIDE)

Herb, Alice; Lazar, Eliot J. Ethics committees and end–of–life decision making. *In:* Zucker, Marjorie B.; Zucker, Howard D., eds. Medical Futility and the Evaluation of Life–Sustaining Interventions. New York, NY: Cambridge University Press; 1997: 110–122.
(ALLOWING TO DIE; ETHICISTS AND ETHICS COMMITTEES)

Herbert, Wray. How the nature vs. nurture debate shapes public policy -- and our view of ourselves. *U.S. News and World Report.* 1997 Apr 21; 122(15): 72–74, 77–80.
(BEHAVIORAL GENETICS)

Herbert, Wray; Sheler, Jeffery L.; Watson, Traci. The world after cloning. *U.S. News and World Report.* 1997 Mar 10; 122(9): 59–63.
(CLONING)

Hern, H. Eugene; Koenig, Barbara A.; Moore, Lisa Jean; Marshall, Patricia A. The difference that culture can make in end–of–life decisionmaking. *Cambridge Quarterly of Healthcare Ethics.* 1998 Winter; 7(1): 27–40.
(INFORMED CONSENT; PROFESSIONAL PATIENT RELATIONSHIP; TERMINAL CARE; TRUTH DISCLOSURE)

Herrick, Charlotte A. see **Doolittle, Norma O.**

Hersey, Jonathan. Enigma of the unborn mother: legal and ethical considerations of aborted fetal ovarian tissue and ova transplantations. *UCLA Law Review.* 1995 Oct; 43(1): 159–207.
(FETUSES; ORGAN AND TISSUE DONATION)

Hervé, C. see **Moutel, G.**

Hervé, Christian see **Auguste, Valérie**

Hervé, Christian see **Howard, Philip J.**

Hervé, Christian see **Pochard, Frédéric**

Herve, Ritva see **Töyry, Eeva**

Herwaldt, Loreen A. Ethical aspects of infection control. *Infection Control and Hospital Epidemiology.* 1996 Feb; 17(2): 108–113.
(PATIENT CARE; PROFESSIONAL ETHICS)

Hesse, Katherine A. Ethical issues and terminal management of the old old. *Journal of Geriatric Psychiatry.* 1995; 28(1): 75–95.
(ALLOWING TO DIE; PATIENT CARE/AGED; TERMINAL CARE)

Hessel, K. see **Naber, D.**

Hettinger, Ned. Patenting life: biotechnology, intellectual property, and environmental ethics. *Boston College Environmental Affairs Law Review.* 1995 Winter; 22(2): 267–305.
(GENETIC INTERVENTION; PATENTING LIFE FORMS)

Heyd, David. Are we our descendants' keepers? *In:* Agius, Emmanuel; Busuttil, Salvino, eds. Germ–Line Intervention and Our Responsibilities to Future Generations. Boston, MA: Kluwer Academic; 1998: 131–145.
(GENETIC INTERVENTION)

Heyd, David. *Human Genome Research and the Challenge of Contingent Future Persons: Toward an Impersonal Theocentric Approach to Value,* by Jan Christian Heller. [Book review essay]. *Bioethics.* 1998 Apr; 12(2): 173–176.
(GENETIC INTERVENTION; GENOME MAPPING)

Hiatt, Howard see **Berwick, Donald**

Hiatt, Jonathan R. see **Wenger, Neil S.**

Hicks, Carolyn. Ethics in midwifery research. *In:* Frith, Lucy, ed. Ethics and Midwifery: Issues in Contemporary Practice. Boston, MA: Butterworth–Heinemann; 1996: 237–257.
(HUMAN EXPERIMENTATION; NURSING ETHICS)

Hicks, Fiona see **Dunphy, Kilian**

Hiday, Virginia A. see **Swartz, Marvin S.**

Hiday, Virginia Aldigé. Involuntary commitment as a psychiatric technology. *International Journal of Technology Assessment in Health Care.* 1996 Fall; 12(4): 585–603.
(INVOLUNTARY COMMITMENT; PATIENT CARE/MENTALLY DISABLED)

Higgins, R.M.; West, N.; Edmunds, M.E.; Dukes, D.C.; Kashi, H.; Jurewicz, A.; Lam, F.T. Effect of a strict HLA matching policy on distribution of cadaveric kidney transplants to Indo–Asian and white European recipients: regional study. *BMJ (British Medical Journal).* 1997 Nov 22; 315(7119): 1354–1355.
(ORGAN AND TISSUE TRANSPLANTATION; RESOURCE ALLOCATION/BIOMEDICAL TECHNOLOGIES; SELECTION FOR TREATMENT)

Higginson, I. see **Shaw, M.**

Higgs, Roger. Shaping our ends: the ethics of respect in a well–led NHS. *British Journal of General Practice.* 1997 Apr; 47(417): 245–249.
(PROFESSIONAL PATIENT RELATIONSHIP)

Higgs, Roger see **Ashcroft, Richard**

Higgs, Roger see **Boyd, Kenneth M.**

Hilberman, Mark; Kutner, Jean; Parsons, Debra; Murphy, Donald J. Marginally effective medical care: ethical analysis of issues in cardiopulmonary resuscitation (CPR). *Journal of Medical Ethics.* 1997 Dec; 23(6): 361–367.
(RESUSCITATION ORDERS; SELECTION FOR TREATMENT)

Hill, Marcia see **Anderson, Gail**

Hill, T. Patrick. A religious voice for bioethics? *NCCE News (Veterans Health Administration National Center for Clinical Ethics).* 1997 Winter–Spring; 5(1): 1–2, 9–10.
(BIOETHICS)

Hillary, Kristine see **McNeilly, Dennis P.**

Hilts, Philip J. Experiments on children are reviewed: research involved now–banned drug. [News]. *New York Times.* 1998 Apr 15: B3.
(HUMAN EXPERIMENTATION/MINORS; HUMAN EXPERIMENTATION/SPECIAL POPULATIONS)

Himmelstein, David U.; Woolhandler, Steffie. Bound to gag. [Editorial]. *Archives of Internal Medicine.* 1997 Oct 13; 157(18): 2033.
(HEALTH CARE/ECONOMICS)

Hingson, Ralph see **Stein, Michael D.**

Hinohara, Shigeaki. Facing death the Japanese way -- customs and ethos. *In:* Hoshino, Kazumasa, ed. Japanese and Western Bioethics: Studies in Moral Diversity. Boston, MA: Kluwer Academic; 1997: 145–154.
(TERMINAL CARE)

Hirtle, Marie. Genetic screening and research revisited. *In:* Knoppers, Bartha Maria, ed. Human DNA: Law and Policy: International and Comparative Perspectives. Proceedings of the First International Conference on DNA Sampling and Human Genetic Research: Ethical, Legal, and Policy Aspects, held in Montreal, Canada, 6–8 Sep 1996. Boston, MA: Kluwer Law International; 1997: 333–340.

(GENETIC RESEARCH; GENETIC SCREENING; HUMAN EXPERIMENTATION/INFORMED CONSENT; INFORMED CONSENT)

Hirtle, Marie see **Luther, Lori**

Ho, Suzanne C. see **Hui, Elsie**

Hobbs, M. Nielsen. US Public Health Service sets out plan for xenotransplantation. [News]. *Lancet.* 1998 Jan 31; 351(9099): 343.
(ORGAN AND TISSUE TRANSPLANTATION)

Hobson, Sarah. Legal aspects of dementia. [Letter]. *Lancet.* 1997 May 17; 349(9063): 1482.
(INVOLUNTARY COMMITMENT/FOREIGN COUNTRIES)

Hobson, Sarah see **Bradley, Peter M.**

Hobson, Sarah Jane. The ethics of compulsory removal under section 47 of the 1948 National Assistance Act. *Journal of Medical Ethics.* 1998 Feb; 24(1): 38–43.
(INVOLUNTARY COMMITMENT/FOREIGN COUNTRIES)

Hochhauser, Mark. Some overlooked aspects of consent form readability. *IRB: A Review of Human Subjects Research.* 1997 Sep–Oct; 19(5): 5–9.
(HUMAN EXPERIMENTATION/INFORMED CONSENT)

Hodgson, Jane E. Abortion procedures and abortifacients. *In:* Edwards, Rem B., ed. Advances in Bioethics. Volume 2: New Essays on Abortion and Bioethics. Greenwich, CT: JAI Press; 1997: 75–106.
(ABORTION)

Hodgson, John. Dolly opens a farm full of possibilities. [News]. *Nature Biotechnology.* 1997 Apr; 15(4): 306.
(CLONING)

Hodgson, John. Rights of the terminally ill patient. *Annals of Health Law.* 1996; 5: 169–191.
(ALLOWING TO DIE/LEGAL ASPECTS; EUTHANASIA/LEGAL ASPECTS; TREATMENT REFUSAL)

Hoefler, James M. Managing Death: The First Guide for Patients, Family Members, and Care Providers on Forgoing Treatment at the End of Life. Boulder, CO: Westview Press; 1997. 206 p.
(ALLOWING TO DIE; TERMINAL CARE)

Hoefnagels, Willibrord H.L. see **Olde Rikkert, Marcel G.M.**

Hoeldtke, Nathan J. see **Calhoun, Byron C.**

Hoenig, Leonard J. see **Freedman, Monroe H.**

Hoffenberg, R.; Lock, M.; Tilney, N.; Casabona, C.; Daar, A.S.; Guttmann, R.D.; Kennedy, I.; Nundy, S.; Radcliffe–Richards, J.; Sells, R.A. Should organs from patients in permanent vegetative state be used for transplantation? [For the International Forum for Transplant Ethics]. *Lancet.* 1997 Nov 1; 350(9087): 1320–1321.
(DETERMINATION OF DEATH; ORGAN AND TISSUE DONATION)

Hoffenberg, R. see **Kennedy, I.**

Hoffenberg, R. see **Radcliffe–Richards, J.**

Hoffenberg, R. see **Steinberg, M.A.**

Hoffenberg, Raymond see **Price, John**

Hoffmann, Diane E. Managing the persistent patient with chronic pain. [Case study and commentary]. *HEC (HealthCare Ethics Committee) Forum.* 1997 Dec; 9(4): 365–372.
(HEALTH CARE/ECONOMICS; PATIENT CARE)

Hofmans, K. see **Bonduelle, M.**

Hogan, Carlton see **Schüklenk, Udo**

Hoge, Steven K. APA resource document: I. The professional responsibilities of psychiatrists in evolving health care systems. *Bulletin of the American Academy of Psychiatry and the Law.* 1996; 24(3): 393–406.
(HEALTH CARE/ECONOMICS; PATIENT CARE/MENTALLY DISABLED; RESOURCE ALLOCATION)

Hoge, Steven K. APA resource document: II. Regulatory guidelines for protecting the interests of psychiatric patients in emerging health care systems. *Bulletin of the American Academy of Psychiatry and the Law.* 1996; 24(3): 407–418.
(HEALTH CARE/ECONOMICS; RESOURCE ALLOCATION)

Hoge, Steven K.; Gutheil, Thomas G.; Kaplan, Eric. The right to refuse treatment under Rogers v. Commissioner: preliminary empirical findings and comparisons. *Bulletin of the American Academy of Psychiatry and the Law.* 1987 Jun; 15(2): 163–169.
(TREATMENT REFUSAL/MENTALLY DISABLED)

Hoggett, Brenda. Mentally incapacitated adults and decision–making: the Law Commission's project. *In:* Grubb, Andrew, ed. Decision–Making and Problems of Incompetence. New York, NY: Wiley; 1994: 27–40.
(INFORMED CONSENT/MENTALLY DISABLED)

Hogle, Linda F. see **Koenig, Barbara A.**

Hoijtink, Herbert see **Alpert, Hillel R.**

Holden, Constance, ed. All quiet on the bioethics front. [News]. *Science.* 1998 Jul 10; 281(5374): 169.
(BIOETHICS; ETHICISTS AND ETHICS COMMITTEES)

Holden, Constance. Tricky ethics of tissue samples. [News]. *Science.* 1998 Mar 13; 279(5357): 1621.
(BIOMEDICAL RESEARCH; ORGAN AND TISSUE DONATION)

Holden, Constance. UN weighs in on cloning. [News]. *Science.* 1997 Nov 21; 278(5342): 1407.
(CLONING)

Holland, Jimmie see **Portenoy, Russell K.**

Holland, Paul V. Consent for transfusion: is it informed? *Transfusion Medicine Reviews.* 1997 Oct; 11(4): 274–285.
(INFORMED CONSENT)

Hollinger, Joan Heifetz. From coitus to commerce: legal and social consequences of noncoital reproduction. *University of Michigan Journal of Law Reform.* 1985 Summer; 18(4): 865–932.
(REPRODUCTIVE TECHNOLOGIES)

Holm, Søren. A life in the shadow: one reason why we should not clone humans. *Cambridge Quarterly of Healthcare Ethics.* 1998 Spring; 7(2): 160–162.
(CLONING)

Holm, Søren. Embryology, ethics of. *In:* Chadwick, Ruth, ed. Encyclopedia of Applied Ethics, Volume 2. San Diego, CA: Academic Press; 1998: 39–45.
(FETUSES)

Holm, Søren. Ethical Problems in Clinical Practice –– A Study of the Ethical Reasoning of Health Care Professionals. Copenhagen: University of Copenhagen; 1996. 258 p.
(BIOETHICS; PROFESSIONAL ETHICS)

Holm, Søren. The medical hierarchy and perceived influence on technical and ethical decisions. *Journal of Internal Medicine.* 1995 May; 237(5): 487–492.
(ALLOWING TO DIE)

Holm, Søren; Evans, Martyn. Product names, proper claims? More ethical issues in the marketing of drugs. *BMJ (British Medical Journal).* 1996 Dec 21–28; 313(7072): 1627–1629.
(PATIENT CARE/DRUGS)

Holmberg, Anders see **White, W.D.**

Holmes–Farley, S. Rebecca. CRG files amicus brief in workplace privacy and discrimination case. [News]. *GeneWATCH.* 1997 Feb; 10(4–5): 1, 4.
(GENETIC SCREENING)

Holosko, Michael J.; Feit, Marvin D., eds. Health and Poverty. New York, NY: Haworth Press; 1997. 252 p.
(HEALTH CARE/ECONOMICS)

Holstein, Martha. Reflections on death and dying. *Academic Medicine.* 1997 Oct; 72(10): 848–855.
(TERMINAL CARE)

Holstein, Martha B. Ethics and Alzheimer's disease: widening the lens. *Journal of Clinical Ethics.* 1998 Spring; 9(1): 13–22.
(PATIENT CARE/MENTALLY DISABLED)

Holt, Bev. Recruitment, selection and compensation of volunteers for phase I studies. *In:* Close, Bryony; Combes, Robert; Hubbard, Anthony; Illingworth, John, eds. Volunteers in Research and Testing. Bristol, PA: Taylor and Francis; 1997: 59–66.
(HUMAN EXPERIMENTATION)

Holt, Janet. Screening and the perfect baby. *In:* Frith, Lucy, ed. Ethics and Midwifery: Issues in Contemporary Practice. Boston, MA: Butterworth–Heinemann; 1996: 140–155.
(ABORTION; PRENATAL DIAGNOSIS)

Holt, S.C. see **Bebeau, M.J.**

Holt, Stanley C. see **Bebeau, Muriel J.**

Holtug, Nils. Altering humans –– the case for and against human gene therapy. *Cambridge Quarterly of Healthcare Ethics.* 1997 Spring; 6(2): 157–174.
(GENE THERAPY)

Holtzman, Neil A. The gene: harnessing the gene and remaking the world, by Jeremy Rifkin. [Book review essay]. *JAMA.* 1998 Aug 12; 280(6): 575.

(GENETIC INTERVENTION; GENETIC RESEARCH)

Holtzman, Neil A.; Murphy, Patricia D.; Watson, Michael S.; Barr, Patricia A. Predictive genetic testing: from basic research to clinical practice. *Science.* 1997 Oct 24; 278(5338): 602–605.
(GENETIC SCREENING; GENETIC SERVICES)

Holtzman, Neil A.; Shapiro, David. The new genetics: genetic testing and public policy. *BMJ (British Medical Journal).* 1998 Mar 14; 316(7134): 852–856.
(GENETIC SCREENING)

Holtzman, Neil A. see **Bernhardt, Barbara A.**

Holtzman, Neil A. see **Finkelstein, Daniel**

Homenko, Donna F. Overview of ethical issues perceived by allied health professionals in the workplace. *Journal of Allied Health.* 1997 Summer; 26(3): 97–103.
(BIOETHICS/EDUCATION; PROFESSIONAL ETHICS/EDUCATION)

Homer, Lou see **White, Jocelyn C.**

Honberg, Ron see **Shamoo, Adil E.**

Hood, Catherine A.; Hope, Tony; Dove, Phillip. Videos, photographs, and patient consent. *BMJ (British Medical Journal).* 1998 Mar 28; 316(7136): 1009–1011.
(CONFIDENTIALITY; INFORMED CONSENT)

Hood, Leroy; Rowen, Lee. Genes, genomes, and society. *In:* Rothstein, Mark A., ed. Genetic Secrets: Protecting Privacy and Confidentiality in the Genetic Era. New Haven, CT: Yale University Press; 1997: 3–30.
(GENOME MAPPING)

Hook, C. Christopher. Genetic testing and confidentiality. *In:* Kilner, John F.; Pentz, Rebecca D.; Young, Frank E., eds. Genetic Ethics: Do the Ends Justify the Genes? Grand Rapids, MI: W.B. Eerdmans; 1997: 124–135.
(CONFIDENTIALITY; GENETIC SCREENING)

Hooker, Ellen Z. Can your research subjects read your study's informed consent form? *SCI Nursing.* 1995 Jun; 12(2): 57–58.
(HUMAN EXPERIMENTATION/INFORMED CONSENT)

Hooper, S.C.; Vaughan, K.J.; Tennant, C.C.; Perz, J.M. Preferences for voluntary euthanasia during major depression and following improvement in an elderly population. *Australian Journal on Ageing.* 1997 Feb; 16(1): 3–7.
(EUTHANASIA/ATTITUDES)

Hopcroft, Thomas. Civil commitment of minors to mental institutions in the Commonwealth of Massachusetts. [Note]. *New England Journal on Criminal and Civil Confinement.* 1995 Summer; 21(2): 543–574.
(INVOLUNTARY COMMITMENT/MINORS)

Hope, Anthony see **Ashcroft, Richard**

Hope, Tony. Aging, research and families. [Editorial]. *Journal of Medical Ethics.* 1997 Oct; 23(5): 267–268.
(HUMAN EXPERIMENTATION/SPECIAL POPULATIONS; INFORMED CONSENT/MENTALLY DISABLED; PATIENT CARE/AGED; PATIENT CARE/MENTALLY DISABLED)

Hope, Tony. Ethics and law for medical students: the core

curriculum. [Editorial]. *Journal of Medical Ethics.* 1998 Jun; 24(3): 147–148.
(BIOETHICS/EDUCATION; MEDICAL ETHICS/EDUCATION)

Hope, Tony see **Hood, Catherine A.**

Hope, Tony see **Savulescu, Julian**

Hopf, G. see **Langer, Anatoly**

Hopkins, Patrick D. Bad copies: how popular media represent cloning as an ethical problem. *Hastings Center Report.* 1998 Mar–Apr; 28(2): 6–13.
(CLONING)

Hoppe, Ruth B. see **Ubel, Peter A.**

Horan, Michael A. see **Mead, Gillian E.**

Horn, David G. Social Bodies: Science, Reproduction, and Italian Modernity. Princeton, NJ: Princeton University Press; 1994. 189 p.
(REPRODUCTION)

Hornblum, Allen M. Acres of Skin: Human Experiments at Holmesburg Prison -- A True Story of Abuse and Exploitation in the Name of Medical Science. New York, NY: Routledge; 1998. 297 p.
(FRAUD AND MISCONDUCT; HUMAN EXPERIMENTATION/SPECIAL POPULATIONS)

Hornblum, Allen M. They were cheap and available: prisoners as research subjects in twentieth century America. *BMJ (British Medical Journal).* 1997 Nov 29; 315(7120): 1437–1441.
(FRAUD AND MISCONDUCT; HUMAN EXPERIMENTATION/SPECIAL POPULATIONS)

Horner, J. Stuart. Medical ethics, history of. *In:* Chadwick, Ruth, ed. Encyclopedia of Applied Ethics, Volume 3. San Diego, CA: Academic Press; 1998: 165–175.
(MEDICAL ETHICS)

Hornstein, Mark D. see **Trad, Fouad S.**

Horton, Larry. Changing cultural and political attitudes toward research with animals. *In:* Eder, G.; Kaiser, E.; King, F.A., eds. The Role of the Chimpanzee in Research. Symposium, Vienna, Austria, May 22–24, 1992. New York, NY: Karger; 1994: 7–17.
(ANIMAL EXPERIMENTATION)

Horton, Richard. Doctors, the General Medical Council, and Bristol. *Lancet.* 1998 May 23; 351(9115): 1525–1526.
(FRAUD AND MISCONDUCT; PATIENT CARE)

Horton, Richard. ICRF: from mayhem to meltdown. *Lancet.* 1997 Oct 11; 350(9084): 1043–1044.
(BIOMEDICAL RESEARCH; HUMAN EXPERIMENTATION/FOREIGN COUNTRIES)

Horton, Richard. Sponsorship, authorship, and a tale of two media. *Lancet.* 1997 May 17; 349(9063): 1411–1412.
(BIOMEDICAL RESEARCH)

Horton, Richard. The unmasked carnival of science. [Commentary]. *Lancet.* 1998 Mar 7; 351(9104): 688–689.
(BIOMEDICAL RESEARCH)

Horton, Richard. Will the UK COPE? [Letter]. *Lancet.*

1997 Jul 26; 350(9073): 234.
(BIOMEDICAL RESEARCH; FRAUD AND MISCONDUCT)

Horwich, Terri Finesmith see **Andrews, Lori**

Hosaka, Takashi see **Berger, Douglas**

Hoshino, Kazumasa. Bioethics in the light of Japanese sentiments. *In:* Hoshino, Kazumasa, ed. Japanese and Western Bioethics: Studies in Moral Diversity. Boston, MA: Kluwer Academic; 1997: 13–23.
(ORGAN AND TISSUE DONATION; PATIENTS' RIGHTS; PROFESSIONAL PATIENT RELATIONSHIP; TRUTH DISCLOSURE)

Hoshino, Kazumasa. Japanese and Western Bioethics: Studies in Moral Diversity. Boston, MA: Kluwer Academic; 1997. 243 p.
(BIOETHICS)

Hotovy, Lisa A. see **Sigmon, Sandra T.**

Housman, David E. see **Bird, Stephanie J.**

Houtepen, Rob. The social construction of euthanasia and medical ethics in the Netherlands. *In:* DeVries, Raymond; Subedi, Janardan, eds. Bioethics and Society: Constructing the Ethical Enterprise. Upper Saddle River, NJ: Prentice Hall; 1998: 117–144.
(BIOETHICS; EUTHANASIA; MEDICAL ETHICS)

Howard, Philip J.; Cole, A.P.; Grassin, Marc; Pochard, Frédéric; Hervé, Christian; White, Margaret. End-of-life decisions in Dutch paediatric practice. [Letters]. *Lancet.* 1997 Sep 13; 350(9080): 816–817.
(ALLOWING TO DIE/INFANTS; EUTHANASIA)

Howe, Edmund G. Biological drivenness: a relative indication for paternalism. *Journal of Clinical Ethics.* 1997 Fall; 8(3): 307–312.
(TREATMENT REFUSAL)

Howe, Edmund G. Caring for patients with dementia: an indication for "emotional communism". *Journal of Clinical Ethics.* 1998 Spring; 9(1): 3–11.
(PATIENT CARE/MENTALLY DISABLED; PROFESSIONAL PATIENT RELATIONSHIP)

Howe, Edmund G. Commentary: "missing" patients by seeing only their cultures. *Journal of Clinical Ethics.* 1998 Summer; 9(2): 191–193.
(PATIENT CARE)

Howe, Edmund G. Deceiving patients for their own good. *Journal of Clinical Ethics.* 1997 Fall; 8(3): 211–216.
(PATIENT CARE/MENTALLY DISABLED)

Howe, Edmund G. Deconstructing equity, autonomy, and ethical analysis. *Journal of Clinical Ethics.* 1998 Summer; 9(2): 99–107.
(PROFESSIONAL PATIENT RELATIONSHIP)

Howe, Edmund G. Everyday heroes, part 2: should careproviders ever be Quintilian? *Journal of Clinical Ethics.* 1997 Summer; 8(2): 115–123.
(ETHICISTS AND ETHICS COMMITTEES)

Howe, Edmund G. "Possible mistakes." *Journal of Clinical Ethics.* 1997 Winter; 8(4): 323–328.
(PATIENT CARE; TRUTH DISCLOSURE)

Howe, Edmund G. Resisting the siren: commentary. *Journal of Clinical Ethics.* 1998 Summer; 9(2): 207–208.
(BIOETHICS)

Howe, K.R. Medical students' evaluations of different levels of medical ethics teaching: implications for curricula. *Medical Education.* 1987 Jul; 21(4): 340–349.
(MEDICAL ETHICS/EDUCATION)

Howell, Nancy R. Abortion and religion. *In:* Edwards, Rem B., ed. Advances in Bioethics. Volume 2: New Essays on Abortion and Bioethics. Greenwich, CT: JAI Press; 1997: 125–149.
(ABORTION/RELIGIOUS ASPECTS)

Hoyte, Patrick see **McFadzean, J.**

Hsu, Irene; DuChane, Janeen; Veatch, Robert M. Recommendation of treatment that would allow parole -- Scenario; Position 1: pharmacist should recommend the hormonal treatment; Position 2: pharmacist should not recommend the hormonal treatment; Analysis and commentary. *American Journal of Health–System Pharmacy.* 1995 Apr 15; 52(8): 829–833.
(BEHAVIOR CONTROL; PATIENT CARE/DRUGS; SELECTION FOR TREATMENT)

Huang, Fu–Yuan see **Jan, Sheau–Wen**

Huang, Lian–Hua see **Jan, Sheau–Wen**

Hubbard, Anthony see **Close, Bryony**

Huber, Ruth; Evans, Virginia Cox. Trust in physicians to honor death related instructions. *Omega: A Journal of Death and Dying.* 1997–1998; 36(1): 9–21.
(ADVANCE DIRECTIVES; ALLOWING TO DIE/ATTITUDES; PROFESSIONAL PATIENT RELATIONSHIP; TERMINAL CARE)

Huda, N.E. see **Kazim, E.**

Huff, Steven see **Corley, Mary C.**

Huffine, Carol see **Slome, Lee**

Hughes, David; Griffiths, Lesley. "But if you look at the coronary anatomy...": risk and rationing in cardiac surgery. *Sociology of Health and Illness.* 1996 Mar; 18(2): 172–197.
(RESOURCE ALLOCATION/BIOMEDICAL TECHNOLOGIES; SELECTION FOR TREATMENT)

Hughes, Jonathan. Xenografting: ethical issues. *Journal of Medical Ethics.* 1998 Feb; 24(1): 18–24.
(ORGAN AND TISSUE TRANSPLANTATION)

Hughes, Katharine Kostbade; Dvorak, Eileen McQuaid. The use of decision analysis to examine ethical decision making by critical care nurses. *Heart and Lung.* 1997 May–Jun; 26(3): 238–248.
(NURSING ETHICS)

Hughes, Vivian see **Parkins, K.J.**

Hui, Elsie; Ho, Suzanne C.; Tsang, June; Lee, S.H.; Woo, Jean. Attitudes toward life-sustaining treatment of older persons in Hong Kong. *Journal of the American Geriatrics Society.* 1997 Oct; 45(10): 1232–1236.
(ALLOWING TO DIE/ATTITUDES; RESUSCITATION ORDERS)

Huibers, A.K. see **van Thiel, G.J.M.W.**

Human Genome Organization. HUGO Statement on Patenting Issues Related to Early Release of Raw Sequence Data. London: HUGO; 1997 May. 2 p.
(GENOME MAPPING; PATENTING LIFE FORMS)

Human Rights Watch Women's Rights Project. Abortion policy and restrictions on women's rights in post–communist Poland. *In: its* The Human Rights Watch Global Report on Women's Human Rights. New York, NY: Human Rights Watch; 1995 Aug: 451–456.
(ABORTION/FOREIGN COUNTRIES; ABORTION/LEGAL ASPECTS)

Human Rights Watch Women's Rights Project. The abortion debate and violations of civil liberties in Ireland. *In: its* The Human Rights Watch Global Report on Women's Human Rights. New York, NY: Human Rights Watch; 1995 Aug: 444–451.
(ABORTION/FOREIGN COUNTRIES; ABORTION/LEGAL ASPECTS)

Humber, James M.; Almeder, Robert F., eds. Alternative Medicine and Ethics. Totowa, NJ: Humana Press; 1998. 220 p.
(PATIENT CARE)

Humphrey, Heather see **Humphrey, Michael**

Humphrey, Michael; Humphrey, Heather. New trends in human reproduction. *In: their* Families with a Difference: Varieties of Surrogate Parenthood. New York, NY: Routledge; 1988: 149–166, 182–183.
(REPRODUCTIVE TECHNOLOGIES)

Humphrey, Michael; Humphrey, Heather. Parenthood by donor insemination. *In: their* Families with a Difference: Varieties of Surrogate Parenthood. New York, NY: Routledge; 1988: 131–148, 181–182.
(ARTIFICIAL INSEMINATION)

Humphreys, Martin; Brockman, Bea. DNA profiling of detained patients. [Letter]. *Lancet.* 1998 Mar 7; 351(9104): 760.
(DNA FINGERPRINTING)

Humphreys, Martin; Ryman, Ann. Knowledge of emergency compulsory detention procedures among general practitioners in Edinburgh: sample survey. *BMJ (British Medical Journal).* 1996 Jun 8; 312(7044): 1462–1463.
(INVOLUNTARY COMMITMENT/FOREIGN COUNTRIES)

Humphry, Derek. Final Exit: The Practicalities of Self–Deliverance and Assisted Suicide for the Dying. Second Edition. New York, NY: Dell Trade Paperback; 1996. 206 p.
(EUTHANASIA; SUICIDE)

Hungary. Law No. 79 of 17 December 1992 on the protection of the life of the fetus. *International Digest of Health Legislation.* 1993; 44(2): 249–253.
(ABORTION/FOREIGN COUNTRIES; ABORTION/LEGAL ASPECTS)

Hunkeler, David see **Badoux, John C.**

Hunt, Geoffrey. The human condition of the professional: discretion and accountability. *Nursing Ethics.* 1997 Nov; 4(6): 519–526.
(FRAUD AND MISCONDUCT; PROFESSIONAL ETHICS)

Hunt, Geoffrey, ed. Whistleblowing in the Health Service: Accountability, Law and Professional Practice. London: Edward Arnold; 1995. 170 p.
(FRAUD AND MISCONDUCT; HEALTH CARE/FOREIGN COUNTRIES)

Hunter, Jeff S. see **Murphy, G. Don**

Huraib, S. see **Aswad, Saleh**

Hurley, Ann C.; Volicer, Ladislav; Rempusheski, Veronica F.; Fry, Sara T. Reaching consensus: the process of recommending treatment decisions for Alzheimer's patients. *Advances in Nursing Science.* 1995 Dec; 18(2): 33–43.
(PATIENT CARE/MENTALLY DISABLED; TERMINAL CARE)

Hurry, Stephanie. Termination of pregnancy — a nurse's right to choose. *British Journal of Theatre Nursing.* 1997 Oct; 7(7): 18–22.
(ABORTION; NURSING ETHICS)

Hurt, Valerie see **Moreno, Jonathan D.**

Hurwitz, Brian; Richardson, Ruth. Swearing to care: the resurgence in medical oaths. *BMJ (British Medical Journal).* 1997 Dec 20–27; 315(7123): 1671–1674.
(MEDICAL ETHICS/CODES OF ETHICS; PROFESSIONAL ETHICS/CODES OF ETHICS)

Huston, Kathleen. Ethical decisions in treating battered women. *Professional Psychology: Research and Practice.* 1984 Dec; 15(6): 822–832.
(PATIENT CARE; PROFESSIONAL PATIENT RELATIONSHIP)

Hutchens, Michael P. Grave robbing and ethics in the 19th century. *JAMA.* 1997 Oct 1; 278(13): 1115.
(FRAUD AND MISCONDUCT; MEDICAL ETHICS)

Hutchinson, S. see **Brawn, W.J.**

Hutchinson, Sally A. see **Andrews, Sam**

Hyde, Henry J. The acceptable time. *Human Life Review.* 1997 Spring; 23(2): 75–78.
(ABORTION/LEGAL ASPECTS)

Hyde, Henry J. see **Sills, E. Scott**

Hyman, Lawrence see **Thies, Winthrop Drake**

I

Ibrahim, Youssef M. Algeria to permit abortions for rape victims. [News]. *New York Times.* 1998 Apr 14: A6.
(ABORTION/FOREIGN COUNTRIES)

IJesselmuiden, Carel B.; Faden, Ruth R. Medical research and the principle of respect for persons in non–Western cultures. *In:* Vanderpool, Harold Y., ed. The Ethics of Research Involving Human Subjects: Facing the 21st Century. Frederick, MD: University Publishing Group; 1996: 281–301.
(HUMAN EXPERIMENTATION/FOREIGN COUNTRIES; HUMAN EXPERIMENTATION/INFORMED CONSENT)

Ikels, Charlotte. Kidney failure and transplantation in China. *Social Science and Medicine.* 1997 May; 44(9): 1271–1283.
(ORGAN AND TISSUE DONATION)

Ikemoto, Lisa C. Destabilizing thoughts on surrogacy legislation. [Commentary]. *University of San Francisco Law Review.* 1994 Spring; 28(3): 633–645.
(REPRODUCTION; SURROGATE MOTHERS)

Illingworth, John see Close, Bryony

Illingworth, Patricia. Warning: AIDS health promotion programs may be hazardous to your autonomy. *In:* Overall, Christine and Zion, William P., eds. Perspectives on AIDS: Ethical and Social Issues. New York, NY: Oxford University Press; 1991: 138–154.
(AIDS; BEHAVIOR CONTROL; PUBLIC HEALTH)

Illinois. Appellate Court, First District, Sixth Division. Doe v. Noe. *North Eastern Reporter, 2d Series.* 1997 Dec 26 (date of decision). 690: 1012–1023.
(AIDS/HEALTH PERSONNEL)

Illinois. Appellate Court, Fourth District. In re Branning. *North Eastern Reporter, 2d Series.* 1996 Dec 18 (date of decision). 674: 463–472.
(ELECTROCONVULSIVE THERAPY; INFORMED CONSENT/MENTALLY DISABLED)

Imber, Jonathan B. Medical publicity before bioethics: nineteenth–century illustrations of twentieth–century dilemmas. *In:* DeVries, Raymond; Subedi, Janardan, eds. Bioethics and Society: Constructing the Ethical Enterprise. Upper Saddle River, NJ: Prentice Hall; 1998: 16–37.
(BIOETHICS; ETHICISTS AND ETHICS COMMITTEES)

Inciardi, James A.; Surratt, Hilary L.; Saum, Christine A. Prenatal cocaine use and the prosecution of pregnant addicts. *In: their* Cocaine–Exposed Infants: Social, Legal, and Public Health Issues. Thousand Oaks, CA: Sage Publications; 1997: 62–85.
(FETUSES; PRENATAL INJURIES)

Indudhara, R.; Singh, S.K.; Minz, M. Opinion poll regarding knowledge, attitudes, and suggestions for developing a cadaver donor program. *Transplantation Proceedings.* 1992 Oct; 24(5): 2069.
(ORGAN AND TISSUE DONATION; ORGAN AND TISSUE TRANSPLANTATION)

Infante, Marie C. see Rushton, Cindy Hylton

Inglis, Steven R. see Lescale, Keith B.

Ingram, Kellie K. see Marson, Daniel

Ingram, Miranda. Russia delays HIV testing for foreigners. [News]. *BMJ (British Medical Journal).* 1995 Aug 12; 311(7002): 407.
(AIDS/TESTING AND SCREENING)

Inoshita, Osamu see Asai, Atsushi

Institute for Science, Law, and Technology Working Group see Andrews, Lori

Institute of Health Services Management (Great Britain). Code of professional practice of the Institute of Health Services Management. *Nursing Ethics.* 1998 Jan; 5(1): 75–77.
(PROFESSIONAL ETHICS/CODES OF ETHICS)

Institute of Medicine see Potts, John T.

Institute of Medicine. Committee on Care at the End of Life see Field, Marilyn J.

International Council of Nurses. International Council of Nurses Code for Nurses: Ethical Concepts Applied to Nursing. [Pamphlet]. Available from the International Council of Nurses, Geneva, Switzerland; 1989. 7 p.
(NURSING ETHICS/CODES OF ETHICS)

International Federation of Gynecology and Obstetrics. Recommendations on ethical issues in obstetrics and gynecology. [Official statement]. *Bulletin of Medical Ethics.* 1997 Nov; No. 133: 8–9.
(CONTRACEPTION; REPRODUCTION)

International Federation of Gynecology and Obstetrics. Committee for the Study of Ethical Aspects of Human Reproduction. Recommendations on Ethical Issues in Obstetrics and Gynecology. London: FIGO; 1997 Jul. 117 p.
(PATIENT CARE; REPRODUCTION)

International Federation of Gynecology and Obstetrics. Committee for the Study of Ethical Aspects of Human Reproduction see Schenker, Joseph G.

Inui, Thomas S. see McCurdy, Layton

Irvin, Susan M. The great dilemma [AIDS]. *Nursing Standard.* 1995 Sep 27–Oct 3; 10(1): 50–53.
(AIDS/HEALTH PERSONNEL; AIDS/TESTING AND SCREENING)

Irving, Dianne N.; Shamoo, Adil E. Washouts/relapses in patients participating in neurobiological research studies in schizophrenia. *In:* Shamoo, Adil E., ed. Ethics in Neurobiological Research with Human Subjects: The Baltimore Conference on Ethics. Amsterdam: Gordon and Breach; 1997: 119–127.
(HUMAN EXPERIMENTATION/RESEARCH DESIGN; HUMAN EXPERIMENTATION/SPECIAL POPULATIONS)

Irving, Miles; Berwick, Donald M.; Rubin, Peter; Treasure, Tom. Five times: coincidence or something more serious? [Article and commentaries]. *BMJ (British Medical Journal).* 1998 Jun 6; 316(7146): 1736–1740.
(FRAUD AND MISCONDUCT; PATIENT CARE)

Irwin, Charles E. see Ford, Carol A.

Isaacson, Jeanne see Gertner, Eric J.

Iserson, Kenneth V. Bioethical dilemmas in emergency medicine and prehospital care. [Revised]. *In:* Monagle, John F.; Thomasma, David C., eds. Health Care Ethics: Critical Issues for the 21st Century. Gaithersburg, MD: Aspen Publishers; 1998: 138–145.
(PATIENT CARE)

Iserson, Kenneth V. Staring at our future. *Cambridge Quarterly of Healthcare Ethics.* 1997 Spring; 6(2): 243–244.
(HEALTH CARE/ECONOMICS)

Iserson, Kenneth V.; Jarrell, Bruce E. Financial relationships with patients. *In:* McCullough, Laurence B.; Jones, James W.; Brody, Baruch A., eds. Surgical Ethics. New York, NY: Oxford University Press; 1998: 322–341.
(HEALTH CARE/ECONOMICS)

Iserson, Kenneth V.; Kastre, Tammy Y. Are emergency departments really a "safety net" for the medically indigent? *American Journal of Emergency Medicine.* 1996 Jan; 14(1): 1–5.
(HEALTH CARE/ECONOMICS)

Iserson, Kenneth V.; Klepper, Howard; Andereck, William S. Sperm donation from a comatose, dying man. [Case study and commentaries]. *Cambridge Quarterly of Healthcare Ethics.* 1998 Spring; 7(2): 209–217.
(ARTIFICIAL INSEMINATION)

Ishikawa, Yoshihiro see Berger, Douglas

Ivanovski, Ninoslav; Stojkovski, Ljupco; Cakalaroski, Koco; Masin, Georgi; Djikova, Sonja; Polenakovic, Momir. Renal transplantation from paid, unrelated donors in India — it is not only unethical, it is also medically unsafe. [Letter]. *Nephrology, Dialysis, Transplantation.* 1997 Sep; 12(9): 2028–2029.
(ORGAN AND TISSUE DONATION)

Iwatsuki, Shunzaboro see Marsh, J. Wallis

J

Jackson, Anthony. Wrongful life and wrongful birth: the English conception. *Journal of Legal Medicine.* 1996 Sep; 17(3): 349–381.
(WRONGFUL LIFE)

Jackson, Jennifer. Determining incompetence: problems with the function test. *In:* Grubb, Andrew, ed. Decision–Making and Problems of Incompetence. New York, NY: Wiley; 1994: 53–65.
(TREATMENT REFUSAL/MENTALLY DISABLED)

Jackson, Jennifer see Edwards, S.J.L.

Jacobs, Joseph J. Alternative medicine and medical futility. *In:* Zucker, Marjorie B.; Zucker, Howard D., eds. Medical Futility and the Evaluation of Life–Sustaining Interventions. New York, NY: Cambridge University Press; 1997: 65–70.
(PATIENT CARE)

Jacobs, R. Genetic screening — uses, potential abuses and ethical issues. *Occupational Medicine.* 1997 Aug; 47(6): 367–370.
(GENETIC SCREENING)

Jacobsen, Barbara see Evans, Lois K.

Jacobsen, Geir; Hals, Arild. Medical investigators' views about ethics and fraud in medical research. *Journal of the Royal College of Physicians of London.* 1995 Sep–Oct; 29(5): 405–409.
(BIOMEDICAL RESEARCH; FRAUD AND MISCONDUCT; HUMAN EXPERIMENTATION/ETHICS COMMITTEES; HUMAN EXPERIMENTATION/FOREIGN COUNTRIES; HUMAN EXPERIMENTATION/RESEARCH DESIGN)

Jacobson, Jay A.; Francis, L.P.; Battin, Margaret P.; Green, David J.; Grammes, C.; VanRiper, J.; Gully, J. Dialogue to action: lessons learned from some family members of deceased patients at an interactive program in seven Utah hospitals. *Journal of Clinical Ethics.* 1997 Winter; 8(4): 359–371.
(ETHICISTS AND ETHICS COMMITTEES; TERMINAL CARE)

Jaeger, Ami see Andrews, Lori

Jaffe, Allan S.; Landau, William M. Death after death: the presumption of informed consent for cardiopulmonary resuscitation — ethical paradox and clinical conundrum. *Neurology.* 1993 Nov; 43(11): 2173–2178.
(ALLOWING TO DIE)

Jaffe, Norman; van Eys, Jan; Gehan, Edmund; Link, Michael P.; Vietti, Teresa J. Response to "Is it ethical not to conduct a prospectively controlled trial of adjuvant chemotherapy in osteosarcoma?" [Letter and response]. *Cancer Treatment Reports.* 1983 Jul–Aug; 67(7–8): 743–745.
(HUMAN EXPERIMENTATION/RESEARCH DESIGN)

Jain, Renu; Thomasma, David C.; Ragas, Rasa. Response to "Ethics and drug infants," by Michelle Oberman (*CQ* Vol. 6, No. 2): points of variance. *Cambridge Quarterly of Healthcare Ethics.* 1998 Winter; 7(1): 94–96.
(ALLOWING TO DIE/INFANTS)

Jakobovits, Yoel. Male infertility: halakhic issues in investigation and management. *In:* Feldman, Emanuel; Wolowelsky, Joel B., eds. Jewish Law and the New Reproductive Technologies. Hoboken, NJ: Ktav; 1997: 115–138.
(PATIENT CARE; REPRODUCTIVE TECHNOLOGIES)

James, Barbara. Animals in experiments. *In: her* Animal Rights. Hove, East Sussex, Eng.: Wayland; 1990: 20–26.
(ANIMAL EXPERIMENTATION)

James, Ron see Klotzko, Arlene Judith

Jamieson, Dale. Experimenting on animals: a reconsideration. *Between the Species.* 1985 Summer; 1(3): 4–11.
(ANIMAL EXPERIMENTATION)

Jamison, Kay Redfield see Kahn, Mary Jo Ellis

Jamison, Tena. Should God be practicing medicine? *Human Rights.* 1995 Summer; 22(3): 10–13.
(HEALTH CARE; REPRODUCTION)

Jan, Sheau–Wen; Chen, Chih–Ping; Huang, Lian–Hua; Huang, Fu–Yuan; Lan, Chung–Chi. Attitudes toward maternal serum screening in Chinese women with positive results. *Journal of Genetic Counseling.* 1996 Dec; 5(4): 169–180.
(GENETIC COUNSELING; GENETIC SCREENING; PRENATAL DIAGNOSIS)

Janeway, Penny see Berwick, Donald

Janhonen, Sirpa see Latvala, Eila

Janssen, Piet J. see Dierckx de Casterlé, Bernadette

Janssens, Rien M.J.P.A. see ten Have, Henk A.M.J.

Jarrell, Bruce E. see Iserson, Kenneth V.

Jayaraman, K.S. Indian guidelines allow limited gene screening. [News]. *Nature.* 1998 Jan 8; 391(6663): 115.
(GENETIC SCREENING)

Jayaraman, K.S. Inquiry looks into Indian cancer deaths. [News]. *Nature.* 1997 Dec 18–25; 390(6661): 653.
(FRAUD AND MISCONDUCT; HUMAN EXPERIMENTATION/FOREIGN COUNTRIES; HUMAN EXPERIMENTATION/INFORMED CONSENT; HUMAN EXPERIMENTATION/SPECIAL POPULATIONS)

Jayaraman, K.S. Policing ethical codes in India proves tough. [News]. *Nature.* 1997 Oct 16; 389(6652): 663.
(HUMAN EXPERIMENTATION/FOREIGN COUNTRIES)

Jecker, Nancy S.; Allen, Margaret D. Surgery and other medical specialties. *In:* McCullough, Laurence B.; Jones, James W.; Brody, Baruch A., eds. Surgical Ethics. New York, NY: Oxford University Press; 1998: 280–301.
(PATIENT CARE)

Jecker, Nancy S.; Jonsen, Albert R. Managed care: a house of mirrors. *Journal of Clinical Ethics.* 1997 Fall; 8(3): 230–241.
(HEALTH CARE/ECONOMICS)

Jeena, Prakash M. see **Bhagwanjee, Satish**

Jefferson, Larry S. see **Sachdeva, Ramesh C.**

Jehu, Derek. Patients as Victims: Sexual Abuse in Psychotherapy and Counselling. New York, NY: Wiley; 1994. 241 p.
(FRAUD AND MISCONDUCT; PROFESSIONAL PATIENT RELATIONSHIP)

Jelen, Ted G. see **Cook, Elizabeth Adell**

Jennett, Bryan. Managing patients in a persistent vegetative state since *Airedale NHS Trust v. Bland. In:* McLean, Sheila A.M., ed. Death, Dying and the Law. Brookfield, VT: Dartmouth; 1996: 19–28.
(ALLOWING TO DIE/LEGAL ASPECTS)

Jennings, Bruce. Autonomy and difference: the travails of liberalism in bioethics. *In:* DeVries, Raymond; Subedi, Janardan, eds. Bioethics and Society: Constructing the Ethical Enterprise. Upper Saddle River, NJ: Prentice Hall; 1998: 258–269.
(BIOETHICS)

Jennings, Maggy; Silcock, Sheila. Benefits, necessity and justification in animal research. *ATLA: Alternatives to Laboratory Animals.* 1995 Nov–Dec; 23(6): 828–836.
(ANIMAL EXPERIMENTATION)

Jennings, Margaret see **Balls, Michael**

Jennings, Patricia see **Beeson, Diane**

Jens, Walter see **Küng, Hans**

Jensen, Roy A. see **Page, David L.**

Jeyaratnam, J. see **Koh, D.**

Jobe, Kathleen A. see **Olson, Carin M.**

Johannes, Laura see **Stecklow, Steve**

Johannes Wier Foundation. Assistance in Hunger Strikes: A Manual for Physicians and Other Health Personnel Dealing with Hunger Strikers. Amersfoort, the Netherlands: Johannes Wier Foundation for Health and Human Rights; 1995. 44 p.
(FORCE FEEDING)

Johns, Jeanine L. Advance directives and opportunities for nurses. *Image: The Journal of Nursing Scholarship.* 1996 Summer; 28(2): 149–153.
(ADVANCE DIRECTIVES)

Johnson, Alan G. Surgery as a placebo. *Lancet.* 1994 Oct 22; 344(8930): 1140–1142.
(PATIENT CARE)

Johnson, Anne M. see **De Cock, Kevin M.**

Johnson, Dirk. Eccentric's hubris set off global frenzy over cloning. [News]. *New York Times.* 1998 Jan 24: A1, A11.
(CLONING)

Johnson, J. Rock see **Shamoo, Adil E.**

Johnson, James R. see **Gurewich, Victor**

Johnson, John P. see **Fanos, Joanna H.**

Johnson, Karen M. see **Elliott, Thomas E.**

Johnson, Linda; Potter, Robert Lyman. Professional and public community projects for developing medical futility guidelines. *In:* Zucker, Marjorie B.; Zucker, Howard D., eds. Medical Futility and the Evaluation of Life-Sustaining Interventions. New York, NY: Cambridge University Press; 1997: 155–167.
(ALLOWING TO DIE; TERMINAL CARE)

Johnson, Martin H. Should egg donors be paid? The culture of unpaid and voluntary egg donation should be strengthened. *BMJ (British Medical Journal).* 1997 May 10; 314(7091): 1401–1402.
(ORGAN AND TISSUE DONATION; REPRODUCTIVE TECHNOLOGIES)

Johnson, Michael H. see **Ford, Helen L.**

Johnson, Timothy. Shattuck lecture -- medicine and the media. *New England Journal of Medicine.* 1998 Jul 9; 339(2): 87–92.
(BIOMEDICAL RESEARCH)

Johnson, Walter see **Veglia, Geremia**

Johnston, S.R.D.; Broadley, K.; Henson, G.; Fisher, C.; Henk, M.; Gore, M.E.; Hammond, Robert; Weijer, Charles. Management of metastatic melanoma during pregnancy. [Case study and commentaries]. *BMJ (British Medical Journal).* 1998 Mar 14; 316(7134): 848–851.
(ABORTION; FETUSES; PATIENT CARE)

Johnstone, Megan-Jane. Bioethics: A Nursing Perspective. Second Edition. Philadelphia, PA: W.B. Saunders; 1994. 574 p.
(BIOETHICS; NURSING ETHICS)

Jones, Anne Hudson. From principles to reflective practice or narrative ethics? Commentary on Carson. *In:* Carson, Ronald A.; Burns, Chester R., eds. Philosophy of Medicine and Bioethics: A Twenty-Year Retrospective and Critical Appraisal. Boston, MA: Kluwer Academic; 1997: 193–195.
(BIOETHICS)

Josefson, Deborah. U.S. sees first legal case of physician assisted suicide. [News]. *BMJ (British Medical Journal).* 1998 Apr 4; 316(7137): 1037.
(SUICIDE)

Josefson, Deborah. US admits radiation experiments on 20,000 veterans. [News]. *BMJ (British Medical Journal).* 1997 Sep 6; 315(7108): 566.
(HUMAN EXPERIMENTATION/SPECIAL POPULATIONS)

Josefson, Deborah. US journal embroiled in another conflict of interest scandal. [News]. *BMJ (British Medical Journal).* 1998 Jan 24; 316(7127): 251.
(FRAUD AND MISCONDUCT; PUBLIC HEALTH)

Josefson, Deborah. US scientist plans human cloning clinic. [News]. *BMJ (British Medical Journal).* 1998 Jan 17; 316(7126): 167.
(CLONING)

Juengst, Eric T. Ethics of prediction: genetic risk and the physician–patient relationship. *Genome Science and Technology.* 1995; 1(1): 21–36.
(GENETIC COUNSELING; GENETIC SCREENING)

Juengst, Eric T. Groups as gatekeepers to genomic research: conceptually confusing, morally hazardous, and practically useless. *Kennedy Institute of Ethics Journal.* 1998 June; 8(2): 183–200.
(GENETIC RESEARCH; HUMAN EXPERIMENTATION/INFORMED CONSENT)

Juengst, Eric T. Prenatal diagnosis and the ethics of uncertainty. [Revised]. *In:* Monagle, John F.; Thomasma, David C., eds. Health Care Ethics: Critical Issues for the 21st Century. Gaithersburg, MD: Aspen Publishers; 1998: 15–28.
(PRENATAL DIAGNOSIS)

Juengst, Eric T. Respecting human subjects in genome research: a preliminary policy agenda. *In:* Vanderpool, Harold Y., ed. The Ethics of Research Involving Human Subjects: Facing the 21st Century. Frederick, MD: University Publishing Group; 1996: 401–429.
(CONFIDENTIALITY; GENETIC RESEARCH; GENOME MAPPING; INFORMED CONSENT)

Juengst, Eric T. Should we treat the human germ–line as a global human resource? *In:* Agius, Emmanuel; Busuttil, Salvino, eds. Germ–Line Intervention and Our Responsibilities to Future Generations. Boston, MA: Kluwer Academic; 1998: 85–102.
(GENE THERAPY)

Julian–Arnold, Gianna see **Sprunger, Suzanne A.**

Jung, Christine see **Wolff, Gerhard**

Jung, Patricia Beattie. What price fertility? *In:* Wildes, Kevin Wm., ed. Infertility: A Crossroad of Faith, Medicine, and Technology. Boston, MA: Kluwer Academic; 1997: 167–180.
(REPRODUCTIVE TECHNOLOGIES; RESOURCE ALLOCATION/BIOMEDICAL TECHNOLOGIES)

Junkerman, Charles; Schiedermayer, David. Practical Ethics for Students, Interns, and Residents: A Short Reference Manual. Second Edition. Frederick, MD: University Publishing Group; 1998. 73 p.
(BIOETHICS; MEDICAL ETHICS)

Jurchak, Martha. Clinical ethics consultants: survey and practice. *In:* Monagle, John F.; Thomasma, David C., eds. Health Care Ethics: Critical Issues for the 21st Century. Gaithersburg, MD: Aspen Publishers; 1998: 471–483.
(ETHICISTS AND ETHICS COMMITTEES)

Jurewicz, A. see **Higgins, R.M.**

Jürgens, Ralf; Palles, Michael. HIV Testing and Confidentiality: A Discussion Paper. Montreal: Canadian HIV/AIDS Legal Network; 1997. 317 p.
(AIDS/CONFIDENTIALITY; AIDS/TESTING AND SCREENING)

K

Kääriäinen, Helena. Genetic studies in populations. *In:* Knoppers, Bartha Maria, ed. Human DNA: Law and Policy: International and Comparative Perspectives. Proceedings of the First International Conference on DNA Sampling and Human Genetic Research: Ethical, Legal, and Policy Aspects, held in Montreal, Canada, 6–8 Sep 1996. Boston, MA: Kluwer Law International; 1997: 177–188.
(GENETIC RESEARCH; GENETIC SCREENING; HUMAN EXPERIMENTATION/INFORMED CONSENT)

Kadane, Joseph B., ed. Bayesian Methods and Ethics in a Clinical Trial Design. New York, NY: Wiley; 1996. 318 p.
(HUMAN EXPERIMENTATION/RESEARCH DESIGN)

Kadish, Sidney P. see **White, W.D.**

Kadlec, Josef V.; McPherson, Richard A. Ethical issues in screening and testing for genetic diseases. *Clinics in Laboratory Medicine.* 1995 Dec; 15(4): 989–999.
(GENETIC SCREENING)

Kahn, Axel. Cloning, dignity and ethical revisionism. [Letter]. *Nature.* 1997 Jul 24; 388(6640): 320.
(CLONING)

Kahn, D. see **Pike, Roseanne E.**

Kahn, Jeffrey P.; Mastroianni, Anna C.; Sugarman, Jeremy. Beyond Consent: Seeking Justice in Research. New York, NY: Oxford University Press; 1998. 190 p.
(HUMAN EXPERIMENTATION)

Kahn, Jeffrey P.; Mastroianni, Anna C.; Sugarman, Jeremy. Changing claims about justice in research: an introduction and overview. *In:* Kahn, Jeffrey P.; Mastroianni, Anna C.; Sugarman, Jeremy, eds. Beyond Consent: Seeking Justice in Research. New York, NY: Oxford University Press; 1998: 1–10.
(HUMAN EXPERIMENTATION/SPECIAL POPULATIONS)

Kahn, Jeffrey P.; Mastroianni, Anna C.; Sugarman, Jeremy. Implementing justice in a changing research environment. *In:* Kahn, Jeffrey P.; Mastroianni, Anna C.; Sugarman, Jeremy, eds. Beyond Consent: Seeking Justice in Research. New York, NY: Oxford University Press; 1998: 166–173.
(HUMAN EXPERIMENTATION)

Kahn, Jeffrey P. see **Sugarman, Jeremy**

Kahn, Katherine L. see **Wenger, Neil S.**

Kahn, Mary Jo Ellis; Jamison, Kay Redfield; Collins, Francis S. Protecting our 'family secrets'. *Washington Post.* 1997 Jul 31: A15.
(GENETIC RESEARCH; GENETIC SCREENING)

Kahn, Mary Jo Ellis see **Geller, Gail**

Kahtan, Susannah see **Richmond, Caroline**

Kaiji, Fumie see **Asai, Atsushi**

Kairys, David. The law of clinical testing with human subjects: legal implications of the new and existing methodologies. *In:* Kadane, Joseph B., ed. Bayesian Methods and Ethics in a Clinical Trial Design. New York, NY: Wiley; 1996: 223–249.
(HUMAN EXPERIMENTATION/RESEARCH DESIGN)

Kairys, David see **Moore, Dale**

Kaiser, Jocelyn. Archive available for genetic studies. [News]. *Science.* 1997 Nov 21; 278(5342): 1389.
(CONFIDENTIALITY; GENETIC RESEARCH)

Kaiser, Jocelyn. Bangkok study adds fuel to AIDS ethics debate. [News]. *Science.* 1997 Nov 28; 278(5343): 1553.
(AIDS/HUMAN EXPERIMENTATION; HUMAN EXPERIMENTATION/RESEARCH DESIGN)

Kaiser, Jocelyn. British editors form misconduct panel. [News]. *Science.* 1997 Aug 1; 277(5326): 627.
(BIOMEDICAL RESEARCH; FRAUD AND MISCONDUCT)

Kaiser, Jocelyn. Fisher wins $2.75 million settlement. [News]. *Science.* 1997 Sep 5; 277(5331): 1425.
(BIOMEDICAL RESEARCH; FRAUD AND MISCONDUCT)

Kaiser, Jocelyn. Flap on NEJM board over ethics articles. [News]. *Science.* 1997 Oct 10; 278(5336): 211.
(AIDS/HUMAN EXPERIMENTATION; HUMAN EXPERIMENTATION/FOREIGN COUNTRIES; HUMAN EXPERIMENTATION/RESEARCH DESIGN; HUMAN EXPERIMENTATION/SPECIAL POPULATIONS)

Kaiser, Jocelyn. Furor over company deal roils AMA. [News]. *Science.* 1997 Oct 3; 278(5335): 26.
(HEALTH CARE/ECONOMICS; PROFESSIONAL ETHICS)

Kaiser, Jocelyn. Privacy rules set no new research curbs. [News]. *Science.* 1997 Sep 19; 277(5333): 1757.
(BIOMEDICAL RESEARCH; CONFIDENTIALITY/LEGAL ASPECTS)

Kaiser, Jocelyn. Tobacco consultants find letters lucrative. [News]. *Science.* 1998 Aug 14; 281(5379): 895, 897.
(BIOMEDICAL RESEARCH)

Kaiser, Jocelyn. UNAIDS to weigh vaccine ethics. [News]. *Science.* 1997 Sep 19; 277(5333): 1751.
(AIDS/HUMAN EXPERIMENTATION; HUMAN EXPERIMENTATION/FOREIGN COUNTRIES; IMMUNIZATION)

Kaiser, Jocelyn. UNESCO drafts bioethics declaration. [News]. *Science.* 1997 Oct 3; 278(5335): 23.
(GENETIC INTERVENTION; GENOME MAPPING)

Kalaça, Cagri; Akin, Ayse. The issue of sex selection in Turkey. *Human Reproduction.* 1995 Jul; 10(7): 1631–1632.
(SEX PRESELECTION)

Kalb, Claudia. How old is too old? *Newsweek.* 1997 May 5; 79(18): 64.
(REPRODUCTIVE TECHNOLOGIES; SELECTION FOR TREATMENT)

Kale, Rajendra see **Bhagwanjee, Satish**

Kallgren, Carl A.; Tauber, Robert T. Undergraduate research and the institutional review board: a mismatch or happy marriage? *Teaching of Psychology.* 1996 Feb; 23(1): 20–25.
(BEHAVIORAL RESEARCH/ETHICS COMMITTEES)

Kalra, Jagmohan see **Narasimhan, Parthas**

Kamisar, Yale. The reasons so many people support physician–assisted suicide -- and why these reasons are not convincing. *Issues in Law and Medicine.* 1996 Fall; 12(2): 113–131.
(SUICIDE)

Kamm, Frances M. Physician–assisted suicide, euthanasia, and intending death. *In:* Battin, Margaret P.; Rhodes, Rosamond; Silvers, Anita, eds. Physician Assisted Suicide: Expanding the Debate. New York, NY: Routledge; 1998: 28–62.
(ALLOWING TO DIE; EUTHANASIA; SUICIDE)

Kandel, Randy Frances. Which came first: the mother or the egg? A kinship solution to gestational surrogacy. *Rutgers Law Review.* 1994 Fall; 47(1): 165–239.
(SURROGATE MOTHERS)

Kandela, Peter. Gulf countries to reconsider organ transplantation. [News]. *Lancet.* 1997 Aug 23; 350(9077): 574.
(ORGAN AND TISSUE DONATION)

Kane, Gregory C.; Leone, Frank T.; Rowane, Joseph; Fish, James E. Nationwide perspective on the use of a formal ethics curriculum during critical care fellowship training. [Letter]. *Academic Medicine.* 1998 Jan; 73(1): 103.
(BIOETHICS/EDUCATION; MEDICAL ETHICS/EDUCATION)

Kane, John M.; Borenstein, Michael. The use of placebo controls in psychiatric research. *In:* Shamoo, Adil E., ed. Ethics in Neurobiological Research with Human Subjects: The Baltimore Conference on Ethics. Amsterdam: Gordon and Breach; 1997: 207–213.
(HUMAN EXPERIMENTATION/RESEARCH DESIGN; HUMAN EXPERIMENTATION/SPECIAL POPULATIONS)

Kane, John M. see **Carpenter, William T.**

Kane, Rosalie A. Ethical and legal issues in long–term care: food for futuristic thought. *Journal of Long–Term Care Administration.* 1993 Fall; 21(3): 66–74.
(PATIENT CARE/AGED)

Kane, Rosalie A.; Caplan, Arthur L.; Urv–Wong, Ene K.; Freeman, Iris C.; Aroskar, Mila A.; Finch, Michael. Everyday matters in the lives of nursing home residents: wish for and perception of choice and control. *Journal of the American Geriatrics Society.* 1997 Sep; 45(9): 1086–1093.
(PATIENT CARE/AGED)

Kaplan, Carl A. see **De Ville, Kenneth**

Kaplan, Edward H. Israel's ban on use of Ethiopians'

blood: how many infectious donations were prevented? *Lancet.* 1998 Apr 11; 351(9109): 1127–1128.
(AIDS; BLOOD DONATION)

Kaplan, Eric see **Hoge, Steven K.**

Kaplan, Karen Orloff. Not quite the last word: scenarios and solutions. *In:* Zucker, Marjorie B.; Zucker, Howard D., eds. Medical Futility and the Evaluation of Life–Sustaining Interventions. New York, NY: Cambridge University Press; 1997: 179–192.
(ALLOWING TO DIE)

Kaplan, Richard S.; Tuennerman, Jill A. Advance directives. [Letter]. *Journal of the American Geriatrics Society.* 1997 Sep; 45(9): 1156–1157.
(ADVANCE DIRECTIVES)

Kaplan, Robert M. see **Schneiderman, Lawrence J.**

Kapp, Marshall B. Medicolegal, employment, and insurance issues in APOE genotyping and Alzheimer's disease. *Annals of the New York Academy of Sciences.* 1996 Dec 16; 802: 139–148.
(GENETIC SCREENING)

Kapp, Marshall B. Our Hands Are Tied: Legal Tensions and Medical Ethics. Westport, CT: Auburn House; 1998. 175 p.
(PATIENT CARE)

Kapp, Marshall B. Persons with dementia as "liability magnets": ethical implications. *Journal of Clinical Ethics.* 1998 Spring; 9(1): 66–70.
(BEHAVIOR CONTROL; PATIENT CARE/MENTALLY DISABLED)

Kaptchuk, Ted J. Powerful placebo: the dark side of the randomised controlled trial. *Lancet.* 1998 Jun 6; 351(9117): 1722–1725.
(HUMAN EXPERIMENTATION/RESEARCH DESIGN)

Kark, Pieter see **Berger, Jeffrey T.**

Kark, Pieter see **Rosner, Fred**

Karlawish, Jason H.T.; Lantos, John. Community equipoise and the architecture of clinical research. *Cambridge Quarterly of Healthcare Ethics.* 1997 Fall; 6(4): 385–396.
(HUMAN EXPERIMENTATION/RESEARCH DESIGN)

Karlawish, Jason H.T.; Sachs, Greg A. Research on the cognitively impaired: lessons and warnings from the emergency research debate. *Journal of the American Geriatrics Society.* 1997 Apr; 45(4): 474–481.
(HUMAN EXPERIMENTATION/REGULATION; HUMAN EXPERIMENTATION/SPECIAL POPULATIONS)

Kash, Kathryn M. see **Portenoy, Russell K.**

Kashi, H. see **Higgins, R.M.**

Kaspar, Larita see **Smith, Martin L.**

Kass, Leon R.; Lund, Nelson. Courting death: assisted suicide, doctors, and the law. *Commentary.* 1996 Dec; 102(6): 17–29.
(SUICIDE)

Kass, Leon R. see **Thies, Winthrop Drake**

Kass, Nancy. Gender and research. *In:* Kahn, Jeffrey P.; Mastroianni, Anna C.; Sugarman, Jeremy, eds. Beyond Consent: Seeking Justice in Research. New York, NY: Oxford University Press; 1998: 67–87.
(HUMAN EXPERIMENTATION/SPECIAL POPULATIONS)

Kass, Nancy see **Gordon, Valery M.**

Kass, Nancy E. The implications of genetic testing for health and life insurance. *In:* Rothstein, Mark A., ed. Genetic Secrets: Protecting Privacy and Confidentiality in the Genetic Era. New Haven, CT: Yale University Press; 1997: 299–316.
(GENETIC SCREENING)

Kassirer, Jerome see **Angell, Marcia**

Kassirer, Jerome P. Managing care -- should we adopt a new ethic? [Editorial]. *New England Journal of Medicine.* 1998 Aug 6; 339(6): 397–398.
(HEALTH CARE/ECONOMICS; MEDICAL ETHICS)

Kassirer, Jerome P.; Angell, Marcia. The high price of product endorsement. [Editorial]. *New England Journal of Medicine.* 1997 Sep 4; 337(10): 700.
(HEALTH CARE/ECONOMICS)

Kassirer, Jerome P.; Rosenthal, Nadia A. Should human cloning research be off limits? [Editorial]. *New England Journal of Medicine.* 1998 Mar 26; 338(13): 905–906.
(CLONING)

Kastre, Tammy Y. see **Iserson, Kenneth V.**

Katajisto, Jouko see **Leino–Kilpi, Helena**

Katz, Katheryn D. see **Moore, Dale**

Katz, Michael see **Garcia, Jario E.**

Katz, Murray S. see **Somerville, Margaret A.**

Katz, Sheila Moriber. Medical education and managed care: keeping pace. *Journal of the American Geriatrics Society.* 1998 Mar; 46(3): 381–384.
(HEALTH CARE/ECONOMICS)

Katz, Stephen J. see **Love, Susan M.**

Kaufert, Joseph M.; O'Neil, John D.; Koolage, William W. The cultural and political context of informed consent for Native Canadians. *Arctic Medical Research.* 1991; (Suppl.): 181–184.
(INFORMED CONSENT)

Kaufert, Patricia see **Mustard, Cameron A.**

Kaufman, Kenneth see **Roth, Loren**

Kavanaugh, John F. Partial truths. *America.* 1997 Apr 5; 176(11): 24.
(ABORTION)

Kaveny, M. Cathleen. Assisted suicide, the Supreme Court, and the constitutive function of the law. *Hastings Center Report.* 1997 Sep–Oct; 27(5): 29–34.
(SUICIDE)

Kay, Jerald see **Roman, Brenda**

Kaye, Celia see Lowenthal, Barbara

Kazem, R.; Thompson, L.A.; Hamilton, M.P.;
Templeton, A. Current attitudes towards egg donation
among men and women. *Human Reproduction.* 1995 Jun;
10(6): 1543–1548.
(ORGAN AND TISSUE DONATION; REPRODUCTIVE
TECHNOLOGIES)

Kazim, E.; al-Rukaimi, M.; Fernandez, H.; Raizada,
S.N.; Mustafa, M.J. Railey; Huda, N.E. Buying a
kidney: the easy way out? *Transplantation Proceedings.*
1992 Oct; 24(5): 2112–2113.
(ORGAN AND TISSUE DONATION; ORGAN AND TISSUE
TRANSPLANTATION)

Kearney, Edmund M. Ethical dilemmas in the treatment
of adolescent gang members. *Ethics and Behavior.* 1998;
8(1): 49–57.
(PATIENT CARE/MENTALLY DISABLED; PATIENT
CARE/MINORS)

Keay, Timothy J. Approximating ethical research content.
In: Shamoo, Adil E., ed. Ethics in Neurobiological
Research with Human Subjects: The Baltimore
Conference on Ethics. Amsterdam: Gordon and
Breach; 1997: 149–153.
(HUMAN EXPERIMENTATION/INFORMED CONSENT;
HUMAN EXPERIMENTATION/SPECIAL POPULATIONS;
INFORMED CONSENT/MENTALLY DISABLED)

Kee, F. see Gaffney, B.

Keeler, William. The problem with human cloning.
Origins. 1998 Feb 26; 27(36): 597, 599–601.
(CLONING)

Keenan, James F. Moral horizons in health care:
reproductive technologies and Catholic identity. *In:*
Wildes, Kevin Wm., ed. Infertility: A Crossroad of Faith,
Medicine, and Technology. Boston, MA: Kluwer
Academic; 1997: 53–71.
(REPRODUCTIVE TECHNOLOGIES)

Keleti, Daniel see Somerville, Margaret A.

Kellett, John M.; Curtis, David. Suspension of nurse who
gave drug on consultant's instructions. [Letters]. *BMJ
(British Medical Journal).* 1997 Apr 5; 314(7086):
1043–1044.
(BEHAVIOR CONTROL; FRAUD AND MISCONDUCT)

Kelley, James L. Psychiatric Malpractice: Stories of
Patients, Psychiatrists, and the Law. New Brunswick,
NJ: Rutgers University Press; 1996. 229 p.
(PATIENT CARE/MENTALLY DISABLED)

Kelly, Brian J.; Varghese, Francis T. Assisted suicide
and euthanasia: what about the clinical issues? *Australian
and New Zealand Journal of Psychiatry.* 1996 Feb; 30(1):
3–8.
(EUTHANASIA; SUICIDE; TERMINAL CARE)

Kelly, Christine Kuehn. Patient-centered ethics
reclaiming center stage. *Annals of Internal Medicine.* 1997
Aug 15; 127(4): I–45.
(PROFESSIONAL PATIENT RELATIONSHIP)

Kelly, David F. Alternatives to physician-assisted suicide.
American Journal of Otolaryngology. 1995 May–Jun; 16(3):
181–185.
(ALLOWING TO DIE; SUICIDE; TERMINAL CARE)

Kelly, Grant. Patient data, confidentiality, and electronics:
identifiable data should no longer be freely available
within the NHS. [Editorial]. *BMJ (British Medical
Journal).* 1998 Mar 7; 316(7133): 718–719.
(CONFIDENTIALITY)

Kelly, John H.; Emanuel, Linda. Doing what's best for
patients: 1957 and 1997. [Letter and response]. *JAMA.*
1997 Oct 1; 278(13): 1061–1062.
(MEDICAL ETHICS)

Kelly, Susan E.; Marshall, Patricia A.; Sanders, Lee
M.; Raffin, Thomas A.; Koenig, Barbara A.
Understanding the practice of ethics consultation: results
of an ethnographic multi-site study. *Journal of Clinical
Ethics.* 1997 Summer; 8(2): 136–149.
(ETHICISTS AND ETHICS COMMITTEES)

Kelner, Merrijoy see Singer, Peter A.

Kemp, Martin. Hyde's horrors. *Nature.* 1998 May 21;
393(6682): 219.
(BEHAVIORAL RESEARCH)

Kemp, Virginia H. The role of critical care nurses in the
ethical decision-making process. *Dimensions of Critical
Care Nursing.* 1985 Nov–Dec; 4(6): 354–359.
(ALLOWING TO DIE)

Kempton, Susan see Domino, George

Kendrick, Kevin. Should nurses always tell the truth?
Honesty versus deception in healthcare. *Professional
Nurse (London).* 1994 Jul; 9: 674–677.
(NURSING ETHICS; TRUTH DISCLOSURE)

Kennedy, I.; Sells, R.A.; Daar, A.S.; Guttmann, R.D.;
Hoffenberg, R.; Lock, M.; Radcliffe-Richards, J.;
Tilney, N. The case for "presumed consent" in organ
donation. [For the International Forum for Transplant
Ethics]. *Lancet.* 1998 May 30; 351(9116): 1650–1652.
(ORGAN AND TISSUE DONATION)

Kennedy, I. see Hoffenberg, R.

Kennedy, I. see Radcliffe-Richards, J.

Kennedy Institute of Ethics (Georgetown University).
Bioethics Information Retrieval Project. Bioethics
Thesaurus. 1998 Edition. Washington, DC: The Institute;
1998. 91 p.
(BIOETHICS)

Kennedy, Randy. Doctor is arraigned in assisted suicide:
veterinarian is said to admit role in terminally ill friend's
death. [News]. *New York Times.* 1998 Oct 15: B3.
(SUICIDE)

Kennedy, Susan Lorraine see Kopala, Beverly

Kenny, Nuala P. The CMA Code of Ethics: more room
for reflection. [Editorial]. *Canadian Medical Association
Journal.* 1996 Oct 15; 155(8): 1063–1065.
(MEDICAL ETHICS/CODES OF ETHICS)

Kent, Alastair. Ethical aspects of the legal protection of
biotechnological inventions and the principle of
non-ownership of the human body. *Bulletin of Medical
Ethics.* 1997 Jan; No. 124: 32–33.
(PATENTING LIFE FORMS)

Kent, Bridie; Owens, R. Glynn. Conflicting attitudes to corneal and organ donation: a study of nurses' attitudes to organ donation. *International Journal of Nursing Studies.* 1995 Oct; 32(5): 484–492.
(ORGAN AND TISSUE DONATION)

Kent–First, Marijo Greene see Levy, Michael J.

Kent, Heather. Medical, health–science students bring different perspectives to interdisciplinary ethics course. *Canadian Medical Association Journal.* 1997 May 1; 156(9): 1317–1318.
(BIOETHICS/EDUCATION)

Kenwright, Simon see Allmers, Henning

Keown, John. Life and death in Dublin. *Cambridge Law Journal.* 1996 Mar; 55(1): 6–8.
(ALLOWING TO DIE/LEGAL ASPECTS)

Keown, John. The euthanasia debate in Britain. *International Journal of Bioethics.* 1997 Mar–Jun; 8(1–2): 55–63.
(EUTHANASIA/LEGAL ASPECTS)

Keran, Christopher see Bernat, James L.

Kerbeshian, Jacob see Burd, Larry

Kern, Donald see Markson, Lawrence

Kerns, Alice Fleury. Better to lay it out on the table rather than do it behind the curtain: hospitals need to obtain consent before using newly deceased patients to teach resuscitation procedures. [Comment]. *Journal of Contemporary Health Law and Policy.* 1997 Spring; 13(2): 581–612.
(INFORMED CONSENT; MEDICAL ETHICS/EDUCATION)

Kerns, Thomas A. Ethical Issues in HIV Vaccine Trials. New York, NY: St. Martin's Press; 1997. 249 p.
(AIDS/HUMAN EXPERIMENTATION; IMMUNIZATION)

Kerns, Thomas A. Jenner on Trial: An Ethical Examination of Vaccine Research in the Age of Smallpox and the Age of AIDS. Lanham, MD: University Press of America; 1997. 98 p.
(HUMAN EXPERIMENTATION; IMMUNIZATION)

Kerr, Anne; Cunningham–Burley, Sarah; Amos, Amanda. Eugenics and the new genetics in Britain: examining contemporary professionals' accounts. *Science, Technology, and Human Values.* 1998 Spring; 23(2): 175–198.
(EUGENICS; GENETIC RESEARCH)

Kerridge, Ian; Lowe, Michael; Henry, David. Ethics and evidence based medicine. *BMJ (British Medical Journal).* 1998 Apr 11; 316(7138): 1151–1153.
(HEALTH CARE)

Kessel, Anthony S. see David, T.J.

Kestenbaum, David. Cloning plan spawns ethics debate. [News]. *Science.* 1998 Jan 16; 279(5349): 315.
(CLONING)

Kestenbaum, David. Groups vie for space chimp colony. [News]. *Science.* 1998 May 22; 280(5367): 1186.
(ANIMAL EXPERIMENTATION)

Ketsararat, Witaya see Robb, Merlin L.

Keville, Terri D. The invisible woman: gender bias in medical research. *Women's Rights Law Reporter.* 1994; 15: 123–142.
(HEALTH; HUMAN EXPERIMENTATION/SPECIAL POPULATIONS)

Kevles, Daniel J. Diamond v. Chakrabarty and beyond: the political economy of patenting life. *In:* Thackray, Arnold, ed. Private Science: Biotechnology and the Rise of the Molecular Sciences. Philadelphia, PA: University of Pennsylvania Press; 1998: 65–79.
(PATENTING LIFE FORMS)

Kevles, Daniel J. In the Name of Eugenics: Genetics and the Uses of Human Heredity. With a New Preface by the Author. Cambridge, MA: Harvard University Press; 1995. 426 p.
(EUGENICS)

Keyes, Denis W. see Coon, Stephanie M.

Keyserlingk, Edward W. Expanding the scope of clinical ethics: making informed consent healthier in the hospital context. *International Journal of Bioethics.* 1997 Mar–Jun; 8(1–2): 127–130.
(INFORMED CONSENT)

Keyserlingk, Edward W. Medical oaths and codes. *In:* Chadwick, Ruth, ed. Encyclopedia of Applied Ethics, Volume 3. San Diego, CA: Academic Press; 1998: 155–163.
(MEDICAL ETHICS/CODES OF ETHICS)

Keyserlingk, Edward W. Quality of life decisions and the hopelessly ill patient: the physician as moral agent and truth teller. *In:* Hoshino, Kazumasa, ed. Japanese and Western Bioethics: Studies in Moral Diversity. Boston, MA: Kluwer Academic; 1997: 103–116.
(ALLOWING TO DIE; TRUTH DISCLOSURE)

Khambaroong, Chirasak see Robb, Merlin L.

Khushf, George. A radical rupture in the paradigm of modern medicine: conflicts of interest, fiduciary obligations, and the scientific ideal. [Book review essay]. *Journal of Medicine and Philosophy.* 1998 Feb; 23(1): 98–122.
(HEALTH CARE/ECONOMICS)

Khushf, George. Administrative and organizational ethics. *HEC (HealthCare Ethics Committee) Forum.* 1997 Dec; 9(4): 299–309.
(ETHICISTS AND ETHICS COMMITTEES; PROFESSIONAL ETHICS)

Khushf, George. Bioethics and the Pentecostal traditions: Christianity as an alternative healing system. *In:* Lustig, B. Andrew, ed.; Center for Medical Ethics and Health Policy (Houston, TX). Bioethics Yearbook, Volume 5: Theological Developments in Bioethics, 1992–1994. Boston, MA: Kluwer Academic; 1997: 123–141.
(BIOETHICS)

Khushf, George. Embryo research: the ethical geography of the debate. *Journal of Medicine and Philosophy.* 1997 Oct; 22(5): 495–519.
(EMBRYO AND FETAL RESEARCH; FETUSES; PERSONHOOD)

Khushf, George. The scope of organizational ethics:

editor's introduction. *HEC (HealthCare Ethics Committee) Forum.* 1998 Jun; 10(2): 127–135.
(HEALTH CARE; PROFESSIONAL ETHICS)

Khushf, George; Gifford, Robert. Understanding, assessing, and managing conflicts of interest. *In:* McCullough, Laurence B.; Jones, James W.; Brody, Baruch A., eds. Surgical Ethics. New York, NY: Oxford University Press; 1998: 342–366.
(HEALTH CARE/ECONOMICS)

Khushf, George see **Brett, Allan S.**

Kielstein, Rita. Clinical and ethical challenges of genetic markers for severe human hereditary disorders. *In:* Becker, Gerhold K., ed. Changing Nature's Course: The Ethical Challenge of Biotechnology. Hong Kong: Hong Kong University Press; 1996: 61–70.
(GENETIC COUNSELING)

Kiernan, Vincent. Truth is no longer its own reward. [News]. *New Scientist.* 1997 Mar 1; 153(2071): 11.
(BIOMEDICAL RESEARCH)

Kigotho, Anderson Wachira. Another HIV-1 trial loses placebo control. [News]. *Lancet.* 1997 Dec 20–27; 350(9094): 1831.
(AIDS/HUMAN EXPERIMENTATION; HUMAN EXPERIMENTATION/FOREIGN COUNTRIES; HUMAN EXPERIMENTATION/RESEARCH DESIGN; HUMAN EXPERIMENTATION/SPECIAL POPULATIONS)

Kilner, John F.; Pentz, Rebecca D.; Young, Frank E., eds. Genetic Ethics: Do the Ends Justify the Genes? Grand Rapids, MI: W.B. Eerdmans; 1997. 291 p.
(GENETIC INTERVENTION)

Kimsma, Gerrit see **Quill, Timothy E.**

Kimura, Rihito. Death, dying, and advance directives in Japan: sociocultural and legal points of view. *In:* Sass, Hans-Martin; Veatch, Robert M.; Kimura, Rihito, eds. Advance Directives and Surrogate Decision Making in Health Care: United States, Germany, and Japan. Baltimore, MD: Johns Hopkins University Press; 1998: 187–208.
(ADVANCE DIRECTIVES; ALLOWING TO DIE/LEGAL ASPECTS; EUTHANASIA/LEGAL ASPECTS; TERMINAL CARE)

Kimura, Rihito see **Sass, Hans-Martin**

King, Ariel R. see **Dickens, Bernard M.**

King, David. Ethics and the oncomouse. *GenEthics News.* 1995 Sep–Oct; No. 8: 7.
(PATENTING LIFE FORMS)

King, David. Eugenic tendencies in modern genetics. *In:* Doherty, Peter; Sutton, Agneta, eds. Man-Made Man: Ethical and Legal Issues in Genetics. Dublin, Ireland: Open Air; 1997: 71–82.
(EUGENICS)

King, David. Is knowledge always good? *GenEthics News.* 1996 May-Jun; No. 12: 6–7.
(GENETIC SCREENING)

King, David. No to genetic engineering of humans! *GenEthics News.* 1995 Nov-Dec; No. 9: 7.
(GENETIC INTERVENTION)

King, Leslie; Meyer, Madonna Harrington. The politics of reproductive benefits: U.S. insurance coverage of contraceptive and infertility treatments. *Gender and Society.* 1997 Feb; 11(1): 8–30.
(CONTRACEPTION; HEALTH CARE/ECONOMICS; REPRODUCTIVE TECHNOLOGIES)

King, Nancy M.P. see **Churchill, Larry R.**

King, Patricia A. Embryo research: the challenge for public policy. *Journal of Medicine and Philosophy.* 1997 Oct; 22(5): 441–455.
(EMBRYO AND FETAL RESEARCH)

King, Patricia A. Race, justice, and research. *In:* Kahn, Jeffrey P.; Mastroianni, Anna C.; Sugarman, Jeremy, eds. Beyond Consent: Seeking Justice in Research. New York, NY: Oxford University Press; 1998: 88–110.
(FRAUD AND MISCONDUCT; HUMAN EXPERIMENTATION/SPECIAL POPULATIONS)

King, Patricia A.; Wolf, Leslie E. Lessons for physician-assisted suicide from the African-American experience. *In:* Battin, Margaret P.; Rhodes, Rosamond; Silvers, Anita, eds. Physician Assisted Suicide: Expanding the Debate. New York, NY: Routledge; 1998: 91–112.
(HEALTH CARE; SUICIDE)

King, Peter see **Cleaton-Jones, Peter E.**

Kinirons, Mark see **Stewart, Kevin**

Kinlaw, Kathy. Is it ethical to provide futile care? *Journal of the Medical Association of Georgia.* 1990 Nov; 79(11): 839–842.
(ALLOWING TO DIE/INFANTS)

Kinmonth, Ann Louise; Reinhard, John; Bobrow, Martin; Pauker, Susan. The new genetics: implications for clinical services in Britain and the United States. *BMJ (British Medical Journal).* 1998 Mar 7; 316(7133): 767–770.
(GENETIC SERVICES; HEALTH CARE/FOREIGN COUNTRIES)

Kinn, Sue. The relationship between clinical audit and ethics. *Journal of Medical Ethics.* 1997 Aug; 23(4): 250–253.
(HEALTH CARE)

Kinney, Joanna H. Restricting donative choice: fetal tissue transplantation and respect for human life. *Journal of Law and Health.* 1995–1996; 10(2): 259–285.
(FETUSES; ORGAN AND TISSUE DONATION)

Kinsella, T. Douglas; Verhoef, Marja J. Assisted suicide: opinions of Alberta physicians. *Clinical and Investigative Medicine.* 1995 Oct; 18(5): 406–412.
(EUTHANASIA/ATTITUDES; SUICIDE)

Kinsella, T. Douglas see **Godard, Béatrice**

Kinsella, T. Douglas see **Verhoef, Marja J.**

Kinzer, Donna J. see **Goldfarb, James**

Kipnis, Kenneth. Confessions of an expert ethics witness. *Journal of Medicine and Philosophy.* 1997 Aug; 22(4): 325–343.
(BIOETHICS; ETHICISTS AND ETHICS COMMITTEES)

Kirby, Dahlian. Transsexualism. *In:* Chadwick, Ruth, ed. Encyclopedia of Applied Ehtics, Volume 4. San Diego, CA: Academic Press; 1998: 409–412.
(PATIENT CARE)

Kircher, T. see **Naber, D.**

Kirk, Maggie. Commercial gene testing: the need for professional and public debate. *British Journal of Nursing.* 1997 Oct 9–22; 6(18): 1043–1047.
(GENETIC SCREENING; GENETIC SERVICES)

Kirkland, Larry R. see **Kowalski, Edgar P.**

Kirsch, Irving; Rosadino, Michael J. Do double–blind studies with informed consent yield externally valid results? An empirical test. *Psychopharmacology (Berlin).* 1993; 110(4): 437–442.
(BEHAVIORAL RESEARCH/INFORMED CONSENT; BEHAVIORAL RESEARCH/RESEARCH DESIGN)

Kirschner, Kristi see **Blanck, Peter**

Kischer, C. Ward. The media and human embryology. *Linacre Quarterly.* 1998 May; 65(2): 33–42.
(FETUSES)

Kishino, Minako see **Asai, Atsushi**

Kitwood, Tom. Toward a theory of dementia care: ethics and interaction. *Journal of Clinical Ethics.* 1998 Spring; 9(1): 23–34.
(PATIENT CARE/MENTALLY DISABLED; PROFESSIONAL PATIENT RELATIONSHIP)

Kjellstrand, Carl see **Roberts, John**

Klasing, Murphy S. Death of an unborn child: jurisprudential inconsistencies in wrongful death, criminal homicide, and abortion cases. *Pepperdine Law Review.* 1995; 22(3): 933–979.
(ABORTION/LEGAL ASPECTS; FETUSES; PERSONHOOD)

Klein, Donald F. Response to Rothman and Michels on placebo–controlled clinical trials. *Psychiatric Annals.* 1995 Jul; 25(7): 401–403.
(HUMAN EXPERIMENTATION/RESEARCH DESIGN)

Klein, Rudolf. Competence, professional self regulation, and the public interest. *BMJ (British Medical Journal).* 1998 Jun 6; 316(7146): 1740–1742.
(FRAUD AND MISCONDUCT; PATIENT CARE)

Klein, Rudolph; Day, Patricia; Redmayne, Sharon. Managing Scarcity: Priority Setting and Rationing in the National Health Service. Philadelphia, PA: Open University Press; 1996. 161 p.
(HEALTH CARE/ECONOMICS; HEALTH CARE/FOREIGN COUNTRIES; RESOURCE ALLOCATION; SELECTION FOR TREATMENT)

Kleinman, Arthur. Anthropology of bioethics. *In: his* Writing at the Margin: Discourse Between Anthropology and Medicine. Berkeley, CA: University of California Press; 1995: 41–67, 268–269.
(BIOETHICS)

Kleinman, Arthur. Intimations of solidarity? The popular culture responds to assisted suicide. *Hastings Center Report.* 1997 Sep–Oct; 27(5): 34–36.
(SUICIDE)

Klepper, Howard see **Iserson, Kenneth V.**

Klinge, Ineke see **van Berkel, Dymphie**

Klingle, Renee Storm see **Young, Marti**

Klingmann, Ingrid. The European dimension. *In:* Close, Bryony; Combes, Robert; Hubbard, Anthony; Illingworth, John, eds. Volunteers in Research and Testing. Bristol, PA: Taylor and Francis; 1997: 169–175.
(HUMAN EXPERIMENTATION/ETHICS COMMITTEES; HUMAN EXPERIMENTATION/FOREIGN COUNTRIES)

Klock, Susan see **Andrews, Lori**

Klonis, Leah K. see **Tysinger, James W.**

Klotzko, Arlene Judith. Dolly, cloning, and the public misunderstanding of science: a challenge for us all. [Editorial]. *Cambridge Quarterly of Healthcare Ethics.* 1998 Spring; 7(2): 115–116.
(CLONING)

Klotzko, Arlene Judith. Medical miracle or medical mischief? The saga of the McCaughey septuplets. *Hastings Center Report.* 1998 May–Jun; 28(3): 5–8.
(REPRODUCTIVE TECHNOLOGIES)

Klotzko, Arlene Judith. Science fictions: cloning is bad and septuplets are good. *Washington Post.* 1997 Dec 14: C3.
(CLONING; REPRODUCTIVE TECHNOLOGIES)

Klotzko, Arlene Judith. The debate about Dolly. *Bioethics.* 1997 Oct; 11(5): 427–438.
(CLONING)

Klotzko, Arlene Judith; Bulfield, Grahame; Campbell, Keith; James, Ron; Wilmut, Ian. Voices from Roslin: the creators of Dolly discuss science, ethics, and social responsibility. [Interview]. *Cambridge Quarterly of Healthcare Ethics.* 1998 Spring; 7(2): 121–140.
(CLONING; GENETIC INTERVENTION)

Kmietowicz, Zosia. MRC cleared of unethical research practices. [News]. *BMJ (British Medical Journal).* 1998 May 30; 316(7145): 1628.
(FRAUD AND MISCONDUCT; HUMAN EXPERIMENTATION/FOREIGN COUNTRIES)

Kmietowicz, Zosia. Woman dies two months after food withdrawal. [News]. *BMJ (British Medical Journal).* 1997 May 24; 314(7093): 1503.
(ALLOWING TO DIE)

Knaus, William A. see **Teno, Joan**

Knaus, William A. see **Teno, Joan M.**

Knepper, Kathleen. The importance of establishing competence in cases involving the involuntary administration of psychotropic medications. *Law and Psychology Review.* 1996 Spring; 20: 97–137.
(TREATMENT REFUSAL/MENTALLY DISABLED)

Knight, James A. Ethics of care in caring for the elderly. *Southern Medical Journal.* 1994 Sep; 87(9): 909–917.
(PATIENT CARE/AGED)

Knoppers, Bartha M. see **de Wachter, Maurice A.M.**

Knoppers, Bartha Maria, ed. Human DNA: Law and Policy: International and Comparative Perspectives. Proceedings of the First International Conference on DNA Sampling and Human Genetic Research: Ethical, Legal, and Policy Aspects, held in Montreal, Canada, 6–8 Sep 1996. Boston, MA: Kluwer Law International; 1997. 455 p.
(GENETIC RESEARCH; GENETIC SCREENING)

Knoppers, Bartha Maria see **Bernard, Claire**

Koch, Hans–Georg. The decision to aid dying and related legal issues: advance directives and durable powers of attorney under German law. *In:* Sass, Hans–Martin; Veatch, Robert M.; Kimura, Rihito, eds. Advance Directives and Surrogate Decision Making in Health Care: United States, Germany, and Japan. Baltimore, MD: Johns Hopkins University Press; 1998: 114–135.
(ADVANCE DIRECTIVES; ALLOWING TO DIE/LEGAL ASPECTS)

Koch, Karen E. see **Davis, Kenneth M.**

Koch, Tom. Principles and purpose: the patient surrogate's perspective and role. *Cambridge Quarterly of Healthcare Ethics.* 1997 Fall; 6(4): 461–469.
(PATIENT CARE)

Koch, Tom; Ridgley, Mark. Distanced perspectives: AIDS, anencephaly, and AHP [Analytic Hierarchy Process]. *Theoretical Medicine and Bioethics.* 1998 Jan; 19(1): 47–58.
(ALLOWING TO DIE/INFANTS; BIOETHICS; PERSONHOOD)

Kodish, Eric; Wiesner, Georgia L.; Mehlman, Maxwell; Murray, Thomas. Genetic testing for cancer risk: how to reconcile the conflicts. *JAMA.* 1998 Jan 21; 279(3): 179–181.
(GENETIC SCREENING)

Kodish, Eric see **Daugherty, Christopher**

Koenig, Barbara A.; Hogle, Linda F. Organ transplantation (re)examined? Commentary. *Medical Anthropology Quarterly.* 1995 Sep; 9(3): 393–397.
(ORGAN AND TISSUE DONATION; ORGAN AND TISSUE TRANSPLANTATION)

Koenig, Barbara A. see **Barnes, Donelle M.**

Koenig, Barbara A. see **Hern, H. Eugene**

Koenig, Barbara A. see **Kelly, Susan E.**

Koenig, Barbara A. see **Marshall, Patricia A.**

Koenig, Robert. Panel calls falsification in German case 'unprecedented.' [News]. *Science.* 1997 Aug 15; 277(5328): 894.
(BIOMEDICAL RESEARCH; FRAUD AND MISCONDUCT)

Koenig, Robert. Panel proposes ways to combat fraud. [News]. *Science.* 1997 Dec 19; 278(5346): 2049–2050.
(BIOMEDICAL RESEARCH; FRAUD AND MISCONDUCT)

Koenig, Robert. Switzerland: voters reject antigenetics initiative. [News]. *Science.* 1998 Jun 12; 280(5370): 1685.
(GENETIC INTERVENTION)

Koenig, Wolfgang see **Schüppel, Reinhart**

Koffman, Jonathan. There must be a better way. [Personal view]. *BMJ (British Medical Journal).* 1998 Jun 27; 316(7149): 1989–1990.
(TERMINAL CARE)

Koh, D.; Jeyaratnam, J. Biomarkers, screening and ethics. *Occupational Medicine.* 1998 Jan; 48(1): 27–30.
(GENETIC SCREENING; OCCUPATIONAL HEALTH)

Kohrman, Arthur F. see **Bartholome, William G.**

Kohut, Nitsa; Sam, Mehran; O'Rourke, Keith; MacFadden, Douglas K.; Salit, Irving; Singer, Peter A. Stability of treatment preferences: although most preferences do not change, most people change some of their preferences. *Journal of Clinical Ethics.* 1997 Summer; 8(2): 124–135.
(ADVANCE DIRECTIVES)

Kok, Gerjo see **Verheggen, Frank W.S.M.**

Kokiko, Jeannine; Watts, Dorraine D. Ethical decision making in the emergency department: the R.O.L.E. acronym for four areas of consideration. *Journal of Emergency Nursing.* 1995 Jun; 21(3): 219–222.
(PATIENT CARE)

Kolata, Gina. Clinics selling embryos made for 'adoption'. [News]. *New York Times.* 1997 Nov 23: 1, 34.
(REPRODUCTIVE TECHNOLOGIES)

Kolata, Gina. Clone: The Road to Dolly, and the Path Ahead. New York, NY: William Morrow; 1998. 276 p.
(CLONING)

Kolata, Gina. Genetic testing falls short of public embrace. [News]. *New York Times.* 1998 Mar 27: A16.
(GENETIC SCREENING)

Kolata, Gina. Scientists face new ethical quandaries in baby–making. [News]. *New York Times.* 1997 Aug 19: C1, C8.
(EMBRYO AND FETAL RESEARCH; REPRODUCTIVE TECHNOLOGIES)

Kolata, Gina. Tough tactics are used over animals in the lab. [News]. *New York Times.* 1998 Mar 24: E1, E6.
(ANIMAL EXPERIMENTATION)

Kollée, L.A.A. see **van der Heide, A.**

Kondratowicz, Diane M. Approaches responsive to reproductive technologies: a need for critical assessment and directions for further study. *Cambridge Quarterly of Healthcare Ethics.* 1997 Spring; 6(2): 148–156.
(REPRODUCTIVE TECHNOLOGIES)

Kondro, Wayne. Alberta retreats over sterilisation compensation. [News]. *Lancet.* 1998 Mar 21; 351(9106): 892.
(STERILIZATION/MENTALLY DISABLED)

Kondro, Wayne. Canada still seeking research code of ethics. [News]. *Lancet.* 1997 Sep 13; 350(9080): 794.
(HUMAN EXPERIMENTATION/FOREIGN COUNTRIES)

Kondro, Wayne. Canada's privacy legislation warning. [News]. *Lancet.* 1997 Oct 11; 350(9084): 1085.
(CONFIDENTIALITY/LEGAL ASPECTS)

Kondro, Wayne. Canadian AIDS doctor convicted of physician–assisted suicide. [News]. *Lancet.* 1998 Jan 10; 351(9096): 121.
(SUICIDE)

Kondro, Wayne. Leaked document indicates Canada's future stance on human research. [News]. *Lancet.* 1998 Jun 20; 351(9119): 1868.
(HUMAN EXPERIMENTATION/FOREIGN COUNTRIES)

Kondro, Wayne. "Mercy killing" takes centre stage in Canada. [News]. *Lancet.* 1997 Nov 15; 350(9089): 1458.
(EUTHANASIA/LEGAL ASPECTS)

Kondro, Wayne. Murder–or–mercy case tested in Canada. [News]. *Lancet.* 1997 May 17; 349(9063): 1458.
(ALLOWING TO DIE/LEGAL ASPECTS; EUTHANASIA/LEGAL ASPECTS)

Kondro, Wayne. New rules on human subjects could end debate in Canada. [News]. *Science.* 1998 Jun 5; 280(5369): 1521.
(BEHAVIORAL RESEARCH/FOREIGN COUNTRIES; BEHAVIORAL RESEARCH/REGULATION; HUMAN EXPERIMENTATION/FOREIGN COUNTRIES; HUMAN EXPERIMENTATION/REGULATION)

Konen, Joseph C. Whose life is it anyway? [Editorial]. *Archives of Family Medicine.* 1997 Jan–Feb; 6(1): 77–78.
(PATIENT CARE)

Königova, Radana see **Pondělíček, Ivo**

Konishi, Emiko. Nurses' attitudes towards developing a do not resuscitate policy in Japan. *Nursing Ethics.* 1998 May; 5(3): 218–227.
(RESUSCITATION ORDERS)

Koolage, William W. see **Kaufert, Joseph M.**

Kopaczynski, Germain. Catholic identity in health care and the relevance of the 1994 Ethical and Religious Directives for Catholic Health Care Services. *Linacre Quarterly.* 1997 May; 64(2): 26–35.
(HEALTH CARE)

Kopala, Beverly; Kennedy, Susan Lorraine. Requests for assisted suicide: a nursing issue. *Nursing Ethics.* 1998 Jan; 5(1): 16–26.
(SUICIDE)

Kopelman, Arthur E. see **Kopelman, Loretta M.**

Kopelman, Loretta M. Female circumcision and genital mutilation. *In:* Chadwick, Ruth, ed. Encyclopedia of Applied Ethics, Volume 2. San Diego, CA: Academic Press; 1998: 249–259.
(HEALTH)

Kopelman, Loretta M. Medical futility. *In:* Chadwick, Ruth, ed. Encyclopedia of Applied Ethics, Volume 3. San Diego, CA: Academic Press; 1998: 185–196.
(ALLOWING TO DIE)

Kopelman, Loretta M. Medicine's challenge to relativism: the case of female genital mutilation. *In:* Carson, Ronald A.; Burns, Chester R., eds. Philosophy of Medicine and Bioethics: A Twenty-Year Retrospective and Critical Appraisal. Boston, MA: Kluwer Academic; 1997: 221–237.
(BIOETHICS; HEALTH)

Kopelman, Loretta M.; Lannin, Donald R.; Kopelman, Arthur E. Preventing and managing unwarranted biases against patients. *In:* McCullough, Laurence B.; Jones, James W.; Brody, Baruch A., eds. Surgical Ethics. New York, NY: Oxford University Press; 1998: 242–254.
(PATIENT CARE; PROFESSIONAL PATIENT RELATIONSHIP)

Kopfensteiner, Thomas R. A response to Leslie Griffin's essay. *In:* Wildes, Kevin Wm.; Mitchell, Alan C., eds. Choosing Life: A Dialogue on *Evangelium Vitae.* Washington, DC: Georgetown University Press; 1997: 174–178.
(ABORTION/RELIGIOUS ASPECTS)

Kopytoff, Barbara. Explorations in the law of surrogacy. [Commentary]. *University of San Francisco Law Review.* 1994 Spring; 28(3): 593–602.
(SURROGATE MOTHERS)

Korein, Julius. Ontogenesis of the brain in the human organism: definitions of life and death of the human being and person. *In:* Edwards, Rem B., ed. Advances in Bioethics. Volume 2: New Essays on Abortion and Bioethics. Greenwich, CT: JAI Press; 1997: 1–74.
(DETERMINATION OF DEATH/BRAIN DEATH; FETUSES; PERSONHOOD)

Koren, Gideon see **Ondrusek, Nancy**

Koren, Gideon see **Somerville, Margaret A.**

Korenman, Stanley G.; Berk, Richard; Wenger, Neil S.; Lew, Vivian. Evaluation of the research norms of scientists and administrators responsible for academic research integrity. *JAMA.* 1998 Jan 7; 279(1): 41–47.
(BIOMEDICAL RESEARCH; FRAUD AND MISCONDUCT; PROFESSIONAL ETHICS)

Kortmann, Frank see **Verweij, Marcel**

Kosalko, Joanne see **Smith, Martin L.**

Kotva, Carol S. see **Kotva, Joseph J.**

Kotva, Joseph J.; Kotva, Carol S. Was this consent informed? *American Journal of Nursing.* 1997 May; 97(5): 23.
(INFORMED CONSENT)

Kovac, Carl. Abortion stirs up controversy in Hungary. [News]. *BMJ (British Medical Journal).* 1998 Apr 4; 316(7137): 1038.
(ABORTION/FOREIGN COUNTRIES)

Kovac, Carl. Anonymous AIDS testing in Hungary to end. [News]. *BMJ (British Medical Journal).* 1997 Sep 6; 315(7108): 567.
(AIDS/CONFIDENTIALITY; AIDS/TESTING AND SCREENING)

Kovac, Carl. Tissue trade in Hungary is investigated. [News]. *BMJ (British Medical Journal).* 1998 Feb 28; 316(7132): 647.
(ORGAN AND TISSUE DONATION)

Koval, Joseph C.; Rousseau, Paul; Coulehan, Jack. The man with stars inside. [Letter and response]. *Annals of Internal Medicine.* 1997 Dec 15; 127(12): 1137–1138.
(SUICIDE; TERMINAL CARE)

Koven, Suzanne J. The ungifted physician. [A piece of

my mind]. *JAMA*. 1998 May 27; 279(20): 1607.
(PROFESSIONAL PATIENT RELATIONSHIP)

Kowalski, Edgar P.; Kowalski, Susan D.; Kirkland, Larry R.; Falasca, Gerald F.; Bancroft, Elizabeth A.; Batavia, Andrew I. Disability and physician–assisted suicide. [Letters and response]. *New England Journal of Medicine*. 1997 Dec 18; 337(25): 1852–1853.
(SUICIDE)

Kowalski, Susan D. Assisted suicide: is there a future? Ethical and nursing considerations. *Critical Care Nursing Quarterly*. 1996 May; 19(1): 45–54.
(ALLOWING TO DIE; EUTHANASIA; SUICIDE)

Kowalski, Susan D. see Kowalski, Edgar P.

Kozyrskyj, Anita see Mustard, Cameron A.

Krakauer, Eric L. see Berkowitz, Sheldon T.

Kramar, Giulia see Roy, David J.

Kravitz, Melva. Informed consent: must ethical responsibility conflict with professional conduct? *Nursing Management*. 1985 Nov; 16(11): 34A–34H.
(INFORMED CONSENT)

Krebs, D. Rules and ethics concerning assisted procreation established by the government in Germany. *Journal of Assisted Reproduction and Genetics*. 1996 Mar; 13(3): 193–195.
(EMBRYO AND FETAL RESEARCH; REPRODUCTIVE TECHNOLOGIES)

Kriegsman, D.M.W. see Muller, M.T.

Krim, Todd M. Beyond *Baby M*: international perspectives on gestational surrogacy and the demise of the unitary biological mother. *Annals of Health Law*. 1996; 5: 193–226.
(SURROGATE MOTHERS)

Krimsky, Sheldon; Rothenberg, L.S. Financial interest and its disclosure in scientific publications. *JAMA*. 1998 Jul 15; 280(3): 225–226.
(BIOMEDICAL RESEARCH)

Kristjanson, Linda J. see Degner, Lesley F.

Krotki, Karol P. see O'Brien, Linda A.

Kuboki, Tomifusa see Berger, Douglas

Kuczewski, Mark. Bioethics' consensus on method: *who could ask for anything more*? *In:* Nelson, Hilde Lindemann, ed. Stories and Their Limits: Narrative Approaches to Bioethics. New York, NY: Routledge; 1997: 134–149.
(BIOETHICS)

Kuczewski, Mark G. Fragmentation and Consensus: Communitarian and Casuist Bioethics. Washington, DC: Georgetown University Press; 1997. 177 p.
(BIOETHICS)

Kuehne, Dale S. see Godfrey, Nelda S.

Kuehnle, Kathryn. Ethics and the forensic expert: a case

study of child custody involving allegations of child sexual abuse. *Ethics and Behavior*. 1998; 8(1): 1–18.
(PROFESSIONAL ETHICS)

Kuhse, Helga. A nursing ethics of care? Why caring is not enough. *In:* Morscher, Edgar; Neumaier, Otto; Simons, Peter, eds. Applied Ethics in a Troubled World. Boston, MA: Kluwer Academic; 1998: 127–142.
(NURSING ETHICS)

Kuhse, Helga. Caring: Nurses, Women and Ethics. Malden, MA: Blackwell; 1997. 296 p.
(NURSING ETHICS; TERMINAL CARE)

Kuhse, Helga. Confidentiality and the AMA's [Australian Medical Association] new code of ethics: an imprudent formulation? *Medical Journal of Australia*. 1996 Sep 16; 165(6): 327–329.
(CONFIDENTIALITY; MEDICAL ETHICS/CODES OF ETHICS)

Kuhse, Helga. From intention to consent: learning from experience with euthanasia. *In:* Battin, Margaret P.; Rhodes, Rosamond; Silvers, Anita, eds. Physician Assisted Suicide: Expanding the Debate. New York, NY: Routledge; 1998: 252–266.
(ALLOWING TO DIE; EUTHANASIA; SUICIDE)

Kuhse, Helga; Singer, Peter. Choosing the sex, race and sexual orientation of our children. [Editorial]. *Bioethics*. 1998 Jan; 12(1): iii–v.
(SEX DETERMINATION; SEX PRESELECTION)

Kuhse, Helga; Singer, Peter. Cloning our way to Armageddon? [Editorial]. *Bioethics*. 1997 Oct; 11(5): iii–v.
(CLONING)

Kuhse, Helga; Singer, Peter. On the ethics of bringing people into existence. [Editorial]. *Bioethics*. 1998 Apr; 12(2): iii–v.
(CLONING; REPRODUCTION)

Kuhse, Helga; Singer, Peter; Rickard, Maurice; Cannold, Leslie; van Dyk, Jessica. Partial and impartial ethical reasoning in health care professionals. *Journal of Medical Ethics*. 1997 Aug; 23(4): 226–232.
(PROFESSIONAL ETHICS)

Kumar, A. see Bugeja, G.

Kumar, Sanjay. Hope, but little cheer, for India's revised code of ethics. [News]. *Lancet*. 1998 Jan 31; 351(9099): 347.
(HUMAN EXPERIMENTATION/FOREIGN COUNTRIES)

Kumar, Sanjay. India to ban use of quinacrine for sterilisation. [News]. *Lancet*. 1998 Mar 28; 351(9107): 968.
(HUMAN EXPERIMENTATION/FOREIGN COUNTRIES; HUMAN EXPERIMENTATION/SPECIAL POPULATIONS; STERILIZATION)

Kumar, Sanjay. Sterilisation by quinacrine comes under fire in India. [News]. *Lancet*. 1997 May 17; 349(9063): 1460.
(HUMAN EXPERIMENTATION/FOREIGN COUNTRIES; HUMAN EXPERIMENTATION/SPECIAL POPULATIONS; STERILIZATION)

Küng, Hans; Jens, Walter. A dignified dying: a plea for personal responsiblity. London: SCM Press; 1995. 132 p.
(EUTHANASIA/LEGAL ASPECTS; EUTHANASIA/RELIGIOUS

ASPECTS)

Kunzel, Carol see Sadowsky, Donald

Kurit, Doris see Goldfarb, James

Kurjak, Asim see Chervenak, Frank A.

Kurokawa, Kiyoshi see Asai, Atsushi

Kurt, Edward J. see Byrne, Paul A.

Kussin, Peter see Weeks, Jane C.

Kussin, Peter see Wenger, Neil S.

Kutner, Jean see Hilberman, Mark

Kuttner, Robert. Must good HMOs go bad? First of two parts: the commercialization of prepaid group health care. *New England Journal of Medicine.* 1998 May 21; 338(21): 1558–1563.
(HEALTH CARE/ECONOMICS)

Kuttner, Robert. Must good HMOs go bad? Second of two parts: the search for checks and balances. *New England Journal of Medicine.* 1998 May 28; 338(22): 1635–1639.
(HEALTH CARE/ECONOMICS)

Kuuppelomäki, Merja; Lauri, Sirkka. Ethical dilemmas in the care of patients with incurable cancer. *Nursing Ethics.* 1998 Jul; 5(4): 283–293.
(TERMINAL CARE; TRUTH DISCLOSURE)

L

La Puma, John. Managed Care Ethics: Essays on the Impact of Managed Care on Traditional Medical Ethics. New York, NY: Hatherleigh Press; 1998. 208 p.
(HEALTH CARE/ECONOMICS)

La Puma, John. Physicians' conflicts of interest in post–marketing research: what the public should know, and why industry should tell them. *In:* Vanderpool, Harold Y., ed. The Ethics of Research Involving Human Subjects: Facing the 21st Century. Frederick, MD: University Publishing Group; 1996: 203–219.
(HUMAN EXPERIMENTATION/INFORMED CONSENT; PATIENT CARE/DRUGS)

La Puma, John. Should medical ethics be part of public relations? *Managed Care.* 1997 Sep; 6(9): 111–112.
(HEALTH CARE)

La Vigne, Gregory; Hassenfeld, Irwin N. The ethics of alcoholism treatment and rehabilitation. *In:* Shelton, Wayne N.; Edwards, Rem B., eds. Advances in Bioethics. Volume 3: Values, Ethics, and Alcoholism. Greenwich, CT: JAI Press; 1997: 81–101.
(PATIENT CARE/MENTALLY DISABLED)

Labib, Karim. Don't leave dignity out of the cloning debate. [Letter]. *Nature.* 1997 Jul 3; 388(6637): 15.
(CLONING)

Ladd, Rosalind Ekman; Forman, Edwin N. Pediatric ethics rounds: an evaluation -- the impact of ethics rounds on clinical decision–making is worthy of further exploration. *Rhode Island Medical Journal.* 1985 Oct; 68(10): 455–458.

(MEDICAL ETHICS/EDUCATION)

Lader, Malcolm see Henn, Fritz A.

LaFleur, William see Ravindra, Ravi

LaFollette, Hugh; Shanks, Niall. The origin of speciesism. *Philosophy.* 1996 Jan; 71(275): 41–61.
(ANIMAL EXPERIMENTATION)

LaFollette, Marcel C. The pathology of research fraud: the history and politics of the US experience. *Journal of Internal Medicine.* 1994 Feb; 235(2): 129–135.
(BIOMEDICAL RESEARCH; FRAUD AND MISCONDUCT)

Lafrance, W. André; Singer, Peter A. Is it ethical to forgo treatment? [Letter and response]. *Canadian Medical Association Journal.* 1997 Dec 15; 157(12): 1740–1741.
(ALLOWING TO DIE; TERMINAL CARE)

Lagnado, Lucette. Columbia urges ethics officers at its hospitals. [News]. *Wall Street Journal.* 1997 Dec 12: B6.
(ETHICISTS AND ETHICS COMMITTEES)

Lagnado, Lucette see Pasztor, Andy

Lahr, J. Gregory. What is the method to their "madness?" Experimental treatment exclusions in health insurance policies. [Comment]. *Journal of Contemporary Health Law and Policy.* 1997 Spring; 13(2): 613–636.
(HEALTH CARE/ECONOMICS; HUMAN EXPERIMENTATION)

Lai, Kwan Kew see FitzGibbon, Scott

Lake, John see Neuberger, James

Lalos, Othon see Daniels, Ken

Lam, F.T. see Higgins, R.M.

Lamb, David. Death, medical aspects of. *In:* Chadwick, Ruth, ed. Encyclopedia of Applied Ethics, Volume 1. San Diego, CA: Academic Press; 1998: 727–734.
(DETERMINATION OF DEATH)

Lamb, David. Ethics of fetal tissue transplants. *In:* Frith, Lucy, ed. Ethics and Midwifery: Issues in Contemporary Practice. Boston, MA: Butterworth–Heinemann; 1996: 156–169.
(FETUSES; ORGAN AND TISSUE DONATION)

Lambe, Neil see Grubb, Andrew

Lambert, Sally A. see McAliley, Lauren G.

Lamberton, Victoria see Markson, Lawrence

Lamberts, Robert J.; MacKie, Palmer; Loehrer, Patrick J. Physician–assisted suicide and euthanasia: a house staff debate. *Indiana Medicine.* 1995 May–Jun; 88(3): 192–195.
(SUICIDE)

Lamke, Celia. Distributive justice and HIV disease in intensive care. *Critical Care Nursing Quarterly.* 1996 May; 19(1): 55–64.
(AIDS; RESOURCE ALLOCATION/BIOMEDICAL TECHNOLOGIES; SELECTION FOR TREATMENT)

Lammers, Stephen E.; Verhey, Allen, eds. On Moral

Medicine: Theological Perspectives in Medical Ethics. Second Edition. Grand Rapids, MI: Eerdmans; 1998. 1,004 p.
(BIOETHICS)

Lamont, Tara see **Entwistle, Vikki A.**

Lan, Chung–Chi see **Jan, Sheau–Wen**

Land, Walter; Cohen, B. Postmortem and living organ donation in Europe: transplant laws and activities. *Transplantation Proceedings.* 1992 Oct; 24(5): 2165–2167.
(ORGAN AND TISSUE DONATION)

Land, Walter see **Gutmann, Thomas**

Landau, William M. see **Jaffe, Allan S.**

Landefeld, C. Seth see **Ubel, Peter A.**

Landi, Francesco see **Bernabei, Roberto**

Lane, Arline; Dubler, Nancy Neveloff. The health care agent: selected but neglected. *Bioethics Forum.* 1997 Summer; 13(2): 17–21.
(ADVANCE DIRECTIVES; INFORMED CONSENT)

Laney, James T. Ethics in health care: what do we have to do? What should we do? *Journal of the Medical Association of Georgia.* 1990 Nov; 79(11): 829–833.
(HEALTH CARE)

Langer, Anatoly; Hopf, G. Early stopping of trials. [Letters]. *Lancet.* 1997 Sep 20; 350(9081): 890–891.
(HUMAN EXPERIMENTATION/RESEARCH DESIGN)

Langer, Dennis H. Children's legal rights as research subjects. *Journal of the American Academy of Child Psychiatry.* 1985 Sep; 24(5): 653–662.
(HUMAN EXPERIMENTATION/MINORS; INFORMED CONSENT/MINORS)

Langston, J. William; Palfreman, Jon. The Case of the Frozen Addicts: Working at the Edge of the Mysteries of the Human Brain. New York, NY: Vintage Books; 1996. 309 p.
(EMBRYO AND FETAL RESEARCH; FETUSES; ORGAN AND TISSUE DONATION; ORGAN AND TISSUE TRANSPLANTATION)

Lanken, Paul N. Ethical considerations in pulmonary intensive care. *In:* Fishman, Alfred P., ed. Pulmonary Rehabilitation. New York, NY: Marcel Dekker; 1996: 289–308.
(ALLOWING TO DIE)

Lanken, Paul N. see **Asch, David A.**

Lankin, Kenneth M. see **DeGroot, Leslie J.**

Lannin, Donald R. see **Kopelman, Loretta M.**

Lantos, John see **Karlawish, Jason H.T.**

Lantos, John see **Meadow, William**

Lantos, John D. Was the UK collaborative ECMO trial ethical? *Paediatric and Perinatal Epidemiology.* 1997 Jul; 11(3): 264–268.
(BIOMEDICAL TECHNOLOGIES; HUMAN EXPERIMENTATION/FOREIGN COUNTRIES; HUMAN EXPERIMENTATION/MINORS; HUMAN EXPERIMENTATION/RESEARCH DESIGN; PATIENT CARE/MINORS)

Lantos, John D. see **Casarett, David J.**

Lapane, Kate see **Bernabei, Roberto**

LaPann, Karin see **O'Brien, Linda A.**

Larcher, Victor F.; Lask, Bryan; McCarthy, Jean M. Paediatrics at the cutting edge: do we need clinical ethics committees? *Journal of Medical Ethics.* 1997 Aug; 23(4): 245–249.
(ETHICISTS AND ETHICS COMMITTEES)

Laros, Russell see **Segal, Arthur I.**

Larsen, P. Munkholm see **Rasmussen, P. Elmegaard**

Larson, Edward J. "In the finest, most womanly way": women in the Southern eugenics movement. *American Journal of Legal History.* 1995 Apr; 39(2): 119–147.
(EUGENICS)

Larson, Edward J.; Amundsen, Darrel W. A Different Death: Euthanasia and the Christian Tradition. Downers Grove, IL: InterVarsity Press; 1998. 288 p.
(EUTHANASIA/RELIGIOUS ASPECTS; SUICIDE)

Lask, Bryan see **Larcher, Victor F.**

Latham, Stephen R. see **Andrews, Lori B.**

Latham, Stephen R. see **Baker, Robert**

Latta, Richard A. see **Nakchbandi, Inaam A.**

Latvala, Eila; Janhonen, Sirpa; Moring, Juha. Ethical dilemmas in a psychiatric nursing study. *Nursing Ethics.* 1998 Jan; 5(1): 27–35.
(BEHAVIORAL RESEARCH/SPECIAL POPULATIONS)

Lau, Hong Sang see **de Boer, Anthonius**

Laurence, D.R. Wills, living wills and enduring powers of attorney. *Journal of the Royal College of Physicians of London.* 1995 Nov–Dec; 29(6): 488–489.
(ADVANCE DIRECTIVES)

Lauri, Sirkka see **Kuuppelomäki, Merja**

Laurie, Graeme T. Biotechnology and intellectual property: a marriage of inconvenience? *In:* McLean, Sheila A.M., ed. Contemporary Issues in Law, Medicine and Ethics. Brookfield, VT: Dartmouth; 1996: 237–267.
(BIOMEDICAL RESEARCH; PATENTING LIFE FORMS; RECOMBINANT DNA RESEARCH)

Lavery, James V. see **Singer, Peter A.**

Lawrence, Robert S. see **Woolf, Steven H.**

Lawson, Craig M. see **Robbennolt, Jennifer K.**

Layde, Peter see **Phillips, Russell S.**

Lazar, Eliot J. see **Herb, Alice**

Lazarus, Jeremy A. Ethical issues in doctor–patient sexual relationships. *Psychiatric Clinics of North America.* 1995

Mar; 18(1): 55–70.
(FRAUD AND MISCONDUCT; PROFESSIONAL PATIENT RELATIONSHIP)

Le Bris, Sonia. National Ethics Bodies: Report. Strasbourg, France: Council of Europe Press; 1993. 77 p.
(ETHICISTS AND ETHICS COMMITTEES)

Le Grand, Julian see New, Bill

Le Roux, Nadège see Pochard, Frédéric

Leader, Leo R. see Durna, Eva M.

Leahy, Joseph see White, W.D.

Leaning, Jennifer. Human rights and medical education. [Editorial]. BMJ (British Medical Journal). 1997 Nov 29; 315(7120): 1390–1391.
(MEDICAL ETHICS/EDUCATION; PROFESSIONAL PATIENT RELATIONSHIP)

Leary, Warren E. Panel urges H.I.V. tests for all pregnant women. [News]. New York Times. 1998 Oct 15: A22.
(AIDS/TESTING AND SCREENING)

Leavine, Barbara Ann. Court–ordered cesareans: can a pregnant woman refuse? Houston Law Review. 1992 Spring; 29(1): 185–218.
(FETUSES; TREATMENT REFUSAL)

Lebacqz, Karen. Difficult difference. Cambridge Quarterly of Healthcare Ethics. 1998 Winter; 7(1): 17–26.
(BIOETHICS)

Lebacqz, Karen. Fair shares: is the genome project just? In: Peters, Ted, ed. Genetics: Issues of Social Justice. Cleveland, OH: Pilgrim Press; 1998: 82–107.
(GENOME MAPPING)

Lebacqz, Karen. Genes, justice, and clones. In: Cole–Turner, Ronald, ed. Human Cloning: Religious Responses. Louisville, KY: Westminister John Knox Press; 1997: 49–57.
(CLONING; REPRODUCTION)

Lebacqz, Karen. Genetic privacy: no deal for the poor. In: Peters, Ted, ed. Genetics: Issues of Social Justice. Cleveland, OH: Pilgrim Press; 1998: 239–254.
(CONFIDENTIALITY; GENETIC SCREENING)

LeBeau, Shane O. see Sehgal, Ashwini R.

Lederman, Richard see Smith, Martin L.

Lee, George F. see Segal, Arthur I.

Lee, Luke T. Population: the human rights approach. Colorado Journal of International Environmental Law and Policy. 1995 Summer; 6(2): 327–344.
(POPULATION CONTROL)

Lee, Melinda A. see Tilden, Virginia P.

Lee, Nick. Spotlight on South African medical profession. [News]. Lancet. 1997 Jul 5; 350(9070): 39.
(FRAUD AND MISCONDUCT; TORTURE)

Lee, S.H. see Hui, Elsie

Legemaate, Johan; Gevers, J.K.M. Physician–assisted suicide in psychiatry: developments in the Netherlands. Cambridge Quarterly of Healthcare Ethics. 1997 Spring; 6(2): 175–188.
(EUTHANASIA/LEGAL ASPECTS; SUICIDE)

Leggatt, Margaret see Furlong, Mark

Lehrman, Sally. Call for human subjects monitoring body. [News]. Nature. 1997 Jul 24; 388(6640): 313.
(HUMAN EXPERIMENTATION/REGULATION)

Lehrman, Sally. Clinton backs congressional efforts on genetic discrimination. [News]. Nature. 1997 Jul 17; 388(6639): 216.
(CONFIDENTIALITY)

Lehrman, Sally. Coalition to pursue ethnic concerns over gene research. [News]. Nature. 1998 Apr 2; 392(6675): 428.
(GENETIC RESEARCH)

Lehrman, Sally. Genetic testing for Alzheimer's disease 'not appropriate.' [News]. Nature. 1997 Oct 30; 389(6654): 898.
(GENETIC SCREENING)

Lehrman, Sally. University settles with patients over trade in 'stolen' embryos. [News]. Nature. 1997 Jul 31; 388(6641): 411.
(FRAUD AND MISCONDUCT; IN VITRO FERTILIZATION)

Leikin, Sanford L. Beyond proforma consent for childhood cancer research. Journal of Clinical Oncology. 1985 Mar; 3(3): 420–428.
(HUMAN EXPERIMENTATION/INFORMED CONSENT; HUMAN EXPERIMENTATION/MINORS)

Leino–Kilpi, Helena; Nyrhinen, Tarja; Katajisto, Jouko. Patients' rights in laboratory examinations: do they realize? Nursing Ethics. 1997 Nov; 4(6): 451–464.
(PATIENTS' RIGHTS)

Lemaire, F.; Blanch, L.; Cohen, S.L.; European Society of Intensive Care Medicine. Working Group on Ethics. Informed consent for research purposes in intensive care patients in Europe –– part I: an official statement of the European Society of Intensive Care Medicine. Intensive Care Medicine. 1997 Mar; 23(3): 338–341.
(HUMAN EXPERIMENTATION/FOREIGN COUNTRIES; HUMAN EXPERIMENTATION/INFORMED CONSENT; HUMAN EXPERIMENTATION/SPECIAL POPULATIONS)

Lemaire, F.; Blanch, L.; Cohen, S.L.; European Society of Intensive Care Medicine. Working Group on Ethics. Informed consent for research purposes in intensive care patients in Europe –– part II: an official statement of the European Society of Intensive Care Medicine. Intensive Care Medicine. 1997 Apr; 23(4): 435–439.
(HUMAN EXPERIMENTATION/FOREIGN COUNTRIES; HUMAN EXPERIMENTATION/INFORMED CONSENT; HUMAN EXPERIMENTATION/SPECIAL POPULATIONS)

Lemieux–Charles, Louise see Meslin, Eric M.

Lemonick, Michael D. The new revolution in making babies. Time. 1997 Dec 1; 150(23): 40–46.
(REPRODUCTIVE TECHNOLOGIES)

Lewin, David I. Animal welfare group seeks ban on MAbs from mouse ascites. [News]. *Journal of NIH Research.* 1997 Jul; 9(7): 22–23.
(ANIMAL EXPERIMENTATION)

Lewin, Tamar. A new technique makes abortions possible earlier. [News]. *New York Times.* 1997 Dec 21: 1, 30.
(ABORTION)

Lewin, Tamar. Abortion fell again in 1995, U.S. says, but rose in some areas last year. [News]. *New York Times.* 1997 Dec 5: A14.
(ABORTION)

Lewin, Tamar. Debate distant for many having abortions. [News]. *New York Times.* 1998 Jan 17: A1, A9.
(ABORTION/ATTITUDES)

Lewins, Frank. Bioethics for Health Professionals: An Introduction and Critical Approach. South Melbourne, VIC: MacMillan Education Australia; 1996. 154 p.
(BIOETHICS)

Lewis, George see Forrow, Lachlan

Lewis, Marcia A.; Tamparo, Carol D. Medical Law, Ethics, and Bioethics for Ambulatory Care. Fourth Edition. Philadelphia, PA: F.A. Davis; 1998. 295 p.
(BIOETHICS; PATIENT CARE; PROFESSIONAL ETHICS)

Lewis, Shon see Fallowfield, Lesley

Lewison, Helen. Choices in childbirth: areas of conflict. *In:* Frith, Lucy, ed. Ethics and Midwifery: Issues in Contemporary Practice. Boston, MA: Butterworth-Heinemann; 1996: 36–50.
(PATIENT CARE)

Lewith, George T. Ethical problems in evaluating complementary medicine. *Bulletin of Medical Ethics.* 1996 Aug; No. 120: 17–20.
(HUMAN EXPERIMENTATION/FOREIGN COUNTRIES; HUMAN EXPERIMENTATION/RESEARCH DESIGN)

Lewkonia, Raymond M. see Verhoef, Marja J.

Lewthwaite, Barbara; Erickson-Nesmith, Sharon. Needs assessment for healthcare ethics education. *HEC (HealthCare Ethics Committee) Forum.* 1998 Mar; 10(1): 86–101.
(BIOETHICS/EDUCATION; ETHICISTS AND ETHICS COMMITTEES)

Li, C.C. see Guo, Sun-Wei

Li, Frederick P. see Patenaude, Andrea Farkas

Liaschenko, Joan see Davis, Anne J.

Lichtblau, Leonard see Elliott, Thomas E.

Licks, Sandra see Teno, Joan M.

Lidz, Charles W. see Roth, Loren

Liebaers, I. see Bonduelle, M.

Light, Donald W. The real ethics of rationing. *BMJ (British Medical Journal).* 1997 Jul 12; 315(7100): 112–115.
(HEALTH CARE/FOREIGN COUNTRIES; RESOURCE

ALLOCATION)

Light, Donald W.; McGee, Glenn. On the social embeddedness of bioethics. *In:* DeVries, Raymond; Subedi, Janardan, eds. Bioethics and Society: Constructing the Ethical Enterprise. Upper Saddle River, NJ: Prentice Hall; 1998: 1–15.
(BIOETHICS)

Lilford, R.J. see Edwards, S.J.L.

Linas, Benjamin P. see Sulmasy, Daniel P.

Lind, Stuart E. Financial issues and incentives related to clinical research and innovative therapies. *In:* Vanderpool, Harold Y., ed. The Ethics of Research Involving Human Subjects: Facing the 21st Century. Frederick, MD: University Publishing Group; 1996: 185–202.
(HUMAN EXPERIMENTATION)

Lind, Stuart E. see Sazama, Kathleen

Lindee, M. Susan see Nelkin, Dorothy

Lindley, Richard I. Thrombolytic treatment for acute ischaemic stroke: consent can be ethical. *BMJ (British Medical Journal).* 1998 Mar 28; 316(7136): 1005–1007.
(HUMAN EXPERIMENTATION/INFORMED CONSENT; HUMAN EXPERIMENTATION/RESEARCH DESIGN)

Lindon, James Lee. Consequences of End-of-Life Physician Orders: Economic and Hospital Policy Implications. Ann Arbor, MI: University Microfilms International; 1993. 108 p.
(RESUSCITATION ORDERS)

Lindsay, R.C.L. see Adair, John G.

Lindsay, Ronald A. Assisted suicide: will the Supreme Court respect the autonomy rights of dying patients? *Free Inquiry.* 1996–1997 Winter; 17(1): 4–5.
(SUICIDE)

Linehan, Elizabeth A. see Churchill, Larry R.

Link, Michael P. see Jaffe, Norman

Link, Ronald C. Recent American developments in the right to die: the *Cruzan* case, living wills, durable powers and family consent statutes. *In:* Grubb, Andrew, ed. Decision-Making and Problems of Incompetence. New York, NY: Wiley; 1994: 127–172.
(ADVANCE DIRECTIVES; ALLOWING TO DIE/LEGAL ASPECTS)

Lipp, Allyson. An enquiry into a combined approach for nursing ethics. *Nursing Ethics.* 1998 Mar; 5(2): 122–138.
(NURSING ETHICS)

Lippman, Abby. The politics of health: geneticization versus health promotion. *In:* Sherwin, Susan, et al. The Politics of Women's Health: Exploring Agency and Autonomy. Philadelphia, PA: Temple University Press; 1998: 64–82.
(GENETIC SCREENING; HEALTH)

Lipsitz, Lewis see Bernabei, Roberto

Lipton, Eric. In houses of healing, an uneasy alliance: worried by church rules, hospital may end union with

Loff, Bebe; Cordner, Stephen. Abortion bills introduced to Western Australian parliament. [News]. *Lancet.* 1998 Mar 21; 351(9106): 892.
(ABORTION/FOREIGN COUNTRIES)

Logmans, A.; Verhoeff, A.; Bol Raap, R.; Creighton, F.; van Lent, M.; Raphael, D.D.; Bhugra, Dinesh; Paterson–Brown, Sara; Webb, Elspeth; Ross, Lainie Friedman. Should doctors reconstruct the vaginal introitus of adolescent girls to mimic the virginal state? [Article and commentaries]. *BMJ (British Medical Journal).* 1998 Feb 7; 316(7129): 459–462.
(PATIENT CARE)

Logue, Barbara J. Physician–assisted suicide: a social science perspective on international trends. *In:* McLean, Sheila A.M., ed. Death, Dying and the Law. Brookfield, VT: Dartmouth; 1996: 95–112.
(EUTHANASIA)

Logue, Gerald see **Wear, Stephen**

Lomax, Karen J.; Garthwaite, Thomas L. VHA's mission: institutional integrity, non–abandonment and VHA special emphasis programs. *HEC (HealthCare Ethics Committee) Forum.* 1997 Jun; 9(2): 182–193.
(HEALTH CARE)

Lomax, Karen J. see **Reagan, James E.**

Lombardo, Paul A. Medicine, eugenics, and the Supreme Court: from coercive sterilization to reproductive freedom. *Journal of Contemporary Health Law and Policy.* 1996 Fall; 13(1): 1–25.
(EUGENICS; REPRODUCTION; STERILIZATION/MENTALLY DISABLED)

London, D. see **Addis, G.J.**

London, Nancy L.; London, W. Thomas. A case of self–experimentation. [Editorial]. *Cancer Epidemiology, Biomarkers and Prevention.* 1997 Jul; 6(7): 475–476.
(HUMAN EXPERIMENTATION)

London, W. Thomas see **London, Nancy L.**

Loneck, Barry. How particular social environments affect alcoholics. *In:* Shelton, Wayne N.; Edwards, Rem B., eds. Advances in Bioethics. Volume 3: Values, Ethics, and Alcoholism. Greenwich, CT: JAI Press; 1997: 171–205.
(PATIENT CARE)

Long, Aishlinn see **Long, Ann**

Long, Ann; Long, Aishlinn; Smyth, Angus. Suicide: a statement of suffering. *Nursing Ethics.* 1998 Jan; 5(1): 3–15.
(PATIENT CARE; PROFESSIONAL PATIENT RELATIONSHIP; SUICIDE)

Long, Ann see **Baxter, Rosario**

Longenecker, J. Craig see **Nakchbandi, Inaam A.**

Loscalzo, John J.; Cooper, David J.; Arena, Francis P.; Llovera, Ingrid. Do families understand "do not resuscitate" orders? *Oncology.* 1996 Apr; 10(4): 504, 507, 511.
(RESUSCITATION ORDERS)

Losekoot, M. see **DudokdeWit, A.C.**

Louhiala, Pekka see **Hemminki, Elina**

Louis, Karen Seashore see **Campbell, Eric G.**

Love, Susan M.; Tuckfelt, Mark; Nicklin, David; Durand, Andre Mark; Katz, Stephen J.; Asch, David A.; Ubel, Peter A. Rationing by any other name. [Letters and response]. *New England Journal of Medicine.* 1997 Nov 6; 337(19): 1395–1396.
(HEALTH CARE/ECONOMICS; RESOURCE ALLOCATION)

Löw, Reinhard. Anthropology as the basis of bioethics. *In:* Becker, Gerhold K., ed. Changing Nature's Course: The Ethical Challenge of Biotechnology. Hong Kong: Hong Kong University Press; 1996: 147–157.
(BIOETHICS)

Lowe, Michael see **Kerridge, Ian**

Lowenthal, Barbara; Getz, Marjorie; Kaye, Celia. The special educator and the hospital ethics committee. Available from the ERIC Document Reproduction Service, DYNCORP I&ET, 7420 Fullerton Rd., Suite 110, Springfield, VA 22153–2852; Document No. ED320338; EC231146; 1990 Feb. 40 p.
(ALLOWING TO DIE/INFANTS; ETHICISTS AND ETHICS COMMITTEES; PATIENT CARE/MINORS)

Lowes, Lesley. Paediatric nursing and research ethics: is there a conflict? *Journal of Clinical Nursing.* 1996 Mar; 5(2): 91–97.
(HUMAN EXPERIMENTATION/MINORS)

Lowrance, William W. Privacy and Health Research: A Report to the U.S. Secretary of Health and Human Services. Washington, DC: U.S. Department of Health and Human Services, Office of the Assistant Secretary for Planning and Evaluation; 1997 May. 80 p.
(BIOMEDICAL RESEARCH; CONFIDENTIALITY)

Lublin, Nancy. Pandora's Box: Feminism Confronts Reproductive Technology. Lanham, MD: Rowman and Littlefield; 1998. 189 p.
(REPRODUCTIVE TECHNOLOGIES)

Lucas, Alan. Should industry sponsor research? Collaborative research with infant formula companies should not always be censored. *BMJ (British Medical Journal).* 1998 Aug 1; 317(7154): 337–338.
(BIOMEDICAL RESEARCH)

Lucassen, Emy. Prenatal genetic testing: the need for legislation. *In:* Doherty, Peter; Sutton, Agneta, eds. Man–Made Man: Ethical and Legal Issues in Genetics. Dublin, Ireland: Open Air; 1997: 98–112.
(GENETIC SCREENING; PRENATAL DIAGNOSIS)

Lucente, Frank E. see **Moreno, Jonathan D.**

Lucey, Michael R.; Beresford, Thomas P. Ethical considerations regarding orthotopic liver transplantation for alcoholic patients. *In:* Shelton, Wayne N.; Edwards, Rem B., eds. Advances in Bioethics. Volume 3: Values, Ethics, and Alcoholism. Greenwich, CT: JAI Press; 1997: 119–129.
(ORGAN AND TISSUE TRANSPLANTATION; RESOURCE ALLOCATION/BIOMEDICAL TECHNOLOGIES; SELECTION FOR TREATMENT)

Lukawski, Jolanta E. see **Gertner, Eric J.**

Lumb, Philip D. see **Groudine, Scott**

Luna, Aurelio see **Osuna, Eduardo**

Lund, Nelson see **Kass, Leon R.**

Lund, Nelson see **Thies, Winthrop Drake**

Lundberg, George D. see **Flanagin, Annette**

Lundberg, George D. see **Relman, Arnold S.**

Lundmark, Thomas. Surgery by an unauthorized surgeon as a battery. *Journal of Law and Health.* 1995–1996; 10(2): 287–296.
(INFORMED CONSENT)

Lupton, Deborah. Consumerism, reflexivity, and the medical encounter. *Social Science and Medicine.* 1997 Aug; 45(3): 373–381.
(PROFESSIONAL PATIENT RELATIONSHIP)

Lupton, Deborah. The Imperative of Health: Public Health and the Regulated Body. Thousand Oaks, CA: Sage Publications; 1995. 181 p.
(BEHAVIOR CONTROL; PUBLIC HEALTH)

Lurie, Nicole see **Borowsky, Steven J.**

Lusthaus, Evelyn W. Involuntary euthanasia and current attempts to define persons with mental retardation as less than human. *Mental Retardation.* 1985 Jun; 23(3): 148–154.
(ALLOWING TO DIE/INFANTS; EUTHANASIA; PERSONHOOD)

Lustig, Andrew; Scardino, Peter. Elective patients. *In:* McCullough, Laurence B.; Jones, James W.; Brody, Baruch A., eds. Surgical Ethics. New York, NY: Oxford University Press; 1998: 133–151.
(INFORMED CONSENT; PATIENT CARE)

Lustig, B. Andrew, ed.; Center for Medical Ethics and Health Policy (Houston, TX). Bioethics Yearbook, Volume 5: Theological Developments in Bioethics, 1992–1994. Boston, MA: Kluwer Academic; 1997. 301 p.
(BIOETHICS)

Lustig, B. Andrew. Recent trends in theological bioethics. *In:* Lustig, B. Andrew, ed.; Center for Medical Ethics and Health Policy (Houston, TX). Bioethics Yearbook, Volume 5: Theological Developments in Bioethics, 1992–1994. Boston, MA: Kluwer Academic; 1997: 1–9.
(BIOETHICS)

Luther, Lori; Hirtle, Marie. Genetic diversity –– a clash of world views? *In:* Knoppers, Bartha Maria, ed. Human DNA: Law and Policy: International and Comparative Perspectives. Proceedings of the First International Conference on DNA Sampling and Human Genetic Research: Ethical, Legal, and Policy Aspects, held in Montreal, Canada, 6–8 Sep 1996. Boston, MA: Kluwer Law International; 1997: 275–280.
(GENETIC RESEARCH; GENOME MAPPING)

Lützén, Kim; Evertzon, Mats; Nordin, Conny. Moral sensitivity in psychiatric practice. *Nursing Ethics.* 1997 Nov; 4(6): 472–482.

(MEDICAL ETHICS; PROFESSIONAL PATIENT RELATIONSHIP)

Lützén, Kim; Nordin, Conny. Structuring moral meaning in psychiatric nursing practice. *Scandinavian Journal of Caring Sciences.* 1993; 7(3): 175–180.
(NURSING ETHICS; PATIENT CARE/MENTALLY DISABLED)

Lyman, Karen A. Living with Alzheimer's disease: the creation of meaning among persons with dementia. *Journal of Clinical Ethics.* 1998 Spring; 9(1): 49–57.
(PATIENT CARE/MENTALLY DISABLED)

Lynch, Abbyann, ed. The Good Pediatrician: An Ethics Curriculum for Use in Canadian Pediatrics Residency Programs. Teacher's Handbook. [Looseleaf format]. Toronto, ON: Department of Bioethics, Hospital for Sick Children; 1996. 348 p.
(MEDICAL ETHICS/EDUCATION; PATIENT CARE/MINORS)

Lynn, Joanne. Legal and ethical issues in palliative health care. *Seminars in Oncology.* 1985 Dec; 12(4): 476–481.
(TERMINAL CARE)

Lynn, Joanne. Measuring Quality of Care at the End of Life: A Statement of Principles. *Journal of the American Geriatrics Society.* 1997 Apr; 45(4): 526–527.
(TERMINAL CARE)

Lynn, Joanne; Cohn, Felicia; Pickering, John H.; Smith, Joel; Stoeppelwerth, Ali M.; American Geriatrics Society. American Geriatrics Society on physician–assisted suicide: brief to the United States Supreme Court. *Journal of the American Geriatrics Society.* 1997 Apr; 45(4): 489–499.
(PATIENT CARE/AGED; SUICIDE; TERMINAL CARE)

Lynn, Joanne; Teno, Joan. A care provider perspective on advance directives and surrogate decision making for incompetent adults in the United States. *In:* Sass, Hans–Martin; Veatch, Robert M.; Kimura, Rihito, eds. Advance Directives and Surrogate Decision Making in Health Care: United States, Germany, and Japan. Baltimore, MD: Johns Hopkins University Press; 1998: 3–33.
(ADVANCE DIRECTIVES; INFORMED CONSENT)

Lynn, Joanne; Wilkinson, Anne; Cohn, Felicia; Jones, Stanley B. Capitated risk–bearing managed care systems could improve end-of-life care. *Journal of the American Geriatrics Society.* 1998 Mar; 46(3): 322–330.
(HEALTH CARE/ECONOMICS; TERMINAL CARE)

Lynn, Joanne see **Ayers, Elise**

Lynn, Joanne see **Burke, James**

Lynn, Joanne see **Goodlin, Sarah J.**

Lynn, Joanne see **Phillips, Russell S.**

Lynn, Joanne see **Rudberg, Mark A.**

Lynn, Joanne see **Teno, Joan**

Lynn, Joanne see **Teno, Joan M.**

Lynn, Joanne see **Tsevat, Joel**

Lynn, Joanne see **Weeks, Jane C.**

M

McAliley, Lauren G.; Lambert, Sally A.; Ashenberg, Margaret D.; Dull, Susan M. Therapeutic relations decision making: the Rainbow framework. *Pediatric Nursing.* 1996 May–Jun; 22(3): 199–203, 210.
(PROFESSIONAL PATIENT RELATIONSHIP)

McAlpine, Heather. Critical reflections about professional ethical stances: have we lost sight of the major objectives? *Journal of Nursing Education.* 1996 Mar; 35(3): 119–126.
(NURSING ETHICS)

McArdle, Robert see **Mattson, Margaret E.**

McCabe, E. see **Clafferty, R.A.**

McCabe, Jennifer see **Westfall, John M.**

McCabe, Jennifer see **Wolf, Bruce L.**

McCall Smith, R.A. see **Mason, John Kenyon**

McCall, Timothy B. see **Gurewich, Victor**

McCanna, Tony. A practical advance directive survey. *Bioethics Forum.* 1997 Summer; 13(2): 44–46.
(ADVANCE DIRECTIVES)

McCarrick, Pat Milmoe, comp. Bibliography [advance directives]. *In:* Sass, Hans–Martin; Veatch, Robert M.; Kimura, Rihito, eds. Advance Directives and Surrogate Decision Making in Health Care: United States, Germany, and Japan. Baltimore, MD: Johns Hopkins University Press; 1998: 279–302.
(ADVANCE DIRECTIVES)

McCarthy, Charles R. Challenges to IRBs in the coming decades. *In:* Vanderpool, Harold Y., ed. The Ethics of Research Involving Human Subjects: Facing the 21st Century. Frederick, MD: University Publishing Group; 1996: 127–144.
(HUMAN EXPERIMENTATION/ETHICS COMMITTEES; HUMAN EXPERIMENTATION/REGULATION)

McCarthy, Charles R. The evolving story of justice in federal research policy. *In:* Kahn, Jeffrey P.; Mastroianni, Anna C.; Sugarman, Jeremy, eds. Beyond Consent: Seeking Justice in Research. New York, NY: Oxford University Press; 1998: 11–31.
(HUMAN EXPERIMENTATION)

McCarthy, Charles R. The rights of human research subjects and the necessity of conducting animal research as illuminated by the Nuremberg Code and the Declaration of Helsinki. *In:* Eder, G.; Kaiser, E.; King, F.A., eds. The Role of the Chimpanzee in Research. Symposium, Vienna, Austria, May 22–24, 1992. New York, NY: Karger; 1994: 1–6.
(ANIMAL EXPERIMENTATION; HUMAN EXPERIMENTATION)

McCarthy, Jean M. see **Larcher, Victor F.**

McCarthy, Michael. AIDS doctors push for live–virus vaccine trials. *Lancet.* 1997 Oct 11; 350(9084): 1082.
(AIDS/HEALTH PERSONNEL; AIDS/HUMAN EXPERIMENTATION; IMMUNIZATION)

McCarthy, Michael. Conflict of interest highlighted in debate on calcium–channel blockers. [News]. *Lancet.* 1998 Jan 17; 351(9097): 191.
(BIOMEDICAL RESEARCH; HEALTH CARE/ECONOMICS; PATIENT CARE/DRUGS)

McCarthy, Michael. US panel urges caution in study of human genetic differences. [News]. *Lancet.* 1997 Nov 1; 350(9087): 1306.
(GENOME MAPPING)

McCarthy, Robert L. see **Richardson, James D.**

McCartney, James J. Mergers and sterilization: ethics in the board room. *HEC (HealthCare Ethics Committee) Forum.* 1997 Sep; 9(3): 284–292.
(STERILIZATION)

McCauley, Shelagh E. see **White, W.D.**

Macchiarini, Paolo see **Daar, A.S.**

McCloskey, Elizabeth Leibold see **Cohen, Cynthia B.**

McClure, Mary Ann. Infertility. *In:* Chadwick, Ruth, ed. Encyclopedia of Applied Ethics, Volume 2. San Diego, CA: Academic Press; 1998: 673–678.
(REPRODUCTIVE TECHNOLOGIES)

McConnell, Carolyn see **Smith, Martin L.**

McCormick, Richard A. A Catholic perspective on access to healthcare. *Cambridge Quarterly of Healthcare Ethics.* 1998 Summer; 7(3): 254–259.
(HEALTH CARE/RIGHTS)

McCormick, Richard A. The end of Catholic hospitals? *America.* 1998 Jul 4; 179(1): 5–6, 8–10, 12.
(HEALTH CARE/ECONOMICS)

McCotter, Patricia I. see **Tripp, Glenn**

McCullough, L.B. see **Chervenak, F.A.**

McCullough, Laurence B. Molecular medicine, managed care, and the moral responsibilities of patients and physicians. *Journal of Medicine and Philosophy.* 1998 Feb; 23(1): 3–9.
(BIOETHICS; HEALTH CARE/ECONOMICS; MEDICAL ETHICS)

McCullough, Laurence B. Preventive ethics, managed practice, and the hospital ethics committee as a resource for physician executives. *HEC (HealthCare Ethics Committee) Forum.* 1998 Jun; 10(2): 136–151.
(ETHICISTS AND ETHICS COMMITTEES; HEALTH CARE/ECONOMICS)

McCullough, Laurence B.; Jones, James W.; Brody, Baruch A. Informed consent: autonomous decision making of the surgical patient. *In:* McCullough, Laurence B.; Jones, James W.; Brody, Baruch A., eds. Surgical Ethics. New York, NY: Oxford University Press; 1998: 15–37.
(INFORMED CONSENT)

McCullough, Laurence B.; Jones, James W.; Brody, Baruch A., eds. Surgical Ethics. New York, NY: Oxford University Press; 1998. 396 p.
(MEDICAL ETHICS; PATIENT CARE)

McCullough, Laurence B. see **Chervenak, Frank A.**

McCullough, Laurence B. see Doukas, David J.

McCullough, Laurence B. see Lescale, Keith B.

McCullough, Laurence B. see Simms, Madeleine

McCullough, Laurence B. see Skupski, Daniel W.

McCurdy, David B. Personhood, spirituality, and hope in the care of human beings with dementia. *Journal of Clinical Ethics*. 1998 Spring; 9(1): 81–91.
(PATIENT CARE/MENTALLY DISABLED; PERSONHOOD)

McCurdy, Layton; Goode, Leslie D.; Inui, Thomas S.; Daugherty, Robert M.; Wilson, Donald E.; Wallace, Andrew G.; Weinstein, Bruce M.; Copeland, Edward M. Fulfilling the social contract between medical schools and the public. *Academic Medicine*. 1997 Dec; 72(12): 1063–1070.
(MEDICAL ETHICS/EDUCATION)

McDaniel, Charlotte. Development and psychometric properties of the Ethics Environment Questionnaire. *Medical Care*. 1997 Sep; 35(9): 901–914.
(PROFESSIONAL ETHICS)

McDaniel, Charlotte. Organizational culture and ethics work satisfaction. *Journal of Nursing Administration*. 1995 Nov; 25(11): 15–21.
(NURSING ETHICS)

McDevitt, Denis. Human volunteers in research: a physician's overview. *In:* Close, Bryony; Combes, Robert; Hubbard, Anthony; Illingworth, John, eds. Volunteers in Research and Testing. Bristol, PA: Taylor and Francis; 1997: 33–39.
(HUMAN EXPERIMENTATION)

McDonagh, Eileen L. Breaking the Abortion Deadlock: From Choice to Consent. New York, NY: Oxford University Press; 1996. 280 p.
(ABORTION/LEGAL ASPECTS)

MacDonald, Deborah J. see Bove, Catherine M.

Macdonald, F.J. see Steinberg, M.A.

Macdonald, K.G. see Taylor, K.M.

MacDonald, S.M. see Steinberg, M.A.

McDonald, Valerie see Michie, Susan

MacDougall, Jamie C. Adam and the implant. *Hastings Center Report*. 1998 Jul–Aug; 28(4): 47.
(PATIENT CARE/MINORS)

McDowell, B. Joan see Silverman, Myrna

McEnhill, Marilyn see Rushton, Cindy Hylton

Macer, Darryl. Bioethics and genetics in Asia and the Pacific: is universal bioethics possible? *In:* Becker, Gerhold K., ed. Changing Nature's Course: The Ethical Challenge of Biotechnology. Hong Kong: Hong Kong University Press; 1996: 171–184.
(GENETIC INTERVENTION)

Macer, Darryl. What can bioethics offer to Japanese culture? *Nichibunken Newsletter*. 1993 Aug; No. 15: 3–6.

(BIOETHICS)

Macer, Darryl R.J. Bioethics and genetic diversity from the perspective of UNESCO and non–governmental organizations. *In:* Knoppers, Bartha Maria, ed. Human DNA: Law and Policy: International and Comparative Perspectives. Proceedings of the First International Conference on DNA Sampling and Human Genetic Research: Ethical, Legal, and Policy Aspects, held in Montreal, Canada, 6–8 Sep 1996. Boston, MA: Kluwer Law International; 1997: 265–273.
(GENETIC RESEARCH; GENOME MAPPING)

Macer, Darryl R.J. Views of euthanasia for sufferers of genetic disease: comments on the Felon [Féron] case. [Letter]. *American Journal of Medical Genetics*. 1995 Sep 25; 58(4): 379–380.
(EUTHANASIA)

Macer, James A. see Segal, Arthur I.

McEvoy, Adrianne see Wear, Stephen E.

McEwen, Jean E. DNA data banks. *In:* Rothstein, Mark A., ed. Genetic Secrets: Protecting Privacy and Confidentiality in the Genetic Era. New Haven, CT: Yale University Press; 1997: 231–251.
(DNA FINGERPRINTING; GENETIC RESEARCH)

McEwen, Jean E. DNA sampling and banking: practices and procedures in the United States. *In:* Knoppers, Bartha Maria, ed. Human DNA: Law and Policy: International and Comparative Perspectives. Proceedings of the First International Conference on DNA Sampling and Human Genetic Research: Ethical, Legal, and Policy Aspects, held in Montreal, Canada, 6–8 Sep 1996. Boston, MA: Kluwer Law International; 1997: 407–421.
(DNA FINGERPRINTING; GENETIC RESEARCH; ORGAN AND TISSUE DONATION)

MacFadden, Douglas K. see Kohut, Nitsa

McFadzean, J.; Monson, J.P.; Watson, J.D.; Coakley, J.H.; Hoyte, Patrick; Caplan, Arthur L.; Hansen–Flaschen, John. The dilemma of the incapacitated patient who has previously refused consent for surgery. [Case study and commentaries]. *BMJ (British Medical Journal)*. 1997 Dec 6; 315(7121): 1530–1532.
(INFORMED CONSENT; TREATMENT REFUSAL)

McGaha, Annette see Wedding, Danny

McGann, John R. To care for the dying. *Origins*. 1997 Mar 20; 26(39): 640–648.
(ALLOWING TO DIE/RELIGIOUS ASPECTS; SUICIDE; TERMINAL CARE)

McGee, Ellen M. Can suicide intervention in hospice be ethical? *Journal of Palliative Care*. 1997 Spring; 13(1): 27–33.
(SUICIDE; TERMINAL CARE/HOSPICES)

McGee, Glenn, ed. The Human Cloning Debate. Berkeley, CA: Berkeley Hills Books; 1998. 270 p.
(CLONING)

McGee, Glenn. Therapeutic clinical ethics. *HEC (HealthCare Ethics Committee) Forum*. 1997 Sep; 9(3): 276–279.
(BIOETHICS; ETHICISTS AND ETHICS COMMITTEES)

McGee, Glenn; Arruda, Monica. A crossroads in genetic counseling and ethics. *Cambridge Quarterly of Healthcare Ethics.* 1998 Winter; 7(1): 97–100.
(GENETIC COUNSELING)

McGee, Glenn; Wilmut, Ian. Cloning and the adoption model. *In:* McGee, Glenn, ed. The Human Cloning Debate. Berkeley, CA: Berkeley Hills Books; 1998: 93–105.
(CLONING)

McGee, Glenn see Fox, Mark D.

McGee, Glenn see Light, Donald W.

McGleenan, Tony. Genetic technology, legal regulation of. *In:* Chadwick, Ruth, ed. Encyclopedia of Applied Ethics, Volume 2. San Diego, CA: Academic Press; 1998: 451–462.
(GENETIC INTERVENTION)

McGough, Helen. OPRR and FDA propose revised expedited review categories. *IRB: A Review of Human Subjects Research.* 1998 Jan–Feb; 20(1): 9, 11.
(HUMAN EXPERIMENTATION/ETHICS COMMITTEES; HUMAN EXPERIMENTATION/REGULATION)

McGuffin, Peter see Daniels, Jo

McGuire, John; Nieri, Deborah; Abbott, David; Sheridan, Kathleen; Fisher, Randy. Do Tarasoff principles apply in AIDS-related psychotherapy? Ethical decision making and the role of therapist homophobia and perceived client dangerousness. *Professional Psychology: Research and Practice.* 1995 Dec; 26(6): 608–611.
(AIDS/CONFIDENTIALITY; AIDS/HEALTH PERSONNEL)

McGurn, William. Princeton defends its philosopher of infanticide. *Wall Street Journal.* 1998 Nov 13: W17.
(ETHICISTS AND ETHICS COMMITTEES)

McHaffie, Hazel. Researching sensitive issues. *In:* Frith, Lucy, ed. Ethics and Midwifery: Issues in Contemporary Pratice. Boston, MA: Butterworth-Heinemann; 1996: 258–273.
(BEHAVIORAL RESEARCH)

Macilwain, Colin. NIH urged to address chimp care 'crisis'. [News]. *Nature.* 1997 Jul 17; 388(6639): 218.
(ANIMAL EXPERIMENTATION)

Macilwain, Colin. Scientists defy their ethics codes and take gifts from industry. [News]. *Nature.* 1998 Apr 2; 392(6675): 427.
(BIOMEDICAL RESEARCH)

McInturff, Bronwyn see Marson, Daniel C.

McKenny, Gerald P. An anthropological bioethics: hermeneutical or critical? Commentary on Elliott. *In:* Carson, Ronald A.; Burns, Chester R., eds. Philosophy of Medicine and Bioethics: A Twenty-Year Retrospective and Critical Appraisal. Boston, MA: Kluwer Academic; 1997: 213–220.
(BIOETHICS)

McKenny, Gerald P. Technology, authority and the loss of tradition: the roots of American bioethics in comparison with Japanese bioethics. *In:* Hoshino, Kazumasa, ed. Japanese and Western Bioethics: Studies

in Moral Diversity. Boston, MA: Kluwer Academic; 1997: 73–87.
(BIOETHICS)

McKenny, Gerald P. To Relieve the Human Condition: Bioethics, Technology, and the Body. Albany, NY: State University of New York Press; 1997. 279 p.
(BIOETHICS)

MacKenzie, Debora. Genes sans frontiéres. *New Scientist.* 1997 Mar 1; 153(2071): 50.
(RECOMBINANT DNA RESEARCH/REGULATION)

McKeown, Carole see Michie, Susan

MacKie, Palmer see Lamberts, Robert J.

McKinnon, Wendy C.; Baty, Bonnie J.; Bennett, Robin L.; Magee, Monica; Neufeld–Kaiser, Whitney A.; Peters, Kathryn F.; Sawyer, Jill C.; Schneider, Katherine A. Predisposition genetic testing for late-onset disorders in adults: a position paper of the National Society of Genetic Counselors. [Policy statement]. *JAMA.* 1997 Oct 15; 278(15): 1217–1220.
(GENETIC COUNSELING; GENETIC SCREENING)

Mackler, Aaron L. Cases and principles in Jewish bioethics: toward a holistic model. *In:* Dorff, Elliot N.; Newman, Louis E., eds. Contemporary Jewish Ethics and Morality: A Reader. New York, NY: Oxford University Press; 1995: 177–193.
(BIOETHICS)

Macklin, Ruth. Genetics and reproductive technologies. *In:* Borchert, Donald M., ed. The Encyclopedia of Philosophy. Supplement. New York, NY: Simon and Schuster and Macmillan; 1996: 217–220.
(GENETIC INTERVENTION; REPRODUCTIVE TECHNOLOGIES)

Macklin, Ruth. Human cloning? Don't just say no. *U.S. News and World Report.* 1997 Mar 10; 122(9): 64.
(CLONING)

Macklin, Ruth. Justice in international research. *In:* Kahn, Jeffrey P.; Mastroianni, Anna C.; Sugarman, Jeremy, eds. Beyond Consent: Seeking Justice in Research. New York, NY: Oxford University Press; 1998: 131–146.
(HUMAN EXPERIMENTATION/FOREIGN COUNTRIES; HUMAN EXPERIMENTATION/SPECIAL POPULATIONS)

Macklin, Ruth; White, Gladys B. Assisted reproductive technologies, ads, and ethics: philosophical, ethical, and clinical perspectives on the use of advertising in reproductive medicine. [Conference report]. *Women's Health Issues.* 1997 May–Jun; 7(3): 127–131.
(REPRODUCTIVE TECHNOLOGIES)

Macklin, Ruth see Goldworth, Amnon

McLachlan, Hugh V. Defending commercial surrogate motherhood against Van Niekerk and Van Zyl. *Journal of Medical Ethics.* 1997 Dec; 23(6): 344–348.
(SURROGATE MOTHERS)

McLaren, Anne; European Commission. Group of Advisers on the Ethical Implications of Biotechnology. Ethical aspects of cloning techniques: opinion of the Group of Advisers on the Ethical Implications of Biotechnology of the European Commission. [Statement and commentary]. *Cambridge*

Quarterly of Healthcare Ethics. 1998 Spring; 7(2): 187–193.
(CLONING)

McLean, G.R. see **Cleaton–Jones, Peter E.**

McLean, Sheila A.M., ed. Contemporary Issues in Law, Medicine and Ethics. Brookfield, VT: Dartmouth; 1996. 277 p.
(BIOETHICS)

McLean, Sheila A.M., ed. Death, Dying and the Law. Brookfield, VT: Dartmouth; 1996. 185 p.
(ADVANCE DIRECTIVES; ALLOWING TO DIE; EUTHANASIA; SUICIDE; TERMINAL CARE)

McLean, Sheila A.M. Law at the end of life: what next? *In:* McLean, Sheila A.M., ed. Death, Dying and the Law. Brookfield, VT: Dartmouth; 1996: 49–66.
(ALLOWING TO DIE/LEGAL ASPECTS; EUTHANASIA/LEGAL ASPECTS)

McLean, Sheila A.M. Letting die or assisting death: how should the law respond to the patient in a persistent vegetative state? *In:* Petersen, Kerry, ed. Intersections: Women on Law, Medicine and Technology. Brookfield, VT: Ashgate; 1997: 167–184.
(ALLOWING TO DIE/LEGAL ASPECTS)

McLean, Sheila A.M. Transplantation and the 'nearly dead': the case of elective ventilation. *In:* McLean, Sheila A.M., ed. Contemporary Issues in Law, Medicine and Ethics. Brookfield, VT: Dartmouth; 1996: 143–162.
(ADVANCE DIRECTIVES; ORGAN AND TISSUE DONATION)

MacLellan, D.G. see **Hardy, K.J.**

McMahon, William M. see **Botkin, Jeffrey R.**

McManus, Robert see **Millard, Charles E.**

MacMaster, Paul see **Neuberger, James**

McMillan, John. Competence to Consent, by Becky Cox White. [Book review essay]. *Theoretical Medicine and Bioethics.* 1998 Apr; 19(2): 161–166.
(INFORMED CONSENT)

McMillan, Margaret P. Banking on cord blood. [Editorial]. *Journal of Obstetric, Gynecologic and Neonatal Nursing.* 1996 Feb; 25(2): 115.
(BLOOD DONATION)

McNeill, Paul. Paying people to participate in research: why not? A response to Wilkinson and Moore. *Bioethics.* 1997 Oct; 11(5): 390–396.
(HUMAN EXPERIMENTATION)

McNeilly, Dennis P.; Hillary, Kristine. The hospice decision: psychosocial facilitators and barriers. *Omega: A Journal of Death and Dying.* 1997; 35(2): 193–217.
(TERMINAL CARE/HOSPICES)

MacPherson, Peter. Is this where we want to go? *Hastings Center Report.* 1997 Nov–Dec; 27(6): 17–22.
(HEALTH CARE/ECONOMICS)

McPherson, Richard A. see **Kadlec, Josef V.**

MacQuitty, Jonathan J. The real implications of Dolly. *Nature Biotechnology.* 1997 Apr; 15(4): 294.

(CLONING)

Macready, Norra. US doctors lie to help patients. [News]. *BMJ (British Medical Journal).* 1997 Jul 19; 315(7101): 148.
(FRAUD AND MISCONDUCT; HEALTH CARE/ECONOMICS)

Macready, Norra. US state rules that a viable fetus is a person. [News]. *BMJ (British Medical Journal).* 1997 Dec 6; 315(7121): 1488.
(FETUSES; PERSONHOOD; PRENATAL INJURIES)

Madden, Robert G. Civil commitment for substance abuse by pregnant women? A view from the front lines. *Politics and the Life Sciences.* 1996 Mar; 15(1): 56–59.
(INVOLUNTARY COMMITMENT; PRENATAL INJURIES)

Madder, Hilary. Existential autonomy: why patients should make their own choices. *Journal of Medical Ethics.* 1997 Aug; 23(4): 221–225.
(PROFESSIONAL PATIENT RELATIONSHIP)

Magee, Monica see **McKinnon, Wendy C.**

Maggiore, Quirino see **Maiorca, Rosario**

Magis, Carlos see **Schüklenk, Udo**

Magnusson, R.S. Australian HIV/AIDS legislation: a review for doctors. *Australian and New Zealand Journal of Medicine.* 1996 Jun; 26(3): 396–406.
(AIDS)

Magnusson, Roger S. Testing for HIV without specific consent: a short review. *Australian and New Zealand Journal of Public Health.* 1996 Feb; 20(1): 57–60.
(AIDS/TESTING AND SCREENING; INFORMED CONSENT)

Mahler, Ch. see **Prosor, Ron**

Mahlmeister, Laura. When cost-saving strategies are unacceptable. *Pediatric Nursing.* 1996 Mar–Apr; 22(2): 130–132.
(HEALTH CARE/ECONOMICS; NURSING ETHICS)

Mahowald, Mary B. An overview of the Human Genome Project and its implications for women. *Women's Health Issues.* 1997 Jul–Aug; 7(4): 206–208.
(GENOME MAPPING)

Mahowald, Mary B. Gender justice in genetics. *Women's Health Issues.* 1997 Jul–Aug; 7(4): 230–233.
(GENETIC SERVICES)

Mahowald, Mary B. see **Harris, Cathleen M.**

Maidment, Anita see **Neuberger, James**

Maiorca, Rosario; Maggiore, Quirino; Mordacci, Roberto; Tonini, Ersilio; Biagi, Enzo; Bissoni, Giovanni; Davison, Sandy; Mallik, Netar. Ethical problems in dialysis and transplantation. *Nephrology, Dialysis, Transplantation.* 1996; 11(Suppl. 9): 100–112.
(BIOMEDICAL TECHNOLOGIES; ORGAN AND TISSUE TRANSPLANTATION)

Mair, Jane. Maternal/foetal conflict: defined or defused? *In:* McLean, Sheila A.M., ed. Contemporary Issues in Law, Medicine and Ethics. Brookfield, VT: Dartmouth; 1996: 79–97.
(FETUSES; PRENATAL INJURIES; TREATMENT REFUSAL)

Maislin, Greg see **Evans, Lois K.**

Maislin, Greg see **O'Brien, Linda A.**

Major, E. see **Briggs, J.D.**

Mallik, Netar see **Maiorca, Rosario**

Malnick, Stephen D.H. see **Prosor, Ron**

Malone, Ruth E.; Workman, Stephen. Caring for "difficult" patients. [Letters]. *Hastings Center Report.* 1998 Jul–Aug; 28(4): 4.
(TREATMENT REFUSAL)

Maloney, Dennis M. Federal agency's final rule says informed consent forms must be dated. [News]. *Human Research Report.* 1996 Dec; 11(12): 1–2.
(HUMAN EXPERIMENTATION/INFORMED CONSENT; HUMAN EXPERIMENTATION/REGULATION)

Mamlin, Lorrie A. see **Ferguson, Jeffrey A.**

Manca di Villahermosa, S. see **Elli, M.**

Manciet, Gerard see **Gromb, Sophie**

Mandel, I.D. On being a scientist in a rapidly changing world. *Journal of Dental Research.* 1996 Feb; 75(2): 841–844.
(BIOMEDICAL RESEARCH; PROFESSIONAL ETHICS)

Mander, Rosemary. Failure to deliver: ethical issues relating to epidural analgesia in uncomplicated labour. *In:* Frith, Lucy, ed. Ethics and Midwifery: Issues in Contemporary Practice. Boston, MA: Butterworth–Heinemann; 1996: 51–71.
(PATIENT CARE/DRUGS)

Mann, Patricia S. Meanings of death. *In:* Battin, Margaret P.; Rhodes, Rosamond; Silvers, Anita, eds. Physician Assisted Suicide: Expanding the Debate. New York, NY: Routledge; 1998: 11–27.
(SUICIDE)

Manni, Corrado. Palliative medicine and Christian eschatology. *Dolentium Hominum: Church and Health in the World.* 1996; 31(11th Yr., No. 1): 173–177.
(TERMINAL CARE)

Mansheim, Bernard J. What care should be covered? *Kennedy Institute of Ethics Journal.* 1997 Dec; 7(4): 331–336.
(HEALTH CARE/ECONOMICS)

Manson, JoAnn E. see **Angell, Marcia**

Mansour, Paul. Turkish doctors collude in torture. [News]. *BMJ (British Medical Journal).* 1997 Mar 8; 314(7082): 699.
(FRAUD AND MISCONDUCT; TORTURE)

Mansour, Ragaa T. see **Serour, Gamal I.**

Mao, Xin; Wertz, Dorothy C. China's genetic services providers' attitudes towards several ethical issues: a cross-cultural survey. *Clinical Genetics.* 1997 Aug; 52(2): 100–109.
(ABORTION/FOREIGN COUNTRIES; GENETIC COUNSELING; SEX DETERMINATION)

Maranto, Gina. Quest for Perfection: The Drive to Breed Better Human Beings. New York, NY: Scribner; 1996. 335 p.
(EUGENICS; REPRODUCTIVE TECHNOLOGIES)

Mardesic, Tonko; Rezacova, Jitka; Ventruba, Pavel. The practice of assisted reproduction in the Czech Republic. *Journal of Assisted Reproduction and Genetics.* 1996 Mar; 13(3): 195–196.
(REPRODUCTIVE TECHNOLOGIES)

Marenco, Marc see **Foster, George E.**

Mariner, Wendy K. Mortal Peril: Our Inalienable Right to Health Care? by Richard A. Epstein. [Book review essay]. *JAMA.* 1998 Jan 28; 279(4): 330–331.
(HEALTH CARE/ECONOMICS; HEALTH CARE/RIGHTS)

Marks, Lee Ann see **Jones, Melinda**

Markson, Lawrence; Clark, Jack; Glantz, Leonard; Lamberton, Victoria; Kern, Donald; Stollerman, Gene. The doctor's role in discussing advance preferences for end-of-life care: perceptions of physicians practicing in the VA. *Journal of the American Geriatrics Society.* 1997 Apr; 45(4): 399–406.
(ADVANCE DIRECTIVES)

Marquis, Don. Abortion. *In:* Borchert, Donald M., ed. The Encyclopedia of Philosophy. Supplement. New York, NY: Simon and Schuster Macmillan; 1996: 1–3.
(ABORTION)

Marquis, Don. The weakness of the case for legalising physician–assisted suicide. *In:* Battin, Margaret P.; Rhodes, Rosamond; Silvers, Anita, eds. Physician Assisted Suicide: Expanding the Debate. New York, NY: Routledge; 1998: 267–278.
(SUICIDE)

Marrero, Ursula see **Finkelstein, Beth S.**

Marritt, Clive. Local research ethics committees: a view from the Department of Health. *In:* Close, Bryony; Combes, Robert; Hubbard, Anthony; Illingworth, John, eds. Volunteers in Research and Testing. Bristol, PA: Taylor and Francis; 1997: 53–58.
(HUMAN EXPERIMENTATION/ETHICS COMMITTEES; HUMAN EXPERIMENTATION/FOREIGN COUNTRIES)

Marsden, Rachel see **Savulescu, Julian**

Marsh, Frank H. Abortion and the law: the Supreme Court, privacy, and abortion. *In:* Edwards, Rem B., ed. Advances in Bioethics. Volume 2: New Essays on Abortion and Bioethics. Greenwich, CT: JAI Press; 1997: 107–123.
(ABORTION/LEGAL ASPECTS)

Marsh, Frank H. see **Cebik, L.B.**

Marsh, J. Wallis; Dvorchik, Igor; Casavilla, Adrian; Fung, John J.; Iwatsuki, Shunzaboro. Should reimbursement be denied for liver transplantation in patients with hepatocellular carcinoma? [Letter]. *JAMA.* 1997 Jul 16; 278(3): 203–205.
(ORGAN AND TISSUE TRANSPLANTATION)

Marshall, Eliot. AIDS therapy: controversial trial offers hopeful result. [News]. *Science.* 1998 Feb 27; 279(5355): 1299.

(AIDS/HUMAN EXPERIMENTATION; HUMAN
EXPERIMENTATION/FOREIGN COUNTRIES; HUMAN
EXPERIMENTATION/RESEARCH DESIGN; HUMAN
EXPERIMENTATION/SPECIAL POPULATIONS)

Marshall, Eliot. Biomedical groups derail fast-track
anticloning bill. [News]. *Science.* 1998 Feb 20; 279(5354):
1123–1124.
(CLONING)

Marshall, Eliot. Medline searches turn up cases of
suspected plagiarism. [News]. *Science.* 1998 Jan 23;
279(5350): 473–474.
(BIOMEDICAL RESEARCH; FRAUD AND MISCONDUCT)

Marshall, Eliot. Need a reagent? Just sign here. [News].
Science. 1997 Oct 10; 278(5336): 212–213.
(BIOMEDICAL RESEARCH)

Marshall, Eliot. NIH examines standards for consent.
[News]. *Science.* 1998 Jun 12; 280(5370): 1688.
(HUMAN EXPERIMENTATION/ETHICS COMMITTEES;
HUMAN EXPERIMENTATION/INFORMED CONSENT)

Marshall, Eliot. 'Playing chicken' over gene markers.
[News]. *Science.* 1997 Dec 19; 278(5346): 2046–2048.
(GENOME MAPPING)

Marshall, Eliot. Review boards: a system 'in jeopardy'?
[News]. *Science.* 1998 Jun 19; 280(5371): 1830–1831.
(HUMAN EXPERIMENTATION/ETHICS COMMITTEES;
HUMAN EXPERIMENTATION/REGULATION)

Marshall, Eliot. Whose DNA is it, anyway? [News].
Science. 1997 Oct 24; 278(5338): 564–567.
(GENETIC RESEARCH; GENOME MAPPING)

Marshall, Eliot; Pennisi, Elizabeth. Hubris and the
human genome. [News]. *Science.* 1998 May 15; 280(5366):
994–995.
(GENOME MAPPING)

Marshall, Mary Faith; Smith, C.D. Confidentiality in
surgical practice. *In:* McCullough, Laurence B.; Jones,
James W.; Brody, Baruch A., eds. Surgical Ethics. New
York, NY: Oxford University Press; 1998: 38–56.
(CONFIDENTIALITY)

Marshall, Mary Faith see **Webb, Sally L.**

Marshall, Patricia A. Boundary crossings: gender and
power in clinical ethics consultations. *In:* Sargent,
Carolyn F.; Brettell; Caroline B., eds. Gender and
Health: An International Perspective. Upper Saddle
River, NJ: Prentice Hall; 1996: 205–226.
(ETHICISTS AND ETHICS COMMITTEES; ORGAN AND
TISSUE TRANSPLANTATION; PROFESSIONAL PATIENT
RELATIONSHIP)

**Marshall, Patricia A.; Koenig, Barbara A.; Barnes,
Donelle M.; Davis, Anne J.** Multiculturalism,
bioethics, and end-of-life care: case narratives of Latino
cancer patients. *In:* Monagle, John F.; Thomasma, David
C., eds. Health Care Ethics: Critical Issues for the 21st
Century. Gaithersburg, MD: Aspen Publishers; 1998:
421–431.
(ADVANCE DIRECTIVES)

Marshall, Patricia A. see **Hern, H. Eugene**

Marshall, Patricia A. see **Kelly, Susan E.**

**Marshall, Tom; St. Leger, Moya Frenz; Woodroffe,
Caroline; Bowling, Ann.** Rationing health care.
[Letters]. *BMJ (British Medical Journal).* 1997 Jun 28;
314(7098): 1901–1902.
(HEALTH CARE/FOREIGN COUNTRIES; RESOURCE
ALLOCATION)

Marson, Daniel; Ingram, Kellie K. Competency to
consent to treatment: a growing field of research:
commentary. *Journal of Ethics, Law, and Aging.* 1996
Fall–Winter; 2(2): 59–63.
(INFORMED CONSENT)

**Marson, Daniel C.; Hawkins, Lauren; McInturff,
Bronwyn; Harrell, Lindy E.** Cognitive models that
predict physician judgments of capacity to consent in
mild Alzheimer's disease. *Journal of the American
Geriatrics Society.* 1997 Apr; 45(4): 458–464.
(INFORMED CONSENT/MENTALLY DISABLED)

**Marson, Daniel C.; McInturff, Bronwyn; Hawkins,
Lauren; Bartolucci, Alfred; Harrell, Lindy E.**
Consistency of physician judgments of capacity to
consent in mild Alzheimer's disease. *Journal of the
American Geriatrics Society.* 1997 Apr; 45(4): 453–457.
(INFORMED CONSENT/MENTALLY DISABLED)

Marta, Jan. Toward a bioethics for the twenty-first
century: a Ricoeurian poststructuralist narrative
hermeneutic approach to informed consent. *In:* Nelson,
Hilde Lindemann, ed. Stories and Their Limits:
Narrative Approaches to Bioethics. New York, NY:
Routledge; 1997: 198–212.
(INFORMED CONSENT)

**Marteau, Theresa; Michie, Susan; Drake, Harriet;
Bobrow, Martin.** Public attitudes towards the selection
of desirable characteristics in children. *Journal of Medical
Genetics.* 1995 Oct; 32(10): 796–798.
(GENETIC INTERVENTION)

Marteau, Theresa see **Drake, Harriet**

Marteau, Theresa see **Michie, Susan**

Marteau, Theresa M.; Croyle, Robert T. The new
genetics: psychological responses to genetic testing. *BMJ
(British Medical Journal).* 1998 Feb 28; 316(7132):
693–696.
(GENETIC COUNSELING; GENETIC SCREENING)

Marteau, Theresa M. see **Michie, Susan**

Martin, David see **Silverman, Myrna**

Martin, Douglas K.; Singer, Peter A.; Siegler, Mark.
Ethical considerations in liver transplantation. *In:* Boyer,
J.L.; Ockner, R.K., eds. Progress in Liver Diseases, Vol.
XII. Philadelphia, PA: Saunders; 1994: 215–229.
(ORGAN AND TISSUE DONATION; ORGAN AND TISSUE
TRANSPLANTATION)

Martin, Douglas K. see **Ferguson, Jeffrey A.**

Martin, Douglas K. see **Singer, Peter A.**

Martin, Geoffrey W. Communication breakdown or ideal
speech situation: the problem of nurse advocacy. *Nursing
Ethics.* 1998 Mar; 5(2): 147–157.
(PROFESSIONAL PATIENT RELATIONSHIP)

Matthews, Eric. Paternalism, care and mental illness. *In:* Grubb, Andrew, ed. Decision–Making and the Problem of Incompetence. New York, NY: Wiley; 1994: 103–114.
(TREATMENT REFUSAL/MENTALLY DISABLED)

Matthews, Mary see **Pozda, Richard**

Matthews, Merrill. Would physician–assisted suicide save the healthcare system money? (Or, is Jack Kevorkian doing all of us a favor?). *In:* Battin, Margaret P.; Rhodes, Rosamond; Silvers, Anita, eds. Physician Assisted Suicide: Expanding the Debate. New York, NY: Routledge; 1998: 312–322.
(HEALTH CARE/ECONOMICS; SUICIDE; TERMINAL CARE)

Mattox, Kenneth L.; Engelhardt, H. Tristram. Emerging patients: serious moral choices with limited time, information, and patient participation. *In:* McCullough, Laurence B.; Jones, James W.; Brody, Baruch A., eds. Surgical Ethics. New York, NY: Oxford University Press; 1998: 78–96.
(PATIENT CARE)

Mattson, Margaret E.; Curb, J. David; McArdle, Robert; Aspirin Myocardial Infarction Study (AMIS) Research Group; Beta–Blocker Heart Attack Trial (BHAT) Research Group. Participation in a clinical trial: the patients' point of view. *Controlled Clinical Trials.* 1985 Jun; 6(2): 156–167.
(HUMAN EXPERIMENTATION)

May, Carl see **Chapple, Alison**

May, Thomas see **Agich, George J.**

May, William E. *Donum Vitae*: Catholic teaching concerning homologous *in vitro* fertilization. *In:* Wildes, Kevin Wm., ed. Infertility: A Crossroad of Faith, Medicine, and Technology. Boston, MA: Kluwer Academic; 1997: 73–92.
(IN VITRO FERTILIZATION)

May, William E. The call to holiness and health care as service. *Linacre Quarterly.* 1997 May; 64(2): 66–73.
(PROFESSIONAL PATIENT RELATIONSHIP)

Mayer, Dan; Thibodeau, Lorraine. Ethical issues in alcohol–related emergencies and emergency care of alcoholic and intoxicated patients. *In:* Shelton, Wayne N.; Edwards, Rem B., eds. Advances in Bioethics. Volume 3: Values, Ethics, and Alcoholism. Greenwich, CT: JAI Press; 1997: 287–308.
(PATIENT CARE)

Mayer, Teresa see **Mustard, Cameron A.**

Mayo, Kelly. Social responsibility in nursing education. *Journal of Holistic Nursing.* 1996 Mar; 14(1): 24–43.
(NURSING ETHICS/EDUCATION)

Mayor, Susan. Pregnant women should routinely be offered HIV tests. [News]. *BMJ (British Medical Journal).* 1998 May 2; 316(7141): 1333.
(AIDS/TESTING AND SCREENING)

Mazen, Noël–Jean. Human DNA on trial in French law. *In:* Knoppers, Bartha Maria, ed. Human DNA: Law and Policy: International and Comparative Perspectives. Proceedings of the First International Conference on DNA Sampling and Human Genetic Research: Ethical, Legal, and Policy Aspects, held in Montreal, Canada, 6–8 Sep 1996. Boston, MA: Kluwer Law International; 1997: 43–54.
(BIOMEDICAL TECHNOLOGIES; ORGAN AND TISSUE DONATION; PATENTING LIFE FORMS)

Mazur, Dennis J. How older patient preferences are influenced by consideration of future health outcomes. *Journal of the American Geriatrics Society.* 1997 Jun; 45(6): 725–728.
(ALLOWING TO DIE; PATIENT CARE/AGED; TREATMENT REFUSAL)

Mbidde, Edward. Bioethics and local circumstances. [Editorial]. *Science.* 1998 Jan 9; 279(5348): 155.
(AIDS/HUMAN EXPERIMENTATION; HUMAN EXPERIMENTATION/FOREIGN COUNTRIES)

Mead, Gillian E.; Pendleton, Neil; Pendleton, Deborah E.; Horan, Michael A.; Bent, Nuala; Rabbit, Patrick. High technology medical interventions: what do older people want? [Letter]. *Journal of the American Geriatrics Society.* 1997 Nov; 45(11): 1409–1411.
(BIOMEDICAL TECHNOLOGIES; PATIENT CARE/AGED)

Meador, Kimford J. see **Burt, R.A.P.**

Meadow, William; Reimshisel, Tyler; Lantos, John. Birth weight–specific mortality for extremely low birth weight infants vanishes by four days of life: epidemiology and ethics in the neonatal intensive care unit. *Pediatrics.* 1996 May; 97(5): 636–643.
(PATIENT CARE/MINORS)

Mehlman, Maxwell see **Kodish, Eric**

Mehlman, Maxwell J.; Botkin, Jeffrey R. Access to the Genome: The Challenge to Equality. Washington, DC: Georgetown University Press; 1998. 152 p.
(GENETIC INTERVENTION; GENETIC SERVICES; GENOME MAPPING; RESOURCE ALLOCATION)

Mehlman, Maxwell J.; Durchslag, Melvyn R.; Neuhauser, Duncan. When do health care decisions discriminate against persons with disabilities? *Journal of Health Politics, Policy and Law.* 1997 Dec; 22(6): 1385–1411.
(HEALTH CARE/ECONOMICS; SELECTION FOR TREATMENT)

Mehta, Cyrus see **Taylor, Kathryn M.**

Mehuron, Kate. "Undemocratic afflictions": a feminist response to the AIDS epidemic. *In:* DiQuinzio, Patrice; Young, Iris Marion, eds. Feminist Ethics and Social Policy. Bloomington, IN: Indiana University Press; 1997: 208–225.
(AIDS; HEALTH CARE)

Meier, Diane E. Voiceless and vulnerable: dementia patients without surrogates in an era of capitation. [Editorial]. *Journal of the American Geriatrics Society.* 1997 Mar; 45(3): 375–377.
(INFORMED CONSENT/MENTALLY DISABLED)

Meier, Diane E.; Emmons, Carol–Ann; Wallenstein, Sylvan; Quill, Timothy; Morrison, R. Sean; Cassel, Christine K. A national survey of physician–assisted suicide and euthanasia in the United States. *New England Journal of Medicine.* 1998 Apr 23; 338(17): 1193–1201.
(EUTHANASIA/ATTITUDES; SUICIDE)

Meier, Diane E. see Baskin, Shari A.

Meier, Diane E. see Hendin, Herbert

Meier, Diane E. see Miller, Franklin G.

Meier, Diane E. see Morrison, R. Sean

Meier, Diane E. see Quill, Timothy E.

Meier, Diane E. see White, W.D.

Meisel, Alan. Legal issues in decision making for incompetent patients: advance directives and surrogate decision making. *In:* Sass, Hans–Martin; Veatch, Robert M.; Kimura, Rihito, eds. Advance Directives and Surrogate Decision Making in Health Care: United States, Germany, and Japan. Baltimore, MD: Johns Hopkins University Press; 1998: 34–65.
(ADVANCE DIRECTIVES; ALLOWING TO DIE/LEGAL ASPECTS; INFORMED CONSENT)

Meisel, Alan see Roth, Loren

Melby, V. see Steele, A.

Meldrum, David R.; Gardner, David K. Two–embryo transfer -- the future looks bright. [Editorial]. *New England Journal of Medicine.* 1998 Aug 27; 339(9): 624–625.
(IN VITRO FERTILIZATION)

Mellsop, Graham. Issues in psychiatric ethics. *New Zealand Medical Journal.* 1983 Aug 10; 96(737): 616–619.
(MEDICAL ETHICS)

Melton, L. Joseph. The threat to medical–records research. *New England Journal of Medicine.* 1997 Nov 13; 337(20): 1466–1470.
(BIOMEDICAL RESEARCH; CONFIDENTIALITY)

Melzer, David. New drug treatment for Alzheimer's disease: lessons for healthcare policy. *BMJ (British Medical Journal).* 1998 Mar 7; 316(7133): 762–764.
(HUMAN EXPERIMENTATION/SPECIAL POPULATIONS; PATIENT CARE/DRUGS; PATIENT CARE/MENTALLY DISABLED)

Melzer, David. Patent protection for medical technologies: why some and not others? *Lancet.* 1998 Feb 14; 351(9101): 518–519.
(BIOMEDICAL TECHNOLOGIES)

Mendelson, Danuta. The concept of medical confidentiality in Australian and Jewish law. *In:* Jewish Law Annual. Volume Twelve. Amsterdam, Netherlands: Harwood Academic Publishers; 1997: 217–249.
(CONFIDENTIALITY; CONFIDENTIALITY/LEGAL ASPECTS)

Mendelssohn, David C. see Singer, Peter A.

Mendez, R.; Aswad, S.; Dessouki, A.; Mendez, R.G.; Obispo, E.; Gavazov, M.; Cicciarelli, J. Difficulties of foreigners seeking transplantation in the United States. *Transplantation Proceedings.* 1992 Oct; 24(5): 2075–2076.
(ORGAN AND TISSUE TRANSPLANTATION)

Mendez, R.G. see Mendez, R.

Menge, Alan C. see Ohl, Dana A.

Mengel, Norma see Foglio, John

Menkes, David B. Hazardous drugs in developing countries. [Editorial]. *BMJ (British Medical Journal).* 1997 Dec 13; 315(7122): 1557–1558.
(PATIENT CARE/DRUGS)

Menzel, Paul T. The moral duty to contribute and its implications for organ procurement policy. *Transplantation Proceedings.* 1992 Oct; 24(5): 2175–2178.
(ORGAN AND TISSUE DONATION)

Menzel, Paul T. see Arnold, Denis G.

Meran, Johannes Gobertus; Poliwoda, Hubert. Clinical perspectives on advance directives and surrogate decision making. *In:* Sass, Hans–Martin; Veatch, Robert M.; Kimura, Rihito, eds. Advance Directives and Surrogate Decision Making in Health Care: United States, Germany, and Japan. Baltimore, MD: Johns Hopkins University Press; 1998: 95–113.
(ADVANCE DIRECTIVES)

Merchant, Jennifer. Biogenetics, artificial procreation, and public policy in the United States and France. *Technology in Society.* 1996; 18(1): 1–15.
(EMBRYO AND FETAL RESEARCH; GENETIC RESEARCH; PRENATAL INJURIES; REPRODUCTIVE TECHNOLOGIES; WRONGFUL LIFE)

Merrick, Janna C. Pregnancy and substance abuse: education or mandatory treatment? *Politics and the Life Sciences.* 1996 Mar; 15(1): 59–60.
(INVOLUNTARY COMMITMENT; PRENATAL INJURIES)

Merriken, Karen; Overcast, Thomas D. Governmental regulation of heart transplantation and the right to privacy. *Journal of Contemporary Law.* 1985; 11(2): 481–514.
(ORGAN AND TISSUE TRANSPLANTATION)

Merz, Jon F. see Cho, Mildred K.

Meslin, Eric M. Oxford Radcliffe Hospital Clinical Ethics Project 1994–1995: final report and recommendations. Oxford Radcliffe Hospital, Clinical Ethics Project, Stable Block, Manor House, Headley Way, Headington, Oxford, England OX3 9DZ; 1995 Jun 12. 53 p.
(ETHICISTS AND ETHICS COMMITTEES)

Meslin, Eric M.; Lemieux–Charles, Louise; Wortley, Jacinth Tracey. An ethics framework for assisting clinician–managers in resource allocation decision making. *Hospital and Health Services Administration.* 1997 Spring; 42(1): 33–48.
(RESOURCE ALLOCATION)

Meslin, Eric M. see Alexandrov, Andrei V.

Meslin, Eric M. see Etchells, Edward

Meslin, Eric M. see Weijer, Charles

Mesman, Jessica see Gallagher, Eugene B.

Messer, Donald E. see Geis, Sally B.

Metcalfe, D. see Blennerhassett, Mitzi

Meyer, Cheryl L. The Wandering Uterus: Politics and the Reproductive Rights of Women. New York, NY:

New York University Press; 1997. 226 p.
(REPRODUCTION; REPRODUCTIVE TECHNOLOGIES)

Meyer, Joanne M. see **Sherman, Stephanie L.**

Meyer, Madonna Harrington see **King, Leslie**

Meystre, Chantal J.N.; Burley, Neil M.J.; Ahmedzai, Sam. What investigations and procedures do patients in hospices want? Interview based survey of patients and their nurses. *BMJ (British Medical Journal).* 1997 Nov 8; 315(7117): 1202–1203.
(TERMINAL CARE/HOSPICES)

Mezey, Mathy; Mitty, Ethel; Rappaport, Michael; Ramsey, Gloria. Implementation of the Patient Self–Determination Act (PSDA) in nursing homes in New York City. *Journal of the American Geriatrics Society.* 1997 Jan; 45(1): 43–49.
(ADVANCE DIRECTIVES)

Micetich, Kenneth. The IRB: current and future challenges. *In:* Monagle, John F.; Thomasma, David C., eds. Health Care Ethics: Critical Issues for the 21st Century. Gaithersburg, MD: Aspen Publishers; 1998: 265–276.
(HUMAN EXPERIMENTATION/ETHICS COMMITTEES)

Michel, Vicki. Reflections on cultural difference and advance directives. *Bioethics Forum.* 1997 Summer; 13(2): 22–26.
(ADVANCE DIRECTIVES)

Michels, Joop see **van Weel, Chris**

Michie, Susan; McDonald, Valerie; Bobrow, Martin; McKeown, Carole; Marteau, Theresa. Parents' responses to predictive genetic testing in their children: report of a single case study. *Journal of Medical Genetics.* 1996 Apr; 33(4): 313–318.
(GENETIC SCREENING)

Michie, Susan; Marteau, Theresa M.; Bobrow, Martin. Genetic counselling: the psychological impact of meeting patients' expectations. *Journal of Medical Genetics.* 1997 Mar; 34(3): 237–241.
(GENETIC COUNSELING)

Michie, Susan see **Marteau, Theresa**

Michielsen, Paul. Informed or presumed consent legislative models. *In:* Chapman, Jeremy R.; Deierhoi, Mark; Wight, Celia, eds. Organ and Tissue Donation for Transplantation. New York, NY: Oxford University Press; 1997: 344–360.
(INFORMED CONSENT; ORGAN AND TISSUE DONATION)

Michigan. Commission on Death and Dying. Final Report of the Michigan Commission on Death and Dying. Lansing, MI: The Commission; 1994 Jun. 1 v.
(SUICIDE)

Mick, Rosemarie see **Daugherty, Christopher**

Miedema, Felicia see **Pozda, Richard**

Milch, Robert see **Wear, Stephen**

Miles, J.A.R. Organ transplants in China: use of organs from executed prisoners. *New Zealand Medical Journal.*

1995 May 10; 108(999): 178.
(ORGAN AND TISSUE DONATION)

Miles, Steven H. The Oregon Death with Dignity Act: A Guidebook for Health Care Providers, edited by Kathleen Haley and Melinda Lee. [Book review essay]. *JAMA.* 1998 Jul 22–29; 280(4): 387–388.
(SUICIDE)

Miles, Steven H. see **Christensen, Kate**

Millard, Charles E.; McManus, Robert. The enigma of today's physician. *Linacre Quarterly.* 1997 May; 64(2): 89–93.
(HEALTH CARE)

Miller, A.S.; Hagihara, A. Organ transplanting in Japan: the debate begins. *Public Health.* 1997 Nov; 111(6): 367–372.
(ORGAN AND TISSUE DONATION; ORGAN AND TISSUE TRANSPLANTATION)

Miller, Alan S. see **Hagihara, Akihito**

Miller, Anthony B. The public health basis of cancer screening: principles and ethical aspects. *In:* Miller, A.B., ed. Advances in Cancer Screening. Boston, MA: Kluwer Academic; 1996: 1–7.
(MASS SCREENING)

Miller, Barbara. Germany remains split on animal testing. [News]. *Nature.* 1998 Feb 12; 391(6668): 624.
(ANIMAL EXPERIMENTATION)

Miller, Deborah J. see **Sulmasy, Daniel P.**

Miller, Franklin G. Dedicatory essay on John C. Fletcher [and] Bibliography of publications by John C. Fletcher. *Journal of Contemporary Health Law and Policy.* 1996 Fall; 13(1): ix–xxxii.
(BIOETHICS; ETHICISTS AND ETHICS COMMITTEES)

Miller, Franklin G.; Caplan, Arthur L.; Fletcher, John C. Dealing with Dolly: inside the National Bioethics Advisory Commission. *Health Affairs.* 1998 May–Jun; 17(3): 264–267.
(CLONING; ETHICISTS AND ETHICS COMMITTEES)

Miller, Franklin G.; Fins, Joseph J.; Bacchetta, Matthew D. Clinical pragmatism: John Dewey and clinical ethics. *Journal of Contemporary Health Law and Policy.* 1996 Fall; 13(1): 27–51.
(BIOETHICS)

Miller, Franklin G.; Meier, Diane E. Voluntary death: a comparison of terminal dehydration and physician–assisted suicide. *Annals of Internal Medicine.* 1998 Apr 1; 128(7): 559–562.
(SUICIDE; TERMINAL CARE)

Miller, Franklin G. see **Fins, Joseph J.**

Miller, Franklin G. see **Fletcher, John C.**

Miller, Franklin G. see **Silvers, Anita**

Miller, Hugh. DNA blueprints, personhood, and genetic privacy. *Health Matrix.* 1998 Summer; 8(2): 179–221.
(CONFIDENTIALITY; GENETIC SCREENING; PERSONHOOD)

Miller, John D. A political review of alternative

surrogacy proposals. [Commentary]. *University of San Francisco Law Review*. 1994 Spring; 28(3): 627–632.
(SURROGATE MOTHERS)

Miller, Judith. The Deschamps Report: controls for clinical research in Quebec. *International Journal of Bioethics*. 1997 Mar–Jun; 8(1–2): 79–85.
(HUMAN EXPERIMENTATION/FOREIGN COUNTRIES; HUMAN EXPERIMENTATION/REGULATION)

Miller, Marvin D. Terminating the "Socially Inadequate": The American Eugenicists and the German Race Hygienists, California to Cold Spring Harbor, Long Island to Germany. Commack, NY: Malamud-Rose; 1996. 289 p.
(EUGENICS; STERILIZATION)

Miller, Pam. Ethical issues in neonatal intensive care. *In:* Frith, Lucy, ed. Ethics and Midwifery: Issues in Contemporary Practice. Boston, MA: Butterworth–Heinemann; 1996: 123–139.
(ALLOWING TO DIE/INFANTS; BIOMEDICAL TECHNOLOGIES; SELECTION FOR TREATMENT)

Miller, Patrick. Struggle. [Personal narrative]. *Bioethics Forum*. 1997 Spring; 13(1): 41–45.
(TERMINAL CARE)

Miller, Randolph A.; Goodman, Kenneth W. Ethical challenges in the use of decision–support software in clinical practice. *In:* Goodman, Kenneth W., ed. Ethics, Computing, and Medicine: Informatics and the Transformation of Health Care. New York, NY: Cambridge University Press; 1998: 102–115.
(BIOMEDICAL TECHNOLOGIES; PATIENT CARE)

Miller, Tracy E. Managed care regulation: in the laboratory of the states. *JAMA*. 1997 Oct 1; 278(13): 1102–1109.
(HEALTH CARE/ECONOMICS)

Miller, Tracy E.; Coleman, Carl H.; Cugliari, Anna Maria. Treatment decisions for patients without surrogates: rethinking policies for a vulnerable population. *Journal of the American Geriatrics Society*. 1997 Mar; 45(3): 369–374.
(ETHICISTS AND ETHICS COMMITTEES; INFORMED CONSENT)

Milliez, J.; Sureau, C. Pre-implantation diagnosis and the eugenics debate: our responsibility to future generations. *In:* Shenfield, F.; Sureau, C., eds. Ethical Dilemmas in Assisted Reproduction. New York, NY: Parthenon Pub. Group; 1997: 57–66.
(EUGENICS; PRENATAL DIAGNOSIS)

Millstein, Susan G. see **Ford, Carol A.**

Milner, Claire Alida. Gulf war guinea pigs: is informed consent optional during war? [Comment]. *Journal of Contemporary Health Law and Policy*. 1996 Fall; 13(1): 199–232.
(HUMAN EXPERIMENTATION/INFORMED CONSENT; HUMAN EXPERIMENTATION/SPECIAL POPULATIONS; WAR)

Milton, P. see **Hardy, K.J.**

Mindes, Paula. Tuberculosis quarantine: a review of legal issues in Ohio and other states. [Note]. *Journal of Law and Health*. 1995–1996; 10(2): 403–428.
(PUBLIC HEALTH)

Minkoff, Howard; O'Sullivan, Mary Jo. The case for rapid HIV testing during labor. *JAMA*. 1998 Jun 3; 279(21): 1743–1744.
(AIDS/TESTING AND SCREENING)

Minogue, Brendan P.; Palmer–Fernández, Gabriel; Reagan, James E., eds. Reading Engelhardt: Essays on the Thought of H. Tristram Engelhardt, Jr. Boston, MA: Kluwer Academic; 1997. 312 p.
(BIOETHICS)

Minow, Martha. Beyond state intervention in the family: for Baby Jane Doe. *University of Michigan Journal of Law Reform*. 1985 Summer; 18(4): 933–1014.
(ALLOWING TO DIE/INFANTS; ALLOWING TO DIE/LEGAL ASPECTS)

Mintz, Benjamin. Analyzing the OPTN [Organ Procurement and Transplant Network] under the state action doctrine –– can UNOS's organ allocation criteria survive strict scrutiny? *Columbia Journal of Law and Social Problems*. 1995 Spring; 28(3): 339–396.
(ORGAN AND TISSUE TRANSPLANTATION; RESOURCE ALLOCATION/BIOMEDICAL TECHNOLOGIES; SELECTION FOR TREATMENT)

Minz, M. see **Indudhara, R.**

Mirvis, David M. Managed care, managing ethics. [Editorial]. *Journal of the American Geriatrics Society*. 1998 Mar; 46(3): 389–390.
(HEALTH CARE/ECONOMICS)

Mirvis, David M.; Chang, Cyril F.; Morreim, E. Haavi. Protecting older people while managing their care. [Editorial]. *Journal of the American Geriatrics Society*. 1997 May; 45(5): 645–646.
(HEALTH CARE/ECONOMICS; PATIENT CARE/AGED)

Misbin, Robert I. see **Portenoy, Russell K.**

Missa, Jean–Noël. Psychosurgery and physical brain manipulation. *In:* Chadwick, Ruth, ed. Encyclopedia of Applied Ethics, Volume 3. San Diego, CA: Academic Press; 1998: 735–744.
(PSYCHOSURGERY)

Mitchell, Peter. Drug industry lobbies against European research–data directive. [News]. *Lancet*. 1997 May 10; 349(9062): 1378.
(BIOMEDICAL RESEARCH; CONFIDENTIALITY)

Mitchell, Peter. Edinburgh doctor struck off because of clinical–trial fraud. [News]. *Lancet*. 1997 Jul 26; 350(9073): 273.
(FRAUD AND MISCONDUCT)

Mitchell, Peter. France gets smart with health à la carte. [News]. *Lancet*. 1998 Mar 7; 351(9104): 736.
(CONFIDENTIALITY)

Mitchell, Peter. Shared decision–making poses problems for UK. [News]. *Lancet*. 1997 May 3; 349(9061): 1306.
(PROFESSIONAL PATIENT RELATIONSHIP)

Mitchinson, Wendy. Agency, diversity, and constraints: women and their physicians, Canada, 1850–1950. *In:* Sherwin, Susan, et al. The Politics of Women's Health: Exploring Agency and Autonomy. Philadelphia, PA: Temple University Press; 1998: 122–149.
(PROFESSIONAL PATIENT RELATIONSHIP; REPRODUCTION)

Mitchinson, Wendy. 'It's not society that's the problem, it's women's bodies': a historical view of medical treatment of women. *In:* Petersen, Kerry, ed. Intersections: Women on Law, Medicine and Technology. Brookfield, VT: Ashgate; 1997: 25–48.
(HEALTH)

Mitrius, Janice V. see **Davis, Helen R.**

Mittwoch, Ursula. This womb for hire? *New Scientist.* 1997 Jun 28; 154(2088): 46.
(SURROGATE MOTHERS)

Mitty, Ethel see **Mezey, Mathy**

Miura, Yasuhiko see **Asai, Atsushi**

Mnookin, Seth. Department of Defense DNA registry raises legal, ethical issues. *GeneWATCH.* 1996 Aug; 10(1): 1, 3, 11.
(DNA FINGERPRINTING)

Moffic, H. Steven. The Ethical Way: Challenges and Solutions for Managed Behavioral Healthcare. San Francisco, CA: Jossey-Bass; 1997. 234 p.
(HEALTH CARE/ECONOMICS; PATIENT CARE/MENTALLY DISABLED)

Mohler, R. Albert. The brave new world of cloning: a Christian worldview perspective. *In:* Cole-Turner, Ronald, ed. Human Cloning: Religious Responses. Louisville, KY: Westminister John Knox Press; 1997: 91–105.
(CLONING; EUGENICS)

Mohr, Wanda K. Ethics, nursing, and health care in the age of "re-form". *N and HC Perspectives on Community.* 1996 Jan–Feb; 17(1): 16–21.
(HEALTH CARE/ECONOMICS; NURSING ETHICS)

Mollica, Richard F. Human rights reflections in daily medical practice. [Editorial]. *Medical Journal of Australia.* 1996 Dec 2–16; 165(11–12): 594–595.
(FRAUD AND MISCONDUCT; PATIENT CARE)

Momeyer, Richard W. see **Savulescu, Julian**

Monaco, Grace Powers see **Burt, R.A.P.**

Monagle, John F.; Thomasma, David C., eds. Health Care Ethics: Critical Issues for the 21st Century. Gaithersburg, MD: Aspen Publishers; 1998. 614 p.
(BIOETHICS)

Mongoven, Ann. Federal hearings on liver transplant allocation and donation. *In:* BioLaw: A Legal and Ethical Reporter on Medicine, Health Care, and Bioengineering. Special Sections 2(12). Frederick, MD: University Publications of America; 1997 Dec: S:373–S:389.
(ORGAN AND TISSUE DONATION; ORGAN AND TISSUE TRANSPLANTATION; RESOURCE ALLOCATION/BIOMEDICAL TECHNOLOGIES; SELECTION FOR TREATMENT)

Monson, J.P. see **McFadzean, J.**

Montello, Martha. Narrative competence. *In:* Nelson, Hilde Lindemann, ed. Stories and Their Limits: Narrative Approaches to Bioethics. New York, NY: Routledge; 1997: 185–197.
(BIOETHICS; MEDICAL ETHICS)

Montgomery, Jonathan. Health care law and ethics: abortion; fertility; maternity care; selective treatment of the newborn; transplantation; terminal care and euthanasia. *In: his* Health Care Law. New York, NY: Oxford University Press; 1997: 357–456.
(ABORTION/FOREIGN COUNTRIES; ABORTION/LEGAL ASPECTS; ALLOWING TO DIE/LEGAL ASPECTS; ORGAN AND TISSUE DONATION; PATIENT CARE; REPRODUCTIVE TECHNOLOGIES)

Montgomery, Jonathan. The position of the patient: consent to treatment; confidentiality and access to health care records; care for children; mental health; research. *In: his* Health Care Law. New York, NY: Oxford University Press; 1997: 225–356.
(CONFIDENTIALITY/LEGAL ASPECTS; HUMAN EXPERIMENTATION/FOREIGN COUNTRIES; INFORMED CONSENT; INFORMED CONSENT/MENTALLY DISABLED; INFORMED CONSENT/MINORS)

Monti, Chantal LeGris see **de Wachter, Maurice A.M.**

Moodley, Prushini see **Bhagwanjee, Satish**

Moore, Andrew see **Wilkinson, Martin**

Moore, Dale; Popp, A. John; Katz, Katheryn D.; Kairys, David. Commentary I [and] Commentary II on "The law of clinical testing with human subjects," [and] Author's response. *In:* Kadane, Joseph B., ed. Bayesian Methods and Ethics in a Clinical Trial Design. New York, NY: Wiley; 1996: 251–266.
(HUMAN EXPERIMENTATION/RESEARCH DESIGN)

Moore, Francis D. see **Murray-Garcia, Jann**

Moore, Lisa Jean see **Hern, H. Eugene**

Moore, Sally see **Schick, Ida Critelli**

Moore, William P. see **Beisecker, Analee E.**

Mor, Vince see **Phillips, Charles D.**

Mor, Vincent see **Bernabei, Roberto**

Morain, William D. Patently unethical. [Editorial]. *Annals of Plastic Surgery.* 1996 Mar; 36(3): 334.
(BIOMEDICAL TECHNOLOGIES; HEALTH CARE/ECONOMICS)

Moran, Tracy see **Barnes, Donelle M.**

Mordacci, Roberto; Sobel, Richard. Health: a comprehensive concept. *Hastings Center Report.* 1998 Jan–Feb; 28(1): 34–37.
(HEALTH)

Mordacci, Roberto see **Maiorca, Rosario**

Moreland, Michael P. see **Paris, John J.**

Moreno, Jonathan D., ed. Arguing Euthanasia: The Controversy Over Mercy Killing, Assisted Suicide, and the "Right to Die." New York, NY: Simon and Schuster; 1995. 251 p.
(EUTHANASIA; SUICIDE)

Moreno, Jonathan D. Convenient and captive populations. *In:* Kahn, Jeffrey P.; Mastroianni, Anna C.; Sugarman, Jeremy, eds. Beyond Consent: Seeking Justice in Research. New York, NY: Oxford University Press;

1998: 111–130.
(HUMAN EXPERIMENTATION/SPECIAL POPULATIONS)

Moreno, Jonathan D. Reassessing the influence of the Nuremberg Code on American medical ethics. *Journal of Contemporary Health Law and Policy.* 1997 Spring; 13(2): 347–360.
(HUMAN EXPERIMENTATION)

Moreno, Jonathan D.; Caplan, Arthur L.; Wolpe, Paul Root. Informed consent. *In:* Chadwick, Ruth, ed. Encyclopedia of Applied Ethics, Volume 2. San Diego, CA: Academic Press; 1998: 687–697.
(INFORMED CONSENT)

Moreno, Jonathan D.; Hurt, Valerie. How the Atomic Energy Commission discovered "informed consent." *In:* DeVries, Raymond; Subedi, Janardan, eds. Bioethics and Society: Constructing the Ethical Enterprise. Upper Saddle River, NJ: Prentice Hall; 1998: 78–93.
(HUMAN EXPERIMENTATION/INFORMED CONSENT)

Moreno, Jonathan D.; Lucente, Frank E. Patients who are family members, friends, colleagues, family members of colleagues. *In:* McCullough, Laurence B.; Jones, James W.; Brody, Baruch A., eds. Surgical Ethics. New York, NY: Oxford University Press; 1998: 198–215.
(MEDICAL ETHICS; PROFESSIONAL PATIENT RELATIONSHIP)

Moretti, Anna. Advocating for the dying: the view of family and friends. *Bioethics Forum.* 1997 Summer; 13(2): 27–31.
(ALLOWING TO DIE)

Moretti, Anna see **Prip, William**

Morgan, Christopher see **Currie, Craig**

Morgan, Derek. Health rights, ethics and justice: the opportunity costs of rhetoric. *In:* McLean, Sheila A.M., ed. Contemporary Issues in Law, Medicine and Ethics. Brookfield, VT: Dartmouth; 1996: 15–27.
(HEALTH CARE/FOREIGN COUNTRIES; HEALTH CARE/RIGHTS; PATIENTS' RIGHTS; RESOURCE ALLOCATION)

Morgan, Kathryn Pauly. Contested bodies, contested knowledges: women, health, and the politics of medicalization. *In:* Sherwin, Susan, et al. The Politics of Women's Health: Exploring Agency and Autonomy. Philadelphia, PA: Temple University Press; 1998: 83–121.
(HEALTH; HEALTH CARE)

Morgan, Thomas R. see **Davison, B. Joyce**

Morgenlander, Keith H.; Greenwald, Devra E. Psychiatric DRGs: the legal and ethical impact. [Editorial]. *QRB/Quality Review Bulletin.* 1985 Jun; 11(6): 175–179.
(HEALTH CARE/ECONOMICS; PATIENT CARE/MENTALLY DISABLED)

Mori, Takahide. Egg donation should be limited to women below 60 years of age. *Journal of Assisted Reproduction and Genetics.* 1995 Apr; 12(4): 229–230.
(REPRODUCTIVE TECHNOLOGIES; SELECTION FOR TREATMENT)

Moring, Juha see **Latvala, Eila**

Morley, Colin; Shabde, Neela; Craft, Alan W. Concerns about using and interpreting covert video surveillance. [Article and commentary]. *BMJ (British Medical Journal).* 1998 May 23; 316(7144): 1603–1605.
(PATIENT CARE/MINORS)

Morone, James A. Enemies of the people: the moral dimension to public health. *Journal of Health Politics, Policy and Law.* 1997 Aug; 22(4): 993–1020.
(PUBLIC HEALTH)

Moros, Daniel A.; Rhodes, Rosamond. Putting universal healthcare on the religious agenda. [Editorial]. *Cambridge Quarterly of Healthcare Ethics.* 1998 Summer; 7(3): 233–234.
(HEALTH CARE/ECONOMICS)

Morreim, E. Haavi. At the intersection of medicine, law, economics, and ethics: bioethics and the art of intellectual cross-dressing. *In:* Carson, Ronald A.; Burns, Chester R., eds. Philosophy of Medicine and Bioethics: A Twenty-Year Retrospective and Critical Appraisal. Boston, MA: Kluwer Academic; 1997: 299–325.
(HEALTH CARE/ECONOMICS; PATIENT CARE; RESOURCE ALLOCATION)

Morreim, E. Haavi. Bioethics, expertise, and the courts: an overview and an argument for inevitability. *Journal of Medicine and Philosophy.* 1997 Aug; 22(4): 291–295.
(BIOETHICS; ETHICISTS AND ETHICS COMMITTEES)

Morreim, E. Haavi. Medicine's monopoly: from trust busting to trust. *In:* Minogue, Brendan P.; Palmer-Fernández, Gabriel; Reagan, James E., eds. Reading Engelhardt: Essays on the Thought of H. Tristram Engelhardt, Jr. Boston, MA: Kluwer Academic; 1997: 45–75.
(HEALTH CARE/ECONOMICS)

Morreim, E. Haavi. Revenue streams and clinical discretion. *Journal of the American Geriatrics Society.* 1998 Mar; 46(3): 331–337.
(HEALTH CARE/ECONOMICS; PROFESSIONAL PATIENT RELATIONSHIP)

Morreim, E. Haavi see **Mirvis, David M.**

Morris, David C. Older adults' perceptions of Dr. Kevorkian in Middletown, U.S.A. *Omega: A Journal of Death and Dying.* 1997; 35(4): 405–412.
(SUICIDE)

Morris, Jane see **Baskin, Shari A.**

Morris, Joan K. see **Templeton, Allan**

Morris, John N. see **Phillips, Charles D.**

Morris, Kelly. UK GMC finds lack of consent merits serious–misconduct judgment. [News]. *Lancet.* 1998 Mar 28; 351(9107): 966.
(FRAUD AND MISCONDUCT; INFORMED CONSENT/MINORS)

Morris, Kelly. UK misconduct case raises informed–consent issues. [News]. *Lancet.* 1998 Mar 21; 351(9106): 885.
(FRAUD AND MISCONDUCT; INFORMED CONSENT/MINORS)

Morris, Kelly see **Wehrwein, Peter**

Morris, Peter J. Pig transplants postponed: until we know

more about graft rejection, physiology, and infectivity. [Editorial]. *BMJ (British Medical Journal)*. 1997 Jan 25; 314(7076): 242.
(ORGAN AND TISSUE TRANSPLANTATION)

Morrison, James; Wickersham, Peter. Physicians disciplined by a state medical board. *JAMA.* 1998 Jun 17; 279(23): 1889–1893.
(FRAUD AND MISCONDUCT)

Morrison, Mary F.; DeMichele, Sarah Gelbach. How culture and religion affect attitudes toward medical futility. *In:* Zucker, Marjorie B.; Zucker Howard D., eds. Medical Futility and the Evaluation of Life–Sustaining Interventions. New York, NY: Cambridge University Press; 1997: 71–84.
(ALLOWING TO DIE/RELIGIOUS ASPECTS; DETERMINATION OF DEATH)

Morrison, R. Sean; Zayas, Luis H.; Mulvihill, Michael; Baskin, Shari A.; Meier, Diane E. Barriers to completion of healthcare proxy forms: a qualitative analysis of ethnic differences. *Journal of Clinical Ethics.* 1998 Summer; 9(2): 118–126.
(ADVANCE DIRECTIVES)

Morrison, R. Sean see **Baskin, Shari A.**

Morrison, R. Sean see **Hendin, Herbert**

Morrison, R. Sean see **Meier, Diane E.**

Morrison, R. Sean see **White, W.D.**

Morrissey, James M. Informed consent: the New York approach. *New York State Journal of Medicine.* 1985 May; 85(5): 210–213.
(INFORMED CONSENT)

Morrissey, John see **Stadler, Holly A.**

Morrow, Elizabeth. Attitudes of women from vulnerable populations toward physician–assisted death: a qualitative approach. *Journal of Clinical Ethics.* 1997 Fall; 8(3): 279–289.
(EUTHANASIA/ATTITUDES; SUICIDE)

Morse, Diane S. see **Epstein, Ronald M.**

Morton, David. A comparison of the controls regarding the ethical judgements on animal and human research. *In:* Close, Bryony; Combes, Robert; Hubbard, Anthony; Illingworth, John, eds. Volunteers in Research and Testing. Bristol, PA: Taylor and Francis; 1997: 109–116.
(ANIMAL EXPERIMENTATION)

Morton, David B. Advances in refinement in animal experimentation over the past 25 years. *ATLA: Alternatives to Laboratory Animals.* 1995 Nov–Dec; 23(6): 812–822.
(ANIMAL EXPERIMENTATION)

Morton, David B. see **Balls, Michael**

Morton, David B. see **Orlans, F. Barbara**

Morton, Kelly R. see **Orr, Robert D.**

Morton, Oliver; Williams, Nigel. First Dolly, now headless tadpoles. [News]. *Science.* 1997 Oct 31; 278(5339): 798.

(CLONING)

Moseley, Kathryn L.; Truesdell, Sandra. A noncompliant patient? [Case study]. *Journal of Clinical Ethics.* 1997 Summer; 8(2): 176–177.
(PROFESSIONAL PATIENT RELATIONSHIP; TREATMENT REFUSAL)

Mosenkis, Ari. Genetic screening for breast cancer susceptibility: a Torah perspective. *Journal of Halacha and Contemporary Society.* 1997 Fall; No. 34: 5–26.
(GENETIC SCREENING; MASS SCREENING)

Mosher, Janet see **Bell, Marilynne**

Moskop, John C.; Smith, Michael L.; De Ville, Kenneth. Ethical and legal aspects of teratogenic medications: the case of isotretinoin. *Journal of Clinical Ethics.* 1997 Fall; 8(3): 264–278.
(PATIENT CARE/DRUGS; PRENATAL INJURIES; WRONGFUL LIFE)

Moskowitz, Ellen see **Boyle, Philip J.**

Moskowitz, Ellen H. Can government ever protect fetuses from substance abuse? *Politics and the Life Sciences.* 1996 Mar; 15(1): 61–63.
(INVOLUNTARY COMMITMENT; PRENATAL INJURIES)

Moskowitz, Ellen H. Clinical responsibility and legal liability in managed care. *Journal of the American Geriatrics Society.* 1998 Mar; 46(3): 373–377.
(HEALTH CARE/ECONOMICS)

Motulsky, Arno G. see **Spiegler, Gerard E.**

Moulton, Jeffrey see **Slome, Lee**

Mount, Balfour. Morphine drips, terminal sedation, and slow euthanasia: definitions and facts, not anecdotes. [Commentary]. *Journal of Palliative Care.* 1996 Winter; 12(4): 31–37.
(EUTHANASIA; TERMINAL CARE)

Moutel, G.; Leroux, N.; Hervé, C. Analysis of a survey of 36 French research committees on intracytoplasmic sperm injection. *Lancet.* 1998 Apr 11; 351(9109): 1121–1123.
(HUMAN EXPERIMENTATION/ETHICS COMMITTEES; HUMAN EXPERIMENTATION/FOREIGN COUNTRIES; REPRODUCTIVE TECHNOLOGIES)

Mowbray, Carol T.; Freddolino, Paul P.; Rhodes, Genice L.; Greenfield, Arnold L. Evaluation of a patient rights protection system: public policy implications. *Administration in Mental Health.* 1985 Summer; 12(4): 264–283.
(PATIENTS' RIGHTS/MENTALLY DISABLED)

Muckart, David J.J. see **Bhagwanjee, Satish**

Mudur, Ganapati. Ban on payment to donors causes blood shortage in India. [News]. *BMJ (British Medical Journal).* 1998 Jan 17; 316(7126): 172.
(BLOOD DONATION)

Mudur, Ganapati. India to ban female sterilisation with malaria drug. [News]. *BMJ (British Medical Journal).* 1998 Mar 28; 316(7136): 958.
(STERILIZATION)

Mudur, Ganapati. India to control foreign research

involving Indian patients. [News]. *BMJ (British Medical Journal).* 1997 Jan 18; 314(7075): 165.
(HUMAN EXPERIMENTATION/FOREIGN COUNTRIES; HUMAN EXPERIMENTATION/REGULATION)

Mudur, Ganapati. Indian study of women with cervical lesions called unethical. [News]. *BMJ (British Medical Journal).* 1997 Apr 12; 314(7087): 1065.
(FRAUD AND MISCONDUCT; HUMAN EXPERIMENTATION/FOREIGN COUNTRIES; HUMAN EXPERIMENTATION/INFORMED CONSENT; HUMAN EXPERIMENTATION/SPECIAL POPULATIONS)

Muehleman, Thomas; Pickens, Bruce K.; Robinson, Franklin. Informing clients about the limits to confidentiality, risks, and their rights: is self–disclosure inhibited? *Professional Psychology: Research and Practice.* 1985 Jun; 16(3): 385–397.
(CONFIDENTIALITY/MENTAL HEALTH; INFORMED CONSENT/MENTALLY DISABLED)

Mueller, Bryan see **Degner, Lesley F.**

Muir, J. Cameron see **Paris, John J.**

Mulhauser, Lynda C. see **Allen, Jill S. Fonda**

Mulkay, Michael. The Embryo Research Debate: Science and the Politics of Reproduction. New York, NY: Cambridge University Press; 1997. 212 p.
(EMBRYO AND FETAL RESEARCH)

Müller–Hill, Benno see **Deichmann, Ute**

Muller, M.T.; Onwuteaka–Philipsen, B.D.; Kriegsman, D.M.W.; van der Wal, G. Voluntary active euthanasia and doctor–assisted suicide: knowledge and attitudes of Dutch medical students. *Medical Education.* 1996 Nov; 30(6): 428–433.
(EUTHANASIA/ATTITUDES; SUICIDE)

Muller, Martien T.; van der Wal, Gerrit; van Eijk, Jacques Th.M.; Ribbe, Miel W. Active euthanasia and physician–assisted suicide in Dutch nursing homes: patients' characteristics. *Age and Ageing.* 1995 Sep; 24(5): 429–433.
(EUTHANASIA; SUICIDE)

Muller, Martien T. see **Onwuteaka–Philipsen, Bregje D.**

Multiple Organ Retrieval and Exchange (M.O.R.E.) Program of Ontario. Task Force on Presumed Consent [and] Board of Directors. Organ Procurement Strategies: A Review of the Ethical Issues and Challenges. [Report]. Toronto, ON: Multiple Organ Retrieval and Exchange (M.O.R.E.) Program of Ontario; 1994 Nov. 31 p.
(INFORMED CONSENT; ORGAN AND TISSUE DONATION)

Mulvihill, Michael see **Morrison, R. Sean**

Munetz, Mark R.; Roth, Loren H. Informing patients about tardive dyskinesia. *Archives of Internal Medicine.* 1985 Sep; 42(9): 866–871.
(INFORMED CONSENT/MENTALLY DISABLED; PATIENT CARE/DRUGS)

Murakami, Masayoshi see **Hagihara, Akihito**

Muram, David; Aiken, Margaret M.; Strong, Carson. Children's refusal of gynecologic examinations for suspected sexual abuse. *Journal of Clinical Ethics.* 1997 Summer; 8(2): 158–164.
(TREATMENT REFUSAL/MINORS)

Muramoto, Osamu. Medical ethics in the treatment of Jehovah's Witnesses. [Letter]. *Archives of Internal Medicine.* 1998 May 25; 158(10): 1155–1156.
(TREATMENT REFUSAL)

Murashige, Kate H. Genome research and traditional intellectual property protection –– a bad fit? *Risk: Health, Safety and Environment.* 1996 Summer; 7(3): 231–238.
(GENETIC RESEARCH)

Murch, Randall S.; Budowle, Bruce. Are developments in forensic applications of DNA technology consistent with privacy protections? *In:* Rothstein, Mark A., ed. Genetic Secrets: Protecting Privacy and Confidentiality in the Genetic Era. New Haven, CT: Yale University Press; 1997: 212–230.
(DNA FINGERPRINTING)

Murden, Robert A. see **Beisecker, Analee E.**

Murdoch, Ian see **Brawn, W.J.**

Murphy, Denis. Ireland faces a "first". *Human Life Review.* 1997 Spring; 23(2): 45–52.
(ABORTION/FOREIGN COUNTRIES)

Murphy, Donald J. The economics of futile interventions. *In:* Zucker, Marjorie B.; Zucker, Howard D., eds. Medical Futility and the Evaluation of Life–Sustaining Interventions. New York, NY: Cambridge University Press; 1997: 123–135.
(HEALTH CARE/ECONOMICS; RESOURCE ALLOCATION/BIOMEDICAL TECHNOLOGIES; SELECTION FOR TREATMENT; TERMINAL CARE)

Murphy, Donald J. see **Hilberman, Mark**

Murphy, Donald P. see **Teno, Joan**

Murphy, Donald P. see **Teno, Joan M.**

Murphy, Elizabeth see **Jones, Roger**

Murphy, G. Don; Schenkenberg, Tom; Hunter, Jeff S.; Battin, Margaret P. Advance directives: a computer assisted approach to assuring patients' rights and compliance with PSDA (Patient Self–Determination Act) and JCAHO standards. *HEC (HealthCare Ethics Committee) Forum.* 1997 Sep; 9(3): 247–255.
(ADVANCE DIRECTIVES)

Murphy, James J. see **Paris, John J.**

Murphy, Patricia. Nursing's role in the assisted suicide debate. [Editorial]. *American Journal of Nursing.* 1997 Jun; 97(6): 80.
(SUICIDE)

Murphy, Patricia D. see **Holtzman, Neil A.**

Murphy, Peter J. see **DeGroot, Leslie J.**

Murphy, Timothy F. AIDS. *In:* Chadwick, Ruth, ed. Encyclopedia of Applied Ethics, Volume 1. San Diego, CA: Academic Press; 1998: 111–122.
(AIDS)

Murphy, Timothy F. Gay Science: The Ethics of Sexual Orientation Research. New York, NY: Columbia University Press; 1997. 268 p.
(BEHAVIORAL GENETICS; BEHAVIORAL RESEARCH/SPECIAL POPULATIONS)

Murray, Clare see **Cook, Rachel**

Murray, David M. see **Elliott, Thomas E.**

Murray–Garcia, Jann; Vietzke, Wesley M.; Wittkopp, George F.; Yarmolinsky, Adam; Moore, Francis D.; Emanuel, Linda. Professionalism vs commercialism in managed care: the need for a National Council on Medical Care. [Letters and responses]. *JAMA.* 1997 Jul 2; 278(1): 20–22.
(HEALTH CARE/ECONOMICS)

Murray, Thomas see **Kodish, Eric**

Murray, Thomas H. Genetic exceptionalism and "future diaries": is genetic information different from other medical information? *In:* Rothstein, Mark A., ed. Genetic Secrets: Protecting Privacy and Confidentiality in the Genetic Era. New Haven, CT: Yale University Press; 1997: 60–73.
(GENETIC SCREENING)

Murray, Thomas H. Genetic screening in the workplace: ethical issues. *Journal of Occupational Medicine.* 1983 Jun; 25(6): 451–454.
(GENETIC SCREENING; OCCUPATIONAL HEALTH)

Murray, Thomas H. What do we mean by "narrative ethics"? *In:* Nelson, Hilde Lindemann, ed. Stories and Their Limits: Narrative Approaches to Bioethics. New York, NY: Routledge; 1997: 3–17.
(BIOETHICS)

Murrell, Trevor see **Grubb, Andrew**

Murton, F. see **Hallowell, N.**

Musa, Donald see **Silverman, Myrna**

Muscari, Mary E. When can an adolescent give consent? *American Journal of Nursing.* 1998 May; 98(5): 18–19.
(INFORMED CONSENT/MINORS)

Muskin, Philip R. Care, support, and concern for noncompliant patients. *Journal of Clinical Ethics.* 1997 Summer; 8(2): 178–180.
(PROFESSIONAL PATIENT RELATIONSHIP; TREATMENT REFUSAL)

Muskin, Philip R. The request to die: role for a psychodynamic perspective on physician–assisted suicide. *JAMA.* 1998 Jan 28; 279(4): 323–328.
(SUICIDE)

Mustafa, M.J. Railey see **Kazim, E.**

Mustard, Cameron A.; Kaufert, Patricia; Kozyrskyj, Anita; Mayer, Teresa. Sex differences in the use of health care services. *New England Journal of Medicine.* 1998 Jun 4; 338(23): 1678–1683.
(HEALTH CARE/ECONOMICS; HEALTH CARE/FOREIGN COUNTRIES)

Mutka, Riitta see **Töyry, Eeva**

Muyskens, James. Should receiving depend upon willingness to give? *Transplantation Proceedings.* 1992 Oct; 24(5): 2181–2184.
(ORGAN AND TISSUE DONATION; ORGAN AND TISSUE TRANSPLANTATION; SELECTION FOR TREATMENT)

N

Naber, D.; Kircher, T.; Hessel, K. Schizophrenic patients' retrospective attitudes regarding involuntary psychopharmacological treatment and restraint. *European Psychiatry.* 1996; 11(1): 7–11.
(PATIENT CARE/DRUGS; PATIENT CARE/MENTALLY DISABLED; TREATMENT REFUSAL/MENTALLY DISABLED)

Nagel, Thomas see **Dworkin, Ronald**

Najman, J. see **Steinberg, M.A.**

Najman, J.M. see **Steinberg, M.A.**

Najman, Jake see **Cartwright, Colleen**

Nakata, Kazumi see **Asai, Atsushi**

Nakchbandi, Inaam A.; Longenecker, J. Craig; Ricksecker, M. Ann; Latta, Richard A.; Healton, Cheryl; Smith, David G. A decision analysis of mandatory compared with voluntary HIV testing in pregnant women. *Annals of Internal Medicine.* 1998 May 1; 128(9): 760–767.
(AIDS/TESTING AND SCREENING)

Namihira, Emiko. The characteristics of Japanese concepts and attitudes with regard to human remains. *In:* Hoshino, Kazumasa, ed. Japanese and Western Bioethics: Studies in Moral Diversity. Boston, MA: Kluwer Academic; 1997: 61–69.
(PERSONHOOD)

Napper, Stan A.; Hale, Paul N. Teaching of ethics in biomedical engineering. *IEEE Engineering in Medicine and Biology Magazine.* 1993 Dec; 12(4): 100–105.
(BIOMEDICAL TECHNOLOGIES)

Naqvi, Ali Anwar. Ethical issues in renal transplantation in developing countries. [Editorial]. *JPMA: Journal of the Pakistan Medical Association.* 1995 Sep; 45(9): 233–234.
(ORGAN AND TISSUE DONATION)

Narasimhan, Parthas; Kalra, Jagmohan; Warde, Padraig; Gospodarowicz, Mary. Ethical questions on the testicular seminoma study. [Letter and response]. *Journal of Clinical Oncology.* 1996 Feb; 14(2): 684.
(HUMAN EXPERIMENTATION/RESEARCH DESIGN)

Nash, Jean E. see **Botkin, Jeffrey R.**

Nassiry, Ladan see **Bernard, Claire**

Nathanson, Vivienne. Humanitarian action: the duty of all doctors. [Editorial]. *BMJ (British Medical Journal).* 1997 Nov 29; 315(7120): 1389–1390.
(MEDICAL ETHICS)

National Childbirth Trust (Great Britain) see **Association for Improvements in the Maternity Services (Great Britain)**

National Council for Hospice and Specialist Palliative

Care Services. Voluntary euthanasia: the Council's view. *Nursing Ethics.* 1998 Jul; 5(4): 371–374.
(EUTHANASIA; TERMINAL CARE)

National Kidney Foundation. Implementing Advance Directives: Suggested Guidelines for Dialysis Facilities. [Pamphlet]. New York, NY: National Kidney Foundation; 1993 Dec. 16 p.
(ADVANCE DIRECTIVES)

National Legal Center for the Medically Dependent and Disabled, Inc. Amicus Curiae Brief of the Ethics and Advocacy Task Force of the Nursing Home Action Group in Support of the Commonwealth of Pennsylvania, Attorney General, in re: Daniel Joseph Fiori, an Adjudged Incompetent, No. 0006 E.D. Appeal Docket 1995. Filed in the Supreme Court of Pennsylvania; 1995 Mar 16. 42 p.
(ALLOWING TO DIE/LEGAL ASPECTS)

National Rehabilitation Association see **American Association on Mental Deficiency**

National Research Council. Committee on Human Genome Diversity. Human rights and human genetic-variation research. *In: its* Evaluating Human Genetic Diversity. Washington, DC: National Academy Press; 1997: 55–68.
(GENETIC RESEARCH)

National Research Council. Committee on Maintaining Privacy and Security in Health Care Applications of the National Information Infrastructure. For the Record: Protecting Electronic Health Information. Washington, DC: National Academy Press; 1997. 264 p.
(CONFIDENTIALITY)

National Science Teachers Association. Code of Practice on Use of Animals in Schools. [Position statement]. Issued by the National Science Teachers Association, 1742 Connecticut Avenue, N.W., Washington, DC 20009; 1985 Jul. 2 p.
(ANIMAL EXPERIMENTATION)

Natowicz, Marvin R.; Ard, Catherine. The commercialization of clinical genetics: an analysis of interrelations between academic centers and for-profit clinical genetics diagnostics companies. *Journal of Genetic Counseling.* 1997 Sep; 6(3): 337–355.
(GENETIC SCREENING; GENETIC SERVICES)

Naumburg, Elizabeth H. see **Franks, Peter**

Neel, James V. Looking ahead: some genetic issues of the future. *Perspectives in Biology and Medicine.* 1997 Spring; 40(3): 328–347.
(GENETIC RESEARCH; POPULATION CONTROL)

Neeleman, J.; van Os, J. Ethical issues in European psychiatry. *European Psychiatry.* 1996; 11(1): 1–6.
(MEDICAL ETHICS)

Neeley, G. Steven. Legal and ethical dilemmas surrounding prayer as a method of alternative healing for children. *In:* Humber, James M.; Almeder, Robert F., eds. Alternative Medicine and Ethics. Totowa, NJ: Humana Press; 1998: 163–194.
(TREATMENT REFUSAL/MINORS)

Neff–Smith, Martha; Giles, Scott; Spencer, Edward M.; Fletcher, John C. Ethics program evaluation: the Virginia Hospital Ethics Fellows example. *HEC (HealthCare Ethics Committee) Forum.* 1997 Dec; 9(4): 375–388.
(BIOETHICS/EDUCATION; ETHICISTS AND ETHICS COMMITTEES)

Nelkin, Dorothy. Genetics, God, and sacred DNA. *Society.* 1996 May–Jun; 33(4): 22–25.
(GENETIC INTERVENTION)

Nelkin, Dorothy; Lindee, M. Susan. Cloning in the popular imagination. *Cambridge Quarterly of Healthcare Ethics.* 1998 Spring; 7(2): 145–149.
(CLONING)

Nelkin, Dorothy; Lindee, M. Susan. "Genes made me do it": the appeal of biological explanations. *Politics and the Life Sciences.* 1996 Mar; 15(1): 95–97.
(BEHAVIORAL GENETICS)

Nelkin, Dorothy see **Andrews, Lori**

Nelmig, Linda see **Beisecker, Analee E.**

Nelson, Christine A. see **Tilden, Virginia P.**

Nelson, Hilde see **Foglio, John**

Nelson, Hilde Lindemann, ed. Stories and Their Limits: Narrative Approaches to Bioethics. New York, NY: Routledge; 1997. 284 p.
(BIOETHICS)

Nelson, J. Robert see **Sechriest, Kay**

Nelson, James Lindemann. Reasons and feelings, duty and dementia. *Journal of Clinical Ethics.* 1998 Spring; 9(1): 58–65.
(PATIENT CARE/MENTALLY DISABLED)

Nelson, James Lindemann. The meaning of the act: reflections on the expressive force of reproductive decision making and policies. *Kennedy Institute of Ethics Journal.* 1998 June; 8(2): 165–182.
(ABORTION; PRENATAL DIAGNOSIS)

Nelson, Kenrad E. see **Robb, Merlin L.**

Nelson, Lawrence J. Editor's introduction [conscience]. *HEC (HealthCare Ethics Committee) Forum.* 1998 Mar; 10(1): 2–8.
(ETHICISTS AND ETHICS COMMITTEES)

Nelson, Paul. Bioethics and the Lutheran Communion. *In:* Lustig, B. Andrew, ed.; Center for Medical Ethics and Health Policy (Houston, TX). Bioethics Yearbook, Volume 5: Theological Developments in Bioethics, 1992–1994. Boston, MA: Kluwer Academic; 1997: 143–169.
(BIOETHICS)

Nelson, Robert M. Children as research subjects. *In:* Kahn, Jeffrey P.; Mastroianni, Anna C.; Sugarman, Jeremy, eds. Beyond Consent: Seeking Justice in Research. New York, NY: Oxford University Press; 1998: 47–66.
(HUMAN EXPERIMENTATION/MINORS)

Nelson, William A.; Wlody, Ginger Schafer. The

evolving role of ethics advisory committees in VHA. *HEC (HealthCare Ethics Committee) Forum.* 1997 Jun; 9(2): 129–146.
(ETHICISTS AND ETHICS COMMITTEES)

Nelson, William A. see **Reagan, James E.**

Nemes, Joanne M. see **Lenke, Roger R.**

Nennstiel, Marianne E. see **Phillips, Charles D.**

Neri, Demetrio. Eugenics. *In:* Chadwick, Ruth, ed. Encyclopedia of Applied Ethics, Volume 2. San Diego, CA: Academic Press; 1998: 161–173.
(EUGENICS; GENETIC INTERVENTION)

Nespoli, Luigi see **Burgio, Giuseppe Roberto**

Netherlands. Law of 17 November 1994 (Stb. 837) amending the Civil Code and certain other laws in connection with the adoption of provisions concerning the agreement to carry out procedures in the field of medicine. *International Digest of Health Legislation.* 1995; 46(2): 196–199.
(INFORMED CONSENT)

Netherlands. Health Council. Standing Committee on Medical Ethics and Health Law. Sex Selection for Non–Medical Reasons. Report of a Committee of the Health Council of the Netherlands. The Hague: Health Council of the Netherlands; 1995. 48 p.
(SEX DETERMINATION; SEX PRESELECTION)

Neuberger, James; Adams, David; MacMaster, Paul; Maidment, Anita; Speed, Mark. Assessing priorities for allocation of donor liver grafts: survey of public and clinicians. *BMJ (British Medical Journal).* 1998 Jul 18; 317(7152): 172–175.
(ORGAN AND TISSUE TRANSPLANTATION; RESOURCE ALLOCATION/BIOMEDICAL TECHNOLOGIES; SELECTION FOR TREATMENT)

Neuberger, James; Lake, John. Allocating donor livers. [Editorial]. *BMJ (British Medical Journal).* 1997 Apr 19; 314(7088): 1140–1141.
(ORGAN AND TISSUE TRANSPLANTATION; RESOURCE ALLOCATION/BIOMEDICAL TECHNOLOGIES; SELECTION FOR TREATMENT)

Neuberger, Julia. Death on camera. [Medicine and the media]. *BMJ (British Medical Journal).* 1998 Apr 4; 316(7137): 1100.
(TERMINAL CARE)

Neufeld–Kaiser, Whitney A. see **McKinnon, Wendy C.**

Neuhauser, Duncan see **Finkelstein, Beth S.**

Neuhauser, Duncan see **Mehlman, Maxwell J.**

Neumann, Peter J. Should health insurance cover IVF? Issues and options. *Journal of Health Politics, Policy and Law.* 1997 Oct; 22(5): 1215–1239.
(HEALTH CARE/ECONOMICS; IN VITRO FERTILIZATION; RESOURCE ALLOCATION/BIOMEDICAL TECHNOLOGIES)

New, Bill; Le Grand, Julian. Rationing in the NHS: Principles and Pragmatism. London: King's Fund Publishing; 1996. 77 p.
(HEALTH CARE/FOREIGN COUNTRIES; RESOURCE ALLOCATION)

New Hampshire. Surrogacy. *New Hampshire Revised Statutes Annotated.* 1995 Nov 1 (date effective). Sects. 168–13:1 to 168–13:31. 18 p.
(SURROGATE MOTHERS)

New Jersey. Superior Court, Appellate Division. Safer v. Estate of Pack. *Atlantic Reporter, 2d Series.* 1996 Jul 11 (date of decision). 677: 1188–1193.
(GENETIC COUNSELING)

New York. Health care agents and proxies. *McKinney's Consolidated Laws of New York Annotated.* 1994 Mar 28 (date effective). Sects. 2980 to 2992. 26 p.
(ADVANCE DIRECTIVES)

New York Academy of Medicine see **Barondess, Jeremiah A.**

New York. Court of Appeals. North Shore University Hospital v. Rosa. *North Eastern Reporter, 2d Series.* 1995 Oct 24 (date of decision). 657: 483–486.
(AIDS)

New York State Task Force on Life and the Law. Assisted Reproductive Technologies: Analysis and Recommendations for Public Policy. New York, NY: The Task Force; 1998 Apr. 474 p.
(REPRODUCTIVE TECHNOLOGIES)

New York. Supreme Court, Appellate Division, Second Department. Hecht v. Kaplan. *New York Supplement, 2d Series.* 1996 Jun 17 (date of decision). 645: 51–54.
(INFORMED CONSENT)

New York. Supreme Court, Queens County. In re Long Island Jewish Medical Center. *New York Supplement, 2d Series.* 1996 Feb 28 (date of decision). 641: 989–992.
(ALLOWING TO DIE/INFANTS; DETERMINATION OF DEATH/BRAIN DEATH)

New York. Supreme Court, Queens County. Grand Jury. DNR Procedures: Purple Dots Revisited. Report of the Special January Third Additional 1983 Grand Jury Concerning "Do Not Resuscitate" Procedures at a Certain Hospital in Queens County. *Connecticut Medicine.* 1985 Jun; 49(6): 367–376.
(RESUSCITATION ORDERS)

Newman, Joel D. Ethics committee offers criteria. *UNOS Update.* 1997 Jan–Feb: 8.
(ORGAN AND TISSUE TRANSPLANTATION; SELECTION FOR TREATMENT)

Newman, Lucile F. Framing the ethical issues in new reproductive technologies. *Health Care for Women International.* 1987; 8(4): 287–292.
(REPRODUCTIVE TECHNOLOGIES)

Newman, Stephen A. Human cloning and the family: reflections on cloning existing children. *New York Law School Journal of Human Rights.* 1997 Spring; 13(3): 523–530.
(CLONING)

Ng, P. see **Taylor, K.M.**

Nicholas, Barbara; Gillett, Grant. Doctors' stories, patients' stories: a narrative approach to teaching medical ethics. *Journal of Medical Ethics.* 1997 Oct; 23(5): 295–299.
(MEDICAL ETHICS/EDUCATION)

Nicholas, Richard A. see Westfall, John M.

Nicholas, Richard A. see Wolf, Bruce L.

Nichols, Rhea see Braun, Kathryn L.

Nicholson, Richard. The greater the ignorance, the greater the dogmatism. *Hastings Center Report.* 1998 May–Jun; 28(3): 4.
(INFORMED CONSENT/MINORS)

Nicholson, Richard see Alderson, Priscilla

Nicholson, Richard H. Seeking harmony in discord. [News]. *Hastings Center Report.* 1998 Jan–Feb; 28(1): 7.
(HUMAN EXPERIMENTATION/ETHICS COMMITTEES; HUMAN EXPERIMENTATION/FOREIGN COUNTRIES)

Nichter, Mark see Ventres, William

Nicklin, David see Love, Susan M.

Nielsen, V.G. see Rasmussen, P. Elmegaard

Nieri, Deborah see McGuire, John

Niermeijer, M.F. see DudokdeWit, A.C.

Niermeijer, M.F. see Tibben, A.

Nightingale, Charles see Philipson, Sandra J.

Nightingale, Stuart L. New [FDA] rules require financial disclosure. [News]. *JAMA.* 1998 Apr 1; 279(13): 984.
(HEALTH CARE/ECONOMICS; HUMAN EXPERIMENTATION/REGULATION)

NIH–DOE Working Group on Ethical, Legal, and Social Implications of Human Genome Research. Task Force on Genetic Testing. Interim Principles. Issued by the Task Force, 550 N. Broadway, Suite 511, Baltimore, MD 21205; 1997 Mar 11. 42 p.
(GENETIC SCREENING; GENETIC SERVICES)

Nikku, Nina; Eriksson, Bengt Erik. Preventive medicine. *In:* Chadwick, Ruth, ed. Encyclopedia of Applied Ethics, Volume 3. San Diego, CA: Academic Press; 1998: 643–648.
(HEALTH CARE; PUBLIC HEALTH)

Niklasson, Aimon see Wennerholm, Ulla–Britt

Nilges, Richard G. see Byrne, Paul A.

Nilsson, Lars see Wennerholm, Ulla–Britt

Nilstun, Tore; Ohlsson, Rolf. Should health care be rationed by age? *Scandinavian Journal of Social Medicine.* 1995 Jun; 23(2): 81–84.
(HEALTH CARE; RESOURCE ALLOCATION; SELECTION FOR TREATMENT)

Nippert, Irmgard see Cohen, Pamela E.

Nisand, I.; Shenfield, F. Multiple pregnancies and embryo reduction: ethical and legal issues. *In:* Shenfield, F.; Sureau, C., eds. Ethical Dilemmas in Assisted Reproduction. New York, NY: Parthenon Pub. Group; 1997: 67–75.
(ABORTION)

Nisker, J.A.; Jones, M. The ethics of sex selection. *In:* Shenfield, F.; Sureau, C., eds. Ethical Dilemmas in Assisted Reproduction. New York, NY: Parthenon Pub. Group; 1997: 41–50.
(SEX DETERMINATION)

Nisker, Jeffrey A. In quest of the perfect analogy for using in vitro fertilization patients as oocyte donors. *Women's Health Issues.* 1997 Jul–Aug; 7(4): 241–247.
(REPRODUCTIVE TECHNOLOGIES)

Njikam Savage, Olayinka Margaret. Secrecy still the best policy: donor insemination in Cameroon. *Politics and the Life Sciences.* 1995 Feb; 14(1): 87–88.
(ARTIFICIAL INSEMINATION; CONFIDENTIALITY)

Noble, Denis; Vincent, Jean–Didier. The Ethics of Life. Paris: Unesco; 1997. 238 p.
(ANIMAL EXPERIMENTATION; BIOETHICS; BIOMEDICAL RESEARCH)

Nobutomo, Koichi see Hagihara, Akihito

Nolan, Mike see Behi, Ruhi

Noll, John O.; Haugan, Mark L. Informed consent to psychotherapy: current practices at university–affiliated psychology training clinics. *Law and Psychology Review.* 1985 Spring; 9: 57–66.
(INFORMED CONSENT/MENTALLY DISABLED)

Noonpakdee, Wilai T. see Deepandung, Attajinda

NOP Consumer Market Research. Euthanasia (Fieldwork: 31 March–5 April 1993): A Report Produced for [the] Voluntary Euthanasia Society. Issued by NOP [National Opinion Poll] Consumer Market Research, London; 1993 Apr. 13 p.
(EUTHANASIA/ATTITUDES; EUTHANASIA/LEGAL ASPECTS)

Norberg, Astrid see Udén, Giggi

Norberg, Siv see Udén, Giggi

Nordgren, Anders. Ethics and imagination: implications of cognitive semantics for medical ethics. *Theoretical Medicine and Bioethics.* 1998 Apr; 19(2): 117–141.
(BIOETHICS)

Nordin, Conny see Lützén, Kim

Nørgaard–Pederson, Bent. Use of stored samples from the Danish PKU register. *In:* Knoppers, Bartha Maria, ed. Human DNA: Law and Policy: International and Comparative Perspectives. Proceedings of the First International Conference on DNA Sampling and Human Genetic Research: Ethical, Legal, and Policy Aspects, held in Montreal, Canada, 6–8 Sep 1996. Boston, MA: Kluwer Law International; 1997: 303–311.
(GENETIC RESEARCH; GENETIC SCREENING)

Norris, John W. see Alexandrov, Andrei V.

Norris, Patrick F. Palliative care and killing: understanding ethical distinctions. *Bioethics Forum.* 1997 Fall; 13(3): 25–30.
(ALLOWING TO DIE; EUTHANASIA; SUICIDE; TERMINAL CARE)

Norton, Peter G. see Ferris, Lorraine E.

Nortvedt, Per. Sensitive judgement: an inquiry into the foundations of nursing ethics. *Nursing Ethics.* 1998 Sep; 5(5): 385–392.
(NURSING ETHICS; PROFESSIONAL PATIENT RELATIONSHIP)

Norup, Michael. Attitudes towards abortion in the Danish population. *Bioethics.* 1997 Oct; 11(5): 439–449.
(ABORTION/ATTITUDES; ABORTION/FOREIGN COUNTRIES)

Norup, Michael. Limits of neonatal treatment: a survey of attitudes in the Danish population. *Journal of Medical Ethics.* 1998 Jun; 24(3): 200–206.
(ALLOWING TO DIE/INFANTS)

Novack, Dennis H. see **Farber, Neil J.**

Nowakowski, Loretta H. Confidentiality and customary practices. *Journal of Professional Nursing.* 1985 Mar–Apr; 1(2): 86–89.
(CONFIDENTIALITY)

Nozick, Robert see **Dworkin, Ronald**

Nundy, S. see **Hoffenberg, R.**

Nutton, Vivian. What's in an oath? *Journal of the Royal College of Physicians of London.* 1995 Nov–Dec; 29(6): 518–524.
(MEDICAL ETHICS/CODES OF ETHICS)

Nylenna, Magne. Details of patients' consent in studies should be reported. [Letter]. *BMJ (British Medical Journal).* 1997 Apr 12; 314(7087): 1127–1128.
(HUMAN EXPERIMENTATION/INFORMED CONSENT)

Nyman, Deborah J.; Sprung, Charles L. International perspectives on ethics in critical care. *Critical Care Clinics.* 1997 Apr; 13(2): 409–415.
(BIOMEDICAL TECHNOLOGIES; PATIENT CARE)

Nyrhinen, Tarja see **Leino–Kilpi, Helena**

O

Oberman, Michelle. Response to "Discontinuing life support in an infant of a drug addicted mother: whose decision is it?" by Renu Jain and David C. Thomasma. *Cambridge Quarterly of Healthcare Ethics.* 1997 Spring; 6(2): 235–239.
(ALLOWING TO DIE/INFANTS)

Oberman, Michelle. Women, fetuses, physicians, and the state: pregnancy and medical ethics in the 21st century. *In:* Monagle, John F.; Thomasma, David C., eds. Health Care Ethics: Critical Issues for the 21st Century. Gaithersburg, MD: Aspen Publishers; 1998: 67–78.
(PRENATAL INJURIES; TREATMENT REFUSAL)

Obernberger, Scott. When love and abuse are not mutually exclusive: the need for government intervention. *Issues in Law and Medicine.* 1997 Spring; 12(4): 355–381.
(TREATMENT REFUSAL/MINORS)

Obispo, E. see **Mendez, R.**

O'Brien, L.M. see **Parkins, K.J.**

O'Brien, Linda A.; Siegert, Elisabeth A.; Grisso, Jeane Ann; Maislin, Greg; LaPann, Karin; Evans, Lois

K.; Krotki, Karol P. Tube feeding preferences among nursing home residents. *Journal of General Internal Medicine.* 1997 Jun; 12(6): 364–371.
(ALLOWING TO DIE/ATTITUDES; PATIENT CARE/AGED)

O'Brien, Mary K. see **Farber, Neil J.**

O'Brien, Ralph G. see **Shepardson, Laura B.**

O'Callaghan, John J. see **Goldberg, Allen I.**

O'Connor, Bonnie see **Gelo, Florence**

O'Connor, Mary Ann see **Teno, Joan M.**

O'Connor, Nancy K.; Cheng, Tsung O.; Hendin, Herbert; Rutenfrans, Chris; Zylicz, Zbigniew. Physician–assisted suicide and euthanasia in the Netherlands: lessons from the Dutch. [Letters and response]. *JAMA.* 1997 Sep 10; 278(10): 817–818.
(EUTHANASIA)

O'Day, Steven J. see **Weeks, Jane C.**

Oddi, Samuel. The tort of interference with the right to die: the wrongful living cause of action. *Georgetown Law Journal.* 1986 Dec; 75(2): 625–665.
(ALLOWING TO DIE/LEGAL ASPECTS; WRONGFUL LIFE)

Odell, J.A. see **Pike, Roseanne E.**

Odenbach, Erwin. Respect for the patient's privacy. *Dolentium Hominum: Church and Health in the World.* 1996; 31(11th Yr., No. 1): 119–123.
(CONFIDENTIALITY)

O'Donnell, Christopher J. see **Giugliano, Robert P.**

O'Dowd, Mary Alice see **Berger, Douglas**

O'Fallon, Judith Rich. Policies for interim analysis and interim reporting of results. [Article and discussion]. *Cancer Treatment Reports.* 1985 Oct; 69(10): 1101–1106.
(HUMAN EXPERIMENTATION/RESEARCH DESIGN)

O'Flynn, Norma; Spencer, John; Jones, Roger. Consent and confidentiality in teaching in general practice: survey of patients' views on presence of students. *BMJ (British Medical Journal).* 1997 Nov 1; 315(7116): 1142.
(CONFIDENTIALITY; MEDICAL ETHICS/EDUCATION)

Ofstein, Abigail see **Furnham, Adrian**

Ogilvie, Alan D. Colombia is confused over legalisation of euthanasia. [News]. *BMJ (British Medical Journal).* 1997 Jun 28; 314(7098): 1852.
(EUTHANASIA/LEGAL ASPECTS)

Ogle, Richard D. see **Feldstein, Bruce D.**

Ogloff, James R.P. see **Bass, Larry J.**

O'Hare, Daniel see **Portenoy, Russell K.**

Ohi, Gen. Advance directives and the Japanese ethos. *In:* Sass, Hans-Martin; Veatch, Robert M.; Kimura, Rihito, eds. Advance Directives and Surrogate Decision Making in Health Care: United States, Germany, and Japan. Baltimore, MD: Johns Hopkins University Press; 1998: 175–186.

(ADVANCE DIRECTIVES; TRUTH DISCLOSURE)

Ohi, Gen. Ethos and its changes: a commentary on 'facing death the Japanese way — customs and ethos'. *In:* Hoshino, Kazumasa, ed. Japanese and Western Bioethics: Studies in Moral Diversity. Boston, MA: Kluwer Academic; 1997: 155–159.
(TRUTH DISCLOSURE)

Ohio. Court of Appeals, Hamilton County. Anderson v. St. Francis–St. George Hospital. *North Eastern Reporter, 2d Series.* 1992 Nov 18 (date of decision). 614: 841–847.
(RESUSCITATION ORDERS; TREATMENT REFUSAL; WRONGFUL LIFE)

Ohl, Dana A.; Park, John; Cohen, Carl; Goodman, Karen; Menge, Alan C. Procreation after death or mental incompetence: medical advance or technology gone awry? *Fertility and Sterility.* 1996 Dec; 66(6): 889–895.
(ORGAN AND TISSUE DONATION; REPRODUCTIVE TECHNOLOGIES)

Ohlsson, Rolf see **Nilstun, Tore**

Oken, Martin M. see **Elliott, Thomas E.**

Okonofua, Friday E. The case against new reproductive technologies in developing countries. *British Journal of Obstetrics and Gynaecology.* 1996 Oct; 103(10): 957–962.
(REPRODUCTIVE TECHNOLOGIES)

Olde Rikkert, Marcel G.M.; van den Bercken, John H.L.; ten Have, Henk A.M.J.; Hoefnagels, Willibrord H.L. Experienced consent in geriatrics research: a new method to optimize the capacity to consent in frail elderly subjects. *Journal of Medical Ethics.* 1997 Oct; 23(5): 271–276.
(HUMAN EXPERIMENTATION/INFORMED CONSENT; HUMAN EXPERIMENTATION/SPECIAL POPULATIONS)

Oldham, John M. see **Haimowitz, Stephan**

Oleszczuk, Thomas A. see **Smith, Theresa C.**

Olivarez, Margie see **Self, Donnie J.**

Olive, David L. see **Greenfeld, Dorothy A.**

Oliver, John. Voluntary euthanasia commands majority support. [Letter]. *BMJ (British Medical Journal).* 1995 Aug 19; 311(7003): 510.
(EUTHANASIA/ATTITUDES)

Ollila, Eeva; Hemminki, Elina. Does licensing of drugs in industrialized countries guarantee drug quality and safety for Third World countries? The case of Norplant licensing in Finland. *International Journal of Health Services.* 1997; 27(2): 309–328.
(CONTRACEPTION; HUMAN EXPERIMENTATION/FOREIGN COUNTRIES; PATIENT CARE/DRUGS)

Olson, Carin M.; Glass, Richard M.; Thacker, Stephen B.; Stroup, Donna F. Ethical issues in studying submissions to a medical journal. *JAMA.* 1998 Jul 15; 280(3): 290–291.
(BIOMEDICAL RESEARCH)

Olson, Carin M.; Jobe, Kathleen A.; Rennie, Drummond; Yank, Veronica. Reporting institutional review board approval and patient consent. [Letter and response]. *JAMA.* 1997 Aug 13; 278(6): 477.
(HUMAN EXPERIMENTATION/ETHICS COMMITTEES; HUMAN EXPERIMENTATION/INFORMED CONSENT)

Olsthoorn–Heim, Els see **Gevers, Sjef**

Olszewski, Nancy A. see **Olver, Ian N.**

Olver, Ian N.; Turrell, Susan J.; Olszewski, Nancy A.; Willson, Kristyn J. Impact of an information and consent form on patients having chemotherapy. *Medical Journal of Australia.* 1995 Jan 16; 162(2): 82–83.
(INFORMED CONSENT; PATIENT CARE/DRUGS)

O'Mathúna, Dónal P. The case of human growth hormone. *In:* Kilner, John F.; Pentz, Rebecca D.; Young, Frank E., eds. Genetic Ethics: Do the Ends Justify the Genes? Grand Rapids, MI: W.B. Eerdmans; 1997: 203–217.
(GENETIC INTERVENTION)

Ondrusek, Nancy; Abramovitch, Rona; Pencharz, Paul; Koren, Gideon. Empirical examination of the ability of children to consent to clinical research. *Journal of Medical Ethics.* 1998 Jun; 24(3): 158–165.
(HUMAN EXPERIMENTATION/INFORMED CONSENT; HUMAN EXPERIMENTATION/MINORS; INFORMED CONSENT/MINORS)

O'Neil, John see **Degner, Lesley F.**

O'Neil, John D. see **Kaufert, Joseph M.**

O'Neill, Patrick see **Seitz, Joanne**

Ong, Bie Nio. The lay perspective in health technology assessment. *International Journal of Technology Assessment in Health Care.* 1996 Summer; 12(3): 511–517.
(BIOMEDICAL TECHNOLOGIES)

Ono, Yutaka see **Berger, Douglas**

Onwuteaka–Philipsen, B.D.; van der Wal, G. Cases of euthanasia and physician assisted suicide among AIDS patients reported to the Public Prosecutor in North Holland. *Public Health.* 1998 Jan; 112(1): 53–56.
(AIDS; EUTHANASIA; SUICIDE)

Onwuteaka–Philipsen, B.D. see **Muller, M.T.**

Onwuteaka–Philipsen, Bregje D.; Muller, Martien T.; van der Wal, Gerrit. Euthanasia and old age. *Age and Ageing.* 1997 Nov; 26(6): 487–492.
(EUTHANASIA; SUICIDE)

Onwuteaka–Philipsen, Bregje D.; Muller, Martien T.; van der Wal, Gerrit; van Eijk, Jacques Th.M.; Ribbe, Miel W. Active voluntary euthanasia or physician–assisted suicide? *Journal of the American Geriatrics Society.* 1997 Oct; 45(10): 1208–1213.
(EUTHANASIA/ATTITUDES; SUICIDE)

Oosthuizen, C. see **Viljoen, D.**

Oppenheimer, Gerald M.; Padgug, Robert A. Health care financing. *In:* Chadwick, Ruth, ed. Encyclopedia of Applied Ethics, Volume 2. San Diego, CA: Academic Press; 1998: 539–549.
(HEALTH CARE/ECONOMICS)

Orentlicher, David. Genetic privacy in the physician–patient relationship. *In:* Rothstein, Mark A., ed. Genetic Secrets: Protecting Privacy and Confidentiality in the Genetic Era. New Haven, CT: Yale University Press; 1997: 77–91.
(CONFIDENTIALITY)

Orentlicher, David. Practice guidelines: a limited role in resolving rationing decisions. *Journal of the American Geriatrics Society.* 1998 Mar; 46(3): 369–372.
(HEALTH CARE/ECONOMICS; RESOURCE ALLOCATION)

Orentlicher, David. The Supreme Court and physician–assisted suicide -- rejecting assisted suicide but embracing euthanasia. *New England Journal of Medicine.* 1997 Oct 23; 337(17): 1236–1239.
(EUTHANASIA/LEGAL ASPECTS; SUICIDE; TERMINAL CARE)

Orentlicher, David. The Supreme Court and terminal sedation: an ethically inferior alternative to physician–assisted suicide. *In:* Battin, Margaret P.; Rhodes, Rosamond; Silvers, Anita, eds. Physician Assisted Suicide: Expanding the Debate. New York, NY: Routledge; 1998: 301–311.
(ALLOWING TO DIE/LEGAL ASPECTS; EUTHANASIA; SUICIDE)

Orentlicher, David see **Curran, William J.**

Orlans, F. Barbara. Ethical decision making about animal experiments. *Ethics and Behavior.* 1997; 7(2): 163–171.
(ANIMAL EXPERIMENTATION)

Orlans, F. Barbara; Beauchamp, Tom L.; Dresser, Rebecca; Morton, David B.; Gluck, John P. The Human Use of Animals: Case Studies in Ethical Choice. New York, NY: Oxford University Press; 1998. 330 p.
(ANIMAL EXPERIMENTATION)

Orlans, F. Barbara see **Freedman, Monroe H.**

Orlans, F. Barbara see **Gluck, John P.**

Orlowski, James P.; Smith, Martin L.; Van Zwienen, Jan. Medical decisions concerning the end of life in children in the Netherlands. [Letter]. *American Journal of Diseases of Children.* 1993 Jun; 147(6): 613–614.
(EUTHANASIA)

Orme, Michael. The risks of studies in healthy volunteers. *In:* Close, Bryony; Combes, Robert; Hubbard, Anthony; Illingworth, John, eds. Volunteers in Research and Testing. Bristol, PA: Taylor and Francis; 1997: 99–107.
(HUMAN EXPERIMENTATION)

O'Rourke, Keith see **Kohut, Nitsa**

O'Rourke, Keith see **Stelfox, Henry Thomas**

O'Rourke, Kevin. Euthanasia and assisted suicide: a response to Edmund Pellegrino. *In:* Wildes, Kevin Wm.; Mitchell, Alan C., eds. Choosing Life: A Dialogue on *Evangelium Vitae.* Washington, DC: Georgetown University Press; 1997: 259–261.
(ALLOWING TO DIE/RELIGIOUS ASPECTS)

O'Rourke, Kevin D. Catholic healthcare as "leaven": to penetrate and renew society, Catholic healthcare must meet five requirements. *Health Progress.* 1997 Mar–Apr; 78(2): 34–38, 43.
(HEALTH CARE)

O'Rourke, Kevin D. Withdrawal of life support: mistaken assumptions. *Health Progress.* 1996 Nov–Dec; 77(6): 60–61, 65.
(ALLOWING TO DIE/RELIGIOUS ASPECTS)

O'Rourke, Kevin D. see **Ashley, Benedict M.**

Orr, Robert D.; Morton, Kelly R.; deLeon, Dennis M.; Fals, Juan C. Evaluation of an ethics consultation service: patient and family perspective. *American Journal of Medicine.* 1996 Aug; 101(2): 135–141.
(ETHICISTS AND ETHICS COMMITTEES)

Orr, Robert D.; Pang, Norman; Pellegrino, Edmund D.; Siegler, Mark. Use of the Hippocratic oath: a review of twentieth century practice and a content analysis of oaths administered in medical schools in the U.S. and Canada in 1993. *Journal of Clinical Ethics.* 1997 Winter; 8(4): 377–388.
(MEDICAL ETHICS/CODES OF ETHICS; MEDICAL ETHICS/EDUCATION)

Ort, Sharon I. see **Greenfeld, Dorothy A.**

Osborne, Judith A. Incarcerating Hippocrates. *Legal Medical Quarterly.* 1984–1985; 8–9: 1–8.
(HEALTH CARE/FOREIGN COUNTRIES)

Oscherwitz, Tom; Tulsky, Jacqueline Peterson; Roger, Steve; Sciortino, Stan; Alpers, Ann; Royce, Sarah; Lo, Bernard. Detention of persistently nonadherent patients with tuberculosis. *JAMA.* 1997 Sep 10; 278(10): 843–846.
(PUBLIC HEALTH)

O'Sullivan, Joan see **Thomas, A. Mathew**

O'Sullivan, Joan L. see **Shamoo, Adil E.**

O'Sullivan, Mary Jo see **Minkoff, Howard**

Osuna, Eduardo; Pérez–Cárceles, Maria D.; Esteban, Miguel A.; Luna, Aurelio. The right to information for the terminally ill patient. *Journal of Medical Ethics.* 1998 Apr; 24(2): 106–109.
(TERMINAL CARE; TRUTH DISCLOSURE)

Otlowski, Margaret. Voluntary Euthanasia and the Common Law. New York, NY: Oxford University Press; 1997. 564 p.
(EUTHANASIA/LEGAL ASPECTS; SUICIDE)

O'Toole, Erin M. HIV–specific crime legislation: targeting an epidemic for criminal prosecution. *Journal of Law and Health.* 1995–1996; 10(1): 183–208.
(AIDS)

Overall, Christine; Zion, William P., eds. Perspectives on AIDS: Ethical and Social Issues. New York, NY: Oxford University Press; 1991. 179 p.
(AIDS)

Overbay, Jane Dring. Parental participation in treatment decisions for pediatric oncology ICU patients. *Dimensions of Critical Care Nursing.* 1996 Jan–Feb; 15(1): 16–24.
(INFORMED CONSENT/MINORS; PROFESSIONAL PATIENT RELATIONSHIP)

Overcast, Thomas D. see Merriken, Karen

Owen, Mike see Daniels, Jo

Owens, R. Glynn see Kent, Bridie

Owens, Steve see Gore, Albert

Oye, Robert K. see Phillips, Russell S.

Oye, Robert K. see Wenger, Neil S.

Ozar, David T. An alternative rationale for informed consent by human subjects. *American Psychologist.* 1983 Feb; 38(2): 230–232.
(HUMAN EXPERIMENTATION/INFORMED CONSENT)

Ozar, David T. The social obligations of health care practitioners. [Revised]. *In:* Monagle, John F.; Thomasma, David C., eds. Health Care Ethics: Issues Critical for the 21st Century. Gaithersburg, MD: Aspen Publishers; 1998: 378–391.
(HEALTH CARE/ECONOMICS; PROFESSIONAL PATIENT RELATIONSHIP)

Ozar, David T. Three models of professionalism and professional obligation in dentistry. *Journal of the American Dental Association.* 1985 Feb; 110(2): 173–177.
(PROFESSIONAL PATIENT RELATIONSHIP)

P

Paavilainen, Eija; Astedt-Kurki, Päivi; Paunonen, Marita. Ethical problems in research on families who are abusing children. *Nursing Ethics.* 1998 May; 5(3): 200–205.
(BEHAVIORAL RESEARCH)

Pace, Brian P. see Flanagin, Annette

Pace, Nicholas A. Law and ethics at the end of life: the practitioner's view. *In:* McLean, Sheila A.M., ed. Death, Dying and the Law. Brookfield, VT: Dartmouth; 1996: 3–18.
(ALLOWING TO DIE; TERMINAL CARE)

Packer, Samuel. Medical ethics and the excimer laser. [Editorial]. *Archives of Ophthalmology.* 1997 May; 115(5): 666–667.
(HEALTH CARE/ECONOMICS)

Packer, Samuel see Rosner, Fred

Padgug, Robert A. see Oppenheimer, Gerald M.

Page, Andrea see Durfy, Sharon J.

Page, David L.; Jensen, Roy A.; Geller, Gail; Botkin, Jeffrey R. Genetic testing and informed consent. [Letter and response]. *JAMA.* 1997 Sep 10; 278(10): 821–822.
(GENETIC RESEARCH; GENETIC SCREENING; INFORMED CONSENT)

Palazanni, Laura. Genetic engineering and human nature. *In:* Doherty, Peter; Sutton, Agneta, eds. Man-Made Man: Ethical and Legal Issues in Genetics. Dublin, Ireland: Open Air; 1997: 46–57.
(GENETIC INTERVENTION)

Palermo, George B. The plight of the deinstitutionalized chronic schizophrenic: ethical considerations. [Revised].

In: Monagle, John F.; Thomasma, David C., eds. Health Care Ethics: Critical Issues for the 21st Century. Gaithersburg, MD: Aspen Publishers; 1998: 164–176.
(PATIENT CARE/MENTALLY DISABLED)

Palfreman, Jon see Langston, J. William

Palles, Michael see Jürgens, Ralf

Palmer-Fernández, Gabriel see Minogue, Brendan P.

Pan-European Consultation on HIV/AIDS in the Context of Public Health and Human Rights, Prague, 26–27 Nov 1991. HIV/AIDS in the Context of Public Health and Human Rights: Report of a Pan-European Consultation. London: International Association of Rights and Humanity, on behalf of the World Health Organization Regional Office for Europe; 1993[?]. 65 p.
(AIDS)

Pandya, Kishan J. see Cleeland, Charles S.

Pang, Mei-che Samantha. Information disclosure: the moral experience of nurses in China. *Nursing Ethics.* 1998 Jul; 5(4): 347–361.
(INFORMED CONSENT; NURSING ETHICS; TERMINAL CARE; TRUTH DISCLOSURE)

Pang, Mei-che Samantha; Wong, Kwok-shing Thomas. Cultivating a moral sense of nursing through model emulation. *Nursing Ethics.* 1998 Sep; 5(5): 424–440.
(NURSING ETHICS/EDUCATION)

Pang, Norman see Orr, Robert D.

Pang, W.S. see Sahadevan, S.

Papadatou, Danai see Wrenn, Robert L.

Papp, Z. see Simms, Madeleine

Parascandola, Mark. Animal research. *In:* Chadwick, Ruth, ed. Encyclopedia of Applied Ethics, Volume 1. San Diego, CA: Academic Press; 1998: 151–160.
(ANIMAL EXPERIMENTATION)

Parens, Erik. Is better always good? The enhancement project. [Project on the Prospect of Technologies Aimed at the Enhancement of Human Capacities and Traits]. *Hastings Center Report.* 1998 Jan–Feb; 28(1): S1–S17.
(BIOMEDICAL TECHNOLOGIES; GENETIC INTERVENTION; HEALTH; HEALTH CARE; PATIENT CARE/DRUGS)

Parens, Erik. Tools from and for democratic deliberations. *Hastings Center Report.* 1997 Sep–Oct; 27(5): 20–22.
(CLONING)

Parens, Erik. What differences make a difference? [Editorial]. *Cambridge Quarterly of Healthcare Ethics.* 1998 Winter; 7(1): 1–6.
(BIOETHICS; PROFESSIONAL PATIENT RELATIONSHIP)

Paris, John J. Autonomy and physician-assisted suicide. *America.* 1997 May 17; 176(17): 11–14.
(EUTHANASIA/RELIGIOUS ASPECTS; SUICIDE)

Paris, John J.; Bell, Anthony J.; Murphy, James J. Pediatric brain death: dead is dead. *Journal of Perinatology.* 1995 Jan–Feb; 15(1): 67–70.
(DETERMINATION OF DEATH/BRAIN DEATH)

Paris, John J.; Moreland, Michael P. A Catholic perspective on physician–assisted suicide. *In:* Battin, Margaret P.; Rhodes, Rosamond; Silvers, Anita, eds. Physician Assisted Suicide: Expanding the Debate. New York, NY: Routledge; 1998: 324–333.
(SUICIDE)

Paris, John J.; Muir, J. Cameron; Reardon, Frank E. Ethical and legal issues in intensive care. *Journal of Intensive Care Medicine.* 1997 Nov–Dec; 12(6): 298–309.
(BIOMEDICAL TECHNOLOGIES; TERMINAL CARE)

Paris, John J.; Poorman, Mark. When religious beliefs and medical judgments conflict: civic polity and the social good. *In:* Zucker, Marjorie B.; Zucker, Howard D., eds. Medical Futility and the Evaluation of Life–Sustaining Interventions. New York, NY: Cambridge University Press; 1997: 85–97.
(ALLOWING TO DIE/RELIGIOUS ASPECTS)

Paris, Peter J. A view from the underside. *In:* Cole-Turner, Ronald, ed. Human Cloning: Religious Responses. Louisville, KY: Westminister John Knox Press; 1997: 43–48.
(CLONING)

Park, John see **Ohl, Dana A.**

Parkash, Ravi; Burge, Frederick. The family's perspective on issues of hydration in terminal care. *Journal of Palliative Care.* 1997 Winter; 13(4): 23–27.
(ALLOWING TO DIE/ATTITUDES; TERMINAL CARE)

Parker, Camilla see **Dolan, Bridget**

Parker, David L. see **Rich, Ann**

Parker, Lisa S. Beauty and breast implantation: how candidate selection affects autonomy and informed consent. *In:* DiQuinzio, Patrice; Young, Iris Marion, eds. Feminist Ethics and Social Policy. Bloomington, IN: Indiana University Press; 1997: 255–273.
(BIOMEDICAL TECHNOLOGIES; INFORMED CONSENT; SELECTION FOR TREATMENT)

Parker, M.H. see **Steinberg, M.A.**

Parker, S. see **Taylor, E.M.**

Parkins, K.J.; Poets, C.F.; O'Brien, L.M.; Stebbens, V.A.; Southall, D.P.; Savulescu, Julian; Hughes, Vivian. Effect of exposure to 15% oxygen on breathing patterns and oxygen saturation in infants: interventional study. [Article, commentaries, and response]. *BMJ (British Medical Journal).* 1998 Mar 21; 316(7135): 887–894.
(HUMAN EXPERIMENTATION/MINORS)

Parnham, Michael J. Animal experimentation. *In: his* Ethical Issues in Drug Research: Through a Glass Darkly. Washington, DC: IOS Press; 1996: 97–114.
(ANIMAL EXPERIMENTATION)

Parnham, Michael J. Ethical Issues in Drug Research: Through a Glass Darkly. Washington, DC: IOS Press; 1996. 155 p.
(BIOMEDICAL RESEARCH; PATIENT CARE/DRUGS)

Parrott, Robert H., et al.; American Academy of Pediatrics. Council on Research. Proposed guidelines on genetic engineering. *Pediatrics.* 1985 Jun; 75(6): 1159.
(GENETIC INTERVENTION; RECOMBINANT DNA RESEARCH/REGULATION)

Parsons, Debra see **Hilberman, Mark**

Parsons, Evelyn; Bradley, Don; Clarke, Angus. Disclosure of Duchenne muscular dystrophy after newborn screening. *Archives of Disease in Childhood.* 1996 Jun; 74(6): 550–553.
(GENETIC SCREENING; TRUTH DISCLOSURE)

Parsons, Mary E. see **Pinch, W.J. Ellenchild**

Pascual-Leone, Alvaro see **Green, Ronald M.**

Passchier, J. see **DudokdeWit, A.C.**

Passik, Steven D. see **Chochinov, Harvey Max**

Pasztor, Andy; Lagnado, Lucette. Ethics czar aims to heal Columbia. [News]. *Wall Street Journal.* 1997 Nov 26: B1, B6.
(FRAUD AND MISCONDUCT; HEALTH CARE/ECONOMICS)

Patel, Tara. Row over sterilisation divides India. [News]. *New Scientist.* 1997 Apr 5; 154(2076): 4.
(HUMAN EXPERIMENTATION/FOREIGN COUNTRIES; HUMAN EXPERIMENTATION/SPECIAL POPULATIONS; STERILIZATION)

Patenaude, Andrea Farkas; Basili, Laura; Fairclough, Diane L.; Li, Frederick P. Attitudes of 47 mothers of pediatric oncology patients toward genetic testing for cancer predisposition. *Journal of Clinical Oncology.* 1996 Feb; 14(2): 415–421.
(GENETIC SCREENING)

Paterson-Brown, Sara see **Amu, Olubusola**

Paterson-Brown, Sara see **Logmans, A.**

Paterson, I.C.M. Consent to treatment: somebody's moved the goalposts. *Clinical Oncology (Royal College of Radiologists).* 1994; 6(3): 179–182.
(INFORMED CONSENT)

Paton, Calum. Necessary conditions for a socialist health service. *Health Care Analysis.* 1997 Sep; 5(3): 205–216.
(HEALTH CARE/ECONOMICS; HEALTH CARE/FOREIGN COUNTRIES)

Patrick, Donald L. see **Pearlman, Robert A.**

Patterson, Bradford see **Taylor, Kathryn M.**

Patterson, Elizabeth G. Human rights and human life: an uneven fit. *Tulane Law Review.* 1994 Jun; 68(6): 1527–1561.
(DETERMINATION OF DEATH/BRAIN DEATH; FETUSES; PERSONHOOD)

Patterson, Elizabeth G.; Andrews, Arlene Bowers. Civil commitment for pregnant substance abusers: is it appropriate and is it enough? *Politics and the Life Sciences.* 1996 Mar; 15(1): 64–66.
(INVOLUNTARY COMMITMENT; PRENATAL INJURIES)

Patterson, W. Bradford; Emanuel, Ezekiel J.; Blumenthal, David. Physician–drug company conflict of interest. *Journal of Clinical Oncology.* 1996 Jan; 14(1): 316–320.
(HEALTH CARE/ECONOMICS; PATIENT CARE/DRUGS)

Patterson, W. Bradford see **Emanuel, Ezekiel J.**

Pattullo, Edward L. Governmental regulation of the investigation of human subjects in social research. *Minerva.* 1985 Winter; 23(4): 521–533.
(BEHAVIORAL RESEARCH/REGULATION)

Pauker, Susan see **Kinmonth, Ann Louise**

Paul, Diane. From eugenics to medical genetics. *In:* Marcus, Alan I.; Cravens, Hamilton, eds. Health Care Policy in Contemporary America. University Park, PA: Pennsylvania State University Press; 1997: 96–116.
(EUGENICS; GENETIC COUNSELING)

Paul, Diane B. Culpability and compassion: lessons from the history of eugenics. *Politics and the Life Sciences.* 1996 Mar; 15(1): 99–100.
(BEHAVIORAL GENETICS; EUGENICS)

Paulson, Richard J. Ethical considerations involving oocyte donation and gestational surrogacy. *Seminars in Reproductive Endocrinology.* 1995 Aug; 13(3): 225–230.
(REPRODUCTIVE TECHNOLOGIES; SURROGATE MOTHERS)

Paunonen, Marita see **Paavilainen, Eija**

Payne–James, Jason; Dean, Peter; Wall, Ian. Medicolegal Essentials in Healthcare. New York, NY: Churchill Livingstone; 1996. 177 p.
(BIOETHICS)

Payne, John see **Sechriest, Kay**

Pear, Robert. Presidential panel sees no need for a law on patient's rights. [News]. *New York Times.* 1998 Mar 13: A17.
(HEALTH CARE/ECONOMICS; PATIENTS' RIGHTS)

Pear, Robert. Proposal to test drugs in children meets resistance. [News]. *New York Times.* 1997 Nov 30: 1, 28.
(HUMAN EXPERIMENTATION/MINORS; HUMAN EXPERIMENTATION/REGULATION)

Pear, Robert. States pass laws to regulate uses of genetic testing. [News]. *New York Times.* 1997 Oct 18: A1, A9.
(CONFIDENTIALITY/LEGAL ASPECTS; GENETIC SCREENING)

Pearlman, Robert A.; Cole, William G.; Patrick, Donald L.; Starks, Helene E.; Cain, Kevin C. Advance care planning: eliciting patient preferences for life–sustaining treatment. *Patient Education and Counseling.* 1995 Sep; 26(1–3): 353–361.
(ADVANCE DIRECTIVES)

Pearson, Marjorie L. see **Wenger, Neil S.**

Pearson, Roger. Heredity and Humanity: Race, Eugenics and Modern Science. Washington, DC: Scott–Townsend; 1996. 162 p.
(EUGENICS; GENETIC RESEARCH)

Pearson, Steven D.; Sabin, James E.; Emanuel, Ezekiel J. Ethical guidelines for physician compensation based on capitation. *New England Journal of Medicine.* 1998 Sep 3; 339(10): 689–693.
(HEALTH CARE/ECONOMICS)

Pechura, Constance M. Fetal and embryo research: a changing scientific, political, and ethical landscape. *In:* Vanderpool, Harold Y., ed. The Ethics of Research Involving Human Subjects: Facing the 21st Century. Frederick, MD: University Publishing Group; 1996: 371–400.
(EMBRYO AND FETAL RESEARCH; ORGAN AND TISSUE DONATION)

Peel, John. After the embryo, the fetus? *Ethics and Medicine.* 1986; 2(2): 19–22.
(EMBRYO AND FETAL RESEARCH)

Peeper, E. Quinn see **Lescale, Keith B.**

Pegels, Carl C. see **Wear, Stephen E.**

Pelias, Mary Z. see **Sherman, Stephanie L.**

Pellegrino, Edmund D. Bioethics as an interdisciplinary enterprise: where does ethics fit in the mosaic of disciplines? *In:* Carson, Ronald A.; Burns, Chester R., eds. Philosophy of Medicine and Bioethics: A Twenty-Year Retrospective and Critical Appraisal. Boston, MA: Kluwer Academic; 1997: 1–23.
(BIOETHICS)

Pellegrino, Edmund D. Emerging ethical issues in palliative care. [Contempo 1998]. *JAMA.* 1998 May 20; 279(19): 1521–1522.
(TERMINAL CARE)

Pellegrino, Edmund D. Ethical issues in managed care: a Catholic Christian perspective. *Christian Bioethics.* 1997 Mar; 3(1): 55–73.
(HEALTH CARE/ECONOMICS)

Pellegrino, Edmund D. Evangelium Vitae, euthanasia, and physician–assisted suicide: John Paul II's dialogue with the culture and ethics of contemporary medicine. *In:* Wildes, Kevin Wm.; Mitchell, Alan C., eds. Choosing Life: A Dialogue on *Evangelium Vitae.* Washington, DC: Georgetown University Press; 1997: 236–253.
(EUTHANASIA/RELIGIOUS ASPECTS; SUICIDE)

Pellegrino, Edmund D. Managed care at the bedside: how do we look in the moral mirror? *Kennedy Institute of Ethics Journal.* 1997 Dec; 7(4): 321–330.
(HEALTH CARE/ECONOMICS; PROFESSIONAL PATIENT RELATIONSHIP; RESOURCE ALLOCATION)

Pellegrino, Edmund D. Praxis as a keystone for the philosophy and professional ethics of medicine: the need for an arch–support: commentary on Toulmin and Wartofsky. *In:* Carson, Ronald A.; Burns, Chester R., eds. Philosophy of Medicine and Bioethics: A Twenty-Year Retrospective and Critical Appraisal. Boston, MA: Kluwer Academic; 1997: 69–84.
(MEDICAL ETHICS)

Pellegrino, Edmund D. The autopsy: some ethical reflections on the obligations of pathologists, hospitals, families, and society. *Archives of Pathology and Laboratory Medicine.* 1996 Aug; 120(8): 739–742.
(MEDICAL ETHICS)

Pellegrino, Edmund D. The false promise of beneficent killing. *In:* Emanuel, Linda L., ed. Regulating How We Die: The Ethical, Medical, and Legal Issues Surrounding Physician–Assisted Suicide. Cambridge, MA: Harvard University Press; 1998: 71–91, 269–274.
(EUTHANASIA; SUICIDE)

Pellegrino, Edmund D.; Caplan, Arthur L.; Goold, Susan Dorr. Doctors and ethics, morals and manuals. *Annals of Internal Medicine.* 1998 Apr 1; 128(7): 569–571.
(MEDICAL ETHICS/CODES OF ETHICS)

Pellegrino, Edmund D.; Thomasma, David C. Edmund D. Pellegrino on the future of bioethics. [Interview]. *Cambridge Quarterly of Healthcare Ethics.* 1997 Fall; 6(4): 373–375.
(BIOETHICS)

Pellegrino, Edmund D. see **Orr, Robert D.**

Pellegrino, Edmund D. see **Sharpe, Virginia A.**

Pence, Gregory E., ed. Classic Works in Medical Ethics: Core Philosophical Readings. Boston, MA: McGraw–Hill; 1998. 399 p.
(BIOETHICS)

Pence, Gregory E., ed. Flesh of My Flesh: The Ethics of Cloning Humans: A Reader. Lanham, MD: Rowman and Littlefield; 1998. 154 p.
(CLONING)

Pence, Gregory E. Who's Afraid of Human Cloning? Lanham, MD: Rowman and Littlefield; 1998. 181 p.
(CLONING)

Pencharz, Paul see **Ondrusek, Nancy**

Pendergast, Mary K. Testimony of Mary K. Pendergast before the Subcommittee on Human Resources, Committee on Government Reform and Oversight, U.S. House of Representatives [re FDA regulation of human experimentation]. *In:* BioLaw: A Legal and Ethical Reporter on Medicine, Health Care, and Bioengineering. Special Sections, 2(11). Frederick, MD: University Publications of America; 1997 Nov: S355–S371.
(HUMAN EXPERIMENTATION/REGULATION)

Pendleton, Deborah E. see **Mead, Gillian E.**

Pendleton, Neil see **Mead, Gillian E.**

Pennings, Guido. Should donors have the right to decide who receives their gametes? *Human Reproduction.* 1995 Oct; 10(10): 2736–2740.
(ORGAN AND TISSUE DONATION; REPRODUCTIVE TECHNOLOGIES)

Pennisi, Elizabeth. After Dolly, a pharming frenzy. [News]. *Science.* 1998 Jan 30; 279(5351): 646–648.
(CLONING; GENETIC INTERVENTION)

Pennisi, Elizabeth. NRC OKs long–delayed survey of human genome diversity. [News]. *Science.* 1997 Oct 24; 278(5338): 568.
(GENOME MAPPING)

Pennisi, Elizabeth. The lamb that roared. [News]. *Science.* 1997 Dec 19; 278(5346): 2038–2039.
(CLONING)

Pennisi, Elizabeth see **Marshall, Eliot**

Pennsylvania. Court of Common Pleas, Dauphin County. Rideout v. Hershey Medical Center. *Dauphin County Reports.* 1995 Dec 29 (date of decision). 115: 472–498.
(ALLOWING TO DIE/LEGAL ASPECTS)

Pennsylvania. Superior Court. Huddleston v. Infertility Center of America. *Atlantic Reporter, 2d Series.* 1997 Aug 20 (date of decision). 700: 453–462.
(SURROGATE MOTHERS)

Pennsylvania. Supreme Court, E.D. In re Fiori. *Atlantic Reporter, 2d Series.* 1996 Apr 2 (date of decision). 673: 905–914.
(ALLOWING TO DIE/LEGAL ASPECTS)

Penticuff, Joy Hinson. Nursing perspectives in bioethics. *In:* Hoshino, Kazumasa, ed. Japanese and Western Bioethics: Studies in Moral Diversity. Boston, MA: Kluwer Academic; 1997: 49–60.
(NURSING ETHICS; PROFESSIONAL PATIENT RELATIONSHIP)

Pentz, Rebecca D. Expanding into organizational ethics: the experience of one clinical ethics committee. *HEC (HealthCare Ethics Committee) Forum.* 1998 Jun; 10(2): 213–219.
(ETHICISTS AND ETHICS COMMITTEES; RESOURCE ALLOCATION)

Pentz, Rebecca D. see **Kilner, John F.**

Peppin, John F. An Engelhardtian analysis of interactions between pharmaceutical sales representatives and physicians. *Journal of Medicine and Philosophy.* 1997 Dec; 22(6): 623–641.
(PATIENT CARE/DRUGS)

Peppin, John F. The Christian physician in the non–Christian institution: objections of conscience and physician value neutrality. *Christian Bioethics.* 1997 Mar; 3(1): 39–54.
(MEDICAL ETHICS; PATIENT CARE)

Peppin, Patricia. Power and disadvantage in medical relationships. *Texas Journal of Women and the Law.* 1994 Spring; 3(2): 221–263.
(PROFESSIONAL PATIENT RELATIONSHIP)

Peretz, Paul; Schroedel, Jean Reith. The road not to travel: a comment on Deborah Mathieu's proposal to mandate outpatient treatment for pregnant substance abusers. *Politics and the Life Sciences.* 1996 Mar; 15(1): 67–69.
(INVOLUNTARY COMMITMENT; PRENATAL INJURIES)

Pérez–Cárceles, Maria D. see **Osuna, Eduardo**

Pergament, Eugene. A clinical geneticist perspective of the patient–physician relationship. *In:* Rothstein, Mark A., ed. Genetic Secrets: Protecting Privacy and Confidentiality in the Genetic Era. New Haven, CT: Yale University Press; 1997: 92–107.
(CONFIDENTIALITY; GENETIC COUNSELING)

Pergament, Eugene see **Andrews, Lori**

Perkins, Henry S.; Supik, Josie D.; Hazuda, Helen P. Cultural differences among health professionals: a case illustration. *Journal of Clinical Ethics.* 1998 Summer; 9(2): 108–117.
(INFORMED CONSENT; PATIENT CARE; TREATMENT REFUSAL)

Perkins, Henry S. see **Berkowitz, Sheldon T.**

Perlin, Terry M. Who will I be? Stephen G. Post's *The*

Moral Challenge of Alzheimer's kAlzheimerl Disease. [Book review essay]. *Journal of Ethics, Law, and Aging.* 1996 Fall–Winter; 2(2): 85–86.
(PATIENT CARE/MENTALLY DISABLED; PERSONHOOD)

Perlmutter, Marty see **Webb, Sally L.**

Perone, Anne M. see **Byrne, Paul A.**

Perry, Seymour. Reports from the Health Council of the Netherlands: sex selection for nonmedical reasons. *International Journal of Technology Assessment in Health Care.* 1996 Fall; 12(4): 756–759.
(SEX DETERMINATION; SEX PRESELECTION)

Perz, J.M. see **Hooper, S.C.**

Peters, Charles see **Weir, Robert F.**

Peters, David A. Risk classification, genetic testing, and health care: a conflict between libertarian and egalitarian values? *In:* Peters, Ted, ed. Genetics: Issues of Social Justice. Cleveland, OH: Pilgrim Press; 1998: 205–217.
(GENETIC SCREENING)

Peters, Kathryn F. see **McKinnon, Wendy C.**

Peters, Ted. Cloning shock: a theological reaction. *In:* Cole–Turner, Ronald, ed. Human Cloning: Religious Responses. Louisville, KY: Westminister John Knox Press; 1997: 12–24.
(CLONING)

Peters, Ted. Designer genes and selective abortion. *In: his* For the Love of Children: Genetic Technology and the Future of the Family. Louisville, KY: Westminster John Knox Press; 1996: 85–118, 193–199.
(ABORTION; ABORTION/RELIGIOUS ASPECTS; FETUSES; GENETIC SCREENING; PERSONHOOD)

Peters, Ted. For the Love of Children: Genetic Technology and the Future of the Family. Louisville, KY: Westminster John Knox Press; 1996. 227 p.
(REPRODUCTION; REPRODUCTIVE TECHNOLOGIES)

Peters, Ted, ed. Genetics: Issues of Social Justice. Cleveland, OH: Pilgrim Press; 1998. 262 p.
(GENETIC INTERVENTION; GENOME MAPPING)

Peters, Ted. Surrogate motherhood: an ethical puzzle. *In: his* For the Love of Children: Genetic Technology and the Future of the Family. Louisville, KY: Westminster John Knox Press; 1996: 58–84, 189–193.
(SURROGATE MOTHERS)

Peters, Ted F. On the gay gene: back to original sin again? *Dialog: A Journal of Theology.* 1994 Winter; 33(1): 30–38.
(BEHAVIORAL GENETICS)

Petersen, K. see **Andersen, C. Yding**

Petersen, Kerry, ed. Intersections: Women on Law, Medicine and Technology. Brookfield, VT: Ashgate; 1997. 246 p.
(BIOETHICS)

Petersen, Kerry. Medical negligence and wrongful birth actions: Australian developments. *Journal of Medical Ethics.* 1997 Oct; 23(5): 319–322.
(ABORTION/FOREIGN COUNTRIES; ABORTION/LEGAL ASPECTS; WRONGFUL LIFE)

Petersen, Kerry. Private decisions and public scrutiny: sterilisation and minors in Australia and England. *In:* McLean, Sheila A.M., ed. Contemporary Issues in Law, Medicine and Ethics. Brookfield, VT: Dartmouth; 1996: 57–77.
(STERILIZATION/MENTALLY DISABLED)

Peterson, Andrew M.; Schwarz, Lewis R.; Veatch, Robert M. Asking a pharmacist to resign for making an error. [Case study and commentaries]. *American Journal of Health–System Pharmacy.* 1996 Apr 1; 53(7): 760–763.
(PROFESSIONAL ETHICS)

Peterson, Christa see **Bass, Larry J.**

Peterson, Eric D. see **Barnhart, J. Marie**

Peterson, James C. Ethical standards for genetic intervention. *In:* Kilner, John F.; Pentz, Rebecca D.; Young, Frank E., eds. Genetic Ethics: Do the Ends Justify the Genes? Grand Rapids, MI: W.B. Eerdmans; 1997: 193–202.
(GENETIC INTERVENTION)

Peterson, Joan see **Viola, Raymond A.**

Peterson, Lynn M. see **Weeks, Jane C.**

Pettifor, Jean L. see **Bass, Larry J.**

Pfaadt, Mary Joyce see **Duffy, Barbara**

Pfeffer, Naomi. Consumers' viewpoint. *In:* Close, Bryony; Combes, Robert; Hubbard, Anthony; Illingworth, John, eds. Volunteers in Research and Testing. Bristol, PA: Taylor and Francis; 1997: 23–31.
(HUMAN EXPERIMENTATION/FOREIGN COUNTRIES)

Phanuphak, Praphan. Ethical issues in studies in Thailand of the vertical transmission of HIV. *New England Journal of Medicine.* 1998 Mar 19; 338(12): 834–835.
(AIDS/HUMAN EXPERIMENTATION; HUMAN EXPERIMENTATION/FOREIGN COUNTRIES; HUMAN EXPERIMENTATION/RESEARCH DESIGN; HUMAN EXPERIMENTATION/SPECIAL POPULATIONS)

Phanuphak, Praphan; Vermund, Sten H. Ethical issues for perinatal HIV trials in developing countries. [Editorial]. *Pediatric AIDS and HIV Infection.* 1996 Aug; 7(4): 236–238.
(AIDS/HUMAN EXPERIMENTATION; HUMAN EXPERIMENTATION/FOREIGN COUNTRIES)

Pharmaceutical Research and Manufacturers of America. Ethical Principles on GENOMICS. [Statement]. Washington, DC: Pharmaceutical Research and Manufacturers of America; 1996 May 16. 1 p.
(GENETIC INTERVENTION)

Phelps, Ruth–Ann. VHA policy–related clinical ethical issues. *HEC (HealthCare Ethics Committee) Forum.* 1997 Jun; 9(2): 159–168.
(BIOETHICS)

Philip, Donald J. Ethics of managed care: implications for group practice. *Medical Group Management Journal.* 1997 Nov–Dec; 44(6): 55–56, 58, 60–64, 66.
(HEALTH CARE/ECONOMICS)

Philipson, Elliot H. see **Philipson, Sandra J.**

Philipson, Sandra J.; Doyle, Mary Anne; Gabram, Sheryl G.A.; Nightingale, Charles; Philipson, Elliot H. Informed consent for research: a study to evaluate readability and processability to effect change. *Journal of Investigative Medicine.* 1995 Oct; 43(5): 459–467.
(HUMAN EXPERIMENTATION/INFORMED CONSENT)

Phillips, Charles D.; Hawes, Catherine; Mor, Vince; Fries, Brant E.; Morris, John N.; Nennstiel, Marianne E. Facility and area variation affecting the use of physical restraints in nursing homes. *Medical Care.* 1996 Nov; 34(11): 1149–1162.
(BEHAVIOR CONTROL; PATIENT CARE/AGED)

Phillips, Jennifer M. Reducing postmortem examination refusal by families of research subjects. *IRB: A Review of Human Subjects Research.* 1997 Sep–Oct; 19(5): 10–11.
(ADVANCE DIRECTIVES; HUMAN EXPERIMENTATION/INFORMED CONSENT)

Phillips, Michael see Sansone, Paulette

Phillips, Pat. Views of assisted suicide from several nations. *JAMA.* 1997 Sep 24; 278(12): 969–970.
(SUICIDE)

Phillips, Russell S.; Wenger, Neil S.; Teno, Joan; Oye, Robert K.; Youngner, Stuart; Califf, Robert; Layde, Peter; Desbiens, Norman; Connors, Alfred F.; Lynn, Joanne. Choices of seriously ill patients about cardiopulmonary resuscitation: correlates and outcomes. [For the SUPPORT Investigators]. *American Journal of Medicine.* 1996 Feb; 100(2): 128–137.
(RESUSCITATION ORDERS)

Phillips, Russell S. see Teno, Joan

Phillips, Russell S. see Teno, Joan M.

Phillips, Russell S. see Tsevat, Joel

Phillips, Russell S. see Weeks, Jane C.

Phillips, Russell S. see Wenger, Neil S.

Phillips, Stephanie G. see Flanagin, Annette

Pickens, Bruce K. see Muehleman, Thomas

Pickering, John H. see Lynn, Joanne

Pickering, Neil. Imaginary restrictions. *Journal of Medical Ethics.* 1998 Jun; 24(3): 171–175.
(MEDICAL ETHICS/EDUCATION; PROFESSIONAL PATIENT RELATIONSHIP)

Pierce, Susan Foley. A model for conceptualizing the moral dynamic in health care. *Nursing Ethics.* 1997 Nov; 4(6): 483–495.
(MEDICAL ETHICS; NURSING ETHICS; PATIENT CARE)

Pieri, Lorenzo see Williams, Christopher J.

Pierro, Agostino; Spitz, Lewis. Informed consent in clinical research: the crisis in paediatrics. [Letter]. *Lancet.* 1997 Jun 7; 349(9066): 1703.
(HUMAN EXPERIMENTATION/INFORMED CONSENT; HUMAN EXPERIMENTATION/MINORS)

Pierson, Vicky Howell. Missouri's parental consent law and teen pregnancy outcomes. *Women and Health.* 1995; 22(3): 47–58.
(ABORTION/MINORS)

Pike, Jon. Strikes. *In:* Chadwick, Ruth, ed. Encyclopedia of Applied Ethics, Volume 4. San Diego, CA: Academic Press; 1998: 239–247.
(HEALTH CARE/ECONOMICS)

Pike, Roseanne E.; Odell, J.A.; Kahn, D. Public attitudes to organ donation in South Africa. [Abstract]. *Transplantation Proceedings.* 1992 Oct; 24(5): 2102.
(ORGAN AND TISSUE DONATION)

Pillsbury, S. Gainer see Segal, Arthur I.

Pinch, W.J. Ellenchild; Parsons, Mary E. Moral orientation of elderly persons: considering ethical dilemmas in health care. *Nursing Ethics.* 1997 Sep; 4(5): 380–393.
(PATIENT CARE/AGED)

Pinch, Winifred J., et al. Allocation of scarce resources: critical care nursing dilemmas. [Case studies and commentaries]. *Dimensions of Critical Care Nursing.* 1985 May–Jun; 4(3): 164–173.
(RESOURCE ALLOCATION/BIOMEDICAL TECHNOLOGIES; SELECTION FOR TREATMENT)

Pinch, Winifred J. Is caring a moral trap? *Nursing Outlook.* 1996 Mar–Apr; 44(2): 84–88.
(NURSING ETHICS)

Pinch, Winifred J. Research and nursing: ethical reflections. *N and HC Perspectives on Community.* 1996 Jan–Feb; 17(1): 26–31.
(HUMAN EXPERIMENTATION/SPECIAL POPULATIONS)

Pinching, Anthony J. see Boyd, Kenneth M.

Pinkerton, JoAnn V.; Finnerty, James J.; Sosnowski, J. Richard. Resolving the clinical and ethical dilemma involved in fetal–maternal conflicts. [Article and discussion]. *American Journal of Obstetrics and Gynecology.* 1996 Aug; 175(2): 289–295.
(FETUSES; TREATMENT REFUSAL)

Pinkerton, JoAnn V. see Rorty, Mary V.

Pinkus, Rosa Lynn. Politics, paternalism, and the rise of the neurosurgeon: the evolution of moral reasoning. *Medical Humanities Review.* 1996 Fall; 10(2): 20–44.
(MEDICAL ETHICS; PATIENT CARE)

Pinnock, C.A. see Scott, P.V.

Piotrowski, Joseph J.; Akhrass, Rami; Alexander, J.J.; Yuhas, J.P.; Brandt, C.P.; Glover, John L. Rupture of known abdominal aortic aneurysms: an ethical dilemma. [Article and commentaries]. *American Surgeon.* 1995 Jul; 61(7): 556–559.
(PATIENT CARE/AGED; SELECTION FOR TREATMENT)

Pisani, F. see Elli, M.

Pizzulli, Francis see Andrews, Lori

Plackowski, Linda C. Ethics in the Work Environment: Applied Bioethics in the Hospital for Delta's Nursing Students. Springfield, VA: ERIC Document Reproduction Service; 1993 Jul. 15 p.

(NURSING ETHICS/EDUCATION)

Plant, Martin; Plant, Moira; Vernon, Bryan. Ethics, funding and alcohol research. *Alcohol and Alcoholism.* 1996 Jan; 31(1): 17–25.
(BEHAVIORAL RESEARCH; BIOMEDICAL RESEARCH; PROFESSIONAL ETHICS)

Plant, Moira see **Plant, Martin**

Plante, Thomas G. Training child clinical predoctoral interns and postdoctoral fellows in ethics and professional issues: an experimental model. *Professional Psychology: Research and Practice.* 1995 Dec; 26(6): 616–619.
(PROFESSIONAL ETHICS/EDUCATION)

Plotnikoff, Gregory A. Spirituality, religion, and the physician: new ethical challenges in patient care. *Bioethics Forum.* 1997 Winter; 13(4): 25–30.
(PATIENT CARE)

Pluhar, Evelyn. On the genetic manipulation of animals. *Between the Species.* 1985 Summer; 1(3): 13–18.
(GENETIC INTERVENTION)

Pochard, Frédéric; Grassin, Marc; Le Roux, Nadège; Hervé, Christian. Medical secrecy or disclosure in HIV transmission: a physician's ethical conflict. [Letter]. *Archives of Internal Medicine.* 1998 Aug 10–24; 158(14–15): 1716, 1719.
(AIDS/CONFIDENTIALITY)

Pochard, Frédéric see **Howard, Philip J.**

Podgers, James. Stepping carefully: [ABA] House of Delegates declines to endorse physician–assisted suicide. [Meeting report]. *ABA Journal: The Lawyer's Magazine.* 1997 Sep; 83: 94.
(SUICIDE)

Poets, C.F. see **Parkins, K.J.**

Poikonen, John; Haupt, Bridget A.; Veatch, Robert M. Preferential service for a powerful physician — Scenario; Position 1: pharmacist should serve physician immediately; Position 2: pharmacist should make physician wait; Analysis and commentary. *American Journal of Health–System Pharmacy.* 1996 Nov 1; 53(21): 2614–2618.
(PATIENT CARE/DRUGS; PROFESSIONAL ETHICS)

Pokorski, Robert J. A test for the insurance industry. *Nature.* 1998 Feb 26; 391(6670): 835–836.
(CONFIDENTIALITY; GENETIC SCREENING)

Poland. Law of 7 January 1993 on family planning, protection of human fetuses, and the conditions under which pregnancy termination is permissible. *International Digest of Health Legislation.* 1993; 44(2): 253–255.
(ABORTION/FOREIGN COUNTRIES; ABORTION/LEGAL ASPECTS)

Polenakovic, Momir see **Ivanovski, Ninoslav**

Poliwoda, Hubert see **Meran, Johannes Gobertus**

Polkinghorne, John. Cloning and the moral imperative. *In:* Cole-Turner, Ronald, ed. Human Cloning: Religious Responses. Louisville, KY: Westminister John Knox Press; 1997: 35–42.

(CLONING)

Pollán, Javier see **Bradley, Peter**

Poltawska, Wanda. The responsibility of the medical doctor and the life of the patient. *Dolentium Hominum: Church and Health in the World.* 1996; 31(11th Yr., No. 1): 137–140.
(MEDICAL ETHICS)

Ponděliček, Ivo; Königova, Radana. The problem of euthanasia and dysthanasia in burns. *Burns, Including Thermal Injury.* 1983 Sep; 10(1): 61–63.
(ALLOWING TO DIE)

Ponder, Bruce. Genetic testing for cancer risk. *Science.* 1997 Nov 7; 278(5340): 1050–1054.
(GENETIC SCREENING)

Poniatowski, Larry see **Worth–Staten, Patricia A.**

Pontén, Jan see **Wigzell, Hans**

Poorman, Mark see **Paris, John J.**

Popp, A. John see **Moore, Dale**

Porath, A. see **Frisho–Lima, P.**

Porsius, Arijan see **de Boer, Anthonius**

Porta, Fulvio see **Burgio, Giuseppe Roberto**

Portenoy, Russell K. Morphine infusions at the end of life: the pitfalls in reasoning from anecdote. [Commentary]. *Journal of Palliative Care.* 1996 Winter; 12(4): 44–46.
(EUTHANASIA; TERMINAL CARE)

Portenoy, Russell K.; Coyle, Nessa; Kash, Kathryn M.; Brescia, Frank; Scanlon, Colleen; O'Hare, Daniel; Misbin, Robert I.; Holland, Jimmie; Foley, Kathleen M. Determinants of the willingness to endorse assisted suicide: a survey of physicians, nurses, and social workers. *Psychosomatics.* 1997 May–Jun; 38(3): 277–287.
(SUICIDE)

Porter, Jean. Human need and natural law. *In:* Wildes, Kevin Wm., ed. Infertility: A Crossroad of Faith, Medicine, and Technology. Boston, MA: Kluwer Academic; 1997: 93–106.
(REPRODUCTIVE TECHNOLOGIES)

Porter, John. Reason, law and medicine: anencephalics as organ donors. *In:* McLean, Sheila A.M., ed. Contemporary Issues in Law, Medicine and Ethics. Brookfield, VT: Dartmouth; 1996: 163–178.
(ORGAN AND TISSUE DONATION)

Portillo, Carmen J. see **Barnes, Donelle M.**

Post, Edward R. see **Davis, Fran**

Post, Linda Farber; Dubler, Nancy Neveloff. Palliative care: a bioethical definition, principles, and clinical guidelines. *Bioethics Forum.* 1997 Fall; 13(3): 17–24.
(TERMINAL CARE)

Post, Stephen G. Baboon livers and the human good. *Archives of Surgery.* 1993 Feb; 128(2): 131–133.

D., eds. Medical Futility and the Evaluation of Life–Sustaining Interventions. New York, NY: Cambridge University Press; 1997: 136–154.
(ALLOWING TO DIE/LEGAL ASPECTS)

Pritchard, Jane. Codes of ethics. *In:* Chadwick, Ruth, ed. Encyclopedia of Applied Ethics, Volume 1. San Diego, CA: Academic Press; 1998: 527–533.
(PROFESSIONAL ETHICS/CODES OF ETHICS)

Pritchard, Jane. Ethical decision–making and the positive use of codes. *In:* Frith, Lucy, ed. Ethics and Midwifery: Issues in Contemporary Practice. Boston, MA: Butterworth–Heinemann; 1996: 189–204.
(NURSING ETHICS)

Privitera, Salvatore. Moral reasoning in bioethics and posterity. *In:* Agius, Emmanuel; Busuttil, Salvino, eds. Germ–Line Intervention and Our Responsibilities to Future Generations. Boston, MA: Kluwer Academic; 1998: 27–33.
(GENETIC INTERVENTION)

Proctor, Christopher J. Should industry sponsor research? Tobacco industry research: collaboration, not confrontation, is the best approach. *BMJ (British Medical Journal).* 1998 Aug 1; 317(7154): 333–334.
(BIOMEDICAL RESEARCH)

Proimos, J. see **Bach, F.H.**

Prokes, Mary Timothy. Technology and the lived body. *In: her* Toward a Theology of the Body. Grand Rapids, MI: W.B. Eerdmans; 1996: 104–117.
(BIOMEDICAL TECHNOLOGIES; PERSONHOOD)

Prosor, Ron; Malnick, Stephen D.H.; Mahler, Ch.; Summerfield, Derek. Medical ethics: the Israeli Medical Association. [Letters and response]. *Lancet.* 1997 Aug 30; 350(9078): 669–670.
(TORTURE)

Proud, Jean. Ethical issues concerning ultrasound in pregnancy. *In:* Frith, Lucy, ed. Ethics and Midwifery: Issues in Contemporary Practice. Boston, MA: Butterworth–Heinemann; 1996: 72–85.
(PRENATAL DIAGNOSIS)

Provisional Commission for the Study on Brain Death and Organ Transplantation (Japan). Important Considerations with Respect to Brain Death and Organ Transplants, January 22, 1992. Tokyo: the Commission; translation issued by the Osaka Kidney Foundation; 1994 Jun. 39 p.
(DETERMINATION OF DEATH/BRAIN DEATH; ORGAN AND TISSUE DONATION; ORGAN AND TISSUE TRANSPLANTATION)

Pruchnicki, Alec. First, do no harm (pending prior approval). [Irony]. *New England Journal of Medicine.* 1997 Nov 27; 337(22): 1627–1628.
(HEALTH CARE/ECONOMICS)

Prunier, Edward see **White, W.D.**

Przygoda, Pablo see **Bradley, Peter**

Purtilo, David T. see **Purtilo, Ruth**

Purtilo, Ruth; Shaw, Byers W.; Arnold, Robert. Obligations of surgeons to non-physician team members

and trainees. *In:* McCullough, Laurence B.; Jones, James W.; Brody, Baruch A., eds. Surgical Ethics. New York, NY: Oxford University Press; 1998: 302–321.
(PATIENT CARE)

Purtilo, Ruth; Sonnabend, Joseph; Purtilo, David T. Confidentiality, informed consent and untoward social consequences in research on a "new killer disease" (AIDS). *Clinical Research.* 1983 Oct; 31(4): 462–472.
(AIDS/CONFIDENTIALITY; AIDS/HUMAN EXPERIMENTATION; HUMAN EXPERIMENTATION/INFORMED CONSENT)

Purtilo, Ruth see **Arnold, Robert M.**

Putnam, Constance E. Who talks? Who listens? Who decides? Doctors and patients in discourse. *In:* van Eemeren, Frans H.; Grootendorst, Rob; Blair, J. Anthony; Willard, Charles A., eds. Special Fields and Cases: Proceedings of the Third ISSA [International Society for the Study of Argumentation] Conference on Argumentation, Volume IV. Amsterdam: International Centre for the Study of Argumentation; 1995: 412–423.
(PROFESSIONAL PATIENT RELATIONSHIP)

Pyers, Greg; Gott, Robert. Fertility Rights: The IVF Debate. Carlton, VIC, Australia: CIS Publishers; 1993. 49 p.
(EMBRYO AND FETAL RESEARCH; IN VITRO FERTILIZATION; REPRODUCTIVE TECHNOLOGIES)

Q

Qiu, Ren–Zong. Germ–line engineering as the eugenics of the future. *In:* Agius, Emmanuel; Busuttil, Salvino, eds. Germ–Line Intervention and Our Responsibilities to Future Generations. Boston, MA: Kluwer Academic; 1998: 105–116.
(EUGENICS; GENE THERAPY)

Quah, Stella R. Social and ethical aspects of organ donation. *Transplantation Proceedings.* 1992 Oct; 24(5): 2097–2098.
(ORGAN AND TISSUE DONATION)

Quattrone, Madelyn S. see **George, James E.**

Quill, Timothy see **Meier, Diane E.**

Quill, Timothy E. A physician's position on physician–assisted suicide. [Hearing testimony]. *Bulletin of the New York Academy of Medicine.* 1997 Summer; 74(1): 114–118.
(SUICIDE)

Quill, Timothy E.; Dresser, Rebecca; Brock, Dan W. The rule of double effect — a critique of its role in end–of–life decision making. *New England Journal of Medicine.* 1997 Dec 11; 337(24): 1768–1771.
(TERMINAL CARE)

Quill, Timothy E.; Kimsma, Gerrit. End–of–life care in the Netherlands and the United States: a comparison of values, justifications, and practices. *Cambridge Quarterly of Healthcare Ethics.* 1997 Spring; 6(2): 189–204.
(ALLOWING TO DIE; EUTHANASIA; SUICIDE; TERMINAL CARE)

Quill, Timothy E.; Lo, Bernard; Brock, Dan W. Palliative options of last resort: a comparison of voluntarily stopping eating and drinking, terminal sedation, physician–assisted suicide, and voluntary active

euthanasia. *JAMA.* 1997 Dec 17; 278(23): 2099–2104.
(ALLOWING TO DIE; EUTHANASIA; SUICIDE; TERMINAL CARE)

Quill, Timothy E.; Meier, Diane E.; Block, Susan D.; Billings, J. Andrew. The debate over physician–assisted suicide: empirical data and convergent views. *Annals of Internal Medicine.* 1998 Apr 1; 128(7): 552–558.
(SUICIDE; TERMINAL CARE)

Quinn, Kevin P. Assisted suicide and equal protection: in defense of the distinction between killing and letting die. *Issues in Law and Medicine.* 1997 Fall; 13(2): 145–171.
(ALLOWING TO DIE/LEGAL ASPECTS; SUICIDE)

Quintana, Octavi. Human tissue banks in Europe. *In:* Knoppers, Bartha Maria, ed. Human DNA: Law and Policy: International and Comparative Perspectives. Proceedings of the First International Conference on DNA Sampling and Human Genetic Research: Ethical, Legal, and Policy Aspects, held in Montreal, Canada, 6–8 Sep 1996. Boston, MA: Kluwer Law International; 1997: 423–427.
(GENETIC RESEARCH; ORGAN AND TISSUE DONATION)

Qunibi, Wajeh; Abulrub, Daad; Shaheen, Faisal; El-Din, A.B. Shehab; Alfurayh, Osman; Almeshari, Khalid. Attitudes of commercial renal transplant recipients toward renal transplantation in India. *Clinical Transplantation.* 1995 Aug; 9(4): 317–321.
(ORGAN AND TISSUE TRANSPLANTATION)

R

Rabbinical Assembly. Committee on Jewish Law and Standards. Jewish Medical Directives for Health Care. New York, NY: The Assembly; 1994 Jan. 16 p.
(ADVANCE DIRECTIVES)

Rabbit, Patrick see **Mead, Gillian E.**

Rachels, James. The principle of agency. *Bioethics.* 1998 Apr; 12(2): 150–161.
(BIOETHICS)

Rachels, Stuart. Is it good to make happy people? *Bioethics.* 1998 Apr; 12(2): 93–110.
(REPRODUCTION)

Radcliffe-Richards, J.; Daar, A.S.; Guttmann, R.D.; Hoffenberg, R.; Kennedy, I.; Lock, M.; Sells, R.A.; Tilney, N. The case for allowing kidney sales. [For the International Forum for Transplant Ethics]. *Lancet.* 1998 Jun 27; 351(9120): 1950–1952.
(ORGAN AND TISSUE DONATION)

Radcliffe-Richards, J. see **Hoffenberg, R.**

Radcliffe-Richards, J. see **Kennedy, I.**

Radin, Margaret Jane. Contested Commodities: The Trouble with Trade in Sex, Children, Body Parts, and Other Things. Cambridge, MA: Harvard University Press; 1996. 279 p.
(ORGAN AND TISSUE DONATION; SURROGATE MOTHERS)

Radin, Margaret Jane. What, if anything, is wrong with baby selling? *Pacific Law Journal.* 1995 Jan; 26(2): 135–145.
(SURROGATE MOTHERS)

Rae, Scott B. Parental rights and the definition of motherhood in surrogate motherhood. *Southern California Review of Law and Women's Studies.* 1994 Spring; 3(2): 219–277.
(SURROGATE MOTHERS)

Rae, Scott B. Prenatal genetic testing, abortion, and beyond. *In:* Kilner, John F.; Pentz, Rebecca D.; Young, Frank E., eds. Genetic Ethics: Do the Ends Justify the Genes? Grand Rapids, MI: W.B. Eerdmans; 1997: 136–145.
(ABORTION/RELIGIOUS ASPECTS; GENETIC SCREENING; PRENATAL DIAGNOSIS)

Raffin, Thomas A. see **Kelly, Susan E.**

Rafkin, Harry S.; Rainey, Thomas. Physicians and medical futility: experience in the critical care setting. *In:* Zucker, Marjorie B.; Zucker, Howard D., eds. Medical Futility and the Evaluation of Life–Sustaining Interventions. New York, NY: Cambridge University Press; 1997: 24–35.
(ALLOWING TO DIE)

Rafter, Nicole Hahn. Creating Born Criminals. Urbana, IL: University of Illinois Press; 1997. 284 p.
(BEHAVIORAL GENETICS; EUGENICS)

Rafuse, Jill. Revised Code of Ethics wins CMA approval. [News]. *Canadian Medical Association Journal.* 1996 Oct 15; 155(8): 1148–1149.
(MEDICAL ETHICS/CODES OF ETHICS)

Ragas, Rasa see **Jain, Renu**

RAGE (Radiotherapy Action Group Exposure) National [Great Britain]. All treatment and trials must have informed consent. [Personal view]. *BMJ (British Medical Journal).* 1997 Apr 12; 314(7087): 1134–1135.
(FRAUD AND MISCONDUCT; HUMAN EXPERIMENTATION/FOREIGN COUNTRIES; HUMAN EXPERIMENTATION/INFORMED CONSENT; HUMAN EXPERIMENTATION/SPECIAL POPULATIONS)

Ragoné, Helena see **Franklin, Sarah**

Räikkä, Juha. Freedom and a right (not) to know. *Bioethics.* 1998 Jan; 12(1): 49–63.
(GENETIC COUNSELING; TRUTH DISCLOSURE)

Rainey, Thomas see **Rafkin, Harry S.**

Raithatha, Nick see **Bradley, Peter**

Raizada, S.N. see **Kazim, E.**

Rajendran, Sasha see **Amu, Olubusola**

Ramogida, C. The views of the patients. *In:* Shenfield, F.; Sureau, C., eds. Ethical Dilemmas in Assisted Reproduction. New York, NY: Parthenon Pub. Group; 1997: 83–85.
(REPRODUCTIVE TECHNOLOGIES)

Ramsay, Lawrence E. see **Senn, Stephen**

Ramsay, M.P. see **Taylor, E.M.**

Ramsay, Sarah. UK public consulted on ethics of human cloning. [News]. *Lancet.* 1998 Feb 7; 351(9100): 427.
(CLONING)

Ramsay, Sarah. UK woman wins right to refuse caesarean section. [News]. *Lancet.* 1998 May 16; 351(9114): 1499.
(FETUSES; TREATMENT REFUSAL)

Ramsey, Gloria see **Mezey, Mathy**

Randall, Fiona. Why causing death is not necessarily morally equivalent to allowing to die -- a response to Ferguson. *Journal of Medical Ethics.* 1997 Dec; 23(6): 373–376.
(ALLOWING TO DIE/LEGAL ASPECTS; EUTHANASIA/LEGAL ASPECTS)

Rankine, James J. Most patients don't read the BMJ. [Personal view]. *BMJ (British Medical Journal).* 1998 Mar 28; 316(7136): 1026–1027.
(CONFIDENTIALITY; INFORMED CONSENT)

Rao, Narasinga see **Balentine, Jerry**

Raphael, D.D. see **Logmans, A.**

Rapin, M. The ethics of intensive care. [Editorial]. *Intensive Care Medicine.* 1987; 13(5): 300–303.
(ALLOWING TO DIE; SELECTION FOR TREATMENT)

Rapp, Suzanne see **Sullivan, Mark**

Rappaport, Michael see **Mezey, Mathy**

Rasheed, H.Z.A. Organ donation and transplantation -- a Muslim viewpoint. *Transplantation Proceedings.* 1992 Oct; 24(5): 2116–2117.
(ORGAN AND TISSUE DONATION)

Rasmussen, P. Elmegaard; Larsen, P. Munkholm; Nielsen, V.G.; Riis, P. Does physicians' knowledge of costing related to clinical decision making change the consumption of resources despite unchanged medical standards? *Scandinavian Journal of Gastroenterology.* 1985; 20(4): 401–406.
(HEALTH CARE/ECONOMICS; HEALTH CARE/FOREIGN COUNTRIES; RESOURCE ALLOCATION/BIOMEDICAL TECHNOLOGIES)

Ratain, M.J. see **Daugherty, C.K.**

Ratain, Mark J. see **Daugherty, Christopher**

Rathbone, Gillian see **Dunphy, Kilian**

Ravetz, J. see **Brunner, E.J.**

Ravindra, Ravi; Roach, Geshe Michael; LaFleur, William; Simmer-Brown, Judith; Gross, Rita M.; Weitsman, Sojun Mel. Buddhists on cloning. *In:* McGee, Glenn, ed. The Human Cloning Debate. Berkeley, CA: Berkeley Hills Books; 1998: 227–230.
(CLONING)

Rawlins, Richard see **Talbot, D.**

Rawls, John see **Dworkin, Ronald**

Ray, Peter N. see **Clarke, Joe T.R.**

Raymond, James I. see **Brett, Allan S.**

Rayner, Claire. A new ethics committee. *Bulletin of Medical Ethics.* 1997 May; No. 128: 20–21.
(ETHICISTS AND ETHICS COMMITTEES)

Read, William Allan. Hospital's Role in Resuscitation Decisions. [Booklet]. Chicago, IL: Hospital Research and Educational Trust; 1983. 14 p.
(RESUSCITATION ORDERS)

Reagan, James E.; Lomax, Karen J.; Nelson, William A. Clinical ethics in the Veterans Health Administration. *HEC (HealthCare Ethics Committee) Forum.* 1997 Jun; 9(2): 120–128.
(BIOETHICS; ETHICISTS AND ETHICS COMMITTEES)

Reagan, James E. see **Minogue, Brendan P.**

Reardon, Frank E. see **Paris, John J.**

Reaves, Randolph P. see **Bass, Larry J.**

Reding, Douglas see **Weeks, Jane C.**

Redmayne, Sharon see **Klein, Rudolph**

Reed, Richard see **Ventres, William**

Rees, Gareth see **Cressey, David M.**

Rees, Grover Joseph see **Sills, E. Scott**

Regan, Tom. The rights of humans and other animals. *Ethics and Behavior.* 1997; 7(2): 103–111.
(ANIMAL EXPERIMENTATION)

Reich, Elsa; Zanko, Andrea; Heimler, Audrey. Testing for HD in twins. [Letter and response]. *Journal of Genetic Counseling.* 1996 Mar; 5(1): 47–51.
(GENETIC COUNSELING; GENETIC SCREENING)

Reichman, Edward. The rabbinic conception of conception: an exercise in fertility. *In:* Feldman, Emanuel; Wolowelsky, Joel B., eds. Jewish Law and the New Reproductive Technologies. Hoboken, NJ: Ktav; 1997: 1–35.
(ARTIFICIAL INSEMINATION; REPRODUCTION)

Reichman, Lee B. Defending the public's health against tuberculosis. [Editorial]. *JAMA.* 1997 Sep 10; 278(10): 865–867.
(PUBLIC HEALTH)

Reid, Margaret see **Drake, Harriet**

Reilly, Philip R. Laws to regulate the use of genetic information. *In:* Rothstein, Mark A., ed. Genetic Secrets: Protecting Privacy and Confidentiality in the Genetic Era. New Haven, CT: Yale University Press; 1997: 369–391.
(CONFIDENTIALITY; GENETIC SCREENING)

Reilly, Philip R. see **Wertz, Dorothy C.**

Reiman, Jeffrey. On euthanasia and health care. *In: his* Critical Moral Liberalism: Theory and Practice. Lanham, MD: Rowman and Littlefield; 1997: 211–219.
(EUTHANASIA; HEALTH CARE; RESOURCE ALLOCATION)

Reimshisel, Tyler see **Meadow, William**

Reinders, Hans S. see **d'Oronzio, Joseph C.**

Reinhard, John see Kinmonth, Ann Louise

Reinhardt, Uwe E. Wanted: a clearly articulated social ethic for American health care. *JAMA.* 1997 Nov 5; 278(17): 1446–1447.
(HEALTH CARE/ECONOMICS; RESOURCE ALLOCATION)

Reinhardt, Uwe E. see Altman, Stuart H.

Reinhardt, Uwe E. see Yaes, Robert J.

Reisman, Joseph M. Physicians and surgeons as inventors: reconciling medical process patents and medical ethics. [Comment]. *High Technology Law Journal.* 1995; 10(2): 355–403.
(BIOMEDICAL TECHNOLOGIES)

Reisner, Michelle; Damato, Anthony N. Attitudes of physicians regarding physician–assisted suicide. *New Jersey Medicine.* 1995 Oct; 92(10): 663–666.
(SUICIDE)

Reiss, Michael. Biotechnology. *In:* Chadwick, Ruth, ed. Encyclopedia of Applied Ethics, Volume 1. San Diego, CA: Academic Press; 1998: 319–333.
(BIOMEDICAL TECHNOLOGIES; GENE THERAPY; GENETIC INTERVENTION; RECOMBINANT DNA RESEARCH)

Reiss, Michael J. Is it right to patent DNA? *Bulletin of Medical Ethics.* 1997 Jan; No. 124: 21–24.
(PATENTING LIFE FORMS)

Reitemeier, Paul J. Musings on medical mistakes: a four–piece ensemble in search of an orchestra. *Journal of Clinical Ethics.* 1997 Winter; 8(4): 353–358.
(BIOETHICS; ETHICISTS AND ETHICS COMMITTEES; PATIENT CARE; TRUTH DISCLOSURE)

Reitman, James S. The debate on assisted suicide –– redefining morally appropriate care for people with intractable suffering. *Issues in Law and Medicine.* 1995 Winter; 11(3): 299–329.
(SUICIDE; TERMINAL CARE)

Reitman, James S. The dilemma of "medical futility": a "wisdom model" for decisionmaking. *Issues in Law and Medicine.* 1996 Winter; 12(3): 231–264.
(ALLOWING TO DIE)

Reitman, James S. see Calhoun, Byron C.

Relman, Arnold S. The economic future of health care: *False Hopes: Why America's Quest for Perfect Health Is a Recipe for Failure,* by Daniel Callahan, and *Life without Disease: The Pursuit of Medical Utopia,* by William B. Schwartz. [Book review essay]. *New England Journal of Medicine.* 1998 Jun 18; 338(25): 1855–1856.
(HEALTH CARE/ECONOMICS; RESOURCE ALLOCATION)

Relman, Arnold S.; Lundberg, George D. Business and professionalism in medicine at the American Medical Association. *JAMA.* 1998 Jan 14; 279(2): 169–170.
(HEALTH CARE/ECONOMICS)

Rempusheski, Veronica F. see Hurley, Ann C.

Renfrew, Mary J. see Entwistle, Vikki A.

Rennie, Drummond. Dealing with research misconduct in the United Kingdom: an American perspective on research integrity. *BMJ (British Medical Journal).* 1998 Jun 6; 316(7146): 1726–1728.
(BIOMEDICAL RESEARCH; FRAUD AND MISCONDUCT)

Rennie, Drummond see DeGroot, Leslie J.

Rennie, Drummond see Flanagin, Annette

Rennie, Drummond see Olson, Carin M.

Resta, Robert G. Eugenics and nondirectiveness in genetic counseling. *Journal of Genetic Counseling.* 1997 Jun; 6(2): 255–258.
(EUGENICS; GENETIC COUNSELING)

Rétfalvi, Teréz see Bass, Larry J.

Reynolds, D.J.M. see Talbot, D.

Reynolds, Fiona see Basketter, David

Rezacova, Jitka see Mardesic, Tonko

Rhoden, Nancy K. Treatment dilemmas for imperiled newborns: why quality of life counts. *Southern California Law Review.* 1985 Sep; 58(6): 1283–1347.
(ALLOWING TO DIE/INFANTS; ALLOWING TO DIE/LEGAL ASPECTS)

Rhodes, Genice L. see Mowbray, Carol T.

Rhodes, Rosamond. Futility and the goals of medicine. *Journal of Clinical Ethics.* 1998 Summer; 9(2): 194–205.
(ALLOWING TO DIE)

Rhodes, Rosamond. Genetic links, family ties, and social bonds: rights and responsibilities in the face of genetic knowledge. *Journal of Medicine and Philosophy.* 1998 Feb; 23(1): 10–30.
(GENETIC COUNSELING; GENETIC SCREENING; TRUTH DISCLOSURE)

Rhodes, Rosamond. Physicians, assisted suicide, and the right to live or die. *In:* Battin, Margaret P.; Rhodes, Rosamond; Silvers, Anita, eds. Physician Assisted Suicide: Expanding the Debate. New York, NY: Routledge; 1998: 165–176.
(EUTHANASIA; SUICIDE)

Rhodes, Rosamond see Battin, Margaret P.

Rhodes, Rosamond see Moros, Daniel A.

Ribbe, Miel W. see Muller, Martien T.

Ribbe, Miel W. see Onwuteaka–Philipsen, Bregje D.

Rice, John see Sherman, Stephanie L.

Rich, Ann; Parker, David L. Reflection and critical incident analysis: ethical and moral implications of their use within nursing and midwifery education. *Journal of Advanced Nursing.* 1995 Dec; 22(6): 1050–1057.
(NURSING ETHICS/EDUCATION)

Rich, Ben A. A legacy of silence: bioethics and the culture of pain. *Journal of Medical Humanities.* 1997 Winter; 18(4): 233–259.
(BIOETHICS; PATIENT CARE; TERMINAL CARE)

Rich, Ben A. Advance directives: the next generation. *Journal of Legal Medicine.* 1998 Mar; 19(1): 63–97.

Robertson, B.A. see **Henley, L.**

Robertson, John A. Ethical and legal issues in human embryo donation. *Fertility and Sterility.* 1995 Nov; 64(5): 885–894.
(REPRODUCTIVE TECHNOLOGIES)

Robertson, John A. Human cloning and the challenge of regulation. *New England Journal of Medicine.* 1998 Jul 9; 339(2): 119–122.
(CLONING)

Robertson, John A. Innovations in infertility treatment and the rush to market. *Women's Health Issues.* 1997 May–Jun; 7(3): 162–166.
(REPRODUCTIVE TECHNOLOGIES)

Robertson, John A. Liberty, identity, and human cloning. *Texas Law Review.* 1998 May; 76(6): 1371–1456.
(CLONING; REPRODUCTION)

Robertson, John A. Meaning what you sign. *Hastings Center Report.* 1998 Jul–Aug; 28(4): 22–23.
(FETUSES; IN VITRO FERTILIZATION)

Robertson, John A. see **Annas, George J.**

Robertson, John A. see **Goldworth, Amnon**

Robertson, John A. see **Jones, Howard**

Robinowitz, Jane see **Eng, Christine M.**

Robinson, Franklin see **Muehleman, Thomas**

Robinson, Sarah see **Grubb, Andrew**

Robinson, Walter see **Blustein, Jeffrey**

Robson, Philip. Cannabis as medicine: time for the phoenix to rise? [Editorial]. *BMJ (British Medical Journal).* 1998 Apr 4; 316(7137): 1034–1035.
(PATIENT CARE/DRUGS)

Robson, S.C. see **Bach, F.H.**

Roche, Patricia (Winnie). Caveat venditor: protecting privacy and ownership interests in DNA. *In:* Knoppers, Bartha Maria, ed. Human DNA: Law and Policy: International and Comparative Perspectives. Proceedings of the First International Conference on DNA Sampling and Human Genetic Research: Ethical, Legal, and Policy Aspects, held in Montreal, Canada, 6–8 Sep 1996. Boston, MA: Kluwer Law International; 1997: 33–41.
(CONFIDENTIALITY/LEGAL ASPECTS; GENETIC RESEARCH; GENETIC SCREENING)

Rodgers, Bruce D.; Rodgers, Diane E. Abortion: the seduction of medicine. *Liberty, Life and Family.* 1996; 2(2): 285–308.
(ABORTION)

Rodgers, Diane E. see **Rodgers, Bruce D.**

Rodgers, Sanda see **Flagler, Elizabeth**

Rodriguez, Eduardo. The Human Genome Project and eugenics. *Linacre Quarterly.* 1998 May; 65(2): 73–82.
(EUGENICS; GENETIC SCREENING)

Rodriguez, Eric see **Silverman, Myrna**

Rodwin, Marc A. Conflicts of interest and accountability in managed care: the aging of medical ethics. *Journal of the American Geriatrics Society.* 1998 Mar; 46(3): 338–341.
(HEALTH CARE/ECONOMICS)

Roeper, Burkhardt. Germany approves DNA tests for visas. [News]. *Nature.* 1998 Feb 19; 391(6669): 723.
(DNA FINGERPRINTING; GENETIC SCREENING)

Roger, Steve see **Oscherwitz, Tom**

Rogers, Arthur. Britain denies prevarication over human-cloning ban. [News]. *Lancet.* 1997 Oct 18; 350(9085): 1151.
(CLONING)

Rogers, Arthur. Europe takes steps to outlaw human cloning. [News]. *Lancet.* 1997 Oct 4; 350(9083): 1012.
(CLONING)

Rogers, Arthur. Europe-wide blood-donor system debated. [News]. *Lancet.* 1998 Apr 11; 351(9109): 1112.
(BLOOD DONATION)

Rogers, Arthur. European drug industry concerned over proposed clinical-trial legislation. [News]. *Lancet.* 1997 Nov 29; 350(9091): 1609.
(HUMAN EXPERIMENTATION/FOREIGN COUNTRIES; HUMAN EXPERIMENTATION/REGULATION)

Rogers, Arthur. European Parliament approves intellectual property rights directive. [News]. *Lancet.* 1997 Jul 26; 350(9073): 272.
(GENETIC INTERVENTION; PATENTING LIFE FORMS)

Rogers, Arthur. European Union approves gene-patent directive. [News]. *Lancet.* 1998 May 16; 351(9114): 1500.
(PATENTING LIFE FORMS)

Rogers, Connie S. see **Davis, Fran**

Rogers, Jill Cellars see **Begleiter, Michael L.**

Rohan, Kelly J. see **Sigmon, Sandra T.**

Roizen, Michael F. see **Sandberg, Warren S.**

Roleff, Tamara L., ed. Biomedical Ethics: Opposing Viewpoints. San Diego, CA: Greenhaven Press; 1998. 252 p.
(BIOETHICS; GENETIC INTERVENTION; GENETIC RESEARCH; ORGAN AND TISSUE DONATION; REPRODUCTIVE TECHNOLOGIES)

Roll-Hansen, Nils see **Broberg, Gunnar**

Rolleston, Francis; Armour, Catherine; Stipich, Nina. Developing a Tri-Council code of conduct for research involving humans. *International Journal of Bioethics.* 1997 Mar–Jun; 8(1–2): 67–70.
(HUMAN EXPERIMENTATION/FOREIGN COUNTRIES; HUMAN EXPERIMENTATION/REGULATION)

Rollin, Bernard E. Laws relevant to animal research in the United States. *In:* Tuffery, A.A., ed. Laboratory Animals: An Introduction for Experimenters. Second Edition. New York, NY: Wiley; 1995: 67–86.
(ANIMAL EXPERIMENTATION)

Rom, Mark Carl. Fatal Extraction: The Story Behind the Florida Dentist Accused of Infecting His Patients with HIV and Poisoning Public Health. San Francisco, CA: Jossey–Bass Publishers; 1997. 226 p.
(AIDS/HEALTH PERSONNEL; PUBLIC HEALTH)

Roman, Brenda; Kay, Jerald. Residency education on the prevention of physician–patient sexual misconduct. *Academic Psychiatry.* 1997 Spring; 21(1): 26–34.
(FRAUD AND MISCONDUCT; PROFESSIONAL PATIENT RELATIONSHIP)

Rooney, Anne L. see **Duffy, Barbara**

Rooney, Brenda L. see **Hammes, Bernard J.**

Rorty, Mary V.; Pinkerton, JoAnn V. Elective fetal reduction: the ultimate elective surgery. *Journal of Contemporary Health Law and Policy.* 1996 Fall; 13(1): 53–77.
(ABORTION)

Rosadino, Michael J. see **Kirsch, Irving**

Rose, John C. Animals in research: an investigator's perspective. *Pharos.* 1985 Fall; 48(4): 19–22.
(ANIMAL EXPERIMENTATION)

Rose, Mary R.; Fischer, Karla. Do authorship policies impact students' judgments of perceived wrongdoing? *Ethics and Behavior.* 1998; 8(1): 59–79.
(BEHAVIORAL RESEARCH; FRAUD AND MISCONDUCT)

Rose, Teresa see **Stadler, Holly A.**

Rosen, Jeffrey. What right to die? *New Republic.* 1996 Jun 24; 214(26): 28–31.
(SUICIDE)

Rosen, Linda. Reporting incompetent or unethical behavior: an ethical and legal dilemma. *Today's OR Nurse.* 1985 Oct; 7(10): 36–37.
(FRAUD AND MISCONDUCT)

Rosenberg, Esther see **Schneiderman, Lawrence J.**

Rosenbloom, Lewis; Sullivan, Peter B. The ethics and implications of treatment programmes for disabled children with feeding difficulties. *In:* Sullivan, Peter B.; Rosenbloom, Lewis, eds. Feeding the Disabled Child. New York, NY: Cambridge University Press; 1996: 151–156.
(PATIENT CARE/MINORS)

Rosenfeld, Azriel. Generation, gestation, and Judaism. *In:* Feldman, Emanuel; Wolowelsky, Joel B., eds. Jewish Law and the New Reproductive Technologies. Hoboken, NJ: Ktav; 1997: 36–45.
(SURROGATE MOTHERS)

Rosenfeld, Barry D. see **Chochinov, Harvey Max**

Rosenkoetter, Marlene Merifield. A code of ethics for nurse educators. *Nursing Outlook.* 1983 Sep–Oct; 31(5): 288.
(NURSING ETHICS/CODES OF ETHICS; NURSING ETHICS/EDUCATION)

Rosenthal, Elisabeth. For one-child policy, China rethinks iron hand. [News]. *New York Times.* 1998 Nov 1: 1, 20.

(POPULATION CONTROL)

Rosenthal, Gary E. see **Shepardson, Laura B.**

Rosenthal, Nadia A. see **Kassirer, Jerome P.**

Roses, Allen D. see **Thomas, A. Mathew**

Rosin, Arnold J.; Sonnenblick, Moshe. Autonomy and paternalism in geriatric medicine: the Jewish ethical approach to issues of feeding terminally ill patients, and to cardiopulmonary resuscitation. *Journal of Medical Ethics.* 1998 Feb; 24(1): 44–48.
(ALLOWING TO DIE/RELIGIOUS ASPECTS; RESUSCITATION ORDERS; TERMINAL CARE)

Rosner, Fred. Euthanasia. *In:* Dorff, Elliot N.; Newman, Louis E., eds. Contemporary Jewish Ethics and Morality: A Reader. New York, NY: Oxford University Press; 1995: 350–362.
(ALLOWING TO DIE/RELIGIOUS ASPECTS; EUTHANASIA/RELIGIOUS ASPECTS)

Rosner, Fred. Informing the patient of a fatal illness. [Letter]. *Archives of Internal Medicine.* 1986 Feb; 146(2): 413.
(TRUTH DISCLOSURE)

Rosner, Fred. Involuntary confinement for tuberculosis control: the Jewish view. *Mount Sinai Journal of Medicine.* 1996 Jan; 63(1): 44–48.
(PUBLIC HEALTH)

Rosner, Fred. Medical confidentiality in Judaism. *Journal of Halacha and Contemporary Society.* 1997 Spring; No. 33: 5–15.
(CONFIDENTIALITY)

Rosner, Fred; Kark, Pieter; Packer, Samuel. Oregon's health care rationing plan. *Journal of General Internal Medicine.* 1996 Feb; 11(2): 104–108.
(HEALTH CARE/ECONOMICS; RESOURCE ALLOCATION)

Rosner, Fred; Widroff, Jacob. Physician's fees in Jewish law. *In:* Jewish Law Annual. Volume Twelve. Amsterdam, Netherlands: Harwood Academic Publishers; 1997: 115–126.
(HEALTH CARE/ECONOMICS)

Rosner, Fred see **Berger, Jeffrey T.**

Ross, Lainie F. see **Hall, Spencer A.**

Ross, Lainie Friedman. Health care decisionmaking by children: is it in their best interest? *Hastings Center Report.* 1997 Nov–Dec; 27(6): 41–45.
(INFORMED CONSENT/MINORS; TREATMENT REFUSAL/MINORS)

Ross, Lainie Friedman see **Logmans, A.**

Ross, Lainie Friedman see **Sells, Robert A.**

Ross, Lena B.; Roy, Manisha, eds. Cast the First Stone: Ethics in Analytic Practice. Wilmette, IL: Chiron Publications; 1995. 146 p.
(FRAUD AND MISCONDUCT; PROFESSIONAL ETHICS; PROFESSIONAL PATIENT RELATIONSHIP)

Ross, Michael W. The ethics of experiments on higher animals. *Social Science and Medicine.* 1981; 15F: 51–60.
(ANIMAL EXPERIMENTATION; BEHAVIORAL RESEARCH)

(GENETIC RESEARCH; GENETIC SCREENING)

Roy, Ina. Philosophical perspectives. *In:* McGee, Glenn, ed. The Human Cloning Debate. Berkeley, CA: Berkeley Hills Books; 1998: 41–66.
(CLONING)

Roy, Manisha see **Ross, Lena B.**

Royal Australasian College of Surgeons. Code of Ethics. *Archives of Surgery.* 1996 Aug; 131(8): 900–901.
(MEDICAL ETHICS/CODES OF ETHICS)

Royal, Michael C. see **Goldstein, Barry**

Royal Pharmaceutical Society of Great Britain. Medicines, Ethics and Practice: A Guide for Pharmacists. Number 17. London: The Society; 1996 Oct. 124 p.
(PATIENT CARE/DRUGS; PROFESSIONAL ETHICS/CODES OF ETHICS)

Royce, Sarah see **Oscherwitz, Tom**

Rozin, Paul see **Brandt, Allan M.**

Rozmiarek, Harry. Animal welfare regulations and accreditation by the American Association for Accreditation of Laboratory Animal Care: impact on chimpanzees in research. *In:* Eder, G.; Kaiser, E.; King, F.A., eds. The Role of the Chimpanzee in Research. Symposium, Vienna, Austria, May 22–24, 1992. New York, NY: Karger; 1994: 26–33.
(ANIMAL EXPERIMENTATION)

Rubenfeld, Gordon D. see **Curtis, J. Randall**

Rubenstein, Donald S. Response to "Dimensions and classification of genetic interventions in the human genome," by Matthew D. Bacchetta and Gerd Richter (*CQ* Vol. 5, No. 3): misinterpretations and misrepresentations. *Cambridge Quarterly of Healthcare Ethics.* 1998 Winter; 7(1): 90–93.
(GENE THERAPY)

Rubenstein, Leonard S. see **Levy, Robert M.**

Rubenstein, William B.; Eisenberg, Ruth; Gostin, Lawrence O. The Rights of People Who Are HIV Positive: The Authoritative ACLU Guide to the Rights of People Living with HIV Disease and AIDS. Carbondale, IL: Southern Illinois University Press; 1996. 384 p.
(AIDS)

Rubin, Peter see **Irving, Miles**

Rubin, Susan B. When Doctors Say No: The Battleground of Medical Futility. Bloomington, IN: Indiana University Press; 1998. 191 p.
(ALLOWING TO DIE)

Rubin, Susan B. see **Zoloth-Dorfman, Laurie**

Rucquoi, Jodi see **Saxton, Marsha**

Rudberg, Mark A.; Teno, Joan M.; Lynn, Joanne; American Geriatrics Society. Ethics Committee. Developing and implementing measures of quality of care at the end of life: a call for action. *Journal of the American Geriatrics Society.* 1997 Apr; 45(4): 528–530.

(TERMINAL CARE)

Ruffin, Mack T. see **Doukas, David J.**

al-Rukaimi, M. see **Kazim, E.**

Rundall, Patti. Should industry sponsor research? How much research in infant feeding comes from unethical marketing? *BMJ (British Medical Journal).* 1998 Aug 1; 317(7154): 338–339.
(BIOMEDICAL RESEARCH)

Runkle, Deborah; Granger, Ellen. Animal rights: teaching or deceiving kids. [Editorial]. *Science.* 1997 Sep 5; 277(5331): 1419.
(ANIMAL EXPERIMENTATION)

Rush, Sharon Elizabeth. Breaking with tradition: surrogacy and gay fathers. *In:* Meyers, Diana Tietjens; Kipnis, Kenneth; Murphy, Cornelius F., eds. Kindred Matters: Rethinking the Philosophy of the Family. Ithaca, NY: Cornell University Press; 1993: 102–142.
(REPRODUCTION; SURROGATE MOTHERS)

Rushton, Cindy Hylton; Armstrong, Linda; McEnhill, Marilyn. Establishing therapeutic boundaries as patient advocates. *Pediatric Nursing.* 1996 May–Jun; 22(3): 185–189.
(PROFESSIONAL PATIENT RELATIONSHIP)

Rushton, Cindy Hylton; Infante, Marie C. Keeping secrets: the ethical and legal challenges. *Pediatric Nursing.* 1995 Sep–Oct; 21(5): 479–482.
(CONFIDENTIALITY)

Rushton, Cindy Hylton; Russell, Kathleen. The language of miracles: ethical challenges. *Pediatric Nursing.* 1996 Jan–Feb; 22(1): 64–67.
(ALLOWING TO DIE/RELIGIOUS ASPECTS)

Ruskin, Andrew. Capitation: the legal implications of using capitation to affect physician decision-making processes. *Journal of Contemporary Health Law and Policy.* 1997 Spring; 13(2): 391–421.
(HEALTH CARE/ECONOMICS; PATIENT CARE)

Russell, Claire see **Balls, Michael**

Russell, Jan see **Smith, Katharine V.**

Russell, Kathleen see **Rushton, Cindy Hylton**

Russell, Phillip K. Development of vaccines to meet public health needs: incentives and obstacles. *Risk: Health, Safety and Environment.* 1996 Summer; 7(3): 239–252.
(IMMUNIZATION)

Russell, Steven; Gilson, Lucy. User fee policies to promote health service access for the poor: a wolf in sheep's clothing? *International Journal of Health Services.* 1997; 27(2): 359–379.
(HEALTH CARE/ECONOMICS)

Russell, William M.S. see **Balls, Michael**

Russian Federation. Law of 2 July 1992 of the Russian Federation on psychiatric care and the safeguarding of citizens' rights in the dispensing of such care. *International Digest of Health Legislation.* 1993; 44(2): 267–281.

Christian bioethics. *Christian Bioethics.* 1997 Mar; 3(1): 20–38.
(PATIENT CARE)

Salomon, Daniel R. see **Daar, A.S.**

Saltzman, Steven L. see **Ehleben, Carole M.**

Sam, Mehran see **Kohut, Nitsa**

Samet, Jeffrey H. see **Stein, Michael D.**

Samet, Jonathan M.; Bailey, Linda A. Environmental population screening. *In:* Rothstein, Mark A., ed. Genetic Secrets: Protecting Privacy and Confidentiality in the Genetic Era. New Haven, CT: Yale University Press; 1997: 197–211.
(CONFIDENTIALITY; GENETIC RESEARCH)

Sampson, Mark T. Revised liver policy approved. *UNOS Update.* 1997 Jan–Feb: 5–7.
(ORGAN AND TISSUE TRANSPLANTATION; RESOURCE ALLOCATION/BIOMEDICAL TECHNOLOGIES; SELECTION FOR TREATMENT)

Samuel, Steven E. see **Gorton, Gregg E.**

Samuels, Patricia see **Harris, Yvonne**

Sandberg, Elisabeth H. see **Sandberg, Warren S.**

Sandberg, Warren S.; Carlos, Ruth; Sandberg, Elisabeth H.; Roizen, Michael F. The effect of educational gifts from pharmaceutical firms on medical students' recall of company names or products. *Academic Medicine.* 1997 Oct; 72(10): 916–918.
(HEALTH CARE/ECONOMICS; MEDICAL ETHICS/EDUCATION; PATIENT CARE/DRUGS)

Sandel, Michael J. The hard questions: last rights. *New Republic.* 1997 Apr 14; 216(16): 27.
(SUICIDE)

Sanders, Lee M. see **Kelly, Susan E.**

Sanfilippo, Alfred. Optimizing the quality of health care through better communication: case conferences. *HEC (HealthCare Ethics Committee) Forum.* 1997 Sep; 9(3): 256–263.
(ETHICISTS AND ETHICS COMMITTEES)

Sanson–Fisher, Rob W. see **Girgis, Afaf**

Sansone, Paulette; Phillips, Michael. Advance directives for elderly people: worthwhile cause or wasted effort? *Social Work.* 1995 May; 40(3): 397–401.
(ADVANCE DIRECTIVES; ALLOWING TO DIE/ATTITUDES)

Sansone, Paulette; Schmitt, Louise. Assessing values: the neglected dimension in long–term care. *HEC (HealthCare Ethics Committee) Forum.* 1997 Sep; 9(3): 264–275.
(ADVANCE DIRECTIVES)

Santalahti, Päivi see **Hemminki, Elina**

Sapin, Emmanuel. The horizons of fetal medicine and its ethical consequences. *Dolentium Hominum: Church and Health in the World.* 1996; 31(11th Yr., No. 1): 155–158.
(FETUSES; PRENATAL DIAGNOSIS)

Sapru, R.P. Ethical concerns in modern medical practice. *Indian Heart Journal.* 1997 Jul–Aug; 49(4): 441–445.
(HEALTH CARE/FOREIGN COUNTRIES; MEDICAL ETHICS; PATIENT CARE)

Sargent, Carolyn F.; Brettell, Caroline B., eds. Gender and Health: An International Perspective. Upper Saddle River, NJ: Prentice Hall; 1996. 370 p.
(HEALTH; HEALTH CARE)

Sasakabe, Sumiko see **Asai, Atsushi**

Sass, Hans–Martin. Advance directives. *In:* Chadwick, Ruth, ed. Encyclopedia of Applied Ethics, Volume 1. San Diego, CA: Academic Press; 1998: 41–49.
(ADVANCE DIRECTIVES)

Sass, Hans–Martin. Images of killing and letting–die, of self–determination and beneficence: the ethical debate on advance directives and surrogate decision making in Germany. *In:* Sass, Hans–Martin; Veatch, Robert M.; Kimura, Rihito, eds. Advance Directives and Surrogate Decision Making in Health Care: United States, Germany, and Japan. Baltimore, MD: Johns Hopkins University Press; 1998: 136–172.
(ADVANCE DIRECTIVES; ALLOWING TO DIE)

Sass, Hans–Martin, comp. Model forms of advance directives and advance care documents. *In:* Sass, Hans–Martin; Veatch, Robert M.; Kimura, Rihito, eds. Advance Directives and Surrogate Decision Making in Health Care: United States, Germany, and Japan. Baltimore, MD: Johns Hopkins University Press; 1998: 223–278.
(ADVANCE DIRECTIVES)

Sass, Hans–Martin. Moral risk assessment in biotechnology. *In:* Becker, Gerhold K., ed. Changing Nature's Course: The Ethical Challenge of Biotechnology. Hong Kong: Hong Kong University Press; 1996: 127–144.
(GENETIC INTERVENTION)

Sass, Hans–Martin; Veatch, Robert M.; Kimura, Rihito, eds. Advance Directives and Surrogate Decision Making in Health Care: United States, Germany, and Japan. Baltimore, MD: Johns Hopkins University Press; 1998. 311 p.
(ADVANCE DIRECTIVES)

Satcher, David see **Varmus, Harold**

Satel, Sally L. Science by quota: P.C. medicine. *New Republic.* 1995 Feb 27; 212(9): 14, 16.
(HUMAN EXPERIMENTATION/SPECIAL POPULATIONS)

Sauer, Mark V. Should egg donors be paid? Exploitation or a woman's right? *BMJ (British Medical Journal).* 1997 May 10; 314(7091): 1403.
(ORGAN AND TISSUE DONATION; REPRODUCTIVE TECHNOLOGIES)

Saum, Christine A. see **Inciardi, James A.**

Saunders, Donald E. see **Brett, Allan S.**

Saunders, Douglas M. see **Bowen, Jennifer R.**

Saunders, Michael see **Savulescu, Julian**

Savage, Wendy. Taking liberties with women: abortion,

sterilization, and contraception. *International Journal of Health Services.* 1982; 12(2): 293–308.
(CONTRACEPTION; STERILIZATION)

Savetsky, Jacqueline see **Stein, Michael D.**

Savolainen, Pirkko see **Töyry, Eeva**

Savulescu, Julian. Consequentialism, reasons, value and justice. *Bioethics.* 1998 Jul; 12(3): 212–235.
(HEALTH CARE; RESOURCE ALLOCATION; SELECTION FOR TREATMENT)

Savulescu, Julian; Chalmers, Iain; Blunt, Jennifer. Does setting good practice standards for research ethics committees increase their legal liability? [Letter]. *BMJ (British Medical Journal).* 1997 Jun 21; 314(7097): 1833.
(HUMAN EXPERIMENTATION/ETHICS COMMITTEES)

Savulescu, Julian; Marsden, Rachel; Hope, Tony; Saunders, Michael; Carlyle, Ruth; Gough, Pippa; Annas, George J. Respect for privacy and the case of Mr. K. [Article and commentaries]. *BMJ (British Medical Journal).* 1998 Mar 21; 316(7135): 921–924.
(PATIENTS' RIGHTS)

Savulescu, Julian; Momeyer, Richard W. Should informed consent be based on rational beliefs? *Journal of Medical Ethics.* 1997 Oct; 23(5): 282–288.
(INFORMED CONSENT; TREATMENT REFUSAL)

Savulescu, Julian see **Blunt, Jennifer**

Savulescu, Julian see **Parkins, K.J.**

Sawada, Kiyomi see **Asai, Atsushi**

Sawyer, Jill C. see **McKinnon, Wendy C.**

Saxton, Marsha; Anderson, Betsy; Blatt, Robin J.R.; Ayers, Karen; Finnegan, Joanne; Thayer, Barbara; Ciarleglio, Leslie; Rucquoi, Jodi. Prenatal diagnosis and pregnancy options. *Genetic Resource.* 1991; 6(1): 31–42.
(GENETIC COUNSELING; PRENATAL DIAGNOSIS)

Sayers, Gwen M.; Schofield, Irene; Aziz, Michael. An analysis of CPR decision-making by elderly patients. *Journal of Medical Ethics.* 1997 Aug; 23(4): 207–212.
(RESUSCITATION ORDERS)

Sayles, Linda see **Corley, Mary C.**

Sazama, Kathleen; Lind, Stuart E. Cord blood stem cells belong to the infant, not to the mother. [Letter and response]. *Transfusion.* 1995 Nov–Dec; 35(11): 967.
(BLOOD DONATION)

Scandinavian Nursing Cooperative. Etiska riklinjer för omvårdnadsforskning i Norden [Ethical guidelines for nursing research]. *Vard i Norden.* 1987 Autumn; 7(3–4): 429–430.
(HUMAN EXPERIMENTATION; NURSING ETHICS)

Scanlon, Colleen; Glover, Jacqueline. A professional code of ethics: providing a moral compass for turbulent times. *Oncology Nursing Forum.* 1995 Nov–Dec; 22(10): 1515–1521.
(NURSING ETHICS/CODES OF ETHICS)

Scanlon, Colleen see **Portenoy, Russell K.**

Scanlon, Thomas see **Dworkin, Ronald**

Scardino, Peter see **Lustig, Andrew**

Schaffner, Kenneth F. Ethically optimizing clinical trials. *In:* Kadane, Joseph B., ed. Bayesian Methods and Ethics in a Clinical Trial Design. New York, NY: Wiley; 1996: 19–63.
(HUMAN EXPERIMENTATION/RESEARCH DESIGN)

Schaffner, Kenneth F. see **Block, Marian R.**

Schaffner, Kenneth F. see **Thomas, A. Mathew**

Schapira, A. see **Frisho–Lima, P.**

Schechter, Clyde see **Eng, Christine M.**

Scheckle, Darren see **Goldworth, Amnon**

Schemo, Diana Jean. Death's new sting in Brazil: removal of organs. [News]. *New York Times.* 1998 Jan 15: A4.
(ORGAN AND TISSUE DONATION)

Schenkenberg, Tom. Salt Lake City VA Medical Center's first 150 ethics committee case consultations: what we have learned (so far). *HEC (HealthCare Ethics Committee) Forum.* 1997 Jun; 9(2): 147–158.
(ETHICISTS AND ETHICS COMMITTEES)

Schenkenberg, Tom see **Murphy, G. Don**

Schenker, Joseph G.; International Federation of Gynecology and Obstetrics. Committee for the Study of Ethical Aspects of Human Reproduction. Report of the FIGO Committee for the Study of Ethical Aspects of Human Reproduction. *International Journal of Gynaecology and Obstetrics.* 1997 Jun; 57(3): 333–337.
(ALLOWING TO DIE/INFANTS; GENETIC INTERVENTION; REPRODUCTION)

Scherger, Joseph E. see **Somerville, Margaret A.**

Schick, Ida Critelli; Moore, Sally. Ethics committees identify four key factors for success. *HEC (HealthCare Ethics Committee) Forum.* 1998 Mar; 10(1): 75–85.
(ETHICISTS AND ETHICS COMMITTEES)

Schiedermayer, David. Holding Owen. *Journal of Clinical Ethics.* 1997 Winter; 8(4): 349–352.
(PATIENT CARE; PROFESSIONAL PATIENT RELATIONSHIP)

Schiedermayer, David see **Junkerman, Charles**

Schiermeier, Quirin. Gene therapist accused of fraud to seek redress in German court. [News]. *Nature.* 1997 Sep 11; 389(6647): 105.
(BIOMEDICAL RESEARCH; FRAUD AND MISCONDUCT)

Schiermeier, Quirin. Swiss researchers facing 'anti-transgenics' vote. [News]. *Nature.* 1997 Jul 24; 388(6640): 315.
(GENETIC INTERVENTION)

Schiermeier, Quirin. Switzerland seeks to head off ban on use of transgenic animals. [News]. *Nature.* 1998 Jan 22; 391(6665): 312.
(GENETIC INTERVENTION)

Schiller, Nina Glick see **Levin, Betty Wolder**

Schirm, Victoria; Stachel, Luisa. The values history as a nursing intervention to encourage use of advance directives among older adults. *Applied Nursing Research.* 1996 May; 9(2): 93–96.
(ADVANCE DIRECTIVES)

Schlomann, Pamela see **Gallagher, Eugene B.**

Schlossberger, Eugene; Hecker, Lorna. HIV and family therapists' duty to warn: a legal and ethical analysis. *Journal of Marital and Family Therapy.* 1996 Jan; 22(1): 27–40.
(AIDS/CONFIDENTIALITY; CONFIDENTIALITY/MENTAL HEALTH)

Schmidt, Terri A. When public health competes with individual needs. *Academic Emergency Medicine.* 1995 Mar; 2(3): 217–222.
(PUBLIC HEALTH)

Schmidt, Volker H. Selection of recipients for donor organs in transplant medicine. *Journal of Medicine and Philosophy.* 1998 Feb; 23(1): 50–74.
(ORGAN AND TISSUE TRANSPLANTATION; RESOURCE ALLOCATION/BIOMEDICAL TECHNOLOGIES; SELECTION FOR TREATMENT)

Schmitt, Louise see **Sansone, Paulette**

Schneider, Carl E. Hard cases. *Hastings Center Report.* 1998 Mar–Apr; 28(2): 24–26.
(EUTHANASIA/LEGAL ASPECTS)

Schneider, Katherine see **Geller, Gail**

Schneider, Katherine A. see **McKinnon, Wendy C.**

Schneiderman, Lawrence J. Commentary: bringing clarity to the futility debate: are the cases wrong? *Cambridge Quarterly of Healthcare Ethics.* 1998 Summer; 7(3): 273–278.
(ALLOWING TO DIE)

Schneiderman, Lawrence J.; Kaplan, Robert M.; Rosenberg, Esther; Teetzel, Holly. Do physicians' own preferences for life–sustaining treatment influence their perceptions of patients' preferences? A second look. *Cambridge Quarterly of Healthcare Ethics.* 1997 Spring; 6(2): 131–137.
(ALLOWING TO DIE/ATTITUDES; INFORMED CONSENT)

Schofield, David J. see **Davis, Kenneth M.**

Schofield, Irene see **Sayers, Gwen M.**

Schooler, Nina R. see **Carpenter, William T.**

Schotsman, Paul. Debating euthanasia in Belgium. [News]. *Hastings Center Report.* 1997 Sep–Oct; 27(5): 46–47.
(EUTHANASIA)

Schroedel, Jean Reith see **Peretz, Paul**

Schroten, Egbert; European Commission. Group of Advisers on the Ethical Implications of Biotechnology. Ethical aspects of genetic modification of animals: opinion of the Group of Advisers on the Ethical Implications of Biotechnology of the European Commission. [Statement and commentary]. *Cambridge*

Quarterly of Healthcare Ethics. 1998 Spring; 7(2): 194–198.
(GENETIC INTERVENTION)

Schüklenk, Udo; del Rio, Carlos; Magis, Carlos; Chokevivat, Vichai. AIDS in the developing world. *In:* Chadwick, Ruth, ed. Encyclopedia of Applied Ethics, Volume 1. San Diego, CA: Academic Press; 1998: 123–127.
(AIDS)

Schüklenk, Udo; Hogan, Carlton. AIDS clinical trials: ethical and design issues. *International Journal of Bioethics.* 1997 Sep; 8(3): 127–132.
(AIDS/HUMAN EXPERIMENTATION; HUMAN EXPERIMENTATION/RESEARCH DESIGN)

Schüklenk, Udo see **Chadwick, Ruth**

Schulman, Kevin A. see **Sulmasy, Daniel P.**

Schultz, Weijmar see **Wilbers, Doaitse**

Schüppel, Reinhart; Büchele, Gisela; Batz, Lothar; Koenig, Wolfgang; Berger, Abi. Sex differences in selection of pacemakers: retrospective observational study. [Article and commentary]. *BMJ (British Medical Journal).* 1998 May 16; 316(7143): 1492–1495.
(SELECTION FOR TREATMENT)

Schwartz, Jack. State regulation of managed care: fragments of reform. *Kennedy Institute of Ethics Journal.* 1997 Dec; 7(4): 345–351.
(HEALTH CARE/ECONOMICS)

Schwartz, Lewis M. An essay on the moral status question. *In:* Edwards, Rem B., ed. Advances in Bioethics. Volume 2: New Essays on Abortion and Bioethics. Greenwich, CT: JAI Press; 1997: 267–301.
(ABORTION; FETUSES; PERSONHOOD)

Schwartz, Paul M. European data protection law and medical privacy. *In:* Rothstein, Mark A., ed. Genetic Secrets: Protecting Privacy and Confidentiality in the Genetic Era. New Haven, CT: Yale University Press; 1997: 392–417.
(CONFIDENTIALITY; GENETIC SCREENING)

Schwartz, Paul M. Protection of privacy in health care reform. *Vanderbilt Law Review.* 1995 Mar; 48(2): 295–347.
(CONFIDENTIALITY/LEGAL ASPECTS)

Schwarz, Lewis R. see **Peterson, Andrew M.**

Sciortino, Stan see **Oscherwitz, Tom**

Scoglio, Stefano. Abortion and the new privacy paradigm. *In: his* Transforming Privacy: A Transpersonal Philosophy of Rights. Westport, CT: Praeger; 1998: 153–185.
(ABORTION/LEGAL ASPECTS)

Scotcher, D. see **Hartley, N.E.**

Scott, P.V.; Pinnock, C.A.; Stone, Peter G.; Blogg, Colin E. Local research ethics committees. [Letters]. *BMJ (British Medical Journal).* 1997 Jul 5; 315(7099): 60–61.
(HUMAN EXPERIMENTATION/ETHICS COMMITTEES)

Scott–Ram, Nicholas. Ethics and the directive for the

legal protection of biotechnological inventions. *Bulletin of Medical Ethics.* 1997 Jan; No. 124: 25–28.
(PATENTING LIFE FORMS)

Scritchfield, Shirley A. The infertility enterprise: IVF and the technological construction of reproductive impairments. *In:* Wertz, Dorothy C., ed. Research in the Sociology of Health Care: A Research Annual. Volume 8. Greenwich, CT: JAI Press; 1989: 61–97.
(IN VITRO FERTILIZATION; REPRODUCTIVE TECHNOLOGIES)

Scutchfield, F. Douglas; Benjamin, Regina. The role of the medical profession in physician discipline. [Editorial]. *JAMA.* 1998 Jun 17; 279(23): 1915–1916.
(FRAUD AND MISCONDUCT)

Sechriest, Kay; Payne, John; Jordan, Lynn; Nelson, J. Robert. Confronting the right to die: caught between a patient's will and a doctor's order. [Case study and commentaries]. *Journal of Christian Nursing.* 1985 Fall; 2(4): 5–10.
(ADVANCE DIRECTIVES; RESUSCITATION ORDERS)

Seedat, Y.K. see **Bhagwanjee, Satish**

Seedhouse, David. Against medical ethics: a response to Cassell. *Journal of Medical Ethics.* 1998 Feb; 24(1): 13–17.
(BIOETHICS/EDUCATION; MEDICAL ETHICS/EDUCATION)

Seedhouse, David. Health Promotion: Philosophy, Prejudice and Practice. New York, NY: Wiley; 1997. 202 p.
(HEALTH)

Seedhouse, David. What's the difference between health care ethics, medical ethics and nursing ethics? [Editorial]. *Health Care Analysis.* 1997 Dec; 5(4): 267–274.
(BIOETHICS; MEDICAL ETHICS; NURSING ETHICS)

Seedhouse, David see **Shotton, Leila**

Seedhouse, David see **van Schie, Tejo**

Seelye, Katharine Q. Advocates of abortion rights report a rise in restrictions. [News]. *New York Times.* 1998 Jan 15: A16.
(ABORTION/LEGAL ASPECTS)

Segal, Arthur I.; Macer, James A.; Pillsbury, S. Gainer; Laros, Russell; Lee, George F.; Rizkallah, Tawfik. Physician attitudes toward human immunodeficiency virus testing in pregnancy. [Article and commentaries]. *American Journal of Obstetrics and Gynecology.* 1996 Jun; 174(6): 1750–1756.
(AIDS/TESTING AND SCREENING)

Segar, Douglas S. see **Ferguson, Jeffrey A.**

Segers, Mary C.; Byrnes, Timothy A., eds. Abortion Politics in American States. Armonk, NY: M.E. Sharpe; 1995. 279 p.
(ABORTION/LEGAL ASPECTS)

Sehgal, Ashwini R.; LeBeau, Shane O.; Youngner, Stuart J. Dialysis patient attitudes toward financial incentives for kidney donation. *American Journal of Kidney Diseases.* 1997 Mar; 29(3): 410–418.
(ORGAN AND TISSUE DONATION)

Seiden, Dena J. Ethics for hospital administrators. *Hospital and Health Services Administration.* 1983 Mar–Apr; 28(2): 81–89.
(PROFESSIONAL ETHICS)

Seifert, Franz; Torgersen, Helge. How to keep out what we don't want: an assessment of 'Sozialverträglichkeit' under the Austrian Genetic Engineering Act. *Public Understanding of Science.* 1997 Oct; 6(4): 301–327.
(GENETIC INTERVENTION)

Seitz, Joanne; O'Neill, Patrick. Ethical decision-making and the Code of Ethics of the Canadian Psychological Association. *Canadian Psychology.* 1996 Feb; 37(1): 23–30.
(PROFESSIONAL ETHICS/CODES OF ETHICS)

Sekela, Michael; Berk, Martin R.; Gallagher, Eugene B.; Blomquist, Glenn C.; Thompson, John S.; Engelberg, Joseph. Cardiac transplantation: costs and ethics. *Hospital Practice (Office Edition).* 1996 Feb 15; 31(2): 127–130, 133–134, 136, 139.
(ORGAN AND TISSUE TRANSPLANTATION; RESOURCE ALLOCATION/BIOMEDICAL TECHNOLOGIES)

Self, Donnie J.; Olivarez, Margie. Retention of moral reasoning skills over the four years of medical education. *Teaching and Learning in Medicine.* 1996; 8(4): 195–199.
(MEDICAL ETHICS/EDUCATION)

Self, Donnie J.; Skeel, Joy D. The moral reasoning of HEC members. *HEC (HealthCare Ethics Committee) Forum.* 1998 Mar; 10(1): 43–54.
(ETHICISTS AND ETHICS COMMITTEES)

Sells, R.A. see **Hoffenberg, R.**

Sells, R.A. see **Kennedy, I.**

Sells, R.A. see **Radcliffe-Richards, J.**

Sells, Robert A. Consent for organ donation: what are the ethical principles? *Transplantation Proceedings.* 1993 Feb; 25(1): 39–41.
(INFORMED CONSENT; ORGAN AND TISSUE DONATION)

Sells, Robert A. The case against buying organs and a futures market in transplants. *Transplantation Proceedings.* 1992 Oct; 24(5): 2198–2202.
(ORGAN AND TISSUE DONATION)

Sells, Robert A. Toward an affordable ethic. *Transplantation Proceedings.* 1992 Oct; 24(5): 2095–2096.
(ORGAN AND TISSUE DONATION)

Sells, Robert A.; Ross, Lainie Friedman; Woodle, E. Steven; Siegler, Mark. Paired-kidney-exchange programs. [Letter and response]. *New England Journal of Medicine.* 1997 Nov 6; 337(19): 1392–1393.
(ORGAN AND TISSUE DONATION)

Selz, Michael. Birth business: industry races to aid infertile. [News]. *Wall Street Journal.* 1997 Nov 26: B1, B12.
(REPRODUCTIVE TECHNOLOGIES)

Senn, Stephen; Ramsay, Lawrence E. Are placebo run ins justified? [Article and commentary]. *BMJ (British Medical Journal).* 1997 Apr 19; 314(7088): 1191–1193.
(HUMAN EXPERIMENTATION/INFORMED CONSENT; HUMAN EXPERIMENTATION/RESEARCH DESIGN)

Sensibaugh, Christine Cregan; Allgeier, Elizabeth Rice.

Factors considered by Ohio juvenile court judges in judicial bypass judgments: a policy–capturing approach. *Politics and the Life Sciences.* 1996 Mar; 15(1): 35–47.
(ABORTION/LEGAL ASPECTS; ABORTION/MINORS)

Seppänen, Marja see **Töyry, Eeva**

Serour, Gamal I. Islamic developments in bioethics. *In:* Lustig, B. Andrew, ed.; Center for Medical Ethics and Health Policy (Houston, TX). Bioethics Yearbook, Volume 5: Theological Developments in Bioethics, 1992–1994. Boston, MA: Kluwer Academic; 1997: 171–188.
(BIOETHICS)

Serour, Gamal I.; Aboulghar, Mohamed A.; Mansour, Ragaa T. Reproductive health care policies around the world: bioethics in medically assisted conception in the Muslim world. *Journal of Assisted Reproduction and Genetics.* 1995 Oct; 12(9): 559–565.
(REPRODUCTIVE TECHNOLOGIES)

Service, Robert F., ed. Research to continue on infected chimps. [News]. *Science.* 1998 Aug 14; 281(5379): 909.
(ANIMAL EXPERIMENTATION)

Sethia, B. see **Brawn, W.J.**

Sethuraman, K.R. see **Gitanjali, B.**

Sevenhuijsen, Selma. Feminist ethics and public health care policies: a case study on the Netherlands. *In:* DiQuinzio, Patrice; Young, Iris Marion, eds. Feminist Ethics and Social Policy. Bloomington, IN: Indiana University Press; 1997: 49–76.
(HEALTH CARE/FOREIGN COUNTRIES)

Severyn, Kristine M. Jacobson v. Massachusetts: impact on informed consent and vaccine policy. *Journal of Pharmacy and Law.* 1996; 5(2): 249–274.
(IMMUNIZATION)

Sfikas, Peter M. Does the dentist have an ethical duty to report child abuse? *Journal of the American Dental Association.* 1996 Apr; 127(4): 521–523.
(CONFIDENTIALITY/LEGAL ASPECTS)

Sgreccia, Elio see **Habgood, John**

Shabde, Neela see **Morley, Colin**

Shaha, Maya. Racism and its implications in ethical–moral reasoning in nursing practice: a tentative approach to a largely unexplored topic. *Nursing Ethics.* 1998 Mar; 5(2): 139–146.
(PROFESSIONAL PATIENT RELATIONSHIP)

Shaheen, Faisal see **Qunibi, Wajeh**

Shalala, Donna E. Health care information and privacy. *Health Matrix.* 1998 Summer; 8(2): 223–232.
(CONFIDENTIALITY)

Shalit, Ruth. When we were philosopher kings: the rise of the medical ethicist. *New Republic.* 1997 Apr 28; 216(17): 24–28.
(ETHICISTS AND ETHICS COMMITTEES)

Shamoo, Adil E. Ethical considerations in medication–free research on the mentally ill. *In:* Shamoo, Adil E., ed. Ethics in Neurobiological Research with Human

Subjects: The Baltimore Conference on Ethics. Amsterdam: Gordon and Breach; 1997: 195–199.
(HUMAN EXPERIMENTATION/SPECIAL POPULATIONS)

Shamoo, Adil E., ed. Ethics in Neurobiological Research with Human Subjects: The Baltimore Conference on Ethics. Amsterdam: Gordon and Breach; 1997. 335 p.
(HUMAN EXPERIMENTATION/SPECIAL POPULATIONS)

Shamoo, Adil E.; Johnson, J. Rock; Honberg, Ron; Flynn, Laurie. NAMI's standards for protection of individuals with severe mental illnesses who participate as human subjects in research. *In:* Shamoo, Adil E., ed. Ethics in Neurobiological Research with Human Subjects: The Baltimore Conference on Ethics. Amsterdam: Gordon and Breach; 1997: 325–328.
(HUMAN EXPERIMENTATION/SPECIAL POPULATIONS)

Shamoo, Adil E.; O'Sullivan, Joan L. The ethics of research on the mentally disabled. *In:* Monagle, John F.; Thomasma, David C., eds. Health Care Ethics: Critical Issues for the 21st Century. Gaithersburg, MD: Aspen Publishers; 1998: 239–250.
(HUMAN EXPERIMENTATION/SPECIAL POPULATIONS)

Shamoo, Adil E. see **Irving, Dianne N.**

Shanahan, Timothy; Wang, Robin. Abortion. *In: their* Reason and Insight: Western and Eastern Perspectives on the Pursuit of Moral Wisdom. Belmont, CA: Wadsworth; 1996: 359–395.
(ABORTION)

Shanahan, Timothy; Wang, Robin. Suicide and euthanasia. *In: their* Reason and Insight: Western and Eastern Perspectives on the Pursuit of Moral Wisdom. Belmont, CA: Wadsworth; 1996: 396–425.
(ALLOWING TO DIE; EUTHANASIA; SUICIDE)

Shanks, Niall see **LaFollette, Hugh**

Shanner, Laura. Teaching women's health issues in a government committee: the story of a successful policy group. *Women's Health Issues.* 1997 Nov–Dec; 7(6): 393–399.
(EMBRYO AND FETAL RESEARCH; ETHICISTS AND ETHICS COMMITTEES; HEALTH)

Shannon, Michael C. Educating practitioners for ethical decision–making: current problems and future concerns. *In:* Haddad, Amy Marie, ed. Teaching and Learning Strategies in Pharmacy Ethics. Second Edition. New York, NY: Pharmaceutical Products Press; 1997: 101–109.
(PROFESSIONAL ETHICS/EDUCATION)

Shannon, Thomas A. Fetal status: sources and implications. *Journal of Medicine and Philosophy.* 1997 Oct; 22(5): 415–422.
(FETUSES; PERSONHOOD)

Shannon, Thomas A. Genetics, ethics, and theology: the Roman Catholic discussion. *In:* Peters, Ted, ed. Genetics: Issues of Social Justice. Cleveland, OH: Pilgrim Press; 1998: 144–179.
(GENETIC INTERVENTION; REPRODUCTION)

Shannon, Thomas A. Response to Khushf. *Journal of Medicine and Philosophy.* 1997 Oct; 22(5): 525–527.
(FETUSES; PERSONHOOD)

Shapiro, David. Cloning, dignity and ethical reasoning. [Letter]. *Nature.* 1997 Aug 7; 388(6642): 511.
(CLONING)

Shapiro, David see **Holtzman, Neil A.**

Shapiro, Joseph P. Death be not swift enough: fraud fighters begin to probe the expense of hospice care. [News]. *U.S. News and World Report.* 1997 Mar 24; 122(11): 34–35.
(FRAUD AND MISCONDUCT; TERMINAL CARE/HOSPICES)

Shapiro, Kenneth J. see **Gluck, John P.**

Shapiro, Martin F. see **Wenger, Neil S.**

Shapiro, Michael H. How (not) to think about surrogacy and other reproductive innovations. [Commentary]. *University of San Francisco Law Review.* 1994 Spring; 28(3): 647–680.
(SURROGATE MOTHERS)

Shapiro, Robyn see **Andrews, Lori**

Sharav, Vera Hassner. Independent family advocates challenge the fraternity of silence. *In:* Shamoo, Adil E., ed. Ethics in Neurobiological Research with Human Subjects: The Baltimore Conference on Ethics. Amsterdam: Gordon and Breach; 1997: 175–181.
(FRAUD AND MISCONDUCT; HUMAN EXPERIMENTATION/SPECIAL POPULATIONS)

Sharland, Gurleen see **Brawn, W.J.**

Sharp, David. Gene tests offered to UK public. [News]. *Lancet.* 1997 Oct 4; 350(9083): 1013.
(GENETIC SCREENING; GENETIC SERVICES)

Sharp, Lesley A. Organ transplantation as a transformative experience: anthropological insights into the restructuring of the self. *Medical Anthropology Quarterly.* 1995 Sep; 9(3): 357–389.
(ORGAN AND TISSUE DONATION; ORGAN AND TISSUE TRANSPLANTATION; PERSONHOOD)

Sharp, Lesley A. see **Joralemon, Donald**

Sharpe, Gilbert see **Etchells, Edward**

Sharpe, Neil F. Presymptomatic testing for Huntington disease: is there a duty to test those under the age of eighteen years? [Letter]. *American Journal of Medical Genetics.* 1993 Apr 15; 46(2): 250–253.
(GENETIC SCREENING)

Sharpe, Virginia A. The politics, economics, and ethics of "appropriateness". *Kennedy Institute of Ethics Journal.* 1997 Dec; 7(4): 337–343.
(HEALTH CARE/ECONOMICS; PATIENT CARE; RESOURCE ALLOCATION)

Sharpe, Virginia A.; Faden, Alan I. Medical Harm: Historical, Conceptual, and Ethical Dimensions of Iatrogenic Illness. New York, NY: Cambridge University Press; 1998. 280 p.
(PATIENT CARE)

Sharpe, Virginia A.; Pellegrino, Edmund D. Medical ethics in the courtroom: a reappraisal. *Journal of Medicine and Philosophy.* 1997 Aug; 22(4): 373–379.
(ETHICISTS AND ETHICS COMMITTEES)

Shashindran, C.H. see **Gitanjali, B.**

Shatz, David. Concepts of autonomy in Jewish medical ethics. *In:* Jewish Law Annual. Volume Twelve. Amsterdam, Netherlands: Harwood Academic Publishers; 1997: 3–43.
(ALLOWING TO DIE/RELIGIOUS ASPECTS; INFORMED CONSENT)

Shaw, A.B. Ensuring equity and quality of care for elderly people: a critique of the College report. *Journal of the Royal College of Physicians of London.* 1995 Mar–Apr; 29(2): 89–91.
(PATIENT CARE/AGED; RESOURCE ALLOCATION; SELECTION FOR TREATMENT)

Shaw, Byers W. see **Arnold, Robert M.**

Shaw, Byers W. see **Purtilo, Ruth**

Shaw, James E. see **Smith, Thomas J.**

Shaw, Linda K. see **Barnhart, J. Marie**

Shaw, M.; Tomlinson, D.; Higginson, I. Survey of HIV patients' views on confidentiality and non–discrimination policies in general practice. *BMJ (British Medical Journal).* 1996 Jun 8; 312(7044): 1463–1464.
(AIDS/CONFIDENTIALITY)

Sheaft, Rod. The Need for Healthcare. New York, NY: Routledge; 1996. 228 p.
(HEALTH CARE/FOREIGN COUNTRIES)

Sheehan, Myles N. Intergenerational justice: is it possible? *In:* Monagle, John F.; Thomasma, David C., eds. Health Care Ethics: Critical Issues for the 21st Century. Gaithersburg, MD: Aspen Publishers; 1998: 353–365.
(RESOURCE ALLOCATION)

Sheldon, Sally; Wilkinson, Stephen. Conjoined twins: the legality and ethics of sacrifice. *Medical Law Review.* 1997 Summer; 5(2): 149–171.
(PATIENT CARE; SELECTION FOR TREATMENT)

Sheldon, Tony. Dutch doctor refuses to treat smokers. [News]. *BMJ (British Medical Journal).* 1998 Jan 24; 316(7127): 250.
(SELECTION FOR TREATMENT)

Sheldon, Tony. Dutch face disclosure of medical records. [News]. *BMJ (British Medical Journal).* 1998 Feb 21; 316(7131): 572.
(CONFIDENTIALITY)

Sheldon, Tony. Dutch GP in euthanasia case will not go to prison. [News]. *BMJ (British Medical Journal).* 1997 Apr 19; 314(7088): 1148.
(EUTHANASIA/LEGAL ASPECTS)

Sheldon, Tony. Row over force feeding of patients with Alzheimer's disease. [News]. *BMJ (British Medical Journal).* 1997 Aug 9; 315(7104): 327.
(ALLOWING TO DIE)

Sheler, Jeffery L. see **Herbert, Wray**

Shelly, Judith Allen see **Salladay, Susan Anthony**

Shelman, Keith see **Yaes, Robert J.**

Shelton, Robert L. Biomedical ethics in Methodist traditions. *In:* Lustig, B. Andrew, ed.; Center for Medical Ethics and Health Policy (Houston, TX). Bioethics Yearbook, Volume 5: Theological Developments in Bioethics, 1992–1994. Boston, MA: Kluwer Academic; 1997: 189–220.
(BIOETHICS)

Shelton, Wayne N. Justice and alcoholism. *In:* Shelton, Wayne N.; Edwards, Rem B., eds. Advances in Bioethics. Volume 3: Values, Ethics, and Alcoholism. Greenwich, CT: JAI Press; 1997: 131–152.
(ORGAN AND TISSUE TRANSPLANTATION; RESOURCE ALLOCATION/BIOMEDICAL TECHNOLOGIES; SELECTION FOR TREATMENT)

Shelton, Wayne N.; Edwards, Rem B., eds. Advances in Bioethics. Volume 3: Values, Ethics, and Alcoholism. Greenwich, CT: JAI Press; 1997. 314 p.
(PATIENT CARE)

Shenfield, F. Justice and access to fertility treatments. *In:* Shenfield, F.; Sureau, C., eds. Ethical Dilemmas in Assisted Reproduction. New York, NY: Parthenon Pub. Group; 1997: 7–14.
(REPRODUCTIVE TECHNOLOGIES; RESOURCE ALLOCATION/BIOMEDICAL TECHNOLOGIES; SELECTION FOR TREATMENT)

Shenfield, F.; Sureau, C., eds. Ethical Dilemmas in Assisted Reproduction. New York, NY: Parthenon Pub. Group; 1997. 96 p.
(REPRODUCTIVE TECHNOLOGIES)

Shenfield, F.; Sureau, C. Ethics of embryo research. *In:* Shenfield, F.; Sureau, C., eds. Ethical Dilemmas in Assisted Reproduction. New York, NY: Parthenon Pub. Group; 1997: 15–21.
(EMBRYO AND FETAL RESEARCH)

Shenfield, F. see **Nisand, I.**

Shenfield, F. see **Van Steirteghem, A.**

Shenkin, Henry A. see **Bradley, Peter M.**

Shepardson, Laura B.; Youngner, Stuart J.; Speroff, Theodore; O'Brien, Ralph G.; Smyth, Kathleen A.; Rosenthal, Gary E. Variation in the use of do–not–resuscitate orders in patients with stroke. *Archives of Internal Medicine.* 1997 Sep 8; 157(16): 1841–1847.
(RESUSCITATION ORDERS)

Shepherd, John Robert. Marriage and Mandatory Abortion among the 17th–Century Siraya. Arlington, VA: American Anthropological Association; 1995. 99 p.
(ABORTION/FOREIGN COUNTRIES)

Shepherd, Jonathan see **Dale, Ruth**

Sheppard, J. see **Brunner, E.J.**

Sheppard, Julie. Patent and be damned! *Bulletin of Medical Ethics.* 1997 Jan; No. 124: 16–17.
(PATENTING LIFE FORMS)

Sher, Geoffrey; Feinman, Michael. Accountability, representation, and advertising. *Women's Health Issues.* 1997 May–Jun; 7(3): 153–161.
(REPRODUCTIVE TECHNOLOGIES)

Sher, Geoffrey see **Jones, Howard**

Sher, Ruben. AIDS treatment and bioethics in South Africa. *In:* Chadwick, Ruth, ed. Encyclopedia of Applied Ethics, Volume 1. San Diego, CA: Academic Press; 1998: 129–135.
(AIDS)

Sheridan, Kathleen see **McGuire, John**

Sherlock, Kevin. The Scarlet Survey: An Accounting from Courthouses, Health Agencies, Police Blotters, and Morgues Across America of Women and Girls Exploited by Abortion on Demand. Akron, OH: Brennyman Books; 1997. 272 p.
(ABORTION)

Sherman, Stephanie L.; DeFries, John C.; Gottesman, Irving I.; Loehlin, John C.; Meyer, Joanne M.; Pelias, Mary Z.; Rice, John; Waldman, Irwin. Behavioral genetics '97 -- ASHG statement: recent developments in human behavioral genetics: past accomplishments and future directions. *American Journal of Human Genetics.* 1997 Jun; 60(6): 1265–1275.
(BEHAVIORAL GENETICS; BEHAVIORAL RESEARCH; GENETIC RESEARCH)

Sherry, Stephen F. The incentive of patents. *In:* Kilner, John F.; Pentz, Rebecca D.; Young, Frank E., eds. Genetic Ethics: Do the Ends Justify the Genes? Grand Rapids, MI: W.B. Eerdmans; 1997: 113–123.
(PATENTING LIFE FORMS; RECOMBINANT DNA RESEARCH)

Sherwin, Susan. A relational approach to autonomy in health care. *In:* Sherwin, Susan, et al. The Politics of Women's Health: Exploring Agency and Autonomy. Philadelphia, PA: Temple University Press; 1998: 19–47.
(HEALTH CARE; PATIENT CARE)

Sherwin, Susan. Cancer and women: some feminist ethics concerns. *In:* Sargent, Carolyn F.; Brettell, Caroline B., eds. Gender and Health: An International Perspective. Upper Saddle River, NJ: Prentice Hall; 1996: 187–204.
(PATIENT CARE)

Sherwin, Susan, et al. The Politics of Women's Health: Exploring Agency and Autonomy. Philadelphia, PA: Temple University Press; 1998. 321 p.
(HEALTH; HEALTH CARE)

Sherwin, Susan see **Baylis, Françoise**

Shi, Da–pu; Yu, Lin. The conflict between the advancement of medical science and technology and traditional Chinese medical ethics. *In:* Becker, Gerhold K., ed. Changing Nature's Course: The Ethical Challenge of Biotechnology. Hong Kong: Hong Kong University Press; 1996: 111–118.
(BIOETHICS; BIOMEDICAL TECHNOLOGIES)

Shickle, Darren. Privacy versus public right to know. *In:* Chadwick, Ruth, ed. Encyclopedia of Applied Ethics, Volume 3. San Diego, CA: Academic Press; 1998: 661–669.
(CONFIDENTIALITY)

Shickle, Darren. Resource allocation. *In:* Chadwick, Ruth, ed. Encyclopedia of Applied Ethics, Volume 3. San Diego, CA: Academic Press; 1998: 861–873.

(HEALTH CARE/ECONOMICS; RESOURCE ALLOCATION)

Shickle, Darren see **Edgar, Andrew**

Shields, Alexandra E. see **Altman, Stuart H.**

Shiell, Alan. Health outcomes are about choices and values: an economic perspective on the health outcomes movement. *Health Policy.* 1997 Jan; 39(1): 5–15.
(HEALTH CARE/ECONOMICS)

Shifman, Pinhas. New reproductive technologies and Jewish law. *In:* Jewish Law Annual. Volume Twelve. Amsterdam, Netherlands: Harwood Academic Publishers; 1997: 127–136.
(REPRODUCTIVE TECHNOLOGIES)

El–Shihabi, R. see **Aswad, Saleh**

Shildrick, Margrit. Leaky Bodies and Boundaries: Feminism, Postmodernism and (Bio)ethics. New York, NY: Routledge; 1997. 252 p.
(BIOETHICS; REPRODUCTIVE TECHNOLOGIES)

Shinn, Roger L. Between Eden and Babel. *In:* Cole–Turner, Ronald, ed. Human Cloning: Religious Responses. Louisville, KY: Westminister John Knox Press; 1997: 106–118.
(CLONING)

Shinn, Roger L. Genetics, ethics, and theology: the ecumenical discussion. *In:* Peters, Ted, ed. Genetics: Issues of Social Justice. Cleveland, OH: Pilgrim Press; 1998: 122–143.
(GENE THERAPY; GENETIC INTERVENTION)

Shinn, Roger Lincoln. The New Genetics: Challenges for Science, Faith, and Politics. Wakefield, RI: Moyer Bell; distributed in North America by Publishers Group West, Emeryville, CA; 1996. 175 p.
(GENE THERAPY; GENETIC INTERVENTION; GENOME MAPPING)

Shmaefsky, Brian R. see **Veglia, Geremia**

Shore, David see **Skirboll, Lana**

Short, Lynette see **Corley, Mary C.**

Shortell, Stephen M.; Waters, Teresa M.; Clarke, Kenneth W.B.; Budetti, Peter P. Physicians as double agents: maintaining trust in an era of multiple accountabilities. *JAMA.* 1998 Sep 23–30; 280(12): 1102–1108.
(HEALTH CARE/ECONOMICS)

Shotton, Leila. The ethics of teaching nursing ethics. *Health Care Analysis.* 1997 Sep; 5(3): 259–263.
(NURSING ETHICS/EDUCATION)

Shotton, Leila; Seedhouse, David. Practical dignity in caring. *Nursing Ethics.* 1998 May; 5(3): 246–255.
(PATIENT CARE)

Shuck, Jerry M. see **Youngner, Stuart J.**

Shulkes, A. see **Hardy, K.J.**

Shulman, Richard H. see **Thies, Winthrop Drake**

Shultz, Marjorie Maguire. Legislative regulation of

surrogacy and reproductive technology. [Commentary]. *University of San Francisco Law Review.* 1994 Spring; 28(3): 613–625.
(SURROGATE MOTHERS)

Shuman, Daniel W. The origins of the physician–patient privilege and professional secret. *Southwestern Law Journal.* 1985 Jun; 39(2): 661–687.
(CONFIDENTIALITY/LEGAL ASPECTS)

Shuman, Daniel W. see **Weiner, Myron F.**

Shuman, Joel see **Hauerwas, Stanley**

Shuster, Evelyne. Fifty years later: the significance of the Nuremberg Code. *New England Journal of Medicine.* 1997 Nov 13; 337(20): 1436–1440.
(HUMAN EXPERIMENTATION/REGULATION)

Shuster, Evelyne. The Nuremberg Code: Hippocratic ethics and human rights. *Lancet.* 1998 Mar 28; 351(9107): 974–977.
(HUMAN EXPERIMENTATION)

Shuttleworth, John Sterling. Ethical issues of cost in long-term care. *Journal of the Medical Association of Georgia.* 1990 Nov; 79(11): 843–845.
(BEHAVIOR CONTROL; HEALTH CARE/ECONOMICS; PATIENT CARE/AGED)

Sibbald, Bonnie see **Buetow, Stephen**

Sidel, Victor see **Forrow, Lachlan**

Sidel, Victor W. see **Forrow, Lachlan**

Sidley, Pat. AIDS drug scandal in South Africa continues. [News]. *BMJ (British Medical Journal).* 1998 Mar 14; 316(7134): 800.
(AIDS/HUMAN EXPERIMENTATION; FRAUD AND MISCONDUCT; HUMAN EXPERIMENTATION/FOREIGN COUNTRIES)

Sidley, Pat. Doctors involved in South Africa's biological warfare programme. [News]. *BMJ (British Medical Journal).* 1998 Jun 20; 316(7148): 1852.
(FRAUD AND MISCONDUCT; WAR)

Sidley, Pat. South Africa Truth Commission calls doctors to account for their actions during the apartheid era. [News]. *BMJ (British Medical Journal).* 1997 Jun 28; 314(7098): 1850.
(FRAUD AND MISCONDUCT; TORTURE)

Sidley, Pat. South African court rules against rationing decision. [News]. *BMJ (British Medical Journal).* 1997 Feb 8; 314(7078): 396.
(RESOURCE ALLOCATION/BIOMEDICAL TECHNOLOGIES)

Sidley, Pat. South African row over denial of dialysis. [News]. *BMJ (British Medical Journal).* 1997 Dec 13; 315(7122): 1562.
(RESOURCE ALLOCATION/BIOMEDICAL TECHNOLOGIES)

Sidley, Pat. South Africa's doctors apologise for apartheid years. [News]. *BMJ (British Medical Journal).* 1995 Jul 15; 311(6998): 148.
(FRAUD AND MISCONDUCT)

Sidley, Pat. South Africa's liberal abortion laws challenged. [News]. *BMJ (British Medical Journal).* 1998

Jun 6; 316(7146): 1696.
(ABORTION/FOREIGN COUNTRIES; ABORTION/LEGAL
ASPECTS)

Siegel–Itzkovich, Judy. Doctors banned from drug
company trip. [News]. *BMJ (British Medical Journal)*.
1998 Aug 8; 317(7155): 370.
(HEALTH CARE/ECONOMICS; HEALTH CARE/FOREIGN
COUNTRIES)

Siegel–Itzkovich, Judy. Palestinian man shackled in
Jerusalem hospital. [News]. *BMJ (British Medical
Journal)*. 1997 Sep 6; 315(7108): 568.
(HEALTH CARE/FOREIGN COUNTRIES; PATIENT CARE)

Siegert, Elisabeth A. see **O'Brien, Linda A.**

Siegler, M. see **Daugherty, C.K.**

Siegler, Mark. Liver transplantation using living donors.
Transplantation Proceedings. 1992 Oct; 24(5): 2223–2224.
(ORGAN AND TISSUE DONATION; ORGAN AND TISSUE
TRANSPLANTATION)

Siegler, Mark see **Andrews, Lori**

Siegler, Mark see **Daugherty, Christopher**

Siegler, Mark see **Heilicser, Bernard**

Siegler, Mark see **Jonsen, Albert R.**

Siegler, Mark see **Martin, Douglas K.**

Siegler, Mark see **Orr, Robert D.**

Siegler, Mark see **Sells, Robert A.**

**Sigmon, Sandra T.; Rohan, Kelly J.; Dorhofer, Diana;
Hotovy, Lisa A.; Trask, Peter C.; Boulard, Nina.**
Effects of consent form information on self–disclosure.
Ethics and Behavior. 1997; 7(4): 299–310.
(BEHAVIORAL RESEARCH/INFORMED CONSENT;
BEHAVIORAL RESEARCH/SPECIAL POPULATIONS)

**Silberfeld, Michel; Grundstein–Amado, Rivka;
Stephens, Derek; Deber, Raisa.** Family and
physicians' views of surrogate decision–making: the roles
and how to choose. *International Psychogeriatrics*. 1996
Winter; 8(4): 589–596.
(INFORMED CONSENT/MENTALLY DISABLED)

Silberner, Joanne. Keeping confidence. *Hastings Center
Report*. 1997 Nov–Dec; 27(6): 8.
(CONFIDENTIALITY/LEGAL ASPECTS)

Silberner, Joanne. Remodelling IRBs. *Hastings Center
Report*. 1998 Jul–Aug; 28(4): 5.
(HUMAN EXPERIMENTATION/ETHICS COMMITTEES)

Silberner, Joanne. Seeding the cloning debate. *Hastings
Center Report*. 1998 Mar–Apr; 28(2): 5.
(CLONING)

Silcock, Sheila see **Jennings, Maggy**

**Sills, E. Scott; Strider, William; Hyde, Henry J.;
Anker, Deborah; Rees, Grover Joseph; Davis, Owen
K.** Gynaecology, forced sterilisation, and asylum in the
USA. *Lancet*. 1998 Jun 6; 351(9117): 1729–1730.
(STERILIZATION)

Silove, E.D. see **Brawn, W.J.**

Silva, J. Arturo see **Leong, Gregory B.**

Silver, Lee M. Cloning, ethics, and religion. *Cambridge
Quarterly of Healthcare Ethics*. 1998 Spring; 7(2):
168–172.
(CLONING)

Silver, Lee M. Remaking Eden: Cloning and Beyond in
a Brave New World. New York, NY: Avon Books; 1997.
317 p.
(CLONING; REPRODUCTIVE TECHNOLOGIES)

Silver, Melanie H. Wilson. Patients' rights in England
and the United States of America: *The Patient's Charter*
and the New Jersey Patient Bill of Rights: a comparison.
Journal of Medical Ethics. 1997 Aug; 23(4): 213–220.
(HEALTH CARE/FOREIGN COUNTRIES; PATIENTS' RIGHTS)

Silverman, Henry. The role of emotions in decisional
competence, standards of competency, and altruistic acts.
Journal of Clinical Ethics. 1997 Summer; 8(2): 171–175.
(ETHICISTS AND ETHICS COMMITTEES; INFORMED
CONSENT/MENTALLY DISABLED; ORGAN AND TISSUE
DONATION)

**Silverman, Myrna; McDowell, B. Joan; Musa, Donald;
Rodriguez, Eric; Martin, David.** To treat or not to
treat: issues in decisions not to treat older persons with
cognitive impairment, depression, and incontinence.
Journal of the American Geriatrics Society. 1997 Sep; 45(9):
1094–1101.
(PATIENT CARE/AGED; SELECTION FOR TREATMENT)

Silvers, Anita. Disability rights. *In:* Chadwick, Ruth, ed.
Encyclopedia of Applied Ethics, Volume 1. San Diego,
CA: Academic Press; 1998: 781–796.
(HEALTH)

Silvers, Anita. Protecting the innocents from
physician–assisted suicide: disability discrimination and
the duty to protect otherwise vulnerable groups. *In:*
Battin, Margaret P.; Rhodes, Rosamond; Silvers, Anita,
eds. Physician Assisted Suicide: Expanding the Debate.
New York, NY: Routledge; 1998: 133–148.
(SUICIDE)

Silvers, Anita; Miller, Franklin G.; Davis, Dena. An
open future. [Letters and response]. *Hastings Center
Report*. 1997 Sep–Oct; 27(5): 5.
(GENETIC COUNSELING)

Silvers, Anita see **Battin, Margaret P.**

Silvers, J.B. see **Finkelstein, Beth S.**

Silvestrini, Bruno. Respect for life and biomedical
research. *Dolentium Hominum: Church and Health in the
World*. 1996; 31(11th Yr., No. 1): 159–162.
(BIOMEDICAL RESEARCH)

Simes, R. John see **Stern, Jerome M.**

Simini, Bruno. Italian surrogate "twins." *Lancet*. 1997 Nov
1; 350(9087): 1307.
(SURROGATE MOTHERS)

Simini, Bruno. Italy's assisted–reproduction clinics face
restriction. [News]. *Lancet*. 1998 Jun 13; 351(9118): 1796.
(REPRODUCTIVE TECHNOLOGIES)

Simini, Bruno. New ethical guidelines issued by the Vatican. [News]. *Lancet.* 1997 Sep 20; 350(9081): 874.
(BIOETHICS)

Simini, Bruno. Public warned about HIV–1–positive prostitute in Italy. [News]. *Lancet.* 1998 Feb 21; 351(9102): 580.
(AIDS/CONFIDENTIALITY)

Simini, Bruno. Revolutionary swap of baby organs ends badly. [News]. *Lancet.* 1998 Feb 14; 351(9101): 503.
(ORGAN AND TISSUE DONATION; ORGAN AND TISSUE TRANSPLANTATION)

Simmer-Brown, Judith see Ravindra, Ravi

Simmons, Paul D. Baptist–Evangelical medical ethics. *In:* Lustig, B. Andrew, ed.; Center for Medical Ethics and Health Policy (Houston, TX). Bioethics Yearbook, Volume 5: Theological Developments in Bioethics, 1992–1994. Boston, MA: Kluwer Academic; 1997: 221–257.
(BIOETHICS)

Simms, Madeleine; Chervenak, Frank A.; McCullough, Laurence B.; Campbell, Stuart; Papp, Z.; Gávai, M.; Görbe, É.; Sirisena, Jayantha. Is third trimester abortion justified? [Letters and responses]. *British Journal of Obstetrics and Gynaecology.* 1996 Feb; 103(2): 187–189.
(ABORTION)

Simon, Norma P. see Bass, Larry J.

Simon, Robert I. Psychiatrists' duties in discharging sicker and potentially violent inpatients in the managed care era. *Psychiatric Services.* 1998 Jan; 49(1): 62–67.
(HEALTH CARE/ECONOMICS; PATIENT CARE/MENTALLY DISABLED)

Simonson, Carol L.S. Teaching caring to nursing students. *Journal of Nursing Education.* 1996 Mar; 35(3): 100–104.
(NURSING ETHICS/EDUCATION)

Simpson, Joe Leigh; Carson, Sandra A. Multifetal reduction in high-order gestations: a nonelective procedure? [Editorial]. *Journal Of The Society For Gynecologic Investigation.* 1996 Jan–Feb; 3(1): 1–2.
(ABORTION)

Simpson, John see Brawn, W.J.

Sims, Andrew see Williams, Christopher J.

Sinclair, Carole see Bass, Larry J.

Sinclair, Daniel B. Jewish law in the state of Israel. *In:* Jewish Law Annual. Volume Twelve. Amsterdam, Netherlands: Harwood Academic Publishers; 1997: 253–266.
(BIOETHICS)

Sines, David see Baxter, Rosario

Singer, Eleanor. Public reactions to some ethical issues of social research: attitudes and behavior. *Journal of Consumer Research.* 1984 Jun; 11: 501–509.
(BEHAVIORAL RESEARCH/INFORMED CONSENT)

Singer, Maxine see Berg, Paul

Singer, Maxine F. Genetics and the law: a scientist's view. *Yale Law and Policy Review.* 1985 Spring; 3(2): 315–335.
(GENETIC INTERVENTION; GENETIC RESEARCH; RECOMBINANT DNA RESEARCH)

Singer, Peter. On comparing the value of human and nonhuman life. *In:* Morscher, Edgar; Neumaier, Otto; Simons, Peter, eds. Applied Ethics in a Troubled World. Boston, MA: Kluwer Academic; 1998: 93–104.
(PERSONHOOD)

Singer, Peter see Kuhse, Helga

Singer, Peter A.; Martin, Douglas K.; Lavery, James V.; Thiel, Elaine C.; Kelner, Merrijoy; Mendelssohn, David C. Reconceptualizing advance care planning from the patient's perspective. *Archives of Internal Medicine.* 1998 Apr 27; 158(8): 879–884.
(ADVANCE DIRECTIVES)

Singer, Peter A. see Etchells, Edward

Singer, Peter A. see Kohut, Nitsa

Singer, Peter A. see Lafrance, W. André

Singer, Peter A. see Martin, Douglas K.

Singh, S.K. see Indudhara, R.

Sinsheimer, Robert L. see Wright, Susan

Sirisena, Jayantha see Simms, Madeleine

Sirmon, Maryella D. The combative patient: ethical issues in patient selection for chronic dialysis. *Seminars in Dialysis.* 1996 Jan–Feb; 9(1): 56–60.
(BIOMEDICAL TECHNOLOGIES; SELECTION FOR TREATMENT)

Sirovatka, Paul see Skirboll, Lana

Sittisombut, Nopporn see Robb, Merlin L.

Sivberg, Bengt. Self-perception and value system as possible predictors of stress. *Nursing Ethics.* 1998 Mar; 5(2): 103–121.
(NURSING ETHICS/EDUCATION)

Sizemore, James Paul. Alabama's confidentiality quagmire: psychotherapists, AIDS, mandatory reporting, and *Tarasoff. Law and Psychology Review.* 1995 Spring; 19: 241–257.
(AIDS/CONFIDENTIALITY)

Skeel, Joy D. see Self, Donnie J.

Skirboll, Lana; Shore, David; Baruchin, Andrea; Sirovatka, Paul. National Institute of Mental Health human subject activities. *In:* Shamoo, Adil E., ed. Ethics in Neurobiological Research with Human Subjects: The Baltimore Conference on Ethics. Amsterdam: Gordon and Breach; 1997: 201–206.
(HUMAN EXPERIMENTATION/SPECIAL POPULATIONS)

Skolnick, Andrew A. Advisory committee report recommends that US make amends for human radiation experiments. [News]. *JAMA.* 1995 Sep 27; 274(12): 933.
(FRAUD AND MISCONDUCT; HUMAN EXPERIMENTATION)

Skolnick, Andrew A. End-of-life care movement

growing. *JAMA*. 1997 Sep 24; 278(12): 967–969.
(MEDICAL ETHICS/EDUCATION; TERMINAL CARE)

Skolnick, Andrew A. MediCaring Project to demonstrate, evaluate innovative end-of-life program for chronically ill. [News]. *JAMA*. 1998 May 20; 279(19): 1511–1512.
(TERMINAL CARE)

Skolnick, Andrew A. Opposition to law officers having unfettered access to medical records. *JAMA*. 1998 Jan 28; 279(4): 257–259.
(CONFIDENTIALITY/LEGAL ASPECTS)

Skovmand, Kaare. First-ever fertilisation bill passed in Denmark. [News]. *Lancet*. 1997 Jun 7; 349(9066): 1678.
(REPRODUCTIVE TECHNOLOGIES)

Skupski, Daniel W.; Chervenak, Frank A.; McCullough, Laurence B. Routine obstetric ultrasound examination: a clinical and ethical evaluation. *In:* Chervenak, Frank A.; Kurjak, Asim, eds. Current Perspectives on the Fetus as a Patient. New York, NY: Parthenon Publishing Group; 1996: 203–212.
(MASS SCREENING; PRENATAL DIAGNOSIS)

Slavin, Stuart see **Wilkes, Michael S.**

Sledge, William H.; Feinstein, Alvan R. A clinimetric approach to the components of the patient–physician relationship. *JAMA*. 1997 Dec 17; 278(23): 2043–2048.
(PROFESSIONAL PATIENT RELATIONSHIP)

Slifkin, Robert F.; Charytan, Chaim. Ethical issues related to the provision or denial of renal services to non–citizens. [Case commentaries on ethical issues in dialysis]. *Seminars in Dialysis*. 1997 May–Jun; 10(3): 173–175.
(BIOMEDICAL TECHNOLOGIES; SELECTION FOR TREATMENT)

Sloan, Jeffrey A. see **Degner, Lesley F.**

Sloan, Laura Curry. Constitutional law — state impediments to abortion funding — National Education Association of Rhode Island v. Garrahy. [Note]. *University of Kansas Law Review*. 1985 Winter; 34(2): 387–409.
(ABORTION/FINANCIAL SUPPORT; ABORTION/LEGAL ASPECTS)

Sloan, Rebecca S. see **Gallagher, Eugene B.**

Slome, Lee; Moulton, Jeffrey; Huffine, Carol; Gorter, Robert; Abrams, Donald. Physicians' attitudes toward assisted suicide in AIDS. *Journal of Acquired Immune Deficiency Syndromes*. 1992; 5(7): 712–718.
(AIDS/HEALTH PERSONNEL; SUICIDE)

Slowther, Anne; Underwood, Martin. Is there a demand for a clinical ethics advisory service in the UK? [Letter]. *Journal of Medical Ethics*. 1998 Jun; 24(3): 207.
(ETHICISTS AND ETHICS COMMITTEES)

Smalley, M. Gene. Jehovah's Witnesses: help with bioethical issues. *In:* Lustig, B. Andrew, ed.; Center for Medical Ethics and Health Policy (Houston, TX). Bioethics Yearbook, Volume 5: Theological Developments in Bioethics, 1992–1994. Boston, MA: Kluwer Academic; 1997: 259–267.
(BIOETHICS)

Smith, Allyne L. In the world but not of it: managing the conflict between Christian and institution. *Christian Bioethics*. 1997 Mar; 3(1): 74–84.
(HEALTH CARE)

Smith, Anthony M.; Edmonds, Polly; Davies, Andrew; Thorns, Andrew. More openness needed in palliative care. [Letters]. *BMJ (British Medical Journal)*. 1998 Jan 31; 316(7128): 390–391.
(EUTHANASIA; TERMINAL CARE)

Smith, C.D. see **Marshall, Mary Faith**

Smith, Carol A. Use of involuntary outpatient commitment in community care of the seriously and persistently mentally ill patient. *Issues in Mental Health Nursing*. 1995 May–Jun; 16(3): 275–284.
(INVOLUNTARY COMMITMENT; PATIENT CARE/MENTALLY DISABLED)

Smith, Cheryl K. Safeguards for physician–assisted suicide: the Oregon Death with Dignity Act. *In:* McLean, Sheila A.M., ed. Death, Dying and the Law. Brookfield, VT: Dartmouth; 1996: 69–93.
(SUICIDE)

Smith, David G. see **Nakchbandi, Inaam A.**

Smith, David H. Religion and the use of animals in research: some first thoughts. *Ethics and Behavior*. 1997; 7(2): 137–147.
(ANIMAL EXPERIMENTATION)

Smith, David H. see **Granbois, Judith A.**

Smith, Douglas. The limits of human studies. *In:* Close, Bryony; Combes, Robert; Hubbard, Anthony; Illingworth, John, eds. Volunteers in Research and Testing. Bristol, PA: Taylor and Francis; 1997: 135–143.
(HUMAN EXPERIMENTATION/FOREIGN COUNTRIES; HUMAN EXPERIMENTATION/SPECIAL POPULATIONS)

Smith, George P. Final Exits: Safeguarding Self–Determination and the Right to Be Free from Cruel and Unusual Punishment. Chicago, IL: Northwestern University Medical School; 1997. 15 p.
(ALLOWING TO DIE)

Smith, Herbert L. see **Tu, Ping**

Smith, J. Clay. The precarious implications of DNA profiling. *University of Pittsburgh Law Review*. 1994 Spring; 55(3): 865–888.
(DNA FINGERPRINTING)

Smith, Jane A.; Boyd, Kenneth M. Ethics and laboratory animals: can the use of animals in experiments be justified? *In:* Tuffery, A.A., ed. Laboratory Animals: An Introduction for Experimenters. Second Edition. New York, NY: Wiley; 1995: 1–13.
(ANIMAL EXPERIMENTATION)

Smith, Joel see **Lynn, Joanne**

Smith, Karen L.; Braslow, Judith B. Public attitudes toward organ and tissue donation. *In:* Chapman, Jeremy R.; Deierhoi, Mark; Wight, Celia, eds. Organ and Tissue Donation for Transplantation. New York, NY: Oxford University Press; 1997: 34–45.
(ORGAN AND TISSUE DONATION)

Smith, Katharine V.; Russell, Jan. Ethical issues experienced by HIV–infected African–American women. *Nursing Ethics.* 1997 Sep; 4(5): 394–402.
(AIDS)

Smith, Ken R. see **Botkin, Jeffrey R.**

Smith, Martin L.; Stagno, Susan J.; Dolske, Michelle; Kosalko, Joanne; McConnell, Carolyn; Kaspar, Larita; Lederman, Richard. Induction procedures for psychogenic seizures: ethical and clinical considerations. *Journal of Clinical Ethics.* 1997 Fall; 8(3): 217–229.
(PATIENT CARE/MENTALLY DISABLED)

Smith, Martin L. see **Orlowski, James P.**

Smith, Melanie K. see **Finkelstein, Daniel**

Smith, Michael L. see **Moskop, John C.**

Smith, Peggie see **Andrews, Lori**

Smith, Richard. All doctors are problem doctors: doctors worldwide must do better with managing problem colleagues. [Editorial]. *BMJ (British Medical Journal).* 1997 Mar 22; 314(7084): 841–842.
(FRAUD AND MISCONDUCT)

Smith, Richard. Beyond conflict of interest: transparency is the key. [Editorial]. *BMJ (British Medical Journal).* 1998 Aug 1; 317(7154): 291–292.
(BIOMEDICAL RESEARCH; FRAUD AND MISCONDUCT)

Smith, Richard. Conflict of interest in clinical research: opprobium or obsession? [Letter]. *Lancet.* 1997 Jun 7; 349(9066): 1703.
(BIOMEDICAL RESEARCH)

Smith, Richard. Don't treat shackled patients: and keep trying to understand what the Nuremberg trials taught us. [Editorial]. *BMJ (British Medical Journal).* 1997 Jan 18; 314(7075): 164.
(PATIENT CARE)

Smith, Richard. Informed consent: edging forwards (and backwards). [Editorial]. *BMJ (British Medical Journal).* 1998 Mar 28; 316(7136): 949–951.
(BIOMEDICAL RESEARCH; CONFIDENTIALITY; INFORMED CONSENT)

Smith, Richard. Misconduct in research: editors respond -- the Committee on Publication Ethics (COPE) is formed. [Editorial]. *BMJ (British Medical Journal).* 1997 Jul 26; 315(7102): 201–202.
(BIOMEDICAL RESEARCH; FRAUD AND MISCONDUCT)

Smith, Richard. Renegotiating medicine's contract with patients: the GMC is leading the way. [Editorial]. *BMJ (British Medical Journal).* 1998 May 30; 316(7145): 1622–1623.
(PATIENT CARE)

Smith, Richard. The need for a national body for research misconduct: nothing less will reassure the public. [Editorial]. *BMJ (British Medical Journal).* 1998 Jun 6; 316(7146): 1686–1687.
(BIOMEDICAL RESEARCH; FRAUD AND MISCONDUCT)

Smith, Richard see **Berwick, Donald**

Smith, Roberta A. see **Rye, Patricia D.**

Smith, Sam. Postmodernity and a hypertensive patient: rescuing value from nihilism. *Journal of Medical Ethics.* 1998 Feb; 24(1): 25–31.
(PROFESSIONAL PATIENT RELATIONSHIP)

Smith, Theresa C.; Oleszczuk, Thomas A. No Asylum: State Psychiatric Repression in the Former USSR. New York, NY: New York University Press; 1996. 289 p.
(INVOLUNTARY COMMITMENT/FOREIGN COUNTRIES)

Smith, Thomas J.; Desch, Christopher E.; Hackney, Mary Helen; Shaw, James E. How long does it take to get a "do not resuscitate" order? *Journal of Palliative Care.* 1997 Spring; 13(1): 5–8.
(RESUSCITATION ORDERS)

Smith, Thomas J.; Swisher, Karen. Telling the truth about terminal cancer. [Editorial]. *JAMA.* 1998 Jun 3; 279(21): 1746–1748.
(TERMINAL CARE; TRUTH DISCLOSURE)

Smith, Wesley J. "Inevitable" assisted suicide?: don't bet your life. *Human Life Review.* 1997 Spring; 23(2): 61–74.
(EUTHANASIA; SUICIDE)

Smurl, James F. Do ethical decisions leave you wondering: "Did I do the right thing?" Ethical decision making for everyday nursing problems. *Nursing Life.* 1983 May–Jun; 3(3): 48–53.
(NURSING ETHICS)

Smyer, Michael see **Dellasega, Cheryl**

Smyth, Angus see **Long, Ann**

Smyth, Kathleen A. see **Shepardson, Laura B.**

Snapper, John W. Responsibility for computer–based decisions in health care. *In:* Goodman, Kenneth W., ed. Ethics, Computing, and Medicine: Informatics and the Transformation of Health Care. New York, NY: Cambridge University Press; 1998: 43–56.
(BIOMEDICAL TECHNOLOGIES; HEALTH CARE)

Sneiderman, Barney; Verhoef, Marja. Patient autonomy and the defence of medical necessity: five Dutch euthanasia cases. *Alberta Law Review.* 1996; 34(2): 374–415.
(EUTHANASIA/LEGAL ASPECTS; SUICIDE)

Snowdon, Claire; Garcia, Jo; Elbourne, Diana. Reactions of participants to the results of a randomised controlled trial: exploratory study. *BMJ (British Medical Journal).* 1998 Jul 4; 317(7150): 21–26.
(HUMAN EXPERIMENTATION/MINORS; HUMAN EXPERIMENTATION/RESEARCH DESIGN)

Snyder, Jack W. Making Medical Spending Decisions: The Law, Ethics, and Economics of Rationing Mechanisms, by Mark A. Hall. [Book review essay]. *Journal of Legal Medicine.* 1998 Mar; 19(1): 143–150.
(HEALTH CARE/ECONOMICS; RESOURCE ALLOCATION)

Snyder, Jack W. see **Berkowitz, Jonathan M.**

Snyder, Lois; Tooker, John. Obligations and opportunities: the role of clinical societies in the ethics of managed care. *Journal of the American Geriatrics Society.* 1998 Mar; 46(3): 378–380.
(HEALTH CARE/ECONOMICS)

Cambridge University Press; 1997: 168–178.
(ALLOWING TO DIE)

Spielman, Bethany see **Agich, George J.**

Spielmann, Horst see **Balls, Michael**

Spike, Jeffrey. A paradox about capacity, alcoholism, and noncompliance. *Journal of Clinical Ethics.* 1997 Fall; 8(3): 303–306.
(ADVANCE DIRECTIVES; TREATMENT REFUSAL)

Spike, Jeffrey. Iatrogenic liver failure, transplantation, and prisoners. *Journal of Clinical Ethics.* 1997 Winter; 8(4): 398–404.
(ORGAN AND TISSUE TRANSPLANTATION; SELECTION FOR TREATMENT)

Spike, Jeffrey. What's love got to do with it? The altruistic giving of organs. *Journal of Clinical Ethics.* 1997 Summer; 8(2): 165–170.
(ETHICISTS AND ETHICS COMMITTEES; INFORMED CONSENT/MENTALLY DISABLED; ORGAN AND TISSUE DONATION)

Spiker, Duane G. see **Roth, Loren**

Spiro, Howard M. see **Freedman, Monroe H.**

Spital, Aaron. Do U.S. transplant centers encourage emotionally related kidney donation? *Transplantation.* 1996 Feb 15; 61(3): 374–377.
(ORGAN AND TISSUE DONATION)

Spital, Aaron. Ethical and policy issues in altruistic living and cadaveric organ donation. *Clinical Transplantation.* 1997 Apr; 11(2): 77–87.
(ORGAN AND TISSUE DONATION)

Spital, Aaron L. Unrelated living donors: should they be used? *Transplantation Proceedings.* 1992 Oct; 24(5): 2215–2217.
(ORGAN AND TISSUE DONATION)

Spitz, Lewis see **Pierro, Agostino**

Spriggs, Merle. Autonomy in the face of a devastating diagnosis. *Journal of Medical Ethics.* 1998 Apr; 24(2): 123–126.
(TRUTH DISCLOSURE)

Sprigler, Gail B. When the truth hurts. *Plastic Surgical Nursing.* 1996 Spring; 16(1): 51–53, 56.
(INFORMED CONSENT; TRUTH DISCLOSURE)

Spritz, Norton. Physicians and medical futility: experience in the setting of general medical care. *In:* Zucker, Marjorie B.; Zucker, Howard D., eds. Medical Futility and the Evaluation of Life-Sustaining Interventions. New York, NY: Cambridge University Press; 1997: 36–47.
(ALLOWING TO DIE)

Sprung, Charles L.; Eidelman, Leonid A.; Steinberg, Avraham. Is the patient's right to die evolving into a duty to die?: Medical decision making and ethical evaluations in health care. *Journal of Evaluation in Clinical Practice.* 1997 Feb; 3(1): 69–75.
(ALLOWING TO DIE)

Sprung, Charles L. see **Nyman, Deborah J.**

Sprunger, Suzanne A.; Julian–Arnold, Gianna. Promoting and managing genome innovation. *Risk: Health, Safety and Environment.* 1996 Summer; 7(3): 197–200.
(GENETIC RESEARCH)

Spudis, Edward V. Non-simultaneous deaths of parallel personhoods crashing through a Denver S & L. [Poetry]. *Journal of Clinical Ethics.* 1998 Summer; 9(2): 206.
(BIOETHICS)

Spurgeon, David. Canadian doctor calls for more education on abortion. [News]. *BMJ (British Medical Journal).* 1997 Nov 15; 315(7118): 1251.
(ABORTION/FOREIGN COUNTRIES)

Spurgeon, David. Trials sponsored by drug companies: review ordered. [News]. *BMJ (British Medical Journal).* 1998 Sep 5; 317(7159): 618.
(BIOMEDICAL RESEARCH; HUMAN EXPERIMENTATION/REGULATION)

Stachel, Luisa see **Schirm, Victoria**

Stadler, Holly A.; Morrissey, John; Rose, Teresa; Haley, Sarah; Trojahn, Carrie; Hampton, Stephanie. Patient capacity and judicial decisionmaking. *HEC (HealthCare Ethics Committee) Forum.* 1997 Sep; 9(3): 197–211.
(INFORMED CONSENT)

Stagno, Susan J. see **Smith, Martin L.**

Stallings, Rebecca Y. see **Sulmasy, Daniel P.**

Stallsworth, Paul T., ed. The Right Choice: Pro-Life Sermons from Elizabeth Achtemeier [and Others]. Nashville, TN: Abingdon Press; 1997. 118 p.
(ABORTION/RELIGIOUS ASPECTS)

Stanley, Teresa. Who is the moral agent? *AORN Journal (Association of Operating Room Nurses).* 1984 Sep; 40(3): 331, 334–335.
(NURSING ETHICS)

Starks, Helene E. see **Pearlman, Robert A.**

Statham, H. see **Hallowell, N.**

Stead, Eugene A. Cognitive brain death: the major ethical issue of our time. [Editorial]. *Journal of the Medical Association of Georgia.* 1990 Nov; 79(11): 814–815.
(ALLOWING TO DIE)

Stebbens, V.A. see **Parkins, K.J.**

Stecklow, Steve; Johannes, Laura. Drug makers relied on clinical researchers who now await trial. [News]. *Wall Street Journal.* 1997 Aug 15: A1, A6.
(FRAUD AND MISCONDUCT; HUMAN EXPERIMENTATION/REGULATION)

Steel, Knight see **Bernabei, Roberto**

Steel, R. Knight see **Burke, James**

Steele, A.; Melby, V. Nurses' knowledge and beliefs about AIDS: comparing nurses in hospital, community and hospice settings. *Journal of Advanced Nursing.* 1995 Nov; 22(5): 879–887.
(AIDS/HEALTH PERSONNEL)

Stefanek, Michael see **Bernhardt, Barbara A.**

Steiber, Steven R. Right to die: public balks at deciding for others. *Hospitals.* 1987 Mar 5; 61(5): 72.
(ALLOWING TO DIE/ATTITUDES)

Steigrad, Stephen J. see **Durna, Eva M.**

Stein, Edward. Choosing the sexual orientation of children. *Bioethics.* 1998 Jan; 12(1): 1–24.
(ABORTION; SEX DETERMINATION; SEX PRESELECTION)

Stein, Michael D.; Freedberg, Kenneth A.; Sullivan, Lisa M.; Savetsky, Jacqueline; Levenson, Suzette M.; Hingson, Ralph; Samet, Jeffrey H. Sexual ethics: disclosure of HIV–positive status to partners. *Archives of Internal Medicine.* 1998 Feb 9; 158(3): 253–257.
(AIDS)

Steinberg, Avraham. Informed consent: ethical and halakhic considerations. *In:* Jewish Law Annual. Volume Twelve. Amsterdam, Netherlands: Harwood Academic Publishers; 1997: 137–152.
(INFORMED CONSENT)

Steinberg, Avraham see **Sprung, Charles L.**

Steinberg, M.A.; Cartwright, C.M.; MacDonald, S.M.; Najman, J.M.; Williams, G.M. Self–determination in terminal care: a comparison of GP and community members' responses. *Australian Family Physician.* 1997 Jun; 26(6): 703–705, 707.
(ADVANCE DIRECTIVES; TERMINAL CARE)

Steinberg, M.A.; Cartwright, C.M.; Najman, J.; MacDonald, S.M.; Williams, G. Healthy Ageing, Healthy Dying: Community and Health Professional Perspectives on End-of-Life Decision-Making. Report to the Research and Development Grants Advisory Committee of the Department of Human Services and Health. Brisbane, QLD: University of Queensland Medical School, Department of Social and Preventive Medicine; 1996 Feb. 116 p.
(TERMINAL CARE)

Steinberg, M.A.; Cartwright, C.M.; Parker, M.H.; Najman, J.M. Patient Self–Determination in Terminal Care: Phase 2. Designing "Useful" Advance Directives and Proxies. Report to the Commonwealth Department of Human Services and Health, Research and Development Grants Program. Brisbane, QLD: University of Queensland Medical School, Department of Social and Preventive Medicine; 1997 May. 130 p.
(ADVANCE DIRECTIVES)

Steinberg, M.A.; Parker, M.H.; Cartwright, C.M.; Macdonald, F.J.; Del Mar, C.B.; Williams, G.M.; Hoffenberg, R. End–of–Life Decision–Making: Perspectives of General Practitioners and Patients. Report to the General Practice Evaluation Programme of the Department of Human Services and Health. Brisbane, QLD: University of Queensland Medical School, Department of Social and Preventive Medicine; 1996 Jul. 1 v.
(TERMINAL CARE)

Steinberg, Margaret see **Cartwright, Colleen**

Stelfox, Henry Thomas; Chua, Grace; O'Rourke, Keith; Detsky, Allan S. Conflict of interest in the debate over calcium–channel antagonists. *New England Journal of Medicine.* 1998 Jan 8; 338(2): 101–105.
(HEALTH CARE/ECONOMICS; PATIENT CARE/DRUGS)

Stell, Lance K. Physician–assisted suicide: to decriminalize or legalize, that is the question. *In:* Battin, Margaret P.; Rhodes, Rosamond; Silvers, Anita, eds. Physician Assisted Suicide: Expanding the Debate. New York, NY: Routledge; 1998: 225–251.
(ALLOWING TO DIE; ALLOWING TO DIE/LEGAL ASPECTS; SUICIDE)

Stell, Lance K. Self–Interest and Universal Health Care: Why Well–Insured Americans Should Support Coverage for Everyone, by Larry J. Churchill. [Book review essay]. *Theoretical Medicine and Bioethics.* 1998 Apr; 19(2): 183–191.
(HEALTH CARE/ECONOMICS; RESOURCE ALLOCATION)

Stempsey, William E. End–of–life decisions: Christian perspectives. *Christian Bioethics.* 1997 Dec; 3(3): 249–261.
(ALLOWING TO DIE/RELIGIOUS ASPECTS; EUTHANASIA/RELIGIOUS ASPECTS; SUICIDE)

Stempsey, William E. Paying people to give up their organs: the problem with commodification of body parts. *Medical Humanities Review.* 1996 Fall; 10(2): 45–55.
(ORGAN AND TISSUE DONATION)

Stempsey, William E. The battle for medical marijuana in the war on drugs. *America.* 1998 Apr 11; 178(12): 14–16.
(PATIENT CARE/DRUGS)

Steneck, Nicholas H. Role of the institutional animal care and use committee in monitoring research. *Ethics and Behavior.* 1997; 7(2): 173–184.
(ANIMAL EXPERIMENTATION)

Stent, Gunther S. see **Martin, Judith**

Stephens, Derek see **Silberfeld, Michel**

Stephens, Martin L. see **Balls, Michael**

Stephenson, Joan. Ethics group drafts guidelines for control of genetic material and information. [News]. *JAMA.* 1998 Jan 21; 279(3): 184.
(CONFIDENTIALITY; GENETIC RESEARCH; ORGAN AND TISSUE DONATION)

Stephenson, Joan. Private venture galvanizes public effort on Human Genome Project. [News]. *JAMA.* 1998 Jun 24; 279(24): 1933, 1935.
(GENOME MAPPING)

Sterling, John see **Foster, George E.**

Stern, Jerome M.; Simes, R. John. Publication bias: evidence of delayed publication in a cohort study of clinical research projects. *BMJ (British Medical Journal).* 1997 Sep 13; 315(7109): 640–645.
(BIOMEDICAL RESEARCH)

Sternberg, S. Release of study ends drug fracas. [News]. *Science News.* 1997 Apr 19; 151(16): 236.
(BIOMEDICAL RESEARCH)

Stevens, M. see **Tibben, A.**

Stevens, M.L. Tina. Redefining death in America, 1968.

Caduceus. 1995 Winter; 11(3): 207–219.
(DETERMINATION OF DEATH/BRAIN DEATH; ORGAN AND TISSUE DONATION)

Stewart, F.E. *JAMA* 100 years ago: is it ethical for medical men to patent medical inventions? [Reprint]. *JAMA.* 1997 Sep 10; 278(10): 816.
(BIOMEDICAL TECHNOLOGIES; HEALTH CARE/ECONOMICS)

Stewart, Kevin. Discussing cardiopulmonary resuscitation with patients and relatives. *Postgraduate Medical Journal.* 1995 Oct; 71(840): 585–589.
(RESUSCITATION ORDERS)

Stewart, Kevin; Wagg, Adrian; Kinirons, Mark. When can elderly patients be excluded from discussing resuscitation? *Journal of the Royal College of Physicians of London.* 1996 Mar–Apr; 30(2): 133–135.
(RESUSCITATION ORDERS)

Stillwell, Susan B. Ethical Issues in Critical Care Nursing. [Videorecording]. St. Louis, MO: Mosby; 1995. 1 videocassette; 36 min.; sd.; color; 1/2 in.; VHS.
(NURSING ETHICS)

Stipich, Nina see **Rolleston, Francis**

Stobo, John. Who should manage care? The case for providers. *Kennedy Institute of Ethics Journal.* 1997 Dec; 7(4): 387–389.
(HEALTH CARE/ECONOMICS; RESOURCE ALLOCATION)

Stocking, Carol see **Daugherty, Christopher**

Stocking, Carol see **Heilicser, Bernard**

Stoeppelwerth, Ali M. see **Lynn, Joanne**

Stojkovski, Ljupco see **Ivanovski, Ninoslav**

Stokes, William S. see **Balls, Michael**

Stolberg, Sheryl Gay. F.D.A. stand on cloning raises even more questions. [News]. *New York Times.* 1998 Jan 21: A14.
(CLONING)

Stolberg, Sheryl Gay. U.S. orders sickest to be given priority on donated organs. [News]. *New York Times.* 1998 Mar 27: A16.
(ORGAN AND TISSUE TRANSPLANTATION; RESOURCE ALLOCATION/BIOMEDICAL TECHNOLOGIES; SELECTION FOR TREATMENT)

Stolberg, Sheryl Gay. U.S. publishes first guide to treatment of infertility. [News]. *New York Times.* 1997 Dec 19: A22.
(REPRODUCTIVE TECHNOLOGIES)

Stolinsky, David C. see **Thies, Winthrop Drake**

Stollerman, Gene see **Markson, Lawrence**

Stone, John. The medical ethics program at Emory. [Editorial]. *Journal of the Medical Association of Georgia.* 1990 Nov; 79(11): 811–812.
(MEDICAL ETHICS/EDUCATION)

Stone, Peter G. see **Scott, P.V.**

Stone, Peter G. see **Talbot, D.**

Strain, James J.; Snyder, Stephen L.; Drooker, Martin. Conflict resolution: experience of consultation–liaison psychiatrists. *In:* Zucker, Marjorie B.; Zucker, Howard D., eds. Medical Futility and the Evaluation of Life–Sustaining Interventions. New York, NY: Cambridge University Press; 1997: 98–109.
(ALLOWING TO DIE; PROFESSIONAL PATIENT RELATIONSHIP; TREATMENT REFUSAL)

Straker, Gillian. Ethical issues in working with children in war zones. *In:* Apfel, Roberta J.; Simon, Bennett, eds. Minefields in Their Hearts: The Mental Health of Children and Communal Violence. New Haven, CT: Yale University Press; 1996: 18–32.
(PATIENT CARE/MENTALLY DISABLED; PATIENT CARE/MINORS; WAR)

Strasser, Mark. Dependence, reliance and abortion. *Philosophical Quarterly.* 1985 Jan; 35(138): 73–82.
(ABORTION; FETUSES)

Straughan, Donald W. see **Balls, Michael**

Strauss, Anselm L. see **Wiener, Carolyn L.**

Strauss, Evelyn. The tissue issue: losing oneself to science? *Science News.* 1997 Sep 20; 152(12): 190–191.
(BIOMEDICAL RESEARCH; HUMAN EXPERIMENTATION/INFORMED CONSENT; ORGAN AND TISSUE DONATION)

Strauss, Michelle see **DeRenzo, Evan G.**

Strauss, Misha see **Bernhardt, Barbara A.**

Straw, Peggy. Consumer representation on IRBs -- how it should be done. *In:* Shamoo, Adil E., ed. Ethics in Neurobiological Research with Human Subjects: The Baltimore Conference on Ethics. Amsterdam: Gordon and Breach; 1997: 187–190.
(HUMAN EXPERIMENTATION/ETHICS COMMITTEES; HUMAN EXPERIMENTATION/SPECIAL POPULATIONS)

Strickland, Ruth Ann. The incivility of mandated drug treatment through civil commitments. *Politics and the Life Sciences.* 1996 Mar; 15(1): 70–72.
(INVOLUNTARY COMMITMENT; PRENATAL INJURIES)

Strider, William see **Sills, E. Scott**

Strijbis, Anne–Margreet see **Stronks, Karien**

Strong, Carson. Cloning and infertility. *Cambridge Quarterly of Healthcare Ethics.* 1998 Summer; 7(3): 279–293.
(CLONING)

Strong, Carson. Response to Khushf. *Journal of Medicine and Philosophy.* 1997 Oct; 22(5): 521–523.
(FETUSES; PERSONHOOD)

Strong, Carson. The moral status of preembryos, embryos, fetuses, and infants. *Journal of Medicine and Philosophy.* 1997 Oct; 22(5): 457–478.
(FETUSES; PERSONHOOD)

Strong, Carson see **Muram, David**

Stronks, Karien; Strijbis, Anne–Margreet; Wendte,

Johannes F.; Gunning–Schepers, Louise J. Who should decide? Qualitative analysis of panel data from public, patients, healthcare professionals, and insurers on priorities in health care. *BMJ (British Medical Journal)*. 1997 Jul 12; 315(7100): 92–96.
(HEALTH CARE/FOREIGN COUNTRIES; RESOURCE ALLOCATION)

Stroup, Donna F. see Olson, Carin M.

Strumpf, Neville E. see Evans, Lois K.

Struve, James K. The consultation: a patient's request to be referred for an abortion sends this physician into an ethical tailspin. *Minnesota Medicine*. 1996 Aug; 79(8): 12–13.
(ABORTION)

Stryker, Jeff. Ethical issues in HIV disease research. *In:* Cohen, P.T.; Sande, Merle A.; Volberding, Paul A., eds. The AIDS Knowledge Base: A Textbook on HIV Disease from the University of California, San Francisco, and the San Francisco General Hospital. Second Edition. Boston, MA: Little, Brown; 1994: 11.5–1 to 11.5–6.
(AIDS/HUMAN EXPERIMENTATION)

Stryker, Jeff. Ethical issues in public health policy toward HIV disease. *In:* Cohen, P.T.; Sande, Merle A.; Volberding, Paul A., eds. The AIDS Knowledge Base: A Textbook on HIV Disease from the University of California, San Francisco, and the San Francisco General Hospital. Second Edition. Boston, MA: Little, Brown; 1994: 11.6–1 to 11.6–4.
(AIDS; PUBLIC HEALTH)

Stryker, Jeff. Ethical issues in the use of tests for HIV infection. *In:* Cohen, P.T.; Sande, Merle A.; Volberding, Paul A., eds. The AIDS Knowledge Base: A Textbook on HIV Disease from the University of California, San Francisco, and the San Francisco General Hospital. Second Edition. Boston, MA: Little, Brown; 1994: 11.4–1 to 11.4–5.
(AIDS/TESTING AND SCREENING)

Stryker, Jeff. Ethical issues in treating competent patients with HIV disease. *In:* Cohen, P.T.; Sande, Merle A.; Volberding, Paul A., eds. The AIDS Knowledge Base: A Textbook on HIV Disease from the University of California, San Francisco, and the San Francisco General Hospital. Second Edition. Boston, MA: Little, Brown; 1994: 11.2–1 to 11.2–5.
(AIDS; ALLOWING TO DIE; SUICIDE)

Stryker, Jeff. Ethical issues in treating incompetent patients with HIV disease. *In:* Cohen, P.T.; Sande, Merle A.; Volberding, Paul A., eds. The AIDS Knowledge Base: A Textbook on HIV Disease from the University of California, San Francisco, and the San Francisco General Hospital. Second Edition. Boston, MA: Little, Brown; 1994: 11.3–1 to 11.3–4.
(ADVANCE DIRECTIVES; AIDS)

Stryker, Jeff. Health care workers and HIV disease: an ethical overview. *In:* Cohen, P.T; Sande, Merle A.; Volberding, Paul A., eds. The AIDS Knowledge Base: A Textbook on HIV Disease from the University of California, San Francisco, and the San Francisco General Hospital. Second Edition. Boston, MA: Little, Brown; 1994: 11.1–1 to 11.1–6.
(AIDS/HEALTH PERSONNEL)

Stryker, Jeff see Bayer, Ronald

Stubblefield, Phillip. Self-administered emergency contraception -- a second chance. [Editorial]. *New England Journal of Medicine*. 1998 Jul 2; 339(1): 41–42.
(CONTRACEPTION)

Studdard, P. Albert see Tierney, William M.

Stumper, O. see Brawn, W.J.

Suarez–Almazor, Maria E.; Belzile, Michelle; Bruera, Eduardo. Euthanasia and physician–assisted suicide: a comparative study of physicians, terminally ill cancer patients, and the general population. *Journal of Clinical Oncology*. 1997 Feb; 15(2): 418–427.
(EUTHANASIA/ATTITUDES; SUICIDE)

Subedi, Janardan see DeVries, Raymond

Sugarman, Jeremy; Harland, Robert. Acute yet non-emergent patients. *In:* McCullough, Laurence B.; Jones, James W.; Brody, Baruch A., eds. Surgical Ethics. New York, NY: Oxford University Press; 1998: 116–132.
(INFORMED CONSENT; PATIENT CARE; TREATMENT REFUSAL)

Sugarman, Jeremy; Mastroianni, Anna C.; Kahn, Jeffrey P., eds. Ethics of Research with Human Subjects: Selected Policies and Resources. Frederick, MD: University Publishing Group; 1998. 244 p.
(HUMAN EXPERIMENTATION/REGULATION)

Sugarman, Jeremy see Gordon, Valery M.

Sugarman, Jeremy see Kahn, Jeffrey P.

Sullivan, Lisa M. see Stein, Michael D.

Sullivan, Lucy G. Euthanasia: wrong problem, wrong answer. *Medical Journal of Australia*. 1996 Nov 18; 165(10): 558–560.
(ALLOWING TO DIE)

Sullivan, Mark; Rapp, Suzanne; Fitzgibbon, Dermot; Chapman, C. Richard. Pain and the choice to hasten death in patients with painful metastatic cancer. *Journal of Palliative Care*. 1997 Autumn; 13(3): 18–28.
(ALLOWING TO DIE/ATTITUDES; EUTHANASIA/ATTITUDES; SUICIDE; TERMINAL CARE)

Sullivan, Mark D.; Ganzini, Linda; Youngner, Stuart J. Should psychiatrists serve as gatekeepers for physician–assisted suicide? *Hastings Center Report*. 1998 Jul–Aug; 28(4): 24–31.
(SUICIDE)

Sullivan, Peter B. see Rosenbloom, Lewis

Sulmasy, Daniel P.; Linas, Benjamin P.; Gold, Karen F.; Schulman, Kevin A. Physician resource use and willingness to participate in assisted suicide. *Archives of Internal Medicine*. 1998 May 11; 158(9): 974–978.
(SUICIDE)

Sulmasy, Daniel P.; Marx, Eric S. A computerized system for entering orders to limit treatment: implementation and evaluation. *Journal of Clinical Ethics*. 1997 Fall; 8(3): 258–263.
(RESUSCITATION ORDERS; TERMINAL CARE)

Sulmasy, Daniel P.; Terry, Peter B.; Weisman, Carol S.; Miller, Deborah J.; Stallings, Rebecca Y.; Vettese, Margaret A.; Haller, Karen B. The accuracy of substituted judgments in patients with terminal diagnoses. *Annals of Internal Medicine.* 1998 Apr 15; 128(8): 621–629.
(ALLOWING TO DIE/ATTITUDES; INFORMED CONSENT; TERMINAL CARE)

Sulmasy, Daniel P. see **Burke, James**

Summerfield, Derek. Medical ethics: the Israeli Medical Association. *Lancet.* 1997 Jul 5; 350(9070): 63–64.
(TORTURE)

Summerfield, Derek see **Blachar, Yoram**

Summerfield, Derek see **Prosor, Ron**

Sumner, L.W. A third way. *In:* Dwyer, Susan; Feinberg, Joel, eds. The Problem of Abortion. Third Edition. Belmont, CA: Wadsworth; 1997: 98–117.
(ABORTION)

Sumner, L.W. Moderate views of abortion. *In:* Edwards, Rem B., ed. Advances in Bioethics. Volume 2: New Essays on Abortion and Bioethics. Greenwich, CT: JAI Press; 1997: 203–226.
(ABORTION)

Supanich, Barbara; Brody, Howard. Ethical issues concerning physician–assisted death. *In:* Monagle, John F.; Thomasma, David C., eds. Health Care Ethics: Critical Issues for the 21st Century. Gaithersburg, MD: Aspen Publishers; 1998: 302–310.
(EUTHANASIA; SUICIDE)

Supik, Josie D. see **Perkins, Henry S.**

Surbone, Antonella. The patient–doctor–family relationship: at the core of medical ethics. *In:* Baider, Lea; Cooper, Cary L.; Kaplan De-Nour, Atara, eds. Cancer and the Family. New York, NY: Wiley; 1996: 389–405.
(PROFESSIONAL PATIENT RELATIONSHIP)

Surbone, Antonella; Zwitter, Matjaž, eds. Communication with the Cancer Patient: Information and Truth. New York, NY: New York Academy of Sciences; 1997. 540 p.
(PROFESSIONAL PATIENT RELATIONSHIP; TRUTH DISCLOSURE)

Sureau, C. see **Milliez, J.**

Sureau, C. see **Shenfield, F.**

Sureau, C. see **Van Steirteghem, A.**

Surratt, Hilary L. see **Inciardi, James A.**

Suter, Sonia M. Value neutrality and nondirectiveness: comments on "Future directions in genetic counseling." *Kennedy Institute of Ethics Journal.* 1998 Jun; 8(2): 161–163.
(GENETIC COUNSELING)

Sutton, Agneta. The new genetics and traditional Hippocratic medicine. *In:* Doherty, Peter; Sutton, Agneta, eds. Man-Made Man: Ethical and Legal Issues in Genetics. Dublin, Ireland: Open Air; 1997: 58–70.
(GENE THERAPY; GENETIC SCREENING)

Sutton, Agneta see **Doherty, Peter**

Sutton, Graham C. Will you still need me, will you still screen me, when I'm past 64? Breast screening policy is based on ageism. [Editorial]. *BMJ (British Medical Journal).* 1997 Oct 25; 315(7115): 1032–1033.
(MASS SCREENING; PATIENT CARE/AGED; SELECTION FOR TREATMENT)

Suzuki, David. A personal journey through genetics and civil rights. *Science.* 1998 Sep 18; 281(5384): 1796–1797.
(EUGENICS)

Swanson, Jeffrey see **Swartz, Marvin S.**

Swartz, Marvin S.; Burns, Barbara J.; George, Linda K.; Swanson, Jeffrey; Hiday, Virginia A.; Borum, Randy; Wagner, H. Ryan. The ethical challenges of a randomized controlled trial of involuntary outpatient commitment. *Journal of Mental Health Administration.* 1997 Winter; 24(1): 35–43.
(BEHAVIORAL RESEARCH/RESEARCH DESIGN; BEHAVIORAL RESEARCH/SPECIAL POPULATIONS; INVOLUNTARY COMMITMENT)

Swazey, Judith P.; Bird, Stephanie J. Teaching and learning research ethics. *Professional Ethics.* 1995 Spring–Summer; 4(3–4): 155–178.
(BIOMEDICAL RESEARCH; PROFESSIONAL ETHICS/EDUCATION)

Sweden. Ministry of Health and Social Affairs. The Swedish Transplant Act. [Pamphlet]. Stockholm: Ministry of Health and Social Affairs; 1997. 52 p.
(FETUSES; ORGAN AND TISSUE DONATION)

Swee, David E. Health care system reform and the changing physician–patient relationship. *New Jersey Medicine.* 1995 May; 92(5): 313–317.
(HEALTH CARE/ECONOMICS; PROFESSIONAL PATIENT RELATIONSHIP)

Sweet, Matthew P.; Bernat, James L. A study of the ethical duty of physicians to disclose errors. *Journal of Clinical Ethics.* 1997 Winter; 8(4): 341–348.
(PATIENT CARE; TRUTH DISCLOSURE)

Swisher, Karen see **Smith, Thomas J.**

Swiss Academy of Medical Sciences; Swiss Academy of Sciences. Ethical principles and guidelines for scientific experiments on animals [revised edition]. *ATLA: Alternatives to Laboratory Animals.* 1997 May–Jun; 25(3): 379–384.
(ANIMAL EXPERIMENTATION)

Swiss Academy of Sciences see **Swiss Academy of Medical Sciences**

Szczygiel, Anthony H. see **Wear, Stephen E.**

T

Taber, S.M. see **Thomas, G.**

Tadd, Win. Nurses' ethics. *In:* Chadwick, Ruth, ed. Encyclopedia of Applied Ethics, Volume 3. San Diego, CA: Academic Press; 1998: 367–380.
(NURSING ETHICS)

Taddio, Anna see **Somerville, Margaret A.**

Takahashi, Yoshitomo see **Berger, Douglas**

Talbot, D.; Reynolds, D.J.M.; Stone, Peter G.; Blogg, Colin E.; Rawlins, Richard; Barton, Andrew. Local research ethics committees. [Letters and response]. *BMJ (British Medical Journal).* 1997 Nov 29; 315(7120): 1464–1465.
(HUMAN EXPERIMENTATION/ETHICS COMMITTEES; HUMAN EXPERIMENTATION/FOREIGN COUNTRIES)

Talbot, Margaret. The egg women. *New Republic.* 1998 Mar 16; 218(11): 42.
(REPRODUCTIVE TECHNOLOGIES)

Tamburini, Joan Killion. Lessons on a minimally acceptable quality of life. *Bioethics Forum.* 1997 Summer; 13(2): 38–41.
(ADVANCE DIRECTIVES)

Tamparo, Carol D. see **Lewis, Marcia A.**

Tanabe, Noboru see **Asai, Atsushi**

Tanenbaum, Sandra J. Say the right thing: communication and physician accountability in the era of medical outcomes. *In:* Boyle, Philip J., ed. Getting Doctors to Listen: Ethics and Outcomes Data in Context. Washington, DC: Georgetown University Press; 1998: 204–223.
(HEALTH CARE/ECONOMICS; PATIENT CARE; PROFESSIONAL PATIENT RELATIONSHIP)

Tankersley, E. Susan see **Brockett, Patrick L.**

Tanne, Janice Hopkins. US hospital mergers threaten reproductive services. [News]. *BMJ (British Medical Journal).* 1997 Nov 22; 315(7119): 1330.
(CONTRACEPTION; HEALTH CARE)

Tännsjö, Torbjörn. Compulsory sterilisation in Sweden. *Bioethics.* 1998 Jul; 12(3): 236–249.
(EUGENICS; REPRODUCTION; STERILIZATION)

Tattersall, Martin see **Blennerhassett, Mitzi**

Tauber, Robert T. see **Kallgren, Carl A.**

Tauer, Carol A. Donum Vitae: dissenting opinions on the "simple case" of in vitro fertilization. *In:* Wildes, Kevin Wm., ed. Infertility: A Crossroad of Faith, Medicine, and Technology. Boston, MA: Kluwer Academic; 1997: 125–146.
(IN VITRO FERTILIZATION)

Tauer, Carol A. Embryo research and public policy: a philosopher's appraisal. *Journal of Medicine and Philosophy.* 1997 Oct; 22(5): 423–439.
(EMBRYO AND FETAL RESEARCH; IN VITRO FERTILIZATION)

Taylor, E.M.; Parker, S.; Ramsay, M.P. Patients' receipt and understanding of written information about a resuscitation policy: report from New Zealand. *Bioethics.* 1998 Jan; 12(1): 65–76.
(RESUSCITATION ORDERS)

Taylor, K.M.; Macdonald, K.G.; Bezjak, A.; Ng, P.; DePetrillo, A.D. Physicians' perspective on quality of life: an exploratory study of oncologists. *Quality of Life Research.* 1996 Feb; 5(1): 5–14.
(PATIENT CARE)

Taylor, Kathryn M.; Mehta, Cyrus; Patterson, Bradford; Anderson, Jim. The doctor's dilemma: physician participation in randomized clinical trials. [Article and discussion]. *Cancer Treatment Reports.* 1985 Oct; 69(10): 1095–1100.
(HUMAN EXPERIMENTATION/RESEARCH DESIGN)

Taylor, Robert M.; American Academy of Neurology. Ethics and Humanities Subcommittee. Palliative care in neurology. [Position statement]. *Neurology.* 1996 Mar; 46(3): 870–872.
(TERMINAL CARE)

Taylor, Susan L. Quandary at the crossroads: paternalism versus advocacy surrounding end-of-treatment decisions. *American Journal of Hospice and Palliative Care.* 1995 Jul–Aug; 12(4): 43–46.
(PROFESSIONAL PATIENT RELATIONSHIP; TERMINAL CARE)

te Meerman, Gerard J. see **Dankert-Roelse, Jeannette E.**

te Velde, E.R.; van Baar, A.L.; van Kooij, R.J. Concerns about assisted reproduction. *Lancet.* 1998 May 23; 351(9115): 1524–1525.
(REPRODUCTIVE TECHNOLOGIES)

Teasdale, Thomas A. see **Ghusn, Husam F.**

Tedeschi, Christopher M. Foetal tissue transplantation research: scientific progress and the role of special interest groups. *Minerva.* 1995 Spring; 33(1): 45–66.
(EMBRYO AND FETAL RESEARCH; ORGAN AND TISSUE DONATION)

Teetzel, Holly see **Schneiderman, Lawrence J.**

Teitelman, Michael. Not in the house: arguments for a policy of excluding physician–assisted suicide from the practice of hospital medicine. *In:* Battin, Margaret P.; Rhodes, Rosamond; Silvers, Anita, eds. Physician Assisted Suicide: Expanding the Debate. New York, NY: Routledge; 1998: 203–222.
(SUICIDE)

Templeton, A. see **Kazem, R.**

Templeton, Allan; Morris, Joan K. Reducing the risk of multiple births by transfer of two embryos after in vitro fertilization. *New England Journal of Medicine.* 1998 Aug 27; 339(9): 573–577.
(IN VITRO FERTILIZATION)

Ten, C.L. The use of reproductive technologies in selecting the sexual orientation, the race, and the sex of children. *Bioethics.* 1998 Jan; 12(1): 45–48.
(SEX DETERMINATION; SEX PRESELECTION)

ten Have, Henk. From synthesis and system to morals and procedure: the development of philosophy of medicine. *In:* Carson, Ronald A.; Burns, Chester R., eds. Philosophy of Medicine and Bioethics: A Twenty-Year Retrospective and Critical Appraisal. Boston, MA: Kluwer Academic; 1997: 105–123.
(BIOETHICS)

ten Have, Henk see **de Witte, Joke I.**

ten Have, Henk A.M.J.; Janssens, Rien M.J.P.A. Regulating euthanasia in the Netherlands: ethics committees for review of euthanasia? *HEC (HealthCare Ethics Committee) Forum.* 1997 Dec; 9(4): 393–399.
(ETHICISTS AND ETHICS COMMITTEES; EUTHANASIA; TERMINAL CARE)

ten Have, Henk A.M.J. see **Olde Rikkert, Marcel G.M.**

Tennant, C.C. see **Hooper, S.C.**

Teno, Joan; Lynn, Joanne; Connors, Alfred F.; Wenger, Neil; Phillips, Russell S.; Alzola, Carlos; Murphy, Donald P.; Desbiens, Norman; Knaus, William A. The illusion of end-of-life resource savings with advance directives. [For the SUPPORT Investigators]. *Journal of the American Geriatrics Society.* 1997 Apr; 45(4): 513–518.
(ADVANCE DIRECTIVES; HEALTH CARE/ECONOMICS; TERMINAL CARE)

Teno, Joan; Lynn, Joanne; Wenger, Neil; Phillips, Russell S.; Murphy, Donald P.; Connors, Alfred F.; Desbiens, Norman; Fulkerson, William; Bellamy, Paul; Knaus, William A. Advance directives for seriously ill hospitalized patients: effectiveness with the Patient Self-Determination Act and the SUPPORT intervention. [For the SUPPORT Investigators]. *Journal of the American Geriatrics Society.* 1997 Apr; 45(4): 500–507.
(ADVANCE DIRECTIVES; RESUSCITATION ORDERS)

Teno, Joan see **Lynn, Joanne**

Teno, Joan see **Phillips, Russell S.**

Teno, Joan M.; Licks, Sandra; Lynn, Joanne; Wenger, Neil; Connors, Alfred F.; Phillips, Russell S.; O'Connor, Mary Ann; Murphy, Donald P.; Fulkerson, William J.; Desbiens, Norman; Knaus, William A. Do advance directives provide instructions that direct care? [For the SUPPORT Investigators]. *Journal of the American Geriatrics Society.* 1997 Apr; 45(4): 508–512.
(ADVANCE DIRECTIVES; ALLOWING TO DIE)

Teno, Joan M. see **Goodlin, Sarah J.**

Teno, Joan M. see **Rudberg, Mark A.**

Teno, Joan M. see **Wenger, Neil S.**

Teo, Bernard. Organ donation and transplantation: a Christian viewpoint. *Transplantation Proceedings.* 1992 Oct; 24(5): 2114–2115.
(ORGAN AND TISSUE DONATION; ORGAN AND TISSUE TRANSPLANTATION)

ter Meulen, Rudd H.J. see **Berghmans, Ron L.P.**

Terrence Higgins Trust (Great Britain). Living Will Project. Advance directives and AIDS. *In:* Grubb, Andrew, ed. Decision-Making and Problems of Incompetence. New York, NY: Wiley; 1994: 187–196.
(ADVANCE DIRECTIVES; AIDS)

Terry, Peter B. see **Sulmasy, Daniel P.**

Thacker, Stephen B. see **Olson, Carin M.**

Thal, Anne E. see **Churchill, Larry R.**

Thayer, Barbara see **Saxton, Marsha**

Thibodeau, Lorraine see **Mayer, Dan**

Thiel, Elaine C. see **Singer, Peter A.**

Thiel, G. Emotionally related living kidney donation: pro and contra. *Nephrology, Dialysis, Transplantation.* 1997 Sep; 12(9): 1820–1824.
(ORGAN AND TISSUE DONATION)

Thielman, Samuel B. Psychiatry and social values: the American Psychiatric Association and immigration restriction, 1880–1930. *Psychiatry.* 1985 Nov; 48(4): 299–310.
(EUGENICS)

Thies, Winthrop Drake; Groth, Philip; Hyman, Lawrence; Shulman, Richard H.; Broaddus, Barbara; Greisdorf, Eliezer; Stolinsky, David C.; Astarita, Joseph; Kass, Leon R.; Lund, Nelson. Assisted suicide. [Letters and response]. *Commentary.* 1997 Apr; 103(4): 3–7.
(SUICIDE)

Thiringer, Klara see **Wennerholm, Ulla–Britt**

Thobaben, James R. A United Methodist approach to end-of-life decisions: intentional ambiguity or ambiguous intentions. *Christian Bioethics.* 1997 Dec; 3(3): 222–248.
(ALLOWING TO DIE/RELIGIOUS ASPECTS; EUTHANASIA/RELIGIOUS ASPECTS; SUICIDE)

Thomas, A. Mathew; Cohen, Gene; Cook-Deegan, Robert M.; O'Sullivan, Joan; Post, Stephen G.; Roses, Allen D.; Schaffner, Kenneth F.; Green, Ronald M. Alzheimer testing at Silver Years. *Cambridge Quarterly of Healthcare Ethics.* 1998 Summer; 7(3): 294–307.
(GENETIC SCREENING; PATIENT CARE/AGED)

Thomas, A. Mathew see **Green, Ronald M.**

Thomas, G.; Ryall, M.; Taber, S.M. Ethical dilemmas in transplantation. *Transplantation Proceedings.* 1992 Oct; 24(5): 2099.
(ORGAN AND TISSUE TRANSPLANTATION)

Thomasma, David C. Ensuring a good death. *Bioethics Forum.* 1997 Winter; 13(4): 7–17.
(ALLOWING TO DIE; TERMINAL CARE)

Thomasma, David C. The ethics of managed care: challenges to the principles of relationship-centered care. *Journal of Allied Health.* 1996 Summer; 25(3): 233–246.
(HEALTH CARE/ECONOMICS)

Thomasma, David C., ed. The Influence of Edmund D. Pellegrino's Philosophy of Medicine. Boston, MA: Kluwer Academic; 1997. 215 p.
(BIOETHICS; MEDICAL ETHICS; PROFESSIONAL PATIENT RELATIONSHIP)

Thomasma, David C.; Loewy, Erich H. A dialogue on species-specific rights: humans and animals in bioethics. *Cambridge Quarterly of Healthcare Ethics.* 1997 Fall; 6(4): 435–444.
(PERSONHOOD)

Thomasma, David C. see Jain, Renu

Thomasma, David C. see Monagle, John F.

Thomasma, David C. see Pellegrino, Edmund D.

Thompson, Carolyn R. HIV and the blood supply: assessing MANTRA [mandatory notification of transfusion alternatives] legislation. *Politics and the Life Sciences.* 1995 Aug; 14(2): 221–228.
(AIDS; INFORMED CONSENT)

Thompson, James N. Moral imperatives for academic medicine. *Academic Medicine.* 1997 Dec; 72(12): 1037–1042.
(HEALTH CARE/ECONOMICS; MEDICAL ETHICS/EDUCATION)

Thompson, John S. see Sekela, Michael

Thompson, L.A. see Kazem, R.

Thomson, Alex N. see Coverdale, John H.

Thomson, Elizabeth J. Genetic counselling. *In:* Kilner, John F.; Pentz, Rebecca D.; Young, Frank E., eds. Genetic Ethics: Do the Ends Justify the Genes? Grand Rapids, MI: W.B. Eerdmans; 1997: 146–155.
(GENETIC COUNSELING)

Thomson, Elizabeth J. Sampling issues in clinical impact of genetic testing and counselling studies. *In:* Knoppers, Bartha Maria, ed. Human DNA: Law and Policy: International and Comparative Perspectives.
Proceedings of the First International Conference on DNA Sampling and Human Genetic Research: Ethical, Legal, and Policy Aspects, held in Montreal, Canada, 6–8 Sep 1996. Boston, MA: Kluwer Law International; 1997: 313–317.
(GENETIC RESEARCH; GENETIC SCREENING)

Thomson, Judith Jarvis see Dworkin, Ronald

Thorns, Andrew see Smith, Anthony M.

Thorogood, J. see Briggs, J.D.

Thwaites, Richard see Brawn, W.J.

Tibben, A.; Stevens, M.; de Wert, G.M.W.R.; Niermeijer, M.F.; van Duijn, C.M.; van Swieten, J.C. Preparing for presymptomatic DNA testing for early onset Alzheimer's disease/cerebral haemorrhage and hereditary Pick disease. *Journal of Medical Genetics.* 1997 Jan; 34(1): 63–72.
(GENETIC COUNSELING; GENETIC SCREENING)

Tibben, A. see DudokdeWit, A.C.

Tibboel, Dick see Caniano, Donna A.

Tiberius, Richard G.; Cleave-Hogg, Doreen. A data base for curriculum design in medical ethics. *Journal of Medical Education.* 1984 Jun; 59(6): 512–513.
(MEDICAL ETHICS/EDUCATION)

Tierney, William see Ubel, Peter A.

Tierney, William M.; Weinberger, Morris; Greene, James Y.; Studdard, P. Albert. Jehovah's Witnesses and blood transfusion: physicians' attitudes and legal precedents. *Southern Medical Journal.* 1984 Apr; 77(4): 473–478.
(TREATMENT REFUSAL)

Tierney, William M. see Dexter, Paul R.

Tierney, William M. see Ferguson, Jeffrey A.

Tilden, Virginia P.; Tolle, Susan W.; Lee, Melinda A.; Nelson, Christine A. Oregon's physician-assisted suicide vote: its effect on palliative care. *Nursing Outlook.* 1996 Mar–Apr; 44(2): 80–83.
(SUICIDE; TERMINAL CARE)

Tilney, N. see Hoffenberg, R.

Tilney, N. see Kennedy, I.

Tilney, N. see Radcliffe-Richards, J.

Timpson, Joanne. Abortion: the antithesis of womanhood? *Journal of Advanced Nursing.* 1996 Apr; 23(4): 776–785.
(ABORTION)

Tindall, Brett; Forde, Sally; Ross, Michael W.; Goldstein, David; Barker, Steven; Cooper, David A. Effects of two formats of informed consent on knowledge amongst persons with advanced HIV disease in a clinical trial of didanosine. *Patient Education and Counseling.* 1994 Dec; 24(3): 261–266.
(AIDS/HUMAN EXPERIMENTATION; HUMAN EXPERIMENTATION/INFORMED CONSENT)

Tipton, Robert M. see Bass, Larry J.

Tisone, G. see Elli, M.

Titmuss, Richard M. The Gift Relationship: From Human Blood to Social Policy. Original Edition with New Chapters Edited by Ann Oakley and John Ashton. New York, NY: New Press; 1997. 360 p.
(BLOOD DONATION)

Toaff, Elio. Judaism. *Dolentium Hominum: Church and Health in the World.* 1996; 31(11th Yr., No. 1): 78–81.
(MEDICAL ETHICS; REPRODUCTIVE TECHNOLOGIES)

Tobias, J.S. Changing the BMJ's position on informed consent would be counterproductive. *BMJ (British Medical Journal).* 1998 Mar 28; 316(7136): 1001–1002.
(HUMAN EXPERIMENTATION/INFORMED CONSENT)

Tokyay, R. see Haberal, Mehmet

Toledo-Pereyra, Luis H. The problem of organ donation in minorities: some facts and incomplete answers. *Transplantation Proceedings.* 1992 Oct; 24(5): 2162–2164.
(ORGAN AND TISSUE DONATION)

Tolle, Susan W. Care of the dying: clinical and financial lessons from the Oregon experience. [Editorial]. *Annals of Internal Medicine.* 1998 Apr 1; 128(7): 567–568.
(TERMINAL CARE)

Tolle, Susan W. see Tilden, Virginia P.

Tolle, Susan W. see Ubel, Peter A.

Toma, Tudor P. Romania adopts new transplant law.

[News]. *BMJ (British Medical Journal).* 1997 Jun 21; 314(7097): 1784.
(ORGAN AND TISSUE DONATION)

Tomlinson, D. see **Shaw, M.**

Tomlinson, G.E. see **Mason R.O.**

Tomlinson, Tom. Inducements for donation: benign incentives or risky business? *Transplantation Proceedings.* 1992 Oct; 24(5): 2204–2206.
(ORGAN AND TISSUE DONATION)

Tomossy, George F.; Weisstub, David N. The reform of adult guardianship laws: the case of non–therapeutic experimentation. *International Journal of Law and Psychiatry.* 1997 Winter; 20(1): 113–139.
(HUMAN EXPERIMENTATION/FOREIGN COUNTRIES; HUMAN EXPERIMENTATION/INFORMED CONSENT; INFORMED CONSENT/MENTALLY DISABLED)

Tonelli, Mark. Beyond living wills. *Bioethics Forum.* 1997 Summer; 13(2): 6–12.
(ADVANCE DIRECTIVES; TERMINAL CARE)

Tong, Rosemarie. The ethics of care: a feminist virtue ethics of care for healthcare practitioners. *Journal of Medicine and Philosophy.* 1998 Apr; 23(2): 131–152.
(BIOETHICS)

Tonini, Ersilio see **Maiorca, Rosario**

Tonti–Filippini, Nicholas. Revising brain death: cultural imperialism? *Linacre Quarterly.* 1998 May; 65(2): 51–72.
(DETERMINATION OF DEATH/BRAIN DEATH)

Tooker, John see **Snyder, Lois**

Tooley, Michael. Value, obligation and the asymmetry question. *Bioethics.* 1998 Apr; 12(2): 111–124.
(REPRODUCTION)

Toombs, S. Kay. Taking the body seriously. [Book review essay]. *Hastings Center Report.* 1997 Sep–Oct; 27(5): 39–43.
(BIOETHICS)

Topolski, James see **Wedding, Danny**

Torgersen, Helge see **Seifert, Franz**

Torgerson, David J. see **Giuffrida, Antonio**

Torraco, Stephen F. Veritatis Splendor and the ethics of organ transplants. *Linacre Quarterly.* 1997 May; 64(2): 52–57.
(ORGAN AND TISSUE DONATION)

Torrey, E. Fuller. Out of the Shadows: Confronting America's Mental Illness Crisis. New York, NY: Wiley; 1997. 244 p.
(HEALTH CARE; PATIENT CARE/MENTALLY DISABLED)

Toulmin, Stephen. The primacy of practice: medicine and postmodernism. *In:* Carson, Ronald A.; Burns, Chester R., eds. Philosophy of Medicine and Bioethics: A Twenty–Year Retrospective and Critical Appraisal. Boston, MA: Kluwer Academic; 1997: 41–53.
(MEDICAL ETHICS)

Tournaye, H. see **Van Steirteghem, A.**

Tovanabutra, Sodsai see **Robb, Merlin L.**

Tovey, Philip. Narrative and knowledge development in medical ethics. *Journal of Medical Ethics.* 1998 Jun; 24(3): 176–181.
(MEDICAL ETHICS)

Towner, Henry. In re Martin. [Note]. *Issues in Law and Medicine.* 1996 Winter; 12(3): 267–271.
(ALLOWING TO DIE/LEGAL ASPECTS)

Townsend, Ricard see **DePalma, Judith A.**

Töyry, Eeva; Herve, Ritva; Mutka, Riitta; Savolainen, Pirkko; Seppänen, Marja. Ethics in health care management: developing an instrument to assess humane caring. *Nursing Ethics.* 1998 May; 5(3): 228–235.
(PATIENT CARE)

Tracy, Kathryn Bayard; Post, Stephen G.; Whitehouse, Peter J. Genetic testing for Alzheimer disease. [Letter and response]. *JAMA.* 1997 Sep 24; 278(12): 978–979.
(GENETIC SCREENING)

Trad, Fouad S.; Hornstein, Mark D.; Barbieri, Robert L. *In vitro* fertilization: a cost–effective alternative for infertile couples? *Journal of Assisted Reproduction and Genetics.* 1995 Aug; 12(7): 418–421.
(IN VITRO FERTILIZATION)

Trappenburg, Margo J. Defining the medical sphere. *Cambridge Quarterly of Healthcare Ethics.* 1997 Fall; 6(4): 416–434.
(HEALTH CARE/RIGHTS; RESOURCE ALLOCATION)

Trask, Peter C. see **Sigmon, Sandra T.**

Traynor, Richard J. see **Byrne, Paul A.**

Treasure, Tom see **Irving, Miles**

Treffert, Darold A. The obviously ill patient in need of treatment: a fourth standard for civil commitment. *Hospital and Community Psychiatry.* 1985 Mar; 36(3): 259–264.
(INVOLUNTARY COMMITMENT)

Tribble, Jack L. see **Austin, Christopher P.**

Tripathi, K.D. see **Gitanjali, B.**

Tripp, Glenn; McCotter, Patricia I. Ethics committee consultation: a case. *HEC (HealthCare Ethics Committee) Forum.* 1997 Dec; 9(4): 389–392.
(ALLOWING TO DIE; ETHICISTS AND ETHICS COMMITTEES)

Trnobranski, Philippa H. The decision to prolong life: ethical perspectives of a clinical dilemma. *Journal of Clinical Nursing.* 1996 Jul; 5(4): 233–240.
(ALLOWING TO DIE)

Trojahn, Carrie see **Stadler, Holly A.**

Trotter, Griffin. The Loyal Physician: Roycean Ethics and the Practice of Medicine. Nashville, TN: Vanderbilt University Press; 1997. 299 p.
(MEDICAL ETHICS)

Truesdell, Sandra see **Moseley, Kathryn L.**

Truog, Robert see **Goldworth, Amnon**

Tsang, June see **Hui, Elsie**

Tschudin, Verena. Myths, magic and reality in nursing ethics: a personal perspective. *Nursing Ethics.* 1998 Jan; 5(1): 52–58.
(NURSING ETHICS)

Tsevat, Joel; Dawson, Neal V.; Wu, Albert W.; Lynn, Joanne; Soukup, Jane R.; Cook, E. Francis; Vidaillet, Humberto; Phillips, Russell S. Health values of hospitalized patients 80 years or older. [For the HELP Investigators]. *JAMA.* 1998 Feb 4; 279(5): 371–375.
(HEALTH; PATIENT CARE/AGED)

Tsuchida, Tomoaki. A differing perspective on advance directives. *In:* Sass, Hans–Martin; Veatch, Robert M.; Kimura, Rihito, eds. Advance Directives and Surrogate Decision Making in Health Care: United States, Germany, and Japan. Baltimore, MD: Johns Hopkins University Press; 1998: 209–221.
(ADVANCE DIRECTIVES)

Tsuguya, Fukui see **Asai, Atsushi**

Tu, Ping; Smith, Herbert L. Determinants of induced abortion and their policy implications in four counties in North China. *Studies in Family Planning.* 1995 Sep–Oct; 26(5): 278–286.
(ABORTION/FOREIGN COUNTRIES)

Tucker, Bonnie Poitras. Deaf culture, cochlear implants, and elective disability. *Hastings Center Report.* 1998 Jul–Aug; 28(4): 6–14.
(PATIENT CARE/MINORS; TREATMENT REFUSAL/MINORS)

Tuckfelt, Mark see **Love, Susan M.**

Tuennerman, Jill A. see **Kaplan, Richard S.**

Tuffs, Annette. Central ethics committee formed in Germany. [News]. *Lancet.* 1995 Aug 12; 346(8972): 433.
(ETHICISTS AND ETHICS COMMITTEES)

Tulsky, Jacqueline Peterson see **Oscherwitz, Tom**

Tulsky, James A.; Cassileth, Barrie R.; Bennett, Charles L. The effect of ethnicity on ICU use and DNR orders in hospitalized AIDS patients. *Journal of Clinical Ethics.* 1997 Summer; 8(2): 150–157.
(AIDS; BIOMEDICAL TECHNOLOGIES; RESUSCITATION ORDERS; TERMINAL CARE)

Tulsky, James A. see **Gertner, Eric J.**

Tunisia. Decree No. 94–1939 of 19 September 1994 laying down the functions, composition, and working procedures of the National Committee on Medical Ethics. *International Digest of Health Legislation.* 1995; 46(2): 201.
(ETHICISTS AND ETHICS COMMITTEES)

Turcotte, Jeremiah G. Supply, demand, and ethics of organ procurement: the medical perspective. *Transplantation Proceedings.* 1992 Oct; 24(5): 2140–2142.
(ORGAN AND TISSUE DONATION; ORGAN AND TISSUE TRANSPLANTATION)

Turcotte, Jeremiah G. Transplantation: a frontier for bioethics and bioscience. *In:* Phillips, Michael G., ed. Organ Procurement, Preservation and Distribution in Transplantation. Second Edition. Richmond, VA: UNOS; 1996: 13–22.
(ORGAN AND TISSUE TRANSPLANTATION)

Turcotte, Jeremiah G. see **Benjamin, Martin**

Turcotte, Jeremiah G. see **Burdick, James F.**

Turiel, Judith Steinberg. Beyond Second Opinions: Making Choices About Fertility Treatment. Berkeley, CA: University of California Press; 1998. 393 p.
(REPRODUCTIVE TECHNOLOGIES)

Turiel, Judy see **Goldworth, Amnon**

Turillazzi, Emanuela see **Fineschi, Vittorio**

Turner, Leigh. A sheep named Dolly. [Editorial]. *Canadian Medical Association Journal.* 1997 Apr 15; 156(8): 1149–1150.
(CLONING)

Turner, Leigh. An anthropological exploration of contemporary bioethics: the varieties of common sense. *Journal of Medical Ethics.* 1998 Apr; 24(2): 127–133.
(BIOETHICS)

Turner, Leigh. The greening of bioethics: corporate funding of bioethics research. *Cambridge Quarterly of Healthcare Ethics.* 1998 Summer; 7(3): 326–328.
(BIOETHICS; ETHICISTS AND ETHICS COMMITTEES)

Turrell, Susan J. see **Olver, Ian N.**

Twycross, Robert. Palliative care. *In:* Chadwick, Ruth, ed. Encyclopedia of Applied Ethics, Volume 3. San Diego, CA: Academic Press; 1998: 419–433.
(TERMINAL CARE/HOSPICES)

Tyler, Audrey; Ball, David; Clarke, Angus. Genetic testing in the classroom. [Letter]. *BMJ (British Medical Journal).* 1995 Jul 29; 311(7000): 330.
(GENETIC SCREENING)

Tynan, Michael see **Brawn, W.J.**

Tysinger, James W.; Klonis, Leah K.; Sadler, John Z.; Wagner, James M. Teaching ethics using small–group, problem–based learning. *Journal of Medical Ethics.* 1997 Oct; 23(5): 315–318.
(MEDICAL ETHICS/EDUCATION)

U

U.S. Congress. House. A bill to amend the Animal Welfare Act to strengthen the annual reporting requirements of research facilities conducting animal experimentation or testing and to improve the accountability of animal experimentation programs of the Department of Defense [Animal Experimentation Right to Know Act]. H.R. 4971, 103d Cong., 2d Sess. Introduced by Robert G. Torricelli; 1994 Aug 16. 6 p.
(ANIMAL EXPERIMENTATION)

U.S. Congress. House. A bill to amend the Fair Labor Standards Act of 1938 to restrict employers in obtaining, disclosing, and using of genetic information. H.R. 3477, 104th Cong., 2d Sess. Introduced by Joseph P. Kennedy;

1996 May 16. 3 p.
(CONFIDENTIALITY/LEGAL ASPECTS; GENETIC
SCREENING)

U.S. Congress. House. A bill to amend title 10, United
States Code, to limit the collection and use by the
Department of Defense of individual genetic identifying
information for the purpose of identification of remains,
other than when the consent of the individual concerned
is obtained. H.R. 2873, 104th Cong., 2d Sess. Introduced
by Joseph P. Kennedy; 1996 Jan 24. 2 p.
(DNA FINGERPRINTING; GENETIC SCREENING)

U.S. Congress. House. A bill to prohibit insurance
providers from denying or canceling health insurance
coverage, or varying the premiums, terms, or conditions
for health insurance coverage on the basis of genetic
information or a request for genetic services, and for
other purposes [Genetic Information Nondiscrimination
in Health Insurance Act of 1995]. H.R. 2748, 104th
Cong., 1st Sess. Introduced by Louise McIntosh
Slaughter; 1995 Dec 7. 8 p.
(GENETIC SCREENING)

U.S. Congress. House. A bill to protect the privacy of
health information in the age of genetic and other new
technologies, and for other purposes [Medical Privacy
in the Age of New Technologies Act of 1996]. H.R.
3482, 104th Cong., 2d Sess. Introduced by Jim
McDermott; 1996 May 16. 73 p.
(CONFIDENTIALITY/LEGAL ASPECTS)

**U.S. Congress. House. Committee on Government
Reform and Oversight. Subcommittee on Human
Resources.** Oversight of NIH and FDA: Bioethics and
the Adequacy of Informed Consent. Hearing, 8 May
1997. Washington, DC: U.S. Government Printing
Office; 1997.
(ETHICISTS AND ETHICS COMMITTEES; HUMAN
EXPERIMENTATION/INFORMED CONSENT; HUMAN
EXPERIMENTATION/REGULATION)

**U.S. Congress. House. Committee on Science.
Subcommittee on Technology.** Biotechnology and the
Ethics of Cloning: How Far Should We Go? Hearing,
5 Mar 1997. Washington, DC: U.S. Government Printing
Office; 1997. 59 p.
(CLONING)

**U.S. Congress. House. Committee on Science.
Subcommittee on Technology.** Review of the
President's Commission's Recommendations on Cloning.
Hearing, 12 Jun 1997. Washington, DC: U.S.
Government Printing Office; 1997. 227 p.
(CLONING)

**U.S. Congress. House. Committee on Science.
Subcommittee on Technology.** Technological
Advances in Genetics Testing: Implications for the
Future. Hearing, 17 Sep 1996. Washington, DC: U.S.
Government Printing Office; 1996. 191 p.
(GENETIC SCREENING)

**U.S. Congress. House. Committee on the Judiciary.
Subcommittee on the Constitution.** Partial-Birth
Abortion. Hearing, 15 Jun 1995. Washington, DC: U.S.
Government Printing Office; 1995. 142 p.
(ABORTION/LEGAL ASPECTS)

U.S. Congress. Senate. A bill to amend Title 18, United
States Code, to ban partial-birth abortions [Partial-Birth
Abortion Ban Act of 1995]. S. 939, 104th Cong., 1st Sess.
Introduced by Robert C. Smith and Phil Gramm; 1995
Jun 19. 3 p.
(ABORTION/LEGAL ASPECTS)

U.S. Congress. Senate. A bill to establish limitation with
respect to the disclosure and use of genetic information,
and for other purposes [Genetic Privacy and
Nondiscrimination Act of 1995]. S. 1416, 104th Cong.,
1st Sess. Introduced by Mark O. Hatfield; 1995 Nov 15.
7 p.
(CONFIDENTIALITY/LEGAL ASPECTS; GENETIC
SCREENING)

U.S. Congress. Senate. A bill to establish limitations on
health plans with respect to genetic information, and for
other purposes [Genetic Fairness Act of 1996]. S. 1600,
104th Cong., 2d Sess. Introduced by Diane Feinstein;
1996 Mar 7. 7 p.
(GENETIC SCREENING)

U.S. Congress. Senate. A bill to prohibit discrimination
against individuals and their family members on the basis
of genetic information, or a request for genetic services
[Genetic Information Nondiscrimination in Health
Insurance Act of 1997]. S. 89, 105th Cong., 1st Sess.
Introduced by Olympia Snowe; 1997 Jan 21. 15 p.
(GENETIC SCREENING)

U.S. Congress. Senate. A bill to prohibit the restriction
of certain types of medical communications between a
health care provider and a patient [Patient Right to
Know Act]. S. 449, 105th Cong., 1st Sess. Introduced
by Jon Kyl; 1997 Mar 17. 8 p.
(HEALTH CARE/ECONOMICS)

U.S. Congress. Senate. A bill to provide for the
establishment of a Commission to Promote a National
Dialogue on Bioethics. S. 1595, 105th Cong., 2d Sess.
Introduced by Bill Frist; 1998 Feb 2. 9 p.
(BIOETHICS; ETHICISTS AND ETHICS COMMITTEES)

**U.S. Congress. Senate. Committee on Labor and
Human Resources.** Human Subjects Research:
Radiation Experimentation. Hearing, 13 Jan 1994
(Waltham, MA). Washington, DC: U.S. Government
Printing Office; 1994. 61 p.
(FRAUD AND MISCONDUCT; HUMAN
EXPERIMENTATION/SPECIAL POPULATIONS)

**U.S. Congress. Senate. Committee on Labor and
Human Resources.** Women's Health: Ensuring Quality
and Equity in Biomedical Research. Hearing, 29 Jun
1992. Washington, DC: U.S. Government Printing
Office; 1992. 48 p.
(BIOMEDICAL RESEARCH; HEALTH; HUMAN
EXPERIMENTATION/SPECIAL POPULATIONS)

**U.S. Congress. Senate. Committee on Labor and
Human Resources. Subcommittee on Public Health
and Safety.** Ethics and Theology: A Continuation of
the National Discussion on Human Cloning. Hearing,
17 Jun 1997. Washington, DC: U.S. Government
Printing Office; 1997. 69 p.
(CLONING)

**U.S. Congress. Senate. Committee on Labor and
Human Resources. Subcommittee on Public Health
and Safety.** Scientific Discoveries in Cloning:
Challenges for Public Policy. Hearing, 12 Mar 1997.
Washington, DC: U.S. Government Printing Office;

1997. 87 p.
(CLONING)

U.S. Court of Appeals, Eighth Circuit. Krauel v. Iowa Methodist Medical Center. *Federal Reporter, 3d Series.* 1996 Sep 11 (date of decision). 95: 674–681.
(REPRODUCTIVE TECHNOLOGIES)

U.S. Court of Appeals, Fifth Circuit. Deramus v. Jackson National Life Insurance Company. *Federal Reporter, 3d Series.* 1996 Aug 7 (date of decision). 92: 274–283.
(AIDS)

U.S. Court of Appeals, Ninth Circuit. Lee v. State of Oregon. *Federal Reporter, 3d Series.* 1997 Feb 27 (date of decision). 107: 1382–1397.
(SUICIDE)

U.S. Court of Appeals, Ninth Circuit. Mayfield v. Dalton. *Federal Reporter, 3d Series.* 1997 Mar 27 (date of decision). 109: 1423–1427.
(DNA FINGERPRINTING)

U.S. Court of Appeals, Sixth Circuit. Brotherton v. Cleveland. *Federal Reporter, 2d Series.* 1991 Jan 18 (date of decision). 923: 477–484.
(INFORMED CONSENT; ORGAN AND TISSUE DONATION)

U.S. Court of Appeals, Third Circuit. United States v. Ward. *Federal Reporter, 3d Series.* 1997 Nov 13 (date of decision). 131: 335–343.
(AIDS/TESTING AND SCREENING)

U.S. Department of Health and Human Services. Confidentiality of Individually Identifiable Health Information: Recommendations of the Secretary of Health and Human Services, Pursuant to Section 264 of the Health Insurance Portability and Accountability Act of 1996. U.S. Government Printing Office; downloaded from Web site: http://aspe.os.hhs.gov/admnsimp/index.htm; 1997 Sep 11. 50 p.
(CONFIDENTIALITY/LEGAL ASPECTS)

U.S. Department of Health and Human Services. Health Insurance in the Age of Genetics. Report: Executive Summary. *In:* BioLaw: A Legal and Ethical Reporter on Medicine, Health Care, and Bioengineering. Special Sections, 2(9). Frederick, MD: University Publications of America; 1997 Sep: S265–S277.
(GENETIC SCREENING)

U.S. Department of Health and Human Services. Departmental Appeals Board. Research Integrity Adjudications Panel. Mikulas Popovic, M.D., Ph.D. [Docket No. A–93–100; Decision No. 1446. 1993 Nov 3 (date of decision)]. Washington, DC: U.S. Department of Health and Human Services; 1993 Nov 3. 79+ p.
(BIOMEDICAL RESEARCH; FRAUD AND MISCONDUCT)

U.S. District Court, D. Hawaii. Mayfield v. Dalton. *Federal Supplement.* 1995 Sep 8 (date of decision). 901: 300–306.
(DNA FINGERPRINTING)

U.S. District Court, D. Montana, Great Falls Division. Armstrong v. Mazurek. *Federal Supplement.* 1995 Sep 29 (date of decision). 906: 561–569.
(ABORTION/LEGAL ASPECTS)

U.S. District Court, D. South Dakota, W.D. Planned Parenthood, Sioux Falls Clinic v. Miller. *Federal Supplement.* 1994 Aug 22 (date of decision). 860: 1409–1421.
(ABORTION/LEGAL ASPECTS)

U.S. District Court, D. Utah, C.D. Utah Women's Clinic, Inc. v. Graham. *Federal Supplement.* 1995 Jun 20 (date of decision). 892: 1379–1385.
(ABORTION/FINANCIAL SUPPORT; ABORTION/LEGAL ASPECTS)

U.S. District Court, W.D. Michigan, S.D. Mauro v. Borgess Medical Center. *Federal Supplement.* 1995 May 4 (date of decision). 886: 1349–1356.
(AIDS/HEALTH PERSONNEL)

U.S. Federal Bureau of Investigation. Legislative Guidelines for DNA Databases [and] Text of the DNA Identification Act (1994), as Enacted: Subtitle C –– DNA Identification [and] Statutes and Legislation Regarding Mandatory Submission of Blood Samples for DNA Identification Purposes, July 1996. Quantico, VA: Federal Bureau of Investigation; 1991. 51 p.
(DNA FINGERPRINTING)

U.S. General Accounting Office. Managed Care: Explicit Gag Clauses Not Found in HMO Contracts, but Physician Concerns Remain. Report to Congressional Requesters. Washington, DC: U.S. General Accounting Office; 1997 Aug. 23 p.
(HEALTH CARE/ECONOMICS; PATIENT CARE)

U.S. General Accounting Office. NIH–Funded Research: Therapeutic Human Fetal Tissue Transplantation Projects Meet Federal Requirements. Report to the Chairmen and Ranking Minority Members, Committee on Labor and Human Resources, U.S. Senate, and Committee on Commerce, House of Representatives. Washington, DC: U.S. General Accounting Office; 1997 Mar. 8 p.
(EMBRYO AND FETAL RESEARCH; ORGAN AND TISSUE DONATION)

U.S. General Accounting Office. Patient Self–Determination Act: Providers Offer Information on Advance Directives but Effectiveness Uncertain. Report to the Ranking Minority Member, Subcommittee on Health, Committee on Ways and Means, House of Representatives. Washington, DC: U.S. General Accounting Office; 1995 Aug 28. 48 p.
(ADVANCE DIRECTIVES)

U.S. National Center for Human Genome Research. ELSI 1990–1995: A Review of the Ethical, Legal, and Social Implications Research Program and Related Activities. Bethesda, MD: U.S. National Center for Human Genome Research; 1996 Apr 12. 17 p.
(GENETIC SCREENING; GENOME MAPPING)

U.S. National Institutes of Health. Guidelines for research involving recombinant DNA molecules. *Federal Register.* 1983 Jun 1; 48(106): 24556–24581.
(RECOMBINANT DNA RESEARCH/REGULATION)

U.S. National Institutes of Health. Recombinant DNA research: proposed actions under the guidelines; notice. *Federal Register.* 1996 Nov 22; 61(227): 59726–59742.
(GENE THERAPY; HUMAN EXPERIMENTATION/ETHICS COMMITTEES; HUMAN EXPERIMENTATION/REGULATION)

U.S. Supreme Court. Bragdon v. Abbott. *Supreme Court*

Reporter. 1998 Jun 25 (date of decision). 118: 2196–2218.
(AIDS/HEALTH PERSONNEL)

Ubel, Peter A.; Arnold, Robert M.; Gramelspacher, Gregory P.; Hoppe, Ruth B.; Landefeld, C. Seth; Levinson, Wendy; Tierney, William; Tolle, Susan W. Acceptance of external funds by physician organizations: issues and policy options. *Journal of General Internal Medicine.* 1995 Nov; 10(11): 624–630.
(HEALTH CARE/ECONOMICS)

Ubel, Peter A.; Asch, David A. Semantic and moral debates about hastening death: a survey of bioethicists. *Journal of Clinical Ethics.* 1997 Fall; 8(3): 242–249.
(ALLOWING TO DIE; ETHICISTS AND ETHICS COMMITTEES; EUTHANASIA; SUICIDE)

Ubel, Peter A.; DeKay, M.; Baron, J.; Asch, D.A. Public preferences for efficiency and racial equity in kidney transplant allocation decisions. *Transplantation Proceedings.* 1996 Oct; 28(5): 2997–3002.
(ORGAN AND TISSUE TRANSPLANTATION; RESOURCE ALLOCATION/BIOMEDICAL TECHNOLOGIES; SELECTION FOR TREATMENT)

Ubel, Peter A.; Goold, Susan Dorr. 'Rationing' health care: not all definitions are created equal. *Archives of Internal Medicine.* 1998 Feb 9; 158(3): 209–214.
(HEALTH CARE; RESOURCE ALLOCATION)

Ubel, Peter A.; Loewenstein, George. Distributing scarce livers: the moral reasoning of the general public. *Social Science and Medicine.* 1996 Apr; 42(7): 1049–1055.
(ORGAN AND TISSUE TRANSPLANTATION; RESOURCE ALLOCATION/BIOMEDICAL TECHNOLOGIES; SELECTION FOR TREATMENT)

Ubel, Peter A.; Loewenstein, George. Public perceptions of the importance of prognosis in allocating transplantable livers to children. *Medical Decision Making.* 1996 Jul–Sep; 16(3): 234–241.
(ORGAN AND TISSUE TRANSPLANTATION; RESOURCE ALLOCATION/BIOMEDICAL TECHNOLOGIES; SELECTION FOR TREATMENT)

Ubel, Peter A.; Loewenstein, George. The efficacy and equity of retransplantation: an experimental survey of public attitudes. *Health Policy.* 1995 Nov; 34(2): 145–151.
(ORGAN AND TISSUE TRANSPLANTATION; RESOURCE ALLOCATION/BIOMEDICAL TECHNOLOGIES; SELECTION FOR TREATMENT)

Ubel, Peter A. see **Love, Susan M.**

UCLA Clinical Research Center. Statement of the UCLA Clinical Research Center. *In:* Shamoo, Adil E., ed. Ethics in Neurobiological Research with Human Subjects: The Baltimore Conference on Ethics. Amsterdam: Gordon and Breach; 1997: 173–174.
(HUMAN EXPERIMENTATION/RESEARCH DESIGN; HUMAN EXPERIMENTATION/SPECIAL POPULATIONS)

Udén, Giggi; Norberg, Astrid; Norberg, Siv. The stories of physicians, registered nurses and enrolled nurses about ethically difficult care episodes in surgical care. *Scandinavian Journal of Caring Sciences.* 1995; 9(4): 245–253.
(MEDICAL ETHICS; NURSING ETHICS; PATIENT CARE)

Uhlmann, Michael M., ed. Last Rights? Assisted Suicide and Euthanasia Debated. Washington, DC: Ethics and Public Policy Center; Grand Rapids, MI: W.B. Eerdmans; 1998. 667 p.
(ALLOWING TO DIE; EUTHANASIA; SUICIDE)

Underwood, C.R. Of ethics –– of right and wrong. [Editorial]. *Journal of the Medical Association of Georgia.* 1990 Nov; 79(11): 800–803.
(MEDICAL ETHICS)

Underwood, Martin see **Slowther, Anne**

United Methodist Church. Faithful Witness on Today's Issues: Genetic Science. [Pamphlet]. Washington, DC: General Board of Church and Society; 1992. 23 p.
(GENETIC INTERVENTION; ORGAN AND TISSUE DONATION)

United Network for Organ Sharing (UNOS). Ethics Committee. Ethics of organ transplantation from living donors. *Transplantation Proceedings.* 1992 Oct; 24(5): 2236–2237.
(ORGAN AND TISSUE DONATION)

United Network for Organ Sharing (UNOS). Ethics Committee. General principles for allocating human organs and tissues. *Transplantation Proceedings.* 1992 Oct; 24(5): 2227–2235.
(ORGAN AND TISSUE TRANSPLANTATION; RESOURCE ALLOCATION/BIOMEDICAL TECHNOLOGIES; SELECTION FOR TREATMENT)

University of Texas. M.D. Anderson Cancer Center. Ethical principles for allocating clinical resources. *HEC (HealthCare Ethics Committee) Forum.* 1998 Jun; 10(2): 220–221.
(RESOURCE ALLOCATION)

Urv–Wong, Ene K. see **Kane, Rosalie A.**

Utzeri, G. see **Elli, M.**

V

Valderrábano, Fernando. Cadaver transplantation as an ethical and cost-effective alternative to living donor transplantation: the Spanish experience. *Transplantation Proceedings.* 1992 Oct; 24(5): 2103–2105.
(ORGAN AND TISSUE DONATION; ORGAN AND TISSUE TRANSPLANTATION)

Valeri, M. see **Elli, M.**

van Baar, A.L. see **te Velde, E.R.**

van Berkel, Dymphie; Klinge, Ineke. Gene technology: also a gender issue: views of Dutch informed women on genetic screening and gene therapy. *Patient Education and Counseling.* 1997 May; 31(1): 49–55.
(GENE THERAPY; GENETIC SCREENING)

van de Wiel, Harry B.M. see **Wilbers, Doaitse**

Vandekieft, Gregg K. see **Brody, Howard**

van Delden, J.J.M. see **van Thiel, G.J.M.W.**

van Delden, Johannes J.M. Do-not-resuscitate decisions. *In:* Chadwick, Ruth, ed. Encyclopedia of Applied Ethics, Volume 1. San Diego, CA: Academic Press; 1998: 839–847.
(RESUSCITATION ORDERS)

van den Bercken, John H.L. see **Olde Rikkert, Marcel**

G.M.

Vandenbroucke, Jan P. Maintaining privacy and the health of the public should not be seen as in opposition. [Editorial]. *BMJ (British Medical Journal).* 1998 May 2; 316(7141): 1331–1332.
(BIOMEDICAL RESEARCH; CONFIDENTIALITY/LEGAL ASPECTS)

van der Arend, Arie J.G. An ethical perspective on euthanasia and assisted suicide in the Netherlands from a nursing point of view. *Nursing Ethics.* 1998 Jul; 5(4): 307–318.
(EUTHANASIA; SUICIDE)

van der Burg, Wibren. Slippery slope arguments. *In:* Chadwick, Ruth, ed. Encyclopedia of Applied Ethics, Volume 4. San Diego, CA: Academic Press; 1998: 129–142.
(BIOETHICS; EUTHANASIA)

van der Heide, A.; van der Maas, P.J.; Kollée, L.A.A. End-of-life decisions in Dutch paediatric practice. [Letter]. *Lancet.* 1997 Dec 6; 350(9092): 1711.
(ALLOWING TO DIE/INFANTS; EUTHANASIA)

van der Kamp, Margot D.O. see **Balls, Michael**

van der Maas, P.J. see **van der Heide, A.**

van der Maas, Paul J. End of life decisions in mentally disabled people: protecting vulnerable life does not mean prolonging it regardless of suffering. [Editorial]. *BMJ (British Medical Journal).* 1997 Jul 12; 315(7100): 73.
(ALLOWING TO DIE; EUTHANASIA)

van der Maas, Paul J.; Emanuel, Linda L. Factual findings. *In:* Emanuel, Linda L., ed. Regulating How We Die: The Ethical, Medical, and Legal Issues Surrounding Physician-Assisted Suicide. Cambridge, MA: Harvard University Press; 1998: 151–174, 300–307.
(EUTHANASIA; SUICIDE)

van der Poel, Cornelius J. Ethical aspects in palliative care. *American Journal of Hospice and Palliative Care.* 1996 May–Jun; 13(3): 49–55.
(TERMINAL CARE)

van der Wal, G. see **Muller, M.T.**

van der Wal, G. see **Onwuteaka–Philipsen, B.D.**

van der Wal, Gerrit see **Haverkate, Ilinka**

van der Wal, Gerrit see **Muller, Martien T.**

van der Wal, Gerrit see **Onwuteaka–Philipsen, Bregje D.**

van der Westhuizen, S. see **Viljoen, D.**

Vanderpool, Harold Y., ed. The Ethics of Research Involving Human Subjects: Facing the 21st Century. Frederick, MD: University Publishing Group; 1996. 531 p.
(HUMAN EXPERIMENTATION)

Vanderpool, Harold Y. What's happening in research ethics? Commentary on Brody. *In:* Carson, Ronald A.; Burns, Chester R., eds. Philosophy of Medicine and Bioethics: A Twenty-Year Retrospective and Critical

Appraisal. Boston, MA: Kluwer Academic; 1997: 287–297.
(BIOMEDICAL RESEARCH; ETHICISTS AND ETHICS COMMITTEES; HUMAN EXPERIMENTATION)

van Duijn, C.M. see **Tibben, A.**

van Dyk, Jessica see **Kuhse, Helga**

van Eijk, Jacques Th.M. see **Muller, Martien T.**

van Eijk, Jacques Th.M. see **Onwuteaka–Philipsen, Bregje D.**

van Eys, Jan see **Jaffe, Norman**

van Haeringen, A. see **DudokdeWit, A.C.**

van Kooij, R.J. see **te Velde, E.R.**

van Lent, M. see **Logmans, A.**

van Os, J. see **Neeleman, J.**

VanRiper, J. see **Jacobson, Jay A.**

van Schie, Tejo; Seedhouse, David. The importance of care. *Health Care Analysis.* 1997 Dec; 5(4): 283–291.
(HEALTH CARE/ECONOMICS)

Van Steirteghem, A.; Tournaye, H.; Sureau, C.; Shenfield, F. Ethical considerations of intracytoplasmic sperm injection. *In:* Shenfield, F.; Sureau, C., eds. Ethical Dilemmas in Assisted Reproduction. New York, NY: Parthenon Pub. Group; 1997: 51–56.
(REPRODUCTIVE TECHNOLOGIES)

Van Steirteghem, A. see **Bonduelle, M.**

Van Steirteghem, André. Outcome of assisted reproductive technology. [Editorial]. *New England Journal of Medicine.* 1998 Jan 15; 338(3): 194–195.
(REPRODUCTIVE TECHNOLOGIES)

van Swieten, J.C. see **Tibben, A.**

van Thiel, G.J.M.W.; van Delden, J.J.M.; de Haan, K.; Huibers, A.K. Retrospective study of doctors' "end of life decisions" in caring for mentally handicapped people in institutions in the Netherlands. *BMJ (British Medical Journal).* 1997 Jul 12; 315(7100): 88–91.
(ALLOWING TO DIE; EUTHANASIA; TERMINAL CARE)

van Weel, Chris; Michels, Joop. Dying, not old age, to blame for costs of health care. *Lancet.* 1997 Oct 18; 350(9085): 1159–1160.
(HEALTH CARE/ECONOMICS; PATIENT CARE/AGED; TERMINAL CARE)

van Zutphen, Bert F.M. see **Balls, Michael**

Van Zwienen, Jan see **Orlowski, James P.**

Varghese, Francis T. see **Kelly, Brian J.**

Varmus, Harold; Satcher, David. Ethical complexities of conducting research in developing countries. *New England Journal of Medicine.* 1997 Oct 2; 337(14): 1003–1005.
(AIDS/HUMAN EXPERIMENTATION; HUMAN

EXPERIMENTATION/FOREIGN COUNTRIES; HUMAN EXPERIMENTATION/RESEARCH DESIGN; HUMAN EXPERIMENTATION/SPECIAL POPULATIONS)

Vaughan, K.J. see **Hooper, S.C.**

Vaught, Wayne see **Gelo, Florence**

Vawter, Dorothy E. see **Burt, R.A.P.**

Vawter, Dorothy E. see **Culhane–Pera, Kathleen A.**

Vazquez, Ma. Suarez. Technology and human dignity. *Dolentium Hominum: Church and Health in the World.* 1996; 33(11th Yr., No. 3): 29–34.
(PATIENT CARE; PROFESSIONAL PATIENT RELATIONSHIP)

Veatch, Robert M. Autonomy and communitarianism: the ethics of terminal care in cross–cultural perspective. *In:* Hoshino, Kazumasa, ed. Japanese and Western Bioethics: Studies in Moral Diversity. Boston, MA: Kluwer Academic; 1997: 119–129.
(ALLOWING TO DIE)

Veatch, Robert M. Case analysis in ethics instruction. *In:* Haddad, Amy Marie, ed. Teaching and Learning Strategies in Pharmacy Ethics. Second Edition. New York, NY: Pharmaceutical Products Press; 1997: 111–125.
(PROFESSIONAL ETHICS/EDUCATION)

Veatch, Robert M. Ethical dimensions of advance directives and surrogate decision making in the United States. *In:* Sass, Hans–Martin; Veatch, Robert M.; Kimura, Rihito, eds. Advance Directives and Surrogate Decision Making in Health Care: United States, Germany, and Japan. Baltimore, MD: Johns Hopkins University Press; 1998: 66–91.
(ADVANCE DIRECTIVES; ALLOWING TO DIE/LEGAL ASPECTS; INFORMED CONSENT; TREATMENT REFUSAL)

Veatch, Robert M., ed. Ethical issues in the changing health care system. *In:* Jonsen, Albert R.; Veatch, Robert M.; Walters, LeRoy, eds. Source Book in Bioethics: A Documentary History. Washington, DC: Georgetown University Press; 1998: 407–504.
(CONFIDENTIALITY; INFORMED CONSENT; ORGAN AND TISSUE DONATION; ORGAN AND TISSUE TRANSPLANTATION)

Veatch, Robert M. From Nuremberg through the 1990s: the priority of autonomy. *In:* Vanderpool, Harold Y., ed. The Ethics of Research Involving Human Subjects: Facing the 21st Century. Frederick, MD: University Publishing Group; 1996: 45–58.
(HUMAN EXPERIMENTATION/INFORMED CONSENT)

Veatch, Robert M. Technology assessment: inevitably a value judgment. *In:* Boyle, Philip J., ed. Getting Doctors to Listen: Ethics and Outcomes Data in Context. Washington, DC: Georgetown University Press; 1998: 180–195.
(BIOMEDICAL TECHNOLOGIES)

Veatch, Robert M., ed. The ethics of death and dying. *In:* Jonsen, Albert R.; Veatch, Robert M.; Walters, LeRoy, eds. Source Book in Bioethics: A Documentary History. Washington, DC: Georgetown University Press; 1998: 111–252.
(ALLOWING TO DIE; ALLOWING TO DIE/LEGAL ASPECTS; DETERMINATION OF DEATH)

Veatch, Robert M. The place of care in ethical theory.

Journal of Medicine and Philosophy. 1998 Apr; 23(2): 210–224.
(BIOETHICS)

Veatch, Robert M. Who should manage care? The case for patients. *Kennedy Institute of Ethics Journal.* 1997 Dec; 7(4): 391–401.
(HEALTH CARE/ECONOMICS; RESOURCE ALLOCATION)

Veatch, Robert M. see **Ashley, Benedict M.**

Veatch, Robert M. see **Burdick, James F.**

Veatch, Robert M. see **Goldstein, Barry**

Veatch, Robert M. see **Hsu, Irene**

Veatch, Robert M. see **Jonsen, Albert R.**

Veatch, Robert M. see **Peterson, Andrew M.**

Veatch, Robert M. see **Poikonen, John**

Veatch, Robert M. see **Sass, Hans–Martin**

Veglia, Geremia; Shmaefsky, Brian R.; Johnson, Walter. Public Attitudes Toward Human Genetic Manipulation: A Revitalization of Eugenics? Available from ERIC Document Reproduction Service, DYNCORP I&ET, 7420 Fullerton Rd., Suite 110, Springfield, VA 22153–2852; Document No. ED327408; SE051655; 1990. 26 p.
(EUGENICS; GENETIC INTERVENTION)

Veitch, P.S. see **Briggs, J.D.**

Venn–Treloar, Josephine. Nuchal translucency -- screening without consent. [Personal view]. *BMJ (British Medical Journal).* 1998 Mar 28; 316(7136): 1027.
(INFORMED CONSENT; PRENATAL DIAGNOSIS)

Ventres, William; Nichter, Mark; Reed, Richard; Frankel, Richard. Do–not–resuscitate discussions: a qualitative analysis. *Family Practice Research Journal.* 1992; 12(2): 157–169.
(PROFESSIONAL PATIENT RELATIONSHIP; RESUSCITATION ORDERS)

Ventruba, Pavel see **Mardesic, Tonko**

Vere, Duncan. Volunteers: the susceptible and the disadvantaged. *In:* Close, Bryony; Combes, Robert; Hubbard, Anthony; Illingworth, John, eds. Volunteers in Research and Testing. Bristol, PA: Taylor and Francis; 1997: 67–80.
(HUMAN EXPERIMENTATION/SPECIAL POPULATIONS)

Verheggen, Frank W.S.M.; Jonkers, Ruud; Kok, Gerjo. Patients' perceptions on informed consent and the quality of information disclosure in clinical trials. *Patient Education and Counseling.* 1996 Nov; 29(2): 137–153.
(HUMAN EXPERIMENTATION/INFORMED CONSENT)

Verhey, Allen. A Protestant perspective on access to healthcare. *Cambridge Quarterly of Healthcare Ethics.* 1998 Summer; 7(3): 247–253.
(HEALTH CARE/ECONOMICS; RESOURCE ALLOCATION)

Verhey, Allen. A Protestant perspective on ending life: faithfulness in the face of death. *In:* Battin, Margaret

P.; Rhodes, Rosamond; Silvers, Anita, eds. Physician Assisted Suicide: Expanding the Debate. New York, NY: Routledge; 1998: 347–361.
(SUICIDE)

Verhey, Allen. Bioethics in the Reformed tradition. *In:* Lustig, B. Andrew, ed.; Center for Medical Ethics and Health Policy (Houston, TX). Bioethics Yearbook, Volume 5: Theological Developments in Bioethics, 1992–1994. Boston, MA: Kluwer Academic; 1997: 269–282.
(BIOETHICS)

Verhey, Allen. Commodification, commercialization, and embodiment. *Women's Health Issues.* 1997 May–Jun; 7(3): 132–142.
(PERSONHOOD; REPRODUCTIVE TECHNOLOGIES)

Verhey, Allen. Theology after Dolly. *Christian Century.* 1997 Mar 19–26; 114(10): 285–286.
(CLONING; REPRODUCTION)

Verhey, Allen see Goldworth, Amnon

Verhey, Allen see Lammers, Stephen E.

Verhoef, Marja see Sneiderman, Barney

Verhoef, Marja J.; Lewkonia, Raymond M.; Kinsella, T. Douglas. Ethical issues concerning current human DNA banking practices in Canada: three perspectives. *In:* Knoppers, Bartha Maria, ed. Human DNA: Law and Policy: International and Comparative Perspectives. Proceedings of the First International Conference on DNA Sampling and Human Genetic Research: Ethical, Legal, and Policy Aspects, held in Montreal, Canada, 6–8 Sep 1996. Boston, MA: Kluwer Law International; 1997: 393–405.
(GENETIC RESEARCH; HUMAN EXPERIMENTATION/ETHICS COMMITTEES)

Verhoef, Marja J. see Kinsella, T. Douglas

Verhoeff, A. see Logmans, A.

Verma, Ishwar C. Ethical concerns in genome diversity studies in developing countries. *In:* Knoppers, Bartha Maria, ed. Human DNA: Law and Policy: International and Comparative Perspectives. Proceedings of the First International Conference on DNA Sampling and Human Genetic Research: Ethical, Legal, and Policy Aspects, held in Montreal, Canada, 6–8 Sep 1996. Boston, MA: Kluwer Law International; 1997: 257–263.
(GENETIC RESEARCH; GENOME MAPPING)

Vermund, Sten H. see Phanuphak, Praphan

Vernon, Bryan see Plant, Martin

Verweij, Marcel; Kortmann, Frank. Moral assessment of growth hormone therapy for children with idiopathic short stature. *Journal of Medical Ethics.* 1997 Oct; 23(5): 305–309.
(PATIENT CARE/MINORS; SELECTION FOR TREATMENT)

Veterans Affairs National Headquarters. Bioethics Committee. Ethical Issues in Long-Term Care: Committee Report. Issued by the VA National Center for Clinical Ethics, White River Junction, VT 05009; 1996 May. 30 p.
(PATIENT CARE/AGED)

Veterans Affairs National Headquarters. Bioethics Committee. Ethics Advisory Committees: Committee Report. Issued by the VA National Center for Clinical Ethics, White River Junction, VT 05009; 1996 May. 8 p.
(ETHICISTS AND ETHICS COMMITTEES)

Veterans Affairs National Headquarters. Bioethics Committee. Physician–Assisted Suicide: Committee Report. Issued by the VA National Center for Clinical Ethics, White River Junction, VT 05009; 1996 May. 5 p.
(SUICIDE; TERMINAL CARE)

Vettese, Margaret A. see Sulmasy, Daniel P.

Viafora, Corrado see Dell'Oro, Roberto

Vickrey, Barbara G. see Bernat, James L.

Vidaillet, Humberto see Tsevat, Joel

Vietti, Teresa J. see Jaffe, Norman

Vietzke, Wesley M. see Murray–Garcia, Jann

Viljoen, D.; Oosthuizen, C.; van der Westhuizen, S. Patient attitudes to prenatal screening and termination of pregnancy at Groote Schuur Hospital: a two year prospective study. *East African Medical Journal.* 1996 May; 73(5): 327–329.
(ABORTION/ATTITUDES; ABORTION/FOREIGN COUNTRIES; PRENATAL DIAGNOSIS)

Vincent, Jean–Didier see Noble, Denis

Vines, Gail. Genetics: let the public decide. [News]. *BMJ (British Medical Journal).* 1997 Apr 5; 314(7086): 1055.
(GENETIC INTERVENTION; GENETIC RESEARCH)

Viola, Raymond A.; Wells, George A.; Peterson, Joan. The effects of fluid status and fluid therapy on the dying: a systematic review. *Journal of Palliative Care.* 1997 Winter; 13(4): 41–52.
(TERMINAL CARE)

Virginia. Status of children of assisted conception. *Code of Virginia Annotated.* 1997 Jul 1 (date effective). Sects. 20–156 to 20–165. 11 p.
(REPRODUCTIVE TECHNOLOGIES; SURROGATE MOTHERS)

Virnig, Beth A.; Caplan, Arthur L. Required request: what difference has it made? *Transplantation Proceedings.* 1992 Oct; 24(5): 2155–2158.
(ORGAN AND TISSUE DONATION)

Vivian, Jesse C.; Brushwood, David B. Legal cases that raise ethical issues. *In:* Haddad, Amy Marie, ed. Teaching and Learning Strategies in Pharmacy Ethics. Second Edition. New York, NY: Pharmaceutical Products Press; 1997: 1–17.
(PROFESSIONAL ETHICS/EDUCATION)

Vogel, Gretchen. Genetic enhancement: from science fiction to ethics quandary. [News]. *Science.* 1997 Sep 19; 277(5333): 1753–1754.
(GENE THERAPY; GENETIC RESEARCH)

Vogel, Gretchen. Xenotransplants: no moratorium on clinical trials. [News]. *Science.* 1998 Jan 30; 279(5351): 648.

(HUMAN EXPERIMENTATION/REGULATION; ORGAN AND TISSUE TRANSPLANTATION)

Volicer, Ladislav. Hospice care for dementia patients. [Editorial]. *Journal of the American Geriatrics Society.* 1997 Sep; 45(9): 1147–1149.
(TERMINAL CARE/HOSPICES)

Volicer, Ladislav see **Hurley, Ann C.**

Volk, Robert J.; Cantor, Scott B.; Spann, Stephen J.; Cass, Alvah R.; Cardenas, Melchor P.; Warren, Michael M. Preferences of husbands and wives for prostate cancer screening. *Archives of Family Medicine.* 1997 Jan–Feb; 6(1): 72–76.
(MASS SCREENING; PATIENT CARE)

von Fragstein, Martin see **Ashcroft, Richard**

W

Wachbroit, Robert. Genetic encores: the ethics of human cloning. *Philosophy and Public Policy.* 1997 Fall; 17(4): 1–7.
(CLONING)

Wachbroit, Robert. Health and disease, concepts of. *In:* Chadwick, Ruth, ed. Encyclopedia of Applied Ethics, Volume 2. San Diego, CA: Academic Press; 1998: 533–538.
(HEALTH)

Wachbroit, Robert. The question not asked: the challenge of pleiotropic genetic tests. *Kennedy Institute of Ethics Journal.* 1998 Jun; 8(2): 131–144.
(GENETIC SCREENING; TRUTH DISCLOSURE)

Wacks, Raymond. Sacrificed for science: are animal experiments morally defensible? *In:* Becker, Gerhold K., ed. Changing Nature's Course: The Ethical Challenge of Biotechnology. Hong Kong: Hong Kong University Press; 1996: 37–57.
(ANIMAL EXPERIMENTATION)

Wade, Nicholas. F.B.I. set to open its DNA database for fighting crime: some fear for privacy. [News]. *New York Times.* 1998 Oct 12: A1, A15.
(DNA FINGERPRINTING)

Wade, Nicholas. Scientists cultivate cells at root of human life: hope for transplants and gene therapy –– ethics at issue. [News]. *New York Times.* 1998 Nov 6: A1, A24.
(EMBRYO AND FETAL RESEARCH; ORGAN AND TISSUE DONATION)

Wadman, Meredith. Backing for anti-cloning bill reopens embryo debate. [News]. *Nature.* 1997 Aug 7; 388(6642): 505.
(CLONING; EMBRYO AND FETAL RESEARCH)

Wadman, Meredith. Bid to give legal protection to laboratory mice in US. [News]. *Nature.* 1998 May 7; 393(6680): 6.
(ANIMAL EXPERIMENTATION)

Wadman, Meredith. Business booms for guides to biology's moral maze. [News]. *Nature.* 1997 Oct 16; 389(6652): 658–659.
(BIOETHICS; ETHICISTS AND ETHICS COMMITTEES)

Wadman, Meredith. Cancer 'cure' article stirs up hot debate. [News]. *Nature.* 1998 May 14; 393(6681): 104–105.
(BIOMEDICAL RESEARCH)

Wadman, Meredith. Cloning for research 'should be allowed.' [News]. *Nature.* 1997 Jul 3; 388(6637): 6.
(CLONING)

Wadman, Meredith. Company aims to beat NIH human genome efforts. [News]. *Nature.* 1998 May 14; 393(6681): 101.
(GENOME MAPPING)

Wadman, Meredith. Controversy flares over AIDS prevention trials in Third World. [News]. *Nature.* 1997 Oct 30; 389(6654): 894.
(AIDS/HUMAN EXPERIMENTATION; HUMAN EXPERIMENTATION/FOREIGN COUNTRIES; HUMAN EXPERIMENTATION/RESEARCH DESIGN; HUMAN EXPERIMENTATION/SPECIAL POPULATIONS)

Wadman, Meredith. Ethical terms set for breast cancer test. [News]. *Nature.* 1997 Nov 27; 390(6658): 324.
(GENETIC SCREENING)

Wadman, Meredith. FDA turns down moratorium demand on xenotransplants. [News]. *Nature.* 1998 Jan 29; 391(6666): 423.
(HUMAN EXPERIMENTATION/REGULATION; ORGAN AND TISSUE TRANSPLANTATION)

Wadman, Meredith. Gene marker database stirs up debate. [News]. *Nature.* 1998 Feb 19; 391(6669): 726.
(GENOME MAPPING)

Wadman, Meredith. Genome panel defends researchers' –– and families' –– interests. [News]. *Nature.* 1998 Feb 26; 391(6670): 826.
(CONFIDENTIALITY; GENETIC RESEARCH; GENOME MAPPING)

Wadman, Meredith. Germline gene therapy 'must be spared excessive regulation.' [News]. *Nature.* 1998 Mar 26; 392(6674): 317.
(GENE THERAPY)

Wadman, Meredith. 'Group debate' urged for gene studies. [News]. *Nature.* 1998 Jan 22; 391(6665): 314.
(GENETIC RESEARCH; HUMAN EXPERIMENTATION/INFORMED CONSENT; ORGAN AND TISSUE DONATION)

Wadman, Meredith. Jewish leaders meet NIH chiefs on genetic stigmatization fears. [News]. *Nature.* 1998 Apr 30; 392(6679): 851.
(GENETIC RESEARCH; GENETIC SCREENING)

Wadman, Meredith. Mentally disabled research subjects 'need protection.' [News]. *Nature.* 1997 Oct 16; 389(6652): 652.
(FRAUD AND MISCONDUCT; HUMAN EXPERIMENTATION/SPECIAL POPULATIONS)

Wadman, Meredith. National Institutes of Health sets up its own bioethics panel. [News]. *Nature.* 1997 Dec 18–25; 390(6661): 651.
(BIOETHICS; ETHICISTS AND ETHICS COMMITTEES)

Wadman, Meredith. Population explosion raises alarm over lab animal health. [News]. *Nature.* 1998 Feb 12; 391(6668): 623.
(ANIMAL EXPERIMENTATION)

Wadman, Meredith. Privacy bill under fire from researchers. [News]. *Nature.* 1998 Mar 5; 392(6671): 6.
(CONFIDENTIALITY/LEGAL ASPECTS; HUMAN EXPERIMENTATION/REGULATION)

Wadman, Meredith. Row erupts over child aggression study. [News]. *Nature.* 1998 Apr 23; 392(6678): 747.
(BEHAVIORAL RESEARCH/MINORS; BEHAVIORAL RESEARCH/SPECIAL POPULATIONS; HUMAN EXPERIMENTATION/MINORS; HUMAN EXPERIMENTATION/SPECIAL POPULATIONS)

Wadman, Meredith. Seed sows further doubts on cloning. [News]. *Nature.* 1998 Jan 15; 391(6664): 218–219.
(CLONING)

Wadman, Meredith. Unesco text will target gene techniques. [News]. *Nature.* 1997 Aug 7; 388(6642): 508.
(CLONING; GENE THERAPY)

Wadman, Meredith. US dispute over live AIDS vaccine trials. [News]. *Nature.* 1997 Oct 2; 389(6650): 426.
(AIDS/HUMAN EXPERIMENTATION; HUMAN EXPERIMENTATION/SPECIAL POPULATIONS; IMMUNIZATION)

Wadman, Meredith. US Senate bills on cloning under fire from researchers. [News]. *Nature.* 1998 Feb 12; 391(6668): 623.
(CLONING)

Wadman, Meredith. US to tighten protection of medical data. [News]. *Nature.* 1997 Aug 14; 388(6643): 611.
(CONFIDENTIALITY/LEGAL ASPECTS)

Wadman, Meredith. $100m payout after drug data withheld. [News]. *Nature.* 1997 Aug 21; 388(6644): 703.
(BIOMEDICAL RESEARCH; FRAUD AND MISCONDUCT; HEALTH CARE/ECONOMICS; PATIENT CARE/DRUGS)

Wadman, Meredith see **Dickson, David**

Wagg, Adrian see **Stewart, Kevin**

Wagner, H. Ryan see **Swartz, Marvin S.**

Wagner, James M. see **Tysinger, James W.**

Wainwright, Paul; Cain, Paul. Using clients: a response to Paul Cain. [Commentary and response]. *Nursing Ethics.* 1998 Jul; 5(4): 363–369.
(CONFIDENTIALITY; INFORMED CONSENT; NURSING ETHICS/EDUCATION)

Waisburd, Marina see **Dexter, Paul R.**

Waldman, Irwin see **Sherman, Stephanie L.**

Waldner, Rosmarie see **Badoux, John C.**

Walker, Gail C. The right to die: healthcare workers' attitudes compared with a national public poll. *Omega: A Journal of Death and Dying.* 1997; 35(4): 339–345.
(ALLOWING TO DIE/ATTITUDES; EUTHANASIA/ATTITUDES; SUICIDE)

Walker, Leslie see **Bradley, Elizabeth**

Wall, Ian see **Payne-James, Jason**

Wall, James M. A time to be born. *Christian Century.* 1997 May 14; 114(16): 467–468.

(REPRODUCTIVE TECHNOLOGIES)

Wallace, A. see **Hartley, N.E.**

Wallace, Andrew G. see **McCurdy, Layton**

Wallace, David see **Williams, Peter**

Wallace, Robert B. see **Wildes, Kevin Wm.**

Wallace, Ruth; Wiegand, Frances; Warren, Connie. Beneficence toward whom? Ethical decision-making in a maternal-fetal conflict. *AACN Clinical Issues in Critical Care Nursing.* 1997 Nov; 8(4): 586–594.
(FETUSES; PATIENT CARE)

Wallach, Edward see **Agard, Ellen**

Wallenstein, Sylvan see **Hendin, Herbert**

Wallenstein, Sylvan see **Meier, Diane E.**

Wallerstein, Claire. Philippines considers euthanasia bill. [News]. *BMJ (British Medical Journal).* 1997 Jun 7; 314(7095): 1644.
(EUTHANASIA/LEGAL ASPECTS)

Walls, Lesley L. see **Foster, George E.**

Wallston, Barbara Strudler see **Rye, Patricia D.**

Wallston, Kenneth A. see **Rye, Patricia D.**

Walsh, Joseph T. see **Zweig, Franklin M.**

Walsh, Pat see **Cressey, David M.**

Walsh, Pat see **Grubb, Andrew**

Walters, James W. What Is a Person? An Ethical Exploration. Urbana, IL: University of Illinois Press; 1997. 187 p.
(ORGAN AND TISSUE DONATION; PERSONHOOD)

Walters, LeRoy, ed. Ethical issues arising from human reproductive technologies and arrangements. *In:* Jonsen, Albert R.; Veatch, Robert M.; Walters, LeRoy, eds. Source Book in Bioethics: A Documentary History. Washington, DC: Georgetown University Press; 1998: 335–406.
(REPRODUCTIVE TECHNOLOGIES)

Walters, LeRoy, ed. Ethical issues in human genetics. *In:* Jonsen, Albert R.; Veatch, Robert M.; Walters, LeRoy, eds. Source Book in Bioethics: A Documentary History. Washington, DC: Georgetown University Press; 1998: 253–333.
(GENE THERAPY; GENETIC INTERVENTION; GENETIC SCREENING; GENOME MAPPING)

Walters, LeRoy. Research and experimentation: a response to Kevin Wildes's essay. *In:* Wildes, Kevin Wm.; Mitchell, Alan C., eds. Choosing Life: A Dialogue on *Evangelium Vitae.* Washington, DC: Georgetown University Press; 1997: 206–209.
(BIOMEDICAL RESEARCH; EMBRYO AND FETAL RESEARCH)

Walters, LeRoy see **Jonsen, Albert R.**

Walters, LeRoy B. Behavioural and germ-line genetic

research. *In:* Kilner, John F.; Pentz, Rebecca D.; Young, Frank E., eds. Genetic Ethics: Do the Ends Justify the Genes? Grand Rapids, MI: W.B. Eerdmans; 1997: 104–112.
(BEHAVIORAL GENETICS; GENE THERAPY; GENETIC INTERVENTION)

Walzer, Michael. The hard questions: feed the face. *New Republic.* 1997 Jun 9; 216(23): 29.
(SUICIDE)

Wang, Robin see **Shanahan, Timothy**

Warburton, Nigel. Freedom to box. *Journal of Medical Ethics.* 1998 Feb; 24(1): 56–60.
(PUBLIC HEALTH)

Ward–Collins, Diana. "Noncompliant": isn't there a better way to say it? *American Journal of Nursing.* 1998 May; 98(5): 27–31.
(PROFESSIONAL PATIENT RELATIONSHIP)

Warde, Padraig see **Narasimhan, Parthas**

Warden, John. Crack down on drug inducements. [News]. *BMJ (British Medical Journal).* 1997 Aug 2; 315(7103): 273.
(HEALTH CARE/ECONOMICS; HEALTH CARE/FOREIGN COUNTRIES)

Warden, John. Surrogacy to be reviewed in United Kingdom. [News]. *BMJ (British Medical Journal).* 1997 Jun 21; 314(7097): 1782.
(SURROGATE MOTHERS)

Warden, John. Xenotransplantation moves ahead in UK. [News]. *BMJ (British Medical Journal).* 1998 Aug 8; 317(7155): 365.
(ORGAN AND TISSUE TRANSPLANTATION)

Warnock, Mary. Informed consent -- a publisher's duty. *BMJ (British Medical Journal).* 1998 Mar 28; 316(7136): 1002–1003.
(HUMAN EXPERIMENTATION/INFORMED CONSENT)

Warnock, Mary. The regulation of technology. *Cambridge Quarterly of Healthcare Ethics.* 1998 Spring; 7(2): 173–175.
(CLONING)

Warren, Connie see **Wallace, Ruth**

Warren, Mark J. see **Bursztajn, Harold**

Warren, Mary Anne. Abortion and human rights. *In: her*: Moral Status: Obligations to Persons and Other Living Things. New York, NY: Oxford University Press; 1997: 201–223.
(ABORTION)

Warren, Mary Anne. Euthanasia and the moral status of human beings. *In: her*: Moral Status: Obligations to Persons and Other Living Things. New York, NY: Oxford University Press; 1997: 185–200.
(ALLOWING TO DIE; EUTHANASIA; SUICIDE)

Warren, Mary Anne. Moral Status: Obligations to Persons and Other Living Things. New York, NY: Oxford University Press; 1997. 265 p.
(BIOETHICS; PERSONHOOD)

Warren, Michael M. see **Volk, Robert J.**

Wartofsky, Marx W. What can the epistemologists learn from the endocrinologists? Or is the philosophy of medicine based on a mistake? *In:* Carson, Ronald A.; Burns, Chester R., eds. Philosophy of Medicine and Bioethics: A Twenty–Year Retrospective and Critical Appraisal. Boston, MA: Kluwer Academic; 1997: 55–68.
(MEDICAL ETHICS)

Warwick, Ruth. Anonymity for unrelated bone marrow donors should remain. [Letter]. *BMJ (British Medical Journal).* 1997 Aug 30; 315(7107): 548–549.
(CONFIDENTIALITY; ORGAN AND TISSUE DONATION)

Warwick, Ruth. Collections of cord blood. [Letter]. *Lancet.* 1997 Jul 26; 350(9073): 297.
(BLOOD DONATION)

Washington. Supreme Court. Seeley v. State. *Pacific Reporter, 2d Series.* 1997 Jul 24 (date of decision). 940: 604–632.
(PATIENT CARE/DRUGS)

Washington. Supreme Court. State v. Olivas. *Pacific Reporter, 2d Series.* 1993 Aug 12 (date of decision). 856: 1076–1094.
(DNA FINGERPRINTING)

Wasserman, David. Research into genetics and crime: consensus and controversy. *Politics and the Life Sciences.* 1996 Mar; 15(1): 107–109.
(BEHAVIORAL GENETICS; GENETIC RESEARCH)

Wasserman, Eric M. see **Green, Ronald M.**

Wassertheil–Smoller, Sylvia see **Barnhart, J. Marie**

Watchko, Jon see **Frader, Joel E.**

Watchko, Jon F. Decision making on critically ill infants by parents. *American Journal of Diseases of Children.* 1983 Aug; 137(8): 795–798.
(ALLOWING TO DIE/INFANTS)

Water, Brent. One flesh? Cloning, procreation, and the family. *In:* Cole–Turner, Ronald, ed. Human Cloning: Religious Responses. Louisville, KY: Westminister John Knox Press; 1997: 78–90.
(CLONING; REPRODUCTION)

Waters, Teresa M. see **Shortell, Stephen M.**

Waters, W.E. Ethics and epidemiological research. *International Journal of Epidemiology.* 1985 Mar; 14(1): 48–51.
(BIOMEDICAL RESEARCH; HUMAN EXPERIMENTATION)

Watkins, William D. see **Fournier, Keith A.**

Watler, Crosbie L.; Gervais, Laurent; Cameron, Stewart. Lessons from Amy. [Letters and response]. *Canadian Medical Association Journal.* 1997 Jul 1; 157(1): 13–14.
(SUICIDE; TREATMENT REFUSAL)

Watson, Alastair J.M. see **Blunt, Jennifer**

Watson, J.D. see **McFadzean, J.**

go–ahead reawakens ethics debate. [News]. *Lancet.* 1998 Jun 13; 351(9118): 1789.
(AIDS/HUMAN EXPERIMENTATION; IMMUNIZATION)

Weijer, Charles. Film and narrative in bioethics: Akira Kurosawa's *Ikiru. In:* Nelson, Hilde Lindemann, ed. Stories and Their Limits: Narrative Approaches to Bioethics. New York, NY: Routledge; 1997: 113–122.
(BIOETHICS)

Weijer, Charles. Research methods and policies. *In:* Chadwick, Ruth, ed. Encyclopedia of Applied Ethics, Volume 3. San Diego, CA: Academic Press; 1998: 853–860.
(HUMAN EXPERIMENTATION)

Weijer, Charles; Dickens, Bernard; Meslin, Eric M. Bioethics for clinicians: 10. Research ethics. *Canadian Medical Association Journal.* 1997 Apr 15; 156(8): 1153–1157.
(HUMAN EXPERIMENTATION)

Weijer, Charles see **Alibhai, Shabbir M.H.**

Weijer, Charles see **Johnston, S.R.D.**

Weil, Peter A. Opinions of health care executives on access to care. *Hospital and Health Services Administration.* 1987 Nov; 32(4): 421–437.
(HEALTH CARE/ECONOMICS)

Weil, Vivian; Arzbaecher, Robert. Ethics and relationships in laboratories and research communities. *Professional Ethics.* 1995 Spring–Summer; 4(3–4): 83–125.
(BIOMEDICAL RESEARCH; FRAUD AND MISCONDUCT; PROFESSIONAL ETHICS)

Weinberger, Morris see **Ferguson, Jeffrey A.**

Weinberger, Morris see **Tierney, William M.**

Weindling, Paul. Weimar eugenics: the Kaiser Wilhelm Institute for Anthropology, Human Heredity and Eugenics in social context. *Annals of Science.* 1985 May; 42(3): 303–318.
(EUGENICS)

Weiner, Myron F.; Shuman, Daniel W. The privilege study. *Archives of General Psychiatry.* 1983 Sep; 40(9): 1027–1030.
(CONFIDENTIALITY/MENTAL HEALTH)

Weinstein, Bruce D. Teaching pharmacy ethics: the case study approach. *In:* Haddad, Amy Marie, ed. Teaching and Learning Strategies in Pharmacy Ethics. Second Edition. New York, NY: Pharmaceutical Products Press; 1997: 18–31.
(PATIENT CARE/DRUGS; PROFESSIONAL ETHICS/EDUCATION)

Weinstein, Bruce M. see **McCurdy, Layton**

Weinstock, Robert see **Leong, Gregory B.**

Weir, Robert F. Differing perspectives on consent, choice and control. *In:* Knoppers, Bartha Maria, ed. Human DNA: Law and Policy: International and Comparative Perspectives. Proceedings of the First International Conference on DNA Sampling and Human Genetic Research: Ethical, Legal, and Policy Aspects, held in Montreal, Canada, 6–8 Sep 1996. Boston, MA: Kluwer

Law International; 1997: 91–107.
(GENETIC RESEARCH; HUMAN EXPERIMENTATION/INFORMED CONSENT; ORGAN AND TISSUE DONATION)

Weir, Robert F.; Peters, Charles. Affirming the decisions adolescents make about life and death. *Hastings Center Report.* 1997 Nov–Dec; 27(6): 29–40.
(ADVANCE DIRECTIVES; INFORMED CONSENT/MINORS; TERMINAL CARE; TREATMENT REFUSAL/MINORS)

Weisman, Carol S. see **Sulmasy, Daniel P.**

Weiss, Gail. Sex–selective abortion: a relational approach. *In:* DiQuinzio, Patrice; Young, Iris Marion, eds. Feminist Ethics and Social Policy. Bloomington, IN: Indiana University Press; 1997: 274–290.
(ABORTION)

Weiss, Lawrence D. Private Medicine and Public Health: Profit, Politics, and Prejudice in the American Health Care Enterprise. Boulder, CO: Westview Press; 1997. 220 p.
(HEALTH CARE)

Weiss, Rick. Bioethics group divided over research on mentally ill. [News]. *Washington Post.* 1998 Nov 16: A6.
(HUMAN EXPERIMENTATION/REGULATION; HUMAN EXPERIMENTATION/SPECIAL POPULATIONS)

Weiss, Rick. Demand for organs fosters aggressive collection methods. [News]. *Washington Post.* 1997 Nov 24: A1, A16.
(ORGAN AND TISSUE DONATION)

Weiss, Rick. Patent sought on making of part–human creatures: scientist seeks to touch off ethics debate. [News]. *Washington Post.* 1998 Apr 2: A12.
(GENETIC INTERVENTION; PATENTING LIFE FORMS)

Weiss, Rick. Research ethics panel urges new regulations to protect mentally ill. [News]. *Washington Post.* 1998 Nov 18: A11.
(HUMAN EXPERIMENTATION/REGULATION; HUMAN EXPERIMENTATION/SPECIAL POPULATIONS)

Weiss, Robin A. Transgenic pigs and virus adaptation. *Nature.* 1998 Jan 22; 391(6665): 327–328.
(ORGAN AND TISSUE TRANSPLANTATION)

Weisstub, David N. see **Tomossy, George F.**

Weisz, Victoria see **Robbennolt, Jennifer K.**

Weitsman, Sojun Mel see **Ravindra, Ravi**

Welch, Robyn Perlman. Characteristics related to DNR orders for pediatric ICU patients. *Dimensions of Critical Care Nursing.* 1996 May–Jun; 15(3): 142–149.
(RESUSCITATION ORDERS)

Welie, Jos V.M. Placebo treatment. *In:* Chadwick, Ruth, ed. Encyclopedia of Applied Ethics, Volume 3. San Diego, CA: Academic Press; 1998: 493–502.
(PATIENT CARE/DRUGS)

Wellman, Carl. The inalienable right to life and the durable power of attorney. *Law and Philosophy.* 1995; 14(2): 245–269.
(ADVANCE DIRECTIVES; ALLOWING TO DIE; TREATMENT REFUSAL)

Wells, Frank O. Management of research misconduct -- in practice. *Journal of Internal Medicine.* 1994 Feb; 235(2): 115–121.
(BIOMEDICAL RESEARCH; FRAUD AND MISCONDUCT)

Wells, George A. see **Viola, Raymond A.**

Wells, John S.G. Health care rationing: nursing perspectives. *Journal of Advanced Nursing.* 1995 Oct; 22(4): 738–744.
(HEALTH CARE/FOREIGN COUNTRIES; RESOURCE ALLOCATION)

Wendte, Johannes F. see **Stronks, Karien**

Wenger, Neil see **FitzGerald, John**

Wenger, Neil see **Teno, Joan**

Wenger, Neil see **Teno, Joan M.**

Wenger, Neil see **Weeks, Jane C.**

Wenger, Neil S.; Greengold, Nancy L.; Oye, Robert K.; Kussin, Peter; Phillips, Russell S.; Desbiens, Norman A.; Liu, Honghu; Hiatt, Jonathan R.; Teno, Joan M.; Connors, Alfred F. Patients with DNR orders in the operating room: surgery, resuscitation, and outcomes. [For the SUPPORT Investigators]. *Journal of Clinical Ethics.* 1997 Fall; 8(3): 250–257.
(RESUSCITATION ORDERS; SELECTION FOR TREATMENT)

Wenger, Neil S.; Pearson, Marjorie L.; Desmond, Katherine A.; Kahn, Katherine L. Changes over time in the use of do not resuscitate orders and the outcomes of patients receiving them. *Medical Care.* 1997 Apr; 35(4): 311–319.
(RESUSCITATION ORDERS)

Wenger, Neil S.; Shapiro, Martin F. Consent and discontent. *Canadian Medical Association Journal.* 1997 Dec 15; 157(12): 1691–1692.
(HUMAN EXPERIMENTATION/INFORMED CONSENT)

Wenger, Neil S. see **Korenman, Stanley G.**

Wenger, Neil S. see **Phillips, Russell S.**

Wennergren, Margareta see **Wennerholm, Ulla–Britt**

Wennerholm, Ulla–Britt; Albertsson–Wikland, Kerstin; Bergh, Christina; Hamberger, Lars; Niklasson, Aimon; Nilsson, Lars; Thiringer, Klara; Wennergren, Margareta; Wikland, Matts; Borres, Magnus P. Postnatal growth and health in children born after cryopreservation as embryos. *Lancet.* 1998 Apr 11; 351(9109): 1085–1090.
(REPRODUCTIVE TECHNOLOGIES)

Wera–arpachai, Manu see **Robb, Merlin L.**

Werber, Stephen J. Ancient answers to modern questions: death, dying, and organ transplants -- a Jewish law perspective. *Journal of Law and Health.* 1996–1997; 11(1–2): 13–44.
(ALLOWING TO DIE/RELIGIOUS ASPECTS; DETERMINATION OF DEATH; EUTHANASIA/RELIGIOUS ASPECTS; ORGAN AND TISSUE DONATION; RESUSCITATION ORDERS; SUICIDE)

Werhane, Patricia; Doering, Jeffrey. Conflicts of interest and conflicts of commitment. *Professional Ethics.* 1995 Spring–Summer; 4(3–4): 47–81.
(BIOMEDICAL RESEARCH; FRAUD AND MISCONDUCT; PROFESSIONAL ETHICS)

Werner, D. Leonard. Informed consent in optometric institutions. *Journal of the American Optometric Association.* 1994 Jun; 65(6): 423–426.
(INFORMED CONSENT)

Werner, D. Leonard see **Foster, George E.**

Werner, Michael J.; American College of Physicians. Understanding the fraud and abuse laws: guidance for internists. *Annals of Internal Medicine.* 1998 Apr 15; 128(8): 678–684.
(FRAUD AND MISCONDUCT; HEALTH CARE/ECONOMICS)

Werpehowski, William. Persons, practices, and the conception argument. *Journal of Medicine and Philosophy.* 1997 Oct; 22(5): 479–494.
(FETUSES; PERSONHOOD)

Wertz, Dorothy C. International research in bioethics: the challenges of cross–cultural interpretation. *In:* DeVries, Raymond; Subedi, Janardan, eds. Bioethics and Society: Constructing the Ethical Enterprise. Upper Saddle River, NJ: Prentice Hall; 1998: 145–165.
(GENETIC COUNSELING)

Wertz, Dorothy C. Provider gender and moral reasoning: the politics of an "ethics of care." *Journal of Genetic Counseling.* 1994 Jun; 3(2): 95–112.
(GENETIC COUNSELING)

Wertz, Dorothy C. Society and the not–so–new genetics: what are we afraid of? Some future predictions from a social scientist. *Journal of Contemporary Health Law and Policy.* 1997 Spring; 13(2): 299–346.
(CONFIDENTIALITY; GENETIC COUNSELING; GENETIC SERVICES)

Wertz, Dorothy C.; Reilly, Philip R. Laboratory policies and practices for the genetic testing of children: a survey of the Helix network. *American Journal of Human Genetics.* 1997 Nov; 61(5): 1163–1168.
(GENETIC SCREENING; GENETIC SERVICES)

Wertz, Dorothy C. see **Cohen, Pamela E.**

Wertz, Dorothy C. see **Mao, Xin**

West, N. see **Higgins, R.M.**

Westall, Jessica. Shackling of prisoners denounced. [News]. *BMJ (British Medical Journal).* 1997 Feb 8; 314(7078): 393.
(BEHAVIOR CONTROL; PATIENT CARE)

Westergaard, L.G. see **Andersen, C. Yding**

Westfall, John M.; McCabe, Jennifer; Nicholas, Richard A. Personal use of drug samples by physicians and office staff. *JAMA.* 1997 Jul 9; 278(2): 141–143.
(HEALTH CARE/ECONOMICS; PATIENT CARE/DRUGS)

Westfall, John M. see **Wolf, Bruce L.**

Westmoreland, Glenda R. see **Ferguson, Jeffrey A.**

Wetle, Terrie see **Bradley, Elizabeth**

Wexler, David B. Some therapeutic jurisprudence implications of the outpatient civil commitment of pregnant substance abusers. *Politics and the Life Sciences.* 1996 Mar; 15(1): 73–75.
(INVOLUNTARY COMMITMENT; PRENATAL INJURIES)

Weymuller, Ernest A. A consideration of ethical issues in the design of clinical trials. *American Journal of Otolaryngology.* 1996 Jan–Feb; 17(1): 2–11.
(HUMAN EXPERIMENTATION/RESEARCH DESIGN)

Whedon, Marie see **Goodlin, Sarah J.**

Wheeler, Sondra Ely. Stewards of Life: Bioethics and Pastoral Care. Nashville, TN: Abingdon Press; 1996. 126 p.
(BIOETHICS)

Whidden, Phillip see **Hedley, A.J.**

Whitbeck, Caroline. Research ethics. *In:* Chadwick, Ruth, ed. Encyclopedia of Applied Ethics, Volume 3. San Diego, CA: Academic Press; 1998: 835–843.
(BIOMEDICAL RESEARCH; FRAUD AND MISCONDUCT)

White, Caroline. Call for research misconduct agency. [News]. *BMJ (British Medical Journal).* 1998 Jun 6; 316(7146): 1695.
(BIOMEDICAL RESEARCH; FRAUD AND MISCONDUCT)

White, Caroline. Lethal injection is medicalising execution. [News]. *BMJ (British Medical Journal).* 1998 Jan 31; 316(7128): 328.
(CAPITAL PUNISHMENT)

White, Gillian E. see **Coverdale, John H.**

White, Gladys B. Philosophical ethics and nursing -- a word of caution. *In:* Chinn, Peggy L., ed. Advances in Nursing Theory Development. Rockville, MD: Aspen Systems Corp.; 1983: 35–46.
(NURSING ETHICS)

White, Gladys B. see **Macklin, Ruth**

White, Jocelyn C.; Dunn, Patrick M.; Homer, Lou. A practical instrument to evaluate ethics consultations. *HEC (HealthCare Ethics Committee) Forum.* 1997 Sep; 9(3): 228–246.
(ETHICISTS AND ETHICS COMMITTEES)

White, Margaret see **Howard, Philip J.**

White, Mary Terrell. Decision-making through dialogue: reconfiguring autonomy in genetic counseling. *Theoretical Medicine and Bioethics.* 1998 Jan; 19(1): 5–19.
(GENETIC COUNSELING)

White, Mary Terrell. "Respect for autonomy" in genetic counseling: an analysis and a proposal. *Journal of Genetic Counseling.* 1997 Sep; 6(3): 297–313.
(GENETIC COUNSELING)

White, Robert J. Ethical issues in pediatric surgical research. *America.* 1997 Feb 8; 176(4): 17–20.
(HUMAN EXPERIMENTATION/MINORS)

White, Robert J. Partial-birth abortion: a neurosurgeon speaks. *America.* 1997 Oct 18; 177(11): 4–5.
(ABORTION)

White, Robert J. see **Goldworth, Amnon**

White, W.D.; Prunier, Edward; Holmberg, Anders; Leahy, Joseph; Kadish, Sidney P.; McCauley, Shelagh E.; Morrison, R. Sean; Meier, Diane E.; Cassel, Christine K. Clinical problem solving: when too much is too little. [Letters and response]. *New England Journal of Medicine.* 1997 May 15; 336(20): 1458–1459.
(TERMINAL CARE)

Whitehouse, Peter see **Dresser, Rebecca**

Whitehouse, Peter J. Readdressing our moral relationship to nonhuman creatures: commentary on "A dialogue on species-specific rights: humans and animals in bioethics." *Cambridge Quarterly of Healthcare Ethics.* 1997 Fall; 6(4): 445–448.
(BIOETHICS; PERSONHOOD)

Whitehouse, Peter J. see **Tracy, Kathryn Bayard**

Whiteis, David G. Unhealthy cities: corporate medicine, community economic underdevelopment, and public health. *International Journal of Health Services.* 1997; 27(2): 227–242.
(HEALTH CARE/ECONOMICS; PUBLIC HEALTH; RESOURCE ALLOCATION)

Whitfield, Adrian see **Dolan, Bridget**

Whitley, Liz see **Foglio, John**

Whitman, Jeffrey P. Reclaiming the medical profession: the military profession as a model. *Professional Ethics.* 1995 Spring; 4(1): 3–22.
(HEALTH CARE/ECONOMICS; MEDICAL ETHICS; PROFESSIONAL ETHICS; RESOURCE ALLOCATION; WAR)

Wickersham, Peter see **Morrison, James**

Widroff, Jacob see **Rosner, Fred**

Wiegand, Frances see **Wallace, Ruth**

Wiener, Carolyn L.; Strauss, Anselm L., eds. Where Medicine Fails. Fifth Edition. New Brunswick, NJ: Transaction Publishers; 1997. 407 p.
(HEALTH CARE/ECONOMICS)

Wiesing, Urban. Medical ethics, use of historical evidence in. *In:* Chadwick, Ruth, ed. Encyclopedia of Applied Ethics, Volume 3. San Diego, CA: Academic Press; 1998: 177–184.
(MEDICAL ETHICS)

Wiesner, Georgia L. see **Kodish, Eric**

Wigzell, Hans; Pontén, Jan. Refutation of investigation commissioned by Karolinska Institute. [Letter]. *Lancet.* 1998 May 16; 351(9114): 1510–1511.
(BIOMEDICAL RESEARCH; FRAUD AND MISCONDUCT)

Wikland, Matts see **Wennerholm, Ulla-Britt**

Wilbers, Doaitse; Willibrord, C.M.; Schultz, Weijmar; van de Wiel, Harry B.M. Sexual contact between

doctors and patients. *In:* Lens, Peter; van der Wal, Gerrit, eds. Problem Doctors: A Conspiracy of Silence. Washington, DC: IOS Press; 1997: 75–85.
(FRAUD AND MISCONDUCT; PROFESSIONAL PATIENT RELATIONSHIP)

Wilcke, Jon Torgny R. Late onset genetic disease: where ignorance is bliss, is it folly to inform relatives? *BMJ (British Medical Journal).* 1998 Sep 12; 317(7160): 744–747.
(GENETIC COUNSELING)

Wilcox, Clyde see **Cook, Elizabeth Adell**

Wilcox, Patti M. see **Bernhardt, Barbara A.**

Wildes, Keven Wm. Institutional identity, integrity, and conscience. *Kennedy Institute of Ethics Journal.* 1997 Dec; 7(4): 413–419.
(BIOETHICS; HEALTH CARE/ECONOMICS)

Wildes, Kevin Wm. Healthy skepticism: the emperor has very few clothes. *Journal of Medicine and Philosophy.* 1997 Aug; 22(4): 365–371.
(BIOETHICS; ETHICISTS AND ETHICS COMMITTEES)

Wildes, Kevin Wm. In the service of life: Evangelium Vitae and medical research. *In:* Wildes, Kevin Wm.; Mitchell, Alan C., eds. Choosing Life: A Dialogue on *Evangelium Vitae.* Washington, DC: Georgetown University Press; 1997: 186–198.
(BIOMEDICAL RESEARCH; EMBRYO AND FETAL RESEARCH)

Wildes, Kevin Wm. *In vitro* fertilization: secular moral authority, biomedicine, and the role of the state. *In:* Wildes, Kevin Wm., ed. Infertility: A Crossroad of Faith, Medicine, and Technology. Boston, MA: Kluwer Academic; 1997: 181–194.
(BIOETHICS)

Wildes, Kevin Wm., ed. Infertility: A Crossroad of Faith, Medicine, and Technology. Boston, MA: Kluwer Academic; 1997. 243 p.
(REPRODUCTIVE TECHNOLOGIES)

Wildes, Kevin Wm. Redesigning the human genome: are there constraints from nature? *In:* Agius, Emmanuel; Busuttil, Salvino, eds. Germ–Line Intervention and Our Responsibilities to Future Generations. Boston, MA: Kluwer Academic; 1998: 35–49.
(BIOETHICS; GENE THERAPY)

Wildes, Kevin Wm. Sanctity of life: a study in ambiguity and confusion. *In:* Hoshino, Kazumasa, ed. Japanese and Western Bioethics: Studies in Moral Diversity. Boston, MA: Kluwer Academic; 1997: 89–101.
(ALLOWING TO DIE/RELIGIOUS ASPECTS; BIOETHICS)

Wildes, Kevin Wm.; Wallace, Robert B. Relationships with payers and institutions that manage and deliver patient services. *In:* McCullough, Laurence B.; Jones, James W.; Brody, Baruch A., eds. Surgical Ethics. New York, NY: Oxford University Press; 1998: 367–383.
(HEALTH CARE/ECONOMICS; PROFESSIONAL PATIENT RELATIONSHIP; RESOURCE ALLOCATION)

Wildes, Kevin Wm. see **Godfrey, Nelda S.**

Wilfond, Benjamin see **Geller, Gail**

Wilfond, Benjamin S. see **Blustein, Jeffrey**

Wilke, Joanne. From a survivor: the emotional experience of genetic testing. [Personal narrative]. *Journal of Psychosocial Nursing and Mental Health Services.* 1995 Apr; 33(4): 28–37.
(GENETIC SCREENING)

Wilkes, Michael S.; Slavin, Stuart. Heart transplantation selection criteria: attitudes of ethnically diverse medical students. *Journal of Clinical Ethics.* 1998 Summer; 9(2): 147–155.
(ORGAN AND TISSUE TRANSPLANTATION; RESOURCE ALLOCATION/BIOMEDICAL TECHNOLOGIES; SELECTION FOR TREATMENT)

Wilkie, Patricia see **Williamson, Charlotte**

Wilkie, Tom; Graham, Elizabeth. Power without responsibility: media portrayals of Dolly and science. *Cambridge Quarterly of Healthcare Ethics.* 1998 Spring; 7(2): 150–159.
(CLONING)

Wilkinson, Anne see **Lynn, Joanne**

Wilkinson, Martin; Moore, Andrew. Inducement in research. *Bioethics.* 1997 Oct; 11(5): 373–389.
(HUMAN EXPERIMENTATION)

Wilkinson, Stephen see **Sheldon, Sally**

Wilks, Ian. The debate over risk–related standards of competence. *Bioethics.* 1997 Oct; 11(5): 413–426.
(INFORMED CONSENT)

Willer, Roger A., ed. Genetic Testing and Screening: Critical Engagement at the Intersection of Faith and Science. Minneapolis, MN: Kirk House Publishers; 1998. 210 p.
(GENETIC SCREENING)

Williams, A. Susan. Investigating abortion. *In: her* Women and Childbirth in the Twentieth Century: A History of the National Birthday Trust Fund 1928–93. Phoenix Mill, Gloucestershire, Eng.: Sutton; 1997: 99–123, 286–289.
(ABORTION/FOREIGN COUNTRIES)

Williams, Carter Catlett; Finch, Caleb E. Physical restraint: not fit for woman, man, or beast. [Editorial]. *Journal of the American Geriatrics Society.* 1997 Jun; 45(6): 773–775.
(BEHAVIOR CONTROL; PATIENT CARE/AGED)

Williams, Christopher J.; Pieri, Lorenzo; Sims, Andrew; Russon, Lynne; Alison, Dawn. Does palliative care have a role in treatment of anorexia nervosa? We should strive to keep patients alive [and] Palliative care does not mean giving up. *BMJ (British Medical Journal).* 1998 Jul 18; 317(7152): 195–197.
(ALLOWING TO DIE; PATIENT CARE/MENTALLY DISABLED)

Williams, F.G. Consent for transfusion. [Editorial]. *BMJ (British Medical Journal).* 1997 Aug 16; 315(7105): 380–381.
(INFORMED CONSENT)

Williams, G. see **Steinberg, M.A.**

Williams, G.M. see **Steinberg, M.A.**

Williams, Gail see Cartwright, Colleen

Williams, Gail see Price, John

Williams, Ged see Cartwright, Colleen

Williams, Glanville. The Gillick saga [and] The Gillick saga -- II. *New Law Journal*. 1985 Nov 22, Nov 29; 135(6230 and 6231): 1156–1158, 1179–1182.
(CONTRACEPTION/MINORS)

Williams, Janet K.; Lessick, Mira. Genome research: implications for children. *Pediatric Nursing*. 1996 Jan–Feb; 22(1): 40–46.
(GENE THERAPY; GENETIC RESEARCH; GENETIC SCREENING)

Williams, John R. The new code of ethics of the Canadian Medical Association. *International Journal of Bioethics*. 1997 Mar–Jun; 8(1–2): 119–122.
(MEDICAL ETHICS/CODES OF ETHICS)

Williams, Nigel. Editors call for misconduct watchdog. [News]. *Science*. 1998 Jun 12; 280(5370): 1685–1686.
(BIOMEDICAL RESEARCH; FRAUD AND MISCONDUCT)

Williams, Nigel. Editors seek ways to cope with fraud. [News]. *Science*. 1997 Nov 14; 278(5341): 1221.
(BIOMEDICAL RESEARCH; FRAUD AND MISCONDUCT)

Williams, Nigel. European Parliament backs new biopatent guidelines. [News]. *Science*. 1997 Jul 25; 277(5325): 472.
(GENETIC INTERVENTION; PATENTING LIFE FORMS)

Williams, Nigel. Paving the way for British xenotransplants. [News]. *Science*. 1998 Aug 7; 281(5378): 767.
(ORGAN AND TISSUE TRANSPLANTATION)

Williams, Nigel see Morton, Oliver

Williams, Peter; Wallace, David. Unit 731: The Japanese Army's Secret of Secrets. London: Hodder and Stoughton; 1989. 366 p.
(FRAUD AND MISCONDUCT; HUMAN EXPERIMENTATION/FOREIGN COUNTRIES; HUMAN EXPERIMENTATION/SPECIAL POPULATIONS; WAR)

Williams, Susan G. Research considerations: family opinions about elderly relatives in research. *Journal of Gerontological Nursing*. 1992 Dec; 18(12): 3–8.
(HUMAN EXPERIMENTATION/INFORMED CONSENT; HUMAN EXPERIMENTATION/SPECIAL POPULATIONS)

Williamson, Charlotte. Not gaining patients' consent in trials is deceitful. [Letter]. *BMJ (British Medical Journal)*. 1996 Jun 8; 312(7044): 1479.
(HUMAN EXPERIMENTATION/INFORMED CONSENT)

Williamson, Charlotte; Wilkie, Patricia. Teaching medical students in general practice: respecting patients' rights. [Editorial]. *BMJ (British Medical Journal)*. 1997 Nov 1; 315(7116): 1108–1109.
(CONFIDENTIALITY; INFORMED CONSENT; MEDICAL ETHICS/EDUCATION; PATIENT CARE)

Williamson, P. see Hartley, N.E.

Willibrord, C.M. see Wilbers, Doaitse

Willson, Kristyn J. see Olver, Ian N.

Wilmshurst, Peter. Scientific imperialism: if they won't benefit from the findings, poor people in the developing world shouldn't be used in research. [Editorial]. *BMJ (British Medical Journal)*. 1997 Mar 22; 314(7084): 840–841.
(HUMAN EXPERIMENTATION/FOREIGN COUNTRIES)

Wilmut, Ian see Klotzko, Arlene Judith

Wilmut, Ian see McGee, Glenn

Wilson, Donald E. see McCurdy, Layton

Wilson, Donna. A report of an investigation of end-of-life care practices in health care facilities and the influences on those practices. *Journal of Palliative Care*. 1997 Winter; 13(4): 34–40.
(BIOMEDICAL TECHNOLOGIES; TERMINAL CARE)

Wilson, Donna M. Administrative decision making in response to sudden health care agency funding reductions: is there a role for ethics? *Nursing Ethics*. 1998 Jul; 5(4): 319–329.
(HEALTH CARE/ECONOMICS; HEALTH CARE/FOREIGN COUNTRIES; PROFESSIONAL ETHICS)

Wilson, John Robert. Clinical Trial Informed Consent: Outsiders and the Love-Justice Correlation. Ann Arbor, MI: University Microfilms International; 1992. 200 p.
(HUMAN EXPERIMENTATION/INFORMED CONSENT)

Wilson, Keith G. see Chochinov, Harvey Max

Wilson, Kerr. Volunteer studies using the Health and Safety Laboratory exposure chamber. *In:* Close, Bryony; Combes, Robert; Hubbard, Anthony; Illingworth, John, eds. Volunteers in Research and Testing. Bristol, PA: Taylor and Francis; 1997: 129–134.
(HUMAN EXPERIMENTATION/FOREIGN COUNTRIES)

Wilson, Kumanan; Cook, Deborah J. Economics and the intensive care unit: a conflict of interests? *Journal of Critical Care*. 1997 Sep; 12(3): 147–151.
(HEALTH CARE/ECONOMICS; RESOURCE ALLOCATION/BIOMEDICAL TECHNOLOGIES)

Winikoff, Beverly see Ewart, Wendy R.

Winslade, William J. Humanistic problem solving: the case of Mr. T. *Journal of Clinical Ethics*. 1997 Winter; 8(4): 389–397.
(INFORMED CONSENT; TREATMENT REFUSAL/MENTALLY DISABLED)

Winslade, William J. Intellectual cross-dressing: an eccentricity or a practical necessity? Commentary on Morreim. *In:* Carson, Ronald A.; Burns, Chester R., eds. Philosophy of Medicine and Bioethics: A Twenty-Year Retrospective and Critical Appraisal. Boston, MA: Kluwer Academic; 1997: 327–334.
(HEALTH CARE/ECONOMICS)

Winslade, William J. see Jonsen, Albert R.

Winston, Robert. The promise of cloning for human medicine: not a moral threat but an exciting challenge. [Editorial]. *BMJ (British Medical Journal)*. 1997 Mar 29; 314(7085): 913–914.
(CLONING)

Winzelberg, Gary S. see Goodlin, Sarah J.

Wisconsin. Court of Appeals. In re Guardianship of Ruth E.J. *North Western Reporter, 2d Series.* 1995 Sep 6 (date of decision). 540: 213–217.
(ELECTROCONVULSIVE THERAPY; INFORMED CONSENT/MENTALLY DISABLED)

Wisconsin. Supreme Court. State v. Kruzicki. *North Western Reporter, 2d Series.* 1997 Apr 22 (date of decision). 561: 729–749.
(BEHAVIOR CONTROL; FETUSES; PERSONHOOD; PRENATAL INJURIES)

Wise, Jacqui. Bills on human cloning are full of loopholes. [News]. *BMJ (British Medical Journal).* 1998 Feb 21; 316(7131): 573.
(CLONING)

Wise, Jacqui. British public wants free health care, whatever the cost. [News]. *BMJ (British Medical Journal).* 1998 May 16; 316(7143): 1478.
(HEALTH CARE/FOREIGN COUNTRIES)

Wise, Jacqui. Doctors fight US company patent on umbilical cord blood. [News]. *BMJ (British Medical Journal).* 1997 Apr 19; 314(7088): 1146.
(BLOOD DONATION; PATENTING LIFE FORMS)

Wise, Jacqui. Japan to allow organ transplants. [News]. *BMJ (British Medical Journal).* 1997 May 3; 314(7090): 1298.
(DETERMINATION OF DEATH/BRAIN DEATH; ORGAN AND TISSUE DONATION)

Wise, Jacqui. Karolinska professor broke research rules. [News]. *BMJ (British Medical Journal).* 1997 Sep 6; 315(7108): 563.
(FRAUD AND MISCONDUCT)

Wise, Jacqui. New authority to monitor xenotransplantation experiments. [News]. *BMJ (British Medical Journal).* 1997 Jan 25; 314(7076): 247.
(HUMAN EXPERIMENTATION/FOREIGN COUNTRIES; HUMAN EXPERIMENTATION/REGULATION; ORGAN AND TISSUE TRANSPLANTATION)

Wise, Jacqui. Research suppressed for seven years by drug company. [News]. *BMJ (British Medical Journal).* 1997 Apr 19; 314(7088): 1145.
(BIOMEDICAL RESEARCH)

Wise, Jacqui. When life saving treatment should be withdrawn in children. [News]. *BMJ (British Medical Journal).* 1997 Oct 4; 315(7112): 834.
(ALLOWING TO DIE)

Wiseman, Virginia. Caring: the neglected health outcome? or input? *Health Policy.* 1997 Jan; 39(1): 43–53.
(HEALTH CARE/ECONOMICS; PATIENT CARE)

Wist, E.A. see **Bremnes, R.M.**

Wiswell, Thomas E. see **Somerville, Margaret A.**

Wittkopp, George F. see **Murray-Garcia, Jann**

Wlody, Ginger Schafer see **Nelson, William A.**

Wolf, Bruce L.; Westfall, John M.; McCabe, Jennifer; Nicholas, Richard A. Drug samples: benefit or bait? [Letter and response]. *JAMA.* 1998 Jun 3; 279(21): 1698–1699.
(HEALTH CARE/ECONOMICS; PATIENT CARE/DRUGS)

Wolf, Leslie E. see **King, Patricia A.**

Wolf, Susan. Facing assisted suicide and euthanasia in children and adolescents. *In:* Emanuel, Linda L., ed. Regulating How We Die: The Ethical, Medical, and Legal Issues Surrounding Physician-Assisted Suicide. Cambridge, MA: Harvard University Press; 1998: 92–119, 274–294.
(EUTHANASIA; SUICIDE)

Wolf, Susan M. Ban cloning? Why NBAC is wrong. *Hastings Center Report.* 1997 Sep–Oct; 27(5): 12–15.
(CLONING; ETHICISTS AND ETHICS COMMITTEES)

Wolfe, Sidney M. see **Dehlendorf, Christine E.**

Wolff, Gerhard; Jung, Christine. Nondirectiveness and genetic counseling. *Journal of Genetic Counseling.* 1995 Mar; 4(1): 3–25.
(GENETIC COUNSELING)

Wolff, Gerhard see **Cohen, Pamela E.**

Wolinsky, Fredric D. see **Dexter, Paul R.**

Wolinsky, Howard. Steps still being taken to undo damage of "America's Nuremberg." [News]. *Annals of Internal Medicine.* 1997 Aug 15; 127(4): I43–I44.
(FRAUD AND MISCONDUCT; HUMAN EXPERIMENTATION/SPECIAL POPULATIONS)

Woliver, Laura R. Policies to assist pregnant women and children should include a complete assessment of the realities of women's lives. *Politics and the Life Sciences.* 1996 Mar; 15(1): 75–77.
(INVOLUNTARY COMMITMENT; PRENATAL INJURIES)

Wolowelsky, Joel B. see **Feldman, Emanuel**

Wolpe, Paul Root. The triumph of autonomy in American bioethics: a sociological view. *In:* DeVries, Raymond; Subedi, Janardan, eds. Bioethics and Society: Constructing the Ethical Enterprise. Upper Saddle River, NJ: Prentice Hall; 1998: 38–59.
(BIOETHICS)

Wolpe, Paul Root see **Moreno, Jonathan D.**

Wong, Kwok-shing Thomas see **Pang, Mei-che Samantha**

Wongchoosri, Suchint see **Robb, Merlin L.**

Woo, Jean see **Hui, Elsie**

Wood, Joseph Patrick. Emergency physicians' obligations to managed care patients under COBRA. *Academic Emergency Medicine.* 1996 Aug; 3(8): 794–800.
(HEALTH CARE/ECONOMICS; SELECTION FOR TREATMENT)

Woodle, E. Steven see **Sells, Robert A.**

Woodroffe, Caroline see **Marshall, Tom**

Woodrow, Philip. Exploring confidentiality in nursing practice. *Nursing Standard.* 1996 May 1; 10(32): 38–42.
(CONFIDENTIALITY)

Woodruff, Roger K. see **Chan, Arlene**

Woods, David. AMA launches institute for ethics. [News]. *BMJ (British Medical Journal).* 1997 Mar 29; 314(7085): 920.
(ETHICISTS AND ETHICS COMMITTEES)

Woody, Robert Henley. Dubious and bogus credentials in mental health practice. *Ethics and Behavior.* 1997; 7(4): 337–345.
(FRAUD AND MISCONDUCT)

Woolf, Steven H. Should we screen for prostate cancer? Men over 50 have a right to decide for themselves. [Editorial]. *BMJ (British Medical Journal).* 1997 Apr 5; 314(7086): 989–990.
(MASS SCREENING)

Woolf, Steven H.; Lawrence, Robert S. Preserving scientific debate and patient choice: lessons from the Consensus Panel on Mammography Screening. *JAMA.* 1997 Dec 17; 278(23): 2105–2108.
(MASS SCREENING)

Woolfrey, Joan. What happens now? Oregon and physician–assisted suicide. *Hastings Center Report.* 1998 May–Jun; 28(3): 9–17.
(SUICIDE)

Woolfrey, Joan. What price reproductive potential? *Hastings Center Report.* 1998 Jan–Feb; 28(1): 47.
(REPRODUCTION)

Woolhandler, Steffie see **Himmelstein, David U.**

Workman, Stephen see **Malone, Ruth E.**

World Health Assembly. Ethical Criteria for Medicinal Drug Promotion. Geneva: World Health Organization; 1988. 16 p.
(PATIENT CARE/DRUGS)

World Health Organization. Ethical, social and legal aspects of genetic technology in medicine [and] Conclusions and recommendations. *In:* Control of Hereditary Diseases: Report of a WHO Scientific Group. Geneva: World Health Organization; 1996: 73–81.
(GENETIC SCREENING)

World Health Organization. Genetic counselling. *In:* Control of Hereditary Diseases: Report of a WHO Scientific Group. Geneva: World Health Organization; 1996: 50–58.
(GENETIC COUNSELING)

World Medical Association. Ethical issues concerning patients with mental illness. [Policy statement]. *Bulletin of Medical Ethics.* 1996 Aug; No. 120: 11.
(MEDICAL ETHICS; PATIENT CARE/MENTALLY DISABLED)

World Medical Association. Family planning and the right of a woman to contraception. [Official statement]. *Bulletin of Medical Ethics.* 1997 Nov; No. 133: 9–10.
(CONTRACEPTION)

Worth–Staten, Patricia A.; Poniatowski, Larry. Advance directives and patient rights: a Joint Commission perspective. *Bioethics Forum.* 1997 Summer; 13(2): 47–50.
(ADVANCE DIRECTIVES; PATIENTS' RIGHTS)

Worthley, John Abbott. The Ethics of the Ordinary in Healthcare: Concepts and Cases. Chicago, IL: Health Administration Press; 1997. 332 p.
(HEALTH CARE; PROFESSIONAL ETHICS)

Worthy, Jane see **Davis, Fran**

Wortley, Jacinth Tracey see **Meslin, Eric M.**

Wreen, Michael. Nihilism, relativism, and Engelhardt. *Theoretical Medicine and Bioethics.* 1998 Jan; 19(1): 73–88.
(BIOETHICS)

Wrenn, Robert L.; Levinson, Dan; Papadatou, Danai. End of Life Decisions: Guidelines for the Health Care Provider. Tucson, AZ: University of Arizona College of Medicine, Arizona Health Services Center; 1996. 44 p.
(TERMINAL CARE)

Wright, D.S. Workplace urine screening for drug abuse. [Letter]. *Journal of Medical Ethics.* 1997 Jun; 23(3): 191.
(MASS SCREENING; OCCUPATIONAL HEALTH)

Wright, J.G.C. see **Brawn, W.J.**

Wright, Susan; Sinsheimer, Robert L. Recombinant DNA and biological warfare. *Bulletin of the Atomic Scientists.* 1983 Nov; 39(9): 20–26.
(RECOMBINANT DNA RESEARCH; WAR)

Wu, Albert W. see **Finkelstein, Daniel**

Wu, Albert W. see **Tsevat, Joel**

Wurzbach, Mary Ellen. Long–term care nurses' ethical convictions about tube feeding. *Western Journal of Nursing Research.* 1996 Feb; 18(1): 63–76.
(ALLOWING TO DIE/ATTITUDES)

Wynne, Jane see **David, T.J.**

Y

Yaes, Robert J.; Dveirin, Keith; Shelman, Keith; Reinhardt, Uwe E. Contempo 1997: economics. [Letters and response]. *JAMA.* 1997 Oct 8; 278(14): 1149–1150.
(HEALTH CARE/ECONOMICS)

Yager, James D. see **Balls, Michael**

Yamazaki, Fumio. A thought on terminal care in Japan. *In:* Hoshino, Kazumasa, ed. Japanese and Western Bioethics: Studies in Moral Diversity. Boston, MA: Kluwer Academic; 1997: 131–134.
(TERMINAL CARE)

Yank, Veronica see **Olson, Carin M.**

Yarborough, Mark. The reluctant retained witness: alleged sexual misconduct in the doctor/patient relationship. *Journal of Medicine and Philosophy.* 1997 Aug; 22(4): 345–364.
(ETHICISTS AND ETHICS COMMITTEES; FRAUD AND MISCONDUCT; PROFESSIONAL PATIENT RELATIONSHIP)

Yarmolinsky, Adam see **Murray–Garcia, Jann**

Yearley, Steven see **Entwistle, Vikki A.**

Yedidia, Michael J.; Berry, Carolyn A.; Barr, Judith

K. Changes in physicians' attitudes toward AIDS during residency training: a longitudinal study of medical school graduates. *Journal of Health and Social Behavior.* 1996 Jun; 37(2): 179–191.
(AIDS/HEALTH PERSONNEL)

Yee, Yale H. Criminal DNA data banks: revolution for law enforcement or threat to individual privacy? [Note]. *American Journal of Criminal Law.* 1995 Winter; 22(2): 461–490.
(CONFIDENTIALITY/LEGAL ASPECTS; DNA FINGERPRINTING)

Yellin, Paul B.; Fleischman, Alan R. DNR in the DR? *Journal of Perinatology.* 1995 May–Jun; 15(3): 232–236.
(ALLOWING TO DIE/INFANTS; RESUSCITATION ORDERS)

Yesley, Michael S. Genetic privacy, discrimination, and social policy: challenges and dilemmas. *Microbial and Comparative Genomics.* 1997; 2(1): 19–35.
(GENETIC SCREENING)

Yokota, Masako see **Asai, Atsushi**

Young, Christopher J. Emergency! Says who?: analysis of the legal issues concerning managed care and emergency medical services. [Comment]. *Journal of Contemporary Health Law and Policy.* 1997 Spring; 13(2): 553–579.
(HEALTH CARE/ECONOMICS)

Young, Frank E. Genetic therapy. *In:* Kilner, John F.; Pentz, Rebecca D.; Young, Frank E., eds. Genetic Ethics: Do the Ends Justify the Genes? Grand Rapids, MI: W.B. Eerdmans; 1997: 171–182.
(GENE THERAPY)

Young, Frank E. see **Kilner, John F.**

Young, Ian F. Medical ethics in relation to transfusion medicine. *Transfusion Medicine Reviews.* 1996 Jan; 10(1): 23–30.
(BLOOD DONATION)

Young, Marti; Klingle, Renee Storm. Silent partners in medical care: a cross–cultural study of patient participation. *Health Communication.* 1996; 8(1): 29–53.
(PROFESSIONAL PATIENT RELATIONSHIP)

Young, Simon N.; Annable, Lawrence; Canadian College of Neuropsychopharmacology. The use of placebos in psychiatry: a response to the draft document prepared by the Tri–Council Working Group. [Position paper]. *Journal of Psychiatry and Neuroscience.* 1996 Jul; 21(4): 235–238.
(HUMAN EXPERIMENTATION/RESEARCH DESIGN; HUMAN EXPERIMENTATION/SPECIAL POPULATIONS)

Younger–Lewis, Catherine. Genital mutilation may raise awkward issues for MDs after birth. [News]. *Canadian Medical Association Journal.* 1997 Oct 15; 157(8): 1013.
(HEALTH; PATIENT CARE)

Youngner, Julius S. The scientific misconduct process: a scientist's view from the inside. *JAMA.* 1998 Jan 7; 279(1): 62–64.
(BIOMEDICAL RESEARCH; FRAUD AND MISCONDUCT)

Youngner, Stuart see **Phillips, Russell S.**

Youngner, Stuart J. Psychological impediments to

procurement. *Transplantation Proceedings.* 1992 Oct; 24(5): 2159–2161.
(ORGAN AND TISSUE DONATION)

Youngner, Stuart J.; Shuck, Jerry M. Advance directives and the determination of death. *In:* McCullough, Laurence B.; Jones, James W.; Brody, Baruch A., eds. Surgical Ethics. New York, NY: Oxford University Press; 1998: 57–77.
(ADVANCE DIRECTIVES; DETERMINATION OF DEATH; RESUSCITATION ORDERS)

Youngner, Stuart J. see **Aulisio, Mark P.**

Youngner, Stuart J. see **Sehgal, Ashwini R.**

Youngner, Stuart J. see **Shepardson, Laura B.**

Youngner, Stuart J. see **Sullivan, Mark D.**

Yount, Lisa. How should health care be allocated? [Juvenile literature]. *In: her* Issues in Biomedical Ethics. San Diego, CA: Lucent Books; 1998: 17–35, 99–101.
(HEALTH CARE/ECONOMICS; RESOURCE ALLOCATION)

Yount, Lisa. Issues in Biomedical Ethics. [Juvenile literature]. San Diego, CA: Lucent Books; 1998. 128 p.
(BIOETHICS)

Yount, Lisa. Should animals be used in medical research and testing? [Juvenile literature]. *In: her* Issues in Biomedical Ethics. San Diego, CA: Lucent Books; 1998: 56–74, 102–104.
(ANIMAL EXPERIMENTATION)

Yount, Lisa. Should doctors ever hasten patients' deaths? [Juvenile literature]. *In: her* Issues in Biomedical Ethics. San Diego, CA: Lucent Books; 1998: 36–55, 101–102.
(ALLOWING TO DIE/LEGAL ASPECTS; EUTHANASIA/LEGAL ASPECTS; SUICIDE)

Yount, Lisa. Should human genes be altered? [Juvenile literature]. *In: her* Issues in Biomedical Ethics. San Diego, CA: Lucent Books; 1998: 75–93, 104–105.
(CLONING; GENE THERAPY; GENETIC INTERVENTION)

Yovich, John L.; Matson, Phillip L. Legislation on the practice of assisted reproduction in Western Australia. *Journal of Assisted Reproduction and Genetics.* 1996 Mar; 13(3): 197–200.
(REPRODUCTIVE TECHNOLOGIES)

Yu, Lin see **Shi, Da–pu**

Yuhas, J.P. see **Piotrowski, Joseph J.**

Yutrzenka, Barbara A. see **Dracy, David L.**

Z

Zager, Shirley see **Andrews, Lori**

Zagrodsky, Jason D. see **Giugliano, Robert P.**

Zaman, Syed; Battcock, Timothy. Doctors need to know more about advance directives. [Letter]. *BMJ (British Medical Journal).* 1998 Jul 11; 317(7151): 146–147.
(ADVANCE DIRECTIVES)

Zanko, Andrea see **Heimler, Audrey**

Zanko, Andrea see **Reich, Elsa**

Zayas, Luis H. see **Morrison, R. Sean**

Zeman, Adam. Persistent vegetative state. *Lancet.* 1997 Sep 13; 350(9080): 795–799.
(ALLOWING TO DIE; PATIENT CARE)

Zerwekh, Joyce V. Do dying patients really need IV fluids? *American Journal of Nursing.* 1997 Mar; 97(3): 26–31.
(TERMINAL CARE)

Zheng, Chang–Jiang see **Guo, Sun–Wei**

Zhou, Xiao–Hua see **Dexter, Paul R.**

Zieselman, Kimberly see **Levy, Michael J.**

Zigmond, Michael J. see **Fischer, Beth A.**

Zilinskas, Raymond A. Bioethics and biological weapons. [Editorial]. *Science.* 1998 Jan 30; 279(5351): 635.
(WAR)

Zimbelman, Joel. Technology assessment, ethics and public policy in biotechnology: the case of the Human Genome Project. *In:* Becker, Gerhold K., ed. Changing Nature's Course: The Ethical Challenge of Biotechnology. Hong Kong: Hong Kong University Press; 1996: 85–108.
(GENOME MAPPING)

Zimring, Franklin E. The genetics of crime: a skeptic's vision of the future. *Politics and the Life Sciences.* 1996 Mar; 15(1): 105–106.
(BEHAVIORAL GENETICS)

Zinberg, Randi see **Eng, Christine M.**

Zinkernagel, Rolf M. Gene technology and democracy. [Editorial]. *Science.* 1997 Nov 14; 278(5341): 1207.
(GENETIC INTERVENTION)

Zinn, Christopher. Australian doctor builds "coma machine." [News]. *BMJ (British Medical Journal).* 1997 May 24; 314(7093): 1503.
(SUICIDE)

Zinn, Christopher. Australian doctors renew battle over euthanasia. [News]. *BMJ (British Medical Journal).* 1996 Jun 8; 312(7044): 1437.
(EUTHANASIA/LEGAL ASPECTS; SUICIDE)

Zinn, Christopher. Australian orphans were used as guinea pigs. [News]. *BMJ (British Medical Journal).* 1997 Jun 21; 314(7097): 1783.
(FRAUD AND MISCONDUCT; HUMAN EXPERIMENTATION/FOREIGN COUNTRIES; HUMAN EXPERIMENTATION/MINORS; IMMUNIZATION)

Zinn, Christopher. Australian voluntary euthanasia law is overturned. [News]. *BMJ (British Medical Journal).* 1997 Apr 5; 314(7086): 994.
(EUTHANASIA/LEGAL ASPECTS; SUICIDE; TERMINAL CARE)

Zion, William P. see **Overall, Christine**

Zlotkin, Stanley see **Rowell, Mary**

Zoeteweij, M.W. see **DudokdeWit, A.C.**

Zohar, Noam J. A Jewish perspective on access to healthcare. *Cambridge Quarterly of Healthcare Ethics.* 1998 Summer; 7(3): 260–265.
(HEALTH CARE/ECONOMICS; RESOURCE ALLOCATION)

Zohar, Noam J. Allocating medical resources: global planning and immediate obligations. *In: his* Alternatives in Jewish Bioethics. Albany, NY: State University of New York Press; 1997: 143–152.
(RESOURCE ALLOCATION)

Zohar, Noam J. Alternatives in Jewish Bioethics. Albany, NY: State University of New York Press; 1997. 165 p.
(BIOETHICS)

Zohar, Noam J. Death: natural process and human intervention. *In: his* Alternatives in Jewish Bioethics. Albany, NY: State University of New York Press; 1997: 37–68.
(EUTHANASIA/RELIGIOUS ASPECTS; SUICIDE)

Zohar, Noam J. Jewish deliberations on suicide: exceptions, toleration, and assistance. *In:* Battin, Margaret P.; Rhodes, Rosamond; Silvers, Anita, eds. Physician Assisted Suicide: Expanding the Debate. New York, NY: Routledge; 1998: 362–372.
(SUICIDE)

Zohar, Noam J. Parenthood: natural fact and human society. *In: his* Alternatives in Jewish Bioethics. Albany, NY: State University of New York Press; 1997: 69–84.
(REPRODUCTIVE TECHNOLOGIES)

Zoloth–Dorfman, Laurie. Mapping the normal human self: the Jew and the mark of otherness. *In:* Peters, Ted, ed. Genetics: Issues of Social Justice. Cleveland, OH: Pilgrim Press; 1998: 180–202.
(EUGENICS; GENOME MAPPING)

Zoloth–Dorfman, Laurie; Rubin, Susan B. Insider trading: conscience and critique in bioethics. *HEC (HealthCare Ethics Committee) Forum.* 1998 Mar; 10(1): 24–33.
(ETHICISTS AND ETHICS COMMITTEES)

Zoloth–Dorfman, Laurie; Rubin, Susan B. "Medical futility": managed care and the powerful new vocabulary for clinical and public policy discourse. *Healthcare Forum Journal.* 1997 Mar–Apr; 40(2): 28, 30–33.
(ALLOWING TO DIE; HEALTH CARE/ECONOMICS; RESOURCE ALLOCATION)

Zoloth–Dorfman, Laurie; Rubin, Susan B. Navigators and captains: expertise in clinical ethics consultation. [Book review essay]. *Theoretical Medicine.* 1997 Dec; 18(4): 421–432.
(BIOETHICS; ETHICISTS AND ETHICS COMMITTEES)

Zribi, Ahmed. Medical ethics and Islam. *Dolentium Hominum: Church and Health in the World.* 1996; 31(11th Yr., No. 1): 82–85.
(BIOETHICS; MEDICAL ETHICS)

Zucker, Arthur. Law and ethics: [assisted suicide]. *Death Studies.* 1997 Jan–Feb; 21(1): 107–110.
(SUICIDE)

Zucker, Arthur. Law and ethics: experimentation; assisted

suicide. *Death Studies.* 1997 Mar–Apr; 21(2): 221–225.
(HUMAN EXPERIMENTATION; SUICIDE)

Zucker, Howard D. see **Zucker, Marjorie B.**

Zucker, Marjorie B.; Zucker, Howard D., eds. Medical Futility and the Evaluation of Life–Sustaining Interventions. New York, NY: Cambridge University Press; 1997. 201 p.
(ALLOWING TO DIE; TERMINAL CARE)

Zuger, Abigail. Ever elusive, privacy slips from grasp of patients. *New York Times.* 1998 Nov 3: F7.
(CONFIDENTIALITY)

Zumpano–Canto, Joe. Nonconsensual sterilization of the mentally disabled in North Carolina: an ethics critique of the statutory standard and its judicial interpretation. *Journal of Contemporary Health Law and Policy.* 1996 Fall; 13(1): 79–111.
(STERILIZATION/MENTALLY DISABLED)

Zurlo, Joanne see **Balls, Michael**

Zwart, Frédérique. A very special day. [Personal narrative on voluntary euthanasia]. *BMJ (British Medical Journal).* 1997 Jul 26; 315(7102): 260.
(EUTHANASIA)

Zweig, Franklin M.; Walsh, Joseph T.; Freeman, Daniel M. Courts and the challenges of adjudicating genetic testing's secrets. *In:* Rothstein, Mark A., ed. Genetic Secrets: Protecting Privacy and Confidentiality in the Genetic Era. New Haven, CT: Yale University Press; 1997: 332–351.
(CONFIDENTIALITY; GENETIC SCREENING)

Zwitter, Matjaž see **Surbone, Antonella**

Zylicz, Zbigniew see **O'Connor, Nancy K.**

ANONYMOUS

A ban on cells that could heal. [Editorial]. *New York Times.* 1998 Nov 7: 14.
(EMBRYO AND FETAL RESEARCH; ORGAN AND TISSUE DONATION)

A challenge to genetic transparency. [Editorial]. *Nature.* 1998 May 21; 393(6682): 195.
(GENOME MAPPING)

A force of nature? Human need could prove too strong for any ban on cloning. [Editorial]. *New Scientist.* 1998 Jan 17; 156(2117): 3.
(CLONING)

A time for responsibility. [Editorial]. *Nature.* 1997 Dec 4; 390(6659): 427.
(BIOMEDICAL RESEARCH)

A triumph of hope.... [Editorial]. *New Scientist.* 1997 May 31; 154(2084): 3.
(CLONING)

A woman who died may become a mother. [News]. *New York Times.* 1997 Dec 7: 33.
(REPRODUCTIVE TECHNOLOGIES)

Aetna to charge extra for in vitro fertilization. [News]. *New York Times.* 1998 Jan 15: A15.
(IN VITRO FERTILIZATION; REPRODUCTIVE TECHNOLOGIES)

An H.M.O., Catholic–run, bars coverage for abortions. [News]. *New York Times.* 1997 Nov 17: B5.
(ABORTION/FINANCIAL SUPPORT; ABORTION/RELIGIOUS ASPECTS)

Banking Our Genes. [Videorecording]. Eunice Kennedy Shriver Center; available for sale from Fanlight Productions, 47 Halifax St., Boston, MA 02130, 800–937–4113; 1995. 1 videocassette; 33 min.; sd.; color; 1/2 in.; VHS.
(DNA FINGERPRINTING; GENETIC RESEARCH)

Breast cancer: research without consent. [News]. *Journal of Medical Ethics.* 1997 Dec; 23(6): 372.
(HUMAN EXPERIMENTATION/FOREIGN COUNTRIES; HUMAN EXPERIMENTATION/INFORMED CONSENT)

British guidelines set out standards for genetic tests. [News]. *Nature.* 1997 Oct 2; 389(6650): 427.
(GENETIC SCREENING; GENETIC SERVICES)

Changing the U.S. transplant system. [Editorial]. *Lancet.* 1998 Jul 11; 352(9122): 79.
(ORGAN AND TISSUE TRANSPLANTATION; RESOURCE ALLOCATION/BIOMEDICAL TECHNOLOGIES)

Chinese deny organ trafficking. [News]. *Lancet.* 1998 Mar 28; 351(9107): 967.
(ORGAN AND TISSUE DONATION)

Chinese doctors speak out against forced organ donation. [News]. *BMJ (British Medical Journal).* 1998 Mar 28; 316(7136): 956.
(ORGAN AND TISSUE DONATION)

Convict DNA bank unconstitutional? [News]. *Science.* 1998 Aug 21; 281(5380): 1121.
(DNA FINGERPRINTING)

Cooling down over cloning. [Editorial]. *Lancet.* 1998 Jan 17; 351(9097): 151.
(CLONING)

Crack–using woman admits guilt in death of her fetus. [News]. *New York Times.* 1997 Dec 3: A33.
(PRENATAL INJURIES)

Crossing the line: Richard Seed may not win a place in history for cloning humans, but someone probably will. [News]. *New Scientist.* 1998 Jan 17; 156(2117): 4.
(CLONING)

D.C. hospital must pay $400,000 for forced test and denial of care. [News]. *AIDS Policy and Law.* 1997 May 2; 12(8): 1, 8–9.
(AIDS/TESTING AND SCREENING)

Diane Blood and the HFEA. *Bulletin of Medical Ethics.* 1997 Jan; No. 124: 2.
(ARTIFICIAL INSEMINATION)

Doctor assisted suicide needs to be discussed. [BMA Annual Meeting, July 1998]. *BMJ (British Medical Journal).* 1998 Jul 18; 317(7152): 214.
(SUICIDE)

Doctors' involvement in death penalty is morally wrong. [BMA Annual Meeting, July 1998]. *BMJ (British Medical Journal).* 1998 Jul 18; 317 (7152): 215–216.

(CAPITAL PUNISHMENT)

Doctors not obliged to accede to patients' requests to die. [BMA Annual Meeting, July 1998]. *BMJ (British Medical Journal).* 1998 Jul 18; 317(7152): 217–218.
(ALLOWING TO DIE)

Dolly clone institute wins research funding reprieve. [News]. *Nature.* 1998 Jan 1; 391(6662): 10.
(CLONING)

Double trouble: Unesco should think again before endorsing an outright condemnation of human cloning. [Editorial]. *Nature.* 1997 Aug 7; 388(6642): 501.
(CLONING)

Dutch GPs often fail to honor euthanasia requests. [News]. *BMJ (British Medical Journal).* 1997 Jan 18; 314(7075): 166.
(EUTHANASIA/ATTITUDES)

Dutch GPs to be offered advice on euthanasia. [News]. *BMJ (British Medical Journal).* 1997 Jun 21; 314(7097): 1782.
(EUTHANASIA)

Editorial [mass vaccination]. *Bulletin of Medical Ethics.* 1996 Jan; No. 114: 1.
(IMMUNIZATION)

Electroconvulsive therapy. *Medical Journal of Australia.* 1985 Sep 2; 143(5): 190–191.
(ELECTROCONVULSIVE THERAPY)

European Directory of Bioethics, 1996. Second Edition. Secaucus, NJ: Lavoisier; distributed by Springer Verlag; 1996. 703 p.
(BIOETHICS; ETHICISTS AND ETHICS COMMITTEES)

FDA seeks public comment on informed consent rules in combat situations. [News]. *Hastings Center Report.* 1997 Sep–Oct; 27(5): 43.
(HUMAN EXPERIMENTATION/INFORMED CONSENT; HUMAN EXPERIMENTATION/SPECIAL POPULATIONS; WAR)

Flawed US proposals on patients' privacy. [Editorial]. *Lancet.* 1997 Sep 20; 350(9081): 823.
(CONFIDENTIALITY/LEGAL ASPECTS)

French Academy split on cloning policy. [News]. *Nature.* 1997 Jul 3; 388(6637): 11.
(CLONING)

From the editors [the future of bioethics]. *Cambridge Quarterly of Healthcare Ethics.* 1997 Fall; 6(4): 365–369.
(BIOETHICS)

Full exposure: eternal vigilance over reproductive technology is better than banning it. [Editorial]. *New Scientist.* 1998 Jan 31; 157(2119): 3.
(REPRODUCTIVE TECHNOLOGIES)

Genethics in the mid–1990s. [News]. *GenEthics News.* 1996 Jul/Aug; 13: 6–7.
(GENETIC INTERVENTION)

Good manners for the pharmaceutical industry. [Editorial]. *Lancet.* 1997 Jun 7; 349(9066): 1635.
(HUMAN EXPERIMENTATION/RESEARCH DESIGN)

Guidelines are urged in using organs of heart–dead patients. [News]. *New York Times.* 1997 Dec 21: 38.
(ORGAN AND TISSUE DONATION)

Halt the xeno–bandwagon. [Editorial]. *Nature.* 1998 Jan 22; 391(6665): 309.
(ORGAN AND TISSUE TRANSPLANTATION)

Hard cases, bad laws: is patching human genes any more immoral than patenting nerve gases? [Editorial]. *New Scientist.* 1997 Jul 12; 155(2090): 3.
(PATENTING LIFE FORMS)

Hospital must notify third party if it suspects patient has HIV [Garcia v. Santa Rosa Health Care Corp.]. *AIDS Policy and Law.* 1996 Jul 26; 11(13): 13.
(AIDS)

How not to run a scientifically successful country. [Editorial]. *Nature.* 1998 Apr 23; 392(6678): 741.
(GENETIC INTERVENTION)

Hubris, benefits and minefields of human cloning. [Editorial]. *Nature.* 1998 Jan 15; 391(6664): 211.
(CLONING)

Human Genetics Advisory Commission meets. [News; title supplied]. *Gene Therapy.* 1997 Apr; 4(4): 271.
(CONFIDENTIALITY; GENETIC SCREENING)

Human rights begin at home. [Editorial]. *BMJ (British Medical Journal).* 1997 Nov 29; 315(7120): 1387.
(FRAUD AND MISCONDUCT; HUMAN EXPERIMENTATION/SPECIAL POPULATIONS; TORTURE)

Informed consent needed before HIV testing of pregnant mothers: CMA. [News]. *Canadian Medical Association Journal.* 1997 Apr 15; 156(8): 1108.
(AIDS/TESTING AND SCREENING)

Integrity in Scientific Research. [Videorecording]. American Association for the Advancement of Science; available for sale from Science Integrity Videos, AAAS Directorate for Science and Policy Programs, 1200 New York Ave., NW, Washington, DC 20005, 202–326–6600; 1996. 5 videocassettes; 44 min. (8–10 min. each); sd.; color; 1/2 in.; VHS.
(BIOMEDICAL RESEARCH; FRAUD AND MISCONDUCT)

Jack Kevorkian. [News; title supplied]. *BMJ (British Medical Journal).* 1997 Nov 1; 315(7116): 1116.
(ORGAN AND TISSUE DONATION; SUICIDE)

Japan says forced sterilizations merit no payments, no apology. [News]. *New York Times.* 1997 Sep 18: A12.
(STERILIZATION)

Knowing your genes. [Editorial]. *Lancet.* 1997 Oct 4; 350(9083): 969.
(GENETIC SCREENING; GENETIC SERVICES)

Light in dark places. [Editorial]. *Nature.* 1997 Oct 23; 389(6653): 767.
(BIOETHICS)

LREC resigns unanimously [Basingstoke Local Research Ethics Committee]. [News]. *Bulletin of Medical Ethics.* 1997 May; No. 128: 3–6.
(HUMAN EXPERIMENTATION/ETHICS COMMITTEES; HUMAN EXPERIMENTATION/FOREIGN COUNTRIES)

MPs call for tough controls on human genetics. [News]. *GenEthics News.* 1995 Jul–Aug; No. 7: 1, 3.
(GENETIC INTERVENTION; GENETIC SCREENING)

Murder charge against Dutch nursing home dropped. [News]. *BMJ (British Medical Journal).* 1997 Sep 13;

315(7109): 624.
(ALLOWING TO DIE/LEGAL ASPECTS)

National Ethical Consultative Committee for the Life and Health Sciences in France issues opinion entitled "Genetics and medicine: from prediction to prevention." *International Digest of Health Legislation.* 1996; 47(2): 263–265.
(GENETIC SCREENING)

New code of medical ethics issued in Italy. [News]. *International Digest of Health Legislation.* 1993; 44(2): 353–354.
(MEDICAL ETHICS/CODES OF ETHICS; PROFESSIONAL ETHICS/CODES OF ETHICS)

New US regulatory framework emerges for genetics. [News]. *Nature Biotechnology.* 1997 Apr; 15(4): 300.
(ETHICISTS AND ETHICS COMMITTEES; GENOME MAPPING)

Opportunity for depth in Chinese eugenics debate. [Editorial]. *Nature.* 1998 Mar 12; 392(6672): 109.
(EUGENICS)

Owning genes. [Editorial]. *Wall Street Journal.* 1998 May 14: A22.
(PATENTING LIFE FORMS)

Perils in free market genomics. [Editorial]. *Nature.* 1998 Mar 26; 392(6674): 315.
(GENE THERAPY; GENETIC RESEARCH)

Philosophers reflect on suicide. [Editorial]. *America.* 1997 Apr 5; 176(11): 3.
(ALLOWING TO DIE; SUICIDE)

Physicians divided on assisted suicide. *Iowa Medicine.* 1996 Jul–Aug; 86(6): 238–239.
(SUICIDE)

Pragmatism in codes of research ethics. [Editorial]. *Lancet.* 1998 Jan 24; 351(9098): 225.
(HUMAN EXPERIMENTATION/FOREIGN COUNTRIES; HUMAN EXPERIMENTATION/RESEARCH DESIGN)

Progress on patents, but more action is needed. [Editorial]. *Nature.* 1997 Jul 24; 388(6640): 309.
(PATENTING LIFE FORMS)

Publication of experimental animal research: ethical aspects. [Editorial]. *Veterinary Quarterly.* 1985 Apr; 7(2): 81–83.
(ANIMAL EXPERIMENTATION)

Pushing ethical pharmaceuticals direct to the public. [Editorial]. *Lancet.* 1998 Mar 28; 351(9107): 921.
(PATIENT CARE/DRUGS)

Referendum's challenge to transgenic research [Switzerland]. [Editorial]. *Nature.* 1997 Sep 11; 389(6647): 103.
(GENETIC INTERVENTION; RECOMBINANT DNA RESEARCH/REGULATION)

Research without consent in South Africa. [News; title supplied]. *BMJ (British Medical Journal).* 1997 Jun 28; 314(7098): 1850.
(FRAUD AND MISCONDUCT; HUMAN EXPERIMENTATION/FOREIGN COUNTRIES; OCCUPATIONAL HEALTH)

Suit says patient was denied heart surgery because of HIV. [News]. *AIDS Policy and Law.* 1997 May 16; 12(9): 3.
(AIDS/HEALTH PERSONNEL)

Swiss to vote on genetic engineering. [News]. *ATLA: Alternatives to Laboratory Animals.* 1997 May–Jun; 25(3): 220–221.
(GENETIC INTERVENTION)

Task force finalizes genetic testing recommendations. [News]. *Nature Biotechnology.* 1997 Apr; 15(4): 300.
(GENETIC SCREENING)

Thanks for the advice. [Editorial]. *Nature Biotechnology.* 1997 Apr; 15(4): 293.
(ETHICISTS AND ETHICS COMMITTEES; GENETIC INTERVENTION)

The means to an end. [Editorial]. *New Scientist.* 1997 Oct 25; 156(2105): 3.
(ANIMAL EXPERIMENTATION)

The screening muddle. [Editorial]. *Lancet.* 1998 Feb 14; 351(9101): 459.
(MASS SCREENING)

Thinking about cloning. [Editorial]. *Nature Biotechnology.* 1997 Apr.; 15(4): 293.
(CLONING)

To clone or not to clone? [News]. *Christian Century.* 1997 Mar 19–26; 114(10): 286–288.
(CLONING)

Tracking H.I.V. infections in New York. [Editorial]. *New York Times.* 1998 Jan 15: A20.
(AIDS/CONFIDENTIALITY)

Trading trust for blood money. [Editorial]. *Lancet.* 1995 Sep 30; 346(8979): 855.
(BLOOD DONATION; CONFIDENTIALITY)

Trust and the bioethics industry. [Editorial]. *Nature.* 1997 Oct 16; 389(6652): 647.
(BIOETHICS)

Widow allowed to export husband's sperm. [News]. *BMJ (British Medical Journal).* 1997 Mar 8; 314(7082): 696.
(ARTIFICIAL INSEMINATION)